Oxford Textbook of

Palliative Nursing

Oxford Textbook of

Palliative Nursing

SIXTH EDITION

EDITED BY

Tara A. Albrecht, PhD, ACNP-BC, ACHPN, RN

Associate Professor
Specialty Director, Palliative Care
Duke University, School of Nursing

Vanessa Battista, DNP, MBA, CPNP-PC, CHPPN, FPCN, FAAN

Senior Nursing Director, Palliative Care
Fellowship Director, Palliative Care Adult Nurse Practitioner Fellowship
Dana-Farber Cancer Institute

Abraham A. Brody, PhD, RN, FAAN, FPCN

Mathy Mezey Professor of Geriatric Nursing, Professor of Medicine, Associate Director, HIGN
New York University Rory Meyers College of Nursing

Heather Coats, PhD, APRN-BC, FAAN, FPCN

Director of Research, Hospice and Palliative Nurses Association
Associate Professor
College of Nursing
Director of Palliative Care Inquiry for Interprofessional Palliative Care Certificate/MS-Palliative Care/Community Hospice and Palliative Medicine Fellowship
Department of General Internal Medicine, School of Medicine
University of Colorado, Anschutz Medical Campus

OXFORD
UNIVERSITY PRESS

OXFORD
UNIVERSITY PRESS

Oxford University Press is a department of the University of Oxford. It furthers the University's objective of excellence in research, scholarship, and education by publishing worldwide. Oxford is a registered trade mark of Oxford University Press in the UK and in certain other countries.

Published in the United States of America by Oxford University Press
198 Madison Avenue, New York, NY 10016, United States of America.

CIP data is on file at the Library of Congress

This material is not intended to be, and should not be considered, a substitute for medical or other professional advice. Treatment for the conditions described in this material is highly dependent on the individual circumstances. And, while this material is designed to offer accurate information with respect to the subject matter covered and to be current as of the time it was written, research and knowledge about medical and health issues is constantly evolving and dose schedules for medications are being revised continually, with new side effects recognized and accounted for regularly. Readers must therefore always check the product information and clinical procedures with the most up-to-date published product information and data sheets provided by the manufacturers and the most recent codes of conduct and safety regulation. The publisher and the authors make no representations or warranties to readers, express or implied, as to the accuracy or completeness of this material. Without limiting the foregoing, the publisher and the authors make no representations or warranties as to the accuracy or efficacy of the drug dosages mentioned in the material. The authors and the publisher do not accept, and expressly disclaim, any responsibility for any liability, loss or risk that may be claimed or incurred as a consequence of the use and/ or application of any of the contents of this material.

ISBN 978–0–19–765746–1

DOI: 10.1093/med/9780197657461.001.0001

Printed by Integrated Books International, United States of America

FSC MIX Paper FSC® C183721

The manufacturer's authorised representative in the EU for product safety is Oxford University Press España S.A. of El Parque Empresarial San Fernando de Henares, Avenida de Castilla, 2 – 28830 Madrid (www.oup.es/en or product.safety@oup.com). OUP España S.A. also acts as importer into Spain of products made by the manufacturer.

Dedication

The sixth edition of the Oxford Textbook of Palliative Nursing is dedicated to Betty Ferrell, PhD, MSN, RN, CHPN, FAAN, FPCN, and Judith (Judy) Paice, PhD, RN, FAAN, FASCO, co-editors of the two previous editions of the textbook. It was Dr. Ferrell, along with Nessa Coyle PhD, RN, who served as co-editor of the first four editions of the book, who had the original vision for a first of its kind textbook, written primarily by nurses for nurses, as a beacon for the field of palliative nursing. Dr. Judith Paice joined them for the 4th edition, adding her invaluable wisdom to the text.

Betty and Judy have impacted the field of palliative nursing in innumerable and immeasurable ways through an enormous collective body of scholarly and clinical work. They have both spent years at the bedside and in the clinic caring for patients and have done research that has contributed not only to the development of the field but also to passing on this knowledge to others. Their work has had an immense direct impact on nurses throughout the world and has literally shaped palliative nursing in the way we know it today.

Betty created the End-of-Life Nursing Education Consortium (ELNEC), which marks its 25th Anniversary this year (2025), and has been taught in a train the trainer model in over 115 countries to over 48,034 nurses and other health professionals who have gone on to teach an innumerate number of others. Her research has taught us about attending to suffering and enhancing quality of life and has had a profound impact on teaching other nurses how to do this work well. Judy is recognized for her many contributions to the field, most notably her research and expertise in pain management, as well as her leadership and advancements in education of others in how to mitigate suffering through careful attention to clinical symptomatology.

It is not an exaggeration to say that we are standing on the shoulders of giants as we humbly and gratefully accept the passing of the torch from Betty and Judy for this next edition. Palliative nursing would not exist were in not for the tremendous contributions of these two women and we are so fortunate to have both of them as our mentors, teachers, and friends. We thank them for all they have done to foster the growth of the palliative care field and for entrusting us with the important task of bringing to life the next edition of this invaluable text. On behalf of all palliative nurses, we thank you, Betty and Judy, and dedicate the 6th edition to you.

Tara Albrecht
Vanessa Battista
Ab Brody
Heather Coats

Contents

Preface xi
Acknowledgments xiii
List of Contributors xv

PART I
General Principles

1. **Introduction to Palliative Care** 3
   Tara A. Albrecht, Heather Coats, and Vanessa Battista
2. **Role of Nursing in Palliative Care** 5
   Michelle Webb
3. **Public Policy for Palliative Care** 10
   Marian Grant
4. **Principles of Patient and Family Assessment** 17
   Shannon L. S. Petros
5. **Palliative Nursing Communication** 27
   Constance Dahlin and Janice Linton
6. **Advance Care Planning** 49
   Shigeko Izumi
7. **Value-Based Care** 59
   Rory B. Farrand and Aparna Gupta
8. **Interdisciplinary Palliative Care Teams: Specialists in Delivering Palliative Care** 66
   Rebekah Malloy, Jessica Bullington, Catherine Rogers, and Adrienne Norquist
9. **Enhancing Team Effectiveness** 77
   Katrina Bezak and Kimberly Chow
10. **The Ethos of Palliative Nursing** 83
    Mark Lazenby and Michael Anthony Moore

PART II
Symptom Assessment and Management in Adult and Older Adult Populations

11. **Pain Management** 89
    Judith A. Paice and Martin Galligan
12. **Dyspnea and Cough** 104
    Rebecca Disler, Susanne McDevitt, and DorAnne Donesky
13. **Anorexia and Cachexia** 119
    Elizabeth E. Schack and Elizabeth Capano
14. **Nausea and Vomiting** 130
    David Collett
15. **Dysphagia, Hiccups, and Other Oral Symptoms** 142
    Rachel Klinedinst, Brenna McCarty, and Barton Bobb
16. **Bowel Management: Constipation, Obstruction, Diarrhea, and Ascites** 150
    Serena Snow and Cameron Jennings
17. **Medically Administered Nutrition and Hydration** 165
    Jennifer A. Tschanz and Carmen N. Spalding
18. **Urinary Tract Disorders in Palliative Care** 178
    Susan D. Bruce
19. **Lymphedema Management** 185
    Mei R. Fu, Charles P. Tilley, Jeanna M. Arbesfeld-Qiu, Rubén Martín Payo, and Catherine S. Finlayson
20. **Palliative Wound, Ostomy, and Continence Care** 198
    Charles P. Tilley, Kim Cavallito, Lindsay Alvarez, and Mei R. Fu
21. **Pruritus, Fever, and Sweats** 227
    Angel Smothers, Amanda Kitzmiller, and Diana Niland
22. **Neurological Disorders** 235
    Lauren Massimo and Brianna Morgan

23. **Acute Delirium** 243
Shih-Yin Lin and Donna E. McCabe

24. **Anxiety and Depression** 251
Katharine Adelstein and Elizabeth Archer-Nanda

25. **Fatigue** 264
Stephanie Gilbertson-White and Nayung Youn

26. **Insomnia** 273
Patricia Carter

27. **Complementary and Integrative Therapies in Palliative Care** 280
Mary-Anne Meyer and Melinda Ring

PART III
Psychosocial and Spiritual Care Across Lifespan

28. **Cultural Considerations in Palliative Care** 293
Carrie L. Cormack and Aminah Fraser-Rahim

29. **Supporting Families and Family Caregivers in Palliative Care** 308
Tamryn F. Gray and J. Nicholas Odom

30. **Hope and Meaning in Illness** 328
Anessa M. Foxwell and Darcy Alimenti

31. **Sexuality and Sexual Function in Serious Illness** 341
Christina M. Wilson and Marloe V. Esch

32. **Ethical Considerations in Palliative Care** 349
Phyllis B. Whitehead and Mark G. Swope

33. **Addressing Spiritual, Religious, and Existential Needs in Palliative Care** 367
Elizabeth Johnston Taylor and William E. Rosa

PART IV
Pediatric Palliative Care

34. **Pain Management in Pediatric Palliative Care** 377
Juliana H. O'Brien and Gina Santucci

35. **Symptom Management in Pediatric Palliative Care** 387
Camara van Breemen and Nadine Lusney

36. **Values and Perspectives Influencing Goals of Care and Decision-Making in Pediatric Palliative Care** 399
Christina McDaniel and Jordan M. Desai

37. **Communication Components for Determining Goals of Care and Advance Care Planning in Pediatric Palliative Care** 408
Deborah Lafond and Kathy Perko

38. **Ethical Considerations in Pediatric Palliative Care** 422
Hilary Carroll McGuire and Nicole Fernandez

39. **Pediatric Spiritual Assessment and Care** 429
Dianne Richoux and Judy Zeringue

40. **Palliative Care in the Perinatal Setting: Neonatal Intensive Care Unit and Labor and Delivery Unit** 436
Cheryl Ann Thaxton, Kathleen Ellis, and Andrea Biondi

41. **Considerations for Adolescents in Pediatric Palliative Care** 447
Lauren Greco and Faith Kinnear

42. **Pediatric Hospice Perspectives** 454
Alice Bass and Rebecca Turner

43. **Nursing Care for the Pediatric Patient at the End of Life** 467
Jenna Freitas and Chelsea Heneghan

44. **Grief and Bereavement in Perinatal and Pediatric Palliative Care** 479
Kathie Kobler, Rana Limbo, and Betty Davies

PART V
Issues in Populations of the Seriously Ill

45. **Pulmonary-Palliative Care** 495
Patricia A. Maani-Fogelman and Jennifer Wescoe-Singley

46. **Palliative Care in Heart Failure** 505
Rachel D. Wells, Avery C. Bechthold, Keith M. Swetz, and J. Nicholas Odom

47. **Palliative Care for People Living with HIV** 519
Jacquelyn Slomka

48. **Palliative Approaches to Dementia Care** 528
Tatiana Sadak and Soo Borson

49. **Palliative Care for Persons with Cirrhosis and Their Family Caregivers** 540
Louise Babikow, Christopher D. Woodrell, and Lissi Hansen

50. **Palliative Care for Persons Living with Advanced Kidney Disease** 549
Kate Sciacca and Marissa Finger

51. **Palliative Care for Persons Living with a Hematologic Malignancy** 556
Ashley Leak Bryant, Lorinda A. Coombs, Samantha Mayo, Argin Malakian, and Tara A. Albrecht

52. **Palliative Care for Persons Living with Cancer** 566
Denice R. Economou, Alissa A. Ulanday, and Eden R. Brauer

PART VI
Care Near the End of Life

53. **Urgent Syndromes at the End of Life** 579
Christina Feindt and Kelli Gershon

54. **Sedation for Refractory Symptoms** 593
Sandra Perrotta

55. **Withdrawal or Cessation of Life-Sustaining Therapies: Mechanical Ventilation, Hemodialysis, Cardiac Devices** 599
Margaret L. Campbell, Alvin H. Moss, and Sarah E. Schroeder

56. **Palliative Care and Requests for Assistance in Dying** 605
Kaveri Roy and Sarah Rossmassler

57. **Planning for Death** 616
Reiko Asano

58. **Grief and Bereavement** 623
Inge B. Corless and Dunui Pupudulou

PART VII
Mode of Palliative Care Delivery

59. **Hospice and Community-Based Palliative Care** 639
Karen F. Hyden, Maura Lipp, and Tammy Stokes

60. **Telehealth, Telephonic Care, and Remote Patient Monitoring** 647
Laraine Ann Chiu, Jennifer Curtis, and Inez Brandon

61. **Palliative Care Nursing in the Outpatient Setting** 656
Nancy A. Robertson and Ami K. Goodnough

62. **Long-Term Care** 662
Melissa McClean and Joan G. Carpenter

63. **Palliative Care in the Emergency Department** 670
Rebecca Wright and Benjamin Roberts

64. **Hospital-Based Palliative Care** 679
Barbara Reville and Anessa M. Foxwell

65. **The Intensive Care Unit** 688
Jennifer McAdam, Céline Gélinas, and Kathleen Turner

PART VIII
Considerations for Person and Family-Centered Palliative Care

66. **Addressing Health Inequalities, Social Determinants of Health, and Underrepresented Individuals in Palliative Care** 701
Binu Koirala, Rebecca Wright, Patricia M. Davidson, Marlena C. Fisher, Katie E. Nelson, Benjamin Roberts, Danetta H. Sloan, and David S. Wu

67. **Affirmative Palliative Care for LGBTQIA+ Patients and Their Families** 711
Kailey E. Roberts, William E. Rosa, Noelle Marie Javier, Pierce DiMauro, Joshua C. Eyer, and Kristin G. Cloyes

68. **Palliative Care in the Setting of Substance Use Disorder** 720
Peggy Compton, Yu-Ping Chang, and Salimah H. Meghani

69. **Palliative Care in the Setting of Serious Mental Illness** 733
Lindsey C. Wright

70. **Rural Palliative Care** 742
Richard A. Taylor, J. Nicholas Odom, Erin R. Currie, Chunhong Xiao, and Marie A. Bakitas

71. **Palliative Care for Older Adults** 750
Laura Tycon Moreines and Lauren Hunt

72. **Global Palliative Care in Low- and Middle-Income Countries** 759
Virginia LeBaron, Thuý Ly Nguyễn, and Usha Thapa

PART IX
Special Considerations for Palliative Care Nurses

73. **Occupational Stress, Burnout, and Self-Care in Palliative Nursing** 771
Erica Frechman and Patricia Wright

74. **Palliative Care and Social Media** 777
Dana Hansen and Amy Petrinec

75. **Career Advancement in Palliative Care** 785
Katherine Stackhouse

76. **Nursing Education** 791
Andra Davis and Megan Lippe

77. **Nursing Research** 801
Micah A. Skeens, Amy R. Newman, and Kathleen E. Montgomery

78. **Developing and Implementing Quality Improvement Programs across Settings** 807
Sean M. Reed

Index 813

Preface

The first edition of the *Oxford Textbook of Palliative Nursing* was published in 2001 and contributed to defining the emerging field of palliative care. The textbook set a cornerstone for the field, identifying elements of patient and family care and the role of nurses who deliver the care.

The subsequent editions evolved at a rapid speed, parallel to the growth of the field as palliative nursing extended across populations and settings of care and recognized new areas of need. The first five editions were led by the two of us, Betty Ferrell and Judith Paice, and our colleague Nessa Coyle. In many ways, the textbook was akin to the expression of "building the plane while flying it" as we were writing about a field very young in its existence but motivated by the need to create a comprehensive resource for nurses.

This sixth edition of the textbook is a major step in the evolution of palliative nursing. The plane is built, and the "wings" and destinations are entering new dimensions. The contents of this edition mirror the expansion of palliative care into new populations, such as those patients living with pulmonary, cardiac, liver, renal, and hematologic diseases. This edition's section on pediatric palliative care is reflective of the phenomenal growth in care of children.

This sixth edition is a combination of the roots that ground us in the foundation of palliative nursing as well as the new growth, the new branches and leaves of a solid tree. The section on end-of-life care reminds us of Florence Nightingale's founding of the nursing profession, committed to caring for the basic needs of the seriously ill and injured and the promise of biopsychosocial and spiritual care. Reading this edition should also stir within each of us the passion and advocacy for the most underserved. Pioneers of our field, including Florence Wald, founder of the first hospice in the United States, and Dame Cicely Saunders of St. Christopher's Hospice in the United Kingdom, spoke passionately of the need for compassionate and competent care of the most vulnerable. How pleased they would be to see this edition with chapters on health inequalities, LGBTQIA+ communities, and care of those with substance use disorders or serious mental illness and those in rural communities.

This sixth edition also represents "handing off the torch" as we have passed on our role as textbook editors to four colleagues and leaders of our field, Tara Albrecht, Vanessa Battista, Ab Brody, and Heather Coats. It is a privilege to pass this torch as we are inspired by these new leaders and the many chapter authors who are taking our discipline to a new level. As founding editors of the textbook, to see the birth of a new field and its maturation to the status of palliative care now as an undeniable field of patient care is a privilege beyond words. We offer our greatest thanks to the authors of these chapters and to the new editors of this textbook. Our field is in very capable hands, and this sixth edition is a roadmap for the future.

Betty R. Ferrell, PhD, RN, MA, CHPN, FAAN, FPCN
Judith Paice, PhD, RN, FAAN

Acknowledgments

We acknowledge all the authors of the 78 chapters in the sixth edition of the *Oxford Textbook of Palliative Nursing*. Each author's expertise and effort are the foundation to this sixth edition, a project that would not have been possible without their contributions. We would also like to give special thanks to Stacy Zhao whose administrative support was invaluable to the processes required to produce this textbook. We will be forever grateful to Marta Moldvai, our Oxford University Press editor, who helped guide us every step of the way. Lastly, we would like to express our deep appreciation and respect to Betty Ferrell and Judy Paice for entrusting us with this textbook to which they have devoted many years of time and expertise to ensure that all nurses have access to the palliative care knowledge they require and deserve.

Contributors

Katharine Adelstein, PhD, PMHNP-BC, ANP-BC
Assistant Professor
Psychiatric/Mental Health Nurse Practitioner Co-Track Coordinator
University of Louisville School of Nursing
Louisville, KY

Tara A. Albrecht, PhD, ACNP-BC, ACHPN, RN
Associate Professor
Specialty Director, Palliative Care
Duke University, School of Nursing
Durham, NC

Darcy Alimenti, MSN, CRNP, ACHPN
Nurse Practitioner
Palliative Care Nurse Practitioner
Home Based Palliative Care Practice
Main Line Health
Radnor, PA

Lindsay Alvarez, MSN, APRN, FNP-BC, CWOCN

Elizabeth Archer-Nanda, DNP, PMHCNS-BC, APRN
Clinical Director
Norton Healthcare
Louisville, KY

Reiko Asano, PhD, RN
Assistant Professor
The Catholic University of America
Conway School of Nursing
Washington, DC

Louise Bablkow, CRNP, MScR
Nurse Practitioner, Master of Science in Research
Penn Medicine Lancaster General Hospital
Lancaster, PA

Marie A. Bakitas, DNSc, CRNP, NP-C, AOCN, ACHPN, FAAN
Professor
Associate Director, Center for Palliative and Supportive Care
The University of Alabama at Birmingham School of Nursing
Birmingham, AL

Alice Bass, MSN, APRN-CNP, CPNP-PC, FPCN
Nursing Professional Practice Specialist
Center for Nursing Excellence
Nurse Practitioner, Informatics, Advanced Illness, Management (AIM) Team
Nationwide Children's Hospital
Columbus, OH

Vanessa Battista, DNP, MBA, CPNP-PC, CHPPN, FPCN, FAAN
Senior Nursing Director, Palliative Care
Dana-Farber Cancer Institute
Boston, MA

Katrina Bezak, DNP, MBA, APRN, FNP-BC
Regional Director of Oncology Services
Karmanos Cancer Center
Charlevoix, MI

Avery C. Bechthold, PhD, RN
Post-doctoral Fellow
The University of Alabama at Birmingham
Birmingham, AL

Jeanna M. Arbesfeld-Qiu, ABMD-PhD Candidate
Harvard Medical School
Boston, MA

Andrea Biondi, DNP, RN, NNP, CPNP
Assistant Professor School of Nursing
MGHIHP
Charlestown, MA

Barton Bobb, MSN, FNP-BC, ACHPN
Palliative Nurse Practitioner
Virginia Commonwealth University Health System
Richmond, VA

Soo Borson, MD
Deputy Editor, Journal of the American Geriatrics Society
Co-Lead,BOLD Center of Excellence on Early Detection of Dementia
Professor of Clinical Family Medicine, USC Keck School of Medicine
Professor Emerita of Psychiatry and Behavioral Sciences, University of Washington School of Medicine

Inez Brandon, MSN RN-C

Eden R. Brauer, PhD, MSN, RN
Assistant Professor
UCLA School of Nursing
Los Angeles, CA

Susan D. Bruce, MSN, RN, AOCNS
Oncology Clinical Nurse Specialist
Duke Cancer Center Raleigh
Raleigh, NC

Ashley Leak Bryant, PhD, RN, OCN, FAAN
Frances Hill Fox Distinguished Professor
Senior Associate Dean, Office of Strategy and Global Affairs Co-Director, PAHO/WHO Collaborating Center in Quality and Safety
Assistant Director, Cancer Research Training and Education Coordination
UNC Lineberger Comprehensive Cancer Center

Jessica Bullington, BSN, RN, CHPN
Palliative Care Program Specialist
Medical University of South Carolina
Charleston, SC

Margaret L. Campbell, PhD, RN, FPCN
Wayne State University, College of Nursing
Detroit, MI

Elizabeth Capano, AGPCNP-BC, ACHPN
Weill Cornell Medicine
Division of Geriatrics and Palliative Medicine
New York, NY

Joan G. Carpenter, PhD, CRNP, ACHPN, FPCN
Assistant Professor
University of Maryland School of Nursing
Organizational Systems and Adult Health
Baltimore, MD
Nurse Practitioner
Coastal Hospice and Palliative Care
Salisbury, MD

Patricia Carter, PhD, RN, CNS
Professor, PhD Program Director
School of Nursing Graduate Studies
The University of Texas Medical Branch
Galveston, TX

Kim Cavallito, BA, BSN, MS, FNP-BC, CWCN
Calvary Hospital
Nurse Practitioner
Hospital for Special Surgery
Wound Care Nurse Practitioner
New York, NY

Yu-Ping Chang, PhD, RN, FGSA, FIAAN, FAAN
Professor and Associate Dean for Research and Scholarship
Patricia H. and Richard E. Garman Endowed Professor
The State University of New York at Buffalo School of Nursing
Buffalo, NY

Laraine Ann Chiu, MSN, APRN, AGACNP-BC
Nurse Practitioner
NYU Langone Health
New York, NY

Kimberly Chow, DNP, MBA, APRN, ANP-BC, ACHPN
Director of Advanced Practice Providers
Lightyear Health
Walnut Creek, CA

Kristin G. Cloyes, PhD, MN, RN
Professor, School of Nursing Ph.D. Program Director, School of Nursing
Elnora E. Thomson Distinguished Professor, School of Nursing
Oregon Health and Science University

Heather Coats, PhD, APRN-BC, FAAN, FPCN
Director of Research
Hospice and Palliative Nurses Association
Pittsburgh, PA
Associate Professor
College of Nursing, University of Colorado Anschutz Medical Campus
Aurora, CO
Director of Palliative Care Inquiry
School of Medicine, University of Colorado Anschutz Medical Campus
Aurora CO

David Collett, MSN, APRN, AGACNP-BC, ACHPN
Nurse Practitioner
Icahn School of Medicine at Mount Sinai
New York, NY

Peggy Compton, RN, PhD, FAAN
Professor and Van Ameringen Endowed Chair
Department of Family and Community Health
University of Pennsylvania School of Nursing
Philadelphia, PA

Lorinda A. Coombs, PhD, MSN, FNP-BC, AONCP
Assistant Professor
Lineberger Comprehensive Cancer Center
University of North Carolina Chapel Hill
School of Nursing
Chapel Hill, NC

Inge B. Corless, PhD, RN, FNAP, FAAN
Professor Emerita
MGH Institute of Health Professions
Boston, MA

Carrie L. Cormack, DNP, APRN, CPNP, CHPPN
Associate Professor
College of Nursing
Medical University of South Carolina
Charleston, SC

Erin R. Currie, PhD, RN
Assistant Professor
Family, Community, and Health Systems Department
The University of Alabama at Birmingham School of Nursing
Birmingham, AL

Jennifer Curtis, BSN, RN, CHPN
Registered Nurse, Home Care
NYU Langone Health
New York, NY

Constance Dahlin, MSN, ANP-BC, ACHPN, FPCN, FAAN
Palliative Nurse Practitioner
MGB Salem Hospital
Salem, MA
Consultant
Center to Advance Palliative Care
New York, NY
Faculty
School of Graduate Studies, Palliative Care
University of Maryland, Baltimore
Baltimore, MD

Patricia M. Davidson, RN PhD
Vice Chancellors Fellow
University of New South Wales, Sydney Australia
Dean Emerita
Johns Hopkins School of Nursing,
Baltimore, MD

Betty Davies, RN, PhD, CT, FAAN
Professor and Senior Scholar
School of Nursing
University of Victoria
Victoria, Canada

Andra Davis, PhD, MN, RN
Associate Professor
School of Nursing and Health Innovations
University of Portland,
Portland, OR

Jordan M. Desai, MS, LISW- CP

Pierce DiMauro, DNP, AGACNP-BC
Palliative Nurse Practitioner
Columbia University Irving Medical Center
New York, NY

Rebecca Disler, PhD, MSc (Research), PDAN (Crit Care), BSc, BN, RN, ATSF, FThorSoc
Associate Professor
Australian Research Council Discovery Early Career Researcher Award Fellow (DECRA)
School of Translational Medicine
Monash University Australia

DorAnne Donesky, PhD, ANP-BC, ACHPN, ATS, FHPN
Professor of Clinical Nursing—Emeritus
University of California, San Francisco
Nurse Practitioner
Inpatient palliative care team
Queen of the Valley Medical Center
Napa, CA

Denice R. Economou, PhD, CNS, CHPN
Associate Adjunct Professor
UCLA School of Nursing
Los Angeles, CA

Amanda Kitzmiller, MSN, APRN, FNP-BC, CNE
Clinical Education Assistant Professor
West Virginia University School of Nursing
Morgantown, WV

Kathleen Ellis, PhD, RN, CCRN, CNE
Nurse Scientist
Children's Health
Dallas, TX

Marloe V. Esch, DNP, RN, APNP, AGCNS-BC, OCN, CSC

Joshua C. Eyer, PhD
Director, Southern Regional Drug Data Research Center
Institute of Data & Analytics
Culverhouse College of Business
The University of Alabama
Tuscaloosa, AL

Rory B. Farrand, MS, MA, MSN, APRN-BC
Senior Palliative Care Consultant
Confidis Consulting
Finleyville, PA

Christina Feindt, DNP, MBA, FNP-C

Nicole Fernandez, DNP, MPH, CPNP
Nurse Practitioner
Pediatric Advanced Care Team
Memorial Sloan Kettering Cancer Center
New York, NY

Marissa Finger, DNP, APRN, CNP-BC

Catherine S. Finlayson, PhD, RN, OCN
Associate Professor
Lienhard School of Nursing
Pace University
Pleasantville, NY

Marlena C. Fisher, PhD, RN, CNL
Nursing Inquiry Program Coordinator
Center for Nursing Inquiry
Johns Hopkins Hospital
Baltimore, MD

Anessa M. Foxwell, PhD, MSN, MBE, APRN, ACHPN, FPCN
NewCourtland Center for Transitions and Health, Predoctoral Fellow
Leonard Davis Institute for Health Economics, Associate Fellow
Clinical Practices of the University of Pennsylvania, Nurse Practitioner
University of Pennsylvania School of Nursing
Philadelphia, PA

Aminah Fraser-Rahim, DNP, APRN, CPNP
Pediatric Palliative Nurse Practitioner
Medical University of South Carolina
Shawn Jenkins Children's Hospital
Charleston, SC

Erica Frechman, PhD, AGPCNP-BC, ACHPN, NEA-BC, FPCN
Assistant Professor of Internal Medicine
Section on Gerontology and Geriatric Medicine
Atrium Health Wake Forest Baptist
Winston-Salem, NC

Jenna Freitas, MSN, RN, CPNP
Nurse Practitioner
Pediatric Advanced Care Team
Boston Children's Hospital
Boston, MA

Mei R. Fu, PhD, RN, FAAN
The Dorothy and Dale Thompson Missouri Endowed Professor in Nursing
Associate Dean for Research
School of Nursing and Health Studies
University of Missouri-Kansas City
ansas City, MO

Martin Galligan, FHEA, RN, MSc, PGCLTHE, PgCert Clin Res, NMP
Lecturer Practitioner
NIHR Doctoral Research Fellow
The Royal Marsden School
London

Céline Gélinas, RN, PhD
Professor
Ingram School of Nursing
McGill University
Montreal, Canada

Kelli Gershon, MSN, FNP-BC, ACHPN
Carelon Palliative Care

Stephanie Gilbertson-White, PhD, RN, FAAN
Associate Professor
Director, PhD Program
University of Iowa
College of Nursing
Iowa City, IA

Ami K. Goodnough, DNP, NP-C, ACHPN, RN
Adjunct Clinical Faculty, Masters in Palliative Care
University of Colorado Anschutz Medical Campus
Anschutz, CO
Regional Director Clinical Care and Wellness, Wheaton Franciscans
Wheaton, IL

Marian Grant, DNP, APRN, ACNP-BC, ACHPN, FPCN
Senior Regulatory Advisor
The Coalition to Transform Advanced Care
Washington, DC

Tamryn F. Gray, PhD, RN, MSN, MPH
Pronouns: She/Her
Assistant Professor
UNC School of Nursing
Chapel Hill, NC

Lauren Greco, MSN, RN CHPPN
Education and Professional Development Administrator, Palliative Care
Dana-Farber Cancer Institute
Boston, MA

Aparna Gupta, DNP, EMBA, FACHE, CPHQ, ANP-BC
Vice President, Quality
National Hospice and Palliative Care Organization
Alexandria, VA

Dana Hansen, PhD, APRN, ACHPN
Assistant Professor
Kent State University College of Nursing
Kent, OH

Lissi Hansen, PhD, RN
Professor
Oregon Health & Science University School of Nursing
Portland, OR

Chelsea Heneghan, DNP, MBA, CPNP
Nurse Practitioner
Pediatric Advanced Care Team
Boston Children's Hospital
Boston, MA

Lauren Hunt, PhD, RN, FNP-BC
Associate Professor
Philip R. Lee Institute for Health Policy Studies
Department of Epidemiology and Biostatistics
Atlantic Senior Fellow, Global Brain Health Studies
University of California
San Francisco, CA

Karen F. Hyden, PhD, MSN/Ed, APN-BC, ACHPN
Licensed Clinical Pastoral Counselor
Senior Director of Compassionate Care
Evergreen Nephrology
Nashville, TN

Shigeko Izumi, PhD, RN, FPCN
Associate Professor
Oregon Health & Science University School of Nursing
Portland, OR

Cameron Jennings, MSN, APRN, FNP-BC, PHCNS-BC, ACHPN
Nurse Practitioner, Palliative & Hospice Care
Central Virginia VA Health Care System
Richmond, VA

Noelle Marie Javier, MD
Associate Professor
Department of Geriatrics and Palliative Medicine
Icahn School of Medicine at Mount Sinai
New York, NY

Faith Kinnear, CPNP-AC, MSN, BSN
Assistant Professor Palliative Care/Critical Care Medicine
Baylor College of Medicine/Texas Children's Hospital
Houston, TX

Rachel Klinedinst, DNP, AGACNP-BC, CRNP, ACHPN
Palliative Care
Hospital of the University of Pennsylvania
Philadelphia, PA

Kathie Kobler, PhD, APRN, PCNS-BC, CHPPN, FPCN
APN Coordinator
Center for Fetal Care
Perinatal Palliative Care
Advocate Children's Hospital
Park Ridge, IL

Binu Koirala
Assistant professor
Johns Hopkins School of Nursing
Baltimore, MD

Deborah Lafond, DNP, PPCNP-BC, CPON, CHPPN, FPCN, FAPHON, FAAN
Chief Executive Officer
PANDA Education Consultants, PLLC
Lakeland, Florida
Palliative Care Educator Emeritus
Children's National Hospital
Washington, DC

Mark Lazenby, PhD, APRN, FAAN
Associate Professor of Nursing
Yale University School of Nursing
Associate Professor of Religion and Health
Yale University Divinity School
New Haven, CT

Virginia LeBaron, PhD, APRN, ACHPN, FAANP, FAAN
Kluge-Schakat Associate Professor of Compassionate Care
University of Virginia School of Nursing
Charlottesville, VA

Rana Limbo, PhD, RN, CPLC, FAAN
Director Emerita and Co-founder
Resolve Through Sharing
Gundersen Medical Foundation
La Crosse, WI

Shih-Yin Lin, PhD, MPH, MM
Senior Research Scientist
NYU Rory Meyers College of Nursing
New York, NY

Janice Linton, DNP, APRN, ANP-BC, CCRN, ACHPN

Maura Lipp, MD
Chair of Ethics, Medical Director of Respiratory Care, Pulmonary/Critical Care Physician
Maury Regional Medical Center
Columbia, TN

Megan Lippe, PhD, MSN, RN, ANEF, FPCN, FAAN
Associate Professor
School of Nursing
UT Health San Antonio
San Antonio, TX

Nadine Lusney, BScN, RN, MN, CHPCN
Clinical Nurse Specialist
Director of Clinical Knowledge
Practice and Innovation
Vancouver

Patricia A. Maani-Fogelman, DNP, ACHPN, FNPC
Division of Pulmonary, Critical Care, and Sleep Medicine
Geisinger Health System
Danville, PA

Argin Malakian, RN, MN, PhD(c)
Clinical Nurse Specialist
Department of Supportive Care
Princess Margaret Cancer Centre,
University Health Network
Toronto, ON, Canada

Rebekah Malloy, RN, BSN, CCRN, CHPN
Director of Clinical Engagement
Compassion and Choices
Littleton, CO

Lauren Massimo, PhD, CRNP
Assistant Professor
University of Pennsylvania, School of Nursing
Philadelphia, PA

Samantha Mayo, PhD, RN
Assistant professor
Lawrence Bloomberg Faculty of Nursing
University of Toronto
Toronto

Jennifer McAdam, RN, PhD
Professor
School of Nursing
Samuel Merritt University
Oakland, CA

Donna E. McCabe, DNP, GNP-BC, PMHNP-BC
Clinical Associate Professor
NYU Rory Meyers College of Nursing
New York, NY

Brenna McCarty, MSN, AGACNP-BC, ACHPN, RN
Palliative Care Nurse Practitioner
VCU Health System
Richmond, VA

Melissa McClean, MSN, CRNP, ANP-BC, ACHPN, CNE
Clinical Instructor
University of Maryland School of Nursing
Organizational Systems and Adult Health
Baltimore, MD

Christina McDaniel, RN, MSN, CHPPN, DNP
Clinical Instructor
MUSC College of Nursing
Charleston, SC

Susanne McDevitt, DNP, ACNP-BC
Adjunct Monash Nursing and Midwifery, Nurse Practitioner
Pulmonary Hypertension Program
University of Michigan Health System

Hilary Carroll McGuire, DNP, FNP-BC, ACHPN
Nurse Practitioner
Supportive Oncology Collaborative and Palliative Care
Dana-Farber Cancer Institute
Boston, MA

Salimah H. Meghani, PhD, MBE, RN, FAAN
Carol E. Ware Endowed Professor in Mental Health Nursing
Department of Biobehavioral Health Sciences
University of Pennsylvania School of Nursing
Philadelphia, PA

Mary-Anne Meyer, APN/CNP
Advance Practice Nurse
Integrative Primary Care
Osher Center for Integrative Medicine
Northwestern Medicine
Master of Science in Nursing
Rush University
Chicago, IL

Kathleen E. Montgomery
Assistant Professor, School of Nursing
University of Wisconsin-Madison
Madison, WI

Michael Anthony Moore, BA, RN
Yale University School of Nursing
New Haven, CT

Laura Tycon Moreines, MSN, FNP-BC, ACHPN
Graduate Student
Rory Meyers College of Nursing
New York University
New York, NY

Brianna Morgan, MSN, CRNP, ACHPN*
Predoctoral Fellow
University of Pennsylvania School of Nursing
Philadelphia, PA

Alvin H. Moss, MD
Professor of Medicine
Divisions of Nephrology, Geriatrics, and Palliative Medicine
West Virginia University School of Medicine
Morgantown, WV

Katie E. Nelson, PhD, MSN, RN
Assistant Scientist, Department of International Health
Johns Hopkins Bloomberg School of Public Health
Baltimore, MD

Amy R. Newman, PhD, RN, CPNP-PC
Associate Professor, College of Nursing
Marquette University
Milwaukee, WI

Thuý Ly Nguyễn , RN, PhD
Hanoi, Vietnam

Diana Niland, PhD, FNP-BC
Assistant Professor
West Virginia University, School of Nursing Keyser Campus
Keyser, WV

Adrienne Norquist, MSN, ACNP-BC, ACHPN
Nurse Practitioner
Hoag Memorial Hospital Presbyterian
Newport Beach, CA

Juliana H. O'Brien, MSN, FNP-BC
Division of Palliative and Supportive Care
Nemours/Alfred I. DuPont Hospital for Children
Wilmington, DE

J. Nicholas Odom, PhD, RN, ACHPN, FPCN, FAAN
Associate Professor and Doreen C. Harper Endowed Chair
Director of Caregiver and Bereavement Support Services, UAB Center for Palliative and Supportive Care
University of Alabama at Birmingham School of Nursing
Birmingham, AL

Judith A. Paice, PhD, RN, FAAN
Director, Cancer Pain Program
Division of Hematology-Oncology
Northwestern University
Feinberg School of Medicine
Chicago, IL

Danai Papadatou, PhD
Professor Emerita of Clinical Psychology School of Health Sciences
Department of Nursing National and Kapodistrian University of Athens
Athens, Greece

Rubén Martín Payo, PhD
Departamento de Medicina
Facultad de Medicina y Ciencias de la Salud
Universidad de Oviedo/Instituto de Investigación Sanitaria del Principado de Asturias

Kathy Perko, MS, PPCNP-BC, CPON, CHPPN, CPLC, FPCN, FAPHON
Pediatric Palliative Care Certificate Track Director
Palliative Care Training Center
University of Washington
Seattle, WA
Chief Operating Officer
PANDA Education Consultants, PLLC
Lakeland, FL

Sandra Perrotta, DNP, APRN, FNP-C, ACHPN
Professor Emerita of Clinical Psychology
School of Health Sciences, Dept. of Nursing, National and Kapodiostrian University of Athens
Athens, Greece

Shannon L. S. Petros, DNP, CNP, ACHPN
Nurse Practitioner, Palliative Medicine

Amy Petrinec, PhD, RN
Assistant Professor
Kent State University College of Nursing
Kent, OH

Sean M. Reed, PhD, APRN, ACNS-BC, ACHPN, AHN-BC, FCNS, SGAHN
Assistant Professor
College of Nursing
University of Colorado
Aurora, CO

Barbara Reville, DNP, ANP
Faculty
Harvard Medical School Center for Palliative Care
Center for Visual Arts in Health Care Brigham and Women's Hospital
Boston, MA

Dianne Richoux, MSN, RN, CPN
Assistant Professor of Nursing
School of Nursing
Nicholls State University
Thibodaux, LA

Melinda Ring, MD, FACP, ABOIM
Director, Osher Center for Integrative Medicine
Northwestern Medicine
Drs. Pat and Carl Greer Distinguished Physician in Integrative Medicine
Clinical Associate Professor of Medicine and Medical Social Sciences
Northwestern University Feinberg School of Medicine
Chicago, IL

Benjamin Roberts, AGACNP-BC, ACHPN
Palliative Care Program
Division of General Internal Medicine
Johns Hopkins Bayview Medical Center
Baltimore, MD

Kailey E. Roberts, PhD
Assistant Professor
Ferkauf Graduate School of Psychology
Yeshiva University
Bronx, NY

Nancy A. Robertson, MSN, ANP-BC, ACHPN
Palliative Care Nurse Practitioner
University of Colorado Masters of Palliative Care Faculty
Anschutz Medical Campus
Aurora, CO

Catherine Rogers, LMSW, APHSW-C
Palliative Care Social Worker
Medical University of South Carolina
Charleston, SC

William E. Rosa, PhD, MBE, NP-BC, FAANP, FAAN, FPCN
Assistant Attending Behavioral Scientist
Department of Psychiatry and Behavioral Sciences
Memorial Sloan Kettering Cancer Center
New York, NY

Sarah Rossmassler DNP, AGPCNP, ANP-BE, ACHPN
Assistant Professor
School of Nursing, MGH Institute of Health Professions
Boston, MA

Kaveri Roy, DNP, RN, CNE
Distinguished Teaching Assistant Professor
School of Nursing, MGH Institute of Health Professions
Boston, MA

Tatiana Sadak, PhD, PMHNP, MAH, RN, FAAN, FNYAM, FGSA
Deputy Dean, Professor
Director of Dementia Palliative Education Network
Yale School of Nursing
Orange, CT

Gina Santucci, MSN, FNP, APN-BC
Assistant Professor/ Nurse Practitioner
Baylor College of Medicine/Texas Children's Hospital
Department of Pediatrics Section on Pediatric Palliative Care
Houston, TX

Elizabeth E. Schack, GNP-BC, CNS, ACHPN

Sarah E. Schroeder, PhD, ACNP-BC, MSN RN
Division of Mechanical Circulatory Support
Bryan Heart
Lincoln, NE

Kate Sciacca, AGACNP-BC
Senior Manager, Palliative Medicine
Brigham and Women's Hospital
Boston, MA

Micah A. Skeens, PhD APRN FAAN
Principal Investigator
Center for Biobehavioral Health
Nationwide Children's Hospital
Columbus, OH

Danetta H. Sloan, PhD, MSW, MA
Associate Research Professor
Johns Hopkins University, Bloomberg School of Public Health
Baltimore, MD

Jacquelyn Slomka, PhD, RN
Independent Scholar and Consultant
Cleveland, OH

Angel Smothers, DNP, APRN, FNP-BC, CNEcl
Associate Dean for Community Engagement
Clinical Associate Professor
West Virginia University School of Nursing
Morgantown, WV

Serena Snow, FNP-BC
Division of Gastroenterology
National Jewish Health®
Denver, CO

Carmen N. Spalding, PhD, RN

Katherine Stackhouse, DNP, RN, FNP-C, ACHPN
Assistant Professor of Clinical Nursing
Division of Nursing
DeSales University
Center Valley, PA

Tammy Stokes, MSN, RN-BC, CHPN
Director of Palliative Care
Maury Regional Medical Center
Columbia, TN

Keith M. Swetz, MD, MA, FACP, FAAHPM, HMDC
Professor of Medicine
The University of Alabama at Birmingham Heersink School of Medicine
Birmingham, AL

Mark G. Swope, PhD, MBE, MDiv
Director of Bioethics
Carilion Clinic
Assistant Professor
Virginia Tech Carilion School of Medicine
Roanoke, VA

Richard A. Taylor, DNP, CRNP, APN-BC
Assistant Professor
Acute, Chronic and Continuing Care Department
The University of Alabama at Birmingham School of Nursing
Birmingham, AL

Elizabeth Johnston Taylor, PhD, RN, FAAN
Professor
School of Nursing
Loma Linda University
Loma Linda, CA

Usha Thapa, RN, MSN
Lecturer
B.P Koirala Memorial Cancer Hospital Nursing College
Bharatpur, Nepal

Cheryl Ann Thaxton, DNP, APRN, CPNP, FNP-BC, CHPPN, FPCN, FAANP, FAAN
Associate Dwuean, Professor, & Graduate Education Chair
College of Nursing | UNT Health Science Center
Fort Worth, TX

Charles P. Tilley, PhD, ANP-BC, ACHPN, CWOCN, CHSE
Associate Professor
Quinnipiac University School of Nursing
Hamdon, CT

Jennifer A. Tschanz, MSN, RN, FNP, AOCNP
Oncology Nurse Practitioner
Virginia Oncology Associates
Norfolk, VA

Kathleen Turner
Rev. Kathleen Turner, RN, CCRN
Clinical Nurse III (ret.)
Medical-Surgical ICU
UCSF Medical Center
San Francisco, CA

Rebecca Turner, BSN, RN, CHPPN
Hospice and Home-based Palliative Care RN Clinical Leader
Nationwide Children's Homecare and Hospice
Columbus, OH

Alissa A. Ulanday, MSN, BSN, AGACNP-BC, ACHPN
Palliative Care Nurse Practitioner
Ronald Reagan UCLA Medical Center
Los Angeles, CA

Camara van Breemen, MN, NP(F)
Canuck Place Children's Hospice
Vancouver, Canada.
Faculty of Medicine, University of British Columbia
Vancouver, Canada.
BC Children's Hospital
Vancouver, Canada.

Michelle Webb, DNP, RN, CHPCA
Assistant Clinical Professor
Duke University School of Nursing
Durham, NC

Rachel D. Wells, PhD, RN, CNL
Assistant Professor; Mixed Methods Consultant
University of Alabama at Birmingham School of Nursing
Birmingham, AL

Jennifer Wescoe-Singley, M.Ed., NCC
Executive Director, Wescoe Foundation for Pulmonary Fibrosis
Wescoe Foundation for Pulmonary Fibrosis
Coopersburg, PA

Phyllis B. Whitehead, PhD, APRN/CNS, ACHPN, PMGT-BC, FCNS, FAAN
Clinical Ethicist
Clinical Nurse Specialist - Palliative Medicine/Pain Management
Carilion Clinic
Associate Professor
Virginia Tech Carilion School of Medicine
Roanoke, VA

Christina M. Wilson, PhD, WHNP-BC
Nurse Practitioner and Investigator
Virginia Gynecologic Oncology, Sarah Cannon Cancer Institute at Henrico Doctors' Hospital
Henrico, VA

Christopher D. Woodrell, MD, MS, FAAHPM
Associate Professor
Brookdale Department of Geriatrics and Palliative Medicine
Icahn School of Medicine at Mount Sinai
New York, NY
Staff Physician
Geriatric Research, Education and Clinical Center
James J. Peters Veterans Affairs Medical Center
Bronx, NY

Lindsey C. Wright, MS, MSN PMHNP-BC, ACHPN
Nurse Practitioner
Palliative Care Supportive Oncology
Laura and Isaac Perlmutter Cancer Center
New York University Langone Health
New York, NY

Patricia Wright, PhD, MBA, MSN, CRNP, ACNS-BC, CNE, CHPN, CPH, FPCN
Professor of Nursing
The University of Scranton
Scranton, PA

Rebecca Wright, PhD, BSc (Hons), RN
Assistant Professor
Johns Hopkins School of Nursing
Baltimore, MD

David S. Wu, MD, FAAHPM
Associate Professor of Clinical Medicine
Johns Hopkins School of Medicine
Baltimore, MD

Chunhong Xiao
The University of Alabama at Birmingham School of Nursing
Birmingham, AL

Nayung Youn, MSN, APN
Research Assistant, College of Nursing
University of Iowa
Iowa city, IA

Judy Zeringue
Palliative Care Nurse Navigator/Spiritual Care
Pelican Krewe Children's Hospital
Founding Member of LCMC Health
New Orleans, LA

PART I
General Principles

1

Introduction to Palliative Care

Tara A. Albrecht, Heather Coats, and Vanessa Battista

Key Points

- The delivery of palliative and hospice care continues to evolve to meet the complex needs of diverse persons living with serious illness and their families.
- Knowledge of palliative care principles and skills is essential for all nurses caring for both patients and families facing serious illness.
- Properly assessing and managing the symptoms of chronic and advanced disease ensures that patients have the best quality of life possible during their illness journey.
- Psychosocial support and spiritual care are a fundamental part of palliative care that supports patients and families and helps them find hope and meaning in illness and in death.

Brief History of Palliative Care as a Specialty

Though the core principles of palliative care are an integral part of quality nursing care, palliative care is an evolving specialty within healthcare. It arose out of the hospice movement initiated by Dame Cicely Saunders in 1948 in England, with the goal of bringing the benefits of hospice to patients/persons earlier in the diagnosis of a serious illness. There have been several key events over the past few decades that have helped to facilitate the standardization and integration of palliative care for patients living with serious illness(es). Given nursing's foundation of providing patient advocacy and holistic, person-centered care, it is not surprising that the nursing profession has been a leader in the development of the hospice and palliative care specialty.

For example, in 1986 the Hospice and Palliative Nursing Association was established. Two years later the American Academy of Hospice and Palliative Medicine was established. Then in 1990, the World Health Organization recognized palliative care as a specialty that focused on reducing the suffering and on quality of life for patients diagnosed with serious illness(es). Nurses also played an important role in carrying out the recommendations put forth in the Institute of Medicine's 2014 report *Dying in America: Improving Quality and Honoring Individual Preferences Near the End of Life*, which was a pivotal document that suggested transformational change in end-of-life care delivery models, communication in the clinical setting, and advance care planning. It also discussed the importance of reform of palliative care policies and payment systems, professional education, and coordinated and comprehensive person- and family-centered care.[1,2] The Hospice and Palliative Nursing Association first offered national board certifications for hospice registered nurses in 1993. In 1999, this certification was expanded to include both hospice and palliative care registered nurses. In 2003, the certifications were expanded again, and a national certification for the Advanced Certified Hospice and Palliative Care Nurse was added. In 2011, the first exam for pediatric registered nurses was offered, resulting in the national certification of the Certified Hospice and Palliative Pediatric Nurse credential.[3]

The first edition of this textbook was published in 2001, further supporting the growth and development of the hospice and palliative nursing specialty. Shortly thereafter, in 2008, the American Board of Medical Specialties offered the first subspecialty certificate in hospice and palliative medicine for physicians. This brief chronological summary of the advances in hospice and palliative care illustrates how far this specialty has come in the little over three decades since its formal inception.

Palliative Care Nursing

Hospice and palliative care nursing is a highly specialized field of nursing, supporting the best quality of life for patients and their families through the management of symptoms, as well as psychological, social, and spiritual needs. Delivering high-quality palliative care requires refined communication skills, astute clinical assessments, critical thinking, and interdisciplinary collaboration. The delivery of high-quality specialty palliative care takes special training and time to refine each of the skills necessary to deliver this type of specialized care. That said, like other specialties in healthcare, all nurses should possess primary palliative care skills to support the delivery of palliative care to all persons living with serious illness(es) for whom they provide care. By ensuring that nurses are prepared to deliver either primary or specialized palliative care, the needs and quality of life for diverse persons living with serious life-threatening illnesses and their families will be supported.

Goal and Purpose of Textbook

This sixth edition of the textbook includes many changes. First and foremost, the biggest change includes new editors. We recognize that we have big shoes to fill. Each of us is deeply honored to serve in this capacity and takes the responsibility of providing a textbook that the readers will value and respect very seriously. For this reason, we spent a lot of time considering not only the updates that should be included in this textbook but what we envisioned as the overall purpose and goal of this textbook. The goal of this textbook is to serve as a guide to help nurses answer real-world questions as they advocate and care for persons living with a serious illness and their families across the life span. With this goal in mind, we have included several new chapters to support the delivery of palliative care to diverse populations. Ultimately, we hope that this textbook will be the predominant evidence-based resource for nurses to advocate for and deliver high-quality primary and specialty palliative care to persons living with serious illness and their families across the life span and in various settings.

REFERENCES

1. Meghani SH, Hinds PS. Policy brief: The Institute of Medicine report Dying in America: improving quality and honoring individual preferences near the end of life. *Nurs Outlook*. 2015;63(1):51–59.
2. Institute of Medicine. *Committee on approaching death: addressing key end-of-life issues*. National Academies Press; 2015.
3. Hospice & Palliative Nurses Association. Accessed January 28, 2024. Hospice and Palliative Credentialing Center (HPCC) History. https://www.advancingexpertcare.org/hpcc/why-certification/hpcc-history/.

2

Role of Nursing in Palliative Care

Michelle Webb

Key Points

- The role of palliative nursing within the larger healthcare system is evolving as transformation of the system continues and the nursing profession charts a path toward health equity.
- Palliative nursing can play a leadership role in transforming serious illness care through education, practice, research, advocacy, and nurse-led models of palliative care.
- Palliative nurses function in diverse roles and healthcare settings reflecting a broad scope of practice, varied levels of education and training, and changing needs and demographics of those who need serious illness care.
- For patients and caregivers to benefit optimally from palliative care, palliative nursing care must be made available throughout the illness trajectory and in all healthcare systems and community settings.

Case Study: Palliative Care across the Continuum

Ann had been successfully living independently in her family's ancestral home for nearly 25 years. She never married and was one of six siblings, all now deceased. Ann retired at the age of 62 after having worked over 25 years in a manufacturing company and maintained a small circle of close friends and a semi-active lifestyle as she became an older adult. At the age of 87, she was injured in a car collision, which resulted in a displaced comminuted tibia fracture. After this accident, she stopped driving, and her life became increasingly confined to her home and limited outings to the grocery store, church, hair salon, and routine medical appointments. Her social circle and activities simultaneously decreased, and she became totally dependent upon relatives living nearby for transportation.

At the age of 91, Ann experienced a gradual onset of symptoms over a 6-month period including increased weakness, anorexia, and gradual but significant weight loss. Her medical history at that time was positive for essential hypertension, a history of peptic ulcer disease, Type 2 diabetes, and mild cognitive decline. While nothing remarkable was discovered at her annual physical exam, a few days later, she sustained a fall in her home and lay on the floor of her bedroom for several hours before being discovered by family. What followed was a brief stay in the hospital, treatment for severe iron-deficiency anemia and mild rhabdomyolysis secondary to remaining immobile post-fall, and a month-long stay in a rehabilitation facility.

After discharge from the rehabilitation facility, she returned to her home, only to sustain a second fall 2 weeks post-discharge with no serious injury. At the time of the fall, she was also experiencing acute shortness of breath. She was subsequently readmitted to the hospital and diagnosed with acute congestive heart failure. She required aggressive medical treatment in the hospital intensive care unit (ICU) for her symptoms, including supplemental oxygen. The hospital-based palliative care team was consulted during this admission. The recommendation was made by her hospital care team that she no longer live independently in the family home and consider moving to an assisted living facility. Ann insisted on continuing to live alone and was resistant to receiving additional healthcare services in her home because "there are too many people coming in and out of my house." She briefly had been seen by a palliative care nurse practitioner (NP) as well as an interdisciplinary home health team but often refused visits because of her desire for privacy.

Prior to her hospitalization, Ann had begun to rely heavily on relatives who lived nearby for meals, mild to moderate assistance with most activities of daily living, and medication management. Care was being provided by numerous family and professional caregivers and was not well coordinated between the primary physician, the home healthcare team, and the palliative care NP. The most recent hospitalization affirmed a need for improved serious illness care management, care coordination, and long-term planning in the event of continued functional decline. The team and the family were preparing for the possibility that Ann would be unable to remain safely in the home as her cardiac disease progressed. This case study will be examined throughout this chapter to illustrate and elucidate the role of palliative nursing in myriad settings and to outline functional practices associated with the diverse roles palliative nurses play within healthcare systems.

The Role of Palliative Nursing

Palliative nursing has been described as both a philosophy of care and an evidence-based nursing practice that includes "the assessment, diagnosis, and treatment of human responses to actual or potential life-threatening illnesses within the context of a dynamic caring relationship with the patient and family" with the goal of reducing or relieving suffering and optimizing health.[1] The principles of palliative nursing firmly align with the humanitarian ethos, professional values, and code of ethics for the nursing profession.[1] Palliative care is any treatment or intervention intended to "palliate," that is, to "alleviate (a disease or its symptoms) without effecting cure; to relieve or ease physical or emotional suffering temporarily."[2] Palliative care aims to relieve or reduce pain or other distressing symptoms caused by serious or life-threatening illness.

"Palliative nursing" is a broad umbrella term for nursing care delivered to individuals who are seriously ill, including those receiving hospice care at the end of life. "Non-hospice palliative care" is an emerging term that has been used to reflect the broader scope of palliative care that the specialty represents.[3] Palliative care may be provided at any point in the presence of serious and life-threatening illness. While healthcare insurance plans often limit access, many patients can benefit from receiving palliative care concurrent with treatment aimed at curing or slowing the progression of their disease. Hospice care is a specific type of palliative care that focuses on quality of life and symptom management for patients with serious illness and an estimated life expectancy of 6 months or less. All hospice care is palliative in that the focus is on controlling symptoms, but not all palliative care includes hospice.[4]

Palliative nurses function in a variety of roles and settings with a broad scope of intervention that is not confined to specific diagnoses, prognoses, age groups, or populations. Palliative nursing applies the holistic approach characteristic of the palliative model of care, an approach that is interdisciplinary and interprofessional, individualizes care, and co-creates a goal-concordant care experience for patients and families that addresses their unique personal, cultural, spiritual, and physical needs while promoting high quality of life. Palliative nurses play a crucial role in early identification, accurate assessment, and treatment of pain and other physical, psychosocial, or spiritual symptoms. Annually, an estimated 40 million people need palliative care globally, with 78% of those persons living in low- to middle-income countries. Worldwide, "only 14% of people who need palliative care receive it."[5] People worldwide are living longer. The World Health Organization projects that by 2050, two-thirds of people over the age of 60 will be living in low- and middle-income countries.[6] The pace of aging of the world's population and the rising burden of noncommunicable diseases (e.g., cardiovascular and respiratory diseases, cancer, diabetes) and some communicable diseases will contribute to a growing need for palliative care. As the need for palliative care continues to increase globally, the expansion and development of the global nursing workforce to promote universal access to palliative care are crucial.[7] Palliative care has been identified as an essential component of healthcare reform in the United States, and the specialty of palliative nursing has been issued a call to action and must play a leadership role in transforming serious illness care through education, practice, research, advocacy, and nurse-led models of care.[8,9]

The American Nurses Association and the Hospice and Palliative Nurses Association convened the Palliative and Hospice Nursing Professional Issues Panel and identified five focus areas in a "Call for Action: Nurses Lead and Transform Palliative Care."[9] The primary recommendation of the "Call for Action" is that "seriously ill and injured patients, families, and communities should receive quality palliative care in all care settings; a goal to be achieved by the delivery of primary palliative nursing by every nurse regardless of setting.[9] Primary palliative care (also known as "generalist or 'basic" palliative care") is care that is delivered by "disease-oriented"[10(p.27)] healthcare professionals (e.g., nurses, physicians, social workers, chaplains, and others) who have not received specialized training or obtained certification in palliative care but have developed palliative care knowledge and core competencies needed to effectively serve seriously ill patients and their families and caregivers.[9,10] By contrast, specialist palliative care is provided by an interdisciplinary team whose members have undergone recognized specialist palliative care training.[10] Therefore, all nurses must be equipped to practice primary palliative care, which includes symptom management, interprofessional communication, collaboration, and advocacy.

The Evolving Role of the Palliative Nurse

The role of nursing in palliative care continues to evolve in response to the growing number and changing demographics of individuals and families with need for and access to essential serious illness care.[9-16] Notable shifts have been observed in the epidemiology and patterns of care at the end of life including rising complexity and shifts in care patterns and sites of death.[12,13] One of the major tenets underlying palliative care as outlined in the *Clinical Practice Guidelines for Quality Palliative Care* is the expectation of equitable access to quality palliative care services across geography, health settings, patient populations, and conditions.[16] As such, palliative nurses will continue to be needed to fulfill the roles of direct care provider, care coordinator, leader of the interdisciplinary team, educator, policymaker, and nurse scientist.

Efforts to advance nursing science and translate research and new evidence into palliative care practice improvements that benefit patients, families, and communities will be vital to the design of future palliative nursing models. Palliative nursing in the mid-21st century may require periodic role realignment to ensure an effective response to evolving patient, family, community, and global needs for palliative care. The demand for both primary and specialist palliative nurses to provide direct care will persist because patients who need palliative care can be encountered anywhere within health systems and communities. While nurses are the largest group in the healthcare workforce, knowledge deficits remain relative to delivering quality palliative care.[9] The case study outlined earlier in this chapter will be used to illustrate the impact of palliative nursing on care outcomes in various settings and to further elucidate the care nurses perform throughout the healthcare system.

Palliative Nursing in the Hospital Setting

The integration of both primary and specialist palliative nursing into the care provided to hospitalized patients is a clinical imperative. Quality care for seriously ill and dying persons in the acute care setting cannot be delivered without increasing engagement of palliative care specialists. The need for palliative nursing was never more evident than during the global COVID-19 pandemic that began in 2019. Rosa et al.[17]14 concluded that critical care nurse engagement of palliative care should be prioritized and strategically integrated as usual and customary care to be provided beyond times of crisis. Primary palliative care is and has always been "critical" care for the seriously ill and should be provided as appropriate for every patient and family with specialist services being sought where indicated.[17]The nurse in the hospital setting is ideally positioned to ensure timely assessment of the patient's need for palliative care. Hospital nurses should be educated and trained to deliver primary palliative nursing and to identify when secondary palliative care is needed.

Beyond the direct and indirect primary and specialist palliative care services that nurses deliver to patients and their families, the scope of palliative nursing extends into providing the support and knowledge needed to create healthy work environments that enhance nurses' moral agency.[17] Institutional support is needed to define and create a culture that supports nurses caring for themselves as they provide palliative care. Members of hospital-based palliative care teams and nurse leaders can collaborate to design education and support services that nurses need to prevent burnout and to develop additional services that families need to prevent caregiver fatigue and associated negative outcomes for patients. Service innovations that promote sustainable caregiving and the creation of community resources may be needed that extend beyond the hospital's walls.[15,16] The theoretical and evidence-based frameworks encompassed in palliative nursing can greatly inform the development of these services.

In the case study exemplar, Ann's need for specialist palliative care services was identified through collaboration between her assigned primary nurse and a hospital nurse case manager. As in her previous hospitalization, the hospital-based palliative care consult team was consulted. The palliative care team worked with the ICU team and attending hospitalist to ensure the delivery of goal-concordant care, support and engage the family, facilitate advance care planning, and develop a discharge plan that aligned with the patient's wish to return home and continue to live as independently as possible. Ultimately, Ann was discharged with a plan for support from a home healthcare team, a community-based palliative care NP, and recommended options for continued support of family caregivers.

Palliative Nursing in the Home Setting

Most actual palliative care (hospice and non-hospice palliative care) happens at home. Non-hospice palliative care is most often delivered in the outpatient setting or as a consultation service during short-term hospital admissions. Although the non-hospice palliative care team is most often based in a hospital or clinic, it is becoming more common for it to be based in the outpatient setting in the home.[17] Hospice care is most commonly provided in the place that patients and families call home.[18]

The provision of palliative nursing in the home setting presents unique opportunities and challenges for those receiving care in the home and their family caregivers.[19,20] Many people with serious illness are impacted by social determinants of health[21–23] and need both healthcare and social supports such as access to food, housing, personal care, transportation, and financial support. The practice of home palliative nursing incorporates multidimensional evidence-based interventions that aim to: (1) facilitate safe, effective transitions from the hospital setting to home; (2) prevent avoidable hospital readmissions; (3) deliver safe, effective patient- and family-centered care that addresses patients' and families' holistic needs and promotes optimal quality of life; and (4) provide equitable access to service for those living at home with advancing serious illness, including the use of innovative and emerging models for delivering high-quality palliative care to underserved and historically excluded populations.[21] Notable disparities persist in access to palliative care in rural areas and among communities of color, veterans, and LGBTQIA+ persons across all settings[24-30]; and the role of palliative nursing is to engage in activities to close the disparity gap and deliver culturally competent, individualized, equitable care.

For Ann, upon discharge, the palliative care NP assumed the role of care coordinator[6] to ensure consistency in the care approach and support effective communication and interprofessional collaboration among all healthcare professionals. The palliative care NP was a natural point of contact for the patient and the family as well as other healthcare providers (individuals and organizations) and provided an additional layer of medical support for safe home care management of Ann's care. The palliative care NP built relationships with other professionals and between the nurse and the family and maintained an awareness of the interdisciplinary plan for care of the patient in her home and the role of each healthcare provider involved in the care. This allowed the palliative care NP to make key recommendations for reducing the symptom burden for Ann. One example was the recommendation that the required labs ordered for monitoring the response and any potential negative outcomes associated with the ordered medication regimen be drawn by the home care registered nurse. This addressed not only transportation challenges that were faced by family caregivers but also the physical challenges that Ann, who was now confined mostly to the home and using supplemental oxygen, was experiencing. At this point, Ann was unable to leave home without a considerable and taxing effort. The positive impact on the quality of life from this intervention by the palliative care NP for Ann and her family was significant.

Palliative Nursing in the Long-Term Care Setting

Long-term care settings such as nursing homes and assisted living facilities are becoming a common site for delivering palliative care. The need for palliative care in these settings is often identified at the nexus of the curative and palliative phase of serious illness.[31,32] The role of the palliative nurse in the long-term care setting is comparable to that in all other healthcare settings and serves to provide early recognition and treatment of symptoms; assure continuity in care; advocate for and respect residents' wishes and care; offer environmental and psychosocial support to patients, families, and facility staff; keep the family informed and educated; and establish a partnership with the patient and family to ensure that the quality of palliative care meets their unique psychosocial, spiritual, and cultural needs.[30,31] Gaps in the quality of palliative care delivered in long-term care facilities are well known and replete in the extant evidence base. These gaps in the literature highlight the need for ongoing education and coordination of care planning and intervention with long-term care facility staff. Workforce shortages in these settings often severely limit access to primary palliative care services, and practice-based research initiatives have demonstrated some success with the creation of specialized palliative care registered nurse roles as part of efforts to reduce potentially avoidable hospitalizations.[32] Nurses with specialized palliative care education, training, and competency should also lead in the design of evidence-based educational interventions to enhance the primary palliative care skills of nursing home staff as well as the design of innovative nurse-led models for the delivery of palliative care.[30] As in all other healthcare settings, the advance practice registered nurse (APRN) can apply advanced knowledge and expertise in medical management, psychosocial support, communication, care coordination, and education to the care of persons with serious illness in nursing homes.[33]

The case study provides a clear, illustrative example of the impact of the APRN on the care experience and outcomes for Ann and her family during her month-long stay in a skilled nursing facility. Ann was admitted after her first hospitalization for skilled rehabilitation services that included daily physical therapy, occupational therapy, and continuous skilled nursing support to address her medical problems and provide close monitoring of her response to medical treatment. Ann's medical problems included uncontrolled hypertension, poorly controlled diabetes, slowly resolving iron-deficiency anemia with anorexia, and generalized weakness. The APRN visited Ann three times weekly and served as the primary contact with the family, ensuring they remained informed of changes to the medical plan of care; provided close monitoring for new, uncontrolled symptoms; and initiated palliative intervention for medication side effects. The APRN facilitated critical advance care planning discussions with the patient and her family that led to the creation of written advance directives that would guide the care throughout the stay in the skilled nursing facility and clarified the patient's wishes for care in case of a life-threatening event and cardiopulmonary arrest. The family came to rely upon the APRN as the first point of contact for understanding the current medical treatment plan and for ensuring goal-concordant care was delivered by all members of the nursing care team post-discharge from the facility.

Conclusion

The role of palliative nursing within the larger healthcare system will continue to evolve and grow as transformation of the healthcare system continues and the nursing profession charts a path toward health equity. Palliative nurses must play a leadership role in transforming serious illness care through education, practice, research, advocacy, and nurse-led models of palliative care. Palliative nurses perform diverse roles and functions in varied healthcare settings, reflecting a broad scope of practice and varied levels of education and training. In the future, palliative nursing will be guided by the changing needs and demographics of those who need serious illness care.

For patients and caregivers (families, friends, and all others who provide support to patients) to benefit optimally from palliative care, palliative nursing care must be made available throughout the illness trajectory and in all healthcare systems and community settings. The implications for palliative nursing education, leadership, practice, health policy, and research are significant as the role of the palliative nurse continues to expand to ensure excellence in the delivery of palliative care and optimal outcomes for those facing serious and life-threatening illness.

REFERENCES

1. Lynch M, Dahlin C, Hultman T, Coakley EE. Palliative care nursing: defining the discipline? *J Hosp Palliat Nurs.* 2011;13(2):106–111. https://doi.org/10.1097/NJH.0b013e3182075b6e.
2. Oxford University Press. *Oxford English Dictionary* (online version). Oxford University Press; 2022. https://www.oed.com/.
3. Beasley A, Bakitas MA, Edwards R, Kavalieratos D. Models of non-hospice palliative care: a review. *Ann Palliat Med.* 2019;8(suppl 1):S15–S21. https://doi.org/10.21037/apm.2018.03.11.
4. Association AL. Understanding Palliative Care: It's Not What You Think. Accessed January 17, 2025. https://www.lung.org/blog/understanding-palliative-care
5. World Health Organization. Palliative Care. Accessed October 2, 2022. https://www.who.int/news-room/fact-sheets/detail/palliative-care.
6. World Health Organization. Ageing and Health. Accessed March 17, 2023. https://www.who.int/news-room/fact-sheets/detail/ageing-and-health.
7. World Health Organization. Noncommunicable Diseases. Accessed March 17, 2023. https://www.who.int/news-room/fact-sheets/detail/noncommunicable-diseases.
8. Rosa WE, Parekh de Campos A, Abedini NC, et al. Optimizing the global nursing workforce to ensure universal palliative care access and alleviate serious health-related suffering worldwide. *J Pain Symptom Manage.* 2022;63(2):e224–e236. https://doi.org/10.1016/j.jpainsymman.2021.07.014.
9. American Nurses Association, Hospice and Palliative Nurses Association. *American Nurses Association Professional Issues Panel|Call for Action: Nurses Lead and Transform Palliative Care;* 2017. https://www.nursingworld.org/get-involved/share-your-expertise/pro-issues-panel/palliative-and-hospice-nursing-panel/
10. Institute of Medicine. *Dying in America: Improving Quality and Honoring Individual Preferences near the End of Life.* National Academies; 2015. Accessed October 2, 2022. https://doi.org/10.17226/18748.
11. National Academies of Sciences, Engineering, and Medicine; National Academy of Medicine; Committee on the Future of Nursing 2020–2030; Flaubert JL, Le Menestrel S, Williams DR, et al., editors. The Future of Nursing 2020–2030: Charting a Path to Achieve Health Equity. Washington (DC): National Academies Press (US); 2021 May 11. Summary. Available from: https://www.ncbi.nlm.nih.gov/books/NBK573919/
12. Morin L, Aubry R, Frova L, et al. Estimating the need for palliative care at the population level: a cross-national study in 12 countries. *Palliat Med.* 2017;31(6):526–536. https://doi.org/10.1177/0269216316671280.
13. Aldridge MD, Bradley EH. Epidemiology and patterns of care at the end of life: rising complexity, shifts in care patterns and sites of death. *Health Aff (Millwood).* 2017;36(7):1175–1183. Accessed October 3, 2022. https://www.healthaffairs.org/doi/10.1377/hlthaff.2017.0182.
14. Hawley P. Barriers to access to palliative care. *Palliat Care.* 2017;10:1178224216688887. doi:10.1177/1178224216688887
15. Zhou K, Fu J. Evolution of oncology and palliative nursing in meeting the changing landscape of cancer care. *J Healthc Eng.* 2022:3831705. https://doi.org/10.1155/2022/3831705.
16. National Consensus Project for Quality Palliative Care, National Coalition for Hospice and Palliative Care. Clinical Practice Guidelines for Quality Palliative Care. 4th ed. National Coalition for Hospice and Palliative Care; 2018. Accessed October 1, 2022. https://www.nationalcoalitionhpc.org/ncp/.
17. Rosa WE, Ferrell BR, Wiencek C. Increasing critical care nurse engagement of palliative care during the COVID-19 pandemic. *Crit Care Nurse.* 2020;40(6):e28–e36. https://doi.org/10.4037/ccn2020946.
18. National Hospice and Palliative Care Organization. *NHPCO Facts and Figures 2024 Edition*; 2024:21. https://www.nhpco.org/wp-content/uploads/NHPCO-Facts-Figures-2024.pdf.

19. Delaney MC. Caring for the caregivers: evaluation of the effect of an eight-week pilot mindful self-compassion (MSC) training program on nurses' compassion fatigue and resilience. *PLoS One*. 2018;13(11):e0207261. https://doi.org/10.1371/journal.pone.0207261.
20. Law S, Ormel I, Babinski S, Kuluski K, Quesnel-Vallée A. "Caregiving is like on the job training but nobody has the manual": Canadian caregivers' perceptions of their roles within the healthcare system. *BMC Geriatr*. 2021;21(1):404. https://doi.org/10.1186/s12877-021-02354-z.
21. Cohn J, Corrigan J, Lynn J, et al. Community-based models of care delivery for people with serious illness. *NAM Perspectives*. 2017;7(4). https://doi.org/10.31478/201704b.
22. Social Determinants of Health. Accessed January 17, 2025. https://www.who.int/health-topics/social-determinants-of-health#tab=tab_1
23. Artiga S, Hinton E. *Beyond Health Care: The Role of Social Determinants in Promoting Health and Health Equity*. Kaiser Family Foundation. May 10, 2018. Accessed October 2, 2022. https://www.kff.org/racial-equity-and-health-policy/issue-brief/beyond-health-care-the-role-of-social-determinants-in-promoting-health-and-health-equity/
24. Pesut B, Hooper B, Jacobsen M, Nielsen B, Falk M, O'Connor BP. Nurse-led navigation to provide early palliative care in rural areas: a pilot study. *BMC Palliat Care*. 2017;16(1):37. https://doi.org/10.1186/s12904-017-0211-2.
25. Estrada LV, Agarwal M, Stone PW. Racial/ethnic disparities in nursing home end-of-life care: a systematic review. *J Am Med Dir Assoc*. 2021;22(2):279–290.e1. https://doi.org/10.1016/j.jamda.2020.12.005.
26. Rosa, WE, Roberts KE, Braybrook D, et al. Palliative and end-of-life care needs, experiences, and preferences of LGBTQ+ individuals with serious illness: a systematic mixed-methods review. *Palliat Med*. 2023:37(4):460–474. doi:10.1177/0269216322114426
27. Haviland K, Walters CB, Newman S. Barriers to palliative care in sexual and gender minority patients with cancer: a scoping review of the literature. *Health Soc Care Community*. 2021;29(2):305–318. doi:10.1111/hsc.13126
28. Kondo K, Low A, Everson T, et al. Health disparities in veterans: a map of the evidence. *Med Care*. 2017;55(9, suppl 2):S9–S15. https://doi.org/10.1097/MLR.0000000000000756.
29. Collons D, Florez N, Petrillo L, Dhawan N, Gray TF. Palliative care for all? An assessment of racial and ethnic disparities research with solutions. *J Pain Symptom Manage*. 2023;66(4):e521e523. doi:10.1016/j.jpainsymman.2023.06.014
30. Gonella S, Basso I, De Marinis MG, Campagna S, Di Giulio P. Good end-of-life care in nursing home according to the family carers' perspective: a systematic review of qualitative findings. *Palliat Med*. 2019;33(6):589–606. https://doi.org/10.1177/0269216319840275.
31. Hickman SE, Parks M, Unroe KT, Ott M, Ersek M. The role of the palliative care registered nurse in the nursing facility setting. *J Hosp Palliat Nurs*. 2020;22(2):152–158. https://doi.org/10.1097/NJH.0000000000000634.
32. Ersek M, Unroe KT, Carpenter JG, Cagle JG, Stephens CE, Stevenson DG. High-quality nursing home and palliative care-one and the same. *J Am Med Dir Assoc*. 2022;23(2):247–252. https://doi.org/10.1016/j.jamda.2021.11.027.
33. Battista V, Sciacca K. Professional standards and the role of the advanced practice registered nurse in hospice and palliative care. *J Hosp Palliat Nurs*. 2023;25(5):249. doi:10.1097/NJH.0000000000000968

3

Public Policy for Palliative Care

Marian Grant

Key Points

- This chapter will review the basics of federal health policies that affect people living with serious illness.
- It will highlight specific policy issues that affect access to palliative care and ways the field is working to address them.
- It will help nurses learn how they can advocate for better care for their patients via public policy advocacy.

Case Study

Juanita is a new nurse working on the palliative care service of an academic medical center. She has always thought of policy only in terms of the ones at her hospital. However, she heard a lecture about palliative care public policy and now realizes that some of the issues she consistently runs into are actually policy-related. For instance, she repeatedly has patients who are interested in hospice but then do not want to stop palliative or curative treatment to get it. Or they want hospice, but their families cannot provide the 24/7 care it would require at home; and they cannot afford to pay for room and board at a nursing home with a hospice overlay. She also has patients who need opioid medication for pain management yet cannot easily access that in the community. She also hears of other hospital and community-based palliative care programs that are struggling financially and use only providers like physicians or nurse practitioners versus a full interdisciplinary team (IDT). This chapter will use this case study and Juanita's perspective throughout to bring palliative care public policy to life.

Medicare

Medicare Basics

The federal government's Medicare program is the foundation of health policy in the United States. Medicare is the federal health insurance program for people 65 years of age and older, certain younger people with disabilities, and those with end-stage renal disease on dialysis.[1] Medicare covered 65 million beneficiaries in 2020[2] and does not pay for all of beneficiaries' covered medical costs, and many other costs/services are not covered at all, such as vision, dental, hearing, or long-term care. See Table 3.1 for key Medicare facts.

People on Medicare have to pay premiums, deductibles, and copays, so while the federal government pays much of beneficiaries' medical care, it is not free to them. Medicare is overseen by the Centers for Medicare & Medicaid Services (CMS).

Juanita heard her grandmother talk about the different "parts" of Medicare using letters when she recently enrolled in Medicare. Table 3.2 explains what those four parts are, what they cover, and how they are funded.

Medicare Part A is what all people get when they enroll in Medicare at age 65.[3] Part A pays for hospitalization and things like hospice. Part B is something people can elect and then pay for additionally. Juanita remembers hearing of patients who had Part A coverage for hospitalization but not Part B, and that made post-discharge medical follow-up hard for them. Part C, Medicare Advantage (MA), and Part D are things people can also sign up and pay for; and MA will be covered later in this chapter.

How Medicare Operates

Medicare is a very large federal agency with thousands of employees at locations across the country. Medicare leaders are political appointees who change every time there is a new presidential administration, while the staff below them can continue across administrations.

Medicare is subject to federal laws, regulations, the federal budget, presidential executive orders, watchdog and advocacy

Table 3.1 Key Medicare facts

Element	Information
People eligible	People 65+ Certain younger people with disabilities Those with end-stage renal disease on dialysis
Number of beneficiaries	65 million
Budget	\$689 billion
% Total health spending	20%

Source: Reference 1.

Table 3.2 The parts of Medicare

Part	Cover	Funding
A	Hospitalization, hospice, home health, skilled nursing facility after hospitalization but not long-term care	Payroll tax, trust fund
B	Office visits, preventive services, durable medical equipment	Premiums cover only 80%, need supplemental
C	Medicare Advantage, full range services	Premiums
D	Prescription drug	Premiums

Source: Reference 3.

organizations, and congressional oversight via groups like the Office of the Inspector General. Ongoing Medicare operations are frequently delegated to government contractors. There is a federal Medicare Payment Advisory Commission, MedPAC, that monitors Medicare payment and reports annually to Congress. Hospice payment policy is a topic they review annually.

Medicare consists of traditional Medicare, using a fee-for-service (FFS) payment system,[4] where a provider is paid for each particular medical service provided, and MA.[5] MA is run by private health insurance companies, and its membership is steadily growing as MA offers more benefits and lower premium prices. As a result, almost half of Medicare beneficiaries are currently covered through MA,[6] and it is projected that more than half will be by 2023. MA uses a star rating system to help people know which plans to sign up for; the more stars a plan has, the better their scores on selected quality measures.[7]

The significance of MA to palliative care is that MA plans can offer different things than traditional Medicare, such as supplemental benefits for chronic illness, which includes services to reduce the functional or psychological impact of health conditions or reduce available emergency or healthcare utilization; home-based palliative care is an example of such a supplemental benefit.[8] Some palliative care programs have successfully negotiated relationships with MA plans via fixed monthly payments for MA members to receive palliative care services; quality bonuses when selected performance measures are achieved; a 2-month palliative care "bundle" for enrolled members, requiring a minimum number of in-home visits; and/or fixed monthly payment plus shared savings and losses.[9] Juanita now wonders if another palliative program in her area that is delivering palliative care at home is doing so via such an MA arrangement.

Medicare Payment

Even though Medicare cares for only older and some people with qualifying disabilities in the United States, it is the largest US healthcare payer, representing 12% of the federal budget and 20% of national health expenditures ($689 billion in 2021).[2] As such, it sets benefits, rates, and policies for the healthcare industry, and private insurance company or payer negotiations are often tied to Medicare's fees. This is important for palliative care since MA can pay for some aspects of palliative care, while traditional Medicare's FFS does not pay for comprehensive palliative care. For example, FFS pays for services of only some healthcare providers on the IDT like physicians, nurse practitioners, or physician assistants but not nurses or social workers. It also only pays for certain medical interventions, like symptom management or advance care planning, but not family or spiritual support. FFS is one reason why many palliative care teams may have only or mostly billable providers and why they focus generally on those services that are billable, as opposed to things like providing family and spiritual support which are not billable services. So, a fundamental aspect of Medicare payment works against the kind of holistic, interdisciplinary care people with serious illness really need.

Fortunately, there is recognition that FFS payment tends to promote more interventions rather than quality care, or volume over value; and there is now a shift to paying for value, or "value-based"[10] or "accountable" care. (Please see Chapter 7 for more information on value-based care.) Medicare is committed to making value-based its dominant payment method by the mid 2020s[11] and is steadily rolling out regulatory changes to do so. Accountable care organizations (ACOs) are another example of value-based payment where networks of providers, hospitals, or clinics try to improve and coordinate care while being paid bonuses for meeting quality targets or penalties for not.[12] Some palliative care programs contract with ACOs to care for populations with complex or chronic illnesses, and palliative care can help ACOs meet their quality targets.[13] Juanita now wonders if her area has such ACOs, and if her team might explore whether they would be open to using them to provide palliative care services to their patients.

New Medicare Serious Illness Models

In addition to shifting to value-based payment, Medicare tests new care delivery models via the Center for Medicare and Medicaid Innovation (CMMI) established in the 2009 Affordable Care Act.[14] The goal of this center is to test new demonstration models to improve care and/or reduce cost, and CMMI can expand any models that are deemed successful. To date, few models have been expanded, and there have been only two pertinent models for serious illness, covered below.

Medicare Care Choices Model

This model, also known as "concurrent care," was tested from 2016 to 2021 with the goal of allowing those with advanced cancer, chronic obstructive pulmonary disease, congestive heart failure, or human immunodeficiency virus/acquired immunodeficiency syndrome (HIV/AIDS) to get hospice care along with disease-modifying treatment. This test was prompted by the fact that the traditional Medicare Hospice Benefit (MHB) does not pay for concurrent care and instead requires people to forego disease-modifying treatment in favor of getting only hospice care. While that made sense in the early 1980s when hospice was first introduced, it makes less sense now when there is more curative and palliative treatment that can meaningfully extend the lives of people with terminal illness. However, the government needs strong evidence to change the MHB, and the Medicare Care Choices Model (MCCM) was a way to get that evidence. Many in the hospice field were very excited about testing this concept, and more hospices participated in the model than were anticipated. Encouragingly, MCCM was one of only six—out of more than 50 CMMI models—that generated statistically significant savings for Medicare. Results showed nearly $6,000 net savings per patient, and family caregiver experience was also greatly improved under this model.[15]

Unfortunately, MCCM was limited in its impact: it still required a 6-month prognosis for enrollment, and patients with only a few selected diagnoses were included. While the financial results showed savings, not enough people were enrolled to have a large enough sample to change the federal MHB.[16] Participating hospices saw that offering concurrent care, like offering palliative care, increased the number of people who enrolled in hospice and for longer, which has encouraged many hospices to try to do this on their own outside of MCCM. Importantly, a provision in the 2009 Affordable Care Act allows concurrent care for pediatric hospice patients,[17] although it has taken several years to develop such programs and they mostly exist in major pediatric medical centers. However, the success of the concurrent care model in pediatrics is another data point suggesting that it would work for adults as well. Juanita wonders if the children's hospital in her area offers concurrent pediatric and hospice care and if some of the local hospices her patients go to are still allowing, and paying for, some types of concurrent care.

MA Value-Based Insurance Design (Hospice Carve-In)

This more recent test may be another way to improve access to hospice care. Historically, MA plans do not cover hospice care. Therefore, people enrolled in MA who opt for hospice have to disenroll from their MA plan, and their providers, and go back into traditional Medicare to receive hospice services. This transition has been a barrier to smooth hospice enrollment, so the MA value-based insurance design test will study allowing MA plans to also offer hospice services. The model also requires that MA plans provide concurrent hospice and curative care for at least 1 month in addition to "appropriate" palliative care services.[18] This is another way to test palliative and concurrent care, and the model will run from 2021 to 2024. Juanita learned that none of the hospices in her area are participating in this model and hopes the results will again be positive.

Medicaid

Medicaid is another government health coverage program for 82 million Americans including eligible low-income adults, children, pregnant women, older adults, and people with disabilities. See Table 3.3 for key Medicaid facts.

It is funded jointly by the states and the federal government and administered by the states per federal requirements.[20] Whereas Medicare is limited in only being able to pay for medical services, Medicaid can also pay for social services like nutrition and transport, family caregiver support, and other helpful services in the community. However, because it is state-based, Medicaid eligibility and services vary by state, and what can be generous services in one state may not be covered in another.[21] Juanita fortunately lives in a state that has more generous services than the other states nearby.

Medicaid is an additional way to provide palliative care services to those getting governmental health coverage. Several states have either passed legislation to require palliative care services for their Medicaid programs or are in the process of applying for Medicaid waivers to do so. In California, legislation passed in 2018 that mandated that the state's Medicaid program include palliative care for those with advanced illness,[22] prompting the development of a statewide palliative care infrastructure. This has taken several years to get started but now offers palliative care services delivered by various providers including hospitals and hospices across that large state. Hawaii is in the process of applying to the federal government to amend its state Medicaid plan to add palliative care.[23] Illinois was able to pass legislation in 2021 requiring palliative care for children in that state's Medicaid program.[24] The learning from California is that once this infrastructure gets built, these services are available for non-Medicaid populations and so could be offered to others living with serious illness. Other states are studying these pioneering examples, and the hope is that over the next few years, more states will have similar Medicaid palliative care benefits and programs. Juanita has heard that her state has just passed legislation to start a palliative care workgroup that will deliver a report to the state that could include plans to pursue a Medicaid benefit there.

Table 3.3 Key 2021 Medicaid facts

Element	Information
People eligible	Eligible low-income adults (varies by state) Children Pregnant women Certain older adults People with disabilities
Number of enrollees	82 million
Budget	$662 billion
% Total health spending	17%

Source: Reference 19.

Serious Illness Population Definition

There has been a shift in health policy toward a population health focus. Population health provides "the health outcomes of a group of individuals, including the distribution of such outcomes within the group."[25] In order to provide population health, however, federal and state programs need to be able to define the specific population receiving care. Defining the population of those people living with cancer or heart failure is not difficult as data in Medicare or insurance claims information is easily available for those groups. Such data is not available for those with serious illness. Those individuals have a wide range of acute or chronic illnesses and can vary in age from neonates to the very old and receive care in a wide range of settings. Therefore, to promote public policies that would deliver better care to those with serious illness, the palliative care field needed to develop a definition of that population. This effort resulted in the serious illness definition[26] shown in Box 3.1.

This definition has been widely adopted by the field, including by the National Committee for Quality Assurance and the National Quality Forum (NQF). Juanita has heard about this definition and has seen it used in presentations to explain serious illness.

Box 3.1 Serious Illness Population Definition

A health condition that carries a high risk of mortality and either negatively impacts a person's daily function, or quality of life, or excessively strains their family caregivers.

Source: Reference 26 (p. S-7).

Quality Measurement

Quality in CMMI models, MA, or value-based arrangements is dependent on performance on validated measures. These measures must be endorsed by the NQF, the federal body responsible for endorsing such measures.[27] Measures need a strong evidence base to be endorsed by the NQF, which has been hard for young fields like palliative care to develop. However, in 2017, Medicare funded a palliative care measure development project led by the American Academy of Hospice and Palliative Medicine, in partnership with the National Coalition for Hospice and Palliative Care and the RAND Corporation.[28] The two measures developed were (1) the percentage of patients with a recent outpatient palliative care visit who reported feeling heard and understood and (2) those who reported getting the help they wanted for their pain.[28] These are patient-reported measures, considered a better gauge of quality than process measures, and are assessed at the level of the palliative care provider and team. They also fill a gap in measuring the quality of communication and symptom management, important aspects of all healthcare, not just palliative care. Patients were included in the development of these measures, and these measures have now gone through the NQF review and endorsement process and have been officially endorsed[29] for use in 2023 Medicare programs and beyond.

Other Pertinent Policy Areas

Advance Care Planning

Chapter 6 will cover advance care planning (ACP) more thoroughly, but it is important to understand that there are policy aspects of this process that affect its access and use. ACP's policy history is tied to the passage of the Patient Self-Determination Act in 1990, which confirmed people's constitutional right to determine their final healthcare.[30] Since then, federal and state policies have been implemented to promote aspects of ACP and the legal documents, advance directives, that are part of this process. (Medical orders like physicians' orders for life sustaining treatment are technically not advance directives, although they also use state-based forms.) At present, all states have laws or regulations around advance directives, and most have state-specific forms.[31] On the federal level CMS defines ACP as "a face-to-face service between a physician (or other qualified health care professional) and a patient to discuss the patient's health care wishes if they become unable to make decisions about their care."[32] These discussions may review advance directives with or without completing the relevant legal forms.

In 2016, CMS created billing codes for ACP[32] to encourage clinicians to have these important conversations. The codes pay for having these discussions in any clinical setting but can only be used by a physician, nurse practitioner, or physician assistant. They also carry a 20% cost-sharing (copay/deductible) for the patient, as is the case for all other Medicare Part B services. The only time there is no cost-sharing is when ACP is done as part of a Medicare annual wellness visit (AWV). However, ACP often occurs outside of an AWV, such as with palliative care and other specialists, during other primary care visits, or in the hospital; and in those situations, the 20% cost-sharing is charged, which can be as much as $40 depending on the specialist or setting. Data from 2017[33] showed a total of $104.5 million in ACP cost-sharing, which is a lot of money from patients.

A 2020 federal report on ACP identified this cost-sharing as a key barrier to ACP access,[34] and a 2021 study of ACP billing code usage showed that communities of color engage less often in ACP as part of an AWV and therefore are charged cost-sharing more often.[35] This is clearly an equity issue, with ACP cost-sharing disproportionately affecting populations who often also lack access to preventive care. Other evidence shows ACP is already less likely to occur among these groups,[36] so adding a financial cost further reduces access to this important service. Concerns about potential patient financial burden from cost-sharing even prevent some providers from billing these codes.[37]

Palliative care policy groups are trying to add other clinicians, like licensed clinical social workers, to the list of those who can be paid by Medicare for ACP. They are also trying to remove the 20% patient cost-sharing. Unfortunately, Medicare lacks the authority to make these changes on its own, so organizations are now working with Congress on federal legislation[38] to allow that. This is an example of a clinical issue (limited members of the team being able to bill for ACP, and patients being charged for it) that has prompted public policy action.

Palliative nurses and others on the IDT could also do ACP, although adding them as billable providers is unlikely for the foreseeable future as they are not billable providers for anything yet in Medicare, while licensed clinical social workers already are for behavioral health.[39] Another way to allow more members of the IDT to do ACP is via value-based contracts since those usually pay a set amount per month per patient from which the palliative care IDT can have whoever is most appropriate handle ACP. This is another reason Juanita thinks her palliative care team should explore such value-based options since she and the team's social worker are often asked to help with ACP.

More recently, CMS funded an effort to make advance directives interoperable across clinical settings.[40] Currently, the paper advance directive form has to go with the patient from the hospital to rehab or hospice or wherever, and scanned images of these documents have not been easy to access in the electronic health record. Technical experts have been working with clinicians to develop technical standards[41] so that information from advance directives could be more easily digitized and shared across settings. It will still take years for this to finally be available, but it is encouraging that the federal government saw this opportunity and has allocated resources for it.

Opioid Public Policies

The opioid overdose epidemic in the United States was problematic before the COVID-19 pandemic and has gotten even worse because of it.[42] Healthcare providers and the general public are now very aware of the risks of opioid misuse. However, palliative care nurses know that these are important medications for many living with serious illness and that, taken appropriately, they can increase function and quality of life. Unfortunately, several public policy efforts have made access to these medications worse. Following are some of the key policy efforts palliative nurses should be aware of.

Centers for Disease and Prevention Control Clinical Practice Guideline for Prescribing Opioids for Pain

The Centers for Disease Control and Prevention (CDC) issued recommendations in 2016 for prescribing opioids for pain.[43] These were specifically for chronic, not acute, pain and only for the primary care setting, not the hospital or cancer center. From the beginning, they excluded or were not for patients on hospice, receiving palliative care, or with cancer. Based on what is now known to be lower-quality evidence, these recommendations included a daily morphine equivalent dose limit of 90 mg and prescribing short courses of opioids versus using them in the long term and discontinuing opioids whenever possible. Unfortunately, these recommendations were quickly taken up by states and parts of the federal government that passed laws and regulations limiting things like how many days an opioid prescription could cover, making opioid refills harder to access by requiring patients to see their providers in person again and/or encouraging opioid discontinuation, resulting in some providers cutting back significantly or not prescribing these medications entirely. In reality, the populations the recommendations excluded, such as those with cancer, getting palliative care, or in hospice, were sometimes incorrectly included in these restrictions; and the impact on those living with chronic or cancer pain was sometimes tragic.[44]

The misuse of the recommendations was so bad it prompted the CDC to issue a 2019 caution[45] to point out (1) the misuse of the recommendations for populations outside of the guideline's scope, such as those with cancer or receiving palliative care or hospice; (2) the misapplication of the guideline's dosage recommendation that resulted in hard limits or "cutting off" opioids; and (3) misunderstanding the recommendations when abruptly tapering or stopping long-term opioid use. In 2022, the CDC updated the opioid guideline based on public input.[46] The revised recommendations are more careful about these issues and sensitive to those who need these medications,[46] and major palliative care associations wrote to support that approach.

Medicare Part D Opioid Overutilization Program

This chapter mentioned Part D early on as a Medicare program for beneficiaries to access medications. In 2013, before the CDC guideline but when the consequences of opioid misuse were becoming clear, Medicare created a program to monitor those participating in Part D drug plans as a way to identify Medicare beneficiaries at risk for opioid misuse.[47] Unfortunately, this program did not exclude those people receiving palliative care, one of the excluded populations in the 2016 CDC opioid guideline. CMS fixed this in 2018 when the palliative care field pointed that error out, and the monitoring program now also excludes those on palliative care in addition to people with cancer or receiving hospice.[48]

Hospital Patient Survey

CMS requires that hospitals regularly survey patients on their inpatient experience, and previous surveys included questions about whether their pain was adequately managed. In 2017, again due to concerns about opioid misuse, all the pain questions from the hospital survey were removed[49]; and now patients are no longer asked about a key aspect of hospitalization.

Public Policy and Health Equity

Evidence consistently shows those from historically underresourced communities who also have serious illness experience poorer care[50] and access. While Chapter 66 will cover this topic more thoroughly, it is worth mentioning equity in this chapter since public policy plays a role in perpetuating inequality. Inequity in healthcare goes very far back, with hospitals, clinics, and providers being historically limited to caring for specific racial groups[51] and poorer individuals often not having any access to healthcare or health insurance before programs like Medicare and Medicaid, established only in 1965.[52]

While some of those 1965 policy changes theoretically increased access to healthcare, it is known that structural racism and implicit bias continue to reduce the care and quality many in historically underresourced groups receive. For instance, consider the MHB. Hospice was designed to be mostly delivered in the person's home, which presumes both the dying person has a physical home and someone to provide care for them there. Juanita knows families who cannot undertake this due to tenuous or multiple jobs where they do not get any time off and cannot telework. While respite care can be provided, that is limited to only a few days and means the hospice patient is now in a facility that may be difficult to get to if the family has transportation or financial issues.

Current hospice policy, as noted earlier in this chapter, also requires people to forego disease-modifying treatment, something that is hard to ask of communities that have never gotten adequate healthcare in the first place. The requirement of a 6-month prognosis can also be difficult for those who have not gotten preventive or basic primary care earlier in their lives and who may get diagnosed only in the last stage of illness, when they may have days instead of months left to live. And the hospice visits at home are usually by non-physician clinicians, which may feel like lesser-quality care to those who have long struggled to see physicians for their care. None of this was intended in the MHB, yet the consequence is that African American and Hispanic individuals have historically lower hospice enrollment of 33%–35% for those groups versus 49% for White patients.[53]

ACP is another example of unintended policy inequity. The state focus on signed documents is problematic for groups who have been misled into signing disadvantageous documents in the past and are now rightly suspicious of them. National research done in 2019 found that almost half of those surveyed were reluctant to engage in ACP as they do not believe their wishes will be honored or do not trust doctors or the healthcare system. As a result, the group that typically completes advance directives is Caucasian, is more highly educated, and has a higher income. Unfortunately, this is a group already used to voicing their preferences and having them heard and honored. Efforts to engage people in ACP have to recognize these attitudinal and trust barriers and be sensitive to cultural norms that may, as is true for some Native Americans, for instance, resist planning for death out of fear that that will make it happen.[54] Juanita is aware of efforts in some local churches to promote ACP conversations in a safer and more trusted environment.

Case Study Conclusion

Juanita has become much more aware of the importance of public policy and how it affects the composition and work of her team and possible future program expansion options. She has become a member of the national Hospice and Palliative Nurses Association and has volunteered to help with policy work for her state chapter. When she runs into clinical barriers, she now asks herself if they are policy-related; and when they are, that renews her commitment to helping overcome them with better policy.

Chapter Key Conclusions

The care of those living with serious illness is affected by numerous federal and state public policies. Some policy issues affect access to palliative care that the field is working to overcome.

Armed with this policy understanding, nurses can advocate for better care for their patients via public policy advocacy.

REFERENCES

1. Centers for Medicare & Medicaid Services. Medicare Program—General Information. Accessed September 13, 2022. https://www.cms.gov/Medicare/Medicare-General-Information/MedicareGenInfo.
2. Kaiser Family Foundation. The Facts about Medicare Spending. June 7, 2022. Accessed September 13, 2022. https://www.kff.org/interactive/medicare-spending/.
3. Medicare Interactive. The parts of Medicare (A, B, C, D). Accessed September 13, 2022. https://www.medicareinteractive.org/get-answers/medicare-basics/medicare-coverage-overview/original-medicare.
4. HealthCare.gov. Fee for Service—Glossary. Accessed September 13, 2022. https://www.healthcare.gov/glossary/fee-for-service.
5. Medicare. Medicare Advantage Plans Cover All Medicare Services. Accessed September 4, 2020. https://www.medicare.gov/what-medicare-covers/what-medicare-health-plans-cover/medicare-advantage-plans-cover-all-medicare-services.
6. Freed M, Damico A. 2022. Medicare Advantage in 2024: Enrollment Update and Key Trends. Kaiser Family Foundation. August 25, 2022. Accessed September 13, 2022. https://www.kff.org/medicare/issue-brief/medicare-advantage-in-2024-enrollment-update-and-key-trends/.
7. Centers for Medicare & Medicaid Services. CMS Releases 2022 Medicare Advantage and Part D Star Ratings to Help Medicare Beneficiaries Compare Plans. October 8, 2021. Accessed September 13, 2022. https://www.cms.gov/newsroom/press-releases/cms-releases-2022-medicare-advantage-and-part-d-star-ratings-help-medicare-beneficiaries-compare.
8. Coleman K. Reinterpretation of "Primarily Health Related" for Supplemental Benefits. Centers for Medicare & Medicaid Services. April 27, 2018. Accessed October 5, 2020. https://www.nahc.org/wp-content/uploads/2018/05/HPMS-Memo-Primarily-Health-Related-4-27-18.pdf.
9. Brandt K. Medicare Reimbursement for Palliative Care. California State University Shiley Haynes Institute for Palliative Care. August 23, 2016. Accessed December 28, 2022. https://csupalliativecare.org/medicare-reimbursement/.
10. Centers for Medicare & Medicaid Services. CMS' Value-Based Programs. Accessed September 8, 2020. https://www.cms.gov/Medicare/Quality-Initiatives-Patient-Assessment-Instruments/Value-Based-Programs/Value-Based-Programs.
11. Health Care Payment Learning & Action Network. Accessed September 4, 2020. https://hcp-lan.org/.
12. Centers for Medicare & Medicaid Services. Accountable Care Organizations (ACOs). Accessed February 2, 2025 at https://www.cms.gov/priorities/innovation/innovation-models/aco
13. Sinclair S, Silvers A. FAQs on the New Seriously Ill Population (SIP) Alternative Payment Model Option Center for Advanced Palliative Care. November 1, 2019. Accessed February 2, 2025. https://www.capc.org/blog/faqs-new-seriously-ill-population-sip-alternative-payment-model-option/
14. Kaiser Family Foundation. "What Is CMMI?" and 11 Other FAQs about the CMS Innovation Center. February 27, 2018. Accessed September 8, 2020. https://www.kff.org/medicare/fact-sheet/what-is-cmmi-and-11-other-faqs-about-the-cms-innovation-center/.
15. CMS Announces One-Year Extension of Medicare Care Choices Model, NHPCO Responds. Accessed February 3, 2025. https://ehospice.com/usa_posts/cms-announces-one-year-extension-of-medicare-care-choices-model/.
16. Centers for Medicare & Medicaid Services. Medicare Care Choices Model Fourth Annual Report. Accessed December 28, 2022. https://innovation.cms.gov/data-and-reports/2022/mccm-fg-fourth-annrpt.
17. Mary J. Labyak Institute for Innovation. *Pediatric Concurrent Care*. National Hospice and Palliative Care Organization; 2012.
18. Centers for Medicare & Medicaid Services. VBID Model Hospice Benefit Component Overview. Accessed February 7, 2023. https://innovation.cms.gov/innovation-models/vbid-hospice-benefit-overview.
19. Williams E. Medicaid Enrollment & Spending Growth: FY 2021 & 2022. Kaiser Family Foundation. October 27, 2021. Accessed September 14, 2022. https://www.kff.org/medicaid/issue-brief/medicaid-enrollment-spending-growth-fy-2021-2022/.
20. Medicaid.gov. Medicaid. Accessed September 13, 2022. https://www.medicaid.gov/medicaid/index.html.
21. Center on Budget and Policy Priorities. Policy Basics: Introduction to Medicaid. April 14, 2020. Accessed January 11, 2023. https://www.cbpp.org/research/health/introduction-to-medicaid.
22. California Department of Health Care Services. Palliative Care and SB 1004. Accessed September 4, 2020. https://www.dhcs.ca.gov/provgovpart/Pages/Palliative-Care-and-SB-1004.aspx.
23. Coalition to Transform Advanced Care. Hawai'i's New Managed Medicaid Benefit for Community-Based Palliative Care. July 28, 2021. Accessed September 13, 2022. https://thectac.org/asset/blog/hawaiis-new-managed-medicaid-benefit-for-community-based-palliative-care/.
24. Illinois General Assembly. Illinois Pediatric Palliative Care Act. Accessed September 13, 2022. https://www.ilga.gov/legislation/ilcs/ilcs3.asp?ActID=3247&ChapterID=28.
25. Silberberg M, Martinez-Bianchi V, Lyn MJ. What is population health? *Prim Care*. 2019;46(4):475–484. https://doi.org/10.1016/j.pop.2019.07.001.
26. Kelley AS, Bollens-Lund E. Identifying the population with serious illness: the "denominator" challenge. *J Palliat Med*. 2018;21(suppl 2):S7–S16. https://doi.org/10.1089/jpm.2017.0548.
27. National Quality Forum. Measuring Performance. Accessed September 13, 2022. https://www.qualityforum.org/measuring_performance/measuring_performance.aspx.
28. National Coalition For Hospice and Palliative Care. MACRA Funds Development of Palliative Care Measures. Accessed September 13, 2022. https://www.nationalcoalitionhpc.org/qualitymeasures/.
29. Good News: The "Felt Heard and Understood" Quality Measure at Last NQF Endorsement Step. Coalition to Transform Advanced

Care. August 25, 2022. Accessed January 11, 2023. https://thectac.org/asset/blog/good-news-the-felt-heard-and-understood-quality-measure-at-last-nqf-endorsement-step/.

30. Teoli D, Ghassemzadeh S. Patient Self-Determination Act. In: *StatPearls*. StatPearls Publishing; 2022. Accessed September 13, 2022. http://www.ncbi.nlm.nih.gov/books/NBK538297/
31. CaringInfo. Download and Complete Your State or Territories' Advance Directive Form. Accessed September 13, 2022. https://www.caringinfo.org/planning/advance-directives/by-state/.
32. Centers for Medicare & Medicaid Services. MLN Factsheet. Advance Care Planning. Accessed February 7, 2023. https://www.cms.gov/outreach-and-education/medicare-learning-network-mln/mlnproducts/downloads/advancecareplanning.pdf.
33. Grant M, Freeland D, Jones LA, Singh S. The Equity Issue with Advance Care Planning Cost Sharing. Health Affairs Forefront. March 16, 2022. https://doi.org/10.1377/forefront.20220314.309752.
34. He F, Gasdaska A, Friedman H, et al. *Advance Care Planning among Medicare Fee-for-Service Beneficiaries and Practitioners: Final Report*. Office of the Assistance Secretary for Planning and Evaluation; 2020. Accessed March 18, 2021. https://aspe.hhs.gov/pdf-report/advance-care-planning-among-medicare-fee-service-beneficiaries-and-practitioners-final-report.
35. Palmer MK, Jacobson M, Enguidanos S. Advance care planning for Medicare beneficiaries increased substantially, but prevalence remained low. *Health Aff (Millwood)*. 2021;40(4):613–621. https://doi.org/10.1377/hlthaff.2020.01895.
36. Hong M, Yi EH, Johnson KJ, Adamek ME. Facilitators and barriers for advance care planning among ethnic and racial minorities in the U.S.: a systematic review of the current literature. *J Immigr Minor Health*. 2018;20(5):1277–1287. https://doi.org/10.1007/s10903-017-0670-9.
37. Ladin K, Bronzi OC, Gazarian PK, et al. Understanding the use of Medicare procedure codes for advance care planning: a national qualitative study. *Health Aff (Millwood)*. 2022;41(1). https://doi.org/10.1377/hlthaff.2021.00848.
38. Mark R. Warner, US senator from the Commonwealth of Virginia. Warner, Collins & Blumenauer Introduce Bipartisan, Bicameral Legislation to Expand Access to Advance Care Planning. September 16, 2022. Accessed January 11, 2023. https://www.warner.senate.gov/public/index.cfm/2022/9/warner-collins-blumenauer-introduce-bipartisan-bicameral-legislation-to-expand-access-to-advance-care-planning.
39. National Association of Social Workers. Accessed September 13, 2022. https://www.socialworkers.org.
40. Coalition to Transform Advanced Care. 4 Things to Know about CMS' PACIO Advance Directive Interoperability Project. June 16, 2021. Accessed September 13, 2022. https://thectac.org/asset/blog/4-things-to-know-about-cms-pacio-advance-directive-interoperability-project/
41. HealthIT. PACIO Advance Directives Project Update. Accessed January 8, 2023. http://www.healthit.gov/isa/uscdi-data-class/advance-directives.
42. Ghose R, Forati AM, Mantsch JR. Impact of the COVID-19 pandemic on opioid overdose deaths: a spatiotemporal analysis. *J Urban Health Bull N Y Acad Med*. 2022;99(2):316–327. https://doi.org/10.1007/s11524-022-00610-0.
43. CDC guideline for prescribing opioids for chronic pain—United States, 2016. *MMWR Recomm Rep*. 2016;65(1):1–49. https://doi.org/10.15585/mmwr.rr6501e1er.
44. Dowell D, Haegerich T, Chou R. No shortcuts to safer opioid prescribing. *N Engl J Med*. 2019;380(24):2285–2287. https://doi.org/10.1056/NEJMp1904190.
45. CDC Newsroom. CDC Advises against Misapplication of the Guideline for Prescribing Opioids for Chronic Pain. January 1, 2016. Accessed September 13, 2022. https://www.cdc.gov/media/releases/2019/s0424-advises-misapplication-guideline-prescribing-opioids.html.
46. Centers for Disease Control and Prevention. Process for Updating the Opioid Prescribing Guideline. April 15, 2022. Accessed September 13, 2022. https://www.cdc.gov/opioids/guideline-update/index.html.
47. Centers for Medicare & Medicaid Services. Medicare Part D Overutilization Monitoring System (OMS) Summary. November 3, 2015. Accessed January 8, 2023. https://www.cms.gov/newsroom/fact-sheets/medicare-part-d-overutilization-monitoring-system-oms-summary.
48. A Prescriber's Guide to Medicare Prescription Drug Part D Opioid Policies. Medicare Learning Network. 2024. Accessed September 13, 2022. https://www.cms.gov/files/document/mln2886155-prescribers-guide-medicare-prescription-drug-part-d-opioid-policies.pdf.
49. American Society of Anesthesiologists. CMS Removes Pain Management Questions from HCAHPS Survey. November 7, 2016. Accessed September 13, 2022. https://www.asahq.org/advocacy-and-asapac/fda-and-washington-alerts/washington-alerts/2016/11/cms-removes-pain-management-questions-from-hcahps-survey.
50. Center to Advance Palliative Care. Project Equity: Improving Health Equity for People with Serious Illness. Accessed September 13, 2022. https://www.capc.org/project-equity-improving-health-equity-for-people-with-serious-illness/.
51. Yearby R, Clark B, Figueroa JF. Structural racism in historical and modern US health care policy. *Health Aff (Millwood)*. 2022;41(2):187–194. https://doi.org/10.1377/hlthaff.2021.01466.
52. Centers for Medicare & Medicaid Services. CMS' Program History. Accessed September 13, 2022. https://www.cms.gov/About-CMS/Agency-Information/History.
53. Chapter 11: Hospice services. Accessed September 13, 2022. https://www.medpac.gov/wp-content/uploads/2022/03/Mar22_MedPAC_ReportToCongress_Ch11_SEC.pdf.
54. Kwak J, Cho YI, Lee YS, Noh H, Roh S. Differences in advance care planning between American Indian and White older adults. *Res Gerontol Nurs*. 2019;12(1):34–43. https://doi.org/10.3928/19404921-20181212-02.

4

Principles of Patient and Family Assessment

Shannon L. S. Petros

Key Points

- Comprehensive assessment of the patient and family by the palliative nurse is essential to planning and implementing an effective plan of care by the interdisciplinary palliative care team.
- Assessment involves input from the patient, family, and all members of the interdisciplinary team with information shared verbally as well as in the patient's health records.
- Ongoing, detailed, and comprehensive assessment is needed to identify the complex and changing needs and goals of patients facing chronic or life-threatening illness and those of their families.

Introduction

Skilled and thorough nursing assessment of patients and families within the realm of palliative care is essential to the interdisciplinary team's (IDT's) ability to determine an effective treatment plan. The palliative nurse will expand on the fundamental skills they have obtained as a generalist within the physical, psychosocial, and spiritual components that make up a patient's and family's being. The National Coalition for Hospice and Palliative Care's *Clinical Practice Guidelines for Quality Palliative Care* emphasizes the importance of a comprehensive assessment of patients and families within each of the eight domains of palliative care (Structure and Processes of Care; Physical Aspects of Care; Psychological and Psychiatric Aspects of Care; Social Aspects of Care; Spiritual, Religious, and Existential Aspects of Care; Cultural Aspects of Care; Care of the Patient Nearing the End of Life; and Ethical and Legal Aspects of Care). Domain 1: Structure and Processes of Care identifies that within the interdisciplinary palliative team, nurses are at the center of not only the initial assessment of the patient and family but also reassessments throughout the disease process.[1]

The first step required of the palliative nurse is to look inward and assess any beliefs, values, and even implicit bias they may have that will in turn affect their care of patients and families. A systematic review of the literature regarding nursing competencies in the field of palliative care identified that self-awareness regarding attitudes, feelings, and beliefs about death and caring for the dying is key to providing care for patients and families.[2] Research has also suggested a positive correlation between self-awareness, communication ability, and caring ability of nursing students, suggesting that the greater the self-awareness, the greater the ability to care for their patients.[3]

One of the tools the palliative nurse, as well as their generalist nursing counterparts, may find useful is the validated Implicit Association Test (IAT) developed by scientists at Harvard University, University of Washington, and University of Virginia. For over 20 years, researchers have been utilizing this tool to help people bring awareness to their own prejudice, stereotypes, and other group biases. This self-assessment can be explored at www.implicit.harvard.edu.[4]

Box 4.1 includes questions that additionally may be important for the palliative nurse to reflect upon regarding their own attitudes and beliefs.

Box 4.1 Topics of Self-Inquiry for the Palliative Nurse

What do I believe about . . . ?

- what quality of life is to me versus my patient
- suffering
- patient autonomy and paternalism in healthcare
- treating pain and the use of opioids and other adjuvant medications for symptom management
- death and dying
- advance directives (e.g., healthcare power of attorney documentation, living will)
- code status (delineations dependent on the state of practice)
- organ donation
- funerals, burial, and cremation
- cultures other than my own
- the use of advanced life support including, but not limited to:
  - cardiopulmonary resuscitation (CPR)
  - intubation, ventilator support, and tracheostomies
  - artificial nutrition and hydration in a terminal condition or at the end of life (e.g., enteral feeding via nasogastric or percutaneous endoscopic gastrostomy tube or total parenteral nutrition)
  - medications that could hasten death (opioids, benzodiazepines, barbiturates)

Case Study: Mary

Mary is a 56-year-old cisgender female who identifies strongly as a woman of African descent and someone who adheres firmly to her Jehovah's Witness beliefs. After having progressively worsening lower-abdominal pain for several months, she was determined to have metastatic uterine cancer. Her husband of 32 years recently died from metastatic lung cancer. She has three children, two sons and a daughter. She currently provides care to her 4-year-old granddaughter 5 days a week so that her youngest son may work. Mary had not worked during her marriage, and since the death of her husband 6 months ago, she has begun to worry about her financial ability to maintain her bills in the absence of his income.

Review of the Electronic Health Record

Before meeting a patient or family member, the palliative nurse must prepare for the initial encounter. This is done by reviewing the patient's electronic health record (EHR). EHRs are now widely used across settings in which palliative care is administered, including the hospital or inpatient hospice facility, long-term care, outpatient offices, and even agencies providing care in the home. It is important to note that some components of a patient's information may still be at least initially stored in paper format and that review of the paper medical chart must take place as well (e.g., a patient brings in a copy of their advance directives, and it has yet to be scanned into the EHR). Thorough review of the EHR can be particularly important in establishing trust and rapport with the patient and their family as they recognize the skill and expertise the palliative nurse has. In addition, it may facilitate lessening the number of questions required of a patient who may have a diminished capacity for prolonged conversation due to fatigue, dyspnea, or pain. Preparation prior to the initial visit may take considerably longer than subsequent review of the EHR with future assessments and visits.

The palliative nurse should review the following information, as available, in the EHR:

Referral information: Whether the patient was referred for palliative services from another healthcare provider and, if so, the date of the referral and the reason given by the referrer for the consult can be determined. This may provide insight into the patient's and family's current needs as well as facilitate collaboration among the palliative nurse and the other professionals on the patient's care team.

Demographic information: The patient's name and identification number, age, date of birth, gender/preferred pronouns, ethnicity, primary language, and occupation can be found. The patient's address and phone number may become important for discharge planning, the completion of advance directives, as well as providing the palliative nurse a general idea of resources, or lack of, in the patient's hometown. Whether or not the patient is a veteran should be noted.

Primary point of contact, surrogate decision maker, and advanced directives: There may be documented contacts in the EHR, but the palliative nurse should be mindful that entered relationships may be inaccurate. These contacts may provide a starting point for familial relationships, such as if the patient has a spouse, significant other, children (adults and minors), parents, or other friends. Although the Health Insurance Portability and Accountability Act (HIPAA) requires protection of personal health information, some patients' identities, whether per their request or on their behalf, are subject to an extra level of security, such as those who are incarcerated, abused persons, and public figures.

Laws regarding advance directives and orders for code status are specific to each state, so the palliative nurse must be familiar with their state laws regarding advance directives and code status delineations. The palliative nurse may find scanned into the EHR healthcare power of attorney (HCPOA) documentation, living wills, durable do-not-resuscitate orders, and Physician Orders for Life-Sustaining Treatment (POLST) documents. The palliative nurse must be scrupulous in review of these documents, ensuring that they are valid (e.g., not missing signatures) or are not financial only in nature. The patient may also have documentation that exists but has not yet been scanned into the record. Close attention must be paid to the labeling of a patient's HCPOA as the patient's legal next of kin (LNOK; in the absence of legal HCPOA documentation) may be entered incorrectly as such by another member of the team. It is also possible that the LNOK or guardian (for pediatric patients) may be incorrectly identified.

Identification of the patient's appropriate surrogate medical decision maker is of utmost importance, particularly when the patient has not been determined to have the capacity to make certain medical decisions. The palliative nurse may need to engage other members of the palliative IDT, such as social work and chaplaincy, should there be difficulty in designating or locating the appropriate surrogate.

Some EHRs may note the patient's status as a registered organ donor or not as well.

- *Religious affiliation*: The patient's stated religious affiliation, if identified by the patient, may be documented.
- *Insurance coverage*: Patient care within the context of the US healthcare system is often limited by the patient's resources. For example, certain insurance agencies may have restricted medication formularies. Individuals with certain Medicaid plans may have long-term care coverage; otherwise, out-of-pocket expenses may be required by the patient and family. Earlier identification of a patient's veteran status and level of service connection may also indicate available benefits with the Veterans Administration. Assistance from the palliative social worker may be especially helpful in identifying current and future resources available.
- *Health history, recent and past*: The palliative nurse should note the patient's diagnosis, history of the present illness, past medical and surgical history, and family and social history. They will search for previous assessment of the patient's physical condition, functional status, and review of systems/reported symptoms. The use and whereabouts of hearing aids, eyeglasses, and dentures and the placement of ports, central lines, pacemakers, defibrillators, and implants should be noted. The initial findings of diagnostic studies and treatment plans/response to administered therapies may also be noted. Specialist consultation notes by the other

involved services and the recent progress notes, including other medical services and ancillary services, such as case management, dietary, respiratory therapy, physical and occupational therapy, and speech therapy, should be reviewed.

- *Medications*: The palliative nurse should review the patient's drug allergies and medications as listed in the EHR (home use and inpatient use), including over-the-counter and herbal preparations. Prescription monitoring programs (PMPs) now exist, acting as databases for the filling of controlled-substance prescriptions. Links to these sites may be built in directly to the EHR. In states where cannabis is legalized for medicinal use, this will be noted as well. Controlled substances administered at a skilled nursing facility, long-term care facility, or clinic assisting with medication for opioid use disorder may not be located within the PMP. Depending on the reasoning for the palliative consultation and the patient's current needs, the prescribing and use of medications for the control of symptoms including pain, dyspnea, anxiety, appetite, nausea, bowel function, and sleep should be noted. Comparing a patient's home medication regimen to what is currently ordered in an inpatient setting may bring to light the discontinuation, intentional or unintentional, of medications that may exacerbate symptom burden or precipitate withdrawal (e.g., opioid or benzodiazepines). Supplements and other herbal remedies utilized at home may not be documented, but the presence or absence of this information will inform the assessment to follow.
- *Diagnostic test results*: Objective information such as current vital signs and the results of diagnostic tests is important not only to understand the patient's current state but also to understand trends that inform the trajectory of the patient's illness and current symptoms. Trends in vital signs can indicate improving or declining status related to infections, oxygenation, and hemodynamic stability. A review of laboratory and diagnostic results, such as creatinine clearance may inform the palliative nurse that the patient's current degree of renal impairment could put the patient at risk for the rapid accumulation of morphine metabolites, leading to neurotoxicity. Similarly, the identification of a prolonged QT interval may aid the palliative nurse in identifying symptom management medications that may put the patient at risk for arrhythmias. Radiology and pathology reports may provide further information about the etiology of symptoms and the severity and trajectory of the patient's illness. The palliative nurse may also note the results of urine drug screening, providing information regarding their assessment of the patient, particularly if drugs used illicitly are noted to be present.
- *Complementary therapies*: The palliative nurse should note the reported use of, or pending referrals for, any complementary therapies such as music or art therapy, massage, aromatherapy, acupuncture, reiki, medical cannabis/herbal supplements, and guided imagery and medication, to name a few.

The palliative nurse may have gathered an extensive amount of information regarding the patient at this time, and if not, they have identified key points to address in the upcoming assessment of the patient and family. The review of the EHR should continue to consider the holistic nature of the patient and family as guided by the eight domains of palliative care.

The Initial Encounter

Having a meaningful initial encounter between the palliative nurse and the patient/family is vitally important to the establishment of a therapeutic and trusting relationship moving forward.[5] In recent years, due to the COVID-19 global pandemic, initial encounters with the patient may not be face to face depending on isolation protocols. Similarly, the initial encounter with the family may be via phone or video conference. The palliative nurse is challenged with the task of establishing rapport and trust, while demonstrating respect and compassion, in the too common setting of physical and distance barriers.

The palliative nurse may be meeting the patient and their family at any point during the disease process. While the nurse, in addition to the palliative IDT, may wish to establish their therapeutic relationship with the patient at the time of diagnosis, palliative is often asked to get involved in a patient's care late in their disease progression or at the end of life. The setting where the initial encounter occurs may also vary, such as during hospital admission or a home visit.

The palliative nurse can facilitate trust and establish rapport with patients and their families by:

- Reviewing the EHR in preparation of the encounter as discussed previously. In an inpatient or facility setting, they may want to find the nurse who is caring for the patient first and ask about any issues the patient had overnight or thus far during the day.
- If the patient is alert, the palliative nurse should introduce themself to the patient, explaining their role and verifying how the patient wishes to be addressed. Any other people in the room should be identified, as well as their relationship to the patient.
- The palliative nurse should ask permission to proceed with the encounter in the presence of the visitors or ask if the patient wishes to have someone present with them, whether in person or via speaker phone/video chat.
- The palliative nurse should take a seat near the patient, being respectful of the patient's cultural norms for physical closeness and eye contact.
- If the patient is not alert, and staff and family have identified that the patient has not requested to sleep at this time, the palliative nurse should attempt to arouse them. The ability or inability to do so should be corroborated with information from the EHR and collaboration with other caregivers and may be important to the assessment of the patient's current clinical condition or response to treatments.

The palliative nurse's ability to not only perform an effective assessment but also begin to establish rapport and develop a therapeutic relationship will be determined by their communication skills. Chapter 5, "Palliative Nursing Communication," will guide the palliative nurse through essential learnings about effective communication. Many validated tools to facilitate communication with patients and families exist, including the COMFORT, SPIKE, and NURSE models.

The palliative nurse should also assess the need for a medical interpreter. When working with a medical interpreter, the palliative nurse should be mindful to speak directly to the patient or family member, not the interpreter. They should speak slowly and pause often so that the interpreter may accurately convey the information to the patient and family. A family member should not be used as an interpreter for major explanations or decision-making about healthcare. Medical interpretation can occur with an on-site face-to-face interpreter, a telephone-based interpreter, or a video-based interpreter over the internet.

Case Study: Mary at Diagnosis: Uterine Cancer

Mary had irregular menstrual cycles her whole life, so when she began to have more erratic vaginal bleeding, she did not immediately deem it abnormal. In addition to her vaginal bleeding, she began to have some lower-abdominal pain and worsening fatigue. Again, she attributed these symptoms to the grief from the death of her husband as well as the increasing demands of caring for her 4-year-old granddaughter. After feeling that she may faint after bending over to pick up her granddaughter's toys, she decided to make an appointment with her gynecologist. After a physical exam in the office, including vitals showing that she was hypotensive, Mary was emergently transferred to the Emergency Department. She was admitted for shock secondary to acute blood loss. Imaging and biopsy confirmed uterine cancer. Mary's gynecologic oncologist placed a referral to the palliative care team to assist with assessment of her symptoms and development of a plan of care moving forward.

The palliative care assessment goals for Mary and her family at the time of diagnosis are to:

- Assess Mary's and her family's understanding of her current diagnosis and evaluate for cultural and spiritual beliefs that may impact her treatment plan moving forward (e.g., Mary's deep Jehovah's Witness faith has informed her decision not to receive blood products).
- Assess Mary's current clinical condition and reported symptoms, including her previous versus current functional status, control of her abdominal pain on admission, and presence of anxiety and depressive symptoms.
- Assess Mary's and her family's need for resources including, but not limited to, financial barriers to her well-being at home as well as ability to adhere to recommended treatment plans. Consider the changing dynamics among the family as Mary may no longer be able to provide care for her granddaughter, impacting her son's ability to work.
- Assess available spiritual support including the need for chaplaincy referral or connection to a professional in her faith community.
- Assess for previous completion of advance directives or desire to complete.

Introduction to Physical Assessment

Physical assessment can provide supportive information regarding patients expressing physical symptoms but also their previous and current functional status. The palliative nurse may be the first member of the palliative IDT to notice changes in a patient's condition throughout their illness progression. The palliative nurse will continue to utilize their physical exam skills as learned during their nursing training. At the initial encounter or during major changes in the patient's health condition, the palliative nurse may perform a full "head-to-toe" assessment that encompasses all organ systems. Alternatively, the palliative nurse may determine that a focused physical assessment is appropriate. For example, a patient's or family's report of new-onset nausea/vomiting may prompt the palliative nurse to perform a detailed abdominal exam, while they may forego an assessment of the cranial nerves. As the palliative nurse furthers their expertise as a specialist, their critical thinking skills will inform the needed evaluation of the patient.

The palliative nurse may also have access to prior physical assessments that may be useful in determining physical changes that have occurred from pre-diagnosis to time of diagnosis or from one illness stage to another. In the above example regarding new-onset nausea/vomiting, if the palliative nurse were to determine an absence of bowel sounds on exam, that would perhaps precipitate prompt notification of the patient's surgical oncologist or discussion with the patient's hospice attending as this may be an indicator of an acute complication or of transition during the dying process. The palliative nurse completes the physical assessment by obtaining objective data by inspection, auscultation, palpation, and percussion. Box 4.2 provides information to guide the physical assessment, whether

Box 4.2 Physical Examination

General: Observe patient disposition, acute distress, arousability, manner of dress, posture, body language, diaphoresis

Vital Signs: Temperature, heart rate, respiratory rate, SpO_2, O_2 rate, O_2 delivery device, ventilator parameters, blood pressure, pain rating

HEENT:

1. Head: Observe for shape and evidence of trauma.
2. Eyes: Observe pupils bilaterally for shape and reaction to light and accommodation, sclera, icterus, discharge, tearing, glasses, contacts.
3. Ears: Observe external ear, ear canal, cerumen, discharge, hearing aids.
4. Nose: Observe for inflammation, obstruction, discharge.
5. Neck: Palpate cervical lymph nodes for stiffness.
6. Throat: Observe for jugular vein distention, thyroid location; palpate sublingual lymph nodes; observe oropharynx, dentition, dental hygiene, dry or cracked lips.

Respiratory: Observe chest expansion, use of accessory muscles; palpate for tenderness; auscultate breath sounds in all lobes anterior/posterior, appreciate adventitious sounds, rales, rhonchi, wheezing

Cardiovascular: Observe posture, edema, cyanosis, cardiac assist devices; auscultate heart sounds; palpate peripheral pulses (radial, pedal) bilaterally

Gastrointestinal: Observe for distention, abdominal ascites, ostomy, rectal tube, stool; auscultate bowel sounds; palpate superficially and deep; observe for rebound tenderness or guarding; percuss for margins of abdominal organs

Genitourinary: Observe for presence of urine, volume, color; palpate for bladder distention, foley or suprapubic catheter

Musculoskeletal: Observe for spontaneous movements of extremities, muscle strength, joint range of motion, spinal flexibility, temperature, deformities; compare bilaterally

Neurological: Observe for level of consciousness, orientation, grossly intact cranial nerves II–XII, sensation in all extremities, cerebellar reflexes, tremors, Romberg, gait

Psychiatric: Observe for mood, affect, anxiety, disordered speech, language, delirium, hallucinations, memory, attention span

Integumentary: Observe for rashes, bruising, wounds, discoloration, mottling, lesions, nevi venous access ports, complexion

Box 4.3 Review of Systems

General: weight changes, changes in sleeping pattern and energy level, fevers, chills, or sweats

Organ systems including: head, eyes, ears, nose, throat (HEENT); respiratory; cardiovascular; gastrointestinal; genitourinary; musculoskeletal; endocrine; immune; hematology/oncology; skin and hair; and neurological

Pain: acute, chronic

P—Precipitates/Palliates: What happened when first noticed? What brings it on? What makes it better?

Q—Quality: Aching, burning, cramping, deep, stabbing, throbbing

R—Region/Radiation: Where is the location of the pain? To where does the pain radiate?

S—Severity: Pain scale, 0 = no pain, 10 = worst ever. Is the level of pain acceptable? Is the pain getting worse, getting better, or staying the same?

T—Timing: Onset, constant or episodic, frequency, duration

U—Understanding: What do you think it means?

head-to-toe in nature or focused. The palliative nurse will want to ensure they are explaining their actions during the assessment to the patient or family.

In addition to the physical assessment, the palliative nurse will perform a review of systems. Box 4.3 provides some guidance for this review. They will need to ensure they are avoiding nursing jargon or medical terminology that may be unfamiliar to the patient and family. Knowledge of the underlying disease process and of the side effects of treatment assists the palliative nurse in focusing re-assessments on those body systems most likely to be affected. Even during the assessment, the palliative nurse may already be formulating a plan for possible nursing interventions and therapies that might be used to address disease progression and symptoms before they occur or worsen.

The *Clinical Practice Guidelines for Quality Palliative Care*, Domain 2: Physical Aspects of Care[1] describes the importance of the utilization of validated assessment tools such as Provocation, Quality, Region (or Radiation), Severity (or Scale), and Timing (PQRST). The palliative nurse should both regularly perform and document their findings as this will allow the palliative IDT to determine the efficacy of current symptom management regimens as well as changes in the patient's clinical condition. The palliative nurse should also pay special attention to patients who may have challenges with communicating their needs or symptoms, whether that is related to delirium, cognitive impairment, or even mechanical interference due to intubation or tracheostomy.[1] The patient's cultural or spiritual views may also impact their willingness to report symptoms experienced. The palliative nurse will cultivate skill in observing for nonverbal signs of distressing symptoms including, but not limited to, a furrowed brow, restlessness, and moaning.

In addition to the palliative nurse's physical exam and review of systems, a thorough functional assessment is imperative in assisting with the collection of information to support prognostication. Accurate prognostication can be one of the most vital pieces of information in regard to patients and their surrogate decision makers' determination of goals of care and planning for end of life. The functional assessment will include the patient's ability to complete both their activities of daily living (ADLs) and instrumental ADLs (IADLs). ADLs include tasks such as toileting, bathing, dressing, feeding, and transferring/ambulation. IADLs include shopping, meal preparation, doing laundry, cleaning, and managing finances. The nurse may choose to utilize a validated tool, such as the Palliative Performance Scale (PPS) to synthesize the information as determined by their physical assessment and interview with the patient and family.[6] Literature has shown that the PPS, while created for use with patients with cancer only, has been validated in patients with noncancer diagnoses as well.[7] Familiarity with the Eastern Cooperative Oncology Group (ECOG) Performance Status Scale may also be helpful as this scoring will be noted frequently by oncology colleagues in regard to patients' eligibility for systemic cancer therapies.[8] See Table 4.1 for scale details of the comparison between PPS and ECOG scoring. The palliative nurse's assessment of PPS during the initial encounter may be compared to the score determined through interview of how they were doing prior. Ongoing evaluation of the patient's PPS will be a helpful tool in further conversations regarding disease trajectory and prognosis.[8]

Patients with life-threatening diagnoses, cancer or other illnesses, may have elected to discontinue disease-directed therapies or withdraw life-prolonging interventions. One of the goals of the palliative nurse at this time is to determine the current physical symptoms that are most distressing to the patient and family and to prepare or advocate for possible palliative interventions. When suspected that the patient is in the active dying phase, the palliative care nurse will want to observe for signs and symptoms of the dying process. This will both assist the palliative nurse in providing education to the patient's family and further advocate and plan for appropriate palliative interventions to alleviate any uncontrolled symptoms. The physical assessment and review of the EHR at this time are crucial to identifying potentially missed devices, such as an implanted defibrillator, for which prompt deactivation may be most consistent with the patient's and family's goals.

While every dying process is unique, certain predictive factors have been identified as particularly helpful in identifying the patient who is imminently dying. The palliative nurse may find more accuracy in continuing to utilize the PPS as well as identifying the presence of breathing patterns such as Cheyne-Stokes. While the palliative nurse may note the presence of respiratory secretions, peripheral cyanosis, and decreased or lack of urinary output on their physical exam, the PPS and presence of Cheyne-Stokes may be the most pertinent signs of impending death.[9] Further guidance will be provided to the palliative nurse in how they support the patient and family at this time in Chapter 57, "Planning for Death."

Astute physical exams by the palliative nurse are not only crucial to the development and evolution of a patient's symptom management plan but may also prompt imperative advance care planning conversations about the patient's wishes. Inquiries regarding the eligibility and desire for hospice services may also arise as the patient nears the end of life. It is important to mention that there are some patients whose diseases may be cured, who go into long remissions, who become chronically ill, or who recover from an exacerbation of a chronic illness. Due to their symptom burden, not limited just to the physical realm, these individuals may require some degree of palliative care for the rest of their lives.

Table 4.1 Comparison of the Palliative Performance Scale (PPS) and Eastern Cooperative Oncology Group (ECOG) scales

PPS					
PPS level	Ambulation	Activity and evidence of disease	Self-care	Intake	Conscious level
100%	Full	Normal activity and work No evidence of disease	Full	Normal	Full
90%	Full	Normal activity and work Some evidence of disease	Full	Normal	Full
80%	Full	Normal activity with effort Some evidence of disease	Full	Normal or reduced	Full
70%	Reduced	Unable to do normal job/work Significant evidence of disease	Full	Normal or reduced	Full
60%	Reduced	Unable to do hobbies/house work Significant evidence of disease	Occasional assistance necessary	Normal or reduced	Full or confusion
50%	Mainly sit/lie	Unable to do any work Extensive disease	Considerable assistance required	Normal or reduced	Full or confusion
40%	Mainly in bed	Unable to do most activity Extensive disease	Mainly assistance	Normal or reduced	Full or drowsy ± confusion
30%	Totally bed-bound	Unable to do any activity Extensive disease	Total care	Normal or reduced	Full or drowsy ± confusion
20%	Totally bed-bound	Unable to do any activity Extensive disease	Total care	Minimal to sips	Full or drowsy ± confusion
10%	Totally bed-bound	Unable to do any activity Extensive disease	Total care	Mouth care only	Drowsy or coma ± confusion
0%	Dead	–	–	–	–
ECOG Performance Status Scale					
Grade	**ECOG Performance Status**				
0	Fully active, able to carry on all pre-disease performance without restriction				
1	Restricted in physically strenuous activity but ambulatory and able to carry out work of a light or sedentary nature				
2	Ambulatory and capable of all self-care but unable to carry out any work activities; up and about more than 50% of waking hours				
3	Capable of only limited self-care; confined to bed or chair more than 50% of waking hours				
4	Completely disabled; cannot carry on any self-care; totally confined to bed or chair				
5	Dead				

Source: References 6 and 11.

Introduction to Psychosocial Assessment

Research has shown that nurses value their ability to recognize through assessment the psychosocial and spiritual needs of the patient and family and that this is crucial to the provision of high-quality palliative care.[2] The holistic and comprehensive nature of palliative care determines the vital importance of assessing for psychosocial distress, or well-being, of the individual with chronic or life-threatening illness.

Depending on the patient's unique experience, they may require that their physical needs, such as alleviation of pain or dyspnea, be met before they are able to further delve into the psychosocial domain. However, a patient experiencing total pain may require an equal emphasis on the alleviation of psychological–social–spiritual distress as on their physical distress. In addition to the physiological etiology of a patient's pain, the palliative nurse may identify psychological, spiritual, and social factors that may increase their report of pain. These exacerbating factors may include the unknown regarding the efficacy of treatment, fear regarding the nature of the treatment or a hospitalization, or the dynamics of and interactions they have with their healthcare team.[10] Cicely Saunders, the founder of hospice care, first identified the concept of total pain, defined as the overall distress (emotional, social, spiritual) caused when pain is not alleviated, impacting both functional and cognitive aspects of the patient.[11]

The *Clinical Practice Guidelines for Quality Palliative Care*, Domain 4: Social Aspects of Care[1] highlights that the palliative nurse and other members of the palliative IDT must engage in the psychosocial assessment in a developmentally and culturally sensitive manner. The Joint Commission defines "cultural competency" as healthcare workers' ability to show respect for patients' cultural, spiritual, and psychosocial values and has determined it vital to understanding patients' and families' expectations about care.[12] A person's culture is defined by their values, beliefs, customs, and behaviors.[5] A systematic review of the literature on the core themes of palliative nurses' competencies also identified that cultural competency is essential to the care of the patient and family.[2]

Box 4.4 provides topics of discussion and evaluation as well as prompts to questions for the palliative nurse to consider including in their assessment recommended in Domain 3: Psychological and Psychiatric Aspects of Care and Domain 4: Social Aspects of Care in the *Clinical Practice Guidelines for Quality Palliative Care*.[1]

Box 4.4 Assessment of Psychosocial Aspects

The palliative nurse should:

- Identify who is in the patient's family or support system. The quality or nature of these relationships may also be elicited. A risk or concern for abuse may be identified, prompting further screening.
- Assess for changes in employment or enrollment in school. With these changes, there may be concern about financial insecurity (i.e., unable to pay bills, utilities, prescribed medications).
- Determine what the patient's living arrangements are. Identify who the patient lives with and what home modifications may be needed. Determine if transportation is now a barrier.
- Assess for the effect of the illness on intimacy and sexual expression.
- Identify the patient's and family's coping strategies.
- Determine the presence of emotional distress, anxiety, or depression. Elicit any history of psychological/psychiatric diagnoses.
- Assess for a history of or current substance use disorder.
- Identify the patient's and family's health literacy and what their preferred method of learning information is.

A systematic review of the literature extracting common themes among available palliative assessment tools identified that the recognition of depressive and anxiety symptoms is imperative as these are the two most commonly reported problems for patients receiving palliative care. In addition, loneliness and fear were highlighted as important psychological symptoms to be mindful of recognizing. Additional social factors reported by palliative care patients included the need for support and maintaining family and social relations.[5] The palliative nurse may wish to incorporate validated assessment tools such as the nine-item Patient Health Questionnaire and seven-item General Anxiety Disorder scale, which both measure depressive and anxiety symptoms. Chapter 24, "Anxiety and Depression" will provide detailed guidance of both the assessment of anxiety and depression as well as treatment strategies.

Grief, both that of patients and families, will be a normal reaction to loss that the palliative nurse will observe for. The palliative nurse should have a basic understanding of the kinds of grief patients and families may experience including anticipatory grief, uncomplicated grief, complicated grief, disenfranchised grief, and unresolved grief. The palliative nurse may identify a need for referral to other members of the palliative IDT, such as social work or chaplaincy, and to a behavioral health professional. More detailed information and useful tools on grief and bereavement are available in Chapter 44, "Grief and Bereavement in Perinatal and Pediatric Palliative Care."

The palliative nurse's psychosocial assessment at the initial encounter will also include an evaluation of the patient's current resuscitation status and desire for advance care planning and completion of advance directives. A component of this will require that the advanced practice nurse, physician, or other appropriate palliative IDT member be able to assess capacity for decision-making based on their scope of practice. Capacity for medical decision-making is time-limited and situation-/question-specific, meaning, for example, that during a particular assessment the patient can demonstrate capacity for decision-making regarding HCPOA appointment but not resuscitation status. At a subsequent visit, the patient's ability to demonstrate capacity may change completely.[13] A general understanding of this concept will allow the palliative nurse to understand the necessity of including LNOK/surrogate decision makers.

The palliative nurse will continue to assess the need for changes in the resuscitation status and plan of care throughout the disease course. Depending on the importance placed on quality of life by the patient and family, the nurse may assess whether the patient feels they have been able to maintain an acceptable quality of life during disease-directed treatment and therapies. If quality of life is no longer acceptable, further conversations about the need for transition of the focus of care are warranted. Chapter 29, "Supporting Families and Family Caregivers in Palliative Care," will provide further information on how to assess needs of caregivers, continuing to practice with palliative care's foundation of being not only patient but also family-centered. Chapter 57, "Planning for Death," will provide more details on the psychosocial assessment of the patient and family during the active dying phase.

Case Study: Mary after Treatment

After 6 months of disease-directed therapies and several hospitalizations for uncontrolled symptoms or complications of therapies, Mary shared with her family and healthcare team that her goals have changed. With support of the palliative care team, Mary voiced a desire to transition to a comfort-focused plan of care. Mary expressed being at peace with this decision, feeling that she was able to survive to her granddaughter's fifth birthday and that her son was able to establish affordable caregiving for his daughter that allowed him to still work. After a visit from a church elder in her Jehovah's Witness community, Mary requested to forego heroic measures at the end of life, including the initiation of artificial nutrition and hydration. With the education of the palliative care team, Mary and her family were agreeable to a referral to a hospice agency in their hometown.

The goals of the palliative care nursing assessment after Mary's treatments have ended are to:

- Establish Mary's wishes with respect to her plan of care moving forward. Assist with the completion of advance directives or do not-resuscitate orders as appropriate.
- Facilitate the need for spiritual support, should Mary feel this is needed, to evaluate her wishes and ensure they are in line with her faith practices.
- Determine the need for a family conference if Mary would find this helpful not only to share her wishes with her family but begin planning for her absence after death.
- Assess for eligibility for hospice enrollment and facilitate referral if appropriate.

Introduction to Spiritual Assessment

Spirituality and the assessment of a patient's and family's spiritual concerns is an essential element of high-quality palliative care.[1] Assessing the spiritual needs of patients and families is not solely the responsibility of the chaplain, clergy, or other officially designated professional. All members of the palliative IDT share the responsibility of identifying and being sensitive to spiritual concerns. The ability of the palliative nurse to identify a patient's spiritual concerns improves the quality of palliative care throughout the illness trajectory. The relief of suffering is frequently identified as one of the main goals of the palliative nurse and IDT throughout the disease process and at the end of life. As defined by Cassell (1999), suffering, as subjectively identified by the patient, is a "specific state of distress that occurs when the intactness or integrity of the person is threatened or disrupted."[14(p531)] As discussed previously, the palliative nurse's spiritual assessment may identify the presence of total pain that the patient may be experiencing.

Patients facing serious illness and at the end of life may experience numerous spiritual concerns. A spiritual assessment or history does not just evaluate the patient's and family's interaction or lack thereof with a religious organization. The patient and their family may identify as spiritual but not religious. Spirituality is defined by consensus in the palliative community as "a dynamic and intrinsic aspect of humanity through which persons seek ultimate meaning, purpose, and transcendence, and experience relationship to self, family, others, community, society, nature, and the significant or sacred. Spirituality is expressed through beliefs, values, traditions, and practices."[15 (p. 646)] Therefore, the palliative nurse's assessment must contain the many aspects of spirituality. A patient-centered approach to the spiritual assessment is required as it is ultimately up to the patient to determine the extent of information that they are willing to disclose regarding their spirituality.

There are many tools that have been developed to assist the clinician's assessment and integration of the patient's spirituality in their care. The Open Invite mnemonic can guide the palliative nurse to "open the door" to conversation by inquiring about any faith practices the patient may have and then "inviting" the patient to further discuss how spirituality affects their health and medical decision-making.[16] The FICA Spiritual History Tool was developed to assist the clinician's integration of patient's spirituality into their care.[17] Research specifically using the FICA Spiritual History Tool as an intervention among the palliative patient population has shown the tool to be useful.[17] The HOPE mnemonic, standing for sources of hope, organized religion, personal spirituality and practices, and effects on medical care and end-of-life issues, is another framework that can guide the palliative nurse in their assessment.[18] A further dive into the spiritual assessment of the patient and their family can be found in Chapter 33, "Addressing Spiritual, Religious, and Existential Needs in Palliative Care."

Consistent with the timing and recurrence of the physical and psychosocial assessments, the palliative nurse will want to perform a spiritual assessment when the patient undergoes a significant change in their clinical condition.[1] The palliative nurse should also consider the inclusion of the spiritual assessment when engaging in conversations regarding advance care planning or with the completion of advanced directives.[19] The literature has shown that the consistent incorporation of patients' spirituality in their care improves both mental and physical health in disease processes such as chronic obstructive pulmonary disease, cardiovascular disease, renal disease, and cancer.[20,21,22]

The *Clinical Practice Guidelines for Quality Palliative Care*, within Domain 5: Spiritual, Religious, and Existential Aspects of Care, encourages the identification of spiritual distress and urgent needs for referral to a chaplain.[1] Box 4.5 notes a few aspects of the spiritual assessment that the palliative nurse and palliative chaplain may touch upon.[1]

Box 4.5 Aspects of the Spiritual Assessment

The palliative nurse, within their spiritual assessment, may:

- Identify the patient's hopes and values, as well as where they find meaning and purpose.
- Determine any existential concerns the patient or family may be having, including the presence of a lack of meaning, questioning one's own existence, or questioning the meaning of their suffering.
- Assess if there is concern about their relationship to God or their higher power.
- Identify concerns about death and the afterlife.

The available standardized tools will also assist the palliative nurse in identifying if the patient or family would benefit from or desires the support of a person within their own faith community such as a priest, pastor, rabbi, imam, counselor, or spiritual advisor. Meaningful rituals, such as communion, special prayers, anointing, and other ceremonies, may be requested by the patient and family. The palliative nurse should ask about spiritual practices that may impact a recommended or standard plan of treatment, such as dietary restrictions, not receiving blood products, or not being touched by a person of the opposite gender. Similarly, the identification of beliefs and how the dying process is viewed will be helpful in guiding the palliative IDT both in caring for the dying patient as well as in understanding the practices the family will carry out once the patient has died.[1,16,17,18]

Case Study: Mary's Death

After meeting with the hospice agency, Mary elected for enrollment and voiced a desire to die at home. With the support of her palliative and hospice teams, her children were able to apply for leave-of-absence benefits, which allowed them to provide 24-hour care at home. Mary's faith community also assisted with caregiving and were particularly helpful for providing vigil shifts when Mary was felt to have minutes to hours to live. The hospice nurse not only performed frequent assessments of Mary's dying process but also noted symptoms that prompted adjustments to her medication regimen. Mary ultimately died peacefully, surrounded by her three children, as one of her church elders provided prayer.

The goals of the palliative nursing assessment during Mary's active dying phase are to:

- Evaluate Mary for uncontrolled symptoms that would inform changes in her symptom management regimen.
- Assess the family for desire and readiness to learn about the dying process.
- Assess for any unmet spiritual needs and provide the appropriate referral to assist with alleviating this distress.
- Evaluate the family's well-being as they are faced with becoming Mary's full-time caregivers.
- Inquire about the family's desire for bereavement services through hospice, educating them about services to support children facing loss.

Box 4.6 Best-Practice Tip

Clinicians may find the use of an abbreviated symptom assessment form helpful to track the efficacy of palliative care interventions. The utilization of validated tools such as the Edmonton Symptom Assessment Scale or the Integrated Palliative care Outcome Scale can assist the palliative nurse to quickly assess for both physical and emotional symptoms.[23,24] These tools, used in conjunction with the Palliative Performance Scale addressing functionality of the patient and prognosis, can provide the palliative nurse and the rest of the interdisciplinary team with a brief but fruitful view of the patient's current clinical condition, response to treatments, and areas of distress to focus interventions.

Conclusion: Principles of Patient and Family Assessment

A comprehensive palliative care nursing assessment of the patient and family occurs throughout the trajectory of the illness and is a holistic view that includes the physical, psychosocial, and spiritual domains. Patient and family assessment provides the foundation for patient and family goal-setting, shared decision-making in determining a plan of care, and evaluating the effectiveness of interventions. Box 4.6 offers a best-practice tip for assessing patients. The role of the palliative nurse is essential to the completion of a comprehensive assessment. As the palliative nurse becomes more experienced in their specialist role, their assessment may both expand in the amount of knowledge gathered and build a trusting and compassionate foundation for the patient and family's experience with palliative care through the end of life.

Acknowledgments

The contributions of the authors of previous versions of this chapter as well as the guidance and mentorship from Kate Dean-Haldet, PhD, PMHCNS, and Tommy Petros, MD, are greatly appreciated and hereby acknowledged.

REFERENCES

1. National Coalition for Hospice and Palliative Care. *Clinical Practice Guidelines for Quality Palliative Care*. 4th ed. National Coalition for Hospice and Palliative Care; 2018. Accessed September 25, 2022. https://www.nationalcoalitionhpc.org/wp-content/uploads/2020/07/NCHPC-NCPGuidelines_4thED_web_FINAL.pdf.
2. Hökkä M, Martins Pereira S, Pölkki T, Kyngäs H, Hernández-Marrero P. Nursing competencies across different levels of palliative care provision: a systematic integrative review with thematic synthesis. *Palliat Med*. 2020;34(7):851–870. https://doi.org/10.1177/0269216320918798.
3. Li T, Jiang T, Shi G, Song C, Shi T. Correlation between self-awareness, communication ability and caring ability of undergraduate nursing students/a cross-sectional study. *Nurse Educ Today*. 2022;116:105450. https://doi.org/10.1016/j.nedt.2022.105450.
4. Project Implicit. *Implicit Associations Test*. Project Implicit; 2011. Accessed September 20, 2022. www.implicit.harvard.edu.
5. Goni-Fuste B, Crespo I, Monforte-Royo C, Porta-Sales J, Balaguer A, Pergolizzi D. What defines the comprehensive assessment of needs in palliative care? An integrative systematic review. *Palliat Med*. 2021;35(4):651–669. https://doi.org/10.1177/0269216321996985.
6. Oken MM, Creech RH, Tormey DC, et al. Toxicity and response criteria of the Eastern Cooperative Oncology Group. *Am J Clin Oncol*. 1982;5(6):649–655.
7. Baik D, Russell D, Jordan L, Dooley F, Bowles KH, Masterson Creber RM. Using the Palliative Performance Scale to estimate survival for patients at the end of life: a systematic review of the literature. *J Palliat Med*. 2018;21(11):1651–1661. https://doi.org/10.1089/jpm.2018.0141.
8. Anderson F, Downing GM, Hill J, Casorso L, Lerch N. Palliative Performance Scale (PPS): a new tool. *J Palliat Care*. 1996;12(1):5–11.
9. White N, Harries P, Harris AJ, et al. How do palliative care doctors recognise imminently dying patients? A judgement analysis. *BMJ Open*. 2018;8(11):e024996. https://doi.org/10.1136/bmjopen-2018-024996.
10. Lin J, Hsieh RK, Chen JS, et al. Satisfaction with pain management and impact of pain on quality of life in cancer patients. *Asia Pac J Clin Oncol*. 2020;16(2):e91–e98. https://doi.org/10.1111/ajco.13095.
11. Saunders C. The evolution of the hospices. In: Mann RD, ed. *The History of the Management of Pain: From Early Principles to Present Practice*. CRC Press; 1988:167–178.
12. Joint Commission. *Cultural Diversity*. 2016. Accessed September 20, 2022. https://docslib.org/doc/413531/the-joint-commission-cultural-diversity
13. Marron JM, Kyi K, Appelbaum PS, Magnuson A. Medical decision-making in oncology for patients lacking capacity. *ASCO Educ Book*. 2020;40:1–11. https://doi.org/10.1200/EDBK_280279.
14. Cassell EJ. Diagnosing suffering: a perspective. *Ann Intern Med*. 1999;131(7):531–534. https://doi.org/10.7326/0003-4819-131-7-199910050-00009.
15. Puchalski CM, Vitillo R, Hull SK, Reller N. Improving the spiritual dimension of whole person care: reaching national and international consensus. *J Palliat Med*. 2014;17(6):642–656. https://doi.org/10.1089/jpm.2014.9427.
16. Saguil A, Phelps K. The spiritual assessment. *Am Fam Physician*. 2012;86(6):546–550.
17. Borneman T, Ferrell B, Puchalski CM. Evaluation of the FICA tool for spiritual assessment. *J Pain Symptom Manage*. 2010;40(2):163–173. https://doi.org/10.1016/j.jpainsymman.2009.12.019.
18. Cadge W, Bandini J. The evolution of spiritual assessment tools in healthcare. *Society*. 2015;52:430–437.
19. Rerucha CM, Salinas R Jr, Shook J, Duane M. House calls. *Am Fam Physician*. 2020;102(4):211–220.
20. Koenig HG. Research on religion, spirituality, and mental health: a review. *Can J Psychiatry*. 2009;54(5):283–291. https://doi.org/10.1177/070674370905400502.
21. Gergianaki I, Kampouraki M, Williams S, Tsiligianni I. Assessing spirituality: is there a beneficial role in the management of COPD? *NPJ Prim Care Respir Med*. 2019;29(1):23. https://doi.org/10.1038/s41533-019-0134-x.
22. Abu HO, Ulbricht C, Ding E, et al. Association of religiosity and spirituality with quality of life in patients with cardiovascular disease: a systematic review. *Qual Life Res*. 2018;27(11):2777–2797. https://doi.org/10.1007/s11136-018-1906-4.

23. Asano R, Anderson KM, Koirala B, Abshire M, Himmelfarb CD, Davidson PM. The Edmonton Symptom Assessment Scale in heart failure: a systematic review. *J Cardiovasc Nurs.* 2022;37(4):341–349. https://doi.org/10.1097/JCN.0000000000000835.

24. Murtagh FE, Ramsenthaler C, Firth A, et al. A brief, patient- and proxy-reported outcome measure in advanced illness: validity, reliability and responsiveness of the Integrated Palliative care Outcome Scale (IPOS). *Palliat Med.* 2019;33(8):1045–1057. https://doi.org/10.1177/0269216319854264.

5

Palliative Nursing Communication

Constance Dahlin and Janice Linton

Key Points

- The foundation of quality palliative care is effective communication that assures an individualized, respectful approach to care, from diagnosis to death, with regard to values, preferences, and beliefs.
- Nursing's role in communication is ensuring patient and family caregiver education to ensure informed decision-making.
- The art of nursing communication involves the therapeutic use of self, presence, silence, and listening to facilitate a patient-focused and family-centered process.
- The science of communication is a learned skill that establishes the nurse–patient relationship, comprised of 20% verbal and 80% nonverbal characteristics.
- Essential nursing communication includes gathering and imparting information and providing support and reassurance, as dictated by the individual needs of patients and families.
- Nurses' presence at times of delivery of illness communication including serious news, poor prognosis, or discussing the transition to hospice cannot be overemphasized.
- Nurses' communication around goals of care or life-sustaining therapies is grounded in nursing standards and scope of practice.
- Interprofessional team collaboration is the backbone of palliative care and includes effective communication and conflict negotiation.

Introduction

The art and science of palliative nursing is grounded on effective communication.[1] Nurses have an important role in patient care, particularly in palliative care communication.[2–4] Often, a nurse is the patient's first healthcare contact and spends the most time with the patient at the bedside. As the most trusted member of the healthcare team for two decades,[5] they have an essential role in advocating for and implementing an individualized, respectful approach to care, from diagnosis to death, with regard to values, preferences, and beliefs. They are consistently available and present to coordinate care and support the patients and family caregivers.[6] Moreover, nurses are essential to interprofessional collaboration to ensure optimal communication among the team, patient, and family as well as better patient outcomes.[3]

Frequently, nurses may question the limits of their scope of practice within communication and patient care.[6] The American Nurses Association's (ANA) *Nursing Scope and Standards of Practice* communication standard states that the nurse "communicates effectively in all areas of professional practice."[7] To do so, the nurse assesses their own communication skills and effectiveness that demonstrate caring, respect, deep listening, authenticity, and trust. This also includes the nurse's responsibility to assess communication ability, utilize alternate strategies for difficulties, convey accurate information, maintain interprofessional team communication, and demonstrate continuous improvement of communication skills.

The ANA *Code of Ethics* delineates the nurse's obligation to promote patient self-determination through the assessment of patient understanding of information and the implications of all potential decisions. Nurses support patient autonomy through patient decision-making, particularly around complex, difficult, decisions.[8,9] Specifically, they assist patients to define their goals and wishes as well as to express their cultural and religious practices and preferences.

Case Study

Lee was a critical care registered nurse (RN) with 3 years of direct care patient experience on an intensive care unit (ICU). On this unit, patients were on average 65 years old and often readmitted with multiple exacerbations from chronic progressive illnesses including congestive heart failure, chronic obstructive pulmonary disease, and complicated Parkinson's disease, with many discharges to skilled nursing facilities (SNFs). Over this time, Lee's nursing skills progressed from advanced beginner to clinically competent, and he was beginning to mentor and preceptor novice RNs.

One patient with several admissions, Winston Smith, a long-term care resident, was a 70-year-old man living with Parkinson's and stage II renal disease. He had been married to his wife for 50 years; she recently died of breast cancer. Mr. Smith had been a project manager for a construction company. He loved figuring out how to organize people and material delivery to create a timeline for the construction of buildings. He had three children who adored him.

Because Lee had cared for Mr. Smith on four previous admissions, he knew him well. To the nursing staff, Mr. Smith appeared more withdrawn. With Lee, he would discuss his grandchildren's academic and sports success. He also talked about the difficulty of his wife's "last days." He expressed how much he missed her and how sad he was that they were not together. He looked forward to being together someday. Lee also developed a rapport with Mr. Smith's adult children—Sondra, Matthew, and Jonah. He learned that when Mr. Smith felt mistrustful of various health team members, he would defer to his children to speak on his behalf.

Communication as the Foundation of Palliative Nursing

Communication is a central aspect of patient- and family-centered care, with the needs of the patient and family guiding the care.[10] Communication drives many critical aspects of care—information-sharing; active listening; identification of values, goals, and healthcare preferences; and decision-making—and communication facilitates support and collaboration.[11] Effective communication provides clarity to patients and families living with serious illnesses. Effective communication offers accurate information in sensitive, simple, and straightforward language that patients can understand.

Good communication provides the basis and foundation for a meaningful nurse–patient relationship and a therapeutic base for palliative care.[1,2,11] Specific nursing behaviors focus on the promotion of information-sharing, disclosure, reassurance, presence, facilitation, and dignity.[12,13] Indeed, emotional intelligence may promote more effective communication. Characteristics of emotional intelligence include self-reflection, self-awareness, problem-solving, and interprofessional collaboration in nursing.[14]

Communication Overview

Communication may seem straightforward, yet it is a complex, continual transactional process that occurs between persons where information, feelings, and meaning are conveyed through verbal and nonverbal messages. Multiple goals theory describes every message as possessing two levels of meaning, the content level and the relationship level. Communication interaction is seen as the exchange of ideas around a task, as well as the exchange of ideas around a relationship.[15] In professional contexts, the levels from mutual goals theory can be referred to as "task" and "relationship" levels.[15]

Message content generally concerns the tasks of communication—for example, instructing, diagnosing, managing, directing, encouraging, and supporting. Task communication may involve a nurse instructing a patient on how to use an incentive spirometer. "Relationship" refers both to how people interpret the content of messages and how they understand their shared connection—for example, open-ended questioning. A nurse asking a patient, "What is your pain level today?" is inquiring to obtain information about the patient's pain. Still, the relationship level of meaning is determined by the nurse's tone and authentic presence. If the nurse is documenting in the electronic health record while asking a question, without eye contact, or if they are standing in the hallway rather than at the bedside, the patient will likely interpret this as a matter of routine communication rather than a genuine inquiry. As a result, no relational components are developed within the exchange.

While the content level of a message is conveyed by stated words, the relational level generally is manifested by nonverbal communication and reflected in the nurse–patient connection. *Nonverbal communication* includes physical demeanor and paralinguistics, both of which influence perception.[16] *Artifacts*, the presence of physical objects, and the environmental setting can be barriers to developing relationships with patients and families.[16] These objects include bedrails, bedside tables, computers, and other medical equipment that reduce the emotional connection during the conversation. A nurse sitting in proximity to a patient can greatly enhance patient-centered communication and connection compared to a nurse standing behind a computer screen. *Vocalics*, the variety of ways that words are spoken, including volume, pitch, accent, rate of speech, use of pauses, and tone, are essential components of nonverbal communication.[16] The cadence of the voice communicates and connects on a relational level. *Proxemics*, the way space and distance are used during communication and whether or not it is respected and acknowledged during nursing work, can impact relational communication.[16] Finally, *haptics*, or the use of touch, can be task-related but can also convey relational messages of warmth and caring.[16]

Until recently, the undergraduate nursing curriculum included limited education specific to communication, let alone the philosophy of palliative care.[4,17,18] The result is nurses often feel unprepared in communication skills.[17] Yet, nurses rank communication as the most important competency. Many nurses fear using the wrong language or words or causing emotional distress or added sadness that they may feel unequipped to manage. Other nurses struggle with not having permission from the clinical team to discuss serious illness, and they have reservations about showing emotions with patients and families during times of distress.[19–22]

Nursing Communication

The nursing metaparadigms include person, environment, health, and nursing.[23] Nursing communication is person-centered, seeing the patient as the person who experiences the illness or condition, as well as the family who supports the patient.[7,24,25] Opportunities for communication exist throughout the delivery of hands-on, task-related, patient care, discussion of illness trajectory, delivering serious news, assessment of spiritual and religious concerns, and participation in interprofessional collaboration.[20,26] There are multiple settings, such as rehabilitation, long-term, correctional, psych-mental health or veteran's facilities, outpatient clinics, homeless shelters, and group homes, where nursing care can occur. Regardless of the clinical setting, without effective communication, patients may experience undue suffering, ineffective symptom control, and poor quality of life (QOL).[27,28]

Nurse interactions have been described within the following categories: supporting, caring, collaborating, reassuring, fostering hope, and advocating for the patient.[29] Research speaks to the various aspects of communication: nonverbal, verbal, active listening, timelines, presence, eliciting preferences, and facilitating communication choices.[30] Emotional intelligence has a valuable role in the nurse's perception and sensitivity, where self-awareness fosters connections to their own emotions, thoughts, and responses to

Table 5.1 Important communication themes for patients and families

Aspects of communications	Theme	Example statements from patients and families
HOW	Nonverbal	Positive: "Well she sat down and looked right at me, she reached out to me a couple of times to reassure me or to communicate with compassion about how I was feeling, she just listened really intently and responded to specific questions that I asked." Negative: "My dad was always aware the nurse was rushed because she asked questions while looking at the computer."
	Verbal	Positive: "They spoke to you. They didn't speak down to you; they spoke directly about the problem."
	Active listening	Positive: "I'm not quite sure how to explain this but they definitely had more of an empathetic approach and showed that in their art of listening and dialogue."
	Location	Negative: "I don't think you should ever tell somebody that their mother is dying standing in a hall corridor."
WHEN	Frequent	Positive: "We generally saw the doctors at least once a day if not more, and obviously the nurses were coming in every hour."
		Positive: "They were really good with my mother. If we needed to speak with them, they were always available."
	Team initiated	Positive: "Even just stopping me in the hall when I was in visiting my mom showed me they cared. Just having a quick chat, talking about progress, her current state, and talking about his insight into the day's activities and sort of what the next steps were going to be."
WHAT	Who is and will be involved in care	Positive: "We would always see who was on staff every day, the name would be posted which was great."
	Progress and results	Positive: "There was a lot of one-on-one explanations of the care that was being received by my mom and a lot of stuff sort of outside of that that provided more general information about the path that I was going to be going down with my mom. That was useful, I don't know how I would have started this process without having that information."
	Discharge plan	Negative: "To be honest it would have been the final meeting just to have an overview of everything. I think honestly that would have made the experience a 10 [out of 10]."

Source: References 1 and 33.

a patient's health journey.[31,32] A thematic analysis revealed important aspects of communication for patients and families as "how" the health team communicated, "when" or the timeliness of the communication, and "what" was communicated (Table 5.1).[33]

Palliative Nursing

Depending on the setting, nurses are often the first to establish a patient–clinician relationship and the first to identify issues for patients living with a life-threatening illness.[34] Nurses create a therapeutic relationship and accompany the patient through the illness journey with their constant presence. They may be best situated to elicit the patient's hopes, worries, dreams, regrets, and fears of being a burden; and they can advocate for the patient's values, preferences, and wishes.[34–36] Therapeutic relationship and patient advocacy require nursing education and empowerment through the use of open-ended questions.[37]

Patients and families want their healthcare professionals to support hope and provide honest conversations. Focusing on QOL offers hope and meaning to support what matters most to the patient. Being hopeful of the possibility of "miracles" and being honest can prepare for the probability of dying. See Chapter 7, "Value Based Care," and Chapter 30, "Hope and Meaning in Illness," for further discussion of promoting QOL as well as supporting hope and meaning for patients. Honesty can be achieved through open dialogue and determining patient readiness to both discuss serious illness and receive unfavorable news. Additionally, honest discussion of possible outcomes on the spectrum of recovery, whether complete, modified, or for a limited time, helps the patient to prepare for what the future may look like with the current illness.

Nurses promote and optimize the health and functionality of their patients, prevent illness and injury, alleviate suffering, treat the patient's response to the illness, and advocate for patients' and families' desired outcomes.[7] Palliative nursing practice is evidence-based nursing practice that includes "the assessment, diagnosis, and treatment of human responses to actual or potential life-limiting illnesses within the context of a dynamic caring relationship with the patient and family, in order to reduce or relieve suffering and optimize health."[38(p109)] All nurses practice aspects of primary palliative care.[39] Availability, authentic presence, empathy, respect, active listening, welcoming voice tone and facial expression, language of comfort, encouragement, humor, as well as the use of touch are various communication modalities that promote relief of physical, emotional, spiritual, cultural, and psychological distress.[40]

The nurse characteristics preferred by patients and families include both verbal and nonverbal communication modalities. In one study, families of patients admitted to acute care settings report high satisfaction in delivery of care and competency but low scores in compassionate communication, specifically a lack of clarity and consistency in communication.[41] Studies report satisfactory communication as determinants in shared decision-making as well as essential factors of quality of care that are fundamental in establishing patient–clinician relationships.[42,43] The most beneficial nurse behaviors for families are (1) keeping family informed, (2) providing assurance, (3) being a compassionate presence, (4) facilitating final acts, and (5) honoring dignity.[30]

Nurse-to-patient communication is multifaceted. The daily flow of nurse–patient interaction is often aimed at accomplishing clinical tasks. This occurs in a conversational manner, where pleasantries are exchanged and information on the plan of care for the day; medications, procedural schedules, and dietary options are disseminated. A major facet includes the nursing process: assessment, nursing diagnosis, planning, implementation, and evaluation.

The nurse approaches the patient in an open manner to assess the physical, psychological, spiritual, cultural, and emotional aspects of care and treatment. Within this process, the nurses allow the patient to determine treatment effectiveness.

The most complex facet of nurse–patient communication occurs in the existential realm. Patients at their sickest and most vulnerable periods in their illness journey may question their existence. Communication at this level is sensitive and often nuanced because the existential aspects of end of life include the perception of suffering, disclosure about the past, and a search for meaning and purpose.[27] Exploration of existential suffering can help clinicians work through nonpathological causes of symptom burden and help the patient with a life-threatening illness cope and experience a better QOL.

Palliative care provides skilled communication at critical junctions of a patient's illness. Depending on the illness trajectory, such communication may occur over a long or a short period of time. Since a significant number of patients who die have a chronic illness, there are usually many opportunities for communication.[44] Within the nurse–patient relationship, Perrin describes the three phases as introductory (initial), middle (working), and termination (ending) (see Table 5.2).[45] The introductory phase of communication occurs when the nurse and the patient learn about each other's styles. The middle phase involves establishing a working relationship in which the work of nursing is done, such as pain and symptom management and discussions about the meaning of life, legacy, and family closure. The termination phase happens when the nurse and the patient discontinue the relationship either because the patient or nurse is leaving the healthcare system or because the patient is dying.

The *introductory* or *initial phase* of communication in the nurse–patient relationship starts at the time of diagnosis and meeting the nurse as a member of the care team. During this period, the nurse assesses the patient's learning styles and information needs, and the patient determines the nurse's style.[45] The tasks for the nurse include exploring the patient's understanding of their illness, eliciting personality and coping styles, and identifying pertinent documents related to the delegation of surrogate decision makers, advance directives, or out-of-hospital medical orders for life-sustaining treatments. Assessing learning style includes discerning the patient's ability to learn and understand the seriousness of the illness. These abilities vary according to the age and cognitive development of the patient, as well as both educational and health literacy, numeracy (capacity for numerical thought and expression), and primary language. For children and some older adults, the family or support unit is primarily involved in both the information-gathering process and ongoing communication with the health team.

The *middle* or *working phase* often extends over the course of the illness while the patient receives pharmacological, nonpharmacological, and integrative therapies for their serious illness. The patient and family establish trust with the nurse, who provides presence and reassurance.[45] The nurse gains insight into patient and family coping, perception of care, and concerns about the illness and possible outcomes. Nurse–patient communication during the middle phase sets the tone for critical communication tasks if the termination phase leads to end-of-life care. Communication, meeting care needs, hospital environment, dignity and respect, and support for relatives were the themes identified in one study of end-of-life care from the perspective of bereaved families.[46] Therefore, discussions concerning serious illness require nursing presence. Because of the nurse–patient relationship established in the introductory and middle phases, the nurse is able to offer their perspectives of care and facilitate ongoing discussions using language and shared information that was similar to language used in initial discussions.

As the patient enters the later stage of advanced illness, the termination phase begins. The nurse–patient relationship is discontinued in the *termination* or *ending phase*. It should be noted that termination may also occur if the patient changes practice settings or the nurse transitions to another position. Communication focuses on support of decision-making, assurance of comfort from pain and symptom burden, delivery of information about the dying process, and guidance in anticipatory grieving. During this last stage, the nurse offers continued presence and reassurance in monitoring comfort and providing intensive caring to both the patient and family.[45] The family caregiver's burden is often overlooked, but it is a major aspect of the illness experience.[47] Both the nurse and

Table 5.2 Stages of the nurse–patient relationship

Stage	Initial or introductory phase	Working or middle phase	Termination or ending phase
Nurse tasks	1. Exploring patient/family understanding of illness 2. Determining personality, coping, and learning styles 3. Eliciting presence of advance care planning	1. Monitoring patient response to illness 2. Providing clinical care 3. Delivering treatment 4. Offering illness/treatment	1. Saying goodbye 2. Telling the patient what they meant to you or taught you 3. Assisting with the transition
Patient tasks	Establishing trust and understanding with the nurse	1. Establishing care plan in collaboration with the team 2. Participating in care 3. Providing information on response to therapy	1. Saying goodbye 2. Showing appreciation to nurse and other staff 3. Articulating needs with transition

Source: References 1 and 45.

the patient work toward closure as the patient moves toward the end of life. Immediately following the death, the nurse provides family support with the goal of promoting a healthy grief and bereavement process.

Communication Barriers

Communication barriers exist for the patient, the family, and the nurse. For the patient, psychological emotions such as anger, fear, sadness, lack of trust, and helplessness hinder communication. Patients may feel that any discussion will cause too much distress for themselves and/or their families. Some patients fear that discussing the illness will induce a worsening or progression of their illness. For some patients, communication is not an area of comfort or value, so they may have little interest in processing feelings or information.

Health inequities have played a major role in communication barriers. This is specifically true when patients and families are culturally, ethnically, spiritually, and racially diverse from the health team.[48] One hindrance to comprehensive communication is the lack of assessment of patients' health literacy, particularly when the team uses healthcare language and jargon instead of lay language (Table 5.3).[49] Social determinants of health have implications in effective communication. Physical surroundings such as semiprivate rooms with neighboring patients, background verbal noise, alarms from equipment and monitors, lighting, and inadequate seating can also be seen as barriers to communication. Age, gender differences, physiological limitations such as pain or anxiety, speech or hearing deficits, or endotracheal tubes are additional barriers to communication.[50]

Family and Caregiver Barriers

Several family and caregiver-related communication barriers exist which affect communication exchange.[51] In order to maintain hope, families tend to overestimate the possibility of a cure. They also fear future regrets if they do not pursue or demand further curative treatment. Families or caregivers may also find it too painful to talk about the advanced state of their loved one's illness. Such discussion may trigger anticipatory grief and the feeling of impending loss. Additionally, families and caregivers may not understand the full extent of the illness and may not know what to discuss. Finally, it is common that family members have little knowledge of the patient's treatment values, beliefs, and preferences. Therefore, their ability to fully participate in decision-making in the context of the patient's preferences is limited.[52] Given all these issues, nurses must attend to the family and caregivers to assure quality care for the patient.[53]

Circumstantial barriers are conditions that can impede nurses' ability to deliver optimal care.[54] These include time, appointment schedules, patient's condition, and settings of care. Time, a circumstantial barrier, is always an issue, in terms of attending to a patient or the time available to deeply discuss an issue. The scheduling of patients using layered appointments and tests may allow for little reflective time or time for meaningful discussion.[55] Another circumstantial challenge is the patient's waxing and waning clinical condition. Rapid changes in the patient's condition may prevent full discussion of health details, considerations of viable treatment options or risks, and burden of interventions. Barriers to goals-of-care discussions include family members' or patients' difficulty in accepting a poor prognosis, difficulty understanding the limitations and complications of treatments, disagreement among family members, and patients' lack of decision-making capacity.[56] Care settings may be another circumstantial barrier, in which there is a lack of privacy such as open treatment suites for chemotherapy, renal care, heart failure, or in urgent care settings, making it unconducive to a sensitive conversation about health information. Families may be uninformed and receive mixed messages. Additionally, situations where information exchange must occur virtually (telephone or video) prevent the nurse from "reading" the family's nonverbal communication.

Nursing Communication Barriers

Nursing communication barriers to patient-centered care include four categories: institutional and healthcare system–related, communication-related, environment-related, and personal and behavior-related barriers.[57] A healthcare organization or system's policy and leadership styles often set the precedent for how and what information nurses can communicate to and with families. Differences in the use of language and cultural norms between the nurse and patient may impede communication. For instance, nonverbal cues, such as head nodding or eye gaze, convey different meanings across cultures. Environmental barriers include various technologies (computers, medical equipment, medical gloves, gowns, and masks) which create physical and psychological barriers between nurses and patients. Finally, professional barriers include a nurse's lack of comfort with caring for the patient of different racial, ethnic, and religious backgrounds. This discomfort can be perceived as disrespectful, disregarding, and disingenuous, ultimately tarnishing the nurse–patient relationship.[57]

Table 5.3 Translation of healthcare language to lay language

Concept	Healthcare language	Lay language
Surrogate decision maker	You assign a durable power of attorney.	You choose or designate someone to make decisions for you when you cannot, or you are unable.
Articulate values and preferences	You state your values and preferences.	You tell us what your beliefs are.
Life-sustaining/Life-supporting/ life-prolonging	We put you on a ventilator and pressors to support life.	You have a tube put in your throat and are placed on a breathing machine to help your lungs work. You are given medications to help your heart to work to prolong your life.
Resuscitation	We perform chest compressions and intubation	Your chest and ribs are squeezed to get your heart restarted, and a tube is inserted into your throat to keep you breathing.

Other barriers include lack of education and training in palliative nursing,[4] difficulty in prognostication, and the perceived reluctance of the patient or family to engage in important conversations. A new nurse's death anxiety may cripple their ability to bring up issues related to end of life.[58] New nurses may experience dread or fear at the mere thought of death or communicating anything to do with dying with the patient or family.[59] Alternatively, there may be concerns about whether the nurse has a scope of practice or authority to initiate any serious illness conversations, discuss diagnosis or prognosis, as well as introduce or discuss palliative care. Finally, even though communication and information-sharing fall under the nursing scope of practice and advocacy for both RNs and advanced practice RNs (APRNs), many nurses express discomfort with serious illness communication and focus on maintaining hope instead of talking about prognosis.[60]

Consequently, nurses may employ avoidance behaviors regarding communication. Varying types of moral anguish, moral injury, moral distress, moral uncertainty, moral dilemma, and moral conflict can also lead to avoidance behaviors.[61,62] A nurse may focus more on quantitative data such as lab results and vital signs and avoid exploring the patient's feelings about their worsening illness. The nurse may also focus on each hospitalization as an isolated episodic event instead of an ongoing trajectory of decline, an outlook that may prevent the patient from expressing previous concerns. The nurse may default to a conversation that provides improbable reassurance, such as "Things will be okay now" or "There is medication for that."

The nurse may try to allay the patient's worry with statements such as "I'll do the worrying for you because worrying just makes you anxious." These statements dismiss the emotion and hinder conversation about fears, worries, and concerns. Another way of avoidance behavior nurses employ is deferring with statements such as "Talk with your doctor, the social worker, the chaplain when they make rounds." Patients and families want to remain positive when facing a life-threatening illness, so nurses and physicians avoid any discussion about death and dying to support the patient's desire; this, however, prevents vital information-sharing and shared decision-making when death is imminent.

Communication Approaches

Case Study Continued: Imparting information

One day, Mr. Smith was admitted from the long-term setting to the hospital for shortness of breath and fever. Workup included laboratory blood draws—complete blood count, complete metabolic profile, urinalysis, chest X-ray, and coronavirus polymerase chain reaction (PCR). It was necessary to communicate this tenuous clinical course with the family.

Lee notified Matthew, the older son, about Mr. Smith's vital signs, chest X-ray findings of fluid on his lungs, initial negative COVID result, necessary medications, and the high probability of discharge to SNF, similar to his previous hospital admissions. Within 36 hours after admission, Mr. Smith developed acute respiratory failure and confusion. He was emergently intubated, without family notification.

Lee felt responsible to communicate with Mr. Smith's family—Sondra, Matthew, and Jonah. They were upset with the lack of discussion about treatment options in respect to goals of care and developed a mistrust of the medical team. Lee made it a point to provide daily virtual updates and provide acknowledgment of their continued caring for their father.

The context of communication influences the process and outcomes of interactions. Because of the rapidly changing complexity of healthcare, different methods of communication may be utilized. Of course, timing is always the first consideration and may dictate the communication method as urgent, less urgent, and routine. Quill and colleagues defined "urgent" situations that necessitate immediate communication.[63] These include the following scenarios: (1) the patient is facing imminent death; (2) the patient is talking about wanting to die; (3) the patient or family is inquiring about hospice; (4) the patient has recently been hospitalized for severe, progressive illness; and (5) the patient is experiencing severe suffering and a short prognosis. Less urgent situations include (1) the discussion of prognosis, particularly if life expectancy is thought to be between 6 and 12 months; (2) the discussion of potential treatment options with a low probability of success; and (3) the discussion of hopes and fears. More "routine" palliative communication includes circumstances when stability or recovery is predicted.[64]

Telehealth

Due to social determinants of health, the changing work environment, and transient lifestyles of families, in-person meetings may not be possible. Telehealth (telephone, video technology, protected website, and e-mail communications) has opportunities and challenges for both the patient and family and the healthcare team.[65,66] Telehealth in palliative care has been growing over recent years and is an important tool. Many lessons were learned from the COVID-19 pandemic when visitor restrictions impacted in-person meetings.[67] Nurses can provide two types of telehealth calls. One type is a clinical call, which includes an assessment of the patient and family. The second type reflects the growing role of care management/coordinator/navigator calls to check in to see if the patient and family have enough medications, equipment, and support, which may trigger a clinical assessment. It is more common that family meetings occur by telephone compared to video technology.[67] When there is an established nurse–patient relationship, delivering serious news by telehealth has the same worries or concerns about how the information will be received, but there is often a lower level of anxiety given the nurse–patient connection.[65] See Chapter 60, "Telehealth, Telephonic Care, and Remote Patient Monitoring," for more information and discussion on the role of the nurse.

Core Elements of Nurse Communication

Imparting Information

A primary role of the nurse is to impart information about the illness, medications, and treatments. However, nuanced scopes of practice for RNs and APRNs mean the language used may differ. By the nature of their scope of practice, APRNs may offer diagnosis, prognosis, and treatment options. The task of imparting information is complex because providing information alone is not enough. Rather, information must be provided within the context of educational level, developmental level, literacy level, numeracy level, and primary language, along with psychological state and other social determinants of care.[68] To impart medical information, the nurse must address both personal and organizational health literacy. Personal health literacy addresses the patient's ability to find, understand, and use the information to make medically informed decisions, while organizational health literacy emphasizes the organization's responsibility to equitably address health literacy.[69] Given that many palliative care discussions are based on "what may happen," it is essential for nurses to tailor their communication to the individual health literacy level of patients and families to promote understanding.[70]

Nurses are responsible for providing health literacy support, but nurses report a high degree of difficulty communicating with patients who exhibit low literacy levels. There are tools and techniques that can be utilized to ensure that nurses communicate effectively and meet patients' health literacy needs.[71–73] Techniques such as chunking (providing small amounts of information) and checking (assessing for understanding) are recommended communication strategies to address health literacy needs.[71] Another strategy is the teach-back method, which involves asking patients to share their understanding of instructions or information discussed in a teaching session. Other actions include adding more time to patient encounters, using effective communication with simpler language, tailoring information, as well as consideration of messaging content.[74] Finally, using analogies and culturally appropriate metaphors can address low health literacy barriers. While assessing health literacy is a core nursing skill, nurses need ongoing education to assess, communicate, and connect with patients who exhibit low health literacy. Boston University's Health Literacy Tool Shed offers over 200 tools specific to certain illnesses, languages, and ages.[75]

Case Study Continued: Gathering Information

Lee discussed the current clinical course and plan of care with the ICU team. Lee understood the family dynamic from previous hospitalizations and had a rapport with Mr. Smith's daughter Sondra. Lee knew that Mr. Smith had fears and concerns about being "kept alive by machines" because he felt these interventions caused his wife distress and left him traumatized when she died. Lee knew that Sondra, however, believed that everything should be done to give her father more time. Matthew and Jonah often reserved their opinions, deferring to their father and sister.

Lee's nurse–patient relationship with Mr. Smith and his family was still strong; therefore, a virtual call with the intensivist, Dr. May, and all of Mr. Smith's children was arranged. Before initiating the call Lee clarified their role and the purpose of the conference call, which was to gather information from the family about how they would make decisions about his care going forward.

During the virtual visit, Lee reintroduced himself to the family and introduced the intensivist, Dr. May, and the social worker, Larry. The goal of the call was to provide an update on Mr. Smith's condition and gather information to consider next steps. Sondra, Matthew, and Jonah conveyed their understanding of their father's admission, as well as their understanding of his chronic medical conditions. However, it became apparent that there was a lack of understanding of the progressive nature of Parkinson's and associated recurrent pneumonias. Lee asked what was important to Mr. Smith and what was important to the family. Dr. May furthered the discussion by stating that honoring Mr. Smith's values and beliefs was important with the potential for emergent respiratory decline and the need to make urgent decisions about life-sustaining treatments.

Information-Gathering

The next role of the nurse is to gather information. The most effective tool in gathering information from patients and families is the use of open-ended questions. Open-ended questions promote both the opportunity to listen and hear the richness of the patient's words and perspective. While listening to the patient's narrative, the nurse can observe nonverbal communication. This allows the nurse to benefit from the expression of values, priorities of care, coping, life priorities, and spiritual concerns. Closed-ended questions include yes-or-no questions or limited-response questions and leading questions. The use of closed-ended questions, which usually focus on physical symptoms or history questions, limits the patient's response, thereby inhibiting elaboration, explanations, and clarifications of various topics.[34] Within the time constraints of clinical care, a nurse may not have enough time for a long conversation. However, a few key questions set the tone of a caring relationship and present a conversation starter (Box 5.1).

Often, important questions are asked, but as the patient or family starts to answer, the nurse interrupts and moves the conversation on. Studies report that a patient has about 11 seconds to speak before a clinician interrupts.[76] When the nurse asks an open-ended question, it is essential to allow for silence and pauses and to wait for and listen to the answer. Otherwise, distraction, unresponsiveness, or lack of acknowledgment is invalidating to the patient and/or family. Resentment may also result if the patient has shared something intimate without receiving acknowledgment of its significance.

Box 5.1 Useful Open-Ended Questions to Initiate Discussions

What concerns or worries you about your illness?
What concerns or worries you about your treatment?
What are you most worried about?
How are you coping with your illness?
What are your hopes in terms of your illness and treatment?
How is treatment going for you? How are things going for you?
Who are the most important people to you?
What relationships are the most important to you?
Who are the people who provide you support?
What matters most to you?
What gives you meaning in your life?
What gives you joy in your life?
What provides you with the strength to live or cope with each day?
Is there any important or unfinished business you need to attend to?

Source: Revised from Reference 35.

Listening

Listening is an active process that requires concentrated presence and attention. Focused listening allows understanding of the patient's journey within the disease trajectory and how the patient is processing information. During the listening process, the nurse focuses on the patient's story attentively, without interrupting, noting their specific word choices and concerns. One helpful technique is to begin the discussion by asking an open-ended question, such as "What brought you to the hospital?" or "Can you tell me about what has been going on?" Specifically, the nurse observes both the verbal and nonverbal content in the patient's responses, focusing on both what is said and what is left unsaid. In addition, the nurse notes speech patterns, tone, rapidity, and coherency. Concurrently, the nurse observes nonverbal expressions including emotion and accompanying physical movement. All these observations will determine distress in the physical, psychological, spiritual, cultural, and emotional dimensions of care as well as which areas are a priority to address.

The nurse's use of silence is paramount. It allows the nurse to be fully present in the moment rather than mentally preparing answers or replies. Correspondingly, the nurse uses reflection to convey empathy. The nurse clarifies what has been heard by such comments as "Hmm" or "Tell me more." By acknowledging the patient's responses and exploring their meaning in a compassionate and supportive way, the nurse encourages the patient to explain difficult or serious issues and concerns.[77] There may be times when the patient is silent. In this circumstance, it is appropriate for the nurse to just sit quietly, letting the patient reflect on the moment and the current situation. It is after these moments of silence that a patient may reveal sensitive information, concerns, thoughts, or past history (trauma, abuse, or illicit behaviors). The patient's revelation of information may be at a deeper level because they have been given the opportunity and permission to reveal such information.

There are several strategies for palliative nursing communication. They include Ask-Tell-Ask, SPIKES, SOLER, and NURSE and are explained in Box 5.2. Any of these strategies is effective, and their use will depend on the expertise and communication style of the nurse.

Eliciting Sensitive Aspects of Care: Culture, Religion, Ethics

Case Study Continued: Cultural Aspects of Care

Lee continued to work with Mr. Smith. Larry, the social worker, did a social assessment and learned that Mr. Smith was worried about being a financial burden and emotional burden on his children. While he understood his increased care needs, Mr. Smith did not enjoy living in the long-term care setting, despite the loving care he received. The chaplain did a spiritual assessment and learned that Mr. Smith was a devout Christian. He believed in life after death but felt God had his plan. He did not feel strongly about having all measures to sustain his life, especially in light of his wife's breast cancer experience. He had stated after watching his wife suffer through treatments and his wife's death, he wanted to "go quietly."

Mr. Smith's daughter, Sondra, wanted all medical measures to keep her father alive; Matthew and Jonah were quiet. Sondra stated she wanted to understand the cause of her father's respiratory decline and how it was being addressed. Her brothers tried to help her understand the broad picture of their father's overall health. Although they all loved him dearly, the sons advocated that the care honor Mr. Smith's values and wishes.

Cultural awareness or cultural sensitivity includes issues pertaining to religious, spiritual, cultural, ethnic, racial, gender, and language issues. There is diversity in communication customs and norms among various cultures. These may include deference to healthcare professionals, preference for the gender of health professionals, or the appropriateness of discussing certain topics. Attending to culture is a very important aspect of communication, necessitating an appreciation of verbal cues and the interpretation of nonverbal cues. In many situations, beneficence takes precedence over autonomy. Disclosure and nondisclosure must be viewed within the context of the patient and the family, with an understanding of and respect for their values and beliefs.

Box 5.2 Communication Strategies

Ask-Tell-Ask	SPIKES[19]	SOLER[20]	NURSE[20]
The nurse asks a question	S—listening skills	Squarely sit opposite the patient	Name—"You sound scared"
The patient then responds with both statements and questions	P—patient perception of the current situation	Open body posture	Understand—"I cannot imagine how hard it must be to think that your father's condition is worsening"
The nurse then responds to the content of the discussion	I—an invitation to provide information	Leaning in to demonstrate empathy	Respect—"The entire ICU team respects how much you all have been at your father's bedside"
The nurse closes by asking a final question to determine patient understanding	K—offering knowledge or the facts	Eye contact as appropriate	Support—"We are here to support you and your family through this"
	E—emotional exploration and empathy	Relaxed positioning	Explore—"Tell me more about what worries you"
	S—summary		

ICU, intensive care unit.

Box 5.3 Cultural Assessment Questions

Where were you born?
Where were you raised?
How does this affect you about health and illness?
Are there any cultural considerations or beliefs important to your care?
Are you spiritual or religious?
How should spirituality or religion be addressed in your healthcare?
Are there any important rituals that are important to your healthcare?
How do you describe your medical condition/illness?
What do you know about your medical condition/illness?
What do you want to know about your medical condition/illness?
What worries you most about your condition and its treatment?
How have you treated your medical condition/illness?
Who else, if anyone, do you want to know about your medical condition/illness?
Who else, if anyone, should we talk to about your medical condition/illness, treatment options, and the disease process?
Who is responsible for making healthcare decisions for you if you are unable or do not want to?
Are there other important people in your community involved in your healthcare?
Are there other people in your community whom we should include in your healthcare?

Source: Adapted from Reference 35.

To be culturally sensitive, a nurse must be "self-aware of their own culture, cultural biases, and assumptions."[48] Understanding one's own background serves as a starting point for the nurse. Palliative nurses cultivate cultural self-awareness by recognizing how their own cultural values, beliefs, biases, and practices inform their perceptions of patients, families, and colleagues.[48] This includes reflection and examination of one's ethical values and beliefs by reflecting on ethnicity and its effect on health, illness, and death; religion and its role in death, dying, and afterlife beliefs; and individual communication patterns.

Eliciting health information and understanding of illness is essential to care. It is imperative for the nurse to assess the patient's and family's religion and culture and how it affects healthcare. In some cultures, there are social norms about whether or not the patient should know their health information, especially if the patient is seriously ill. An assessment includes how much, if any, information a patient wants to know as well as what and how much information is conveyed, which may be dictated by culture and ethnicity. It is important for the healthcare team to understand any religious or cultural practices that will affect health decisions and utilize assessment tools to garner discussions about cultural and religious concerns (Box 5.3).[78] For instance, some religions or cultures do not allow surgical removal of organs or blood transfusions; others may not allow pain medications. See Chapter 28, "Cultural Considerations in Palliative Care," for further discussion of culture in the care of individuals with serious illness.

Information Needs of Patients and Families

To best provide supportive care to patients and families, it is necessary to understand their information and communication needs. Patients require information about treatment options, management of symptoms, support from family and friends, fulfillment of family or cultural expectations, attaining meaning, and maintaining dignity and control. Correspondingly, the communication needs of the patient include disease specifics, rationale for care, being listened to, and the opportunity to participate in important discussions. The role of the nurse is to assess the patient's knowledge and concerns in these areas, offer reinforcement of health information, and facilitate information exchange with the rest of the care team. The nurse also guides the patient in understanding the care plan, clarifies team responsibility for specific aspects of care, and provides support in the process.[49]

For full participation in the patient's care, family communication is essential. The communication needs of the family and other caregivers depend on their role in the family system, age, decision-making ability, and other rules within and specific to the family. Family caregivers/members are not always aware of the information they might need, may avoid relevant information, and may not express their information needs.[79] Families also need to understand how the interprofessional team works, including the individual team members involved in care, their roles in the plan of care, what influences the plan of care, and the site of care.[80] The most frequently reported information need among patients and families receiving palliative care is about pain management.

Patients with chronic, progressive illnesses often endure periods of exacerbation and remission. The clinical course of one or more exacerbations may present with more complex symptoms and pathology, subsequently requiring more medical intervention that may or may not result in reversible conditions. Each episodic illness is seen as an isolated condition by the patient and family and often presents as a crisis when the patient ends up in a critical care unit. As families endure the situational crisis of a loved one in a critical care unit, they move through phases of hovering, information-seeking, tracking, and garnering resources. During the hovering phase, worry and anxiety center on the medical condition and critical care environment. In the information-seeking phase, the family asks multiple questions but often finds limited information-sharing from clinicians, and this amplifies the hovering phase. The family then moves to the tracking phase, where they evaluate the delivery of care and clinicians. Finally, families move into the phase of garnering resources to seek tangible support to meet their emotional needs.[81]

Nurses are information providers and communication facilitators, educating patients and family caregivers about illness and procedures, challenging family members to consider the consequences of treatment, and encouraging awareness about a patient's decline over time.[82] As an information provider and communication facilitator, the nurse offers reassurance of the patient's comfort, support in coping with the patient's condition, explanations of the evolving care plan, and delineation of the current aspect of clinical care. Moreover, families may be very involved in the patient's care but have multiple home and work obligations. Therefore, it may be difficult for family members to participate directly in meetings at the bedside, which may necessitate frequent nursing updates about care. Finally, families may experience a high level of stress resulting from their need for constant updates of information. The nurse's role is to acknowledge and validate the family's stress and emotions. Families who are able to talk about the disease are able to support a patient's preferences for care, navigate the practical demands of care, and come to terms with challenging issues.[83]

Conflict in palliative care arises from mismatched expectations and suboptimal communication.[84] When family members begin to have concerns about the patient's quality of care, this is an indication that they are insufficiently prepared for the patient's death and/or are having difficulty understanding and accepting the prognosis.[83] A common circumstance occurs when either the family member or the patient requests that the other party not be informed about the extent of the seriousness of the situation. If the family is protecting the patient, the nurse should explore the family's reason for withholding information. Such requests may include spiritual beliefs, cultural issues, fear of death, fear that the patient will lose hope and give up their fight, or discomfort with any such discussions. Each concern requires a different approach.

If there is a spiritual or cultural issue, the nurse must explore the family's spiritual dimension and cultural mores.[78,85,86] If the family states they are fearful, the nurse can explain that most patients want to know their diagnosis so that they can participate in life-closure activities and determine how to spend their final days. Most importantly, the nurse must assess the patient and determine whether they prefer to know health information and how much health information. Finally, in this situation, the nurse must attend to their own integrity. To the family who requests that topics be avoided, the nurse should respond that they will not necessarily introduce such topics; however, they will be honest and respond to the patient if they bring up such topics.

When the patient is trying to protect the family, the principles of autonomy and confidentiality are paramount. In this situation, the nurse should explore the reasons the patient is withholding information from the family. Often, there may be a past personal history or event rooted in shame, guilt, or lack of acceptance of a lifestyle. The nurse can first provide a therapeutic presence in allowing the patient to process this. Additional social work and/or spiritual care support may be necessary. If appropriate, the nurse should explain that if the family is to be involved in caregiving, it is helpful for them to have a full understanding of the patient's illness and comorbid conditions. The patient ultimately has the right to allow or limit information, and the nurse must honor this.

Another challenge is family dynamics. Serious illness results in either effective coping, where the family comes together, or ineffective coping, where the family falls apart. Assessment of both the patient and family reveals consistency in perspectives of family coping. Patient support may be suboptimal if there is inconsistent structure to support the ill person or if family members are overburdened by care. Family members may report distress and dissatisfaction as a result of lack of clear, consistent family–clinician commination and poor emotional support from the health team. Family dynamics are impacted by conflicted relationships due to divorce or separation; psychological, physical, or sexual abuse; neglect; substance abuse; and past violence. These situations are fraught with drama and divert the focus away from the patient. The nurse must understand that they cannot fix these problems and focus instead on the tangible health issues at hand. In addition, these situations necessitate interprofessional collaboration, including assistance from social workers, mental health specialists, and/or addiction specialists.

Care or Family Meetings

Care or family meetings are a wonderful but underutilized tool. These meetings promote respectful and sensitive delivery of information in a timely, thorough, current, comprehensive, and accurate fashion. The patient may or may not attend depending on their condition, decision-making capacity, and preference for involvement. It can be helpful to hear consistent messages. For the family, it is a time to meet the various team members and understand their roles. Patient and family care meetings create open dialogue about the understanding of the illness; the current medical crisis; the most likely, least likely, and probable outcomes; as well as the risks, burdens, and benefits of treatment options. The care or family meeting also provides clinicians an opportunity to collaboratively formulate a plan of care that is consistent with the goals and wishes of the patient and family.[35,63]

Scheduled meeting times are imperative to allow the patient to prepare emotionally and psychologically for any potential news. There are several types of meetings that occur within the context of palliative care: information meetings, advance care planning (ACP) meetings, serious news discussions, and code status discussions.[35,87]

These meetings help form a working relationship between the patient, the family, and the care team. There may be no particular agenda other than to convey information about the patient's current status or the nature of the illness and its symptoms. The first meeting gives the family the opportunity to narrate their observation of the patient's day-to-day as they live with the illness. Often, from this narrative the clinician gets a picture of the steady decline typically associated with chronic illnesses. This is later incorporated in follow-up meetings to clarify symptom burden, declining functional state, or worsening disease state that leads to death.

Other topics include predictions about the course of illness and treatment options, symptom management, medications, and post-hospital care needs.

No matter the reason for a care or family meeting, there are guidelines for holding a meeting. Before calling a care or family meeting, it is important to maximize the effective use of time by clarifying the meeting's goal. A pre-meeting should be held to clarify the messages to be conveyed and determine who should lead the meeting; the leader may not necessarily be the physician.[84,87] Organizational cultures may dictate which clinician may lead family meetings. However, nurses may be the best to lead such meetings due to their proximity to bedside clinical care, particularly in the home, long-term care setting, and hospital. Nurses are highly accessible and responsive in the daily delivery of hands-on care, allowing them to facilitate the initial conversation as focal to the continuity of care.[81] This allows them to advocate and coordinate family-centered communication. For more complex or contentious families, having a team meeting specifically to plan strategies to deal with a challenging family is time well spent. Consideration should be given to the attendance of essential healthcare clinicians.

There is a stepwise approach to conducting a care or family meeting: (1) finding an appropriate, private space for the meeting; (2) introducing all the participants at the meeting; (3) using open-ended questions to establish patient (and family) illness

Box 5.4 The Care or Family Meeting

Pre-meeting planning	1. Conduct clinician pre-meeting to assure consistency of message and process. 2. Clarify goals of meeting with patient and family caregivers as well as staff. 3. Decide on the essential people to attend the meeting—patient, family caregivers, and healthcare professionals.
The care or family meeting encounter	1. Arrange an appropriate setting. 2. Introduce all participants in room and their relationship to patient's care. 3. Review goal of meeting. 4. Elicit patient/family understanding of care to date. 5. Review current medical condition. 6. Attend to questions. 7. Review options for care. 8. Elicit response from patient if they have decision-making capacity. 9. Elicit response from family in terms of what patient would choose for themself if they could.
Summary	1. Review plan. If agreement, then decision. If no agreement, what follow-up is planned? 2. Document meeting—who attended, what was discussed, and plan.

Source: References 35, 87, 88, 91, and 92.

understanding; (4) determining how the patient wishes the information to be presented; (5) presenting information in a straightforward manner, using understandable language, in small quantities, and with pauses for processing and questions to assess understanding; (6) responding to emotions; (7) clarifying goals of care and treatment priorities; and (8) establishing a plan.[11,84,88] These steps are categorized as the pre-meeting planning, the family meeting encounter, and summary (Box 5.4). It is essential that culture, health literacy, and linguistic literacy are considered within meetings.

Several steps are important to the success of care meetings. After introductions have been done, the goal(s) of the meeting can be stated. Then, using open-ended questions, the patient can be asked about their understanding of the medical condition and situation. This is followed by ascertaining the patient's worries and fears, how much information the patient wants to know, which individual(s) the patient wants to be informed about concerning clinical issues, and who will be involved in their care.[35,63,84,88] Additionally, it is important to determine patient and family understanding of the illness and their values, preferences, and beliefs, along with their informational needs for the decision-making patient who is hesitant to express emotional concerns and who may need prompting or an invitation to speak. The designated meeting leader then offers a summary of the planned care. The next part of the meeting addresses questions and issues that require clarification. After this discussion, the leader summarizes the issues and develops a plan of care in collaboration with the patient and family.[35,84,87] One of the most important, yet often neglected, tasks after the meeting is documentation. The names and titles of the people who attended, the issues discussed, and the decisions made should be recorded in the medical record.

One model, the PARTNER trial (Pairing Re-engineered ICU Teams with Nurse-Driven Emotional Support and Relationship-Building), was implemented as a family support intervention where nurses were trained in advanced communication skills to engage with patients and families in the ICU. PARTNER nurses met daily with families, and family meetings were arranged with the medical team within 48 hours of admission to the ICU for those patients who met the criteria.[89]

Scheduled Meetings and Nursing Presence

Nurses play an essential role in these meetings because they are often responsible for organizing the meeting. Before the meeting, the nurse may assess the patient's physical, emotional, and psychological concerns to be conveyed in a meeting. This information can assist the team in planning discussion points at the scheduled meeting. After the meeting, the nurse can follow up and reinforce the information communicated.

Nursing presence at any discussions—particularly when important information is conveyed—cannot be overemphasized. The team may need education regarding nursing's pivotal role in patient advocacy, particularly in supporting the patient after receiving serious news.[90] If a primary nurse is not able to participate in important discussions, a nursing colleague may participate to offer a nursing perspective. If this is not possible, it is essential that the team review the specifics of the conversation with the nurse—in particular, the news delivered, the phrasing used, and the patient's response. This allows the nurse to provide collaborative follow-up support. Sometimes the nurse may be reticent and wait to be invited rather than being proactive in participating and facilitating discussions. This reticence can cause the nurse to feel uninformed and undervalued, ultimately leading to ineffective care.

The nurse may facilitate the initial conversation by serving as a reference point for the patient and family in conveying important concerns or worries gleaned from previous interactions. Often this occurs at the beginning of the meeting and personalizes the discussions to the specific needs of the patient and family. In addition, the nurse may act as a translator between the medical team and the patient, facilitating information-sharing, interpreting information and medical jargon in language the patient understands, and ensuring that the members of the care team understand the patient's words and language. Early assessment and conversation about coping skills are paramount to the flow of the meeting (Box 5.5). If the patient/family agrees to

Box 5.5 Questions to Address Patients' and Families' Coping

How have you/your family coped with crises or difficult or hard situations in the past?
Have you/your family been through something like this before?
How did you/your family react/cope?
Can you identify/anticipate any potential areas of concern for you and your family?
Have you told your family what you would want in terms of life-prolonging treatments?
Did the patient ever tell you what they wanted for themselves in terms of life-prolonging treatments?
Is there anyone you need to see? Is there anyone you think the patient would like to see?
Who is supporting you now? Is there anyone you'd like us to call?
Who could you call if things became more serious, difficult, or hard? Who would you call if you needed emotional support?

Source: Revised from Reference 35.

the plan, the meeting can end with a synopsis of the meeting and the decisions made. The meeting may be derailed in the setting of ineffective coping. Ineffective coping in the face of a medical crisis may manifest as personal and misdirected anger, abandonment, despair, hyper-vigilant faith, and overbearing tendencies. If the misdirected anger appears to be derailing the care or family meeting where the focus is no longer on the goals and best interest of the patient, then termination and rescheduling of the meeting is strongly recommended. It may be necessary to set ground rules about appropriate behavior. After the completion of such a meeting, these family members may be offered resources and referrals to help with their own individual grief and coping.

Advance Care Planning

ACP is a comprehensive process of discussions to determine the patient's values, goals, fears, and concerns while also developing the core topics for patient education, including the right to high-quality pain control and symptom management. There are three discrete elements of ACP: designation of a healthcare durable power of attorney, completion of an advance directive, and out-of-hospital resuscitation orders. The National Consensus Project's *Clinical Practice Guidelines for Quality Palliative Care* describes how person-centered goals, preferences, and choices form the basis for the plan of care.[44] Nurses can perform ACP and use the information to create a plan of care and continue to advocate for the patient.[4,9,39] See Chapter 6, "Advance Care Planning," on the nurse's role in ACP.

Ongoing Discussions of Goals of Care

Case Study Continued: Goals of Care

Mr. Smith continued to require ventilatory support and antibiotics for several days. After 4 days, another meeting was arranged when Lee was working. The team described how Mr. Smith's condition was more tenuous, and he was now somnolent. A chest X-ray revealed worsening atypical pneumonia, a PCR test revealed Mr. Smith was now positive for coronavirus, and his laboratory blood tests revealed poor renal function trending toward acute-on-chronic renal failure. A vasopressor was started to stabilize his blood pressure.

Lee ensured optimal skin and oral hygiene for Mr. Smith. To create an atmosphere of calm, the lights were dimmed and the TV had low-volume religious music. Lee moved the monitor and IV machines to the head of the bed to allow the family to get close to their dad. Sondra arrived first, looking visibly distressed. Lee met her at the nurse's station, exchanged greetings, and walked her to her father's room. Sondra expressed gratitude that Lee was the nurse for the day and voiced, "At least, Dad will have comfort and trust your presence since he knows you." Sons Matthew and Jonah arrived shortly afterward.

Lee explained everything going on to them. Sondra asked, "What has happened to my dad; he was fine 36 hours ago." She struggled to see her father's decline. Matthew gently interjected, "Dad has been sick a long time, and he is tired." Lee allowed them to sit in silence for a bit and then asked, "What are you seeing when you look at your dad?" Within the silence, the tears flowed from all the children.

Eventually, Sondra spoke, "My dad went downhill so quickly this time, and it seems like several other things are going bad with him. How did we get here?" Because this was the first time her father had multiple consultants as part of his care team, she wanted to hear from all clinicians. She wanted someone to give her hope. Jonah replied, "We are so glad we got to have time with Dad and Mom. And we are grateful to be here at this time." Matthew said, "It is time to let him go on his own terms." After supporting the family in their decision, Lee allowed the family to have time alone with their father.

The patient's priorities and needs shift, resulting in a changing and evolving care plan. Many palliative care specialists have emphasized the importance of systematic meetings to discuss the patient's concerns. In particular, the early introduction of such conversations in the disease process promotes better outcomes.[63,86] These outcomes include more informed choices, better palliation of symptoms, and more opportunity for the resolution of important issues. It is within the nurse's practice in all settings to have these conversations, and there are new models evolving for nurses leading communication across the community.[91,92]

Nurses may be particularly helpful in advocating for patients when they are unable to speak for themselves. In these cases, the nurse may assist the surrogate decision maker to convey the patient's wishes by inquiring more about the patient's personal history. Asking the patient a question such as "Are there things that would be left undone if you were to die sooner rather than later?" stimulates thought and discussion about dying and important life-closure issues, such as healing broken relationships and completing financial transactions. However, a nurse may ask this in a different way, such as "Are there things you need to do in case things do not go as well as we hope?" Encouraging patients to hope for the best outcome while preparing for the possibility that treatment may not work—"hope for the best, prepare for the worst"—is helpful in guiding the patient. Again, the advocacy role facilitates the provision of all essential information the patient needs to make choices. This includes managing care at home and support structures for family caregivers. Box 5.6 offers

Box 5.6 Questions for Discussion about Ongoing Care

How do you spend your days?
What is an average day like for you?
If you were not ill, how would you like to spend your time?
How has your condition/disease interfered with your daily activities?
What practical problems/issues have occurred as a result of your illness?
Which symptoms bother you the most?
How are things with family and friends?
Have you been feeling worried, sad, or frightened about your illness?
Do you have a preference for where you spend your time, at home, in the hospital, or at health appointments?

Source: Revised from Reference 21.

questions for ongoing care. See Chapter 30, "Hope and Meaning in Illness," for ensuring hope and meaning for individuals with serious illness.

Serious News Discussions

In palliative care, serious news includes a poor disease diagnosis, recurrence, disease progression, lack of further curative treatments, lack of any treatments to stabilize disease, transition to comfort care, and a short prognosis. Serious news encompasses "any news that drastically and negatively alters the patient's view of their future."[28] Nurses working in inpatient care settings, especially critical care nurses, are particularly prone to serious news disclosures as they develop relationships with patients and families in a constantly changing environment.[93]

Nurses, particularly APRNs, along with their physician colleagues, communicate a wide range of serious illness news to patients. However, RNs may feel uncomfortable in meaningful conversations because they may perceive lack of permission, authority, or scope of practice within their organization.[9] They may also lack communication skills, communication education, or role modeling in effective communication.[4,9] RNs may inform patients about cancellations or delays in treatments, confirmation of a serious or life-threatening illness, decrease in QOL, and care-setting options. APRNs may provide diagnosis and prognosis.

Deciding who delivers the serious news may depend on multiple factors: the relationship of the patient with the team, the clinician the patient most trusts, and, sometimes, institutional culture or practice guidelines. Serious news discussions are emotionally charged events both for the patient and family and for the nurse and require continuous assessment of patient understanding, fears, and information preferences.[93,94] Coyle and Sculco beautifully describe the emotional setting of delivering serious news for the clinician and the patient:

> Is it possible for any news, transmitted by a [clinician] to a patient, to be "good news" in the face of advancing disease that is not responsive to chemotherapy? The [clinician] is in a position of having to give information that the patient does not want to hear, and yet the patient needs to have the information in order to make necessary life decisions. Does it matter how the information is given when medical information itself can remove hope for continued existence? In a way, both parties—the [clinician] and the patient—are engaged in a communication dance of vulnerability. The [clinician] is vulnerable because he/she must deliver the facts, whatever they may be, and the patient is vulnerable because he/she doesn't want to hear any more bad news.[95(p210)]

Many palliative care team members are part of this communication dance. Patients with advanced diseases generally want to have this information. Paradoxically, however, although patients may want information, clinicians may be reluctant to initiate such a discussion.[96] Physicians may avoid telling the patient too much because they want to avoid feelings of failure. While the principle of delivering serious news in the context of the patient's and family's understanding is essential, a large underlying factor is the relationship of the caregiver with the patient and family and their understanding of the condition and its trajectory.

Devastating news can come in many forms for patients and families, and nurses cannot expect to anticipate with accuracy what news will be considered difficult or challenging. When information is not as good as hoped, as interpreted by a patient and a family caregiver, a nurse's compassionate presence does not mean having the right answers or all the answers but rather just means "being there" for patients. Mindful presence in serious news disclosures can attend to the spiritual, religious, and existential aspects of care. Nurses are often charged with regularly exploring and assessing patient fears, beliefs, preferences, and desires. Simply providing therapeutic presence and talking about these concerns is noted as very meaningful to patients and families.[97]

Recommended steps for family meetings about serious news focus on the following: (1) ensuring privacy and adequate time, (2) assessing patients' understanding, (3) providing information about diagnosis and prognosis simply and honestly, (4) avoiding the use of euphemisms, (5) encouraging expression of feelings, (6) being empathetic, (7) giving a broad but realistic time frame regarding prognosis, and (8) arranging review or follow-up.[87] Other points are summarized in Box 5.7.

It is essential to provide accurate, hopeful information. When the patient asks whether they can partake in some activity that may or may not be in a realistic time frame, the nurse can respond, "I wish that were possible, but I am worried it won't happen." Or "I hope that you can do that, too, but if you can't, here is what we can do in the meantime." The issue of abandonment should be deliberately addressed. This can be achieved with such words as "I wish things were different. But no matter what, I will be there to support you in your decisions and promote your quality of life." This allays the fear that even though the patient can no longer tolerate treatment, clinicians will continue caring for them.

Prognosis

Another common and difficult question is the patient's response to such news with the question "How long do I have to live?" Responding to and acknowledging such a question normalizes the discussion around death and dying. The nurse may choose to answer in several ways, depending on their comfort in these discussions. One response is "Are you asking for a specific timeline?" Here, the nurse is trying to ascertain whether the patient is asking about dying or is thinking of a certain event that they wish to live to experience. Another response is "How long do you think you have to live?" This allows patients to voice concerns about time and offer their own impression of their remaining time. The patient may say "Not long, but I wanted to see how long you thought," thus comparing input

Box 5.7 Delivering Serious News

1. Prepare for the meeting:
   Determine with the patient whom they want present.
   Determine with the team which healthcare clinicians should be present.
2. Create a comfortable, quiet setting with seating for all participants and free of interruptions.
   Obtain interpreter as needed.
3. Clarify and clearly state your and the patient's goals for the meeting.
4. Determine what the patient and family know about the patient's condition and what they have been told.
5. Provide the foundation of a brief overview of the patient's course and condition for understanding of the entire group.
6. Give a warning of the news to come:
   "Unfortunately, I have some serious news to share with you." "I wish I had better news." "This isn't the information I expected."
7. Pause.
8. Deliver the serious news.
9. Sit quietly and allow the patient and family to absorb the information.
10. Wait for the patient to respond.
11. After being silent, check in with the patient such as by saying:
    "I have just told you some serious news. Do you feel comfortable sharing your thoughts about this?" This may help the patient verbalize concerns.[28]
12. Listen carefully and acknowledge the patient's and family's emotions, such as by reflecting on both the meaning and the effect of their responses. Give an opportunity for questions and comments.
13. Provide a summary and give description of follow-up.

Source: Revised from Reference 35.

from different members of the team. A third response may be along the lines of "Why are you asking that question now?," "What makes you ask that question now?," or "Why do you ask?" This invites the patient to share their fears and concerns about dying. The nurse may also reflect on serious information with "I imagine it is very frightening not knowing what will happen and when. Do you have particular fears and concerns?"

Finally, if the anticipated survival time is short or the nurse is uncomfortable, they may reply "What has the team told you?" In this case, the patient may state that the team has given a certain estimate of time, or the patient may be seeking validation of the prediction.

When it is appropriate to offer a timeline, it is helpful to give a range of time rather than exact times. Instead of the specific time of 2 weeks or 6 months, it is more helpful to say "weeks to months." This prevents the patient or family from making a calendar and ticking off the days until death. In those cases, if the patient surpasses the exact time, there is often anger about the countdown. However, when death is imminent, it is helpful to say "hours to days." It is also useful to explain what supports that timeline, such as significant changes, signs and symptoms of dying, or rapid disease progression. This allows the patient and family to prepare for their final time together.

Discussion of Life-Sustaining Treatments

Often when patients are critically ill and have advanced disease, the healthcare team seeks clarification on the use or continuation of life-sustaining measures. Life-sustaining measures may include vasopressors to help the heart pump more efficiently and effectively, dialysis for kidney failure, antibiotics for infections, and medically administered nutrition and hydration. "Code status" is commonly defined as the use, or limitation of use, of life-sustaining therapy in the event of clinical deterioration of respiratory function and/or cardiac arrest. Major life-sustaining measures within cardiopulmonary resuscitation (CPR) include invasive ventilator support consisting of nasotracheal or endotracheal intubation, noninvasive ventilator support (continuous positive airway pressure, bilevel positive airway pressure), and defibrillation (cardiac electroshock). The use, continuation, and discontinuation of life-sustaining measures are all necessary aspects to these discussions. The significant role of nurses in providing information and family guidance during challenging decision-making about life-sustaining measures cannot be overemphasized. Specifically, they may act as interpreters in these meetings. Medical vernacular language such as "full code" or "no code" and "Do you want everything done?" can be ambiguous at best. These terms simply indicate whether or not to perform a procedure, offering little insight into the patient's goals of care. By educating the patient about the actual intervention and likely outcome, a nurse may be able to reassure the patient.[98]

According to the position statement *Nursing Care and Do Not Resuscitate (DNR) Decisions*, "Nurses advocate for and play an active role in initiating discussions about resuscitation with patients, families, and members of the health care team."[99] The team can offer the patient and family a plan that focuses on aggressive pain and symptom management, psychological support, and better QOL. They can then ask for agreement from the patient and family, thereby allowing the patient and family to assent to a plan. "Assent" means the family agrees to the plan without having to take on the burden of choosing a specific option. "Consent" means the family is offered a range of options, and they choose which option. By assenting, the burden of the decision is removed from the family and placed on the care team. For many families, this feels like less of a burden because the team makes the difficult decision. It may still be the same plan, but the team has allowed the patient and family to "unshoulder" the burden or weight of the decision.

Nurses are often ideally positioned to contribute to conversations about serious illness care and decisions, including maintaining a focus on a patient's preferences and establishing mechanisms to respect the patient's autonomy.[100] There are often circumstances when the patient and family convey their overwhelming sense of pressure or responsibility about the decisions they are being asked to make. When this occurs, often the responsibility of making such a decision is too great for patients and families. They may feel that by making a choice to refuse resuscitation, they are "pulling the plug." In these situations, nurses can take an active role in creating an interprofessional care plan as described by ANA's position statement *Nurses' Roles and Responsibilities in Providing Care and Support at the End of Life*: "Nurses are obligated to provide comprehensive and compassionate end-of-life care ... taking measure within their scope of practice ... to optimize patients' comfort and families' understanding and adaptation."[100] See Chapter 55, "Withdrawal or Cessation of Life-Sustaining Therapies."

This discussion is similar to other care or family meetings. The recommended steps include (1) establishing an appropriate setting; (2) asking the patient and family what they understand of the patient's condition; (3) finding out what the patient expects for the future; (4) discussing resuscitation within the context of the patient's condition; (5) eliciting the patient's understanding of the present condition and thoughts of the future, including the context in which resuscitation would be considered; (6) responding to concerns and emotions; and (7) developing a plan. To dispel concerns of abandonment, it is particularly important to reassure the patient, family, and surrogate that even though CPR will not be performed, all beneficial care will be actively provided. See Chapter 55, "Withdrawal or Cessation of Life-Sustaining Therapies," for more discussion of discontinuation of life-sustaining therapies and the role of the nurse.

Conversations about Medically Administered Hydration and Nutrition

Numerous cultures place great social and cultural importance on drinking and eating. When patients are not able to take food or fluid by mouth, medically administered hydration and nutrition may be provided through the gastrointestinal tract using a nasogastric or gastric tube or may be administered intravenously. This treatment has benefits—prolonging life, treating delirium, giving energy—as well as burdens—continued aspiration pneumonia, infection at the insertion site, edema, and diarrhea.[101] Many people believe that not eating and drinking causes great physical suffering. Medically administered hydration and nutrition may alleviate any guilt felt by patients and family caregivers arising out of the feeling that they had not "tried everything." Also, for some cultures, intravenous fluids and nutrition may be necessary to prevent any sense of hastening death. Therefore, it is necessary to discuss the potential benefits and burdens of both instituting and withholding medically administered hydration and nutrition.[101] The rationales for and against these procedures are discussed in Chapter 32, "Ethical Considerations in Palliative Care."

Conversations about the Transition to Palliative Care or Hospice

The transition in care away from curative-directed therapies is often an emotional time for patients, families, and clinicians alike. Patients may feel a sense of sadness, anger, denial, and loss of control to the disease. Families may finally come to terms with the reality of the situation or the serious nature of the illness. Physicians may feel a sense of failure for not curing the disease and frustration with the lack of any further medical options. Nurses may feel grief from the impending termination of the patient and family relationship. The focus of care shifts from curing the disease—from physical cure to emotional and psychological healing.

The nurse has a central role to empower the patient at this time. This is accomplished by a continued dialogue about hopes, preferences, and QOL. Each situation is individual and cannot be determined by an algorithm or recipe approach; personalizing the experience promotes emotional healing. Guidelines for initiating conversations during the last phase of life include (1) focusing on the patient's unique illness experience, (2) discussing issues of closure, (3) promoting discussions about pain and symptom management at the end of life, (4) addressing and planning for the preferred site of death and who will provide care for them, (5) facilitating home health and hospice arrangements, and (6) promoting a respectful death. Box 5.8 offers questions to open exploration of changing goals.

Nurses offer information to patients and families about resources and transitions of care. This includes hospice, home health, and other community-based healthcare resources, when such resources are consistent with the patient's and family's values, beliefs, preferences, and goals of care. A direct nursing approach is helpful, stating "We are no longer able to cure or control your disease. We would like to optimize your quality of life, manage pain and symptoms to avoid suffering, and promote optimal functioning. There are expert nurses who care for patients with advanced illnesses, helping you avoid the hospital. We will work with them to care for you at home." This allows the patient and family to understand that they will continue to be cared for and not feel abandoned. Such discussions lend themselves to completing legal and financial business. This allows for life closure in preparation for death and legacy work. Usually, this also includes attending to psychological–emotional–spiritual work. For the family, such discussions promote preparation and planning for a home death and strategies for sustainability in caregiving.

The nurse is then responsible for the coordination and communication of the plan. The nurse promotes continuity of care and continued support in the home. The hospice, palliative, or home care nurse must educate the patient and family about necessary caregiving skills concerning medications, equipment, and personal care.

Box 5.8 Questions for Changing Goals of Care

What do you understand about your disease and current condition?
What do you understand about further treatment?
What are some of the concerns you have at this time?
What is most important to you now and as you think about the future?
What, if anything, are you worried about or afraid of?
Given the severity of your illness, what is most important for you to achieve?
What are your most important goals if your health worsens or your disease progresses?
Have you given any thought to what kinds of treatment you would want (and not want) if you become unable to speak for yourself in the future?
We want to focus on maximal comfort and optimal functioning with as much support as possible. Is that okay?
How is your family handling your illness and its change?
How is your family coping with your changing condition?
Are there topics you need help in discussing with them?
Would it be helpful to have us talk to them with you about changes in goals?

Source: Revised from Reference 35.

Communication at Transition to Death

Case Study Continued: Care at End of Life

Sondra, Matthew, and Jonah stayed with their father a bit in quiet reminiscence. Then they decided to quickly arrange an extended family video conference within Mr. Smith's room to allow for the larger family to join together to share stories, hymns, and prayers. They asked for a visit from the chaplain to have a blessing. They asked for Lee to provide support.

Within the hour, a video call was held with family close by and far and those old and young. People shared pictures, stories, songs, and favorite scripture. After an hour, everyone had participated, and a final prayer was said. Mr. Smith appeared comfortable and peaceful. Sondra, Matthew, and Jonah expressed their gratitude to all their extended family for joining them and returned to their vigil. Mr. Smith died within a few hours. Lee was privileged to provide final care to Mr. Smith's body and supported the children to wash Mr. Smith's face, hands, and feet. Sondra, Matthew, and Jonah left the floor emotionally exhausted but grateful for the respectful death of their father. The team debriefed Mr. Smith's death at rounds. They sent a bereavement card to Sondra, Matthew, and Jonah; and the chaplaincy department provided bereavement follow-up.

When cure is no longer possible, there is the potential instead for physical comfort and psychological healing. Simple presence, listening, and attending to the basic humanity of the dying patient may be one of the nurse's most powerful contributions. Nurses help reduce anxiety and help prepare patients and families just by describing the dying process. As appropriate, the explanation includes the actual physiological and biological process of dying in simple language. The alleviation of pain and symptoms is based on a patient's previously stated preferences regarding a desired level of alertness. This may include discussion about the withdrawal of ineffective and/or burdensome medical treatments, including preferences concerning medically administered hydration and nutrition.

Often, a patient considers the meaning of their life or performs a life review. This facilitates healing in recognition of personal purpose and meaning, resolution of past conflicts, attaining forgiveness and reconciliation, and achievement of personal integration and inner peace. Additional strategies to help relieve emotional and spiritual suffering include guided imagery, music, reading, and art that focuses on healing.[102] All this may include the collaboration of social workers, volunteers, music and art therapists, and chaplain colleagues, as well as child life specialists for children.

The nurse's therapeutic presence with the patient in their state of vulnerability and decline can be profound. Here, the nurse consciously and nonjudgmentally listens and bears witness to the patient, encouraging any expression of emotion, doubts, or regrets. The simple acts of visitation, presence, and attention can be potent healing affirmations—a sacramental gesture received by the dying person who may be feeling helpless, diminished, and fearful that they have little to offer others. The willingness to demonstrate concern to the patient far outweighs any technique or expertise in the art of listening.

During the dying process, the nurse guides care while promoting healthy bereavement within the family. One fundamental nursing task is role modeling for families. Specifically, the nurse demonstrates the art of being present to the dying person. Simply encouraging the family to engage in loving, physical contact, such as holding hands, embracing, or lying next to the patient can be healing. It may help the patient in their transition and may help the survivors in their anticipatory grief. For families who want to be present at the time of death, explaining that patients often wait until they are alone to die may prevent the family from feeling a sense of guilt if they are not present at the time of death. Allowing the family to be with the patient after death may help the surviving family members grieve the loss of their loved one.

After death, the nurse offers continued presence, support, and information. The nurse informs the family of the process of certifying death and may assist the family in informing others about the death. Awareness of anticipatory grief and bereavement guides care at this time. Bereaved families are often in most need of having someone to listen to them. Such activities, including telling the story of the loved one's illness, with details of the days and weeks around the death of their loved one, and sharing memories of the loved one, are therapeutic. The nurse may offer information for burial or funeral services as well as grief services. When the family is ready to leave their loved one, the nurse assures respect for the body and explains the process of postmortem care. The nurse then facilitates communication of the death to the team.

Team Communication and Collaboration

Collaboration within an interprofessional team is a vital force in working with patients with serious illnesses. Hanson and Carter describe collaboration as a "dynamic interpersonal process in which two or more individuals make a commitment to each other to interact authentically and constructively to solve problems and to learn from one another to accomplish identified goals, purposes, or outcomes. The individuals recognize and articulate the shared values that make this commitment possible."[103(p300)] Good communication ensures better collaboration, ensures comprehensive care, and assures safety and quality.[104] Collaboration enables the well-being and sustainability of the team.

However, teams are social systems and have their own dynamics, just as a family does. In effect, the team can be a "work family." With good leadership, role delineation, and flexibility, interprofessional teams have the capacity to work well, creating a synergy that promotes positive outcomes.[104] If working effectively, the team's identity as a palliative care team supersedes each individual member's discipline. There are necessary qualities to promote effective collaborative teams. First, the participation of all members is essential; the degree of involvement may depend on the issues of the patient and family. Each member's role should be well defined and respected. Good communication and negotiation are necessary to delineate roles. Second, each team member should have a voice in team processes. Third, the team's mission and goals should be periodically reviewed to assure that all members are working on the same premise. Team members share information and work both independently and together to develop goals. Each team member should be committed to quality care. Fourth, each team member should understand their role in patient care and maintain the process of the group. Leadership is shared among team members depending on the task at hand. This means that there must be respect for different styles, trust in clinical competence, and compassion for each other.[102, 105, 106] Periodic reviews of these guidelines will ensure the team's effectiveness and efficiency.

Effective teams promote collaboration through good team equity, communication, organization, coordination, and competency. This teamwork will be characterized by different environmental and organizational cultures, which dictate the nature of the teamwork as collaborative, deferential, or hierarchical. It is also variable depending on a nurse's role and level of practice. Part of teamwork is the development of working relationships and understanding differing communication styles. This necessitates the following[107]:

1. Recognition of individual and interprofessional team member contributions.

2. Respect for and acknowledgment of the competence and expertise of team members.
3. Understanding of the value of interprofessional work, equitable opportunities for leadership, professional development, and academic work.
4. Clear definition of roles, responsibilities, and tasks.
5. Well-defined reporting structures for both work functions and practice.
6. Scheduled communication among team members and meeting times.
7. Skilled leadership to manage different levels of nursing experience: novices, intermediate practitioners, and experts.
8. Evaluation processes for quality of care and team effectiveness.
9. Psychological and spiritual support for team.
10. Ethical and legal resources for the team.
11. Respect for patients as individuals.

There is a negative process to teamwork as well. Barriers to effective teamwork include lack of training, hierarchical team structures, organizational rules, value based on reimbursement, practice based on authority, and lack of psychological safety or safe spaces to discuss different perspectives.[108,109] Ineffective leadership results in a lack of a shared mission and vision. Moreover, team attitude can have an effect on care. There has been an emerging arrogance among palliative care team members that "they know best, are the most caring, effective, and ethical." This can cause negative feelings among other healthcare colleagues, who may feel they are just as caring and committed to patient care.

Poor communication results in poor care, negative outcomes, conflicts, and, ultimately, team demoralization.[104,110] If roles and responsibilities have not been clearly delineated, nurses may feel restrained to broach and discuss certain topics with patients and families, defaulting to the physician, who may prefer that these discussions occur at the nursing level. Consequently, a lack of clear roles between nurse and physician can leave patients and families with no communication about their illness, treatment, or prognosis. Ongoing discussions between physician and nurse occur more as a task-focused discussion about patient assessment and response to treatment.[111] Nurses also play an important role in mediating communication between physician and patient and family.[110,112]

Much has been written about how conflict among team members results in poor practices. Eight problematic team behaviors are (1) overwhelming the patient,[112] (2) making the patient part of the team,[103] (3) squelching the voice of individual team members, (4) lack of accountability, (5) team process trumping client outcome, (6) orthodoxy and groupthink,[113,114,115] (7) overemphasis on health and safety goals, and (8) squandering of resources. All of these issues can occur at various times within the palliative care team and necessitate good communication and conflict resolution. Examples of these problems include the following:

1. *Overwhelming the patient and family*[113]: This occurs in several ways in terms of timing, information, and presence. One is overwhelming the patient with too much information. An example is when the patient and family have just heard serious news. Then the palliative care or hospice team enters to "fix" everything before the patient and family have had time to absorb and integrate the information. Another overwhelming experience is a high ratio of healthcare professionals in family meetings. The patient or family may feel outnumbered and disempowered to raise individual issues or concerns.
2. *Making the patient part of the team*[102]: Patients are told that they are part of the decision-making team and are asked for input. The boundaries about what decisions they can or cannot make are ambiguous, especially if they disagree. Moreover, as the patient declines, they may not really be able to participate in decision-making.
3. *Squelching the voice of individual team members*: The team may explicitly express that everyone's input is equal when, implicitly, that is not the case. Nonphysician voices may be dismissed, minimized, marginalized, or overturned by physicians when there is disagreement. Another example occurs when, in trying to advocate for a certain unpopular perspective, a team member's opinion may be discounted as "not really understanding the situation," being "no longer objective," or being "too close to the situation."
4. *Lack of accountability*: This is often a challenge when there are too many healthcare consultants working with the primary team. Sometimes, with everyone on the palliative care team working on the same issues, no one takes responsibility for the overall care of the patient. In addition, there may be cases where a primary team is detached but asks for input from the palliative care team, but nothing is implemented. Or there may be too many consultants, and the patient receives many mixed opinions with no clear advocate.
5. *Team process having higher value than client outcome*: Healthcare professionals often have certain ideas or feelings about what is right or wrong and how things are done. The challenge is to allow an open process to occur and not to limit it to one particular pathway simply because that is the way it is always done. Patients and families are unique in their needs and do not always follow algorithms.
6. *Orthodoxy and groupthink*: A group can become insular and not incorporate new ideas.[113,114] The team becomes unable to assess itself, and obvious problems are overlooked. In advanced illness situations, this often happens in relation to the dying process. A nurse may understand that the patient is dying, but other health professionals look for a specific symptom and treat it. The team may think the nurse is "giving up," rather than admit the patient is dying.
7. *Overemphasis on health and safety goals*: This occurs when the care plan itself takes precedence over the patient's needs or choices. This is often seen in the discharge process when the healthcare team disagrees with the patient's lifestyle choices. So, the team resorts to making a plan based on their "safety agenda" rather than a patient's choice.
8. *Squandering of resources*: The needs of patients are missed, especially in the dying phase, resulting in implementation of high-cost interventions with low impact on the patient's overall care.

The Nurse and The Physician

Among the team, nurses work the most closely with physicians, either implementing medical orders or following care plans. However, nurses and physicians differ in their communication styles. Nurses tend to be more narrative or qualitative and to emphasize more process and reflection. Physicians tend to be more quantitative and want facts and numbers. Neither style is better than the other; rather, both styles are essential in patient- and family-centered holistic care. Nurses become frustrated with physician communication when physicians seem inattentive or are unwilling to discuss goals of care. On the other hand, physicians report frustration when nurses share disorganized information, include extraneous or irrelevant information, or delay in getting to the point.[116]

The goal of a communication interaction between the nurse and the physician dictates whether reflection or facts are needed. If the contact is about information-sharing, the nurse may need to present details, albeit short and brief. If a treatment change is warranted, the nurse provides supporting evidence. For example, if calling about pain and symptoms, the nurse should know the medications the patient is taking, when they were last taken, the patient's pain scores, and should offer a suggested plan. Or if calling about a patient's change in code status or goals of care, it is important that the nurse offer the rich narrative of the context of the conversation so that the physician may have an effective follow-up conversation.

Quality communication between physician and nurse includes delineating communication roles, reviewing topics to be discussed with the patient and family and by whom, fostering an active communicative role for nurses rather than blindly following physicians' requests, and limiting their own communication with others.[103] When nurses receive authorization or permission from physicians to communicate with patients and families about designated topics or to participate in delivering serious news, it removes a barrier to nurse communication, which promotes better patient outcomes and patient safety.[104]

Conflict Resolution

Conflict is a situation in which two or more people or parties disagree. This can occur due to different perspectives of care, different patient goals, different values, different ethics, or different role expectations. *Task communication* for teams involves gathering information from each other about clinical care of the patient and family, while *relational team communication* emerges from the general support that team members share regarding workplace stress, coping, and burnout.

Nurses on the front line deal with conflict all the time. This may occur between a patient and a nurse, between a nurse and a doctor, between an APRN and an RN, or between two healthcare teams. Conflict is inevitable and healthy for palliative teams, secondary to different perspectives, different experiences, length of time in palliative care, and the sense of urgency to alleviate symptoms. If managed well, it helps people look at different perspectives and can allow for creativity and positive movement. If dismissed or ignored, it can breed demoralization and negativity.

Nurses deal with conflict differently depending on their level of practice, practice site, and experience. Often, nurses avoid conflict if they constantly have difficulty dealing with a team member who will not talk about disagreements. However, in palliative care, the goal should be collaboration in which all problems are discussed and mutual solutions are reached.

Several methods are available to resolve conflict: negotiation, accommodation, and collaboration. What differentiates these approaches are the perceived power differences. Conflict resolution occurs through a process (see Box 5.9). This involves looking at the facts of a conflict, the feelings of a conflict, and the identity in the conflict.[117] First, the nurse identifies the source of the conflict, reviewing the facts of what happened and what the impact was. Second, the nurse reflects on the emotional aspect of the conflict—these are the feelings. Then, the nurse addresses the goal of conflict resolution in terms of what they hope to accomplish as it relates to the patient and/or family. Sometimes, this may require looking at the role each clinician has at stake and then thinking about what is best for the patient.

There are several steps in meeting with a team member about a conflict. Be curious about your colleague's perspective by learning

Box 5.9 Effective Conflict Negotiation

1. Reflection of the conflict

A. Identify the conflict—the facts

Review the conflict with the other person:
What happened? This is looking at objective data.
What emotions contributed to conflict? This is looking at subjective data.

Consider:
What impact has the situation had on you?
How did you contribute to the problem?

B. Identify the goal of conflict resolution

Clarify:
What do you hope to accomplish by resolving the conflict? This is your motivation.
What is the best way to address the conflict or broader issue around the conflict?
What is at stake for you?

2. Negotiation of the conflict

A. Address the conflict with the other person.

Consider:
When and what is the best way to raise the conflict or broader issue around the conflict?
What is the best way to achieve the purpose of a resolution?

B. Identify each individual's purpose to conflict resolution—the feelings

Review:
Where do you and the other person share purposes?
Where do you and the other person's interests differ?

C. Exploration of the conflict

Discuss:
What is the other person's perspective? Listen to the other individual and explore the story.
What are the other person's feelings? Acknowledge feelings behind story and paraphrase them.
Does the other person understand or want to understand your perspective? This is emotional intelligence.
Ask other individual to "listen to you as you share your version of the events and your intentions."

D. Problem-solve, with patient's best interest as goal

Invent options to meet each side's most important concerns and interests.
Decide tack of resolution: avoidance, collaborate, compromise.
Use objective criteria or palliative care standards (National Consensus Project's *Clinical Practice Guidelines*) for what should happen.
Determine approach for future communication.

Source: Revised from Reference 35.

their story. In doing so, the two parties share their common purposes and differing interests. Express your views, including statements of feelings, and take the time to listen. This leads to exploration of the conflict and letting each party tell their perspective while acknowledging feelings and each party's version of the events. Among the hardest things to learn to say are "I am sorry," "I was wrong," and "You could be right." It is not necessary for the nurse to feel pressured to agree instantly. Rather, it is important to discuss the range of the issues. Problem-solve together, with the common goal being the patient's well-being, and decide on a tack of resolution.

Conclusion

Communication in palliative nursing is the essential tool by which nurses deliver care. Effective communication sets the foundation on which the care plan is established and guides the care. Patient- and family-centered care necessitates effective nurse communication to impart communication, gather information, and provide a therapeutic presence. Nurses have a direct role in conversations regarding serious illness ranging from information-sharing about diagnosis and treatment, counseling about serious illness care choices, determining values and preferences, supporting patients and families in conversations about serious news, and facilitating transitions to palliative and hospice care. The art of nursing communication is based on the use of physical presence, listening, silence, therapeutic presence, and emotional intelligence. The science of nursing communication involves skills in verbal and nonverbal communication and the application of communication strategies to promote effective, quality care. For more effective care, communication is essential in interprofessional team collaboration and conflict. To be effective and confident, nurses need education and to practice communication skills in situations specific to patients with serious illnesses.[6,118,119] Moreover, these should be individualized to the scope and language of nurses to promote a better patient experience and better patient outcomes.[3]

REFERENCES

1. Dahlin C. Communication in palliative nursing. In: Wittenberg E, Ferrell B, Goldsmith J, et al., eds. *Textbook of Palliative Communication*. Oxford University Press; 2016:54–62.
2. Izumi S. Advance care planning: the nurses' role. *Am J Nurs.* 2017;117(6):56–61. https://doi.org/10.1097/01.NAJ.0000520255.65083.35.
3. Bennett F, O'Conner-Von S. Communication interventions to improve goal-concordant care of seriously ill patients: an integrative review. *J Hosp Palliat Nursing.* 2020;22(1):40–48. https://doi.org/10.1097/NJH.0000000000000606.
4. Head BA, Song MK, Wiencek C, Nevidjon B, Fraser D, Mazanec P. Palliative nursing summit: nurses leading change and transforming care: the nurse's role in communication and advance care planning. *J Hosp Palliat Nurs.* 2018;20(1):23–29. https://doi.org/10.1097/NJH.0000000000000406.
5. Walker A. Nursing Ranked as the Most Trusted Profession for 23nd year in a Row. Nurse.org. News. January 14, 2025. Accessed January 17, 2025. https://nurse.org/articles/nursing-ranked-most-honest-profession.
6. Sekse R, Hunskår, I, Ellingsen, S. The nurse's role in palliative care: A qualitative meta-synthesis. *J Clin Nurs.* 2018;27(1–2):e21–e38. https://doi.org/10.1111/jocn.13912.
7. American Nurses Association. *Nursing: Scope and Standards of Practice*. 4th ed. American Nurses Association; 2021.
8. American Nurses Association. *Code of Ethics for Nurses with Interpretive Statements*. American Nurses Association; 2015.
9. Hagan TL, Xu J, Lopez RP, Bressler T. Nursing's role in leading palliative care: A call to action. *Nurse Educ Today.* 2018;61:216–219.
10. Ali M. Communication skills 1: benefits of effective communication for patients. *Nurs Times.* 2017;113(12):18–19.
11. Dahlin C. Communication in palliative care: an essential competency for nurses. In: Ferrell BR, Coyle N, eds. *Oxford Textbook of Palliative Nursing*. 3rd ed. Oxford University Press; 2010:107–133.
12. Clayton MF, Hulett J, Kaur K, Reblin M, Wilson A, Ellington L. Nursing support of home hospice caregivers on the day of patient death. *Oncol Nurs Forum.* 2017;44(4):457–464. https://doi.org/10.1188/17.ONF.457-464.
13. Chochinov HM, McClement S, Hack T, Thompson G, Dufault B, Harlos M. Eliciting personhood within clinical practice: effects on patients, families, and health care providers. *J Pain Symptom Manage.* 2015;49(2):974–980.e972.
14. Kaiafas KN. Emotional intelligence and role-modeling nursing's soft skills. *J Christ Nurs.* 2021;38(4):240–243.
15. du Pré A, Foster E. Transactional communication. In: Wittenberg E, Ferrell B, Goldsmith J, et al., eds. *Textbook of Palliative Care Communication*. Oxford University Press; 2016:14–21.
16. Wanko Keutchafo EL, Kerr J, Jarvis MA. Evidence of nonverbal communication between nurses and older adults: a scoping review. *BMC Nurs.* 2020;19:53.
17. White K, Coyne P, Lee J. Nurses' perceptions of educational gaps in delivering end-of-life care. *Oncol Nurs Forum.* 2011;38(6):711–717.
18. White KR, Roczen ML, Coyne PJ, Wiencek C. Acute and critical care nurses' perceptions of palliative care competencies: a pilot study. *J Contin Educ Nurs.* 2014;45(6):265–277.
19. Peereboom K, Coyle N. Facilitating goals-of-care discussions for patients with life-limiting disease—communication strategies for nurses. *J Hosp Palliat Nurs.* 2012;14(4):251–258.
20. Northfield S, Nabauer M. The caregiving journey for family members of relatives with cancer: how do they cope? *Clin J Oncol Nurs.* 2010;14(5):567–577.
21. Moir C, Roberts R, Perry J, Tivis L. Communicating with patients and their families about palliative and end of life: comfort and educational needs of staff RNs. *Int J Palliat Nurs.* 2015;21(3):109–112.
22. Hendricks-Ferguson V, Sawin KJ, Montgomery K, et al. Novice nurses' experiences with palliative and end-of-life communication. *J Pediat Oncol Nurs.* 2015;32(4):240–252.
23. Roy C. Key issues in nursing theory: developments, challenges, and future directions. *Nurs Res.* 2018;67(2):81–92.
24. Regan S, Kanter E. Learning the patient's story. *Semin Oncol Nurs.* 2017;33(5):467–474.
25. Schellinger SE, Anderson EW, Frazer MS, Cain CL. Patient self-defined goals: essentials of person-centered care for serious illness. *Am J Hosp Palliat Care.* 2018;35(1):159–165.
26. Malloy P, Virani R, Kelly K, Munevar C. Beyond bad news: communication skills of nurses in palliative care. *J Hosp Palliat Nursing.* 2010;12(3):166–174.
27. Ferrell BR, Coyle N. *The Nature of Suffering and the Goals of Nursing*. Oxford University Press; 2008.
28. Buckman R. *Practical Plans for Difficult Conversations in Medicine*. Johns Hopkins University Press; 2010.

29. Williams B, Lewis D, Burgio KL, Goode P. "Wrapped in their arms"—next-of-kin's perceptions of how hospital nursing staff support family presence before, during, and after the death of a loved one. *J Hosp Palliat Nurs*. 2012;14(8):541–550.
30. Prince-Paul M, Kelley C. Mindful communication: being present. *Semin Oncol Nurs*. 2017;33(5):475–482.
31. Pollak KI, Childers JW, Arnold RM. Applying motivational interviewing techniques to palliative care communication. *J Palliat Med*. 2011;14(5):587–592.
32. Raghubir AE. Emotional intelligence in professional nursing practice: a concept review using Rodgers's evolutionary analysis approach *Int J Nurs Sci*. 2018;5(2):126–130. Published correction appears in *Int J Nurs Sci*. 2020;8(1):4.
33. Huang SC, Morgan A, Peck V, Khoury L. Improving communications with patients and families in geriatric care. The how, when, and what. *J Patient Exp*. 2021;8:8:23743735211034047.
34. Dahlin C, Coyne P. End of life: reflecting on things that matter. *Semin Oncol Nurs*. 2017;33(5):483–488.
35. Dahlin C, Wittenberg-Lyles E. Communication in palliative care: an essential competency for nurses. In: Ferrell B, Paice J, eds. *Oxford Textbook of Palliative Nursing*. 5th ed. Oxford University Press; 2019:55–78.
36. Delgado-Guay MO, De La Cruz MG, Epner DE. "I don't want to burden my family": handling communication challenges in geriatric oncology. *Ann Oncol*. 2013;24(suppl 7):vii30–35.
37. Johnsson A, Wagman P, Boman Å, Pennbrant S. What are they talking about? Content of the communication exchanges between nurses, patients and relatives in a department of medicine for older people—an ethnographic study. *J Clin Nurs*. 2018;27(7–8):e1651–e1659.
38. Lynch M, Dahlin C, Hultman T, Coakley E. Palliative care nursing—defining the discipline? *J Hosp Palliat Nurs*. 2011;13(2):106–111.
39. American Nurses Association, Hospice and Palliative Nurses Association. *A Call for Action—Nurses Lead and Transform Palliative Care*. American Nurses Association; 2017.
40. Martins C, Basto M. Relieving the suffering of end of life patients: a grounded theory study. *J Hosp Palliat Nurs*. 2011;13(3):161–171.
41. Carlson EB, Spain DA, Muhtadie L, McDade-Montez L, Macia KS. Care and caring in the intensive care unit: family members' distress and perceptions about staff skills, communication, and emotional support. *J Crit Care*. 2015;30(3):557–561.
42. Nejati B, Lin CC, Aaronson NK, et al. Determinants of satisfactory patient communication and shared decision making in patients with multiple myeloma. *Psychooncology*. 2019;28(7):1490–1497.
43. Jóhannesdóttir S, Hjörleifsdóttir E. Communication is more than just a conversation: family members' satisfaction with end-of-life care. *Int J Palliat Nurs*. 2018;24(10):483–491.
44. National Consensus Project for Quality Palliative Care. *Clinical Practice Guidelines for Quality Palliative Care*. 4th ed. National Coalition for Hospice and Palliative Care; 2018.
45. Perrin K. Communicating with seriously ill and dying patients, their families, and their health practitioners. In: Matzo M, Witt Sherman D, eds. *Palliative Care Nursing—Quality Care at the End of Life*. 4th ed. Springer Publishing Company; 2015:169–188.
46. Donnelly S, Prizeman G, Coimín DÓ, Korn B, Hynes G. Voices that matter: end-of-life care in two acute hospitals from the perspective of bereaved relatives. *BMC Palliat Care*. 2018;17(1):117.
47. Freidemann MI, Buckwalter KC. Family caregiver role and burden related to gender and family relationships. *J Fam Nurs*. 2014;20(3):313–336.
48. Dahlin C, DePace N, Ford J, Maani-Fogelman P, Chow K. Promoting health equity: palliative nurses on the frontlines. *J Hosp Palliat Nurs*. 2022;24(4):218–224.
49. Wittenberg E, Ferrell B, Kanter E, Buller H. Nurse communication challenges with health literacy assessment. *Clin J Oncol Nurs*. 2018;22(1):53–61.
50. Norouzinia R, Aghabarari M, Shiri M, Karimi M, Samami E. Communication barriers perceived by nurses and patients. *Glob J Health Sci*. 2015;8(6):65–74.
51. Wittenberg E, Kravits K, Goldsmith J, Ferrell B, Fujinami B. Validation of a model of family caregiver communication types and related caregiver outcome. *Palliat Support Care*. 2016;15(1):3–11.
52. Wittenberg E, Ferrell B, Koczywas M, Del Ferraro C. Communication coaching: a case study of family caregiver burden. *Clin J Oncol Nurs*. 2017;21(2):219–225.
53. Banerjee S, Manna R, Coyle N, et al. Oncology nurses' communication challenges with patients and families: a qualitative study. *Nurse Educ Pract*. 2016;16(1):193–201.
54. Wittenberg-Lyles E, Goldsmith J, Platt CS. Palliative care communication. *Semin Oncol Nurs*. 2014;30(4):280–286.
55. McCourt R, Power JJ, Glackin M. General nurses' experiences of end-of-life care in the acute hospital setting: a literature review. *Int J Palliat Nurs*. 2013;19(10):510–516.
56. You JJ, Downar J, Fowler RA, et al. Barriers to goals of care discussions with seriously ill hospitalized patients and their families: a multicenter survey of clinicians. *JAMA Intern Med*. 2015;175(4):549–556.
57. Kwame A, Petrucka P. A literature-based study of patient-centered care and communication in nurse–patient interactions: barriers, facilitators, and the way forward. *BMC Nurs*. 2021;20(1):158.
58. Peters L, Cant R, Payne S. How death anxiety impacts nurses' caring for patients at the end of life: a review of literature. *Open Nurs J*. 2013;7:14–21.
59. Travers A, Taylor V. What are the barriers to initiating end-of-life conversations with patients in the last year of life? *Int J Palliat Nurs*. 2016;22(9):454–462.
60. Kalowes P. Improving end-of-life care prognostic discussions: role of advanced practice nurses. *AACN Adv Crit Care*. 2015;26(2):151–166.
61. Godshall M. Coping with moral distress during COVID-19. *Nursing*. 2021;51(2):55–58.
62. Altaker KW, Howie-Esquivel J, Cataldo JK. Relationships among palliative care, ethical climate, empowerment, and moral distress in intensive care unit nurses. *Am J Crit Care*. 2018;27(4):295–302.
63. Quill TE. Initiating end-of-life discussions with seriously ill patients: addressing the "elephant in the room." *JAMA*. 2000;284(19):2502–2507.
64. Quill TE, Arnold RM, Platt F. "I wish things were different": expressing wishes in response to loss, futility, and unrealistic hopes. *Ann Intern Med*. 2001;135(7):551–555.
65. Kyle K, Dahlin C. The palliative APRN in telehealth. In: Dahlin C, Coyne P, eds. *Advanced Practice Palliative Nursing*. 2nd ed. Oxford University Press; 2023:208–215.
66. Steindal SA, Nes AAG, Godskesen TE, et al. Patients' experiences of telehealth in palliative home care: scoping review. *J Med Internet Res*. 2020;22(5):e16218.
67. Piscitello GM, Fukushima CM, Saulitis AK, et al. Family meetings in the intensive care unit during the coronavirus disease 2019 pandemic. *Am J Hosp Palliat Care*. 2021;38(3):305–312.
68. Asare M, Flannery M, Kamen C. Social determinants of health: a framework for studying cancer health disparities and minority participation in research. *Oncol Nurs Forum*. 2017;44(1):20–23.

69. Office of Disease Prevention and Health Promotion. Health Literacy in Healthy People 2030. 2023. Accessed January 17, 2025. https://health.gov/healthypeople/priority-areas/health-literacy-healthy-people-2030.
70. Chou WYS, Gaysynsky A, Persoskie A. Health literacy and communication in palliative care. In: Wittenberg E, Ferrell B, Goldsmith J, et al., eds. *Textbook of Palliative Care Communication*. Oxford University Press; 2016:90–101.
71. Christensen D. The impact of health literacy on palliative care outcomes. *J Hosp Palliat Nurs*. 2017;18(6):544–549.
72. Badaczewski A, Bauman L, Blank A, et al. Relationship between teach-back and patient-centered communication in primary care pediatric encounters. *Patient Educ Couns*. 2017;100(7):1345–1352.
73. Ballard D, Hill J. The nurse's role in health literacy of patients with cancer. *Clin J Oncol Nurs*. 2016;20(3):232–234.
74. Roodbeen R, Vreke A, Boland G, et al. Communication and shared decision-making with patients with limited health literacy; helpful strategies, barriers and suggestions for improvement reported by hospital-based palliative care providers. *PLoS One*. 2020;15(6):e0234926.
75. Boston University. Boston Medical. New Health Literacy Tool Shed. 2023. Accessed January 17, 2025. https://www.bumc.bu.edu/healthliteracyconference/toolshed-new/
76. Singh Ospina N, Phillips K, Rodriguez-Gutierrez R, et al. Eliciting the patient's agenda—secondary analysis of recorded clinical encounters. *J Gen Intern Med*. 2019;34(1):36–40.
77. Boyle D, Barbour S, Anderson W, et al. Palliative care in the ICU: implications for an oncology–critical care nursing partnership. *Semin Oncol Nurs*. 2017;33(5):544–554.
78. Ellington L, Billitteri J, Reblin M, Clayton M. Spiritual care communication in cancer patients. *Semin Oncol Nurs*. 2017;33(5):517–525.
79. Alzougool B, Chang S, Gray K. The effects of informal carers' characteristics on their information needs: the information needs state approach. *Inform Health Soc Care*. 2017;42(3):261–273.
80. Boreale K. Communication. In: Coyne PJ, Bobb B, Plakovic K, eds. *Conversations in Palliative Care: Questions and Answers with the Experts*. 4th ed. Hospice and Palliative Nurses Association; 2017:33–45.
81. Linton J. Reducing stress and anger among family members. *Crit Care Nurse*. 2020;40(6):72–74.
82. Hanson J, Grant M, Wittenberg E. Families. In: Coyne P, Bobb B, Plakovic K, eds. *Conversations in Palliative Care—Questions with the Experts*. 4th ed. Hospice and Palliative Nurses Association; 2017:55–66.
83. Francois K, Lobb E, Barclay S, Forbat L. The nature of conflict in palliative care: a qualitative exploration of the experiences of staff and family members. *Patient Educ Couns*. 2017;100(8):1459–1465.
84. Rabow M, Hauser J, Adams J. Supporting family caregivers at the end of life—"they don't know what they don't know." *JAMA*. 2004;291(4):483–489.
85. Nuebauer K, Dixon W, Coronoa R, Boudurtha. Cultural humility In: Wittenberg E, Ferrell B, Goldsmith J, et al., eds. *Textbook of Palliative Care Communication*. Oxford University Press; 2016:79–89.
86. Cormack C, Mazanec P, Panke J. Cultural considerations in palliative care. In: Ferrell BR, Paice JA, eds. *Oxford Textbook of Palliative Nursing*. 5th ed. Oxford University Press; 2019:469–482.
87. Glajchen M, Goehring A. The family meeting in palliative care: role of the oncology nurse. *Semin Oncol Nurs*. 2017;33(5):489–497.
88. Neff P, Lyckholm L, Smith T. Truth or consequences: what to do when the patient doesn't want to know. *J Clin Oncol*. 2002;21(9):3035–3037.
89. White DB, Angus DC, Shields A-M, et al. A randomized trial of a family-support intervention in intensive care units. *N Engl J Med*. 2018;378(25):2365–2375.
90. Newman AR. Nurses' perceptions of diagnosis and prognosis-related communication. *Cancer Nurs*. 2016;39:E48–E60.
91. Lally K, Fulton A, Baxter K, Rochon T, Durcharme C, Adams KM. Expanding the serious illness care team: the conversation nurse model. In. *Health Affairs Forefront* blog. December 18, 2018. Accessed January 17, 2025. https://www.healthaffairs.org/content/forefront/expanding-serious-illness-care-team-conversation-nurse-model.
92. Lally K, Tuya Fulton A, Ducharme C, Scott R, Filpo J. Using nurse care managers trained in the serious illness conversation guide to increase goals-of-care conversations in an accountable care organization. *J Palliat Med*. 2020;23(1):112–115.
93. Warnock C, Tod A, Foster J, Soreny C. Breaking bad news in inpatient clinical settings: role of the nurse. *J Adv Nurs*. 2010;66(7):1543–1555.
94. Bumb M, Keefe J, Miller L, Overcash J. Breaking bad news: an evidence-based review of communication models for oncology nurses. *Cin J Oncol Nurs*. 2017;21(5):573–580.
95. Coyle N, Sculco L. Communication and patient/physician relationship: phenomenological inquiry. *J Support Oncol*. 2003;1(3):206–215.
96. Abbaszadeh A, Ehsani S, Begjani J, et al. Nurses' perspectives on breaking bad news to patients and their families: a qualitative content analysis. *J Med Ethics Hist Med*. 2014;7(18):7–18.
97. Visser A, Wysmans M. Improving patient education by an in-service communication training for health care providers at a cancer ward: communication climate, patient satisfaction and the need of lasting implementation. *Patient Educ Couns*. 2010;78(3):402–408.
98. Adams A, Mannix T, Harrington A. Nurses' communication with families in the intensive care unit—a literature review. *Nurs Crit Care*. 2017;22(2):70–80.
99. American Nurses Association. *Position Statement—Nursing Care and Do Not Resuscitate (DNR) Decisions*. American Nurses Association; 2020.
100. American Nurses Association. *Position Statement—Nurses' Roles and Responsibilities in Providing Care and Support at the End of Life*. Vol. 2017. American Nurses Association; 2016.
101. Ramirez C, Dahlin C. Discontinuing medically administered nutrition. *Am Nurse*. 2022;17(5):14–18. Accessed January 17, 2025. https://www.myamericannurse.com/discontinuing-medically-administered-nutrition-manh/.
102. Fage-Butler MA, Jense NM. Patient- and family-centered written communication in the palliative care setting. In: Wittenberg E, Ferrell B, Goldsmith J, et al., eds. *Textbook of Palliative Care Communication*. Oxford University Press; 2016:102–110.
103. Hanson C, Carter M. Collaboration. In: Hamric A, Hanson C, Tracy MF, O'Grady E, eds. *Advanced Practice Nursing—An Integrative Approach*. 5th ed. Elsevier Saunders; 2014:299–327.
104. Mitchell P, Wynia R, Golden B, et al. *Core Principles & Values of Effective Team-Based Health Care*. Institute of Medicine; 2012.
105. Crawford G, Price S. Team working: palliative care as a model of interdisciplinary practice. *Med J Aust*. 2003;179(suppl. 6):s32–s34.
106. Lindeke L, Sieckert A. Nurse–physician workplace collaboration. *Online J Issues Nurs*. 2005;10(1):5.
107. Altilio T, Dahlin C, Remke SS, Tucker R, Weissman D. *Strategies for Maximizing the Health/Function of Palliative Care Teams: A Resource Monograph from the Center to Advance Palliative Care*

(CAPC). Center to Advance Palliative Care; 2014. Accessed January 17, 2025. https://www.capc.org/documents/download/98/

108. Wittenberg E, Goldsmith J, Ferrell B, Platt CS. Enhancing communication related to symptom management through plain language. *J Pain Symptom Manage*. 2015;50(5):707–711.
109. Ho A, Jameson K, Pavlish C. An exploratory study of interprofessional collaboration in end-of-life decision-making beyond palliative care settings. *J Interprof Care*. 2016;30(6):795–803.
110. American Association of Critical Care Nurses. *ACCN Standards for Establishing and Sustaining Healthy Work Environments—A Journey to Excellence*. 2nd ed. American Association of Critical Care Nurses; 2016. Accessed January 17, 2025. https://www.aacn.org/WD/HWE/Docs/HWEStandards.pdf.
111. Blackwood B, Junk C, Lyons JD, McAuley DF, Rose L. Role responsibilities in mechanical ventilation and weaning in pediatric intensive care units: a national survey. *Am J Crit Care*. 2013;22(3):189–197.
112. Manojlovich M, Antonakos CL, Ronis DL. Intensive care units, communication between nurses and physicians, and patients' outcomes. *Am J Crit Care*. 2009;18(1):21–30.
113. Israilov S, Cho H. How co-creation helped address hierarchy, overwhelmed patients, and conflicts of interest in health care quality and safety. *AMA J Ethics*. 2017;19(11):1139–1145. https://doi.org/10.1001/journalofethics.2017.19.11.mhst1-1711.
114. DiPierro K, Lee H, Pain KJ, Durning SJ, Choi JJ. Groupthink among health professional teams in patient care: a scoping review. *Med Teach*. 2022;44(3):309–318. https://doi.org/10.1080/0142159X.2021.1987404.
115. Forbes Coaches Council. 10 Effects of Groupthink and How to Avoid Them. November 4, 2016; Accessed January 17, 2025. https://www.forbes.com/sites/forbescoachescouncil/2016/11/04/10-effect-of-groupthink-and-how-to-avoid-them/?sh=4992c07f4cef.
116. Foronda C, MacWilliams B, McArthur E. Interprofessional communication in healthcare: an integrative review. *Nurse Educ Pract*. 2016;19:36–40. https://doi.org/10.1016/j.nepr.2016.04.005.
117. Stone D, Patton B, Heen S. *Difficult Conversations: How to Discuss What Matters Most*. 2nd ed. Penguin Books; 2010.
118. Coyle N, Manna R, Shen M, et al. Discussing death dying, and end-of-life goals of care: a communication skills training module for oncology nurses. *Clin J Oncol Nurs*. 2015;19:697–712. https://doi.org/10.1188/15.CJON.697-702.
119. Delgado SA. Increasing nurses' palliative care communication skills. *Am J Crit Care*. 2017;26(5):372. https://doi.org/10.4037/ajcc2017427.

6

Advance Care Planning

Shigeko Izumi

Key Points

- Advances in medical technology have made extension of life possible and various end-of-life treatment options available; however, patients frequently lack decision-making capacity at the time they need to make end-of-life decisions for themselves.
- Family members and healthcare providers often do not know what end-of-life care patients want. They experience psychological distress during and after making end-of-life decisions for patients when they do not know patients' preferences.
- Advance care planning is a process that facilitates patient reflection and sharing their life goals, values, and preferences for end-of-life care if they are not capable of making their own decisions.
- Patients can share their thoughts with family members, significant others, and healthcare providers, thereby allowing them to be better prepared to make end-of-life decisions for the patients that align with their values, goals, and preferences.
- Advance care planning is a central tenet of person-centered care. There is an urgent need to build standard systems that assist all patients with advance care planning and deliver care that aligns with their values.

Introduction

The goal of healthcare is to provide care patients need and want to receive.[1] However, providing care patients need and want is difficult if the care team does not know the patients' goals, values, and preferences. Advance care planning (ACP) is a process to share a person's goals, values, and preferences to plan for future healthcare so that family members, surrogate decision-makers, and healthcare providers can make decisions that align with the goals and values of patients when they become unable to make decisions or express preferences.[2] While ACP is increasingly recognized as essential to deliver patient-centered and high-quality care, how to implement it in practice, facilitate the conversations, and use it to guide end-of-life decision-making remain challenging.[3,4] This chapter provides background for the evolving concept of ACP, the process and use in practice, and the nurse's role in ACP for adult patients. Please see Chapter 37 regarding ACP in pediatric and young adult populations.

Contextual Background of ACP

Advances in medical technology have made the extension of life possible and various end-of-life treatment options available.[5] To date, when patients face life-threatening illness or injury, several treatment options may be available, including cardiopulmonary resuscitation (CPR), mechanical ventilation, artificial nutrition to extend life, experimental treatments aimed at achieving a cure, and palliative care focusing on comfort and improving quality of life. With these options available and current healthcare aiming to deliver patient-centered care, many healthcare professionals want to know what treatment patients want or do not want. Patients and their families are increasingly expected to participate in decision-making, sharing what types of care they want to receive. However, a gap remains between what end-of-life care people want and what they actually receive.

While a national survey of Medicare beneficiaries shows that 86% of people prefer to spend their last days at home rather than in a hospital and that they do not want life-prolonging treatments that make them feel worse,[6,7] over one-third of US decedents died in a hospital in 2018.[8] Studies also show increases in intensive care unit (ICU) use in the last 30 days of life and increases in the number of healthcare transitions in the last few months of life.[9,10] Multiple healthcare transitions, including going into and out of the ICU during the end stage of their lives, imply that patients' health status fluctuates during this time; and they have to make multiple healthcare decisions as to where and what kind of care they receive.

Changes in treatment and care site transitions as conditions change are common and appropriate if each decision reflects the patient's preferences and goals of care at that moment. However, because the default medical treatment for seriously ill patients is still "do everything to save a life," some transitions that happen in the last few months, weeks, or days may be driven by this default and may not reflect the patient's preferences based on well-informed decision-making.[11] Furthermore, approximately 70% of patients needing to make end-of-life care decisions are unable to participate in the discussions as they lose decision-making capacity or the ability to express their preferences.[12,13] Therefore, it is important that family members and healthcare providers have conversations to know what is important to patients and what end-of-life care they want to receive while patients are still capable of expressing their preferences.

Patients and families expect that healthcare professionals will initiate these conversations at the right time,[14,15] while many clinicians hesitate to initiate the conversations because they perceive they are not adequately trained to facilitate such conversations, do not want to take hope away from patients, or do not have time to engage in lengthy end-of-life care discussions.[16] Family members who are expected to assume the surrogate decision-maker role also often do not know the patient's preferences or values. Family members and loved ones who are asked to make decisions for critically ill patients without having prior conversations struggle and experience strong emotions such as anxiety, depression, and guilt during and after rendering a decision, which contributes to long-lasting psychological suffering.[17,18] Having ACP conversations with patients prior to the decision-making is shown to be associated with less decisional conflict and less psychological burden for surrogate decision-makers.[19]

Evolving Concept of ACP

Definitions of ACP

The definition of ACP that is broadly used currently was developed based on consensus by multidisciplinary international ACP experts[2] (see Box 6.1). Key points of the current ACP definition are:

1) ACP is a process, not a one-time event.
2) ACP includes continuous conversations to understand and share values, goals, and preferences of the person for future medical care.
3) ACP can start at any age or stage of life.

The concept of ACP has evolved over the last three decades, and the focus and approaches to ACP have shifted.[20] Because of shifts in the concept, there is some confusion about what ACP is and how to facilitate it. In the following sections, historical perspectives, clinical issues, and evidence that have driven the shift of focus and emerging trends of ACP will be discussed.

Shift of Focus from Legal Forms to Conversations

The original concept of ACP emerged from some high-profile court cases in the 1970s where the withdrawal of life-sustaining treatments from patients whose treatment preferences were unknown was challenged. Then ACP, in the form of having a written document expressing their end-of-life treatment choices, became part of healthcare practice when the Patient Self-Determination Act (PSDA) passed in 1990.[21] The PSDA requires hospitals, nursing homes, and other healthcare institutions to provide patients an explanation of their right to make decisions about their healthcare, ask whether the patient has an advance directive (AD), and provide information about ADs if patients do not have one.[22] Although the PSDA was intended to educate patients about their healthcare decision-making rights and encourage them to make decisions and document their preferences in a legal form, it became one of many routine admission questions to check off without any follow-up interventions and lost its original intention to educate and encourage patients to think about and express their treatment preferences.[23,24]

Over the last few decades after the enactment of the PSDA, completion rates of ADs or living wills, written forms that document a person's preference regarding life-sustaining treatments, remains low at around 20%–30%.[4,25–30] In addition, the usefulness of written ADs to guide end-of-life decision-making and promote better end-of-life care has been questioned.[31] Even if patients have completed an AD, family members may not know of its existence, and the document may not be available or accessible when decisions need to be made. Patients' treatment preferences may change over the course of their life and illness. Treatment choices that were documented in an AD years ago when patients were healthy may not reflect what they want in the current situation. Treatment preferences that are based on hypothetical scenarios may not reflect treatment options available in the actual situation.[32] ACP focusing on completion of a form that expresses a patient's preferred life-sustaining treatment has not been effective, and situations where family members and healthcare professionals have to make difficult end-of-life care decisions without knowing the patient's preferences continue.

Many persons complete an AD or a living will without sharing it with anybody. Some persons complete ADs with a lawyer as part of their will and estate planning without talking with family members or healthcare professionals. Although statements written in isolation may provide some information regarding the person's preferences, it is often difficult to interpret what they mean and when to apply if they were not shared and discussed with family members/surrogate decision-makers, and healthcare professionals. Having conversations with family members and significant others about what treatments they would want or not want at the end of life and why would be a great opportunity for patients to reflect their values and share them with others. In conversations, surrogate decision-makers can ask patients to clarify what they mean, what is important for them, and how they want decisions to be made.[32] Recognizing the limitations of ACP forms and the benefit of discussions, the focus of ACP has shifted from completing written forms to encouraging conversations where patients share what matters to them so that people who need to make decisions on their behalf know their goals and values and make decisions accordingly.

Shift of Focus from Treatment Choices to Patients' Values

Specific treatments (e.g., CPR, tube feedings) patients want or do not want at the end of life may be useful information. However, treatment options they need to make decisions about near the end of life are complex, fluid, and unpredictable.[33,34] Treatments they want to receive in their actual end-of-life situation could be different from what they imagined based on hypothetical situations in the past.

Box 6.1 Consensus Definition of Advance Care Planning

Advance care planning is a process that supports adults at any age or stage of health in understanding and sharing their personal values, life goals, and preferences regarding future medical care. The goal of advance care planning is to help ensure that people receive medical care that is consistent with their values, goals, and preferences during serious and chronic illness.

Source: Reference 2.

Persons' priorities and preferences could change as their health conditions and life circumstances change over the course of their lives. Surrogate decision-makers may need to make decisions that were not indicated in the AD (e.g., use of antibiotic medications, whether to go to hospital). The prognosis and availability of treatments may be much more uncertain than these hypothetical situations (e.g., acute respiratory exacerbation due to COVID-19).[35,36] Because no one can predict what types of decisions need to be made in what circumstances, experts recommend that knowing the person's life goals and values could be more helpful to guide end-of-life decision-making rather than preferences for specific treatments.[2,34] By knowing what outcomes patients value most, such as "being able to talk and play with her grandsons matters most to my mother" or "being able to go to the bathroom by himself is the most important thing for my husband," surrogates may be better prepared to participate with clinicians in making the best possible treatment decisions that align with patients' goals and values. This shift in focus of ACP from asking patients to make premature end-of-life care treatment choices to learning about patients' goals and values is a critical point all clinicians engaged in ACP should keep in mind.

Trends to Make ACP Upstream and Inclusive

There is a trend in ACP practice to expand the reach upstream and to be more inclusive. Starting ACP conversations when patients are critically ill is often too late to elicit their goals and values because patients may be too sick, or patients and their family members may be in crisis and not able to think clearly about their goals and values. The trend is to move the start of ACP conversations earlier to the time of diagnosis of a life-limiting illness, or even as an annual health maintenance activity for healthy adults. With an illness such as dementia, patients may lose their decision-making capacity even before entering the terminal stage of illness. In these situations, the recommendation is to start ACP conversations at the time of diagnosis.[37] To promote early ACP conversations and reach out to persons while they are still relatively healthy and before needing healthcare, there are movements to bring ACP to communities where persons live. There are faith communities promoting and assisting congregations to have ACP conversations.[38,39] There also are increasing efforts to implement ACP as routine conversations among residents, families, and staff in nursing homes and residential care settings.[40–43]

In addition to upstreaming the target of who should have ACP, there are emerging efforts to make ACP more inclusive and acceptable by diverse populations. The rate of ACP completion among racial/ethnic minorities and marginalized populations such as those with lower socioeconomic status or health literacy and those in the LGBTQ community is much lower than that in the general population.[44-48] Blacks, Latinos, Asians, and Indigenous populations are less likely to engage in ACP than White Americans.[49,50] Certain cultural values in different groups may contribute to a lower degree of acceptance and participation in ACP. Mistrust in the healthcare system rooted in historical trauma could be another reason for less ACP participation by patients from marginalized populations. Some researchers have reported that clinicians may have preconceived perceptions or biases and avoid having ACP conversations with patients from marginalized populations.[51,52] In response to the increasing awareness about ACP disparities, there are efforts to make ACP more culturally and linguistically inclusive.[53–56]

Trend for System and Team Approach for ACP

Given the complexity and longitudinal nature of ACP over patient illness trajectories, a systematic approach to implement ACP is recommended. Educating individual clinicians about ACP and conversation facilitation skills alone is not enough to make ACP a routine practice.[57,58] For ACP to happen consistently as routine practice, the process needs to be built into the system-level workflow of practice, and all involved clinicians need to know their roles and be accountable.[57,59]

The process of ACP includes identifying patients for ACP, securing time and reminding clinicians to have ACP conversations, documenting the ACP conversations, and tracking and following up as needed.[57,58] It requires electronic health record systems that accommodate documentation, tracking, and communication of ACP.[34,60,61] To enhance the effectiveness and share the process of ACP, a team approach for ACP is gaining interest. Traditionally, ACP conversations with patients were facilitated mostly by individual healthcare providers (e.g., physicians and advanced practice providers) whose scope of practice includes prognostication and medical decision-making. As the focus of ACP shifts from treatment decisions to learning about patient goals and values and assisting patients and surrogates to prepare for future decision-making, the roles other clinicians, such as registered nurses, clinical licensed social workers, and chaplains, could play in ACP are being recognized.[62–66] Teamwork and collaboration with other team members allow for the distribution of various tasks related to ACP among team members and make more timely and high-quality ACP possible for patients. Team membership, roles, and functions of team members vary broadly by practice. Team members who are best positioned to identify patients, to have ACP conversations, or to communicate with patients' surrogates differ by team. Engaging all team members in discussions and planning for how to incorporate ACP processes in their workflow and clarifying who does what would be key for the successful implementation of ACP by interprofessional teams.[66]

Process, Tools, and Strategies to Facilitate ACP

ACP conversations should start well before the time of end-of-life decision-making, ideally while persons are healthy. ACP conversations should be revisited as the person's health and life situations change. As the person becomes ill and gets closer to the end of life, the focus of ACP conversations could be narrower and more specific. Figure 6.1 is a model showing the continuum of ACP along with health trajectory.[67] This model illustrates ACP activities across a continuum from healthy to ill and frail to end of life. Because these activities and conversations happen over the person's life course and likely in different settings, it is rare that a same clinician is involved in the entire process of ACP over the person's life. Whatever the setting a clinician encounters with a patient, the clinician needs to be able to discern where on the ACP continuum the patient is (i.e., what ACP activities the patient has done before) and what ACP activity they should initiate given where the patient is on the health trajectory at the moment. This model can be used to ascertain how to address ACP appropriately for the patient's health trajectory. In the following section, the process, tools, and strategies for nurses to facilitate ACP along with the continuum of the ACP model will be described.

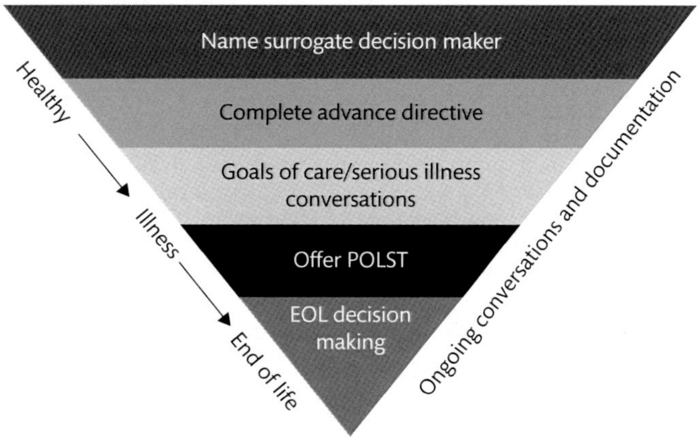
Name surrogate decision maker
Complete advance directive
Goals of care/serious illness conversations
Offer POLST
EOL decision making
Healthy
Illness
End of life
Ongoing conversations and documentation

Figure 6.1 Continuum of advance care planning (modified by the author). EOL, end of life; POLST, Portable Orders for Life-Sustaining Treatment.
Source: Reference 67.

Naming the Surrogate Decision Maker

Because acute illness or injury where a person loses decision-making capacity could happen to anybody, it is recommended to ask all patients to name a surrogate decision-maker and document it in the health record. Even healthy patients admitted to a hospital for elective surgery may need someone to make decisions for them while they are under anesthesia. Case 6.1 is an example of how not knowing the patient's surrogate decision-maker resulted in less-than-optimal decisions that were not concordant with the patient's preferences.

Case 6.1: Not Knowing the Right Surrogate Decision Maker Impaired the Decision-Making

Ms. Jackson is a 24-year-old obstetric patient who was admitted to a hospital for an elective cesarean section. During the procedure, she experienced massive blood loss necessitating an emergent decision about hysterectomy. Because the patient was unconscious and a decision needed to be made, the physicians reached out to Ms. Jackson's mother, who was present in the waiting area and was listed as her "emergency contact" in the electronic health record. The mother consented for the hysterectomy, and the procedure was completed. After the surgery, the patient was upset because she wanted her fiancé with whom she was going to make future family plans to make the decision, not her mother. Asking patients about their surrogate decision-makers was not a requirement before a procedure in this hospital, and the surrogate decision-maker section in the health record was left empty.

A surrogate decision-maker is someone patients trust to make healthcare decisions and to speak for them in the event they are unable to speak for themselves. A surrogate decision-maker is also called a "healthcare proxy," a "durable power of attorney for healthcare," a "healthcare agent," or a "healthcare representative." Most states and many healthcare organizations have policies about who would be the surrogate decision-maker for incapacitated patients. If a patient does not appoint a surrogate before they lose capacity, decision-making falls to the patient's next of kin according to state law, usually in the following order: spouse, adult children, parents, adult siblings, and adult grandchildren.

Box 6.2 Important Characteristics for Patients to Consider When They Are Selecting Their Surrogate Decision Maker

The surrogate decision maker should be someone who:
✓ You can trust to speak for you
✓ You can talk to about your values, goals, and preferences
✓ Is willing to accept the role
✓ Is able to follow your wishes (not what they wish for you)
✓ Is able to speak up on your behalf
✓ Is able to make decisions in stressful situations

Patients can name the surrogate decision-maker out of order of the state law or name someone other than the next of kin, but it needs to be documented in a legal form such as an AD or healthcare proxy to be valid. In Case 6.1, the patient's mother was not only the emergency contact person and present in the waiting area but also the legally valid next of kin to be the surrogate decision-maker. Because the patient was not asked and did not name her fiancé as her surrogate decision-maker in a legal document, her fiancé was not contacted when the decision had to be made while she was under anesthesia. Today's family structures and personal relationships are diverse and complex. If the surrogate decision-maker a patient trusts is not the conventional next of kin, it is important to advise the patients to legally name the surrogate decision-maker. After this incident, the hospital in the case implemented a procedure to ask all patients to identify a surrogate decision-maker and document it in the medical record at the time of admission.

Speaking up on behalf of a patient and making healthcare decisions in a high-stress situation is very difficult and a great responsibility. Box 6.2 shows how nurses can describe the role of surrogate decision-maker to patients and assist them to select the right person as their surrogate decision-maker. Additional resources guiding the selection of surrogate decision-makers are shown in the Table 6.1.

Completing Advance Directives

Advance Directives (AD) are written documents that describe a person's treatment preferences in end-of-life care and legally name a surrogate decision-maker. In some states, surrogate decision-makers are appointed using a special form (e.g., healthcare proxy, healthcare power of attorney) separate from an AD form. The section for treatment preferences in an AD is also called "living will," where persons express what life-sustaining treatment (e.g., CPR, tube feeding) they would or would not want in terminal conditions.

Thinking and making decisions about future end-of-life care is an overwhelming task. In addition, emerging critiques point out the limited usefulness of a completed AD document alone in guiding end-of-life decision-making, as discussed in the previous section. Yet, the process of completing an AD creates an opportunity to prompt persons to reflect on their goals and values and talk about them with their loved ones and surrogates. Resources to guide laypersons in having these conversations and formulating ADs are shown in Table 6.1.

Keeping ADs in a safety deposit vault or a lawyer's office without telling anybody does not serve its purpose. Nurses should advise persons who have completed ADs to (1) give copies to their surrogate decision-makers, other family members, and friends who are likely to be involved at the time of decision-making; (2) inform

Table 6.1 Resources and tools for advance care planning (ACP)

ACP activities	
Naming surrogate decision makers	• The Conversation Project: Website provides materials for laypersons to support their conversations about goals and values with their loved ones including tips to select surrogate decision makers. Free. (https://theconversationproject.org/wp-content/uploads/2017/03/ConversationProject-ProxyKit-English.pdf)
Completing advance directives	• The Conversation Project: Website provides a toolkit for laypersons to support their conversations about goals and values with their loved ones. Free. (https://theconversationproject.org/) • PREPARE™ for Your Care: A web-based guide that helps people plan for and make decisions about their future care. The website include step-by-step video instructions for patients to complete advance directives and the Easy-to-Read Advance Directive. Free. (https://prepareforyourcare.org/en/welcome) • Five Wishes: This organization provides a form "Five Wishes" in which persons can write their wishes related to their end-of-life care. This form is regarded as a formal advance directive/living will in some US states. One form is free for a person. (https://www.fivewishes.org/) • Respecting Choices®: This program provides training to healthcare professionals to facilitate ACP conversations with patients in different stages of health (First Step, Next Step, and Advanced Step). First Step ACP facilitation training is for healthcare professionals to be an ACP facilitator to assist healthy persons to think about and document advance directives. Training program for fee. (https://respectingchoices.org/)
Goals-of-care conversations	• Respecting Choices®: This program provides training to healthcare professionals to facilitate ACP conversations with patients in different stages of health (First Step, Next Step, and Advanced Step). Next Step training is to have goals-of-care conversations with patients living with serious illnesses. Cost to enroll to the training. (https://respectingchoices.org/) • Serious Illness Care Program: This program provides training to healthcare professionals to facilitate serious illness conversations and strategies to implement serious illness care program in healthcare organizations. Most of the materials are licensed under the Creative Commons and free. (https://www.ariadnelabs.org/serious-illness-care/) • VitalTalk: This program provides communication skill training to healthcare professionals to have difficult conversations delivering bad news, exploring patient preferences, and making shared decisions with patients who are seriously ill with a limited prognosis. Cost to enroll in the training. (www.vitaltalk.org)
Portable medical order for life-sustaining treatment	• POLST: This website provides information about a portable medical order regarding life-sustaining treatments for specific states. (http://polst.org/about-the-national-polst-paradigm/what-is-polst/) • Respecting Choices®: This program provides training to healthcare professionals to facilitate ACP conversations with patients in different stages of health (First Step, Next Step, and Advanced Step). Advanced Step ACP facilitation training is for healthcare professionals to have conversations about life-sustaining treatment preferences to complete POLST form. Training program for fee. (https://respectingchoices.org/)

POLST, Portable Orders for Life-Sustaining Treatment.

their families and close friends about their surrogate decision-maker and wishes; (3) keep a copy of the AD where it can be easily found; and (4) take a copy with them if they go to a hospital or nursing home.

ACP is an ongoing conversation, and completing an AD should not be a one-time event. Nurses can take the role of reminding patients to revisit their AD and continue the ACP conversation because nurses often attend to patients when they are at health or life transitions. For example, a hospital nurse can ask a patient whether they have an AD or have had ACP conversations prior to the first hospital admission for chemotherapy after a cancer diagnosis and assist the patient to revisit their prior AD or conversations as their health conditions and priority and values may change. A primary care clinic nurse can ask all patients who come for annual wellness visits whether they have an AD and remind them to revisit it regularly and revise it as needed. By talking about ACP and encouraging patients to revisit ADs as part of regular medical encounters, nurses can educate patients that ACP is a lifelong conversation and should happen long before the end of life. This normalizes ACP as part of routine practice for everyone.

Having Goals-of-Care Conversations

When patients become ill, more focused conversations need to occur. The aim of such conversations is for clinicians to understand patients' goals and values as their health conditions decline so that patients, surrogates, and healthcare professionals can be prepared to make decisions that align medical treatments with patients' goals and values when the time comes. This conversation does not need to be about end-of-life care only. It could be used to discuss and decide treatments that would be best for the patient who is newly diagnosed with early-stage cancer or heart failure that is gradually progressing. The underlying tenet is that patients should receive care that is consistent with their goals and values at any time in the illness trajectory. Thus, each treatment decision should be made based on candid conversations, ensuring that the treatment goals align with the patients' goals and values at that moment in time.

It also could be a conversation with patients where poor prognosis may be looming and (re)visiting patients' goals and values in the context of the specific illness trajectory is needed. This conversation is usually triggered by clinicians when they see patients with advanced stage illness and want to explore patients' goals and values to guide potential future end-of-life care decisions before it becomes too late. Nurses who work closely and have a trusting relationship with patients are often in a great position to facilitate conversations soliciting patients' goals and values and aligning them with treatment choices. However, many nurses believe that they are not well prepared to facilitate these goals-of-care conversations. There are established programs to train healthcare professionals to have meaningful goals-of-care conversations with their patients (see Table 6.1). These training programs provide frameworks, strategies, opportunities to practice communication skills, and some useful language to facilitate goals-of-care conversations. Please see Chapters 5 and 37 for more information about specific communication strategies.

Medical Orders for Life-Sustaining Treatment

Portable Orders for Life-Sustaining Treatment (POLST; also called Medical Orders for Life-Sustaining Treatment [MOLST or MOST] in some states) is a medical order form that instructs healthcare providers such as paramedics/emergency medical technicians (EMTs) and emergency department clinicians what life-sustaining treatments the patient should or should not receive. In advanced stages of illness, sudden deterioration of health conditions (e.g., cardiac arrest, shortness of breath) and loss of decisional capacity could happen. When patients or family members call for an ambulance, come to an emergency department, or are admitted to hospitals due to worsening conditions, clinicians who make the decisions related to life-sustaining treatment in these situations are likely ones who do not know the patient's goals and values. A POLST is a tool translating patients' preferences about life-sustaining treatments into standing medical orders so that clinicians in these emergency situations can deliver the treatment that aligns with the patients' goals and values by following the POLST. A POLST should be based on ACP conversations with the patient about what life-sustaining treatment would align with their goals and values. Both ADs and POLST are useful tools to document and communicate patients' values and preferences for end-of-life care but have different functions. Table 6.2 summarizes the differences between ADs and POLST.

A POLST paradigm is adopted in many states. Although details may vary slightly by states, the POLST form usually includes preferences for CPR, different levels of medical interventions (comfort measures only, limited treatment, or full treatment), and a signature by the ordering healthcare provider. The POLST form should be completed based on informed shared decision-making between patients and healthcare providers. The POLST form must be signed by a healthcare provider, who is accountable for the medical orders. State law identifies which healthcare providers are authorized to sign medical orders.

POLST forms should be portable and stay with patients. If patients live at home, POLST should be posted in a visible location (e.g., refrigerator door). If patients are transported to a nursing home, emergency department, or hospital, the POLST should go with the patient. In Oregon, where POLST was originally developed, there is a statewide POLST registry. Through this registry, clinicians (including EMTs outside of hospitals) can access their patients' POLST online as needed and have increased accessibility and availability of this medical order in emergency situations.

Use of ACP in End-of-Life Decision-Making

The four activities shown in the continuum of the ACP model (Figure 6.1) aim to prepare patients and their families and surrogate decision-makers for the time of end-of-life decision-making. In that sense, the activity of actual decision-making of end-of-life care (the bottom triangle of the model) is not part of *advance care planning*. However, healthcare professionals who engage in ACP conversations with patients as well as who are involved in the decision-making need to understand how to use the ACP to make in-the-moment decisions that respect patients' goals and values.[32,68] When a person becomes unable to make their own decisions, all prior ACP conversations and documents of these conversations will help those present in the decision-making (i.e., family, friends, and the healthcare team) feel prepared to make the best decisions for the patient.

When healthcare professionals see a patient who is seriously ill, their default response is to save the patient's life. But if that is not what the patient wants, making attempts to save the patient's life may not be quality care for that patient. Some healthcare professionals equate providing life-extending treatment despite patients' expressed preference against it to making a medical error.[69] To avoid the medical error of delivering care that patients do not want, clinicians in the moment of decision-making need to inquire whether the patient has done the work of ACP and elicit the patient's treatment preferences instead of automatically assuming routine life-sustaining procedures. Clinicians involved in end-of-life decision-making need to identify the surrogate decision-makers the patient has named, work with the surrogate decision-makers to elicit the patient's goals and values, and assist them in making end-of-life care decisions that honor the patient's values. In Case 6.2, a social worker in a family conference asks whether the patient has an AD, and a registered nurse asks the family what matters most to the patient and describes what the choice of tracheostomy may mean for his life. This is an example of how clinicians can assist surrogates and family members make the best decisions for patients using prior ACP conversations.

Table 6.2 Differences between advance directives and POLST

Advance directives	POLST
For anyone 18 years or older, if completed for themselves; may exist for those younger than 18 years of age if completed by legal guardian	Most appropriate for those who are frail or seriously ill
Legal document completed by patients with instructions for the end-of-life treatments they prefer	Medical orders for life-sustaining treatments based on discussions between a patient and a healthcare provider
Does not guide emergency personnel because it is NOT a medical order	Provides medical orders for emergency and other medical personnel
No need for healthcare provider's signature	Needs healthcare provider's signature
Appoints a surrogate decision maker Needs patient's and surrogate decision maker's signatures	May not identify surrogate decision maker Patient's and/or surrogate decision maker's signature is recommended but not required
No registry available Patients and/or family members need to bring a copy of it when needed	POLST registry may be available POLST stays with patient

POLST, Portable Orders for Life-Sustaining Treatment.

Case 6.2: Facilitating End-of-Life Decision-Making Based on ACP

Mr. Sanchez is an 83-year-old widower living with chronic obstructive pulmonary disease and heart failure. He was the main caregiver for his wife before she died from breast cancer several years ago. Seeing his wife's end-of-life care, he completed an AD indicating his oldest daughter as the surrogate decision-maker and no CPR and no tube feedings when he becomes terminally ill.

His condition deteriorated over several years, and he was hospitalized for pneumonia and exacerbated shortness of breath. He was temporarily on a ventilator, and a family conference was called to determine the goals of care and discuss treatment options. Mr. Sanchez has three adult daughters and one son living in the area, and all of them attended the family conference. A hospitalist, a nurse, and a medical social worker in the unit attended the conference. Although Mr. Sanchez had been admitted to this hospital two times before, none of the clinicians had met with him previously. The hospitalist described his current condition and treatment options including a tracheostomy for long-term ventilation. The social worker asked if he had an AD, and the oldest daughter showed his AD to the team. Because there was no indication about his preference regarding tracheostomy in his AD, the hospitalist asked the oldest daughter whether he would want to have a tracheostomy or not. The son responded, "Of course, so he can live." The hospitalist described, "Yes, the breathing machine will help him to continue breathing. But his lungs are very weak. He may not be able to regain the ability to breathe by himself without a machine even though his pneumonia may get better." The nurse asked, "Have any of you talked with your father about what matters to him most?" The oldest daughter said, "My dad always says having dinner with the whole family at the table makes him very happy. Being there with us and his grandkids is what matters to him." Then the nurse described that with a tracheostomy and breathing machine he will not be able to sit at the table and have dinner together with his whole family. After a few moments of silence, the oldest daughter said, "I don't think my dad wants to be like that," and all the other children nodded in agreement. The family members asked more questions about what other treatment options meant and what he would be able to do or not. At the end of the conference, the family decided to keep him on a ventilator without tracheostomy for 3 days, hoping his condition would get better after recovering from pneumonia. After 3 days of trial, his condition improved, and the ventilator was removed. He was discharged to his oldest daughter's home with hospice services. He died 14 days after the discharge. During this time, he was able to sit at the table with his entire family for his grandson's birthday and another Sunday dinner together.

Roles and Responsibilities of Nurses in ACP

The American Nurses Association's position statement[70] asserts that nurses are responsible for facilitating the process of informed healthcare decision-making for patients. ACP is a central tenet of person-centered care, and it is a form of facilitating informed shared decision-making for end-of-life care by assisting patients to reflect on and communicate their values. The Hospice & Palliative Nurses Association position statement asserts that nurses must take a leading role in ACP through the education of patients, families, and other healthcare professionals and its implementation in everyday practice.[71] As described in prior sections, ACP should occur across the various stages of patients' health, and all patients that nurses encounter in practice should have the opportunity to plan and prepare for future health situations.

Case 6.3: ACP Conversation at Hospital Admission Made a Difference

Nurses in a bone marrow transplant (BMT) unit in an academic medical center were conducting a quality-improvement project to ask all patients to name surrogate decision-makers and encourage them to have ADs within 48 hours of admission to their unit. On admission, a patient with a new diagnosis of blood cancer told the nurse that she wanted her two best friends to be her surrogate decision-makers instead of her family. She explained that her ex-husband was a primary support but not the decision-maker, and her daughter was using substances and unreliable. The nurse involved a social worker to assist this patient in completing an AD appointing her friends as surrogate decision-makers.

Two weeks later, this patient was dying unexpectedly in the ICU. At the bedside was her ex-husband and daughter who wanted "to do everything." ICU nurses saw the AD and contacted the social worker in the BMT unit who spoke with the patient's surrogate decision-makers, her friends, by phone. The surrogate decision-makers had had previous conversations with the patient about the end-of-life care she wanted. The decision was made to not intubate and not continue aggressive life support. The patient's ex-husband and daughter were upset that they were not the decision-makers, but the patient's end-of-life wishes were honored because she had talked about these issues previously and had an AD. This patient died 5 minutes after aggressive treatment was stopped, and she was comfortable as she died with her daughter holding her hand.

In Case 6.3, the patient was not expected to die during this hospital stay, but nurses asked who the patient trusted to be her surrogate decision-maker and encouraged her to have conversations with the surrogates. The nurse's early ACP conversation in the BMT unit with the patient to plan for end-of-life decision-making enabled the ICU care team to provide the care the patient wanted. Nurses are responsible for educating their patients about the importance of ACP and assisting them in making appropriate plans. Nurses working in ambulatory care settings could educate patients who come in for annual wellness visits or regular follow-up visits about the importance of identifying surrogate decision-makers and encourage them to start the conversations with their families in case of an unpredictable event such as a car accident. Reviewing ACP can be a part of routine health maintenance similar to immunizations. Nurses seeing patients with chronic illness can assist them in thinking about what is important to them and encourage them to have conversations with healthcare providers to make informed shared decisions about treatments that are consistent with their values.

When patients are planning for future treatment by completing ADs or POLST forms, nurses can explain what the potential implications of CPR or tube feedings are and assist them in having meaningful conversations with healthcare providers and in making well-informed decisions. When patients and their families are in situations where end-of-life care decisions need to be made, nurses should advocate for patients by getting healthcare teams to attend to patients' values, goals, and preferences, ensuring that patients receive the care they want.[72]

In addition to responsibilities as registered nurses, advance practice nurses need to be familiar with the process of ACP that is appropriate to their specialty role and patient population. The specialty role may include communication, documentation of information and forms, and possibly billing for the ACP conversation to make the ACP facilitation sustainable in their practice.[73] Additional training to facilitate serious illness conversations including prognosis and treatment decisions may be needed. Models describing the process of ACP and tools introduced in the prior sections could be useful to advance practice nurses' planning and implementation of ACP.

Summary

ACP is gaining recognition as an essential component of quality end-of-life care, and both the public and healthcare professionals are increasingly aware of its importance. While the concept of ACP is broadly accepted as good practice, confusion about what ACP entails exists, and implementation of ACP in routine practice in many care settings remains challenging. In addition, evidence showing what and how ACP improves the quality of care patients receive is still limited.

Essential components of ACP such as knowing a person's values, goals, and preferences; facilitating conversations with patients, families, and healthcare providers for informed shared decision-making; and advocating for provision of care that is consistent with a patient's values are core principles of nursing. Nurses, particularly palliative nurses who have expertise in these areas, take a leading role in ACP by educating patients, families, and other healthcare professionals and advocating for its implementation in everyday practice.

REFERENCES

1. Office of Disease Prevention and Health Promotion, Office of the Secretary, US Department of Health and Human Services. Healthy People 2030. https://health.gov/healthypeople/objectives-and-data/browse-objectives/health-care#:~:text=High%2Dquality%20health%20care%20helps,health%20care%20services%20they%20need.
2. Sudore RL, Lum HD, You JJ, et al. Defining advance care planning for adults: a consensus definition from a multidisciplinary Delphi panel. *J Pain Symptom Manage.* 2017;53:821–832. https://doi.org/10.1016/j.jpainsymman.2016.12.331.
3. Fulmer T, Escobedo M, Berman A, Koren MJ, Hernandez S, Hult A. Physicians' views on advance care planning and end-of-life care conversations. *J Am Geriatr Soc.* 2018;66(6):1201–1205. https://doi.org/10.1111/jgs.15374.
4. Yadav KN, Gabler NB, Cooney E, et al. Approximately one in three US adults completes any type of advance directive for end-of-life care. *Health Aff (Millwood).* 2017;36(7):1244–1251. https://doi.org/10.1377/hlthaff.2017.0175.
5. Institute of Medicine. *Dying in America: Improving Quality and Honoring Individual Preferences Near the End of Life.* National Academies Press; 2014.
6. Burge F, Lawson B, Johnston G, Asada Y, McIntyre PF, Flowerdew G. Preferred and actual location of death: what factors enable a preferred home death? *J Palliat Med.* 2015;18(12):1054–1059. https://doi.org/10.1089/jpm.2015.0177.
7. Aldridge MD, Bradley EH. Epidemiology and patterns of care at the end of life: rising complexity, shifts in care patterns and sites of death. Article. *Health Aff (Millwood).* 2017;36(7):1175–1183. https://doi.org/10.1377/hlthaff.2017.0182
8. QuickStats: Percentage of Deaths by Place of Death—National Vital Statistics System, United States, 2000–2018. *MMWR Morb Mortal Wkly Rep.* 2020;69(19):611. https://www.cdc.gov/mmwr/volumes/69/wr/mm6919a4.htm
9. Palan Lopez R, Mitchell SL, Givens JL. Preventing burdensome transitions of nursing home residents with advanced dementia: it's more than advance directives. *J Palliat Med.* 2017;20(11):1205–1209. https://doi.org/10.1089/jpm.2017.0050.
10. Wang X, Teno JM, Gozalo PL, Dosa D, Thomas KS, Bélanger E. State variation in potentially burdensome transitions among assisted living residents at the end of life. *JAMA Intern Med.* 2021;182(2):229–231. https://doi.org/10.1001/jamainternmed.2021.7260.
11. Barnato AE. Challenges in understanding and respecting patients' preferences. *Health Aff (Millwood).* 2017;36(7):1252–1257. https://doi.org/10.1377/hlthaff.2017.0177.
12. Silveira MJ, Kim SYH, Langa KM. Advance directives and outcomes of surrogate decision making before death. *N Engl J Med.* 2010;362(13):1211–1218. https://doi.org/10.1056/NEJMsa0907901
13. Torke AM, Sachs GA, Helft PR, et al. Scope and outcomes of surrogate decision making among hospitalized older adults. *JAMA Intern Med.* 2014;174(3):370–377. https://doi.org/10.1001/jamainternmed.2013.13315.
14. De Vleminck A, Batteauw D, Demeyere T, Pype P. Do non-terminally ill adults want to discuss the end of life with their family physician? An explorative mixed-method study on patients' preferences and family physicians' views in Belgium. *Fam Pract.* 2018;35(4):495–502. https://doi.org/10.1093/fampra/cmx125.
15. Song M-K, Ward SE, Fine JP, et al. Advance care planning and end-of-life decision making in dialysis: a randomized controlled trial targeting patients and their surrogates. *Am J Kidney Dis.* 2015;66(5):813–822. https://doi.org/10.1053/j.ajkd.2015.05.018.
16. Griffin S, Cubanski J, Neuman T, Jankiewicz A, Rousseau D; for the Kaiser Family Foundation. Medicare and end-of-life care. *JAMA.* 2016;316(17):1754. https://doi.org/10.1001/jama.2016.15577.
17. Brinkman-Stoppelenburg A, Rietjens JAC, Van Der Heide A. The effects of advance care planning on end-of-life care: a systematic review. *Palliat Med.* 2014;28(8):1000–1025. https://doi.org/10.1177/0269216314526272.
18. Houben CH, Spruit MA, Groenen MT, Wouters EF, Janssen DJ. Efficacy of advance care planning: a systematic review and meta-analysis. *J Am Med Dir Assoc.* 2014;15(7):477–89. https://doi.org/10.1016/j.jamda.2014.01.008.
19. Chiarchiaro J, Buddadhumaruk P, Arnold RM, White DB. Prior advance care planning is associated with less decisional conflict among surrogates for critically ill patients. *Ann Am Thorac Soc.* 2015;12(10):1528–33. https://doi.org/10.1513/AnnalsATS.201504-253OC.

20. Sabatino CP. The evolution of health care advance planning law and policy. *Milbank Q*. 2010;88(2):211–239. https://doi.org/10.1111/j.1468-0009.2010.00596.x.
21. Kelley K. The Patient Self-Determination Act. A matter of life and death. *Physician Assist*. 1995;19(3):49–60.
22. American Bar Association. Law for Older Americans: Health Care Advance Directives. March 18, 2013. https://www.americanbar.org/groups/public_education/resources/law_issues_for_consumers/patient_self_determination_act/.
23. Castillo LS, Williams BA, Hooper SM, Sabatino CP, Weithorn LA, Sudore RL. Lost in translation: the unintended consequences of advance directive law on clinical care. *Ann Intern Med*. 2011;154(2):121–128. https://doi.org/10.7326/0003-4819-154-2-201101180-00012.
24. Hammes BJ, Rooney BL. Death and end-of-life planning in one midwestern community. *Arch Intern Med*. 1998;158(4):383–390. https://doi.org/10.1001/archinte.158.4.383.
25. Teno J, Lynn J, Wenger N, et al. Advance directives for seriously ill hospitalized patients: effectiveness with the Patient Self-Determination Act and the SUPPORT intervention. *J Am Geriatr Soc*. 1997;45(4):500–507. https://doi.org/10.1111/j.1532-5415.1997.tb05178.x.
26. Gamertsfelder EM, Seaman JB, Tate J, Buddadhumaruk P, Happ MB. Prevalence of advance directives among older adults admitted to intensive care units and requiring mechanical ventilation. *J Gerontol Nurs*. 2016;42(4):34–41. https://doi.org/10.3928/00989134-20151124-02.
27. Huang IA, Neuhaus JM, Chiong W. Racial and ethnic differences in advance directive possession: role of demographic factors, religious affiliation, and personal health values in a national survey of older adults. *J Palliat Med*. 2016;19(2):149–156. https://doi.org/10.1089/jpm.2015.0326.
28. Rao JK, Anderson LA, Lin FC, Laux JP. Completion of advance directives among U.S. consumers. *Am J Prev Med*. 2014;46(1):65–70. https://doi.org/10.1016/j.amepre.2013.09.008.
29. Silveira MJ, Wiitala W, Piette J. Advance directive completion by elderly Americans: a decade of change. *J Am Geriatr Soc*. 2014;62(4):706–710. https://doi.org/10.1111/jgs.12736.
30. Tjia J, Dharmawardene M, Givens JL. Advance directives among nursing home residents with mild, moderate, and advanced dementia. *J Palliat Med*. 2018;21(1):16–21. https://doi.org/10.1089/jpm.2016.0473.
31. Morrison SR. Advance directives/care planning: clear, simple, and wrong. *J Palliat Med*. 2020;23(7):878–879. https://doi.org/10.1089/jpm.2020.0272.
32. Sudore RL, Fried TR. Redefining the "planning" in advance care planning: preparing for end-of-life decision making. *Ann Intern Med*. 2010;153(4):256–261. https://doi.org/10.7326/0003-4819-153-4-201008170-00008.
33. Morrison RS, Meier DE, Arnold RM. What's wrong with advance care planning? *JAMA*. 2021;326(16):1575–1576. https://doi.org/10.1001/jama.2021.16430.
34. Bernacki RE, Block SD. Communication about serious illness care goals: a review and synthesis of best practices. *JAMA Intern Med*. 2014;174(12):1994–2003. https://doi.org/10.1001/jamainternmed.2014.5271.
35. Heyland DK. Advance care planning (ACP) vs. advance serious illness preparations and planning (ASIPP). *Healthcare*. 2020;8(3):218. https://doi.org/10.3390/healthcare8030218.
36. Sanders JJ, Curtis JR, Tulsky JA. Achieving goal-concordant care: a conceptual model and approach to measuring serious illness communication and its impact. *J Palliat Med*. 2018;21(suppl 2):S17–s27. https://doi.org/10.1089/jpm.2017.0459.
37. Dixon J, Karagiannidou M, Knapp M. The effectiveness of advance care planning in improving end-of-life outcomes for people with dementia and their carers: a systematic review and critical discussion. *J Pain Symptom Manage*. 2018;55(1):132–150.e1. https://doi.org/10.1016/j.jpainsymman.2017.04.009.
38. Alameda County Care Alliance Advanced Illness Care Program. The Value & Power of Relationships. https://www.care-alliance.org/our-story.
39. Sloan DH, Gray TF, Harris D, et al. Church leaders and parishioners speak out about the role of the church in advance care planning and end-of-life care. *Palliat Support Care*. 2021;19(3):322–328. https://doi.org/10.1017/s1478951520000966.
40. Aasmul I, Husebo BS, Sampson EL, Flo E. Advance care planning in nursing homes—improving the communication among patient, family, and staff: results from a cluster randomized controlled trial (COSMOS). *Front psychol*. 2018;9:2284. https://doi.org/10.3389/fpsyg.2018.02284.
41. Gilissen J, Pivodic L, Wendrich-van Dael A, et al. Implementing advance care planning in routine nursing home care: the development of the theory-based ACP+ program. *PLoS One*. 2019;14(10):e0223586. https://doi.org/10.1371/journal.pone.0223586.
42. Mitchell SL, Volandes AE, Gutman R, et al. Advance care planning video intervention among long-stay nursing home residents: a pragmatic cluster randomized clinical trial. *JAMA Intern Med*. 2020;180(8):1070–1078. https://doi.org/10.1001/jamainternmed.2020.2366.
43. Hickman SE, Unroe KT, Ersek M, et al. Systematic advance care planning and potentially avoidable hospitalizations of nursing facility residents. *J Am Geriatr Soc*. 2019;67(8):1649–1655. https://doi.org/10.1111/jgs.15927.
44. Choi S, McDonough IM, Kim M, Kim G. The association between the number of chronic health conditions and advance care planning varies by race/ethnicity. *Aging Ment Health*. 2020;24(3):453–463. https://doi.org/10.1080/13607863.2018.1533521.
45. Reich AJ, Perez S, Fleming J, et al. Advance care planning experiences among sexual and gender minority people. *JAMA Netw Open*. 2022;5(7):e2222993. https://doi.org/10.1001/jamanetworkopen.2022.22993.
46. Jia Z, Yeh IM, Lee CH, Yeung AS, Tulsky JA, Leiter RE. Barriers and facilitators to advance care planning among Chinese patients with advanced cancer and their caregivers. *J Palliat Med*. 2022;25(5):774–782. https://doi.org/10.1089/jpm.2021.0404.
47. Sudore RL, Landefeld CS, Perez-Stable EJ, Bibbins-Domingo K, Williams BA, Schillinger D. Unraveling the relationship between literacy, language proficiency, and patient-physician communication. *Patient Educ Couns*. 2009;75(3):398–402. https://doi.org/10.1016/j.pec.2009.02.019.
48. Sanders JJ, Robinson MT, Block SD. Factors impacting advance care planning among African Americans: results of a systematic integrated review. *J Palliat Med*. 2016;19(2):202–227. https://doi.org/10.1089/jpm.2015.0325.
49. Jones T, Luth EA, Lin SY, Brody AA. Advance care planning, palliative care, and end-of-life care interventions for racial and ethnic underrepresented groups: a systematic review. *J Pain Symptom Manage*. 2021;62(3):e248–e260. https://doi.org/10.1016/j.jpainsymman.2021.04.025.
50. Rosa WE, Izumi S, Sullivan DR, et al. Advance care planning in serious illness: a narrative review. *J Pain Symptom*

Manage. 2023;65(1):e63–e78. https://doi.org/10.1016/j.jpainsymman.2022.08.012.
51. Ashana DC, D'Arcangelo N, Gazarian PK, et al. "Don't talk to them about goals of care": understanding disparities in advance care planning. *J Gerontol A Biol Sci Med Sci*. 2022;77(2):339–346. https://doi.org/10.1093/gerona/glab091.
52. Periyakoil VS, Neri E, Kraemer H. No easy talk: a mixed methods study of doctor reported barriers to conducting effective end-of-life conversations with diverse patients. *PLoS One*. 2015;10(4):e0122321. https://doi.org/10.1371/journal.pone.0122321.
53. Lillie KM, Dirks LG, Curtis JR, Candrian C, Kutner JS, Shaw JL. Culturally adapting an advance care planning communication intervention with American Indian and Alaska Native people in primary care. *J Transcult Nurs*. 2020;31(2):178–187. https://doi.org/10.1177/1043659619859055.
54. Elk R, Emanuel L, Hauser J, Bakitas M, Levkoff S. Developing and testing the feasibility of a culturally based tele-palliative care consult based on the cultural values and preferences of southern, rural African American and White community members: a program by and for the community. *Health Equity*. 2020;4(1):52–82. https://doi.org/10.1089/heq.2019.0120.
55. Sanders JJ, Johnson KS, Cannady K, et al. From barriers to assets: rethinking factors impacting advance care planning for African Americans. *Palliat Support Care*. 2019;17(3):306–313. https://doi.org/10.1017/s147895151800038x.
56. Sun A, Bui Q, Tsoh JY, et al. Efficacy of a church-based, culturally tailored program to promote completion of advance directives among Asian Americans. *J Immigr Minor Health*. 2017;19(2):381–391. https://doi.org/10.1007/s10903-016-0365-7.
57. Lakin JR, Koritsanszky LA, Cunningham R, et al. A systematic intervention to improve serious illness communication in primary care. *Health Aff (Millwood)*. 2017;36(7):1258–1264. https://doi.org/10.1377/hlthaff.2017.0219.
58. Briggs L, Hammes BJ, Anderson S. *Respecting Choices: Advance Care Planning Facilitator Certification Manual*. Gundersen Lutheran Medical Foundation; 2015.
59. Hammes BJ, Rooney BL, Gundrum JD. A comparative, retrospective, observational study of the prevalence, availability, and specificity of advance care plans in a county that implemented an advance care planning microsystem. *J Am Geriatr Soc*. 2010;58(7):1249–1255. https://doi.org/10.1111/j.1532-5415.2010.02956.x.
60. Knutzen KE, Sacks OA, Brody-Bizar OC, et al. Actual and missed opportunities for end-of-life care discussions with oncology patients: a qualitative study. *JAMA Netw Open*. 2021;4(6):e2113193. https://doi.org/10.1001/jamanetworkopen.2021.13193.
61. Kantor MA, Scott BS, Abe-Jones Y, Raffel KE, Thombley R, Mourad M. Ask about what matters: an intervention to improve accessible advance care planning documentation. *J Pain Symptom Manage*. 2021;62(5):893–901. https://doi.org/10.1016/j.jpainsymman.2021.05.007.
62. Epstein AS, Desai AV, Bernal C, et al. Giving voice to patient values throughout cancer: a novel nurse-led intervention. *J Pain Symptom Manage*. 2019;58(1):72–79.e2. https://doi.org/10.1016/j.jpainsymman.2019.04.028.
63. Gabbard J, Pajewski NM, Callahan KE, et al. Effectiveness of a nurse-led multidisciplinary intervention vs usual care on advance care planning for vulnerable older adults in an accountable care organization: a randomized clinical trial. *JAMA Intern Med*. 2021;181(3):361–369. https://doi.org/10.1001/jamainternmed.2020.5950.
64. Clark MA, Ott M, Rogers ML, et al. Advance care planning as a shared endeavor: completion of ACP documents in a multidisciplinary cancer program. *Psychooncology*. 2017;26(1):67–73. https://doi.org/10.1002/pon.4010.
65. Lakin JR, Benotti E, Paladino J, Henrich N, Sanders J. Interprofessional work in serious illness communication in primary care: a qualitative study. *J Palliat Med*. 2019;22(7):751–763. https://doi.org/10.1089/jpm.2018.0471.
66. Izumi SS, Caron D, Guay-Bélanger S, et al. Development and evaluation of serious illness conversation training for interprofessional primary care teams. *J Palliat Med*. 2023;26(9):1198–1206. https://doi.org/10.1089/jpm.2022.0268.
67. Izumi S, Fromme EK. A model to promote clinicians' understanding of the continuum of advance care planning. *J Palliat Med*. 2017;20(3):220–221. https://doi.org/10.1089/jpm.2016.0516.
68. Hickman SE, Lum HD, Walling AM, Savoy A, Sudore RL. The care planning umbrella: the evolution of advance care planning. *J Am Geriatr Soc*. 2023;71(7):2350–2356. https://doi.org/10.1111/jgs.18287.
69. Span P. The patients were saved. That's why the families are suing. *New York Times*. April 11, 2017. https://www.nytimes.com/2017/04/10/health/wrongful-life-lawsuit-dnr.html.
70. American Nurses Association. *Position Statement: Nurses' Roles and Responsibilities in Providing Care and Support at the End of Life*. American Nurses Association; 2016.
71. National Hospice and Palliative Nurses Association. HPNA Position Statement: Advance Care Planning. Accessed January 12, 2025.https://www.advancingexpertcare.org/practice-research/statements-hpna/.
72. Izumi S. Advance care planning: the nurse's role. *Am J Nurs*. 2017;117(6):56–61.
73. Pelland K, Morphis B, Harris D, Gardner R. Assessment of first-year use of Medicare's advance care planning billing codes. *JAMA Intern Med*. 2019;179(6):827–829. https://doi.org/10.1001/jamainternmed.2018.8107.

7

Value-Based Care

Rory B. Farrand and Aparna Gupta

Key Points

- Value-based care (VBC) is a healthcare delivery model where providers are paid based on the health outcomes and quality of care of their patients, rather than the amount or type of services they deliver
- Stakeholders who will be impacted by VBC include all players (payers, providers, patients/families) across all settings of care. Hospice and palliative care providers are not immune from the shift from volume to value and are, in fact, well poised to support VBC delivery payment approaches.
- Documentation and data empower VBC teams to reduce costs and improve healthcare outcomes and operational performance.

Introduction

Today's healthcare environment is ever seeking measured improvement in a person's health outcomes, without exceeding costs related to achieving that improvement.[1] One way payers such as Medicare are seeking improved value is through innovative approaches to care, including supportive models such as those exemplified by palliative care.[2] Our population is aging, and today older adults are living with more chronic illnesses than ever before.[3] Additionally, the whole of our population is affected by longstanding systemic inequities, disparities stemming from social determinants of health or poor health outcomes related to not having access to quality primary (or specialty) care. Following the early years of the COVID-19 pandemic, the US health sector saw a 9.7% increase in total national healthcare spending, driving the costs upward of $4 trillion.[4] At the same time, the United States spends the most on healthcare[5,6] without a comparable increase in patient-centered outcomes. As these costs rise, healthcare delivery systems and payers continue to seek opportunities to curb spending while also attempting to ensure that beneficiaries receive the care and services they need to stay healthy, happy, and productive. Following the introduction of the Affordable Care Act much attention has been focused on value-based care (VBC), or care delivered under value-based contracts with the goal of achieving the "triple aim." The goals of the triple aim are to provide better care for individuals (which can improve the overall health of identified populations), improve the care experience for patients, and lower costs of care.[7] Despite these noble intentions, for many provider organizations, translating the premise of VBC into practice can be challenging.

From Volume to Value

At its core, VBC is a healthcare delivery concept under which providers—hospitals, labs, physicians, advanced practice providers, and others—are paid/incentivized based on the health *outcomes* of their patients and the quality of services rendered, in contrast to reimbursement based on volume. Positive patient outcomes include better managed chronic disease burden and use of evidence-based practice to promote healthy behaviors—ideally to prevent health-related conditions before they become problems. This proactive, rather than reactive, approach also emphasizes a team-based model for care; an example is that patients can be enrolled in patient-centered medical homes, which are not actually physical locations but describe an approach to care led by patients' primary care providers (PCPs). A patient's interprofessional care team may include expected members such as physicians or nurses but can also include social workers, chaplains, case managers, mental health specialists, pharmacists, dieticians, educators, psychologists, health coaches, administrators, and even others. Not all team members may be providing direct clinical care; however, they do work collaboratively with patients and caregivers to help identify and address each individual's healthcare needs. The idea is to engage patients and to help them solve problems and better manage their total health. Within the framework of this model, patient data is shared, and care is coordinated across providers/settings, which can limit or even reduce unwanted services and procedures.

Accountable care organizations (ACOs) are a variation on this approach specifically for Medicare beneficiaries. Providers work together to provide the most effective care for the lowest cost, and again, there is an emphasis on both collaborative teamwork and sharing of data. The most advanced types of VBC, often called "next-generation" models, are showing the greatest potential for improved outcomes and lower costs.[8] Next-generation models include ACO products, which can be comprised of integrated groups of doctors, hospitals, and other healthcare providers that work together to provide high-quality coordinated care. Sometimes joint ventures (JVs) form where two organizations, such as a health system and an insurance company, partner to form a new company and a new health plan.

Another approach to VBC payment reimbursement may take the form of capitation, where providers take on financial responsibility for the health and well-being of the patient population they serve. One of the earliest examples of this approach is the hospice model of care. Hospice providers are paid a per-diem rate, which covers all professional services, ancillary supplies, and equipment defined by the Medicare Hospice Benefit that relate to the patient's terminal illness and that are documented in the plan of care. There is no need for a patient to defer hospice care due to financial concerns. The per-diem rate varies by level of care and by the location where the service is delivered. All hospices in the local market receive the same per-diem rate from Medicare for the same level of service. The per-diem rate includes the program medical director's general supervisory services and the team physician's participation in developing the patient's plan of care.

The Centers for Medicare & Medicare Services (CMS), a state, and a health plan can also engage in capitation to provide comprehensive, coordinated care. With this approach, the health plan is given a lump sum (prospective payment) for each member based on what the health plan predicts is the likely amount spent for that member.[9] Commercial health plans have also demonstrated how capitation approaches (over fee-for-service models) better incentivize physicians to prioritize preventive care to keep patients healthy and out of hospitals. Patients with more significant medical issues cost more to care for, so providers are incentivized to keep patients healthy and to prevent illness.[10]

A further extension of a capitated model includes shared savings and shared risk, where payers establish a budget for costs associated with delivering care for a group of individuals. If providers can deliver care below that budget target, they can share in the savings; however, if their costs exceed the budget, due to shared risk, providers would be responsible to pay for those additional costs.[11] Hospice and palliative care providers are well poised to engage in certain payment demonstration models that are aimed at primary care practices that are already taking on risk. This is because improving care for high-need, high-cost individuals with multiple chronic conditions and complex social needs is a growing priority for policymakers, payers, and health systems. The new High Needs ACO Realizing Equity, Access, and Community Health program shifts the emphasis of care delivery from what will be reimbursed toward services that will bring downstream value. ACOs are looking for high-quality hospice providers to expand access to palliative care that reduces cost and improves patient experience for their members.

This shift from fee-for-service to VBC has significantly changed the way healthcare is delivered and, of course, reimbursed, as outlined. In addition to how providers choose to negotiate payments, they may be able to earn incentives for providing high-quality, efficient care. VBC differs from the traditional fee-for-service model where providers are paid separately for each medical service rendered. While quality care can be provided under all the available payment approaches, it is the difference in how providers are paid, paired with the way patient care is managed, that provides the opportunity for health improvements and savings in a VBC environment.

The Stakeholders

There is hardly a segment of the healthcare continuum that is not impacted by the shift to VBC. While the pandemic highlighted some significant challenges in the US healthcare system, it also helped elevate concerns that have been at the forefront of patients' minds, namely those related to treatment for mental health and issues related to chronic disease management. Quality outcomes related to these, as well as other, concerns may help patients improve their health if the program in which they receive their healthcare coverage is enrolled under a value-based arrangement. One of the advantages of VBC approaches is how the models support patients so that they are not left to navigate the healthcare system on their own. The care team supports patients throughout their healthcare journey; prevention, wellness, as well as identification of strategies to better coordinate care across the continuum are all equally important priorities, especially for those managing chronic conditions.

Payers are other stakeholders in the shift to VBC, whether the payer is Medicare, Medicaid, or a commercial insurer. Previously, the focus on volume likely contributed to the ballooning of healthcare costs in the United States. The 2020 National Health Expenditures report, prepared by the CMS, notes that private health insurer spending was $1.15 trillion in 2020, making up 28% of the total national spending. The next highest tier of dollars spent was by Medicare (making up 20%), which amounted to $829.5 billion, while Medicaid spending came in at $671.2 billion.[4] The report also noted that the three largest categories of where these dollars were spent was on hospital care, physician and clinical services, as well as retail prescription drugs. Whether through paycheck deduction for our employer-sponsored health plans or by contributing part of earnings in taxes, all taxpayers end up shouldering the burdens of these expenditures. Reports[6,12] comparing the health system performance of several high-income countries find that, among them, the United States spends far and away the most on healthcare but, despite this outlay of dollars, ranks at the bottom for performance as well as for access, equity, and healthcare outcomes. Other countries in these reports included Australia, Canada, France, Germany, the Netherlands, New Zealand, Norway, Sweden, Switzerland, and the United Kingdom.[6,12]

Providers are not immune to the shift toward VBC. With disease burden in the United States listed as the highest among developed countries, 6 in 10 American adults have at least one chronic condition—high blood pressure, diabetes, mental illness—and 4 in 10 are managing more than one condition.[13] According to the Centers for Disease Control and Prevention, 90% of healthcare dollars are spent each year for people with chronic and mental health conditions.[14]

Patients experiencing serious illness are the last group of stakeholders who are impacted by VBC. Patients who have multiple chronic illnesses are frequent utilizers of emergency departments for care and are more frequently hospitalized[15] (with longer stays); this stresses an already overburdened care system plagued by staffing shortages, clinician burnout, and intensive, sometimes futile interventions, especially for patients at the end of life.[16] With VBC approaches, providers may find that their patients are healthier and more satisfied with their care and that their practices are more efficient and possibly even more profitable if they can reap benefits from shared savings. Additionally, palliative care interventions are associated with a decrease in total healthcare costs, a reduction in healthcare resource utilization, and improvements in patient (and caregiver) reported outcomes,[17] especially when delivered in the home setting.[18]

VBC and Collaboration across Care Settings

Many Americans are used to a healthcare system that takes care of people once they are already sick; however, within VBC, the focus on the triple aim is to improve the healthcare experience, improve the health of individuals and populations, and reduce the costs of healthcare.[7] To do this, VBC models aim to move beyond reactive, sickness-focused care and instead adopt a proactive, team-oriented, and data-driven approach to keeping people healthy.[19] However, clinicians who practice in inpatient/hospital settings generally do not interact with patients when they are well. For VBC to be effective, clinicians, including those who practice in acute care settings, need to consider changes to their practice patterns; VBC models will also need to align incentives for practitioners of emergency medicine, as well as for other hospital-based clinicians, to drive desirable behaviors. Historically, productivity-based reimbursement is ingrained in many hospital settings, so reimbursement tied to quality outcomes will require some adjustment to all the parties involved.

Outpatient settings should partner with patients to drive responsible behaviors that lead to good outcomes and can help avoid complications of chronic illness. A focus on maintaining health can help keep people from becoming patients in the first place, which eases burdens on our healthcare systems. VBC arrangements are not limited to clinicians; early VBC arrangements included purchasers of drugs or medical devices. The goals of these arrangements were to improve access to effective but possibly costly products by linking coverage of and/or payment for services to specified desirable outcomes.

Nursing facilities may elect to engage with CMS' Skilled Nursing Facility (SNF) Value-Based Purchasing program,[20] which awards incentive payments to encourage SNFs to improve the quality of care they deliver to Medicare beneficiaries receiving care in those settings. Currently the program looks at a single measure: all-cause readmissions. It is easy to understand how this success using this measure can help to control costs to Medicare but also improve quality of life for patients. The program is funded by a small percentage withheld from Medicare Part A payments, and then the program redistributes a portion of this to SNFs as incentive payments.[20]

While assisted living facilities do not typically engage in value-based contracts, home-based care providers, including home health agencies, may be impacted by these emerging models of care. Home-based care providers are uniquely positioned to support VBC outcomes due to their unfiltered look at how patients actually live with their serious illness conditions. Home health aides, nurses, and other clinicians seeing patients in their homes can use tools such as those developed by INTERACT (e.g., STOP and WATCH); such tools can identify the earliest changes in patients and help them to address concerns early, when many conditions are easier to manage.[21] Patient monitoring technology that uploads data or provides alerts in real time also have considerable value. Home health providers can partner with PCP groups to help avoid unnecessary hospitalizations by helping patients understand and adhere to their plan of care, as well as to provide education and guidance related to changes of condition.

Innovation related to how to best utilize how healthcare dollars are spent can also be found in the Veteran's Health Administration (VHA).[22] The VHA's Center for Care and Payment Innovation has launched pilot programs to introduce value-based payments within the VHA. These pilots focus on proactive identification of high-risk, high-need veterans to address both serious illness challenges and health equity issues; however, the sheer size of this system as well as the unique needs of the nation's veterans have been just a few of the challenges related to adopting VBC approaches. As with all other value-based approaches in healthcare, another hurdle related to implementation of VBC has been related to data sharing. As already outlined, one of the critical areas of VBC is the sharing of data to improve outcomes; and while a large system like the VHA has many platforms that may take time to fully mature to the complex VBC environment, clinicians in the system can focus on incremental changes intended to improve outcomes and continue to focus on high-quality care to veterans, including those with serious illness.

A publication[23] looking at care provided within correctional settings identified several high-priority needs to reduce mortality of those persons in custody. While some may question why this setting is included here, the reality is that many incarcerated persons enter facilities in already poor health; additionally, they struggle with mental illness, disease, and addiction in disproportionate numbers compared to the rest of the population.[23,24] Florence Nightingale's environmental theory of nursing has one core principle: that nursing is "the act of utilizing the environment of the patient to assist that patient in their recovery"[25(p1)]; the reality for persons in custody is that the settings in which they are confined can actually be detrimental to overall health and safety in a variety of ways. Given this perspective, the types of living conditions found in correctional settings may exacerbate certain preexisting conditions; and, coupled with the fact that there has been growth in incarceration rates, it can be extrapolated that those settings house significant numbers of generally unhealthy (as well as seriously ill) individuals for longer periods of time.[23] Many of these individuals are also aging and may develop a serious illness over the course of their incarceration. Incarcerated persons have been reported to have high pain and symptom burdens and generally poorer health outcomes than peers who are not incarcerated.[24] Add rising health costs to the equation, the combined result generally represents a significant taxpayer burden. While there are no specific pilots or projects related to VBC and the providers of care to this population, it is the authors' opinions that several of the priorities outlined in the publication equate to those outlined in the triple aim, which makes this setting a good match for value-based approaches to care. Additionally, incorporating palliative care and hospice within the correctional system will ensure that even incarcerated persons can receive holistic symptom management and are not denied their right to compassionate end-of-life care, which benefits not only those incarcerated individuals but their families and even society.[24]

Case Study: VBC in Action

Hal is a 47-year-old with chronic kidney disease (CKD) living in Philadelphia, Pennsylvania, and has been receiving his medical care from and is supported by a team within his local accountable care network. Not long ago, Hal was admitted to the hospital with shortness of breath and swelling in both legs, indications that the symptoms of his disease were not controlled. CKD affects about 15% of adults in the United States, and it can be both a very burdensome as well as expensive disease that becomes costlier as the disease progresses toward kidney failure.[26] Despite patients with advanced CKD and/or end-stage renal disease generally having low admission rates to hospice, research indicates that multidisciplinary care programs upstream from end-of-life care can be an effective way to slow the progression of kidney disease. Slowing the progression can ideally reduce the need for dialysis and other costly interventions while also extending life expectancy.[27]

As Hal's care was provided through an ACO, which is a previously discussed approach to VBC, he worked closely with a nurse case manager who conducted a comprehensive assessment to identify gaps in his and his partner's understanding about his CKD and then also provided specific, achievable goals to help improve his symptoms/health. The case manager made a referral to a dietician, who answered Hal's questions about a kidney-friendly diet and made numerous practical suggestions about how to make smarter choices.

As Hal's illness progressed and he eventually required hemodialysis, he struggled to adapt to how this affected his ability to work a traditional job with regular hours; thus, Hal and his partner both were increasingly worried about financial security. The ACO case manager suggested that Hal consider enrolling in a palliative care program that was affiliated with their group. The case manager referred Hal to a palliative care social worker (PCSW). Despite initial hesitation due to a misunderstanding of how palliative care differs from hospice, Hal accepted the referral, and the PCSW helped Hal wade through the often complicated process of applying for disability support. The PCSW also recognized symptoms of increased depression and anxiety and provided counseling and support to keep him making positive choices, despite feeling discouraged and overwhelmed. The primary care physician and nurse practitioner worked with Hal's nephrologist to get his physical symptoms under control, which helped Hal feel better and able to continue his dialysis treatments Through the combined efforts of his multidisciplinary team, Hal had fewer symptom-related crises and was empowered to reach out for help/support as necessary. This meant Hal was more knowledgeable about self-management and recognized changes in his condition earlier, before they became problems; thereby, he was not routinely seeking care though his emergency department. His commitment to optimal health while living with a serious illness and the support he received from his care team helped him to obtain a spot on a kidney transplant waitlist.

In VBC, Patients Are Part of the Team

Patients like Hal may spend only a few hours each year in their providers' care and countless hours where they are responsible for their own self-care. When education and communication are robust and information is shared freely across care teams, patients experience enhanced trust and engagement. This helps both patients (and caregivers) feel more empowered to take better care of themselves between visits, as well as to relay concerns or issues back to their care teams. All of these are essential elements for the success of prevention strategies and care management programs. Evidence shows that care teams involved in VBC may have a number of positive outcomes, including improved quality of care and patient satisfaction; and providers may benefit from shared savings resulting from lower healthcare expenditures within the population they serve.[28] These teams recognize that involving patients in conversations about treatment plans and medications, that is, engaging them in shared decision-making, helps patients to achieve their desired outcomes; more importantly, when care teams are aware of patients' goals for their own health, they are less likely to recommend interventions or procedures which are not aligned with those stated goals.[29] Also, it takes a community to transform a population: resources like nutritionists, social workers, in-home liaisons, and mental health counselors are likely to be tapped to address unmet needs and to help patients meet their goals.

Documentation and Data: The "Secret Sauce" That Empowers VBC Teams to Improve Outcomes and Performance

The current world is a digital world with extraordinary access to a wealth of information. Healthcare, with robust electronic health records (EHRs) or electronic medical records (EMRs), has the ability to receive, analyze, and share healthcare data across settings of care. Ideally, this facilitates communication and collaboration by connecting patients and their healthcare teams with actionable clinical information. Members of the care teams within ACOs and JVs, for example, all have rapid access to the same data, providing the best opportunity to deliver the right treatment at the right time. Extended members of the patient's care team can use this information to identify gaps in care and proactively reach out to patients who are due for a primary care visit or a preventive screening. Actionable information of this sort can help patients and caregivers who may be having difficulty managing conditions or struggling with the treatment plan, for example, when the patient has not filled a prescription or lagged in making an appointment for follow-up care.

Innovations in remote patient monitoring or other types of technologies allow patients to capture and share self-generated data, which empowers patients to be active participants in maintaining their health and can boost engagement and collaboration within the extended care team.[30] EMRs/EHRs may send patients information to help them better understand their conditions and medications and encourage them to stick to established treatment plans. Wearable technology, such as those which exist on many smart watches, collects important health data individuals can use to track their own health; gamification can help incentivize patients to beat their own personal best achievements. Patients who may use features like electrocardiogram monitoring or fall alerts may elect to share that captured data with their healthcare team, and this may allow them to intervene quickly as appropriate. Of course, telemedicine can improve outcomes and lower costs for patients who would not otherwise seek needed care through traditional means. This can be especially helpful in mental health care where stigma still keeps many from seeking services.

What is exciting about VBC models of care is a newfound embrace of the idea that health is more than the absence of disease. Asking about and collecting data related to social drivers of health (the communal, physical, and economic conditions of the environments where people live, work, and age) puts people on a path to improve equity and access to care as many of the causes of healthcare disparities are attributable to increased costs and poor outcomes.[31] Populations and individuals who may benefit from initiatives that address food insecurity, housing instability, poor access to healthcare, low health literacy/education, as well as needs for transportation and employment opportunities may find opportunities to address these issues if their provider/payer is participating in VBC arrangements.[32,33] Some payers have taken the initiative to develop community gardens or have proposed affordable housing initiatives and other programs (e.g., access to ride-shares) that provide greater access to local healthcare. This kind of holistic care delivery provides all individuals of a population, and the community at large, the best opportunities to be healthier.

How Does All of This Add Up to Improved Outcomes?

Patient-centered outcomes are the north star for every provider and payer interaction. The eventual desired goal is optimization of cost and resources, along with continued improvement in healthcare outcomes. The healthcare outcomes may appear to be different and will need to be individualized for every consumer, community, and family. For example, health outcomes in chronic disease are reflected differently than health outcomes in the presence of low health literacy or those that are along the chronic illness and end-of-life continuum. When the focus of each healthcare professional and part of the healthcare system becomes improved outcomes, then more people receive preventive services like colonoscopies, mammograms, and flu vaccinations. Individuals have a better experience navigating the healthcare system. Not only that, but health risk factors and early disease are more rapidly detected and addressed. Chronic diseases, like high blood pressure, diabetes, and kidney disease are more likely to be under control. There are fewer emergency room visits, hospitalizations, and readmissions, which in turn leads to a more satisfactory patient/family experience and reduced healthcare cost. Healthcare is coordinated and efficient, data and technology are utilized effectively, and patients are engaged in care. Hospice, a value-based approach to care from its inception, and palliative care delivered upstream from hospice are both focused on patients' goals, wishes, and what matters most to them as they receive care. According to the Center to Advance Palliative Care, palliative care drives high satisfaction and positive patient experiences, with 93% of people who have received palliative care being likely to recommend it to others. Additionally, palliative care markedly improves quality of life and symptom burden as much as 66%, with these results lasting months after an initial palliative care consultation. While these results are reason enough to incorporate palliative care into population health approaches, the concurrent reduction in healthcare expenditures and utilizations across settings of care (whether inpatient, outpatient, skilled nursing, or home) is how palliative care demonstrates its value.[34]

VBC and Healthcare Cost

The concept of VBC requires the pivotal role of a proactive, data-driven approach, which also means that providers, patients, and payers (e.g., insurance companies) are better aligned with the goals of keeping patients healthy and keeping costs down over time. Management and optimization of any health risk factors and identification of early-stage disease are important for patients and less expensive than late-stage interventions and hospitalizations. Thus, well-managed chronic conditions incur fewer costs compared to uncontrolled conditions that often progress at an unpredictable rate. Enhanced care coordination and data sharing can also help streamline administrative processes and reduce wasted spending.

Healthcare cost savings can be generated from multiple sources like early detection and proactively addressing risk factors; enhanced patient engagement and better management of chronic conditions; standardization of care and utilization of specialty centers of excellence; better use of evidence-based decision-making, leading to personalized treatment plans; informed referrals and best site of service, such as utilizing walk-in clinics and urgent care sites rather than emergency rooms, when appropriate; improved care coordination, fewer complications, and hospitalizations; fewer unnecessary or duplicative tests and procedures; and prescribing of generic medications when possible.

A recent study from NORC at the University of Chicago[35] found that, in the last year of life, the total costs of care to Medicare for beneficiaries who used hospice was 3.1% lower than those who did not. In 2019, the last year data was not affected by the pandemic, Medicare spending for those who received hospice care was $3.5 billion less for hospice patients compared to those who received no hospice care. The research also showed that even when patients were in hospice for longer periods, of 6 months or more, cost savings to Medicare were achieved. Considering that only 52% of Medicare's 2019 decedents were enrolled in hospice, increased adoption of the practice would generate even more Medicare savings. Again, while savings for payers are important, patients and families can also experience less financial strain by having more days wherever they may call home (as compared to in-hospital days) during their end-of-life journeys.[36]

Keeping It Simple: Effective Messaging of VBC for Patients and Families

While providers and healthcare professionals often understand VBC in the context of care delivery, the concept may get lost in the message to consumers and patients. Keeping the focus of care delivery on optimized and evidence-based pathways as well as the best possible patient experience is an easy and effective message that can be standardized at the workflow level. It is important for providers to share the same or similar messaging when communicating the importance of VBC. Do not assume that the patient knows what quality metrics, data collection, and outcome-driven care mean. An assessment of health literacy and level of engagement in self-care is important for the provider to understand what kind of educational resources would be beneficial for the patient to understand and to be an engaged partner in value-based, person-driven care. A sole focus on reducing cost and minimizing healthcare services (where necessary) is not the best way to explain VBC and may lead to resistance or doubts from the patient, who may be seeking the best care possible during acute or chronic illness. Rather, a focus on high-quality, healthcare outcome–driven, efficient, and timely care, as well an optimum patient experience, will motivate the patient and the family to engage productively as best as possible.

Barriers to Implementing VBC

Knowledge management (KM), time constraints, and lack of buy-in are the biggest barriers to implementing VBC. KM has become a core logistic support activity for the healthcare organization (HCO), providing the communication essential for care; defining, acquiring, and maintaining performance measures; and supporting learning activities.[37] These activities require financial resources, education, staff training, and a continuous focus on quality innovation as well as clinical excellence.

While a robust use of KM requires resources from every part of the HCO, effective KM also delivers efficiency for the provider and a data-driven, streamlined manner of billing, coding, reimbursement, and evaluation of quality metrics. A data-driven approach provides the information providers need at their fingertips for closing preventative gaps, meeting quality thresholds, and leading the HCO toward shared savings and VBC where applicable. On the other hand, HCOs that do not focus on KM and data management will likely struggle with provider time management, efficient data collection and evaluation, and managing quality measures.

In the absence of effective and timely internal data collection, providers do not have the visibility that is needed at the point of care for customizing treatment plans and engaging the patient meaningfully. Finally, a lack of buy-in and commitment to VBC at all levels of the organization, from the board of directors to the front line, is a barrier to effective implementation of VBC. A laser focus on evidence-based care pathways; standardized workflows; data collection, monitoring, and analysis; as well as periodic evaluation of population healthcare outcomes is necessary for a VBC model to be implemented. To deliver on what patients and families expect from their care, nurses (registered nurses and advanced practice nurses) must be able to practice at the fullest scope of their licensure; when this is done reports have shown that those settings of care score higher on value-based measures and patient satisfaction rates.[38] All departments of the organizations must be synchronized and tuned in as vital parts of the VBC mechanism for effective implementation of care that is consistent, high-quality, and focused on healthcare outcomes.

Conclusion

The health of the individual consumer as well as the population is dependent not only on the clinical knowledge of the provider but also on how well the HCO and the provider are focused on the outcomes of care delivery. Safe, effective, efficient, timely, and equitable care can be delivered when the provider, payer, and patient are focused on the results and quality of care delivered. This means that the traditional fee-for-service model of care is no longer sufficient for improving the health of communities and optimizing the patient experience. CMS and private insurers alike are focused on quality metrics (the "how" of care delivery) as well as outcomes (the "what" of care delivery). Thus, the most ideal environment for a provider is one where there is a focus on and commitment to collecting data, implementing consistent workflows, and improving quality of care. In a VBC model, when high-quality, low-cost care is delivered, the value of care goes up, which results in shared savings for the organization and a better, patient-centered care experience for the consumer and the family. The role of the nurse and/or nurse practitioner is central to success in understanding the basics and changing rules of VBC but also in understanding how incentives and penalties work, how the message needs to be communicated to patients, and the vital role of KM at the point of care.

REFERENCES

1. Teisberg E, Wallace S, O'Hara S. Defining and implementing value-based health care: a strategic framework. *Acad Med.* 2020;95(5):682–685. https://doi.org/10.1097/ACM.0000000000003122.
2. Centers for Medicare and Medicaid Services. Palliative Care Projects: Synthesis of Evaluation Results 2012–2021 Findings at a Glance. December 2022. Accessed May 31, 2023. https://www.cms.gov/priorities/innovation/data-and-reports/2022/palliative-care-synthesis-2012-2021-aag.
3. Pennsylvania State University. Older Adults More Likely to Have Multiple Health Ailments Than Prior Generations. Science Daily. June 13, 2022. Accessed September 7, 2022. https://www.sciencedaily.com/releases/2022/06/220613111944.htm.
4. Centers for Medicare and Medicaid Services. National Health Spending in 2020 Increases due to Impact of COVID-19 Pandemic. December 15, 2021. Accessed September 7, 2022. https://www.cms.gov/newsroom/press-releases/national-health-spending-2020-increases-due-impact-covid-19-pandemic#:~:text=Major%20payer%20spending%20in%202020%20was%20as%20follows%3A.
5. Organisation for Economic Co-operation and Development. Health at a Glance 2021: OECD Indicators. November 9, 2021. Accessed September 7, 2022. https://doi.org/10.1787/ae3016b9-en.
6. Schneider EC, Sarnak DO, Squires D, Shah A, Doty M. Mirror, *Mirror 2017: International Comparison Reflects Flaws and Opportunities for Better U.S. Health Care.* Commonwealth Fund. July 14, 2017. Accessed September 19, 2022. https://doi.org/10.26099/0mh5-a632.
7. Institute for Healthcare Improvement. IHI Triple Aim Initiative. Accessed January 16, 2025. https://www.ihi.org/improvement-areas/improvement-area-triple-aim-and-population-health.
8. NORC at the University of Chicago. *Fifth Evaluation Report—Next Generation Accountable Care Organization (NGACO) Model Evaluation.* November 2022. Accessed May 31, 2023. https://innovation.cms.gov/data-and-reports/2022/nextgenaco-fifthevalrpt.
9. Centers for Medicare and Medicaid Services. Capitated Model. March 30, 2023. Accessed May 31, 2023. https://www.cms.gov/Medicare-Medicaid-Coordination/Medicare-and-Medicaid-Coordination/Medicare-Medicaid-Coordination-Office/FinancialAlignmentInitiative/CapitatedModel.

10. Morse S. UnitedHealth Study Shows Capitation Model Works to Improve Value-Based Care. Healthcare Finance. August 14, 2020. Accessed May 31, 2023. https://www.healthcarefinancenews.com/news/unitedhealth-study-shows-capitation-model-works-improve-value-based-care#:~:text=UnitedHealth%20study%20shows%20capitation%20model%20works%20to%20improve,%28HEDIS%29%20related%20to%20preventive%20care%20and%20chronic%20conditions.
11. Urban Institute. Payment Methods and Benefit Designs: How They Work and How They Work Together to Improve Health Care. April 2016. Accessed May 31, 2023. https://www.urban.org/sites/default/files/2016/05/03/08_shared_savings.pdf#:~:text=A%20fundamental%20difference%20between%20global%20capitation%20and%20shared,or%20per%20diems%20for%20hospitals%2C%20and%20so%20on.
12. Kurani N, Wager E. How Does the Quality of the US Health System Compare to Other Countries? Health System Tracker. September 30, 2021. Accessed October 12, 2022. https://www.healthsystemtracker.org/chart-collection/quality-u-s-healthcare-system-compare-countries/#item-start.
13. Buttorff C, Ruder T, Bauman M. *Multiple Chronic Conditions in the United States*. RAND Corporation; 2017. Accessed October 12, 2022. https://www.rand.org/content/dam/rand/pubs/tools/TL200/TL221/RAND_TL221.pdf.
14. Centers for Disease Control and Prevention. Health and Economic Costs of Chronic Diseases. March 23, 2023. Accessed June 1, 2023. https://www.cdc.gov/chronicdisease/about/costs/index.htm#ref1.
15. Harris LJ, Graetz I, Podila PS, Wan J, Waters TM, Bailey JE. Characteristics of hospital and emergency care super-utilizers with multiple chronic conditions. *J Emerg Med*. 2016;50(4):e203–e214. https://doi.org/10.1016/j.jemermed.2015.09.002.
16. Singh R, Volner K, Marlowe D. Provider burnout. In: *StatPearls*. StatPearls Publishing; June 21, 2022.
17. Luta X, Ottino B, Hall P, et al. Evidence on the economic value of end-of-life and palliative care interventions: a narrative review of reviews. *BMC Palliat Care*. 2021;20:89. https://doi.org/10.1186/s12904-021-00782-7.
18. Bernstein RH, Singh LA. A value-based payment model for palliative care: an analysis of savings and return on investment. *J Ambul Care Manage*. 2019;42(1):66–73. https://doi.org/10.1097/JAC.0000000000000259.
19. Institute of Medicine. *Best Care at Lower Costs: The Path to Continuously Learning Health Care in America*. National Academies Press; 2013.
20. Centers for Medicare & Medicaid Services. The Skilled Nursing Facility Value Based Purchasing (SNF VBP) Program. 2023. Accessed January 10, 2023. https://www.cms.gov/Medicare/Quality-Initiatives-Patient-Assessment-Instruments/Value-Based-Programs/SNF-VBP/SNF-VBP-Page.
21. Briggs Healthcare. INTERACT Stop and Watch Early Warning Tool. Accessed June 1, 2023. https://www.briggshealthcare.com/INTERACT-Stop-and-Watch-Early-Warning-Tool#:~:text=The%20INTERACT%C2%AE%20Stop%20and%20Watch%20Early%20Warning%20Tool,and%20communicating%20the%20possible%20change%20to%20nursing%20staff.
22. Veteran's Administration Center for Care and Payment Innovation. Advancing a Value-Based Health Care System for All Veterans. Accessed June 1, 2023. https://www.innovation.va.gov/careandpayment/index.html.
23. Russo J. Caring for Those in Custody. National Institute of Justice. August 1, 2019. Accessed October 2, 2022. https://nij.ojp.gov/topics/articles/caring-those-custody.
24. Burles M, Holtslander L, Peternelj-Taylor C. Palliative and hospice care in correctional facilities: integrating a family nursing approach to address relational barriers. *Cancer Nurs*. 2021;44(1):29–36. https://doi.org/10.1097/NCC.0000000000000754.
25. Gonzalo A. Florence Nightingale: Environmental Theory and Biography. Nurseslabs. January 12, 2023. Accessed May 31, 2023. https://nurseslabs.com/florence-nightingales-environmental-theory/#environmental_theory.
26. Centers for Disease Control and Prevention. Chronic Kidney Disease in the US, 2021 2021. Accessed September 18, 2022. https://www.cdc.gov/kidneydisease/publications-resources/ckd-national-facts.html.
27. Lin E, Chertow GM, Yan B, Malcolm E, Goldhaber-Fiebert JD. Cost-effectiveness of multidisciplinary care in mild to moderate chronic kidney disease in the United States: a modeling study. *PLoS Med*. 2018;15(3):e1002532. https://doi.org/10.1371/journal.pmed.1002532.
28. Song Z, Ji Y, Safran DG, Chernew ME. Health care spending, utilization, and quality 8 years into global payment. *N Engl J Med*. 2019;381(3):252–263. https://doi.org/10.1056/NEJMsa1813621.
29. Abijade B. Assessing the patient's needs and planning effective care. *Br J Nurs*. 2021;30(20):1166–1171. https://www.britishjournalofnursing.com/content/clinical/assessing-the-patients-needs-and-planning-effective-care.
30. Omboni S, McManus RJ, Bosworth HB, et al. Evidence and recommendations on the use of telemedicine for the management of arterial hypertension: an international expert position paper. *Hypertension*. 2020;76(5):1368–1383. https://doi.org/10.1161/HYPERTENSIONAHA.120.15873.
31. Agency for Healthcare Research and Quality. National Healthcare Quality and Disparities Reports. March 2023. Accessed June 1, 2023. https://www.ahrq.gov/research/findings/nhqrdr/index.html.
32. Russi C, Goodman A. How Focusing on Social Determinants of Health Can Help Plans Advance Value-Based Care. ZS. July 11, 2021. Accessed June 1, 2023. https://www.zs.com/insights/how-focusing-on-sdoh-can-help-plans-advance-vbc#:~:text=Programs%20to%20address%C2%A0SDOH%20can%20include%20a%20range%20of,be%20tackled%20to%20help%20VBC%20models%20to%20thrive.
33. Centers for Disease Control and Prevention. Social Determinants of Health at CDC. December 8, 2022. Accessed June 1, 2023. https://www.cdc.gov/about/sdoh/index.html.
34. Center to Advance Palliative Care. Palliative Care Ensures Value. 2019. Accessed June 1, 2023. https://www.capc.org/documents/download/245/.
35. NORC at the University of Chicago. Value of Hospice in Medicare. March 2023. Accessed June 1, 2023. https://www.nhpco.org/wp-content/uploads/Value_Hospice_in_Medicare.pdf.
36. Roberts B, Robertson M, Ojukwu EI, Wu DS. Home based palliative care: known benefits and future directions. *Curr Geriatr Rep*. 2021;10(4):141–147. https://doi.org/10.1007/s13670-021-00372-8.
37. White KR, Griffith JR. *The Well-Managed Healthcare Organization*. 7th ed. Health Administration Press and Association of University Programs in Health Administration; 2010.
38. National Advisory Council on Nurse Education and Practice. *Promoting Nursing Leadership in the Transition to Value-Based Care*. 2019. Accessed June 1, 2023. https://www.hrsa.gov/sites/default/files/hrsa/advisory-committees/nursing/reports/2019-fifteenthreport.pdf.

8

Interdisciplinary Palliative Care Teams: Specialists in Delivering Palliative Care

Rebekah Malloy, Jessica Bullington, Catherine Rogers, and Adrienne Norquist

Key Points

- Palliative care attends to the physical, psychological, social, and spiritual domains of quality of life, providing specialty care by an interdisciplinary team of specialists for patients with serious and life-threatening illness and their families.
- The roles of the interdisciplinary palliative care team members are unique within their specialty; however, there are many instances in which team members' roles may overlap.
- There are four major models of team-based palliative care—inpatient consult teams, ambulatory care teams, community-based palliative care teams, and hospice teams—with each model providing interdisciplinary expertise in the delivery of quality palliative care across the serious illness trajectory.
- A highly functioning palliative care team requires that its members share the mission and vision of the team, share leadership accountability, and display trust and respect for each other.

Introduction

Palliative care is a medical specialty that provides relief of debilitating symptoms and stress related to serious illness and specializes in assessment and management of the physical, psychological, social, and spiritual needs of patients and their families.[1] At its core, palliative care is provided by interdisciplinary teams (IDTs), bringing together specialists from nursing, medicine, social work, chaplaincy, child life, pharmacy, volunteer services, and other specialties, as appropriate. These teams are increasing across the United States. According to a 2019 report from the Centers to Advance Palliative Care, 72% of hospitals in the United States with 50 beds or more have a palliative care team.[2] Today, palliative care is recognized as a subspecialty with over 7,600 board-certified physicians and more than 18,000 palliative care certified nurses.[2] In addition, palliative care certification is available to social workers, chaplains, physician assistants, and pharmacists.[2] Members of the palliative care team work not as individual disciplines but as a team, with a shared vision and mission to improve patient and family quality of life (QOL).[3]

Over the past two decades, the United States has witnessed a remarkable growth in palliative care services with the expansion of four major care delivery models.[1] The most frequently utilized interdisciplinary model of palliative care was initiated in the early 1990s in acute care settings as a consult service, assisting patients hospitalized with serious illness. This inpatient consult service provided specialty care in the hospital setting, with or without a dedicated palliative care unit.[4] In the early 2000s, research began to demonstrate that patients benefited from having specialty palliative care services available in ambulatory care settings. This second model for palliative care started in oncology clinics and has expanded to other outpatient specialties such as cardiovascular and neuromuscular clinics caring for those with chronic serious illness.[4,5] Most recently, the third model of palliative care delivery, community-based palliative care (CBPC) and home-based palliative care, has arisen out of a significant need to focus on the delivery of palliative care to those in the home, including assisted living and long-term care facilities. It is notable that home-based palliative care fills a gap in home care by providing numerous vital services, particularly to the frail and elderly. Home-based palliative care allows patients to receive excellent care and support for those who want to remain at home and are not yet ready for home hospice services.[6] Community-based palliative care (CBPC can be delivered in person or via telehealth in areas of limited access. Telehealth has increased, especially since the beginning of the COVID-19 pandemic.[7]

Finally, the fourth model of palliative care delivery is hospice care. Hospice services are the initial model of interdisciplinary-based palliative care, which began in the United States in the 1970s in response to a need to improve care to patients at the end of life and their families.[8] Hospice is regulated by federal programs (i.e., Medicare, Medicaid, and Veterans Affairs) in the United States, as a separate system of care for those with a "terminal illness," with a life expectancy of 6 months or less, who choose to forgo disease-focused treatment(s).[1,3,9] Hospice is palliative care that focuses on comfort measures at the end of life and not alongside disease-modifying therapies. Whereas palliative care is appropriate at any

Table 8.1 Models of palliative care

	Inpatient consult service	Ambulatory palliative care	Community-based palliative care	Hospice care
Team	Interdisciplinary team: physician, nurse; access to SW, and chaplaincy as available and as needed	Interdisciplinary team: physician, nurse; access to outpatient SW, chaplaincy as available and as needed	APRN or physician: requests are made for additional team members, if available	Interdisciplinary team: physicians, nurses, SW, chaplain, volunteers, nursing assistants, and bereavement coordinators
Eligibility	From diagnosis of serious illness across disease trajectory	From diagnosis of serious illness across disease trajectory	From diagnosis of serious illness across disease trajectory	Patients of all ages who have a prognosis of survival of 6 months or less if the disease follows its usual course; must forgo Medicare coverage for curative treatment related to the terminal illness
Delivery site	Consult services go to patients and families in the ICU, ER, and hospital units	Outpatient clinic setting; can be embedded in specialty clinics (heart failure) or in a designated palliative care clinic; ideally, space is allocated for conferencing with patients and families	In patient's home, including assisted living, long-term care facilities; may also use telehealth resources	Most hospice care is delivered in the patient's home; other sites include assisted living, long-term care facilities, residential hospice facilities, inpatient hospice units, and hospice-contracted inpatient beds
Reimbursement	Physician and APRN bill insurance or Medicare Part B for inpatient care	Physician and APRN bill for outpatient specialty visit	Physician and APRN bill insurance for specialty provider care	Team care is bundled and covered by Medicare hospice benefit or commercial insurance hospice benefit, modeled after Medicare; Medicaid coverage varies by state

APRN, advanced practice registered nurse; ER, emergency room; ICU, intensive care unit; SW, social work.

stage of serious illness, hospice benefits are used when life expectancy is 6 months or less and the patient either forgoes disease-modifying therapy or there are no further treatment options. These two services can cause great confusion to the public, yet educating patients and families, as well as other healthcare providers, remains a top priority (Table 8.1).

The focus of this chapter is on the IDT that provides specialty palliative care, regardless of the model of care delivery. The chapter emphasizes each team member's essential role in the provision of quality palliative care and how the team collaborates with the patient and family to ensure that the patient's goals of care are respected and honored. A complex case study will demonstrate the various roles of the team and their unique contributions to quality palliative care for both a patient and their family. This chapter will also discuss the four major models of palliative care in more depth and the current benefits and challenges of each model. An introduction to the development of a palliative care team and the importance of maintaining a healthy, functional team will be presented throughout the chapter.

The Interdisciplinary Palliative Care Team

According to the National Consensus Project (NCP) guidelines, palliative care "provides relief from pain and other symptoms, supports quality of life, and is focused on patients with serious advanced illness and their families." Palliative care is appropriate at any age and any stage of serious illness and can be delivered across the healthcare continuum including in the home, nursing homes, long-term acute care facilities, acute care hospitals, long-term acute care hospitals, and outpatient clinics.[3] The spectrum of palliative care can be delivered by a patient's primary care provider or specialist with primary palliative care training or by palliative care specialist when symptoms are more complex and difficult to manage.

Within Domain 1 of the NCP *Guidelines for Quality Palliative Care*, Structure and Processes of Care, there are 10 guidelines, each with its own criteria, that relate directly to the palliative care delivery model and the IDT.[3] These guidelines are important not only for the development of the palliative care team but also for sustaining the IDT by evaluating their ability to meet these criteria on a regular basis and revise processes as necessary. Quality structure and processes of care are critical to the sustainability of the palliative care IDT. Communication and collaboration within the team are essential. It is not unusual for there to be some overlap in the roles of these IDT members, but collaboration and communication among team members ensure a well-functioning team and improve the overall patient and family outcomes.

Role of the Team Members

Chaplain

According to Domain 5 of the NCP *Guidelines for Quality Palliative Care*,[3] spiritual care is an essential component of a palliative care team; however, only 44% of palliative care teams with complete IDTs report only a part-time chaplain.[10]

Spirituality is

> recognized as a fundamental aspect of compassionate, patient- and family-centered palliative care. It is a dynamic and intrinsic aspect of humanity, through which individuals seek meaning, purpose, and transcendence and experience relationships to self, family, others, community, society, and the significant or sacred. Spirituality is expressed through beliefs, values, traditions, and practices.[3]

Although it is the responsibility of all IDT members to recognize spiritual distress and attend to the patient's and the family's spiritual needs within their scope of practice, the palliative care chaplain can complete a comprehensive spiritual assessment and initiate appropriate interventions for those needing spiritual support.[2,3,11]

The primary role of the chaplain on a palliative care team is to support and/or accommodate the spiritual and religious needs of patients, families, and staff. Chaplains provide support across cultures and faiths by offering a nonjudgmental presence. Chaplains can be called on simply to talk, using religious or nonreligious language; or they can be called on to address specific religious needs, such as providing sacraments or other rituals that provide existential comfort. The goal of the chaplain is to aid in restoring identity, meaning, and/or connection to those who invite a chaplain's care. The palliative care chaplain builds on the traditional hospital chaplaincy role by assisting the team in symptom assessment, especially existential distress, eliciting goals of care, advance care planning, and supportive complex decision-making.[12] Chaplains may achieve a certification acknowledging their advanced spiritual care for those facing the end of life in palliative care with the Board Certified Chaplain—Palliative Care & Hospice Advanced Certification.[13]

Palliative Care Nurse

It is not unusual for a large palliative care team to include both registered nurses (RNs) and advanced practice RNs (APRNs). Nurses are trained to focus on the holistic needs of the person, providing supportive care for the physical, psychological, social, and spiritual needs of patients and families and advocating for those needs. While APRNs see patient consults for symptom management and goals of care in both inpatient and outpatient settings, RNs and specialty palliative care nurses (PCNs) can have a variety of roles on the team in both settings. PCNs use expert communication skills,[14] listening to patients and their families and exploring the patients' values, goals of care, and communication preferences. The PCN on the team also contributes to pain and symptom assessment and management, is skilled in pharmacological and nonpharmacological approaches to pain and symptoms, and has expertise in equianalgesia.

The PCN collaborates with the team to develop a plan to aggressively treat pain and symptoms, to reassess interventions, and to evaluate and report the efficacy to both the palliative team and other collaborating healthcare providers involved in the patient's care. PCNs can help with consult triage, care coordination, and support for bedside nurses (from help with end-of-life needs to facilitating symptom management protocols that may be less familiar to staff). The PCN has a major role in coordinating care among all healthcare providers involved in the patient's care. The nurse collaborates with the IDT to identify which team members should be involved in the patient's care based on the patient's acuity (e.g., physical, psychological, social, and/or spiritual needs) and with the patient's other healthcare providers across clinical settings (e.g., inpatient, ambulatory care, and hospice) to keep them informed of the plan of care and to ensure that the patient's values and wishes are honored.

Another key role of the PCN is education for patients and families experiencing serious illness and other healthcare professionals unfamiliar with palliative care.[15] It is often the PCN who initiates and leads debriefing of the staff who have faced challenges in caring for a patient, discussing what went well, what could have been done differently, and lessons learned for the future.

Board certification in this nursing specialty is available for RNs in both adult and pediatric populations (certified hospice and palliative nurse and certified hospice and palliative pediatric nurse), as well as for APRNs (advanced certified hospice and palliative nurse). These certifications are offered through the nursing organization the Hospice and Palliative Credentialing Center.[16]

Advanced Practice Registered Nurse

Specialty trained and board-certified master's or doctorally prepared APRNs are valuable members of the palliative care team.[17] As nurses, they can fulfill the role described for the specialty PCN; additionally, they are licensed providers who can determine and order appropriate diagnostic testing and pharmacologic interventions for patients with serious illness (the APRN scope of practice may vary by state). They receive additional training in communication and advance care planning, and many play a leadership role on the palliative care team. Fellowships and specialty certifications in palliative care are also available to APRNs.[15]

Physician

The palliative care physician brings to the palliative care team their clinical expertise in facilitating difficult conversations, as well as their knowledge of medical diagnosis, disease course, and prognostication. Medical management by a board-certified hospice and palliative medicine physician provides patients with evidence-based interventions for complex pain and symptom management. The American Academy of Hospice and Palliative Medicine recognizes the specialty of palliative medicine and offers board certification for physicians completing a fellowship in hospice and palliative medicine.[18] Hospice and palliative fellowships attract physicians from many primary specialties, including emergency medicine, pediatrics, oncology, family and internal medicine.

In addition to specialty medical management, the palliative care physician is helpful in addressing issues and concerns that the primary team or other specialists may have by clarifying information and advocating for the patient's goals and wishes. The physician participates in discharge planning by assessing the appropriateness of nursing home placement and the need for a rehabilitation facility, transitional care facility, and/or hospice. Physicians often fill the role of program director and advocate for clinical and team needs.

Social Worker

Major aspects of the social worker role in caring for patients with serious illness are to assess the needs, strengths, and resources of the patient and family; build on their strengths; enhance their connections to their resources and supports; and connect them with new resources to meet emotional, legal, and financial needs.[19] Social workers are trained to understand complex family dynamics and are skilled at integrating cultural considerations into care, communicating with patients and families, and advocating for patient preferences.[20] Additionally palliative care social workers (PCSWs) often have more flexibility to offer individual counseling and psychotherapy to patients and families in both the inpatient and ambulatory settings.[21] Depending on the policies of the institution where they are employed, the state in which they reside, and the level of licensure, social workers may be able to contribute to the financial health of a palliative care program by billing for therapy and advanced care planning.[21] While the PCSW will follow the patient and family throughout the illness, various primary/generalist social workers may also be involved in other clinic visits or hospitalizations.

Clear communication between the other social workers and nurse case managers involved in a patient's care is crucial to ensure the continuity of care and avoid duplication of effort.[19]

Palliative Care Bereavement Coordinator

The role of bereavement coordinator is not a part of every palliative care program, although bereavement care is part of quality palliative care.[3,4] Bereavement coordinators help to identify and follow up with families at risk for complicated grief. They send cards and resources to bereaved families and make regular calls to those at risk for or exhibiting signs of complicated grief. Often, they coordinate memorial/celebration of life services for family and staff. Many palliative care teams ask that their social worker or chaplain assist in this role.

Volunteers

Some palliative care teams include volunteers to offer additional support and services to patients and families, as recommended in Domain 1 of the NCP *Guidelines for Quality Palliative Care*.[3] Volunteers require supplementary palliative care training to meet the unique needs of patients with serious illness and their families. The value of volunteers should never be underestimated as the extra support they offer covers many domains and is an additional workforce that most institutions cannot afford to hire. Potential volunteer roles in palliative care include supportive visitation, end-of-life vigil and respite for families, memory-making or legacy work, pet therapy, and even volunteer facilitated complementary therapies.

For any volunteer program to thrive, particularly a specialized one, someone must be dedicated to training, guiding, and supporting these volunteers. Volunteer coordinators are an important addition to palliative care teams. Recruitment, selection, and orientation of volunteers vary among institutions, some having centralized volunteer departments to help with this onboarding process, while others may rely solely on volunteer coordinators for these duties. Palliative care volunteer coordinators identify volunteers who have interests and skills that match the needs of patients and families cared for by the team. Furthermore, coordinators provide support to these volunteers who give the gift of their time and presence to patients and families during extremely difficult times.[22] Palliative care volunteers should always have access to the coordinator for debriefing and, if possible, to the chaplain or social worker for grief and bereavement support and as well as moral distress.[23]

Ancillary Disciplines/Consultants

Ancillary disciplines and consultants will vary depending on the practice setting (e.g., home vs. inpatient); this refers to services often needed by palliative patients that usually fall outside of the core palliative care team's roles. According to the NCP *Guidelines for Quality Palliative Care*,[3] other disciplines may be included on the patient's team as needed. These ancillary disciplines are consulted for their expertise in areas of need that have been identified by the palliative care team.

Examples of these ancillary disciplines include ethics consultation, art and music therapy, recreational therapy, pet therapy, child life, nursing assistants, dieticians, occupational therapy, respiratory therapy, pharmacy, physical therapy, massage therapy, psychology, and speech and language therapy.[3] In addition, complementary and alternative therapies such as acupuncture or reiki, if available, may be utilized to address pain and symptom management if available through trained volunteers or staff.[24]

Case Study: Demonstrating the Unique Contributions of IDT Members

Jane Smith, a 40-year-old married woman with two young children, was diagnosed with a rapidly progressing neurodegenerative disease, amyotrophic lateral sclerosis. Jane and her husband, Robert, were both working parents at the time of her diagnosis. She and her family were given the devastating news that her life expectancy was 1–5 years and that her ability to live as she had would change dramatically as her disease progressed. Jane worried how her husband would manage caring for their children, John and Sarah, as well as her elderly mother. Early in her diagnosis, the palliative care team was introduced to Jane and her family. Jane learned that this team would help provide support to her and her family across the disease trajectory, as well as manage any symptoms she developed along the way.

Six months post-diagnosis, Jane developed pneumonia that resulted in respiratory distress, intubation, and admission to an intensive care unit (ICU). She was weaned from the ventilator after a few weeks and moved to an acute medical unit for further recovery. Unfortunately, her disease began to progress more rapidly, affecting her ability to walk and care for herself independently. Due to the financial burden of her 24/7 care needs, she was transferred to a long-term care unit within the hospital. She remained on this unit another 6 months until she contracted COVID-19 (SARS-CoV-2), was transferred to the ICU, and eventually died from the infection.

Throughout Jane's hospitalization, the inpatient palliative care team continued to care for her. They provided consistency and care coordination as she changed from one unit to the next. The team was able to assess her changing goals as her illness advanced. Following her intubation in the ICU, Jane stated that she did not wish to go back on a ventilator ever again. She felt very strongly about this decision, even though her husband was hesitant to relinquish this potentially life-prolonging intervention. As her illness advanced, Jane's decisions centered around prolonging her time with her family but stopped short of wanting aggressive resuscitative measures. Unfortunately, due to COVID-19 isolation precautions, her family was unable to be present with her during her final days and hours of life. The palliative care team was pivotal in Jane's care during those final moments, not only to tend to her symptoms but also to facilitate a connection between her and her family as they could not be at her bedside. In this case study, you will see how the palliative care team helped Jane by advocating for her goals of care and framed her decisions with her family and staff in the context of her desired QOL.

The following paragraphs detail how each team member addressed patient and family needs throughout the illness.

Palliative Care Chaplain

The chaplain became acquainted with Jane while participating in morning rounds as a member of the palliative care team. She reviewed her pertinent background information in the medical record and consulted with the bedside RN to gain insight into the patient's mood, recent medical events, and any observed interactions with family before going to her room.

On the first meeting, the chaplain identified herself and inquired whether Jane desired a chaplain visit. She welcomed a visit but immediately in the conversation identified herself as "not religious," although her husband, Robert, was an active member of a local faith organization. The chaplain offered affirmation of Jane's experiences with structured religion and invited further broadening of the discussion as to the things that she felt gave her life meaning and connection. Jane stated that she found greatest meaning when she was engaged in her children's lives and, therefore, was experiencing anxiety due to loss of involvement with them because of her current hospitalization. She also stated that she was struggling with loss of autotomy as she was becoming more dependent on others for many aspects of her care.

The chaplain employed active listening to assist the patient in identifying and celebrating ways that her influence continues to play a role in her children's development, exploring ways she could feel less isolated, and allowing emotional space for the patient to safely express her fears and frustrations. At the conclusion of the visit, Jane expressed that she felt less anxious and thanked the chaplain for the opportunity to give voice to her existential struggles. She also indicated that she was open to follow-up visits and invited the chaplain to return when her husband was present so that he could also feel supported. Immediately after the visit, the chaplain documented a detailed spiritual assessment in the patient's medical record and a follow-up plan and consulted with the other members of the palliative care team. The chaplain continued to provide support throughout Jane's hospitalization and at the end of life was a familiar presence at her bedside to provide words of comfort and to facilitate a video conference call to Robert and their children.

PCN

The PCN became actively involved in Jane's care during her ICU admission. The PCN completed a thorough physical assessment, paying close attention to Jane's pain and other distressing symptoms. The PCN then gathered information from the ICU team regarding Jane's condition, sharing changes, concerns regarding the progression of disease, and treatment options with the rest of the palliative care team. From there, the PCN coordinated a formal family meeting with Jane, her family, and the palliative care team to discuss concerns, changes in condition, and goals of care and to provide emotional support to Jane and her family. After Jane was successfully extubated, the nurse ensured that all members of the IDT and other healthcare providers were aware that Jane did not want to be reintubated and documented her conversation with Jane in the electronic medical record.

Knowing that care preferences can change over time, the PCN continued to check in with Jane and her family. The PCN provided a mindful presence to allow Jane and her family to process difficult information and concerns. Although Jane's husband disagreed with her decision not to be reintubated, the PCN allowed Jane's husband to express his distress and assisted him in reframing expectations for Jane's care through her eyes.

Throughout the trajectory of Jane's hospitalization, the PCN assisted in assessing, planning, intervening, and reassessing Jane's pain and symptoms. Recognizing that Jane's distress was not only physical but also spiritual and emotional pain, the PCN collaborated with the chaplain and social workers to ensure that Jane's needs were being addressed. As Jane's disease progressed, she expressed that she did not want to die at home and was aware that it would be too difficult for the family to provide the level of nursing care she needed 24/7. Although hospice services were offered, she preferred not to die in her home. The PCN documented these wishes and remained involved by providing ongoing support to ensure Jane's comfort until her death.

Palliative Care Physician

The palliative care physician met Jane for the first time at the time of diagnosis, in the neurology clinic, and then again as an inpatient when she was admitted to the hospital. In both instances, it was critical to assess her understanding of her disease and its progressive, life-limiting nature, treatment options, and symptoms, as well as her need for psychological, social, and spiritual support.

Management of her dyspnea and pain was critical during her hospitalization. The palliative care physician worked with the team and respiratory therapy to develop a plan to keep Jane as comfortable as possible. Specific conversations with Jane and her husband during her hospital admission included a discussion about the eventual respiratory failure that results from this disease and the treatment options available when that time comes. A discussion of reintubation and tracheostomy—the risks, benefits, and burdens—as well as expectations that accompany each option was presented during her hospitalization. QOL and patient values were at the center of these conversations.

During Jane's stay in the long-term care unit, the palliative care physician continued the conversation about goals of care and began to discuss end-of-life planning. That conversation included a discussion of eating for pleasure, despite its aspiration risks. For her, the comfort and pleasure associated with eating was always worth the risk.

Once Jane returned to the ICU setting and continued to decline clinically, she confirmed her desire to die in the hospital instead of at home. The physician confirmed Jane's desire to continue comfort-focused interventions and, given the progression of her disease and severity of symptoms, initiated general inpatient hospice benefits to ensure her comfort while remaining in a familiar environment.

Palliative Care Social Worker

The PCSW, along with the palliative care team physician, met Jane, Robert, and Jane's mother at the neurology clinic to provide emotional support to them after Jane's diagnosis of a devastating life-limiting illness. The PCSW acknowledged that the grieving of the loss of their life together had already begun and offered support groups locally and online that could help the family, as well as tips on communicating and supporting the children as Jane's disease progressed.

During the psychosocial assessment, it was clear that a strength for Jane and Robert was that their friends, neighbors, and faith community were eager to offer assistance in any way they could. Jane and Robert shared that they had always been uncomfortable accepting help, even prior to this diagnosis, and were so overwhelmed that they did not know what help to ask for. The PCSW provided support and attempted to normalize their feelings of being overwhelmed by the flood of offers to assist. Together Jane, Robert, and the PCSW thought through options to help Jane and Robert define what their needs were and better manage offers of help. Jane and Robert felt that an online tool to create a care calendar that they could update with needs and where family and friends could sign up for certain tasks would be the most helpful to them. The PCSW helped them to identify free online resources and encouraged Jane and Robert to identify a neighbor who could monitor the website and manage updates.

To ensure continuity of care, the PCSW met with Jane when she was initially admitted to the hospital. During that assessment, Jane's primary worry was that she was nearing the end of long-term disability from her job, which would also mean that her health insurance would terminate. The PCSW counseled Jane and Robert on starting the application process for Social Security Disability either online or by making an appointment at their local Social Security office. During this conversation, the PCSW also introduced the concept of completing advance directives, encouraged Jane and Robert to complete estate planning, and provided a list of experts in the community who could respond quickly to their needs.

When Jane was admitted to the ICU with an aspiration event, the PCSW met with Robert and Jane's mother for support. The PCSW also provided hospital resources to Robert about how to prepare their children to visit Jane in the ICU. The PCSW offered support and validation for Robert as he struggled to find the best answers for his children when they asked if they would ever be able to speak with their mother again. Additionally, the PCSW connected him with a child life specialist (CLS) who could offer further education and information on explaining Jane's condition to their children. After Jane's continued decline in the long-term care unit left her unable to feed herself but wanting to eat in spite of the risk of aspiration pneumonia, the PCSW supported Robert as he made the final decisions regarding Jane's care, including no reintubation, which was respecting Jane's previous stated advanced directives.

As Jane's death became imminent, the PCSW reconnected Robert with the CLS for assistance in communicating with their children that Jane was dying. Robert was provided a list of grief resources (counselors, groups, camps, websites, and a book list) for him and the children. The chaplain and the PCSW made certain that Jane's room was peaceful and provided support to the family throughout Jane's last days.

The palliative care team held a debriefing session, led by the PCSW and chaplain, for staff the week after her death. They, too, were grieving the loss of this vibrant woman whose independence they had grown to admire. Nine months later, at the hospital's bereavement service, which Jane's entire family attended, Robert shared with the PCSW the bereavement cards he received quarterly from the palliative care team. He shared how these helped him realize that others were still thinking of Jane. He enrolled the children in a grief camp in the coming months, and together they attended a grief support group at their church regularly, which helped them to know that they were not alone in their grief.

Volunteers

The Smith family benefited from the presence of palliative care volunteers throughout the course of Jane's hospitalization. When Jane was initially admitted to the ICU, palliative care volunteers provided supportive visits to her family and brought the children coloring books and other activities to use while visiting at the hospital. As Jane improved and was no longer intubated, volunteers were able to communicate with her directly and provide supportive visits when her family members were at school or at work.

The palliative care volunteers continued this supportive relationship as Jane transferred to other units within the hospital. Their continued visitation furnished a consistent, nonclinical relationship based on providing compassionate presence, active listening, and comfort. Over time, the volunteers provided many services to both Jane and her family, including helping her with journaling and assisting her with composing letters and cards for her children to receive after she was gone. As Jane's illness progressed and her family struggled to cope with their inevitable loss, a volunteer assisted with legacy work for her children, making memory stones with Jane's fingerprint. Jane's children were able to carry these stones with her fingerprint in their pockets wherever they went, feeling a tangible connection with their mother.

Ancillary Disciplines Consulted

Ethics Consultation

After Jane's transfer to a long-term care unit within the hospital, staff grew concerned about her ability to swallow food and drink. Both her family and staff worried she might aspirate again and questioned whether they should continue to provide comfort feeding. Jane made it clear to everyone that eating was an important aspect of her life and that she did not want life support if she aspirated. Due to the distress of family and the staff taking care of Jane, an ethics consult was called to help clarify the situation. Through the ethics consultation, it was determined that because her wishes were well known and documented in her advance directive, there was no conflict with feeding her. Family also joined the ethics consultation to note recommendations and to affirm that they would carry out Jane's wishes.

Respiratory Therapy

Respiratory therapy was involved throughout Jane's hospitalization, from intubation in the ICU to her final hours of life. Respiratory therapists worked with Jane on maintaining her lung function and airway clearance for as long as possible and tailored their interventions to support her wishes of no reintubation. They made recommendations to the medical team to administer corticosteroids and other bronchodilators in her final days of life to ensure that she would not endure dyspnea in the last hours of her life.

Physical and Occupational Therapy

Physical and occupational therapists were involved in Jane's care plan from her time of diagnosis to help preserve her functional status, safety, and ability to perform activities of daily living independently for as long as possible.

Speech–Language Pathology

Speech–language pathologists worked to prolong Jane's ability to speak, eat, and drink by teaching her exercises and compensatory strategies as the disease progressed. Understanding her desire to continue eating and not be reintubated, they worked to educate Jane, her family, and the staff on foods and techniques to reduce the risk of aspiration events.

Registered Dietitian/Nutritionist

As Jane grew weaker, the registered dietitian/nutritionist (RDN) was consulted for supplemental nutrition via percutaneous endoscopic gastrostomy (PEG) tube. Although Jane did not desire most forms of life support, receiving supplemental nutrition via a PEG tube supported her goal to have as much quality time with her family as possible. The RDN recommended nocturnal feedings with comfort meals during the day. Upon Jane's final days in the acute care setting, the RDN worked with the palliative care team to reassure her husband that supplemental nutrition was no longer necessary and that feedings at this juncture would actually do her harm. In conjunction with ethics consultants, the RDN and palliative care ensured that proper documentation of Jane's wishes and medical status was in line with state law regarding this discontinuation of tube feeds as this can vary state to state.

CLS

CLSs have training in the emotional and developmental needs of children facing illness and expertise in pediatric bereavement and coping strategies. CLSs supported Jane's children during the ICU experience and helped both parents prepare the children for Jane's decline and impending death.

Palliative Care Bereavement Coordinator

The bereavement coordinator followed up with Jane's family through telephone calls and cards for 12 months following her death. The bereavement coordinator provided resources to help the children, such as bereavement camps and support groups designed for children, as well as resources for Jane's husband. In addition, the bereavement coordinator provided staff debriefings to promote staff grieving and coping. At the yearly remembrance ceremony, Jane's family and staff were reconnected.

Case Study: Summary

By having access to a palliative care team that addressed physical, psychological, social, and spiritual needs and coordinated all necessary services, Jane had the opportunity for the best possible outcomes in the face of her illness. But what made her wishes a potential reality was the communication between her palliative care team and her other healthcare providers. Without assessment, reassessment, and collaboration between disciplines and services, it would not have been possible to tailor her care based upon what was most important to Jane and her family. A strong palliative care team, comprising a physician, nurse, social worker, and chaplain, as well as other interprofessional colleagues, can support a patient like Jane by honoring her wishes, providing aggressive pain and symptom management, and offering support and grief counseling and spiritual care for existential distress.

Palliative Care Delivery Models

Inpatient Palliative Care Consult Team

Inpatient palliative care consult services have tripled since the year 2000 in hospitals with 50 or more beds. In 2020, 83% of hospitals this size had a palliative care team.[25] Most consult services usually include a basic team of board-certified palliative care physicians, nurses, and advanced practice providers (APRN, Physician Assistant, Clinical Nurse Specialist). Ideally palliative care trained social workers and chaplains are also dedicated to the palliative care IDT; however, in some institutions, the palliative care providers utilize the institution's primary team social workers and hospital chaplains to support patients referred for palliative care. Providers on the palliative care IDT (physicians and many APRNs) bill for their consulting services, similar to other specialty consult services.[26] Research has demonstrated that inpatient palliative care services decrease hospital costs, ICU admissions, and emergency room visits as well as improve patient satisfaction, alleviate symptom burden, improve hospice utilization, and improve QOL.[8,26–28]

Palliative care is appropriate for patients throughout the continuum of potentially life-limiting illnesses.[25]

For patients who are newly diagnosed with a serious illness, the palliative care team assists in providing information regarding the illness trajectory and treatment options and serves as a conduit of communication between the patient, family, healthcare providers, therapy services, and community resources (i.e., home health, veterans' benefits, ambulatory palliative care, or hospice services). For inpatient consults that arise later in the disease process, the palliative care team is often asked for assistance in facilitating advance care planning conversations, including when it may be time to focus on comfort care and when hospice may be most appropriate.

For the first time in over half a century, more patients are dying at home rather than in a hospital.[29] Patients may come to the decision that they do not want more diagnostic tests, procedures, or disease-modifying treatments, all of which increase their time spent in observation units or inpatient settings. Instead, they may choose to spend the last chapter of their life outside of the hospital, in whatever environment they consider home. However, for some dying at home, while preferred, may not be possible.[29] It is in these situations that inpatient palliative care teams are invaluable. Inpatient palliative care teams are skilled at eliciting a patient's and family's values, thus aiding them with care decisions that reflect their personal values and preferences.

For patients who are actively dying in acute care settings, a consultation with the palliative care team helps identify the patient's goals and preferences for end-of-life care. The palliative care team's role is to not only support and uphold the patient's goals of care but also to provide support to the family and the primary team as well as expert symptom management recommendations. If the acute care facility has a palliative care unit, transfer to that unit that is staffed with skilled PCNs providing 24/7 care can provide the best possible care for the patient and family who are unable to return home or uncomfortable returning home with hospice care.

Ambulatory Palliative Care Teams

The landmark study by Temel et al. demonstrated that outpatient palliative care not only improves QOL for patients with advanced lung cancer but also increases length of life.[4] For patients who are not admitted to the hospital and are undergoing life-prolonging treatments, ambulatory palliative care, if available, can assist with pain and symptom management while continuing conversations regarding goals of care. Outpatient palliative care usually occurs in ambulatory care centers or specialty clinics. Ambulatory palliative care teams have been shown to improve patient and family satisfaction and ensure that care is consistent with patient wishes.[5,49] In addition, outpatient palliative care improves early access to palliative care, improves symptom management, and has decreased the utilization of hospital resources, especially emergency room visits.[5,49] During an outpatient palliative care visit, patients can be assessed by many members of the IDT in a single setting and, depending on patient and family need, during one visit.[5,30]

The IDT may look different depending on where an ambulatory palliative care clinic is located. A standalone clinic may employ nurses, medical assistants, physicians, nurse practitioners, social workers, psychologists, or chaplains. Alternatively, an outpatient palliative care clinic may be embedded within another clinic, most commonly cancer centers.[31] In an embedded clinic the IDT may include oncology nurses, oncology providers, palliative care providers, as well as other clinic staff.[5]

CBPC Teams

Although palliative care is predominantly tied to a hospital system, CBPC is rapidly growing and bringing services to patients outside of the hospital, wherever they call home.[3] CBPC is distinct from hospice in the population that it serves. Patients enrolled with a CBPC either do not yet meet the criteria for the hospice benefit or are choosing to proceed with disease-modifying therapies even though their prognosis may be less than 6 months. CBPC agencies provide care in not only the patient's home but also their assisted living, skilled nursing facility, or transitional housing center. One of the primary benefits of bringing this care into a patient's residence is the decreased visit burden and the associated stress of transportation to and from a clinic setting. One study found that patients seen at home by CBPC agencies were often older, less functional, and mostly referred for care planning versus symptom management.[33] When the patient is not eligible for hospice care or does not elect hospice services, CBPC fills a gap that had previously existed in the healthcare system, by offering both symptom management expertise and the opportunity to engage in ongoing goals of care discussions as disease progresses.

Research has shown that patients receiving CBPC tend to be referred to hospice earlier and have an increased median and total length of stay on hospice care.[32] The team is able to offer support in the home, help establish clear goals of care with the patient and family, and provide expertise in pain and symptom management.[34] This model of palliative care delivery is decreasing unwanted hospital, ICU, and emergency room admissions.[35] However, access to CBPC currently is limited in many areas of the country. An additional barrier to accessing CBPC is that visits from palliative care specialists in the home are not always covered by insurance.

Tele-Palliative Care

Telehealth was not a new concept in March 2020; however, the adoption and utilization of telehealth services were accelerated by the COVID-19 pandemic.[36] Telemedicine was first conceived of during the 1970s and was defined as "healing from a distance."[37] Coupled with the flourishing field of palliative care, telemedicine, now more commonly referred to as "telehealth," delivery models aim to bring care to those patients who may have barriers to receiving palliative care services. Patients who are homebound or live in rural areas may not have access to quality palliative care in their traditional hospitals or outpatient settings. Those patients can access palliative care via telehealth for assessment and management of symptoms, as well as discussions of medical decision-making and goals of care. While telehealth is primarily utilized by patients in the community setting, there is a role for specialty palliative care providers that offer teleconsults for patients admitted to hospital or nursing home facilities which lack palliative care practitioners for face-to-face encounters. The interdisciplinary care offered by tele-palliative care is one tool that can be used to close the gap in disparities of care in palliative care.[38–40] However, this delivery model is an area that lacks research and evidence on efficacy. Tele-palliative care represents many opportunities for growth and study that may support its use in filling healthcare gaps and access to this specialty.[39]

The Hospice Team

Hospice care is palliative care for patients and families whose physician has determined are in the final 6 months of life and who choose to forgo disease-modifying treatment.[9] The overall focus of hospice is to provide comfort and improve all domains of QOL—physical, psychological, social, and spiritual—in whatever environment they call home. Hospice care is provided by an IDT including physicians, nurses, social workers, chaplains, hospice aides, volunteers, and other disciplines as needed.

The Medicare Hospice Benefit[9] defines hospice eligibility based on what a patient's prognosis may be. A patient may become hospice-eligible when two doctors certify that there is a prognosis equal to or less than 6 months to live, assuming the disease takes its natural course.[9] The Medicare Hospice Benefit covers the cost for all hospice team services, as well as any medical equipment and all medications related to the patient's serious illness at no additional cost. If a patient does not have insurance but is eligible for and desires hospice care, a Medicare-certified hospice must provide care, regardless of ability to pay.[9] Commercial insurance providers typically include a hospice benefit that will cover hospice services similar to Medicare and Medicaid. However, there may be a maximum dollar amount covered by commercial insurance for hospice services.

The hospice team delivers care whether the patient is living in the home, assisted living, hospital, or long-term care nursing facility. Hospices provide 24/7 coverage in addition to short-term general inpatient hospice care for patients whose symptoms are difficult to control. Hospice also offers short-term respite care for exhausted caregivers caring for the patient in the home.[9] It is important that patients who qualify for hospice-level care and their families are educated about the benefits of hospice care. Many are misinformed, thinking that hospice is a place rather than a palliative care delivery model or that hospice care is only for the final days or weeks of life. Early intervention with hospice care provides the best-quality care, rather than crisis intervention, for all who are eligible for this care.[41]

Building a Palliative Care Team

When considering starting or enhancing a palliative care team, many things need to be taken into consideration. It is critical to identify the vision and goals of the team as well as how they will meet the needs of the institution. These factors will vary based on available resources, mission and size of the institution, administrative priorities, educational requirements (including staff, learner, fellowship needs), and demographics of patient populations. It is also important to consider the overall value that palliative care has from the perspective of institutional core values. Making the case to a healthcare institution about the benefits of palliative care requires understanding the impact palliative care has on a healthcare system as well as the priorities of the institution.[25] Part of the palliative care team mission should include tracking data about improved patient and family satisfaction scores as well as substantial cost savings to the institution, including decreased 30-day readmission rates and decreased length of stay.[42]

The palliative care members included on the team will vary greatly based on institutional requirements and resources as well as the palliative care delivery model (i.e., whether it is an inpatient consult service, an outpatient service, a clinic, or an inpatient unit).[25,43] The leadership within the palliative care team must ensure that all members of the palliative care team share the same vision so that there is no miscommunication about the role each team member may fill as needs evolve. Of equal importance, the vision/mission of a palliative care team must coincide with that of the institution in order to thrive.

Resources for developing a palliative care team and making the case to leadership are readily available.[25,39] Detailed information on how to start and maintain a strong palliative care team is beyond the purview of this chapter but is available from the Center to Advance Palliative Care.[25]

Sustaining a Healthy, Functioning Palliative Care Team

A healthy team is one in which the members respect and appreciate their team members as individuals and the team as a whole unit while sharing similar values, mission, and vision. Team members need clearly delineated roles and must understand that there are many aspects of palliative care that are shared by each discipline.[44,45] There needs to be shared accountability for quality patient and family care, and work and productivity expectations must be transparent.[46]

According to Guideline 1.8 of the NCP *Guidelines for Quality Palliative Care*,[3] the palliative care program must recognize the emotional impact that caring for those with serious illness has on team members. Processes need to be in place to provide support for sustainability.

Burnout and compassion fatigue in hospice and palliative care professionals are significant and on the rise, making retention a problem for some teams.[45] Burnout among palliative care teams has been reported at 38.7%, with higher rates found among nonphysician providers.[46] Proactive team activities for individual and team self-care, resilience strategies, and healthy work environment are critical to success. Some strategies that palliative care teams have adopted to promote sustainability are personal and team wellness programs; regularly scheduled debriefing sessions to vent frustrations, anger, and concerns; and a plan for crisis debriefing.[47] An awareness of the potential for burnout among palliative care teams, coupled with strategies for the prevention and management of burnout is a first step in helping palliative care IDTs provide sustainable palliative care to patients in all stages of illness.

Whenever a team comprises more than one individual, conflict is inevitable. It is important that team members are aware of symptoms of stress and conflict and are comfortable discussing them openly. One study found that effective teams shared common core practices. These core practices include consistent access to expert palliative care resources; strong intra-team communication; the ability to respond rapidly to patient needs; whole-person focused care; preparedness, peace, and fulfillment in the work; and advocacy for patient preferences. These common core practices can be accomplished by teams through different strategies based on the location of the team, the structure of the team, and the patient population.[48] Poorly functioning teams suffer from rivalry, mistrust, and role ambiguity, all of which are toxic to team health.

Team-building activities that encourage trust and mutual respect will help to prevent these challenges from arising.[47] Most importantly, the team needs to keep its focus on its agreed-upon mission and values and care that is in the best interest of the patient and family. Although working as a team adds a layer of challenge, including conflicting work schedules, role overlap, differing opinions, and occasionally conflict, team collaboration allows the palliative team to offer a higher level of service for patients and families while supporting the needs of its individual team members.

Conclusion

Palliative care is best delivered by an IDT that attends to the physical, psychological, social, and spiritual well-being of patients with serious illness and their families, delivering holistic, whole-person care.

The NCP *Guidelines for Quality Palliative Care* give direction for the structure and processes of developing and sustaining palliative care teams.[3] Interdisciplinary professionals bring the expertise and perspective of their discipline to the patient's care plan as well as the collaboration of the team. Sharing unique perspectives and integrating them as a team help to achieve the best possible patient and family outcomes. The models of palliative care delivery vary in their settings, reimbursement, and eligibility; however, the mission and vision for all models of palliative care are focused on the patient and family goals regarding care and QOL. A team that works collaboratively and addresses individual and team wellness will be resilient and sustainable, despite team challenges and changing dynamics of the healthcare system. Most importantly, the team will be rewarded with the professional satisfaction of delivering quality palliative care to all patients and families receiving their ministrations.

REFERENCES

1. Center to Advance Palliative Care. Palliative Care Definition. What Is Palliative Care. 2019. Accessed August 15, 2022. https://www.capc.org/about/palliative-care/.
2. Center to Advance Palliative Care and the National Palliative Care Research Center. America's Care of Serious Illness: A State-by-State Report Card on Access to Palliative Care in Our Nation's Hospitals. September 2019. Accessed August 15, 2022. https://reportcard.capc.org/.
3. National Consensus Project for Quality Palliative Care. *Clinical Practice Guidelines for Quality Palliative Care*. 4th ed. National Coalition for Hospice and Palliative Care; 2018. Accessed August 15, 2022. https://www.nationalcoalitionhpc.org/ncp.

4. Temel JS, Greer JA, Muzikansky A, et al. Early palliative care for patients with metastatic non-small-cell lung cancer. *N Engl J Med.* 2010;363(8):733–742. https://doi.org/10.1056/NEJMoa1000678.
5. Smith AK, Thai JN, Bakitas MA, et al. The diverse landscape of palliative care clinics. *J Palliat Med.* 2013;16(6):661–668. https://doi.org/10.1089/jpm.2012.0469.
6. Ahluwalia SC, Chen C, Raaen L, et al. A systematic review in support of the National Consensus Project Clinical Practice Guidelines for Quality Palliative Care, fourth edition. *J Pain Symptom Manage.* 2018;56(6):831–870. https://doi.org/10.1016/j.jpainsymman.2018.09.008.
7. National Academy of Medicine. *Emerging Stronger from COVID-19. Priorities for Health System Transformation.* National Academies Press; 2022. Accessed October 1, 2022. https://doi.org/10.17226/26657.
8. Connor SR. *Hospice and Palliative Care: The Essential Guide.* Taylor and Francis; 2017.
9. Centers for Medicare & Medicaid Services. Medicare Hospice Benefits. March 2023. Accessed November 28, 2023. https://www.medicare.gov/publications/02154-medicare-hospice-benefits.pdf.
10. Center to Advance Palliative Care. National Palliative Care Registry. 2019. Accessed November 28, 2023. https://www.capc.org/national-palliative-care-registry/.
11. Higgins E, Coyne HL, Rogers CKM, Infanzon J, Velez N, Coyne P. The CASH assessment tool: a window into existential suffering. *J Health Care Chaplain.* 2022;28(4):482–496. https://doi.org/10.1080/08854726.2021.1922980.
12. McCann Klug L. The specialty chaplain on the palliative care team: a narrative review. *Am J Hosp Palliat Med.* 2022;40(9):1021–1028. https://doi.org/10.1177/10499091221134021.
13. Board of Chaplaincy Certification Inc. Becoming Certified. 2023. Accessed November 30, 2023. http://bcci.professionalchaplains.org.
14. Ma JE, Haverfield M, Lorenz KA, et al. Exploring expanded interdisciplinary roles in goals of care conversations in a national goals of care initiative: a qualitative approach. *Palliat Med.* 2021;35(8):1542–1552. https://doi.org/10.1177/02692163211020473.
15. Ferrell B, Paice J. *Oxford Textbook of Palliative Nursing.* 5th ed. Oxford University Press; 2019:3–10.
16. Hospice and Palliative Credentialing Center. Certification. 2023. Accessed November 30, 2023. https://www.advancingexpertcare.org/hpcc/.
17. Dahlin C, Coyne P. *Advanced Practice Palliative Nursing.* 2nd ed. Oxford University Press, 2023:19–33.
18. American Academy of Hospice and Palliative Medicine. Certification for Hospice and Palliative Medicine Specialists. Accessed November 30, 2023. https://aahpm.org/career/certification.
19. Firn J, Preston N, Walshe C. Hospital-based social workers' perceptions of generalist- and specialist-level palliative social work activities. *J Soc Work.* 2021;21(3):416–434. https://doi.org/10.1177/1468017320911507.
20. National Association of Social Workers. Standards for Palliative and End of Life Care. 2004. Accessed December 1, 2023. https://www.socialworkers.org/Practice/NASW-Practice-Standards-Guidelines/Standards-for-Palliative-and-End-of-Life-Care.
21. Altilio T, Otis-Green S, Cagle J. *The Oxford Textbook of Palliative Social Work: Guess Who's Coming to Dinner? The Evolving Identity of Palliative Social Workers.* Oxford University Press; 2022:65–76.
22. Coyne E. How volunteer services can improve and advance palliative care programs. *J Hosp Palliat Nurs.* 2017;19(2):166–169.
23. Coleman H, Sanderson-Thomas A, Walshe C. The impact on emotional well-being of being a palliative care volunteer: an interpretative phenomenological analysis. *Palliat Med.* 2021;36(4):671–679. https://doi.org/10.1177/02692163211064770.
24. Dingley C, Ruckdeschel A, Kotula K, Lekhak N. Implementation and outcomes of complementary therapies in hospice care: an integrative review. *Palliat Care Soc Pract.* 2021;15:263235242110517. https://doi.org/10.1177/26323524211051753.
25. Center to Advance Palliative Care. Growth of Palliative Care in U.S. Hospitals: 2022 Snapshot. March 29, 2022. Accessed October 17, 2022. https://www.capc.org/blog/capc-releases-its-growth-of-palliative-care-in-us-hospitals-2022-snapshot/.
26. Center to Advance Palliative Care. Optimizing Billing Practices. December 20, 2022. Accessed October 17, 2022. https://www.capc.org/toolkits/optimizing-billing-practices/?clickthrough_doc_id=resources.toolkitpage.244&clickthrough_req_id=fjmyQ_puT0Sn28P5KPVgHg&clickthrough_query=billing%20for%20services.
27. Fitzpatrick J, Mavissakalian M, Luciani T, Xu Y, Mazurek A. Economic impact of early inpatient palliative care intervention in a community hospital setting. *J Palliat Med.* 2018;21(7):933–939. https://doi.org/10.1089/jpm.2017.0416.
28. Hui D, Hannon BL, Zimmermann C, Bruera E. Improving patient and caregiver outcomes in oncology: team-based, timely, and targeted palliative care. *CA Cancer J Clin.* 2018;68(5):356–376. https://doi.org/10.3322/caac.21490.
29. Cross SH, Warraich HJ. Changes in the place of death in the United States. *N Engl J Med.* 2019;381(24):2369–2370. https://doi.org/10.1056/nejmc1911892.
30. Yennurajalingam S, Bruera E, eds. *Oxford American Handbook of Hospice and Palliative Medicine and Supportive Care.* Oxford University Press; 2016.
31. Finlay E, Rabow MW, Buss MK. Filling the gap: creating an outpatient palliative care program in your institution. *Am Soc Clin Oncol Educ Book.* 2018;(38):111–121. https://doi.org/10.1200/edbk_200775.
32. Smith GB, Calton B, Rabow MW, et al. Comparing the palliative care needs of patients seen by specialty palliative care teams at home versus in clinic. *J Pain Symtom Manage.* 2021;62(1):28–38.
33. Bull J, Kamal AH, Harker M, et al. Tracking patients in community-based palliative care through the Centers for Medicare & Medicaid Services Healthcare Innovation Project. *J Palliat Med.* 2017;20(11):1231–1236. https://doi.org/10.1089/jpm.2017.0080.
34. Killackey T, Lovrics E, Saunders S, Isenberg SR. Palliative care transitions from acute care to community-based care: a qualitative systematic review of the experiences and perspectives of health care providers. *Palliat Med.* 2020;34(10).1316–1331. https://doi.org/10.1177/0269216320947601.
35. Knighten ML. The business case to care for persons with serious illness using home-based and community-based palliative care. *Nurs Adm Q.* 2022;46(4):309–315. https://doi.org/10.1097/NAQ.0000000000000547.
36. Levoy K, Foxwell A, Rosa WE. Palliative care delivery changes during COVID-19 and enduring implications in oncology nursing: a rapid review. *Curr Opin Support Palliat Care.* 2022;16(3):94–101. https://doi.org/10.1097/spc.0000000000000603.
37. Doraiswamy S, Abraham A, Mamtani R, Cheema S. Use of telehealth during the COVID-19 pandemic: a scoping review. *Journal of Medical Internet Research.* 2020;22(12):e24087. https://doi.org/10.2196/24087.
38. Tang M, Reddy A. Telemedicine and its past, present, and future roles in providing palliative care to advanced cancer patients.

Cancers. 2022;14(8):1884. https://doi.org/10.3390/cancers14081884.

39. Cormi C, Petit M, Auclair J, Bagaragaza E, Colombet I, Sanchez S. Building a telepalliative care strategy in nursing homes: a qualitative study with mobile palliative care teams. *BMC Palliat Care.* 2021;20(1):156. https://doi.org/10.1186/s12904-021-00864-6.
40. Dahlin C, Coyne P. *Advanced Practice Palliative Nursing.* 2nd ed. Oxford University Press; 2023:208–215.
41. Coyne P, Bobb B, Plakovic K, eds. *Conversations in Palliative Care: Questions and Answers with Experts.* 4th ed. Hospice and Palliative Nurses Association; 2017:9–32.
42. Noreika DM, Coyne PJ. Implementing palliative care interdisciplinary teams: consultative versus integrative models. *Crit Care Nurs Clin North Am.* 2015;27(3):297–306. https://doi.org/10.1016/j.cnc.2015.05.006.
43. Ohana S, Shaulov A, Ganz FD. Acute palliative care models: scoping review. *BMJ Support Palliat Care.* 2023;14(e1). https://doi.org/10.1136/spcare-2022-004124.
44. Imes RS, Omilion-Hodges LM, Hester JDB. *Communication and Care Coordination for the Palliative Care Team: A Handbook for Building and Maintaining Optimal Teams.* Springer; 2021.
45. Klarare A, Hansson J, Fossum B, Fürst CJ, Lundh Hagelin C. Team type, team maturity and team effectiveness in specialist palliative home care: an exploratory questionnaire study. *J Interprof Care.* 2018;33(5):504–511. https://doi.org/10.1080/13561820.2018.1551861.
46. Atilio T, Dahlin C, Tucker R, Remke S, Weissman D. Strategies for Maximizing the Health/Function of Palliative Care Teams. Center to Advance Palliative Care; 2019. Accessed August 17, 2022. https://media.capc.org/bootcamp-2019/26-capc-monograph-strategies-for-maximizing-the-health-function-of-palliative-care-teams.pdf
47. Taffurelli C, Barello S, Cervantes Camacho V, Bertuol M, Savarese M, Artioli G. Taking care of dying patients through an "interprofessional ecosystem": a grounded theory study on the experience of an interprofessional team in palliative care. *Scand J Caring Sci.* 2020;35(4). https://doi.org/10.1111/scs.12934.
48. Seow H, Bainbridge D, Brouwers M, Bryant D, Tan Toyofuku S, Kelley ML. Common care practices among effective community-based specialist palliative care teams: a qualitative study. *BMJ Support Palliat Care.* 2017;10(1):e3. https://doi.org/10.1136/bmjspcare-2016-001221.
49. Finlay E, Newport K, Sivendran S, Kilpatrick L, Owens M, Buss MK. Models of outpatient palliative care clinics for patients with cancer. *J Oncol Pract.* 2019;15(4):187–193. https://doi.org/10.1200/JOP.18.00634.

9

Enhancing Team Effectiveness

Katrina Bezak and Kimberly Chow

Key Points

- Palliative care is provided by an interdisciplinary team (IDT) whose members are palliative care specialists able to meet the complex, multidimensional needs of patients and families facing serious illness.
- Palliative care is also an approach to care that attends to the physical, psychological, social, and spiritual domains of quality of life, providing specialty care for patients with serious illness and their families.
- All members of the IDT are responsible for providing varying levels of palliative care for patients and their caregivers, yet many report lack of knowledge and training as well as barriers to referral that include negative stereotypes, patient fear, and prognostic uncertainty.
- Four major models of team-based palliative care—inpatient consult teams, ambulatory care teams, community-based palliative care teams, and hospice teams—leverage both the expertise of the palliative IDT and the trusting and supportive relationships of primary disease management and nursing teams across the serious illness trajectory.
- Nurses interact closely with patients at every point of the care continuum and play one of the most critical roles in palliative care delivery.

Introduction

Palliative care is interdisciplinary care (nursing, medicine, social work, chaplaincy, and other specialties as appropriate) that specializes in assessing and managing the physical, psychological, social, and spiritual needs of patients and families dealing with serious illness.[1] Care focuses on improving the quality of life (QOL) of patients and families and is initiated ideally at the time of a serious illness diagnosis and provided concurrently with disease-oriented treatment, across the serious illness trajectory.[1–4]

There is a wealth of evidence that supports the many benefits of early palliative care referral that include improved symptoms, QOL, and satisfaction with care, as well as decreased resource utilization.[5,6] While the earliest, most influential studies centered around the oncology population, evidence is growing to support palliative care for noncancer serious illness populations such as persons living with cardiovascular and neurodegenerative disorders.[7,8] With a steep increase in demand for palliative care, there are now major shortages in the specialist workforce needed to meet the growing population of patients. Recent literature estimates a workforce gap of approximately 18,000 providers.[9]

Now more than ever, healthcare teams must come together to optimize palliative care for patients and families across disease continuums. This is accomplished by engaging cross-functional teams in continuous bidirectional learning and respectful collaboration, which requires humility and empathy for the unique challenges each care team faces within the context of patient relationships. At the center of these teams are nurses at every point of care who embody the requisite attributes of holistic and healing care for patients, regardless of their diagnosis or prognosis.[10] To understand how palliative care is best offered, nurses must take steps to familiarize themselves with the role of the palliative care interdisciplinary team (IDT), the core aspects of palliative care that primary disease teams are responsible for providing, and how nurses, whether formally trained or not, play one of the most critical roles in palliative care delivery.[11,12]

The focus of this chapter is on enhancing the team approach to palliative care throughout the illness trajectory and across a variety of care delivery models. Essential primary, specialist, and nursing roles in the provision of quality palliative care will be reviewed with an emphasis on how teams collaborate with one another to deliver care that honors and respects patients' goals of care and dignity. A case study to highlight how palliative care can be seamlessly integrated throughout the care continuum will be presented.

The Interdisciplinary Palliative Care Team

Palliative care requires the expertise of a strong IDT to meet the unique and challenging needs of the patients and families they care for daily. The core members of specialist teams often include board-certified physicians, nurses, and advanced practice registered nurses (APRNs). Ideally, social workers and chaplains are also key members of the team; but in some institutions, the palliative care team must use existing institutional resources to support their efforts.[3] In

Table 9.1 Palliative care interdisciplinary team roles

Team member	Definition	Role
Chaplain	Completes a comprehensive spiritual assessment and initiates appropriate interventions for those needing spiritual support	To support and/or accommodate the spiritual and religious needs of patients, families, and staff; to provide support across cultures and faiths by offering a nonjudgmental presence
Palliative care nurse	Adds expert communication skills, knowledge of pain and symptom assessment and management, and expertise in coordination of care Skilled in educating patients, families, and other healthcare professionals about core palliative care concepts	Collaborates with the team to develop a plan to aggressively treat pain and symptoms, to reassess interventions, and to evaluate and report the efficacy to the other healthcare providers involved in the patients' care
Advanced practice registered nurse (APRN)	Specialty-trained licensed provider who receives training in symptom management, medical management, communication, prognostication, and advance care planning	Assess, diagnose, and treat the palliative care needs of patients and provide support for families; can order appropriate diagnostic testing and pharmacologic interventions; often has leadership role on the palliative care team
Physician	Brings the clinical expertise of medical diagnosis, knowledge of the disease course, prognostication, expertise in goals-of-care conversations, and medical management, including pain and symptom management	Also helpful in addressing issues and concerns that the primary team may have, clarifying information, and respecting and advocating for patients' goals and wishes
Social worker	Educated to understand complex family dynamics and skilled at integrating cultural considerations into care, communicating with patients and families, and advocating for patient preferences	Assess the needs, strengths, and resources of the patient and family; build on their strengths; enhance their connections to their resources and supports; and connect them with new resources to meet emotional, legal, and financial needs
Primary disease management team	Have the medical knowledge and expertise of the patient and their chronic healthcare needs Teams include, but are not limited to, physicians, nurses, APRNs, physician assistants, social workers, and case managers	Responsible for providing primary and basic palliative care for patients, which includes symptom management, psychosocial support, and advanced care planning from the earliest visits Provides timely referral to specialist palliative care and helps establish trust between the patient and palliative care partners Remains actively involved with the palliative care needs of patients throughout the care continuum

the pediatric setting, child life specialists are often included as part of the team; and other resources, such as art and music therapists, may also be included in some instances. Interdisciplinary professionals bring their unique discipline's expertise to the patients' plan of care and then collaborate as a team to achieve the best possible patient and family outcomes.[13] Effective teams are ones where each member understands their role and how it complements others' work while minimizing redundancies.

For patients newly diagnosed with a serious illness, the palliative care team assists in providing information regarding the illness trajectory and treatment options and can serve as a conduit of communication between the patient and family, healthcare providers, therapy services, and community resources.[3] Complex symptom management that fluctuates throughout the serious illness journey is another important role played by the palliative care IDT. Symptoms such as disease-related pain highlight how the expertise across all disciplines comes together to assess and treat the psychological, social, spiritual, and physical impacts of disease on the mind and body. Referrals that arise later in the disease process often seek the palliative care IDT's involvement with complicated and uncomplicated advance care planning conversations, including decisions regarding hospice care.[14]

The National Consensus Project's *Guidelines for Quality Palliative Care*[15] give direction and guidelines for the structure and processes of developing and sustaining palliative care teams. Success of palliative care IDTs requires early identification of the team's vision and goals and how they intertwine with and meet the needs of the greater institution. Institutions' emphasis on palliative care can be driven by improvement in hospital mortality, patient-centered symptom management, or reduction in unplanned hospitalizations.[16] Needs will vary based on resources, mission and size of the institution, administrative priorities, educational requirements, demographics of the patient population, and the plan to include learners, as well as the overall value that palliative care has as an institutional core value. The palliative IDT and their roles are summarized in Table 9.1.[4,15–17]

The Role of Primary Disease Management Teams

Primary disease management teams have expertise in the diagnosis and management of specific acute and chronic illnesses (e.g., congestive heart failure, Parkinson's disease). The primary IDT may include, but is not limited to, physicians, nurses, APRNs, physician assistants, social workers, and case managers. Team members often have the closest and longest relationships with patients and their caregivers as they usher patients from diagnosis through either survivorship, disease maintenance, or death.

Despite the known benefits of collaboration between primary disease management teams and palliative care, multiple barriers prevent timely referral to palliative care including negative stereotypes, patient resistance, role confusion, provider's lack of knowledge about palliative care's role, and prognostic uncertainty.[18] Some of the negative stereotypes of palliative care are the association with end-of-life or hospice care, giving up, and disease progression.[18,19] More specifically for patients, the palliative care team is also linked to fear of imminent death, decreased access to services that may or may not be necessary, and abandonment from their primary team.[18]

Palliative care from the earliest stages of disease management, and regardless of prognosis, has proven to be effective in alleviating the physical, psychological, social, and spiritual burdens of illness.

Examples of serious illness populations who can benefit from early integration of palliative care include patients living with chronic kidney disease,[20] heart disease, cancer, chronic obstructive pulmonary disease, Parkinson's, and dementia.[21] Most recently, data from Kuebler[22] shows the benefit of engaging palliative care when caring for patients diagnosed with COVID-19.

Effective palliative care across the healthcare continuum begins with the primary disease management team and requires timely and ongoing collaboration with the palliative care IDT as disease and symptoms progress. One of the primary limitations preventing referral is the lack of functional knowledge about the palliative care referral process.[23] Identified knowledge gaps include unfamiliarity with timing of referral, ability to prognosticate, and understanding of palliative care's role. In a study by Kavalieratos et al.,[24] cardiology providers were unaware of the concurrent palliative care benefits for their patients. Furthermore, some providers were unaware that palliative care referral did not require termination of life-prolonging treatments.[24]

Continuous dialogue and exposure to each other's expertise sets the stage for bidirectional learning, empathy for each team's challenges as they care for patients, and improved care outcomes. The role of the primary disease management team is to address the earliest palliative care needs of their patients which include advance care planning, assessing and clarifying illness understanding, providing psychosocial support, and effectively managing basic illness-related symptoms. Once the primary team reaches the limits of their skill set, their role is to initiate timely referral, provide patient education about palliative care while emphasizing their full support, and remain involved in their patients' care in close collaboration with the palliative IDT.[25] Although there are numerous barriers preventing the partnership between primary disease management teams and palliative care, it is important that all members of the care team are openly communicating, establishing respect for each other, and collaborating to manage the patients' care.

The Nurses' Role in Palliative Care

There is a natural synergy that exists between the field of nursing and the philosophy and practice of palliative care at both the primary and specialist levels.[10] Nurses are educated to focus on the holistic needs of the person, providing and advocating for care that supports the physical, psychological, social, and spiritual needs of patients and families.[12,26] Necessary primary palliative care skills for nurses include understanding the natural illness trajectory of their patient population, basic understanding of how common symptoms are identified and managed, assessing and documenting the core values that drive patient decision-making from diagnosis to death, and understanding the limitations of their primary skills and when to call for specialist support.[10] Nurses must also leverage their trusted position within primary disease management teams to role-model, champion and encourage the implementation of primary palliative care and greater collaboration with specialty palliative care teams.[5,27]

Specialty-trained and board-certified palliative care nurses (PCNs) build on their nursing foundation by adding expert communication skills, knowledge of pain and symptom assessment and management, expertise in coordination of care, and skill in educating patients, families, and other healthcare professionals about palliative care concepts.[11,12] The PCN collaborates with the team to develop a plan to aggressively treat pain and symptoms, to reassess interventions, and to evaluate and report the efficacy to other healthcare providers involved in the patients' care.[3]

PCNs play a major role in coordinating care among all healthcare providers involved in the patients' care. They collaborate with the IDT to identify which team members to involve in the patients' care and are often the one who keeps primary care team informed of the plan of care. Additionally, it is often the PCN who initiates and leads debriefing of the staff who have faced challenges in caring for a patient, discussing what went well, what could have been done differently, and lessons learned for the future.[3]

Palliative Care along the Care Continuum

Over the past two decades, the United States has witnessed a remarkable increase in palliative care services with the expansion of four major care delivery models: inpatient consultation, ambulatory, community-based, and hospice care.[13,14,28] In each model, members work not as individual disciplines and services but as a unified team with a shared vision and mission to improve patient and family QOL. Success requires a deep understanding of how palliative care services directly improve outcomes and how they complement care delivered by primary and other specialist teams. When the palliative care team is fully optimized, the result is care that integrates seamlessly across the disease continuum and with the full collaboration of primary disease management teams.[25,29] Nurses play a critical role in the provision of palliative care both from within the team itself and as caregivers supporting patients and their families at every level of the serious illness trajectory and in every setting. Table 9.2[28–35] details the roles of specialists, primary disease management teams, and nurses in delivering palliative care to patients and families in each care delivery model.

Case Study

Mr. Edwards is an 82-year-old World War II veteran with multiple chronic health conditions, including hypercholesterolemia, hypertension, anxiety, depression, bilateral lower extremity neuropathy, and early-onset dementia. He also suffers from chronic pain as a result of three wounds inflicted from his time in the war. He has been married for 50 years, lives with his wife in their own home, and has five daughters who intermittently help care for him. His wife also has numerous chronic medical conditions that make it difficult for her to care for herself. Mr. Edwards does not regularly follow specialists as he only trusts his primary care provider of 30 years, Dr. Anderson.

Mr. Edwards goes to see Dr. Anderson for a follow-up appointment. He is accompanied by his daughter, who is a pharmacist. She is upset that they have been unable to control his chronic pain. She is also frustrated because he has been more lethargic lately and not participating in physical therapy. She says he appears disengaged with things he used to love. Mr. Edwards becomes frustrated by his daughter's involvement and wants to be able to care for himself. He states that he is in excellent care with Dr. Anderson. He feels his daughter is overreacting to his medical care needs and states that he is not having any issues. Dr. Anderson tries to address the issues

Table 9.2 Team roles across models of palliative care delivery

	Specialist palliative care interdisciplinary team (IDT)	Primary disease management team	Nursing professionals
Inpatient consult	• Serves as consultants in close collaboration with primary teams • Oversees the acute palliative care units (when available) where patients are admitted under and managed by the palliative care team • Consulted for various reasons including advance care planning, moderate to complex symptom management, navigating difficult conversations, end-of-life (EOL) planning, care transitions, and care coordination • Develops a clear understanding of patients' disease status, overall prognosis, and the primary disease management's treatment recommendations • Quickly builds trust and rapport with patients and caregivers • Provides support for patients, caregivers, nurses, and primary teams • Often lead debriefing sessions for complex patient cases	• Admits, stabilizes, and manages patients throughout hospital course • Assesses for and treats common symptoms associated with the specific illness or acute event • Requires clear and effective communication skills to help guide informed decision-making • Quickly builds rapport and trust • Consults and collaborates with members of the IDT • Places referrals for specialty services and incorporates recommendations into the plan of care • Participates in or leads family meetings that address goals of care • Cares for patients at EOL who may not be appropriate to transfer home or to hospice	• Includes bedside nurses, nurse consultants, nurse case managers, and ambulatory nurses • Builds trusting and therapeutic relationships with patients and caregivers as they navigate the challenges of acute illness • First responders to patients' symptoms, administering prescribed treatments, reassessing and communicating effectiveness across care teams • Provides emotional and psychological support • Explores advanced care planning, care goals, and illness understanding • Participates in family meetings • Places referrals for additional support services including chaplaincy, social workers, and volunteers • Advocates for specialist palliative care referral when needed
Ambulatory care	• Introduces palliative care services; builds trusting relationship with patients and caregivers • Develops a clear understanding of patients' disease status, overall prognosis, and the primary disease management team's treatment recommendations • Early and ongoing assessment of patients' illness understanding, values, and goals • Early and ongoing advanced care planning discussions • Early and ongoing assessment and management of disease-related symptoms • Early and ongoing assessment of the cultural, spiritual, and psychological impacts of disease • Maintains close communication and collaboration with primary disease management teams	• Often the patient's and caregiver's first introduction to the healthcare team • Leads early discussions on the natural course of illness and recommended treatment pathways • May refer to other specialist teams but is ultimately responsible for the integration of recommendations into the comprehensive plan of care • Core knowledge and skills in basic symptom management, advanced care planning, and empathic communication are essential • Fundamental knowledge of the palliative care specialty, team-based approach to care, and the appropriate timing of referral • Ongoing collaboration with palliative care IDT across all care delivery models	• Includes nurses in ambulatory primary or specialist clinics, nurse coordinators and treatment nurses (e.g., dialysis, infusion clinic nurses) • Builds trusting and therapeutic relationships with patients and caregivers • Disease experts who educate and support patients and caregivers • First responders to patients' symptoms • Exploring advanced care planning, goals of care, and illness understanding starting at the earliest clinic visits • Advocates for the fluctuating needs of patients to ensure care is aligned with greater goals of care • Provides emotional and psychological support for patients and caregivers • Places referrals for additional support services including chaplaincy, social workers and volunteers • Advocates for specialist palliative care referral when needed
Community-based palliative care (CBPC)	• Offers support and services in the home setting • Often refers patients who are not eligible for or decline hospice care • Helps establish clear goals of care with the patient and family • Provides expert pain and symptom management • Communicates findings and recommendations back to primary disease management teams • Assists with care coordination and community resources	• Places referral for CBPC for patients who would benefit from specialist care but are not eligible for or decline hospice services • Works closely with CBPC team to address the varying needs of patients and caregivers • Communicates updates in disease status and treatment recommendations • Continues to follow patients and oversee care in the ambulatory care setting	• Includes ambulatory nurses from the primary disease management team and community nurses • Facilitates the transition from acute care to community care through preparation, education, and support • Liaise across clinical, organizational, and geographical barriers to become the eyes and ears of the care team within the patients' home environment
Hospice care	• Provided by a palliative care IDT including physicians, nurses, social workers, chaplains, hospice aides, and volunteers • Care provided wherever the patient is living: home, assisted living, hospital, or long-term care nursing facility • Offers 24/7 coverage as well as short-term general inpatient hospice care for patients whose symptoms are difficult to control • Provides short-term respite care for caregivers caring for the patient • EOL and legacy planning • Provides support for patients incrementally addressing the spiritual, psychological, social, and physical distress at EOL	• Refers to hospice services for patients who choose to forego disease-directed treatment or when additional therapies threaten patient safety • Certifies hospice eligibility when there is a prognosis equal to or less than 6 months to live, assuming the disease takes its natural course • May remain the hospice attending of record who responds to the various EOL needs of patients • Patients and caregivers appreciate ongoing involvement and support from primary teams as their illness progresses and they must navigate EOL	• Includes nurses from primary disease management teams who often have the longest and closest relationships with patients and their caregivers • Works alongside hospice teams to ensure patients and caregivers do not feel abandoned during EOL transitions • Collaborates with hospice teams to ensure communication and messaging to patients and caregivers are unified and consistent • Provides updates to other members of the primary disease management team

brought up by his daughter, but this is somewhat limited since labs and other studies that Dr. Anderson ordered months ago still have not been completed. Mr. Edwards denies receiving any phone calls to schedule imaging studies or instructions in previous visits for labs. He continues to insist that he is able to care for himself and manage his own affairs, although finances and what medications he should be taking have always been managed by his wife.

Six weeks later, Mr. Edwards is hospitalized for weakness and confusion. His family are frustrated that they are unable to visit because of COVID-19 guidelines and are wondering why he is declining. His nurse, Molly, has been providing care for Mr. Edwards during his hospital stay and is engaging the family, when possible. She has been giving his medication regularly, helping to bathe him, caring for his newly diagnosed pressure ulcer, and providing comfort when he states he is lonely. During this time, Molly notes that Mr. Edward's mentation and engagement in self-care are improving. However, she does note concerns to the family that, despite his improvements, he is still having difficulty remembering things that occurred during the hospital stay or even earlier that same day.

Because of their close relationship, Dr. Anderson rounds on Mr. Edwards while in the hospital. He is medically stable and cleared for discharge. After suggestion from Molly, Dr. Anderson places an ambulatory palliative care referral for Mr. Edwards, which he initially refuses, stating "Why do I need them? I'm not dying." After Dr. Anderson discusses the many benefits of palliative care to help address Mr. Edward's complicated care needs, he accepts the palliative care referral. He is discharged with palliative care to follow in the outpatient setting. The palliative care IDT partners with Dr. Anderson, Mr. Edwards, and his family to provide pain management, advance care planning, anxiety interventions, and wound care. Mr. Edwards continues to improve from an energy standpoint but also his memory. After 6 months of palliative care, Mr. Edwards is discharged with fully healed pressure ulcers, a stable pain regimen which Dr. Anderson will continue managing, and all diagnostic testing completed. His house has been equipped with all durable medical equipment needed to aid his mobility issues due to neuropathy, and for the first time in 5 years, he has made all his follow-up appointments with Dr. Anderson.

Conclusion

The palliative care needs of patients and their caregivers arise in varying degrees at every stage of illness from diagnosis through death and bereavement. At the earliest stages, individuals with serious illness are trying to understand and cope with how their lives will be affected and how to move forward. Likewise, the new or increased presence of illness-related symptoms is often what triggers patients to seek medical care and must be managed effectively. Primary disease management teams that include nurses as one of the key team members must be skilled in addressing basic palliative care needs, knowledgeable on the benefits of palliative care and when specialist referral is appropriate, and willing to continuously collaborate across teams.[25,29]

Palliative care specialists bring their expertise to patients in essentially all care settings—acute, ambulatory, community, and home hospice—alleviating symptoms and guiding patients and caregivers through some of the most challenging moments they will face. Another vital role specialists take on is educating, collaborating with, and even palliating primary disease management and nursing teams across these same care settings. Patient acuity is rising, and the greater healthcare system is becoming more complex. Teams that work collaboratively and acknowledge each other's roles and expertise with humility and appreciation will be resilient and sustainable. Most importantly, the team will be rewarded with the professional satisfaction of delivering high-quality care to the patients and caregivers in their care.

REFERENCES

1. World Health Organization. Palliative Care. Accessed September 1, 2022. https://www.who.int/news-room/fact-sheets/detail/palliative-care.
2. Ferrell BR, Twaddle ML, Melnick A, Meier DE. National Consensus Project clinical practice guidelines for quality palliative care guidelines, 4th edition. *J Palliat Med.* 2018;21(12): 1684–1689. https://doi.org/10.1089/jpm.2018.0431.
3. Mazanec P, Reimer R, Bullington J, et al. Interdisciplinary palliative care teams. In: Ferrell BR, Paice J, eds. *Oxford Textbook of Palliative Nursing.* 5th ed. Oxford University Press; 2019:89–97.
4. Gorman RD. Integrating palliative care into primary care. *Nurs Clin North Am.* 2016;51:367–379.
5. Desai AV, Klimek VM, Chow K, et al. 1-2-3 Project: a quality improvement initiative to normalize and systematize palliative care for all patients with cancer in the outpatient clinic setting. *J Oncol Pract.* 2018;14(12):e775–e785. https://doi.org/10.1200/JOP.18.00346.
6. Kamal AH, Bausewein C, Casarett DJ, Currow DC, Dudgeon DJ, Higginson IJ. Standards, guidelines, and quality measures for successful specialty palliative care integration into oncology: current approaches and future directions. *J Clin Oncol.* 2020;38(9):987–994. https://doi.org/10.1200/JCO.18.02440.
7. Abedini NC, Guo G, Hummel SL, et al. Factors influencing palliative care referral for hospitalised patients with heart failure: an exploratory, randomised, multi-institutional survey of hospitalists and cardiologist. *BMJ Open.* 2020;10(12):1–8. https://doi.org/10.1136/bmjopen-2020-040857.
8. Hanson LC, Kistler CE, Lavin K, et al. Triggered palliative care for late-stage dementia: a pilot randomized trail. *J Pain Symptom Manage.* 2019;57(1):10–19. https://doi.org/10.1016/j.jpainsymman.2018.10.494.
9. Kamal AH, Bull JH, Swetz KM, Wolf SP, Shanafelt TD, Meyers ER. Future of the palliative care workforce: preview to an impending crisis. *Am J Med.* 2017;130(2):113–114. https://doi.org/10.1016/j.amjmed.2016.08.046.
10. Chow K, Dahlin C. Integration of palliative care and oncology nursing. *Semin Oncol Nurs.* 2018;34(3):192–201. https://doi.org/10.1016/j.soncn.2018.06.001.
11. Ferrell B, Buller H, Paice J, Anderson W, Donesky D. End-of-life nursing and education consortium communication curriculum for interdisciplinary palliative care teams. *J Palliat Med.* 2019;22(9):1082–1091. https://doi.org/10.1089/jpm.2018.0645.
12. Hagen TL, Xu J, Lopez RP, Bressler T. Nursing's role in leading palliative care: a call to action. *Nurse Educ Today.* 2018;61:216–219. https://doi.org/10.1016/j.nedt.2017.11.037.
13. Center to Advance Palliative Care. Accessed September 1, 2022. https://www.capc.org.

14. Hui D, Bruera E. Models of palliative care delivery for patients with cancer. *J Clin Oncol.* 2020;38:852–865. https://doi.org/10.1200/JCO.18.02123.
15. National Consensus Project for Quality Palliative Care. *Clinical Practice Guidelines for Quality Palliative Care.* 4th ed. National Coalition for Hospice and Palliative Care; 2018. https://www.nationalcoalitionhpc.org/ncp-guidelines.
16. Stein GL, Cagle JG, Christ GH. Social work involvement in advance care planning: findings from a large survey of social workers in hospice and palliative care settings. *J Palliat Med.* 2017;20(3):253–259.
17. Kearney G, Fisher L, Groninger H. Integrating spiritual care into palliative consultation: a case study in expanded practice. *J Relig Health.* 2017;56:2308–2316.
18. Parajuli J, Hupcey JE. A systematic review on barriers to palliative care in oncology. *Am J Hosp Palliat Care.* 2021;38(11):1361–1377. https://doi.org/10.1177/1049909120983283.
19. Walter JK, Hill DL, Schall TE, et al. An interprofessional team-based intervention to address barriers to initiating palliative care in pediatric oncology: a multiple-method evaluation of feasibility, acceptability, and impact. *J Pain Symptom Manage.* 2021;62(6):1135–1144. https://doi.org/10.1016/j.jpainsymman.2021.06.008.
20. Ernecoff NC, Bell LF, Arnold RM, et al. Clinicians' perceptions of collaborative palliative care delivery in chronic kidney disease. *J Pain Symptom Manage.* 2022;64(2):168–177. https://doi.org/10.1016/j.jpainsymman.2022.04.167.
21. Bernacki RE, Block SD. Communication about serious illness care goals: a review and synthesis of best practices communication about serious illness care goals communication about serious illness care goals. *JAMA Intern Med.* 2014;174(12):1994–2003. https://doi.org/10.1001/jamainternmed.2014.5271.
22. Kuebler K. COVID-19 and palliative care: primary care symptom management can enhance quality of life and prevent hospitalization. *Am Nurse Today.* 2022;17(7):24–27.
23. Enguidanos S, Cardenas V, Wenceslao M, et al. Health care provider barriers to patient referral to palliative care. *Am J Hosp Palliat Care.* 2021;38(9):1112–1119. https://doi.org/10.1177/1049909120973200.
24. Kavalieratos D, Mitchell EM, Carey TS, et al. "Not the 'grim reaper service'": an assessment of provider knowledge, attitudes, and perceptions regarding palliative care referral barriers in heart failure. *J Am Heart Assoc.* 2014;3(1):e000544. https://doi.org/10.1161/JAHA.113.000544.
25. Periyakoil VS, von Gunten CF, Fischer S, Pantilat S, Quill T. Generalist versus specialist palliative medicine. *J Palliat Med.* 2022;25(2):193–199. https://doi.org/10.1089/jpm.2021.0644.
26. Mazenac P, Ferrell B, Virani R, Alayu J, Ruel NH. Preparing new graduate RNs to provide primary palliative care. *J Contin Educ Nurs.* 2020;51(6):280–286. https://doi.org/10.3928/00220124-20200514-08.
27. Kramer D, Chow K, Davis ME, et al. The acknowledge–normalize–partner (ANP) framework: a novel empathic communication tool for oncology nurses. *Palliat Support Care.* 2023;21(1):12–19. https://doi.org/10.1017/S1478951522000086.
28. Wiencek C, Coyne P. Palliative care delivery models. *Semin Oncol Nurs.* 2014;30(4):227–233.
29. Mitchell S, Maynard V, Lyons V, Jones N, Gardiner C. The role and response of primary healthcare services in the delivery of palliative care in epidemics and pandemics: a rapid review to inform practice and service delivery during the COVID-19 pandemic. *Palliat Med.* 2020;34(9):1182–1192. https://doi.org/10.1177/0269216320947623.
30. Beasley A, Bakitas MA, Edwards R, Kavalieratos D. Models of non-hospice palliative care: a review. *Ann Palliat Med.* 2019;8(suppl 1):S15–S21. https://doi.org/10.21037/apm.2018.03.11.
31. Killackey T, Lovrics E, Saunders S, Isenberg SR. Palliative care transitions from acute care to community-based care: a qualitative systematic review of the experiences and perspectives of health care providers. *Palliat Med.* 2020;34(10):1316–1331. https://doi.org/10.1177/0269216320947601.
32. Bull J, Kamal AH, Harka M, et al. Tracking patients in community-based palliative care through the Centers for Medicare & Medicaid Services Healthcare Innovation Project. *J Palliat Med.* 2017;20(11):1231–1236. https://doi.org/10.1089/jpm.2017.0080.
33. Jackson MJ, Mecklenburg J, Feshzion A. Palliative care at the doorstep: a community-based model. *J Hosp Palliat Nurs.* 2017;19(3):282–286.
34. Nevin M, Hynes G, Smith V. Healthcare providers' views and experiences of non-specialist palliative care in hospitals: a qualitative systematic review and thematic synthesis. *Palliat Med.* 2020;34(5):605–618. https://doi.org/10.1177/0269216319899335.
35. Mueggenburg K. Hospice: care and comfort when it is needed most. In: Coyne P, Bobb B, Plakovic K, eds. *Conversations in Palliative Care: Questions and Answers with the Experts.* 4th ed. Hospice and Palliative Nurses Association; 2017:9–32.
36. Teike Lüthi F, Bernard M, Beauverd M, Gamondi C, Ramelet AS, Borasio GD. IDentification of patients in need of general and specialised PALLiative care (ID-PALL©): item generation, content and face validity of a new interprofessional screening instrument. *BMC Palliat Care.* 2020;19(1):19. https://doi.org/10.1186/s12904-020-0522-6.

10

The Ethos of Palliative Nursing

Mark Lazenby and Michael Anthony Moore

Key Points

- Palliative nursing has an ethos, a moral character, that builds meaning in the context of serious illness and death and dying.
- This moral character is defined by the qualities of a caring relationship.
- Trustworthiness, moral imagination, attending to the beauty of patients' humanity, creating a moral space in which patients can flourish, and being present with them are some of these qualities.

Case Study: The Ethos of Palliative Nursing

In the windowless hospital room lay a man dying of bone-rattling prostate cancer. The stars shined bright on the desert sky, but in this moment misery raked this man's soul. Between shallow, painful breaths, and the interludes of his wife wiping his beady brow, I asked this man to tell me his story. As a child, he was born and grew up a free man, but here lay in sharp contrast, a 61-year-old man in stateless adulthood. His childhood memories are of being with his siblings and friends, running and playing hide-and-seek in the olive trees in his grandparents' orchard. Trees even more ancient than his grandparents stood steady while war after war roiled through. Beneath the cover of night, the teenaged-man forcedly packed what cherished belongings he could carry with him and fled his homeland for a distant country not his own. As he started his trek, the man packed away some olive wood that had lain on the ground outside his house. This wood honored the lineage not just of his grandparents, and their parents, and their parents' parents, but also of all the olive trees that bore witness to his family's history.

The day I stepped into his story, he was dying—not just dying of prostate cancer but of a misery deep and untouchable by hormone therapy, steroids, opiates, or anything that we, as palliative care clinicians, have in our armamentarium to cure. Since I was a foreign, visiting scholar with a flexible schedule, I decided to sit with him and his wife for a few hours. I had nowhere else urgent to be—no beeping alarms, no intravenous line to change, no medications to give to lure me away; I had only time. And so, it was time I gave this man and his wife. My questions began by asking him about how he came to be in this country, the country of his adulthood but not of his childhood—the country of his fleeing-to but not of his rising-up-in. His story brought us to the olive groves that he lay under at night as a mere youth, looking up at the stars, more stars than he could count, stars that, to be sure, were biblical. Those ancient stars, he imparted, were the same stars King David had lain under after his anointing, the very stars that had guided the Magi to Bethlehem, the stars that Saint Paul used to navigate the road to Damascus, and the stars that the Damascenes used to travel to Mecca to go to the Holy Mosque for the Haj. After only a half hour of talking, the man's story arrived at what he wished for his final goodbye to this earth. He wanted to see those stars, the stars that observed biblical history and that had shown upon the olive trees of his youth. These ancient stars were calling him home, to his permanent home, a home beyond wars, borders, religions—a home where his ancestors dwell, a home in the stars.

To aid in his final goodbye, I secured clearance from the cancer center to take him and his wife up to the roof of the hospital one night. His pain notwithstanding, it was an ordeal. No elevator went all the way to the roof, so we had to devise a plan that included four of us carrying him up the last flight of stairs. Another helper worked to hold his urinary catheter as we executed the tactical operation. Prior to moving the patient, we placed a mattress for him to lie upon. We did it—we got him there on a stunning desert night when the stars smiled brilliantly at him. He lay there on the mattress with his wife, indulging in a talkative spurt of energy I had not hitherto seen in him. He looked upon the stars, and, in his native tongue, chattered to his wife. She gripped his hand tight, while tears were visible on her face. She did not wipe them. He could not see them as his eyes remained fixed on the stars. She listened, and cried, and held his hand tight. I understood his chattering enough to hear him say that he was ready to go; he wanted to see his family up there—in the stars. A few days later, the man died. It was a welcomed death as his pain had become unremitting. He had fallen into an obtunded state, but now he was with the stars.

Shortly after he had died, I came in and sat with him and his wife. Again, I was able to offer her time by being with her. She clutched a cross in her hands, and I could hear her praying while moving it between her fingers. The woman fell into deep sobs, convulsing in grief, so I continued to be with her. I spoke no words, but rather, I felt all I could do was witness her incomprehensible and ineffable sadness. And then, without words, she handed me that cross. She opened my clenched fingers and placed it into the palm of my hand.

She looked up at me and said, "He carved it from the olive wood he took with him. I want you to have it. You are his child."

Here I had in my hand the cross this man had carved from the olive wood he had taken with him as he escaped his childhood homeland. During a war that had threatened him and his family, he still made it a point to pack this meaningful olive wood with the few belongings he was able to carry. I meditated on the cross of wood and the symbolism of the fallen branches from the trees that had looked upon his family through the centuries. The stars that had witnessed his familial history bore witness to his religious and biblical history and then, finally, to his death.

Caring for this man and his wife was the job of any palliative nurse. And, in a sense, no palliative nurse deserved such a special gift, but the token of the olive cross honored the relationship of the nurse with the patient's wife and with the patient himself. An ethics of caring is based on the notion that what it means to be a good person—a moral person, that is—has to do with the nature of relationships.[1, 2, 3] With this, what it means to be a good palliative nurse has to do with the nature of the relationships nurses develop with their patients and loved ones. This chapter will describe five qualities that are part of a caring relationship and, within the context of palliative care, form the ethos—the moral character—of palliative nursing. These five qualities are trustworthiness, imagination, beauty, space, and presence.

Trustworthiness

Trustworthiness cuts close to the heart of the ethos of palliative care nursing. Year after year, the public has rated nurses as members of the most trusted of professions.[4] Speculation on the potential reasons for the public's trust is possible, but the most obvious answer is that nurses are, in fact, trustworthy. The contemporary bioethicist Onora O'Neill has convincingly argued that trustworthiness has three components: competence, reliability, and honesty.[5]

Competency is essential for palliative nurses. This is why the Hospice and Palliative Nursing Association and the Hospice and Palliative Credentialing Center have established minimum experience and knowledge standards for achieving and maintaining certification as a hospice and palliative nurse. The contribution of competence to nursing's trustworthiness is so important that nurses work together as a community to ensure that each nurse practices safely. Nurses are each other's keeper, and the keeper of the public's trust, by working together to make sure that nurses do not harm patients. Competence also involves practicing according to the latest evidence. Nursing science contributes to trustworthiness by guiding practicing nurses through the results of rigorous science to help direct the most efficient ways to bring about patients' desired goals of care.

Reliability and competence are first cousins because a reliable nurse must first be competent. However, reliability differs from competence in that, to be reliable, nurses must do what they say they will do and be present when they say they will be present. The moral force of reliability is that patients and families can depend on what nurses say to them.

After listening to the man's stories in the case study, it is clear that the nurse wanted to give the patient a view of the stars before he died. But before the nurse asked the patient whether he wanted to see the stars one last time, the nurse had to have a way to make it happen. The nurse's own reliability and the reliability of the nurse's colleagues and the hospital would have otherwise been at stake. So, before the nurse proposed the idea to the patient and his wife, the nurse would have first had to check with colleagues and nursing administration. The hospital administration's embrace of the idea was dim, but administration understood the importance of the unusual plan for the patient's and his wife's wishes. If the nurse had mentioned the plan to the patient and his wife before the nurse had done this homework, the collective reliability of the nurse, the nurse's colleagues, and the hospital would have been on the line.

The palliative nurse also understands that reliability entwines with *honesty*. A nurse's word, to a large degree, verbalizes her or his reliability. In the context of healthcare, honesty, O'Neill suggests, is not just keeping one's word, but ensuring the absence of deception. When patients and families ask questions for which there is no easy, straightforward answer, it is dishonest for nurses to pretend there is an answer. No medication guarantees a relief of the patient's symptoms—remember that science traffics in probability, whereas treatment plans favor the odds, rather than guarantees, of success. Based on scientific testing, the probability of a medication's efficacy for relieving a symptom may be in the patient's favor, and that is exactly how nurses need to respond to patients' questions. However, in the end, the medication may not relieve the patient's symptom. The medication or treatment may fail to work as science suggests it does. Explaining efficacy of medical options should guide nurse–patient communication and will aid in rationalizing why a palliative care team may have to move on to other modalities to attempt symptom relief. The sake of honesty further demands not deceiving patients and their families. Nurses practice in very few certainties other than the singular idea that each human, including the nurse herself, shall one day die. Honesty with patients and their families rests in nurses acknowledging that there are no certainties. Nurses cannot deceive patients and their families by withholding information or deceiving them with fake certainties. Rather, being present with them in the indeterminacy of pain and suffering and dying is how nurses do not deceive patients and families.

Imagination

The second quality of a caring relationship is imagination. Often, not having straightforward answers to medical and spiritual issues overwhelms those in palliative nursing. All nurses have had patients who, before they die, have one last desire that seems impossible to achieve. These situations demand imaginative thinking. The eighteenth-century philosopher, Immanuel Kant, believed that imagination takes an individual back to "first principles," meaning that imagination brings one back to what matters most and what is most fundamental.[6]

In the case study, imagination was necessary, as the nurse knew that the patient could not be taken back to his grandfather's olive trees; the patient was too sick to transport that far. Whatever the nurse could do for the patient had to be imagined right where the patient was. The nurse's colleagues, the hospital administration, and the nurse had to think new thoughts about how to take the patient back to those memories of lying under the trees and looking up at the stars. They had to use their imaginations to devise a plan to get the patient as close to that experience as possible.

Imagination as described here is deeper than just devising a creative plan to achieve a desired result. Moral imagination means that nurses can *feel with* their patients and their families. This does not mean that, through empathy, nurses must suffer the same as patients and families suffer. However, it does mean that nurses have to feel, or sympathize, with how important goals, beliefs, and practices are to patients and families. Nurses must work to feel the depth of whatever brings their patients meaning, purpose, peace, and comfort as they face serious illness and even death. This feeling—a feeling named here as *compassion*, a feeling of caring for what matters to others who suffer—gives nurses the energy to think creatively about how to help patients and families achieve their goals. Furthermore, compassion aids nurses in being faithful to patients' and families' beliefs and practices when the odds are against them. Compassionate imagination gives one's creative solutions legs, not just by thinking about innovative solutions to achieve patients' and families' goals, but compassionate imagination requires actively working to bring that solution to fruition. By engaging in imaginative solutions to seemingly intractable problems, nurses see the humanity of their patients. Humanity is, after all, beautiful.

Beauty

Beauty is another quality of a caring relationship: seeing the beauty of patients' humanity. The first way to honor patients' beauty is to listen to them. Not only is listening the process of relationships, according to the contemporary moral psychologist Carol Gilligan, but listening is the only way a provider can discover who patients are and what matters to them as they face serious illness.[7] Furthermore, what is distinctive about the beauty of humanity is that humanity can be injured. "Injury," the contemporary scholar of aesthetics, Elaine Scarry, says, is the opposite of beauty.[8] And yet, if, *per impossibile*, someone were invulnerable to injury, by definition he or she would be incapable of being beautiful. Being beautiful is being open to injury, even though injury is a wrong, as Scarry notes. Serious illness is a wrong in that it opens individuals up to injury by directly challenging their humanity. But amid the injury of serious illness, listening to patients is actively restorative. Listening is the succor that restores their humanity in face of the injury of serious illness. While actively listening, the nurse ceases to be the nurse, the healthcare provider, the medication prescriber, the Other; rather, the nurse becomes a person listening to another person, listening to the other's joys and sorrows, reminiscences and regrets, hopes and fears. When actively listening, nurses treat their patients not as patients but as people who, though sick and dying, are alive.

The man dying of prostate cancer, in a country not his own, was foreign to the nurse. The nurse could speak the patient's tongue grammatically, but only a native speaker who had shared the culture and experiences of this patient could so easily share the unspoken symbols of the language. Although the physical language was understood, the underlying humanity brought from the historical culture of the language could have been easily lost in translation without the nurse's actively listening. It was active work for the nurse to sit and listen to the patient's stories through this foreign tongue. Nurses may not immediately fully understand their patients because of a lack of shared experiences or culture. After listening to a few stories, though, surely nurses can find deep commonalities and connections. More profoundly, humanity is shared by all; this is a commonality between nurse and patient; everyone shares the same nature: human nature. When nurses listen deeply enough, they hear their own humanity in others' stories. In hearing one's own humanity in others, one can then feel the compassion that motivates imagination.

The realities of modern nursing, however, conspire against imagination. Nurses do not have time to sit and listen to patients for hours, much less minutes, on end. Nurses are busy, and the demands of the modern hospital, clinic, and hospice restrict their time. That said, nurses also know from experience that it does not take all that long to listen. A few minutes, sitting down, being attentive, not using the precious time with one's own words, but being aware of patients' words and of their emotions as they speak them: this is listening. Present, attentive listening is the kind of listening that restores beauty even as disease and death injure.

Space

In the modern medical industrial complex, patients present to nurses with their humanity injured by serious illness. Some patients present to the nurse dying. The humanity nurses aim to restore through caring relationships may be injured even more by the public spaces of the hospital, the clinic, and the hospice. This includes the machines that make it possible for nurses to deliver quality symptom management. Even when patients present in their homes, nurses bring with them the paraphernalia of the medical complex: the hospital beds and the equipment and machines that would never otherwise be in their homes.

One quality of a caring relationship is to create the space, in the context of the impersonal medical industrial complex, in which patients can still be themselves.[9] Of course, this is not simple. By being trustworthy with their patients, by imagining what needs to be done to fulfill patients' goals, by being faithful to who patients are, and by active listening, nurses open up the space for patients to be who they are—undefined by serious illness. This is part of the reason to become a palliative nurse: to treat patients as the people they are, to provide them the space to be who they are, even as serious illness imperils or takes their lives. For many palliative nurses, it is what sustains them: that moment when they see a smile shine through, a laugh, the confession of fear, the expression of hope, and the stories of a beautiful life. When nurses care that they are trustworthy, imaginative, and listen to find the beauty of their patients' stories, they then open up the space in the context of serious illness for their patients to be present as themselves.

Presence

To be trustworthy with patients, to offer imaginative responses, to listen to stories, to create the space for patients to be themselves in the clinic or their home, nurses must be present. Being present is another quality of a caring relationship. *Presence*, in the context of palliative nursing, is not nurses adopting a power pose by which to assert themselves and their desires upon patients and families. Presence is, rather, being with patients and families not as cases but as people.

When in the presence of other people, nurses respect patients' capacity to make their own decisions and to be in relationships.[10]

The capacity to make decisions is essential to what it means to be a person. There are often circumstances where the nurse may not understand, or even agree with, every decision the patient makes. For instance, the patient's disease may be progressing with every evidence-based treatment already utilized, but the patient still may want to "keep going." There are infinite reasons why a patient may choose a particular decision or course of action, and the patient may need psychological or spiritual support to come to terms with said reasons. A nurse must not take away the patient's capacity and ability to make decisions about his or her own care, lest the nurse take away the patient's personhood. By taking away personhood, the nurse ceases to be in the presence of this human, and, therefore, the ability to be in a caring relationship with this person ceases. For a palliative nurse, this is simply untenable. For palliative nursing, the quality of presence is to be in the presence of a person who makes decisions about his or her own life.

The quality of presence includes respecting people's capacity to be in relationships. Patients have the capacity to choose with whom they want to be in relationship—including the nurse. Remember, patients come with their own histories around relationships, which may include traumatic relationships. Nurses must be open to patients choosing, or not choosing, to be in relationship with them. If the choice is the latter, it does not negate the role of the palliative nurse. It means, rather, that the nature of the nursing arrangement with the patient becomes more task-oriented. Yet, the nurse, through mindful presence, can still look for moments when the patient is open to relationship. It is in these moments that patients and nurses are present with each other and can make meaning in shared experiences.

The authors believe that that is what happened with the man who died of prostate cancer and with the nurse in the case study. The patient opened himself up to having a relationship with the nurse, even though he had only come to know the nurse in the last few days of his life. It is uncertain whether the patient made some meaning out of his and the nurse's relationship, but it seems as if he did. He asked his wife to give the nurse the cross the patient had carved out of the wood he had carried with him from the land from which he had long ago been dispossessed. Nor do we know whether the nurse made meaning out of her relationship with the patient and his wife. This gift of presence, however, gave the nurse the opportunity to become a better person, if only by learning to be open to having a relationship with people who seem far from one. The quality of presence is the quality of being open to the choices of patients, including their choices to make meaning out of illness with the nurse by their side. By being present to them—ready for them to choose to be in relationship—the nurse remains open to her or his own growth.

Palliative nursing demands much from nurses; it taxes emotions and spirits. However, if nurses attend to the qualities of a caring relationship through the five qualities articulated here, then the unexpected creation of meaning in the context of relationships with other people for whom nurses care becomes the ethos that carries nurses through these difficulties. These five qualities of a caring relationship—trustworthiness, imagination, beauty, space, and presence—help guide the palliative nurse to honor the humanity of his or her patients and his or her own humanity, too. There surely are other ways of articulating these and other qualities via serendipitous creativity,[11] which is an openness to the new meaning one can create in caring for the sick and the dying. But this is what the authors take the ethos—the moral character—of palliative nursing to be: that nurses are in caring relationships with their patients.

REFERENCES

1. Lazenby M. *Caring Matters Most: The Ethical Significance of Nursing*. New York: Oxford University Press; 2017.
2. Gilligan C. *In a Different Voice: Psychological Development and Women's Development*. Cambridge, MA: Harvard University Press; 1982.
3. Baier A. *A Progress of Sentiments: Reflections on Hume's Treatise*. Cambridge, MA: Harvard University Press; 1991.
4. Norman J. Americans Rate Healthcare Providers High on Honesty, Ethics. Gallup News Web site. 2016; http://news.gallup.com/poll/200057/americans-rate-healthcare-providers-high-honesty-ethics.aspx. Accessed December 7, 2017.
5. O'Neill O. *A Question of Trust: The BBC Reith Lectures 2002*. Cambridge: Cambridge University Press; 2002.
6. Kant I. *Fundamental Principles of the Metaphysics of Morals*. New York: Liberal Arts Press; 1949.
7. Gilligan C, Eddy J. Listening as a path to psychological discovery: an introduction to the Listening Guide. *Perspect Med Educ*. 2017;6(2):76–81. doi: 10.1007/s40037-017-0335-3.
8. Scarry E. *On Beauty and Being Just: The Tanner Lectures on Human Values 1998*. Princeton, NJ: Princeton University Press; 1999.
9. Butler J. *Notes Toward a Performative Theory of Assembly*. Cambridge, MA: Harvard University Press; 2015.
10. Farley MA. *Compassionate Respect: A Feminist Approach to Medical Ethics and Other Questions*. Mahwah, NJ: Paulist Press; 2002.
11. Kaufman GD. *In Face of Mystery: A Constructive Theology*. Cambridge, MA: Harvard University Press; 1995.

PART II

Symptom Assessment and Management in Adult and Older Adult Populations

11

Pain Management

Judith A. Paice and Martin Galligan

Key Points

- Pain is highly prevalent in palliative care, yet the majority of individuals can obtain good relief with available treatment options.
- An awareness of barriers to adequate pain care allows palliative care nurses to assess for and to plan interventions to overcome these obstacles when caring for patients. Advocacy is a critical role of the palliative care nurse.
- Assessment of pain, including a thorough history and comprehensive physical exam, guides the development of the pharmacological and nonpharmacological treatment plan.
- Treatment options include pharmacological therapies such as non-opioids, opioids, and adjuvant analgesics, along with nonpharmacological, integrative, and interventional therapies; in those with certain illnesses such as cancer, disease-modifying treatments can provide relief.

Of the many symptoms experienced by those with serious illness, pain is one of the most common and most feared. However, this fear is largely unfounded because the majority of patients with serious illness can obtain relief. Nurses are critical members of the palliative care team, particularly in providing pain management. The nurse's role begins with assessment and continues through the development of a plan of care and its implementation. During this process, the nurse provides education and counseling to the patient, family, and other team members. Nurses also are critical for developing institutional policies and monitoring outcomes that ensure good pain management for all patients within their palliative care program. To provide optimal pain control, all healthcare professionals must understand the barriers that prevent good management, the assessment of this syndrome, and the treatments used to provide relief. Effective pain control and alleviation of suffering are highly dependent upon the strength of the clinician, patient, and family communication and relationship. These are key strengths of nursing, at all phases of palliative care.

Case Study

Elaine Adams is a 45-year-old woman with metastatic triple-negative breast cancer, treated with multiple courses of chemotherapy and radiotherapy. She developed low back pain and was found to have a new metastatic lesion at L3. The low back pain radiated to the left buttock and lateral thigh; the low back pain was aching, and the left buttock and leg pain was described as shooting and electrical. She was taking hydrocodone/acetaminophen 10/325 mg two tablets every 4 hours without adequate relief (usually 8–10 tablets per 24 hours). Because of the frequent requests for refills, the oncology team consulted palliative care.

Prevalence of Pain

The prevalence of pain in those with serious illness varies by diagnosis and other factors. Approximately one-third of persons who are actively receiving treatment for cancer and two-thirds of those with advanced malignant disease experience pain.[1] Individuals at particular risk for undertreatment include the elderly, minorities, and women. Almost three-quarters of patients with advanced cancer admitted to the hospital experience pain upon admission. In other studies of patients admitted to palliative care units, pain often is the dominant symptom, along with fatigue and dyspnea. Children with cancer also are at risk for pain and suffering.[2]

Unfortunately, there has been little characterization of the pain prevalence and experience of patients with other life-threatening disorders. However, those working in palliative care are well aware that pain frequently accompanies many serious illnesses, such as human immunodeficiency virus (HIV), multiple sclerosis, amyotrophic lateral sclerosis, end-stage renal disease (ESRD), and, more recently, COVID-19.[3,4] Furthermore, many patients in hospice and palliative care are elderly and more likely to have existing chronic pain syndromes, such as osteoarthritis or low back pain.[5]

Additional research is needed to fully characterize the frequency and the type of pain syndromes seen in patients with serious illness. This information will lead to improved detection, assessment, and, ultimately, treatment. Unfortunately, pain continues to be undertreated, even when prevalence rates and syndromes are well understood. The undertreatment is largely due to barriers related to healthcare professionals, the system, and patients and their families.[6]

Barriers to Pain Relief

Barriers to good pain relief are numerous and pervasive. Often, because of lack of education, misconceptions, or attitudinal issues, these barriers contribute to the significant numbers of patients who do not get adequate pain relief. Careful examination of these barriers provides a guide for changing individual practice, as well as building an institutional plan within the palliative care program to improve pain relief (Box 11.1). Most studies address the barriers associated with cancer pain. Therefore, barriers facing individuals with other disorders commonly seen in palliative care are not well characterized. One might suggest that these individuals are affected to an even greater extent as biases may be more pronounced in those with noncancer diagnoses.

Healthcare Providers

Fears related to opioids held by professionals lead to underuse of these analgesics, and this concern has been exacerbated by the exploding opioid misuse epidemic.[7] Numerous surveys have revealed that physicians, nurses, and pharmacists express concerns about substance use disorder, tolerance, and side effects of morphine and related compounds.[6] Inevitability of pain is also expressed, despite evidence to the contrary. Not surprisingly, lack of attention to pain and its treatment during basic education is frequently cited.[8] The result is a reduction in opioid prescribing that may be leading to unrelieved pain and increased pain-related admissions to the emergency department by those with advanced disease.[9,10] Those of a minority race and those with lower socioeconomic status often receive lower rates of opioid prescribing.[11] Those providing care at the end of life must evaluate their own knowledge and beliefs, including cultural biases, and strive to educate themselves and their colleagues.

Box 11.1 Barriers to Cancer Pain Management

Problems Related to Healthcare Professionals

Inadequate knowledge of pain management
Poor assessment of pain
Concern about regulation of controlled substances
Fear of patients developing substance use disorder
Concern about side effects of analgesics
Concern about patients' becoming tolerant to analgesics
Lack of discussions regarding prognosis and treatment planning

Problems Related to the Healthcare System

Low priority given to cancer pain treatment
Restrictive regulation of controlled substances
Problems of availability of treatment or access to it

- Inadequate reimbursement
- Shortages of medications
- Limited availability of palliative care and pain specialists
- Limited access to specialists for patients with substance use disorder
- Insufficient time

Problems Related to Patients

Reluctance to report pain
Concern about distracting physicians from treatment of underlying disease
Fear regarding the cause of pain (uncertainty or that pain means disease is worse)
Concern about not being a "good" patient
Spiritual/religious beliefs regarding pain and its treatment
Poor health literacy/challenges to adherence to analgesic regimen
Reluctance to take pain medications
Fear of substance use disorder or of being thought of as an "addict"
Worries about unmanageable side effects
Concern about becoming tolerant to pain medications

Healthcare Settings

Lack of availability of opioids is pervasive, affecting not only sparsely populated rural settings but also inner-city pharmacies reluctant to carry these medications. Pain management continues to be a low priority in some healthcare settings, reimbursement for these services is poor, and, as a result, some settings lack qualified professionals with expertise in pain management. All of this is complicated by the cost of analgesic treatments and lack of reimbursement by third-party payers.[12]

Patients and Families

Understanding these barriers will lead the professional to better educate and better counsel patients and their families. Since these fears are insidious, patients and family members or support persons should be asked if they are concerned about substance use disorder and tolerance (often described as becoming "immune" to the drug by laypersons).[12] Stigma regarding opioids is a powerful barrier to effective relief.[13,14] Studies have suggested that these fears lead to undermedication and increased intensity of pain.[15] Concerns about being a "good" patient or belief in the inevitability of cancer pain lead patients to hesitate in reporting pain. In these studies, less educated and older patients were more likely to express these beliefs. Patients seeking active treatment may believe that admitting to pain or other symptoms may reduce their eligibility for clinical trials. Lack of adherence to the medication regimen, complicated by limited understanding, can lead to unrelieved pain. Some patients and family members delay taking opioids, believing they are only for the dying.

At the end of life, patients may need to rely on family members or other support persons to dispense medications. Each person's concerns must be addressed or provision of medication may be inadequate. The interdisciplinary team is essential, with nurses, social workers, chaplains, physicians, volunteers, and others exploring the meaning of pain and possible barriers to good relief. Education, counseling, reframing, and spiritual support are imperative. Nurses are particularly well trained to offer the education and "coaching" that has been shown to provide improved relief. Strategies to provide education and support have included print materials, internet-based programs, telehealth programs, and videoconferencing to educate patients, particularly those in rural areas. Overall, patient education has resulted in modest improvements in pain outcomes.[16]

Effects of Unrelieved Pain

Although many professionals and laypersons fear that opioid analgesics lead to shortened life, there is evolving evidence to the contrary.[17] It is likely that inadequate pain relief hastens death by increasing physiological stress, potentially diminishing immunocompetence, decreasing mobility, worsening proclivities toward pneumonia and thromboembolism, and increasing the work of breathing and myocardial oxygen requirements. Furthermore, pain may lead to spiritual death as the individual's quality of life is impaired through suffering.[18] Therefore, it is the professional and ethical responsibility of clinicians to focus on, and attend to, adequate pain relief for their patients and to properly educate patients and their caregivers about all analgesic therapies, including opioids.

Assessment and Common Pain Syndromes

Comprehensive assessment of pain is imperative. This must be conducted initially, regularly throughout the treatment, and during any changes in the patient's pain state. Table 11.1 addresses the differing qualities of pain (e.g., neuropathic, nociceptive [also called "somatic"], visceral, and "total pain") aligned with examples of syndromes and treatments that may be of benefit. For many individuals with serious illness, a combination of pain types is common.[19–21]

Table 11.1 Pain assessment: relationship to assessment findings and therapy

Pain type	Etiological factors	Distribution	Descriptors	Potential pharmacological interventions	Potential nonpharmacological interventions
Neuropathic	Peripheral or central nervous system injury Nerve involvement by tumor Spinal cord compression Neuralgia (trigeminal, post-herpetic) Peripheral neuropathies (microtubule inhibitors, viral or antiretroviral therapies, diabetes) Post-stroke pain Phantom pain Radiation plexopathy Post-surgical	Symmetrical distribution across one or more dermatomes at the site of pain (e.g., post-herpetic neuralgia), in the area of innervation from the nerve root (e.g., radiculopathy), localized to feet and hands (e.g., chemotherapy-induced peripheral neuropathy) Focal distribution, includes the level of spinal lesion plus area below it (e.g., spinal cord compression) Stroke pain impacting contralateral area of damage	Burning Electrical Numb "Pins and needles" Radiating Shooting Tingling Stabbing	Anticonvulsants Antidepressants Local anesthetics Corticosteroids Nerve blocks Opioids	Exercise Heat/cold Massage Acupuncture Mindfulness TENS Cognitive behavioral therapy
Somatic (nociceptive)	Nociceptor activation or injury to superficial cutaneous and deep musculoskeletal structures Bone or spine metastasis Fractures Arthritis Osteoporosis Immobility Post-surgical Wound pain	Specific to the site of injury because of nociceptive activation Temperature: extremes of hot or cold resulting in tissue damage in a specific area Mechanical: stretching or pressure resulting in tissue damage Chemical: inflammatory cascade because of injury, causing localized pain and swelling	Aching Dull Sore Throbbing Sharp	NSAIDs Acetaminophen Corticosteroids Bisphosphonates Radiation therapy (bone metastasis) Opioids Local anesthetics	Exercise Heat/cold Massage Acupuncture Mindfulness TENS Cognitive behavioral therapy Distraction
Visceral	Bowel obstruction Venous occlusion or ischemia Liver metastasis Ascites Post-abdominal or -thoracic surgery Pancreatitis Cancers in the abdomen and chest	Poorly localized and can present as a more diffuse generalized pain throughout an area of the body Often referred (e.g., liver metastases causing pain in right shoulder)	Bloated Crampy Deep Pressure Squeezing Stretching	NSAIDs Acetaminophen Opioids (use with caution in patients with bowel obstruction) Spinal analgesia	Exercise Heat/cold Massage Acupuncture Mindfulness TENS Cognitive behavioral therapy
Existential pain or pain exacerbated by emotional distress	Suffering Mood disorders Altered coping	Distribution can vary significantly and change site, duration, and intensity Widespread total-body pain Difficult to localize	"Pain all over"	Greater emphasis on team support, spiritual care, and nonpharmacologic strategies; may include antidepressants	Multidisciplinary team: Psychological support Spiritual support Nonpharmacologic strategies

NSAIDs, nonsteroidal anti-inflammatory drugs; TENS, transcutaneous electrical nerve stimulation.
Sources: References 19–21.

A variety of pain assessment tools are available, including for those unable to verbally self-report. Excellent reviews provide in-depth discussions of the use of these instruments.[22,23] An important change in pain assessment has been the increasing emphasis on function; this provides a goal and measurable outcome for the efficacy of analgesic treatment. We often ask patients, "If we can do a better job with pain control, what might you be able to do that you cannot now?" Examples may include returning to work, walking outside, or holding a grandchild. Another change in pain assessment has been the inclusion of risk factors for substance use disorder (see Chapter 68 for comprehensive discussion).

Pharmacological Management of Pain in Advanced Disease

A sound understanding of pharmacotherapy in the treatment of pain is of great importance in palliative care nursing. First, this knowledge allows the nurse to contribute to and fully understand the comprehensive plan of care. Thorough understanding also allows the nurse to recognize, prevent, and assess medication-related adverse effects; to understand drug–drug and drug–disease interactions; and to educate patients and caregivers regarding appropriate medication usage.

This section provides an overview of the most commonly used pharmaceutical agents available in the United States for the treatment of unremitting and recurrent pain associated with advanced disease. The intent of this section is to arm the reader with a fundamental and practical understanding of the medications that are (or should be) available in most contemporary care settings, emphasizing those therapies for which there is clear and convincing evidence of efficacy.

Since patients or family members are not always aware of the names of their medications, or they may bring pills to the hospital or clinic that are not in their original bottles, many web-based resources provide pictures that can assist the nurse in identifying the current analgesic regimen. These can be found at http://www.drugs.com/pill_identification.html or http://www.webmd.com/pill-identification/default.htm. Many of these programs are available as applications for mobile phones and tablets.

Non-opioid Analgesics

Acetaminophen

Acetaminophen has been determined to be one of the safest analgesics for long-term use in the management of mild pain or as a supplement in the management of more intense pain syndromes, yet questions regarding its analgesic efficacy have been raised. Acetaminophen (also abbreviated as "APAP" and referred to as "paracetamol" outside of North America) may be considered an adjunct to any chronic pain regimen. A Cochrane review of oral acetaminophen found no high-quality evidence to support or refute its use alone or in combination with opioids for cancer pain.[24] Reduced dose or avoidance of acetaminophen is recommended in the face of renal insufficiency or liver dysfunction. A complete review of both prescribed as well as over-the-counter (OTC) medications taken by the patient is indicated. Many OTCs contain acetaminophen, and patients may not be aware of the risk of overdose. An intravenous formulation of acetaminophen is currently available and has been studied in a variety of perioperative, postoperative, and acute care settings. Cost issues and lack of clear benefit over oral administration may preclude its use in palliative care.

Nonsteroidal Anti-inflammatory Drugs

Nonsteroidal anti-inflammatory drugs (NSAIDs) affect analgesia by reducing the biosynthesis of prostaglandins, thereby inhibiting the cascade of inflammatory events that cause, amplify, or maintain nociception. These agents also appear to reduce pain by influences on the peripheral or central nervous system independent of their anti-inflammatory mechanism of action. This secondary mode of analgesic efficacy is poorly understood. The "classic" NSAIDs (e.g., aspirin and ibuprofen) are relatively nonselective in their inhibitory effects on the enzymes that convert arachidonic acid to prostaglandins. As a result, gastrointestinal (GI) ulceration, renal dysfunction, and impaired platelet aggregation are common. The cyclooxygenase-2 (COX-2) enzymatic pathway is induced by tissue injury or other inflammation-inducing conditions. It is for this reason that there appears to be less risk of GI bleeding with use of the COX-2-selective NSAID celecoxib, at least during initial months of treatment (Table 11.2).

Although data remains limited, clinical experience suggests that the NSAIDs are useful in the treatment of many pain conditions mediated by inflammation, including those caused by cancer.[25,26] The NSAIDs offer the potential advantage of causing minimal nausea, constipation, sedation, or other effects on mental functioning. Therefore, depending on the cause of pain, NSAIDs may be useful for moderate to severe pain control, either alone or as an adjunct to opioid analgesic therapy. The addition of NSAIDs to opioids has the benefit of potentially allowing reduction of the opioid dose when sedation, confusion, dizziness, or other central nervous system effects of opioid analgesic therapy alone become burdensome.

Decreased renal function and liver failure are relative contraindications for NSAID use. Similarly, platelet dysfunction or other potential bleeding disorders contraindicate use of the nonselective NSAIDs due to their inhibitory effects on platelet aggregation, with resultant prolonged bleeding time. Cardiovascular risk associated with NSAIDs, including myocardial infarction and stroke, has been identified and appears to be higher in those with preexisting risk factors. Cardiovascular risk appears to be dependent upon duration of use, with celecoxib risk associated with 30 days or more of continuous use, while with other NSAIDs, such as ibuprofen, the risk increases within 7 days of use.[27,28] Studies suggest that patients are often unaware of the adverse effects associated with these drugs and may use NSAIDs in a way that increases risk.[29]

Opioid Analgesics

As a pharmacological class, the opioid analgesics represent the most useful agents for the treatment of pain associated with advanced disease. The opioids are nonspecific insofar as they decrease pain signal transmission and perception throughout the nervous system,

Table 11.2 Acetaminophen and selected nonsteroidal anti-inflammatory drugs

Drug	Dose if patient >50 kg	Dose if patient <50 kg
Acetaminophen[a,b]	500–1,000 mg q 4–6 h oral; maximum 4,000 mg/24 h (2,000–3,000 mg if used chronically) 1,000 mg q 6 h IV (given over 15-min infusion); maximum 4,000 mg/24 h	10–15 mg/kg q 4 h (oral) 15 mg/kg q 6 h; maximum 75 mg (IV)
		15–20 mg/kg q 4 h (rectal)
Aspirin[a,b]	4,000 mg/24 h maximum, given q 4–6 h	10–15 mg/kg q 4 h (oral)
		15–20 mg/kg q 4 h (rectal)
Ibuprofen[a,b]	2,400 mg/24 h maximum, given q 6–8 h	10 mg/kg q 6–8 h (oral)
Naproxen[a,b]	1,000 mg/24 h maximum, given q 8–12 h	5 mg/kg q 8 h (oral/rectal)
Choline magnesium trisalicylate[a,c]	2,000–3,000 mg/24 h maximum, given q 8–12 h	25 mg/kg q 8 h (oral)
Indomethacin[b]	75–150 mg/24 h maximum, given q 8–12 h	0.5–1 mg/kg q 8–12 h (oral/rectal)
Ketorolac[d]	30–60 mg IM/IV initially, then 15–30 mg q 6 h bolus IV/IM or continuous IV/SQ infusion; short-term use only (3–5 days)	0.25–1 mg/kg q 6 h short-term use only (3–5 days)
Celecoxib[c,e]	100–200 mg PO up to bid	No data available
Salsalate[c]	1,500 mg PO bid; reduce dose in elderly	No data available

bid, twice a day; IM, intramuscularly; IV, intravenously; PO, orally (per os); q, every; SQ, subcutaneously.

[a] Commercially available in a liquid form.

[b] Commercially available in a suppository form.

[c] Minimal platelet dysfunction.

[d] Potent anti-inflammatory (short-term use only due to gastrointestinal side effects).

[e] Cyclooxygenase-2-selective nonsteroidal anti-inflammatory drug.

regardless of the pathophysiology of the pain. Moderate to severe pain is the main clinical indication for the opioid analgesics.[30] Despite past beliefs that opioids were ineffective for neuropathic pain, these agents have been found to be useful in the treatment of this complex pain syndrome; however, higher doses are usually warranted. Other indications for opioid use include the treatment of dyspnea, reduction in diarrhea, use as an anesthetic adjunct, and use as a form of prophylactic therapy in the treatment of opioid use disorder (e.g., methadone, buprenorphine, or naloxone for those with a history of misuse of opioids).

There is significant inter- and intraindividual variation in clinical responses to the various opioids, so in most cases, a dose-titration approach should be viewed as the best means of optimizing care.[31] This implies that close follow-up is required to determine when clinical endpoints have been reached. Furthermore, idiosyncratic responses may require trials of different agents to determine the most effective drug and route of delivery for any given patient.

Another factor that needs to be considered with opioid analgesics is the potential to accumulate toxic metabolites, especially in the face of decreasing drug clearance and elimination as disease progresses and organ function deteriorates. Due to its neurotoxic metabolite, normeperidine, meperidine use is specifically discouraged for chronic pain management. As well, the mixed agonist–antagonist agents, typified by butorphanol, nalbuphine, and pentazocine, are not recommended for the treatment of chronic pain. They have limited efficacy, and their use may cause an acute abstinence syndrome in patients who are otherwise using pure agonist opioid analgesics.

Morphine

Morphine is most often considered the "gold standard" of opioid analgesics and is used as a measure for dose "equivalence" to determine conversion from one opioid to another or to another route of administration. Although some patients cannot tolerate morphine due to itching, headache, dysphoria, or other adverse effects, common initial dosing effects such as sedation and nausea often resolve within a few days. In fact, one should anticipate these adverse effects, especially constipation, nausea, and sedation, and prevent or treat appropriately (see later discussion). Metabolites of morphine and hydromorphone, morphine-3-glucuronide and hydromorphone-3-glucuronide, respectively, may contribute to myoclonus, seizures, and hyperalgesia (increasing pain), particularly when patients cannot clear these metabolites due to renal impairment.[32]

When patients have dysphagia, several options are available. The 24-hour, long-acting morphine capsule can be broken open and the "sprinkles" placed in applesauce or other soft food. Oral morphine solution can be swallowed, or small volumes (0.5–1 mL) of a concentrated solution (e.g., 20 mg/mL) can be placed in the mouth of patients whose voluntary swallowing capabilities are more significantly limited; the drug gradually enters the GI tract. Buccal uptake of morphine is slow, unpredictable, and insufficient to produce analgesia due to its hydrophilic nature.[33] Furthermore, again due to the hydrophilic nature of morphine, creams, gels, and patches that contain morphine do not cross the skin and therefore do not provide systemic analgesia.[34] Commercially prepared suppositories, compounded suppositories, or microenemas can be used to deliver the drug into the rectum.

Fentanyl

Fentanyl is a highly lipid-soluble opioid that has been administered parenterally, spinally, transdermally, and by nebulizer for the management of dyspnea. Because of its potency, dosing is usually conducted in micrograms.

Transdermal Fentanyl

Transdermal fentanyl, often called the "fentanyl patch," is particularly useful when patients cannot swallow, do not remember to take medications, or have adverse effects to other opioids. Two primary systems are currently available—a reservoir-based patch and a matrix-type patch. These systems exhibit quite similar effects in intact skin, although differences may result when exposed to heat (greater drug permeation at 72 hours in the reservoir system) or to compromised skin (greater permeation seen in the matrix patch).[35] Fever, diaphoresis, cachexia, morbid obesity, liver function, ascites, and the concomitant use of cytochrome P450 3A4 (CYP3A4) inducers may have an impact on the absorption, predictability of blood levels, and clinical effects of transdermal fentanyl. Clinical experience reveals that transdermal fentanyl can be effective even in those patients with few fat stores. Higher doses may be indicated. There is some suggestion that transdermal fentanyl may produce less constipation when compared to long-acting morphine.[36]

Some patients experience decreased analgesic effects after only 48 hours of applying a new patch; a more frequent (q 48 h) patch change should be scheduled. As with all long-acting preparations, breakthrough pain medications should be made available to patients using continuous-release opioids such as the fentanyl patch.[37]

Oxycodone

Oxycodone is a synthetic opioid available in a long-acting formulation, as well as in immediate-release tablets (alone or with acetaminophen, aspirin, or ibuprofen) and liquid. It is approximately as lipid-soluble as morphine but has better oral absorption. The equianalgesic ratio is approximately 20 mg to 30 mg of oral morphine. Side effects appear to be similar to those experienced with morphine. Substances that inhibit CYP3A4, such as the highly active antiretroviral agent ritonavir, the antiviral voriconazole, and even grapefruit juice, have been found to increase oxycodone concentrations.[38] Lower doses of oxycodone may be warranted when CYP3A4 inhibitors are administered.

Methadone

Methadone has several characteristics that make it useful in the management of severe, chronic pain. The half-life of 24 to 60 hours or longer allows prolonged dosing intervals, although for pain control, dosing every 8–12 hours is recommended. Methadone may also bind as an antagonist to the *N*-methyl-D-aspartate (NMDA) receptor, believed to be of particular benefit in neuropathic pain and in preventing hyperalgesia. Additionally, methadone can be given orally, parenterally, and sublingually. Furthermore, methadone is much less costly than comparable doses of proprietary continuous-release formulations, making it potentially more available for patients without sufficient financial resources for more costly drugs.

Despite these advantages, much is unknown about the appropriate dosing ratio between methadone and morphine, as well as the safest and most effective time course for conversion from another opioid to methadone. As a result, a consensus document representing the expert opinions of pain and palliative care clinicians suggests that opioid-naive patients (and those taking less than 60 mg of oral morphine equivalents each day) be started on no more than 7.5 mg of methadone per day with very slow upward titration.[39] For those who are tolerant to opioids with a daily dose of 60–199 mg of morphine equivalents, a ratio of 10:1 should be used to convert to morphine or another opioid.[40] For those receiving 200 mg or more of oral morphine equivalents, the ratio should be 20:1. Regardless of the dose found through conversion, the highest starting dose should be no greater than 30–40 mg per day of methadone.

Methadone should not be used for breakthrough pain dosing or on an as-needed basis. Furthermore, although the long half-life is an advantage, it also increases the potential for drug accumulation before achieving steady-state blood levels, putting patients at risk for oversedation and respiratory depression. For example, it would take 12 days to reach steady state when the half-life is 60 hours. As a result, dose increases should be done no more often than every 5–7 days. Close monitoring of these potentially adverse or even life-threatening effects is required, and most experts suggest that methadone only be prescribed by experienced clinicians.[20,31] Myoclonus has been reported with parenteral methadone use. Of concern for some patients is the prolongation of the QT wave (also called "torsade de pointes") that can occur with methadone administration. Electrocardiographic monitoring may be indicated if consistent with prognosis and goals of care.[39]

Methadone is metabolized by CYP3A4, CYP2D6, and other enzymes. As a result, drugs that induce CYP enzymes accelerate the metabolism of methadone, resulting in reduced serum levels of the drug. This may be demonstrated clinically by shortened analgesic periods or reduced overall pain relief. Examples of these drugs often used in palliative care include several antiretroviral agents, some tyrosine kinase inhibitors, dexamethasone, carbamazepine, phenytoin, and barbiturates.[39,41,42] Drugs that inhibit CYP enzymes slow methadone metabolism, potentially leading to sedation and respiratory depression. These include ketoconazole, omeprazole, and serotonin selective reuptake inhibitor (SSRI) antidepressants such as fluoxetine, paroxetine, and sertraline.

Patients currently receiving methadone as part of a maintenance program for substance use disorder will have developed cross-tolerance to the opioids and, as a result, require higher doses than naive patients. Prescribing methadone for substitution therapy in substance use disorder requires a special license in the United States.

Hydromorphone

Hydromorphone may be a useful alternative when synthetic opioids provide an advantage, although a recent Cochrane review endorsed the need for additional research.[43] It is available in oral tablets, liquids, suppositories, parenteral formulations, and a long-acting formulation. Although hydromorphone-3-glucuronide may accumulate in renal disease, this metabolite is removed when patients are receiving dialysis, providing evidence for the safety of this drug in these patients.[31]

Oxymorphone

Oxymorphone is a semisynthetic opioid that has been available in a parenteral formulation for almost 50 years and more recently in oral immediate-release and extended-release formulations.[44] The safety and efficacy profile in people with cancer is similar to other opioids, such as morphine and oxycodone. The immediate-release formulation has a longer half-life than other immediate-release opioids and may have an advantage for those receiving enteral feeding when other long-acting agents cannot be used.[45]

Other Opioids

Buprenorphine, codeine, hydrocodone, levorphanol, tramadol, and tapentadol are other opioids available in the United States for treatment of pain.

Buprenorphine

This partial agonist, is used for pain control or as part of a medication assisted therapy program for those with opioid misuse disorder or for those with concomitant pain and opioid use disorder.[46] A 7-day buprenorphine patch is approved for moderate to severe pain, and the lowest dose of 5 mcg/hour can be safely used in patients who are opioid-naive. Other formulations include intravenous and sublingual or buccal tablets and films.[47]

Codeine

As a prodrug, codeine must be broken down by the enzyme CYP2D6 to provide analgesia, yet approximately 10% of Caucasians in the United States are poor metabolizers.[48] Conversely, some patients are ultrarapid metabolizers, which can lead to overdose.[49] Recent guidelines suggest care when considering codeine as an analgesic for people with cancer.[30]

Hydrocodone

Immediate-release hydrocodone is only available in combination products, thus limiting dose escalation in palliative care due to concerns regarding excess acetaminophen or other agents. There are single-agent, long-acting hydrocodone products that are administered daily or every 12 hours.[50] The conversion from morphine to hydrocodone is approximately 1.5 (similar to oxycodone).[51]

Levorphanol

Levorphanol has similarities to methadone, including a longer half-life, although it does not affect QTc prolongation and has fewer drug–drug interactions.[52] Availability and lack of awareness, along with limited research, complicate its use.[53]

Tramadol

This weak opioid also has serotonin and norepinephrine reuptake inhibition properties. It is available in immediate- and extended-release formulations. Although effective for mild, nonmalignant, neuropathic pain, a systematic review found insufficient data to support its use for cancer pain.[54] Dose escalation is limited due to potential lowering of the seizure threshold, and clinicians must be alert to the risk of serotonin syndrome. For these reasons, a recent practice guideline recommended caution when used in those with cancer pain.[30]

Tapentadol

Available in immediate- and extended-release formulations, reports suggest tapentadol may be useful in some palliative care settings, particularly in the relief of neuropathic pain.[55,56] Challenges in its use include availability and high cost.

Alternative Routes of Administration for Opioid Analgesics

Many routes of administration are available when patients can no longer swallow or when other dynamics preclude the oral route or favor other routes. These include transdermal, transmucosal (buccal), rectal, enteral, vaginal, epidural, and intrathecal. In a study of cancer patients at 4 weeks, 1 week, and 24 hours before death, the oral route of opioid administration was continued in 62%, 43%, and 20% of patients, respectively. More than half of these patients required more than one route of opioid administration. As patients approached death and oral use diminished, the use of intermittent subcutaneous injections and intravenous or subcutaneous infusions increased.

Thus, in the palliative care setting, non-oral routes of administration must often be available. Enteral feeding tubes can be used to access the gut when patients can no longer swallow. The size of the tube should be considered when administering long-acting morphine or oxycodone "sprinkles" to avoid obstruction of the tube. The rectum, stoma, or vagina can be used to deliver medication. Thrombocytopenia, neutropenia, or painful lesions may preclude the use of these routes. Additionally, delivering medications via these routes can be difficult for family members, especially when the patient is obtunded or unable to assist. As previously discussed, transdermal, transmucosal, or buccal fentanyl are useful alternatives to these techniques.

Parenteral administration includes subcutaneous and intravenous delivery (intramuscular opioid delivery is inappropriate in the palliative care setting). The intravenous route provides rapid drug delivery but requires vascular access, placing the patient at risk for infection and potentially complicating the care provided by family or other loved ones. Subcutaneous boluses have a slower onset and lower peak effect when compared with intravenous boluses. Subcutaneous infusions may total up to 10 mL/hour (although most patients absorb 2 to 3 mL/hour with least difficulty). Volumes greater than 10 mL/hour are poorly absorbed. Hyaluronidase has been reported to speed absorption of subcutaneously administered drugs.

Intraspinal routes, including epidural or intrathecal delivery, may allow administration of drugs, such as opioids, local anesthetics, α-adrenergic agonists, or ziconitide.[57] The equipment used to deliver these medications is complex, requiring specialized knowledge for healthcare professionals and potentially greater caregiver burden.

Preventing and Treating Adverse Effects of Opioid Analgesics

Constipation

Patients in palliative care frequently experience constipation, in part due to opioid therapy. Always begin a prophylactic bowel regimen when commencing opioid analgesic therapy. Recent practice guidelines suggest that conventional laxatives should be considered as first-line treatment and that lifestyle changes (e.g., increased fiber or exercise) have a limited role, and if unrelieved, consider adding specialist medication (e.g., linaclotide, lubiprostone, and prucalopride).[58,59] Several peripherally acting mu-opioid receptor antagonists are available, including subcutaneous and oral formulations (namely methylnaltrexone and naloxegal). For a more comprehensive review of bowel management, refer to Chapter 16.

Sedation

Excessive sedation may occur with the initial exposure to opioids. If sedation persists after 24–48 hours and other correctable causes have been identified and treated if possible, opioid rotation or the addition of psychostimulants may be beneficial. Psychostimulants include dextroamphetamine 2.5–5 mg orally every morning and midday or methylphenidate 5–10 mg orally every morning and 2.5–5 mg midday (although higher doses are frequently used). Adjust both the dose and timing to prevent nocturnal insomnia and monitor for undesirable psychotomimetic effects (such as agitation, hallucinations, and irritability). Little research is available to guide the use of these agents. Modafinil, an agent approved to manage narcolepsy, has been reported to relieve opioid-induced sedation with once-daily dosing. Because of the lack of data regarding these agents, selection of drug and dosing are empirical.

Respiratory Depression

Respiratory depression is rarely a clinically significant problem for opioid-tolerant patients in pain. When respiratory depression occurs in a patient with advanced disease, the cause is usually multifactorial. Therefore, other factors beyond opioids need to be assessed, although opioids are frequently blamed for the reduced respirations. When undesired, depressed consciousness occurs along with a respiratory rate less than 8/minute or hypoxemia (O_2 saturation <90%) associated with opioid use; cautious and slow titration of naloxone, which reverses the effects of the opioids, should be instituted. Excessive administration may cause abrupt opioid reversal with pain and autonomic crisis. In a controlled environment such as an inpatient setting, dilute one ampule of naloxone (0.4 mg/mL) in 10 mL of injectable saline (final concentration 40 mcg/mL) and inject 1 mL every 2–3 minutes while closely monitoring the level of consciousness and respiratory rate. For patients in the home, consider prescribing nasal naloxone (in some states this is mandatory when prescribing an opioid). Educate patients and families regarding appropriate use; often the person experiencing respiratory depression is the opioid-naive child or person inappropriately using the patient's medication. After applying naloxone nasally, call 911 immediately as the duration of effect of naloxone is approximately 30–60 minutes, yet the respiratory depressant effects of the opioid will last much longer.

Nausea and Vomiting

Nausea and vomiting are common with opioids due to activation of the chemoreceptor trigger zone in the medulla, vestibular sensitivity, and delayed gastric emptying; but habituation occurs in most cases within several days. Assess for other treatable causes. Common interventions include antiemetics, opioid switching, and changing the route of the opioid.[60] See Chapter 14 for a thorough discussion of the assessment and treatment of nausea and vomiting.

Myoclonus

Myoclonic jerking can be a neuroexcitatory effect of opioids, occuring more commonly with high-dose opioid therapy, although it has also been reported with lower dosing.[61,62] Opioid rotation and hydration have been reported as beneficial, along with the addition of a benzodiazepine. Clonazepam 0.5–1 mg orally every 6–8 hours, to be increased as needed and tolerated, may be useful in treating myoclonus in patients who are still alert, able to communicate, and take oral preparations. Lorazepam can be given sublingually, if the patient is unable to swallow. Otherwise, parenteral administration of a benzodiazepine, such as midazolam, is indicated if symptoms are distressing.

Pruritus

Pruritus appears to be most common with morphine, in part due to histamine release, but can occur with most opioids. Fentanyl and oxymorphone may be less likely to cause histamine release. Most antipruritic therapies cause sedation, so this side effect must be viewed by the patient as an acceptable trade-off. Antihistamines (such as diphenydramine) are the most common first-line approach to this opioid-induced symptom when treatment is indicated.[63] Ondansetron has been reported to be effective in relieving opioid-induced pruritus, but no randomized controlled studies exist.[64] See Chapter 21 for more information regarding pruritus.

Adjuvant Analgesics

A wide variety of non-opioid medications from several pharmacological classes have been demonstrated to reduce pain caused by various pathological conditions (Table 11.3). As a group, these drugs have been called analgesic "adjuvants," but this is something of a misnomer since they often reduce pain when used alone. However, under most circumstances, when these drugs are indicated for the treatment of moderate to severe neuropathic pain or bone pain, opioid analgesics are used concomitantly to provide adequate pain relief.

Antidepressants

The mechanism of the analgesic effect of tricyclic antidepressants appears to be related to inhibition of norepinephrine and serotonin.[65] The tricyclic antidepressants are generally believed to provide relief from neuropathic pain.[66] Side effects often limit the use of these agents in palliative care. Cardiac arrhythmias, conduction abnormalities, narrow-angle glaucoma, and clinically significant prostatic hyperplasia are relative contraindications to the tricyclic antidepressants. The delay in onset of pain relief, from days to weeks, may preclude the use of these agents for pain relief in end-of-life care. However, their sleep-enhancing and mood-elevating effects may be of benefit.

Both older antidepressants and newer atypical agents have been shown to be effective in relieving neuropathic pain, although there remains little support for the analgesic effect of SSRIs. Atypical antidepressants, venlafaxine and duloxetine, have been shown to reduce neuropathy associated with chemotherapy-induced neuropathy, alone or in combination with gabapentinoids.[67]

Antiepilepsy Drugs

The older antiepilepsy or anticonvulsant drugs, such as carbamazepine and clonazepam, relieve pain by blocking sodium channels. Previously referred to as "membrane stabilizers," these compounds are useful in the treatment of neuropathic pain, especially in those with episodic, lancinating qualities. Gabapentin and pregabalin act at the alpha-2 delta subunit of the voltage-gated calcium channel.[65] Additional evidence supports the use of these agents in neuropathic pain syndromes seen in palliative care, such as thalamic pain, pain due to spinal cord injury, and cancer pain, along with restless leg

Table 11.3 Adjuvant analgesics

Drug class	Daily adult starting dose[a] (range)	Routes of administration	Adverse effects	Indications
Antidepressants	Nortriptyline 10–25 mg	PO	Anticholinergic effects	Neuropathic pain
	Desipramine 10–25 mg	PO		
	Venlafaxine 37.5 mg bid	PO	Nausea, dizziness	
	Duloxetine 30 mg	PO	Nausea	
Anticonvulsants	Clonazepam 0.5–1 mg hs, bid, or tid	PO	Sedation	Neuropathic pain
	Carbamazepine 100 mg q day or tid	PO	Sedation, Aplastic anemia (rare)	
	Gabapentin 100–300 mg tid	PO	Sedation, dizziness	
	Pregabalin 50 mg bid or tid		Sedation, dizziness	
Corticosteroids	Dexamethasone 2–24 mg q day; may give up to 100 mg IV bolus for pain crises	PO/IV/SQ	"Steroid psychosis," dyspepsia	Cerebral edema, spinal cord compression, bone pain, neuropathic pain, visceral pain
	Prednisone 15–30 mg tid	PO		
Local anesthetics	Lidocaine 1–5 mg/kg hourly Lidocaine patch or cream	IV or SQ infusion Topical	Lightheadedness, arrhythmias Skin erythema	Neuropathic pain
N-Methyl-d-aspartate antagonists	Dextromethorphan, effective dose unknown	PO	Confusion	Neuropathic pain
	Ketamine	IV or PO	Cognitive changes	Neuropathic pain Opioid hyperalgesia
Capsaicin	0.025–0.075% cream 8% patch	Topical	Burning	Neuropathic pain
Baclofen	10 mg q day or tid	PO	Muscle weakness, cognitive changes	

bid, twice a day; hs, hour of sleep; IV, intravenously; PO, orally (per os); q, every; SQ, subcutaneously; tid, three times a day.
[a] Pediatric doses for pain control not well established.
Source: Reference 31.

syndrome.[66,68] Both gabapentin and pregabalin require dose reduction in ESRD.[69] Other anticonvulsants have been used with success in treating neuropathies, including lamotrigine, levetiracetam, tiagabine, topiramate, and zonisamide; yet no randomized controlled clinical trials are currently available.

Corticosteroids

Corticosteroids inhibit prostaglandin synthesis and reduce edema surrounding neural tissues. Dexamethasone has been found to reduce postoperative pain and nausea and is particularly useful for relieving painful neuropathic syndromes, including plexopathies, as well as pain associated with stretching of the liver capsule due to metastases.[31] Corticosteroids are also highly effective for treating bone pain due to their anti-inflammatory effects, as well as pain flair after radiation treatment of bone metastases.[70] Dexamethasone has been found to be useful in relieving symptoms associated with malignant intestinal obstruction. Dexamethasone produces the least amount of mineralocorticoid effect, leading to reduced potential for Cushing's syndrome. Dexamethasone is available in oral, intravenous, subcutaneous, and epidural formulations. The standard dose is 2–24 mg/day and can be administered once daily due to the long half-life of this drug. Dexamethasone doses as high as 100 mg may be given with severe pain crises. Intravenous bolus doses should be pushed slowly, to prevent uncomfortable perineal burning and itching.

Local Anesthetics

Local anesthetics work in a manner similar to the older anticonvulsants—by inhibiting the movement of ions across the neural membrane. They are useful for relieving neuropathic pain. Local anesthetics can be given orally, topically, intravenously, subcutaneously, or spinally. Mexiletine has been reported to be useful when anticonvulsants and other adjuvant therapies have failed, although high-quality studies are lacking. Local anesthetic gels and patches have been used to prevent the pain associated with needle stick and other minor procedures. Both gel and patch versions of lidocaine have been shown to reduce the pain of post-herpetic neuropathy. Intravenous or subcutaneous lidocaine at 1–5 mg/kg (maximum 500 mg) administered over 1 hour, followed by a continuous infusion of 1–2 mg/kg/hour has been reported to reduce intractable neuropathic pain in patients in inpatient palliative care and home hospice settings in adults and children.[71]

NMDA Antagonists—Ketamine

Antagonists to NMDA are believed to block the binding of excitatory amino acids, such as glutamate, in the spinal cord. Ketamine, a dissociative anesthetic, is believed to relieve severe neuropathic pain by blocking NMDA receptors. Case reports and small studies suggest that intravenous or oral ketamine can be used in adults and children for the relief of neuropathic pain or to reduce opioid doses.[72] A Cochrane review found insufficient trials conducted to determine safety and efficacy when used in combination with morphine in cancer pain.[73] A randomized, controlled trial of oral ketamine found no difference from placebo when treating cancer-related neuropathic pain.[74] Despite negative results, these investigators suggest there may be a role for ketamine in treating opioid-induced hyperalgesia.

Ketamine is commercially available in the United States only in a parenteral formulation. If the oral route is indicated, a palatable solution can be compounded or the parenteral solution ingested, usually mixed with juice or other liquids to mask the bitter taste. Because the opioid sparing effect is so pronounced, the opioid dose should be reduced by 25%–50% when initiating ketamine. Routine use may be limited by cognitive changes, hallucinations, and other adverse effects, although gradual upward titration may prevent these effects. More research is needed regarding the efficacy of, and adverse effects associated with, the use of ketamine for intractable pain in the palliative care population.

Bisphosphonates

Bisphosphonates, such as pamidronate, zoledronic acid, and ibandronate, inhibit osteoclast-mediated bone resorption. Bisphosphonates treat hypercalcemia and prevent pain related to skeletal events such as metastatic bone disease and multiple myeloma.[75] Denosumab, a RANKL inhibitor, prevents the development of osteoclasts and has been shown to reduce skeletally related events associated with solid tumors, which would reduce pain associated with fractures. A Cochrane review of these agents used to treat bone metastases of breast cancer found some evidence to support pain relief.[75] Another Cochrane review of their use in prostate cancer with bone metastases found no benefit in reducing pain, although there was a reduction in skeletally related events.[76] Toxicities include hypocalcemia, renal dysfunction, and osteonecrosis of the jaw. Clodronate and sodium etidronate appear to provide little or no analgesia.

Case Study—Continued

The palliative care team met with Elaine and conducted a thorough pain, functional, and social assessment. The team also screened for risk for opioid misuse, as they do with each patient; and Elaine was found to have no obvious risk factors for misuse. Her goal was to continue working as an accountant, although this was becoming increasingly difficult as she was having difficulty even getting out of bed most days. She was married, had a supportive wife, and had two teenage sons who were both in high school. Her daily oral morphine milligram equivalence was 100 mg, and opioid prescriptions along with other controlled substances were confirmed during review of the prescription drug monitoring program. Medication review revealed she was supplementing the hydrocodone with ibuprofen 800 mg every 6 hours; she did not previously report this as she thought medications bought OTC did not need to be added to her medication list.

Due to concerns regarding acetaminophen intake, the team added oxycodone extended release 40 mg every 12 hours and continued hydrocodone/acetaminophen 10/325 mg one tablet every 3 hours as needed. She was also started on pregabalin 50 mg twice daily for the neuropathic component of pain, and this dose was gradually increased with benefit. The team recommended stopping ibuprofen at this time as her platelet levels were decreased. A bowel regimen was begun. She and her family were educated about safe use and storage of the medication, and nasal naloxone was prescribed.

Radiation Therapy and Radiopharmaceuticals

Radiotherapy can be enormously beneficial in relieving pain due to bone metastases or other lesions. In some cases, single-fraction external beam therapy can be used to facilitate treatment in debilitated patients. Goals of treatment should be clearly articulated so that patients and family members understand the role of this therapy. Stereotactic body radiation therapy, a targeted therapy that is also referred to as "cyberknife" or "gamma knife radiosurgery," can be effective in selected situations.[77] Radiolabeled agents, also described as radiopharmaceuticals, such as strontium-89 and samarium-153, have been shown to be effective at reducing metastatic bone pain.[78] Thrombocytopenia and leukopenia are relative contraindications since strontium-89 can cause thrombocytopenia in as many as 33% of those treated and leukopenia in up to 10%. Because of the delayed onset and timing of peak effect, only those patients with a projected life span of greater than 3 months should be considered for treatment. Patients should be advised that a transitory pain flare can occur after either external beam therapy or radiolabeled agents; additional analgesics should be provided in anticipation.

Cancer Directed Therapies: Chemotherapy/ Immunotherapy

Therapies that are directed to address tumor burden, such as chemotherapy and immunotherapy, may relieve symptoms such as pain. Patient goals, performance status, sensitivity of the tumor, and potential toxicities must be considered. Examples of symptoms that may improve with chemotherapy include hormonal therapy in breast cancer to relieve chest wall pain due to tumor ulceration, as well as chemotherapy or immunotherapy in lung cancer to relieve dyspnea. However, in a study of patients with stage IV cancers, 69% of those with lung and 81% of those with colorectal cancers did not understand that the chemotherapy was not curative.[79] A prospective trial of palliative chemotherapy given 4 months before death revealed an increased risk of undergoing cardiopulmonary resuscitation, mechanical ventilation, or dying in an intensive care unit.[80] Clear discussions regarding the goals of therapy are warranted.

Other Adjunct Analgesics

Capsaicin

Topical capsaicin is believed to relieve pain by inhibiting the release of substance P. This compound has been shown to be useful in relieving pain associated with post-mastectomy syndrome, post-herpetic neuralgia, and postsurgical neuropathic pain in cancer. A burning sensation experienced by patients is a common reason for discontinuing therapy. A Cochrane review of low-dose topical capsaicin found this therapy unlikely to have meaningful effect, but the high-concentration (8%) topical capsaicin patch was found to be effective in treating HIV-associated and other painful neuropathies.[81,82]

Cannabinoids

There is great interest in the use cannabinoids for the relief of pain in serious illness, particularly as many states have legalized medical marijuana. A thorough discussion of cannabis in palliative care is beyond the scope of this chapter; readers are directed to several review papers.[83,84] Major advances, such as the characterization of the cannabinoid receptors (CB1 and CB2), have increased our understanding of the basic mechanisms of these receptors in pain. Unfortunately, review of existing clinical literature is contradictory, with some studies supporting the role of cannabinoids in relieving neuropathic pain while others demonstrate no reduction in opioid use. Most studies are limited by small sample size and the absence of an effective sham control. Adverse effects include short-term cognitive impairment and hyperemesis syndrome. The potential impact of cannabis on immunotherapy efficacy remains unclear. The International Association for the Study of Pain (IASP) advanced a position statement on cannabis and cannabinoid analgesia after extensive systematic reviews of preclinical and clinical data. This task force concluded that due to the lack of high-quality data, the IASP could not endorse the use of cannabis for pain control and acknowledged the need for additional research.[85]

Interventional Therapies

In addition to previously discussed spinal administration of analgesics, interventional therapies to relieve pain at the end of life can be beneficial, including nerve blocks; vertebroplasty; kyphoplasty, radiofrequency or cyroablation of painful metastases, procedures to drain painful effusions; and other techniques.[86] Few of these procedures have undergone controlled clinical studies. One technique, the celiac plexus block, has been shown to be superior to morphine alone in patients with pain due to unresectable pancreatic cancer, although persistent diarrhea is a potential risk.[87] A complete review of interventional procedures can be found in a variety of sources. The choice of one of these techniques depends on the availability of experts in this area who understand the special needs of palliative care patients, the patient's ability to undergo the procedure, and the patient's and family's goals of care.

Nonpharmacological Therapies

Non-drug therapies, including cognitive behavioral techniques, physical measures, and integrative therapies are critical components of pain control in the palliative care setting. The patient's and caregivers' abilities to participate must be considered when selecting one of these therapies, including their fatigue level, interest, cognitive level, and other factors. Cognitive behavioral therapy often includes strategies to improve coping and relaxation, such as relaxation, guided imagery, mindfulness, music, prayer, reframing, and virtual reality.[88,89] These strategies have been found to be useful in reducing pain and anxiety and improving sleep in those with advanced disease as well as reducing endocrine symptoms in women being treated for breast cancer. Physical measures, such as massage, reflexology, heat, chiropractic, and other techniques, have also been shown to produce relaxation and relieve pain. Integrative therapies include acupuncture, aromatherapy, herbal therapies, and many other techniques formerly called "complementary and integrative therapies."[90] See Chapter 27 for information about these approaches to pain and symptom management. More rigorous research is needed in the palliative care setting regarding all of the non-drug therapies that might enhance pain relief.

Case Study—Continued

The palliative care nurse also wondered about the role of psychological and spiritual distress in contributing to Elaine's pain, so they recommended involvement by the social worker and chaplain on the team. The nurse discussed nonpharmacologic therapies with Elaine and found her to be receptive to breathing exercises guided by an app on her mobile phone. Over time, pain was well managed, allowing Elaine to meet her new goals of being with her family while eating meals.

Principles of Pain Management

Pain is a biopsychosocial and spiritual phenomenon, and this is particularly true in those with life-threatening illnesses. Therefore, multimodal therapies, incorporating pharmacologic, nonpharmacologic, interventional, and integrative therapies, are indicated for the relief of pain in this population. When applied carefully, these treatments provide relief for the majority of patients. A few guidelines[30,31]:

- Pain assessment includes a comprehensive history that includes current and past medication use for pain along with any adverse effects, evaluation of function, understanding of risk factors for substance use disorder, along with a thorough physical examination.
- Consider a multimodal approach when developing a treatment plan based on the etiology and quality of pain.
- Titrate analgesics based on patient goals, requirements for supplemental analgesics, pain intensity, severity of undesirable or adverse drug effects, measures of functionality, sleep, emotional state, and patients'/caregivers' reports of impact of pain on quality of life.
- Opioids should be considered for moderate to severe pain unless contraindicated; start low and increase the dose gradually by approximately 25%–50%, although patient factors such as organ dysfunction must be considered.
- Sustained-release formulations or around-the-clock dosing of immediate-release opioids should be used for continuous pain syndromes.

- Immediate-release formulations should be made available for breakthrough pain. Each breakthrough dose is usually 5%–20% of the 24-hour dose of the sustained-release formulation.
- Cost, convenience, and availability of medications (and other identified issues influencing compliance) are highly practical and important matters that should be taken into account with every prescription.
- Anticipate, prevent, and treat predictable side effects and adverse drug effects.
- Monitor patient status frequently during dose titration.
- Be aware of potential drug–drug and drug–disease interactions.
- Recommend expert pain management and/or palliative care specialty consultation if pain is not adequately relieved within a reasonable amount of time after applying standard analgesic guidelines and interventions.

These basic guidelines and considerations will optimize the pharmacologic management of all patients with pain, particularly those with serious illness.

Case Study—Final Points

Although initially reluctant to discuss advance directives or goals, Elaine now began to accept and seek support, including hospice care. Her family provided support to allow her to remain at home, and she died comfortably with limited pain or symptom burden. Elaine Adams' case illustrates several important points about pain management in palliative care, particularly highlighting the need for ongoing assessment as the patient's condition changes over time. Other key concepts:

- Evaluate acetaminophen and NSAID intake when using combination products; this can be exacerbated by use of OTC agents. Serious adverse effects can occur.
- Opioids are warranted in the treatment of moderate to severe pain; sustained-release medications should be supplemented with immediate-release agents.
- Neuropathic pain requires multimodal therapy, including adjuvant analgesics.
- Use of alternate routes of drug delivery is common in serious illness.
- Safe storage and disposal principles of controlled substances should be taught and implemented in the home; nasal naloxone should be considered in most cases.

Conclusion

Pain control in the palliative care setting is feasible in the majority of patients. Understanding the barriers that limit relief will lead to improved education and other strategies to address these obstacles. Ongoing, skilled assessment captures changes in pain and other symptoms as the patient's condition evolves. Developing comfort and skill with the use of pharmacological and nonpharmacological therapies will enhance pain relief. Together, these efforts will reduce suffering, relieve pain, and enhance the quality of life of those at the end of life.

REFERENCES

1. van den Beuken-van Everdingen MH, Hochstenbach LM, Joosten EA, Tjan-Heijnen VC, Janssen DJ. Update on prevalence of pain in patients with cancer: systematic review and meta-analysis. *J Pain Symptom Manage.* 2016;51(6):1070–1090.e9. https://doi.org/10.1016/j.jpainsymman.2015.12.340.
2. Tutelman PR, Chambers CT, Stinson JN, et al. Pain in children with cancer: prevalence, characteristics, and parent management. *Clin J Pain.* 2018;34(3):198–206. https://doi.org/10.1097/AJP.0000000000000531.
3. da Silva JG, da Rocha Morgan DA, Melo FCM, et al. Level of pain and quality of life of people living with HIV/AIDS pain and quality of life in HIV/AIDS. *AIDS Care.* 2017;29(8):1041–1048. https://doi.org/10.1080/09540121.2016.1274013.
4. Lovell N, Maddocks M, Etkind SN, et al. Characteristics, symptom management, and outcomes of 101 patients with COVID-19 referred for hospital palliative care. *J Pain Symptom Manage.* 2020;60(1):e77–e81. https://doi.org/10.1016/j.jpainsymman.2020.04.015.
5. Coelho T, Paul C, Gobbens RJJ, Fernandes L. Multidimensional frailty and pain in community dwelling elderly. *Pain Med.* 2017;18(4):693–701. https://doi.org/10.1111/pme.12746.
6. Gunnarsdottir S, Sigurdardottir V, Kloke M, et al. A multicenter study of attitudinal barriers to cancer pain management. *Support Care Cancer.* 2017;25(11):3595–3602. https://doi.org/10.1007/s00520-017-3791-8.
7. Paice JA. Under pressure: the tension between access and abuse of opioids in cancer pain management. *J Oncol Pract.* 2017;13(9):595–596. https://doi.org/10.1200/JOP.2017.026120.
8. Silbermann M, Calimag MM, Eisenberg E, et al. Evaluating pain management practices for cancer patients among health professionals: a global survey. *J Palliat Med.* 2022;25(8):1243–1248. https://doi.org/10.1089/jpm.2021.0596.
9. Zhang H, Paice J, Portenoy R, Bruera E, Reid MC, Bao Y. Prescription opioids dispensed to patients with cancer with bone metastasis: 2011–2017. *Oncologist.* 2021;26(10):e1890–e1892. https://doi.org/10.1002/onco.13898.
10. Enzinger AC, Ghosh K, Keating NL, Cutler DM, Landrum MB, Wright AA. US trends in opioid access among patients with poor prognosis cancer near the end-of-life. *J Clin Oncol.* 2021;39(26):2948–2958. https://doi.org/10.1200/JCO.21.00476.
11. Vitzthum LK, Nalawade V, Riviere P, et al. Racial, ethnic, and socioeconomic discrepancies in opioid prescriptions among older patients with cancer. *JCO Oncol Pract.* 2021;17(6):e703–e713. https://doi.org/10.1200/OP.20.00773.
12. Schenker Y, Hamm M, Bulls HW, et al. This is a different patient population: opioid prescribing challenges for patients with cancer-related pain. *JCO Oncol Pract.* 2021;17(7):e1030–e1037. https://doi.org/10.1200/OP.20.01041.
13. Bulls HW, Chu E, Goodin BR, et al. Framework for opioid stigma in cancer pain. *Pain.* 2022;163(2):e182–e189. https://doi.org/10.1097/j.pain.0000000000002343.
14. Azizoddin DR, Knoerl R, Adam R, et al. Cancer pain self-management in the context of a national opioid epidemic: experiences of patients with advanced cancer using opioids. *Cancer.* 2021;127(17):3239–3245. https://doi.org/10.1002/cncr.33532.
15. Furuno JP, Noble BN, Fromme EK, et al. Decreasing trends in opioid prescribing on discharge to hospice care. *J Pain Symptom Manage.* 2021;62(5):1026–1033. https://doi.org/10.1016/j.jpainsymman.2021.03.025.

16. Oldenmenger WH, Geerling JI, Mostovaya I, et al. A systematic review of the effectiveness of patient-based educational interventions to improve cancer-related pain. *Cancer Treat Rev*. 2017;63:96–103. https://doi.org/10.1016/j.ctrv.2017.12.005.
17. Zylberberg HM, Woodrell C, Rustgi SD, et al. Opioid prescription is associated with increased survival in older adult patients with pancreatic cancer in the United States: a propensity score analysis. *JCO Oncol Pract*. 2022;18(5):e659–e668. https://doi.org/10.1200/OP.21.00488.
18. Stilwell P, Hudon A, Meldrum K, Page MG, Wideman TH. What is pain-related suffering? Conceptual critiques, key attributes, and outstanding questions. *J Pain*. 2022;23(5):729–738. https://doi.org/10.1016/j.jpain.2021.11.005.
19. Colloca L, Ludman T, Bouhassira D, et al. Neuropathic pain. *Nat Rev Dis Primers*. 2017;3:17002. https://doi.org/10.1038/nrdp.2017.2.
20. Fallon M, Giusti R, Aielli F, et al. Management of cancer pain in adult patients: ESMO clinical practice guidelines. *Ann Oncol*. 2018;29(suppl 4):iv166–iv191. https://doi.org/10.1093/annonc/mdy152.
21. World Health Organization. *WHO Guidelines for the Pharmacological and Radiotherapeutic Management of Cancer Pain in Adults and Adolescents*. World Health Organization; 2018.
22. Herr K, Coyne PJ, Ely E, Gelinas C, Manworren RCB. ASPMN 2019 position statement: pain assessment in the patient unable to self-report. *Pain Manag Nurs*. 2019;20(5):402–403. https://doi.org/10.1016/j.pmn.2019.07.007.
23. Fink RM, Gallagher E. Cancer pain assessment and measurement. *Semin Oncol Nurs*. 2019;35(3):229–234. https://doi.org/10.1016/j.soncn.2019.04.003.
24. Wiffen PJ, Derry S, Moore RA, et al. Oral paracetamol (acetaminophen) for cancer pain. *Cochrane Database Syst Rev*. 2017;7:CD012637. https://doi.org/10.1002/14651858.CD012637.pub2.
25. Strawson J. Nonsteroidal anti-inflammatory drugs and cancer pain. *Curr Opin Support Palliat Care*. 2018;12(2):102–107. https://doi.org/10.1097/SPC.0000000000000332.
26. Magee DJ, Jhanji S, Poulogiannis G, Farquhar-Smith P, Brown MRD. Nonsteroidal anti inflammatory drugs and pain in cancer patients: a systematic review and reappraisal of the evidence. *Br J Anaesth*. 2019;123(2):e412–e423. https://doi.org/10.1016/j.bja.2019.02.028.
27. Bally M, Beauchamp ME, Abrahamowicz M, Nadeau L, Brophy JM. Risk of acute myocardial infarction with real-world NSAIDs depends on dose and timing of exposure. *Pharmacoepidemiol Drug Saf*. 2018;27(1):69–77. https://doi.org/10.1002/pds.4358.
28. Bally M, Dendukuri N, Rich B, et al. Risk of acute myocardial infarction with NSAIDs in real world use: Bayesian meta analysis of individual patient data. *BMJ*. 2017;357:j1909. https://doi.org/10.1136/bmj.j1909.
29. Cryer B, Barnett MA, Wagner J, Wilcox CM. Overuse and misperceptions of nonsteroidal anti-inflammatory drugs in the United States. *Am J Med Sci*. 2016;352(5):472–480. https://doi.org/10.1016/j.amjms.2016.08.028.
30. Paice JA, Bohlke K, Barton D, et al. Use of opioids for adults with pain from cancer or cancer treatment: ASCO guideline. *J Clin Oncol*. 2023;41(4):914–930.
31. Swarm RA, Paice JA, Anghelescu DL, et al. Adult cancer pain, version 3.2019, NCCN clinical practice guidelines in oncology. *J Natl Compr Canc Netw*. 2019;17(8):977–1007. https://doi.org/10.6004/jnccn.2019.0038.
32. Sande TA, Laird BJ, Fallon MT. The use of opioids in cancer patients with renal impairment-a systematic review. *Support Care Cancer*. 2017;25(2):661–675. https://doi.org/10.1007/s00520-016-3447-0.
33. McCulloch R, Sattar M, Henderson EM, Lane ME, Bluebond-Langner M. Use of buccal morphine in the management of pain in children with life-limiting conditions: results of a laboratory study. *Palliat Med*. 2018;32(2):554–558. https://doi.org/10.1177/0269216317717192.
34. Paice JA, Von Roenn JH, Hudgins JC, Luong L, Krejcie TC, Avram MJ. Morphine bioavailability from a topical gel formulation in volunteers. *J Pain Symptom Manage*. 2008;35(3):314–320. https://doi.org/10.1016/j.jpainsymman.2007.04.016.
35. Schug SA, Ting S. Fentanyl formulations in the management of pain: an update. *Drugs*. 2017;77(7):747–763. https://doi.org/10.1007/s40265-017-0727-z.
36. Hadley G, Derry S, Moore RA, Wiffen PJ. Transdermal fentanyl for cancer pain. *Cochrane Database Syst Rev*. 2013;(10):CD010270. https://doi.org/10.1002/14651858.CD010270.pub2.
37. Ueberall MA, Lorenzl S, Lux EA, Voltz R, Perelman M. Efficacy, safety, and tolerability of fentanyl pectin nasal spray in patients with breakthrough cancer pain. *J Pain Res*. 2016;9:571–585. https://doi.org/10.2147/JPR.S106177.
38. Kim JH, Kim JY, Lee N, Yee J, Gwak HS. The impact of drug interactions on adverse effects of oral oxycodone in male geriatric patients. *J Clin Pharm Ther*. 2020;45(5):976–982. https://doi.org/10.1111/jcpt.13113.
39. McPherson ML, Walker KA, Davis MP, et al. Safe and appropriate use of methadone in hospice and palliative care: expert consensus white paper. *J Pain Symptom Manage*. 2019;57(3):635–645.e4. https://doi.org/10.1016/j.jpainsymman.2018.12.001.
40. Mammana G, Bertolino M, Bruera E, et al. First-line methadone for cancer pain: titration time analysis. *Support Care Cancer*. 2021;29:6335–6341. https://doi.org/10.1007/s00520-021-06211-y.
41. Kharasch ED. Current concepts in methadone metabolism and transport. *Clin Pharmacol Drug Dev*. 2017;6(2):125–134. https://doi.org/10.1002/cpdd.326.
42. Edmonds KP, Saunders IM, Willeford A, Ajayi TA, Atayee RS. Emerging challenges to the safe and effective use of methadone for cancer-related pain in paediatric and adult patient populations. *Drugs*. 2020;80(2):115–130. https://doi.org/10.1007/s40265-019-01234-6.
43. Li Y, Ma J, Lu G, et al. Hydromorphone for cancer pain. *Cochrane Database Syst Rev*. 2021;8(8):CD011108. https://doi.org/10.1002/14651858.CD011108.pub3.
44. Vadivelu N, Chang D, Helander EM, et al. Ketorolac, oxymorphone, tapentadol, and tramadol: a comprehensive review. *Anesthesiol Clin*. 2017;35(2):e1–e20. https://doi.org/10.1016/j.anclin.2017.01.001.
45. Reddy A, Vidal M, Haider A, et al. A retrospective review of the use of oxymorphone immediate release for long term pain control in cancer patients with gastrostomy tubes. *Ann Palliat Med*. 2021;10(3):2662–2667. https://doi.org/10.21037/apm-20-969.
46. Moryl N, Filkins A, Griffo Y, et al. Successful use of buprenorphine-naloxone medication-assisted program to treat concurrent pain and opioid addiction after cancer therapy. *J Opioid Manag*. 2020;16(2):111–118. https://doi.org/10.5055/jom.2020.0557.
47. Quirk K, Stevenson M. Buprenorphine microdosing for the pain and palliative care clinician. *J Palliat Med*. 2022;25(1):145–154. https://doi.org/10.1089/jpm.2021.0378.
48. Linares OA, Fudin J, Schiesser WE, Daly Linares AL, Boston RC. CYP2D6 phenotype-specific codeine population pharmacokinetics.

J Pain Palliat Care Pharmacother. 2015;29(1):4–15. https://doi.org/10.3109/15360288.2014.997854.
49. Racoosin JA, Roberson DW, Pacanowski MA, Nielsen DR. New evidence about an old drug—risk with codeine after adenotonsillectomy. *N Engl J Med*. 2013;368(23):2155–2157. https://doi.org/10.1056/NEJMp1302454.
50. Dhillon S. Hydrocodone bitartrate ER (Hysingla® ER): a review in chronic pain. *Clin Drug Investig*. 2016;36(11):969–980. https://doi.org/10.1007/s40261-016-0466-z.
51. Reddy A, Yennurajalingam S, Desai H, et al. The opioid rotation ratio of hydrocodone to strong opioids in cancer patients. *Oncologist*. 2014;19(11):1186–1193. https://doi.org/10.1634/theoncologist.2014-0130.
52. Reddy A, Ng A, Mallipeddi T, Bruera E. Levorphanol for treatment of intractable neuropathic pain in cancer patients. *J Palliat Med*. 2018;21(3):399–402. https://doi.org/10.1089/jpm.2017.0475
53. Haider A, Reddy A. Levorphanol versus methadone use: safety considerations. *Ann Palliat Med*. 2020;9(2):579–585. https://doi.org/10.21037/apm.2020.02.01.
54. Wiffen PJ, Derry S, Moore RA. Tramadol with or without paracetamol (acetaminophen) for cancer pain. *Cochrane Database Syst Rev*. 2017;5:CD012508. https://doi.org/10.1002/14651858.CD012508.pub2.
55. Homma M, Kokubun H, Okuwaki K, et al. Pharmacokinetic analysis, analgesic effects, and adverse effects of tapentadol in cancer patients with pain. *Biol Pharm Bull*. 2020;43(6):1000–1006. https://doi.org/10.1248/bpb.b20-00084.
56. Kress HG, Coluzzi F. Tapentadol in the management of cancer pain: current evidence and future perspectives. *J Pain Res*. 2019;12:1553–1560. https://doi.org/10.2147/JPR.S191543.
57. Bruel BM, Burton AW. Intrathecal therapy for cancer-related pain. *Pain Med*. 2016;17(12):2404–2421. https://doi.org/10.1093/pm/pnw060.
58. Davies A, Leach C, Caponero R, et al. MASCC recommendations on the management of constipation in patients with advanced cancer. *Support Care Cancer*. 2020;28(1):23–33. https://doi.org/10.1007/s00520-019-05016-4.
59. Rao VL, Micic D, Davis AM. Medical management of opioid-induced constipation. *JAMA*. 2019;322(22):2241–2242. https://doi.org/10.1001/jama.2019.15852.
60. Sande TA, Laird BJA, Fallon MT. The management of opioid-induced nausea and vomiting in patients with cancer: a systematic review. *J Palliat Med*. 2019;22(1):90–97. https://doi.org/10.1089/jpm.2018.0260.
61. Hofmann A, Tangri N, Lafontaine AL, Postuma RB. Myoclonus as an acute complication of low-dose hydromorphone in multiple system atrophy. *J Neurol Neurosurg Psychiatry*. 2006;77(8):994–995. https://doi.org/10.1136/jnnp.2005.076588.
62. Ito S, Liao S. Myoclonus associated with high-dose parenteral methadone. *J Palliat Med*. 2008;11(6):838–841. https://doi.org/10.1089/jpm.2008.0040.
63. Benson JL, Campbell HE, Phillips CN. Opioid-induced pruritus. *Consult Pharm*. 2015;30(4):221–227. https://doi.org/10.4140/TCP.n.2015.221.
64. Rashid S, Trivedi DD, Al-Shathir M, Moulton M, Baumrucker SJ. Is there a role for 5-HT3 receptor antagonists in the treatment of opioid-induced pruritus? *Am J Hosp Palliat Care*. 2018;35(4):740–744. https://doi.org/10.1177/1049909117736062.
65. Kremer M, Salvat E, Muller A, Yalcin I, Barrot M. Antidepressants and gabapentinoids in neuropathic pain: mechanistic insights. *Neuroscience*. 2016;338:183–206. https://doi.org/10.1016/j.neuroscience.2016.06.057.
66. Guan J, Tanaka S, Kawakami K. Anticonvulsants or antidepressants in combination pharmacotherapy for treatment of neuropathic pain in cancer patients: a systematic review and meta-analysis. *Clin J Pain*. 2016;32(8):719–725. https://doi.org/10.1097/AJP.0000000000000310.
67. Matsuoka H, Iwase S, Miyaji T, et al. Additive duloxetine for cancer-related neuropathic pain nonresponsive or intolerant to opioid-pregabalin therapy: a randomized controlled trial (JORTC-PAL08). *J Pain Symptom Manage*. 2019;58(4):645–653. https://doi.org/10.1016/j.jpainsymman.2019.06.020.
68. Davis M, Loprinzi C. Pregabalin for chemotherapy-induced neuropathy: background and rationale for further study. *Support Care Cancer*. 2022;30(11):8845–8853. https://doi.org/10.1007/s00520-022-07317-7.
69. Wilcock A, Charlesworth S, Twycross R, et al. Prescribing non-opioid drugs in end-stage kidney disease. *J Pain Symptom Manage*. 2017;54(5):776–787. https://doi.org/10.1016/j.jpainsymman.2017.08.014.
70. Lim FMY, Bobrowski A, Agarwal A, Silva MF. Use of corticosteroids for pain control in cancer patients with bone metastases: a comprehensive literature review. *Curr Opin Support Palliat Care*. 2017;11(2):78–87. https://doi.org/10.1097/SPC.0000000000000263.
71. Seah DSE, Herschtal A, Tran H, Thakerar A, Fullerton S. Subcutaneous lidocaine infusion for pain in patients with cancer. *J Palliat Med*. 2017;20(6):667–671. https://doi.org/10.1089/jpm.2016.0298.
72. Jonkman K, van de Donk T, Dahan A. Ketamine for cancer pain: what is the evidence? *Curr Opin Support Palliat Care*. 2017;11(2):88–92. https://doi.org/10.1097/SPC.0000000000000262.
73. Bell RF, Eccleston C, Kalso EA. Ketamine as an adjuvant to opioids for cancer pain. *Cochrane Database Syst Rev*. 2017;6:CD003351. https://doi.org/10.1002/14651858.CD003351.pub3.
74. Fallon MT, Wilcock A, Kelly CA, et al. Oral ketamine vs placebo in patients with cancer-related neuropathic pain: a randomized clinical trial. *JAMA Oncol*. 2018;4(6):870–872. https://doi.org/10.1001/jamaoncol.2018.0131.
75. O'Carrigan B, Wong MH, Willson ML, Stockler MR, Pavlakis N, Goodwin A. Bisphosphonates and other bone agents for breast cancer. *Cochrane Database Syst Rev*. 2017;10:CD003474. https://doi.org/10.1002/14651858.CD003474.pub4.
76. Moretti A. What are the efficacy and safety of bisphosphonates and RANK-ligand-inhibitors for men with prostate cancer and bone metastases?—A Cochrane Review summary with commentary. *J Musculoskelet Neuronal Interact*. 2021;21(4):451–454.
77. Amini A, Shinde A, Wong J. Palliative radiation for cancer pain management. *Cancer Treat Res*. 2021;182:145–156. https://doi.org/10.1007/978-3-030-81526-4_10.
78. Bilen MA, Johnson MM, Mathew P, et al. Randomized phase 2 study of bone-targeted therapy containing strontium-89 in advanced castrate-sensitive prostate cancer. *Cancer*. 2015;121(1):69–76. https://doi.org/10.1002/cncr.28971.
79. Weeks JC, Catalano PJ, Cronin A, et al. Patients' expectations about effects of chemotherapy for advanced cancer. *N Engl J Med*. 2012;367(17):1616–1625. https://doi.org/10.1056/NEJMoa1204410.
80. Wright AA, Zhang B, Keating NL, Weeks JC, Prigerson HG. Associations between palliative chemotherapy and adult cancer patients' end of life care and place of death: prospective cohort study. *BMJ*. 2014;348:g1219. https://doi.org/10.1136/bmj.g1219.
81. Derry S, Rice AS, Cole P, Tan T, Moore RA. Topical capsaicin (high concentration) for chronic neuropathic pain in adults. *Cochrane*

Database Syst Rev. 2017;1:CD007393. https://doi.org/10.1002/14651858.CD007393.pub4.

82. Dupoiron D, Jubier-Hamon S, Seegers V, et al. Peripheral neuropathic pain following breast cancer: effectiveness and tolerability of high-concentration capsaicin patch. *J Pain Res*. 2022;15:241–255. https://doi.org/10.2147/JPR.S341378.
83. Worster B, Hajjar ER, Handley N. Cannabis use in patients with cancer: a clinical review. *JCO Oncol Pract*. 2022;18(11):743–749. https://doi.org/10.1200/OP.22.00080.
84. Byars T, Theisen E, Bolton DL. Using cannabis to treat cancer-related pain. *Semin Oncol Nurs*. 2019;35(3):300–309. https://doi.org/10.1016/j.soncn.2019.04.012.
85. IASP Presidential Task Force on Cannabis and Cannabinoid Analgesia. International Association for the Study of Pain Presidential Task Force on Cannabis and Cannabinoid Analgesia position statement. *Pain*. 2021;162(suppl 1):S1–S2. https://doi.org/10.1097/j.pain.0000000000002265.
86. Sadeghi-Naini M, Aarabi S, Shokraneh F, Janani L, Vaccaro AR, Rahimi-Movaghar V. Vertebroplasty and kyphoplasty for metastatic spinal lesions: a systematic review. *Clin Spine Surg*. 2018;31(5):203–210. https://doi.org/10.1097/BSD.0000000000000601.
87. Okita M, Otani K, Gibo N, Matsui S. Systematic review and meta-analysis of celiac plexus neurolysis for abdominal pain associated with unresectable pancreatic cancer. *Pain Pract*. 2022;22(7):652–661. https://doi.org/10.1111/papr.13143.
88. Winger JG, Ramos K, Kelleher SA, et al. Meaning-centered pain coping skills training: a pilot feasibility trial of a psychosocial pain management intervention for patients with advanced cancer. *J Palliat Med*. 2022;25(1):60–69. https://doi.org/10.1089/jpm.2021.0081.
89. Kelleher SA, Fisher HM, Winger JG, et al. Virtual reality for improving pain and pain-related symptoms in patients with advanced stage colorectal cancer: a pilot trial to test feasibility and acceptability. *Palliat Support Care*. 2022;20(4):471–481. https://doi.org/10.1017/S1478951521002017.
90. Yang J, Wahner-Roedler DL, Zhou X, et al. Acupuncture for palliative cancer pain management: systematic review. *BMJ Support Palliat Care*. 2021;11(3):264–270. https://doi.org/10.1136/bmjspcare-2020-002638.

12

Dyspnea and Cough

Rebecca Disler, Susanne McDevitt, and DorAnne Donesky

Key Points

- This chapter discusses the causes, assessment, and management of dyspnea and cough.
- Dyspnea and cough are multidimensional, burdensome symptoms that are often distressing for both patients and family members.
- Dyspnea management incorporates both attention to correction of the physiological defect causing dyspnea and interventions aimed at the common neurological pathway for dyspnea.
- People living with chronic dyspnea or cough should be encouraged to notice what works well for them in managing those symptoms using "*N* of 1" trials and then implement those strategies whenever the symptom recurs.

Case Study Part 1: Patient Living with Idiopathic Pulmonary Fibrosis

Robin was 54 years old when she first noticed that it was difficult to take a deep breath. She was on a ski vacation and attributed it to the elevation. She developed a dry cough that was not responsive to treatment, and 5 years later some abnormalities ("honeycombing") showed up on her chest X-ray. After several false diagnoses, she was told that she had idiopathic pulmonary fibrosis (IPF) and enrolled in a clinical trial of an antifibrotic medication.

At first, the persistent cough did not change much. She felt more fatigue and decreased stamina rather than shortness of breath, but 5 years after diagnosis she first noticed shortness of breath while showering. For the next 7 years, she experienced progressively increasing bouts of dry cough and shortness of breath triggered by less and less activity. The dry cough got longer, more frequent, and intense. She began to use supplemental oxygen, cut down on her volunteer activities, and carried an oximeter with her. Robin's progression and needs will be discussed throughout the chapter.

Source: Adapted from the writing of Robin Curley. Written October 31, 2017. Died November 15, 2017. Used with permission.

Introduction

Breathing is the one vital body function that can be controlled consciously or can continue without any awareness or thought, completely subconsciously, when conscious attention is placed elsewhere. The breath is the focus of many spiritual traditions and serves as a bridge between the conscious and subconscious mind.[1] Attention to the breath as a method to optimize well-being has been documented since ancient times.[2,3] Conscious breathing is used to release stress and tension, build energy, support emotions, manage symptoms, improve physical and mental performance, and facilitate spiritual transformation.[4] Breathing is an important component of many mind–body therapies including yoga, guided imagery, and somatic grounding.[5] The respiratory system is a topic of interest for both popular self-help authors and basic, translational, and clinical researchers who are searching for ways to optimize the health and minimize the symptoms of patients living with serious illness.

We take breath for granted, rarely thinking about it; but when something goes awry, it is the cause of panic and fear. Difficulty breathing feels dangerous and like a sign of impending suffocation in the setting of chronic lung disease.[6] Patients tend to stop their activity if they perceive danger, which leads to deconditioning and increased dyspnea over time in the vicious cycle of inactivity.[7,8] Patients with chronic dyspnea related to severe cardiopulmonary disease may live with dyspnea for many years and experience the stigma of a debilitating invisible disability.[9] Dyspnea correlates with mortality more than other measures such as pulmonary function.[10] Given its impact on depression, mortality, and quality of life (QOL), the importance of dyspnea has been recognized with the description of dyspnea as "the first vital symptom."[11]

The metaphorical significance of dyspnea has been recognized by the Life of Breath project (https://lifeofbreath.webspace.durham.ac.uk/), which explores breath at the intersection of medicine, art, and the humanities—a medical humanities approach. The disciplines of anesthesia and engineering may also supplement the traditional work of pulmonology and palliative care in offering a new perspective on dyspnea management.[12] The purpose of this chapter is to review the current understanding of the pathophysiology, assessment, and management options for people living with serious illness who experience dyspnea and cough.

A *symptom cluster* is the coexistence of two or more concurrent symptoms that may have a common cause.[13] Symptoms can occur because of the disease itself, treatment side effects, or comorbidities.[13] While many clusters exist, in the context of dyspnea and cough, chronic breathlessness, cough, and fatigue have been recognized as a respiratory triad, or "respiratory cluster," in advanced respiratory disease[14,15] and can also be present in lung cancer.[16] Distress related to dyspnea is similarly associated with symptom clusters that include fatigue and nausea.[17] Chronic dyspnea in chronic obstructive pulmonary disease (COPD) has also been strongly associated with anxiety and depression, at times referred to as part of a "psychological symptom cluster."[14] Pain and dyspnea often coexist, frequently in the context of depression and functional impairments.[18] Cough has also been associated with a cough–insomnia-related symptom cluster, that includes cough, dry mouth, poor appetite, and insomnia.[14] While individual symptoms should be addressed, a broad, holistic approach is recommended from the nurse with the interprofessional team (including, e.g., chaplain, social worker, physician, pharmacist, occupational therapist, physiotherapist), particularly when symptoms persist despite optimization of underlying disease.[15] Symptom-specific interventions may benefit the multiple symptoms in a cluster simultaneously, due to a shared common symptom pathway described below.[12,19,20]

Dyspnea Physiology, Measurement, and Interventions

Dyspnea is a multidimensional symptom with an affective component; it is defined by the American Thoracic Society as "an unpleasant subjective experience of discomfort with breathing that worsens as underlying disease processes increase in severity; in its chronic and severe state, it can lead to significant disability, progressive inactivity, social isolation and substantive suffering."[21(p1108)] It is useful to engage a stepped approach to the assessment and management of dyspnea, including (1) addressing reversible underlying causes (e.g., pleural effusion, anemia, or psychological causes such as anxiety) and employing (2) nonpharmacological and (3) pharmacological interventions, as discussed below.

"Breathlessness," "shortness of breath," and "dyspnea" are often used interchangeably when talking about the difficulty of breathing experienced by patients living with serious illness. Other terms include "labored breathing" and "breathing discomfort." Dyspnea can be categorized into three primary groups. "Work" or "effort" is often used to describe the sensation of patients with impaired or fatigued respiratory muscles.[2] "Chest tightness" is used to describe the dyspnea experienced in asthma.[22] "Unsatisfied inspiration" or "air hunger" describes the sensation at the end of exercise or when breathing high levels of carbon dioxide.[23] In addition, breathless patients report anxiety, distress, discomfort, fear, and other negative terms when describing breathing experience.[24] The nomenclature for dyspnea continues to develop. Dyspnea can be acute or chronic, continuous or episodic, with variation in the timing and coping response.[25,26] *Chronic breathlessness syndrome*, previously called "refractory breathlessness," is defined as breathlessness that "persists despite optimal treatment of the underlying pathophysiology and that results in disability."[21(p1109)] This is a distinct syndrome with unique neural activity in the brain which persists after treatment of underlying disease, with an important aspect being heightened breathlessness even at rest. The focus on the persistent nature of this breathlessness, as opposed to episodic crises, is hoped to "advance the palliative understanding and potential interventions associated with the day-in and day-out experience of breathlessness."[21(p1109)]

Patient Experience of Dyspnea

Dyspnea is one of the most distressing symptoms at the end of life[12] and occurs in the majority of patients diagnosed with COPD, lung cancer, or heart failure.[12,27,28] Dyspnea is frequently present in community-dwelling older adults who do not have any of the diagnoses traditionally associated with dyspnea.[29] The trajectory of dyspnea is distinct according to diagnosis; patients with COPD often experience moderate to severe fluctuating dyspnea for months with little change as death approaches,[30] while many patients with cancer experience increasing dyspnea as they approach death, even if the cancer is not in the lungs.[31] When people are living with chronic lung disease, their life can begin to revolve around their breathing needs. The case study details the personal experience of a woman living with IPF. Along with the dyspnea, logistical challenges when living with chronic lung disease and dyspnea include the need for oxygen and coordination with the medical equipment company, learning to use an oximeter, and potential weight gain or loss. Self-care activities focus on managing the physical manifestations of the illness, coping with the psychological effects, minimizing the social burden of the illness, and developing the knowledge and skills necessary to interact wisely with the healthcare team.[25,32,33] Patients often feel stigmatized and blamed for their disease because of the association between smoking and lung disease, and the insidious onset of the disease often interferes with early initial treatment. The uncertainty of the symptom contributes to fear and difficulties with coping.[30] Chronic breathlessness is frightening and distressing for both patient and family,[12,28] but evidence-based multidimensional interventions can provide relief.[15,25,32]

Pathophysiology of Dyspnea

Dyspnea is a complex phenomenon that includes the sensation of respiratory discomfort, an affective response to the sensation, and the impact on physical functioning and daily activities.[34] A beneficial model of breathlessness includes perception of both intensity and unpleasantness, emotional response, and functional consequences. Many factors contribute to the sensation of dyspnea.[7] At its most basic level, the respiratory system is a pump that brings fresh oxygen to the tissues and removes carbon dioxide waste. The pump is activated by a neurological feedback system in communication with the musculature. The prevailing theory is that dyspnea results from a mismatch between respiratory demand and ventilatory mechanics, an imbalance between the demand to breathe and the ability to breathe.[35] The automatic drive to breathe originates in the brainstem and communicates through a feedback system with the lungs and chest wall. When a mismatch occurs between the urge to breathe and actual ventilation, the brainstem communicates through a corollary discharge (see Figure 12.1) with the cortex and limbic regions of the brain, which triggers emotions, memories, abstract thoughts, and the evaluation and affective response to the dyspnea sensation.

Increased respiratory demand can be triggered by multiple factors. Metabolism naturally increases in the setting of exercise or fever, and the built-in reserves of the ventilatory mechanics can easily accommodate those usual demands. Systemic illness such as hyperthyroid, sepsis, or cachexia also stimulates an increased demand on the respiratory system.[10] The muscle wasting of cachexia seen in COPD, heart failure, and cancer is linked to increased sympathetic drive, neurohumoral changes, and inflammation. The resulting skeletal muscle loss is independently associated with dyspnea, and

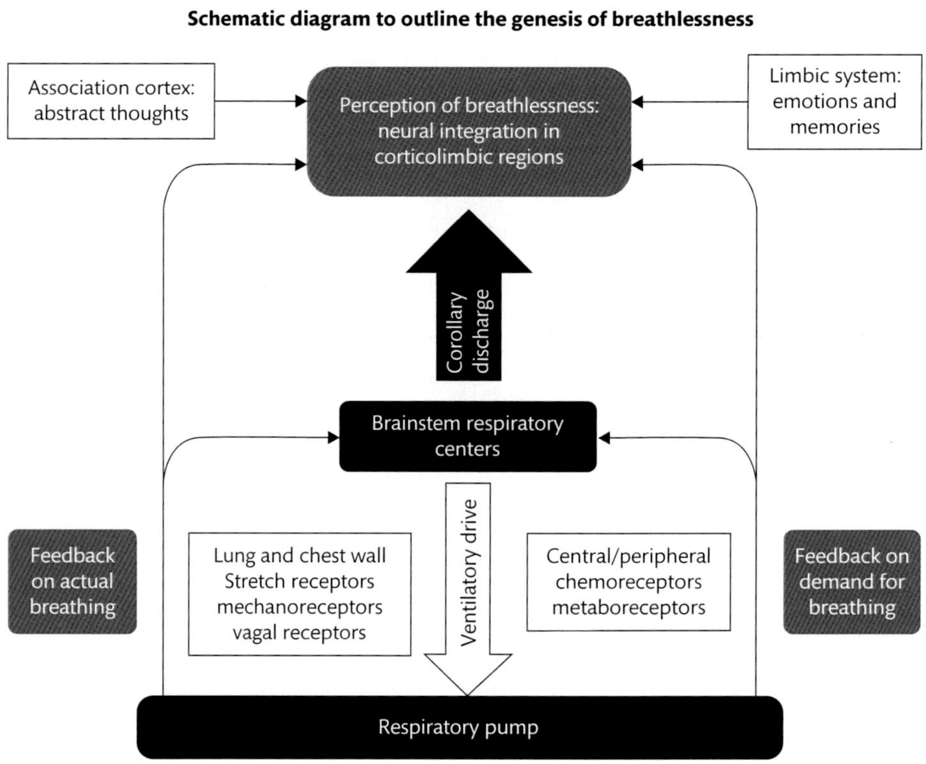

Figure 12.1 Schematic diagram to outline the genesis of breathlessness.
Source: References 12 and 37.

exercise training possibly combined with nutritional supplementation may reverse breathlessness with the associated myopathy, exercise intolerance, and fatigue.[36] A chemical imbalance between oxygen and carbon dioxide in the blood will also increase the respiratory demand. In anemia, the decreased hemoglobin available to carry oxygen prevents the cardiovascular system from supplying adequate oxygen to the tissues.[10] In hypercapnic respiratory failure, the body's respiratory demand to expire carbon dioxide overwhelms its ventilatory capabilities, and carbon dioxide builds up in the blood, leading to life-threatening respiratory acidosis. Neuromuscular disorders increase the workload relative to the body's ability to move the respiratory pump, given reduced muscular strength and/or neurological input. Anything that increases the external workload on the respiratory system will increase respiratory demand and may fatigue the muscles beyond their ability to function. Efforts to reduce respiratory demand should be employed to reduce work of breathing and ease associated breathlessness.

Similarly, problems with airway obstruction, a restrictive defect, vascular problems, or fluid buildup in the air sacs can interfere with ventilation or gas exchange. In these situations, the body is not able to supply enough ventilation to meet the demand.[35] Airway *obstruction* occurs when something is preventing the movement of air, usually on exhalation—this can be caused by mucus buildup or constriction of smooth muscle surrounding the airways, which is often the case with asthma or chronic bronchitis. Obstruction also occurs when the air sacs/alveoli responsible for gas exchange are damaged and no longer able to function, as occurs with emphysema, or filled with fluid due to pneumonia or pulmonary edema. A mechanical obstruction can occur when a tumor or scar tissue blocks either the upper or lower airways. When obstruction continues over time, the lungs may become hyperinflated when exhalation does not match the volume of inhalation, thus reducing the space available in the lung for movement of air—thereby requiring additional effort to expand the lungs. Airway *restriction* can occur because of decreased compliance or stiffness of the lung tissue from a condition such as fibrosis or scarring. The pleural space and lining of the lung may be restricted due to plaque, or the restriction may be external due to obesity, kyphoscoliosis, or neuromuscular disease. *Fluid buildup* or *exudate* due to pneumonia or pulmonary edema may interrupt ventilation and prevent oxygen from entering the alveoli and reaching the capillaries. *Pulmonary edema* occurs when hydrostatic pressure from fluid overload moves fluid from the vascular space into the interstitial space and alveoli.

Any factors that increase the demand to breathe or reduce the body's ventilatory capacity may trigger a sensation of dyspnea. Physical deconditioning may do both and is therefore a primary reason for dyspnea, regardless of whether other causes of dyspnea are present. Physical deconditioning contributes to dyspnea, even in otherwise healthy adults.[7] People with dyspnea often progressively learn to limit their activities to minimize their dyspnea, leading to reduced muscle bulk and increased deconditioning and thus contributing to a vicious cycle of inactivity. This relationship between the perception of the sensation and the affective reaction to the sensation has also been called the "spiral of disability."[7]

Final Common Pathway of Dyspnea

Breathlessness related to the physiology of the lungs, chest, airways, and blood vessels can be addressed by correcting the mismatch between respiratory demand and ventilatory mechanics.[20] When breathlessness remains after the mismatch and/or any specific etiology has been addressed, the breathlessness may be related to central neurological processing and perception, the "final common pathway," a central perception of breathlessness triggered by the corollary discharge (see Figure 12.1).[12,20,37] The emotion-related areas of the insular cortex, anterior cingulate cortex, and amygdala are areas in the brain that are active during breathlessness and during the fear response, as recognized by functional magnetic resonance imaging and positron emission tomography.[7] The final common pathway of dyspnea may contribute to *symptom clusters*, the coexistence of two or more concurrent symptoms that may have a common cause.[19,20]

Measurement of Dyspnea

Like pain, breathlessness is not a single, universal sensation but rather varies in intensity and impact through the experience of distress. Nurses may integrate the use of validated dyspnea assessment tools within patient history, physical examination, and diagnostic testing as indicated. Patient-reported outcomes are the foundation of dyspnea measurement as no physiological correlate has been identified that accurately predicts dyspnea.[38] Dyspnea scales measure one or more of the sensations of respiratory discomfort, an affective response to the sensation, and the impact on physical functioning and daily activities.[34]

The multidimensional sensation of breathlessness has been measured by a range of instruments developed for children, youth, and adults, whether able or unable to self-report. Multidimensional scales[34] are accessible and easy to use for the nurse and interprofessional team and are recommended by the American Thoracic Society to comprehensively evaluate the physical, psychological, social factors associated with dyspnea. Eight psychometrically rigorous instruments have been developed that comprehensively measure one or more specific domains of the sensation of breathlessness (intensity, sensory quality, affective distress).[39] Multidimensional instruments such as the Dyspnea-12 (D-12), Multidimensional Dyspnea Profile (MDP), Cancer Dyspnea Scale (CDS), and the Dyspnea-ALS Scale were developed to evaluate the multiple sensations contributing to breathlessness experiences and identify which dimensions may be modifiable by pharmacological and nonpharmacological interventions.[39] In a systematic review, Williams and colleagues found that the D-12 and MDP were widely used and reliable and valid for measuring multiple dimensions of breathlessness across populations and settings.[40] The D-12 and CDS principally derive a summary score, rather than separation of different components.[41]

Unidimensional scales are available and typically measure the intensity or distress of the sensation as a single aspect, such as the visual analogue scale (VAS), Borg scale, and numeric rating scale (NRS). Unidimensional scales capture the overall intensity of dyspnea at a specific time point, although do not capture information about the quality of the breathing discomfort, including its unpleasantness or associated emotional responses.[41] These tools are easy to implement in a clinical setting and familiar to patients who have often used similar ones. When a brief overview of a variety of symptoms is needed, the commonly used Edmonton Symptom Assessment Survey (ESAS) includes a 10-point NRS for nine symptoms including dyspnea.[42] The Edmonton Symptom Assessment Scale (ESAS) has been validated in many languages other than English.[43–46] The Memorial Symptom Assessment Scale also evaluates the intensity, frequency, and distress of 32 symptoms including dyspnea.[47,48] One aspect to consider in dyspnea measurement is "response shift,"[49] when patients subconsciously decrease activity levels to cope with dyspnea. Consequently, patients' actual dyspnea scores may not change, but further inquiry into their current activity levels in comparison to several years prior may reveal dyspnea as the reason for reduced activity—see *spiral of disability* discussed above. Additionally, attention to a symptom may cause increased distress from that symptom,[50] with additional awareness of dyspnea an unintended consequence of symptom measurement.[36]

Dyspnea Management–Breathing Thinking Functioning Model

The "breathing, thinking, functioning" (BTF) model (Figure 12.2) was developed to guide clinicians, patients, and caregivers in understanding the generation of breathlessness and initial management, with particular reference to nonpharmacological approaches.[12,37] The clinical model proposes three vicious cycles of breathlessness and associated predominant cognitive and behavioral reactions that can increase or decrease the symptom[37] and focuses on three domains, as named: breathing, thinking and functioning. The *Breathing* domain focuses on an ineffective breathing pattern that can trigger the vicious cycle of increased breathlessness.[12] Dysfunctional breathing patterns can cause breathless patients to increase their tidal volume or respiratory rate by recruiting the upper chest and other inspiratory and accessory muscles.[51] Increased reliance on accessory muscles and decreased use of the fatigue-resistant diaphragmatic muscle for respiration can consequently increase breathing effort and exacerbate breathlessness symptoms among patients.[52] The *Thinking* domain is perpetuated through anxiety derived from a rapidly escalating sense of panic, alongside other cognitive problems experienced by patients and caregivers during breathlessness. Anxiety in this context is seen to trigger an increase in patients' respiratory rate, causing muscle tension in both the ventilatory pump and other skeletal muscles.[37] These cognitions can further intensify breathlessness and increase the work of breathing for patients. And finally, the *Functioning* domain describes breathlessness as exacerbated by a decline in patients' physical and mental activity; patients' avoidance of exercise due to fear of triggering breathlessness and/or anxiety initiates a cycle of deconditioning and intensified breathlessness.[12] Patients who remain active may avoid deconditioning and paradoxical increased demand on the respiratory system.[37]

Breathlessness is a commonly frightening and fatiguing experience for patients. A diverse array of effective nonpharmacological interventions exist to relieve patients' breathlessness experiences that are captured in the three domains of the BTF model. Although all three vicious cycles in the model are interconnected, one or two often predominate. Patients' engagement and self-management can be facilitated by directing treatment strategies toward the predominant cycle. Focus on a specific cycle can increase the patient's understanding and prioritization of management strategies and subsequently increase treatment adherence.[12,37]

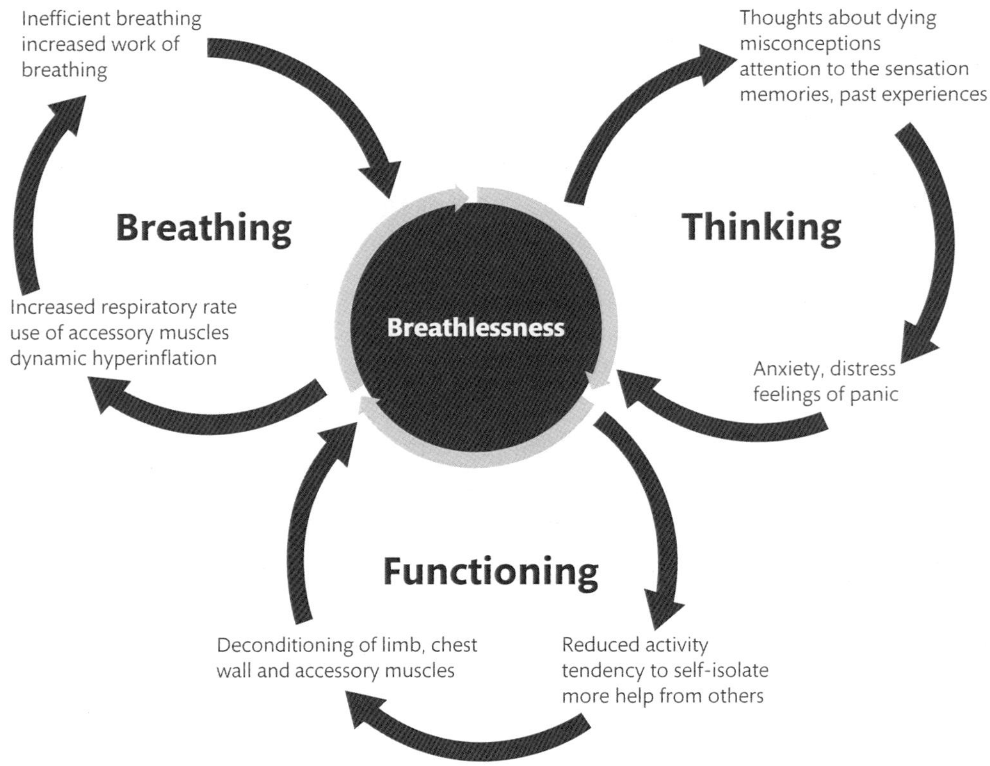

Figure 12.2 The breathing, thinking, functioning clinical model.
Source: Reference 37.

Case Study Part 2: Patient Living with IPF

Robin contracted influenza in the 12 months prior to her death, and she was left with a constant cough and sensation of sputum in her lower lobes. Her oxygen requirements increased considerably, she began to cough uncontrollably while walking, and she began to breathe through her mouth as she did not feel like she could get enough air when breathing through her nose. She developed atrial tachycardia, which caused wide fluctuations in heart rate. She explained to the nurse that during these episodes she found that forcing herself to cough and laying on her bed with her head hanging over the side, below the level of the heart, would help her regain her equilibrium. She used large quantities of guaifenesin, with frequent nose blowing, water, and rest. She further explained that she had started to worry about dying and that her only outings were her multiple medical appointments.

Through discussion, the nurse was able to ascertain that Robin had worsening dyspnea when she was anxious or fatigued but that she had never trialed medication for dyspnea. The nurse then referred her to the palliative care team for assistance with chronic dyspnea and cough management and goals-of-care discussion. In terms of QOL and advance care planning, she conveyed she knew she had a life-limiting illness and was hoping to feel better and live longer with a reasonable QOL. She worried about being a burden to her family and decided to pursue do-not-resuscitate status.

Specific Interventions for Dyspnea

When considering interventional options for patients with dyspnea, the nurse with the interprofessional team must first consider the specific mechanisms of dyspnea as correcting the physiological defect will often improve dyspnea.[36] After optimizing the pathophysiology of the symptom, the nurse with the interprofessional team should seek dyspnea management strategies that ultimately provide relief through the central common pathway of dyspnea. A task force of the Hospice and Palliative Nurses Association reviewed the evidence for dyspnea interventions available through December 2019.[25] This chapter provides updated evidence, including 55 additional articles in PubMed and/or CINAHL published between January 2020 and September 2024, reporting on original research of interventions for patients with serious illness that included dyspnea as an outcome, as summarized in Table 12.1. Interventions are organized according to the levels of evidence adapted from the Oncology Nursing Society's putting evidence into practice classification,[53] including interventions: "Recommended for practice" when effectiveness has been demonstrated by at least two well-conducted randomized controlled trials (RCTs) performed at more than one institution; "Likely to be effective" when supportive evidence includes a single RCT at one institution with fewer than 100 patients; "Balance benefit with harm" where evidence may be associated with potential adverse effects; "Effectiveness not established" when insufficient, noncontrolled, or poor-quality data exists; "Effectiveness unlikely" where no evidence exists or no benefit or unacceptable toxicity is likely; and "Not recommended for practice" when a clear pattern of excessive cost, adverse events, or burden is associated with the intervention.

In addition, the importance of the interprofessional team in breathlessness intervention programs should be noted, with team members offering unique perspectives related to dyspnea management.

Table 12.1 Summary of interventions for dyspnea management

Evidence	Interventions[a]
Recommended for practice	• Oxygen to correct hypoxemia • Pulmonary rehabilitation for COPD • Hand-held fan directed to the face • Activity-pacing • Long-acting bronchodilators for COPD • Breathlessness Intervention programs (e.. multicomponent breathlessness services) • *Breathing management techniques*
Likely to be effective	• Short-acting bronchodilators for COPD • Home-based exercise • *Cognitive behavioural therapy* • Acupoints and acupressure, including TENS • *Inhaled dual phosphodiesterase 3 and 4 inhibitor* • *Noninvasive ventilation* • *Inspiratory muscle training*
Balance benefit with harm	• High-flow nasal oxygen • Nutraceutical: coenzyme Q10 • Acupuncture • Palliative bronchoscopic interventions • *Short-term opioids near end-of-life for non-malignant refractory dyspnea (opioids are not effective for long-term use, as below)* • *Expressive art therapy* • *Biofeedback* • *Qigong, tai chi, yoga* • *Lung conduction (Korean pulmonary rehab) exercise* • *Nitric oxide* • *Inhaler training*
Effectiveness not established	• Oxygen without hypoxemia • Nebulized diuretics • Vaporized cannabis • Heliox • Oral steroids • Mindfulness training • Music therapy • *Thoracic kinesio taping, back massage* • *Mesh nebulizer, nebulized verapamil* • *Manual osteopathic therapy* • *LABA/ICS* • *Daoyin (Chinese pulmonary rehab)* • *Triple versus dual inhaler therapy*
Effectiveness unlikely	• *Mirtazapine* • Epidural methadone • Oxygen without hypoxemia/oxygen near death • *Intranasal or inhaled fentanyl*
Not effective	• *Opioid for chronic breathlessness (long or short-acting)* • *Benzodiazepines* • *Nebulized morphine* • Extended-release morphine in pulmonary hypertension • Oxycodone for chronic breathlessness • Opioids to improve exercise capacity

COPD, chronic obstructive pulmonary disease; ICS, inhaled corticosteroids; LABA, long-acting bronchodilator inhalation therapy that includes a beta agonist; TENS, transcutaneous electrical nerve stimulation.

[a] Additions or adjustments to level of evidence from updated evidence are indicated in italics.

Source: Adapted from Reference 25.

From a nurse perspective, holistic assessment with symptom and self-management education are effective, along with coordination of pharmacological and nonpharmacological intervention. From a physical therapy perspective, physical conditioning, reassurance, positioning, and explanations of the anatomy and physiology related to breathing strategies are effective means to support patients in managing their dyspnea.[54] Occupational therapists use energy conservation and supervised practice to support maintenance of everyday activities.[55–57] Although respiratory therapists, based in the United States, have traditionally practiced in hospital settings, their experience in leading pulmonary rehabilitation (PR) programs demonstrates their expertise in supporting dyspnea management within a whole-person context.[58–60]

Recommended for Practice

There are several recommended strategies that the nurse and interprofessional team may employ. The strongest evidence supports long-acting bronchodilator inhalation therapy that includes a beta agonist (LABA) combined with long-acting muscarinic antagonist (LAMA) for the relief of dyspnea in patients with COPD. The evidence in support of this recommendation has increased substantially since 2020, with nine new published articles supporting LABA/LAMA therapy in various dosages, combinations, and settings.[61–70] The nurse with the interprofessional team should explore these inhaled medications that can be administered by several nebulized and inhalation medication devices; the choice of device should reflect the patient's current capabilities, and optimal technique, as important considerations.[71]

Oxygen therapy to correct hypoxemia has been shown to be beneficial in relieving dyspnea.[25] Supplemental oxygen may even prolong life in patients with hypoxemia,[65] but the mortality benefit is not present in mild hypoxemia at rest (peripheral capillary oxygen saturation [SpO_2] 89%–93%) or during exercise (SpO_2 80%–89% for no more than 5 minutes during a 6-minute walk).[72] Nasal high-flow oxygen therapy may improve lung mechanics and short-term emergency treatment of dyspnea.[73,74] As the end of life approaches and comfort becomes the primary focus, maintaining oxygen saturation is no longer the goal, and a fan or pursed-lip breathing may be more advantageous.[75]

Interprofessional pulmonary rehabilitation (PR) is known to be effective in managing breathlessness. It also shares many similarities with palliative care in its focus on symptom management and QOL. Dyspnea is a complex multifactorial symptom that includes affective and psychological aspects, and therefore complex interventions are often necessary to adequately address the multiple causes and impacts of the symptom. PR combines exercise training, patient education, and psychosocial support in a comprehensive evidence-based intervention for patients with lung disease.[76] PR classes typically meet two or three times per week over a 6- to 12-week interval, with an optional maintenance exercise program indefinitely after initial program completion. The foundation of PR is exercise training, whereas palliative care integrates more of a focus on advance care planning and spiritual dimensions.[77] The beneficial outcomes following PR decline over time, and perhaps palliative care follow-up after PR would support maintenance of PR outcomes.

Directing a fan toward the cheek, near the mouth, has been shown in multiple studies to relieve dyspnea.[25,78] This intervention is attractive because it is inexpensive, readily available, and safe. The mechanism of action is thought to be related to stimulation of the trigeminal nerve, distraction and relaxation, or alteration of the brain's perception of respiratory afferent signals.[78] Five additional recent studies supporting the benefits of breathing strategies have moved breathing management techniques into the highest level of evidence. These breathing strategies tend to focus on pursed-lip breathing, diaphragmatic breathing, progressive muscle relaxation with deep breathing, and the active cycle of breathing technique in a variety of diagnoses including heart failure,[79] COPD,[80–82] cystic fibrosis,[83] and lung cancer.[84]

Likely to Be Effective

Noninvasive ventilation (NIV) is reported to relieve dyspnea in patients with hypercapnic respiratory failure[85] as well as during exercise[86] and as a pre-hospital intervention.[87] High-intensity positive pressures, using the highest inspiratory pressures that the patient can tolerate, may provide more relief and better outcomes than usual low-intensity NIV.[88] While NIV can be helpful, many patients find it difficult to tolerate the mask or participate in activities of daily living such as eating, drinking, speaking, and sleeping when using NIV. Clinicians, including nurses, with skill in adjusting the NIV settings to optimize tolerance and minimize breathlessness are crucial to successful use of NIV. Inspiratory muscle training (IMT) has also been shown to benefit dyspnea in COPD[89,90] and in heart failure.[91,92] In one study, IMT was combined with high-frequency airway oscillation, with no difference between the intervention and sham groups.[93] Other noninvasive mechanical interventions to consider for airway clearance and optimal breathing are oscillatory positive pressure devices such as the Acapella, Flutter, or Aerobika[94]; autogenic drainage[95]; and high-frequency chest wall oscillation.[96]

A study of ensifentrine, an inhaled dual phosphodiesterase 3 and 4 inhibitor, documented improvement in dyspnea as well as QOL ($n = 405$).[97] Stimulation of an acupoint by transcutaneous electrical nerve stimulation (TENS) did not improve dyspnea,[98] although previous studies of TENS with other acupressure points was beneficial for dyspnea relief.[25] In addition, short-acting beta agonist and short-acting muscarinic antagonist inhalers, acupressure, dyspnea self-management programs, and home-based exercise[99] are all likely to be effective in relieving dyspnea.[25]

Balance Benefit with Harm

Interventions that may be considered on an individual basis, balancing benefit with harm, include high-flow nasal oxygen,[100] nitric oxide,[101] inhaler training,[80] palliative bronchoscopic interventions,[25] and complementary and integrative therapies. A variety of noninvasive endoscopic options for reducing lung hyperinflation and the resultant dyspnea are available, including the use of bronchial valves, coil implants, lung sealant, and thermal vapor ablation.[102]

Complementary and Integrative Therapies

Despite the attention that dyspnea management has received in the literature, patients and their families primarily manage and cope with dyspnea to the best of their ability, when not in direct contact with health professionals. Patients report many strategies for managing their symptoms, and very few of those strategies include evidence-based or medically prescribed interventions. Complementary and integrative therapies may be beneficial for people living with breathlessness if the safety profile merits an "*N* of 1" trial with careful consideration of the risk–benefit analysis.[103] Acupuncture and co-enzyme Q10[25] have been tested as useful, along with multiple exercise types, including qigong,[16] tai chi,[104,105] yoga,[106] and Korean lung conduction exercise.[107] Expressive art therapy,[108] biofeedback,[109] and hypnosis[110] have also been studied with promising results. Those therapies studied that have not had effectiveness established include thoracic kinesio taping,[111] manual osteopathic therapy,[112] Daoyin,[113] back massage,[114] and Squill-Oxymel, a Persian dietary supplement.[115]

Most nonpharmacological and complementary therapies for dyspnea management are focused on the central pathway of dyspnea. The concept of "total dyspnea,"[116] which acknowledges the multiple components of distress related to dyspnea and incorporates the meaning of the symptom within a context of whole-person care, provides a rationale for the improvements in dyspnea that can be experienced with interventions that do not have a clear physiologic rationale. Interventions focused on anxiety, depression, and other symptoms commonly found with dyspnea in symptom clusters can be beneficial for improving dyspnea as well.

Not recommended for chronic breathlessness

Opioids are no longer recommended for routine treatment of chronic breathlessness. A 2024 European Respiratory Society guideline, informed by a comprehensive systematic review, recommended against their use in this context and found no meaningful benefit in breathlessness from opioid use over days or weeks at home.[117,118] While earlier studies suggested short-term relief, in largely laboratory environments, more recent evidence does not support ongoing use in daily life. In contrast, adverse effects, including nausea, constipation, sedation, and in some cases hospitalization or death, are common, and concerns about safety, dependence, and stigma further limit their acceptability.

Opioids may still be considered for individuals with advanced respiratory disease and severe refractory breathlessness near the end of life. However, in such cases, clinicians must carefully consider risks, engage in shared decision-making, and align with the person's goals of care.

Benzodiazepines are not recommended for routine management of chronic breathlessness, except in second- or third-line settings or for patients nearing end of life where rapid relief of distress is needed.[119] Risks such as sedation, cognitive impairment, and dependence are particularly concerning in older adults. Mirtazapine has been trialled in this context, but a recent placebo-controlled study in severe COPD and ILD showed no benefit and higher side effects (64% vs 40%), despite being underpowered due to COVID-19.[120] Its routine use is not supported. Anxiolytics or antidepressants should be reserved for select cases, with close monitoring for benefit and harm.

Management of Dyspnea Crisis

"Sudden breathlessness" or "dyspnea crisis" is a term developed for use by patients.[25,121] This describes, in patients with chronic, sustained, and severe resting breathing discomfort, sudden dyspnea episodes that come on quickly and severely and overwhelm a patient's and family's ability to cope or achieve symptom relief.[25,122] These crises often happen in the context of a patient who is living with chronic breathlessness but who does not want to return to the emergency department and undergo intubation and mechanical ventilation. The pattern of dyspnea is unique with each individual and includes both continuous and breakthrough dyspnea.[25,122] The American Thoracic Society's patient education series on sudden breathlessness outlines the *COMFORT* approach for planning patient response during a crisis episode.[28] Nurses and the interprofessional team can use this tool to facilitate patients to

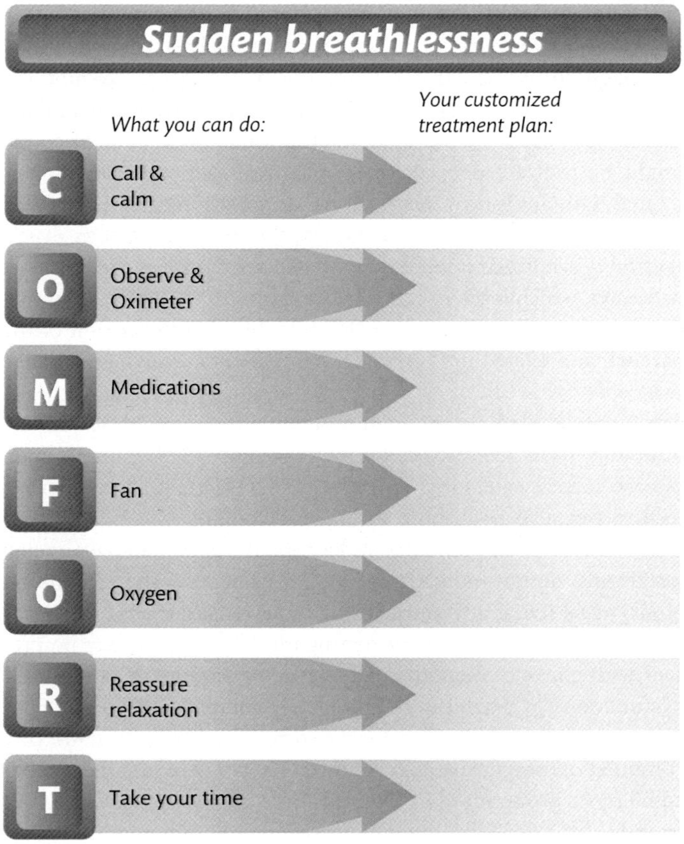

Figure 12.3 COMFORT sudden breathlessness mnemonic.
Source: Reference 28.

develop a personalized plan relative to their own experience.[28] The COMFORT sequence is provided in Figure 12.3, with further information provided in the factsheet accessible through the following link: https://www.atsjournals.org/doi/epdf/10.1164/rccm.20511P22?role=tab. Examples of the information in the sequence include: "F: Fan to face. Also, try opening the window or cooling the room. If driving in a car, open the window or turn on the air conditioner for air to circulate across the face." And "R: Reassure and relax. Slow down! Do things that make the surroundings calm. Examples are looking outside, guided imagery, prayer, or saying a mantra."

Support for Caregivers, Family Members, and Those Close to the Patient with Chronic Breathlessness

Chronic breathlessness is highly distressing for patients and their loved ones. With a rise in home-based care and even death in the home for patients, caregivers are increasingly supporting breathless loved ones at home. With certainty, caregiver distress is highly associated with a patient's level of distress.[123] Nursing interventions should be individualized and consider the patient–caregiver dyad as the focus of care. Caregiver support may include assessment and treatment of anxiety and depression, disease and symptom education, and bereavement support.[124] Additionally, identifying the positive characteristics of caregiving including personal growth and strengthened relationship may be useful.[30] Caregivers' experiences related to breathlessness include "anxiety and emotional distress, isolation, personal restrictions, lack of knowledge and strategies, helplessness and powerlessness, and lack of support or assistance."[124] Farquhar and colleagues describe caregivers as living in an "imploded world," feeling overwhelmed by breathlessness and lack of strategies to manage it.[124] Caregivers also report unmet physical and psychological needs, challenges in patient mood and subsequent loneliness and social isolation, emotional burden, and lack of education on disease process, advance care planning, and financial guidance.[125] Patient dyspnea, depression, and anxiety have been deemed to negatively impact perception of burden among family caregivers playing a role in palliative care.[126] Caregivers for those who are breathless report high levels of unmet needs and burden and fewer rewards to their caring.[127] Nurses with the interprofessional team should educate patients and carers on the potential causes of dyspnea and cough, as well as treatments that may impact the underlying pathology and provide symptomatic benefit. Caregivers are often not acknowledged by healthcare professionals and ideally should be supported as additional clients.[124] Patients living with the support of caregivers have fewer hospital admissions than those living alone.[30] The nurse may need to allay concerns and myths related to use of opioids and anxiolytics for the management of respiratory symptoms.[128] Supporting patients to self-manage may enhance the individual's self-efficacy and impact feelings of helplessness by the patient and caregiver.[129]

Potential online patient and family resources for management of dyspnea include the following:

- Supporting Someone with Breathlessness. 2025. Available from: https://supporting-breathlessness.org.uk.
- Lung Foundation Australia. 2025. Available from: https://lungfoundation.com.au.
- Support for you. Asthma Lung UK. 2025. Available from: https://www.blf.org.uk/support-for-you.
- Lung Disease Information Hub. European Lung Foundation. 2025. Available from: https://europeanlung.org/en/information-hub/.
- Patients. American Thoracic Society. 2025. Available from: https://www.thoracic.org/patients/.
- INSPIRE: Breathing Better. 2025. Available from: https://inspirebreathingbetter.com.
- The COPD Caregiver. 2025. Available from: https://www.copdfoundation.org/Learn-More/I-am-a-Caregiver/The-COPD-Caregiver.aspx.

Case Study Part 3: Patient Living with IPF

The palliative care registered nurse's (RN's) goal was to reduce suffering from dyspnea and cough using a multimodal approach. The RN decided to undertake a dyspnea assessment that included the PQRST mnemonic for pain: provoking/palliative factors, quality and characteristics, relationship to other symptoms, severity by patient report (3 = a lot), and timing. On physical examination, the RN found that Robin appeared frail and anxious with a forward-leaning, slouched posture. Lung sounds were diminished with bibasilar crackles, she was receiving oxygen via nasal cannula, and she used pursed-lip breathing. Nursing care included reinforcing adherence with medications and self-management. Nonpharmacologic interventions directed by the RN in collaboration with the professional team included calm reassurance, sitting upright, breathing training, fan to face, cool compress to forehead, and distraction therapy. Pharmacologic interventions implemented through the RN with the professional team included high-flow supplemental oxygen and Ativan 0.5 mg orally every 6 hours as needed for anxiety related to dyspnea. RN cough strategies included education on meditation, diet modification, cool humidified air, and use of low-dose morphine, prednisone, and dextromethorphan. A bowel regimen was implemented to prevent opioid-induced constipation. The RN included Robin's family in discussions of patient wishes, strategies for dyspnea and cough, and anticipatory grieving.

Cough Physiology, Measurement, and Interventions

Despite cough being a common and distressing symptom that interrupts social situations and is physically exhausting,[130] no treatment interventions are consistently effective. Cough is an important protective mechanism to maintain airway patency and facilitate secretion clearance; however, chronic persistent cough, over time, can affect physical, mental, and social health. Secondary symptoms can include sleep disturbance, fatigue, pain, depression, anxiety, anorexia, vocal quality interference, and urinary incontinence, leading to exhaustion and disrupted QOL.[130] Cough is one of the most common symptoms that spur medical visits. For the nurse with the interprofessional team, management primarily relies on the identification of the underlying cause of the cough; however, once disease-related treatments are optimized, management of persistent cough should focus on symptom management.

Pathophysiology of Cough

The cough reflex in the brainstem protects the airways from mechanical or chemical irritants mediated by sensory nerves in the large and peripheral airways. Voluntary cough and the urge to cough are centered in the cerebral cortex.[131] Early brain imaging evidence suggests that the conscious regulation of cough occurs in brain regions and neural pathways that are separate from the urge to cough. Both the voluntary and the reflex pathways are involved in cough control.[130,132,133] Overlap with the descending inhibitory pathways related to other stimuli may explain why cough is suppressed in the presence of other stimuli. Cough is stimulated by mechanical (touch), biochemical (capsaicin), and neurosensory stimuli.[132] Irritation can be caused by the presence of pathology in the airways, parenchymal inflammation from treatment, heightened cough reflex sensitivity, or comorbidities such as esophagopharyngeal reflux,[130,133] With hypersensitivity, even minimal irritation such as laughing, talking, or temperature changes can lead to cough. Other environmental irritants include smoking and perfume.[130,132–135] Cough is evoked and regulated by multiple peripheral and central neural pathways. Peripheral sensory nerve fibers can detect irritant signals within the airways.[133] Central processing may occur in several brain regions.[132,133,136]

The most common causes of cough are obesity, heart failure, obstructive sleep apnea, esophagopharyngeal reflux, medications, underlying respiratory disease such as asthma, and exposure to environmental, occupational, and/or indoor pollutants including smoking and cold air.[130,135,136] New pathologies have been identified for cough, including chronic cough due to esophageal dysmotility; thus, esophagopharyngeal reflux rather than gastroesophageal reflux disease may cause cough.[130] Other unusual sources of cough might be protracted bacterial bronchitis; basidiomycetes fungus, treated with antifungal medications; cervical spondylosis; and abnormal salivary glands at the base of the tongue.[137] *Cough hypersensitivity syndrome* signifies heightened sensitivity of the neuronal pathways, which leads to excessive coughing.[130,132–134,136–138] Chronic dry cough is very common in IPF, possibly due to traction of the parenchyma related to fibrosis.[134,138] In patients receiving palliative care, opiates have been used in guidelines for symptomatic relief of dry cough.[138] Medications such as angiotensin-converting enzyme inhibitors have been associated with cough.[130,135,136] Chronic lung disease such as interstitial lung disease, COPD/emphysema, or infection can also contribute to chronic cough.[130,133–136,138] Chronic sinusitis and postnasal drip, redefined as "upper airways cough syndrome," do not induce lower airways cough.[130] The recognition of laryngeal irritability and chronic hypersensitivity has led to the idea that cough is a sensory neuropathy,[130,132] which may be present with chronic cough, laryngospasm, or paradoxical vocal cord dysfunction.[137] Cough can be completely voluntary and under conscious control, completely reflexive in response to a stimulus, or a combination of reflexive and voluntary. Reflexive coughing can become more pronounced as a person becomes sensitized to a given stimulus.[132,133] Sensitization is triggered by inflammatory mediators that may be released after exposure to external and noxious stimuli like cold air, gastric fluid, and cigarette smoke.[130,136,137] Cough can be the first sign of lung cancer.[135,136]

Measurement of Cough

Severity, frequency, and disruptiveness are components of cough that should be measured.[132,133,136] VASs are easy to use for each component. Several instruments including the Leicester Cough Questionnaire[139] and the Cough Specific Quality of Life Questionnaire[140] measure the global impact of cough. The seven-item Cough Severity Diary has also been tested in patients with chronic and subacute cough.[141] Objective measurement of cough has been attempted with ambulatory cough monitoring such as the Leicester Cough Monitor and the VitaloJAK; however, distinguishing cough from other sounds has been a complicating factor.[142] Cough hypersensitivity syndrome encompasses chronic idiopathic cough, chronic refractory cough, and sensory neuropathic cough.[130,133] Recent guidelines for unexplained chronic cough provide an assessment algorithm, with recommendation to evaluate sputum eosinophils or exhaled nitric oxide to identify bronchial hyperresponsiveness that might respond to inhaled corticosteroids.[130,133]

Interventions for Cough

As noted above, the nurse with the interprofessional team should first address disease-related and underlying causes of cough, with subsequent adjustment to symptom management with persistent chronic cough. It may be that cough appears to be one entity but actually has multiple causes that have not yet been identified or linked to an effective intervention. The goal for cough treatment is to allow normal cough while blocking pathological cough.[132] Many therapies have been suggested for cough, seemingly because none work very well. The CHEST Expert Cough Panel develops clinical practice guidelines as a living document with continually updated evidence, technologies, and recommendations.[143] Simple strategies that the nurse with the interprofessional team can engage may include pursed-lip breathing; swallowing to diminish the urge to cough; avoiding smoking, mouth breathing, alcohol, and caffeine; and increasing water intake or using steam inhalation.[144,145] However, directing patients to physiotherapy, speech and language therapies, and psychoeducational counseling is the primary management approach, with a lack of evidence for pharmacological treatments. Nonpharmacological speech pathology approaches such as behavioral cough control techniques and vocal hygiene strategies may reduce cough symptoms.[130,144] Complex physiotherapy and speech and language intervention aims to reduce laryngeal irritation and increase voluntary cough control through sputum clearance and cough-reflex hypersensitivity training.[136,144]

Given the age and low level of evidence, recommendations for palliative cough management balance risk with benefit. As above, the first step is to consider disease-directed treatment and review medications to see if any might be exacerbating the cough, as well as evaluation and treatment of any comorbidities that may be contributing to cough. Sodium cromoglycate may be considered in people with IPF, being relatively safe although supported by minimal evidence, but is not effective in patients with refractory chronic cough.[134,137,138] If still unresponsive, opioid derivatives such as morphine, codeine, or dextromethorphan may be considered.[130,132,137] In patients with unexplained cough that has not responded to a trial of inhaled corticosteroids, speech therapy and gabapentin trials are recommended.[144] A recent systematic review of treatments for cough related to the common cold found many treatment options available, but the evidence was not compelling for any of the options, including decongestants, antihistamines, acetylcysteine, nonsteroidal anti-inflammatory drugs, honey, zinc lozenges, over-the-counter antitussives, expectorants, mucolytics, or combination products.[146] The evidence base has not changed since the 2006 guidelines were published, with the majority of the research published before 2000.[147]

Despite limited evidence worldwide surrounding pharmacological treatments, P2X3 receptor antagonists such as the neuromodulator gabapentin have been used to treat chronic refractory cough in adults. A recent systematic review and meta-analysis of gabapentin in refractory cough, reported significant improvement in cough-specific quality of life, and cough frequency and severity.[148] The recommended use of these antitussives to provide a pathway to mediate cough reflex by targeting airway vagal afferent nerve hypersensitization is a promising, novel strategy to address this distressing symptom.[130,132,137] Clinical trials investigating the efficacy and safety of gefapixant, a non-narcotic selective antagonist of the P2X3 receptor, have been initiated in people with refractory and unexplained chronic cough.[130,132,149] To date, evidence demonstrates efficacy at lower doses (50 mg twice daily over a period of 12 weeks) to reduce cough frequency and improve tolerability, cough severity, and QOL in people with refractory chronic cough. Further studies are required to examine longer-term benefits.[149]

For cough in adult patients with lung cancer, a stepped approach is recommended, with the nurse with the interprofessional team starting with identification and treatment of coexisting causes of cough, nonpharmacological cough suppression exercises, endobronchial brachytherapy, and graduated trials of various cough suppressants.[150] Although many substances including glaucine, Chinese herbs, Duopect, moguisteine, pipazethate, guaifenesin, *N*-acetylcysteine, diphenhydramine, loratadine, erythromycin, ipratropium, and inhaled corticosteroids have been tested as antitussives; over-the-counter, symptomatic cough suppressants such as codeine, benzonatate, and dextromethorphan are the only agents shown to treat chronic cough.[132,136] Low-dose slow-release morphine (5–10 mg twice daily)[130,132,136,137] and dextromethorphan both act centrally to inhibit cough reflex.[132,136] Thalidomide has been tested for cough due to anti-inflammatory properties, but the side effects are severe.[138] With recognition that cough may be triggered sensory neuropathically or by laryngeal irritability, neuromodulators used to treat neuropathic pain, such as gabapentin, pregabalin, desipramine, tramadol, or amitriptyline, may be helpful.[130,132,137] Disease-directed treatment for cancer-related cough may also include drainage of pleural effusions, brachytherapy, or photodynamic therapy.[145] A Cochrane review of RCTs for cancer-related cough treatment found minimal evidence but suggested that treatments like butamirate linctus, codeine 60 mg, morphine, dihydrocodeine, cromoglycate, and hydropropizine or levodropropizine may be beneficial.[145]

Case Study Recap

In the month prior to her death, Robin was very short of breath with minimal activities and required 10–15 L/minute O_2 to maintain an oxygen saturation of 90%. She was coughing at least hourly (2–5 min episodes), which she described to the RN as "exhausting" and disruptive to her daily living. She reported feelings of "gasping" and "suffocating," with marked anxiety with episodes of severe dyspnea. Robin used low-dose opioids for dyspnea management but was concerned that her secretions became more difficult to expectorate. On discussion with the RN, the interprofessional team, and her family, Robin ultimately agreed to a home hospice plan of care. Up until the last weeks of her life, she was pleased with her QOL. She appreciated her scooter that gave her mobility (with her oxygen tanks) to attend her grandchildren's soccer games and dance recitals. She enjoyed the opportunity to move nearer her son for the last few years of her life and was satisfied with the "lasting good" she had done in this world.

Conclusion

Dyspnea and cough are burdensome respiratory conditions often present in patients receiving palliative care. While the nurse with the interprofessional team should address disease-related and underlying causes first, a broad, holistic approach is recommended, particularly when symptoms persist despite optimization of treatments. Varied pharmacological and nonpharmacological interventions exist. Given the complexity, people with chronic dyspnea and cough should be encouraged to notice what works well for them in managing their symptoms using "*N* of 1" trials to implement these strategies. It is possible to achieve a positive sensation of breathing and relief from cough at the end of life. Nurses must use all available resources to provide relief for patients and their loved ones with serious illness.

REFERENCES

1. Brule D. *Just Breathe: Mastering Breathwork for Success in Life, Love, Business, and Beyond*. Simon & Schuster; 2017.
2. Mahler DA. Evaluation of dyspnea in the elderly. *Clin Geriatr Med*. 2017;33(4):503–521.
3. Kravitz J. Transformational Breath Foundation. 2022. Accessed October 7, 2022. http://transformationalbreath.com/.
4. Dennis R. *And Breathe: The Complete Guide to Conscious Breathing for Health and Happiness*. Da Capo Press; 2017.
5. Payne P, Levine PA, Crane-Godreau MA. Somatic experiencing: using interoception and proprioception as core elements of trauma therapy. *Front Psychol*. 2015;6:93.
6. Palmer E, Kavanagh E, Visram S, Bourke A-M, Forrest I, Exley C. When should palliative care be introduced for people with progressive fibrotic interstitial lung disease? A meta-ethnography of the experiences of people with end-stage interstitial lung disease and their family carers. *Palliat Med*. 2022;36(8):1171–1185.
7. O'Donnell DE, James MD, Milne KM, Neder JA. The pathophysiology of dyspnea and exercise intolerance in chronic obstructive pulmonary disease. *Clin Chest Med*. 2019;40(2):343–366.
8. Johnson MJ, Hui D, Currow DC. Opioids, exertion, and dyspnea: a review of the evidence. *Am J Hosp Palliat Care*. 2016;33(2):194–200.
9. Macnaughton J. Making breath visible: reflections on relations between bodies, breath and world in the critical medical humanities. *Body Soc*. 2020;26(2):30–54.
10. Chin C, Booth S. Managing breathlessness: a palliative care approach. *Postgrad Med J*. 2016;92(1089):393–400.
11. Currow DC, Johnson MJ. Distilling the essence of breathlessness: the first vital symptom. *Eur Respir J*. 2015;45:1526–1528.
12. Booth S, Johnson MJ. Improving the quality of life of people with advanced respiratory disease and severe breathlessness. *Breathe*. 2019;15(3):198–215.
13. So WK, Law BM, Chan DN, Xing W, Chan CW, McCarthy AL. The effect of nonpharmacological interventions on managing symptom clusters among cancer patients: a systematic review. *Cancer Nurs*. 2020;43(6):E304–E327.
14. Fei F, Siegert RJ, Zhang X, Gao W, Koffman J. Symptom clusters, associated factors and health-related quality of life in patients with chronic obstructive pulmonary disease: a structural equation modelling analysis. *J Clin Nurs*. 2023;32(1–2):298–310.
15. Disler R, Smallwood N, Philip JAM. Advanced respiratory disease: managing symptoms in the last years of life. *Respir Med Today*. 2021;6(2):6–11.
16. Molassiotis A, Vu DV, Ching SSY. The effectiveness of qigong in managing a cluster of symptoms (breathlessness–fatigue–anxiety) in patients with lung cancer: a randomized controlled trial. *Integr Cancer Ther*. 2021;20:15347354211008253.
17. Ekström M, Allingham SF, Eagar K, Yates P, Johnson C, Currow DC. Breathlessness during the last week of life in palliative care: an Australian prospective, longitudinal study. *J Pain Symptom Manage*. 2016;51(5):816–823.
18. Clark N, Fan VS, Slatore CG, et al. Dyspnea and pain frequently co-occur among Medicare managed care recipients. *Ann Am Thorac Soc*. 2014;11(6):890–897.
19. Currow DC, Higginson IJ, Johnson MJ. Breathlessness—current and emerging mechanisms, measurement and management: a discussion from an European Association of Palliative Care workshop. *Palliat Med*. 2013;27(10):932–938.
20. O'Donnell DE, Neder JA. The enigma of dyspnoea in COPD: a physiological perspective. *Respirology*. 2020;25(2):134–136.
21. Mularski RA. Advancing a common understanding and approach to dyspnea management. Consensus proposal for the chronic breathlessness syndrome. *Ann Am Thorac Soc*. 2017;14(7):1108–1110.
22. Chang AS, Munson J, Gifford AH, Mahler DA. Prospective use of descriptors of dyspnea to diagnose common respiratory diseases. *Chest*. 2015;148(4):895–902.
23. Banzett RB, Sheridan AR, Baker KM, Lansing RW, Stevens JP. "Scared to death" dyspnoea from the hospitalised patient's perspective. *BMJ Open Respir Res*. 2020;7(1):e000493.
24. Janssen DJ, Wouters EF, Spruit MA. Psychosocial consequences of living with breathlessness due to advanced disease. *Curr Opin Support Palliat Care*. 2015;9(3):232–237.
25. Campbell ML, Donesky D, Sarkozy A, Reinke LF. Treatment of dyspnea in advanced disease and at the end of life. *J Hosp Palliat Nurs*. 2021;23(5):406–420.
26. Higginson IJ, Reilly CC, Maddocks M. Breathlessness. In: Lindell KO, Danoff SK, eds. *Palliative Care in Lung Disease*. Springer International Publishing; 2021:89–113.
27. Massart A, Hunt DP. Management of refractory breathlessness: a review for general internists. *J Gen Intern Med*. 2021;36(4):1035–1040.
28. Donesky D, Schneidman A, Reinke L, Carrieri-Kohlman V. Sudden breathlessness. *Am J Respir Crit Care Med*. 2022;205(11):P22–P24.
29. Clark N, Fan VS, Slatore CG, et al. Dyspnea and pain frequently co-occur among Medicare managed care recipients. *Ann Am Thorac Soc*. 2014;11(6):890–897.
30. Maddocks M, Lovell N, Booth S, Man WD, Higginson IJ. Palliative care and management of troublesome symptoms for people with chronic obstructive pulmonary disease. *Lancet*. 2017;390(10098):988–1002.
31. Campbell ML. Dyspnea prevalence, trajectories, and measurement in critical care and at life's end. *Curr Opin Support Palliat Care*. 2012;6(2):168–171.
32. Maddocks M, Brighton LJ, Farquhar M, et al. Holistic services for people with advanced disease and chronic or refractory breathlessness: a mixed-methods evidence synthesis. *Health Services and Delivery Research*. 2019;7(22).
33. Clari M, Matarese M, Ivziku D, De Marinis MG. Self-care of people with chronic obstructive pulmonary disease: a meta-synthesis. *Patient*. 2017;10(4):407–427.
34. Parshall MB, Schwartzstein RM, Adams L, et al. An official American Thoracic Society statement: update on the mechanisms, assessment, and management of dyspnea. *Am J Respir Crit Care Med*. 2012;185(4):435–452.
35. O'Donnell DE, Milne KM, James MD, de Torres JP, Neder JA. Dyspnea in COPD: new mechanistic insights and management implications. *Adv Ther*. 2020;37(1):41–60.
36. Currow DC, Higginson IJ, Johnson MJ. Breathlessness—current and emerging mechanisms, measurement and management: a discussion from an European Association of Palliative Care workshop. *Palliat Med*. 2013;27(10):932–938.
37. Spathis A, Booth S, Moffat C, et al. The breathing, thinking, functioning clinical model: a proposal to facilitate evidence-based breathlessness management in chronic respiratory disease. *NPJ Prim Care Respir Med*. 2017;27(1):27.
38. Anzueto A, Miravitlles M. Pathophysiology of dyspnea in COPD. *Postgrad Med*. 2017;129(3):366–374.

39. Williams MT, Johnston KN. Multidimensional measurement of breathlessness: recent advances. *Curr Opin Support Palliat Care.* 2019;13(3):184–192.
40. Williams MT, Lewthwaite H, Paquet C, et al. Dyspnoea-12 and multidimensional dyspnea profile: systematic review of use and properties. *J Pain Symptom Manage.* 2022;63(1):e75–e87.
41. Banzett RB, O'Donnell CR, Guilfoyle TE, et al. Multidimensional dyspnea profile: an instrument for clinical and laboratory research. *Eur Respir J.* 2015;45(6):1681–1691.
42. Hui D, Bruera E. The Edmonton Symptom Assessment System 25 years later: past, present, and future developments. *J Pain Symptom Manage.* 2017;53(3):630–643.
43. Carvajal A, Hribernik N, Duarte E, Sanz-Rubiales A, Centeno C. The Spanish version of the Edmonton Symptom Assessment System-Revised (ESAS-r): first psychometric analysis involving patients with advanced cancer. *J Pain Symptom Manage.* 2013;45(1):129–136.
44. Kwon JH, Nam SH, Koh S, et al. Validation of the Edmonton Symptom Assessment System in Korean patients with cancer. *J Pain Symptom Manage.* 2013;46(6):947–956.
45. Nekolaichuk C, Huot A, Gratton V, Bush SH, Tarumi Y, Watanabe SM. Development of a French version of the Edmonton Symptom Assessment System-Revised: a pilot study of palliative care patients' perspectives. *J Palliat Med.* 2017;20:966–976.
46. Yamaguchi T, Morita T, Nitto A, et al. Establishing cutoff points for defining symptom severity using the Edmonton Symptom Assessment System-Revised Japanese version. *J Pain Symptom Manage.* 2016;51(2):292–297.
47. Chang VT, Hwang SS, Feuerman M, Kasimis BS, Thaler HT. The Memorial Symptom Assessment Scale Short Form (MSAS-SF). *Cancer.* 2000;89(5):1162–1171.
48. Portenoy RK, Thaler HT, Kornblith AB, et al. The Memorial Symptom Assessment Scale: an instrument for the evaluation of symptom prevalence, characteristics and distress. *Eur J Cancer.* 1994;30a(9):1326–1336.
49. Ahmed S, Bourbeau J, Maltais F, Mansour A. The Oort structural equation modeling approach detected a response shift after a COPD self-management program not detected by the Schmitt technique. *J Clin Epidemiol.* 2009;62(11):1165–1172.
50. Hayen A, Herigstad M, Pattinson KT. Understanding dyspnea as a complex individual experience. *Maturitas.* 2013;76(1):45–50.
51. Dempsey JA, Romer L, Rodman J, Miller J, Smith C. Consequences of exercise-induced respiratory muscle work. *Respir Physiol Neurobiol.* 2006;151(2):242–250.
52. Ward ME, Eidelman D, Stubbing DG, Bellemare F, Macklem PT. Respiratory sensation and pattern of respiratory muscle activation during diaphragm fatigue. *J Appl Physiol (1985).* 1988;65(5):2181–2189.
53. Mitchell SA, Friese CR. Decision Rules for Summative Evaluation of a Body of Evidence. Oncology Nursing Society. https://www.ons.org/decision-rules-summative-evaluation-body-evidence.
54. Taylor J. The non-pharmacological management of breathlessness. *End Life J.* 2007;1(1):20–27.
55. Martinsen U, Bentzen H, Holter MK, et al. The effect of occupational therapy in patients with chronic obstructive pulmonary disease: a randomized controlled trial. *Scand J Occup Ther.* 2017;24(2):89–97.
56. Morgan DD, White KM. Occupational therapy interventions for breathlessness at the end of life. *Curr Opin Support Palliat Care.* 2012;6(2):138–143.
57. White KM. The role of the occupational therapist in the care of people living with lung cancer. *Transl Lung Cancer Res.* 2016;5(3):244–246.
58. Hill W, Bendall C. Registered respiratory therapists as force multipliers in interprofessional complex continuing care. *Can J Respir Ther.* 2015;51(3):54.
59. Nickerson JW. A needs assessment to determine the need for respiratory therapy in complex continuing care: a methods paper. *Can J Respir Ther.* 2015;51(3):55.
60. Smith SG, Endee LM, Benz Scott LA, Linden PL. The future of respiratory care: results of a New York State survey of respiratory therapists. *Respir Care.* 2017;62(3):279–287.
61. Beaulieu J, Jensen D, O'Donnell DE, et al. Relieving exertional dyspnea during the 3-min constant speed shuttle test in patients with COPD with indacaterol/glycopyrronium versus tiotropium: the RED trial. *Ther Adv Respir Dis.* 2020;14:1753466620939507.
62. Calverley PM, Hoz Adl, Xue W, Ferguson GT, Miravitlles M. COPD maintenance therapy with tiotropium/olodaterol compared with tiotropium: an analysis in the absence of additional ICS therapy. *COPD.* 2020;17(5):477–484.
63. Chen R, Zhong N, Wang H-Y, et al. Efficacy and safety of glycopyrrolate/formoterol fumarate metered dose inhaler (GFF MDI) formulated using co-suspension delivery technology in Chinese patients with COPD. *Int J Chron Obstruct Pulmon Dis.* 2020;15:43–56.
64. Takahashi K, Uchida M, Kato G, et al. First-line treatment with tiotropium/olodaterol improves physical activity in patients with treatment-naive chronic obstructive pulmonary disease. *Int J Chron Obstruct Pulmon Dis.* 2020;15:2115–2126.
65. Barjaktarevic I, Cooper CB. Supplemental oxygen therapy for patients with chronic obstructive pulmonary disease. *Semin Respir Crit Care Med.* 2015;36(4):552–566.
66. Vogelmeier CF, Jones PW, Kerwin EM, et al. Efficacy of umeclidinium/vilanterol according to the degree of reversibility of airflow limitation at screening: a post hoc analysis of the EMAX trial. *Respir Res.* 2021;22(1):1–11.
67. Muraki M, Kunita Y, Shirahase K, et al. A randomized controlled trial of long-acting muscarinic antagonist and long-acting β2 agonist fixed-dose combinations in patients with chronic obstructive pulmonary disease. *BMC Pulmon Med.* 2021;21(1):1–8.
68. van Geffen WH, Carpaij OA, Westbroek LF, et al. Long-acting dual bronchodilator therapy (indacaterol/glycopyrronium) versus nebulized short-acting dual bronchodilator (salbutamol/ipratropium) in chronic obstructive pulmonary disease: a double blind, randomized, placebo controlled trial. *Respir Med.* 2020;171:106064.
69. Gon Y, Nishi K, Sato K, et al. Efficacy and safety of glycopyrrolate/formoterol fumarate metered dose inhaler delivered using co-suspension delivery technology in Japanese patients with moderate-to-very severe chronic obstructive pulmonary disease. *Respir Investig.* 2021;59(1):135–144.
70. Zhong N, Zheng J, Lee SH, Lipson DA, Du X, Wu S. Efficacy and safety of once-daily inhaled umeclidinium in Asian patients with COPD: results from a randomized, placebo-controlled study. *Int J Chron Obstruct Pulmon Dis.* 2020;15:809–819.
71. Lavorini F, Mannini C, Chellini E, Fontana GA. Optimising inhaled pharmacotherapy for elderly patients with chronic obstructive pulmonary disease: the importance of delivery devices. *Drugs Aging.* 2016;33(7):461–473.
72. Albert RK, Au DH, Blackford AL, et al. A randomized trial of long-term oxygen for COPD with moderate desaturation. *N Engl J Med.* 2016;375(17):1617–1627.

73. Fraser JF, Spooner AJ, Dunster KR, Anstey CM, Corley A. Nasal high flow oxygen therapy in patients with COPD reduces respiratory rate and tissue carbon dioxide while increasing tidal and end-expiratory lung volumes: a randomised crossover trial. *Thorax*. 2016;71(8):759–761.
74. Rittayamai N, Tscheikuna J, Praphruetkit N, Kijpinyochai S. Use of high-flow nasal cannula for acute dyspnea and hypoxemia in the emergency department. *Respir Care*. 2015;60(10):1377–1382.
75. Tiep B, Carter R, Zachariah F, et al. Oxygen for end-of-life lung cancer care: managing dyspnea and hypoxemia. *Expert Rev Respir Med*. 2013;7(5):479–490.
76. Spruit MA, Singh SJ, Garvey C, et al. An official American Thoracic Society/European Respiratory Society statement: key concepts and advances in pulmonary rehabilitation. *Am J Respir Crit Care Med*. 2013;188(8):e13–e64.
77. Reticker AL, Nici L, ZuWallack R. Pulmonary rehabilitation and palliative care in COPD: two sides of the same coin? *Chron Respir Dis*. 2012;9(2):107–116.
78. Kocatepe V, Can G, Oruç Ö. Lung cancer–related dyspnea: the effects of a handheld fan on management of symptoms. *Clin J Oncol Nurs*. 2021;25(6):655–661.
79. Srimookda N, Saensom D, Mitsungnern T, Kotruchin P, Ruaisungnoen W. The effects of breathing training on dyspnea and anxiety among patients with acute heart failure at emergency department. *Int Emerg Nurs*. 2021;56:101008.
80. Ceyhan Y, Tekinsoy Kartin P. The effects of breathing exercises and inhaler training in patients with COPD on the severity of dyspnea and life quality: a randomized controlled trial. *Trials*. 2022;23(1):1–11.
81. Hasanpour Dehkordi A, Ebrahimi-Dehkordi S, Banitalebi-Dehkordi F, Salehi Tali S, Kheiri S, Soleimani Babadi A. The effect of teach-back training intervention of breathing exercise on the level of dyspnea, six-minutes walking test and FEV1/FVC ratio in patients with chronic obstructive pulmonary disease; a randomized controlled trial. *Expert Rev Respir Med*. 2021;15(1):161–169.
82. Neşe A, Samancıoğlu Bağlama S. The effect of progressive muscle relaxation and deep breathing exercises on dyspnea and fatigue symptoms of COPD patients: a randomized controlled study. *Holist Nurs Pract*. 2022;36(4):E18–E26.
83. Mckoy NA, Wilson LM, Saldanha IJ, Odelola OA, Robinson KA. Active cycle of breathing technique for cystic fibrosis. *Cochrane Database Syst Rev*. 2016;7(7):CD007862.
84. Lu H-B, Liu X, Wang Y-Q, et al. Active cycle of breathing technique: a respiratory modality to improve perioperative outcomes in patients with lung cancer. *Clin J Oncol Nurs*. 2022;26(2):176–182.
85. Nava S, Ferrer M, Esquinas A, et al. Palliative use of non-invasive ventilation in end-of-life patients with solid tumours: a randomised feasibility trial. *Lancet Oncol*. 2013;14(3):219–227.
86. Dennis CJ, Menadue C, Schneeberger T, et al. Perceptions of noninvasive ventilation during exercise in noninvasive ventilation-naïve patients with COPD. *Respir Care*. 2022;67(5):543–552.
87. Finn JC, Brink D, Mckenzie N, et al. Prehospital continuous positive airway pressure (CPAP) for acute respiratory distress: a randomised controlled trial. *Emerg Med J*. 2022;39(1):37–44.
88. Altintas N. Update: non-invasive positive pressure ventilation in chronic respiratory failure due to COPD. *COPD*. 2016;13(1):110–121.
89. Koch R, Rodrigues de Lemos Augusto T, Ramos AG, de Tarso Müller P. Inspiratory muscle training potentiates the beneficial effects of proportional assisted ventilation on exertional dyspnea and exercise tolerance in COPD: a proof-of-concept randomized and controlled trial. *COPD*. 2020;17(4):384–391.
90. Saka S, Gurses HN, Bayram M. Effect of inspiratory muscle training on dyspnea-related kinesiophobia in chronic obstructive pulmonary disease: a randomized controlled trial. *Complement Ther Clin Pract*. 2021;44:101418.
91. Hossein Pour AH, Gholami M, Saki M, Birjandi M. The effect of inspiratory muscle training on fatigue and dyspnea in patients with heart failure: a randomized, controlled trial. *Jpn J Nurs Sci*. 2020;17(2):e12290.
92. Katayıfçı N, Güçlü MB, Şen F. A comparison of the effects of inspiratory muscle strength and endurance training on exercise capacity, respiratory muscle strength and endurance, and quality of life in pacemaker patients with heart failure: a randomized study. *Heart Lung*. 2022;55:49–58.
93. Daynes E, Greening N, Singh SJ. Randomised controlled trial to investigate the use of high-frequency airway oscillations as training to improve dyspnoea (TIDe) in COPD. *Thorax*. 2022;77(7):690–696.
94. Barker R, Laverty AA, Hopkinson NS. Adjuncts for sputum clearance in COPD: clinical consensus versus actual use. *BMJ Open Respir Res*. 2017;4(1):e000226.
95. McCormack P, Burnham P, Southern KW. Autogenic drainage for airway clearance in cystic fibrosis. *Cochrane Database Syst Rev*. 2017;10(10):CD009595.
96. Morrison L, Milroy S. Oscillating devices for airway clearance in people with cystic fibrosis. *Paediatr Respir Rev*. 2017;25:30–32.
97. Watz H, Rickard K, Rheault T, Bengtsson T, Singh D. Symptom improvement following treatment with the inhaled dual phosphodiesterase 3 and 4 inhibitor ensifentrine in patients with moderate to severe COPD—a detailed analysis. *Int J Chron Obstruct Pulmon Dis*. 2020;15:2199–2206.
98. Nakano J, Ishii K, Fukushima T, et al. Effects of transcutaneous electrical nerve stimulation on physical symptoms in advanced cancer patients receiving palliative care. *Int J Rehabil Res*. 2020;43(1):62–68.
99. Ma R-C, Zhao Y, Liu X, et al. Multimodal exercise program: a pilot randomized trial for patients with lung cancer receiving surgical treatment. *Clin J Oncol Nurs*. 2021;25(3):E26–E34.
100. Tung L-F, Shen S-Y, Shih H-H, Chen Y-T, Yen C-t, Ho S-C. Effect of high-flow nasal therapy during early pulmonary rehabilitation in patients with severe AECOPD: a randomized controlled study. *Respir Res*. 2020;21(1):1–11.
101. Phillips DB, Brotto AR, Ross BA, et al. Inhaled nitric oxide improves ventilatory efficiency and exercise capacity in patients with mild COPD: a randomized-control cross-over trial. *J Physiol*. 2021;599(5):1665–1683.
102. Herth FJ, Slebos D-J, Criner GJ, Valipour A, Sciurba F, Shah PL. Endoscopic lung volume reduction: an expert panel recommendation—update 2019. *Respiration*. 2019;97(6):548–57.
103. Kamal AH, Maguire JM, Wheeler JL, Currow DC, Abernethy AP. Dyspnea review for the palliative care professional: treatment goals and therapeutic options. *J Palliat Med*. 2012;15(1):106–114.
104. Gilliam EA, Cheung T, Kraemer K, et al. The impact of tai chi and mind-body breathing in COPD: insights from a

qualitative sub-study of a randomized controlled trial. *PLoS One*. 2021;16(4):e0249263.

105. Yeh GY, Litrownik D, Wayne PM, et al. BEAM study (breathing, education, awareness, movement): a randomised controlled feasibility trial of tai chi exercise in patients with COPD. *BMJ Open Respir Res*. 2020;7(1):e000697.
106. Özer Z, Turan GB, Aksoy M. The effects of yoga on dyspnea, sleep and fatigue in chronic respiratory diseases. *Complement Ther Clin Pract*. 2021;43:101306.
107. Lee SW, Lyu YR, Park SJ, et al. The effect of lung-conduction exercise in chronic obstructive pulmonary disease: study protocol for randomized, assessor-blind, multicenter trial. *Medicine (Baltimore)*. 2020;99(18):e19826.
108. Zuo X, Lou P, Zhu Y, et al. Effects of expressive art therapy on health status of patients with chronic obstructive pulmonary disease: a community-based cluster randomized controlled trial. *Ther Adv Respir Dis*. 2022;16:17534666221111876.
109. Kaja R, Vaiyapuri A, Sirajudeen MS, et al. Biofeedback flutter device for managing the symptoms of patients with COPD. *Technol Health Care*. 2020;28(5):477–485.
110. Anlló H, Herer B, Delignières A, et al. Hypnosis for the management of anxiety and dyspnea in COPD: a randomized, sham-controlled crossover trial. *Int J Chron Obstruct Pulmon Dis*. 2020;15:2609–2620.
111. Tomruk M, Keleş E, Özalevli S, Alpaydin AÖ. Effects of thoracic kinesio taping on pulmonary functions, respiratory muscle strength and functional capacity in patients with chronic obstructive pulmonary disease: a randomized controlled trial. *Explore (NY)*. 2020;16(5):332–338.
112. Buran Cirak Y, Yilmaz Yelvar GD, Durustkan Elbasi N. Effectiveness of 12-week inspiratory muscle training with manual therapy in patients with COPD: a randomized controlled study. *Clin Respir J*. 2022;16(4):317–328.
113. Zhou M, Zhang H, Li F, et al. Pulmonary Daoyin as a traditional Chinese medicine rehabilitation programme for patients with IPF: a randomized controlled trial. *Respirology*. 2021;26(4):360–369.
114. Yilmaz CK, Aşiret GD, Çetinkaya F. The effect of back massage on physiological parameters, dyspnoea, and anxiety in patients with chronic obstructive pulmonary disease in the intensive care unit: a randomised clinical trial. *Intensive Crit Care Nurs*. 2021;63:102962.
115. Mohammadi-Araghi M, Eslaminejad A, Karegar-Borzi H, Mazloomzadeh S, Nejatbakhsh F. An add-on treatment for moderate COPD with squill-oxymel (a traditional formulation from *Drimia maritima* (L.) Stearn): a pilot randomized triple-blinded placebo-controlled clinical trial. *Evid Based Complement Alternat Med*. 2022;2022:5024792.
116. Abernethy AP, Wheeler JL. Total dyspnoea. *Curr Opin Support Palliat Care*. 2008;2(2):110–113.
117. Smallwood NE, Pascoe A, Wijsenbeek M, et al. Opioids for the palliation of symptoms in people with serious respiratory illness: a systematic review and meta-analysis. *Eur Respir Rev*. 2024;33(174).
118. Holland AE, Spathis A, Marsaa K, et al. European Respiratory Society clinical practice guideline on symptom management for adults with serious respiratory illness. *Eur Respir J*. 2024;63(6).
119. Verberkt CA, van den Beuken-van MH, Schols JM, et al. Respiratory adverse effects of opioids for breathlessness: a systematic review and meta-analysis. *Eur Respir J*. 2017;50(5).
120. Higginson IJ, Brown ST, Oluyase AO, et al. Mirtazapine to alleviate severe breathlessness in patients with COPD or interstitial lung diseases (BETTER-B): an international, multicentre, double-blind, randomised, placebo-controlled, phase 3 mixed-method trial. *Lancet Respir Med*. 2024;12(10):763–774.
121. Mularski RA, Reinke LF, Carrieri-Kohlman V, et al. An official American Thoracic Society workshop report: assessment and palliative management of dyspnea crisis. *Ann Am Thorac Soc*. 2013;10(5):S98–S106.
122. Donesky D. Management of acute breathlessness in the person with chronic refractory breathlessness. *Curr Opin Support Palliat Care*. 2015;9(3):212–216.
123. Williams AL, McCorkle R. Cancer family caregivers during the palliative, hospice, and bereavement phases: a review of the descriptive psychosocial literature. *Palliat Support Care*. 2011;9(3):315–325.
124. Farquhar M, Penfold C, Benson J, et al. Six key topics informal carers of patients with breathlessness in advanced disease want to learn about and why: MRC phase I study to inform an educational intervention. *PLoS One*. 2017;12(5):e0177081.
125. Klein S, Logan A, Lindell KO. A scoping review of unmet needs of caregivers of patients with pulmonary fibrosis. *Curr Opin Support Palliat Care*. 2021;15(4):226–232.
126. Krug K, Miksch A, Peters-Klimm F, Engeser P, Szecsenyi J. Correlation between patient quality of life in palliative care and burden of their family caregivers: a prospective observational cohort study. *BMC Palliat Care*. 2016;15:4.
127. Malik FA, Gysels M, Higginson IJ. Living with breathlessness: a survey of caregivers of breathless patients with lung cancer or heart failure. *Palliat Med*. 2013;27(7):647–656.
128. Horton R, Rocker G. What is the role of opioids in treatment of refractory dyspnea in advanced chronic obstructive pulmonary disease? In Goldstein NE, Morrison RS, eds. *Evidence-Based Practice of Palliative Medicine*. Saunders; 2012:111–119.
129. Yorke J, Lloyd-Williams M, Smith J, et al. Management of the respiratory distress symptom cluster in lung cancer: a randomised controlled feasibility trial. *Support Care Cancer*. 2015;23(11):3373–3384.
130. Morice AH, Millqvist E, Bieksiene K, et al. ERS guidelines on the diagnosis and treatment of chronic cough in adults and children. *Eur Respir J*. 2020;55(1):1901136.
131. van Manen MJ, Birring SS, Vancheri C, et al. Cough in idiopathic pulmonary fibrosis. *Eur Respir Rev*. 2016;25(141):278–286.
132. Mazzone SB, McGarvey L. Mechanisms and rationale for targeted therapies in refractory and unexplained chronic cough. *Clin Pharmacol Ther*. 2021;109(3):619–636.
133. Mazzone SB, Chung KF, McGarvey L. The heterogeneity of chronic cough: a case for endotypes of cough hypersensitivity. *Lancet Respir Med*. 2018;6(8):636–646.
134. 1van Manen MJG, Wijsenbeek MS. Cough, an unresolved problem in interstitial lung diseases. *Curr Opin Support Palliat Care*. 2019;13(3):143–151.
135. Arinze JT, de Roos EW, Karimi L, Verhamme KMC, Stricker BH, Brusselle GG. Prevalence and incidence of, and risk factors for chronic cough in the adult population: the Rotterdam Study. *ERJ Open Res*. 2020;6(2):00300–2019.

136. Spanevello A, Beghé B, Visca D, Fabbri LM, Papi A. Chronic cough in adults. *Eur J Intern Med*. 2020;78:8–16.
137. Ryan NM, Vertigan AE, Birring SS. An update and systematic review on drug therapies for the treatment of refractory chronic cough. *Expert Opin Pharmacother*. 2018;19(7):687–711.
138. Birring SS, Kavanagh JE, Irwin RS, et al. Treatment of interstitial lung disease associated cough. *Chest*. 2018;154(4):904–917.
139. Ward N. The Leicester Cough Questionnaire. *J Physiother*. 2016;62(1):53.
140. French CT, Irwin RS, Fletcher KE, Adams TM. Evaluation of a cough-specific quality-of-life questionnaire. *Chest*. 2002;121(4):1123–1131.
141. Vernon M, Kline Leidy N, Nacson A, Nelsen L. Measuring cough severity: development and pilot testing of a new seven-item cough severity patient-reported outcome measure. *Ther Adv Respir Dis*. 2010;4(4):199–208.
142. Spinou A, Birring SS. An update on measurement and monitoring of cough: what are the important study endpoints? *J Thorac Dis*. 2014;6(suppl 7):S728–S734.
143. Lewis SZ, Diekemper RL, French CT, Gold PM, Irwin RS. Methodologies for the development of the management of cough: CHEST guideline and expert panel report. *Chest*. 2014;146(5):1395–1402.
144. Slinger C, Mehdi SB, Milan SJ, et al. Speech and language therapy for management of chronic cough. *Cochrane Database Syst Rev*. 2019;7(7):CD013067.
145. Molassiotis A, Bailey C, Caress A, Tan JY. Interventions for cough in cancer. *Cochrane Database Syst Rev*. 2015;5(5):CD007881.
146. Malesker MA, Callahan-Lyon P, Ireland B, Irwin RS. Pharmacologic and nonpharmacologic treatment for acute cough associated with the common cold: CHEST Expert Panel Report. *Chest*. 2017;152(5):1021–1037.
147. Yancy WS Jr, McCrory DC, Coeytaux RR, et al. Efficacy and tolerability of treatments for chronic cough: a systematic review and meta-analysis. *Chest*. 2013;144(6):1827–1838.
148. Xie S, Xie M, Shen Y, Cheng D. Gabapentin for chronic refractory cough: a system review and meta-analysis. *Heliyon*. 2023;9(5).
149. Smith JA, Kitt MM, Morice AH, et al. Gefapixant, a P2X3 receptor antagonist, for the treatment of refractory or unexplained chronic cough: a randomised, double-blind, controlled, parallel-group, phase 2b trial. *Lancet Respir Med*. 2020;8(8):775–785.
150. Molassiotis A, Smith JA, Mazzone P, Blackhall F, Irwin RS. Symptomatic treatment of cough among adult patients with lung cancer: chest guideline and expert panel report. *Chest*. 2017;151(4):861–874.

13

Anorexia and Cachexia

Elizabeth E. Schack and Elizabeth Capano

Key Points

- Anorexia and cachexia are distressing symptoms of advanced and chronic illnesses.
- They are distinct syndromes but clinically difficult to differentiate.
- Metabolic alterations are the primary cause of anorexia/cachexia syndrome.
- Assessment and treatment of anorexia and cachexia include determining whether exogenous etiologies such as nausea and pain are involved and undertaking vigorous treatment of any such etiologies if present.

Case Study: Some Issues Commonly Associated with Anorexia/Cachexia Syndrome

Mr. J is a 67-year-old man with non-small cell lung cancer (metastatic to bone and brain) who was sent from the oncology clinic to the hospital for dehydration, hypotension, and decreased oral intake with significant weight loss. He received his most recent palliative chemotherapy 2 weeks ago and had been tolerating the treatment well. He had been maintaining his weight with nutritional liquid supplements and small, frequent meals. The case will be referred to throughout the chapter to illustrate assessment and management of anorexia/cachexia syndrome (ACS) commonly seen in serious illness.

Introduction

Management of ACS requires a multimodal, interdisciplinary approach utilizing pharmacological, nonpharmacological, and psychosocial interventions. Anorexia is defined as the reduction or loss of desire to eat[1] and is a symptom that accompanies many common illnesses. In acute events, anorexia usually resolves with resolution of the illness, and any weight lost may be replaced with nutritional supplements or increased intake. Unchecked, anorexia leads to insufficient caloric intake and protein-calorie malnutrition. Weight loss from this starvation phenomenon usually involves loss of fat, rather than muscle tissue.[2] Anorexia is common among patients with advanced cancer, and advanced acquired immune deficiency syndrome (AIDS) but also characterizes the clinical course of patients with other chronic progressive diseases, such as chronic obstructive pulmonary disease (COPD), congestive heart failure (CHF), and end-stage renal disease.[3–5] In addition, anorexia can often be seen in older adults and is influenced by multiple physiological changes occurring in late life.[1]

Anorexia and cachexia are two distinct clinical syndromes but are often intertwined in chronic progressive disease. Cachexia is a complex syndrome that usually involves anorexia along with significant weight loss, loss of muscle mass with or without fat wasting, and generalized weakness associated with increased protein catabolism and inflammatory response.[6] The word "cachexia" is derived from the Greek *kakos*, meaning "bad things," and *hexis*, meaning "condition, state of being or appearance"; throughout medical history, cachexia has been associated with the gravely ill.[5,7] The first clinical definition can be traced to Hippocrates earlier than 400 BCE: "The flesh is consumed and becomes water … the abdomen fills with water, the feet and legs swell, the shoulders, clavicles, chest and thighs melt away … the illness is fatal." It is important to differentiate cachexia syndrome from simple anorexia or starvation. Anorexia resulting in decreased intake is usually a component of both phenomena, but cachexia can still be found in the absence of decreased appetite.[8] Anorexia alone does not account for the magnitude of weight loss seen in diseases like cancer, and nutritional supplementation does not restore the lean body mass of cancer ACS.[8] Two separate international groups came together in 2008[6] and 2011[9] to develop operational definitions of cachexia, diagnostic criteria, and classification in the hopes of advancing future clinical practice and outcome measures for future clinical trials. In 2011, Fearon and colleagues provided this definition of cachexia:

> Multifactorial syndrome characterized by an ongoing loss of skeletal mass (with or without loss of fat mass) that cannot be fully reversed by conventional nutritional support and leads to progressive functional impairment. The pathophysiology is characterized by a negative protein and energy balance driven by a variable combination of reduced food intake and abnormal metabolism.[9(p490)]

Cachexia is a devastating multifactorial syndrome; in contrast to the starvation seen in anorexia where lean mass is preserved and adipose tissue is primarily affected, there is loss of skeletal muscle with or without fat loss, significant loss of bone mineral content, and no significant response to nutritional supplements or increased intake.[10,11]

Weight loss, regardless of etiology, has a decidedly negative effect on survival; and loss of lean body mass has an especially deleterious effect. Evidence-based reviews about prognosis reveal a significant correlation between anorexia/cachexia and survival in newly diagnosed cancer patients and in patients with advanced disease. Weight loss is also linked to decreased survival in CHF, COPD, end-stage renal disease, and AIDS.[3,12–14] The term "anorexia/cachexia syndrome" has been used mostly in reference to patients with cancer, and thus the condition is sometimes termed "cancer-related anorexia/cachexia" (C-ACS).[8,15] A classification system for cancer cachexia has been developed with three stages of clinical relevance—pre-cachexia, cachexia, and refractory cachexia[9,16]—with the hope that it will improve ease of cachexia recognition by clinicians through objective and standardized criteria. Varied terminology has been used to describe the syndrome in other disease states: for instance, HIV wasting syndrome, cardiac cachexia, pulmonary cachexia syndrome, rheumatoid cachexia, and, in patients with advanced renal disease, malnutrition-inflammation-cachexia syndrome.[17,18] Table 13.1 lists the various terms used to describe anorexia/cachexia and estimated prevalence in different disease states. The pathophysiology and clinical presentation of ACS overlap in these various diseases even though the underlying metabolic and neurohormonal imbalances may differ. The basic issue of underlying chronic inflammation can be seen in them all.[5] For the purposes of this chapter, the term "ACS" refers to all chronic, advanced disease–related anorexia/cachexia syndromes.

The ACS of all diseases is characterized by a variety of signs and symptoms that represent interference with energy intake (decreased appetite, early satiety, nausea, taste/smell changes, etc.) and nutritional status that include increased metabolic rate, weight loss, hormonal alterations, muscle and adipose tissue wasting, fatigue, and decreased performance status.[8,9,21,22] Whatever the specific disease, the development of ACS poses a significant clinical problem. It is a grave prognostic sign but also has a detrimental effect on quality of life (QOL), as documented by studies of all the preceding major diagnoses. This syndrome leads to serious physical and functional deficits and can be devastating to self-image, social and family relationships, and spiritual well-being.

Table 13.1 Anorexia/cachexia syndrome (ACS) in various disease states

Disease	Terminology	Estimated prevalence: highest in advanced disease
Cancer	Cancer-related ACS	Up to 85%
Congestive heart failure	Cardiac cachexia	16%–36%
Chronic obstructive pulmonary disease	Pulmonary cachexia syndrome	30%–70%
HIV disease	HIV wasting syndrome	10%–35%
Renal disease	MIC: malnutrition-inflammation cachexia syndrome	30%–60%
Rheumatoid arthritis	Rheumatoid cachexia	Up to 32%

Sources: References 2, 5, 7, 15, 17–20.

Pathophysiology of ACS

The basic etiologies of ACS are (1) decreased food intake, (2) metabolic abnormalities, (3) the actions of pro-inflammatory cytokines and other inflammatory mediators, (4) systemic inflammation, (5) neurohormonal dysregulation, (6) tumor by-products, and (7) the catabolic state.[23,24] These result in derangement of function with negative effects on survival and QOL. There is within some of these mechanisms a mutually reinforcing aspect; for example, anorexia leads to fatigue, fatigue increases anorexia, anorexia increases fatigue, and so on.[23] Table 13.2 summarizes the mechanisms and effects of ACS.

ACS can be categorized into two different classes, primary and secondary, depending on its etiology.[26] *Primary* ACS results from endogenous metabolic abnormalities such as cytokine production, which stimulates chronic inflammation and resulting catabolism. The syndrome is called *secondary* if it results from exogenous etiologies caused by symptoms that interfere with the intake or absorption of nutrients. Examples of such interfering symptoms are pain, nausea, intestinal obstruction, and psychosocial distress.[26,27]

Primary ACS

The pathogenesis of primary ACS is multifactorial, complex, and incompletely understood. Accumulating evidence suggests that chronic illness disrupts the homeostatic function of the central nervous system, leading to profound metabolic changes.[27] Peripheral input causes the awareness of threats such as a growing tumor or cardiac or renal failure, and this promotes a catabolic effect, which results in increased energy expenditure, reduced intake, increased muscle breakdown, and loss of adipose tissue.[28] Overall, patients develop an increased metabolic rate for their lean body mass.[28]

Metabolic Alterations

Metabolic alterations are common in cancer and other diseases and are thought to be due in large part to the systemic inflammatory response and stimulation of cytokine production (principally tumor necrosis factor alpha [TNF-α], prostaglandins, interleukin-1 [IL-1], IL-2, IL-6, IL-10, interferon α [IFN-α], and IFN-β).[5,29] Other catabolic tumor-derived factors thought to play a role in cachexia include proteolysis-inducing factor and lipid-mobilizing factor. Major metabolic alterations

Table 13.2 Mechanisms and effects of anorexia/cachexia syndrome

Mechanisms	Effect
Loss of appetite	Generalized host tissue wasting, nausea or "sick feeling," loss of socialization and pleasure at meals
Reduced voluntary motor activity (fatigue)	Skeletal muscle wasting and inanition (fatigue)
Reduced rate of muscle protein synthesis	Skeletal muscle wasting and asthenia (weakness)
Decreased immune response	Increased susceptibility to infections
Decreased response to therapy or treatment intolerability	Earlier demise and increased complications of illness

Sources: References 23 and 25.

include glucose intolerance, insulin resistance, increased lipolysis, increased skeletal muscle catabolism, negative nitrogen balance, and, in some patients, increased basal energy expenditure.[30]

Several different theories regarding the pathophysiology of ACS continue to be studied. The maladaptive activation of oxidative processes that may be seen in chronic illness is also thought to be partially responsible for cachexia syndrome.[31] Recent advances in genomics suggest that specific genetic polymorphisms contribute to the prominent inflammatory component of this problem.[32] The melanocortin system of the hypothalamus, which coordinates appetite and feeding, is influenced by peptide hormones such as leptin and ghrelin. Any chronic illness in severity can have the potential to suppress gonadotropin levels, causing hypogonadism or "nongonadal illness," heightening the wasting in patients.[33] Disturbances in these hormonally regulated feedback loops appear to play a role in ACS. Other potential mediators of ACS include testosterone, insulin-like growth factor-1, myostatin, and adrenal hormones.[5] In sum, the underlying pathophysiological processes of ACS are complex and not yet fully understood. Researchers postulate that the preceding mechanisms play different roles of varying importance in different diseases. The relative importance of these factors and the interplay among them remain unclear. However, irrespective of the underlying mechanism or specific medical illness, patients experience progressive worsening of their clinical condition and, ultimately, shorter survival soon after the development of cachexia.[28]

Secondary ACS

Secondary causes of ACS include exogenous factors that can frequently lead to weight loss, anorexia, fatigue, or other symptoms associated with this wasting syndrome.[26,27]

Physical Symptoms

A number of physical symptoms of advanced disease may contribute to or cause anorexia, including pain, dysgeusia (abnormalities in taste, especially aversion to meat), ageusia (loss of taste), hyperosmia (increased sensitivity to odor), hyposmia (decreased sensitivity to odor), anosmia (absence of sense of smell), stomatitis, dysphagia, odynophagia, dyspnea, hepatomegaly, splenomegaly, gastric compression, delayed emptying, malabsorption, intestinal obstruction, nausea, vomiting, diarrhea, constipation, inanition, asthenia, various infections (see later discussion), and early satiety.[8,10] Alcoholism or other substance dependence (i.e., tobacco, illicit drugs) may also contribute to or cause anorexia and have the potential to heighten other physical symptoms associated with chronic illlnesses.[34] Primary or metastatic disease sites have an effect on appetite, with cancers such as gastric and pancreatic having direct effects on organs of alimentation.[27,35]

In general, people who are seriously ill and/or suffering distressing symptoms have poor appetites. In addition, in cancer, metabolic paraneoplastic syndromes such as hypercalcemia or hyponatremia (syndrome of inappropriate antidiuretic hormone secretion) may cause anorexia or symptoms such as fatigue that contribute to anorexia. Patients with HIV disease may also develop primary muscle disease, leading to weight loss.[36] Many treatments for chronic diseases have deleterious effects on appetite or result in side effects leading to anorexia and/or weight loss.[37] Each of these should be ruled out as a contributing cause of anorexia and, if present, treated as discussed elsewhere in this textbook.

Treatment Side Effects

Many interventions used to treat advanced chronic disease have adverse effects on nutritional status. Cytotoxic drugs and immunotherapies can be emetogenic, cause taste changes, or precipitate other gastrointestinal side effects such as oral stomatitis and diarrhea.[15] Radiotherapy can also lead to significant side effects, including nausea, vomiting, diarrhea, xerostomia, and severe fatigue.[15] Despite the success of highly active antiretroviral therapy in curbing ACS in many patients, the myriad medications involved in the prevention and treatment of AIDS complications can lead to anorexia and malabsorption themselves, and HIV wasting remains a problem.[36] Among patients with advanced renal disease on dialysis, there is a high prevalence of protein-energy malnutrition.[32,38]

Psychological and/or Spiritual Distress

Psychological and spiritual distresses are often overlooked causes of anorexia. The physical effects of the illness and/or treatment coupled with psychological responses (especially anxiety and depression) and spiritual distress may result in little enthusiasm or energy for preparing or eating food.[15] As weight is lost and energy decreases, changes in self-image occur. Appetite and the ability to eat are key determinants of physical and psychological QOL.[39,40] Cultural influences must always be considered. For many patients, the net result of ACS and weight loss constitute a negative-feedback loop of ever-increasing magnitude and suffering in multiple dimensions.[39] Clinicians evaluating patients with anorexia are encouraged to review basic principles for the assessment and management of depression, as covered in detail in Chapter 24. Treatment of underlying depression can improve appetite considerably.

Oral Issues

Special attention should be directed toward the oral cavity of patients with advanced disease. The fit of dentures may change with weight loss, or already poorly fitting dentures may not be as well tolerated in advanced disease. Dental pain may be overlooked in the context of serious illness. Oral and esophageal infections and complications increase with disease progression and immunocompromise. Xerostomia and worsening of tooth decay can occur with radiation therapy to the head and neck region. Basic oral hygiene can often be neglected in the setting of advanced illness. Aphthous ulcers, mucositis, candidiasis, aspergillosis, viral infections (e.g., herpes simplex), and bacterial infections cause oral or esophageal pain and, thus, anorexia.[41]

Assessment

Anorexia and weight loss may begin insidiously with only decreased appetite and slight weight loss, which can accompany virtually any illness. As the disease progresses and comorbid conditions increase in number and severity, anorexia and malnutrition increase, and a mutually reinforcing process may emerge. Cachexia has long been considered a part of advanced disease and end of life. However, skeletal muscle loss may be present earlier in the disease trajectory, and the early stages may be missed in patients with underlying obesity.[42] Early identification is optimal, but further research is needed to more clearly define the benefits of early assessment and intervention on patient outcomes.[43,44]

With ACS common and in many cases inevitable among patients with a serious illness, identifying specific causes is an extremely challenging task. Several international workgroups have proposed guidelines for the definition and classification of anorexia and cachexia.[6,9] More specifically, an international consensus exists on the framework for the definition of cachexia and the diagnostic criteria and classification of cancer cachexia. Future validation of these frameworks should ultimately aid in future study trials, leading to universally accepted guidelines and routine clinical management.[5,9] There have been standardized tools for the general assessment of nutrition status but none specific to ACS for palliative care.[28,45] Nevertheless, anorexia from some etiologies is treatable; hence, assessment of the possible presence of etiologies noted previously is integral to quality palliative care. Assessment parameters are used according to the patient's ability to tolerate and benefit from the assessment.

Assessment parameters should include appetite, nutritional intake, physical examination, and basic nutritional status.[44] Common objective measures used to evaluate nutritional status are consecutive measurements of body weight, anthropometrics, biochemical laboratory measures, and observed assessment of dietary intake.[5] Appetite is a component of several well-validated tools of global symptom assessment, such as the Edmonton Symptom Assessment Scale,[46] the Memorial Symptom Assessment Scale,[47] and the visual analog scale.[48] In addition, simple assessment questions about change in appetite can be transformed into a numerical assessment scale. Intake can be measured retrospectively by recall or prospectively by calorie count. Detailed exploration with appropriate physical examination can identify associated factors (i.e., dysphagia, gastroparesis, nausea, oral issues, or pain). Open-ended questions can be helpful in eliciting specific characteristics of the eating problem.

While there is no single screening tool, there are a variety of methods that can be used to assess nutritional status. Some basic tools to assess nutritional status in the clinical setting include the Subjective Global Assessment for Nutrition (SGA)[45,49] and its modified patient-generated version (PG-SGA),[50,51] the mini-nutritional assessment, the Malnutrition Universal Screening Tool,[52] and the Simplified Nutritional Appetite Questionnaire.[53] The more sophisticated anthropometric and laboratory tests are other tools that can be incorporated into the diagnostic evaluation. However, common lab values may reveal decreased serum albumin, a prognostic indicator of increased morbidity and mortality, as well as changes in several electrolyte and mineral levels.[43] Other patient-rated tools like the Functional Assessment of Anorexia/Cachexia Therapy[17] and its Anorexia/Cachexia Subscale have been developed for clinical trials for orexigenic (appetite-stimulating) agents for cancer- or HIV-related anorexia and are too cumbersome for routine patient evaluation.[48]

Perhaps the most important component of assessment in ACS involves the patient's goals of care. Since palliative care encompasses the entire disease continuum, stage of illness and goals of care should be clearly determined before detailed assessment and intervention are planned or initiated. It is imperative to evaluate the degree of suffering or distress experienced as a result of the ACS. A cost–benefit analysis should be undertaken to determine whether a diagnostic workup is valuable in light of the effort, cost, or discomfort it may incur. At some point in the illness, even basic assessments, such as weight, serve only to decrease the patient's QOL. Assessment parameters are summarized in Box 13.1.

Box 13.1 Assessment Parameters in Anorexia and Cachexia

The patient is likely to report anorexia and/or early satiety.
Weakness (asthenia) and fatigue are present.
Mental status declines, with decreased attention span and ability to concentrate. Depression may increase concurrently.
Inspection/observation may show progressive muscle wasting, loss of strength, and decreased fat. There often is increased total body water, and edema may thus mask some wasting.
Weight may decrease. Weight may reflect nutritional status or fluid accumulation or loss.
Increased weight in the presence of heart disease suggests heart failure.
Triceps skinfold thickness decreases with protein calorie malnutrition (PCM; skinfold thickness and midarm circumference vary with hydration status).
Midarm muscle circumference decreases with PCM.
Serum albumin concentrations decrease as nutritional status declines. Albumin has a half-life of 20 days; hence, it is less affected by current intake than other measures.
Other lab values associated with anorexia/cachexia syndrome include anemia, increased triglycerides, decreased nitrogen balance, and glucose intolerance.

Sources: References 43, 51, 54, and 55.

Assessment also includes a psychosocial evaluation, particularly concerning food, determining usual intake patterns, food likes and dislikes, and the meaning of food or eating to the patient and family. Too often, a family member attaches huge significance to nutritional intake and exerts pressure on the patient to increase intake: "If she would just get enough to eat." Giving sustenance is a fundamental means of caring and nurturing, and it is no surprise that the presence of devastating illness often evokes an almost primitive urge to give food. Assessment should also include an evaluation of the patient and family health literacy level, as well as their desire and preferred means of receiving health information.[56,57]

In some cases the patient is less troubled than the family by poor nutritional intake. Clinicians should explore the meaning of feeding in the context of the family's cultural and religious background and help identify other ways in which the family can participate in caring for the patient.[54]

Case Study

During assessment of nutritional status and weight loss, Mr. J reports changes in taste of foods he used to enjoy. He reports intermittent nausea associated with eating but denies active vomiting. He reports that he has not had a bowel movement in 8 days and noticed that he was feeling full most of the time even with just small amounts of food. Over the past several weeks, he was spending a large portion of his day in bed since the onset of his symptoms, and his wife reports that she needed to use a wheelchair for the first time when she brought him to the oncology clinic. He reports that he has had a poor appetite for many months, and he has lost 8 pounds since his last chemotherapy. Over the last several months he is noted to have a slow decrease in his serum albumin that now is below normal range.

Interventions

The palliative approach to care of the patient with ACS focuses on improving patient comfort and minimizing distress caused by the anorexia and weight loss. Assisting patients and families to adapt to progressive symptoms and alleviating symptoms that may be exacerbating the problem are two foci of interventions. Interventions may combine a variety of approaches, including treatment of secondary (exogenous) causes of anorexia, nutritional support, enteral and parenteral nutrition, pharmacological management, and psychosocial support.[58]

Exogenous/Secondary Symptom Management

The presence of symptoms that may cause or exacerbate secondary anorexia and weight loss should be evaluated and treated as possible. If anorexia is due to an identifiable problem, such as pain, nausea, fatigue, depression, or taste disorder, appropriate interventions as discussed elsewhere in this book should be instituted. The goal here is to identify and manage potentially correctable problems that contribute to low dietary intake.[15]

Nutritional Support

Oral nutritional support, in an attempt to increase intake or to maximize nutritional content, may be helpful, especially early in the disease process or in specific disease states. For example, there is evidence that nutritional supplementation can be effective in patients with COPD.[59] However, C ACS studies have been disappointing. The current evidence continues to reveal that, despite best efforts at improving the quantity and quality of nutrition through conventional nutritional support, it does not improve lean body mass in patients with cancer.[8,15] Unfortunately, there is still no conclusive evidence that nutrition/dietary counseling or other conventional nutritional support has increased survival, led to significant weight gain, or improved QOL for patients with cancer; but the overall risks are low, and patients and families tend to value this support. The literature and studies continue to focus on an interdisciplinary care approach that involves trained dietary specialists, nurses, physicians, physical and speech therapists, pharmacists, social workers, and symptom specialists in order to maximize strategies and provide the most comprehensive care.[15]

Helping family members understand nutritional needs and limitations in terminal situations is essential.[60] Consultation with a nutritionist is usually warranted for the purpose of education and recommendation of appropriate supplements. General guidelines for nutritional interventions include the following[39,54,61–64]:

- The nutritional quality of intake should be evaluated and appropriately modified to improve it. Patients who are not moribund may benefit emotionally from supplementary sources of protein and calories. Clinicians should determine the meaning to the patient and family of giving, taking, and refusing food. Strong and even unconscious beliefs about food are difficult to modify, and many families require education and frequent support in the face of helplessness and frustration related to ever-diminishing intake.
- Culturally appropriate or favored foods should be encouraged. Preserving cultural or social traditions around meals may also be helpful. Families should be encouraged to share mealtime with patients or continue habits such as a glass of wine with meals, if medically appropriate.
- Small meals, on the patient's schedule and according to the taste and whims of the patient, are helpful, at least emotionally, and should be instituted early in the illness so that eating does not become burdensome.
- Foods with different tastes, textures, temperatures, seasonings, degrees of spiciness, degrees of moisture, and colors should be tried; but the family should be cautioned against overwhelming the patient with a constant parade of foods to try. Room temperature and less spicy foods are preferred by many patients.
- Different liquids should also be tried. Cold, clear liquids are usually well tolerated and enjoyed, though cultural constraints may exist. For example, patients with illnesses that are classified as "cold" by some Southeast Asians and Latinos are thought to be harmed by taking drinks or foods that are either cold in temperature or thought to have "cold" properties.
- Measures as basic as timing intake may also be instituted. Patients who experience early satiety, for example, should take the most nutritious part of the meal first. Filling fluids without nutritional value (such as carbonated soda) should be avoided at mealtime. Oral care must be considered an integral part of nutritional support. Hygiene and management of any oral pain are essential in nutritional support. Procedures, treatments, psychological upsets (negative or positive), or other stresses or activities should be limited prior to meals.

Enteral and Parenteral Nutrition

Enteral feeding (via nasoenteric tube, gastrostomy, or jejunostomy) may be indicated in a small subset of terminally ill patients. Many clinicians postulate that there exist certain patients with a good functional status and a relevant secondary (exogenous) component to their ACS who may benefit from invasive nutritional interventions. Examples include patients with head and neck cancer with severe dysphagia who are undergoing radiation therapy, patients with slow-growing tumors causing bowel obstruction, patients undergoing certain surgeries for upper gastrointestinal tract malignancies, or those undergoing bone marrow transplant.[22,61,65] However, the evidence remains insufficient to recommend precise guidelines for specific populations. In general, guidelines recommend against enteral feedings for patients with cancer undergoing routine radiotherapy, chemotherapy, or bone marrow transplantation.[66] Furthermore, despite the common practice of placing percutaneous endoscopic gastrostomy (PEG) tubes in patients with head and neck cancer, insufficient evidence exists that prophylactic PEG placement improves clinical outcomes.[67]

The clinical indications for enteral nutrition in noncancer diagnoses remain controversial, perhaps no more so than in the case of dementia. For patients with dementia, the best available data suggests that tube feeding does not improve QOL, reduce pressure ulcer formation or healing, limit aspiration risk, enhance functional capacity, or increase survival.[68] In these patients, careful hand feeding has been recommended as an alternative. Two nonmalignant conditions warrant consideration of enteral feeding. These include patients with stroke who otherwise have good QOL and patients with early amyotrophic lateral sclerosis.[69,70] In general, patients with poor performance status and poor prognosis are at high risk for mortality from gastrostomy.[57] In these patients, comfort feeding should be the primary focus in maintaining QOL.

The use of parenteral nutrition in ACS has been controversial within the palliative care field; and, in nearly all cases, if the patient has a functioning gut, enteral nutrition is preferred over parenteral nutrition because of the latter's very limited benefit and because the former is associated with lower cost and fewer complications. In palliative care settings, long-term use of parenteral nutrition should be considered only if aligned with goals of care and in those with good underlying functional status, a prognosis of 2–3 months, and in whom enteral feeding is not possible.[67]

Pharmacological Interventions

A plethora of pharmacological studies have targeted C-ACS, and recent work includes other chronic advanced disease. One of the better-studied medications, megestrol acetate (MA), a synthetic progesterone agent, acts to increase appetite and weight gain.[71] Although the mechanisms by which MA operates are not well understood, most hypotheses suggest that the medication acts on cytokines, inhibiting TNF; and it may also increase release of neuropeptide Y in the hypothalamus, resulting in stimulation of the neurons involved in the satiety mechanism.[72] A 2018 meta-analysis of the Cochrane review of 2013 discussed trials that evaluated the efficacy, effectiveness, and safety of MA in palliating ACS in patients with cancer, AIDS, and other underlying pathologies.[73,74] MA improves appetite but has a small effect on weight gain and does not improve QOL.[72,74] Side effects of MA include hypoadrenalism, hypogonadism, and thrombosis and deep vein thrombosis.[74] If MA is selected as the starting agent for your patient (contraindications noted), a short 2-week trial is suggested; and if there is no improvement in the patient's appetite, then it should be discontinued.[5]

Glucocorticoids are widely used in the palliative care setting to address a number of symptoms, including pain, dyspnea, and nausea.[75] In patients with cancer, steroids have been shown to have a limited positive effect on appetite, nutritional intake, and sense of well-being but no demonstrable effect on weight.[28] The varying use of corticosteroids (dexamethasone, methylprednisolone, or betamethasone), dose quantity, treatment duration, and attrition rates in studies make it difficult to draw firm conclusions on which corticosteroid and dosing is safest to use.[76] The majority of the data was collected from research in patients with advanced cancer and not in anorexia related to patients with end-stage nonmalignant disease.[5] The wide range of side effects, especially with longer duration of use, including adrenal suppression, hyperglycemia, and peptic ulceration, may preclude their use in some patients. However, some suggest that corticosteroids may be more suitable for patients with shorter life expectancy, especially if they have other symptoms that may be alleviated by this drug, as just suggested.[28]

While not commonly used by primary palliative care providers, the potential benefits of testosterone (anabolic steroid) supplementation/replacement in hypogonadal men with diagnosed advanced HIV/AIDS or those who have been receiving long-term opioid therapy are noteworthy.[5] The overall benefit of testosterone replacement therapy in hypogonadal men with advanced cancer has not been determined. For providers treating patients who fall into this category, consider working in collaboration with other providers to explore its value and potential benefit if indicated.

Cannabinoids have shown similar positive effects: improved appetite, nausea control, QOL, and mood but without or with limited weight gain.[15,77] While a small and promising Israeli pilot study completed in 2019 demonstrated a weight increase of ≥10% in 17.6% of participants, the attrition rate was a limiting factor in the study's reliability and validity.[78] The US Food and Drug Administration–approved cannabinoids are as follows: dronabinol (approved for treatment of anorexia associated with weight loss in patients with HIV/AIDS and for treatment of chemotherapy-induced nausea and vomiting) and nabilone (currently not available in the United States).[5] Dronabinol also has a newer oral solution formulation called Syndros.[36] Outside the United States, Sativex, a nabiximol, is available in an oromucosal spray containing dronabinol and cannabidiol and approved to relieve spasticity with multiple sclerosis.[5] None of the above medications are currently indicated for cancer-associated cachexia,[77] and they are not able to restore weight loss. Dronabinol, in particular, has been shown to be less effective than Megace against anorexia in clinical trials for advanced cancer.[79] However, the central nervous system side effects, especially in the older population, and difficulty in dosing limit the use of this medication.[80] Commonly used pharmacological options with indications and notable side effects are presented in Table 13.3.

As of October 2022, 37 US states and the District of Columbia have medical marijuana programs, although marijuana remains illegal under federal law.[81,82] Currently, only anecdotal reports and small studies have suggested that marijuana stimulates appetite, encouraging interest in the use of cannabinoids in patients struggling with anorexia/cachexia.[5] However, it is notable that the number of registered clinical trials has increased from 30 in 2013 to 103 in 2021. More than 40% of registered clinical trials in 2021 were phase II and phase III.[83] Hospital and primary care physicians from various specialties encounter inquiries about medical marijuana from their patients. While there may be openness to provide it, there is a wide gap in terms of willingness and confidence based upon perceived lack of evidence-based knowledge and guidelines.[84] Based on the medical and legal concerns, the use of medical marijuana is not included in any domestic treatment guidelines.

Future directions in pharmacological management target various pathways implicated in ACS. Neurohormonal manipulation, cytokine inhibition, and anti-inflammatory interventions all show some promise in clinical trials.[71]

The peptide hormone ghrelin is a circulating mediator of appetite and has been implicated in ACS. Early trials that supplement ghrelin in various illnesses have shown short-term increases in caloric intake in patients with cancer and renal failure and improved lean body mass and exercise capacity in those with COPD and CHF.[8,14] An oral ghrelin mimic, anamorelin, seems to have shown the best progress toward approval after early-phase trials showed increased food intake, appetite, and lean body mass in patients with cancer.[85] In preliminary studies, selective androgen receptor modulators and ghrelin

Table 13.3 Medications commonly used in anorexia/cachexia syndrome

Medication effects and common dosing	Indications	Side effects and considerations
Progestational agents Megestrol acetate 160–800 mg/day	Improves appetite, weight gain, and sense of well-being	Thromboembolic events, glucocorticoid effects, GI upset/problems, heart failure, menstrual abnormalities, tumor flare
Corticosteroids Dexamethasone 3–6 mg/day in divided doses (considered preferable due to its lower mineralocorticoid effect) Prednisone 20–40 mg/day	Improves appetite and sense of well-being	Immunosuppression, masks infection, HTN, myopathy, GI disturbances, dermal atrophy, increased ICP, electrolyte imbalances, anxiety, avoid abrupt cessation
Cannabinoids Dronabinol 5–20 mg/day, use twice daily dosing at 2.5 mg	Increases appetite and decreases anxiety	Hallucinations; somnolence; confusion; dysphoria paranoia, especially in elderly; tachycardia
Metoclopramide 10 mg before meals	Improves gastric emptying, decreases early satiety, improves appetite	Diarrhea, restlessness, fatigue, drowsiness, extrapyramidal side effects

GI, gastrointestinal; HTN, hypertension; ICP, intracranial pressure.
Sources: References 28, 35, 76, 90, 91.

mimetics have an overall positive effect on lean body mass but not on function. As a result, they have not been approved for clinical use.[86]

Thalidomide is a controversial medication of interest to ACS researchers. Previously withdrawn from the market due to its teratogenic side effects, thalidomide is now under study in advanced disease due to its potent antiemetic and TNF and IL-6 inhibitor activity. Although its safety profile remains a concern, this medication may be a useful option.[8]

Other medications under study include melanocortin (thought to decrease circulating TNF); various anabolic steroids, such as growth factor, insulin-like growth factor, and testosterone derivatives; omega-3 polyunsaturated fatty acids (as found in fish oils); the antidepressant mirtazapine; the atypical antipsychotic olanzapine; beta-adrenergic agonists; and anti-inflammatory medications (i.e., cyclooxygenase-2 inhibitors).[8,10,28] While further research continues, these agents have shown some benefit in lab and in limited clinical studies.[87] There is also increasing evidence that, given the multifactorial process involved in ACS, treatments involving combinations of agents may show promise.[15]

Psychosocial Support

Anorexia and cachexia can have a profound impact on the QOL of patients, not only heralding physical decline but also leading to significant emotional and social distress.[88] Weight loss negatively affects patient self-esteem but can cause even more distress and anxiety among family and partners. In a descriptive study by Reid and colleagues,[89] patients viewed wasting as a social stigma and an ominous prognostic sign. However, family held on to beliefs that weight loss was a result of decreased appetite alone. Conflict over food was a common consequence of such dissenting views. Lack of education and a strong symbolic attachment to food increased distress.[27,89] Nurses can play a critical role in assessing patients and family and providing sensitive and culturally appropriate education and support.

Multimodal Approach

The devastating psychosocial consequences, pathophysiological complexities, and treatment resistance of ACS lead inevitably to consideration of a multimodal approach. A summary of what should be included in this approach is given in Box 13.2.

Box 13.2 Components of a Multimodal Approach to Anorexia/Cachexia Syndrome

1. Early and ongoing determination of goals of care
2. Optimal treatment of underlying disease according to goals of care
3. Prevention, recognition, and prompt treatment of exogenous causes
4. Guidance from nutrition specialists
5. Appropriate pharmacological interventions
6. Resistance exercise as appropriate and possible referral to physical therapist
7. Compassionate counseling to patient, family, and significant caregivers with clear, consistent, and empathetic dialogue

Sources: References 15, 27, 54, and 92.

Case Study

During Mr. J's hospital admission, his constipation resolved with enemas and an aggressive bowel regimen, and his hypotension resolved with adequate hydration. Unfortunately, despite these improvements, he reports worsening underlying nausea that interferes with his eating, unrelieved with the Zofran 8 mg he was taking as needed. The nutritionist along with the primary, oncology, and palliative care teams worked closely with Mr. J and his wife to determine his goals and assess his needs moving forward, uncovering educational gaps and promoting management options and support. Mr. J decided that he wanted to trial a short stay at a skilled nursing facility (SNF) to allow a chance to "regain some of my strength with the goal of going home." Mr. J felt that he wanted to continue to work with the oncology team to see what other options he may have despite this setback. The palliative care team initiated low-dose dexamethasone 4 mg/day orally with some slight improvement of the patient's appetite but significant relief of his underlying nausea. Mr. J also reported some improvement of his appetite with dronabinol 5 mg twice daily before meals, which was also initiated with moderate improvement in his appetite. Prior to Mr. J's discharge to an SNF, he was stabilized, and his symptoms were controlled with a clear plan in place and follow-up with outpatient palliative care team within 1 week.

Conclusion

Increasingly, ACS is recognized as a serious aspect of advanced or terminal illness and as an area requiring further research, especially with respect to (1) the pathophysiology of cachexia and (2) increasing treatment options.

Current understanding of ACS includes the following:

- Anorexia and cachexia are distinct syndromes but clinically difficult to differentiate.
- Anorexia is characterized by decreased appetite that may result from a variety of causes (including unmanaged symptoms such as nausea and pain). It results primarily in loss of fat tissue, and the resultant weight loss is reversible.
- Cachexia is a complex metabolic syndrome thought to result from the production of pro-inflammatory cytokines such as TNF and IL-1. In cachexia, there is approximately equal loss of fat and muscle and significant loss of bone mineral content. Weight loss from cachexia does not respond to nutritional interventions.
- In 2011, an international consensus defined cachexia as a multifactorial syndrome characterized by an ongoing loss of skeletal mass (with or without loss of fat mass) that cannot be fully reversed by conventional nutritional support and leads to progressive functional impairment. The pathophysiology is characterized by a negative protein and energy balance driven by a variable combination of reduced food intake and abnormal metabolism.
- Assessment and treatment of ACS include determination of whether exogenous etiologies such as nausea or pain are involved, the vigorous treatment of any such etiologies, and nutritional and psychosocial support if indicated.
- Treatment of cachexia is unsatisfactory, and no single pharmacologic agent successfully treats it, so a multimodal approach as discussed earlier is recommended.

The management of ACS is complicated by numerous obstacles, including lack of clear definitions and guidelines, inconsistency in assessment and management strategies, and knowledge deficits about this complex clinical syndrome in health professionals and caregiving families. The challenge is compounded by the interwoven emotional symbolism of food and nurturance. As palliative care providers, we should strive to support, understand, and translate the developing evidence that guides our care. The complex and potentially devastating impact of this problem demands a holistic response. Palliative care nurses are optimally situated to coordinate and drive the necessary multidisciplinary approach to address anorexia and cachexia in advanced, progressive disease.

REFERENCES

1. Landi F, Picca A, Calvani R, Marzetti E. Anorexia of aging: assessment and management. *Clin Geriatr Med.* 2017;33(3):315–323. https://doi.org/10.1016/j.cger.2017.02.004.
2. Payne C, Wiffen PJ, Martin S. Interventions for fatigue and weight loss in adults with advanced progressive illness. *Cochrane Database Syst Rev.* 2017;4:CD008427. https://doi.org/10.1002/14651858.CD008427.pub3.
3. Molfino A, Kaysen GA, Chertow GM, et al. Validating appetite assessment tools among patients receiving hemodialysis. *J Ren Nutr.* 2016;26(2):103–110. https://doi.org/10.1053/j.jrn.2015.09.002.
4. Lowey SE. Palliative care in the management of patients with advanced heart failure. *Adv Exp Med Biol.* 2018;1067:295–311. https://doi.org/10.1007/5584_2017_115.
5. Bruera E, Dev R. Assessment and Management of Anorexia and Cachexia in Palliative Care. UpToDate. November 5, 2021. Accessed December 4, 2022. https://www.uptodate.com/contents/assessment-and-management-of-anorexia-and-cachexia-in-palliative-care?search=palliative%20care:%20assessment%20and.%20management%20oif%20anorexia%20an%20dcachexia&source=search_result&selectedTitle=2~150&usage_type=default&display_rank=2.
6. Evans WJ, Morley JE, Argilés J, et al. Cachexia: a new definition. *Clin Nutr.* 2008;27(6):793–799. https://doi.org/10.1016/j.clnu.2008.06.013.
7. Peterson SJ, Mozer M. Differentiating sarcopenia and cachexia among patients with cancer. *Nutr Clin Pract.* 2017;32(1):30–39. https://doi.org/10.1177/0884533616680354.
8. Mattox TW. Cancer cachexia: cause, diagnosis, and treatment. *Nutr Clin Pract.* 2017;32(5):599–606. https://doi.org/10.1177/0884533617722986.
9. Fearon K, Strasser F, Anker SD, et al. Definition and classification of cancer cachexia: an international consensus. *Lancet Oncol.* 2011;12(5):489–495. https://doi.org/10.1016/S1470-2045(10)70218-7.
10. Clamon G, Byrne MM, Talbert EE. Inflammation as a therapeutic target in cancer cachexia. *Cancers.* 2022;14(21):5262. https://doi.org/10.3390/cancers14215262.
11. Peixoto da Silva S, Santos JMO, Costa e Silva MP, Gil da Costa RM, Medeiros R. Cancer cachexia and its pathophysiology: links with sarcopenia, anorexia and asthenia. *J Cachexia Sarcopenia Muscle.* 2020;11(3):619–635. https://doi.org/10.1002/jcsm.12528.
12. Erlandson KM, Li X, Abraham AG, et al. Long-term impact of HIV wasting on physical function. *AIDS.* 2016;30(3):445–454. https://doi.org/10.1097/QAD.0000000000000932.
13. Krysztofiak H, Wleklik M, Migaj J, et al. Cardiac cachexia: a well-known but challenging complication of heart failure. *Clin Interv Aging.* 2020;15:2041–2051. https://doi.org/10.2147/CIA.S273967.
14. De Brandt J, Beijers RJHCG, Chiles J, et al. Update on the etiology, assessment, and management of COPD cachexia: considerations for the clinician. *Int J Chron Obstruct Pulmon Dis.* 2022;17:2957–2976. https://doi.org/10.2147/COPD.S334228.
15. Oakvik J, Ready D. Updates in cancer-related symptom management of anorexia and cachexia syndrome. *Semin Oncol Nurs.* 2022;38(1):151254. https://doi.org/10.1016/j.soncn.2022.151254.
16. Ni J, Zhang L. Cancer cachexia: definition, staging, and emerging treatments. *Cancer Manag Res.* 2020;12:5597–5605. https://doi.org/10.2147/CMAR.S261585.
17. Yang Z, Luo Y, Lu H, et al. Validation of the functional assessment of anorexia/cachexia therapy instrument to assess quality of life in maintenance hemodialysis patients with cachexia. *Semin Dial.* 2022;35(4):330–336. https://doi.org/10.1111/sdi.13053.
18. Santo RCE, Fernandes KZ, Lora PS, Filippin LI, Xavier RM. Prevalence of rheumatoid cachexia in rheumatoid arthritis: a systematic review and meta-analysis. *J Cachexia Sarcopenia Muscle.* 2018;9(5):816–825. https://doi.org/10.1002/jcsm.12320.
19. Okoshi MP, Capalbo RV, Romeiro FG, Okoshi K. Cardiac cachexia: perspectives for prevention and treatment. *Arq Bras Cardiol.* 2017;108(1):74–80. https://doi.org/10.5935/abc.20160142.
20. Rahman A, Jafry S, Jeejeebhoy K, Nagpal AD, Pisani B, Agarwala R. Malnutrition and cachexia in heart failure. *JPEN J Parenter Enteral Nutr.* 2016;40(4):475–486. https://doi.org/10.1177/0148607114566854.

21. Jozwiak R, Recka K. The anorexia–cachexia syndrome: definitions, evaluation, and nonpharmacological management #386. *J Palliat Med.* 2020;23(2):287–289. https://doi.org/10.1089/jpm.2019.0498.
22. Arends J, Baracos V, Bertz H, et al. ESPEN expert group recommendations for action against cancer-related malnutrition. *Clin Nutr.* 2017;36(5):1187–1196. https://doi.org/10.1016/j.clnu.2017.06.017.
23. Alesi ER, del Fabbro E. Opportunities for targeting the fatigue–anorexia–cachexia symptom cluster. *Cancer J.* 2014;20(5):325–329. https://doi.org/10.1097/PPO.0000000000000065.
24. Ryan AM, Power DG, Daly L, Cushen SJ, Ní Bhuachalla Ê, Prado CM. Cancer-associated malnutrition, cachexia and sarcopenia: the skeleton in the hospital closet 40 years later. *Proc Nutr Soc.* 2016;75(2):199–211. https://doi.org/10.1017/S002966511500419X.
25. Fearon K, Arends J, Baracos V. Understanding the mechanisms and treatment options in cancer cachexia. *Nat Rev Clin Oncol.* 2013;10(2):90–99. https://doi.org/10.1038/nrclinonc.2012.209.
26. Strasser F, Bruera ED. Update on anorexia and cachexia. *Hematol Oncol Clin North Am.* 2002;16(3):589–617. https://doi.org/10.1016/S0889-8588(02)00011-4.
27. Granda-Cameron C, DeMille D, Lynch MP, et al. An interdisciplinary approach to manage cancer cachexia. *Clin J Oncol Nurs.* 2010;14(1):72–80. https://doi.org/10.1188/10.CJON.72-80.
28. Baracos V, Watanabe SM. Aetiology, classification, assessment and treatment of the anorexia–cachexia syndrome. In: Cherny NI, Fallon MT, Kaasa S, Portenoy RK, Currow DC, eds. *Oxford Textbook of Palliative Medicine.* 6th ed. Oxford University Press; 2021:567–578.
29. Ohnuma T, Ali MA, Adigun R. Anorexia and cachexia. In: *StatPearls.* StatPearls Publishing; 2022. Accessed December 29, 2022. http://www.ncbi.nlm.nih.gov/books/NBK430977/.
30. Argilés JM, Busquets S, Stemmler B, López-Soriano FJ. Cancer cachexia: understanding the molecular basis. *Nat Rev Cancer.* 2014;14(11):754–762. https://doi.org/10.1038/nrc3829.
31. Suzuki H, Asakawa A, Amitani H, Nakamura N, Inui A. Cancer cachexia—pathophysiology and management. *J Gastroenterol.* 2013;48(5):574–594. https://doi.org/10.1007/s00535-013-0787-0.
32. Johns N, Stretch C, Tan BHL, et al. New genetic signatures associated with cancer cachexia as defined by low skeletal muscle index and weight loss. *J Cachexia Sarcopenia Muscle.* 2017;8(1):122–130. https://doi.org/10.1002/jcsm.12138.
33. Giovanelli L, Quinton R. Therapeutic effects of androgens for cachexia. *Best Pract Res Clin Endocrinol Metab.* 2022;36(5):101598. https://doi.org/10.1016/j.beem.2021.101598.
34. Anandarajah G, Mennillo HA, Rachu G, Harder T, Ghosh J. Lifestyle medicine interventions in patients with advanced disease receiving palliative or hospice care. *Am J Lifestyle Med.* 2020;14(3):243–257. https://doi.org/10.1177/1559827619830049.
35. Malec M, Shega JW. Management of gastrointestinal symptoms (nausea, anorexia and cachexia, constipation) in advanced illness. *Med Clin North Am.* 2020;104(3):439–454. https://doi.org/10.1016/j.mcna.2019.12.005.
36. Badowski ME, Yanful PK. Dronabinol oral solution in the management of anorexia and weight loss in AIDS and cancer. *Ther Clin Risk Manag.* 2018;14:643–651. https://doi.org/10.2147/TCRM.S126849.
37. Aversa Z, Costelli P, Muscaritoli M. Cancer-induced muscle wasting: latest findings in prevention and treatment. *Ther Adv Med Oncol.* 2017;9(5):369–382. https://doi.org/10.1177/1758834017698643.
38. Reid J, Noble HR, Slee, A, et al. Distinguishing between cachexia, sarcopenia and protein energy wasting in end-stage renal disease patients on dialysis. *Palliat Med Hosp Care.* 2016;2(2):e11–e13. https://doi.org/10.17140/PMHCOJ-2-e004.
39. Hopkinson JB. Psychosocial impact of cancer cachexia. *J Cachexia Sarcopenia Muscle.* 2014;5(2):89–94. https://doi.org/10.1007/s13539-014-0142-1.
40. Sadeghi M, Keshavarz-Fathi M, Baracos V, Arends J, Mahmoudi M, Rezaei N. Cancer cachexia: diagnosis, assessment, and treatment. *Crit Rev Oncol Hematol.* 2018;127:91–104. https://doi.org/10.1016/j.critrevonc.2018.05.006.
41. Davies AN. Oral care. In: Cherny NI, Fallon MT, Kaasa S, Portenoy RK, Currow DC, eds. *Oxford Textbook of Palliative Medicine.* 6th ed. Oxford University Press; 2021:656–669.
42. Baracos, VE, Arribas, L. Sarcopenic obesity: hidden muscle wasting and its impact for survival and complications of cancer therapy. *Ann Oncol.* 2018;29(suppl 2):ii1–ii9.
43. Berry DL, Blonquist T, Nayak MM, et al. Cancer anorexia and cachexia: screening in an ambulatory infusion service and nutrition consultation. *Clin J Oncol Nurs.* 2018;22(1):63–68. https://doi.org/10.1188/18.CJON.63-68.
44. Del Fabbro E, Jatoi A, Davis M, Fearon K, di Tomasso J, Vigano A. Health professionals' attitudes toward the detection and management of cancer-related anorexia–cachexia syndrome, and a proposal for standardized assessment. *J Community Support Oncol.* 2015;13(5):181–187. https://doi.org/10.12788/jcso.0133.
45. Leuenberger M, Kurmann S, Stanga Z. Nutritional screening tools in daily clinical practice: the focus on cancer. *Support Care Cancer.* 2010;18(suppl 2):S17–27. https://doi.org/10.1007/s00520-009-0805-1.
46. Bruera E, Kuehn N, Miller MJ, Selmser P, Macmillan K. The Edmonton Symptom Assessment System (ESAS): a simple method for the assessment of palliative care patients. *J Palliat Care.* 1991;7(2):6–9.
47. Chang VT, Hwang SS, Kasimis B, Thaler HT. Shorter symptom assessment instruments: the Condensed Memorial Symptom Assessment Scale (CMSAS). *Cancer Invest.* 2004;22(4):526–536. https://doi.org/10.1081/cnv-200026487.
48. Blauwhoff-Buskermolen S, Ruijgrok C, Ostelo RW, et al. The assessment of anorexia in patients with cancer: cut-off values for the FAACT-A/CS and the VAS for appetite. *Support Care Cancer.* 2016;24(2):661–666. https://doi.org/10.1007/s00520-015-2826-2.
49. Detsky AS, McLaughlin JR, Baker JP, et al. What is subjective global assessment of nutritional status? *JPEN J Parenter Enteral Nutr.* 1987;11(1):8–13. https://doi.org/10.1177/014860718701100108.
50. Bauer J, Capra S, Ferguson M. Use of the scored Patient-Generated Subjective Global Assessment (PG-SGA) as a nutrition assessment tool in patients with cancer. *Eur J Clin Nutr.* 2002;56(8):779–785. https://doi.org/10.1038/sj.ejcn.1601412.
51. Kwang AY, Kandiah M. Objective and subjective nutritional assessment of patients with cancer in palliative care. *Am J Hosp Palliat Care.* 2010;27(2):117–126. https://doi.org/10.1177/1049909109353900.
52. Boleo-Tome C, Chaves M, Monteiro-Grillo I, Camilo M, Ravasco P. Teaching nutrition integration: MUST screening in cancer. *Oncologist.* 2011;16(2):239–245.
53. Kruizenga HM, Seidell JC, de Vet HCW, Wierdsma NJ, van Bokhorst-de van der Schueren MAE. Development and validation of a hospital screening tool for malnutrition: the short nutritional assessment questionnaire (SNAQ©). *Clin Nutr.* 2005;24(1):75–82. https://doi.org/10.1016/j.clnu.2004.07.015.

54. Maddocks M, Hopkinson J, Conibear J, Reeves A, Shaw C, Fearon KCH. Practical multimodal care for cancer cachexia. *Curr Opin Support Palliat Care*. 2016;10(4):298–305. https://doi.org/10.1097/SPC.0000000000000241.
55. Mondello P, Mian M, Aloisi C, Famà F, Mondello S, Pitini V. Cancer cachexia syndrome: pathogenesis, diagnosis, and new therapeutic options. *Nutr Cancer*. 2015;67(1):12–26. https://doi.org/10.1080/01635581.2015.976318.
56. Gibbs HD, Ellerbeck EF, Gajewski B, Zhang C, Sullivan DK. The nutrition literacy assessment instrument is a valid and reliable measure of nutrition literacy in adults with chronic disease. *J Nutr Educ Behav*. 2018;50(3):247–257.e1. https://doi.org/10.1016/j.jneb.2017.10.008.
57. Hui D, Dev R, Bruera E. The last days of life: symptom burden and impact on nutrition and hydration in cancer patients. *Curr Opin Support Palliat Care*. 2015;9(4):346–354. https://doi.org/10.1097/SPC.0000000000000171.
58. Swihart DL, Yarrarapu SNS, Martin RL. Cultural religious competence in clinical practice. In: *StatPearls*. StatPearls Publishing; 2022. Accessed March 14, 2023. http://www.ncbi.nlm.nih.gov/books/NBK493216/.
59. Collins PF, Yang IA, Chang YC, Vaughan A. Nutritional support in chronic obstructive pulmonary disease (COPD): an evidence update. *J Thorac Dis*. 2019;11(S17):S2230–S2237. https://doi.org/10.21037/jtd.2019.10.41.
60. Scott D, Reid J, Hudson P, Martin P, Porter S. Health care professionals' experience, understanding and perception of need of advanced cancer patients with cachexia and their families: the benefits of a dedicated clinic. *BMC Palliat Care*. 2016;15(1):100. https://doi.org/10.1186/s12904-016-0171-y.
61. Roeland EJ, Bohlke K, Baracos VE, et al. Management of cancer cachexia: ASCO guideline. *J Clin Oncol*. 2020;38(21):2438–2453. https://doi.org/10.1200/JCO.20.00611.
62. Gaafer OU, Zimmers TA. Nutrition challenges of cancer cachexia. *JPEN J Parenter Enter Nutr*. 2021;45(suppl 2):S16–S25. https://doi.org/10.1002/jpen.2287.
63. Balstad TR, Solheim TS, Strasser F, Kaasa S, Bye A. Dietary treatment of weight loss in patients with advanced cancer and cachexia: a systematic literature review. *Crit Rev Oncol Hematol*. 2014;91(2):210–221. https://doi.org/10.1016/j.critrevonc.2014.02.005.
64. Hopkinson JB. The nursing contribution to nutritional care in cancer cachexia. *Proc Nutr Soc*. 2015;74(4):413–418. https://doi.org/10.1017/S0029665115002384.
65. Cotogni P. Enteral versus parenteral nutrition in cancer patients: evidences and controversies. *Ann Palliat Med*. 2016;5(1):42–49. https://doi.org/10.3978/j.issn.2224-5820.2016.01.05.
66. Arends J, Strasser F, Gonella S, et al. Cancer cachexia in adult patients: ESMO clinical practice guidelines. *ESMO Open*. 2021;6(3):100092. https://doi.org/10.1016/j.esmoop.2021.100092.
67. Bouleuc C, Anota A, Cornet C, et al. Impact on health-related quality of life of parenteral nutrition for patients with advanced cancer cachexia: results from a randomized controlled trial. *Oncologist*. 2020;25(5):e843–e851. https://doi.org/10.1634/theoncologist.2019-0856.
68. Ijaopo EO, Ijaopo RO. Tube feeding in individuals with advanced dementia: a review of its burdens and perceived benefits. *J Aging Res*. 2019;2019:1–16. https://doi.org/10.1155/2019/7272067.
69. Castanheira A, Swash M, De Carvalho M. Percutaneous gastrostomy in amyotrophic lateral sclerosis: a review. *Amyotroph Lateral Scler Frontotemporal Degener*. 2022;23(3–4):176–189. https://doi.org/10.1080/21678421.2021.1946089.
70. Joundi RA, Saposnik G, Martino R, Fang J, Kapral MK. Predictors of direct enteral tube placement after acute stroke. *J Stroke Cerebrovasc Dis*. 2019;28(1):191–197. https://doi.org/10.1016/j.jstrokecerebrovasdis.2018.09.032.
71. Siddiqui JA, Pothuraju R, Jain M, Batra SK, Nasser MW. Advances in cancer cachexia: intersection between affected organs, mediators, and pharmacological interventions. *Biochim Biophys Acta Rev Cancer*. 2020;1873(2):188359. https://doi.org/10.1016/j.bbcan.2020.188359.
72. Argilés JM, Anguera A, Stemmler B. A new look at an old drug for the treatment of cancer cachexia: megestrol acetate. *Clin Nutr*. 2013;32(3):319–324. https://doi.org/10.1016/j.clnu.2013.01.004.
73. Ruiz Garcia V, López-Briz E, Carbonell Sanchis R, Gonzalvez Perales JL, Bort-Marti S. Megestrol acetate for treatment of anorexia–cachexia syndrome. *Cochrane Database Syst Rev*. 2013;2013(3):CD004310. https://doi.org/10.1002/14651858.CD004310.pub3.
74. Ruiz-García V, López-Briz E, Carbonell-Sanchis R, Bort-Martí S, González-Perales JL. Megestrol acetate for cachexia–anorexia syndrome. A systematic review. *J Cachexia Sarcopenia Muscle*. 2018;9(3):444–452. https://doi.org/10.1002/jcsm.12292.
75. Hardy J, Haywood A, Rickett K, Sallnow L, Good P. Practice review: evidence-based quality use of corticosteroids in the palliative care of patients with advanced cancer. *Palliat Med*. 2021;35(3):461–472. https://doi.org/10.1177/0269216320986717.
76. Miller S, McNutt L, McCann MA, McCorry N. Use of corticosteroids for anorexia in palliative medicine: a systematic review. *J Palliat Med*. 2014;17(4):482–485. https://doi.org/10.1089/jpm.2013.0324.
77. Simon L, Baldwin C, Kalea AZ, Slee A. Cannabinoid interventions for improving cachexia outcomes in cancer: a systematic review and meta-analysis. *J Cachexia Sarcopenia Muscle*. 2022;13(1):23–41. https://doi.org/10.1002/jcsm.12861.
78. Bar-Sela G, Zalman D, Semenysty V, Ballan E. The effects of dosage-controlled cannabis capsules on cancer-related cachexia and anorexia syndrome in advanced cancer patients: pilot study. *Integr Cancer Ther*. 2019;18:1534735419881498. https://doi.org/10.1177/1534735419881498.
79. Jatoi A, Windschitl H, Loprinzi C, Sloan JA, Dakhil SR, Maillard JA. Dronabinol versus megestrol acetate versus combination therapy for cancer-associated anorexia: a north central cancer treatment group study. *J Clin Oncol*. 2002;20(2):567–573.
80. Smeltz R. Anorexia and cachexia. In: Dahlin C, Coyne P, Ferrell P, eds. *Advanced Practice Palliative Nursing*. Oxford University Press; 2016:254–259.
81. Rein JL, Wyatt CM. Marijuana and cannabinoids in ESRD and earlier stages of CKD. *Am J Kidney Dis*. 2018;71(2):267–274. https://doi.org/10.1053/j.ajkd.2017.06.020.
82. Ramirez M. Biden pardons federally convicted marijuana users. Here's where marijuana laws stand in each state. *USA Today*. October 6, 2022.
83. Modaresi F, Talachian K. The characteristics of clinical trials on cannabis and cannabinoids: a review of trials for therapeutic or drug development purposes. *Pharm Med*. 2022;36(6):387–400. https://doi.org/10.1007/s40290-022-00447-7.
84. Rønne ST, Rosenbæk F, Pedersen LB, et al. Physicians' experiences, attitudes, and beliefs towards medical cannabis: a systematic literature review. *BMC Fam Pract*. 2021;22(1):212. https://doi.org/10.1186/s12875-021-01559-w.
85. Wakabayashi H, Arai H, Inui A. The regulatory approval of anamorelin for treatment of cachexia in patients with non-small

cell lung cancer, gastric cancer, pancreatic cancer, and colorectal cancer in Japan: facts and numbers. *J Cachexia Sarcopenia Muscle*. 2021;12(1):14–16. https://doi.org/10.1002/jcsm.12675.

86. Hui D. Cancer cachexia: it takes a team to fix the complex machinery. *J Oncol Pract*. 2016;12(11):1172–1173. https://doi.org/10.1200/JOP.2016.017657.
87. Advani SM, Advani PG, VonVille HM, Jafri SH. Pharmacological management of cachexia in adult cancer patients: a systematic review of clinical trials. *BMC Cancer*. 2018;18(1):1174. https://doi.org/10.1186/s12885-018-5080-4.
88. Amano K, Hopkinson J, Baracos V. Psychological symptoms of illness and emotional distress in advanced cancer cachexia. *Curr Opin Clin Nutr Metab Care*. 2022;25(3):167–172. https://doi.org/10.1097/MCO.0000000000000815.
89. Reid J, McKenna H, Fitzsimons D, McCance T. The experience of cancer cachexia: a qualitative study of advanced cancer patients and their family members. *Int J Nurs Stud*. 2009;46(5):606–616. https://doi.org/10.1016/j.ijnurstu.2008.10.012.
90. Loprinzi CL, Michalak JC, Schaid DJ, et al. Phase III evaluation of four doses of megestrol acetate as therapy for patients with cancer anorexia and/or cachexia. *J Clin Oncol*. 1993;11(4):762–767. https://doi.org/10.1200/JCO.1993.11.4.762.
91. Camilleri M, Kuo B, Nguyen L, et al. ACG clinical guideline: gastroparesis. *Am J Gastroenterol*. 2022;117(8):1197–1220. https://doi.org/10.14309/ajg.0000000000001874.
92. McClement S. Cancer cachexia and its impact on patient dignity: what nurses need to know. *Asia Pac J Oncol Nurs*. 2016;3(3):218–219. https://doi.org/10.4103/2347-5625.189808.

14 Nausea and Vomiting

David Collett

Key Points

- Nausea and vomiting are symptoms commonly experienced in advanced disease, often with multifactorial causes.
- Pharmacological and nonpharmacological interventions should be considered when managing the distressful symptoms of nausea and vomiting, with treatment tailored to the individual needs and goals of each patient.
- Nurses play a vital role in symptom assessment, treatment administration, and patient/caregiver education.

Case Study

Ms. L is a 45-year-old female with metastatic colon cancer with peritoneal and lung involvement who presented to the emergency department with abdominal pain, loss of appetite, and severe nausea and vomiting. She reports that her crampy and colicky abdominal pain has been increasing over the past 3 days, and she reports "I just haven't had any good days lately. This is a terrible way to live." She is evaluated by the emergency department team, and the surgical team is consulted.

Introduction

Nausea and vomiting are symptoms commonly experienced by patients with serious illness.[1] These symptoms may be directly or indirectly related to disease and can have a significant impact on both the physiological and psychological well-being of patients.[2] Poorly controlled nausea and vomiting can cause metabolic disturbances, malnutrition, electrolyte imbalances, and impairment of functional ability, as well as unnecessary hospitalizations, emergency room visits, and interruptions in treatments.[3,4]

To date, most of the research on nausea and vomiting focuses on oncology populations, with an emphasis on treatment-induced symptoms in patients receiving disease-directed therapy. Larger organizations including the National Comprehensive Cancer Network, the American Society of Clinical Oncology, and the American Nurses Association have embraced palliative care as part of comprehensive cancer care starting at diagnosis to improve patient outcomes and quality of life (QOL) throughout treatment.[3,5,6] As such, palliative care specialists must work alongside primary teams to ensure the proper palliation of these bothersome symptoms.

Unfortunately, the literature on the prevalence, assessment, and management of nausea and vomiting in the noncancer population is lacking. Advances in healthcare and technology have led to increased survival across various disease populations, with patients now living longer with serious illness and the potential for high symptom burden. More research is needed to better understand the prevalence and etiology of noncancer nausea and vomiting to develop treatment regimens that are disease- and patient-specific.

Given the available evidence, this chapter will use advanced cancer patients as a model for assessment and treatment of nausea and vomiting, which can then be extrapolated for use in other patients with noncancer diseases. Understanding the emetic pathway and main neurotransmitters involved in this process may be one place to start.[7] Methods for proper symptom management, including screening, preventing, assessing, treating, and follow-up, will be explored; and nursing interventions and patient and family education will be highlighted.

Epidemiology of Nausea and Vomiting in Palliative Care

The extent of suffering with any serious illness is largely determined by the presence and intensity of disease-related symptoms. An understanding of symptom prevalence in different diseases will allow clinicians to anticipate problems for the patient, develop plans of care, and educate clinical staff.

The prevalence and severity of nausea and vomiting in the palliative care population have been difficult to capture for various reasons including lack of standardized tools to measure symptoms and the common misconception that nausea and vomiting occur as a single entity when they are, in fact, two individual symptoms. While they should be viewed as independent symptoms, it is common for nausea and vomiting to form a highly distressful *symptom cluster*. Symptom clusters have been described as a stable group of two or more interrelated symptoms that often occur together, and studies have looked at their effects on QOL and treatment approaches.[8,9] Gastrointestinal

(GI)–specific clusters may include nausea, vomiting, appetite loss, and taste change.[8] Understanding the pathophysiology of these clusters may lead to a better and more effective approach to symptom management that targets multiple rather than individual symptoms.

Terminology

The terms "nausea" and "vomiting," often clinically associated, are distinct concepts frequently mistakenly used interchangeably or imprecisely, impacting the ability to assess and measure prevalence and burden.[10] *Nausea* is an unpleasant feeling of the need to vomit experienced in the back of the throat and epigastrium. *Vomiting* is a physical event that results in the forceful expulsion of gastric contents from the stomach through a complex reflex involving the GI tract, diaphragm, and abdominal muscles.[11] The two should always be assessed separately. *Retching* has similar abdominal contractions to vomiting without the actual expulsion of material.[11]

Cancer Population

Prevalence of nausea and vomiting in patients with advanced cancer has been reported between 10% and 70% and is described by patients and caregivers as one of the most worrisome symptoms.[1,12] Research on nausea and vomiting over the past three decades has led to steady improvements in the control of chemotherapy-induced nausea and vomiting (CINV), with the development of 5-hydroxytryptamine3 (5HT3) receptor antagonists (i.e., ondansetron) in the 1990s being one of the most significant advances in symptom management for patients receiving chemotherapy.[13]

Despite these advances, approximately 30%–50% of patients' post-chemotherapy administration will experience nausea, vomiting, or both.[13] Oncology patients may experience these symptoms because of disease and/or treatment. The incidence, prevalence, and severity are primarily related to the emetic potential of the chosen treatment regimen and specific patient variables, with some studies suggesting that female sex, younger age, and/or previous CINV are predisposing factors for CINV.[3]

The data on the prevalence of nausea and vomiting at end-of-life in cancer patients is mixed, and prevalence has been reported to be as high as 70% in the last weeks of life.[11,12] The severity of symptoms is related to cancer type, whether the patient is receiving disease-targeted therapies, and acute issues that may occur with disease progression. One acute complication of some cancers is malignant bowel obstruction (MBO), which is a common cause of morbidity and death in patients with advanced GI and gynecological malignancies. Prevalence of MBO ranges from 25% to 50% in colon cancer, from 16% to 29% in ovarian cancer, and from 6% to 19% in the gastric cancer population.[14] Common clinical signs and symptoms of MBO include nausea, vomiting, lack of stool or flatus, and abdominal pain. An MBO can lead to a significant impact on patients and caregivers, due to the symptom burden and challenging nature of interventions.[15]

Noncancer Population

Nausea and vomiting for patients with noncancer serious illness have received less attention, and available research provides conflicting information. Like the cancer population, drawing firm conclusions regarding the epidemiology of nausea and vomiting in the noncancer population is complicated by methodological difficulties and the lack of standardized symptom definition and reporting.[16,17]

One large retrospective cohort analysis of patients receiving community-based palliative care, 90% with noncancer diagnoses, found that lower palliative performance status was associated with higher scores of pain, depression, nausea, and constipation.[18] Other studies suggest that nausea and/or vomiting are experienced by people with advanced illness, such as AIDS, congestive heart failure, chronic liver disease, and chronic kidney failure, but not as commonly as pain, breathlessness, or fatigue.[17]

Despite the need for additional research, nausea and vomiting are very possible symptoms for patients experiencing serious illness, especially as medical advancements are enabling patients to live with these conditions longer. Symptom management has been noted to be a significant concern for patients with noncancer diagnoses receiving palliative care, and these patients should continue to receive thorough symptom assessments, including for nausea and vomiting.[19]

Physiological Mechanisms of Nausea and Vomiting

Understanding the pathophysiology of nausea and vomiting is important for optimal management of a patient with these symptoms. Having knowledge of the mechanisms allows for a rational selection of pharmacological and nonpharmacological therapies or interventions to address the cause.

Vomiting occurs when the vomiting center, located in the medulla oblongata, is activated by peripheral and central afferent pathways. Peripherally, afferent nerves from the GI tract activate the vomiting center when there is pathology such as mucosal irritation, bowel wall invasion by neoplasm, or activation of stretch receptors. Stretching of the bowel lumen, as well as stretching of the capsule on visceral organs, can activate the afferent neural circuit. The gag reflex occurs when the glossopharyngeal nerve (cranial nerve IX) is stimulated in the pharynx by coughing or other mechanical irritation.[20] Central neural circuits that induce vomiting include the chemoreceptor zone and the cortex. The chemoreceptor trigger zone (CTZ) is a vascular region in the area postrema of the fourth ventricle and is outside of the blood–brain barrier.[21]

Chemical irritants (e.g., medications), electrolyte disturbances (e.g., hypercalcemia), and infections stimulate the CTZ. Vomiting that occurs when our senses of smell, taste, sight, or hearing are stimulated or vomiting associated with fear or anxiety is cortical. The nausea and vomiting that occur with motion sickness or vertigo are mediated by the vestibulocochlear nerve. Vomiting that is prominent in the morning can be associated with increased intracranial pressure (ICP).[22] The neural pathway for nausea and vomiting associated with increased ICP is less understood than other neural pathways to the vomiting center. Figure 14.1 is a conceptual illustration of the emetic pathways.

The afferent pathways and the vomiting center rely on specific neurotransmitters that result in nausea and emesis when there is an appropriate stimulus. For example, enterochromaffin cells in the gut release serotonin when there is mucosal irritation from chemotherapeutic agents. The released serotonin binds to its receptor, and this afferent signal is transmitted to the vomiting center. Previously, it was believed that chemotherapy caused nausea and vomiting primarily by triggering the CTZ. Now, it is understood that irritation of the gut and resultant serotonin activation of the

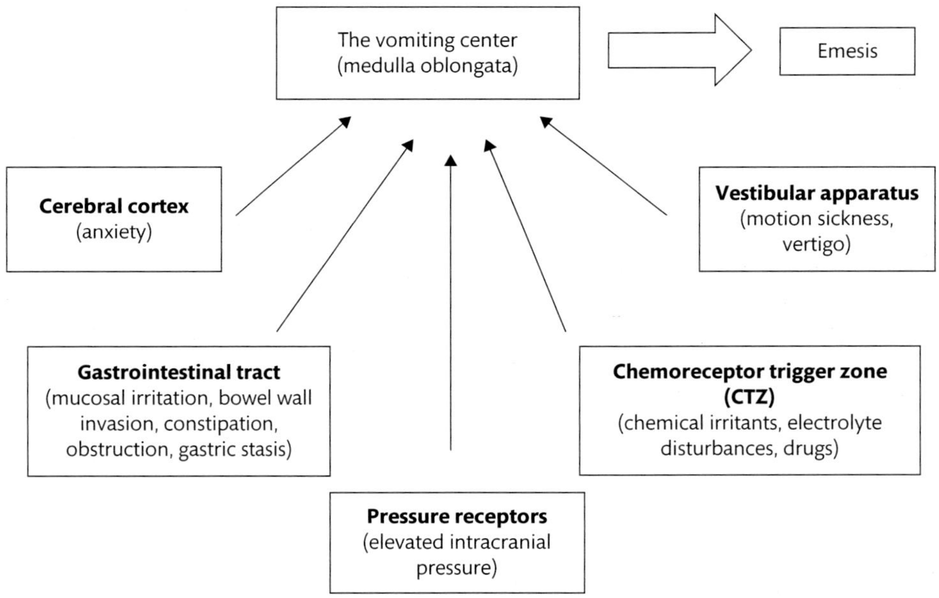

Figure 14.1 Emetic pathways.

peripheral afferent pathway from the gut are important causes, along with central afferent CTZ activation. The neurotransmitters involved in activation of the CTZ are dopamine and serotonin. The vestibular system depends on activation of histamine and acetylcholine to transmit afferent signals to the vomiting center. The vomiting center is rich in serotonin, histamine, and acetylcholine receptors.[21,23,24]

Pharmacologic therapies often target these ligand–receptor actions to prevent nausea and vomiting. Serotonin receptor antagonists, such as ondansetron, are particularly helpful for CINV because they block the activation of the GI afferent loop to the vomiting center, as well as inhibit serotonin action in the CTZ and the vomiting center. Neurokinin-1 (NK1) receptor antagonists, like aprepitant, target the neurokinin receptor NK1 that was more recently discovered to be involved in vomiting. The vomiting center is rich in NK1 receptors, and when the usual ligand, substance P, is attached to the receptor, vomiting is induced.[25]

Causes of Nausea and Vomiting

There are numerous potential causes of nausea and vomiting in patients with cancer. It is helpful to have a thorough understanding of the common causes, which can be subdivided into six clinical syndromes: biochemically/drug-induced, gastric stasis, GI obstruction/irritation, increased ICP, vestibular, and psychological. It is important to remember that common causes may overlap (e.g., drug-induced and psychological causes). These clinical syndromes are presented in Box 14.1.[3,12,22]

Although the potential causes of nausea and vomiting are extensive and the goals of care of the palliative care patient may preclude invasive diagnostic testing, studies have shown that it is possible to determine the underlying causes(s) for targeted therapy.[26] Approach to treatment relies heavily on identifying the symptoms present and any patterns, grasping the physiological mechanisms involved, and determining the underlying etiology, keeping in mind that causes are often multifactorial.[3,12] The skilled clinician will use their assessment to quickly identify any reasonably reversible causes that remain in line with the patient's and family's goals of care.

Assessment of Nausea and Vomiting

The primary goal of emesis control is to prevent nausea and vomiting.[3] When this goal is not achieved, recommendations advocate for a structured approach to assessing and treating these symptoms.[12] Assessment is an important process and the foundation of all treatment-related decisions. It should be an ongoing process that begins with the initial patient contact.

The palliative care specialists' approach to symptom assessment and treatment requires understanding of symptom pathophysiology and possible etiologies, which can be obtained from the patient's history, physical exam, and diagnostic test results. A comprehensive exam is needed to narrow down the list of differential diagnoses while paying special attention to causes that may be reversible.[12]

The history of present illness and review of systems should include questions regarding the pattern of symptoms (e.g., time of onset, duration, volume of vomitus), whether the symptoms occur in tandem or in proximity with other symptoms (e.g., epigastric pain, dysphagia, hiccups, heartburn, or constipation), possible triggers (e.g., medications, radiation therapy, meals, position, smells), and previous remedies attempted (e.g., over-the-counter or prescription medications). The clinician should also consider the functional status of the patient and their overall prognosis as this can help guide treatment decisions.[12]

A physical exam should be comprehensive to assess for possible etiologies. The oral cavity should be assessed for thrush or mucositis. The abdomen should be visually inspected, auscultated, and palpated to assess for physical signs such as abdominal distension or masses, presence or absence of bowel sounds, and organ

Box 14.1 Common Syndromes Involving Nausea and Vomiting in the Palliative Care Population

Biochemically/Drug-Induced
Fluid and electrolyte imbalances (e.g., hypercalcemia, hyponatremia)
Organ failure (e.g., liver, renal)
Chemotherapy
Medications (e.g., opioids, antibiotics, anticonvulsants, antidepressants)
Cannanbinoid hyperemesis syndrome

Gastric Stasis
Carcinoma of stomach
Ascites
Opioid-related
Anticholinergic drugs
Peptic ulcers

Gastrointestinal Obstruction/Irritation
Cancer-related
Esophagitis
Peptic ulcers
Pancreatitis
Gastric distension or compression
Excessive secretions
Delayed gastric emptying
Partial or complete bowel obstruction
Constipation
Biliary obstruction
Intra-abdominal spread (e.g., peritoneal disease)
Adhesions
Treatment-related (e.g., chemotherapy, radiation)
Infection (e.g., cryptosporidiosis)
Medications (e.g., aspirin, NSAIDs)

Increased Intracranial Pressure
Cerebral edema
Intracranial tumor
Intracranial bleeding
Meningeal disease

Vestibular
Opioid-induced
Cerebral metastases
Motion sickness

Psychological
Fear or anxiety
Anticipatory
Disordered eating

NSAIDs, nonsteroidal anti-inflammatory drugs.
Sources: References 3, 12, and 22.

enlargement or ascites.[27] A rectal examination should be performed if there is suspicion of impaction. A neurological exam is also recommended, assessing for increased ICP or other neurological etiologies. Laboratory studies may help rule out organ dysfunction, infection, and electrolyte imbalances; imaging diagnostics should be ordered if indicated to guide treatment decisions. Ultrasound, computed tomography (CT) scan, and magnetic resonance imaging are all imaging modalities that can be useful to further diagnose etiologies (e.g., small bowel obstruction, intracranial causes).[27]

Box 14.2 Rhodes and McDaniel Recommended Criteria for Choosing Instruments to Measure Nausea, Vomiting, and Retching

1. Use self-report tools rather than observational assessment whenever possible
2. Check reliability and validity
3. Look for clarity, precision, cultural sensitivity, and understandable wording
4. Instrument should be in an easy-to-read format
5. Determine and describe the symptoms and components
6. Determine a time frame for recall of the symptom experienced
7. Consider the purpose of the tool, the target population, and whether it is for acute, delayed, or anticipatory nausea and vomiting or for patients with advanced cancer
8. Consider the ease of scoring and type of score

Source: Reference 21.

Information obtained by questionnaires or self-report tools such as diaries or logs is crucial for the identification and management of this symptom complex and for improving the patient's QOL. Rhodes and McDaniel provide clear criteria when trying to choose the appropriate assessment tool for individual patients, summarized in Box 14.2.[21]

There are several tools to assess nausea and vomiting. Some tools provide a global measure, while others measure a single component of nausea and vomiting. Instruments may involve checklists, visual analog scales, patient interviews, or Likert scales; and almost all involve self-report by the patient. The most commonly used tools for nausea and vomiting with reliability and validity reproducible in research studies are shown in Table 14.1.[21,28–32] Global tools, like the Edmonton Symptom Assessment System Revised, incorporate nausea among other commonly experienced symptoms.[1]

Nurses need to use skillful observation along with effective data collection techniques for a comprehensive assessment as they work alongside multidisciplinary teams, including advance practice providers, physicians, and pharmacists. This is especially applicable in populations that may have difficulty communicating symptoms, such as in pediatric populations, long-term care populations, or

Table 14.1 Tools to measure nausea and vomiting

Instrument	Type	Reliability/validity
Visual Analogue Scale	100-mm line, with anchor descriptors at each end	Reliability is a strength
Morrow Assessment of Nausea and Emesis, Rhodes Index of Nausea and Vomiting Form 2	16-item Likert scale (onset, severity–intensity) 8-item Likert scale	Test/retest reliability 0.61–0.78 Split-half reliability 0.83–0.99 Cronbach's alpha 0.98 Construct validity 0.87
Functional Living Index Emesis	18-item Likert scale	Content and criterion validity Internal consistency
Multinational Association for Supportive Care in Cancer Antiemesis Tool	8-item, variable	Content validity Internal consistency

Sources: References 21, 28–32.

patients with limited abilities to communicate. Research has shown that caregiver symptom reports can be helpful when making these assessments.[33]

Pharmacological Management of Nausea and Vomiting

It is essential for the nurse to know the clinical pharmacology of the large and increasing number of antiemetics available for use. This includes understanding of mechanism of action, common side effects, contraindications, monitoring requirements, dosing ranges, and routes of delivery. As with other medications, nurses provide ongoing education to patients and caregivers and help promote safe use of medications. Classes of antiemetics are listed in Box 14.3.

Like the management of chronic pain, patients with chronic nausea may need around-the-clock medications for baseline symptom control, supplemented with rescue dosing. Guidelines for the pharmacological treatment of these symptoms in the palliative care population rely primarily on basic pharmacology and consensus guidelines.[3]

Two approaches to pharmacological treatment are used: a mechanistic approach and an empirical approach.[10–12] The mechanistic approach to treatment uses medications expected to block the relevant receptors in the emetic pathway as inferred from the patient's clinical presentation. For example, a prokinetic agent, like metoclopramide, is chosen when a patient's nausea is related to gastric stasis. Once an appropriate medication is selected, it is titrated to effect, until maximum doses are reached or the patient experiences dose-limiting side effects. If the nausea is not relieved with the first agent, a second agent from another class should be added and similarly titrated.[11,12]

The empirical approach for nausea and vomiting uses trials of antiemetic drug classes or other interventions to evaluate for effect and adjusting based on response.[11] These two approaches have been compared, without significant difference in outcomes.[34] As treatment selection for nausea and vomiting can be challenging for the patient's team, it underscores the need for the nurse to perform quality assessments—including discussing with patients any interventions or medications they have found benefit from in the past, as well as their current regimen.

Prokinetic Agents

Prokinetic agents include metoclopramide, domperidone, cisapride, and macrolide antibiotics. Domperidone and cisapride are recognized as effective prokinetic medications, but neither are available for use in the United States due to QTc prolongation and risk of serious cardiac toxicity.

Box 14.3 Classes of Antiemetics

- Antihistamines and anticholinergics
- Dopamine receptor antagonists
- Serotonin receptor antagonists
- Neurokinin receptor antagonists (substance P)
- Glucocorticoids
- Cannabinoids
- Benzodiazepines
- Prokinetic agents
- Octreotide

Prokinetic medications alleviate nausea and vomiting by stimulating motility of the upper GI tract. Four potential mechanisms for this effect have been proposed: stimulation of serotonin (5HT4) receptors in the gut wall, antagonism of 5HT3 receptors in the CTZ and gut, activation of motilin receptors, and release of the "dopaminergic brake" on gastric emptying. At higher doses, metoclopramide has antiemetic activity due to dopamine (D_2) receptor antagonism in the CTZ. Metoclopramide's activity at the 5HT4 receptor requires acetylcholine as a mediator at the myenteric plexus; thus, in theory, anticholinergic medications can antagonize its effect.[26,35]

Metoclopramide is widely used across palliative care settings and is often favored as first-line treatment of nausea and vomiting.[12,36] This prokinetic agent is often used in the setting of gastric stasis. The central dopamine blockade in the CTZ results in a side-effect profile like antipsychotic medications, including extrapyramidal symptoms (EPS). Other adverse effects include akathisia, serotonin syndrome, and tardive dyskinesia. Due to the risk of tardive dyskinesia, a potentially irreversible condition, the US Food and Drug Administration (FDA) issued a black box warning, with risk increased in use >12 weeks.[37] Reduced doses are recommended for patients with renal impairment or older adults. Metoclopramide is contraindicated in the presence of complete bowel obstruction, GI hemorrhage or perforation, and immediately postoperatively.[27,37]

The macrolide antibiotic erythromycin has also been identified as a prokinetic medication due to its motilin receptor stimulation, and it has been shown to be effective in treating diabetic gastroparesis. Side effects include hepatotoxicity and QTc prolongation, and it is also contraindicated in complete bowel obstruction.[38]

Dopamine Receptor Antagonists: Butyrophenones, Phenothiazines, Atypical Antipsychotics

Butyrophenones

Droperidol and haloperidol are drugs in the butyrophenone class, acting primarily as dopamine antagonists. They achieve their antiemetic effect by binding to the D_2 receptors in the CTZ. There is mixed evidence regarding the use of haloperidol or droperidol for treatment of nausea and vomiting. To date, there have not been any randomized control trials (RCTs) evaluating the effectiveness of these two drugs.[12] One recent RCT found that haloperidol provided relief from nausea (not from disease-directed treatment) for 70% of participants with advanced cancer.[39]

Common side effects of this medication class include sedation, hypotension, anticholinergic effects, dystonias, EPS, QTc prolongation, and, rarely, neuroleptic malignant syndrome.[12,40] Haloperidol is less sedating than antipsychotics of the phenothiazine class. Because of its direct antidopaminergic activity, haloperidol should not be given to patients with Parkinson's disease. The FDA has issued black box warnings for both drugs due to concerns related to prolonged QTc, though this may be less of a concern with lower doses.[3]

Phenothiazines

Phenothiazines include prochlorperazine, chlorpromazine, and levomepromazine. Levomepromazine is not registered for use in the United States. These medications possess a broader spectrum of activity compared to haloperidol, blocking histaminic, muscarinic, serotonergic, and/or alpha-adrenergic receptors in addition to dopamine blockade.[39] One recent RCT found that levomepromazine provided relief from nausea (not from disease-directed treatment) for 70% of participants with advanced cancer.[34] Phenothiazines have numerous side effects including sedation, hypotension, anticholinergic effects, dystonias, EPS, QTc prolongation, leukopenia, and lowered seizure thresholds.[23,37]

Atypical Antipsychotics

Olanzapine is an atypical antipsychotic that blocks dopaminergic, serotonergic, histaminic, and muscarinic receptors. Coverage of multiple receptors allows olanzapine to address nausea and vomiting that are caused by cancer or medications.[41] Consensus has shown that it has been used as a second-line antiemetic for patients with refractory nausea, with efficacy shown in small uncontrolled studies.[12,42] It has been used with advanced cancer patients in multicenter trials.[43] In small case reports, olanzapine was effective in treating nausea refractory to other treatments.[44,45] Reviews have identified RCTs showing its effectiveness for preventing and addressing breakthrough CINV, though not specifically for palliative care.[46,47] Some authors have recommended olanzapine as a first-line monotherapy for nausea and vomiting in palliative care, though it can be included as part of multidrug regimens as well.[41]

Because advanced cancer patients may have multiple causes of nausea and vomiting, olanzapine is well suited for palliative care settings. Olanzapine causes fewer EPS than other antipsychotics and does not usually cause QTc prolongation. Its low cost and once-daily dosing schedule are additional benefits that can reduce financial and medication burden.[41]

Antihistaminic Agents

Antihistaminic agents include promethazine, cyclizine, meclizine, hydroxyzine, and diphenhydramine. Currently, cyclizine is not available for use in the United States. The first generation of piperazine antihistamines have recognized antiemetic properties related to H_1 receptor blockade in the vomiting center, CTZ, and vestibular nuclei.[26] Due to their action in the inner ear, antihistamines are specifically indicated for nausea and vomiting associated with movement, dizziness, or vertigo. Evidence supports antihistamines as a class likely to be beneficial for the treatment of nausea and vomiting in noncancer chronic diseases as well as postoperative nausea and vomiting, with less support for its use in CINV.[37] Diphenhydramine is often used in combination protocols to minimize the development of EPS when dopamine antagonists are used.[26,27]

Cyclizine is an H_1-antihistaminic anticholinergic medication. It achieves its antiemetic effect by decreasing excitability in the inner ear labyrinth, blocking conduction in the vestibular-cerebellar pathways, and directly inhibiting the H_1 receptor in the vomiting center. It is recommended for use when nausea or vomiting is caused by elevated ICP, motion sickness, pharyngeal stimulation, or mechanical bowel obstruction; and it is less sedating than promethazine.[26]

Anticholinergic medications include scopolamine, atropine, and hyoscyamine. Scopolamine (hyoscine) is the most used anticholinergic medication for antiemesis and is a naturally occurring muscarinic antagonist. It achieves its antiemetic effect by blocking the muscarinic receptors in the vestibular nucleus and the vomiting center. A small study has shown sublingual scopolamine to have benefit for nausea for patients with cancer in a palliative care unit.[48]

Anticholinergic medications are specifically indicated for nausea and vomiting associated with movement or dizziness. They are also used with treatment of bowel obstruction if the obstruction cannot be resolved, though it is inferior to other agents, like octreotide.[49] These medications can cause the full range of anticholinergic side effects, including sedation, constipation, urinary retention, blurry vision, xerostomia, and delirium. Older adult patients are particularly sensitive to these side effects.[37] Anticholinergic medications are available in multiple formulations, including transdermal patches, ophthalmic drops that can be administered sublingually, and intravenous and subcutaneous injections, thus offering flexibility of administration in non-hospital settings.[37]

Selective 5HT3 Receptor Antagonists

Serotonin antagonists include ondansetron, granisetron, tropisetron, dolasetron, and palonosetron and achieve their antiemetic effect by antagonizing 5HT3 receptors centrally in the CTZ and vomiting center and peripherally in the gut wall. There is strong evidence to support their use in the prevention of chemotherapy- and radiation-induced nausea and vomiting.[50] Their effect is enhanced by the addition of dexamethasone and recommended by consensus guidelines.[3]

Consensus guidelines recommend their use for chemical causes of nausea and vomiting, vomiting refractory to dopamine antagonists, or when nausea is thought to result from massive release of serotonin from enterochromaffin cells, as seen in bowel obstruction and renal failure. Constipation is the most common side effect, and there is a potential for QT prolongation.[3]

Corticosteroids

Though the mechanism of action that produces the antiemetic effect is not well understood, there is evidence to support the use of corticosteroids, such as dexamethasone, in multidrug prophylactic antiemetic treatment during chemotherapy and radiation therapy.[3] A recent systematic review found low-quality evidence that steroids may provide benefit for nausea that is not due to cancer therapy.[51] Corticosteroids may be used to treat nausea stemming from increased ICP related to intracranial tumors, hypercalcemia of malignancy, or malignant bowel obstruction. Side effects are well documented, with significant adverse effects on nearly all organ systems, especially with long-term use. Short-term adverse effects include hyperglycemia, insomnia, and psychosis.[37]

Benzodiazepines

Benzodiazepines, such as lorazepam or alprazolam, act on the gamma-aminobutyric acid receptors of the cerebral cortex and are often used to treat anticipatory nausea. Lorazepam may be used alone when the intent is to treat anticipatory nausea, due to its temporary amnestic effect, or when anxiety is a contributing factor to nausea or vomiting.[52,53] Sedation, confusion, and dizziness are possible common side effects. Benzodiazepines have been shown to be effective to treat anticipatory nausea in adult patients in combination with psychological techniques.[52–54]

Somatostatin Analogues

Octreotide acetate is a long-acting somatostatin analog (vs. an antiemetic) that inhibits gastric, pancreatic, and intestinal secretions and reduces GI motility. Studies have shown that octreotide may be helpful for nausea and vomiting associated with intestinal obstruction, where it is recommended to be used in conjunction with an antiemetic like haloperidol.[49] Adverse effects may include diarrhea, abdominal pain, and nausea. There are long-acting, depot forms of octreotide available for patients who would benefit from monthly dosing.

Cannabinoids

Cannabis (marijuana) is the best-known cannabinoid, and dronabinol is the plant extract preparation available for prescription use. The semisynthetic agents are nabilone and levonantradol. Cannabinoids are proposed to exert an antiemetic effect by binding specific cannabinoid receptors in the brainstem and to the opioid mu receptor.[55] A recent systematic review found that cannabinoids provided benefit for CINV, though patients reported dizziness, dysphoria, euphoria, and sedation as side effects to therapy.[56]

The evidence to support the use of cannabinoids in advanced cancer is weaker, and recommendations support the ongoing use of metoclopramide or haloperidol as first-line therapy, followed by 5HT3 receptor antagonists or olanzapine as second-line therapy.[55] With the approved use of cannabis-based medications for medical purposes, including cancer-related symptom management, more rigorous studies are needed to support its place in standard guidelines and to determine the risk–benefit ratio.

In recent years, cannabis has become increasingly available for both medical and recreational use. Palliative care nurses should understand their local jurisdictions' latest regulations regarding cannabis and be prepared to address stigmas or concerns by patients.[57] As there are side effects from cannabis, as well as interactions with other drugs, asking patients about use remains important.

Substance P Antagonists (NK1 Receptor Antagonists)

NK1 receptor antagonists, such as aprepitant and fosaprepitant, prevent the binding of substance P to NK1 receptors. Aprepitant is an oral drug that acts as an NK1 antagonist, and its use in preventing and treating CINV has been supported by national guidelines.[3,5,12] Aprepitant is particularly effective when combined with a 5HT3 receptor antagonist, such as ondansetron, and dexamethasone to prevent acute and delayed CINV.[3] Fosaprepitant is an intravenous formulation that is converted to aprepitant within 30 minutes of administration.

NK1 receptor antagonists are currently indicated for acute, not chronic, use, thus limiting their use for patients with advanced cancer who may not be receiving further disease-directed therapies. Aprepitant is generally well tolerated, with some reports of nausea, diarrhea, and anorexia. Patients have reported pain at the injection site with fosaprepitant, as well as fatigue and hiccups.[37]

Case Study: Continued

Ms. L's physical exam was remarkable for abdominal distention and moderate tenderness to palpation. She has tried supportive care at home, taking in fluids and bland food, but reports "it's just hard to keep anything down." In the emergency department, a CT scan of her abdomen showed a partial small bowel obstruction, and she was admitted under a surgical service for further management.

Once admitted, she was placed on a nothing-by-mouth diet and given intravenous fluids, and a nasogastric tube was placed for decompression. After evaluation by the surgical service, it was decided that surgical intervention was not required, and she was managed conservatively. Due to her advanced disease and symptoms, her bedside nurse asked her primary team about consulting palliative care, and a consult was placed. She noted improvement with nasogastric decompression, and she was also given metoclopramide intravenously, which she found benefit from. She also received oxycodone 5 mg orally every 4 hours as needed for pain. Ultimately, her obstruction resolved with conservative management, she was discharged home a few days later, and she was also referred to the outpatient palliative care clinic.

Nonpharmacological Approach to Nausea and Vomiting

Nonpharmacological management of nausea and vomiting plays an important role alongside medical management. Treatments can include simple self-management techniques, integrative therapies, and other palliative interventions. The use of certain nonpharmacological modalities has more recently been adopted into antiemetic guidelines, particularly for the treatment of anticipatory nausea and vomiting. Their use is based on a lower level of evidence but with uniform consensus that the interventions are appropriate.[3,53] Uncontrolled symptoms, whether treatment- or disease-related, possibly interfere with a patient's QOL and willingness to continue with treatments. Understanding nonpharmacological approaches to symptom management and integrating them into usual care are appropriate to minimize the physiological effects of uncontrolled symptoms and their potentially negative effects on QOL.

Self-Management Techniques

Self-management emphasizes patient autonomy in their own care, encourages patients and families to assume the responsibility of managing their condition, and can help promote increased QOL.[58] Self-management theories acknowledge the complexity of living with chronic conditions and the importance of managing these complexities in the context of one's everyday life rather than expecting patients to adhere to a series of prescribed orders that can be generalized across populations. These techniques start with evidence to guide treatment recommendations and are then tailored to meet the individual needs of patients and their families.[58,59]

There are a variety of potentially useful self-management strategies including psychological, cognitive, and behavioral modifications, presented in Box 14.4.[3,60,61] While many of these interventions are not currently backed by strong evidence, they are associated with little harm and should be considered when treating nausea and vomiting in early and advanced disease.

Integrative Medicine

"Integrative medicine" refers to a wide variety of therapies that can be categorized into biological and nonbiological or behavioral interventions.[62] Recommendations are supported by limited data and may suggest a role for integrative therapies for symptomatic

Box 14.4 Self-Management Strategies for Management of Nausea and Vomiting

Dietary Modifications
Eat smaller, more frequent meals
Reduce food aromas and other strong food odors
Avoid spicy, fatty, and highly salty foods
Premedicate with antiemetics prior to meals
Give clear liquids

Environmental Modifications
Avoid the sight and smell of food when not hungry
Provide fresh air
Avoid strong or unpleasant odors
Minimize sights, sounds, or smells that can initiate nausea

Psychological Strategies
Use relaxation and meditation
Practice deep breathing
Use cognitive distraction

Other Strategies
Exercise
Take medications as prescribed

relief of disease-related symptoms, and the effectiveness of these interventions appears to depend on individual preference.[11,26,63] Patients should be educated to exercise caution before initiating certain herbal therapies due to the risk of drug interaction and adverse effects. The primary medical team treating the patient's disease should be made aware of all conventional or integrative modalities of treatment. As many complementary therapies are utilized or gain attention, consulting expert sources is crucial. One recommended resource is the National Institutes of Health's National Center for Complementary and Integrative Health, which provides a database of health topics, herbs, and information designed for health professional reference.[64]

Biological Therapies

Integrative biological therapies include nutritional supplements such as vitamins, minerals, botanicals, probiotics, and antioxidants as well as herbal medicines derived from natural sources. There have been few studies performed on these specific therapies for nausea and vomiting in advanced disease, and there are no expert consensus recommendations to date.[5,65,66]

Among patients with cancer, one herbal remedy frequently discussed is ginger (*Zingiber officinale*). Ginger has been used in Ayurvedic and traditional Chinese medicine to treat GI symptoms such as nausea and excessive flatulence since the sixteenth century. Some studies have found benefit for patients undergoing disease treatment, specifically for CINV, although findings and efficacy remain mixed, with no consensus recommendation.[5,62,67,68]

Reported adverse effects include heartburn, bruising, bleeding, flushing, and rash. Potential adverse effects and herb–drug interactions must be understood before recommending ginger for symptom relief because the herb has been associated with increased risk of bleeding and hypoglycemia, and it is contraindicated with the use of tacrolimus, nonsteroidal anti-inflammatory drugs, blood thinners, and glucose-lowering medications.[69]

Nonbiological Therapies

Some nonbiological therapies recommended in guidelines for the treatment of anticipatory nausea and vomiting include acupuncture/acupressure, progressive muscle relaxation, systematic desensitization, hypnosis, and music therapy. Selected nonbiological integrative therapies are detailed in Table 14.2.[70–82]

Nursing Interventions

Palliative care focuses on improving QOL and provides relief from distressing symptoms associated with the disease or treatment—which include nausea and vomiting.[83] The National Comprehensive Cancer Network's palliative care guidelines recommend aggressive symptom management, clarification of the intent of treatments, anticipation of the needs of patients and their families, and involvement of caregivers in the treatment process when appropriate.[3] Nurses have an essential role—whether it is doing an abdominal exam at the bedside, providing antiemetic guidance over the phone, or asking about the pattern of a patient's nausea during an outpatient assessment. Palliative care is best when delivered as part of an interdisciplinary team, and the palliative care nurse is instrumental in promoting a collaborative approach among team members.[83,84] Nurses in various treatment settings should understand the standards of palliative care, advances in the management of nausea and vomiting, changes to relevant treatment guidelines, and potential side effects of treatments being administered.[85,86]

Just as vital are the roles that the patient and caregivers play in managing nausea and vomiting from disease or treatment. Patients with cancer have reported high information needs regarding self-management of adverse effects.[81] As active participants in their care, they must be provided with the tools needed to practice symptom management and self-care. Personalized education plans and diaries with additional resources can help patients understand how to follow their plan at home and keep track of their symptoms—which can provide the healthcare provider with an understanding of symptom burden.[87] Education must include when and why to take certain antiemetic medications because patients may be given multiple agents, when to escalate symptom reporting to providers, and timelines for follow-up assessment.[88]

Sitting down with the patient to address their overall environment, fears, and concerns is crucial to ensure that the steps to adequately control nausea and vomiting are achieved. Referring patients to other providers, such as palliative care specialists, should occur when symptoms cannot be controlled or if additional support is needed.[88] Earlier involvement of palliative care resources can decrease symptom burden.

Case Study: Continued

In the months after discharge, she continued to be followed in the outpatient palliative care clinic by an interdisciplinary team for symptom management—primarily her nausea. In the outpatient setting, she was trialed on metoclopramide 10 mg orally every 6 hours as needed and ondansetron 4 mg orally every 8 hours as needed but found little relief with either agent. Ms. L had kept a medication log and had regular symptom assessments from the clinic nurse, which

Table 14.2 Nonbiological integrative therapies

Technique	Description	Comments
Acupuncture and acupressure	Insertion of fine needles along specific meridians on body by a trained specialist (acupuncture) or application of pressure on designated points on body (acupressure) For nausea, typically uses the P6 acupoint, on anterior surface of forearm, near wrist	Evidence of benefit for prevention and management of CINV Integration into standards of care limited by lack of quality trials Acupressure techniques can sometimes be performed independently
Aromatherapy	Therapeutic use of essential oils primarily via inhalation of vapors	Studies limited by design, small sample size, varied doses and methods, no clear benefit in postoperative populations
Cognitive distraction	Studied in adults and children Learn to divert attention away from a threatening situation and toward relaxing sensations Uses videos, games, puzzles, counting objects, deep breathing	No side effects Associated with decreased ANV and post-chemotherapy distress
Hypnosis	Behavioral intervention that teaches patients to focus their attention on thoughts or images unrelated to the actual source of distress, often using passive types of muscle relaxation and distraction	Few controlled studies have been performed Somewhat similar to systematic desensitization One of the first psychological techniques used to treat and control anticipatory nausea and vomiting
Massage	Soft tissue manipulation using touch and movement Reduces stress and anxiety while promoting relaxation, which may lead to decreased heart rate, blood pressure, and respiratory rate	Effectiveness not established Variability in episodes of CINV and retching in breast cancer patients
Music therapy	Performed by credentialed professionals Incorporated at any phase of illness Addresses multiple dimensions of QOL First introduced in hospice population in 1980s	Likely to be effective Associated with significant reduction in severity and duration of CINV Perceived effects on autonomic nervous system Less time and energy to implement for patients
Progressive muscle relaxation	Isolation of muscle groups with goal of inducing relaxation when responding to an anxious stimulus	Most effective in reducing nausea after administration of chemotherapy Not as effective with anticipatory nausea Has benefit on not only symptoms but mental mood and anxiety as well
Systematic desensitization	Teaches patient to counter conditioned stimulus that elicits maladaptive response (i.e., nausea)	Most effective for anticipatory nausea Also used to treat fears and phobias, which may develop through similar learned response

ANV, anticipatory nausea and vomiting; CINV, chemotherapy-induced nausea and vomiting; QOL, quality of life.
Sources: References 70–82.

was helpful for the team to track trends for what was or was not effective for her. The team tried an empirical approach and prescribed olanzapine 2.5 mg orally at bedtime, which she found mild relief with—the dose was eventually titrated to 5 mg orally at bedtime, which provided excellent antiemetic benefit. Ms. L was also referred to the clinic's mindfulness coach for self-management strategies, which she also found beneficial.

Conclusion

Nausea and vomiting are prevalent and distressing symptoms experienced by patients in both the cancer and noncancer palliative care populations, and relief should be a focus of all palliative care nurses. Multiple studies and reviews have highlighted the need for more rigorous research on the management of nausea and vomiting, particularly in patients at the end of life and within the noncancer population. Despite this, vigilant assessment, appropriate use and evaluation of pharmacological and nonpharmacological interventions, and appropriate patient and family education and support may avert the need for unnecessary interventions at the end of life and allow for QOL throughout the disease trajectory up until death and through bereavement. Nausea and vomiting profoundly affect all aspects of a person's well-being; adequately managing these symptoms is essential.

REFERENCES

1. Henson LA, Maddocks M, Evans C, Davidson M, Hicks S, Higginson IJ. Palliative care and the management of common distressing symptoms in advanced cancer: pain, breathlessness, nausea and vomiting, and fatigue. *J Clin Oncol.* 2020;38(9):905–914. https://doi.org/10.1200/JCO.19.00470.
2. Verkissen MN, Hjermstad MJ, Van Belle S, Kaasa S, Deliens L, Pardon K. Quality of life and symptom intensity over time in people with cancer receiving palliative care: results from the international European Palliative Care Cancer Symptom study. *PLoS One.* 2019;14(10):e0222988. https://doi.org/10.1371/journal.pone.0222988.
3. National Comprehensive Cancer Network. NCCN Clinical Practice Guidelines in Oncology: Antiemesis. March 2022. Accessed November 11, 2022. https://www.nccn.org/professionals/physician_gls/pdf/antiemesis.pdf.
4. Bruce CM, Smith J, Price A. A study of the incidence and management of admissions for cancer-related symptoms in a district general hospital: the potential role of an acute oncology service. *Clin Oncol.* 2017;29(9):e148–e155. https://doi.org/10.1016/j.clon.2017.03.012.
5. Hesketh PJ, Kris MG, Basch E, et al. Antiemetics: American Society of Clinical Oncology clinical practice guideline update. *J Clin Oncol.* 2017;35(28):3240–3261. https://doi.org/10.1200/JCO.2017.74.4789.

6. American Nurses Association. *Call for Action: Nurses Lead and Transform Palliative Care*. 2017. Accessed January 15, 2025. https://www.nursingworld.org/globalassets/practiceandpolicy/health-policy/palliativecareprofessionalissuespanelcallforaction.pdf.
7. Zhong W, Shahbaz O, Teskey G, et al. Mechanisms of nausea and vomiting: current knowledge and recent advances in intracellular emetic signaling systems. *Int J Mol Sci*. 2021;22(11):5797. https://doi.org/10.3390/ijms22115797.
8. Rha SY, Lee J. Stable symptom clusters and evolving symptom networks in relation to chemotherapy cycles. *J Pain Symptom Manage*. 2021;61(3):544–554. https://doi.org/10.1016/j.jpainsymman.2020.08.008.
9. Rha SY, Lee J. Symptom clusters during palliative chemotherapy and their influence on functioning and quality of life. *Support Care Cancer*. 2017;25(5):1519–1527. https://doi.org/10.1007/s00520-016-3545-z.
10. Kammell A, Marks S. Nausea and Vomiting: Common Etiologies and Management. Palliative Care Network of Wisconsin. September 2021. Accessed November 11, 2022. https://www.mypcnow.org/fast-fact/the-causes-of-nausea-and-vomiting-v-o-m-i-t/.
11. Moorthy GS, Letizia M. The management of nausea at the end of life. *J Hosp Palliat Nurs*. 2018;20(5):442–449. https://doi.org/10.1097/NJH.0000000000000453.
12. Walsh D, Davis M, Ripamonti C, Bruera E, Davies A, Molassiotis A. 2016 Updated MASCC/ESMO consensus recommendations: management of nausea and vomiting in advanced cancer. *Support Care Cancer*. 2017;25(1):333–340. https://doi.org/10.1007/s00520-016-3371-3.
13. Gilmore J, D'Amato S, Griffith N, Schwartzberg L. Recent advances in antiemetics: new formulations of 5HT3-receptor antagonists. *Cancer Manag Res*. 2018;10:1827–1857. https://doi.org/10.2147/CMAR.S166912.
14. Alese OB, Kim S, Chen Z, Owonikoko TK, El-Rayes BF. Management patterns and predictors of mortality among US patients with cancer hospitalized for malignant bowel obstruction: MBO in US patients hospitalized with cancer. *Cancer*. 2015;121(11):1772–1778. https://doi.org/10.1002/cncr.29297.
15. Baddeley E, Mann M, Bravington A, et al. Symptom burden and lived experiences of patients, caregivers and healthcare professionals on the management of malignant bowel obstruction: a qualitative systematic review. *Palliat Med*. 2022;36(6):895–911. https://doi.org/10.1177/02692163221081331.
16. Smedbäck J, Öhlén J, Årestedt K, Alvariza A, Fürst CJ, Håkanson C. Palliative care during the final week of life of older people in nursing homes: a register-based study. *Palliat Support Care*. 2017;15(4):417–424. https://doi.org/10.1017/S1478951516000948.
17. Wajnberg A, Ornstein K, Zhang M, Smith KL, Soriano T. Symptom burden in chronically ill homebound individuals. *J Am Geriatr Soc*. 2013;61(1):126–131. https://doi.org/10.1111/jgs.12038.
18. Kamal AH, Nipp RD, Bull J, Stinson CS, Abernethy AP. Symptom burden and performance status among community-dwelling patients with serious illness. *J Palliat Med*. 2015;18(6):542–544. https://doi.org/10.1089/jpm.2014.0381.
19. Bandeali S, des Ordons AR, Sinnarajah A. Comparing the physical, psychological, social, and spiritual needs of patients with non-cancer and cancer diagnoses in a tertiary palliative care setting. *Palliat Support Care*. 2020;18(5):513–518. https://doi.org/10.1017/S1478951519001020.
20. Vilensky JA, Robertson W, Suárez-Quian CA, eds. *The Clinical Anatomy of the Cranial Nerves: The Nerves of "On Old Olympus Towering Top."* John Wiley & Sons; 2015.
21. Rhodes VA, McDaniel RW. Nausea, vomiting, and retching: complex problems in palliative care. *CA Cancer J Clin*. 2001;51(4):232–248. https://doi.org/10.3322/canjclin.51.4.232.
22. Dietrich B, Ramchandran K, Von Roenn JH. Nausea and vomiting. In: Holland JC, Breitbart WS, Jacobsen PB, Loscalzo MJ, McCorkle R, Butow PN, eds. *Psycho-Oncology*. Oxford University Press; 2015:199–208. https://doi.org/10.1093/med/9780199363315.003.0026.
23. Glare P, Miller J, Nikolova T, Tickoo R. Treating nausea and vomiting in palliative care: a review. *Clin Interv Aging*. 2011;6:243–259. https://doi.org/10.2147/CIA.S13109.
24. Hardy JR, Glare P, Yates P, Mannix KA. Palliation of nausea and vomiting. In: Kaasa S, Cherny N, Fallon M, Currow DC, Portenoy RK, eds. *Oxford Textbook of Palliative Medicine, 5th edn*. Oxford University Press; 2015:661–674. https://doi.org/10.1093/med/9780199656097.003.0202.
25. Schank JR, Heilig M. Substance P and the neurokinin-1 receptor: the new CRF. In: Todd E. Thiele, ed. *International Review of Neurobiology*. Vol 136. Elsevier; 2017:151–175. https://doi.org/10.1016/bs.irn.2017.06.008.
26. Gordon P, LeGrand SB, Walsh D. Nausea and vomiting in advanced cancer. *Eur J Pharmacol*. 2014;722:187–191. https://doi.org/10.1016/j.ejphar.2013.10.010.
27. Collis E, Mather H. Nausea and vomiting in palliative care. *BMJ*. 2015;351:h6249. https://doi.org/10.1136/bmj.h6249.
28. Brearley SG, Clements CV, Molassiotis A. A review of patient self-report tools for chemotherapy-induced nausea and vomiting. *Support Care Cancer*. 2008;16(11):1213–1229. https://doi.org/10.1007/s00520-008-0428-y.
29. Meek R, Graudins A. Visual analog scale rating change cut-offs for detection of improvement in nausea severity. *Emerg Med Australas*. 2019;31(4):673–675. https://doi.org/10.1111/1742-6723.13291.
30. Martin CG, Rubenstein EB, Elting LS, Kim YJ, Osoba D. Measuring chemotherapy-induced nausea and emesis: psychometric properties of a quality of life questionnaire. *Cancer*. 2003;98(3):645–655. https://doi.org/10.1002/cncr.11540.
31. Wood JM, Chapman K, Eilers J. Tools for assessing nausea, vomiting, and retching: a literature review. *Cancer Nurs*. 2011;34(1):E14–E24. https://doi.org/10.1097/NCC.0b013e3181e2cd79.
32. Molassiotis A, Coventry PA, Stricker CT, et al. Validation and psychometric assessment of a short clinical scale to measure chemotherapy-induced nausea and vomiting: the MASCC Antiemesis Tool. *J Pain Symptom Manage*. 2007;34(2):148–159. https://doi.org/10.1016/j.jpainsymman.2006.10.018.
33. Dawber R, Armour K, Ferry P, Mukherjee B, Carter C, Meystre C. Comparison of informal caregiver and named nurse assessment of symptoms in elderly patients dying in hospital using the palliative outcome scale. *BMJ Support Palliat Care*. 2019;9(2):175–182. https://doi.org/10.1136/bmjspcare-2015-000850.
34. Hardy J, Skerman H, Glare P, et al. A randomized open-label study of guideline-driven antiemetic therapy versus single agent antiemetic therapy in patients with advanced cancer and nausea not related to anticancer treatment. *BMC Cancer*. 2018;18(1):510. https://doi.org/10.1186/s12885-018-4404-8.
35. Sanger GJ, Broad J, Andrews PLR. The relationship between gastric motility and nausea: gastric prokinetic agents as treatments. *Eur J Pharmacol*. 2013;715(1–3):10–14. https://doi.org/10.1016/j.ejphar.2013.06.031.
36. Gupta M, Davis M, Walsh D, LeGrand S, Lagman R, Parala-Metz A. Nausea and vomiting in advanced cancer—the Cleveland Clinic

protocol (TH310). *J Pain Symptom Manage*. 2013;45(2):338–339. https://doi.org/10.1016/j.jpainsymman.2012.10.042.
37. Hendren G, Aponte-Feliciano A, Kovac A. Safety and efficacy of commonly used antiemetics. *Expert Opin Drug Metab Toxicol*. 2015;11(11):1753–1767. https://doi.org/10.1517/17425255.2015.1080688.
38. Wickham RJ. Nausea and vomiting: a palliative care imperative. *Curr Oncol Rep*. 2020;22(1):1. https://doi.org/10.1007/s11912-020-0871-6.
39. Hardy J, Skerman H, Franzen K, Foster K, Yates P. A randomised, controlled, double blind study of oral methotrimeprazine versus oral haloperidol in patients with cancer and nausea not related to anticancer therapy. *Ann Oncol*. 2017;28:x156. https://doi.org/10.1093/annonc/mdx676.004.
40. Cox L, Darvill E, Dorman S. Levomepromazine for nausea and vomiting in palliative care. *Cochrane Database Syst Rev*. 2015;2015(11):CD009420. https://doi.org/10.1002/14651858.CD009420.pub3.
41. Bosnjak SM, Dimitrijevic J, Djordjevic F. Cancer and chemotherapy-induced nausea and vomiting: a focus on olanzapine. *Curr Opin Support Palliat Care*. 2016;10(2):180–188. https://doi.org/10.1097/SPC.0000000000000206.
42. MacKintosh D. Olanzapine in the management of difficult to control nausea and vomiting in a palliative care population: a case series. *J Palliat Med*. 2016;19(1):87–90. https://doi.org/10.1089/jpm.2015.0224.
43. Kaneishi K, Nishimura K, Sakurai N, et al. Use of olanzapine for the relief of nausea and vomiting in patients with advanced cancer: a multicenter survey in Japan. *Support Care Cancer*. 2016;24(6):2393–2395. https://doi.org/10.1007/s00520-016-3101-x.
44. Atkinson SR. Olanzapine for intractable nausea and vomiting in palliative care patients not receiving chemotherapy. *J Palliat Med*. 2014;17(5):503–504. https://doi.org/10.1089/jpm.2014.0030.
45. Vig S, Seibert L, Green MR. Olanzapine is effective for refractory chemotherapy-induced nausea and vomiting irrespective of chemotherapy emetogenicity. *J Cancer Res Clin Oncol*. 2014;140(1):77–82. https://doi.org/10.1007/s00432-013-1540-z.
46. Chiu L, Chow R, Popovic M, et al. Efficacy of olanzapine for the prophylaxis and rescue of chemotherapy-induced nausea and vomiting (CINV): a systematic review and meta-analysis. *Support Care Cancer*. 2016;24(5):2381–2392. https://doi.org/10.1007/s00520-016-3075-8.
47. Sutherland A, Naessens K, Plugge E, et al. Olanzapine for the prevention and treatment of cancer-related nausea and vomiting in adults. *Cochrane Database Syst Rev*. 2018;2018(9):CD012555. https://doi.org/10.1002/14651858.CD012555.pub2.
48. Imai K, Ikenaga M, Kodama T, Kanemura S, Tamura K, Morita T. Sublingually administered scopolamine for nausea in terminally ill cancer patients. *Support Care Cancer*. 2013;21(10):2777–2781. https://doi.org/10.1007/s00520-013-1846-z.
49. Davis M, Hui D, Davies A, et al. Medical management of malignant bowel obstruction in patients with advanced cancer: 2021 MASCC guideline update. *Support Care Cancer*. 2021;29(12):8089–8096. https://doi.org/10.1007/s00520-021-06438-9.
50. Ganesh V, Drost L, DeAngelis C, et al. A pilot study with palonosetron in the prophylaxis of radiation-induced nausea and vomiting. *Ann Palliat Med*. 2018;7(2):211–220. https://doi.org/10.21037/apm.2018.03.12.
51. Vayne-Bossert P, Haywood A, Good P, Khan S, Rickett K, Hardy JR. Corticosteroids for adult patients with advanced cancer who have nausea and vomiting (not related to chemotherapy, radiotherapy, or surgery). *Cochrane Database Syst Rev*. 2017;7(7):CD12002. https://doi.org/10.1002/14651858.CD012002.pub2.
52. James A, Nair MM, Abraham DS, Kovoor JS, Jose WM, Reghu R. Effect of lorazepam in reducing psychological distress and anticipatory nausea and vomiting in patients undergoing chemotherapy. *J Pharmacol Pharmacother*. 2017;8(3):112–115. https://doi.org/10.4103/jpp.JPP_54_17.
53. Dupuis LL, Roscoe JA, Olver I, Aapro M, Molassiotis A. 2016 updated MASCC/ESMO consensus recommendations: anticipatory nausea and vomiting in children and adults receiving chemotherapy. *Support Care Cancer*. 2017;25(1):317–321. https://doi.org/10.1007/s00520-016-3330-z.
54. Kamen C, Tejani MA, Chandwani K, et al. Anticipatory nausea and vomiting due to chemotherapy. *Eur J Pharmacol*. 2014;722:172–179. https://doi.org/10.1016/j.ejphar.2013.09.071.
55. Davis MP. Cannabinoids for symptom management and cancer therapy: the evidence. *J Natl Compr Canc Netw*. 2016;14(7):915–922. https://doi.org/10.6004/jnccn.2016.0094.
56. Smith LA, Azariah F, Lavender VT, Stoner NS, Bettiol S. Cannabinoids for nausea and vomiting in adults with cancer receiving chemotherapy. *Cochrane Database Syst Rev*. 2015;2015(11):CD009464. https://doi.org/10.1002/14651858.CD009464.pub2.
57. Clark C. Medical cannabis: the oncology nurse's role in patient education about the effects of marijuana on cancer palliation. *Clin J Oncol Nurs*. 2018;22(1):E1–E6. https://doi.org/10.1188/18.CJON.E1-E6.
58. Schulman-Green D, Brody A, Gilbertson-White S, Whittemore R, McCorkle R. Supporting self-management in palliative care throughout the cancer care trajectory. *Curr Opin Support Palliat Care*. 2018;12(3):299–307. https://doi.org/10.1097/SPC.0000000000000373.
59. Lewis L, Williams AM, Athifa M, Brown D, Budgeon CA, Bremner AP. Evidence-based self-care guidelines for people receiving chemotherapy: do they reduce symptom burden and psychological distress? *Cancer Nurs*. 2015;38(3):E1–E8. https://doi.org/10.1097/NCC.0000000000000154.
60. Wochna Loerzel V, Clochesy J, Geddie P. Using serious games to increase prevention and self-management of chemotherapy-induced nausea and vomiting in older adults with cancer. *Oncol Nurs Forum*. 2020;47(5):567–576. https://doi.org/10.1188/20.ONF.567-576.
61. Cherny NI, Fallon M, Kaasa S, Portenoy RK, Currow D, eds. *Oxford Textbook of Palliative Medicine*. 6th ed. Oxford University Press; 2021.
62. Greenlee H, DuPont-Reyes MJ, Balneaves LG, et al. Clinical practice guidelines on the evidence-based use of integrative therapies during and after breast cancer treatment: integrative therapies during and after breast cancer treatment. *CA Cancer J Clin*. 2017;67(3):194–232. https://doi.org/10.3322/caac.21397.
63. Wu X, Chung VC, Hui EP, et al. Effectiveness of acupuncture and related therapies for palliative care of cancer: overview of systematic reviews. *Sci Rep*. 2015;5(1):16776. https://doi.org/10.1038/srep16776.
64. National Center for Complementary and Integrative Health. Resources for Health Care Providers. November 2022. Accessed November 9, 2022. https://www.nccih.nih.gov/health/providers.
65. Leong M, Smith TJ, Rowland-Seymour A. Complementary and integrative medicine for older adults in palliative care. *Clin Geriatr Med*. 2015;31(2):177–191. https://doi.org/10.1016/j.cger.2015.01.004.

66. Oh B, Butow P, Mullan B, et al. The use and perceived benefits resulting from the use of complementary and alternative medicine by cancer patients in Australia: perceived benefits from the use of CAM. *Asia Pac J Clin Oncol.* 2010;6(4):342–349. https://doi.org/10.1111/j.1743-7563.2010.01329.x.
67. Ryan JL, Heckler CE, Roscoe JA, et al. Ginger (*Zingiber officinale*) reduces acute chemotherapy-induced nausea: a URCC CCOP study of 576 patients. *Support Care Cancer.* 2012;20(7):1479–1489. https://doi.org/10.1007/s00520-011-1236-3.
68. Marx W, McCarthy A, Ried K, et al. The effect of a standardized ginger extract on chemotherapy-induced nausea-related quality of life in patients undergoing moderately or highly emetogenic chemotherapy: a double blind, randomized, placebo controlled trial. *Nutrients.* 2017;9(8):867. https://doi.org/10.3390/nu9080867.
69. Memorial Sloan Kettering Cancer Center. Ginger. June 2022. Accessed November 11, 2022. https://www.mskcc.org/cancer-care/integrative-medicine/herbs/ginger.
70. Garcia MK, McQuade J, Haddad R, et al. Systematic review of acupuncture in cancer care: a synthesis of the evidence. *J Clin Oncol.* 2013;31(7):952–960. https://doi.org/10.1200/JCO.2012.43.5818.
71. Lyman GH, Greenlee H, Bohlke K, et al. Integrative therapies during and after breast cancer treatment: ASCO endorsement of the SIO clinical practice guideline. *J Clin Oncol.* 2018;36(25):2647–2655. https://doi.org/10.1200/JCO.2018.79.2721.
72. Towler P, Molassiotis A, Brearley SG. What is the evidence for the use of acupuncture as an intervention for symptom management in cancer supportive and palliative care: an integrative overview of reviews. *Support Care Cancer.* 2013;21(10):2913–2923. https://doi.org/10.1007/s00520-013-1882-8.
73. Molassiotis A, Russell W, Hughes J, et al. The effectiveness of acupressure for the control and management of chemotherapy-related acute and delayed nausea: a randomized controlled trial. *J Pain Symptom Manage.* 2014;47(1):12–25. https://doi.org/10.1016/j.jpainsymman.2013.03.007.
74. Shin ES, Seo KH, Lee SH, et al. Massage with or without aromatherapy for symptom relief in people with cancer. *Cochrane Database Syst Rev.* 2016;2016(6):CD009873. https://doi.org/10.1002/14651858.CD009873.pub3.
75. Zorba P, Ozdemir L. The preliminary effects of massage and inhalation aromatherapy on chemotherapy-induced acute nausea and vomiting: a quasi-randomized controlled pilot trial. *Cancer Nurs.* 2018;41(5):359–366. https://doi.org/10.1097/NCC.0000000000000496.
76. Hines S, Steels E, Chang A, Gibbons K. Aromatherapy for treatment of postoperative nausea and vomiting. *Cochrane Database Syst Rev.* 2018;3(3):CD007598. https://doi.org/10.1002/14651858.CD007598.pub3.
77. Mao JJ, Wagner KE, Seluzicki CM, et al. Integrating oncology massage into chemoinfusion suites: a program evaluation. *J Oncol Pract.* 2017;13(3):e207–e216. https://doi.org/10.1200/JOP.2016.015081.
78. Carlson LE. Distress management through mind–body therapies in oncology. *JNCI Monogr.* 2017;2017(52):lgx009. https://doi.org/10.1093/jncimonographs/lgx009.
79. Bates D, Bolwell B, Majhail NS, et al. Music therapy for symptom management after autologous stem cell transplantation: results from a randomized study. *Biol Blood Marrow Transplant.* 2017;23(9):1567–1572. https://doi.org/10.1016/j.bbmt.2017.05.015.
80. Karagozoglu S, Tekyasar F, Yilmaz FA. Effects of music therapy and guided visual imagery on chemotherapy-induced anxiety and nausea-vomiting. *J Clin Nurs.* 2013;22(1–2):39–50. https://doi.org/10.1111/jocn.12030.
81. Lotfi-Jam K, Carey M, Jefford M, Schofield P, Charleson C, Aranda S. Nonpharmacologic strategies for managing common chemotherapy adverse effects: a systematic review. *J Clin Oncol.* 2008;26(34):5618–5629. https://doi.org/10.1200/JCO.2007.15.9053.
82. Kapogiannis A, Tsoli S, Chrousos G. Investigating the effects of the progressive muscle relaxation-guided imagery combination on patients with cancer receiving chemotherapy treatment: a systematic review of randomized controlled trials. *Explore (NY).* 2018;14(2):137–143. https://doi.org/10.1016/j.explore.2017.10.008.
83. Oncology Nursing Society. Palliative Care for People with Cancer. November 11, 2022. Accessed November 11, 2022. https://www.ons.org/make-difference/ons-center-advocacy-and-health-policy/position-statements/palliative-care-people.
84. Kamal AH, Bausewein C, Casarett DJ, Currow DC, Dudgeon DJ, Higginson IJ. Standards, guidelines, and quality measures for successful specialty palliative care integration into oncology: current approaches and future directions. *J Clin Oncol.* 2020;38(9):987–994. https://doi.org/10.1200/JCO.18.02440.
85. Pinto S, Caldeira S, Martins JC. A qualitative study about palliative care patients' experiences of comfort: implications for nursing diagnosis and interventions. *J Nurs Educ Pract.* 2017;7(8):37. https://doi.org/10.5430/jnep.v7n8p37.
86. Wheeler MS. Primary palliative care for every nurse practitioner. *J Nurse Pract.* 2016;12(10):647–653. https://doi.org/10.1016/j.nurpra.2016.09.003.
87. Gonella S, Di Giulio P. Delayed chemotherapy-induced nausea and vomiting in the hematology population: a review of the literature. *Clin J Oncol Nurs.* 2015;19(4):438–443. https://doi.org/10.1188/15.CJON.438-443.
88. Bickel KE, McNiff K, Buss MK, et al. Defining high-quality palliative care in oncology practice: an American Society of Clinical Oncology/American Academy of Hospice and Palliative Medicine guidance statement. *J Oncol Pract.* 2016;12(9):e828–e838. https://doi.org/10.1200/JOP.2016.010686.

15

Dysphagia, Hiccups, and Other Oral Symptoms

Rachel Klinedinst, Brenna McCarty, and Barton Bobb

Key Points

- Swallowing problems commonly occur in many advanced disease processes and can cause significant distress and burden on both the patient and the caregiver.
- Management of swallowing difficulties and oral complications in patients with serious illness focuses on preventing functional decline, maximizing quality of life and comfort, and supporting the patient's wishes.
- Oral symptoms and complications often occur concurrently and can impact patients' safety and comfort, as well as their ability to sustain nutrition and hydration and to manage oral medications.
- A multidisciplinary team approach will promote successful treatment with better outcomes and improved relief of symptoms.

Case Study: A Patient with Amyotrophic Lateral Sclerosis

DS is a 68-year-old patient who presents to the hospital with increased oxygen requirements at home and progressive weakness over the past 2 months. They typically use bilevel positive airway pressure at night but now require it during the day as well for management of shortness of breath. An electromyogram was performed, which showed lower motor neuron abnormalities, supporting a new diagnosis of amyotrophic lateral sclerosis (ALS). Additional complications for DS include weak voice, poor cough strength, and dysphagia.

Introduction

Food is a central aspect of life and symbolizes love and community. Participating in the sharing of food and drink is a ritual that adds texture to life through socialization, communication, and enjoyment. Dysphagia, hiccups, and other oral symptoms such as sialorrhea, xerostomia, and dysgeusia are commonly experienced in patients with serious illnesses. These symptoms often occur concurrently, impacting not only a patient's safety and ability to sustain adequate nutrition and hydration but also physical comfort, social well-being, and quality of life. The care and management of dysphagia and oral symptoms focus on the specific disease process and trajectory, while also encompassing the individual's preferences and goals.

Dysphagia

Definition

Dysphagia is defined as difficulty swallowing food or liquid. Swallowing impairments can threaten the safety and efficiency with which oral nutrition and hydration are maintained, as well as affecting patients' ability to manage oral medications. Chronic difficulty swallowing can be both frustrating and frightening for patients and their caregivers. Because nutrition is compromised, generalized weakness, diminished appetite, weight loss, or malnutrition may ensue. Aspiration can also occur, causing pneumonia, fevers, malaise, shortness of breath, and death.[1–3] The development of dysphagia may be pivotal in redirecting care from sustaining life to a palliative focus.[1] Swallowing difficulties and withdrawal from daily activities such as eating and drinking may become increasingly prevalent and may alter social encounters.[2]

Physiology and Pathophysiology of Swallowing

Swallowing, an extremely complex physiological act, involves the passage of food or liquid from the oral cavity through the esophagus and into the stomach, where the process of digestion begins.[3,4] Because humans swallow hundreds of times per day and are largely unaware of the activity, it is remarkable that difficulties do not occur more frequently. The first stage of swallowing, the oral stage, is responsible for readying the bolus (ball of food or liquid) for swallowing.[5,6] It is also during this stage that one takes pleasure from the flavor and texture of food through the chemoreceptors of the tongue and palate. The second stage of swallowing, the pharyngeal stage, lasts approximately 1 second. This stage is the most complex, requiring precise timing and coordination between respiration, airway protection, bolus propulsion, and opening of the cervical esophagus. The esophageal stage of swallowing is the longest phase and involves transport of the bolus from the upper esophageal segment, through the lower esophageal segment, and into the stomach.[4,7]

Etiology of Dysphagia

Dysphagia is a common symptom in patients receiving palliative care. Swallowing difficulties may be the presenting clinical feature or a sign of advancing illness. Understanding the physiological impact of the illness is critical in evaluation of the swallowing disorder and in determining the method of management. Some commonly encountered etiological categories of dysphagia in palliative care include neoplasms, progressive neuromuscular diseases, dementia, and chronic illnesses. Dysphagia can also be a side effect of medications.

Assessment of Dysphagia

For the patient with a serious and life-threatening illness, the goals of the swallowing evaluation are to (1) identify the underlying physiological nature of the disorder, (2) determine reversible conditions that may be a causative or contributing factor,[8] (3) determine interventions that can best alleviate dysphagia and concomitant distress, and (4) collaborate with the patient, family, and caregivers on the safest and most efficacious method of nutrition and hydration. There are numerous tests and procedures to evaluate swallowing function. The correct evaluation is driven by specific patient concerns and goals of care. Nurses can play an integral role throughout this process.

Clinical Examination of Swallowing

Eliciting a description of the patient's complaints about swallowing, current eating habits, appetite, and diet is critical to understanding the physiological basis of the problem. Details of disease progression and prognosis, as well as the patient's level of alertness, positioning, breathing, and ability to follow directions are considered when determining the aggressiveness of a swallowing workup and its treatment. Direct observation of the patient eating, drinking, or taking medications by a perceptive clinician, including the nurse, can yield valuable information about the underlying disorder.

Screening of Swallowing Function

Given the causes of dysphagia and its impact on patients' overall health, outcomes, hospital length of stay, and cost of care,[9] early identification of swallowing dysfunction in high-risk hospitalized patients is paramount.[10,11] Dysphagia screening has been formally recognized in the care of stroke patients for more than a decade.[12] A validated screening protocol to identify potential aspiration risk can be completed by the nurse or a member of the healthcare team who undergoes appropriate training. Screening programs have been shown to improve patient outcomes, including a 55% reduction in cases of pneumonia and a shorter length of stay in many hospitalized patient populations.[9]

Specific clinical predictors of swallowing dysfunction that warrant further instrumental evaluation are provided in Box 15.1.

Box 15.1 Indications of a Swallowing Disorder

Reduced Alertness or Cognitive Impairment

Coma, heavy sedation, dementia, delirium
Inattention during eating
Residual food in the oral cavity after eating
Impulsivity with regard to eating
Playing with food

Signs of Oral-Pharyngeal Dysfunction

Dysarthria or slurred, imprecise speech
Wet-sounding voice
Inability to manage secretions
Drooling or leaking from the lips
Frequent throat clearing, coughing, or choking during or immediately after meals
Voice changes after swallowing
Laborious chewing, multiple swallows per small bites
Residual food in the oral cavity after eating
Nasal regurgitation
Recurrent aspiration pneumonias
Food or fluid noted in tracheotomy tube
Changes in posture or head movements during eating

Signs of Esophageal Dysfunction

Regurgitation or emesis after swallowing
Sour taste in mouth after eating
Solids caught in the chest region
Burping during/after eating
Pain on swallowing

Specific Patient Complaints (Adapted from the EAT-10)

Sensation of food caught in the throat
Coughing and choking while eating
Painful or effortful swallowing
Alterations in attitudes toward eating
Swallowing problem interferes with pleasure when eating or socializing
Shortness of breath while chewing or after meals
Weight loss
Protracted mealtimes or inability to complete a meal
Avoidance of particular foods or fluids
Refusal to eat in the presence of others

Sources: References 3, 4, 13–16.

Management of Dysphagia

The physiologic information obtained from a swallowing assessment helps to determine intervention strategies. The goal of intervention is increasing swallowing safety and efficiency and/or maximizing residual abilities. Often, treatment utilizes a variety of approaches and techniques simultaneously. Management strategies are individualized and only effective when targeting specific impairments in the biomechanics of swallowing, as determined by an objective swallowing evaluation. Consideration of any swallowing intervention should align closely with overall patient preferences, goals of care, and treatment plan. The nurse may be asked to assist with swallow evaluations, followed by implementing compensatory swallowing strategies.

Case Study: Conversations about Artificial Nutrition

DS undergoes a swallow study, which demonstrates that liquid with honey consistency is the safest for their oral intake. The nurse assists DS and their family with education and demonstrates how to implement the recommended dietary changes. Further discussion about alternative nutrition pathways determines that feeding tubes and artificial nutrition are not in line with DS's overall goals of care. Recognizing the quick progression of ALS and the projected prognosis, they would like to pursue comfort-focused care. This includes "pleasure feeding" and liberalizing diet, recognizing the risk of aspiration, dehydration, and malnutrition. A hospice referral is placed to assist with discharge planning, in hopes of continuing care at home.

Compensatory Swallowing Strategies

Alterations in head and neck posture, modifications in food and liquid texture, techniques to improve airway closure, and external cueing to increase sensory awareness and feeding behaviors are considered compensatory in nature. Their effectiveness may be limited in patients with altered cognition or pulmonary complications or for patients who do not have a caregiver who can assist them. Other modifications, such as altering food/liquid consistency, may significantly impact the patient's pleasure with eating.

Postural Modifications

Postural changes during swallowing often have the effect of diverting food or liquid to prevent aspiration or obstruction, but they do not change the swallowing physiology.[3,4] These strategies may be used in isolation or in combination, depending on the nature of the underlying swallowing pathophysiology (see Table 15.1).

Changes in Texture and Consistency of Food

Changes in food texture and liquid consistency play a vital role when managing dysphagia and may be the best option to ensure a patient's comfort or to improve safety and efficiency of oral intake. Diet modifications may include drinking liquids with nectar or honey consistency and/or eating a pureed or minced diet.[17] The nurse should be aware of any recommended changes in food texture and liquid consistency and ensure that they are implemented correctly. Because these alterations can be unappealing, it may be necessary for the nurse to provide emotional support while patients and caregivers adjust to a new diet. See Box 15.2 for suggestions for oral feeding.

Table 15.1 Postural modifications

Postural strategy	Rationale
Chin tuck	Closes larynx, pushes tongue closer to posterior pharyngeal wall, and promotes epiglottic deflection
Head back	Promotes bolus movement through the oral cavity with assistance of gravity
Head tilt to stronger side	Directs bolus down stronger side with assistance of gravity
Head turned to weaker side	Diverts bolus away from weaker side of pharynx, promotes opening of upper esophagus
Head tilt plus chin tuck	Directs bolus down stronger side while increasing closure of larynx
Head rotation plus chin tuck	Diverts bolus away from weaker side while facilitating closure of laryngeal vestibule and vocal folds

Sources: Adapted from References 3 and 4.

Box 15.2 Suggestions for Oral Feeding

1. *Remove distractions at mealtime.* This can help patients focus on swallowing and using compensatory swallowing strategies.
2. *Emphasize heightened awareness of sensory and taste cues.* Using a larger bolus size, increased downward pressure of the spoon on the tongue, and cold or sour foods may alert the patient that food is in the mouth and improve oral sensation and awareness.
3. *Provide feeding utensils.* Patients with hand tremors or weakness that impact self-feeding may be aided with devices such as weighted cuffs or built-up utensils.
4. *Optimize the position of the patient.* Sitting as upright as possible when eating, drinking, or taking medications is typically deemed safest. Reduce the tendency to slump forward or to the side or head extension, which can make the patient more vulnerable to aspiration.
5. *Schedule mealtimes.* Time meals to coincide with increased function and reduced fatigue or sedation from medications.
6. *Consider more frequent, smaller meals with high-calorie supplements.* Increased frequency of small meals may help patients who do not have sufficient efficiency or endurance to complete an entire meal at one time.
7. *Encourage the maximal number of calories for the least amount of effort.* Make every bite count with increased caloric and nutritional value by using cream, oils, and butter; adding sauces; and avoiding calorie-free beverages or foods unless otherwise indicated.
8. *Consider hand-feeding when appropriate.* Hand-feeding allows for continued intimate contact between patient and caregiver.

Airway Clearance Techniques

The ability to effectively cough to clear secretions and aspirated material is essential to reduce pulmonary infections and respiratory difficulties. Supportive airway clearance techniques may be recommended to improve oxygenation and cough function, mobilize secretions in order to combat pulmonary infection, improve swallowing, and strengthen airway clearance. These techniques have been found to decrease length of time on a ventilator, reduce intensive care unit stays, resolve atelectasis/consolidation, and/or improve respiratory mechanics.[18] Supportive treatments can be beneficial as part of the armamentarium of dysphagia management in patients with aspiration risk and/or poor secretion management.

A mechanical insufflator–exsufflator, or cough assist machine, provides positive pressure to maximally inflate the lungs, followed by an abrupt switch to negative pressure. The rapid change from positive to negative pressure simulates a cough, thereby assisting sputum clearance. This can prevent pneumonia and other complications associated with secretion retention.[19] The device can be used with an oral mouthpiece or via tracheostomy tube.

Hiccups

Case Study: New Hiccups in a Patient with ALS

At home, DS develops persistent, intermittent hiccups that affect their ability to talk. Eating is more difficult with hiccups, and the symptom often awakens DS at night, preventing adequate sleep. DS also reports chronic constipation that is no longer responding to the standing bowel regimen. The nurse performs a thorough examination and notes increased abdominal distension. Based on the nurse's assessment, DS is prescribed metoclopramide and lactulose to relieve constipation, as well as baclofen three times daily, which reduces the severity of the hiccups.

Etiology and Pathophysiology

Hiccups, or singultus, are involuntary contractions of the diaphragm and intercostal muscles, which result in sudden inspiration and abrupt closure of the glottis, producing a characteristic "hic" sound. Hiccups originate through a reflex arc composed of afferent neurons, a reflex center in the brain and spinal cord, and efferent neurons that stimulate muscle contraction.[20,21]

Common causes include conditions that affect the phrenic and vagus nerves, such as abdominal or mediastinal tumor compression, or central nervous system disorders like stroke, brain tumors, and neurologic diseases.[21] Other causes of hiccups include sepsis, pericarditis, pneumonia, pleuritis, esophagitis, gastric distension, pancreatitis, and hepatitis.[20] Many medications also trigger hiccups, including steroids, chemotherapeutic agents, dopamine antagonists, megestrol, methyldopa, opioids, benzodiazepines, and muscle relaxants.[22]

Hiccups may begin as benign (lasting only minutes) but can become persistent or even intractable (lasting a month or more).[20] Duration of hiccups may not be as critical as their impact on a patient's quality of life. Prolonged hiccups may cause fatigue, insomnia, anxiety, depression, dehydration, and weight loss due to poor oral intake.[20]

Nursing Assessment of Hiccups

Assessment should begin with a physical exam to identify underlying causes. The nurse should inspect for infections of the mouth and throat, pneumonia or pericarditis, abdominal distention or ascites, and signs of stroke or delirium.[20,23] History should include onset and duration of hiccups, previous episodes, and interference with rest, talking, or oral intake. Inquiry into precipitating factors such as eating, drinking, or positioning may be helpful. Medication review may identify pharmacological triggers.

The nurse should also screen for secondary symptoms, including anorexia due to impaired swallowing, shortness of breath from inability to take deep breaths, fatigue as the result of excess energy use, insomnia from hiccupping all night, heartburn from acid reflux produced by hiccups, and depression or anxiety related to concern that hiccups are untreatable.[20]

Nursing Interventions for Hiccups

Many patients express frustration that the discomfort and disruption caused by hiccups are not taken seriously. Nursing interventions should focus on providing emotional support as well as offering information and suggestions about the broad range of strategies for treating hiccups.

The nurse should recommend nonpharmacological interventions first:[20,24]

- Respiratory maneuvers such as breath-holding, diaphragm compression, or rebreathing into a paper bag
- Nasal and pharyngeal stimulation such as drinking from the far side of a glass, swallowing a spoonful of sugar, sucking a lemon wedge with bitters, or gently touching the soft palate with a cotton applicator
- Vagal stimulation such as ocular or digital rectal massage
- Gastric decompression such as holding oral intake or insertion of a nasogastric tube
- Other measures such as distraction or drinking peppermint water to stimulate the esophagus

If the above measures are ineffective, the nurse may suggest pharmacological interventions.[20,22–24] Gastric distension is a common cause of hiccups, and medications that promote gastric emptying (metoclopramide, simethicone) are the first-line recommendation. For hiccups resulting from muscle spasms due to tumor compression or neurologic disease, muscle relaxants (baclofen, midazolam) may be effective. Steroids such as dexamethasone relieve inflammation that may contribute to hiccups. Other medications to treat hiccups include dopaminergic agents (chlorpromazine, haloperidol), anticonvulsants (gabapentin, pregabalin), calcium channel blockers (lidocaine, nifedipine), antidepressants (amitriptyline, sertraline), and ketamine.

If medications fail to relieve hiccups, the nurse may suggest referral to a pain management specialist for interventional therapies such as phrenic or cervical nerve blocks or radiofrequency ablation.[20,21] For intractable hiccups, palliative sedation may be considered. Decisions about procedural interventions and sedation should include discussion about prognosis, benefits and burdens, and patient goals and preferences.

Other Oral Symptoms

Case Study: Oral Symptoms in a Patient with ALS

DS has been doing well at home, but their spouse reports that oral secretions have become more burdensome. The nurse observes moderate to severe sialorrhea, which often pools and creates excess moisture on DS's neck and clothing. DS reports increased difficulty breathing due to the burden of oral secretions. At times DS reports a foul taste in their mouth, which the nurse recognizes as dysgeusia. A strategy of expectorating secretions and using a portable device for frequent oral suctioning is implemented. DS uses a neck collar to maintain optimal posture for eating. Frequent oral care is provided, including tooth brushing and oral rinses to minimize taste alterations.

Sialorrhea (Excess Oral Secretions)

Etiology and Pathophysiology

Sialorrhea is unintentional and excessive loss of saliva from the mouth, described as drooling. The symptom results from one of two mechanisms: (1) overproduction of saliva or (2) poor oral clearance of saliva.[25,26] Excess saliva production may occur due to oral or dental infections, side effects of medications (e.g., anticonvulsants, anticholinesterase, or lithium), vitamin deficiencies, or gastroesophageal reflux.[25] Inability to clear saliva may be caused by reduced frequency of swallowing, weakness of oropharyngeal or laryngeal muscles, tongue spasticity, poor head posture, or sensory dysfunction.[26] Sialorrhea is common in patients with head and neck cancer or neurologic disease.[25,26]

While distressing on its own, sialorrhea puts patients at risk for additional symptoms, including moisture-related skin breakdown, altered speech, and sleep disruptions.[25,26] In patients with impaired breathing and swallowing, the sensation of choking and inability to clear excess saliva can be anxiety-provoking and may increase the risk of aspiration, poor oxygenation, and pneumonias.[25,26] Prolonged sialorrhea and its sequelae may result in fatigue, embarrassment, social withdrawal, and isolation.[26]

Nursing Assessment of Sialorrhea

Assessment should begin with a physical exam to assess for underlying causes. The nurse should inspect for sores on lips/chin, dental problems, ulcerations of gums or oral mucosa, and changes in head posture or lip/tongue strength and sensation.[25] History should include onset and duration of sialorrhea, provoking factors, and amount/consistency of secretions. Medication review may identify drug therapies that cause hypersalivation.

The nurse should also evaluate the impact of sialorrhea on the patient's functional abilities such as eating, drinking, and speaking. Use of a screening tool such as the Oral Secretion Scale or the Sialorrhea Scoring Scale may aid the nurse in assessing and documenting the extent of sialorrhea.[27]

Nursing Interventions for Sialorrhea

The nurse should encourage self-management of saliva through behavioral techniques such as purposeful swallowing before eating or speaking.[26,28] Assistance with positioning prior to meals or prolonged conversations may be helpful. The nurse should also promote and assist with good oral care and, if indicated, oral suctioning before meals. The patient may benefit from working with a speech therapist to learn strengthening exercises that improve oromotor function and tongue control.[25,28] Physical therapy and supportive neck collars or other orthopedic devices for correction of body and head posture may also be useful.[26,28]

For moderate to severe sialorrhea, pharmacological therapy is indicated and may require a process of trial and error to achieve optimal results.[26] Anticholinergic medications are utilized to block parasympathetic stimulation to the salivary glands and reduce saliva production.[25,26,28] These medications include glycopyrrolate, amitriptyline, benztropine, scopolamine transdermal patch, and atropine or hyoscyamine sublingual drops. The nurse should closely monitor use of these medications in older adults, due to risk of drowsiness and confusion. Other symptoms of anticholinergic agents include thickened respiratory secretions, dry mouth, urinary retention, and blurred vision.

Patients may inquire about botulinum toxin injections, which are an alternative treatment for sialorrhea in motor neuron disease and Parkinson's disease.[26] External beam radiation to the salivary glands is another treatment for refractory hypersalivation or for patients who cannot tolerate botulinum toxin injections.[25,26] Surgical interventions including denervation, excision, or ablation of the salivary glands and ligation or rerouting of the salivary ducts may be an option.[25,26,28] Discussions about procedural interventions should include prognosis, benefits and burdens, and the patient's goals and preferences.

Xerostomia (Dry Mouth)

Etiology and Pathophysiology

Xerostomia is the sensation of oral dryness, which may result from hyposalivation, or a decrease in salivary secretions. However, even with normal salivary gland function and saliva production, many patients with serious illness report subjective xerostomia.[29] Causes of xerostomia include infection, dehydration, endocrine and autoimmune processes, and age-related changes.[30–32] Mouth breathing at the end of life also produces oral dryness.[32]

In patients with cancer, xerostomia may occur due to physiologic changes to the oral mucosa known as "oral mucositis." These changes are strongly associated with chemotherapy and radiation treatments and may include erythema, ulcerations, and soft tissue damage that contribute to dry mouth.[33] Besides chemotherapeutic agents, other medications that induce xerostomia include sedatives, tranquilizers, antihistamines, anti-parkinsonian agents, antiepileptics, muscle relaxants, tricyclic antidepressants, and anticholinergics.[29,30–32] Xerostomia is common in advanced diabetes, renal failure, cardiac disease, liver disease, and autoimmune diseases such as AIDS and Sjögren's syndrome.[31]

Prolonged xerostomia can bring about secondary symptoms, including dental caries; oral pain and burning; lesions of the tongue, lips, gums, and oral mucosa; mouth infections such as candidiasis; taste changes; and bad breath.[29–31] Other problems include swallowing difficulties and alterations in speech.[30,31] Eating may be impaired due to chapped lips, difficulty chewing, and the need for frequent sips of liquid to mobilize food.[29,31]

Nursing Assessment of Xerostomia

Assessment should include a physical examination of the mouth and oral mucosa to identify signs of infection, gum disease, or dental problems. Examine the mouth for ulcers or mucositis, and check the tongue for erythema or fissures. Observe salivary glands for swelling, a sign of obstruction. Oral appliances and dentures should be noted and their fit and condition assessed. Assess for cracked lips, angular cheilitis (lip inflammation), or candidiasis at the corners of the mouth.

History should include onset and duration of xerostomia, any provoking factors, and interference with rest, swallowing, eating, or speech. Medication review may identify drug therapies that potentiate dry mouth. Use of a screening scale such as the OPQRSTUV acronym (onset, provoking/palliating factors, quality, region/radiation, severity time/treatment, understanding, values) may aid in the assessment and documentation of xerostomia.[34]

Nursing Interventions for Xerostomia

Initial interventions for xerostomia should focus on identifying and treating reversible causes. Underlying oral infections such as candida or mucositis should be treated with antifungals (nystatin, fluconazole) and oral rinses that promote healing. Medications that cause or exacerbate dry mouth should be eliminated. If discontinuing the medication is not possible, the nurse may recommend decreasing the dose or modifying the schedule so that it does not coincide with the diurnal decrease in saliva production that occurs after awakening.[24]

If xerostomia is interfering with the patient's ability to eat and drink, the nurse should offer strategies for adequate hydration and

Table 15.2 Nursing interventions for xerostomia

Intervention	Nursing considerations
Oral and dental care	Encourage frequent soft brushing, water jet, denture cleaning, fluoride rinses, and flossing as these can stimulate salivation and prevent oral infections.
Lip protectants	Apply lip balm, petroleum jelly, oils, and salves to protect lips and promote healing. Avoid products containing alcohol, since these can be irritating. For cheilitis at the corners of the mouth, protect with lanolin or KY jelly.
Mouthwashes	Encourage rinsing with peppermint water, oral rinses made with warm water and sodium bicarbonate, or glycerin to replenish moisture. Commercial mouthwashes should be alcohol-free to avoid irritation.
Artificial saliva	Educate patient that saliva substitutes are available over the counter in spray or gel formulas. They are most effective when used regularly every few hours. Many products contain carboxy-methylcellulose or mucin, which are animal products. Consider patient's religious beliefs and dietary preferences when recommending.
Chewing gum, mints	Recommend sugar-free gum/mints to prevent dental caries. Educate on the side effect of diarrhea from sorbitol if excessive sugar-free gum/mints are ingested. Consider the social acceptance of gum chewing, particularly in older populations.
Dietary modifications	Suggest soft-textured foods as they are better tolerated (soup, pudding, yogurt, mashed potatoes, smoothies or shakes). Instruct patient to take fluids with all meals. Add gravies and juices to food to aid swallowing. Apply olive oil to the gums and mucosa to act as a lubricant while eating. Educate patient regarding the avoidance of acidic and spicy foods as these may be painful and irritating. Carbonated drinks (ginger ale) or citrus juices (lemonade, pineapple, papaya) may be refreshing; however, citrus may be too irritating for patients with oral ulcerations.
Hydration	Encourage frequent sips of water or sprays from a small diffuser. Water may be warm or cold based on patient preference.
Procedural interventions	Laser treatment of the salivary glands and tongue is provided in an office setting and may provide more long-lasting relief than other nonpharmacological interventions. A less expensive alternative to laser treatment is electrostimulation of the salivary glands using a battery-powered device. Emerging evidence indicates that acupuncture may provide significant reduction in radiation-induced xerostomia.

Sources: References 24, 35, and 36.

encourage diet modifications that facilitate swallowing. Lip lubrication, small sips of water, and chewing gum or hard candies may improve difficulties in speaking. Humidification via a mask or face tent may help to loosen secretions, moisten the oropharyngeal mucosa, and maximize comfort. Above all, the nurse should encourage regular mouth care, tailored to the individual patient's needs.[35] See Table 15.2 for a summary of nursing interventions for xerostomia.

Medications may be effective at preventing or alleviating xerostomia, particularly when it occurs as a sequela of radiation therapy used to treat cancer. Muscarinic agonists (pilocarpine, bethanechol, cevimeline) work by activating the parasympathetic nerves to stimulate saliva production.[24] Pilocarpine is the most effective of these agents but also carries the greatest likelihood of side effects. In contrast, cevimeline produces fewer unwanted side effects but is generally less effective. With all muscarinic agonists, the nurse should provide education about side effects, including vision changes, sweating, nausea, diarrhea, urinary frequency, rhinitis, bradycardia, and bronchoconstriction. Muscarinic agonists are contraindicated in patients with pulmonary disease and should be used with caution in conjunction with beta-blockers.[29,31,32]

Dysgeusia

Etiology and Pathophysiology

Dysgeusia is an alteration or distortion in the perception of taste, usually described as being unpleasant. Patients may report taste sensations that are abnormally bitter, sour, salty, or metallic.[37] Dysgeusia occurs frequently among patients undergoing chemotherapy or radiation treatments.[38,39] This is likely because the turnover rate of taste bud receptor cells is only about 10 days, rendering them particularly susceptible to damage by cancer therapies that target cells with rapid turnover rates.[38,39]

Taste alterations also affect patients with neurologic diseases such as Parkinson's disease, ALS, multiple sclerosis, and dementia.[37] Other diseases associated with dysgeusia include diabetes, hypothyroidism, heart failure, and kidney or liver disease. Individuals infected with the COVID-19 virus have reported dysgeusia, often accompanied by anosmia (loss of the sense of smell).[37,38] Poor dental hygiene, mucosal or sinus infections, tobacco use, and diet are also risk factors.[37] Many medications cause dysgeusia, including antibiotics, migraine medications, anti-parkinsonian agents, muscle relaxants, angiotensin-converting enzyme inhibitors, antiarrhythmics, statins, diuretics, tricyclic antidepressants, antipsychotics, mood stabilizers, antihistamines, and bronchodilators.[37,40]

Consequences of prolonged dysgeusia include poor appetite, food aversions, decreased oral intake, and subsequent weight loss and malnutrition.[37,38,41] Furthermore, the associated inability to enjoy food and the social aspect of mealtimes may negatively impact overall quality of life.[37,38,41]

Nursing Assessment of Dysgeusia

Patient self-report is the standard in assessing taste disturbances. A physical exam should include oral inspection of teeth, gums, and tongue to identify any ulcerations or infections that may contribute to the symptom. History should include onset and duration of dysgeusia, any provoking factors, and impact on appetite and oral intake. Medication review is key to identify drug therapies that potentiate dysgeusia. The nurse should also assess for secondary symptoms, including weight loss and social withdrawal from mealtimes.

Nursing Interventions for Dysgeusia

Nursing interventions should focus on nonpharmacological approaches. Because taste alterations can dramatically impact appetite and enjoyment of food, the nurse should offer strategies to maintain adequate nutritional intake. Dietary interventions may include eating small, frequent meals; trying recipes that differ from the patient's usual choices; eating strongly flavored foods or conversely eating only bland foods; honoring specific food cravings; eating sugar-free candy before meals; cutting food with lemon; drinking sweetened beverages; using plastic cutlery to minimize metallic taste; and drinking from a straw.[42,43] The nurse should also recommend frequent oral care, including brushing one's teeth and tongue and cleansing the mouth with baking soda, salt rinses, or antibacterial mouthwash.[42]

Some patients report that consuming *Synsepalum dulcificum* (miracle fruit) prior to meals can mask unpleasant flavors and create positive taste changes that make food more appealing.[44] Zinc supplementation may proactively prevent radiation-induced dysgeusia but has a minimal effect on alleviating the symptom once it occurs.[45,46] Other medications such as dronabinol, alpha lipoic acid, biotin, gingko biloba, and glutamate have been suggested in the literature but have little or no evidence supporting their efficacy.[46] The nurse should advise patients who are considering such medications to discuss risks and benefits with their healthcare provider.

Conclusion

Dysphagia, hiccups, and other oral symptoms commonly occur in advanced disease processes and can cause significant burden for both the patient and the caregiver. Swallowing difficulties may not only impede adequate nutrition and hydration but also impact daily activities and social interactions. Symptoms such as hiccups, sialorrhea, xerostomia, and dysgeusia may seem inconsequential and are often overlooked by clinicians. However, these conditions are a visible aspect of a person's well-being.

Nurses are often the first to identify these symptoms and to understand their negative impact. Nursing interventions for dysphagia, hiccups, and oral symptoms in patients with serious illness focus on preventing functional decline, maximizing comfort and quality of life, and supporting the patient's wishes. Oral care is perhaps the most essential intervention for dysphagia, sialorrhea, xerostomia, and dysgeusia. Nurses should address continued oral care as a vital aspect of promoting dignity, comfort, and quality of life for patients with troublesome oral symptoms.

Acknowledgment

The authors would like to acknowledge previous senior author Constance M. Dahlin, whose significant prior contributions remain a foundation for this chapter.

REFERENCES

1. Moreira MJDS, Guimarães MF, Lopes L, Moreti F. Contributions of speech-language pathology in palliative and end-of-life care. *Codas*. 2020;32(4):e20190202.
2. Hui D, dos Santos R, Chisholm GB, Bruera E. Symptom expression in the last seven days of life among cancer patients admitted to acute palliative care units. *J Pain Symptom Manage.* 2015;50(4):488–494.
3. Corbin-Lewis K, Liss JM. *Clinical Anatomy and Physiology of the Swallow Mechanism*. 2nd ed. Cengage Learning; 2015.
4. Logemann JA. *Evaluation and Treatment of Swallowing Disorders*. 2nd ed. Pro-Ed; 1998.
5. Panara K, Ramezanpour Ahangar E, Padalia D. Physiology, swallowing. In: *StatPearls*. StatPearls Publishing; 2022.
6. Bolser DC, Gestreau C, Morris KF, Davenport PW, Pitts TE. Central neural circuits for coordination of swallowing, breathing, and coughing: predictions from computational modeling and simulation. *Otolaryngol Clin North Am*. 2013;46(6):957–964.
7. Goyal RK, Chaudhury A. Physiology of normal esophageal motility. *J Clin Gastroenterol*. 2008;42(5):610–619.
8. Roe J, George R. When a little may be just enough? Caring for people with swallowing difficulties at the end of life, and their caregivers. *Perspect ASHA Spec Interest Groups*. 2016;1(13):89–93.
9. Altman KW, Yu GP, Schaefer SD. Consequence of dysphagia in the hospitalized patient: impact on prognosis and hospital resources. *Arch Otolaryngol Head Neck Surg*. 2010;136(8):784–789.
10. Bassi D, Furkim AM, Silva CA, et al. Identification of risk groups for oropharyngeal dysphagia in hospitalized patients in a university hospital. *Codas*. 2014;26(1):17–27.
11. Leder SB, Suiter DM, Agogo GO, Cooney LM Jr. An epidemiologic study on ageing and dysphagia in the acute care geriatric-hospitalized population: a replication and continuation study. *Dysphagia*. 2016;31(5):619–625.
12. Eltringham SA, Kilner K, Gee M, et al. Impact of dysphagia assessment and management on risk of stroke-associated pneumonia: a systematic review. *Cerebrovasc Dis*. 2018;46(3–4):99–107.
13. Murry T, Carrau RL, Chan K. *Clinical Management of Swallowing Disorders*. 4th ed. Plural Publishing; 2016.
14. Groher M, Crary, M. *Dysphagia: Clinical Management in Adults and Children*. 2nd ed. Elsevier; 2016.
15. Daniels SK, Anderson JA, Willson PC. Valid items for screening dysphagia risk in patients with stroke: a systematic review. *Stroke*. 2012;43(3):892–897.
16. Cheney DM, Siddiqui MT, Litts JK, Kuhn MA, Belafsky PC. The ability of the 10-item Eating Assessment Tool (EAT-10) to predict aspiration risk in persons with dysphagia. *Ann Otol Rhinol Laryngol*. 2015;124(5):351–354.
17. International Dysphagia Diet Standardisation Initiative. What Is the IDDSI Framework? Accessed September 27, 2022. http://iddsi.org/framework/.
18. Strickland SL, Rubin BK, Drescher GS, et al. AARC clinical practice guideline: effectiveness of nonpharmacologic airway clearance therapies in hospitalized patients. *Respir Care*. 2013;58(12):2187–2193.
19. Chatwin M, Toussaint M, Gonçalves MR, et al. Airway clearance techniques in neuromuscular disorders: a state of the art review. *Respir Med*. 2018;136:98–110.
20. Calsina-Berna A, Garcia-Gomez G, Gonzalez-Barboteo J, Porta-Sales J. Treatment of chronic hiccups in cancer patients: a systematic review. *J Palliat Med*. 2012;15(10):1142–1150.
21. Kohse EK, Hollmann MW, Bardenheuer HJ, Kessler J. Chronic hiccups: an underestimated problem. *Anesth Analg*. 2017;125(4):1169–1183.
22. Polito NB, Fellows SE. Pharmacologic interventions for intractable and persistent hiccups: a systematic review. *J Emerg Med*. 2017;53(4):540–549.

23. Moretto EN, Wee B, Wiffen PJ, Murchison AG. Interventions for treating persistent and intractable hiccups in adults. *Cochrane Database Syst Rev*. 2013;2013(1):CD008768.
24. Dahlin C, Cohen A, Goldsmith T. Dysphagia, xerostomia, and hiccups. In: Ferrell BR, Coyle N, Paice JA, eds. *Oxford Textbook of Palliative Nursing*. 4th Ed. Oxford University Press; 2015:191–216.
25. Paine CC, Snider JW. When saliva becomes a problem: the challenges and palliative care for patients with sialorrhea. *Ann Palliat Med*. 2020;9(3):1333–1339.
26. James E, Ellis C, Brassington R, Sathasivam S, Young CA. Treatment for sialorrhea (excessive saliva) in people with motor neuron disease/amyotrophic lateral sclerosis. *Cochrane Database Syst Rev*. 2022;5(5):CD006981.
27. Abdelnour-Mallet M, Tezenas Du Montcel S, Cazzolli PA, et al. Validation of robust tools to measure sialorrhea in amyotrophic lateral sclerosis: a study in a large French cohort. *Amyotroph Lateral Scler Frontotemporal Degener*. 2013;14(4):302–307.
28. McGeachan AJ, McDermott CJ. Management of oral secretions in neurological disease. *Pract Neurol*. 2017;17(2):96–103.
29. Thakkar JP, Lane CJ. Hyposalivation and xerostomia and burning mouth syndrome: medical management. *Oral Maxillofac Surg Clin*. 2022;34(1):135–146.
30. Turner MD. Hyposalivation and xerostomia: etiology, complications, and medical management. *Dent Clin North Am*. 2016;60(2):435–443.
31. Millsop JW, Wang EA, Fazel N. Etiology, evaluation, and management of xerostomia. *Clin Dermatol*. 2017;35(5):468–476.
32. Donaldson M, Goodchild JH. A systematic approach to xerostomia diagnosis and management. *Compend Contin Educ Dent*. 2018;39(suppl 5):1–9.
33. Sroussi HY, Epstein JB, Bensadoun RJ, et al. Common oral complications of head and neck cancer radiation therapy: mucositis, infections, saliva change, fibrosis, sensory dysfunctions, dental caries, periodontal disease, and osteoradionecrosis. *Cancer Med*. 2017;6(12):2918–2931.
34. Cancer Care Ontario. Algorithm: xerostomia in adults with cancer. Accessed October 3, 2022. Xerostomia & salivary hypofunction in adults with cancer. The full link is: https://www.cancercareontario.ca/en/symptom-management/3156.
35. Kvalheim SF, Strand GV. A narrative of oral care in palliative patients. *International J Environ Res Public Health*. 2022;19(10):6306.
36. Ni X, Tian T, Chen D, et al. Acupuncture for radiation-induced xerostomia in cancer patients: a systematic review and meta-analysis. *Integr Cancer Ther*. 2020;19:1534735420980825.
37. Jafari A, Alaee A, Ghods K. The etiologies and considerations of dysgeusia: a review of literature. *J Oral Biosci*. 2021;63(4):319–326.
38. Gaillard D, Barlow LA. A mechanistic overview of taste bud maintenance and impairment in cancer therapies. *Chemical Senses*. 2021;46:bjab011.
39. Togni L, Mascitti M, Vignini A, et al. Treatment-related dysgeusia in oral and oropharyngeal cancer: a comprehensive review. *Nutrients*. 2021;13(10):3325.
40. Mortazavi H, Shafiei S, Sadr S, Safiaghdam H. Drug-related dysgeusia: a systematic review. *Oral Health Prev Dent*. 2018;16(6):499–507.
41. Ponticelli E, Clari M, Frigerio S, et al. Dysgeusia and health-related quality of life of cancer patients receiving chemotherapy: a cross-sectional study. *Eur J Cancer Care*. 2017;26:e1261.
42. Speck RM, DeMichele A, Farrar JT, et al. Taste alteration in breast cancer patients treated with taxane chemotherapy: experience, effect, and coping strategies. *Support Care Cancer*. 2013;21(2):549–555.
43. Rehwaldt M, Wickham R, Purl S, et al. Self-care strategies to cope with taste changes after chemotherapy. *Oncol Nurs Forum*. 2009;36(2):e47–e56.
44. Wilken MK, Satiroff BA. Pilot study of "miracle fruit" to improve food palatability for patients receiving chemotherapy. *Clin J Oncol Nurs*. 2012;16(5):e173–e177.
45. Chi WJ, Myers JN, Frank SJ, et al. The effects of zinc on radiation-induced dysgeusia: a systematic review and meta-analysis. *Support Care Cancer*. 2020;28:1–12.
46. Nagraj SK, George RP, Shetty N, Levenson D, Ferraiolo DM, Shrestha A. Interventions for managing taste disturbances. *Cochrane Database Syst Rev*. 2017;12(12):CD010470.

16

Bowel Management: Constipation, Obstruction, Diarrhea, and Ascites

Serena Snow and Cameron Jennings

Key Points

- Constipation and diarrhea are common symptoms for persons with serious and life-threatening illness and should be assessed and managed to reduce symptom burden and impact on quality of life.
- Malignant bowel obstruction and ascites can be challenging complications that require diligent assessment and an individualized management plan.
- Palliative care for bowel management requires nursing assessment, patient education, pharmacologic management, coaching, and support of individual care goals.

Constipation

Case Study 1: A Patient with Parkinson's Disease

Mr. H is an 81-year-old male with advanced Parkinson's disease. He is started on a short course of opioid analgesia after sustaining a fracture from a fall. During a clinic visit, he mentions that he has not had a bowel movement in 4 days and feels uncomfortable. He has tried increasing fluids and fiber in his diet and is taking over-the-counter stool softeners without relief.

Prevalence and Impact

Constipation is a common symptom worldwide. It is estimated to be experienced by 16% of adults and 33.5% of older adults aged 60 and above.[1] Prevalence is higher among specific populations including community-dwelling older adults, those in long-term care facilities, and persons with advanced cancer.[2–4] For persons with serious and life-threatening illness, constipation can compound overall disease burden. A systematic review of palliative care–related problems affecting adults with nine different disease types found the prevalence of constipation ranging from 4% to 65%.[5]

Definitions

There is no widely agreed-upon definition for constipation. *Oxford Reference* defines constipation as a condition in which bowel evacuations occur infrequently, in which the feces are hard and small, or where passage of the feces causes difficulty or pain.[6] The Rome I criteria were established in 1994 to objectively define clinical or functional constipation. In 2016, the revised Rome IV criteria were published, including new diagnostic criteria for opioid-induced constipation (OIC). Table 16.1 provides an overview of the Rome IV criteria for both chronic constipation and OIC.[7] Given the symptom duration requirements to fulfill the Rome IV criteria for clinical constipation, it may be less useful for applying to persons with life-threatening illness. Dzierżanowski and Larkin propose that constipation in palliative care should include objective and subjective measures within a reasonably short observation period and diagnosed if at least one of the following reaches or surpasses the cutoff value: difficulty in defecation of ≥2 on a 0–4 scale, last bowel movement ≥2 days, and frequency of bowel movement ≤3 times per week.[8]

Pathophysiology and Risk Factors

The normal gastrointestinal (GI) physiology is complicated and involves a combination of fluid regulation and intrinsic and extrinsic neurologic factors. The act of having a bowel movement, or defecation, requires the coordination of neural, muscular, hormonal, and cognitive systems. The process to expel feces from the body is influenced by dietary intake, GI transit time, and stool volume/consistency. While wide variations exist, frequency of defecation is most commonly reported as three bowel movements per day to three bowel movements per week.[9] Risk factors associated with constipation include female sex, increased age, lower socioeconomic status, depression, physical and sexual abuse, and stressful life events.[10] The relationships between the presence of constipation and the gut–brain axis, gut microbiome and permeability, and altered immune function are still being explored.[11]

Constipation can be broken down into primary and secondary causes. Primary causes of functional constipation are categorized as slow-transit constipation, normal-transit constipation, and

Table 16.1 Rome IV diagnostic criteria for constipation

Chronic constipation	**Opioid-induced constipation**
Over the past 3 months with initial onset at least 6 months prior: Two or more of the following are present: • Straining more than 25% of bowel movements • Lumpy/hard stools more than 25% of bowel movements • Sensation of incomplete evacuation more than 25% of bowel movements • Sensation of anorectic obstruction or blockage more than 25% of bowel movements • Manual maneuvers to facilitate more than 25% of bowel movements (e.g., digital evacuation, pelvic floor support) • Fewer than three spontaneous bowel movements per week Additionally: • Loose stools are rarely present without laxative use • Criteria are not met for the diagnosis of irritable bowel syndrome	After initiating, changing, or increasing opioid therapy: Two or more of the following are present: • Straining more than 25% of bowel movements • Lumpy/hard stools more than 25% of bowel movements • Sensation of incomplete evacuation more than 25% of bowel movements • Sensation of anorectic obstruction or blockage more than 25% of bowel movements • Manual maneuvers to facilitate more than 25% of bowel movements (e.g., digital evacuation, pelvic floor support) • Fewer than three spontaneous bowel movements per week Additionally: • Loose stools are rarely present without laxative use

Source: Reference 7.

Table 16.2 Secondary causes of constipation

Type	Examples	
Iatrogenic	Medications Treatment side effects	
Metabolic	Hypercalcemia Hypokalemia Hyponatremia Hypomagnesemia Prolonged hyperglycemia Hyperparathyroidism Hypothyroidism	
Neurologic	Cerebral tumors Multiple sclerosis Parkinson's disease Spinal cord injury Stroke	
Psychologic	Anxiety Depression Psychosomatic conditions	
Pharmacologic	Analgesics	Morphine, oxycodone, ibuprofen
	Antacids	Calcium-containing, aluminum-containing
	Antiemetics	Ondansetron
	Anticonvulsants	Carbamazepine
	Antidepressants	Amitriptyline, phenelzine
	Antihistamines	Diphenhydramine
	Antihypertensives	Verapamil
	Antineoplastics	Vincristine, cyclophosphamide
	Antipsychotics	Chlorpromazine, clozapine, haloperidol
	Antispasmodics	Dicyclomine
	Bile acid sequestrants	Cholestyramine
	Diuretics	Furosemide
	Endocrine agents	Alendronate
	Mineral supplements	Calcium-containing, iron-containing
Structural	Abdominal wall weakness Malignancy Metastases Pelvic floor dysfunction Surgical adhesions Surgical interruption of gastrointestinal tract	

Sources: References 1, 4, and 12.

defecatory evacuation disorders.[12] Secondary causes of constipation are listed in Table 16.2.

OIC

One of the most common causes of constipation in palliative care is opioid-induced bowel dysfunction (OIBD). Higher doses and longer duration of opioid use further increase the risk for OIBD.[13,14] OIBD occurs when the opioid binds to opioid receptors within the gut. OIBD includes the collective GI-related side effects of nausea, vomiting, dry mouth, gastroesophageal reflux, abdominal cramping, bloating, spasm, and constipation. Of these, OIC is the most frequently reported.[15] Unlike most opioid side effects which improve over time, constipation does not.[16] OIC is frequently designated as a subtype of secondary constipation given its own pathophysiology, with a prevalence ranging between 40% and 60%.[4] Enteric mu-receptors are activated in the small intestine and proximal colon, with reduction in peristalsis, increased ileocecal valve tone, shifts in fluid and electrolytes, and increased anal sphincter tone. Combined, this results in harder, drier stools and less effective, less frequent defecation.[16,17]

Assessment

History

A review of past medical, surgical, and social history as well as history of or presenting illness should be completed to identify factors that may be contributing to the constipation. Key elements of constipation assessment are found in Box 16.1. It is important for nurses to inquire about recent change in fluid and oral intake. However, bowel movements are still expected even in the absence of oral intake since food, sloughed cells of the GI tract, and bacteria all contribute to total stool content.

Patients with constipation may report bloating, early satiety, abdominal pain, nausea, vomiting, and malaise. Many scales have been proposed to better understand a patient's symptoms. The Constipation Assessment Scale and the Bowel Function Index are two commonly used screens that are reliable and validated, which both pertain to symptoms over the prior 7 days but differ in administration, rating, and scoring.[14,18] These screens are also practical to

Box 16.1 Key Elements of Constipation Assessment

- Date of last bowel movement
- Frequency of bowel movements
- Effort to move bowels
- Sensation of evaluation (complete or incomplete)
- Stool consistency
- Recent changes in bowel pattern
- Current and previous laxative use
- Urge to defecate (present or absent)
- Stool incontinence or rectal leakage
- Warning signs and symptoms—unintentional weight loss, blood in stool or rectal bleeding, dark/tarry stools, severe nausea or abdominal pain, change in stool caliber, family history of colon cancer
- Importance of regular bowel movement to patient
- Environmental factors affecting bowel movements

Sources: References 4 and 21.

use across different clinical settings. In cases of altered mental status, constipation can be evaluated on an objective basis using observable criteria and caregiver assessment.[8] It is also important to assess for signs and symptoms that could indicate a serious issue (e.g., bloody or melenic stools, severe and intractable nausea or abdominal pain, significant weight loss, concurrent anemia, family history of GI malignancy).[19]

Physical Examination

An abdominal exam should include visual inspection for surgical scars, distension, or skin changes. Auscultation can provide information on whether the bowels are moving, and percussion may be dull over a colon filled with stool versus tympanic over areas filled with gas. A rectal exam should be performed to exclude fecal impaction or diagnose external hemorrhoids, fissures, or ulcerations except with patients who have either thrombocytopenia or neutropenia, which increase the risk of bleeding and infection, respectively. The presence of bloody stool may be suggestive of hemorrhoids, colitis, or tumor. A neurologic examination can identify central nervous system or spinal cord abnormalities that could predispose a patient to constipation and is suggested for patients where a neurologic cause is suspected.[7]

Diagnostic Studies

Constipation is heterogeneous, and no one test provides a pathophysiologic etiology. If a bowel obstruction is not a concern, routine blood tests, radiologic examination, and endoscopy are not recommended.[4,20] Calcium, magnesium, potassium, sodium, glucose, and thyroid levels should be considered if metabolic disorder is suspected. Additional investigation with abdominal radiographs or computed tomography (CT) may be considered to exclude bowel obstruction when aligned with individual care goals.

Nursing Interventions and Supportive Care

The aim of constipation management is to re-establish comfortable bowel habits and alleviate discomfort while honoring patient preferences.[21] Concurrently, the goal is to prevent or relieve complications including early satiety, nausea, vomiting, abdominal distension, abdominal pain, overflow diarrhea, hemorrhoids, anal tears, bowel obstruction, or fecal impaction. Nurses should provide education, coaching, and guidance for patients regarding oral intake, bowel regimen, expectations, and maintenance plan. Optimizing dignity and privacy are essential, especially when use of a bedpan or bedside commode is required.

Regarding food and fluid intake, there is limited evidence that increasing oral fluids helps with constipation except for those with dehydration.[22] Patients can be encouraged to increase their dietary fiber intake, aiming for 20–30 g per day. The increase of fiber should be completed over weeks, not days, to minimize GI discomfort. Whole-fiber foods such as prunes and apricots can also be encouraged for functional constipation.[23] Whole fruits and vegetables have been found to be more effective in increasing daily bowel movements compared to 100% fruit and vegetable juices.[24] Avoidance of fermented dairy products, red meat, and processed foods may also be helpful.[22]

Current evidence does not support the use of exercise to manage constipation, which may be technically challenging and a safety concern for persons with serious illness. Expert opinion suggests that activity be increased as able. More importantly, allowing for privacy, easy access to facilities or commode, and establishing and maintaining a routine (colonic motility is highest in the morning) are simple interventions that can help prevent and improve constipation.[22] Abdominal massage added to a laxative regimen was shown to improve constipation greater than laxative or massage alone, suggesting it may be a helpful adjunct that can be performed by nursing staff or a trained caregiver.[25] Using a defecation posture modification device or footstool helps straighten the anorectal angle and was found to decrease defecatory time, reduce straining, and promote complete evacuation of bowels in healthy study participants.[26] Biofeedback can be effective for persons who have constipation associated with pelvic floor dyssynergia but may not be widely available or practical for persons with serious or life-threatening illness.[2,20] When indicated, manual fecal disimpaction is a nursing intervention that can provide significant relief.

Pharmacologic Management

An initial pharmacologic approach includes avoidance of constipating medications and using alternatives when possible. In patients taking opioids, a prophylactic bowel regimen is recommended unless otherwise contraindicated.[27,28] As opioid doses increase, the bowel regimen should be adjusted accordingly. There are several classes of oral laxatives which are used to improve bowel elimination and often recommended as first-line therapies due to their efficacy and low cost. Nurses are likely to be asked about different medications and their affects. They may also encounter over-the-counter medications used for bowel management during medication reconciliation.

Bulk Laxatives

Bulk laxatives or bulk-forming laxatives such as psyllium and methylcellulose are indicated for patients with mild constipation and irritable bowel syndrome (IBS-C). They are typically not effective as monotherapy in patients with OIC[29] and should be avoided in those with significantly reduced physical activity and poor fluid intake due to increased risk of bowel obstruction.[13] They are likely to only be effective in those with adequate fluid intake and low fiber intake.[17]

Surfactant (Detergent, Emollient, Softener) Laxatives

Stool softeners such as docusate sodium and docusate calcium are surfactant agents that cause hydration and softening of the stool.[2] Surfactants work by decreasing the surface tension of the stool; but while the stool may become softer, surfactants do not induce laxation.

Osmotic Laxatives

Osmotic laxatives retain more fluid in the intestine, therefore hydrating and loosening the stool. Osmotic laxatives include medications such as polyethylene glycol (PEG), lactulose, and magnesium citrate. Although safe and effective, side effects of abdominal bloating and flatulence can occur.[2] Osmotic laxatives should be avoided in patients with suspected or known partial or complete bowel obstruction. Although rare, fluid and electrolyte abnormalities may also result, and laxatives containing magnesium should be avoided in patients with renal dysfunction, while laxatives with sodium should be avoided in patients with congestive heart failure, hypertension, and edema.[30]

PEG is a powder preparation that is mixed with water, is typically well tolerated, and is not absorbed systemically, which significantly reduces the side effect profile. Additionally, studies suggest superiority in stool frequency over lactulose for patients with chronic constipation.[30] Lactulose is an osmotic laxative in liquid form which is also commonly used but can have poor adherence due to common side effects of bloating, flatulence, abdominal discomfort, and hyperglycemia. Sorbitol is another hyperosmotic laxative that is less expensive and less likely to cause nausea and vomiting than lactulose. This should be used cautiously in patients with diabetes, cardiopulmonary disease, or renal disease due to the risks of hyperglycemia and fluid/electrolyte imbalance.[30] Magnesium is a component of many saline laxatives, which are sometimes used for acute evacuation due to rapid onset, typically within 1–6 hours. Use is limited due to increased risk of electrolyte abnormality.

Stimulant Laxatives

Stimulant laxatives such as bisacodyl and sennosides are available over the counter at a low cost and function by stimulating secretion of fluid in the colon and acting as a prokinetic in the colon. Bisacodyl has been shown to help prevent constipation related to opioid use if given prophylactically.[15]

Laxative-refractory constipation implies no response to scheduled use of laxatives from one or more of the above classes of laxatives for at least 4 days.[17] In this case, additional therapies are available. They have proven safe and effective but are often costly and may have limitations in persons with serious and life-threatening illness.

Peripherally Acting Mu Opioid Receptor Antagonists

Peripherally acting mu opioid receptor antagonists (PAMORAs) function by blocking mu opioid receptors in the GI tract, leading to improved peristalsis. Nalmedine, naloxegol, naloxone, and methylnaltrexone are examples of PAMORAs that are sometimes used in the setting of OIC in patients who have chronic noncancer pain.[31] They can help regulate the GI tract but can potentially cause side effects such as abdominal pain, nausea/vomiting, and diarrhea. Rarely, opioid withdrawal can be experienced by the patient, so the nurse should be alert to concurrent opioid use if these medications are used.[31]

Chloride Channel Activators

A common medication in this category, lubiprostone, leads to increased fluid secretion and motility, resulting in improvement in straining, abdominal bloating and discomfort, and severity of constipation.[30,32,33] The nurse should be alert to concern of bowel obstruction and use of methadone, which would affect use of lupirostone.

Guanylate Cyclase-C Receptor Agonists

Examples of medications in this class include linaclotide and plecanatide. Though their use is often limited due to cost, they can provide some relief in visceral hypersensitivity and bloating related to constipation. Common side effects include diarrhea and are also contraindicated in those patients with bowel obstruction.

Selective Serotonin Agonists

Prucalopride is a selective serotonin (5-HT4) receptor agonist used to increase fluid secretion into the intestine, stimulate intestinal motility, and improve gastrointestinal pain. The most common side effects include diarrhea, abdominal bloating, abdominal pain, and diarrhea. The nurse should also be aware that, although uncommon, exacerbation of depression or suicidality could occur due to the increase in serotonin.[2,34–37]

Probiotics

Probiotics are substances that benefit a host by altering the balance of helpful to harmful microorganisms. Some studies have demonstrated alterations in the microbiome of patients with IBS-C and subsequent improvement in stool frequency and consistency with use of certain probiotic strains,[38,39] such as *Bifidobacterium animalis*, *Lactobacillus acidophilus*, and *Lactobacillus casei*.[40]

Case Study 1: Continued

Mr. H has multiple risk factors for constipation, including advanced age, baseline Parkinson's disease, and recent addition of opioid analgesia. Exam shows mild abdominal distension and hypoactive bowel sounds but is otherwise benign. Mr. H is told to add two tablets of sennosides at bedtime, in addition to PEG daily as needed. One week later he reports having regular bowel movements four to five times per week and that his pain and constipation are managed.

Malignant Bowel Obstruction

Case Study 2: A Patient with Ovarian Cancer

Ms. B is a 52-year-old woman with advanced ovarian cancer and prior abdominal surgeries. She is currently receiving palliative chemotherapy. She presents with acute-onset nausea with bilious emesis and abdominal pain. She reports one small, watery bowel movement last night but has not been able to keep down any intake including food, liquids, or medications for the last 2 days.

Definition and Prevalence

Malignant bowel obstruction (MBO) occurs when the physiologic transit and digestive process are interrupted due to involvement of malignancy from cancer or its treatments. Approximately 3%–15% of all patients with cancer will develop MBO.[41] It is most common in patients with GI and gynecologic cancers, affecting 10%–30% of persons with GI malignancies and up to 60% of persons with gynecologic malignancies.[42] MBO may be the presenting symptom of intra-abdominal malignancy or the first sign of tumor recurrence. Symptoms commonly associated with MBO include nausea, emesis, colicky abdominal pain, distension, and obstipation.[42–44] When MBO occurs early and in surgically fit persons, average survival is about 8 months.[42,45] In persons with advanced cancer and inoperable MBO, average survival is 4–5 weeks.[41,42] There has been little change in survival outcomes for MBO over the last decade.[46]

Pathophysiology and Risk Factors

MBO results from mechanical or functional obstruction. Mechanical obstruction is more common and is caused by both intrinsic and extrinsic compression. Functional obstructions may be related to nerve involvement or iatrogenic causes. Obstruction may be partial or complete, unifocal or involving multiple areas of the intestine. About 61% of MBO cases start in the small intestine, 33% in the large intestine, and 20% in both simultaneously.[41,43] Advanced age, male sex, multiple comorbidities, and weight loss are all risk factors for increased mortality.[47]

MBO occurs when intestinal intraluminal pressure is increased, and a vicious cycle develops involving distension, secretions, and contractions. The cycle can lead to fluid and electrolyte disorders, changes in the acid–base balance, and reduced circulatory blood volume.[43] Bacterial overgrowth and translocation contribute to worsening symptoms.[48] Advanced MBO progression can lead to severe infection, multiorgan failure, shock, and death.[43]

Assessment

History

Nurses should inquire about any medications the patient may be taking that slow the gut as well as a history of a bowel obstruction, abdominal surgery, radiation, or chemotherapy. A previous obstruction is important to know as studies have shown that more than half of patients with resolved MBO later develop recurrent obstruction.[41] Early symptoms of periumbilical abdominal pain, anorexia, and large-volume bilious emesis are more commonly associated with small bowel obstruction (SBO). Symptoms associated with large bowel obstruction (LBO) include localized, colicky abdominal pain; marked abdominal distension; and foul small-volume emesis.[42,49] Anorexia and dehydration are often present and occur more frequently in SBO due to nausea with emesis.[49] Obstipation lasting more than 72 hours may signal more definitive obstruction,[42] though loose stools may continue to occur if obstruction is only partial.

Physical Examination

Abdominal examination should include inspection for surgical scars and hernias as well as abdominal distension and any tenderness. Percussion may yield a tympanic sound more indicative of air, or a dull sound is more suggestive of ascites or stool. Auscultation of bowel sounds may yield a hyperactive "tinkling" sound or borborygmi or absent bowel sounds with paralytic ileus.[50] A rectal exam can exclude fecal impaction but should be avoided when the patient has neutropenia or thrombocytopenia.

Diagnostic Studies

Diagnostic testing may be impacted by the patient's tolerability of workup and care goals. Abdominal radiographs have the benefit of low cost, wide availability, low radiation exposure, and speed of obtaining; but accuracy for diagnosis ranges from 50% to 75%.[41] Abdominal CT is the gold standard for diagnosing MBO.[41,51] CT has a sensitivity and a specificity of greater than 90%[41] and can localize obstruction, evaluate completeness, and identify risk factors like carcinomatosis or adhesions. It can also rule out surgical emergencies. Ultrasound, magnetic resonance imaging (MRI), and contrast studies/fluoroscopy are not first-line diagnostic tests for MBO.[51]

Nursing Interventions and Supportive Care

Specific individual factors should be considered when determining management options including age, nutritional status, tumor grade, history of cancer therapies, expected survival time, and treatment expectations.[43] Goals of management should be individualized with consideration of alleviating burdensome symptoms, promoting oral intake, and promoting return to preferred care setting with minimal additional morbidity.[52] A systematic review of persons living with MBO highlighted the need for healthcare providers to address psychosocial distress around interventions, loss of social norms like eating, and the lack of predictability of MBO in addition to managing physical symptoms.[53] The hospitalization of a patient with MBO is a prognostically significant event[45] and should prompt discussion of the patient's priorities and preferences for care. Given the high morbidity and mortality associated with inoperable obstruction, it is reasonable to discuss the option of hospice care, which focuses on quality of life (QOL) and supportive and pharmacologic management of symptoms. Patients should understand that even when obstruction does resolve, there is a high rate of recurrence.[54,55]

Patients who present with MBO are often placed *nil per os* (NPO) to help manage nausea. Intravenous hydration and electrolyte replacement may help improve bowel motility. Nasogastric tube (NGT) decompression is a common early intervention in MBO and is most helpful for patients with SBO with intractable nausea and vomiting. Bowel rest and gastric decompression alone can result in resolution of obstruction without further intervention. Anticipated duration of intervention, practical issues, and body image should be addressed. Complications most commonly include discomfort, epistaxis, or sinusitis. Duration of NGT can contribute to other complications including aspiration, pressure ulcers and necrosis from tube pressure on the nare, and abdominal lining irritation with possible GI bleed.[56] In general, parenteral nutrition is not recommended for patients with MBO and concomitant terminal cachexia and may worsen symptoms by contributing to ascites, worsening pleural effusions, increasing GI secretions, and causing metabolic abnormalities.[57] A Cochrane review was unable to conclude that home parenteral nutrition improves survival or QOL in people with MBO.[58]

Surgical Management

There are no well-defined criteria for surgical candidacy in MBO. Surgical intervention may include lysis of adhesion, tumor debulking, bowel resection with anastomosis, intestinal bypass, or ostomy. Up to 50% of patients who undergo surgical intervention may later reobstruct,[54,55] an important consideration as nurses help support patients and families through their decision-making. A meta-analysis of palliative interventions for MBO in ovarian cancer found that surgery prolonged survival period and relieved symptoms of obstruction but did not impact recurrence rates, and the surgical group had a higher 30-day mortality compared with the non-surgical group.[52]

Procedural Management

A venting gastrostomy tube (VGT) for MBO has been shown to relieve symptoms in 77%–100% of patients.[46] For patients who desire food for oral gratification, VGT may allow the opportunity to enjoy the taste of food, modified for elimination by the tube. A study of older adults with MBO comparing venting gastrostomy, surgery, and medical management found that VGT was associated with fewer readmissions, increased hospice enrollment, and less time in the intensive care unit and inpatient death.[45] In VGTs placed for gastric decompression, it is important to provide education that the goal is to relieve symptoms and not for enteral nutrition.

The percutaneous transesophageal gastrotube (PTEG) was developed as a novel, minimally invasive technique to provide gastric drainage or supplemental nutrition. Use of the PTEG has been limited in North America to date, but for a small cohort of patients in a palliative care setting, PTEG was found to be safe and well tolerated.[59]

The self-expandable metal stent (SEMS) is a procedural intervention that can benefit patients with unifocal obstruction, with obstruction relieved 83%–100% of the time.[60,61] A review on palliative treatment for malignant colorectal obstruction found that SEMS resulted in better short-term outcomes (complications, mortality, QOL), fewer stoma constructions, and shorter duration of hospital stay versus emergency surgery.[62] For single-level LBO in the absence of perforation, SEMS is the preferred management alternative.[48]

Pharmacologic Management

It is important to note that inoperable MBO may resolve in more than a third of patients receiving supportive and pharmacologic management alone.[41] Oral administration of medications is typically avoided in MBO due to risk of worsening nausea and poor absorption. Nurses are likely to use non-oral routes including intravenous (IV), subcutaneous (SC), intramuscular (IM), transdermal (TD), sublingual, and rectal (PR) routes. Nurses should also be aware that in MBO many medications are utilized off-label.

Antiemetics

Steroids, neuroleptics, and serotonin (5-HT3) antagonists are examples of commonly used antiemetics in this situation. Ondansetron, prochlorperazine, promethazine, and cannabis have not been found to be effective antiemetics in MBO management and are not recommended as first- or second-line treatments.[44]

The Multinational Association for Supportive Care in Cancer (MASCC) suggests that steroids can be used for short-term benefit and may help with acute obstruction.[48] Dexamethasone is typically the steroid of choice given lower mineralocorticoid activity, leading to less fluid retention. While the therapeutic trial period is undetermined, it is reasonable to discontinue if there is no response after 4–5 days.[63]

Neuroleptics decrease nausea by acting as central dopamine antagonists.[64] Many experts consider haloperidol, a butyrophenone antipsychotic, a first-line option due to a lower rate of sedation and lower anticholinergic side effects compared to chlorpromazine.[65] MASCC suggest that haloperidol may be an effective antiemetic, especially in the setting of complete MBO. A similar level of evidence suggests that chlorpromazine, a phenothiazide, may also reduce nausea and vomiting in MBO.[48]

Dopamine antagonist prokinetic agents such as metoclopramide can also be considered but with a caveat: use should be avoided in a patient with complete obstruction as it may paradoxically worsen abdominal pain and nausea and increase risk of bowel perforation.[48,65] There is less evidence for olanzapine, a thienobenzodiazeopene (second-generation) antipsychotic to manage symptoms of MBO; but it is suggested that it may reduce nausea and vomiting in MBO.[48]

Studies have suggested that 5-HT3 antagonists may help control emesis when used in combination with dexamethasone,[48] but because constipation is a common side effect, other alternatives are preferred, especially in patients with ileus.

Antisecretory Agents

MASCC guidelines recommend with a strong level and grade of evidence that somatostatin analogues may reduce vomiting in MBO.[48] Octreotide has been studied the most and has the most evidence to support its use for hypersecretion management in MBO.[42] Due to the short half-life and 6–12-hour duration of action, multiple daily doses are needed.[48] An IM depot version can be given every 28 days; however, steady state takes a week to reach, so immediate-release dosing is often given for 6 days after initiation.

Anticholinergics

This is a large group of medications that have antiemetic effects on the vestibular center, as well as antispasmodic and antisecretory effects. Common side effects are dry mouth and urinary retention. Scopolamine is one option and can be administered via continuous IV or SC infusion or more conveniently as a TD patch. Glycopyrrolate is sometimes used instead of scopolamine related to lower risk of potentiating delirium as it poorly crosses the blood–brain barrier.

Laxatives

Per expert consensus, oral osmotic laxatives may be used in managing impaired bowel movements if there is partial obstruction. They are not recommended in the setting of complete MBO and should be avoided. Enemas should not be given in MBO due to increased risk of perforation.[48]

Analgesics

There is no evidence to support the use of opioids for MBO-related pain; more research is needed. Despite this, opioid analgesia is commonly used for pain from MBO.[48] Commonly used non-oral opioid routes include PR, TD, and IV or SC patient-controlled analgesia (PCA). Oral concentrate formulation of opioids given sublingually may provide relief to patients with low opioid requirements since bioavailability is approximately 20%.[66] If indicated, transmucosal immediate-release fentanyl (TIRF) may be used and requires providers to have Risk Evaluation and Mitigation Strategy certification. Neither TD nor TIRF are appropriate for opioid-naive patients.

Case 2: Continued

Ms. B is started on IV hydration and placed NPO. Her CT scan shows carcinomatosis and obstruction of the small bowel, and she is deemed not to be a surgical candidate. She is started on IV dexamethasone and haloperidol for nausea, and her abdominal pain is initially controlled with a PCA. Her nurse provided empathetic listening as she shares concerns about NGT placement and fear about the future. During a goals-of-care discussion, her nurse supports her to share these concerns, and given her desire to focus on QOL and time with family, Ms. B elects transition home with hospice care, with conversion of medications to oral solutions and TD fentanyl patch for pain.

Diarrhea

Case Study 3: A Patient with Lung Cancer

Ms. J is a 63-year-old female with lung cancer being treated with cisplatin. She developed acute diarrhea following antimicrobial treatment of cellulitis. She shares with her nurse that she is having 8–10 bloody stools daily and complains of stool urgency and diffuse abdominal cramping.

Definition

Diarrhea is defined by the World Health Organization (WHO) as three or more loose or liquid stools per day or more frequent stool passage than what an individual considers normal. Acute diarrhea may last for a few hours or days, where persistent diarrhea persists for 14 days or longer.[67] The US Department of Health and Human Services developed *Common Terminology Criteria for Adverse Events* including diarrhea to better define the severity. Criteria grades severity on a scale of 1–5, with grade 5 being the most severe,[68] as shown in Box 16.2.

Box 16.2 National Cancer Institute Common Toxicity Criteria in Diarrhea

Grade 1: Fewer than four bowel movements over baseline per day or mild increase in ostomy output compared to baseline.
Grade 2: Four to six bowel movements over baseline per day or moderate increase in ostomy output compared to baseline, in addition to symptoms limiting instrumental activities of daily living.
Grade 3: Seven or more bowel movements over baseline per day or severe increase in ostomy output compared to baseline, in addition to symptoms interfering with self-care activities of daily living. Hospitalization is indicated.
Grade 4: Urgent intervention indicated as symptoms cause life-threatening consequences.
Grade 5: Death

Source: Reference 68.

Prevalence and Impact

Diarrhea is present in many patients receiving cancer therapies upon entering hospice care. Although it is not as common as constipation within palliative care, it can have physical and psychological implications on patients, significantly impacting QOL and social functioning. In the most severe cases, it can also be life-threatening. Due to the many potential causes, diarrhea can be costly to evaluate and treat, causing strain on resources.[29,69]

Diarrhea frequently results in loss of fluids and electrolytes and can also affect nutritional intake due to loss of appetite. Skin breakdown, abdominal discomfort, rectal discomfort, hemorrhoids, and fatigue may be seen in patients experiencing diarrhea. In severe cases of diarrhea, especially in those already impacted by chemotherapy drugs or life-limiting illnesses, diarrhea can increase morbidity and mortality.

Pathophysiology and Risk Factors

Many patients receiving palliative care may experience a combination of factors, such as medication side effects, changes in diet and oral intake, infection, and psychological changes, that can lead to diarrhea, which is important to consider in evaluation and treatment. Categories of diarrhea include osmotic, secretory, exudative, and functional. Osmotic diarrhea occurs when there is poor absorption of water and/or electrolytes from the colon, causing an increase in intraluminal fluid and looser stool. Secretory diarrhea is a result of an increase of electrolytes being released into the colon, such as with GI infections. Exudative diarrhea is typically associated with damage to the lining of the intestine, such as with inflammatory bowel conditions. GI tract infections can cause diarrhea; thus, this is important to consider as an underlying etiology. Therapies such as chemotherapy and radiation can sometimes lead to diarrhea, as can the underlying stress of serious and life-threatening illness.

Infection-Related Diarrhea

Infectious diarrhea is defined by the WHO as acute watery and bloody diarrhea. This may also be accompanied by fever and vomiting. Common causes include *Clostridium difficile*, *Salmonella enterica*, *Escherichia coli*, and norovirus.[70] Opportunistic infections including cytomegalovirus, herpes simplex virus, *Giardia lamblia*, and *Mycobacterium avium* complex can also lead to diarrhea, especially in those patients with compromised immune systems, including those with acquired immunodeficiency syndrome or undergoing cancer therapies.[71] *C. difficile* infection (CDI) is an important consideration in differential diagnoses of diarrhea as it can be fatal and is easily spread. It can often be prevented by proper hand hygiene and use of personal protective equipment such as gloves and gowns.[70]

Infectious diarrhea can be seen in patients receiving palliative care due to factors such as immunocompromised status, use of antimicrobials, multiple caregivers, and admission to healthcare facilities. Patients with serious illness are often immunocompromised, and infectious diarrhea should be suspected when bloody diarrhea is present. Clinical practice guidelines from the Infectious Diseases Society of America recommend collecting blood and stool samples for cultures and considering empiric treatment with a broad-spectrum antibiotic when there is a high suspicion of infectious diarrhea.[70] If/when infectious diarrhea is confirmed, antibiotic therapy can be initiated.

Infections in the GI tract can cause colitis, limiting absorption of water in the colon and resulting in large-volume fluid loss and dehydration. It is important to monitor fluid status and evaluate for dehydration in the palliative care patient with *any* form of diarrhea and help maintain fluid and electrolyte balance as dehydration is likely to occur.[70]

Clostridioides difficile (known as *Clostridium difficile* until 2016) can be an infectious cause of diarrhea in the palliative care population. It is a bacterium that causes severe diarrhea and can cause pseudomembranous colitis and toxic megacolon. CDI accounted for more than 29,000 deaths in 2011 alone.[72] When a patient has been confirmed to have CDI, washing hands with soap and water is recommended over alcohol-based hand sanitizers as *C. difficile* spores are more effectively removed from the hands with soap and water and more likely to remain on the hands and be transferred when using alcohol-based hand sanitizers alone.[73] Treatment for CDI with antibiotics is recommended, as is rehydration with a reduced-osmolarity oral or nasogastric rehydration solution.[70]

Recommended treatments for CDI include vancomycin, fidaxomicin, and metronidazole.[74–77] There is some research regarding use of probiotics to prevent *C. difficile* as they may protect the lining of the intestine, decrease permeability, and help healthy cells survive, although American College of Gastroenterology guidelines do not currently recommend probiotics for primary prevention of CDI.[72,75,78]

Cancer Associated Diarrhea

Diarrhea can be a side effect of a medication or treatment or an effect of a malignant disease process. Radiation to the abdomen or pelvic regions has been known to cause radiation colitis, radiation enteritis, and radiation proctitis. Patients who are or have been treated for prostate cancer and cervical cancer are likely to experience this due to the location of treatment. Colitis caused by radiation often leads to GI ulcerations and can also cause fistulas, abscesses, perforation, and stricture. Rectal bleeding is not uncommon in the presence of GI ulceration, especially when the rectum is involved; and this can potentially mimic symptoms similar to infectious diarrhea. Corticosteroids, in either oral or rectal administration, can deliver benefit in this setting.[79] The nurse should be aware of use of corticosteroids for treatment as they can lead to additional side effects such as difficulty sleeping, irritability, and appetite changes.

Diarrhea is a common side effect of cancer treatment, estimated to affect up to 80% of patients taking chemotherapy drugs. Irinotecan, 5-fluorouracil, cisplatin, hydroxyurea, and interferon are frequently known to cause diarrhea. Many chemotherapies work by targeting rapidly dividing cancer cells; but unfortunately, they can also affect the rapidly dividing cells of the GI epithelium. This leads to mucositis with resultant secretory and hypermotile diarrhea.[80] Chemotherapy can also alter the normal intestinal microbiota, making a patient more susceptible to infectious diarrhea. The severity of chemotherapy-related diarrhea is directly correlated to dose, with 22% of patients requiring dose reduction, 28% requiring dose delay, and 15% requiring discontinuation of treatment.[81]

Immunotherapy drugs such as ipilimumab, pembrolizumab, and nivolumab stimulate the immune system to act against cancer cells; and diarrhea is one of the most common side effects of these therapies.[79] This is known to vary in frequency depending on the medication and typically increases with multiple therapies. Diarrhea related to immunotherapy drugs occurs in approximately one-third of patients and can significantly impact QOL.[79] A dose reduction or change in immunotherapy may be necessary depending on severity of diarrhea.

Certain cancers including neuroendocrine tumors (NETs) can cause significant diarrhea as most of these tumors originate in the GI tract and can cause secretion of vasoactive peptides and serotonin. The increase of serotonin leads to secretory diarrhea because of increased peristalsis and GI transit time, increased mucus secretion, impaired fluid absorption, and electrolyte disturbance. Diarrhea is a common feature of carcinoid syndrome, often seen in the setting of NETs and may be treated with antidiarrheals and pancreatic enzymes.[82]

Iatrogenic and Other Causes of Diarrhea

In managing the common symptom of constipation seen in patients receiving palliative care, use of laxatives must be monitored closely to avoid rebound diarrhea, which can occur with high use. Medications such as antibiotics and antacids may also be associated with diarrhea. Surgical interventions such as ileal resection or colectomy can lead to short gut syndrome and secretory diarrhea. Malabsorption is another common cause of diarrhea. Carbohydrate malabsorption such as fructose or lactose malabsorption can result in osmotic diarrhea. Biliary or pancreatic disease including pancreatic cancer and pancreatic insufficiency can lead to fat malabsorption with resultant hypermotile diarrhea associated with steatorrhea. Additional causes of diarrhea include inflammatory bowel diseases, such as Crohn's disease and ulcerative colitis, which cause inflammation and ulcerations in the GI tract.

Assessment

History

History should include the frequency of bowel movements, consistency of stool, presence of urgency or incontinence, and presence of blood, mucus, or pus. Other symptoms such as abdominal pain, fevers, nausea, and vomiting should be assessed. Attention should be given to the diet in the days prior to onset of diarrhea, to assess for food poisoning and contamination. It should be noted if the patient has potentially had contact with sick individuals, which could suggest an infectious diarrhea. Past medical history should be reviewed for underlying conditions which may predispose a patient to diarrhea. A recent medication history should be reviewed to identify any prescription or over-the-counter medications with known side effects of diarrhea or for overuse of laxatives.[69]

Physical Examination

Nurses should begin their assessment with evaluation of orthostatic blood pressures, heart rate, skin turgor, and mucus membranes, which may help assess the presence and severity of dehydration. It is also important for nurses to assess for signs of a fever as this may be suggestive of an infection.[69] The abdominal exam should include auscultation and palpation to determine if bowel sounds are hyperactive, normal, or absent and to determine the presence and location of pain or masses. Perineal skin should be examined for evidence of skin breakdown, hemorrhoids, and fissures. In those patients who are not severely neutropenic or thrombocytopenic, a rectal exam may also be performed to assess for abscesses or masses or to obtain a sample of stool for evaluation.[69]

Diagnostic Studies

Diagnostic studies may help identify the underlying cause of diarrhea, although they are not always necessary and can lead to overdiagnosis, increased cost, and increased burden. Decisions on whether laboratory, radiologic, and endoscopic studies should be done are dependent on the presentation of the patient and their symptom severity.[69] Many cases of mild diarrhea can be treated empirically, but testing should be considered in cases where more concerning symptoms are present. Serology testing can help identify the presence of leukocytosis, anemia, systemic inflammation, and thyroid dysfunction. Stool testing may be useful for identifying specific infections, presence of blood, or evidence of GI infection. Imaging studies are often not warranted and are costly, but CT or MRI can be utilized in the setting of abdominal pain to detect enterocolitis, bowel perforation, diverticulitis, pancreatitis, or abscesses.

Prevention, Nursing Interventions, and Supportive Care

Nurses should educate patients regarding known causes of diarrhea. For example, infection is a frequent cause of diarrhea in patients receiving palliative care and can often be prevented by frequent handwashing and good hand hygiene practices.[70] Additionally, education regarding treatment regimens and side effects is important, especially if an agent known to cause diarrhea is initiated. Patients should be given provider contact information to report changes in bowel habits along with other symptoms such as nausea, vomiting, fever, or abdominal pain. For those with mobility challenges, supportive care should include access to accommodations such as bedside commodes and hygiene products to reduce frequent trips to the restroom and improve cleanliness. Use of barrier creams helps reduce skin breakdown. Dietary management can be helpful when managing diarrhea. Lactose can aggravate diarrhea and should be avoided until symptoms improve. The National Cancer Institute also recommends avoiding large meals, alcohol, caffeine, high-sugar foods/drinks, and high-fat foods.[29] It is important for patients with diarrhea to remain well hydrated due to the risk of dehydration, and clear liquids may be the most easily tolerated. Additionally, fiber supplements can cause bulking of the stool, leading to improved stool consistency and decreased frequency.

Pharmacologic Management

Opioid Agonists

Opioid agonists are the first-line pharmacologic option for relief of diarrhea when conservative measures are not sufficient. These medications improve diarrhea by binding to opioid receptors in the GI tract, resulting in reduced peristalsis and increased water reabsorption in the colon.[83,84]

Loperamide and oral hydration are acceptable first-line treatments for patients with mild, uncomplicated diarrhea (grade 1–2) without significant systemic symptoms or concern for infectious or inflammatory etiologies.[69,79] Loperamide is available without prescription at low cost, and dosing can be titrated up to 16 mg daily as needed, although it can lead to constipation or cause paralytic ileus, so patient response must be closely evaluated. It is helpful in cases of IBS, drug/treatment side effect, and dietary indiscretion[69,70] but is not recommended in a patient suspected of having infectious or inflammatory causes.

Diphenoxylate/atropine is a combination drug, with diphenoxylate working as a peripheral opioid agonist and atropine working as an anticholinergic, together reducing GI secretions and peristalsis.

Tincture of opium is also used to slow GI motility but must not be confused with paregoric, which is a less potent alcohol-based tincture.[69]

Adsorbent Agents

These agents add bulk and density to the stool. They include methylcellulose and pectin, which can require large volumes to offer therapeutic effect and can cause abdominal bloating and discomfort.

Anticholinergics

These medications reduce GI secretions and peristalsis and can additionally provide relief of abdominal cramping. Mentioned previously, atropine is an anticholinergic which can be used with diphenoxylate. Scopolamine is another anticholinergic administered TD and can be considered in refractory cases, especially those with concurrent nausea.

Antisecretory Agents

Somatostatin analogues such as octreotide may be considered in severe or persistent diarrhea. It functions by suppressing the release of insulin, glucagon, and vasoactive intestinal peptide. It can also inhibit gastric acid secretion, reduce GI motility, and increase absorption of water and electrolytes.[69] It may be given IV or SC as a first-line treatment in severe chemotherapy-induced diarrhea, second-line treatment for mild diarrhea, or for profuse secretory HIV-related diarrhea. Crofelemer is an antisecretory agent that represents the only US Food and Drug Administration–approved therapy for symptomatic relief of noninfectious diarrhea in patients with HIV on antiretroviral therapy.[85]

Other Antidiarrhea Options

Additional medications can be considered for specific underlying causes of diarrhea. Pancreatic enzymes containing lipase can benefit a patient with pancreatic insufficiency, and bile acid sequestrants can be helpful if there is concern for bile acid malabsorption.

Case Study 3: Continued

Ms. J was tested for *C. difficile* and was positive. Her nurse discussed transmission of CDI and demonstrated appropriate hand hygiene. She also treated her with vancomycin 125 mg four times daily for 10 days. Ms. J was encouraged to maintain adequate hydration and tolerated approximately 64 ounces of clear fluids daily throughout treatment. Her nurse provided a bedside commode to ensure Ms. J's safety while requiring frequent toileting. Her blood pressure remained stable, and she remained afebrile. Diarrhea and hematochezia resolved with treatment, and normal stool frequency returned. She was encouraged to continue good hand hygiene indefinitely.

Ascites

Case Study 4: A Patient with Nonalcoholic Steatohepatitis Cirrhosis

Mr. C is a 68-year-old man with cirrhosis related to nonalcoholic steatohepatitis. He reports increased fatigue over the last few weeks as well as early satiety and breathing discomfort when lying flat. His nurse shares concerns that Mr. C has increased abdominal girth and new yellowing of the skin since his prior clinic visit.

Definition, Prevalence, and Pathophysiology

Ascites is an abnormal collection of fluid within the intraperitoneal cavity. Ascites formation can impact body image and QOL and is often a direct cause of further health-related complications. Ascites may be characterized as Grade 1—mild, Grade 2—moderate, and Grade 3—large ascites.[86] There are multiple etiologies of ascites that can be broken down into conditions associated with portal hypertension, peritoneal disease, and hypoalbuminemia.

Portal hypertension is a condition of resistance to portal blood flow due to structural changes in organs involved or dynamic changes affecting the velocity of blood flow. The pathophysiology of ascites accumulation in the setting of portal hypertension is complex, involving vasodilatation, translocation of circulating bacteria, inflammatory mediators, shifts in pressure, and changes in vascular tone, plasma volume, and capillary permeability.[87]

Liver cirrhosis is the most common cause of ascites related to portal hypertension and represents about 80% of all ascites cases.[88] Nearly half of patients with cirrhosis develop ascites, an event marking poorer prognosis.[89] Of those with cirrhosis who develop ascites, 2-year mortality becomes 50%. When ascites becomes refractory to medical therapy, mortality is 50% within 6–12 months.[90] Other common causes of portal hypertension that can lead to ascites include portal vein thrombosis, heart failure, constrictive pericarditis, and hepatic veno-occlusive disease.[87]

When the peritoneum is damaged, lymphatic drainage is impaired and vascular permeability increases, resulting in accumulation of fluid within the peritoneal cavity.[91] Malignancy with peritoneal carcinomatosis is a common cause of this and represents roughly 10% of all patients with ascites.[88,92] Malignant ascites (MA) is most associated with ovarian cancer, occurring in about one-fourth of cases, but may also be associated with other abdominal and extra-abdominal cancers. Liver metastasis, edema, and low albumin in the setting of MA are indicative of poorer prognosis.[92] Tuberculosis can also damage the peritoneum, representing about 2% of patients with ascites.[88]

Hypoalbuminemia occurs primarily due to loss of oncotic pressure within the cardiovascular system, leading to increased vascular permeability and resulting in peritoneal cavity fluid accumulation. Nephrotic syndrome, severe malnutrition, and protein-losing enteropathies can all increase a patient's risk of developing ascites.[88]

Assessment

History

Nurses collecting a patient history should be sure to inquire about medication use and past medical history. Risk factors for liver or infectious disease should be assessed, including current and past history of alcohol use, hepatitis, hepatocellular carcinoma, or travel to tuberculosis-endemic regions.[93] Additionally, patients should be asked about recent weight gain and edema. Abdominal pain may be accompanied by pelvic or back pain due to carrying additional weight. Important to remember when evaluating your patient is that the hallmark symptom of ascites is abdominal distension. Anorexia and early satiety may develop, as well as nausea and vomiting. Additional symptoms to review are presence of fatigue, dyspnea and orthopnea, urinary frequency, and constipation.[94] In patients with liver disease, pruritus may be present due to hyperbilirubinemia or confusion related to hepatic encephalopathy.

Physical Examination

Exam may demonstrate underlying etiology of ascites, including heart failure, malignancy, and liver disease. An abdominal exam should assess for distension and hepatosplenomegaly. Abdominal percussion may result in a dull tone over the flanks in comparison to tympanic sound more often present in bowel obstruction. At least 1.5 L of fluid must be present to appreciate dullness to percussion, and this in combination with bulging flanks yields a 75% sensitivity and 57% specificity in the diagnosis of ascites.[93] Dullness to percussion may also shift as the patient changes position, a sign more predictive of ascites than presence of a fluid wave.[93]

Diagnostic Studies, Paracentesis, and Laparoscopy

The primary value of obtaining blood tests is to look for conditions that predispose to ascites such as liver dysfunction, renal dysfunction, heart failure, or cancer. Thus, liver function tests, creatinine and blood urea nitrogen, coagulation studies, or brain natriuretic peptide levels may be abnormal. Additionally, abnormal albumin levels may indicate malnutrition.

Any patient who presents with new-onset ascites warrants a diagnostic paracentesis to determine the cause.[88] Analysis of the ascitic fluid includes assessment of neutrophil count, total protein, albumin concentration, and fluid culture. When the cause of ascites is not immediately evident, the serum-ascites albumin gradient can be calculated. The color of the ascitic fluid should be observed, with straw color common in liver cirrhosis. A red blood cell count greater than 10,000/mm^3 in ascitic fluid indicates hemorrhagic ascites, found in 5% of patients with cirrhosis and most associated with a traumatic tap.[89] For a patient with suspected cancer, a positive cytology evaluation of the ascitic fluid is 100% specific for the diagnosis of malignancy but only 60% sensitive.[88] In some situations, diagnostic laparoscopy may allow for detailed visual examination of the intraperitoneal space to look for ascites etiology, as well as the option to take tissue biopsies.[95]

Infectious workup of ascites includes a microscopic analysis to rule out spontaneous bacterial peritonitis (SBP). Presence of more than 250 neutrophils/mm^3 is suggestive of infection.[95] Fungal cultures may also be obtained, with a polymorphonuclear cell count ≥250 cells/mm^3 found in spontaneous fungal peritonitis (SFP).[96]

Nursing Interventions and Supportive Care

Because the presence of ascites in most situations indicates terminal illness, the goal of treatment is palliation of symptoms.[95] Nutritional interventions are considered standard of care; however, evidence to support specific interventions is sparse. Nurses can coach patients on current evidence that supports limiting sodium intake along with a high-calorie, high-protein diet. While data is limited to support specific targets, nurses can coach their patients on restricting dietary sodium to less than 2,000 mg/day. Neither parenteral nutrition nor IV amino acids were found to be effective as stand-alone interventions.[97] Assisting with proper positioning additionally improves discomfort and dyspnea, and physical and occupational therapy can be considered to assist with mobility concerns.

Pharmacologic Management

While nurses may experience giving diuretics for the management of cirrhotic ascites, they should note that diuretics have less efficacy in malignant ascites, providing symptom relief for approximately 40% of cases.[92] The potassium-sparing diuretic spironolactone is the drug of choice. Loop diuretics like furosemide are sometimes used, with limited evidence of utility. Compared with paracentesis plus fluid replacement, aldosterone antagonists plus loop diuretics had a higher rate of decompensation events including hepatic encephalopathy, hepatorenal syndrome, and variceal bleeding.[98]

Other pharmacologic treatments include chemotherapy for patients with chemosensitive malignancies, especially in ovarian and some GI cancers.[99] There are some reports that drainage combined with the chemotherapeutic agent catumaxomab provided increased QOL for longer duration compared to drainage alone among women with gynecologic cancers.[100] Another emerging therapy specifically for malignant ascites is intraperitoneal catumaxomab. More research is needed, but one study found that almost two-thirds of participants were able to receive all four doses in the outpatient setting, with a shorter (3-hour) infusion time.[92]

Antibiotics and antifungals have a role in management of SBP and SFP, respectively. Antibiotic prophylaxis may be indicated after the first episode of SBP as well as in patients with high risk of developing SBP or those who with GI bleeding. Duration of antibiotic prophylaxis in those with serious illness may be indefinite. SFP carries a higher risk of mortality. When indicated, an early course of antifungal therapy is associated with improved outcomes.[96]

Procedural and Surgical Management

Therapeutic Paracentesis

Therapeutic paracentesis is recommended as the first-line treatment for large or grade 3 ascites and in ascites refractory to supportive and pharmacologic interventions.[86] This provides relief of symptoms, albeit temporary, and can be performed on an outpatient basis up to every 2 weeks.[90] To prevent complications from large-volume ascites removal known as "post-paracentesis circulatory dysfunction," plasma volume expansion with albumin infusion is recommended.[86] Rare but life-threatening side effects include a 1% chance of significant bleeding and a 0.4% chance of small bowel perforation.[90] Thus, nursing care should include close monitoring of any clinical changes.

Catheters

Patients requiring frequent paracentesis for symptomatic relief may benefit from an indwelling catheter for ease of fluid removal. A single-cuffed indwelling peritoneal catheter (e.g., PeritX™ or Rocket®) is often used when ascites persists in spite of large-volume bimonthly paracentesis when shunts are contraindicated. These catheters have a high rate of technical success but have complication rates of 9% to 36%,[101] including increased risk of infection the longer they are present, especially after 3 months. Other complications include leakage or cellulitis at the catheter site, occlusion, or fatal hypotension.[92] Qualitative studies show benefit of improved control of ascites, individualized care, and more time at home in addition to the avoidance of travel to and from a medical facility for drainage.[102] Another catheter option is a double-cuffed pigtail peritoneal dialysis catheter (e.g., Tenckhoff®), which allows for drainage of malignant ascites and the option to infuse cytotoxic medications, with an overall low complication rate.[103]

Shunts

Transjugular intrahepatic portosystemic shunt (TIPS) is typically reserved as a second-line option for patients with refractory ascites. For cirrhotic patients, TIPS offers better control of ascites than large-volume paracentesis and can improve QOL but yields a higher risk of severe hepatic encephalopathy; rifaximin prophylaxis has been shown to help for post-TIPS hepatic encephalopathy.[104] Contraindications to this procedure include significant heart failure, pulmonary hypertension, systemic infection, and biliary obstruction. For patients with cirrhosis over the age of 70 who undergo TIPS, mortality is increased. While age should not be an absolute contraindication, careful risk stratification is warranted, including assessment of risk predictors including serum creatinine and sodium levels.[105] Another option is the peritoneovenous (e.g., Denver or Le Veen) shunt. Ascitic fluid is shunted from the intraperitoneal space into the superior vena cava via a pressure gradient. This is sometimes utilized in patients unable to benefit from TIPS or large-volume paracentesis and has a 70% rate of symptom palliation.[95]

Additional Interventions

Liver transplantation may be an option to improve both symptoms and prognosis; however, for many patients, this is not an option due to etiology of the disease, level of illness severity, and comorbid conditions. A newer technology under clinical investigation in the United States is the alfapump®, an implantable, automated medical device that pumps ascitic fluid from the peritoneum into the urinary bladder, where it is excreted.[106]

Hyperthermic intraperitoneal chemotherapy (HIPEC) is a procedure where ascites is removed through drainage tubes and washout of the peritoneal cavity with isothermic saline, followed by intraperitoneal infusion of chemotherapy. Ovarian cancer tends to be more susceptible to this approach than GI cancers.[107] HIPEC is generally well tolerated with less toxicity than systemic chemotherapy but requires hospitalization.

Concentrated ascites reinfusion therapy (CART) involves paracentesis, followed by filtration of ascitic fluid to remove any malignant cells, bacteria, and excess fluid or electrolytes, after which the filtered, concentrated ascites is reinfused.[108] CART has been found to improve symptoms of abdominal distension, dyspnea, and fatigue and increased serum albumin and total protein, with performance status improvement for 17% of patients.[109] Fever is a common adverse effect, and additional prospective studies are warranted.

Case Study 4: Continued

Mr. C undergoes ultrasound, which confirms ascites. His diagnostic paracentesis does not show evidence of bleeding or infection, and his workup is consistent with portal hypertension. The nurse educator coaches him and his family on limiting sodium and increasing protein in his diet. Spironolactone is initiated without significant improvement. Therapeutic paracentesis yields 4 L of straw-colored fluid, improving his comfort for about 2.5 weeks. His nurse establishes a schedule for recurrent paracentesis and provides education on positioning techniques that improve comfort and breathing when lying down.

REFERENCES

1. Forootan M, Bagheri N, Darvishi M. Chronic constipation: a review of literature. *Medicine*. 2018;97(20):e10631. https://doi.org/10.1097/MD.0000000000010631.
2. Lucak S, Lunsford TN, Harris LA. Evaluation and treatment of constipation in the geriatric population. *Clin Geriatr Med*. 2021;37(1):85–102. https://doi.org/10.1016/j.cger.2020.08.007.
3. McIlfatrick S, Muldrew DHL, Beck E, et al. Examining constipation assessment and the management of patients with advanced cancer receiving specialist palliative care: a multi-site retrospective case note review of clinical practice. *BMC Palliat Care*. 2019;18:57. https://doi.org/10.1186/s12904-019-0436-3.
4. Larkin PJ, Cherny NI, La Carpia D, et al. Diagnosis, assessment and management of constipation in advanced cancer: ESMO clinical practice guidelines. *Ann Oncol*. 2018;29(suppl 4):S111–S125. https://doi.org/10.1093/annonc/mdy148.
5. Moens K, Higginson IJ, Harding R. Are there differences in the prevalence of palliative care-related problems in people living with advanced cancer and eight non-cancer conditions? A systematic review. *J Pain Symptom Manage*. 2014;48(4):660–677. https://doi.org/10.1016/j.jpainsymman.2013.11.009.
6. Law J, Martin E, eds. Constipation. In: *Oxford Reference*. Oxford University Press; 2025. Accessed January 8, 2025. https://www.oxfordreference.com/display/10.1093/oi/authority.20110803095633876
7. Lacy BE, Mearin F, Chang L, et al. Bowel disorders. *Gastroenterology*. 2016;150(6):1393–1407. https://doi.org/10.1053/j.gastro.2016.02.031.
8. Dzierżanowski T, Larkin P. Proposed criteria for constipation in palliative care patients: a multicenter cohort study. *J Clin Med*. 2020;10:40. https://doi.org/10.3390/jcm10010040.
9. Heitmann PT, Vollebregt PF, Knowles CH, et al. Understanding the physiology of human defaecation and disorders of continence and evacuation. *Nat Rev Gastroenterol Hepatol*. 2021;18:751–769. https://doi.org/10.1038/s41575-021-00487-5.
10. Barucha AE, Pemberton JH, Locke GE III. American Gastroenterological Association technical review on constipation. *Gastroenterology*. 2013;144:218–238. https://doi.org/10.1053/j.gastro.2012.10.028.
11. Simrén M, Palsson OS, Whitehead WE. Update on Rome IV criteria for colorectal disorders: implications for clinical practice. *Curr Gastroenterol Rep*. 2017;19:15. https://doi.org/10.1007/s11894-017-0554-0.
12. Bharucha AE, Lacy BE. Mechanisms, evaluation, and management of chronic constipation. *Gastroenterology*. 2020;158(5):1232–1249. https://doi.org/10.1053/j.gastro.2019.12.034.
13. Andrews A, Morgan G. Constipation in palliative care: treatment options and consideration for individual patient management. *Int J Palliat Nurs*. 2013;19(6):266–273.
14. Argoff CE, Brennan MJ, Camilleri M, et al. Consensus recommendations on initiating prescription therapies for opioid-induced constipation. *Pain Med*. 2015;16(12):2324–2337.
15. Müller-Lissner S, Bassotti G, Coffin B, et al. Opioid-induced constipation and bowel dysfunction: a clinical guideline. *Pain Med*. 2017;18:1837–1863. https://doi.org/10.1093/pm/pnw255.
16. Davies A, Leach C, Caponero R, et al. MASCC recommendations of the management of constipation in patients with advanced cancer. *Support Care Cancer*. 2020;28:23–33. https://doi.org/10.1007/s00520-019-05016-4.
17. Crockett SD, Greer KB, Heidelbaugh JJ, Falck-Ytter Y, Hanson BJ, Sultan S. American Gastroenterological Association Institute guideline on the medical management of opioid-induced constipation. *Gastroenterology*. 2019;156(1):218–226. https://doi.org/10.1053/j.gastro.2018.07.016.
18. McMillan SC, Tofthagen C, Small B, Karver S, Craig D. Trajectory of medication-induced constipation in patients with cancer. *Oncol Nurs Forum*. 2013;40(3):E92–E100.
19. Davis M, Gamier P. New options in constipation management. *Curr Oncol Rep*. 2015;17(12):55.
20. Paquette IM, Madhulika V, Ternent C, et al. The American Society of Colon and Rectal Surgeons' clinical practice guideline for the evaluation and management of constipation. *Dis Colon Rectum*. 2016;59(6):479–492. https://doi.org/10.1097/DCR.0000000000000599.
21. Larkin PJ, Sykes NP, Centeno C, et al. The management of constipation in palliative care: clinical practice recommendations. *Palliat Med*. 2008;22:796–807. https://doi.org/10.1177.0269216308096908.
22. Fritz D, Pitlick M. Evidence about the prevention and management of constipation: implications for comfort part 1. *Home Healthc Nurse*. 2012;30(9):533–540; quiz 540–532.
23. Gill SK, Rossi M, Bajka B, Whelan K. Dietary fibre in gastrointestinal health and disease. *Nat Rev Gastroenterol Hepatol*. 2021;18(2):101–116. https://doi.org/10.1038/s41575-020-00375-4.
24. Dreher M. Whole fruits and fruit fiber emerging health effects. *Nutrients*. 2018;10:1833. https://doi.org/10.3390/nu10121833.
25. Mokhtare M, Karimi S, Bahardoust M, Sotoudeheian M, Ghazi A, Babaei-Ghazani A. How adding the abdominal massage to polyethylene glycol can improve symptom and quality of life in patients with functional constipation in comparison with each one of the treatment modalities alone: a randomized clinical trial.

Complement Ther Med. 2020;52:102495. https://doi.org/10.1016/j.ctim.2020.102495.
26. Modi RM, Hinton A, Pinkhas D, et al. Implementation of a defecation posture modification device: impact on bowel movement patterns in healthy subjects. *J Clin Gastroenterol*. 2019;53(3):216–219.
27. Clemens KE, Faust M, Jaspers B, Mikus G. Pharmacological treatment of constipation in palliative care. *Curr Opin Support Palliat Care*. 2013;7(2):183–191.
28. Prichard D, Bharucha A. Management of opioid-induced constipation for people in palliative care. *Int J Palliat Nurs*. 2015;21(6):272, 274–280.
29. National Cancer Institute. Gastrointestinal Complications (PDQ®)-Health Professional Version. 2022. Accessed August 22, 2022. https://www.cancer.gov/about-cancer/treatment/side-effects/constipation/gi-complications-hp-pdq.
30. Pitlick M, Fritz D. Evidence about the pharmacological management of constipation, part 2: implications for palliative care. *Home Healthc Nurse*. 2013;31(4):207–218.
31. Wild J, Webster L, Yamada T, Hale M. Safety and efficacy of naldemine for the treatment of opioid-induced constipation in patients with chronic non-cancer pain receiving opioid therapy: a subgroup analysis of patients ≥65 years of age. *Drugs Aging*. 2020;27(4):271–279. https://doi.org/10.1007/s40266-020-00753-2.
32. Rao SSC, Lichtlen P, Habibi S. Effects of lubiprostone, an intestinal secretagogue, on electrolyte homeostasis in chronic idiopathic and opioid-induced constipation. *J Clin Gastroenterol*. 2021;55(6):512–519. https://doi.org/10.1097/MCG.0000000000001385.
33. Holder RM, Rhee D. Novel oral therapies for opioid-induced bowel dysfunction in patients with chronic noncancer pain. *Pharmacotherapy*. 2016;36(3):287–299.
34. Leppert W, Woron J. The role of naloxegol in the management of opioid-induced bowel dysfunction. *Therap Adv Gastroenterol*. 2016;9(5):736–746.
35. Schoenfeld P, Lacy BE, Chey WD, Lembo AJ, Kurtz CB, Reasner DS, et al. Low-dose linaclotide (72μg) for chronic idiopathic constipation: a 12-week, randomized, double-blind, placebo-controlled trial. *Am J Gastroenterol*. 2018;113(1):105–114. https://doi.org/10.1038/ajg.2017.230.
36. Miner PB, Koltun WD, Wiener GJ, De La Portilla M, Prieto B, Shailubhai K, et al. A randomized phase III clinical trial of plecanatide, a uroguanylin analog, in patients with chronic idiopathic constipation. *Am J Gastroenterol*. 2017;112(4):613–621. https://doi.org/10.1038/ajg.2016.611.
37. Vahora IS, Tsouklidis N, Kumar R, et al. How serotonin level fluctuation affects the effectiveness of treatment in irritable bowel syndrome. *Cureus*. 2020;12(8):e9871. https://doi.org/10.7759/cureus.9871.
38. Ohkusa T, Koido S, Nishikawa Y, Sato N. Gut microbiota and chronic constipation: a review and update. *Front Med (Lausanne)*. 2019;6:19. https://doi.org/10.3389/fmed.2019.00019.
39. Martínez-Martínez MI, Calabuig-Tolsá R, Cauli O. The effect of probiotics as a treatment for constipation in elderly people: a systematic review. *Arch Gerontol Geriatr*. 2017;71:142–149. https://doi.org/10.1016/j.archger.2017.04.004.
40. Šola KF, Vladimir-Knežević S, Hrabač P, et al. The effect of multistrain probiotics on functional constipation in the elderly: a randomized controlled trial. *Eur J Clin Nutr*. 2022;76:1675–1681. https://doi.org/10.1038/s41430-022-01189-0.
41. Tuca A, Guell E, Martinez-Losada E, Codorniu N. Malignant bowel obstruction in advanced cancer patients: epidemiology, management, and factors influencing spontaneous resolution. *Cancer Manag Res*. 2012;4:159–169.
42. Fackche NT, Johnston FM. Malignant bowel obstruction. *Adv Surg*. 2021;55:35–48. https://doi.org/10.1016/j.yasu.2021.05.003.
43. Huang X, Xue J, Gao M, et al. Medical management of malignant bowel obstruction. *Ann Pharmacother*. 2021;55(9):1134–1145. https://doi.org/10.1177/1060028020979773.
44. Davis M, Hui D, Davies A, et al. Medical management of malignant bowel obstruction in patients with advanced cancer: 2021 MASCC guideline update. *Support Care Cancer*. 2021;29:8089–8096. https://doi.org/10.1007/s00520-021-06438-9.
45. Lilley EJ, Scott JW, Goldberg JE, et al. Survival, healthcare utilization, and end-of-life care among older adults with malignancy-associated bowel obstruction. *Ann Surg*. 2018;267(4):692–699. https://doi.org/10.1097/SLA.0000000000002164.
46. Shariff F, Bogach J, Guidolin K, Nadler A. Malignant bowel obstruction management over time: are we doing anything new? A current narrative review. *Ann Surg Oncol*. 2022;29:1995–2005. https://doi.org/10.1245/s10434-021-10922-1.
47. Alese OB, Kim S, Chen Z, Owonikoko TK, El-Rayes BF. Management patterns and predictors of mortality among US patients with cancer hospitalized for malignant bowel obstruction. *Cancer*. 2015;121(11):1772–1778.
48. Madariaga A, Lau J, Ghoshal A, et al. MASCC multidisciplinary evidence-based recommendations for the management of malignant bowel obstruction in advanced cancer. *Support Care Cancer*. 2022;30:4711–4728. https://doi.org/10.1007/s00520-022-06889-8.
49. Klein C, Stiel S, Bukki J, Ostgathe C. Pharmacological treatment of malignant bowel obstruction in severely ill and dying patients: a systematic literature review. *Schmerz*. 2012;26(5):587–599.
50. Ferguson HJ, Ferguson CI, Speakman J, Ismail T. Management of intestinal obstruction in advanced malignancy. *Ann Med Surg (Lond)*. 2015;4(3):264–270.
51. Nelms DW, Kann BR. Imaging modalities for evaluation of intestinal obstruction. *Clin Colon Rectal Surg*. 2021;34(4):205–218. https://doi.org/10.1055/s-0041-1729737.
52. Jin M, Shen F, Li M, Chen Y. Palliative treatment for bowel obstruction in ovarian cancer: a meta-analysis. *Arch Gynecol Obstet*. 2020;302:241–248. https://doi.org/10.1007/s00404-020-05545-y.
53. Baddeley E, Mann M, Bravington A, et al. Symptom burden and lived experiences of patients, caregivers and healthcare professionals on the management of malignant bowel obstruction: a qualitative systematic review. *Palliat Med*. 2022;36(6):895–911. https://doi.org/10.1177/02692163221081331.
54. Dalal KM, Gollub MJ, Miner TJ, et al. Management of patients with malignant bowel obstruction and stage IV colorectal cancer. *J Palliat Med*. 2011;14(7):822–828.
55. Santangelo ML, Grifasi C, Criscitiello C, et al. Bowel obstruction and peritoneal carcinomatosis in the elderly. A systematic review. *Aging Clin Exp Res*. 2017;29(suppl 1):73–78.
56. Sigmon DF, An J. Nasogastric tube. In: *StatPearls*. StatPearls Publishing; 2022. Updated May 26, 2022. Accessed August 27, 2022. https://www.ncbi.nlm.nih.gov/books/NBK556063/.
57. Chouhan J, Gupta R, Ensor J, et al. Retrospective analysis of systemic chemotherapy and total parenteral nutrition for the treatment of malignant small bowel obstruction. *Cancer Med*. 2016;5(2):239–247.
58. Sowerbutts AM, Lal S, Sremanakova J, et al. Home parenteral nutrition for people with inoperable malignant bowel obstruction.

Cochrane Database Sys Rev. 2018;8:CD012812. https://doi.org/10.1002/14651858.CD012812.pub2.
59. Selby D, Nolen A, Sittambalam C, Johansen K, Pugash R. Percutaneous transesophageal gastrostomy (PTEG): a safe and well-tolerated procedure for palliation of end-stage malignant bowel obstruction. *J Pain Symptom Manage*. 2019;58(2):306–310. https://doi.org/10.1016/j.jpainsymman.2019.04.031.
60. Abelson JS, Yeo HL, Mao J, Milsom JW, Sedrakyan A. Long-term postprocedural outcomes of palliative emergency stenting vs stoma in malignant large-bowel obstruction. *JAMA Surg*. 2017;152(5):429–435.
61. Atukorale YN, Church JL, Hoggan BL, et al. Self-expanding metallic stents for the management of emergency malignant large bowel obstruction: a systematic review. *J Gastrointest Surg*. 2016;20(2):455–462.
62. Veld J, Umans D, van Halsema E, et al. Self-expandable metal stent (SEMS) placement or emergency surgery as palliative treatment for obstructive colorectal cancer: a systematic review and meta-analysis. *Crit Rev Oncol Hematol*. 2020;155:103110. https://doi.org/10.1016/j.critrevonc.2020.103110.
63. Feuer DJ, Broadley KE. Corticosteroids for the resolution of malignant bowel obstruction in advance gynaecological and gastrointestinal cancer. *Cochrane Database Syst Rev*. 2000;1:CD001219. https://doi.org/10.1002/14651858.CD001219.
64. Murray-Brown F, Dorman S. Haloperidol for the treatment of nausea and vomiting in palliative care patients. *Cochrane Database Syst Rev*. 2015;2015(11):CD006271.
65. Laval G, Marcelin-Benazech B, Guirimand F, et al. Recommendations for bowel obstruction with peritoneal carcinomatosis. *J Pain Symptom Manage*. 2014;48(1):75–91.
66. Reisfield GM, Wilson GR. Rational use of sublingual opioids in palliative medicine. *J Palliat Med*. 2007;10(2):465–475.
67. World Health Organization. Diarrhoea. Updated May 2, 2017. Accessed August 22, 2022. https://www.who.int/health-topics/diarrhoea.
68. US Department of Health and Human Services. *Common Terminology Criteria for Adverse Events (CTCAE)*. Version 5.0. November 27, 2017. Accessed September 9, 2022.https://ctep.cancer.gov/protocoldevelopment/electronic_applications/docs/ctcae_v5_quick_reference_5x7.pdf.
69. Bossi P, Antonuzzo A, Cherny NI, et al. Diarrhoea in adult cancer patients: ESMO clinical practice guidelines. *Ann Oncol*. 2018;29(4):126–142. https://doi.org/10.1093/annonc/mdy145.
70. Shane AL, Mody RK, Crump JA, et al. 2017 Infectious Diseases Society of America clinical guidelines for the diagnosis and management of infectious diarrhea. *Clin Infect Dis*. 2017;65(12):e45–e80. https://doi.org/10.1093/cid/cix669.
71. Reid MJA, Tien PC. Diarrhea in HIV-infected patients. In: Chin RL, Frazee BW, Coralic Z, eds. *Emergency Management of Infectious Diseases*. 2nd ed. Cambridge University Press; 2018:181–187. https://doi.org/10.1017/9781316597095.028.
72. Shen NT, Maw A, Tmanova LL, et al. Timely use of probiotics in hospitalized adults prevents *Clostridium difficile* infection: a systematic review with meta-regression analysis. *Gastroenterology*. 2017;152(8):1889–1900.e9. https://doi.org/10.1053/j.gastro.2017.02.003.
73. Jabbar U, Leischner J, Kasper D, et al. Effectiveness of alcohol-based hand rubs for removal of *Clostridium difficile* spores from hands. *Infect Control Hosp Epidemiol*. 2010;31(6):565–570. https://doi.org/10.1086/652772.
74. Johnson S, Lavergne V, Skinner A, et al. Clinical practice guideline by the Infectious Diseases Society of America (IDSA) and Society for Healthcare Epidemiology of America (SHEA): 2021 focused update guidelines on management of *Clostridioides difficile* infection in adults. *Clin Infect Dis*. 2021;73(5):e1029–e1044. https://doi.org/10.1093/cid/ciab549.
75. Kelly C, Fischer M, Allegretti J, et al. ACG clinical guidelines: prevention, diagnosis, and treatment of *Clostridioides difficile* infections. *Am J Gasteroenterol*. 2021;116(6):1124–1147. https://doi.org/10.14309/ajg.0000000000001278.
76. Cornely OA, Miller MA, Fantin B, Mullane K, Kean Y, Gorbach S. Resolution of *Clostridium difficile*-associated diarrhea in patients with cancer treated with fidaxomicin or vancomycin. *J Clin Oncol*. 2013:31(19):2493–2499. https://doi.org/10.1200/jco.2012.45.5899.
77. Gentry CA, Nguyen PK, Thind S, Kurdgelashvili G, Skrepnek GH, Williams RJ II. Fidaxomicin versus oral vancomycin for severe *Clostridium difficile* infection: a retrospective cohort study. *Clin Microbiol Infect*. 2010:25(8):987–993. https://doi.org/10.1016/j.cmi.2018.12.007.
78. Silva MJ, Carneiro MB, dos Anjos Pultz B, Pereira Silva D, Lopes ME, dos Santos LM. The multifaceted role of commensual microbiota in homeostasis and gastrointestinal diseases. *J Immunol Res*. 2015;2015:321241.
79. O'Reilly M, Mellotte G, Ryan B, O'Connor A. Gastrointestinal side effects of cancer treatments. *Ther Adv Chronic Dis*. 2020;11:1–7. https://doi.org/10.1177/2040622320970354.
80. Andreyev J, Ross P, Donnellan C, et al. Guidance on the management of diarrhoea during cancer chemotherapy. *Lancet Oncol*. 2014;15(10):e447–e460.
81. McQuade RM, Stojanovska V, Abalo R, Bornstein JC, Nurgali K. Chemotherapy-induced constipation and diarrhea: pathophysiology, current and emerging treatments. *Front Pharmacol*. 2016;7:414.
82. Naraev BG, Halland M, Halperin D, et al. Management of diarrhea in patients with carcinoid syndrome. *Pancreas*. 2019;48(8):961–972.
83. von Gunten CF, Gafford E. Treatment of non-pain-related symptoms. *Cancer J*. 2013;19(5):397–404.
84. Pastrana T, Meissner W. Treatment of diarrhea with loperamide in palliative medicine: a systematic review. *Schmerz*. 2013;27(2):182–189.
85. Dikman AE, Schonfeld E, Srisarajivakul NC, Poles MA. Human immunodeficiency virus-associated diarrhea: still an issue in the era of antiretroviral therapy. *Dig Dis Sci*. 2015;60(8):2236–2245.
86. European Association for the Study of the Liver. EASL clinical practice guidelines for the management of patients with decompensated cirrhosis. *J Hepatol*. 2018;69(2):406–460. https://doi.org/10.1016/j.jhep.2018.03.024.
87. Madoff DC, Cornman-Homonoff J, Fortune BE, et al. Management of refractory ascites due to portal hypertension: current status. *Radiology*. 2021;298:493–504. https://doi.org/10.1148/radiol.2021201960.
88. Runyon BA, Montano AA, Akriviadis EA, Antillon MR, Irving MA, McHutchison JG. The serum-ascites albumin gradient is superior to the exudate-transudate concept in the differential diagnosis of ascites. *Ann Intern Med*. 1992;117(3):215–220.
89. Iqbal U, Ahmed Z, Anwar H, et al. Hemorrhagic ascites is associated with reduced survival in cirrhosis: a systematic review and meta-analysis. *Gastroenterol Res*. 2022;15(1):26–32. https://doi.org/10.14740/gr1485.
90. Reinglas J, Amjadi K, Petrcich B, Momoli F, Shaw-Stiffel T. The palliative management of refractory cirrhotic ascites using the PleurX© catheter. *Can J Gastroenterol Hepatol*. 2016;2016:4680543.

91. Wong BC, Cake L, Kachuik L, Amjadi K. Indwelling peritoneal catheters for managing malignancy-associated ascites. *J Palliat Care*. 2015;31(4):243–249.
92. Hodge C, Badgwell BD. Palliation of malignant ascites. *J Surg Oncol*. 2019;120:67–73. https://doi.org/10.1002/jso.25453.
93. Oey RC, van Buuren HR, de Man RA. The diagnostic work-up in patients with ascites: current guidelines and future prospects. *Neth J Med*. 2016;74(8):330–335.
94. Ammouri L, Prommer EE. Palliative treatment of malignant ascites: profile of catumaxomab. *Biologics*. 2010;4:103–110.
95. Adam RA, Adam YG. Malignant ascites: past, present, and future. *J Am Coll Surg*. 2004;198(6):999–1011.
96. Allaire M, Cadranel J, Nguyen TT, et al. Management of infections in patients with cirrhosis in the context of increasing therapeutic resistance: a systematic review. *Clin Res Hepatol Gastroenterol*. 2020; 44:264–274. https://doi.org/10.1016/j.clinre.2019.10.003.
97. Baki J, Brown P, Tapper E. Do nutritional interventions improve the outcomes of patients with cirrhosis and ascites: a systematic review of randomized trials. *Curr Hepatol Rep*. 2020;19(2):71–77. https://doi.org/10.1007/s11901-020-00513-1.
98. Benmassaoud A, Freeman SC, Roccarina D, et al. Treatment for ascites in adults with decompensated liver cirrhosis: a network meta-analysis. *Cochrane Database Syst Rev*. 2020;1:CD013123. https://doi.org/10.1002/14651858.CD013123.pub2.
99. Matsusaki K, Aridome K, Emoto S, et al. Clinical practice guideline for the treatment of malignant ascites: section summary in clinical practice guideline for peritoneal dissemination (2021). *Int J Clin Oncol*. 2022;27:1–6. https://doi.org/10.1007/s10147-021-02077-6.
100. Kietpeerakool C, Rattanakanokchai S, Jampathong N, Srisomboon J, Lumbiganon P. Management of drainage for malignant ascites in gynaecological cancer. *Cochrane Database Syst Rev*. 2019;12:CD007794. https://doi.org/10.1002/14651858.CD007794.pub3.
101. Bleicher J, Lambert LA. A palliative approach to management of peritoneal carcinomatosis and malignant ascites. *Surg Oncol Clin N Am*. 2021;30(3):475–490. https://doi.org/10.1016/j.soc.2021.02.004.
102. Cooper M, Pollard A, Pandey A, et al. Palliative long-term abdominal drains versus large volume paracentesis in refractory ascites due to cirrhosis (REDUCe study): qualitative outcomes. *J Pain Symptom Manage*. 2021;62(2):312–325. https://doi.org/10.1016/j.jpainsymman.2020.12.007.
103. Maleux G, Indesteege I, Laenen A, et al. Tenckhoff tunneled peritoneal catheter placement in the palliative treatment of malignant ascites: technical results and overall clinical outcome. *Radiol Oncol*. 2016;50(2):197–203.
104. Bureau C, Thabut D, Jezequel C, et al. The use of rifaximin in the prevention of over hepatic encephalopathy after transjugular intrahepatic portosystemic shunt. *Ann Intern Med*. 2022;174:633–640. https://doi.org/10.7326/M20-0202.
105. Vizzutti F, Celsa C, Calvaruso V, et al. Mortality after transjugular intrahepatic portosystemic shunt in older adult patients with cirrhosis: a validated prediction model. *Hepatology*. 2023;77(2):476–488. https://doi.org/10.1002/hep.32704.
106. Aagaard NK, Malago M, De Gottardi A, et al. Consensus care recommendations for alfapump® in cirrhotic patients with refractory or recurrent ascites. *BMC Gastroenterol*. 2022;22:111. https://doi.org/10.1186/s12876-022-02173-5.
107. Orgiano L, Pani F, Astara G, et al. The role of "closed abdomen" hyperthermic intraperitoneal chemotherapy (HIPEC) in the palliative treatment of neoplastic ascites from peritoneal carcinomatosis: report of a single-center experience. *Support Care Cancer*. 2016;24(10):4293–4299.
108. Hanafusa N, Isoai A, Ishihara T, et al. Safety and efficacy of cell-free and concentrated ascites reinfusion therapy (CART) in refractory ascites: post-marketing surveillance results. *PLoS One*. 2017;12(5):e0177303.
109. Chen H, Ishihara M, Horita M, et al. Effectiveness of cell-free and concentrated ascites reinfusion therapy in the treatment of malignancy-related ascites: a systematic review and meta-analysis. *Cancers*. 13:4873. https://doi.org/10.3390/cancers13194873.

17 Medically Administered Nutrition and Hydration

Jennifer A. Tschanz and Carmen N. Spalding

Key Points

- For many people, food and drink are synonymous with care, but medically administered nutrition and hydration (MANH) should be considered a medical intervention rather than a basic form of comfort.
- Decreased appetite or inability to tolerate or enjoy food and fluids is a natural sign of advanced disease and can be a source of distress for patients, family, and caregivers.
- Discussions and decisions regarding initiating or withholding MANH at the end of life are guided by goals of care, evaluation of benefits and burden, ethical and cultural considerations, and the beliefs and wishes of the patient and family. These wishes should be documented in an advance directive.
- It is medically and legally acceptable for patients or families to choose to voluntarily refuse any form of nutrition or hydration, commonly called "voluntarily stopping eating and drinking."
- Nurses caring for patients and families faced with the decision to start or withhold or withdraw MANH are responsible for promoting patient autonomy, providing education regarding benefits and burdens of interventions, promoting informed decision-making based on values, and delivering quality care with the rest of the care team.
- It is not recommended to provide MANH at the end of life, particularly for those with end-stage cancer.

Case Study

Ms. K is a 56-year-old woman with a diagnosis of metastatic breast cancer to bone. She had completed several lines of therapy before the cancer was found to have spread to her brain and liver 4 months ago. She completed radiation and decided to forego additional medical treatments due to her declining performance status and desire to spend time with her family and friends as opposed to attending medical appointments. She was referred to a community-based palliative care team. During a visit at home by her palliative care nurse, Ms. K's sister verbalized concern that Ms. K continues to lose weight and tires easily. The sister is worried Ms. K is "starving and dehydrated" and asks if she would consider a feeding tube to "get some energy." Ms. K states she "doesn't feel hungry." Ms. K weighed 130 pounds at intake 4 months ago and now weighs 92 pounds despite adhering to the recommendations for protein shakes, small and frequent meals, steroids, and appetite stimulants. Ms. K is still able to make decisions for herself. The nurse proceeds with a conversation about medically administered nutrition and hydration (MANH).

Introduction

In the context of providing palliative care, decisions to initiate or withhold or withdraw the interventions of MANH can be challenging for the patient, the family, and members of the healthcare team. For patients who are in the last days to weeks of life there is little evidence that nutrition or hydration offers any benefit at this stage of illness. Decreased appetite or inability to tolerate or enjoy food and fluids is often a hallmark of the terminal phase of an illness; however, the starting point is not well defined.[1] In many cultures, providing food and fluids is synonymous with caring, hope, and comfort.[2] Individuals and their families may ask for MANH to address a variety of situations (e.g., fears of starvation, weight loss, and dehydration). Clinicians may recommend medically administered nutrition (MAN) or medically administered hydration (MAH) in specific circumstances (e.g., malnutrition, dehydration, and new onset of delirium). Patients with the ability to clearly make and communicate their choices to others may voluntarily stop eating and drinking as the end of life approaches. As with any palliative care intervention, the nurse needs to understand the patient's illness trajectory and patient and family goals of care, which can be influenced by a person's culture or religion. The nurse also needs to be familiar with the current evidence for MANH for patients with advanced illness as nurses often participate in conversations regarding treatment options and have a critical role in supporting the patient in identifying interventions that best meet their goals.

Natural Fluid Deficits in Advanced Disease

Homeostasis of fluids is achieved in normal individuals by matching daily water intake and fluid loss. This match ultimately provides maintenance and balance for stable composition of body fluids. About 2,500 mL is the average amount of water consumed and lost per day. Fluid can be lost through kidneys, the gastrointestinal (GI) tract, lungs, and skin. Fluid deficits in patients who are seriously ill can have varying etiologies and be multifactorial. Regardless of the cause, the result is a naturally occurring fluid deficit disorder with both hypovolemia and dehydration.

As patients enter the dying process, it is most often characterized by diminished oral intake, progressive fluid deficits, and progressive accumulation of drugs, which can cause new symptoms or exacerbate existing ones (e.g., fatigue, dizziness, myoclonus, sedation, and hallucinations).[3,4] This phenomenon results in a further decline in the ability to drink fluids. During this phase, the evidence suggests diminished awareness, which may decrease the patient's perception of thirst and hunger.[5–7]

Medically Administered Nutrition

MAN is the provision of nutrition that involves non-oral enteral or parenteral delivery of nutrients. Enteral approaches include nasogastric, percutaneous endoscopic gastrostomy (PEG), PEG jejunostomy, or gastrojejunostomy tubes.[3] Parenteral approaches include central or peripheral venous access.

MAN is a medical intervention to address malnutrition. In the advanced stages of cancer and dementia it has been linked to poorer outcomes such as increased mortality, infections, and pressure ulcers.[4,8] Malnutrition occurs when the body does not get the nutrients it needs.[9] Causes of malnutrition include an inadequate diet, mechanical issues with digestion or absorption of nutrients, and specific medical conditions.[8] In patients with a serious illness, specific causes of malnutrition include anorexia, cachexia, and physiological issues. When caring for multimorbid patients with advanced disease there are often a myriad of etiologies for malnutrition and fluid electrolyte imbalances. Hospice and palliative nurses play an integral role around assessment, treatment, support, and ongoing evaluation for patients contemplating MAN. Anorexia manifests with a decrease in appetite, which can lead to a loss of fat tissue. The weight loss that results can be reversible depending on the underlying causes. Many patients with advanced illness experience anorexia.[5] Cancer cachexia is a multifactorial syndrome in which there is loss of skeletal muscle that cannot be completely reversed by nutritional support, resulting in a negative impact on functional status.[10] Mechanical issues include malignant bowel obstruction and dysphagia.

Benefits and Burdens

While the benefits of MAN are clearer in patients who are expected to recover, they are not as clear in patients who have advanced chronic illness or who are seriously ill.[11] The expected benefits include improving a patient's nutritional status to alleviate distressing symptoms resulting from malnutrition; however, MAN in the palliative care setting does not always have a positive impact. In amyotrophic lateral sclerosis (ALS), there are guidelines recommending the use and timing of MAN since malnutrition and weight loss are prognosticators for survival.[12–14] In patients with cancers of the oropharynx or esophagus, MAN may be appropriate earlier in the disease trajectory, especially when the cause of malnutrition is directly related to the inability to maintain intake due to mechanical blockages and acute treatment effects (e.g., mucositis secondary to chemoradiation).[15] For patients in a permanent vegetative state, life expectancy can be extended by months to years.[16] Outside of these clinical diagnoses and settings, studies have indicated that MAN has no effect on prolonging life or improving functional status in advanced illness.[17]

A study looking at whether clinical, functional, or nutritional indices could determine if patients would benefit from MAN found that comorbidity, cognitive function, and social function could predict a patient's success with MAN.[18] This same study found that predictors of the ineffectiveness of MAN on clinical outcomes included severe cognitive impairment and frailty.

While there may be some benefit in certain populations with end-stage diseases, enteral and parenteral feedings are interventions with the potential for associated morbidity and increased suffering. Patients and families worry about anorexia and believe MAN to be beneficial to address both physical and psychosocial symptoms.[19,20] Therefore, it is critical for the nurse caring for these patients and families to not only review the benefits and burdens medically but also to explain the long-term caregiving, financial, social, and emotional impacts of long-term MAN.

Potential complications from the administration of MAN are listed in Table 17.1. Potential additional burdens include complications from tube placement, increased risk of infection or skin excoriation around the tube, worsening bowel and bladder control, and use of mechanical or pharmacologic restraints to preserve access.[8]

Malnutrition, Anorexia, and Cachexia

In many end-stage diseases, weight loss due to malnutrition, anorexia, or cachexia is a common occurrence. In patients with cancer with persistent anorexia and cachexia, MAN has not been shown to reverse the weight loss.[21] It is commonly thought that weight loss may be secondary to the release of cytokines that increase protein degradation.[22] In one study looking at body mass index (BMI) as a specific marker of nutritional status, the provision of MAN helped to stabilize decreases in BMI for patients who were alive at the 3-month follow-up (10 out of 17 patients); however, the study did not

Table 17.1 Potential complications of enteral support

Complication	Symptom	Cause
Aspiration	Coughing	Excess residual
	Fever	Large-bore tube
Diarrhea	Watery stool	Hyperosmotic solution
		Rapid infusion
		Lactose intolerance
Constipation	Hard, infrequent stools	Inadequate fluid
		Inadequate fiber
Dumping syndrome	Dizziness	High volume
		Hyperosmotic fluids

measure quality of life (QOL) for the same population.[23] In the terminal phase of diseases such as cancer, MAN may not be metabolized in a way that would reverse the effects, and the intervention for palliative purposes is rarely recommended.[24,25]

Dysphagia

When a patient has difficulty swallowing, MAN may be considered to ensure that the patient receives adequate nutrition or to reduce the risk for aspiration pneumonia. In certain disease states, such as ALS and dementia, it is a matter of when, not if, dysphagia will occur. For ALS patients, the goal for enteral feeding is to improve the QOL, and the preferred mechanism to deliver MAN is via a PEG tube, if indicated.[26] The onset of dysphagia and the resulting weight loss are indications of when to start MAN in the ALS patient population.[13] Providers may consider initiating enteral feeds to reduce the risk for aspiration pneumonia due to "food going down the wrong way"; however, studies have shown that enteral nutrition does not reduce, and may increase, the risk for aspiration pneumonia.[21,27,28]

Hunger

Families often express concern about their loved one experiencing hunger or have fears about their loved one starving at the end of life, yet patients will often deny sensations of hunger in the terminal phase. Minimal research surrounding this phenomenon exists. One study looking at the incidence of hunger in the seriously ill found that most patients (63%) denied hunger on admission and did not report any hunger during the admission. Of the remaining patients, only 3% (one patient) reported hunger throughout the admission; the others reported feeling hungry, but the hunger disappeared over time. These patients were offered food by mouth as requested, and the small amounts they tolerated satisfied their hunger; no patients were given MAN.[5] In advanced cancer and dementia, hunger is not a symptom often experienced due to the natural disease process.[5,29]

Pressure Ulcers

Patients who are malnourished are at increased risk for pressure ulcers, yet at the end of life there is no evidence to support the use of MAN to treat or prevent pressure ulcers.[21,27,30] One study showed that in patients with dementia, the use of a PEG tube to administer MAN was associated with an increased risk of developing new stage 2 pressure ulcers and a decreased likelihood of the healing of existing pressure ulcers.[31] Potential reasons for this association include risk factors such as increased likelihood of immobility due to the use of restraints that may be used to ensure that feeding tubes are maintained and potential for diarrhea due to the composition of the enteral feeds.[31] Currently, clinicians are advised against using MAN for treatment of pressure ulcers as the complications of artificial feeds (malabsorption, diarrhea) can cause more burden than benefit.[32]

Survival Time

There is no compelling evidence that MAN increases the survival of patients with end-stage diseases.[21,27] For patients with advanced dementia, studies do not indicate that MAN prolongs life.[28] The literature suggests that there is also no indication of improved overall function, prevention of aspiration, or reduced pressure sores.[32,33] One study found a median survival post–feeding tube insertion of 165 days and a 64% mortality rate, with half of those who died doing so within the first 2 months following insertion.[34] Another study compared the impact on survival time of PEG tube insertion or the timing of the insertion and found no impact.[35] Other studies have shown an increase in survival in specific populations. One study compared survival time in dementia patients in Japan who used self-feeding oral intake versus home parenteral nutrition or PEG feeding and found that the groups who used either home parenteral nutrition or PEG feeding survived almost twice as long.[35] In this study, patients were not in the end stage of dementia, which may explain the longer survival time. Another study looked at whether dementia was a risk factor for survival after PEG and found no difference in survival between patients with dementia and patients without dementia who received a PEG tube.[36] The authors did not include the stage of dementia in their analysis. These findings must be interpreted with caution. To date, there has been no high-quality research studying the effect of MAN for palliative care patients, which limits the clinician's ability to make evidence-based recommendations for practice. Further research is warranted.[11]

QOL

There have not been many studies that specifically measure QOL for patients with a serious illness receiving MAN. In a Cochrane review of enteral tube feeding in older adults with advanced dementia, none of the studies reviewed measured QOL. Another Cochrane review found two studies that did not demonstrate improved QOL in both a population with motor neuron disease and one with advanced cancer.[37] One randomized controlled study conducted with patients with advanced cancer cachexia and a functional GI tract demonstrated that parenteral nutrition did not improve QOL or survival over oral feedings.[38] Patients and their families determine the impact of interventions such as MAN on QOL. Some studies have shown that patients and families perceive MAN to have a positive impact on reducing burden from physical and psychosocial symptoms, such as maintaining the fight against the disease, reducing anxiety due to anorexia, and alleviating symptoms. Other studies have looked at the use of MAN and the prevalence of interventions that may be thought to negatively impact QOL, such as the use of restraints. In studies looking at patients with dementia receiving tube feeds, MAN has been correlated with an increased use of restraints, either physical or pharmacological.[39,40] In a study assessing family members' perceptions of the impact of a feeding tube, only 32.9% of the people who responded stated that the intervention improved the patient's QOL.[41]

Summary

MAN has been shown to have a positive impact on survival and nutritional parameters in certain populations, such as earlier in the disease trajectories for ALS and some cancers. However, there is not enough evidence to support a specific recommendation on when or if, in a palliative care population, it is best to use MAN.[39] The individual patient's condition, and the goals of care, needs to be considered to best determine the benefit of employing MAN compared to the burdens of the intervention.

Hydration

MAH is the provision of water or electrolyte solutions by any route other than the mouth. This can be achieved by intravenous (IV), subcutaneous (SC; hypodermoclysis), and rectal (proctoclysis) administration.[41]

Hydration is an intervention used to address situations such as fluid deficits and altered mental status secondary to medication toxicities in advanced disease. Fluid deficit disorders include dehydration and volume depletion. *Dehydration* is intracellular water depletion with hypernatremia (hyperosmolality) and usually presents with symptoms of thirst, anorexia, nausea/vomiting, fatigue, and irritability. Physical findings may include lethargy, confusion, muscle twitching, and hyperreflexia. *Volume depletion* is the loss of intravascular water (with varying sodium levels) and presents with diminished skin turgor/capillary refill and orthostatic hypotension and dizziness.[31] Patients with advanced illness experiencing anorexia may also experience a loss of interest in drinking.[42] During the terminal phase, fluid deficits, similar to malnutrition, may result from anorexia/early satiety, nausea/vomiting, bowel obstruction, dysphagia, and cognitive impairment.[31,43,44]

Some patients and families believe that decreased oral intake and the ensuing dehydration cause suffering. Patients and families are concerned that dehydration may precipitate symptoms of delirium, confusion, myoclonus, somnolence, fatigue, neuromuscular irritability, restlessness, thirst, hunger, and constipation, especially in the presence of opioids, benzodiazepines, and neuroleptics.[45] There is limited information regarding the effects of hydration in addressing these symptoms. Many patients with advanced cancer and their caregivers perceive that hydration provides hope and comfort, improves symptoms and QOL, and fulfills a basic human need for water. Emphasis on the importance of taking the patient's specific diagnosis, wishes, and hopes into consideration when discussions about medically administered hydration arise is imperative.[46]

When considering hydration, it is important to consider where the patient is on the disease trajectory (e.g., acutely ill or in the dying phase) to help establish goals of care. A survey of palliative care physicians in Australia and New Zealand identified palliation of family and patient concern as the most common reason for prescribing artificial hydration, not a physical symptom.[47] Hydration can be used for the temporary relief of symptoms of fluid loss such as nausea, vomiting, diarrhea, and fevers; to decrease fatigue; to improve mental cognition status associated with medication toxicities; and as a respect to cultural and familial beliefs.

Methods of Administration

There are various alternative routes to oral administration to meet the goals of care and wishes of the patient and family. Standard methods for replacement of fluids, similar to nutrition, can be achieved by the use of enteral feeding tubes and parenteral methods, such as SC or IV infusion.

Intravenous access requires a competent vein. Clinicians may use permanent access devices if they have previously been placed or if ongoing hydration is anticipated. *Hypodermoclysis* is the SC infusion of isotonic solution. It does not require special access devices and can be used for patients who have poor venous access for IV placement. The absorption of the SC fluids has been found to be comparable with absorption of IV fluids when administered appropriately.[41,43] *Proctoclysis* is used to administer water or saline into the GI tract via the rectum using a nasogastric tube. Proctoclysis may be appropriate for patients who are unable to eat or drink, who have poor vascular access, and whose skin integrity may be unable to withstand hypodermoclysis. Researchers have found proctoclysis to be safe and economical, but there has been cultural and social reluctance to accept this mode of administration.[45]

There is no consensus regarding the volume or type of fluid replacement. Clinicians make choices based on previous experiences and knowledge of the patient's condition and wishes. Some providers allow the individual to have 1 L/day, even though it may be inadequate replacement. Risks and burdens must be considered (Table 17.2).

Benefits and Burdens

The decision for hydration needs to include an evaluation of goals of care, discussion of the risks and benefits, and timely re-evaluation to determine if goals or symptoms are improving or worsening. Insurance coverage, impact on healthcare benefits, social impact, and maintenance of administration should be carefully evaluated and require input from the other healthcare team members. Risks for overhydration, as evidenced by worsening fluid retention and signs of increased shortness of breath, increased emotional distress, or change in mental status, must be monitored. Advantages of not providing medically administered hydration can include reduced urine output, leading to reduced incontinence and need for catheterization; reduction of GI secretions, leading to decreased incidence of vomiting; and decreased respiratory tract secretions, leading to decreased cough and need for suction.[45]

Table 17.2 Potential complications of routes for medically administered hydration

IV peripheral	IV central	SC hypodermoclysis	Proctoclysis
Pain	Sepsis	Pain	Discomfort
Short duration of access	Hemothorax	Infection	Enema effect
Infection	Pneumothorax	Third-spacing	Accidental dislodgement
Phlebitis	Central vein thrombosis	Tissue sloughing	
	Catheter fragment thrombosis	Local bleeding	
	Air embolus		
	Brachial plexus injury		
	Arterial laceration		

IV, intravenous; SC, subcutaneous.

Factors arguing against initiating hydration include increasing the incidence of pulmonary and peripheral edema and increased respiratory tract secretions, cough, and ascites.[45,46,48] Starting IV hydration can cause pain, be distressing, restrict mobility, hinder family contact, and increase the use of restraints.[5]

Review of the Literature

Dehydration and Fluid Retention

Dehydration can cause unpleasant symptoms such as confusion and restlessness in non–terminally ill patients.[49] These problems are common in the dying. There is limited research regarding the effect of hydration on alleviating dehydration at the end of life. Results can be challenging to interpret due to the ways various studies define and measure dehydration. Findings suggest that providing medically administered hydration may or may not affect physical signs and symptoms of dehydration at the end of life. One study demonstrated no difference in hydration status after 7 days between advanced cancer patients who were given 1,000 mL/day and those given 100 mL/day. The same study also scored four dehydration symptoms (fatigue, myoclonus, sedation, and hallucinations) and noted no difference in the sum of the scores after the 7-day hydration trial.[50] A retrospective chart review study showed that medically administered hydration in the last 48 hours of life had no significant impact on symptoms related to hydration status (e.g., agitation, myoclonus, urinary retention, confusion, congestive cardiac failure, respiratory tract secretions, nausea and vomiting, and ascites).[45] These findings suggest that there is no benefit of hydration during the terminal phase.

Depending on the volume of hydration administered, hydration may increase the risk of developing fluid retention symptoms. In a study that measured the effect of hydration volume on terminally ill cancer patients with abdominal malignancies, dehydration was evaluated based on physical findings that included moisture on the mucous membranes of the mouth, axillary moisture, and sunken eyes within 72 hours of death. Patients in the hydration group who received 1,000 mL or more of MAH per day 1 and 3 weeks before death were found to have less deterioration in dehydration symptoms than the non-hydration group who received on average less than 1,000 mL of MAH over the 3 weeks prior to death. However, the patients who were in the hydration group were noted to have increased symptoms of overhydration such as edema, ascites, and bronchial secretions. No difference was noted between the groups regarding pleural effusion.[50] These findings are similar to those of a study that showed increased dehydration status in the non-hydration group who did not receive hydration and increased fluid retention symptoms of peripheral edema and ascites in the hydration group.[51]

A prevalence of bronchial secretions in the last 48 hours of life was noted more in the large-volume group that received more than 1,000 mL hydration per day compared to those in the small-volume group that received less than 1,000 mL/day.[52] The accumulation of these bronchial secretions at the end of life can contribute to the gurgling sound called the "death rattle." There is limited research regarding the effect of artificial hydration on the death rattle. One prospective observational study in the Netherlands did not find an association between artificial hydration volume and the occurrence of the death rattle.[53] However, a study with abdominal cancer patients measuring hydration volume and the incidence of death rattle showed an increase in prevalence of the death rattle in patients who received more than 500 mL/day than in those who received less than 500 mL/day.[54]

A national guideline for parenteral hydration therapy was established in Japan in 2007 that encouraged respecting patient and family wishes, conducting a comprehensive assessment of the patient's QOL, allowing for total parenteral nutrition to be administered if bowel obstruction was present, and recommending that hydration be decreased to less than 1,000 mL/day if fluid retention signs were present.[55] A study to measure the efficacy of this guideline demonstrated that providing hydration to patients with advanced cancer according to the guidelines led to stable measurements in global QOL, discomfort, most physical symptoms, and fluid retention signs.[56]

Thirst and Dry Mouth

Thirst is thought to be a nonspecific symptom of dehydration. One study looked at interventions for thirst and dry mouth as an alternative to hydration. Researchers found that routine care, defined as offering food and fluids, administering ice chips, and providing mouth care, helped to alleviate these symptoms.[5,52] Dry mouth is treated with an intensive, every 2-hour schedule of mouth care, including hygiene, lip lubrication, and ice chips or popsicles. Elimination of medications that cause dry mouth, such as tricyclic antidepressants and antihistamines, should be considered. Sometimes, drugs that contribute to these symptoms are being administered to palliate other symptoms, such as the opioids for pain and anticholinergics to minimize oral secretions. Mouth breathing can also contribute to dry mouth. *Candida* infection, a frequent cause of dry mouth, can be treated. Agents such as pilocarpine can be used to increase salivation.

In one study, hydration was shown to alleviate symptoms of dry mouth in patients with advanced cancer who have a relatively longer prognosis. It was noted that dry mouth intensity decreased significantly in the group receiving a large volume of hydration (1,000 mL/day or more) compared to those in the small volume group (less than 1,000 mL/day). This same group also experienced a higher incidence of bronchial secretions.[56]

Delirium, Confusion, Agitation

Delirium can be caused by multiple factors including end-organ failure, dehydration, and medications. Symptoms of delirium can be distressing for patients and families. In advanced cancer patients, no significant difference in delirium and agitation was noted in patients receiving more hydration versus less hydration.[50,55]

Medications such as opioids, anticholinergics, antihistamines, and corticosteroids have been known to impact delirium. If delirium is related to the accumulation of opioids, interventions to decrease or rotate opioids and to increase hydration are believed to control the symptoms of hyperactive delirium, such as agitation and hallucinations of opioid-induced neurotoxicity, by assisting with the clearance of toxic opioid metabolites.[56]

"Terminal restlessness" refers to the confusion, agitation, and emotional distress/lability at the end of life. One observational, prospective study in the Netherlands looked at the amount of fluid intake (through oral and IV routes) and opioid use in patients expected to die within hours or days. They observed terminal restlessness was associated with fluid greater than 250 mL/day during the 48–25 hours before death.[53]

Myoclonus

Myoclonus, or involuntary contractions of muscles, is commonly associated with chronic opioid use at the end of life. It has also been reported in cancer patients without opioid use who are experiencing decreased oral intake.[43] There is limited and mixed information regarding the effects of hydration on myoclonus depending on patient setting. Myoclonus was shown to improve in the intervention group who received 1,000 mL normal saline over 4 hours for 2 days versus 100 mL.[57] However, no difference in myoclonus symptoms was noted between patients with advanced abdominal malignancies in the hydration group who were given on average 838 to 1,405 mL/day during the last 3 weeks of life and those in the non-hydration group who received an average of 200 mL/day.

Survival Benefit

There is limited research regarding the survival benefit of hydration. Two studies noted that hydration provided no survival benefit for terminally ill cancer patients with short prognosis.[50,55]

QOL

There is limited research regarding the impact of hydration on QOL in the terminally ill. Research on patients with advanced cancer shows that parenteral hydration of 1,000 mL/day did not improve symptoms associated with QOL over placebo of 100 mL/day.[58] Another study showed that QOL measurements remained stable when hydration was administered according to Japanese guidelines that took into account QOL and symptoms of fluid retention whether patients received small (<1,000 mL/day) or large (>1,000 mL/day) volumes of hydration.[56] In a study that interviewed patients with advanced cancer and their caregivers, both patients and their caregivers perceived hydration as fulfilling the basic human need for water, promoting hope and dignity, and enhancing QOL. Caregivers in the same study reported that hydration improved pain management and that the patient had more energy, better sleeping habits, an improved appetite, and a healthier physical experience. The study did not include information on volumes or duration of hydration.

Quality of Death

A prospective, observational study in Taiwan investigated the relationship between artificial hydration alone on survival, symptoms, and quality of dying in terminal cancer patients. Participants were separated into a hydration group and a non-hydration group who received fluid up to 400 mL/day. Between the two arms, researchers found no difference in dehydration symptom relief and no difference in survival. Researchers did note higher Good Death Scale (GDS) scores in the group who received hydration.[59] The GDS included the following five domains: awareness that one is dying, acceptance of death peacefully, honoring the patient's wishes, death timing, and the degree of physical comfort three days before death. Similarly, researchers further sought to quantify the volume of fluid that could improve GDS scores in terminally ill cancer patients living in Japan, Korea, and Taiwan. It was observed that patients given artificial hydration volumes between 250 and 400 mL/day were found to have better GDS scores than those who did not receive artificial hydration.[60] The authors caution there is no direct causal relationship between artificial hydration and GDS scores and concluded that communication with patients and families about artificial hydration benefits and burdens could better prepare patients and families and lead to a good death.

Summary

Parenteral hydration has been found to be effective in temporary, short-term situations to alleviate symptoms related to dehydration and improve mental cognition. In the palliative care setting, research does not support that parenteral hydration improves signs of dehydration, survival, or QOL. In the setting of delirium related to opioid toxicity, there is mixed evidence supporting hydration and possible opioid rotation to improve delirium symptoms. When deciding to initiate or stop hydration, it is important to assess goals of care, risks and benefits, and the patient's preferences related to their values and needs.

Review of Position Statements and Guidelines

Many professional organizations have published position statements or guidelines on the use of MANH. Common themes across these documents include the following:

- MANH is an intervention that should be evaluated by the patient, family, and care team with careful consideration of its benefits and burdens.[61–64]
- MANH is considered a medical intervention that can be refused, withheld, or withdrawn based on the patient's clinical condition and goals of care.[39,65]
- Decisions about MANH need to reflect the patient's and family's values, beliefs, and culture.[65]

In addition to general position statements regarding MANH, disease-specific recommendations are summarized in Table 17.3.

Decision-Making and MANH

Decisions about the initiation or withholding or withdrawing of MANH are complex.[65] In addition to the review of the clinical evidence regarding the efficacy of MANH to improve symptoms and QOL, it is important to consider ethical principles and legal precedents that highlight the role nurses have in advocating for the patient as well as their responsibilities in respecting patient and family wishes. While the withdrawing of MAN and/or MAH may cause more emotional distress for clinicians as well as for patients and

Table 17.3 Disease-specific guidelines for medically administered nutrition and hydration

Advanced dementia	Feeding tubes are not recommended. Enhance oral feedings by improving the environment and supporting patient-centered approaches.
End-stage cancer	Use of nutritional support for terminally ill cancer patients is not usually indicated.
Amyotrophic lateral sclerosis	Early insertion of a feeding tube is recommended if enteral feeding is determined to be an appropriate intervention.

their families than withholding such treatment, there is no ethical or legal distinction between them.[2] When decision-making is difficult or complicated by a particular goal or value, a short goal-based trial can be offered with the intention of temporary support being emphasized. In this circumstance, the patient should be routinely assessed for adverse effects of the MANH intervention (Table 17.4).

Ethical Issues

Initiating or withholding or withdrawing MANH, like other medical interventions, needs to be done utilizing ethical principles. The three ethical principles that are most relevant in decision-making for MANH are autonomy, beneficence, and nonmaleficence.[66] "Autonomy" refers to the patient's or surrogate's right to self-determination. Respecting autonomy in decisions about MANH means that a patient or family has the choice to accept or refuse the intervention based on their personal values and beliefs.[66] "Beneficence" means "to do good" and implies that nurses must act in the interest of the patient.[66] The nurse has a responsibility to engage the patient and family in a conversation about what "good" looks like, respecting the individual's values and goals for care. For example, a patient with end-stage cancer may be experiencing dysphagia yet still find enjoyment in small sips of liquid. While the risk for aspiration exists in this situation, the nurse would exhibit beneficence by supporting the intake of fluids. "Nonmaleficence" means "to do no harm" and can be exemplified by not administering treatments that increase the risk of suffering and have no benefit or whose benefit is less than their burden.

Legal Precedent

Landmark cases such as the Quinlan case, the Cruzan case, the Barber case, and *Vacco v. Quill* have set the foundation for current decision-making regarding MANH within the healthcare system. Karen Ann Quinlan was 21 years old when she was deemed to be in a persistent vegetative state due to anoxic brain injury. Her father sought guardianship to cease "extraordinary" measures keeping her alive.[67] In this case, the court supported the standard of substituted judgment, enabling her father to speak for her as if she could speak for herself.[68] Nancy Cruzan was thrown from her vehicle in a car accident. Although found by the paramedics with no pulse, they were able to resuscitate her. She was in a coma for several weeks before being determined by her physicians to be in a persistent vegetative state.[69] In her case, the court supported the right to refuse treatment

Table 17.4 Hydration and/or nutrition in advanced illness or end of life: Key studies

Author, year, design	Sample size and characteristics	Variables evaluated	Results	Overall impact of hydration
Nakajima et al. (2013)[48] Observational study	75 terminally ill patients with gastrointestinal malignancy	Hydration score	Dehydration score was higher in non-hydration group (35% vs. 13%, p. 03); edema/ascites/bronchial secretions higher in hydration group (57% vs. 33%, p. 04)	No benefit secondary to adverse effects
Bruera et al. (2013)[50] Randomized controlled trial	129 patients in hospice care	Symptoms for dehydration, delirium, myoclonus, and survival	No difference between treatment and control groups in delirium, dehydration	Negative
Morita et al. (2005)[46] Prospective controlled trial	226 advanced cancer patients (59 hydrated and 167 non-hydrated)	Dehydration and fluid retention symptoms	No significant difference in dehydration or retention symptoms	Negative
Bruera et al. (2005)[57] Randomized controlled trial	60 dehydrated patients with advanced cancer	Symptoms of dehydration	Mixed for sedation and myoclonus Improvement, composite score for fatigue, hallucinations	Mixed
Morita et al. (2001)[7] Observational study	88 terminally ill cancer patients in hospice	Assessment using visual analogue scale on symptoms of thirst	No correlation of thirst scores	Negative
Cerchietti et al. (2000) Randomized controlled trial	42 advanced cancer patients who were dehydrated	Thirst, nausea, delirium and Mini-Mental Status Exam, anguish, mood	No significant differences in groups	Negative
Ellershaw et al. (1995)[6] Observational study	82 cancer patients 2 days before death	Thirst, respiratory secretions, dry mouth	No correlation between hydration status and thirst	Negative
Musgrave et al. (1995) Uncontrolled trial	30 cancer patients in the last day of life	Thirst level	All patients who were alert experienced some level of thirst	Negative
McCann et al. (1994)[5] Uncontrolled trial	32 terminally ill patients who were mentally aware	Thirst, hunger, and dry mouth	63% no hunger, 34% initial hunger only, 62% no thirst or initial thirst	Negative
Waller et al. (1994) Observational study	68 cancer patients within 48 hours of death, 13 received fluids	Consciousness	No correlation in improvement of consciousness and administration of fluids	Negative
Wu et al. (2021)[59] Prospective, observational study	100 terminally ill cancer patients (hydration group received less than 400 mL, non-hydration group)	Higher Good Death Scale (GDS) scores in hydration group	Survival, symptoms (review for more info), GDS No significant difference in survival or symptom between the two groups	
Wu et al. (2022)[60] Observational study	1,530 terminally ill patients on palliative care units	GDS	GDS scores were better for those who received 250–400 mL/day than those without artificial hydration	

for competent individuals. The court also supported the need for "clear and convincing evidence" since she was incompetent and had not previously recorded her wishes. This case helped to support the federal Patient Self-Determination Act passed in 1991 in an effort to help patients document their wishes.[67] The *Vacco v. Quill* case also supported the right to refuse treatment, distinguishing respecting patient wishes from intentionally hastening death.[67] In the Barber case, the court found two physicians who had discontinued MANH to be innocent from charges of murder and conspiracy to commit murder, reinforcing the precept that MANH is considered a medical intervention and not basic care.[67]

Religious and Cultural Issues

To deliver patient-centered care, nurses must recognize the roles that religious or spiritual beliefs and culture, including race and ethnicity, play in patient and family values surrounding food and fluids. Understanding these factors and encouraging discussions about patient values will enable nurses to respect patient autonomy and engage in a dialog of how to meet patient needs regarding nutrition and hydration to maximize beneficence and minimize nonmaleficence while ensuring patient autonomy. Integrating other care team members with experience in this area can be extremely helpful to all stakeholders. In particular, social work and chaplain support will assure that patient and family psychosocial and spiritual needs are met.

Research in religious practices and artificial hydration and nutrition at the end of life is sparse. One study that surveyed physicians about the topic showed that physicians of the Jewish and Muslim faiths were more likely to oppose withholding artificial nutrition and hydration than non-Evangelical Protestants.[70] In another survey, 94% of Islamic physician respondents supported artificial nutrition for patients with a do-not-resuscitate order.[71] These studies sought responses from physicians only and may not be representative of the entire population that practices these religions.

In reviewing the common beliefs of various religious traditions and cultures, it is important to remember that not everyone of a particular faith or a particular culture will have the same beliefs, and nurses should inquire as to how much influence a patient's faith or culture has on their beliefs regarding MANH. Most religions recognize the justification of stopping medical treatment in situations where the treatments cause more harm than benefit; however, in the case of artificial hydration and nutrition, the guidance is less clear. Clinicians should be aware that some religions may view voluntary cessation of hydration and nutrition as an intentional and forbidden shortening of life. Even within religions, there can be varying opinions or interpretations of religious law to guide decisions on whether to initiate or withdraw MANH. Table 17.5 summarizes beliefs by selected religious traditions specific to MANH.

In addition to religious influences, culture affects patient and family perspectives on MANH. Studies have shown variance associated with race in the use of tube feedings, with Caucasians having lower rates than people of other cultural backgrounds.[60] In studies looking at the use of feeding tubes between White subjects compared to African American and Latino subjects, use was consistently higher in the latter groups.[72] Studies have also shown that African Americans have a stronger preference for more intensive care.[73] This study looked at preferences between African American and Caucasian participants using focus groups, assessing for factors that might affect decisions about care at end of life, including MAN. From the qualitative data gathered in the focus groups, the researchers found more similarities than differences in how the two groups thought about food, artificial nutrition, and decision-making at the end of life.[73] The differences were not by category but more on focus within common themes.[73]

In a study looking at what meaning Singaporean Chinese caregivers attributed to feeding, the researchers found three major themes emerge. One theme was a sense of filial piety, where duty to one's family may motivate a push for more aggressive interventions even if the patient is at the end of life. Another theme was the link between providing nutrition and hope. A third theme was that providing food showed caring for their loved one, a theme common across many cultures.[74]

While there is not a large body of research on how differing religious and cultural backgrounds influence individual preferences for MANH, there are resources that nurses can access to learn the information needed to initiate a conversation with a patient on this issue. Whether it is through position statements from religious organizations or talking to leaders within a religious tradition or ethnic community, nurses can seek to understand how these factors play a role in each specific situation with the patient for whom they are caring.

Engaging in Conversations and Goals of Care about MANH

In working with palliative care and terminally ill patients, nurses play a pivotal role in exploring a patient's values and hopes to ensure that care related to the provision of food and fluids is person-centered. Because decisions about MANH are complex, nurses have multiple responsibilities. Nurses need to self-reflect, understand the literature, understand the position statements, understand the prognosis, and thoroughly assess the patient and family unit as a whole prior to making a nursing plan or recommendation.

One of the primary tasks of the nurse is to ensure that a patient's autonomy and dignity are respected in a way that is culturally acceptable to the patient by understanding the patient's values regarding MANH and the broader goals that the individual is hoping to achieve. This task can be best accomplished by promoting early conversations regarding patient and family preferences and having them documented. The focus should be on the patient as the decision maker, even if the patient is not participating in the conversation. While open-ended questions may encourage exploration of knowledge and understanding of patient and family hopes, focused and directed questions regarding preferences may guide patients and families to more concrete goals and decisions. Two important questions to consider in the decision-making process regarding MANH are (1) What are the views and preferences of the patient? and (2) What are the individualized goals of care? Having an evidence-based goals-of-care framework that addresses both

Table 17.5 Various religious beliefs about medically administered nutrition and hydration (MANH)

Religious faith	Beliefs
Buddhism	• Belief that all beings suffer. • Main focus at end of life is on spiritual comfort. • Less focus on extending life through MANH and other interventions. • Voluntarily stopping eating and drinking can be considered an allowable option.[a]
Catholicism[b,c]	• Current position (as of 2011) focuses on "life prolongation based on fundamental human dignity." • Some within the church assert that MANH is not considered a medical technology but is an ordinary measure to preserve life. • Others feel that MANH should be evaluated using the proportionate/disproportionate framework (ordinary vs. extraordinary) on an individual basis. • Catholic healthcare facilities are obligated to offer food and fluids regardless of disease state. • MANH can be considered extraordinary in conditions where the underlying disease would be the cause of death, not the withholding of MANH.
Hinduism[d]	• Withholding or withdrawal of MANH at the very end of life is acceptable. • Some Hindus fast to prepare for death.
Islam[e]	• "Guiding purpose of Islamic law is to protect and preserve religion, life, progeny, intellect, and wealth." • Islamic rules regarding care for terminally ill are based on the principle that one should prevent or avoid injury or harm. • Islamic law permits withdrawal of MANH and allowing the disease to take its natural course. • There can be various beliefs among Muslims, so it is necessary to ascertain the patient's values. • "Islamic law states that palliative care should not shorten a patient's life, but futile treatment is not justified." • "Islamic law forbids passively or actively causing death." • Nutritional support is considered basic care and not medical treatment, leading to a duty to feed patients who are no longer able to feed themselves. • Varied opinion among different Islamic communities regarding withdrawing and withholding MANH.
Judaism[f,g]	• Provision of food and fluids is considered an ordinary measure, not extraordinary. • Withholding food and fluids is not consistent with Jewish law. • Administration of food and fluids, even via IV or feeding tube, is not considered to be artificial. • "The religious authorities hold that [MANH is] ordinary supportive measures rather than heroic."[e] • Terminal dehydration, hospice without provision of MANH, and withdrawing or withholding MANH are not considered aligned with Jewish teaching unless there is proof of *goses* (less than 72 hours until death) and futility of intervention under any denomination of Judaism. • "While the [Israeli] law respects the right of a competent dying patient to refuse nutrition and hydration, it introduces a legal requirement to persuade 'the use of oxygen, nutrition and hydration,' even by artificial means."[f]
Protestantism[d]	• There is diversity in positions regarding MANH across denominations. • Common belief that interventions such as MANH that allow time for repentance may outweigh other burdens of treatment.

[a] Reference 80, [b] Reference 81, [c] Reference 82, [d] Reference 83, [e] Reference 84, [f] Reference 85, [g] Reference 86.

short- and long-term goals and the feasibility of those goals can be helpful. A challenge in performing this task arises when patient and family preferences conflict with a nurse's or healthcare team's preferences for treatment. The focus of discussions should be "Did we do everything to meet the patient's goals?" not "Did we do everything possible?"

Additionally, nurses can empower patients and families by educating them about the normal symptoms of the dying process and the known benefits and burdens of MANH as an intervention to effectively treat symptoms associated with dying. To facilitate informed decision-making, education can focus on symptoms and progression of the normal dying process, available options for MANH, and known benefits and burdens of MANH interventions, as well as the limitations of evidence supporting MANH in managing some symptoms and alternative options to treat distressing symptoms. Studies have shown that the use of decision aids (videos, handouts, information guides, and structured conversations) improved patient's/family members' decision-making in end-stage dementia care. Patients and families should also be informed that MANH can be withheld and withdrawn. If a nurse is unable to provide appropriate information, the nurse should feel comfortable with saying "I do not know" over providing false reassurances.[73] It is recommended that the nurse seek counsel from available resources such as the primary team, the interdisciplinary team, or the palliative care team and then return to the patient and family with information. By providing this care coordination, the channels of communication are opened between individuals caring for the patient and will allow for improved alignment as a team in supporting complex care decisions.

Alternatives to MANH

Voluntary Stopping of Eating and Drinking

One option that a patient with autonomy can choose is to voluntarily stop eating and drinking as a method of hastening death. Voluntary stopping of eating and drinking (VSED) is legally protected when the patient is at the end of their life and can competently make decisions for themselves.[75,76] No one else, not even the medical proxy, can make this decision for the patient. The VSED decision is binding, even if the patient loses capacity during the dying process. Once made, only the autonomous patient can decide to resume eating and drinking if they wish. Patients at the end of life have physiologic changes that can reduce their appetite or ability to eat, so they typically do not experience suffering. Nurses can assist and support patients in decision-making and provide ongoing care for palliation of symptoms that may occur, such as dry mouth.[77] The American Nurses Association issued a position statement that includes the following VSED recommendations: "decisions about accepting or forgoing nutrition and hydration will be honored, including those decisions about artificially delivered as well as VSED, [and] people with decision-making capacity have the right to stop eating and drinking as a means of hastening death."[64(p2)]

VSED is a relatively new and poorly studied phenomenon. Many caregivers are unfamiliar with the practices of VSED, and some healthcare professionals may have moral concerns about it. Further education and research on VSED are needed. Nurses should become educated on the legal, moral, and ethical considerations of VSED and ensure that patients receive care reflective of their known wishes to ensure patient autonomy.

Comfort Feeding Only

Eating and drinking not only sustain our bodies but are also a way many patients' families show they care. Patients at the end of life often have reduced oral intake, which can lead to significant changes to their bodies. When a patient can no longer sustain their body's nutritional status with oral intake, family members can feel compelled to request MANH as either a way to delay death or to align with the patient's or family member's religious or ethical beliefs. The family can feel forced to make a hard decision to either force-feed their loved one or allow them to starve. One option the nurse can discuss is "comfort feeding only" (CFO).[1] The nurse can inform the patient and family of the diminishing need for food and drink at the end of life and, rather than force-food or -drink by mouth or other means, encourage the family to offer small amounts of the patient's favorite food or drink when the patient indicates an interest. This concept is relatively unknown, and many practitioners may be unfamiliar with the terminology, so nurses should become familiar with this terminology and advocate for CFO when it is appropriate for their patient.

Case Study

Ms. K continues to have bouts of dehydration and weight loss. Her weight is now 88 pounds. She reports she has no appetite and eats mostly to "keep her family from worrying" about her. In her online cancer support group, a friend mentioned something about VSED. Ms. K is asking the nurse to give information on what VSED entails.

Initiating and Withdrawing or Withholding MANH

If the decision is made to initiate MANH in a patient to meet the goals of care, the nurse has a responsibility to continually assess the patient's condition, evaluating the impact of the intervention on symptoms and the patient's responses to treatment. MANH can be offered as a time-limited trial to determine whether the patient experiences any benefits from the intervention compared to burdens. As MANH is often instituted during an acute event while in the hospital, nurses can inquire about previous medical history or expressed wishes and promote conversations that look at the bigger picture beyond the acute admission.[78] Nurses in any setting can inform patients and families early in the disease continuum of the progression of the illness and ensure that wishes are elicited and documented by the healthcare team regarding MANH. The nurse needs to facilitate ongoing conversations about MANH to ensure that the role of this therapy continues to meet patient and family goals without excessive burden.

If the decision is made to either withdraw or withhold MANH, the nurse can provide emotional support and assurances that the patient's dignity will be respected with comfort care. If the patient is able, it is OK to gently encourage oral intake if it is compatible with the patient's overall goals. If eating and drinking become too difficult or require too much effort, the patient should not be pressured. Alleviation of symptoms of dry mouth and thirst should be a focus and can include gentle oral cleaning, ice chips or popsicles, moistened sponges, lip moisturizer, and artificial saliva.[58,79] If unable to support a patient's or family's decision regarding MANH for religious or personal reasons, it is the responsibility of the nurse to request a change in assignment and for the healthcare system to ensure that a nurse who is comfortable in these situations can provide patient-centered care when MANH is being withheld or withdrawn.

Case Study

Ms. K is admitted to the palliative care unit for increased agitation and confusion. It is felt she may have hours to days to live. Her chart states she wishes for no extraordinary measures to prolong her life. Comfort-only measures were initiated, and an IV was placed for medication administration. The family is concerned that Ms. K is suffering because of her agitation and confusion. They noted when she was brought to the emergency room a few months ago for confusion related to change in her pain medication, she "perked up" after receiving IV hydration. The family would like to know if Ms. K would benefit from IV fluids at this time.

Conclusion

Food and fluid requirement changes in the terminally ill are frequently multifactorial in etiology and a naturally occurring, expected phenomenon. MANH should be considered an intervention, rather than a basic provision of care. When a patient experiences a decreased desire to eat or drink as part of the end stage of illness, the patient along with the family may struggle to seek interventions to extend life, reduce the impact of possible symptoms such as hunger or dehydration, or fulfill a religious or cultural need at the end of life. Decisions about MANH are complex and must be guided by the ethical principles of autonomy, beneficence, and nonmaleficence. Nurses need to understand the factors, such as religion and culture, which influence a patient's preferences. Nurses need to provide accurate and complete information about the benefits and burdens of MANH to the patient, family, and other care team members. In doing so, nurses will ensure that decisions to initiate, withhold, or withdraw MANH will be patient-centered. When the patient is no longer taking in hydration or nutrition in any form, nurses must be attentive to comfort and support for both the patient and family.

REFERENCES

1. Blum D, Jensen W, Ullrich A, Hlawatsch C, Bokemeyer C, Oechsle K. Tipping point: when patients stop eating and drinking in the last phase of their life. *Clin Nutr ESPEN*. 2020;38:280–282.
2. Cohen MZ, Torres-Vigil I, Burbach BE, De La Rosa A, Bruera E. The meaning of parenteral hydration to family caregivers and patients with advanced cancer receiving hospice care. *J Pain Symptom Manage*. 2012;43(5):855–865.
3. Marian D. Stopping artificial nutrition and hydration and the end of life. 2025. Accessed April 28, 2025. https://www.uptodate.com/contents/stopping-nutrition-and-hydration-at-the-end-of-life?search=Stopping%20artificial%20nutrition%20and%20hydration%20at%20the%20end%20of%20life&source=search_result&selectedTitle=1%7E150&usage_type=default&display_rank=1
4. Bruera E, Belzile M, Watanabe S, Fainsinger RL. Volume of hydration in terminal cancer patients. *Support Care Cancer*. 1996;4:147–150.
5. McCann RM, Hall WJ, Groth-Juncker A. Comfort care for terminally ill patients: the appropriate use of nutrition and hydration. *JAMA*. 1994;272(16):1263–1266.
6. Ellershaw JE, Sutcliffe JM, Saunders CM. Dehydration and the dying patient. *J Pain Symptom Manage*. 1995;10(3):192–197.
7. Morita T, Tei Y, Tsunoda J, Inoue S, Chihara S. Determinants of the sensation of thirst in terminally ill cancer patients. *Support Care Cancer*. 2001;9:177–186.
8. Davies N, Barrado-Martin Y, Vickerstaff V, et al. Enteral tube feeding for people with severe dementia. *Cochrane Database Syst Rev*. 2021;8(8):CD013503.
9. Zieve D, Eltz D. Malnutrition 2021. MedlinePlus. Accessed September 2, 2022. http://www.nlm.nih.gov/medlineplus/ency/article/000404.htm.
10. Fearon K, Strasser F, Anker SD, et al. Definition and classification of cancer cachexia: an international consensus. *Lancet Oncol*. 2011;12:489–495. https://doi.org/10.1016/S1470-2045(10)70218-7.
11. Good P, Richard R, Syrmis W, Jenkins-Marsh S, Stephens J. Medically assisted nutrition for adult palliative care patients. *Cochrane Database Syst Rev*, 2014;4:CD006274.
12. Oliveira ASB, Pereira RDB. Amyotrophic lateral sclerosis (ALS): three letters that change the people's life. For ever. *Arq Neuropsiquiatr*. 2009;67:750–782.
13. Thibodeaux LS, Gutierrez A. Management of symptoms in amyotrophic lateral sclerosis. *Curr Treat Options Neurol*. 2008;10(2):77–85.
14. Morassutti I, Giometto M, Baruffi C, et al. Nutritional intervention for amyotrophic lateral sclerosis. *Minerva Gastroenterol Dietol*. 2012;58(3):253–260.
15. National Comprehensive Cancer Network. NCCN Clinical Practice Guidelines in Oncology: Head and Neck Cancers. NCCN. 2025. Accessed April 28, 2025. https://www.nccn.org/professionals/physician_gls/pdf/head-and-neck.pdf.
16. Bozzetti F, Arends J, Lundholm K, Micklewright A, Zurcher G, Muscaritoli M. ESPEN guidelines on parenteral nutrition: non-surgical oncology. *Clin Nutr*. 2009;28(4):445–454.
17. Borum ML, Lynn J, Zhong Z, et al. The effect of nutritional supplementation on survival in seriously ill hospitalized adults: an evaluation of the SUPPORT data. *J Am Geriatr Soc*. 2000;48(S1):S33–S38.
18. Donini LM, Savina C, Ricciardi LM, et al. Predicting the outcome of artificial nutrition by clinical and functional indices. *Nutrition*. 2009;25(1):11–19.
19. Del Rio M, Shand B, Bonati P, et al. Hydration and nutrition at the end of life: a systematic review of emotional impact, perceptions, and decision-making among patients, family, and health care staff. *Psychooncology*. 2012;21(9):913–921.
20. Orrevall Y, Tishelman C, Permert J, Cederholm T. The use of artificial nutrition among cancer patients enrolled in palliative home care services. *Palliat Med*. 2009;23(6):556–564.
21. Payne C, Wiffen PJ, Martin S. Interventions for fatigue and weight loss in adults with advanced progressive illness. *Cochrane Database Syst Rev*. 2012;1:CD008427.
22. Dunlop RJ, Campbell CW. Cytokines and advanced cancer. *J Pain Symptom Manage*. 2000;20(3):214–232.
23. Grilo A, Santos CA, Fonseca J. Percutaneous endoscopic gastrostomy for nutritional palliation of upper esophageal cancer unsuitable for esophageal stenting. *Arq Gastroenterol*. 2012;49:227–231.
24. August DA, Huhmann MB. ASPEN clinical guidelines: nutrition support therapy during adult anticancer treatment and in hematopoietic cell transplantation. *JPEN J Parenter Enteral Nutr*. 2009;33(5):472–500.
25. National Comprehensive Cancer Network. *NCCN Clinical Practice Guidelines in Oncology: Palliative Care*. National Comprehensive Cancer Network; 2022.
26. EFNS Task Force on Diagnosis and Management of Amyotrophic Lateral Sclerosis. EFNS guidelines on the clinical management of amyotrophic lateral sclerosis (MALS)—revised report of an EFNS task force. *Eur J Neurol*. 2012;19(3):360–375.
27. American Geriatrics Society. American geriatrics society feeding tubes in advanced dementia position statement. J Am Geriatr Soc. 2014, 62(8) 1590–1593.
28. Ticinesi A, Nouvenne A, Lauretani F, et al. Survival in older adults with dementia and eating problems: to PEG or not to PEG? *Clin Nutr*. 2016;35(6):1512–1516.
29. Hutton JL, Baracos VE, Wismer WV. Chemosensory dysfunction is a primary factor in the evolution of declining nutritional status and quality of life in patients with advanced cancer. *J Pain Symptom Manage*. 2007;33:156–165. https://doi.org/10.1016/j.jpainsymman.2006.07.017.
30. Mathus-Vliegen EM. Old age, malnutrition, and pressure sores: an ill-fated alliance. *J Gerontol A Biol Sci Med Sci*. 2004;59(4):M355–M360.
31. Hui D, Dev R, Bruera E. The last days of life: symptom burden and impact on nutrition and hydration in cancer patients. *Curr Opin Support Palliat Care*. 2015;9(1):346.
32. Finucane TE, Bynum JP. Use of tube feeding to prevent aspiration pneumonia. *Lancet*. 1996;348(9039):1421–1424.
33. Finucane TE. Malnutrition, tube feeding and pressure sores: data are incomplete. *J Am Geriatr Soc*. 1995;43(4):447–451.
34. Kuo S, Rhodes RL, Mitchell SL, Mor V, Teno JM. Natural history of feeding-tube use in nursing home residents with advanced dementia. *J Am Med Dir Assoc*. 2009;10(4):264–270.
35. Shintani S. Efficacy and ethics of artificial nutrition in patients with neurologic impairments in home care. *J Clin Neurosci*. 2013;20(2):220–223.
36. Higaki F, Yokota O, Ohishi M. Factors predictive of survival after percutaneous endoscopic gastrostomy in the elderly: is dementia really a risk factor? *Am J Gastroenterol*. 2008;103(4):1011–1016.
37. Good P, Cavenagh J, Mather M, Ravenscroft P. Medically assisted nutrition for palliative care in adult patients. *Cochrane Database Syst Rev*. 2008;4:CD006274.
38. Bouleuc C, Anota A, Cornet C, et al. Impact on health-related quality of life of parenteral nutrition for patients with advanced cancer cachexia: results from a randomized controlled trial. *Oncologist*. 2020;25(5):e843–e851.

39. Teno JM, Mitchell SL, Kuo SK, et al. Decision-making and outcomes of feeding tube insertion: a five-state study. *J Am Geriatr Soc*. 2011;59(5):881–886.
40. Di Giulio P, Toscani F, Villani D, Brunelli C, Gentile S, Spadin P. Dying with advanced dementia in long-term care geriatric institutions: a retrospective study. *J Palliat Med*. 2008;11(7):1023–1028.
41. Vidal M, Hui D, Williams J, Bruera E. A prospective study of hypodermoclysis performed by caregivers in the home setting. *J Pain Symptom Manage*. 2016;52(4):570–574.e579.
42. Krishna LKR, Poulose JV, Goh C. Artificial hydration at the end of life in an oncology ward in Singapore. *Indian J Palliat Care*. 2010;16(3):168.
43. Lybarger EH. Hypodermoclysis in the home and long-term care settings. *J Infus Nurs*. 2009;32(1):40–44.
44. Bruera E, Pruvost M, Schoeller T, Montejo G, Watanabe S. Proctoclysis for hydration of terminally ill cancer patients. *J Pain Symptom Manage*. 1998;15(4):216–219.
45. Gent MJ, Fradsham S, Whyte GM, Mayland CR. What influences attitudes towards clinically assisted hydration in the care of dying patients? A review of the literature. *BMJ Support Palliat Care*. 2015;5(3):223–231.
46. Morita T, Hyodo I, Yoshimi T, et al. Association between hydration volume and symptoms in terminally ill cancer patients with abdominal malignancies. *Ann Oncol*. 2005;16(4):640–647.
47. Oehme J, Sheehan C. Use of artificial hydration at the end of life: a survey of Australian and New Zealand palliative medicine doctors. *J Palliat Med*. 2018;21(8):1145–1151.
48. Nakajima N, Hata Y, Kusumuto K. A clinical study on the influence of hydration volume on the signs of terminally ill cancer patients with abdominal malignancies. *J Palliat Med*. 2013;16(2):185–189.
49. Fritzson A, Tavelin B, Axelsson B. Association between parenteral fluids and symptoms in hospital end-of-life care: an observational study of 280 patients. *BMJ Support Palliat Care*. 2015;5(2):160–168.
50. Bruera E, Hui D, Dalal S, et al. Parenteral hydration in patients with advanced cancer: a multicenter, double-blind, placebo-controlled randomized trial. *J Clin Oncol*. 2013;31(1):111.
51. Fainsinger RL, Bruera E. When to treat dehydration in a terminally ill patient? *Support Care Cancer*. 1997;5:205–211.
52. Yamaguchi T, Morita T, Shinjo T, et al. Effect of parenteral hydration therapy based on the Japanese national clinical guideline on quality of life, discomfort, and symptom intensity in patients with advanced cancer. *J Pain Symptom Manage*. 2012;43(6):1001–1012.
53. Lokker ME, Van der Heide A, Oldenmenger WH, Van der Rijt CC, Van Zuylen L. Hydration and symptoms in the last days of life. *BMJ Support Palliat Care*. 2021;11(3):335–343.
54. Yokomichi N, Morita T, Yamaguchi T. Hydration volume is associated with development of death rattle in patients with abdominal cancer. *J Palliat Med*. 2022;25(1):130–134.
55. Morita T, Bito S, Koyama H, Uchitomi Y, Adachi I. Development of a national clinical guideline for artificial hydration therapy for terminally ill patients with cancer. *J Palliat Med*. 2007;10(3):770–780.
56. Galanakis C, Mayo NE, Gagnon B. Assessing the role of hydration in delirium at the end of life. *Curr Opin Support Palliat Care*. 2011;5(2):169–173.
57. Bruera E, Sala R, Rico MA, et al. Effects of parenteral hydration in terminally ill cancer patients: a preliminary study. *J Clin Oncol*. 2005;23(10):2366–2371.
58. Puntillo K, Arai SR, Cooper BA, Stotts NA, Nelson JE. A randomized clinical trial of an intervention to relieve thirst and dry mouth in intensive care unit patients. *Intensive Care Med*. 2014;40:1295–1302.
59. Wu C-Y, Chen P-J, Ho T-L, Lin W-Y, Cheng S-Y. To hydrate or not to hydrate? The effect of hydration on survival, symptoms and quality of dying among terminally ill cancer patients. *BMC Palliat Care*. 2021;20(1):1–10.
60. Wu CY, Chen PJ, Cheng SY, et al. Association between the amount of artificial hydration and quality of dying among terminally ill patients with cancer: the East Asian Collaborative Cross-Cultural Study to Elucidate the Dying Process. *Cancer*. 2022;128(8):1699–1708.
61. Schwartz DB, Barrocas A, Annetta MG, et al. Ethical aspects of artificially administered nutrition and hydration: an ASPEN position paper. *Nutr Clin Pract*. 2021;36(2):254–267.
62. Hospice and Palliative Nurse Association. Medically Administered Nutrition and Hydration Position Statement 2020. *J Hosp Palliat Nurs*. 2020; 22(3): E13-E16.
63. American Academy of Hospice and Palliative Medicine. Artificial Nutrition and Hydration Near the End of Life. AAHPM. 2025. Accessed on April 28, 2025. https://aahpm.org/advocacy/where-we-stand/anh/
64. American Nurses Association. Nutrition and Hydration at the End of Life Position Statement. ANA. 2017. Accessed April 28, 2025. https://www.nursingworld.org/globalassets/docs/ana/ethics/ps_nutrition-and-hydration-at-the-end-of-life_2017june7.pdf
65. Geppert CM, Andrews MR, Druyan ME. Ethical issues in artificial nutrition and hydration: a review. *JPEN J Parenter Enteral Nutr*. 2010;34(1):79–88.
66. Best C. Introducing enteral nutrition support: ethical considerations. *Nurs Stand*. 2010;24(37):41–45.
67. Vacco v. Quill. Wikipedia. 2022. Accessed October 27, 2022. https://en.wikipedia.org/w/index.php?title=Vacco_v._Quill&oldid=1094871901.
68. Nash RR. Palliative care: Ethic and the law. In: Berger AM, Shuster JLJr, Von Roenn JH, eds. *Principles and Practice of Palliative Care and Supportive Oncology*. 4th ed. Philadelphia, PA: Lippincott Williams & Wilkins; 2013:748–760.
69. Cruzan v. Director, Missouri Department of Health. Wikipedia. 2022 Accessed October 20, 2022. https://en.wikipedia.org/w/index.php?title=Cruzan_v._Director,_Missouri_Department_of_Health&oldid=1105015911.
70. Wolenberg KM, Yoon JD, Rasinski KA, Curlin FA. Religion and United States physicians' opinions and self-predicted practices concerning artificial nutrition and hydration. *J Relig Health*. 2013;52:1051–1065.
71. Ur Rahman M, Abuhasna S, Abu-Zidan FM. Care of terminally-ill patients: an opinion survey among critical care healthcare providers in the Middle East. *Afr Health Sci*. 2013;13(4):893–898.
72. Garrido MM, Harrington ST, Prigerson HG. End-of-life treatment preferences: a key to reducing ethnic/racial disparities in advance care planning? *Cancer*. 2014;120(24):3981–3986.
73. Mahon MM. Clinical decision making in palliative care and end of life care. *Nurs Clin*. 2010;45(3):345–362.
74. Chai HZ, Krishna LKR, Wong VHM. Feeding: what it means to patients and caregivers and how these views influence Singaporean

Chinese caregivers' decisions to continue feeding at the end of life. *Am J Hosp Palliat Med.* 2014;31(2):166–171.

75. Quill TE, Ganzini L, Truog RD, Pope TM. Voluntarily stopping eating and drinking among patients with serious advanced illness—clinical, ethical, and legal aspects. *JAMA Intern Med.* 2018;178(1):123–127.
76. Truog RD, Cochrane TI. Refusal of hydration and nutrition: irrelevance of the "artificial" vs "natural" distinction. *Arch Intern Med.* 2005;165(22):2574–2576.
77. Clarke G, Galbraith S, Woodward J, Holland A, Barclay S. Eating and drinking interventions for people at risk of lacking decision-making capacity: who decides and how? *BMC Med Ethics.* 2015;16(1):1–11.
78. Coyne PJ, Lyckholm LJ. Artificial nutrition for cognitively impaired individuals: strategies to promote appropriate care. *J Hosp Palliat Nurs.* 2010;12(4):263–267.
79. Zehm A, Mullin J, Zhang H. Thirst in palliative care #313. *J Palliat Med.* 2016;19(9):1009–1010.
80. Keown D. End of life: the Buddhist view. *Lancet.* 2005;366(9489):952–955. https://doi.org/10.1016/s0140-6736(05)67323-0.
81. Bradley CT. Roman Catholic doctrine guiding end-of-life care: a summary of the recent discourse. *J Palliat Med.* 2009;12(4):373–377. https://doi.org/10.1089/jpm.2008.0162.
82. Brody H, Hermer LD, Scott LD, Grumbles LL, Kutac JE, McCammon SD. Artificial nutrition and hydration: the evolution of ethics, evidence, and policy. *J Gen Intern Med.* 2011;26(9):1053–1058. https://doi.org/10.1007/s11606-011-1659-z.
83. Heuberger RA. Artificial nutrition and hydration at the end of life. *J Nutr Elderly.* 2010;29(4):347–385. https://doi.org/10.1080/01639366.2010.521020.
84. Alsolamy S. Islamic views on artificial nutrition and hydration in terminally ill patients. *Bioethics.* 2014;28(2):96–99. https://doi.org/10.1111/j.1467-8519.2012.01996.x.
85. Rosner F, Abramson N. Fluids and nutrition: perspectives from Jewish law (halachah). *South Med J.* 2009;102(3):248–250. https://doi.org/10.1097/smj.0b013e318197f536.
86. Ravitsky V. A Jewish perspective on the refusal of life-sustaining therapies: culture as shaping bioethical discourse. *Am J Bioethics.* 2009;9(4):60–62. https://doi.org/10.1080/15265160902790591.

18

Urinary Tract Disorders in Palliative Care

Susan D. Bruce

Key Points

- Urinary dysfunction in palliative care can cause great distress and discomfort for both patients and their caregivers. Nursing management of these issues is a priority and should be matched with the patient's own clinical situation and preferences.
- The causes of urinary dysfunction in the patient receiving palliative care are myriad, including the presence of a malignant tumor, iatrogenic factors, infection, neurological factors, or other comorbidities. Treatment or management strategies that reflect the etiology of the patient's condition should be considered, and this may include the selection of products or devices as well as pharmacological solutions or behavioral interventions.
- Limited evidence exists to support many aspects of nursing management of urinary tract disorders in palliative care, including the insertion of indwelling urethral urinary catheters. As such, nurses are required to work in partnership with patients, families, and other members of the patient's healthcare team, bringing their clinical expertise and interpersonal skills in order to deliver high-quality care.

Introduction

Urinary tract disorders are commonly experienced by patients with serious illnesses receiving palliative care. Urinary tract disorders include urinary retention or obstruction, incontinence, cystitis, hematuria, and other disorders. Each of these disorders commonly causes bothersome and distressing symptoms for patients.

Urinary tract disorders in patients receiving palliative care are most often caused from systemic disease, cancer, or a complication from treatment. Managing urinary tract disorders in patients needs to be a priority for nurses. Our overall goal as nurses caring for patients with urinary tract disorders is to provide person-centered care to reduce distress and discomfort. The symptoms that result from urinary tract dysfunction can cause great distress and discomfort for patients and their caregivers. The challenge is to manage the patient's urinary tract disorder and the accompanying symptoms in a manner that considers their medical situation, emotional state, personal preferences, overall goals of care, and anticipated life expectancy. Thus, management strategies must be individualized for each patient's unique needs.

This chapter provides an overview of the most common urinary tract disorders and a case study of a patient living with a serious illness and reviews evidence-based approaches for nurses to deliver personalized, holistic care to their patients.

Case Study

Brice Allen is a 76-year-old male, who has a history of non-muscle-invasive bladder cancer. He had a transurethral resection of a bladder tumor on September 10, 2021. Immediately after surgery he received intravesical (instilled into the bladder) bacillus Calmette-Guerin (BCG). Mr. Allen's recommendations for follow-up include cystoscopy every 3 months with periodic imaging and induction of BCG with 6 weekly instillations of intravesical therapy followed by maintenance therapy at 3, 6, 12, 18, 24, 30, and 36 months. The goal of this treatment plan would be to minimize treatment burden while attempting to detect recurrence and progression events early. Risks of intravesical therapy include bleeding, infection, pain, cystitis, and bladder shrinkage.

Mr. Allen presents to the emergency room (ER) on December 4, 2022, with complaints of dysuria and gross hematuria with increased blood in his urine with clots. He has been anuric (without urine output) for almost 8 hours. He was seen the day before in the ER for evaluation of hematuria with dark red blood and clots. Urology was consulted and was instructed to return if his symptoms worsened. About 5 months prior to this, Mr. Allen had urinary stents placed and was started on apixiban (5 mg, orally every 12 hours).

Pathophysiology and Risk Factors

The urinary system can be divided into the upper urinary tract and the lower urinary tract. The upper urinary tract comprises the kidneys and the ureters. The lower urinary tract comprises the bladder and the urethra. The kidneys are essential for maintaining water and electrolyte homeostasis within the body. They filter nearly 200 L of fluid from the body's bloodstream every day, which allows toxins, metabolic wastes, and excess ions to leave the body in the form of urine, while returning vital substances to the blood.[1] The two ureters transport the urine produced in the kidneys to the bladder, where it is stored temporarily before being carried through the urethra to the exterior of the body in the process of micturition or urination. There are a number of causes and risk factors that can increase the chances that an individual will experience urinary tract dysfunction. These factors include medical interventions such as medications, treatments, and surgery; infections (i.e., urinary tract infections [UTIs]); impaired and restricted mobility; and bowel dysfunction and physiologic changes that may occur as a result of a tumor growth or neurologic changes. Damage to nerves in the bladder caused by either injury or disease can lead to impaired communication in the nervous system, which ultimately can lead to voiding difficulties. Functional and cognitive decline are other concerns in both aging individuals and those with serious and progressive illnesses. The type of urological dysfunction that occurs depends on the location of the damage; for example, neurological lesions above the pontine micturition center in the brainstem (caused by the presence of a posterior fossa tumor) can lead to lower urinary tract dysfunction, presenting as urinary retention, that can ultimately lead to urinary incontinence.[2] Similarly, a lesion that occurs below the pons in the spinal cord often leads to detrusor-sphincter dyssynergia (lack of coordination between bladder and sphincter) and therefore incomplete evacuation and urinary retention.[3]

Neurological conditions may result in urinary dysfunction. Connections between the micturition center in the brain, the spinal cord, and the peripheral nerves which enervate the bladder and sphincter must be intact for the bladder to enact its dual function of storage and voiding. Abnormalities at any level of the nervous system (i.e., the brain, spinal cord, peripheral nerves) can result in abnormal bladder function. Disruption to these pathways leads to dysfunction, causing voiding difficulties, or urinary retention.

Explanation of Urinary Dysfunction

There are many causes of urinary dysfunction including medications, side effects, and medical conditions, all of which will be discussed and are summarized in Table 18.1. Medications such as sedatives, opioid analgesics, and benzodiazepines may affect the patient's ability to recognize the need to void or to access toileting facilities or products effectively. Diuretics may increase urine production, leading to urinary frequency.

Oncological treatments including tumor invasion, chemotherapy, and radiotherapy can cause bladder irritation, bladder spasm, or hemorrhagic cystitis. Patients living with a serious illness are often at increased risk of bacteria entering the urinary tract and resulting in a UTI. UTIs may cause urinary incontinence[4] or exacerbate existing urinary incontinence, bladder irritation, and/or bladder spasm. Severe pain or dyspnea can impair or prevent a patient's ability to access toileting facilities or products in a timely fashion. In addition, the disease process itself can lead to physical deconditioning, weakness, or exhaustion that puts the patient at risk for falls.

Chronic cognitive impairment such as dementia or acute cognitive impairment such as delirium or confusion may limit a patient's ability to recognize or respond to cues to urinate. Delirium is common in the last weeks or days of life and can be caused by metabolic disturbance, organ failure, certain drugs (including benzodiazepines and opioids), sepsis, hypoxia, and primary or secondary cerebral tumors.[5]

Constipation is common in the palliative care patient due to factors including immobility, dehydration, metabolic factors, intestinal dysmotility, and opioid use.[6] Constipation can have an impact on urinary function as bladder and bowel function are anatomically closely connected.

Disease-related causes include tumor infiltration, blood clots, spinal cord injury, or other neurological conditions. Treatment-related causes include radiation fibrosis, chemotherapy- or radiation-induced cystitis, bladder or other lower abdominal surgery, and medications such as intravesical BCG or mitomycin. Urethral surgery such as prostatectomy or surgery which indirectly affects the urethra such as hysterectomy[7,8] can lead to intrinsic sphincter deficiency and therefore urinary incontinence. Surgery can also cause fibrosis and scarring. Mechanical causes can include the presence of an indwelling catheter or ureteral stent. Infection can be caused by UTIs.

Neurological problems include neurogenic bladder, and "neurogenic lower urinary tract dysfunction" is the term often given to bladder dysfunction caused by neurological damage.[9] Neurological

Table 18.1 Risk factors for urinary tract disorders

Risk factor	Example
Medications	Diuretics; skeletal muscle relaxants; immunosuppressive agents; anticholinergics; anti-arrhythmic; decongestant, opioids; nonsteroidal anti-inflammatory agents; calcium channel blockers[37]
Disease	Diabetes mellitus; neurogenic bladder; spinal cord injury; vulvovaginal atrophy; pelvic and vaginal prolapse[38]
Treatments	Radiation treatments to the pelvis; chemotherapy; immunotherapy[39]
Surgery	Prostatectomy; hysterectomy; bladder cancer surgery; pelvic surgery[39]
Infection	Bacterial (most commonly *Escherichia coli*); fungal; viruses[37]
Impaired/restricted mobility	Bed rest; limited range of motion
Bowel dysfunction	Constipation; irritable bowel disease
Neurological changes	Parkinson's disease; cranial nerve disease; brain tumors; spinal cord tumors; multiple sclerosis; stroke; cauda equina syndrome[40,41]
Cognitive impairment	Alzheimer's disease; dementia; delirium[41]

Disclaimer: Examples are provided, but this is not an exhaustive list of risk factors lesions leading to bladder dysfunction can be caused by multiple factors including, but not limited to, problems with the brain and brainstem, causing brain tumors, dementia, Parkinson's disease, cerebrovascular accident, or traumatic brain injury. Multiple diseases involving the spinal cord can lead to multiple sclerosis, spina bifida, traumatic spinal cord injury, or spinal surgery. Conditions of the peripheral nervous system can result in diabetes, chronic alcohol abuse, chemotherapy-induced peripheral neuropathy, and Guillain-Barré syndrome. A few other known causes include HIV (human immunodeficiency virus) and systemic lupus erythematosus.

Assessment

A thorough history needs to be conducted to help determine the nature of the urinary problem and the severity. A review of current medications the patient is taking can identify medications contributing to the problem. Inquiring how the patient has been managing the problem at home can be telling. You need a history detailing their normal urinary patterns. Be sure to question what makes their symptoms better or worse.

A reduction or cessation in urinary output in any patient receiving palliative care can signal an underlying problem which merits attention and appropriate management. For patients who may be experiencing a urinary tract disorder, nurses must make a distinction between the lack of urine output caused by failure of the kidneys to filter blood and make urine (anuria/oliguria), blockage preventing flow of urine between the upper and lower urinary tracts (urinary stasis), and failure of the bladder to empty (urinary retention).[10] This section will review important considerations during the assessment of your patient.

It is important that an accurate and thorough medical history is collected and physical examination is performed (including using an ultrasound bladder scanner if available). For example, metastatic spinal cord compression develops in approximately 5% of patients with cancer.[11] It is a medical emergency and often presents in the acute setting. It occurs when the spinal cord or cauda equina is compressed (e.g., by direct pressure of a tumor) in such a way that could cause neurological disability. If left untreated, the consequences can be serious, often resulting in irreversible loss of motor and bladder function.[12] Urinary incontinence is a late feature of spinal cord compression, but with cauda equina syndrome, bladder dysfunction in the form of retention or overflow incontinence may present at an earlier stage.[13]

Currently, there are a broad range of generic assessment tools assessing symptoms experienced by individuals receiving palliative care, but currently a specific tool is available to guide continence assessment.[14] Toileting problems can include identifying any potentially modifiable causes and precipitating or relieving factors. It is important to determine the frequency and severity of urinary leakage or toileting difficulties. Nurses need to have current knowledge of containment methods used and their usefulness as well as exploring other alternatives. The impact of urinary tract disorders on the patient's quality of life needs to include a holistic assessment of the individual's experience and preferences for containment methods.

A complete physical examination should include palpation of the abdomen to assess for a distended bladder, tenderness, or pain. In men, a digital rectal examination should be performed to determine an enlarged prostate. Physical examination, particularly in individuals receiving palliative care who are unable to communicate verbally is essential. Restlessness could signal urinary retention. A bladder scan can be useful in identifying urinary retention, which would be suspected if more than 400–500 mL is present in the bladder.

There are additional tests which may be considered to provide further information to help guide care considerations. These tests may include urinalysis, blood tests to evaluate kidney function, urine cytology to look for abnormal cells in the urine, and prostate-specific antigen testing in men.

Returning to our case study, Mr. Allen has continued his intravesical therapy with BCG, the most recent one being November 17, 2022. This is the first one where he developed hematuria. Physical exam was normal. Abdominal exam showed that the abdomen was soft, nontender, and nondistended. All labs were within normal limits (WNL) with the exception of his urinalysis which showed 3+ blood. Mr. Allen's hemoglobin was 16.4, and hematocrit was 47.0, both WNL. White blood cell count was elevated at 12.7, but urinalysis was negative for infection.

Voiding Dysfunction

Urinary retention is the inability to empty the bladder completely. It can be categorized by several factors: complete or partial emptying, acute or chronic duration, painful or not, by underlying cause (obstructive or nonobstructive), and high- or low-pressure. However, urinary retention lacks a clear, widely accepted clinical definition, thus having the potential to lead to both under- and overtreatment. It is caused by one of two disorders: bladder outlet obstruction (in which flow from the urethra is obstructed) or deficient detrusor contraction strength (in which bladder muscle strength is insufficient to effectively empty the bladder),[10] detailed in Table 18.1. Management of urinary retention will depend on the underlying cause. It is important to distinguish between urinary retention and oliguria. Initially, conservative measures should be employed in an attempt to rectify urinary retention. For example, rectal emptying (most commonly by way of a mild laxative rather than by more invasive methods like manual evacuation) should be considered, especially for patients who are constipated or taking medications that are known to cause constipation. For male patients, providing assistance for them to stand to void may facilitate bladder emptying. If these less invasive measures are ineffective, an indwelling or intermittent urinary catheter may be necessary to relieve the presence of urinary retention. The choice between an intermittent and an indwelling urinary catheter will depend on the context of care, including the availability of a caregiver who can catheterize and the preferences of the patient.

The prognosis and goals of care will guide the treatment plan. For example, for patients receiving palliative care an injection of botulism toxin, electrical nerve stimulation, or surgery could be considered. However, in the end-of-life care setting often conservative management is most appropriate. Depending upon the primary urological issue, treatment may include use of indwelling urethral or suprapubic catheter/intermittent catheterization,[9] continence products such as urinary sheaths, toileting assistance, antimuscarinic therapy, and possibly behavioral treatment. Behavioral treatments, such as bladder training, biofeedback, and pelvic floor muscle training (Kegel exercises) can be used to reduce symptoms and improve quality of life. Behavioral therapy, alone or in combination with other interventions, is generally more effective than pharmacological therapies alone in treating urinary symptoms.[15] The benefits of these other more invasive methods will need to be balanced with potential risks to the patient (e.g., UTI introduced by catheterization).

There is little evidence to guide the use of a urinary catheter in palliative and end-of -life care. Despite this, a significant proportion of patients receiving palliative care in an acute or hospice setting are catheterized (up to 79%).[16–18] Insertion of a urinary catheter in the patient receiving palliative care must be carefully considered. Urinary catheterization is often undertaken to relieve distressing bladder symptoms and may provide comfort from retention, keep an incontinent patient dry, and prevent breakdown of the skin from urinary leakage. However, the act of insertion itself may cause distress, and an indwelling catheter may be uncomfortable.[19] In addition, urinary catheters may present problems of their own, including leakage due to bypassing, blockage, and infection.[20–22] Despite potential problems related to catheterization, there are a number of reasons it may be appropriate to insert a urinary catheter in patients receiving palliative care. Specifically, urinary catheterization may be warranted when the goal is to ensure dignity, comfort, and convenience for patients and their caregivers. For example, if the patient is immobile, using a bedside commode is impossible, and/or frequent changes of bed linen caused by episodes of incontinence is distressing, the use of a urinary catheter should be considered. However, urinary incontinence alone is not an indication for urinary catheterization. If an indwelling catheter is inserted, daily assessment should be made as to whether the catheter is still required, and discontinuation of the catheter should be done promptly when it is no longer needed. Intermittent catheterization can be based on the patient's preferences and life expectancy.

Incontinence and Toileting

High rates of toileting (intentional opening of bladder or bowels) problems and incontinence (involuntary loss or leakage of urine) are commonly associated with functional and cognitive decline, often accompanying serious illnesses and their associated treatments. Prevalence varies by diagnosis and proximity to death, with sudden death associated with lowest rates (range 28.6%–37.0%) and frailty or dementia the highest (65.3%–72%) in the last year of life.[23] By the last month of life 67%–89% of people living in nursing homes were found to experience incontinence, and in acute palliative care environments, incontinence increases in the last 7 days of life (30%–65%).[24] However, decreased urine output is associated with a high likelihood of death within 3 days.[24]

Appropriateness of interventions to reduce either the frequency or severity of urinary leakage or the impact of the leakage needs to be considered in conjunction with the individual's cognitive and physical function. In palliative care, there are two main bladder management goals: symptom management, including avoidance of pain or discomfort, and achieving social continence to protect personhood and dignity. Interventions such as dietary modifications or bladder training are likely to be appropriate for patients receiving palliative care. Behavioral interventions such as prompted voiding could support the maintenance of continence for some patients if physical and cognitive functional allows.

Choosing the right toileting aid or containment product can be complex. The individual's physical needs and personal preferences, daily activities, the context of care, and the availability of devices will impact on decision-making. Commodes or urinals are commonly used. Containment products such as absorbent pads or urinary sheaths are appropriate selections. It can be necessary to trial several products to find the one that best meets an individual's needs (see Table 18.2).

Table 18.2 Toileting aids and containment products suitable for patients receiving palliative care

Toileting aids provide an alternative to the toilet for when a patient can voluntarily void urine.	**Bedside commodes** can be used by patients who can safely transfer (with or without support) from bed to commode and back and maintain a seated position but are unable to reach a conventional toilet. Different size designs, from pediatric to bariatric, are available to accommodate different body frames. The commode should be emptied and cleaned after every use to avoid smell. As condition can change rapidly at the end of life, care should be taken to assess the patient's ability to transfer before each use. **Handheld urinals** are available in designs (reusable or disposable) suitable for either men or women and can be useful when mobility is limited. Products for women tend to have a flat end which can be put into position underneath the patient, whereas products for men ("bottles") generally have an aperture to accommodate the penis. Urinals can often be used in a supine or seated position and might help to maintain independence by reducing the need for a caregiver to help with mobility. Different designs are available to help with different limitations, for example, poor grip. **Bedpans** are more commonly used when people wish to move their bowels but are unable to safely or comfortably transfer to a commode or conventional toilet. Bedpans can be uncomfortable and difficult to clean outside hospital environments, and, generally, handheld urinals are preferred for micturition, particularly for men. Some women might prefer a bedpan if handheld urinals do not work well for them.
Containment products are used when the patient cannot comfortably or reliably control voiding. Many people benefit from using a combination of products (e.g., different products for day and night).	**Absorbent products** are the most commonly used containment products to manage urinary incontinence and are available in a wide range of designs and styles, including disposable and washable. Pads should contain leakage and smell, be comfortable, discreet, and easily changed. To get the right pad, assessment must consider level (light, moderate, or heavy) and type of leakage (e.g., urinary only or urinary and fecal), whether the person can stand for product changes (e.g., avoid pull-ups if the person cannot stand), convenience (e.g., washables can work well for heavy leakage but require washing and drying facilities), and individual preferences. Product design requirements are likely to change as functional abilities decline. **Male devices** include urinary sheaths (condom catheters) and body-worn urinals that are attached via tubing to urinary collection bags. Sheaths come in different sizes, styles, and materials (latex or silicone), and men should be carefully measured to ensure a good fit. A new sheath should be fitted at least daily after washing. For men with a retracted penis, an external device that fits to the glans is available. Body-worn urinals can offer an alternative if a sheath is not successful but might not be suitable for men nursed in bed. **Female devices** include external urine management devices that contour to the female perineal area and are kept in place with an adhesive pad secured to the lower abdomen. These devices divert urine away from the skin. Urine is then absorbed into the system and suctioned into a collection cannister. These external devices can facilitate earlier removal of urinary catheters and promote comfort for the patient. The use of **indwelling catheters** is described elsewhere, and indications for use in the terminal phase include urine retention, skin protection, or patient preference for comfort (e.g., frequent product changes cause pain). However, it is important to remember that catheterization is an invasive procedure, and alternatives should be fully explored.

Nurses should be aware that incontinence products are not without issues. For example, urinary sheaths can have leakage, leading to uncomfortable changes of bed linen or trauma to skin or tissue from body-worn devices. Thus, with all of these products, regular careful attention to hygiene and washing should be maintained to minimize harm to skin from the urine,[25] to help maintain comfort, and to avoid unpleasant smells.

Common Bladder Disorders and Emergencies

Bladder Spasms

Bladder discomfort in patients with a serious illness can arise from a number of sources including bladder spasms which are sometimes referred to as "overactive bladder." Bladder spasm occurs when the detrusor muscle contracts suddenly. This can cause intense suprapubic and urethral pain. Bladder spasms can cause significant discomfort for the patient including causing the urge to urinate as well as forcing urine out of the bladder, leading to leakage. Thus, this can be very distressing for the patient.

Treatment for bladder spasm will depend on the cause and preferences of the patient. If the cause is an indwelling catheter, there are several nursing interventions that should be attempted. First, the nurse could change the catheter. The force generated by bladder spasms can overwhelm the drainage capacity of the catheter, resulting in leakage around the catheter. Changing the catheter can help eliminate the problem. Second, the volume of the balloon could be reduced. A catheter balloon may be overinflated or positioned in a way that it is irritating the bladder. Third, the nurse may consider a bladder washout to reverse catheter sludging, although this approach lacks evidence of efficacy to improve or reduce the patient's symptoms.[26] If these nursing interventions cannot be completed or do not resolve the issue, consideration should be made as to whether the catheter could be removed altogether or if intermittent catheterization would be a better alternative.

Pharmacological treatments to reduce bladder spasm or relieve the resulting pain should also be considered. Antimuscarinic drugs such as oxybutynin or tolterodine reduce the sensitivity of the bladder muscle, decreasing bladder contractions.[27] Tricyclic antidepressants such as imipramine and amitriptyline may also help to reduce spasms.[28] Analgesics such as morphine can be used to reduce pain if it is severe. If a UTI is confirmed, antibiotics should be administered.[29] Overactive bladder in the absence of spasm or pain can be managed with the use of a condom catheter, adaptation of the home environment, and effective nursing support, where pharmacological treatments cause significant side effects or are of no therapeutic benefit.[30]

Hemorrhagic Cystitis

Hemorrhagic cystitis occurs when the epithelium of the bladder is damaged, leading to lower urinary tract symptoms including bladder irritation, painful and/or frequent voiding, and hematuria. Oncology patients receiving chemotherapy (particularly cyclophosphamide and ifosfamide, which are excreted through the bladder) and pelvic radiation are at risk for developing hemorrhagic cystitis, and prophylactic measures should be implemented. Bone marrow transplant patients are also at particular risk due to the high levels of chemotherapy they receive as part of their treatment[31] and their consequent susceptibility to BK (abbreviation for the name of first person isolated with the virus) virus–associated hemorrhagic cystitis. Hemorrhagic cystitis can also be caused by an infection. This is an important consideration for both nurses and patients to recognize as consequences can be severe, including urinary outlet obstruction, anemia due to bleeding, or even urosepsis (a severe systemic infection).

Hemorrhagic cystitis is a medical emergency, and the management strategies involve removing the cause of the problem. In the patient who is receiving chemotherapy (e.g., ifosfamide or cyclophosphamide) the treatment needs to stop. If an infection is the cause, antibiotics should be administered. Additionally, interventions to alleviate additional discomfort that may result from the complication such as the administration of analgesics should be considered. There are additional treatment-specific interventions to manage hemorrhagic cystitis that may be considered, depending on the goals of care. Treatments can include intravesical medications, such as hyaluronic acid that serves as a protective barrier to the urothelium. To manage bleeding after radiation treatment to help the heal the bladder tissue, the patient may require hyperbaric oxygen treatments. Surgical options, including cutaneous ureterostomy, cystoscopy, diathermy (electrically induced heat or use of high-frequency electromagnetic currents as a form of physical therapy in surgical procedures), vesical artery embolization, and supravesical urinary diversion, may be used.

Returning to the case study, during Mr. Allen's treatment in the ER, a 24 French three-way urinary catheter was placed by the nurse in preparation for continuous bladder irrigation (CBI). Upon catheter insertion, there was removal of 250 mL of bloody urine, with no clots observed. There is blood noted at the meatus. Preparations are made to admit the patient.

Mr. Allen is admitted to the hospital medicine service with gross hematuria and urinary retention for CBI and close monitoring. His hemoglobin and hematocrit will be rechecked in the evening. His apixaban will be held pending recommendations by cardiology. He will be started on tamsulosin hydrochloride, a drug that targets the smooth muscle receptors of the prostate and urethra. Blocking these receptors relaxes the smooth muscle of the bladder and urethra to improve urine flow.

Prophylactic treatment for patients at risk of developing hemorrhagic cystitis should be a routine part of care. For example, patients who are receiving agents such as cyclophosphamide or ifosfamide should receive aggressive intravenous hydration and the administration of mesna (2-mercaptoethane sodium sulfonate), and continuous bladder irrigation should be part of routine nursing care.

In palliative care, intervention is not necessarily required if there is microscopic hematuria or if gross hematuria does not lead to urinary outlet obstruction or a clinically significant reduction in hematocrit or hemoglobin. For gross hematuria requiring treatment, required nursing actions should include a medication review to check whether the patient is currently taking anticoagulants or nonsteroidal anti-inflammatory agents as these medications may need to be held. Obtaining a urinalysis, either by dipstick or microscopy, can determine infection status and location of bleeding.

If bleeding persists, cystoscopy may be considered but should be carefully balanced with the patient's goals of care. The same may be said for intravenous fluid infusion and transfusion of red blood cells. Catheterization with a large-gauge three-way catheter (22–24 French) and continuous balder irrigation may be necessary if gross bleeding results in clots and obstruction and if the patient can tolerate the catheter.

Urinary Tract Infections

UTIs are not uncommon in individuals with serious illnesses, including those at the end of life. There is an increased prevalence of developing a UTI associated with having an indwelling urinary catheter. Diagnosing a UTI is not always straightforward, and distinguishing between a UTI and an asymptomatic bacteriuria that does not require treatment can be problematic, particularly in older adults or those unable to report symptoms. Consensus guidelines have developed UTI definitions that generally include a urine culture with 10^5 colony-forming units/mL or higher combined with the presence of genitourinary symptoms (i.e., dysuria, suprapubic pain or tenderness, frequency or urgency of urination). UTIs can cause significant discomfort and can result in delirium for patients, especially those nearing the end of life. Unrecognized and untreated UTIs can also lead to sepsis and unwanted admission into acute care settings,[32] so it is important that they are managed appropriately. Treatment guidelines recommend considering narrow-spectrum antibiotics such as trimethoprim or nitrofurantoin as first-line treatments. Broad-spectrum antibiotics (e.g., amoxicillin/clavulanate, quinolones, and cephalosporins) should be avoided as they increase the risk of *Clostridium difficile* infection, methicillin-resistant *Staphylococcus aureus*, and resistant UTIs, which are becoming increasingly problematic. However, UTIs are also one of the most common reasons for using antimicrobials even at the end of life, and unnecessary use should be avoided due to the potential for unwanted side effects (e.g., nausea or allergic reaction) and the burden of antimicrobial resistance. Asymptomatic bacteriuria should not be treated with antibiotics.

Psychosocial Factors and Care Environment

Psychosocial factors are important considerations for the patient who will receive assistance with their bladder problems. Little may be known about patients' preferences for bladder management. It is important to involve the patient and caregiver in this discussion. The burden of care often falls on the patient's caregiver,[33] which can be problematic for both the patient and caregiver. It is essential to maintain privacy during intimate care such as washing, toileting, catheterization, and bowel interventions for the patient and their caregiver. Some patients might worry about having intimate care provided by family members, and needing help with managing bladder emptying can add to a patient's distress. Furthermore, coping with incontinence problems has been demonstrated to greatly add to distress and workload for caregivers,[34] who report feeling unprepared for and unsupported in their role.[35]

When patients and caregivers are involved in day-to-day bladder care, they should be provided with the information, support, and equipment to successfully undertake the role. However, caregivers are often reluctant to seek help for incontinence-related problems.[36] Healthcare professionals should be proactive in openly discussing bladder problems and management strategies. This can alleviate patient and caregiver concerns in protecting dignity, avoiding exhaustion, and maintaining social continence.

Proactive discussions with patients (where possible) and caregivers should include explaining the need for regular assessment, taking into account changing circumstances, listening to patient preferences, establishing the context of care (e.g., who will be caring for the patient), and the likely trajectory of incontinence needs and potential interventions (e.g., provision of bedside commode or absorbent products) that might be beneficial. There are varying palliative care trajectories for patients. They may have a short illness with rapid decline or a long illness with periodic acute episodes that can have an impact on incontinence symptoms encountered and the level of support and information required.

Applying this information to our case study, nursing management will include use of 3-L bags of sterile saline for the CBI. The rate will involve a constant drip for the infusion of the fluid. The urinary catheter drainage bag will need to be emptied frequently due to the volume of fluid infusing into the bladder. The nurse will need to maintain an accurate output to determine the actual amount of urine produced by Mr. Allen. To determine the actual amount of urine, subtract all the 3-L bags of solution from everything emptied from the catheter drainage bag.

The nurse will need to document the color of the urine obtained in the catheter drainage bag (i.e., dark red, cherry red, pale pink, pink-tinged), as well as the presence of clots or debris in the urine. Signs and symptoms that should be reported to the provider include an increase in bleeding, a drop-in hemoglobin and hematocrit, bladder spasms, and decrease in urine output. Mr. Allen was discharged 2 days later when his urine returned to a normal color and he was voiding without difficulty.

Conclusion

Bladder management in a patient receiving palliative care, regardless of the setting, is a complex issue. Previous palliative care studies that looked into bladder care and urinary catheterization have estimated that 57%–71% of hospitalized patients have required urinary catheterization.[1,4,5] Nurses looking after patients with bladder difficulties in the palliative care setting may face barriers including lack of resources or knowledge about products available to assist these patients as well as the psychological and clinical considerations described in this chapter. Knowledge of local policies, procedures, and guidelines is therefore essential, in addition to the general overview provided by this chapter.

Much of the literature on bladder management in the palliative care setting is anecdotal or based on nurse and patient experiences or best practices. No evidence-based guidelines exist on this topic. There is a great need for clinical attention to be focused on improvement in the management of urinary dysfunction in the palliative care setting. Future research on use of urinary catheters, antibiotics, and quality-of-life outcomes in palliative care is warranted.

REFERENCES

1. Marieb EN. *Essentials of Human Anatomy and Physiology*. 11th ed. Pearson; 2014.
2. Wein AJ, Andersson KE, Drake MJ, Dmochowski RR. *Bladder Dysfunction in the Adult: The Basis for Clinical Management*. Humana Press; 2014.

3. Stoffel JT. Detrusor sphincter dyssynergia: a review of physiology, diagnosis, and treatment strategies. *Trans Androl Urol.* 2016;5(1):127–135.
4. Yates A. Incontinence and associated complications: is it avoidable? *Nurse Prescribing.* 2017;15(6):288–295.
5. Hosker CM, Bennett MI. Delirium and agitation at the end of life. *BMJ.* 2016;353:i3085. https://doi.org/10.1136/bmj.i3085.
6. Pritchard D, Bharucha A. Management of opioid-induced constipation for people in palliative care. *Int J Palliat Nurs.* 2016;21(6):272–280.
7. Mohammed Al-Ali B, Ponholzer A, Augustin H, Madersbacher S, Pummer K. The long-term effect of radical prostatectomy on erectile function, urinary continence, and lower urinary tract symptoms: a comparison to age-matched healthy controls. *BioMed Res Int.* 2017;2017:9615080. https://doi.org/10.1155/2017/9615080.
8. Bohlin KS, Ankardal M, Lindkvist H, Milsom I. Factors influencing the incidence and remission of urinary incontinence after hysterectomy. *Am J Obstet Gynecol.* 2017;216(1):53.e1–53.e9. http://dx.doi.org/10.1016/j.ajog.2016.08.034.
9. Krebs J, Wöllner J, Pannek J. Bladder management in individuals with chronic neurogenic lower urinary tract dysfunction. *Spinal Cord.* 2016;54:609–613.
10. Gray M, Sims T. Urinary tract disorders. In: Ferrell BR, Coyle N, Paice J, eds. *Oxford Textbook of Palliative Nursing.* 4th ed. Oxford University Press; 2015:262–279.
11. Madersbacher H, Mürtz G, Stöhrer M. Neurogenic detrusor overactivity in adults: a review on efficacy, tolerability and safety of oral antimuscarinics. *Spinal Cord.* 2013;51:432–441.
12. Chmielowski B, Territo M. *Manual of Clinical Oncology.* 8th ed. Wolters Kluwer; 2017.
13. Harris M. Quality of life in patients with malignant spinal cord compression: a review of evidence-based literature. *Int J Palliat Nurs.* 2016:22(1):37–43.
14. Singer A, Meeker D, Teno J, et al. Symptom trends in the last year of life from 1998 to 2010. A cohort study. *Ann Intern Med.* 2015;162:175–183.
15. Balk EM, Rofeberg VN, Adams G, Trikalinos TA, Kimmel HJ, Jeppson PC. Pharmacologic and nonpharmacologic treatments for urinary incontinence in women. *Ann Intern Med.* 2019;170(7):465–479.
16. Cassidy J, Bisset D, Spence RAJ, Payne M, Morris-Stiff G. *Oxford Handbook of Oncology.* Oxford University Press; 2015.
17. Farrington N, Fader M, Richardson A, Prieto J, Bush H. Indwelling urinary catheter use at the end of life: a retrospective audit. *Br J Nurs.* 2014;23:S4–S10.
18. Pais R, Lee P, Cross S, Gebski V, Aggarwal R. Bladder care in palliative care inpatients: a prospective dual site cohort study. *Palliat Med Rep.* 2020;1:215–258.
19. Gutmanis I, Shadd J, Woolmore-Goodwin S, Whitfield P, Byrne J, Faulds C. Prevalence and indications for bladder catheterization on a palliative care unit: a prospective, observational study. *Palliat Med.* 2014;28(10):1239–1240.
20. Nazarko L. Catheter-associated bladder pain: it's not always infection. *Br J Community Nurs.* 2014;19(1):6–11.
21. Bardsley A. Preventing urinary tract infections in catheter care. *Nurs Resid Care.* 2017;19(5):260–263.
22. Gibney LE. Blocked urinary catheters: can they be better managed? *Br J Nurs.* 2016;25(15):828–833.
23. Stickler DJ. Clinical complications of urinary catheters caused by biofilms: something needs to be done. *J Intern Med.* 2014;276(2):120–129.
24. Hui D, dos Santos, R, Chisholm G, et al. Clinical signs of impending death in cancer patients. *Oncologist.* 2014;19(6):681–687.
25. Wagg A, Chen LK, Johnson T, et al. Incontinence in the frail elderly. In Abrams P, Cardozo L, Wein A, Wagg A, eds. *Incontinence: 6th International Consultation on Incontinence.* European Association of Urology & International Consultation on Urological Diseases; 2017:1309–1441.
26. Beeckman D. A decade of research on incontinence-associated dermatitis (IAD): evidence, knowledge gaps and next steps. *J Tissue Viability.* 2016;26(1):47–56.
27. Shepherd AJ, Mackay WG, Hagen S. Washout policies in long-term indwelling urinary catheterisation in adults. *Cochrane Database Syst Rev.* 2017;3:CD004012.
28. Bardsley A. An overview of urinary incontinence. *Br J Nurs.* 2016;25(18):S14–S21.
29. Kaya H, Aydin GO. An important problem for the individuals with spinal cord injury: neurogenic bladder. *J Neurol Neurosurg Nurs.* 2015; 4(1):35–39.
30. Helde-Frankling M, Bergqvist J, Bergman P, Björkhem-Bergman L. Antibiotic treatment in end-of-life cancer patients: a retrospective observational study at a palliative care centre in Sweden. *Cancers (Basel).* 2016;8:84.
31. Walton A. Managing overactive bladder symptoms in a palliative care setting. *J Palliat Med.* 2014;17(1):118–121.
32. Gonella S, di Pasquale T, Palese A. Preventive measures for cyclophosphamide-related hemorrhagic cystitis in blood and bone marrow transplantation: an Italian multicenter retrospective study. *Clin J Oncol Nurs.* 2014;19(1):E8–E14.
33. Leadership Alliance for the Care of Dying People. *One Chance to Get It Right: Improving People's Experience of Care in the Last Few Days and Hours of Life.* Leadership Alliance for the Care of Dying People; 2014. Accessed October 26, 2017. https://www.gov.uk/government/uploads/system/uploads/attachment_data/file/323188/One_chance_to_get_it_right.pdf.
34. Choice in End of Life Care Programme Board. What's important to me: a review of choice in end of life care. Choice in End of Life Care Programme Board; 2015. Accessed October 26, 2017. http://www.ncpc.org.uk/sites/default/files/CHOICE%20REVIEW_FINAL%20for%20web.pdf.
35. Rossa D, Lamura G. The impact of incontinence management on informal caregivers' quality of life. *Aging Clin Exp Res.* 2015;28(1):89–97. https://doi.org/10.1007/s40520-015-0367-7.
36. Woodman C, Baillie J, Sivell S. The preferences and perspectives of family caregivers towards place of care for their relatives at the end-of-life. A systematic review and thematic synthesis of the qualitative evidence. *BMJ Support Palliat Care.* 2015;6(4):418–429.
37. Dobrek L. Drug-related urinary tract infections. *Wiad Lek.* 2021;74(7):1728–1736.
38. Storme O, Saucedo JT, Garcia-Mora A, Dehesa-Davila M, Naber KG. Risk factors and predisposing conditions for urinary tract infections. *Ther Adv Urol.* 2019;11:19–28.
39. National Cancer Institute. Urinary and Bladder Problems. Accessed June 12, 2023. https://www.cancer.gov/about-cancer/treatment/side-effects/urination-changes.
40. Koitabashi R, Uchida Y. Analysing the relationship between cognition and urine storage function. *Int J Urol Nurs.* 2019;13:51–56.
41. Smith TJ, Andrews V, Cho S, Drinnan N, Dunsmuir W. Bladder problems associated with neurological disease. *InnovAiT.* 2015;8(5):291–297.

19

Lymphedema Management

Mei R. Fu, Charles P. Tilley, Jeanna M. Arbesfeld-Qiu, Rubén Martín Payo, and Catherine S. Finlayson

Key Points

- Lymphedema is a syndrome of abnormal accumulation of lymph fluid and multiple symptoms that is caused by irreversible damage to or congenital malformation of the lymphatic system.
- There is no cure for lymphedema, and management of lymphedema requires daily self-care and changes in lifestyle.
- Strategies to promote lymph fluid flow and prevent infection are essential to reduce the risk of lymphedema and achieve long-term effective lymphedema management.

Case Study

Ms. M is an 84-year-old woman with a history of breast cancer and swelling in the right upper extremity (RUE). Ms. M was diagnosed with lymphedema after sudden onset of pain and swelling in her right arm. Ms. M had a right mastectomy with axillary dissection and hormone therapy, followed by four cycles of chemotherapy. Ms. M self-scored the pain, heaviness, and discomfort in her RUE as 5/10.

Ms. M was left hand–dominant but was able to perform multiple activities with both arms. There was severe mixed pitting and fibrotic, nonpitting edema of the RUE from the fingers to the axilla, extending into the right posterior axilla and right lateral trunk. Skin of the right chest wall was adherent and puckered. Circumferential measurements taken of both upper extremities revealed differences as follows: mid-hand 1.7 cm, wrist 3.8 cm, forearm 8.8 cm, elbow 8.5 cm, upper arm 14.7 cm, and axilla 9.8 cm. Ms. M had impaired range of motion in the RUE as follows: shoulder flexion was 0–120 degrees, shoulder abduction was 0–90 degrees, internal and external rotation were 0–60 degrees, elbow flexion was 0–110 degrees, wrist flexion was 0–10 degrees, and wrist extension was 0–45 degrees.

Ms. M started a 4-week course of lymphedema treatment after she completed external beam radiation treatment to the right chest and axilla. She stated that she did not have any significant burns during the radiation treatment. Lymph drainage followed the right axillo-inguinal collateral lymph pathway, and multilayer, short-stretch compression bandages were applied to the RUE from the fingers to the axilla. Foam chip pads were placed under the compression bandages, and they greatly reduced the fibrotic tissue in the RUE. The wound in the right axilla healed slowly. A custom elastic compression arm-sleeve and glove (compression class 1–20 mm Hg) were ordered for daytime compression, and a ready-to-wear foam and fabric alternative compression sleeve and gauntlet were provided for night compression. Ms. M was instructed in a modified exercise program emphasizing lymphatic breathing exercises. At the end of her 4-week course of treatment Ms. M's RUE exhibited a reduction of 34.7 cm or 47%, comparing it with her unaffected left upper extremity. She self-scored the heaviness and discomfort in her RUE as 3/10, an improvement from 5/10 prior to treatment. At Ms. M's 1-month follow-up, her RUE was stable; her lymphedema continued to be stable for 5 years with follow-up every 6 months.

During her follow-up visit after 5 years, her RUE began to show an increase in edema and pain, causing her difficulty in wearing her compression garments and compression bandaging. Ms. M was placed on oxygen due to shortness of breath. Pulmonary lesions were suspected, and test results were pending. Ms. M lost some of her initial edema reduction, which now measured 28.9 cm/37% at this 3-month follow-up. Ms. M's RUE exhibited a significant increase in swelling: 55 cm from initial baseline measurements. An unusual rash was noted on Ms. M's chest and back at this time. Her daughter was encouraged to have Ms. M seen by her oncologist. The diagnosis of recurrent cancer was made. Ms. M started a course of palliative lymphedema treatment. Multiple open, draining skin lesions were present on the right chest wall, in the right axilla, and on the proximal portion of the right upper arm. Ms. M was in severe pain but refused to take pain medications. She had a difficult time lying on the treatment table due to pain. Modified positioning with Ms. M sitting facing the treatment table with her arms supported on a pillow was used. We encouraged Ms. M to take her pain medications at home prior to coming to treatment. Ms. M experienced severe itching during treatment. She was resistant to taking her opioid pain medications. She began to develop swelling in her lower extremities. Upon questioning, Ms. M's daughter revealed that her mom was not taking her prescribed diuretic (diuretics are not a treatment for lymphedema itself but are helpful in cases of malignant lymphedema or when there are medical comorbidities that require diuretic treatment). She was encouraged to take her medication as prescribed and contacted her oncologist to advise them of this. The custom elastic arm-sleeve and glove she had from her prior course of treatment would no longer fit because of the marked increase in her edema. She was measured for a custom inelastic Velcro adjustable arm-sleeve and gauntlet.

Ms. M's chest lesions began to drain profusely, and her pain worsened significantly as her malignant disease progressed. Her family members were instructed in donning the Velcro compression garments and compression bandaging for home use as tolerated. She was discharged from palliative treatment. Ms. M was admitted to hospice care and expired. Her family was grateful that they were able to assist in Ms. M's care in those last months and felt that having some tools to help control the swelling gave both Ms. M and the family some measure of comfort during this difficult time.

Definitions

Lymphedema is the pathological accumulation of protein-rich lymph fluid in the interstitial tissue spaces due to an imbalance between lymph fluid production and transport, manifested clinically by tissue swelling and other physical symptoms (e.g., pain, heaviness, tightness, tingling).[1–3] *Edema*, a symptom, refers to excessive accumulation of fluid within interstitial tissues and is one of the manifestations of lymphedema. Long-term, neglected edema, such as lower extremity venous insufficiency, can develop into chronic lymphedema. Discerning the difference between edema and lymphedema ensures appropriate treatment.

One or several factors can precipitate an imbalance in extracellular fluid volume. Excess fluids, proteins, immunological cells, and debris in affected tissues can produce chronic inflammation and connective tissue proliferation, including hypertrophy of adipose tissue.[3,4] Some degree of progression usually occurs and can produce subcutaneous and dermal thickening (i.e., fibrosis).[2,4] Lymphedema and edema are contrasted in Table 19.1, which provides definitions, signs and symptoms, and basic pathophysiology.[1,3,4]

Table 19.1 Comparison of edema and lymphedema

	Edema	Lymphedema
Disorder	A symptom of various disorders	A chronic, currently incurable edema
Definition	Swelling caused by excessive fluid in interstitial tissues—due to imbalance between capillary filtration and lymph drainage over time	Swelling (edema) caused by accumulation of lymph fluid within interstitial tissues as a result of lymphatic drainage failure, increased production of lymph fluid over time, or both
Signs and symptoms	Swelling, decreased skin mobility	Swelling, decreased skin mobility
	Tightness, tingling, or bursting	Tightness, heaviness, firmness, tingling, feeling of fullness, or bursting sensations
	Decreased strength and mobility	Decreased strength and mobility
	Discomfort (aching to severe pain)	Discomfort (aching, soreness to severe pain)
	Possible skin color change	Progressive skin changes (color, texture, tone, temperature), impairment in integrity such as blisters, weeping (lymphorrhea), hyperkeratosis, warts, papillomatosis, and elephantiasis
	Pitting scale is often used:	*Pitting scale is NOT used*
	1+ Edema barely detectable	
	2+ Slight indentation with depression	
	3+ Deep indentation for 5–30 s with pressure	
	4+ Area 1.5–2 times greater than normal	
Pathophysiology	Capillary filtration rate exceeds fluid transport capacity	Inadequate lymph transport capacity
		Primary—Inadequately developed lymphatic pathways
	Example: Heart failure, fluid overload, and/or venous thrombosis are common causes of increased capillary pressure, leading to an increased capillary filtration rate that causes edema	*Secondary*—Damage outside lymphatic pathways (obstruction/obliteration)
		Initial sequelae of transport failure:
		Lymphatic stasis → increased tissue fluid → accumulated protein and cellular metabolites → lymphedema
	Note: Timely treatment of the underlying cause or causes usually reduces edema	Further increased tissue water and pressure
		Potential long-term sequelae:
	Prolonged, untreated edema can transition to lymphedema	Macrophages seek to decrease inflammation
		Increased fibroblasts and keratinocytes cause chronic inflammation
		Gradual increase in adipose tissue
		Lymphorrhea (leakage of lymph through skin)
		Gradual skin and tissue thickening and hardening progressing to hyperkeratosis, papillomatosis, and other problems
		Ever-increasing risk of infection and other complications

Source: References 2, 8–10, 14, and 30.

Prevalence and Risk Factors

The world prevalence of edema is unknown, and that of lymphedema is poorly documented. Primary lymphedema, a genetic disorder, is attributed to embryonic developmental abnormalities, which may be sporadic, or part of a syndrome caused by either chromosomal abnormalities (e.g., Turner's syndrome) or inherited single-gene defects.[5,6] Primary lymphedema occurs in about 1 in 6,000 individuals and is more common in women than men, with a 3:1 ratio.[7]

Secondary (acquired) lymphedema results from obstruction or obliteration of lymph nodes or lymphatic vessels.[1,8–10] Cancer, trauma, surgery, severe infections, cardiac disease, poor venous function, immobility, and paralyzing diseases are major causes of secondary lymphedema.[1,8–10] In developing countries, lymphatic filariasis, a parasitic infection transmitted by mosquitoes, is the predominant cause of secondary lymphedema. Mosquitoes transmit filariasis nematodes, which embed in human lymphatics and release inflammatory substances that cause progressive lymphatic damage. It is estimated that the worldwide incidence of filariasis is 863 million in 47 countries.[11] In developed countries, the most common causes of lymphedema are cancer and/or its treatment (e.g., surgery and radiation therapy) that damages the lymphatic system and surrounding soft tissues, resulting in the inability of the lymphatic system to transport lymph fluid from the tissues to the blood vascular system.[1,2,8–10] As a chronic and progressive disease, lymphedema is a significant health issue for many cancer survivors, including people with breast cancer (20%–40%), gynecologic cancer (20%), melanoma (16%), genitourinary cancer (10%), head and neck cancer, and sarcoma (4%).[10,12,13] Risk factors related to cancer treatment include extent of surgery, extent of lymph node resection, and radiation therapy.[14–17] Ms. M in the case study represents at least 20% of breast cancer survivors who develop lymphedema after cancer treatment.

Other major factors of lymphedema risk include inflammation, infection, skin trauma, and higher body mass index (BMI).[2,3,10,14] Cancer survivors who undergo surgery and dissection of lymph nodes and vessels are known to have a compromised lymphatic system, which makes them more vulnerable to infection and impaired lymphatic drainage.[2,10,17–18] Women who had previous infections and skin trauma (e.g. cuts/scratches, sunburn, oil splash or steam burns, insect bites) were more likely to develop lymphedema; weight gain and obesity (BMI >30 kg/m^2) increase lymphedema risk.[10,14–16] Nevertheless, these risk factors only partially explain who develops lymphedema. Lymphedema can and does occur in patients lacking these risk factors. Research on the effect of genetics or genetic variations on secondary lymphedema related to cancer treatment is very limited. However, mutations and genetic variations in lymph-specific growth factors are associated with hereditary lymphedema and secondary lymphedema related to breast cancer, such as vascular endothelial growth factor (VEGF-C, VEGF-D, VEGFR2, VEGFR3) and inflammatory cytokines (interleukin [IL]-4 and IL-13).[17,19,20] Understanding the biological mechanism of lymphedema through the exploration of inherited genetic susceptibility is essential for finding a cure.

Impact

Lymphedema impacts an individual's quality of life (QOL), causing physical discomfort, functional disabilities, impaired occupational roles, poor self-image, decreased self-esteem, interrupted interpersonal relationships, financial burden, and lifestyle changes.[20–23] Physically, lymphedema leads to distressing symptoms such as swelling, firmness, tightness, heaviness, pain, fatigue, numbness, and impaired limb mobility.[9,18,24] In addition, lymphedema predisposes individuals to skin and tissue fibrosis, cellulitis, infections, lymphadenitis, and septicemia.[10,18,22] Prolonged fluid stasis can lead to severe skin and tissue symptoms, sometimes referred to as "elephantiasis." Symptoms include hyperkeratosis (hard, reptile-like skin), warts, and papillomas (engorged and raised lymph vessels on the skin surface).[10,18] Chronic lymphedema is associated with the development of the rare, usually fatal cancer lymphangiosarcoma.[2] Functionally, lymphedema makes it difficult for individuals to accomplish activities of daily living (ADLs).[24,25] A recently published study detailed that patients with lymphedema and lymphatic pain reported impairments in 45% of ADLs and had a significantly increased risk of having difficulty in performing all of the 13 ADLs (i.e., cooking, using a knife, writing/typing, cleaning, vacuuming, laundry, carrying objects, yard work, dressing self, bathing self, driving, making bed, and taking care of children).[24,25] Pain in the late stage of lymphedema and cancer, experienced by Ms. M in the case study, can be devastating to patients in every aspect of ADLs.

Psychologically, individuals feel stigmatized, and some experience loss of sexual attractiveness because of obvious disfigurement, which often elicits emotional distress, social anxiety, depression, and disruption of interpersonal relationships.[21,22,26–27] Disparities among patients with lymphedema are maintained by a lack of cost-effective, accessible, and appropriately adapted supportive care opportunities found at more resourced medical centers.[28,29] This results in a large symptom burden (i.e., lymphatic pain) for patients, providers, and healthcare systems. Routine checkups for lymphedema management, long-term physical therapy, management equipment (compression garments, bandages, special lotions), and repeated cellulitis, infections, and lymphangitis create financial and economic burdens not only for survivors but also for the healthcare system.[27]

Anatomy, Physiology, and Pathophysiology

Edema

Edema is a symptom that results from an imbalance between capillary filtration and lymph drainage. Edema requires treatment of the underlying disorder that is precipitating tissue fluid excess. Precipitators can include cardiac, hepatic, renal, allergic, or hypoproteinemic disease; venous obstruction; and medication complications[30] (see Table 19.1). Chronic edema can develop into secondary lymphedema with sufficient lymphatic damage, such as in chronic venous insufficiency, posttraumatic swelling from significant soft tissue injury, or fractures of the lower extremities.[31]

Lymphedema

A healthy lymphatic system helps regulate the tissue cellular environment, including collecting and returning plasma and proteins.[32,33] Every day, 20%–50% of the total accumulating plasma proteins travel through 2–4 Liter of lymph fluid in a healthy lymphatic system.[32,33] Lymphatics also remove cellular waste products, mutants, and debris; eliminate non-self-antigens; and regulate local immune defense in the process of maintaining homeostasis.[32,33]

Unidirectional vessels traverse from superficial to deep lymphatics through 600–700 lymph nodes, carrying lymph fluid to the venous system at the right or left venous angle of the anterior chest on either side of the neck. Lymph nodes filter, concentrate, and purify lymph fluid, eliminating defective cells, toxins, and bacteria, explaining the increased risk of infection for patients with compromised lymphatics.[32,33] Lymphedema pathology signifies malfunction in any part of the process of collecting, transporting, filtering, and depositing lymph into the venous system. Lymphedema pathophysiology suggests disruption of these processes and is described in Table 19.1.

In brief, lymph fluid is transported initially from the interstitium by the initial lymphatic vessels, moving proximally through progressively larger collecting lymph vessels; filtered through lymph nodes; then drained into the two large lymph-collecting ducts; and finally returned to the venous bloodstream via the left and right subclavian veins. Damage to any structures of the lymphatic system can lead to accumulation of lymph fluid in the affected area. Furthermore, physiological variations in each individual's lymphatic system, such as numbers or sizes of lymph nodes, make it difficult to quantify each individual's risk for lymphedema.

Secondary lymphedema from cancer treatment is caused by trauma to the lymphatic system, mainly from surgery and radiotherapy.[8,12] Surgery creates disruption to the lymphatic system by directly dissecting lymph vessels and removing lymph nodes.[9] Unfortunately, lymph nodes do not regenerate once dissected.[31–33] Formation of scar tissue and tissue fibrosis from surgery create further impairment to lymph flow. The disruption or blockage of the lymphatic system reduces its ability to transport and filter the lymph, resulting in a functional overload and insufficient capability of the lymphatic system to transport the normal volume of lymph.[34] As a result, an abnormal accumulation of lymph fluid occurs, which leads to swelling of the affected area.

Radiation exposure during radiotherapy is also traumatic to the lymphatic system. Radiation impairs the lymphatic system by causing tissue fibrosis surrounding the lymphatic vessels,[9] and it reduces lymphatic transport reserve by increasing long-term changes in basal lymph circulation and lymph flow in the affected area.[9,33] While lymphatic vessels are relatively insensitive to radiotherapy, lymph nodes are radiosensitive to conventional doses of radiotherapy.[33,34] The radiated lymph nodes respond first with lymphocyte depletion, followed by fatty replacement, then by fibrosis.[33,34] As a result, radiation hinders lymph nodes from properly filtering and transporting lymph and alters immune function. Research has not clarified the specific roles of chemotherapy in contributing to lymphedema. In addition to the definite risk from cancer treatment, certain personal risk factors such as weight gain or obesity (BMI >30 kg/m^2), infection, skin trauma, and immobility increase an individual's risk for lymphedema.[8–1014,15] Socioeconomic factors such as financial hardships, being Black, and being of younger age also increase the risk of lymphedema for cancer survivors.[24] Please check YouTube (https://www.youtube.com/watch?v=c-FL1XwDYzs) for the lymphatic system video.

Precision Assessment and Diagnosis

Assessing and diagnosing lymphedema continue to be challenges for research and clinical practice. Several factors contribute to the challenge: lack of universally recognized diagnostic criteria, failure to precisely evaluate symptoms, coexisting conditions, and lack of awareness of lymphedema among healthcare professionals.[17,34,35] Inconsistency in the criteria defining lymphedema and the use of different measures in research have presented tremendous challenges in the assessment and diagnosing of lymphedema.[1,8,9,32,35] Often, lymphedema is diagnosed via provider observation of swelling in clinical practice. Lymphedema can occur in body areas where measuring swelling is difficult, including head, neck, shoulder, breast and thoracic regions, abdomen, lower extremities, foot, and ankle.[1,8,9,32,35] A critical need exists to understand heterogeneity (i.e., different types) of lymphedema phenotype to advance precision phenotype assessment of lymphedema and provide insights to biological mechanisms.

To optimize the precision assessment of heterogeneity of lymphedema phenotypes and ensure accurate diagnosis, it is important for nurses to conduct a careful review of the patient's health history to rule out other medical conditions that may cause similar symptoms, such as recurrent cancer, deep vein thrombosis, chronic venous insufficiency, diabetes, hypertension, and cardiac, hepatic, thyroid, and renal diseases. These alternative diagnoses should be ruled out before establishing a diagnosis of lymphedema and referring the patient for lymphedema therapy. Assessment for infection, thrombosis, or cancer metastasis should be performed at every patient contact.[18,32] Most infections develop subcutaneously, beneath intact skin. Cultures are not recommended because they rarely document a bacterial source and can further increase the risk of infection.[9] Suspected thrombosis or new or recurring cancer requires appropriate diagnostic evaluation (e.g., Doppler ultrasonography, magnetic resonance imaging, positron emission tomography, computed tomographic scanning). Venous ultrasonography is reported to be safer than venography for evaluation of suspected thrombosis in a limb with or at high risk for lymphedema.[9,33] Changes in pain or comfort, increased swelling, skin (color, temperature, condition), or mobility and range of motion are other possible early signs of major complications, such as cancer reoccurrence for Ms. M.[3]

"Best practice"[8] components of lymphedema nursing assessment are displayed in Box 19.1. The first assessment priority is proper diagnosis. For example, a nurse should ask Ms. M, the elderly woman with suspected lymphedema, during the initial contact whether she had a history of cancer and whether she had lymphedema symptoms, such as pain, swelling, heaviness, and impaired range of motion in the affected upper limb. For Ms. M, the results of physical assessment and patient history should indicate possible lymphedema diagnosis that warrants further evaluation to confirm the diagnosis.[32,35] Lymphoscintigraphy (isotope lymphography) can ensure definite lymphedema diagnosis.[32] Lymphography (direct) is now rarely used in lymphedema patients because of its potential to cause lymphatic injury and its inability to clarify function.[32]

Supportive communication is essential for precision assessment. Supportive communication helps to understand the patient's perspectives and gain essential information, including the patient's (1) view of lymphedema, (2) readiness for instruction and treatment, (3) pertinent work and lifestyle, (4) spiritual concerns, (5) illness and adjustment issues, and (6) desired goals. Often the patient's initial goal is cure, which is unattainable. In this situation, the patient needs time to understand the chronicity of lymphedema and to formulate new goals. In Ms. M's situation of cancer reoccurrence and

Box 19.1 Sequential Components of Lymphedema Assessment

- *Ask questions to rule out or address immediate complications* (i.e., infection, thrombosis, severe pain, new or recurrent cancer, significant nonrelated disorders). For example: Have you been diagnosed with cancer? Have you experienced pain or heaviness in your right arm (or leg)?
- *Conduct history and physical examination*
  - Routine physical assessments: vital signs, blood pressure, height and weight, body mass index
  - Past and current health status, including medications and allergies (especially antibiotic allergies and history of infection, trauma, or surgery in affected area)
  - Check for lymphedema symptoms (i.e., swelling, pain, heaviness, aching, soreness, etc.)
  - Current activities of daily living (job, home responsibilities, leisure activities, sleep position, activities that aggravate lymphedema)
  - Current psychological health, support people, view of lymphedema and health
  - History of lymphedema etiology, presentation, duration, and progression
- *Assess patient knowledge of and response to lymphedema, interest in assistance, and goals*
- *Check third-party payer status*
- *Quantification of lymphedema status* (lymphedema signs and symptoms, volume, pain and other neurological symptoms, tissue status, range of motion of nearby joints, site-specific and overall patient function)

severe stage of lymphedema, the nurse should be aware of patient QOL goals for end-of-life palliative care. Nurses' and healthcare providers' understanding of patients' perspectives and knowledge is paramount to ensure optimal patient education, support, multidisciplinary referrals, goal setting, assistance with self-care and palliative care, complication avoidance, and long-term management.[36]

Assessment of Symptoms

Lymphedema is a sign of an impaired lymphatic system.[1–3,9,33] Impairment in the lymphatic system leads to a chronic disease state with multiple associated symptoms, such as heaviness, tightness, firmness, pain, numbness, or impaired mobility.[1,3,9,17,33] Lymphedema symptoms significantly impact patients' daily living function,[24–26] psychological distress,[26] and QOL.[22,23,27]

Symptom assessment is essential since very often observable swelling and measurable volume changes are absent during the initial development of lymphedema.[1,3,10,17] Table 19.2 presents an example of a symptom checklist for breast cancer–related lymphedema.[1,3,17,24–26] Assessing lymphedema symptoms plays an important role in diagnosis until objective measurements capable of detecting latent stages of lymphedema are established in at-risk individuals.[1,3,17,24–26] For example, lymphatic pain is a cardinal sign for an early stage of lymphedema.[3,24–26] Patients who report lymphatic pain are nearly twice as likely to develop lymphedema.[24] Lymphatic pain refers to various pain (e.g., aching or soreness) in the ipsilateral body or upper limb due to a compromised lymphatic system from breast cancer treatment.[24–26] Without timely intervention in this early stage, lymphedema can progress into a chronic condition that no surgical or medical interventions can cure.[8] Limb volume change has significantly increased as breast cancer survivors' reports of swelling, heaviness, tenderness, firmness, tightness, and aching have increased.[3,9,37] A diagnostic cutoff of three symptoms was able to detect breast cancer survivors with lymphedema from healthy women with 94% accuracy, while a diagnostic cutoff of nine symptoms identified survivors with lymphedema with 64% accuracy. As early intervention leads to better clinical outcomes, patients with nine or more symptoms should be evaluated immediately and treated in a timely manner.[9]

Table 19.2 Example of symptom checklist: Breast cancer and lymphedema symptom experience index

The following questions are about symptoms in your affected arm, hand, breast, axilla (under arm), or chest today or in the past month.
Have you had ___? No Yes
1. Limited shoulder movement
2. Limited elbow movement
3. Limited wrist movement
4. Limited finger movement
5. Limited arm movement
6. Hand or arm swelling
7. Breast swelling
8. Chest wall swelling
9. Firmness
10. Tightness
11. Heaviness
12. Toughness or thickness of skin
13. Stiffness
14. Tenderness
15. Hotness/increased temperature
16. Redness
17. Blistering
18. Pain/aching/soreness
19. Numbness
20. Burning
21. Stabbing
22. Tingling (pins and needles)
23. Arm or hand fatigue
24. Arm or hand weakness
Tips for Making Clinical Decisions: **If a patient who previously received surgical treatment for breast cancer, if she/he marks "Yes" for arm swelling alone or for nine or more of the above symptoms, the patient should immediately be referred for further evaluation of lymphedema. Remember, early diagnosis and early treatment often lead to better clinical outcomes.**

Source: Copyright 2006. Contact Mei R. Fu, PhD, RN, FAAN; Telephone: 973-986-1758; e-mail: mf67nyu@gmail.com.

Quantification of Lymphedema

A variety of measurement approaches make quantification of lymphedema a challenge.[8,17,35,38,39] Methods of measuring limb volume or circumference include sequential circumference limb measurement, water displacement, infrared perometry, and bioelectrical impedance.[38–41] Water displacement is seldom used in clinical settings because of spillover and hygienic concerns.[35] The method is contraindicated in patients with open skin lesions. Patients may find it difficult to hold the position for the time needed for the tank overflow to drain. Unfortunately, lymphedema can also occur in the face, neck, shoulder, breast, abdomen, thoracic regions, and genital areas, which presents a challenge for quantification.[42]

Sequential Circumferential Arm Measurements

Measuring limb volume and circumference are the most widely used diagnostic methods. A flexible nonstretch tape measure for circumferences is usually used to assure consistent tension over soft tissue, muscle, and bony prominences.[35,39,43] Measurements are done on both affected and nonaffected limbs at the hand proximal to the metacarpals, wrist, and then every 4 cm from the wrist to the axilla. Limb size and limb volume are calculated based on sequential circumferential arm measurements. The formula often used for calculating limb volume with a presurgery baseline limb volume is: Limb Volume Increase = (Affected Frustum Limb Volume$_{\text{Follow-up}}$/Affected Frustum Limb Volume$_{\text{baseline}}$)/(Contralateral Frustum Limb Volume$_{\text{Follow-up}}$/Contralateral Frustum Limb Volume$_{\text{baseline}}$).[35,39,43] If presurgical baseline limb volume is not available, the following formula can be used: Limb Volume Ratio = Affected Frustum Limb Volume/Contralateral Frustum Limb Volume; Limb Volume Difference = Affected Frustum Limb Volume − Contralateral Frustum Limb Volume.[35,39,43] Arm lymphedema is often arbitrarily defined as 2 cm or more in limb girth or 200 mL or greater difference in limb volume as compared to the unaffected limb or 10% volume increase in the affected limb from presurgery baseline limb volume.[35,39,43] Recent research has shown that among breast cancer survivors, a 5% or greater limb volume increase from presurgical baseline enables detectable differences in QOL and better clinical outcomes with interventions to promote lymph flow[25,37] (Figure 19.1).

Infrared Perometry

The infrared perometer, an optoelectronic device developed to meet the need for a quick, hygienic, and accurate method for volume calculation, works similarly to computer-assisted tomography but makes use of light instead of X-rays (Figure 19.2).[35,37,39] The perometer maps a three-dimensional graph of the affected and unaffected extremities using numerous rectilinear light beams and interfaces with a computer for data analysis and storage. A three-dimensional limb image is generated, and limb volume is calculated automatically. This optoelectronic method has a standard deviation of 8.9 mL (arm), less than 0.5% of limb volume with repeated measuring.[35,37,39] The perometer can be operated by nurses or lymphedema therapists after training.

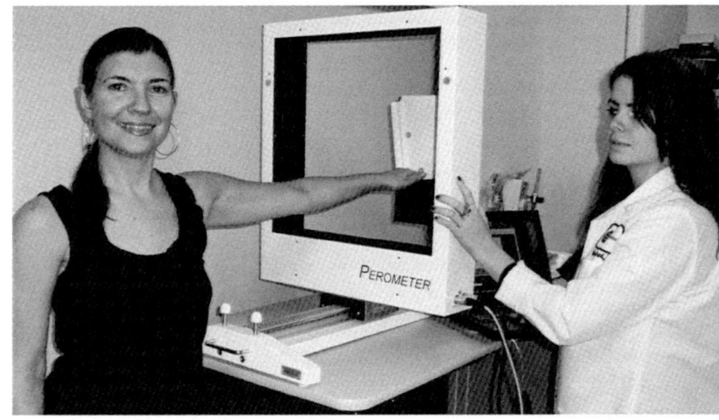

Figure 19.2 Infrared perometer measurement.

Bioelectrical Impedance Analysis

Bioelectrical impedance analysis (BIA) measures impedance or resistance of the extracellular fluid using low-frequency electrical current.[38,40] BIA provides an impedance ratio to calculate a lymphedema index (L-Dex ratio). With the development of lymphedema, the limb impedance decreases, and the L-Dex ratio therefore increases. The L-Dex ratio ranges from −10 to +10. Since approximately 20% of true arm lymphedema cases are still missed by BIA with a cutoff point of greater than +7.1, it is critical for healthcare professionals to incorporate other assessment methods, including self-report, clinical observation, or perometry, to ensure precision assessment of arm lymphedema[38,40] (Figure 19.3).

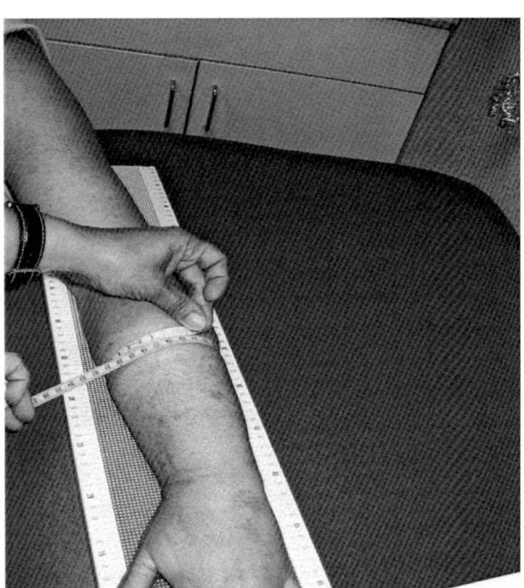

Figure 19.1 Tape measurement.

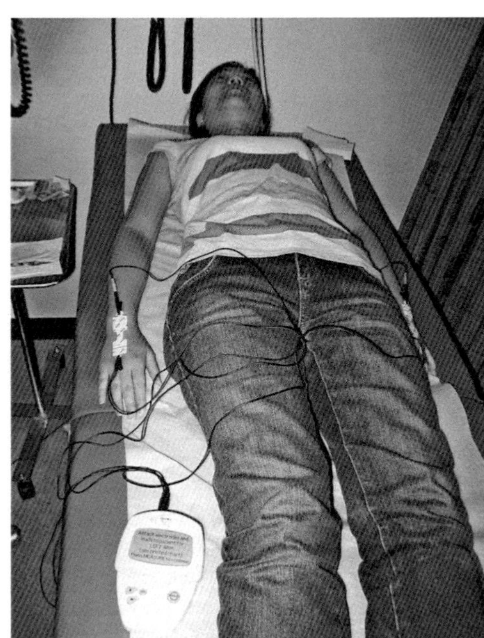

Figure 19.3 Bioelectrical impedance analysis (ImpXCA).

Lymphedema Risk Reduction

The benefits of early nursing intervention in decreasing lymphedema occurrence and severity and lymphedema symptoms in breast cancer survivors have been well documented.[45–51] Nurses can assist high-risk patients by presenting or reinforcing prevention strategies to promote lymph flow, prevent infection, and perform physical exercise safely. Emphasis on self-care rather than rigid rules fosters patient empowerment.[45–50] An empowered patient assumes responsibility for reminding staff to avoid use of the affected arm rather than expecting medical personnel to remember to do so.

Strategies to Promote Lymph Flow

Behavioral strategies to promote lymph flow *based on physiological (lymph fluid accumulation and inflammation) and cognitive principles (low self-efficacy)* are efficacious in lymphedema risk reduction and treating symptoms of pain and swelling. *The-Optimal-Lymph-Flow* (TOLF) is a nonpharmacological, behavioral, nursing intervention that has been extensively tested and demonstrated improvements in pain and swelling related to breast cancer, lymph fluid accumulation, and other important patient-centered outcomes.[45–51] TOLF is an intervention based on physiological–cognitive–behavioral principles that builds patients' self-management skills to promote lymph flow and results in reduced pain, swelling, and lymph fluid level; reversal of mild lymphedema; and improved function and QOL.[45–51] TOLF includes strategies to promote lymph flow: therapeutic lymphatic exercises, healthy diet (i.e., nutrition-balanced, portion-appropriate diet, adequate hydration), and proper sleep. The core TOLF intervention is 8-minute TOLF lymphatic exercises to promote lymph flow (i.e., muscle-tightening deep breathing, muscle-tightening pumping, and limb mobility exercises).[46,52–54] TOLF includes a website that provides patients with TOLF intervention materials, information, and daily assessments used to personalize sessions.[45,47,50] The efficacy of the TOLF intervention to prevent lymph fluid accumulation was demonstrated in a published clinical trial in which over 90% of 140 patients after breast cancer surgery were able to maintain presurgical limb volume.[37] In a published single-arm pilot trial,[46] TOLF was able to reduce lymphedema-related symptoms; reversed mild lymphedema; improved functional impairment; improved social, emotional, and psychological distress; and improved self-perception (all $p < 0.01$). A published single-arm trial focusing on the immediate effects of one dose of TOLF lymphatic exercises[13] demonstrated significant reductions in pain ($Med_{\Delta} = -1.00$, confidence interval $[CI] = [-1.5, -0.1]$, $p = 0.004$), arm/hand swelling ($Med_{\Delta} = -1.00$, $CI = [-1.5, -0.5]$, $p = 0.004$), and lymph fluid levels in bioimpedance L-Dex scores ($M_{\Delta} = -2.68$, $CI = [-4.67, -0.69]$, $p = 0.010$).[46] In a larger, 12-week parallel published randomized clinical trial[47] 120 patients were randomized either into Arm Precaution with Shoulder Mobility exercises (AP) control to improve limb mobility or TOLF intervention to promote lymph flow; significantly fewer patients in the TOLF intervention group reported chronic pain (49% vs. 71%; odds ratio $[OR] = 0.39$, $CI = [0.17, 0.90]$, $p = 0.021$) at the end of the trial. Fifty percent of patients who received the TOLF intervention achieved a complete pain reduction (50% vs. 22%; $OR = 3.56$, $CI = [1.39, 9.76]$, $p = 0.005$) compared to control AP of 22%. Significantly lower median severity scores were found in the TOLF group for chronic pain ($Med_{TOLF} = 0$, interquartile range [IQR] = 0–1 vs. $Med_{AP} = 1$, IQR = 0–2, $p = 0.024$) and general bodily pain ($Med_{TOLF} = 1$, IQR = 0–1.5 vs $Med_{AP} = 1$, IQR = 1–3, $p = 0.040$).[47] Compared to AP control, significantly fewer patients in the TOLF group reported arm/hand swelling ($p = 0.038$), heaviness ($p = 0.027$), redness ($p = 0.033$), and limited movement in shoulder ($p = 0.015$) and arm ($p = 0.025$). The TOLF intervention resulted in a 13% reduction in proportions of patients who took pain medications compared to the AP control, which had a 5% increase; there was a 12% reduction in proportions of patients with ≥5% limb volume differences in the TOLF group and a 5% increase in proportions of patients in the AP group. In a recent clinical trial, the use of TOLF for early intervention demonstrated significant reduction in limb volume, symptoms, and QOL.[50] Given TOLF is efficacious, focused on self-management skills, and welcomed by patients (<10% attrition rate in a variety of trials), TOLF has demonstrated particular benefits for patients who face personal challenges of time, travel, competing demands, and cost for therapist-administered treatment. In addition, a technologically driven delivery model[51–52] makes it easy for community-level implementation to address system barriers of intervention availability, staffing, and therapist.

Prevention of Infection and Skin Trauma

Infection Prevention of infection and skin trauma is vital for lymphedema risk reduction.[10,34,37,44,45] Infection is a significant risk factor and is the most frequent lymphedema complication.[10,18] To prevent infection, nurses and other healthcare providers should always avoid drawing blood from the affected limb as infection risk increases with breaches in skin integrity. Occasional drawing of blood from the limb at risk is necessary for some patients when no other reasonable option exists.[10] Patients can request an experienced phlebotomist and emphasize their increased infection risk. Subcutaneous, intramuscular, or intravenous injections in the limb at risk can cause an allergic or inflammatory response and/or infection that may compromise a weakened lymphatic system. These risks must be compared with the benefit and risk of use of a central venous catheter or suboptimal venipuncture site such as the lower extremity.[10] Diabetes potentially increases breast cancer patients' lymphedema risk when the affected limb is used for continual blood sticks or insulin injections. Patients with bilateral limb risk, especially of the upper extremities, face lifelong decisions regarding adherence to precautions. Nurses should assess and educate patients on signs and symptoms of infection. A recent large and observational study of 567 breast cancer survivors examined the effects of daily-living risks on lymphedema.[10] The study demonstrated that significant odds of lymphedema were associated with infection (OR = 2.58, 95% CI = 1.95-3.42), cuts/scratches (OR = 2.65, 95% CI = 1.97-3.56), sunburn (OR = 1.89, 95% CI = 1.39-3.56), oil splash or steam burns (OR = 2.08, 95% CI = 1.53-3.83), insect bites (OR = 1.59, 95% CI = 1.18-2.13). The study also found the incremental risk of skin trauma, that is having 3, 4, or 5 skin trauma risks significantly increased the odds of lymphedema to 4.31, 5.14, and 6.94 times.

Safe Physical Exercise

In the past, breast cancer survivors were cautioned to restrict exercise as a way to reduce their risk for lymphedema. However, a growing body of evidence suggests that exercise does not necessarily increase lymphedema risk.[8] Research suggests that breast cancer survivors should be encouraged to carry out all postoperative exercises, resume normal precancer activities as tolerated, and be as fit as possible while regularly monitoring their high-risk or affected limb.[8] In addition to the importance of physical exercise in general health, weight control, and QOL, physical exercise can promote lymph fluid drainage through large muscle movement. Nurses should instruct patients to perform physical exercise according to the general exercise guidelines[8,32]: (1) initiate exercise at lower intensity, gradually increasing intensity as tolerated, monitoring the at-risk limb(s) for signs and symptoms of swelling; (2) exercise to the extent that the affected body part is not fatigued; (3) modify physical exercise to reduce the risk of trauma and injury; and (4) use a compression garment during exercise if recommended by healthcare professionals with lymphedema training.

Edema Treatment

Edema treatment focuses on detection and intervention related to the causative factor or factors. Effective treatment stabilizes the interstitial fluid volume.[30] Tissue support and/or gentle compression can be useful in relieving edema that might progress to lymphedema.

Lymphedema Treatment

Lymphedema treatment refers to therapies to help reduce swelling and associated symptoms as well as maintain reductions in swelling, pain, and other lymphedema symptoms achieved through treatment while minimizing lymphedema exacerbations. Treatments include surgery, pharmacological therapy, and complete decongestive therapy (CDT).[8,32] Pharmacological therapy and surgery have limited proven effectiveness. Diuretics are not recommended for the treatment of lymphedema and are proven to be ineffective[8]; however, there are cases where lymphedema is combined with edema caused by other comorbid conditions such as heart or renal failure in which diuretics are part of the medical management of edema caused by the comorbid conditions. Patients may have heard that "diuretics are not a treatment for lymphedema"; nurses should explain to patients the need to continue their diuretics if they have been prescribed to treat hypertension, heart or renal failure, or other comorbid conditions. The case study presents examples of CDT, compression, and lymphedema palliative care.

Surgical Approach

A recent systematic review of research from 2009 to 2014 concludes that the effectiveness of surgical treatment for lymphedema has not been established.[8,43] The various surgical treatment options for lymphedema can be broadly categorized as excisional procedures, liposuction, lymphatic reconstruction, and tissue transfer procedures. In the past decade, significant progress has been made in contemporary surgical treatment for lymphedema, particularly microsurgical procedures (e.g., lymphaticovenous anastomosis, vascularized lymph node transfer, and lymphaticolymphatic bypass). With proper diagnosis and the careful selection of the appropriate procedure, surgical techniques can be used to treat lymphedema in patients when combined with integrated lymphedema therapy.[8,43] However, the efficacy and long-term outcomes of the surgical approaches in this population have yet to be reported. At this point, surgical treatment of lymphedema is reserved primarily for patients who have lymphedema that is refractory to standard treatment modalities.[8,43]

CDT

CDT, or decongestive lymphatic therapy, evolved in Europe when Michael Foldi[8,26,43] combined Vodder's manual lymph drainage (MLD) technique with bandaging, exercises, and specialized skin care. Dr. Foldi described his four-modality lymphedema treatment as "complete decongestive therapy." CDT is the current standard of care for treatment of lymphedema. It consists of an intensive lymphedema therapy (phase I of CDT), followed by an ongoing, individualized maintenance and self-management phase (phase II of CDT).[8,26,43] In the intensive therapy phase, therapists use MLD, compression garments, multilayer short-stretch compression bandaging, remedial exercise, and skin care to reduce visible or palpable swelling.[8,26,43] The duration of the intensive lymphedema therapy phase, averaging about two to three treatments per week for up to 8 weeks, varies with the severity of lymphedema and patient response. Clinically, phase I of CDT ends when swelling has been reduced and symptoms have been controlled. Following the completion of intensive lymphedema therapy, the patient is taught to initiate self-management (phase II of CDT) for control of chronic soft tissue changes and to conduct the individual components of CDT, including self-MLD, skin care, exercises, and application of prescribed compression garments and/or bandages to prevent exacerbation of swelling and symptoms. The self-management phase is a lifelong process; regular checkups with the primary care provider and the lymphedema therapist are necessary.[8,26,43]

Adherence to the prescribed treatment can be difficult because even the most customized garments or sleeves sometimes are uncomfortable, unsightly, and laborious to put on.[8,18] A constellation of complex factors (e.g., physical, financial, aesthetic, time) can influence survivors' adherence with treatment. Lymphedema is a complex condition that needs to be treated by therapists with special training and experience in this field.[53] Lymphology Association of North America (http://www.clt-lana.org/), a multidisciplinary organizations has outlined training requirements for clinicians to gain certification in this field.

Bandages and Garments

Both compression garments and bandages are effective in treating lymphedema by providing proper compression to improve muscle and joint pumps during activity, to aid in moving lymph fluid from the affected area, to prevent the further accumulation of evacuated lymph fluid, and to maintain the results achieved during MLD.[8,54]

Compression bandages and multilayer lymphedema bandaging (MLLB) are effective and flexible forms of compression, particularly in the early stages of lymphedema therapy. MLLB provides external compression. For some patients, MLLB may be used as part of long-term or palliative management. MLLB uses inelastic or low-stretch bandages to produce a massaging effect and stimulate lymph flow and is especially important for patients with severe lymphedema, such as lymphedema complicated by morbid obesity or neglected primary lymphedema. It is also important for patients who choose self- or caregiver-bandaging to enhance comfort or for nighttime compression when they wear a compression garment during the day.[8,34] Foam or other padding is often used under bandages to improve edema reduction, soften fibrosis, and restore normal limb contours. The time, effort, and dexterity required for bandaging can become burdensome, and bandaging is not practical or possible for some patients, necessitating the use of an alternative compression method.[34] MLLB should be avoided for the following conditions: (1) severe arterial insufficiency with an ankle/brachial index of less than 0.6, although modified MLLB with reduced pressures can be used under close supervision; (2) uncontrolled heart failure; and (3) severe peripheral neuropathy.[37] Some components of the MLLB system can be washed and dried according to the manufacturer's instructions and reused. Over time, inelastic bandages will progressively lose their extensibility, which will increase their stiffness. Heavily soiled, cohesive, and adhesive bandages should be discarded after use.[33,34] Patients with lymphedema graduate from bandages to elastic compression garments. Compression garments generally need to be worn throughout the patient's life.

Compression garments are recommended for patients with lymphedema of the extremities.[8] Compression garments may be used in the initial management of patients who have mild upper or lower limb lymphedema with minor pitting, no significant tissue changes, no or minimal shape distortion, or palliative needs.[33,34] Proper fit of the compression garment is imperative. An ill-fitting garment can cause swelling to develop in an area proximal or distal to the end of the garment (i.e., in the hand, in the anterior or posterior axillary/shoulder areas, or in the toes or genital/pubic/buttock/abdominal areas). Patients must be instructed to remove their garment if such swelling, pain, numbness, or muscle cramps occur and consult with their lymphedema specialist regarding revision of the garment to ensure proper fit and function. Gradient compression provides the greatest pressure distally and less pressure proximally; this is optimal for improved lymphatic transport.[55,56] Skin care, exercise or body movement, elevation, and self-lymph drainage should be taught, along with self-monitoring to help relieve lymphedema symptoms in individuals receiving palliative care. Patients should be reassessed 4–6 weeks after initial fitting and then approximately every 3–6 months.[55,56]

Compression garments should be laundered every time they are worn and replaced every 3–6 months. Patients need to moisturize and check their skin daily for signs of irritation/infection. A variety of helpful products exist to assist patients in applying garments, which may be an especially challenging task for elderly and disabled patients. Usually, ridged rubber gloves (dishwashing gloves) facilitate application of garments and extend their longevity. Timely garment replacement (usually every 6 months) is essential for good edema control.[56,57] If a compression garment causes pain, neurological symptoms, or color or temperature changes, it should be removed and the patient instructed to consult with their lymphedema specialist to resolve the problem.

Pneumatic (Mechanical) Pumps: Intermittent Pneumatic Compression Devices

Mechanical pneumatic pumps use electricity to inflate a single-chamber or multichambered sleeve that produces external limb compression. A decreased tissue capillary filtration rate facilitates tissue fluid reduction and, consequently, limb volume decrease.[58,59] A recent systematic review on research from 2009 to 2014 concluded that the effectiveness of pneumatic compression devices (PCDs) on limb volume reduction has not been established; furthermore, adverse events related to PCD use are reported, such as increased swelling of hand and torso, forearm pain, finger numbness, and pain in the axilla and back.[8] After more than 50 years of pump use in lymphedema care and long-established Medicare reimbursement, no guidelines exist, significant complications are reported, and research has not clarified benefit. Clearly, more studies with rigorous design and adequate sample sizes are needed.[8]

Infection Prevention and Treatment

Infection is the most common lymphedema complication.[10] Lymph stasis, decreased local immune response, tissue congestion, and accumulated proteins and other debris foster infection.[2] Traditional signs and symptoms (fever, malaise, lethargy, and nausea) are often present. Decades of literature support prompt oral or intravenous antibiotic therapy.[43] Because streptococci and staphylococci are frequent precipitators, antibiotics must have good skin penetration and cover normal skin flora, as well as gram-positive cocci.[10,43] Early detection and treatment of infections can help prevent the need for intravenous therapy and hospitalization.[10,43] Intravenous antibiotic therapy is recommended for systemic signs of infection or insufficient response to oral antibiotics. Nursing activities include assisting patients in obtaining prompt antibiotic therapy, monitoring and reporting signs and symptoms, and providing instruction regarding high fluid intake, rest, elevation of the infected limb, and avoidance of strenuous activity. Garment-type compression is encouraged as soon as tolerable during infection. Wound care or infectious disease specialists can be helpful in complicated cases. Infection prophylaxis has been highly effective for patients who experience repeated serious infections or inflammatory episodes.[43] Effective edema reduction and control may also help reduce the incidence of lymphedema infection.[43,59]

The feet, which are especially susceptible to fungal infections in lower extremity lymphedema, can exhibit peeling, scaly skin, and toenail changes. Antifungal powders are recommended prophylactically. Antifungal creams should be used at the first sign of fungus. Diabetic-like skin care and use of cotton socks and well-fitted, breathable (leather or canvas), sturdy shoes are beneficial.[43,59]

Lymphedema Management

Edema usually subsides with proper treatment, whereas lymphedema is a lifelong and chronic condition requiring long-term management.[8,10,18,43] Lymphedema management focuses on daily activities and strategies undertaken to decrease the swelling, relieve symptom distress, and prevent acute exacerbations and infections.[8,10,18,43] Components of long-term lymphedema management are listed in Box 19.2 and described throughout the chapter. Long-term

Box 19.2 Components of Long-Term Lymphedema Management

- History, physical examination, and ongoing assessment and support
- Individualized and holistic care coordination
- Multidisciplinary referrals
- Comprehensive initial and ongoing patient instruction
- Ongoing psychosocial support
- Promotion of ongoing optimal self-care management
- Facilitation of appropriate evidence-based, individualized treatment
- Patient and practice outcome measurement
- Access and long-term follow-up and management
- Communication and collaboration with related healthcare providers

management is a process of fostering optimal physical, functional, psychosocial, and spiritual wellness. Spiritual care guidelines have been gradually evolving in nursing for several decades. Spiritual care supports patients' efforts to make meaning out of illness and to redefine themselves in their new state of being. Specific spiritual interventions can include (1) support during the struggle with and exploration of life's ambiguities, (2) acknowledgment of patients' real and potential losses and victories, and (3) guidance in patients' exploration of end-of-life issues and decisions.[8,10,18,43]

Lymphedema management necessitates a multidisciplinary approach.[8,10,18,53,56] Nurses should assess for signs of infection, changes in limb volume or limb size, as well as limb or torso contour, pain, and degree of swelling at each patient visit. Additional inquiries need to be made as for any other symptoms patients may be experiencing because of the lymphedema. Nurses should assess self-care behaviors and encourage patients with lymphedema to wear their compression garment as prescribed. Patients with new-onset or worsening lymphedema should be referred to certified lymphedema therapists for volume reduction treatment. Antibiotics may be prescribed for infections. Certified lymphedema therapists provide assessment and treatment for the swollen limb or area as well as any musculoskeletal impairment that may develop as a consequence of surgery, radiation, and or chemotherapy to treat cancer. In addition, certified lymphedema therapists also design individualized patient education about self-care practices, skin care, wear and care of compression garments, exercise and exercise progression based on individual lymphedema risk factors, and level of fitness. Certified lymphedema therapists have the expertise to recommend home and workplace modifications if needed to reduce risk for injury or overuse of the at-risk or affected limbs. Collecting and reviewing outcomes with patients over time fosters ongoing instruction, complication prevention, sustained lymphedema improvement, and patient empowerment.[8,10,18,43]

Pain and Lymphedema Symptom Management

Approximately 30%–60% of patients with lymphedema post–breast cancer treatment report pain.[3,9,17,24–26] Causes of pain include fluid accumulation, infection, postoperative changes in the axilla, postmastectomy pain syndrome, brachial plexopathy, various arthritic conditions, peripheral entrapment neuropathies, vascular compromise, and cancer recurrence. Sudden onset of pain requires careful assessment for complications. Use of the 0–10 pain scale is recommended for cancer pain assessment. Behavioral interventions (e.g., TOLF) have demonstrated significant effects on pain related to lymphedema and fluid accumulation.[44–50] Pharmacological pain management for end-of life palliative care is important for patients and family, as in Ms. M's case.

Self-Care

Optimal patient self-care typically includes adherence to risk-reduction behaviors, use of compression, weight management, fitness and lymphedema exercises, optimal nutrition and hydration, healthy lifestyle practices, and seeking assistance for lymphedema-related problems.[8,37] Patient empowerment for optimal self-care is a great impetus to long-term management success.[8,32] Evidence from breast cancer patients indicates that weight management, including reduction of BMI or weight, lymphatic exercises (e.g., TOLF Lymphatic Exercise), and manual lymph drainage appear to be an effective means of assisting in the reduction of arm volume during lymphedema treatment.[8,46,47,50,54]

Safe Physical Exercise

Exercise or body movement is an integral part of lymphedema management and risk reduction. Exercise improves muscular strength, cardiovascular function, psychological well-being, and functional capacity.[8] Research evidence from patients with upper extremity lymphedema has clearly shown that exercise (e.g., progressive weightlifting and other resistance exercises) under close supervision is not associated with a worsening of lymphedema or related symptoms. Lymphatic exercises (e.g., TOLF Lymphatic Exercise), and whole-body exercise may help stabilize limb volume and improve joint mobility in the affected area.[8,45–47,50]

Gentle resistance exercise (e.g., TOLF Lymphatic Exercise) stimulates muscle pumps and increases lymph flow; aerobic exercise facilitates changes in intra-abdominal pressure, which facilitates pumping of the thoracic duct.[8,45–47,50] A tailored exercise or body movement program that combines flexibility, resistance, and aerobic exercise may be beneficial in reducing the risk of and controlling lymphedema. General exercise guidelines include the following[8]:

- Start with low- to moderate-intensity exercise.
- Walking, swimming, cycling, and low-impact aerobics are recommended.
- Flexibility exercises should be performed to maintain range of movement.
- Appropriate warming-up and cooling-down phases should be implemented as part of exercise to avoid exacerbation of swelling.
- Compression garments should be worn by individuals with lymphedema during exercise.

Skin Care

Skin care is important for lymphedema risk reduction and management, which optimizes the condition of the skin and prevents infection.[8,10,32,43] Lymphedema can cause skin dryness and irritation, which is increased with long-term use of compression products. Bland, unscented products are recommended for daily cleansing and moisturizing.[8,10,32,43] Low-pH moisturizers, which discourage infection, are recommended for lymphedema because skin and tissue changes increase infection risk. Water-based moisturizers, which are absorbed more readily, are less likely to damage compression products but are not suitable for all patients. Cotton clothing allows ventilation and is absorbent.[10]

Advanced lymphedema can cause several skin complications, including lymphorrhea, lymphoceles, papillomas, and hyperkeratosis. *Lymphorrhea* is leakage of lymph fluid through the skin that occurs when skin cannot accommodate accumulated fluid. Nonadherent dressings, good skin care, and compression are used to alleviate leakage. Compression and good skin care also reduce the occurrence of lymphoceles, papillomas, and hyperkeratosis; these complications reflect skin adaptation to excess subcutaneous lymph.

Unusual Lymphedemas

Palliative care may require the management of unusual and challenging lymphedema sites, such as breast, head, neck, trunk, or

Box 19.3 Lymphedema Secondary to Cancer of the Head and Neck

Lymphedema secondary to head and neck cancer commonly presents following surgery and radiotherapy. Lymphedema is frequently found below the chin in the anterior neck. Difficulty in swallowing and breathing are the major symptoms causing distress from neck lymphedema. Mild swelling often progresses fairly rapidly to firm, nonpitting swelling and thus may often not be recognized or treated as lymphedema.

Quantification of neck edema can be achieved by measuring from the tip of one ear lobe to the tip of the contralateral ear lobe along the line of the chin, and then measuring this distance for every 2-cm (or 4-cm) interval down to the intersection of the neck and chest. Quantifiable outcome measurement over time fosters patient participation and improved long-term outcomes and might be beneficial as substantiation for third-party payers.

Compression supports can be useful after cosmetic facial surgery for neck lymphedema. These products provide gentle compression to the chin using two sets of long, narrow Velcro straps that extend from the chin to the top of the head and to the back of the neck. This size-adjustable "chin strap" provides gentle, size-adjustable compression to the chin and neck. Patients are encouraged to use the product continually for at least several weeks or a month to achieve optimal edema reduction. Although lifelong product use is encouraged for optimal lymph function, some patients have been able to transition to mainly nighttime product use and still maintain acceptable edema control.

Nursing interventions for head and neck lymphedema include:

- Help patients to make an informed decision in a supportive environment.
- Instruction and support in establishment of a lifelong daily self-care regimen including range-of-motion exercises, skin assessment, and application of moisturizers and early, skilled patient complication assistance and use of safe external compression. A written self-care program may foster patient self-care adherence.
- Monitor external neck compression. External neck compression must provide sufficient pressure to stimulate lymphatic function without causing skin irritation/injury or impairment of breathing, eating, or swallowing.
- Encourage the use of daily self-care using manual lymph drainage and exercises for facial, neck, and postural muscles to further improve edema control and posture.
- Document patient outcomes, including interval neck circumferences, skin integrity, pain level, and neck range of motion.

genitals.[54,56,60] MLD, skin-softening techniques, foam chip pads, and external compression (if possible) are recommended.[55,57,60] External compression may be achieved with collars, vests, custom pants or tights, scrotal supports, or spandex-type exercise apparel. The assistance of occupational or physical therapists and a seamstress may be helpful. Nationally, instructional courses are available to provide guidance for managing these difficult lymphedemas. Therapists can obtain professional certification for lymphedema treatment from the Lymphology Association of North America (http://www.clt-lana.org/). Box 19.3 presents detailed information about neck lymphedema from head and neck cancer.

Conclusion

Edema is a symptom usually relieved by addressing the causative factor. Lymphedema is a chronic disorder that requires lifelong management. Oncology nurses and other nurses have increasingly contributed to lymphedema management as they have improved cancer survivorship. Nursing's unique focus and scope of practice are ideally suited to chronic illness management, both at entry and advanced practice levels. To meet the physical and psychological needs of patients, nurses and other healthcare professionals must make efforts to understand the pathophysiology and chronic nature of lymphedema, as well as its physical, functional, and psychosocial impact. Equipped with such knowledge and competencies, nurses can then engage patients in supportive dialogue about risk reduction and lymphedema management. With the advent of precision health that aims at discovering the right treatment for the right patient at the right time, as well as determination of factors contributing to or protecting from common and complex diseases, researchers have started to explore the role of inherited genetic susceptibility and the pathogenesis of lymphedema.[61]

REFERENCES

1. Fu MR, Wang Y, Li C, et al. Machine learning for detection of lymphedema among breast cancer survivors. *mHealth*. 2018;4:17. https://doi.org/10.21037/mhealth.2018.04.02.
2. Carlson J. Lymphedema and subclinical lymphostasis (microlymphedema) facilitate cutaneous infection, inflammatory dermatoses, and neoplasia: a locus minoris resistentiae. *Clin Dermatol*. 2014;32(5):599–615.
3. Fu MR, Aouizerat BE, Yu G, et al. Model-based patterns of lymphedema symptomatology: phenotypic and biomarker characterization. *Curr Breast Cancer Rep*. 2021;13(1):1–18. https://doi.org/10.1007/s12609-020-00397-6.
4. Sano M, Hirakawa S, Sasaki T, et al. Role of subcutaneous adipose tissues in the pathophysiology of secondary lymphedema. *Lymphat Res Biol*. 2022;20(6):593–599. https://doi.org/10.1089/lrb.2021.0054.
5. Bonetti G, Paolacci S, Samaja M, et al. Low efficacy of genetic tests for the diagnosis of primary lymphedema prompts novel insights into the underlying molecular pathways. *Int J Mol Sci*. 2022;23(13):7414. https://doi.org/10.3390/ijms23137414.
6. Smoot B, Kober KM, Paul SM, et al. Potassium channel candidate genes predict the development of secondary lymphedema following breast cancer surgery. *Nurs Res*. 2017;66(2):85–94.
7. Sui Y, Lu Y, Lin M, et al. A family with Milroy disease caused by the *FLT4/VEGFR3* gene variant c.2774 T > A. *BMC Med Genomics*. 2021;14(1):151. https://doi.org/10.1186/s12920-021-00997-w.
8. Armer JM, Ostby PL, Ginex PK, et al. ONS Guidelines™ for cancer treatment-related lymphedema. *Oncol Nurs Forum*. 2020;47(5):518–538. https://doi.org/10.1188/20.ONF.518-538.
9. Fu MR, Axelrod D, Cleland CM, et al. Symptom report in detecting breast cancer-related lymphedema. *Breast Cancer (Dove Med Press)*. 2015;7:345–352. https://doi.org/10.2147/BCTT.S87854.
10. Fu MR, Liu B, Qiu JM, et al. The effects of daily-living risks on breast cancer-related lymphedema. *Ann Surg Oncol*. 2024;31(12):8076–8085. doi:10.1245/s10434-024-15946-x.
11. World Health Organization. Lymphatic Filariasis. March 16, 2022. Accessed February 18, 2023. http://www.who.int/mediacentre/factsheets/fs102/en/.
12. Koelmeyer LA, Gaitatzis K, Dietrich MS, et al. Risk factors for breast cancer–related lymphedema in patients undergoing 3 years of prospective surveillance with intervention. *Cancer*. 2022;128(18):3408–3415. https://doi.org/10.1002/cncr.34377.

13. Cormier J, Askew R, Mungovan K, Xing Y, Ross M, Armer J. Lymphedema beyond breast cancer. *Cancer*. 2010;116(22):5138–5149.
14. Fu MR, Axelrod D, Guth A, et al. The effects of obesity on lymphatic pain and swelling in breast cancer patients. *Biomedicines*. 2021;9(7):818. https://doi.org/10.3390/biomedicines9070818.
15. Fu MR, Axelrod D, Guth A, et al. Patterns of obesity and lymph fluid level during the first year of breast cancer treatment: a prospective study. *J Pers Med*. 2015;5(4):326–340.
16. Shallwani SM, Hodgson P, Towers A. Examining obesity in lymphedema: a retrospective study of 178 new patients with suspected lymphedema at a Canadian hospital-based clinic. *Physiother Can*. 2020;72(1):18–25. https://doi.org/10.3138/ptc-2018-0076.
17. Fu MR, Conley YP, Axelrod D, et al. Precision assessment of heterogeneity of lymphedema phenotype, genotypes and risk prediction. *Breast*. 2016;29:231–240.
18. Deng J, Radina E, Fu MR, et al. Self-care status, symptom burden, and reported infections in individuals with lower-extremity primary lymphedema. *J Nurs Scholarsh*. 2014;47(2):126–134.
19. Leung G, Baggott C, West C, et al. Cytokine candidate genes predict the development of secondary lymphedema following breast cancer surgery. *Lymphat Res Biol*. 2014;12(1):10–22.
20. Miaskowski C, Dodd M, Paul SM, et al. Lymphatic and angiogenic candidate genes predict the development of secondary lymphedema following breast cancer surgery. *PLoS One*. 2013;8(4):e60164.
21. Fu MR, Ridner SH, Hu SH, Stewart B, Cormier JN, Armer JM. Psychosocial impact of lymphedema: a systematic review of literature from 2004 to 2011. *Psychooncology*. 2012;22(7):1466–1484.
22. Shi S, Lu Q, Fu MR, et al. Psychometric properties of the breast cancer and lymphedema symptom experience index: the Chinese version. *Eur J Oncol Nurs*. 2016;20:10–16.
23. Radina ME, Fu MR, Horstman L, Kang Y. Breast cancer–related lymphedema and sexual experiences: a mixed-method comparison study. *Psychooncology*. 2015;24(12):1655–1662.
24. Fitzgerald Jones K, Fu MR, McTernan ML, et al. Lymphatic pain in breast cancer survivors. *Lymphat Res Biol*. 2022;20(5):525–532. https://doi.org/10.1089/lrb.2021.0017.
25. Park JH, Merriman J, Brody A, et al. Limb volume changes and activities of daily living: a prospective study. *Lymphat Res Biol*. 2021;19(3):261–268. https://doi.org/10.1089/lrb.2020.0077.
26. Fu MR, McTernan ML, Qiu JM, et al. Co-occurring fatigue and lymphatic pain incrementally aggravate their negative effects on activities of daily living, emotional distress, and overall health of breast cancer patients. *Integr Cancer Ther*. 2022;21:15347354221089605. https://doi.org/10.1177/15347354221089605.
27. Shih YC, Xu Y, Cormier JN, et al. Incidence, treatment costs, and complications of lymphedema after breast cancer among women of working age: a 2-year follow-up study. *J Clin Oncol*. 2009;27(12):2007–2014.
28. Miller JW, Smith JL, Ryerson AB, Tucker TC, Allemani C. Disparities in breast cancer survival in the United States (2001–2009): findings from the CONCORD-2 study. *Cancer*. 2017;123(suppl 24):5100–5118. https://doi.org/10.1002/cncr.30988.
29. Wielen LM, Gilchrist EC, Nowels MA, Petterson SM, Rust G, Miller BF. Not near enough: racial and ethnic disparities in access to nearby behavioral health care and primary care. *J Health Care Poor Underserved*. 2015;26(3):1032–1047. https://doi.org/10.1353/hpu.2015.0083.
30. Cobbe S, Real S, Slattery S. Assessment, treatment goals and interventions for oedema/lymphoedema in palliative care. *Int J Palliat Nurs*. 2017;23(3):111–119.
31. Raju S, Furrh JB 4th, Neglén P. Diagnosis and treatment of venous lymphedema. *J Vasc Surg*. 2012;55(1):141–149. https://doi.org/10.1016/j.jvs.2011.07.078.
32. Fu MR. Breast cancer–related lymphedema: symptoms, diagnosis, risk reduction, and management. *World J Clin Oncol*. 2014;5(3):241–247. https://doi.org/10.5306/wjco.v5.i3.241.
33. Földi M, Földi E, Clodius L, Neu H. Complications of lymphedema. In: Földi M, Földi E, Kubik S, eds. *Textbook of Lymphology for Physicians and Lymphedema Therapists*. Urgan & Fischer Verlag (Elsevier); 2003.
34. Davies C, Levenhagen K, Ryans K, Perdomo M, Gilchrist L. An executive summary of the clinical practice guideline: diagnosis of upper-quadrant lymphedema secondary to cancer. *Rehabil Oncol*. 2017;35(3):114–118.
35. Fu MR, Deng J, Armer JM, et al. Precision health and precision phenotype assessment of breast cancer–related lymphedema. *Advance Nurses*. 2016;29:231–240.
36. Jeffs E, Ream E, Shewbridge A, et al. Exploring patient perception of success and benefit in self-management of breast cancer–related arm lymphoedema. *Eur J Oncol Nurs*. 2016;20:173–183.
37. Fu MR, Axelrod D, Guth A, et al. Proactive approach to lymphedema risk reduction: a prospective study. *Ann Surg Oncol*. 2014;21(11):3481–3489.
38. Fu MR, Cleland CM, Guth AA, et al. L-Dex ratio in detecting breast cancer-related lymphedema: reliability, sensitivity, and specificity. *Lymphology*. 2013;46(2):85–96.
39. Armer JM, Stewart BR. A comparison of four diagnostic criteria for lymphedema in a post-breast cancer population. *Lymphat Res Biol*. 2005;3(4):208–217. https://doi.org/10.1089/lrb.2005.3.208.
40. Mastick J, Smoot BJ, Paul SM, et al. A comparison of supine versus stand-on bioimpedance devices to assess breast cancer-related lymphedema. *Lymphat Res Biol*. 2021;19(6):553–561. https://doi.org/10.1089/lrb.2020.0058.
41. Mastick J, Smoot BJ, Paul SM, et al. Assessment of arm volume using a tape measure versus a 3D optical scanner in survivors with breast cancer–related lymphedema. *Lymphat Res* Biol. 2022;20(1):39–47. https://doi.org/10.1089/lrb.2020.0119.
42. Deng J, Ridner SH, Wells N, Dietrich MS, Murphy BA. Development and preliminary testing of head and neck cancer related external lymphedema and fibrosis assessment criteria. *Eur J Oncol Nurs*. 2015;19(1):75–80.
43. Wanchai A, Armer J, Stewart B, Lasinski B. Breast cancer–related lymphedema: a literature review for clinical practice. *Int J Nurs Sci*. 2016;3(2):202–207.
44. Fu MR, Axelrod D, Guth AA, et al. Usability and feasibility of health IT interventions to enhance self-care for lymphedema symptom management in breast cancer survivors. *Internet Interv*. 2016;5:56–64.
45. Fu MR, Axelrod D, Guth AA, et al. mHealth self-care interventions: managing symptoms following breast cancer treatment. m*Health*. 2016;2:28.
46. Fu MR, McTernan ML, Qiu JM, et al. The effects of Kinect-enhanced lymphatic exercise intervention on lymphatic pain, swelling, and lymph fluid level. *Integr Cancer Ther*. 2021;20:15347354211026757. https://doi.org/10.1177/15347354211026757.
47. Fu MR, Axelrod D, Guth AA, et al. A web- and mobile-based intervention for women treated for breast cancer to manage chronic pain and symptoms related to lymphedema: results of a

randomized clinical trial. *JMIR Cancer*. 2022;8(1):e29485. https://doi.org/10.2196/29485.

48. Liu F, Li F, Fu MR, et al. Self-management strategies for risk reduction of subclinical and mild stage of breast cancer-related lymphedema: a longitudinal, quasi-experimental study. *Cancer Nurs*. 2021;44(6):E493–E502. https://doi.org/10.1097/NCC.0000000000000919.
49. Fu MR, Axelrod D, Guth AA, et al. Proactive approach to lymphedema risk reduction: a prospective study. *Ann Surg Oncol.* 2014;21(11):3481–3489. https://doi.org/10.1245/s10434-014-3761-z.
50. Du X, Li Y, Fu L, et al. Strategies in activating lymphatic system to promote lymph flow on lymphedema symptoms in breast cancer survivors: a randomized controlled trial. *Front Oncol.* 2022;12:1015387. https://doi.org/10.3389/fonc.2022.1015387.
51. Chiang AT, Chen Q, Wang Y, Fu MR. Kinect-based in-home exercise system for lymphatic health and lymphedema intervention. *IEEE J Transl Eng Health Med.* 2018;6:4100313. https://doi.org/10.1109/JTEHM.2018.2859992.
52. Chiang AT, Chen Q, Wang Y, Fu MR. Motion sequence alignment for a Kinect based in-home exercise system for lymphatic health and lymphedema intervention. *Annu Int Conf IEEE Eng Med Biol Soc.* 2018;2018:2072–2075. https://doi.org/10.1109/EMBC.2018.8512635.
53. Flores AM, Fu MR, Bock KJ, et al. Post-operative care for patients following surgical treatment of lymphedema. *Med Oncol.* 2024;41(11):296. Published 2024 Oct 23. doi:10.1007/s12032-024-02420-7
54. Müller M, Klingberg K, Wertli MM, Carreira H. Manual lymphatic drainage and quality of life in patients with lymphoedema and mixed oedema: a systematic review of randomised controlled trials. *Qual Life Res.* 2018;27(6):1403–1414. https://doi.org/10.1007/s11136-018-1796-5.
55. Lasinski BB, Thrift KM, Squire D, et al. A systematic review of the evidence for complete decongestive therapy in the treatment of lymphedema from 2004 to 2011. *PM R.* 2012;4(8):580–601.
56. Vignes S. Genital lymphedema after cancer treatment: a narrative review. *Cancers (Basel).* 2022;14(23):5809. https://doi.org/10.3390/cancers14235809.
57. Clinckaert A, Callens K, Cooreman A, et al. The prevalence of lower limb and genital lymphedema after prostate cancer treatment: a systematic review. *Cancers (Basel).* 2022;14(22):5667. https://doi.org/10.3390/cancers14225667.
58. Maldonado TS, Rokosh RS, Padberg F, et al. Assessment of quality of life changes in patients with lower extremity lymphedema using an advanced pneumatic compression device at home. *J Vasc Surg Venous Lymphat Disord.* 2021;9(3):745–752. https://doi.org/10.1016/j.jvsv.2020.10.013.
59. Armer JM, Hulett JM, Bernas M, Ostby P, Stewart BR, Cormier JM. Best practice guidelines in assessment, risk reduction management, and surveillance for post-breast cancer lymphedema. *Curr Breast Cancer Rep.* 2013;5(2):134–144.
60. Beck M, Wanchai A, Stewart BR, Cormier JN, Armer J. Palliative care for cancer-related lymphedema: a systematic review. *J Palliat Med.* 2012;15(7):821–827.
61. Fu MR, Kurnat-Thoma E, Starkweather A, et al. Precision health: a nursing perspective. *Int J Nurs Sci.* 2019;7(1):5–12. https://doi.org/10.1016/j.ijnss.2019.12.008. Published correction appears in *Int J Nurs Sci.* 2020;8(1):III.

20

Palliative Wound, Ostomy, and Continence Care

Charles P. Tilley, Kim Cavallito, Lindsay Alvarez, and Mei R. Fu

Key Points

- Palliative wound, ostomy, and continence (WOC) care emphasizes an interprofessional, patient-centered approach to alleviate suffering and promote well-being and quality of life (QOL) through evidence-based WOC care, palliation of symptoms, and preservation or restoration of functional performance.
- Specialist-level WOC nurses ideally possess both specialty certification in hospice and palliative care nursing and WOC nursing at either the baccalaureate or advanced practice level.
- Palliative wound care is a dynamic, interprofessional, patient- and family-centered process that combines the principles of evidence-based wound care with the science of advanced symptom management to preserve or restore functional performance and psychological well-being, thereby promoting QOL.
- Palliative care of the patient with a urinary or fecal diversion or fistula centers on specialist-level WOC nurse guidance to manage advanced symptoms, stoma/fistula pouching complexities, and peristomal/perifistular complications by adapting product selection and patient and caregiver education to the progressive functional decline experienced in serious illness, with a gradual shift of responsibilities to the caregiver.
- Urinary and fecal incontinence management in palliative care centers focuses on promoting continence through meticulous assessment and reduction of barriers to maintaining continence; choosing minimally invasive, highly individualized incontinence interventions adapted to the seriously ill patient's progressive functional decline; prevention of incontinence-associated dermatitis; and preservation of the patient's dignity.

Introduction

The exact prevalence of wound, ostomy, and continence (WOC) issues in hospice and palliative care is unknown. A classic study conducted in 1996 found that 60% of current and 80% of discharged patients in hospice had incontinence, a urinary catheter, an ileostomy, or a colostomy.[1] Another 2008 landmark study of 593 patients with advanced illness found that 53% of patients with cancer and 67% of patients without cancer developed wounds.[2] Pressure injuries (PIs) accounted for 66% of the 43 types of wounds identified, occurred predominately in patients without cancer, and commonly developed on the sacrum/coccyx.[2] Similarly, a 2017 study found that 47% of patients presented to hospice with wounds, up to half of those PIs.[3] Another more recent study in 2020 found a PI incidence of 17.3% in patients with cancer admitted to hospice.[4] Given that in 2019 51.6% of Medicare beneficiaries died while enrolled in hospice[5] and an anticipated population of 83.7 million over the age of 65 by 2050,[6] the projected number of patients with serious illness and WOC maladies is staggering.

The rapidly escalating need for palliative WOC care in those with serious illness is clear; however, this emerging area of palliative nursing remains poorly defined and underresearched. There is no globally accepted definition of palliative WOC nursing; however, it is generally accepted that the overarching goals of palliative WOC nursing are to alleviate suffering and promote quality of life (QOL).[7–9]

There is consensus that palliative WOC care includes (1) expert guidance[7,9]; (2) an interprofessional team approach[7,9]; (3) a center of care that includes both the patient and their caregivers[7–9]; (4) a focus on the prevention of complications, advanced symptom management, and preservation of functional performance and well-being[9]; and (5) person-centered care that prioritizes patients' advance directives and treatment preferences.[9,10]

This chapter will address approaches to WOC-specific assessment, prevention, symptom management, psychosocial support, maximization of functional performance, and product selection. The first section concentrates on the role of the WOC nurse in hospice and palliative settings. The second section covers palliative wound care, including the concepts of skin changes at end of life (SCALE), skin failure, and avoidable versus unavoidable PIs, Kennedy terminal ulcers (KTUs), and Trombley-Brennan terminal tissue injury (TB-TTI); strategies for the prevention, management, and symptom palliation of PIs; medical device–related PIs (MDRPIs), skin tears, and medical adhesive–related skin injuries (MARSIs); chronic critical limb ischemia with gangrene; malignant fungating wounds (MFWs); and less commonly encountered wounds (Marjolin's ulcers, COVID-19 skin manifestations, calciphylaxis, radiation dermatitis). The third part of the chapter will discuss the palliative management of continent and incontinent diversions and fistulas, and the last section will discuss the management of incontinence-associated dermatitis (IAD).

Case Study: WOC Care at the End of Life

This unfolding case study follows a 66-year-old woman with metastatic colorectal cancer, a colostomy, and malignancy-related pain from admission to home hospice through transfer to the inpatient hospice unit for end-of-life care. Upon admission to home hospice, the hospice nurse finds the woman cognitively intact, extremely fatigued, and cachectic, her colostomy nonfunctioning with a poorly fitting pouching system and painful, inflamed skin of the buttocks from constant contact with urine. The nurse also notes several large subcutaneous metastatic abdominal nodules. The patient is bedbound, requires total care, and has 8 home health aide hours daily. The patient's wish is to remain at home, so her sister has agreed to be her primary, live-in caregiver. Her sister has no experience in caregiving and fears she does not have the strength to perform skin care nor the knowledge to care for her sister's colostomy. The hospice nurse practitioner and the WOC nurse were consulted to devise a plan of care that would enable the pair to remain in the patient's apartment for as long as possible.

For the assessment, management and resolution of the patient's nonfunctioning colostomy, peristomal complications, pain, fatigue, and anorexia, see section three, Palliative Care of Continent Diversions, Incontinent Diversions, and Fistulas.

The Role of the Specialist-Level Palliative WOC Nurse

The specialist-level palliative WOC nurse provides expert WOC leadership in hospice and palliative care settings.[10] The evolving role of the specialist-level palliative WOC nurse ideally incorporates the scope and standards of both WOC and palliative nursing.[11,12] Specialist-level palliative WOC nurses may be baccalaureate, master's, or doctoral (PhD, DNP) prepared.[11] They may be registered nurses (RNs) or advance practice RNs (APRNs).[11] Box 20.1 outlines the responsibilities of the WOC nurse on a hospice team or palliative care service.[9–12] All hospice programs should employ or consult with a WOC nurse certified in both hospice and palliative care (CHPN®, ACHPN®) and WOC nursing (CWOCN®). Dual certification ensures specialist-level expertise in caring for those with serious illness and allows nursing professionals to practice palliative WOC care under the full scope of their licensure.[11,12]

Box 20.1 The Specialist-Level Palliative Wound, Ostomy, and Continence (WOC) Nurse Role

Educator

Provides patient and caregiver education

Develops patient and caregiver educational materials

Provides palliative WOC care competency-based staff development

Provides palliative WOC education at the local, national, and international levels

Acts as a WOC Nursing Society preceptor

Clinician

Provides specialist-level palliative WOC care consultation to co-workers

Provides specialist-level palliative WOC care consultation to referring agencies

Supports staff decision-making concerning palliative approaches to WOC care

Researcher

Initiates and supports evidence-based palliative WOC care, including quality improvement projects

Generates and supports original palliative WOC research based on National Institute for Nursing Research and Hospice and Palliative Nursing Association research foci

Mentors PhD or DNP students conducting WOC research or quality improvement projects

Administrator

Acts as chair of the interprofessional palliative wound, ostomy, and continence committee:

a. Leads WOC policy, procedure, and protocol development

Leads WOC supply management:

a. Cost analysis and containment
b. Formulary development
c. Product evaluation

Supports WOC quality improvement:

a. Patient satisfaction
b. Pressure injury prevalence and incidence

Source: Reference 9.

Palliative Wound Care

Palliative wound care is a holistic, integrated approach that emphasizes symptom management, enhancement of psychosocial well-being, integration of patient and family goals, and an interprofessional approach.[7] The concept of palliative wound care is still evolving, with the term first appearing in the literature in the 1980s. Since then, the palliative care and hospice movement has gained international attention, and each subsequent decade has seen a steady increase in both palliative wound care research and evidence-based literature.[7] There is no consensus, and there are few explicit definitions of palliative wound care.[7,9] Palliative wound care is a dynamic, interprofessional, patient- and family-centered process that combines the principles of evidence-based wound care with the science of advanced symptom management to preserve or restore functional performance and psychological well-being, thereby promoting QOL.

Wound-specific symptoms are considered advanced when conventional therapies and symptom management no longer work, exerting a negative impact on physical and psychosocial functioning and QOL.[8,9] Although management of wound-specific symptoms is a priority, it is erroneous to make the assumption that the goals of palliative wound care can never include wound healing.[13] The PALCARE© mnemonic (prognosis, advance care planning, living situation, comprehensive history, assessment, evidence-based recommendations, and education of patient, family, and staff) is a comprehensive framework for developing a holistic, interprofessional,

Box 20.2 A Systematic Approach to Palliative Wound Care: PALCARE©

Prognosis

Hospice diagnosis and Palliative Performance Score
Is the patient's life expectancy weeks or months?
Is the patient in the last hours or days of life?

Advance care planning

Goals of care

- Further hospitalizations (under what circumstances)
- Resuscitation wishes: full code status versus natural death
- Antibiotics: intravenous, oral, topical
- Medically administered nutrition or hydration
- Emergency management clarification (hemorrhage, sepsis)

Advance Directives

Complete MOLST, POLST, healthcare proxy, living will

Living Situation

Caregiver availability
Caregiver participation (willingness)
Caregiver ability (cognitive/physical)
Caregiver reliability
Environment/setting (domiciled vs. undomiciled, running water, shower facilities)
Fiduciary or food insecurity
Consider appropriate hospice level of care

- Inpatient hospice for uncontrolled symptoms
- Hospice home care (symptoms manageable in the community)
- Respite care (caregiver is overwhelmed or unavailable)

Comprehensive History

Non-wound-related symptoms, symptom management, functional performance including activities of daily living
Wound-specific symptoms (pain, odor, exudate, bleeding, pruritis, lymphedema, perceived bulk effect, and wound status), wound-specific symptom management, current and past wound care strategies including frequency of dressing changes
Psychiatric (Patient Health Questionnaire 2, Generalized Anxiety Disorder 7)[14,15]
Social (legal status, insurance, employment, fiduciary/housing/food insecurity)
Spiritual (FICA or HOPE tool)[16]

Assessment

Comprehensive physical assessment
Focused wound assessment
Wound photographs (follow institution policy)
Wound cultures, laboratory studies (as necessary)

Recommendations

Establish wound-specific symptom management and palliative wound care goals
Topical and/or systemic interventions
Referrals: wound, ostomy, and continence nurse (if not already involved), psychiatry, spiritual care, social work, and so forth

Education

Patient, family, caregivers
Staff education
Hospice medical directors, administrators, wound care resource nurses

MOLST, Medical Orders for Life-Sustaining Treatment; POLST, Physician's Orders for Life-Sustaining Treatment.

Source: Reference 9.

patient-centered palliative plan of care for patients with serious illness and complex wounds (see Box 20.2).[9]

Skin Changes at Life's End and Skin Failure

The concepts of SCALE, skin failure, TB-TTI, KTUs, and unavoidable PIs have received growing attention over the past decade as practitioners struggle to define and classify these underresearched phenomena, relying primarily on expert opinion and consensus.[17] SCALE is defined as physiological changes occurring as a result of the dying process that may affect the skin and soft tissues and may manifest as objective changes in skin color, turgor, or integrity or as subjective symptoms such as localized pain.[18] In 2009, an expert panel utilized a modified Delphi process to reach consensus on 10 statements describing the etiology, risk factors, signs and symptoms, and management of SCALE (see Table 20.1).[18]

The skin is the largest organ of the body and is vulnerable to organ dysfunction and failure.[18] Skin failure is a clinical syndrome: "the state in which tissue tolerance is so compromised that cells can no longer survive in zones of physiological impairment such as hypoxia, local mechanical stresses, impaired delivery of nutrients, and buildup of toxic metabolic byproducts."[17(p139)] Skin failure occurs across the illness continuum and may be classified as acute, chronic, or end-stage.[19] Acute skin failure is an event in which critically ill patients experiencing hemodynamic instability become hypoperfused, leading to skin and underlying tissue death.[19] A study of 549 patients in the intensive care unit identified five variables associated with acute skin failure: peripheral arterial disease, respiratory failure,

Table 20.1 SCALE consensus statements

Statement 1	Physiological changes that occur as a result of the dying process may affect the skin and soft tissues and may manifest as objective changes in skin color, turgor, or integrity or as subjective symptoms such as localized pain.
Statement 2	The plan of care and patient response should be clearly documented and reflected in the entire medical record.
Statement 3	Patient-centered concerns should be addressed including pain and activities of daily living.
Statement 4	SCALE area reflection of compromised skin (reduced soft-tissue perfusion, decreased tolerance to external insults, and impaired removal of metabolic wastes).
Statement 5	Expectations around the patient's end-of-life goals and concerns should be communicated among members of the interprofessional team and the patient's circle of care (potential for SCALE, skin breakdown, pressure injuries).
Statement 6	Risk factors, symptoms, and signs associated with SCALE have not been fully elucidated but may include weakness, progressive immobility, suboptimal nutrition, diminished tissue perfusion, impaired immune function, and loss of skin integrity.
Statement 7	A total skin assessment should be performed regularly and document all areas of concern consistent with the wishes and condition of the patient.
Statement 8	Consultation with a qualified healthcare professional is recommended for any skin changes associated with increased pain, signs of infection, skin breakdown, and whenever the patient's circle of care expresses a significant concern.
Statement 9	The probable skin change etiology and goals of care should be determined. The 5 Ps are recommended for determining strategies: prevention, prescription, preservation, palliation, and preference.
Statement 10	Patients and concerned individuals should be educated regarding SCALE and the plan of care.

mechanical ventilation, liver failure, and severe sepsis/septic shock.[20] Chronic skin failure results in skin and underlying tissue death due to hypoperfusion in patients with chronic disease states such as peripheral arterial disease, nephropathy, diabetes, and neurodegenerative disorders.[19] Hypoperfusion concurrent with end of life that leads to skin and underlying tissue death is termed "end-stage skin failure."[19]

KTUs, TB-TTIs, and Avoidable versus Unavoidable PIs

Rapidly developing sacral ulcers in patients with serious illness were first described in 1877 by French physician Jean-Martin Charcot, who termed the wound *decubitus ominosus*, as most patients died shortly thereafter.[21] More recently, terminal wounds over bony prominences (KTUs) and in tissues not prone to pressure (TB-TTIs) have been described parallel to the evolving attributes that define avoidable versus unavoidable PIs.[22,23]

In 1989, the term "Kennedy terminal ulcer" was coined to describe rapidly progressing, full-thickness PIs attributed to end-stage skin failure.[22,23] KTUs are ominous prognostic signs, developing anywhere from 24 hours to 8 weeks prior to death.[22–24] KTUs are associated with five characteristics: sudden onset; sacrococcygeal location; a butterfly or pear shape; purple, red, blue, or black color (often variegated); and irregular borders.[22,24]

TB-TTIs are spontaneously appearing, rapidly evolving, and progressing skin alterations over areas of little to no pressure, such as the thighs, attributed to end-stage skin failure.[25] A study of 166 adult patients in palliative care (mean age 79 years) found the median time from identification of a TB-TTI to death was 1.3 days.[25] The wounds presented over seven different locations on the trunk and upper and lower extremities, both anteriorly and posteriorly; were of varying morphology; and, strikingly, remained intact to time of death.[25] Cancer (18.3%), neurological diseases (16.5%), sepsis (15.2%), and respiratory diseases (14%) were the most common admitting diagnoses.[25] Ninety-one percent of patients had multiple comorbidities.[25] Both KTUs and TB-TTIs are considered unavoidable PIs and do not imply poor quality of end-of-life care.[22–25]

In 2017, the Wound, Ostomy, Continence Nurses Society (WOCN Society) published an updated position paper on avoidable versus unavoidable PIs.[23] The definitions were originally long-term care standards developed by the Centers for Medicare & Medicaid Services but have been broadened and applied to all clinical practice settings by the National Pressure Injury Advisory Panel (NPIAP; formerly known as the National Pressure Ulcer Advisory Panel [NPUAP]).[26] The current definitions are as follows:

Avoidable PI: An avoidable PI can develop when the provider did not do one or more of the following: evaluate the individual's clinical condition and PI risk factors; define and implement interventions consistent with individual needs, individual goals, and recognized standards of practice; monitor and evaluate the impact of the interventions; or revise the interventions as appropriate.

Unavoidable PI: An unavoidable PI can develop even though the provider evaluated the individual's clinical condition and PI risk factors; defined and implemented interventions consistent with individual needs, goals, and recognized standards of practice; monitored and evaluated the impact of the interventions; or revised the approaches as appropriate.

A retrospective study of 20 patients who developed hospital-acquired PIs despite appropriate risk assessment and prevention, identified 10 prevalent physiologic comorbidities: hypoalbuminemia, severe anemia, respiratory failure with intubation, hypoxia with sedation or chemical paralysis, hypotension, infection or sepsis, malignancy, diabetes, renal failure, and/or congestive heart failure.[27] These conditions are included in hospice eligibility criteria and are common comorbidities encountered in those with serious illness. Experts have additionally identified malnourishment, advanced age, dehydration, and obesity as factors contributing to unavoidable PIs,[28] as well as hospitalization in a critical care unit,[27,29,30] corticosteroid use,[31] and treatment with vasopressors.[29]

The NPIAP updated its unavoidable PI position paper in 2020 in light of the COVID-19 pandemic.[32] The NPIAP identified COVID-related hypercoagulation and microvascular occlusion as possible intrinsic factors leading to purpuric lesions that progress rapidly to necrosis, especially over tissues exposed to pressure and shear, including under medical devices.[32] The effects of COVID-19-related microvascular occlusion on tissue may increase nonmodifiable risk to a level impossible to overcome with standard PI prevention.[32]

Wound-Specific Symptoms in Complex and Nonhealing Wounds

A combination of traditional pharmacologic therapies, basic and advanced dressings, debridement, complementary medicine, and cognitive behavioral therapy is used in palliative wound care to manage wound-specific symptoms of pain, pruritus, odor, exudate, bleeding, lymphedema, and perceived bulk effect and wound status.[9,33,34]

Pain: The skin has the most sensory nerve endings of any organ in the body and has special nociceptors that can perceive somatic, neuropathic, or mixed pain caused by mechanical, thermal, or chemical injury.[34–36] Wound-specific pain occurs in up to 84% of patients with PIs, reported both at rest (chronic) and with dressing changes (cyclic).[35] The prevalence of MFW-specific pain is 30.2%–77.3%.[34,37,38] Wound-specific pain in patients with breast MFWs points to a mixed neuropathic and somatic etiology that may be associated with wound location, morphology, size, tissue type, and proximity to other anatomical structures.[38] Several studies of lower extremity wound characteristics identified pain to be the most bothersome wound-specific symptom reported.[39] Box 20.3 lists pathologic and iatrogenic causes of temporary (cyclic—with dressing changes, incident—with isolated procedures such as debridement) and persistent wound pain (chronic—between dressing changes, at night, and at rest).[36]

Non-wound-related and wound-specific pain assessments are guided by the *total pain* concept, which includes physical, psychological, spiritual, and social factors.[41] Use of valid and reliable

Box 20.3 Etiology of Wound Pain

Pathologic

- Direct tumor compression of an organ
- Dermal erosion and exposure of nerve endings
- Damage of nerves related to direct tumor invasion or compression
- Edema secondary to impaired lymphatic drainage or wound infection
- Inflammation secondary to wound infection or periwound moisture-associated skin damage

Iatrogenic

- Manipulation of dressings
- Inappropriate dressing selection
- Adhesive removal
- Wound cleansing or irrigation
- Debridement

Sources: References 35, 36, and 40.

pain assessment tools is recommended, as is exploration of temporary and persistent wound-specific pain etiologies. The total pain approach (see Box 20.4) includes both non-wound-related and wound-specific pain management, interprofessional involvement to address psychosocial or spiritual factors, and specialist-level palliative WOC nurse referral.[9,42]

Pruritus: The etiology of wound-specific pruritus may be either pruritoceptive (cutaneous) or neuropathic (afferent neuronal pathways) and may occur in the wound bed itself, the periwound skin, or both.[9,34,42,43] Wound-specific pruritus has been reported in venous ulcers, burns, MFWs, PIs, and postsurgical wounds.[43] Wound bed pruritus may be part of the normal healing process[44] or due to inflammation, dryness, nerve regeneration,[45] exudate, [34,45] compression garments,[46] or dressings.[34] Periwound pruritus and pain may be caused by periwound moisture-associated skin damage (MASD),[9,34] defined as inflammation and erosion of skin caused by prolonged exposure to wound effluent.[47] The principles of wound-specific pruritus management are similar to those of pain; the nurse must first identify the underlying etiology, if possible. Once identified, a multipronged management approach is recommended, combining systemic and topical antipruritic agents with periwound skin protection. Table 20.2 displays periwound skin protection options.

Odor and exudate: Infection may retard wound healing and contribute to odor, exudate formation, and pain.[34,42] Devitalized tissue enhances bioburden proliferation, contributes to malodor and excessive exudate, and is an impediment to wound healing.[48,49] Whenever possible, infections should be eliminated and necrotic tissue should be removed, two of the four key components of wound bed preparation[48–50] (see Box 20.5).

The degree of aggressiveness in managing infection and the removal of devitalized tissue is guided by the patient's prognosis, advance directives, and preferences. Wound infections at end of life may be treated empirically, by either oral or parenteral routes, with or without concurrent topical antimicrobials, and rarely require cultures. Clinical diagnosis of infection in chronic wounds is more important than qualitative cultures.[40] Surface cultures are controversial, and deep tissue cultures are rarely appropriate in palliative wound care.[9,40] The choice of wound debridement method depends on many factors, as shown in Box 20.6.

Table 20.3 summarizes the common debridement methodologies used in palliative wound care, the advantages and disadvantages of each, and contraindications. Mechanical debridement (wet-to-dry) is nonselective, painful, and labor-intensive and is not recommended in palliative patients.

Odor has been described as one of the most distressing wound-specific symptoms.[34] The source of the malodor may be related to moist

Box 20.4 Total Pain Management

AssessmentAssessment

Physiologic and iatrogenic factors

- Non-wound-related pain (cancer or other underlying disease)
- Wound-specific pain
- Wound care–related pain
  - Frequent dressing manipulation and changes
  - Adherence of dressings to the wound bed during dressing removal
  - Vigorous irrigation or rubbing of fragile tissue with cleansing
  - Medical adhesive-related skin injury
  - Failure to protect periwound skin (periwound moisture-associated skin damage)
  - Failure to address infection or adequately premedicate prior to dressing changes

Psychological and social factors

- Anxiety, depression, grief, and prebereavement issues
- Body image disturbances
- Housing, food, fiduciary insecurities
- Lack of caregiver support

Spiritual factors

- Existential angst

Interventions and Referrals

Physiologic (non-wound-related and wound-specific pain management)

- Adequate systemic pain management with nonpharmacologic interventions, non-opioids, adjuvants, short-acting opioids, long-acting opioids
- Adequate wound-specific pain management with topical opioids (10 mg morphine in 8 g hydrogel),[42] topical anesthetics (2% lidocaine jelly, lidocaine patches periwound)[42]

Physiologic (wound care–related) pain management

- Decrease frequency of dressing changes[9,42]
- Soak dressings before removal with normal saline or tepid tap water
- Cleanse by gentle irrigation, patting, or blotting of wound bed
- Use moisture-retentive, nonadherent foam, petrolatum-based or silicone dressings[9]
- Avoid adhesives; use burn net, mesh undergarments, or postsurgical bras to secure dressings and normalize body image[9] (see **Figure 20.1**)
- If adhesives are necessary, use skin protectants prior to application[9,42]
- Protect periwound skin[9,42] (see **Table 20.2**)
- Use antimicrobial dressings and/or systemic antibiotics to treat infection

Psychosocial pain management

- Referral to social work, psychology, or grief counselor

Spiritual pain management

- Referral to spiritual care

Sources: References 9 and 42.

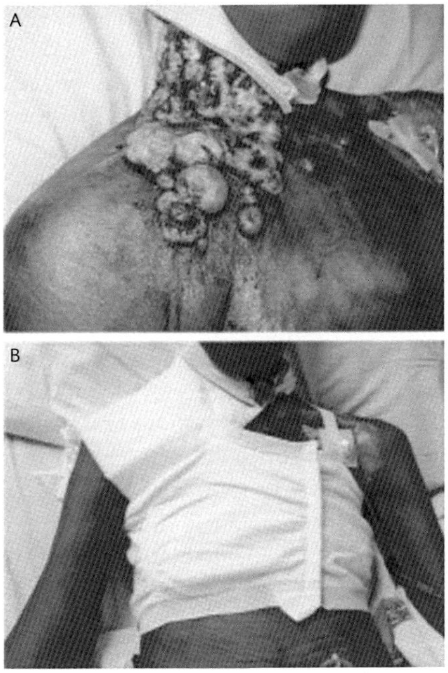

Figure 20.1 Fungating wound of head and neck extending to right chest wall before (A) and after (B) dressing change secured with surgical bra.

Table 20.2 Periwound skin protection

Skin protectant	Description	Consideration	Examples
Liquid polymer acrylates	Liquid polymers that contain solvents that, when they evaporate, form a protective film	Periwound moisture-associated skin damage (MASD) prevention Peristomal/perifistula MASD prevention Preparation of skin attachment sites for drainage tubes, external catheters, surrounding stoma sites, and adhesive dressings	Cavilon™ (3M) No-sting Skin Prep (Smith & Nephew) McKesson Skin Barrier Film (McKesson)
Dimethicone	Silicone-based oil	Modest MASD protection Promotes skin hydration Variable periwound MASD protection	Remedy Olivamine, Dimethicone Moisture Barrier (Medline)
Zinc oxide–based skin protectant	White powder mixed with a cream or ointment base	Periwound MASD protection Incontinence barrier Calazime contains menthol, which cools irritated skin Zinc offers poor skin hydration and does not avoid maceration Messy, difficult to remove Interferes with dressing adhesion and absorption	Remedy Phytoplex Z-Guard Skin Protectant Paste (Medline) Remedy Olivamine Calazime Skin Protectant Paste (Medline) Critic-Aid® Thick Moisture Barrier Paste (Coloplast)
Petrolatum-based skin protectant	Blend of castor seed oil and hydrogenated castor oil	Periwound MASD protection Incontinence barrier Modest skin hydration Messy, difficult to remove Interferes with dressing adhesion and absorption	ConvaTec Sensi-Care Protective Barrier (ConvaTec) Remedy Phytoplex Z-Guard Skin Protectant Paste (Medline)
Combination skin protectants	Blend of dimethicone, petrolatum, or zinc oxide	Zinc oxide with 5% dimethicone Zinc oxide, dimethicone, petrolatum	Sooth & Cool® INZO® (Medline) Triad® Wound Dressing (Coloplast)

Source: Reference 9.

necrotic tissue, bioburden, infection, unchanged or saturated dressings, or old dressings that have not been properly disposed of. Multiple studies have documented the detrimental role wound-specific malodor has on body image, relationships, sexuality, and femininity.[34,51,52] This results in shame, embarrassment, anxiety, and lack of self-confidence, leading to social isolation and diminished QOL.[34,51,52]

The prevalence of malodor in MFWs is 10.4%.[34,37] "Garbage," "rotting flesh," "putrid," and "moldy" are descriptors elicited from patients, family members, and other caregivers, including nurses.[34,37,51] One subject likened the smell to a "cadaver."[34,51,52] Malodor is pervasive; caregivers recall altering their breathing patterns to avoid the smell and having vivid memories decades later.[34]

Prevalence of exudate in MFWs is 14.6%[34,37] and one of the most challenging wound-specific symptoms to manage.[34,52] Exudate may impact psychosocial function and contribute to the development of periwound MASD.[34,52] Patients have described being humiliated and exhausted by heavily exudating wounds, with frequent dressing changes and cleaning of soiled clothing becoming all-consuming.[34,51] Public soiling of their clothing has also forced the women into self-imposed isolation, "safe from scrutiny and negative comments that damaged their identity."[52–54] Management of odor and exudate may require specialist-level palliative WOC nurse consultation. Table 20.4 displays odor- and exudate-absorbent dressings, topical antimicrobial agents, and topical antiseptics used to decrease bioburden and control odor and exudate.[9,40]

Bleeding: Wound-specific bleeding may range from superficial, isolated rupture of microvasculature in the wound bed to erosion of large vessels and hemorrhage. Patients have described bleeding due to direct tumor invasion or friable wound beds as "unpredictable."[51,52] One recalled spontaneous bleeding during a work meeting, the blood camouflaged by her jacket, necessitating an impromptu clothing change.[51] Uncontrolled bleeding has also forced women, in denial or experiencing shame, to seek the medical care they had been avoiding.[51,52] Table 20.5 outlines interventions for controlling bleeding.

Box 20.5 Key Components to Wound Bed Preparation: TIME

Tissue that is nonviable must be debrided.
Infection (or inflammation) must be reduced and managed.
Moisture imbalance or exudate control must be addressed to avoid desiccation or maceration.
Epidermal margins of the wound must be examined for nonadherence.

Source: Reference 50.

Box 20.6 Factors Influencing Choice of Wound Debridement Method

Amount of debris
Available time for debridement
Cost of debridement process
Nature of care setting
Patient allergies
Patient's pain level
Patient's prognosis and treatment plan
Patient's wishes and opinions
Potential patient problems
Maceration of wound
Tissue trauma
Bleeding (hemorrhage)
Presence of infection
Size of wound
Skill of the clinician
Type of debris
Type of exudate
Wound depth and undermining and tunneling

Source: Reference 48.

Table 20.3 Common debridement methodologies in palliative care

Method/definition	Advantages	Disadvantages	Contraindications
Chemical (nonselective) Hypochlorites (e.g., Dakin's solution) Povidone iodine Cadexomer iodine (e.g., Iodosorb, Iodoflex)	Helps debride necrotic tissues slowly Lowers microbial count Cheap and readily available Broad-spectrum antimicrobial May help dry slough for easier debridement Slow release Safe for cellular viability Absorbs exudate Helps with autolytic debridement	Deleterious to healing tissue Possibly irritating to periwound skin and wound edges Stains tissue Deleterious to fibroblasts Safe for fibroblasts Use with caution in patients with thyroid disease	Clean, noninfected wound Clean, noninfected wound Iodine allergy Clean, noninfected wound
Enzymatic (selective) Enzymes that work by degrading and debriding necrotic tissue by digesting and dissolving it Collagenase (Santyl™)	Good for patients who decline sharp debridement or surgery or are on anticoagulants or home care Will not harm normal tissue Can be used in infected wounds, sometimes used with topical antibiotics Cost-effective if used properly	Not effective for advanced cellulitic wounds Require prescriber's order Expensive Cannot be used with other common wound products such as metal ions (e.g., silver) or with topical antiseptics (e.g., Dakin's) Cross-hatching of eschar recommended	Clean, granulating wound Allergies
Autolytic (selective) Use of body's own wound fluid enzymes to liquefy necrotic tissue; fully or semi-occlusive moisture-retentive topical therapy. Hydrogels, alginates, foams, hydrofibers, films	Hydrogels, alginates, foams, and hydrofibers will absorb some wound fluid Maintain moist wound therapy Easy to perform in any care setting Comfortable and soothing Good choice if not a candidate for sharp debridement	Works slowly compared to other methods Requires constant monitoring for infection Hydrocolloid dressing fluid odor often mistaken for "infected" Absorptive dressings can dry out wound bed if not discontinued when appropriate	Dry wound beds are not appropriate for absorptive dressings
Conservative sharp debridement (selective) Use of instruments to remove devitalized tissue from wound bed	Fast and effective Can be performed at the bedside Preferred if debridement is urgent (sepsis) May be performed by specially educated nurses, therapists, and physicians	Analgesia required pre-procedure Require discernment of viable versus nonviable tissue Potential for bacteremia Requires special training and/or licensure	Bleeding disorders Severe immune compromise Ischemic extremity

Source: Reference 48.

Table 20.4 Odor- and exudate-absorbent dressings, topical antimicrobials, and topical antiseptics

Dressings, topical antimicrobials, and topical antiseptics	Examples	Beneficial effects and considerations	Cost
Foams (exudate-absorbent dressings)	Allevyn (Smith & Nephew) Aquacel Foam (Convatec) Tegaderm Foam (3M) Mepilex (Monlynlycke Health Care)	Promotes moist wound environment and does not adhere to tissue Prevents strikethrough Multiple shapes and sizes available to fit difficult dressing sites (i.e., heels) and conforms to the body	5 × 5 box = $$ 5 × 5 box = $$ 6 × 6 box = $$ 6 × 6 box = $$
Calcium alginates (exudate-absorbent dressings)	Algicell (Derma Sciences) Algisite M (Smith & Nephew) Tegaderm High Gelling (3M)	May be used to cover or fill wound bed Dressing material becomes a gel and absorbs any drainage while promoting a moist wound bed May act as a hemostatic agent.	4 × 4 box = $ 4 × 4 box = $ 4 × 4 box = $
Charcoals (odor-absorbent dressings)	CarboFlex (Convatec)	Absorbs small gas molecules and bacterial spores Used as a secondary dressing.	4 × 4 box = $$
Honey (topical antimicrobial)	Activon Tulle (Avancis) Medihoney (Medihoney)	Supersaturated sugar solution with high osmolarity, low water activity Bactericidal, moistens wound and removes necrotic tissue Lowers wound pH to promote healing	4 × 4 box = $ 4 × 4 box = $
Silver (topical antimicrobial)	Aquacel Ag hydrofiber (Convatec) Acticoat 3 (Smith & Nephew) Optifoam Ag (Medline)	Gradual release of silver provides sustained broad-spectrum bactericidal effects	12 box = $$$ 4 × 4 box = $$$ 4 × 4 box = $$
Metronidazole (topical antimicrobial)	1% Flagyl spray 5% Flagyl powder Crushed tablets 0.71% Flagyl gel	Bactericidal, effective against anaerobes	100 mL = $ 57 g = $ 14 tablets = $ 0.71% gel (1 tube, 45 g) = $$
Dakin's solution (sodium hypochlorite; topical antiseptic)	0.25% concentration	Broad-spectrum bactericidal effects and promotes dissolution of necrotic tissue May require twice-daily dressing changes	1 16-oz bottle = $

Prices: $, <$100; $$, >$100; $$$, >$200.

Sources: Reference 9. Data from References 9 and 13, and prices from Wound Care Shop: http://www.woundcareshop.com/. Accessed December 22, 2022.

Table 20.5 Interventions for wound-specific bleeding

Category of bleeding	Interventions	Considerations
Prevention	Dressing selection and wound cleansing	1. Nonadherent dressings are recommended as a contact layer (silicone, foam, or petrolatum-based gauze) 2. Gentle cleansing or irrigation, no rubbing 3. Wet dressings before removal to loosen and prevent adherence to the wound bed
Minor bleeding (controllable at the bedside)	Direct pressure Silver nitrate Epinephrine soaks Calcium alginate	1. Apply local pressure with clean gauze 2. Cauterize with silver nitrate (see **Figure 20.2**) 3. Soak gauze with 1 mg of epinephrine and 1 mL of normal saline (1:1 ratio) applied for 10 minutes of direct pressure to promote local vasoconstriction[9] 4. Pack wound with calcium alginate, acts as a hemostatic agent; may embed itself in the wound and be difficult to extract
Major bleeding (requiring invasive or aggressive interventions)	Vascular intervention Radiation	1. Apply direct pressure until emergency management at a tertiary care hospital is available
Hemorrhage as a terminal event	Comfort measures	1. Dark towels should be readily available and used to contain and absorb blood loss 2. Sedate with a parenteral benzodiazepine and manage pain with a parenteral opioid 3. Cover with blankets (blood loss may lead to hypothermia and cause chills or rigors)

Source: Reprinted with permission from Reference 9.

Goals-of-care discussions surrounding bleeding are integral for the patient with serious illness and a complex, nonhealing wound because interventions may range from the benign (i.e., direct pressure, vitamin K replacement, modification of topical antimicrobial therapy) to aggressive and/or invasive (i.e., vascular interventions for hemorrhage, blood products, radiation).[9] The discontinuation of anticoagulation for patients with atrial fibrillation, deep vein thrombosis, pulmonary embolism, or embolic stroke requires a discussion of risks versus benefits.

Lymphedema: Lymphedema is known to have a negative psychological and social impact on patients.[55] Patients with lymphedema secondary to MFWs of the breast reported a sense of compromised normalcy. Restricted mobility limited wardrobe choices, as did the desire to "hide" the arm swelling due to embarrassment, ultimately restricting access to social support and contributing to isolation.[31,33,54] Chapter 19 provides in-depth information on lymphedema.

Perceived bulk effect. Perceived bulk effect is the patient-reported perception of how noticeable the wound dressing is and the degree to which it alters their appearance and causes distress.[34] This can impact clothing choices, restrict mobility, and result in additional symptoms such as discomfort or pruritus.[34,51,52] Conscious utilization of surgical bras (see Figure 20.1), burn net, and gender-specific absorptive undergarments to secure dressings may help reduce perceived bulk effect.[9]

Perceived wound status: Perceived wound status is the patient-reported perception of the meaning of the wound's appearance and the degree to which it causes distress.[34] Perceived wound status may be associated with disease progression and shortened life span, provoking anxiety and fear.[34,52,54] Studies found that MFWs were constant reminders of advanced and incurable disease, robbing patients of hope as the wound grew in size or new lesions or symptoms appeared.[34,54] Visibility of the tumor provoked fear and conveyed a threat to their body and existence. These patients must be screened for depression and anxiety and referred to social work and/or psychiatry as indicated.[9,14,15]

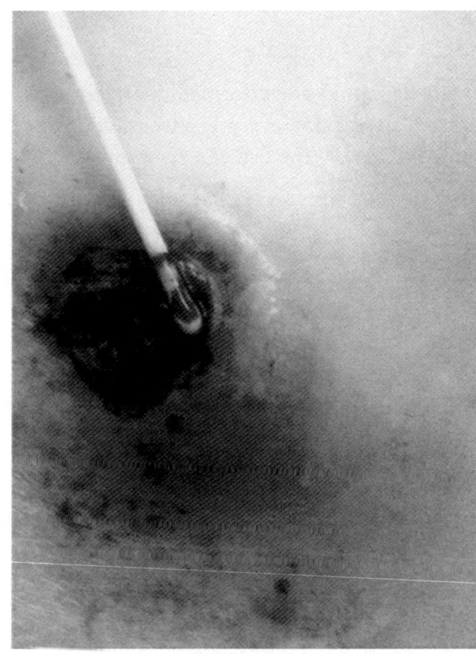

Figure 20.2 Cauterization of bleeding abdominal malignant lesion with silver nitrate sticks at the bedside. The stick is first wet with regular tap water (not normal saline) to activate, then rolled back and forth over the bleeding tissue (results in a pearly gray appearance). Cauterization may be repeated with each dressing change as needed, is relatively inexpensive, and is easy to learn. Assess for stinging or burning and, if uncomfortable, consider alternatives.

Source: Reference 9.

Periwound MASD

MASD is characterized by inflammation of the skin with or without erosion or denudation and a serous exudate.[47,56] MASD causes irritant dermatitis from contact with urine or fecal matter, perspiration, wound exudate, mucus, digestive secretions, respiratory sections, or saliva.[47] Periwound MASD is one of the four subcategories of MASD[47,56] and is a key consideration in palliative wound care.[9]

Heavily exudating wounds may cause an overhydration of the skin and maceration and contain active metabolites leading to further skin breakdown, infections, pain, or pruritus.[47,56,57] Maceration of the skin is described as irritation and damage of the skin adjacent (within a 4-cm periwound border) to a wound caused by supersaturation.[56] Maceration may present as pale, white, or gray wrinkled skin or inflammation; erythema; and swelling, usually associated with pain or pruritus.[56] A study of women with fungating breast wounds found exudate with higher levels of putrescine and the presence of cadaverine to be associated with a higher incidence of periwound MASD and pruritus.[57,58]

Treatment and prevention of periwound MASD start with the selection of an appropriate absorbent dressing (see Table 20.4) and cleansing of the wound bed.[40] Periwound skin protection is the crucial next step in preventing periwound MASD, with several products available (see Table 20.2). Multiple factors should be considered when selecting a skin barrier, including wound location, allergies, and caregiver support.[59–61] A liquid polymer acrylate for upper body, head, and facial wounds is appropriate because there is less mess and no interference with adhesion of dressings.[9] Consider a zinc oxide- or petrolatum-based skin barrier for genital or groin wounds, especially in the presence of fecal or urinary incontinence.[9] A meta-analysis of nonmalignant wounds found film barriers to be superior to placebo in four studies and comparable to zinc oxide– and petrolatum-based products.[59]

Wound Assessment Principles

Wound assessment should be performed upon admission to a hospice or palliative care service, every 1–2 weeks thereafter, and with any change in condition.[40] The use of a systematic approach with a comprehensive assessment tool is recommended (see Box 20.7).[40] Monitoring of the wound (inspection) by less-skilled caregivers (licensed practical nurses, therapists, caregivers, family members, patients) with dressing changes is helpful.[40] The caregiver can report changes or disconcerting findings to the RN or APRN, who then conducts a full assessment (inspection, palpation, interpretation of patterns and trends in the data).[40]

Box 20.7 Systematic Wound Assessment

1. Etiology/type of skin damage
2. Location
3. Stage (pressure injuries [PIs] only)
4. Dimensions: (length [head-to-toe], width [hip-to-hip], depth [use a q-tip], height)
5. Undermining/tunneling (stage III or IV PIs only): Measure undermining by the clock method, noting the deepest part of the undermining; measure depth of sinus tract/tunnel, and give direction by the clock method
6. Wound base description
   Granulation: Pink or beefy red, shiny, moist, granular
   Necrotic tissue: Gray to black and moist
   Eschar: Gray to black and dry/leathery
   Slough: Yellow to white and may be stringy (loose) or appear as a layer over the wound base (adherent)
   Epithelial: New or pink shiny tissue
   If mixed, may approximate tissue type in percentages or use a wound camera with this capability
7. Exudate
   Amount: Scant, moderate, or copious
   Color/consistency: Serous, serosanguineous, purulent, etc.
8. Malodor: Present or not
9. Periwound skin/wound edges
10. Wound-specific pain: (location [wound bed or periwound], severity [rating], duration [constant, intermittent], quality, aggravating or alleviating factors)
    Chronic: Occurs between dressing changes
    Cyclic: Occurs with wound dressing changes
    Incident: Occurs with isolated wound procedures (debriding, wound biopsy, etc.)
11. Infection: Present or not (describe signs or symptoms)

Source: Reference 9.

Pressure Injuries and Medical Device-Related Pressure Injuries

The NPUAP changed the term "pressure ulcer" to "pressure injury" in 2016 to lessen confusion over staging PIs with intact skin versus open ulcers.[62] A PI is localized damage to the skin and/or underlying soft tissue, usually over a bony prominence or related to a medical or other device.[62] PIs in palliative care settings are often unavoidable; interventions to eradicate them in the seriously ill are complicated by the population's frailty, extensive risk factors, and comorbid conditions.[23,25–27,32]

"Medical device–related pressure injury" (MDRPI) describes an etiology of PI due to an external medical device at the location of the PI that mirrors the shape of the device.[63] An MDRPI should be staged using the NPIAP PI staging system (see Table 20.6) unless it involves the mucosal membranes.[63,64] Mucosal injuries should be identified as mucosal membrane device–related PIs.[64] MDRPIs are caused by prolonged pressure from diagnostic devices (temperature-sensing Foley catheters), therapeutic devices (nasogastric tubes, rectal tubes), or nonmedical devices (bed clutter, furniture, equipment).[63,64]

Risk Factors, Risk Assessment, and Risk Reduction

A variety of factors exist in those with advanced and terminal illness that put them at risk for PI development and nonhealing. Risk factors include advanced age, protein-calorie malnutrition, immobility and inactivity, shear, friction, moisture, incontinence, and altered sensory perception.[66–68] Screening tools ascertain patients at risk for PI development through identification of specific risk factors, which then allows for targeted risk reduction interventions. The NPIAP has recommended assessing the risk for new PI development on admission, at regular intervals thereafter, and with any change in condition using a validated risk assessment tool.[66–68] Multiple PI risk assessment tools have been developed. The Norton Scale[69] and the Braden Scale[70] are two of the most widely used tools, despite minimal data on their validation in hospice populations. The Hunters Hill Marie Curie Center Risk Assessment Tool[71] and the Hospice Pressure Ulcer Risk Assessment Scale[72] were specifically developed for and validated in hospice populations. A comparison of the four scales is shown in Table 20.7.

Treatment

Palliative wound care is an emerging field of research. Currently, there are no evidence-based protocols for treating PIs in the terminally ill and dying.[67,68] Seven principles for the palliative management of wounds in the terminally ill have been proposed: preventing wound development and/or deterioration, correcting or treating the underlying cause of the wound, controlling wound-related symptoms, using patient self-assessment, providing psychosocial support, promoting independence, and improving QOL.[67,68]

Palliative wound care combines the wound-specific symptom management previously discussed in this chapter with evidence-based

Table 20.6 National Pressure Injury Advisory Panel pressure injury staging system

Stage	Definition and clinical description	Illustration
Stage 1 Pressure Injury: Nonblanchable erythema of intact skin	Intact skin with a localized area of nonblanchable erythema, which may appear differently in darkly pigmented skin. Changes in sensation, temperature, or firmness may precede the presence of blanchable erythema. Color changes do not include purple or maroon discoloration; these may indicate deep tissue pressure injury.	Stage 1 pressure injury - lightly pigmented 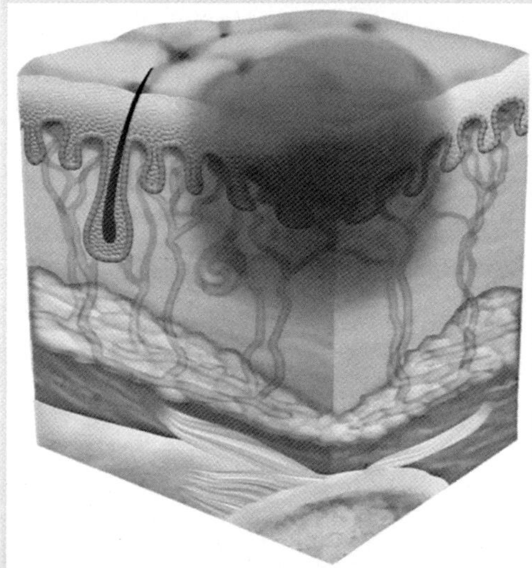
Stage 2 Pressure Injury: Partial-thickness skin loss with exposed dermis	Partial-thickness skin loss with exposed dermis. The wound bed is viable, pink or red, and moist and may also present as an intact or serum-filled blister. Adipose and deeper tissues are not visible, and granulation tissue, eschar, and slough are not present. These injuries commonly result from adverse microclimate and shear in the skin over the pelvis and shear in the heel. This stage should not be used to describe moisture-associated skin damage including incontinence associated dermatitis, intertriginous dermatitis, medical adhesive-related skin injury, or traumatic wounds (skin tears, burns, abrasions).	Stage 2 pressure injury 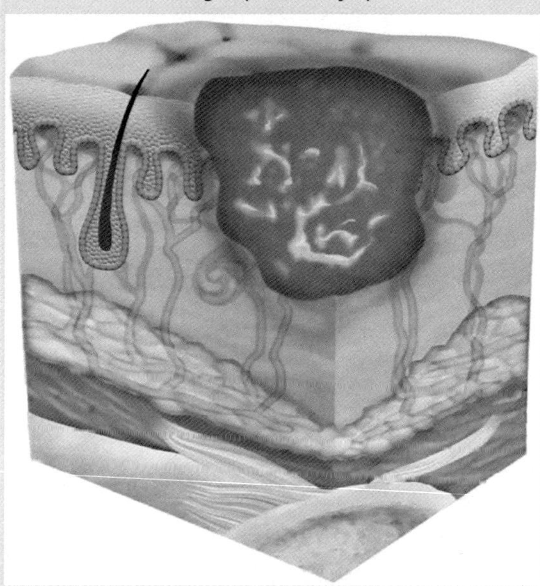
Stage 3 Pressure Injury: Full-thickness skin loss	Full-thickness loss of skin, in which adipose is visible in the ulcer and granulation tissue, and epibole (rolled wound edges) are often present. The depth of tissue damage varies by anatomical location; areas of significant adiposity can develop deep wounds. Slough and/or eschar may be visible, and undermining,[a] tunneling,[b] or sinus tracts[c] may occur. Fascia, muscle, tendon, ligament, cartilage, and/or bone are not exposed.	Stage 3 pressure injury with epibole 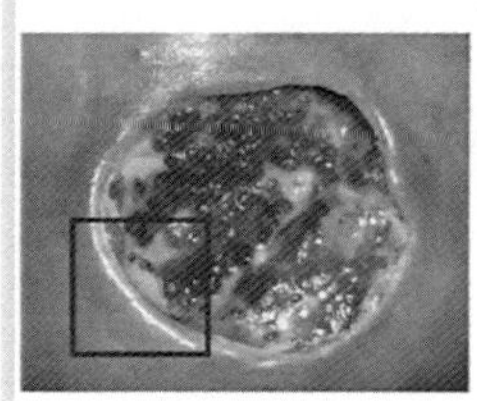 Area of focus 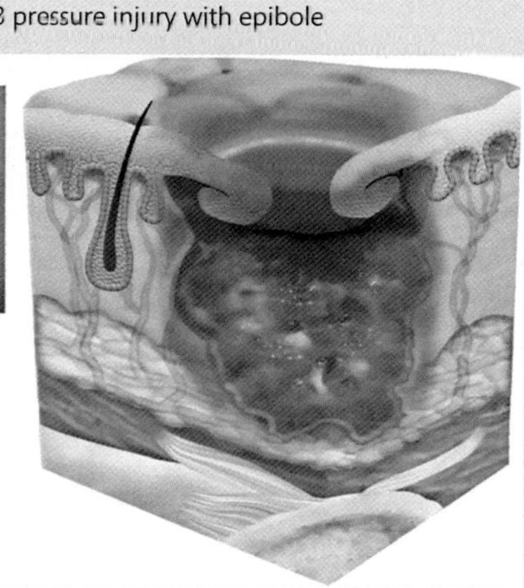

(continued)

Table 20.6 Continued

Stage	Definition and clinical description	Illustration
Stage 4 Pressure Injury: Full-thickness skin and tissue loss	Full-thickness skin and tissue loss with exposed or directly palpable fascia, muscle, tendon, ligament, cartilage, or bone in the ulcer. The depth of tissue damage varies by anatomical location. Slough and/or eschar may be visible, and epibole, undermining,a tunneling,b or sinus tractsc may occur.	Stage 4 pressure injury 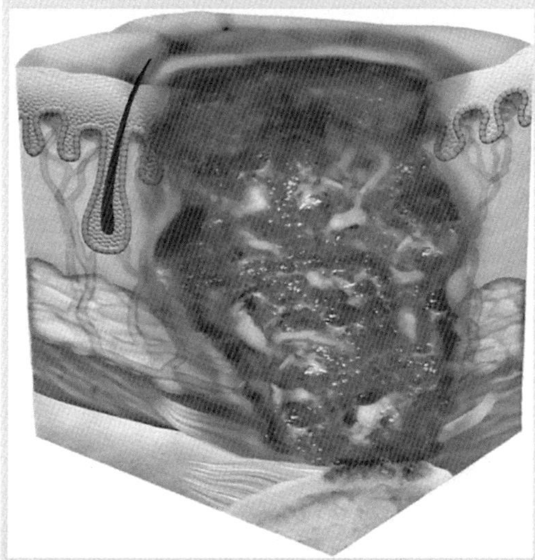
Unstageable Pressure Injury: Obscured full-thickness skin and tissue loss	Full-thickness skin and tissue loss in which the extent of tissue damage within the ulcer cannot be confirmed because it is obscured by slough or eschar. If slough or eschar is removed, a stage 3 or stage 4 pressure injury will be revealed.	Unstageable pressure injury - slough and eschar 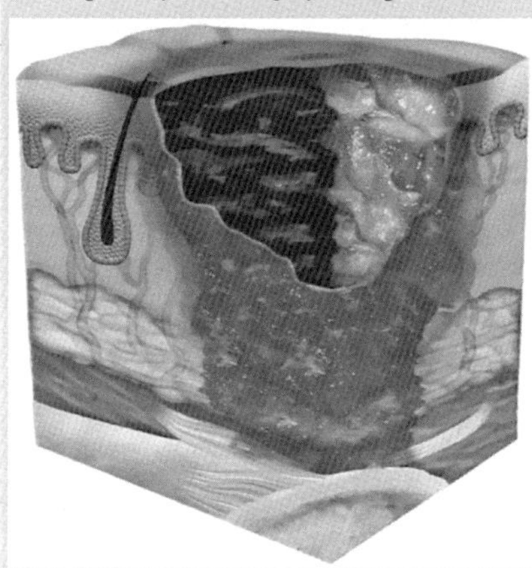
Deep Tissue Pressure Injury: Persistent nonblanchable deep red, maroon, or purple discoloration	Intact or non-intact skin with localized area of persistent nonblanchable deep red, maroon, purple discoloration or epidermal separation revealing a dark wound bed or blood-filled blister. Pain and temperature change often precede skin color changes. Discoloration may appear differently in darkly pigmented skin. This injury results from intense and/or prolonged pressure and shear forces at the bone–muscle interface. The wound may evolve rapidly to reveal the actual extent of tissue injury or may resolve without tissue loss.	Deep tissue pressure injury 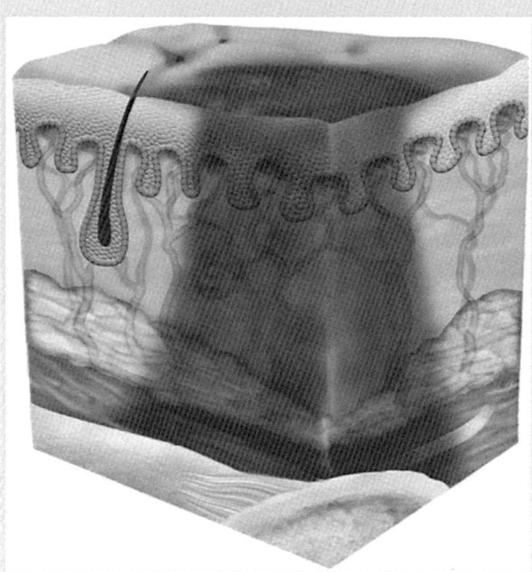

[a] Undermining: Deep tissue (subcutaneous fat and muscle) damage around the wound margin.
[b] Tunneling: Tunnel under the skin surface that does not involve deep tissue.
[c] Sinus tracts: A narrow tract that moves away from the wound margins and downward into the wound.
Sources: References 62 and 65.

Table 20.7 Pressure injury risk assessment tools

Pressure injury risk assessment tool	Year developed	Subscales	Validation in hospice and palliative populations
Norton Scale	1958	Physical condition, mental state, activity, mobility, incontinence	Minimal information on the validation in hospice patients[69]
Braden Scale	1983	Sensory perception, moisture, activity, nutrition, friction/shear, mobility	Minimal information on the validation in hospice patients[70] Braden scores are highly correlated with Karnofsky and Palliative Performance Scale scores
Hunters Hill Marie Curie Center Risk Assessment Tool	2000	Sensation, mobility, moisture, activity in bed, nutrition/weight change, skin condition, friction/shear	Developed specifically for palliative care and validated in hospice patients[71]
Hospice Pressure Ulcer Risk Assessment Scale	2003	Physical activity, mobility, age	Developed specifically for palliative care and validated in hospice patients[72]

Risk reduction interventions include pressure redistribution, skin and incontinence care, and maximizing nutrition and hydration.[66–68] Avoid foam rings, foam cut-outs, or donut-type devices because they concentrate pressure on the surrounding tissue.[66] Table 20.8 summarizes select recommendations from the *WOCN 2016 Guideline for Prevention and Management of Pressure Injuries (Ulcers)* for preventing pressure injuries[66] and palliative care-specific considerations or adaptations. The patient at end of life may not tolerate all recommendations due to symptoms of pain, dyspnea, delirium, or terminal secretions or may make the conscious choice not to participate based on their goals of care and advance directives. The patient's and family's wishes and preferences at end of life must be respected and documented in the patient's medical record and plan of care.

Table 20.8 Risk factors and pressure injury risk reduction strategies in palliative care

Risk factor	Risk reduction intervention	Palliative considerations
Pressure and immobility	1. Minimize/eliminate pressure from medical devices 2. Schedule regular repositioning and turning for bed-bound and chair-bound patients 3. Use heel suspension devices and protective dressings in at-risk patients 4. Utilize support surfaces on beds and chairs to redistribute pressure 5. Place patients at high risk on pressure redistribution surfaces 6. Educate patients and caregivers about the causes and risk factors for developing pressure injuries and ways to minimize the risks	1. Equipment such as bilevel positive airway pressure masks and oxygen tubing may need protective hydrocolloid over the bridge of the nose or padding over the ears 2. Assess and premedicate for pain 20–30 minutes prior to care, patients with uncontrolled symptoms may not tolerate repositioning 3. Introduce the possibility of unavoidable pressure ulcers due to skin failure, assure the family it is not from poor care
Friction/shear	1. Maintain the head-of-bed elevation at/or below 30 degrees 2. Use a 30-degree side-lying position	1. Patient with increased intracranial pressure, ascites, end-stage pulmonary or cardiac disease, or orthopnea may not tolerate 2. May facilitate drainage of secretions
Incontinence	Use incontinence skin barriers to protect and maintain intact skin	Consider Foley placement for those with dyspnea or pain who cannot tolerate frequent skin care
Nutrition	Offer individuals with nutritional and pressure ulcer risks a minimum of 30–35 kcal/kg body weight per day, 1.25–1.5 g of protein/kg body weight per day, and 1 mL of fluid intake per kilocalorie per day	The patient with advanced disease or who is at end of life may not realistically tolerate these nutritional recommendations; dysphagia, odynophagia, anorexia-cachexia syndromes, advanced symptoms, or voluntarily stopping eating and drinking will warrant an individualized plan of care

Source: Adapted from Reference 66.

interventions. Again, the patient's and family's wishes and preferences drive the plan of care. Table 20.9 summarizes select evidence-based treatment recommendations from the *WOCN 2016 Guideline for Prevention and Management of Pressure Injuries (Ulcers)* for the treatment of PIs[66] and palliative care–specific considerations or adaptions. Comfort is of the utmost importance and may supersede wound prevention or care for those who are actively dying or have a condition causing them to have a single position of comfort.[67,68]

Skin Tears and MARSI

Skin tears are wounds caused by shear, friction, and/or blunt force trauma resulting in separation of skin layers.[73,74] A skin tear can be partial-thickness (separation of the epidermis from the dermis) or full-thickness (separation of both the epidermis and dermis from underlying structures).[74] Prevalence of skin tears in palliative populations is 14.3%.[74] Skin tears may increase patient morbidity and mortality[75,76] and are associated with increased pain and decreased QOL.[74,75] There are three classification systems for skin tears: the original 1993 Payne-Martin classification system, the 2007 Skin Tear Audit Research classification system, and, most recently, the 2013 International Skin Tear Advisory Panel (ISTAP) Skin Tear classification system.[73] The ISTAP classifies skin tears as follows: type I, no skin/flap loss; type II, partial skin/flap loss; or type III, total skin/flap loss.[73] The ISTAP Skin Tear classification system has undergone reliability and validity testing in 44 countries and may be used for systematic assessment in clinical practice.[73] Skin tears are a subset of MARSI but have varied etiologies.[74,75]

MARSI is skin damage related to the use of medical adhesive products or devices such as tapes, wound dressings, stoma products, electrodes, medication patches, and wound closure strips.[61] Types of MARSI by etiology include (mechanical) epidermal stripping, tension injury or blister, skin tear, (dermatitis) irritant contact

Table 20.9 Palliative considerations in the treatment of pressure injuries (PIs)

Treatment	Palliative considerations
1. Float the heels completely off the surface with a pillow for stage I or II PIs or a heel suspension device for stage III or IV PIs.	1. Assess patients for uncontrolled symptoms, especially pain, prior to heel suspension; and premedicate 20–30 minutes prior if needed. Patients at end of life may not tolerate heel suspension; follow individual preferences.
2. Turn and reposition the patient regularly and frequently.	2. Assess patients for uncontrolled symptoms, especially pain and dyspnea, prior to turning; and premedicate 20–30 minutes prior if needed. Patients at end of life may not tolerate frequent repositioning, so develop a flexible schedule and follow individual preferences, including their "position of comfort."
3. Utilize support surfaces for patients with pressure injuries that meet the individual's needs and are compatible with the care setting (both seating and lying redistribution).	3. Consider changing the support surface to improve pressure redistribution and comfort.
4. Utilize an individualized bowel/bladder management program for the patient with incontinence.	4. Foley catheters may be preferred to manage urinary incontinence in patients who cannot tolerate toileting due to advanced symptoms (pain, dyspnea).
5. Cleanse the wound and periwound at each dressing change with potable tap water, distilled water, wound cleanser, or normal saline.	5. Use care to remove devitalized tissue to control wound odor.
6. Consider a 2-week course of topical antibiotics for nonhealing, clean PIs.	6. Review the patient's advance directives to discern their willingness to trial antibiotics.
7. Consider the use of topical antiseptics for "maintenance wounds," which are defined as wounds not expected to heal and wounds that are critically colonized.	7. Dakin's solution may sting in the wound and can be irritating to the respiratory system.
8. Use systematic antibiotics in the presence of bacteremia, sepsis, advancing cellulitis, or osteomyelitis.	8. Review the patient's advance directives to discern their willingness to trial antibiotics.
9. Debride the PI of devitalized tissue.	9. Review the patient's advance directives and goals of care. Avoid sharp debridement with fragile tissue that bleeds easily.
10. Implement appropriate treatment of PIs to optimize healing, recognizing that complete healing may be unrealistic in some patients.	10. Use dressings that can remain in place for longer periods of time to promote comfort.
11. Offer individuals with nutritional and pressure ulcer risks a minimum of 30–35 kcal/kg body weight per day, 1.25–1.5 g of protein/kg body weight per day, and 1 mL of fluid intake per kilocalorie per day	11. Allow the patient to ingest fluids and foods of choice. Offer several small meals per day. Adequate nutrition is often not attainable when the patient is unable or declines to eat.

Sources: Adapted from References 66 and 68.

dermatitis, allergic dermatitis, (moisture) maceration, and (inflammatory) folliculitis.[61] MARSI prevalence in hospice and palliative care populations is largely unknown.

Risk Factors and Prevention

Patients with serious illness, including those at the end of life, are most at risk for skin tears and MARSI. Factors that increase the risk for both types of injury are similar. Intrinsic factors include extremes of age, race/ethnicity, dermatologic conditions (eczema, dermatitis), underlying medical conditions (e.g., diabetes, infection, immunosuppression), malnutrition, and dehydration.[74,75] Extrinsic factors include repeated taping, tape/dressing/device removal, photodamage, radiation therapy, maceration, certain medications (long-term corticosteroids, anticoagulants), and drying of the skin due to harsh skin cleansers or excessive bathing.[74,75] Falls, previous skin tears, the presence of edema, and handling during care are additional risk factors

Table 20.10 Preventing skin tears and medical adhesive-related skin injuries (MARSI)

Skin tears	MARSI
1. Assess for risk upon admission and whenever the individual's condition changes 2. Implement a systematic prevention protocol 3. Have individuals at risk wear long sleeves, long pants/trousers, or knee-high socks 4. Provide shin guards to those individuals who experience repeated skin tears to shins 5. Ensure safe patient handling techniques and equipment/environment 6. Involve individuals and families in preventive strategies 7. Educate registered and nonregistered staff and caregivers to ensure proper techniques for providing care without causing skin tears 8. Consult dietitian to ensure adequate nutrition and hydration 9. Keep skin well lubricated by applying hypoallergenic moisturizer at least twice daily 10. Protect individuals at high risk from trauma during routine care and from self-injury	1. Application of adhesive-containing products • Ensure the area is clean and dry • Clip excessive hair • Apply a skin barrier (dry thoroughly) • Apply the adhesive product without tension, pulling, or stretching • Smooth the adhesive product into place • Use gentle, stretchable adhesive products if edema/movement anticipated • If compression needed, stretch the adhesive over the dressing only and press remaining tape onto skin without tension 2. Removal of adhesive-containing products • Loosen edges of the adhesive product • With the fingers of the opposite hand, push the skin down and away from the adhesive • Remove the adhesive product low and slow in the direction of hair growth • Use the stretch and relax technique to remove transparent films • Slowly remove tape strips by each side, toward the wound • Use medical adhesive remover

Sources: Adapted from References 61, 76, and 77.

that contribute to skin tears.[74,75] Not all skin tears are preventable in high-risk patients (multiple comorbidities, multiorgan failure, dementia with aggression), and incurring this type of wound does not necessarily imply poor quality of care.[75,76] Table 20.10 shows interventions to prevent skin tears and MARSI. Additionally, the ISTAP maintains that it is essential to incorporate fall prevention as part of skin tear prevention programs.[76]

Treatment

The best management for both skin tears and MARSI is prevention. When these wounds do occur, it is generally recommended that the practitioner follow evidence-based wound care principles and consult a wound specialist if the wound does not heal within 7 days or deteriorates.[77,78] A dressing should be chosen that (1) maintains constant moisture, (2) suits the local wound environment, (3) protects the periwound skin, (4) controls or manages exudate, (5) controls or manages infection, and (6) optimizes caregiver time.[77,78] Adhesive strips, hydrocolloids, and traditional films are not recommended for either injury.[76–78] Best practices in skin tear management include (1) cleansing with a nontoxic solution, such as normal saline; (2) approximate the skin flap (if possible); (3) control bleeding and remove clots; (4) apply a skin protectant periwound; and (5) apply a hydrogel, foam, soft silicone, or nonadherent dressing.[77,78] These best practices may be considered in the care of MARSI as well. Never secure dressings covering either type of wound with adhesive products; instead utilize burn net, stocking-like products, or cotton gauze wraps.

Chronic Critical Limb Ischemia with Gangrene

Chronic critical limb ischemia is a condition related to arterial occlusive disease that manifests as rest pain, ulceration, or gangrene.[79] Gangrene is the localized death and decomposition of body tissue, resulting from either obstructed circulation or bacterial infection.[80] The three main types of gangrene are wet gangrene, dry gangrene, and gas gangrene.[80] Wound healing is usually not a realistic goal when invasive vascular interventions are not feasible.[79] Palliative wound care goals often include delaying an inevitable amputation.[79,80] Dry gangrene develops slowly, distal to arterial occlusion, with a line of demarcation between viable and gangrenous tissue, and is associated with ischemic pain during early development.[80] As the limb or digit mummifies, the gangrenous appendage becomes painless.[80] Dry gangrene is usually odorless and may be painted with povidone iodine every 48 hours and wrapped with a dry gauze dressing, with caution not to moisten the necrotic tissue to prevent conversion to wet gangrene. A retrospective study of 11 patients showed cadexomer iodine was also an effective palliative dressing that exerted an antimicrobial effect that prevented wet gangrene.[81]

Wet gangrene signals bacterial infection, which can spread quickly to other tissues, causing edema, erythema, pain, and fevers.[80] The tissue becomes discolored, boggy, blistered, and malodorous with exudate. Gas gangrene is characterized by edema, crepitus, and gas on radiographs.[80] *Clostridium perfringens* is a gas-forming organism with an affinity for necrotic tissue that may cause the crepitus in the affected limb.[79,80] Antibiotic treatment should be tailored to the causative organism if consistent with goals of care. Half- or quarter-strength Dakin's solution (sodium hypochlorite) once or twice daily has been used successfully to manage odor and exudate due to its broad-spectrum bactericidal properties.[82] Dakin's solution has been shown to be effective against *C. perfringens*, aerobes, anaerobes, biofilms, and multidrug-resistant organisms.[82] Anecdotally, Dakin's solution also has desiccant properties, drying the wound bed and thereby decreasing exudate.

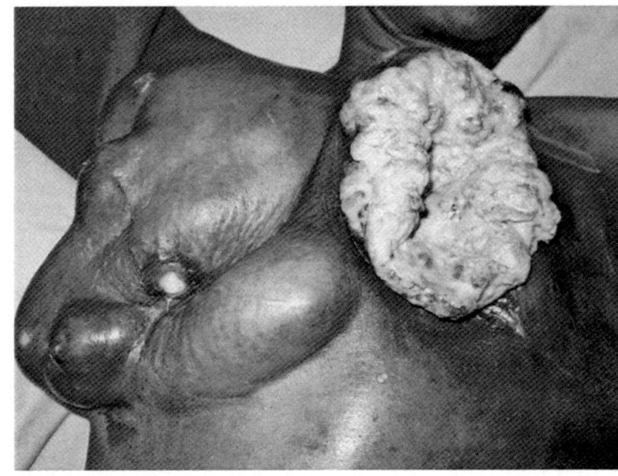

Figure 20.3 Malignant fungating wound of the breast from metastatic breast cancer.

MFWs

MFWs are nonhealing wounds resulting from aggressive proliferation of malignant cells and infiltration of the skin, blood, and lymph vessels by tumors in patients with advanced cancer.[34,83,84] Unchecked local tumor extension inflicts widespread tissue damage and causes disfigurement, loss of vascularity with subsequent tissue hypoxia and necrosis, polymicrobial proliferation, and fungating ulceration of the wound bed (see Figures 20.3 and 20.4).[34,57,83]

MFWs originate from one of three etiologies: primary skin neoplasms, local extension and integumentary erosion from primary tumors or malignancy recurrence, and metastatic cutaneous lesions.[83,85] Characteristically, these wounds have a tendency to expand rapidly; to occur along pathways of least resistance such as surgical incisions, tissue planes, and blood or lymph vessels, and to cause lymphedema secondary to local lymphatic vessel invasion.[85]

MFWs afflict 5%–14.5% of people with advanced cancer, disproportionately affecting women and older adults.[34] MFWs may arise

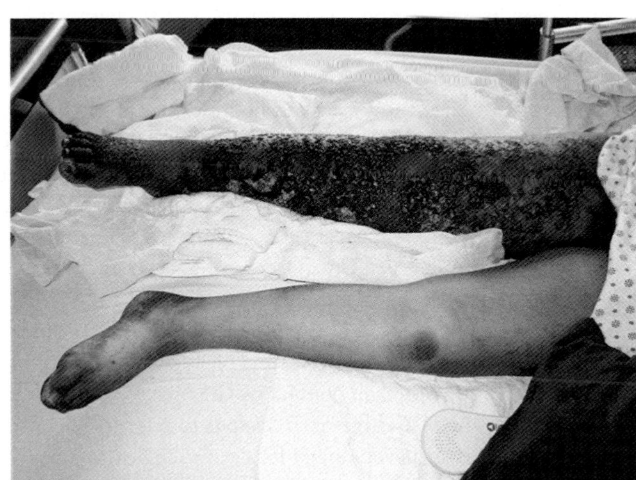

Figure 20.4 Malignant fungating wound of entire right leg with lymphedema from metastatic colon cancer.

from any type of underlying malignancy, but MFWs of the breast are most prevalent (63%), followed by head and neck (24%), then groin, genitals, and back (3%), with all other sites accounting for the remaining 8%.[34,83]

MFWs are visible markers of underlying neoplastic disease and indicate a grave prognosis.[34,83,84] Upon discovery of the cutaneous lesion, average life expectancy ranges from 6 to 12 months.[85] Studies report grimmer survival rates for certain primaries from first appearance of cutaneous metastasis: 6 weeks for genitourinary cancers[86] and 3 months for lung, cervical, or esophageal cancers.[87] Additionally, one study reported a 30% reduction in average survival in patients with multiple sites of metastasis as compared to single-site cutaneous involvement.[88] As life-prolonging treatments continue to evolve and life expectancy increases, it is reasonable to expect the percentage of people with MFWs to rise.

Assessment

Initially, MFWs present as inflammation, peau d'orange skin, smooth raised nodules varying in size and pigmentation, erythematous plaques or patches, areas of alopecia, or violaceous papules.[83,85,86] They rapidly progress to cauliflower-shaped lesions (proliferative) or an ulcerated area (erosive), sometimes forming fistulas or a sinus tract.[88,89] Fungating and ulcerating lesions may be differentiated by morphology, the former protruding and grotesque, the latter cavity-forming, with both prone to bleeding, infection, and malodorous exudate.[90] A survey of nurses reported a variety of MFW morphologies: ulcer (56%), fungating shape (31%), a crust (25%), nodular shape (24%), crater shape (23%), and other (6%).[91] Initial and ongoing skin and wound assessments are essential in monitoring the deterioration of MFWs and for the development of new or worsening wound-specific symptoms.

Psychosocial and Spiritual Aspects of Care

MFWs have a negative impact on psychosocial, physical, and functional health,[34,89] resulting in compromised QOL.[34] Lawton, during her 10-month observational study of hospice patients enduring horrific physical and psychological suffering, introduced the concept of being "unbounded."[54] The state of becoming unbounded was caused by odors, exudate, pain, bleeding, and disfigurement as a result of "the disintegrating, decaying body," with the dying experiencing marginalization, isolation, and loss of self and social identity.[54] Her study notably included patients with MFWs of the head and neck, groin and genitalia, and breast. Studies on femininity demonstrated body image disturbances and a loss of confidence among women with MFWs. Body image has a great impact on psychological well-being because it is associated with one's identity. Surgical bras and mesh undergarments may be used to secure dressings, minimize bulk effect, and normalize appearance.

The hospice team must use timely screening, assessment, interventions, and referrals in addressing the psychosocial and spiritual issues experienced by patients with MFWs. The authors recommend depression, anxiety, and spiritual screening on admission, every 2–4 weeks thereafter, and with each contact by the hospice nurse practitioner or hospice medical director. Decisions to refer to a licensed clinical social worker or psychologist for counseling or to a psychiatrist for evaluation and pharmacologic recommendations should be shared with the patient and family. Those expressing spiritual distress should be referred to spiritual care for intervention.

Wound Care Considerations in MFWs

Topical antimicrobial therapy and absorbent dressings, combined with cleansing and odor-eliminating interventions, have been the mainstay of MFW odor and exudate treatment. However, only one study, identified in a Cochrane Review, provided weak evidence suggesting that silver foam dressings may reduce malodor, indicating an urgent need for further research.[92,93] The effect of topical antimicrobial dressings on microbial resistance, biofilms, and the characterization of microbiomes in MFWs is also largely unknown. Table 20.4 lists topical interventions that may be used to control odor and exudate. Carrying an extra set of clothing in the event of exudate leakage is also suggested.

The cause of bleeding in patients with advanced cancer and MFW is usually multifactorial and may be attributed to the cancer itself, cancer treatment, or the MFW. Goals-of-care discussions surrounding bleeding are an integral part of advance care planning for the patient with MFW because interventions may range from benign to aggressive to comfort (see Table 20.5).[9]

Given the high symptom burden experienced and the incurable nature of their wounds, this population will require aggressive palliative care until death. Developing a pragmatic, patient- and family-centered palliative wound care plan is essential to alleviate suffering. The case study of a woman with stage IV vulvar cancer and a vaginal MFW demonstrates the use of the PALCARE© mnemonic (see Box 20.2) as a framework for developing a holistic, patient-centered, palliative plan of care (see Figure 20.5).

Marjolin's Ulcers, Calciphylaxis, Radiation Dermatitis, and COVID-19 Skin Manifestations

Marjolin's ulcers, calciphylaxis, and radiation dermatitis are wounds less commonly encountered in palliative settings. COVID-19 skin manifestations are a new phenomenon seen in patients with serious illness, including those at the end of life. Each malady has the propensity to cause wound-specific symptoms and intense suffering, presenting unique challenges for the palliative care service or hospice team.

Marjolin's Ulcers

Like MFWs, Marjolin's ulcers have cancerous wound beds; however, their etiology is quite different. Marjolin's ulcers are rare, malignant degenerations that most commonly arise from areas of chronic inflammation or injury, developing over years or even decades (see Box 20.8).[94–96] One recent review found that the average time for malignant transformation is 29 years.[97] The ulcers were first described by French surgeon Jean Nicholas Marjolin in 1784, after observing villous changes arising in a burn scar.[96] Classically, these ulcers transform from their original etiology to a squamous cell carcinoma (SCC), but basal cell carcinomas and malignant melanoma have also been reported.[95] Marjolin's ulcers may arise in nearly any location on the body, but they are most commonly found in the lower extremities.[96] They are associated with a poor prognosis.[97]

Marjolin's ulcers are diagnosed by performing a thorough history and physical (including a detailed wound assessment) and attaining a tissue biopsy.[98] The magnitude of the wound, the clinical presentation, and the patient's goals of care will guide more extensive oncologic workups. These ulcers may not present as a classic SCC but as a characteristic triad of nodule formation, induration,

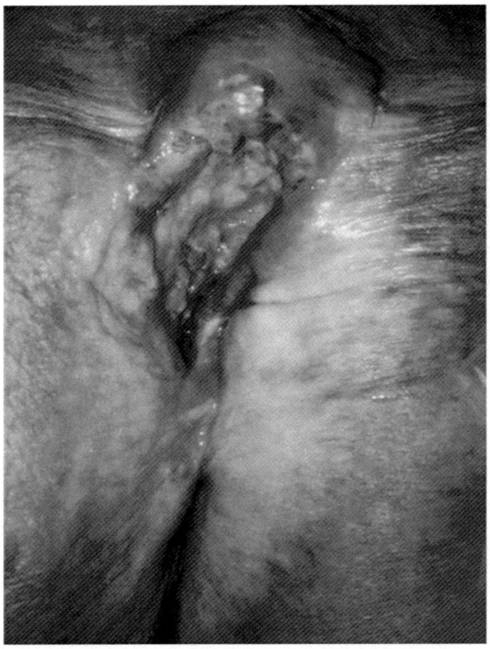

Figure 20.5 Malignant fungating wound (MFW) of the vagina form metastatic vulvar cancer. A synopsis of her hospice care using the PALCARE© framework:

Prognosis: 45-year-old female with metastatic vulvar cancer status post-vulvectomy, radiation, and chemotherapy. She has a life expectancy of 2–4 weeks and a Palliative Performance Score of 30%.

Advance care planning: She has a do-not-resuscitate/do-not-intubate order, declines hospitalization or heroic measures, and will accept oral and/or topical antibiotics.

Living situation: She is transferred to the hospice inpatient unit (IPU) from home with uncontrolled pain, malodor, and excessive exudate from a vaginal MFW. She was self-managing the wound with obstetric pads, showers, and frequent changes of underwear and pants when soiled. Her primary caregiver is overwhelmed and unable to care for her at home.

Comprehensive history: On admission to the IPU, she screened positive for depression and anxiety and complains of painful periwound moisture-associated skin damage (MASD) of the vaginal MFW circumferentially. She additionally complains of wound-specific odor and exudate that stained her underwear and pants two to three times per day. She also complains of intermittent cancer-related abdominal pain not controlled with four to five doses of short-acting opioids daily

Assessment: MFW bed had friable, yellow-pink tissue with moderate, yellow, foul exudate and circumferential periwound maceration and erythema. Odor noted at the door of her room with dressing intact.

Recommendations: She was seen by the hospice nurse (also a wound, ostomy, and continence nurse) who ordered: Wound Care—Cleanse with warm soapy water via a peribottle, pat dry, 1% metronidazole spray to wound bed, petrolatum-based barrier periwound, and abdominal pads held in place by Attends mesh undergarments. Wound-Specific Pain Management—A short-acting opioid was administered a half-hour before wound care and again after completion if needed (MASD and wound-specific pain resolved, odor and exudate were controlled within 3 days). Cancer-Related Pain Management—A long-acting opioid and daily corticosteroids with a short-acting opioid for breakthrough pain were started. (Cancer-related pain was controlled within 48 hours.) Psychosocial—Licensed clinical social worker and rabbi consulted for counseling; mirtazapine started for depression, insomnia, and anorexia; and a short-acting benzodiazepine for anxiety as needed (improvements in sleep and anxiety observed).

E: IPU staff, patient, and her husband were educated about the wound care and pain management plans and psychosocial referrals. The patient was able to participate in her own wound care, but as her health and cognition failed, the staff assumed total responsibility until her death 3 weeks later.

and ulceration suggestive of the diagnosis.[97,98] Other clinical signs may include chronic ulceration greater than 3 months, rolled wound margins, an irregular base or margins, excessive granulation tissue, crusting over, and an increase in size despite appropriate treatment.[97,98] Marjolin's ulcers may also be associated with wound-specific symptoms: bleeding, malodor, purulent exudate, pain, pruritus, and bulk effect.[95]

Box 20.8 Skin Pathologies Giving Rise to Marjolin's Ulcers

Burn scars
Traumatic wounds
Venous ulcers
Pressure injuries
Osteomyelitis
Frostbitten tissue
Snakebites
Leprosy ulcers
Lupus rashes
Urinary fistulas
Irradiated skin
Vaccination sites
Skin graft donor sites
Discoid lupus erythematous
Pilonidal abscess
Hidradenitis suppurativa

Sources: References 96 and 98.

Treatment

Early detection with immediate referral to plastic surgery for biopsy and wide excision with grafting are the key to successful curative treatment.[95,98] Palliative care nurses are likely to encounter Marjolin's ulcers that have either progressed beyond curative treatment or are considered secondary to a more dire diagnosis. Palliative treatment of Marjolin's ulcers follows the same guiding principles of palliative wound care previously discussed in this chapter.

Calciphylaxis

Calciphylaxis is a cutaneous ischemic infarct caused by the occlusion of blood vessels in subcutaneous fat and dermis from calcification both within vessel walls and externally.[99] Calciphylaxis in end-stage renal disease (ESRD) is classified as uremic calciphylaxis, with annual incidence ranging from 0.04% to 4%.[99] Risk factors include ESRD (especially dialysis and renal transplant patients), derangements in calcium and phosphate levels, vitamin K deficiency (40%–50% of patients with calciphylaxis take warfarin), and obesity, diabetes mellitus, and female sex.[99,100]

The most prominent symptom associated with calciphylaxis is pain, usually of mixed ischemic–neuropathic origin, that is often out of proportion to the skin injuries or precedes them.[99] Wound characteristics may include plaques and nodules (most common), livedo reticularis (red–purple marbled discoloration), or ulcers.[99,100] The most frequently affected sites are the thighs and abdomen, but wounds can occur on bilateral lower extremities.[99] Calciphylaxis may affect multiple body areas including the fingers and toes and occasionally even the peristomal skin.[100]

Skin biopsies are rarely indicated to diagnose uremic calciphylaxis. When a patient presents with ESRD and indurated, painful plaques or ulcers on the abdomen or thighs/legs, a clinical diagnosis can be made.

Treatment

Treatment is complex and should be based on goals of care. If possible, the underlying disease process should be managed, electrolyte abnormalities corrected, warfarin discontinued, aggressive pain management initiated, and a palliative wound care plan developed. There are no standard wound care protocols. General wound care principles apply: (1) remove impediments from the wound (loose, hard, calcium deposits and slough), (2) balance wound bed moisture, (3) reduce bioburden (prevent and treat infections), (4) reduce edema, (5) control venous insufficiency, and (6) protect periwound skin.[99,100]

Radiation Dermatitis

Ninety-five percent of patients with cancer receiving radiation therapy will develop some form of radiation dermatitis, which may result in treatment delay, disfigurement, pain, and/or diminished QOL.[101,102] Radiation dermatitis is also known as "radiodermatitis," "radiation burn," "radiation injury," or "radiation-induced skin reaction."[102] Radiation injures rapidly dividing cells of the epidermis (basal layer), underlying dermis, and epidermal appendages: hair follicles, sebaceous glands, and nails.[101,102]

Risk factors for radiation dermatitis include type and dose of radiation, higher total doses of radiation due to cumulative effects, anatomic area irradiated (face, neck, upper back, and chest), concomitant chemotherapy, presence of skin folds, and an increased body mass index.[101]

Skin assessment should be performed prior to the start of radiation and regularly thereafter. Radiation-induced skin changes may be acute (develops within 90 days of treatment initiation) or chronic (develop more than 90 days after treatment initiation, possibly months to years). Acute skin changes may manifest as transient erythema (within first 24 hours) and progress to dry desquamation (see Figure 20.6) or moist desquamation (see Figure 20.7).[101] Dry desquamation is clinically characterized by pruritus, scaling, and flaking of dry skin. Moist desquamation is clinically characterized by dermal erosion, edema, fibrinous exudate, potential bullae formation, and pain.[101] Chronic radiation-induced skin changes may include epidermal thinning, telangiectasias, dyspigmentation, dermal atrophy, fibrosis, and rarely dermal necrosis with ulceration.[101]

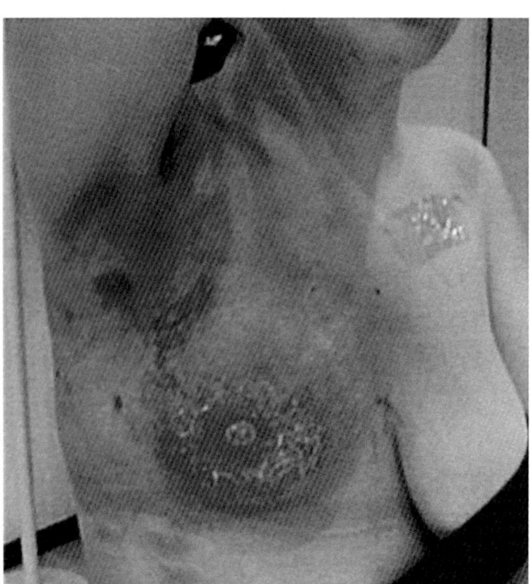

Figure 20.6 Dry desquamation and moderate erythema in a patient with breast cancer undergoing radiation treatment.

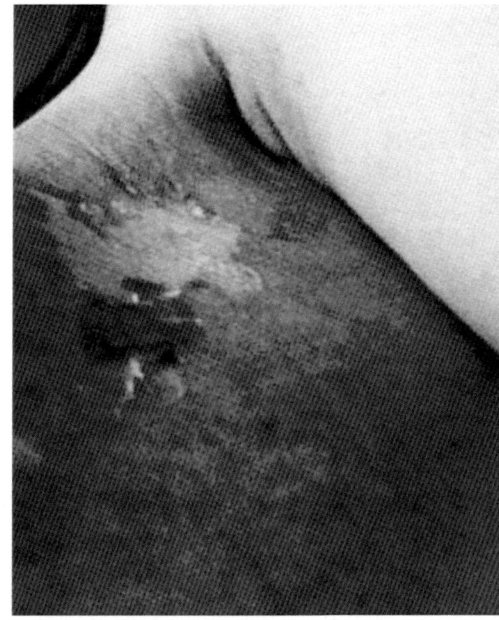

Figure 20.7 Moist desquamation and severe erythema in a patient with breast cancer undergoing radiation treatment.

Treatment

Broadly, goals of treatment should include the promotion of healing, the prevention of infection, and the management of wound-specific symptoms (pain, pruritus, exudate). There is a dearth of evidence supporting specific recommendations in the treatment of acute and chronic radiation dermatitis.[102] General skin care during radiation therapy includes the use of mild soaps and lukewarm water, loose-fitted clothing over the irradiated site, avoiding sun exposure and scratching, and adequate nutrition.[102] Prophylactic use of steroids and silver sulfadiazine or silver nylon dressings have proved effective in the reduction of acute radiation dermatitis.[102,103] Calendula (a catechin), β-sitosterol, hyaluronic acid, epidermal growth factor, statins, and granulocyte-macrophage colony-stimulating factor have weak evidence supporting their effectiveness in acute radiation dermatitis; however, confirmatory studies are needed.[103] Pentoxifylline for the reduction of fibrosis has been used with success in patients with chronic radiation-induced telangiectasia and fibrosis.[104]

COVID-19 Skin Manifestations

The SARS-CoV-2 virus was first identified in December 2019, evolving into the COVID-19 pandemic by March 2020.[105] COVID-19 skin manifestations, on or near bony prominences that are atypical of classic PIs, have been noted; however, their exact etiology and pathology remain unclear.[106] Hypercoagulation with microvascular occlusion, vasculitis, drug sensitivities, and triggering of immune mechanisms have been postulated.[106] Skin manifestations include pseudo-chilblains (COVID toes),[107] purpuric lesions/petechiae, vesicular eruptions, urticarial lesions, morbilliform/maculopapular rashes, and areas of livedo or necrosis.[106,108] Table 20.11 describes the clinical presentation of COVID-19 skin

Table 20.11 COVID-19 skin manifestation characteristics

Cutaneous manifestation	Clinical characteristics	Anatomical location
Pseudo-chilblains (COVID toes)	Itchy or tender/painful erythema-edema with or without red or purple plaques, macules, or nodules	Toes
Vesicular rashes	Clear fluid-filled blisters (<1 cm), isolated or in clusters	May occur on the mucous membranes or skin
Urticaria (hives)	Itchy, raised red or skin-colored welts, may appear rapidly, disappear, reappear	Commonly occur on the trunk, may extend to the extremities
Morbilliform rashes	Erythematous maculopapular rash	Commonly occur on the trunk, may extend to the extremities
Livedoid lesions	Painful red or purple lesions with a branched or irregular pattern, may progress to necrosis	Commonly occur on the lower extremities and feet
Purpuric lesions/petechiae	Rash of red, maroon, or purple spots.	May occur on the mucous membranes or skin

Sources: Adapted from References 106 and 107.

manifestations.[106–108] These skin manifestations may precede other signs and symptoms, may be the only manifestations of the COVID-19 infection, or may appear and progress during the course of the illness.[106–108]

Treatment

Palliative treatment of COVID-19 skin manifestations follows the same guiding principles of palliative wound care previously discussed in this chapter.

Palliative Care of Continent Diversions, Incontinent Diversions, and Fistulas

Palliative care of the patient with a urinary or fecal diversion or fistula centers on specialist-level WOC nurse guidance to manage advanced symptoms, stoma/fistula pouching complexities, and peristomal/perifistular complications by adapting product selection and patient and caregiver education to the progressive functional decline experienced in serious illness, with a gradual shift of responsibilities to the caregiver.

Case Study: WOC Care at the End of Life

The WOC nurse conducted a comprehensive history, which revealed a long- and short-acting opioid pain management plan, though without a bowel regime. The physical exam included digitalization of the patient's stoma, which revealed a fecal impaction, explaining the nonfunctioning colostomy. After consulting with the hospice nurse practitioner, she irrigated the colostomy for a large amount of hard, constipated stool and started a bowel regime (stool softener with stimulant twice a day). She also started a low-dose corticosteroid to combat pain, fatigue, and anorexia. The WOC nurse also discovered peristomal MASD of the inferior peristomal skin from stool leakage, the skin denuded and inflamed. The erosions and inflammation were very painful, and pouch changes distressed both the patient and her sister. Additionally, the peristomal subcutaneous abdominal masses caused uneven abdominal planes, interfering with the two-piece system's seal, causing it to lift and leak.

The WOC nurse used a "crusting" technique (layering no-sting skin protectant with stoma powder) to cover the denuded skin and create a dry surface for the skin barrier to adhere to. She then chose a flexible one-piece pouching system that would fit the uneven contours of the patient's abdomen. She instructed the patient, patient's sister, and nursing staff on the pouch-changing regimen (wear-time goal is 24–45 hours) and the importance of emptying the pouch when it was one-third full to avoid tension on the skin barrier. She recommended premedication with a short-acting opioid 20–30 minutes prior to the pouch change as part of pain management.

For the assessment and management of the patient's IAD and end-of-life care, see the Case Study Resolution.

Continent and Incontinent Fecal and Urinary Diversions

No published research specifically addresses the current prevalence, management, or QOL aspects related to ostomy issues in men, women, and children facing life-limiting illness.[8] An ostomy is a surgically created stoma for the elimination of urine or stool that can be permanent or temporary.[109] Stoma creation is indicated for both malignancy-related (colon, rectal, anal, or bladder cancers) and non-malignancy-related diseases (ulcerative colitis, Crohn's disease, trauma, congenital disorders, diverticular disease, or severe neurogenic bladder).[109] Table 20.12 describes the different continent and incontinent fecal and urinary diversions the palliative care nurse may encounter.[109,110]

Most stomas require a pouching system which maintains peristomal skin health, provides a secure seal, and allows the patient to maintain their functional performance status. Pouching procedures for either one- or two-piece pouching systems can be complex and include essential tasks such as emptying and removing the pouching system, washing and drying the skin, measuring the stoma, putting on a new pouching system, and disposing of the used pouching system.[8,110] As taxing as this process can be for an otherwise "well" person with a stoma, basic ostomy care, supply ordering, pouch disposal, and troubleshooting leakage may present an insurmountable challenge for persons with serious illness.[8] These persons may have vision, cognitive, and/or motor-sensory deficits that worsen as the illness progresses; heavy symptom burdens; and peristomal complications.[8]

Table 20.12 Continent and incontinent fecal and urinary diversions

Type of diversion	Continent or incontinent	Description
Ileostomy	Incontinent (fecal)	A stoma (surgical opening) constructed by bringing the end or loop of the ileum out onto the surface of the skin. A one- or two-piece pouching system is then worn to collect the effluent.[110]
Colostomy	Incontinent (fecal)	A stoma (surgical opening) constructed by drawing the healthy end of the large intestine or colon through an incision in the anterior abdominal wall and suturing it into place. A one- or two-piece pouching system is then worn to collect the effluent. Conversely, colostomy irrigation and a stoma cap may be chosen for patients with distal stomas.[110]
Continent ileostomy (Koch pouch)	Continent (fecal)	The small intestine is connected to an internal, S-shaped reservoir created from a section of the ileum. A one-way valve is constructed through which a Medena catheter (30 Fr) is inserted four to eight times a day to drain the fecal effluent.[109,110]
Urostomy (ileal conduit)	Incontinent (urinary)	The ureters are surgically resected from the bladder and drain the urine into a detached section of the ileum. The end of the ileum is brought out through a stoma in the abdominal wall. The residual small bowel is reanastomosed with the residual terminal ileum. A collection pouch fitted with a belt is then worn snugly against the abdomen and over the stoma to collect the urine.[110]
Ureterostomy	Incontinent (urinary)	One or both ureters are detached from the bladder and brought through the abdominal wall to form a stoma. A collection pouch fitted with a belt is then worn snugly against the abdomen and over the "ureteral buds" or stomas to collect the urine as it passes through the ureters.[110]
Heterotopic continent bladder replacement (Indiana pouch)	Continent (urinary)	Following cystectomy, an ileal or ilio-cecal segment is used to form a reservoir. The ureters are connected to the reservoir. A one-way valve is constructed through which a catheter is inserted four to six times a day and at bedtime to drain the urine.[110]
Orthotopic bladder substitution (neobladder)	Continent (urinary)	Treatment of choice when the intent is curative. This is closest to the natural bladder's urine storage and voiding function. Following cystectomy, a reservoir is created from a section of ileum and situated in the pelvis minor and connected to the patient's urethra. Continence is achieved through the patient's own sphincter.[110]

Assessment

It is essential the hospice nurse perform a meticulous history and physical, including presence of functional performance deficits.[8,110] Stoma assessment must include the stoma etiology, location, type (urinary, fecal, continent, or incontinent), shape (round or oval), and size (using a measuring guide); whether the stoma is budded, flush, or retracted; peristomal skin; and effluent characteristics. The nurse should record the type, size, and product serial number of pouching or intubation supplies, through which company and how the supplies are ordered (phone, internet, hospice formulary, etc.), and current supply inventory and identify who is primarily responsible for stoma care.

Vision Deficits

Vision deficits are common among palliative patients. Compromised eyesight can greatly hinder the ability of the patient with a stoma to measure for or change an appliance, note peristomal complications, or empty the pouch. Ultimately, the potential inability to perform self-care may encroach on the patient's independence, which can negatively influence body image.[8,109,110] Diabetic retinopathy, conjunctival erythema in ESRD, primary brain tumors, MFWs of the head and neck, secondary ocular manifestations of rheumatoid arthritis or multiple sclerosis, chemotherapy-induced ocular toxicities, and surgery or radiation are possible causes of vision deficits in patients with serious illness.[8]

Multiple strategies may be used to address stoma care challenges in patients with visual deficits. Educational materials with large font on blue- or cream-colored paper that reduces glare are suggested.[8,111] Bright lights, readers, and magnifying glasses also may be needed. Audiotapes with step-by-step instructions that can be conveniently played as frequently as the patient with a stoma or caregiver require may be employed.[8,111] In the absence of peripheral neuropathy, focus on the patient's strength and keen sense of touch.[8,111] Changing the ostomy appliance when the stoma is not functioning (i.e., when there is no output) and utilizing a two-piece pouching system are recommended because it is easier to center the skin barrier by feeling the stoma by touch.[8,111] If the patient has an ileal conduit, they may be taught to wick the urine with a tampon or dental wick, both to keep the peristomal skin dry and to help center the skin barrier.[8] Tactile aides also have been developed by Coloplast Corporation (Marietta, GA).

Cognitive Deficits

Many disease processes may cause progressive cognitive deficits in the palliative care population.[8] These patients will eventually experience loss of memory and cognitive skills, as well as physical functional impairment. The palliative care nurse must be vigilant about cognitive decline in patients with stomas; ongoing assessment of cognitive function is critical and early referral to the WOC nurse essential.[8]

Interventions by the WOC nurse must be directed at the patient's level of functioning. Early in the cognitive disease trajectory, it is prudent to identify one or more caregivers willing to learn about and assist with the patient's stoma care. At early stages of memory loss, the patient may need visual reminders to prompt them to empty the pouch, intubate a continent diversion, or order supplies.[8] As memory and cognition diminish, step-by-step instructions, coaching/prompting, or visual aids may be considered.[8] Simple pre-cut or one-piece appliances with Velcro closures may be suggested. Eventually, the caregiver(s) will need to assume total daily care. This will necessitate the development of a teaching plan for either family or staff depending on home care or facility placement. The additional caregiver burden of providing stoma care or diversion intubation should

Table 20.13 Stoma care considerations for patients with motor and sensory deficits

Diagnosis	Pathophysiology	Sequelae	General and stoma-specific considerations
Advanced Parkinson's disease	Depigmentation of the substantia nigra and locus coeruleus with loss of dopaminergic neurons and the appearance of Lewy bodies[112]	Freezing, rigidity, bradykinesia, unilateral resting tremor, cognitive decline, Lewy body dementia, and dyskinesias due to levodopa[112]	• Collaboration with neurology to ensure maximization of dopaminergic agents and limiting side effects. • Loss of hand dexterity could impair the patient's ability to apply and remove a clip, cut a pattern, or empty a pouch. • Cognitive decline necessitates caregiver training early in the disease process.
Advanced multiple sclerosis (MS)	Multifocal plaques of demyelination within the central nervous system.[113] If diagnosed under the age of 40 years, recurring episodes of neurologic impairment followed by periods of spontaneous remission are common.	Spasticity, optic neuritis.[113] Pain syndromes have been reported in up to 76% of MS patients.[113] Dysesthesias are extremely common.	• Spasticity is usually treated with baclofen or tizanidine. • Spasticity and loss of hand dexterity could impair the patient's ability to apply and remove a clip, cut a pattern, or empty a pouch. • Vision deficits and increasingly frequent debilitating "relapses" and "flares" necessitate caregiver training early in the disease process.
Amyotrophic lateral sclerosis	Loss of both upper motor neurons (UMN) in the motor cortex and lower motor neurons (LMN) in the brainstem and spinal cord.[114] Average life span post-diagnosis of 3–5 years.[114]	Spasticity, slow movements, hyperreflexia, and poor dexterity are sequelae of UMN disease. Weakness, atrophy, reduced tone, and hyporeflexia are due to LMN involvement.[114]	• Poor hand dexterity could impair the patient's ability to apply and remove a clip, cut a pattern, or empty a pouch. • Eventual functional quadriplegia necessitates caregiver training early in the disease process.
Stroke	May affect sensory or motor function and often both depending on location and extent of injury. May be ischemic (thrombotic, embolic), hemorrhagic (intracerebral, subarachnoid), or lacunar.[115]	Hemiparesis, ataxia, paresthesia, adhesive capsulitis (frozen shoulder)[115]	• Presents the challenge of caring for a stoma with one, possibly the nondominant, hand. • Inability to feel a clip or flange or to recognize it as such (stereognosis).
Quadriplegia or paraplegia	Spinal cord trauma, spinal stenosis, or cord compression due to primary tumor or metastasis	Injuries from C4 through C7 may affect shoulder and arm musculature, C6 through C8 (forearm extensors and flexors), and C8 through T1 (hand musculature).[116] Total cord transection syndrome results in the loss of all types of sensation and motor function below the level of the lesion.[116]	• May lack the physical coordination to perform majority of gross and/or fine motor skills needed to perform daily stoma care. • Focus on modifying a plan to accommodate abilities. • Cervical quadriplegia necessitates caregiver training early in the disease process.
Peripheral neuropathy	Diseases causing polyneuropathies include diabetes, alcoholism, shingles, HIV/AIDS, hepatitis C, RA, end-stage renal disease, or end-stage liver disease.[117] Chemotherapy-induced peripheral neuropathy (CIPN) is a well-known side effect of cancer treatment.[117]	Symptoms may range in severity from minimal, transient numbness and tingling in the extremities to burning pain and lack of coordination.[117]	• Chemotherapeutic agents responsible for CIPN are the taxanes, vinca alkaloids, and platinum compounds.[117] • May lack the physical coordination to perform majority of gross and/or fine motor skills needed to perform daily stoma care.
Rheumatoid arthritis (RA)	Acute and chronic inflammation in the synovium associated with joint tissue destruction and instability.[118]	Loss of joint mobility and dexterity, as well as crippling pain, accompany RA.[118]	• Be diligent about pain control during acute flares. • Loss of hand dexterity could impair ability to apply and remove a clip, cut a pattern, or empty a pouch.

Source: Reference 8.

be considered and the need for respite care, support groups, or counseling routinely assessed.

Motor and Sensory Deficits

For people living with serious illness, alterations in their physical functioning from the disease process or treatment regimen may lead to motor and/or sensory deficits. Serious rheumatic or neuromuscular illness can affect people with stomas in numerous debilitating and often painful ways, making stoma care challenging or impossible (see Table 20.13).[112–117]

The WOC nurse is consulted to assess the patient's functional status, modify the pouching system, simplify the care routine, and/or teach the caregiver or staff how to care for the stoma.[8] Key to ensuring adherence to the treatment plan and stoma health, as well as to maintaining the patient's autonomy and self-esteem, is the development of a realistic plan of care.[8] For patients with impaired motor skills, Velcro pouches may eliminate the need to use clips, and one-piece appliances may be applied with one hand for easy applications. Moldable technology may be an option for persons with minimal manual dexterity, vision impairment, chronic metacarpal joint pain, or polyneuropathies of the hands. Moldable skin barriers do not need to be cut (eliminating the need to manage scissors or visualize patterns) and fit snugly against the stoma, facilitating adaptation to changing stoma size and shape.[8] Colostomy patients may consider using a disposable, closed-end pouch, thus eliminating the need for a clip, while urostomy patients may need to try various spouts and tabs to find the product easiest for them to use.[110] Occupational therapy may assist in teaching manual skills and recommending needed adaptive devices. If self-care is not possible, transition of care to the family or caregiver must be explored. However, if caregivers are not available, home care agencies or long-term care placement may be necessary.[8]

Peristomal Complications

No statistical data or research directly describes peristomal complication prevalence and incidence in hospice and palliative care settings. Tilley has observed that these issues may be more pronounced or prevalent in the hospice population due to an increase in the frequency and duration of risk factors.[8] The *Peristomal Skin Assessment Guide* is a tool developed by the WOCN Society that provides basic guidance to clinicians on identifying and treating peristomal skin complications, including instructions for patient care and conditions that warrant referral to a WOC nurse.[110,119] Changes in abdominal planes, mucocutaneous separation, peristomal varices (caput medusa), and peristomal MASD are among the most commonly encountered complications and will be discussed next.

Changes in Abdominal Planes

The peristomal plane is the surface area under the solid skin barrier and adhesive of the pouching system, extending out approximately 4 inches by 4 inches from the base of the stoma.[110] Assessing the plane with the patient lying down, sitting, and standing helps the practitioner decide on the type of skin barrier needed.[110] The following factors should be considered when selecting a pouching system: type of ostomy, stoma type and location, abdominal contours, lifestyle, personal preferences, visual acuity, and manual dexterity.[109,110] The skin surrounding the stoma should be assessed for firmness, excessive softness, unevenness caused by subcutaneous tumors, the presence of fungating wounds, and rounded protrusion caused by ascites, scars from prior surgeries, or areas of breakdown or trauma.[8] The type of pouching system included in the plan of care may need to be changed multiple times during the palliative to hospice continuum as the disease process progresses and abdominal tumor burden or ascites increases, weight loss occurs, or malignant bowel obstruction develops.[8]

The skin barrier should mirror the topography of the peristomal plane. In the case of a protruding abdomen or a peristomal plane with creases, wrinkles (as seen with excessive weight loss common to palliative care patients), or scars, a convex pouching system may be considered.[8,110] This system also may be used in patients with uneven planes due to tumors; barrier paste can be used to fill in uneven areas.[8] An extended-wear barrier, left in place for up to 7 days, may be chosen for a patient with a large abdominal tumor burden who is experiencing pain, to decrease frequent changes and discomfort.[8] Premedicating with a short-acting opioid before the wafer change should be included in the plan of care, if indicated.[8] In all cases, the back of the skin barrier should be examined during each pouch change to ascertain undermining by effluent, and the skin should be assessed for peristomal MASD.[110]

Mucocutaneous Separation

Mucocutaneous separation is the complete or partial detachment of the stoma from the surrounding skin (see Figure 20.8).[110,120] Risk factors include smoking, administration of corticosteroids, chemotherapy, abdominal radiation, diabetes, inflammatory bowel disease, infection, malnutrition, stoma necrosis,[110,120] and recurrence of malignancy or any of the chronic, debilitating diseases mentioned throughout this chapter.[8]

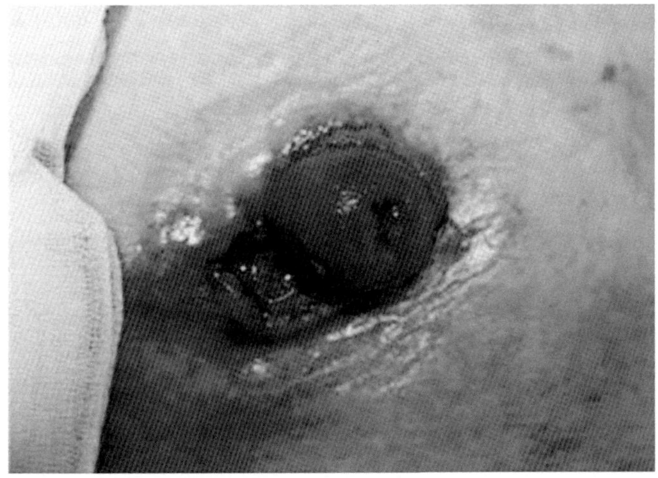

Figure 20.8 Partial mucocutaneous separation.

Corticosteroids, a mainstay in the treatment of pain, dyspnea, cerebral edema, fatigue, and anorexia, are used routinely in palliative care settings. Malnutrition and anorexia/cachexia syndromes may be seen in several serious illnesses such as acquired immune deficiency syndrome, chronic obstructive pulmonary disease, congestive heart failure, dementia, tuberculosis, malaria, chronic kidney disease, liver disease, and rheumatoid arthritis.[121] Cachexia occurs in up to 70% of patients with advanced cancer.[121] Infection and recurrence of disease due to the debilitating nature of chronic illness may be anticipated.

Conservative management is key because, at the end of life, the etiology of the complication most likely will not be correctable.[8] The wound left by the skin separation should be flushed with normal saline or tap water and filled with an absorbent material such as skin barrier powder, skin barrier paste, hydrofiber, or calcium alginates to absorb drainage as well as to prevent excessive soiling from urine or feces.[110,120] The pouching system is then placed over the area to protect from effluent. Consider using a two-piece system with a floating flange to facilitate comfort during pouch removal and reapplication.[120] A convex

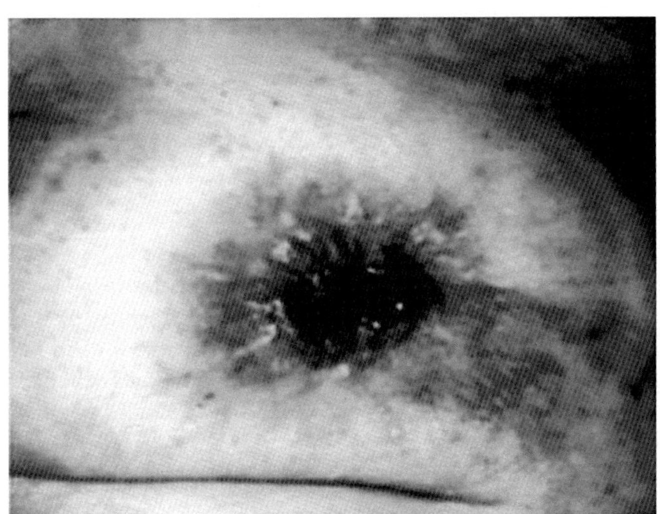

Figure 20.9 Peristomal varices.

pouching system should be avoided because it may cause deeper tissue destruction and impaired healing at the stoma–skin junction.[120]

Peristomal Varices (Caput Medusae)

Peristomal varices occurring at the site of the stoma may be seen in patients with portal hypertension and end-stage liver disease from either malignancy or cirrhosis.[120,122] This condition, often referred to as "caput medusae," accounts for between 1% and 5% of all variceal bleeding.[120,122] A purple hue caused by dilation of mucocutaneous vessels and profuse bleeding may surround the stoma if it is eroded or traumatized (see Figure 20.9). In the case of acute bleeding, apply direct pressure; and if needed, cauterize with silver nitrate, use epi-soaked gauze or gel foam, or suture ligation.[8,120] Educate the caregiver about the need to (1) use skin barriers that are easily removable, (2) use adhesive removers when possible, (3) use flexible pouching devices, and (4) avoid rigid ostomy products and covexity.[120] If unable to stop the bleeding, instruct the caregiver to seek emergency care (if consistent with the patient's advance directives).

Peristomal MASD

Peristomal MASD is defined as inflammation and erosion of skin related to moisture that begins at the stoma–skin junction and extends outward.[60] The etiology of peristomal MASD is prolonged exposure of the peristomal skin to urine or stool, perspiration, an external water source (swimming or bathing), or wound or fistula drainage.[60] The etiology of the skin damage drives the treatment plan and pouching system selection. The ultimate goal is to choose a pouching system that fits closely around the stoma and prevents leakage under the barrier.[60,110] Damaged skin can exude serous fluid and contribute to pouch adherence failure. "Crusting" is a technique that layers no-sting barrier film and stoma powder, forming a dry, protective barrier over denuded skin. The patient with a urostomy should connect the pouch to a bedside drainage bag at night to prevent urine from undermining the skin barrier.[110]

Fistulas

Fistulas negatively impact patients' QOL and present a unique challenge to the palliative care practitioner. A fistula is an abnormal passage or opening between two or more body organs or spaces. Fistulas are named either for the two communicating biological structures or spaces involved or the originating organ (see Table 20.14).[110,122,123] The majority of fistulas arise mainly from the gastrointestinal and genitourinary systems. The etiology of fistula development may be related to postoperative complications or spontaneous events. Surgical adhesions, a foreign body next to the suture line, tension on a suture line, breakdown of intestinal anastomosis, and compromised vascular supply can lead to fistula formation in the surgical patient.[110,122] Spontaneous occurrences may be seen in malignancy (malignant bowel obstruction, tumor invasion), small bowel obstruction, and Crohn's disease, while factors such as infection, poor nutritional status, steroid therapy, and endocrine and metabolic disorders can predispose patients with advanced and terminal illness to fistula development.[110,122] Fistulas occur in 1% of patients with advanced cancer.[110,124] Patients with gastrointestinal malignancies and those who have received pelvic irradiation are at highest risk.[110,124]

Fistulas can be classified in different ways, but the most useful for the palliative care practitioner is by output. Low-output fistulas produce less than 200 cc/day of effluent (most will close spontaneously if they can epithelialize), moderate-output fistulas produce 200–467 cc/day (variable spontaneous closure rates), and high-output fistula produce greater than 467 cc/day (requires surgical therapy to close).[110,124] The goals of care may be palliative if spontaneous closure of the fistula, which usually occurs within 4–7 weeks, cannot be achieved. Factors that inhibit fistula closure include complete disruption of bowel continuity, distal obstruction, foreign body in the fistula tract, epithelialization of the tract, presence of cancer, previous radiation, and Crohn's disease (see Box 20.9).[110,123,124]

Mortality in patients with fistulas is related to fluid and electrolyte imbalances, malnutrition, failed operative closure, cholestatic

Box 20.9 ABC's of Persistent Fistulae

A—Abscess, infection
B—Irritable bowel disease
C—Cancer, Crohn's
D—Distal obstruction
E—Epithelialization of tract
F—Foreign body
G—Gamma (radiation therapy)

Sources: References 123 and 124.

Table 20.14 Fistula terminology

Name	From	To
Enteroatmospheric	Intestine	Open wound base
Enterocolonic	Intestine	Colon
Enterocutaneous	Intestine	Skin
Enterovesical	Intestine	Bladder
Enterovaginal	Intestine	Vagina
Colocutaneous	Colon	Skin
Colovesical	Colon	Bladder
Pancreatic	Pancreas	Skin
Rectovaginal	Rectum	Vagina
Spit fistula (esophagostomy)	Esophagus	Skin
Vesicocutaneous	Bladder	Skin
Vesicovaginal	Bladder	Vagina

Source: Reference 110.

Box 20.10 Commonly Occurring Complications Associated with Fistulas

Sepsis
Malnutrition
Fluid and electrolyte imbalance
Anemia
Acid–base imbalances
Tissue destruction
Pain
Delirium

Table 20.15 Characteristics of fistula effluent

Fistula type	Effluent color	Daily output	pH	Components
Colocutaneous	Brown, tan	1–1.5 L/day	6.8–7.8	Water, mucus, sodium, potassium, and bicarbonate
Enterocutaneous	Bilious, tan, beige	7–8 L/day	6.5–7.5	Water, mucus, potassium, and bicarbonate
Pancreatic	Colorless	670–1,000 mL/day	8.3	Water, bicarbonate, sodium, and potassium
Spit fistula (esophagostomy)	Clear or color of fluids ingested	1–1.5 L/day	7.1–7.5	Water, mucus, amylase

Source: Reference 110.

liver failure, and sepsis.[110,125] Mortality may be as high as 10%–30% in patients with enterocutaneous fistulas.[124,125] Box 20.10 lists frequent complications, some of them life-threatening, associated with fistulas.[124,125]

Diagnosis and Assessment

Fistulogram, a radiographic imaging technique where water-soluble contrast is injected directly into the fistula tract to determine the involved structures, is usually the initial imaging of choice.[110,124,125] This may be followed by an upper gastrointestinal series, a barium enema, a computerized tomography scan, cystoscopy, or an intravenous pyelogram depending on the presenting symptoms. Once diagnosed, meticulous assessment is required to correct potentially distressing or even lethal complications. Comprehensive assessment includes nutrition and hydration status, vital signs, mental/cognitive status, pain assessment, inspection of the surrounding skin or wound bed, the quality and amount of fistula effluent, and electrolyte and acid–base evaluation. The effluent should be assessed for odor, color, consistency, amount, and pH.[110,124,125] Characteristics of the most common types of fistula effluent are displayed in Table 20.15.[110,126]

Palliative Fistula Management

Ostomy pouching techniques are the mainstay of palliative fistula management. Skin cleansing, skin protection, uneven skin surface management, dressing or pouch selection, containment of output, and odor control are essential components to fistula management in those with terminal illness.[124,126] Table 20.16 offers

Table 20.16 Palliative fistula management

Fistula classification	WOCN consult recommended	Pouching/containment system	Odor control
Low-output	No, unless odor is uncontrollable	Skin barrier/skin deficit management Gauze dressings Foam dressings Pediatric pouches Colostomy caps (small closed-end pouches)	Gauze dressing with charcoal Silver foams Pouching Pouch change in a well-ventilated room
Moderate-output	Yes	Skin barrier/skin deficit management Pouches that allow direct visualization and/or access through a valve or door Spit fistulas may benefit from pediatric pouching due to difficult-to-pouch locations Multiple fistulas may be amenable to saddlebagging[a] Enteroatmospheric fistulas may be amenable to troughing[b] or bridging[c]	Pouching Pouch change in a well-ventilated room Internal body deodorants: bismuth, charcoal, peppermint oil
High-output	Yes	Pouches that allow direct visualization and/or access through a valve or door High-output pouching system Spit fistulas may benefit from pediatric pouching due to difficult-to-pouch locations Multiple fistulas may be amenable to saddlebagging[a] Enteroatmospheric fistulas may be amenable to troughing[b] or bridging[c] Negative pressure wound therapy may be considered	Pouching Pouch change in a well-ventilated room Internal body deodorants: bismuth, charcoal, peppermint oil

WOCN, wound, ostomy, and continence nurse.

[a] *Saddlebagging*: Cut fistula openings on the back of two or more cut-to-fit ostomy pouches, off-center. Cleanse skin with warm water, apply skin protectant, and fill deficits with stoma paste. Apply ostomy pouches, adhered to each other in an overlapping "saddlebag" fashion.[127]

[b] *Troughing*: Line the skin surrounding the wound and fistula with a skin barrier wafer, and seal the edge nearest the wound with stoma paste. Place thin film dressings over the anterior aspect of the wound, continuing down to the fistula orifice and posterior aspect of the wound. Then place a cut-to-fit pouch over the opening in the film dressing that exposes the fistula orifice.[127]

[c] *Bridging*: (Prevents fistula output from contaminating the wound site.) Build a "bridge" by consecutively layering small pieces of skin barrier wafers together until it is the same height as the depth of the wound. Using barrier past, adhere the skin barrier "wedge" to the wound bed near the fistula opening. Cut to fit an ostomy pouch around the fistula using the bridge to adhere the pouch. Dress the anterior aspect of the wound.[127]

Sources: References 126 and 127.

management considerations based on fistula output, number of fistula tracts, and location. In addition to these considerations, the type of pouching system should be chosen based on effluent consistency and location.[110,126] Thick pasty output is better managed with a pouch that has an open end and clamp and thin watery effluent with a narrow spigot or tube.[126] Spit fistulas may be better managed with neonatal or pediatric pouches as anatomical structures of the head and neck region present unique challenges. All pouches must be emptied frequently, when one-third to one-half full. WOC consultation for moderate- to high-output fistulas is important to select the appropriate containment system, train staff and caregivers, and contain cost in terms of supplies and human resources. WOC consultation is also necessary if negative pressure wound therapy is chosen for both fistula and wound closure in enteroatmospheric fistulas.

Pharmacologic Management

Management of fistula effluent may require pharmacologic interventions aimed at reducing gastric secretions, gut-slowing, and/or minimizing output.[128–130] Gut-slowing and decreasing the amount of effluent help maintain intact pouching systems and the integrity of perifistula skin and maximize the ability to use the gut for nutrition.[110,128,130]

Reduction of fistula effluent includes the use of histamine-2 receptor antagonists or proton pump inhibitors to decrease gastric acidity and the volume of secretions.[129,130] Gradual titration and stepwise addition of medications such as loperamide, diphenoxylate hydrochloride and atropine sulfate, codeine, tincture of opium, and octreotide may reduce fistula output and slow gastrointestinal motility.[128,130]

Somatostatin is a hormone produced in the hypothalamus and other regions of the brain that inhibits the secretion of nearly all alimentary hormones, thereby enhancing absorption of fluids and electrolytes and inhibiting secretion of gastric acid, pepsin, and bile.[129] In some studies, somatostatin analogues, such as octreotide, have been shown to decrease overall fistula output.[129,130] The efficacy of the role of somatostatin analogues in enterocutaneous and pancreatic fistula closure is, however, inconclusive.[129] Sufficient evidence does exist to use octreotide on a case-by-case basis for patients with moderate- and high-output fistulas.[129,130] WOC nurse consultation is recommended when considering the use of octreotide, typically given subcutaneously as 100 mcg every 8 hours over at least 7 days.[110,129,130] The WOC nurse will monitor for both efficacious and adverse effects, such as abdominal discomfort, nausea, flatulence, diarrhea, and steatorrhea.[110,130]

Nutrition Management

Nutritional support and fluid and electrolyte balance are essential components of fistula management. Malnutrition, dehydration, and electrolyte imbalances should be addressed based on the patient's preferences and goals of care. The gastrointestinal system should be used whenever possible for nutritional support, but intravenous fluid, parenteral electrolyte replacement, and total parenteral nutrition may be necessary. If nutrition can bypass the fistula site, absorption and tolerance are better with use of the intestinal tract; but this is not always possible.[127] Feeding via the fistula itself, termed "fistuloclysis," has been documented using a 14-French tube and semielemental (partially digested) tube feeding formula.[128] WOC nurse and registered dietician consultation is recommended for all patients who warrant fistuloclysis or parenteral nutrition therapy.[110]

Comprehensive management of fistulas in patients with serious illness requires an interprofessional team approach guided by a specialist-level WOC nurse. Odor and effluent containment, perifistular skin protection, and maintenance of adequate nutrition and hydration combined with the prevention of sepsis, anemia, acid–base and electrolyte imbalances, pain, and delirium are essential in maintaining QOL.

Case Study Resolution: WOC Care at the End of Life

The WOC nurse noted during her history that the patient was incontinent of urine and, due to malignancy-related pain, was intermittently uncomfortable when placed on a bedpan and unable to sit on a commode. Upon assessment, the skin of the patient's buttocks was erythematous, in the outline of urine, and minimally weeping with few pinpoint dermal erosions that bled slightly. She declined a Foley catheter, opting for absorbent undergarments. A pH-balanced incontinence cleanser, zinc oxide barrier ointment, and mesh undergarments with absorbent inserts to allow ventilation, maximum wicking, and ease of changing were ordered.

After 6 weeks at home with adequate symptom control, the patient transitioned to active dying; she was minimally responsive with terminal dyspnea and escalating malignancy-related pain. She was transferred to the hospice inpatient unit and started on parenteral opioids, and stoma and incontinence care was shifted to the nursing staff. With her sister at her side, she died peacefully 2 days later.

IAD in Palliative Settings

Urinary and fecal incontinence management in palliative care centers on promoting continence through meticulous assessment and reduction of barriers to maintaining continence, choosing minimally invasive, highly individualized incontinence interventions adapted to the seriously ill patient's progressive functional decline, prevention of IAD, and preservation of the patient's dignity. There is little published research about incontinence in palliative care and hospice settings. The focus of this section is the prevention and management of IAD.

IAD is a form of irritant contact dermatitis that develops from prolonged exposure to urine, stool, or dual incontinence.[131] Repeated exposure to urine in the presence of occlusion or fecal material puts the skin at higher risk.[132] Normally skin has a pH that ranges from 4.5 to 6, forming a protective "acid mantle."[47,132] Raising the skin's pH to alkaline compromises this protective mechanism.[47,132] When ammonia in urine is converted to ammonium by fecal bacteria, skin pH rises. Semi-formed and liquid stool may also raise skin pH as high as 9.2.[131] Liquid stool may contain higher proportions of water and digestive enzymes that contribute to dermal moisture and inflamation.[131,132]

Prevention and Management

Prevention of IAD starts with assessment and identification of fecal and urinary incontinence and elimination of barriers to maintaining continence (immobility, inappropriate containment products). Prevention may entail use of toileting schedules, minimally invasive containment products (absorptive products, fecal pouches, condom catheters, female urinals), or more invasive interventions (indwelling Foley catheters, fecal management systems) on a case-by-case basis. Meticulous skin care of the incontinent patient is also key to preventing IAD.

Management includes the use of a skin moisturizer with humectants and emollients after bathing.[131,132] Perform hygiene after each episode of incontinence using a pH-balanced, no-rinse cleanser, carefully cleaning and drying skin folds and avoiding vigorous scrubbing.[131,132] For intact skin, implement preventive strategies and use a petrolatum-based skin barrier. For IAD with denuded or inflamed skin, implement preventive strategies, use a zinc oxide–based skin barrier, eliminate cutaneous candidiasis, and consider diversion of urine and/or stool using the least invasive intervention possible.[131,132] Only soiled, top layers of zinc oxide– and petrolatum-based barrier products should be removed during incontinence care. Layers of barrier products in contact with skin should be kept intact and superficial layers reinforced with new barrier product after cleansing. See Table 20.2 for skin barrier options.

Conclusion

WOC maladies contribute to suffering and diminished QOL in patients with serious illness. Evidence-based palliative WOC interventions combined with specialist-level WOC nurse consultation are key to providing high-quality palliative and end-of-life care and alleviating suffering. Specialist-level palliative WOC care can once again "bind" the body, alleviate suffering, prevent institutionalization, and palliate the patient's and family's psychological distress at the end of life.[54] Importantly, this chapter underscores the dearth of research in palliative WOC care and the need for rigorous studies in populations with serious illness.

REFERENCES

1. US Department of Health and Human Services, Centers for Disease Control and Prevention, National Center for Health Statistics. *The National Home and Hospice Care Survey; 1996 Summary, Series 13.* Data from National Health Survey No. 141. DHHS Publication (PHS) 99-1712. 1996. Accessed September 2022. https://pubmed.ncbi.nlm.nih.gov/10549237/.
2. Maida V, Corbo M, Doldhykov M, Ennis M, Irani S, Trozzolo L. Wounds in advanced illness: a prevalence and incidence study based on a prospective case series. *Int Wound J.* 2008;5(2):305–314. https://doi.org/10.1111/j.1742-481X.2007.00379.x.
3. Kelechi TJ, Prentice M, Madisetti M, Brunette G, Mueller M. Palliative care in the management of pain, odor, and exudate in chronic wounds at the end of life: a cohort study. *J Hosp Palliat Nurs.* 2017;19(1):17–25. https://doi.org/10.1097/NJH.0000000000000306.
4. Jakobsen TBT, Pittureri C, Seganti P, et al. Incidence and prevalence of pressure ulcers in cancer patients admitted to hospice: a multicentre prospective cohort study. *Int Wound J.* 2020;17(3):641–649. https://doi.org/10.1111/iwj.13317.
5. National Hospice and Palliative Care Organization. *Facts and Figures: Hospice Care in America.* National Hospice and Palliative Care Organization; 2021.
6. Ortman JM, Velkoff VA, Hogan H. US Department of Commerce, Economics and Statistics Administration, US Census Bureau. *An Aging Nation: The Older Population in the United States. Population Estimates and Projections.* P25-1140. 2014. Accessed December 12, 2022. https://www.census.gov/prod/2014pubs/p25-1140.pdf.
7. Emmons KR, Lachman, VD. Palliative wound care: a concept analysis. *J Wound Ostomy Continence Nurs.* 2010;37(6):639–641. https://doi.org/10.1097/WON.0b013e3181f90a4a.
8. Tilley C. Caring for the patient with a fecal or urinary diversion in palliative and hospice settings: a literature review. *Ostomy Wound Manage.* 2012;58(1):24–34.
9. Tilley C, Lipson J, Ramos M. Palliative wound care for malignant wounds at end-of-life. *Nurs Clin North Am.* 2016;48:483–501. https://doi.org/10.1016/j.cnur.2016.05.006.
10. McKinney S, Feeser DL. *Fact Sheet: How Does a Wound, Ostomy and Continence Nurse Fit into Your Palliative/Hospice Team?* Wound, Ostomy and Continence Nurses Society; 2013. Accessed December 12, 2022. https://cdn.ymaws.com/member.wocn.org/resource/resmgr/document_library/How_WOC_Nurse_Fit_into_Palli.pdf.
11. Wound, Ostomy and Continence Nurses Society. *Scope and Standards of Practice.* 2nd ed. WOCN National Office; 2018.
12. Dahlin CM. *Palliative Nursing: Scope and Standards of Practice.* 6th ed. American Nurses Association; 2021.
13. Alvarez O, Kalimski C, Nusbaum J, et al. Incorporating wound healing strategies to improve palliation (symptom management) in patients with chronic wounds. *J Palliat Med.* 2007;10:1158–1189. https://doi.org/10.1089/jpm.2007.9909.
14. Maurer DM, Raymond TJ, Davis BN. Depression: screening and diagnosis. *Am Fam Physician.* 2018;98(8):508–515.
15. Locke AB, Kirst N, Shultz CG. Diagnosis and management of generalized anxiety disorder and panic disorder in adults. *Am Fam Physician.* 2015;91(9):617–624.
16. Blaber M, Jone J, Willis D. Spiritual care: which is the best assessment tool for palliative settings? *Int J Palliat Nurs.* 2015;21(9):430–438. https://doi.org/10.12968/ijpn.2015.21.9.430.
17. Levine JM, Delmore B, Cox J. Skin failure: concept review and proposed model. *Adv Skin Wound Care.* 2022;35(3):139–148. https://doi.org/10.1097/01.ASW.0000818572.31307.7b.
18. Sibbald RG, Krasner DL, Lutz J. SCALE: Skin changes at life's end: final consensus statement: October 1, 2009. *Adv Skin Wound Care.* 2010;23:225–236. https://doi.org/10.1097/01.ASW.0000363537.75328.36.
19. Langemoe DK, Brown G. Skin fails too: acute, chronic, and end-stage skin failure. *Adv Skin Wound.* 2006;19(4):206–211. https://doi.org/10.1097/00129334-200605000-00014.
20. Delmore B, Cox J, Rolnitzky L, Chu A, Stolfi A. Differentiating a pressure ulcer from acute skin failure in the adult critical care patient. *Adv Skin Wound.* 2015;28(11):484–494. https://doi.org/10.1097/01.ASW.0000471876.11836.dc.

21. Levine JM. Historical perspective on pressure ulcers: the decubitus ominosus of Jean-Martin Charcot. *J Am Geriatr Soc.* 2005;53(7):1248–1251. https://doi.org/10.1111/j.1532-5415.2005.53358.x.
22. Latimer S, Walker, RM, Ray-Barruel G, et al. Defining and describing terminal ulcers in adults at end of life: an integrative review. *Adv Skin Wound.* 2022;35(4):225–233. https://doi.org/10.1097/01.ASW.0000798032.98853.95.
23. Schmitt S, Andries MK, Ashmore PM, Brunette G, Judge K. *WOCN Society Position Paper: Avoidable versus Unavoidable Pressure Ulcers (Injuries).* Wound, Ostomy and Continence Nurses Society; 2017.
24. Sarabia-Cobo CM. Poly ulceration patient terminal: Kennedy terminal ulcer (KTU). *J Palliat Care Med.* 2017;7(1):297. https://doi.org/10.4172/2165-7386.1000297.
25. Brennan MR, Thomas L, Kline M. Prelude to death or practice failure? Trombley-Brennan terminal tissue injury update. *Am J Hosp Palliat Med.* 2019;36(11):1016–1019. https://doi.org/10.1177/1049909119838969.
26. Black JM, Edsberg LE, Baharestani MM, et al. Pressure ulcers: avoidable or unavoidable? Results of the National Pressure Ulcer Advisory Panel consensus conference. *Ostomy Wound Manage.* 2011;49(2):24–37. https://pubmed.ncbi.nlm.nih.gov/21350270/.
27. Levine JM, Humphrey S, Lebovits S, Fogel J. The unavoidable pressure ulcer: a retrospective case series. *J Clin Outcomes Manag.* 2009;16(8):1–5.
28. McIntyre L, May R, Marks-Maran D. A strategy to reduce avoidable pressure ulcers. *Nurs Times.* 2012;108(29):14–17.
29. Cox J, Roche S. Vasopressors and development of pressure ulcers in adult critical care patients. *Am J Crit Care.* 2015;24(6):501–510.
30. Cox J, Schallom M. Pressure injuries in critical care: a survey of critical care nurses. *Crit Care Nurse.* 2017;37(5):46–55.
31. Lyder CH, Wang Y, Metersky M, et al. Hospital-acquired pressure ulcers: results from the national Medicare patient safety monitoring system study. *J Am Geriatr Soc.* 2012;57(9):1573–1578.
32. National Pressure Injury Advisory Panel. Unavoidable Pressure Injury during COVID-19 Pandemic: A Position Paper from the National Pressure Injury Advisory Panel. 2020. Accessed December 27, 2022. https://cdn.ymaws.com/npiap.com/resource/resmgr/white_papers/Unavoidable_in_COVID_Pandemi.pdf.
33. Woo KY, Krasner DL, Kennedy B, Wardle D, Moir O. Palliative wound care management strategies for palliative patients and their circles of care. *Adv Skin Wound Care.* 2015; 28(3):130–140.
34. Tilley CP, Fu MR, Van Cleave JH, Crocilla BL, Comfort CP. Symptoms of malignant fungating wounds and functional performance among patients with advanced cancer: an integrative review from 2000 to 2019. *J Palliat Med.* 2020;23(6):848–862. https://doi.org/10.1089/jpm.2019.0617.
35. Woo K, Sibbald G, Fogh K, et al. Assessment and management of persistent (chronic) and total wound pain. *Int Wound J.* 2008;5(2):205–215. https://doi.org/10.1111/j.1742-481X.2008.00483.x.
36. Price P, Fogh K, Glynn C, et al. Managing painful chronic wounds: the wound pain management model. *Int Wound J.* 2007;4(suppl 1):4–15. https://doi.org/10.1111/j.1742-481X.2007.00311.x.
37. Maida V, Ennis M, Kuziemsky C, Trozzolo L. Symptoms associated with malignant wounds: a prospective case series. *J Pain Symptom Manage.* 2009;37: 206–211. https://doi.org/10.1016/j.jpainsymman.2008.01.009.
38. Tamai N, Mugita Y, Ikeda M, Sanada H. The relationship between malignant wound status and pain in breast cancer patients. *Eur J Oncol Nurs.* 2016;24:8–12. https://doi.org/10.1016/j.ejon.2016.05.004.
39. Adeyi A, Muzerengi S, Gupta I. Leg ulcers in older people: a review of management. *Br J Med Practit.* 2009;2(3):21–28.
40. McNichol LL, Ratliff C, Yates S. *Wound Ostomy and Continence Nurses Society Core Curriculum: Wound Management.* 2nd ed. Wolters Kluwer; 2021.
41. Mehta A, Chan L. Understanding of the concept of "total pain." *J Hosp Palliat Nurs.* 2008;10(1):26–32. https://doi.org/10.1097/01.NJH.0000306714.50539.1a.
42. Walsh A, Bradley M, Cavallito K. Management of fungating tumors and pressure ulcers in a patient with stage IV cutaneous malignant melanoma. *J Hosp Palliat Nurs.* 2014;16(4):208–214. https://doi.org/10.1097/njh.0000000000000059.
43. Parnell L. Itching for knowledge about wound and scar pruritus. *Wounds.* 2018;30(1):17–26.
44. Twycross R, Greaves MW, Handwerker H, et al. Itch: scratching more than the surface. *J Wound Care.* 2013;22(9):501–508. https://doi.org/10.1093/qjmed/hcg002.
45. Paul J. Characteristics of chronic wounds that itch. *Adv Skin Wound Care.* 2013;26(7):320–332. https://doi.org/10.1097/01.ASW.0000431203.64591.2f.
46. Stansal A, Lazareth I, Pasturel UM, et al. Compression therapy in 100 consecutive patients with venous leg ulcers. *J Mal Vasc.* 2013;38(4):252–258. https://doi.org/10.1016/j.jmv.2013.05.006.
47. Gray M, Bliss DZ, McNichol L. Moisture-associated skin damage. *J Wound Ostomy Continence Nurs.* 2022;49(2):143–151. https://doi.org/10.1097/WON.0000000000000865.
48. Beitz J. Wound debridement: therapeutic options and care considerations. *Nurs Clin North Am.* 2005;40:233–249. https://doi.org/10.1016/j.cnur.2004.09.004.
49. Barrett S. Wound-bed preparation: a vital step in the healing process. *Br J Nurs.* 2017;26(12):S24–S31. https://doi.org/10.12968/bjon.2017.26.12.S24.
50. Harries RL, Bosanquet DC, Harding KG. Wound bed preparation: TIME for an update. *Int Wound J.* 2016;13(S3):8–14. https://doi.org/10.1111/iwj.12662.
51. Probst S, Arber A, Faithfull S. Coping with an ulcerative breast carcinoma: an interpretive phenomenological study. *J Wound Care.* 2013;22:349–357. https://doi.org/10.12968/jowc.2013.22.7.352.
52. Probst S, Arber A, Faithfull S. Malignant fungating wounds: the meaning of living in an unbounded body. *Eur J Oncol Nurs.* 2013;17:38–42. https://doi.org/10.1016/j.ejon.2012.02.001.
53. Reynolds H, Gethin G. The psychological effects of malignant fungating wounds. *EWMS J.* 2015;15:29–32.
54. Lawton J. Contemporary hospice care: the sequestration of the unbounded body and "dirty dying." *Sociol Health Illn.* 1998;20:121–140. https://doi.org/10.1111/1467-9566.00094.
55. Fu M, Ridner SH, Hu SH, Stewart BR, Cormier JN, Armer JM. Psychosocial impact of lymphedema: a systematic review of literature from 2004–2011. *Psychol Oncol.* 2013;22:1466–1484. https://doi.org/10.1002/pon.3201.
56. Gray M, Black JM, Baharestani MM, et al. Moisture-associated skin damage: overview and pathophysiology. *J Wound Ostomy Continence Nurs.* 2011;38(3):233–241. https://doi.org/10.1097/WON.0b013e318215f798.
57. Tilley CP, Fu MR, Qiu JM, et al. The microbiome and metabolome of malignant fungating wounds: a systematic review of the literature from 1995 to 2020. *J Wound Ostomy Continence Nurs.* 2021;48(2):124–135. https://doi.org/10.1097/WON.0000000000000749.

58. Tamai N, Akase T, Minematsu T, et al. Association between components of exudates and periwound moisture-associated dermatitis in breast cancer patients with malignant fungating wounds. *Biol Res Nurs*. 2016;18(2):199–206. https://doi.org/10.1177/1099800415594452.
59. Schuren J, Becker A, Sibbald RA. Liquid film-forming acrylate for peri-wound protection: a systematic review and meta-analysis (3M Cavilon no-sting barrier film). *Int Wound J*. 2005;2:230–238. https://doi.org/10.1111/j.1742-4801.2005.00131.x.
60. Colwell JC, Ratliff CR, Goldberg M, et al. MASD part 3: peristomal-moisture-associated dermatitis and periwound moisture-associated dermatitis. *J Wound Ostomy Continence Nurs*. 2011;38(5):511–550. https://doi.org/10.1097/WON.0b013e31822acd95.
61. Fumarola S, Allaway R, Callaghan R, et al. International consensus document: overlooked and underestimated: medical adhesive-related skin injuries. *J Wound Care*. 2020;29(suppl 3c):S1–S24. https://doi.org/10.12968/jowc.2020.29.Sup3c.S1.
62. National Pressure Ulcer Advisory Panel. National Pressure Ulcer Advisory Panel (NPUAP) Announces a Change in Terminology from Pressure Ulcer to Pressure Injury and Updates the Stages of Pressure Injury. 2016. Accessed December 18, 2022. doi:10.1097/WON.0000000000000281. https://pmc.ncbi.nlm.nih.gov/articles/PMC5098472/.
63. Pittman J, Gillespie C. Medical device–related pressure injuries. *Crit Care Nurs Clin North Am*. 2020;32:533–542. https://doi.org/10.1016/j.cnc.2020.08.004.
64. Edsberg L, Black J, Goldberg M, et al. Revised National Pressure Ulcer Advisory Panel pressure injury staging system. *J Wound Ostomy Continence Nurs*. 2016;43(6):585–597. https://doi.org/10.1097/WON.0000000000000281.
65. National Pressure Ulcer Advisory Panel. Pressure Injury Staging Illustrations. 2016. Accessed December 20, 2022. http://www.npuap.org/resources/educational-and-clinical-resources/pressure-injury-staging-illustrations/.
66. Wound, Ostomy and Continence Nurses Society-Wound Guidelines Task Force. WOCN 2016 guideline for prevention and management of pressure injuries (ulcers). *J Wound Ostomy Continence Nurs*. 2017;41(3):241–246. https://doi.org/10.1097/WON.0000000000000321.
67. Langemo D, Haesler E, Naylor W, Tippett A, Young T. Evidence-based guidelines for pressure ulcer management at the end of life. *Int J Palliat Nurs*. 2015;21(5):225–232. https://doi.org/10.12968/ijpn.2015.21.5.225.
68. Langemo DK, Black J. Pressure ulcers in individuals receiving palliative care: a national Pressure Ulcer Advisory Panel white paper. *Adv Skin Wound Care*. 2010;23(2):59–72. https://doi.org/10.1097/01.ASW.0000363502.84737.c8.
69. Norton D. Calculating the risk: reflections on the Norton scale. *Decubitus*. 1989;2:24–31.
70. Bergstrom N, Demuth PJ, Braden BJ. A clinical trial of the Braden Scale for predicting pressure sore risk. *Nurs Clin North Am*. 1987;22:417–28.
71. Chaplin J. Pressure sore risk assessment in palliative care. *J Tissue Viability*. 2000;10(1):27–31. https://doi.org/10.1016/s0965-206x(00)80017-0.
72. Henoch I, Gustafsson M. Pressure ulcers in palliative care: development of a hospice pressure ulcer risk assessment scale. *Int J Palliat Care*. 1994;11(6):14–19. https://doi.org/10.12968/ijpn.2003.9.11.11872.
73. Van Tiggelen H, Kottner J, Campbell K, et al. Measurement properties of classifications for skin tears: a systematic review. *Int J Nurs Stud*. 2020;110:12–13. https://doi.org/10.1016/j.ijnurstu.2020.103694.
74. Strazzieri-Pulido K, Pilolo Peres G, Faustino Campanili T, Gouvela Santos, V. Incidence of skin tears and risk factors: a systematic review. *J Wound Ostomy Continence Nurs*. 2017;44(1):29–33. https://doi.org/10.1097/WON.0000000000000288.
75. Serra R, Ielapi N, Barbetta A, Franciscis SD. Skin tears and risk factors assessment: a systematic review on evidence-based medicine. *Int Wound J*. 2017;15(1):38–42. https://doi.org/10.1111/iwj.12815.
76. Stephen-Haynes J, Deeth M. The prevention, assessment and management of skin tears. *Pract Nurse*. 2016;46(6):32–37.
77. Baranoski S, LeBlanc K, Gloeckner M. Preventing, assessing, and managing skin tears: a clinical review. *Am J Nurs*. 2016;116(11):24–30. https://doi.org/10.1097/01.NAJ.0000505581.01967.75.
78. LeBlanc K, Woo K, Christensen D, et al. *Best Practice Recommendations for the Prevention and Management of Skin Tears. Foundations of Best Practice for Skin and Wound Management*. Wounds Canada; 2018. Accessed November 30, 2022. https://www.woundscanada.ca/docman/public/health-care-professional/bpr-workshop/552-bpr-prevention-and-management-of-skin-tears/file.
79. Neschis DG, Hasan HD, Golden MA. Management of Chronic Limb-Threatening Ischemia. UptoDate. November 2022. Accessed December 29, 2022. https://www.uptodate.com/contents/management-of-chronic-limb-threatening-ischemia.
80. Buttolph A, Sapra A. Gangrene. In: *StatPearls*. StatPearls Publishing; 2022.
81. Williams RL. Cadexomer iodine: an effective palliative dressing in chronic critical limb ischemia. *Wounds*. 2009;21(1):1–7.
82. Armstrong DG, Bohn G, Glat P, et al. Expert recommendations for the use of hypochlorous solution: science and clinical application. *Ostomy Wound Manage*. 2015;58(5):S2–S19.
83. Alexander S. Malignant fungating wounds: epidemiology, aetiology, presentation and assessment. *J Wound Care*. 2009;18:273–280. https://doi.org/10.12968/jowc.2009.18.7.43110.
84. Grocott P, Gethin G, Probst S. Malignant wound management in advanced illness: new insights. *Curr Opin Support Palliat Care*. 2013;7:101–105. https://doi.org/10.1097/SPC.0b013e32835c0482.
85. Lookingbill DP, Spangler N, Helm KF. Cutaneous metastases in patients with metastatic carcinoma: a retrospective study of 4020 patients. *J Am Acad Dermatol*. 1993;29:228–236. https://doi.org/10.1016/0190-9622(93)70173-q.
86. Wu JJ, Huang DB, Pang KR, Tyring SK. Cutaneous metastasis to the chest wall from prostate cancer. *Int J Dermatol*. 2006;42:946–948. https://doi.org/10.1111/j.1365-4632.2004.02503.x.
87. Fyrmpas G, Barbetakis N, Efstathiou A, Konstantinidis I, Tsilikas C. Cutaneous metastasis to the face from colonadeno carcinoma. Case report. *Int Semin Surg Oncol*. 2006;3:2. https://doi.org/10.1186/1477-7800-3-2.
88. Saeed S, Keehn CA, Morgan MB. Cutaneous metastasis: a clinical, pathological, and immunohistochemical appraisal. *J Cutaneous Pathol*. 2004;31:419–430. https://doi.org/10.1111/j.0303-6987.2004.00207.x.
89. Alexander S. Malignant fungating wounds: key symptoms and psychosocial issues. *J Wound Care*. 2009b;18:325–329. https://doi.org/10.12968/jowc.2009.18.8.43631.
90. Carville K. *Wound Care Manual*. 5th ed. Silver Chain Nursing Association; 2005.

91. Probst S, Arber A, Faithfull S. Malignant fungating wounds: a survey of nurses' clinical practice in Switzerland. *Eur J Oncol Nurs.* 2009;13:295–298. https://doi.org/10.1016/j.ejon.2009.03.008.
92. Adderley U, Smith R. Topical agents and dressings for fungating wounds. *Cochrane Database Syst Rev.* 2007;2:CD003948. https://doi.org/10.1002/14651858.CD003948.pub2.
93. Kalemikerakis J. Comparison of foam dressings with silver versus foam dressings without silver in the care of malodorous malignant fungating wounds. *J BUON.* 2012;17(3):560–4.
94. Choa R, Rayatt S, Mahtani K. Marjolin's ulcer. *BMJ.* 2015;351:h3997. https://doi.org/10.1136/bmj.h3997.
95. Tobin C, Sanger JR. Marjolin's ulcers: a case series and literature review. *Wounds.* 2014;26(9):248–251.
96. Bowers RF, Young JM. Carcinoma arising in scars, osteomyelitis, and fistulae. *Arch Surg.* 1960;80:564–570. https://doi.org/10.1001/archsurg.1960.01290210032006.
97. Bazaliński D, Przybek-Mita J, Barańska B, Więch P. Marjolin's ulcer in chronic wounds—review of available literature. *Contemp Oncol (Pozn).* 2017;21(3):197–202. https://doi.org/10.5114/wo.2017.70109.
98. Pekarek B, Buck S, Osher L. A comprehensive review on Marjolin's ulcers: diagnosis and treatment. *J Am Coll Clin Wound Spec.* 2011;3(3):57–61. https://doi.org/10.1016/j.jcws.2012.04.001.
99. Chang JJ. Calciphylaxis: diagnosis, pathogenesis, and treatment. *Adv Skin Wound Care.* 2019;32(5):205–215. https://doi.org/10.1097/01.ASW.0000554443.14002.13.
100. Famorca M, Beauchaine D, Angulo N. Management of complex peristomal calciphylaxis. *J Wound Ostomy Continence Nurs.* 2017;41(4):380–383. https://doi.org/10.1097/WON.0000000000000343.
101. Hegedus F, Mathew LM, Schwartz RA. Radiation dermatitis: an overview. *Int J Dermatol.* 2017;56(9):909–914. https://doi.org/10.1111/ijd.13371.
102. Rosenthal A, Israilevich R, Moy R. Management of acute radiation dermatitis: a review of the literature and proposal for treatment algorithm. *J Am Acad Dermatol.* 2019;81(2):558–567. https://doi.org/10.1016/j.jaad.2019.02.047.
103. Singh M, Alavi A, Wong R, Akita S. Radiodermatitis: a review of our current understanding. *Am J Clin Dermatol.* 2016;17:277–292. https://doi.org/10.1007/s40257-016-0186-4.
104. Patel V, McGurk M. Use of pentoxifylline and tocopherol in radiation-induced fibrosis and fibroatrophy. *Br J Oral Maxillofac Surg.* 2017;55(3):235–241. https://doi.org/10.1016/j.bjoms.2016.11.323.
105. World Health Organization. COVID-19 Pandemic. 2022. Accessed December 29, 2022. https://www.who.int/emergencies/diseases/novel-coronavirus-2019.
106. Pontieri-Lewis V, Emmons KR, Scardillo J, et al. COVID-19 skin manifestations: a guide for WOC nursing practice. *J Wound Ostomy Continence Nurs.* 2021;48(5):410–414. https://doi.org/10.1097/WON.0000000000000809.
107. Beuscher TL, Andrews SE. What are COVID toes? A case study. *J Wound Ostomy Continence Nurs.* 2020;47(6):619–621. https://doi.org/10.1097/WON.0000000000000711.
108. Singh C, Tay J, Shoqirat N. Skin and mucosal damage in patients diagnosed with COVID-19: a case report. *J Wound Ostomy Continence Nurs.* 2020;47(5):435–438. https://doi.org/10.1097/WON.0000000000000690.
109. Wound Ostomy and Continence Nursing Society. WOCN Society clinical guideline: management of the adult patient with a fecal or urinary ostomy—an executive summary. *J Wound Ostomy Continence Nurs.* 2018;42(1):50–58. https://doi.org/10.1097/WON.0000000000000396.
110. Carmel JE, Colwell JC, Goldberg MT. *Wound Ostomy and Continence Nurses Society Core Curriculum: Ostomy Management.* 2nd ed. Wolters Kluwer; 2021.
111. Flick V, Woodward S. Teaching tool for the blind or partially sighted. *WCET.* 2000;20:22–23.
112. Hayes MT. Parkinson's disease and parkinsonism. *Am J Med.* 2019:132:802–807. https://doi.org/10.1016/j.amjmed.2019.03.001.
113. Olek MJ. Multiple sclerosis. *Ann Intern Med.* 2021;174(6):ITC81–ITC96. https://doi.org/10.7326/AITC202106150.
114. Hulisz D. Amyotrophic lateral sclerosis: disease state overview. *Am J Manag Care.* 2018;24(15 suppl):S320–S326.
115. Le Danseur M. Stroke rehabilitation. *Crit Care Nurs Clin North Am.* 2020;32(1):97–108. https://doi.org/10.1016/j.cnc.2019.11.004
116. Eisen A. Anatomy and Localization of Spinal Cord Disorders. UpToDate. Updated February 2022. Accessed January 7, 2023. www.uptodate.com/contents/anatomy-and-localization-of-spinal-cord-disorders.
117. Rutkove SB. Overview of Polyneuropathy. UpToDate. Updated February 2022. Accessed January 7, 2023. https://www.uptodate.com/contents/search?search=peripheral%20neuropathy.
118. England BR. Clinical Manifestations of Rheumatoid Arthritis. UptoDate. Updated May, 2022. Accessed January 5, 2023. https://www.uptodate.com/contents/clinical-manifestations-of-rheumatoid-arthritis
119. Wound, Ostomy Continence Nurses Society. *Peristomal Skin Assessment Guide for Consumers.* Accessed March 31, 2020. https://www.wocn.org/what-is-the-peristomal-skin-assessment-guide-for-consumers-and-who-can-benefit-from-it/
120. Wound, Ostomy Continence Nurses Society. *Stoma Complications: Best Practice for Clinicians.* Wound, Ostomy Continence Nurses Society; 2014.
121. Baker Rogers J, Syed K, Minteer JF. Cachexia. In. *StatPearls.* StatPearls; 2022. Accessed December 27, 2022. https://www.ncbi.nlm.nih.gov/books/NBK470208/.
122. Rao NAR. Caput medusae. *ANZ J Surg.* 2022;92(6):1569. https://doi.org/10.1111/ans.17347.
123. Evans M, Anders T. Chronic enterocutaneous fistula: management in the community setting. *Br J Nurs.* 2020;29(12):S38–S42. https://doi.org/10.12968/bjon.2020.29.12.S38.
124. Haack CI, Galloway JR, Srinivasan J. Enterocutaneous fistulas: a look at causes and management. *Curr Surg Rep.* 2014;2:71. https://link.springer.com/content/pdf/10.1007%2Fs40137-014-0071-0.pdf.
125. Wainstein DE, Tungler V, Ravazzola C, Chara O. Management of external small bowel fistulae: challenges and controversies confronting the general surgeon. *Int J Surg.* 2011;9:198–203. https://doi.org/10.1016/j.ijsu.2010.11.009.
126. Hollister Education. Ostomy Care Tips: Fistula Management. Updated 2017. Accessed December 26, 2022. https://www.hollister.com/-/media/files/hollister-clinical-education/hollister-ostomy-care-tip-fistula-management-us-00222.ashx.

127. Seaman S, Bates-Jensen BM. Skin disorders: malignant wounds, fistulas, and stomas. In: Ferrell BR, Coyle N, Paice J, eds. *Oxford Textbook of Palliative Nursing*. 4th ed. Oxford University Press; 2010:325–340.
128. Willcutts K, Mercer D, Zielgler J. Fistuloclysis: an interprofessional approach to nourishing the fistula patient. *J Wound Ostomy Continence Nurs.*2015;39(5):519–550. https://doi.org/10.1097/WON.0000000000000166.
129. Stevens P, Foulkes RE, Hartford-Beynon JS, Delicata R. Systematic review and meta-analysis of the role of somatostatin analogues in the treatment of enterocutaneous fistula. *Eur J Gastroenterol Hepatol.* 2011;23:912–922. https://doi.org/10.1097/MEG.0b013e32834a345d.
130. Gribovskaja-Rupp I, Melton GB. Enterocutaneous fistula: proven strategies and updates. *Clin Colon Rectal Surg.* 2016;29:130–137. https://doi.org/10.1055/s-0036-1580732.
131. Gray M, Giuliano KK. Incontinence-associated dermatitis, characteristics and relationship to pressure injury: a multisite epidemiologic analysis. *J Wound Ostomy Continence Nurs.* 2018;45(1):63–67. https://doi.org/10.1097/WON.0000000000000390.
132. Ermer-Seltun J, Engberg S. *Wound Ostomy and Continence Nurses Society Core Curriculum: Continence Management*, 2nd ed. Wolters Kluwer; 2021.

21

Pruritus, Fever, and Sweats

Angel Smothers, Amanda Kitzmiller, and Diana Niland

Key Points

- Pruritus, fever, and sweats can decrease the quality of life for a patient living with a serious chronic illness.
- Both nonpharmacological and pharmacological interventions could improve these symptoms for patients.
- The underlying pathophysiology for all three symptoms is multifaceted and complicated.

Introduction

In this chapter, emphasis will be placed on three of the symptoms that are commonly seen in patients who are living with a serious chronic illness. Symptom presentation is unique in each patient and can occur individually but also can occur simultaneously.[1] By having a strong knowledge base of the underlying reasons for a symptom, the nurse can help select the best treatment option that will also result in the least number of negative sequelae. Each common symptom—pruritus, fever, and sweats—will be examined individually and then collectively at the end of the chapter. Pruritus is defined as an unpleasant sensation that triggers the need for a mechanical response such as scratching, rubbing, or pressure. Fever has been defined as an elevation of body temperature that is mediated by the hypothalamus in response to exogenous pyrogens and pyrogenic cytokines. Sweats, also known as perspiration, occur when secretions are excreted through sweat glands in the skin. These symptoms that are experienced by patients who are living with a serious chronic illness can vary depending on the diagnosis as well as treatment plan for their diagnosis.[1,2] There are times when symptoms result from a disease, but there are also times when they occur as a side effect of a medication or other treatment modality. Because each patient's response to a serious chronic illness is unique, it is important to have a broad understanding of what the research shows as being effective in the management of symptoms.

Pruritus

Pruritus is estimated to occur in 6% of the palliative care population.[3] Research suggests that smoking and excessive drinking are possible risk factors for pruritus.[3] Pruritus is considered chronic when lasting 6 weeks or longer.[4] This sensation can negatively impact quality of life (QOL) and impair sleep.[5] Pruritus is not a disease but instead a symptom of a disease or of an alteration of physiological functioning of one or more of the body's regulatory systems. Common underlying triggers for pruritus include alteration of liver or biliary duct function, alteration in urinary secretory function, malignancy, human immune deficiency virus (HIV), and medications.[6] Pruritus can further be classified as either peripheral (prurioreceptive) or central (neuropathic). When considering a peripheral cause, the nurse might identify sources such as dermatitis, insect bites, or other skin reactions that could result in itch. On the other hand, with neuropathic causes, identifying the source of the pruritus by nursing assessment is often more difficult. With a neuropathic cause, the underlying source is often renal, biliary, hepatic, or malignancy-related.[5,6] There are additional sources of pruritus, with none of the sources being fully understood. Each of the potential sources will be reviewed in the following sections.

Nursing Assessment of Pruritus

Nursing assessment of a patient with the complaint of "itching" will focus on different aspects using the assessment process. The nurse should start with an assessment of the patient's subjective complaint. This might include the patient explaining in their own words the sensation they are experiencing. Then, the nurse should ask probing questions, such as How long has this been happening? When did this start? Is there anything that makes it worse or better? Has this happened before? Have you used any new soaps or laundry detergents? If so, what helped relieve it?

Next, the nurse should visually assess the areas where the patient is complaining of an itch. Often the sensation is generalized, and the patient is not able to pinpoint a location.[7] The nurse should assess for peripheral or dermatological sources of the itch, including rash, dry skin, or erythema. Afterward, the nurse should discuss with the patient their past medical history to include medications, recent changes in the treatment plan, or past medical diagnoses. Collecting as much information as possible on the patient's complaint will allow for a thorough report to the practitioner who will be potentially prescribing medication or other treatments for the patient.[8]

Case Study: A Hemodialysis Patient with Pruritus

Sam is a 76-year-old patient who was admitted to the hospital post-hemodialysis after a significant drop in blood pressure and heart rate. Sam has a long-term history of the following medical diagnoses: diabetes, hypertension, congestive heart failure, hyperlipidemia, and anxiety disorder. Sam has been receiving hemodialysis 3 days a week for the past 4 years, after developing end-stage renal disease (ESRD) related to long-term uncontrolled diabetes. Sam has a family history of Type 2 diabetes and has struggled since the age of 38 with managing blood glucose levels. During a recent hospital stay, Sam developed severe pruritus and multiple skin abrasions resulting from constant scratching. Sam stated the symptoms were causing great distress and were altering their QOL due to lack of sleep.

The nurse consulted the palliative care team at the hospital where the patient was staying, and the following treatment plan was developed.

1. The underlying source of pruritus was most likely uremic in nature. Patient and family were provided education on this as the potential source of the itching.
2. Nonpharmacological interventions that are supported in the literature were implemented and included cool baths, aloe vera gel, and phototherapy. Medications that are supported in the literature as being helpful in the management of pruritus were reviewed. See Table 21.1.
3. After review of patient's current medication list, which already included gabapentin, it was determined the next medication to try would be cromolyn sodium.

Sam was started on the nonpharmacological interventions as well as on cromolyn sodium and reported improvement in symptoms within 24 hours.

Nonpharmacological Treatment for Pruritus of Varying Origin

Research supports the use of nonpharmacological treatments as a part of a treatment plan for pruritus of any origin. Nonpharmacological treatments shown to be effective in the management of pruritus utilizing skin application include baby oil, aqueous gel with aloe vera, lotion with mud from the Dead Sea, and cream containing sericin.[9,10] There is some evidence to support the effectiveness of phototherapy, which involves an ultraviolet lamp; acupuncture by a trained acupuncturist; and thermal therapy using far-infrared radiation as nonpharmacological treatments for pruritus.[11] Transcutaneous electronic nerve stimulation units have some research support as an effective option for nonpharmacological management of pruritus of varying origins.[12] Nursing interventions that could be utilized to improve comfort for patients who experience pruritus include the following: using lukewarm water for bathing, light cotton bedding and clothing, long-sleeved shirts, short fingernails, and a cool fan.[9,10]

Pharmacological Management of Pruritus of Varying Origins

Pruritus management in palliative care patients can be difficult due to the multiple underlying mechanisms that could be linked to the symptoms. The treatment plan is individualized since there could be overlapping reasons for the symptoms. Therefore, understanding medications that could help manage pruritus in the palliative care population is important. Table 21.1 shows classes of medications that have some research to support them as potential treatment options for patients with varying underlying reasons for pruritus.[13–15]

Pruritus of Uremic Origin

Uremic pruritus (UP) is a common symptom that has been reported in as many as 42%–75% of ESRD patients.[14] For patients who have been adequately dialyzed, the report is the same. UP can be acute, short-term, or chronic in duration.[11] The exact cause of UP is not well understood, but evidence supports the relationship between this symptom in ESRD patients and a chronic inflammatory response involving sensory neurons, specifically unmyelinated C fibers.[8] Some of these sensory nerves respond only to itch, while others respond to both pain and itch; thus, these systems are closely linked. Mediators that have been linked to this response include histamine, endogenous opioids, serotonin, serum thymus, and activation-regulated chemokine levels.[15]

Pharmacological Treatments for UP

Research has supported the effectiveness of pharmacological treatments in the management of pruritus. Because the underlying origins of pruritus are not well understood, the medications to treat it are based on potential underlying causes for the itching sensation in patients. Additional research is needed to assess effectiveness. There is evidence that the upper motor neuron system plays a role in the development of pruritus in renal failure.[16,17]

Gabapentin has been studied and identified as an effective treatment option for UP. Gabapentin is classified as an antiepileptic drug and has been successfully used for many years in the management of nerve-related symptoms including neuropathy, pain, and itch. Because there is a neuronal mechanism that has been identified as a potential source of pruritus, gabapentin has been studied and determined to be effective in managing UP.[5,8]

There is some evidence that mediators released from mast cells play a role in UP. Therefore, cromolyn sodium has been studied as a potential treatment for UP. This medication blocks mast cell degranulation and therefore leads to decreased release of histamine. A study identified a potential role for the medication sertraline in the management of UP. Other selective serotonin reuptake inhibitors have been researched and shown to be effective in UP but do require dose adjustment in ESRD. Sertraline appears to be a better option due to the limited need for dose adjustment with ESRD.[5,6]

Pruritus of Cholestatic Origin

Pharmacologic Treatments for Cholestatic Pruritus

The pathophysiological mechanism of cholestatic pruritus (CP) is still not well defined. Several hypotheses have been raised in the past. The most important one included the participation of bile acids and endogenous opioids.[19] There is evidence supporting the use of medications to mitigate pruritus in patients with CP (Table 21.1). Evidence supports the use of rifampin, which is a class of antibiotic, as a pharmacological treatment of pruritus. Because rifampin has been shown to induce detoxicating hepatic enzymes and, therefore, competitively inhibit the reuptake of bile acids, there is evidence to support that it would lead to a decreased rate of pruritus in patients with CP. In addition, flumecinol, which is a benzhydryl derivative,

Table 21.1 Medications indicated in the management of pruritus

Class of medication	Name of medication	Type of pruritus	Indication
Opioid antagonist[16]	Naltrexone (Revia, Vivitrol)	Cholestatic	Prevents the activation of spinal neurons that can lead to pruritus
K-opioid receptor agonist[16,17]	Nalfurafine hydrochloride (remitch): currently in clinical trials in the United States Approved for use in Japan	Uremic	Prevents the activation of spinal neurons that can lead to pruritus
Selective serotonin reuptake inhibitor[16,17]	Sertraline (Zoloft) Paroxetine (Paxil)	Pruritus of unknown origin	Increases the amounts of serotonin available extracellularly, which can then bind to the postsynaptic cleft, preventing transmission of the itch sensation
Antiepileptic[16,17]	Gabapentin (Neurontin) Pregabalin (Lyrica)	Uremic	May inhibit the transmission of nociceptive sensations to the brain, thereby suppressing pruritus
Antibiotics[16,17]	Rifampicin (Rifadin)	Cholestatic	May change the GI bacterial growth, which may influence the absorption of pruritogens
Immunomodulator[16,17]	Thalidomide (Thalomid)	All origins	May act as a peripheral and central nerve depressant
Benzhydryl derivative[16,17]	Flumecinol (Zixoryn)	Cholestatic	Has been shown to lower serum bilirubin
Anion exchange resin[16,17]	Cholestyramine (Questran)	Cholestatic	Interrupts the enterohepatic circulation of bile
Mast cell stabilizer[16,17]	Cromolyn sodium	All origins	Works by preventing the release of substances in the body that cause inflammation; has also been shown to reduce serum tryptase levels
Leukotriene modifier[16,17]	Montelukast (Singular)	All origins	Prevents the inflammatory response produced by leukotrienes
Hormone/glycoprotein[16,17]	Erythropoietin	All origins	May work to lower the effect of the hormone on plasma histamine concentrations
Binding agent[16,17]	Activated charcoal	Uremic	May work to bind the agents that lead to uremic pruritus
Topical antipruritic/ alkaloid[16,17]	Capsaicin (active component of chili peppers) Gamma-linolenic acid 2.2% cream	All origins	Targets the transient receptor potential vanilloid receptor and counteracts itch by activating pain neurons
Immunosuppressant/ calcineurin inhibitor[16,17]	Tacrolimus (Prograf)	All origins	Works by suppressing the differentiation of Th1 lymphocytes and ensuing interleukin-2 production
Local anesthetic[16]	Pramoxine hydrochloride (Caladryl)	All origins	May work by blocking sodium channels within the neuronal membrane, decreasing conduction
Vitamins/herbal[16]	Ergocalciferol (vitamin D_2, calciferol) Nicotinamide (niacinamide) Omega-3 fatty acids Turmeric (powder of *Curcuma longa* L.) Zinc sulfate	All origins	May have antipyretic effect in uremic causes of pruritus due to impaired vitamin D metabolism that can occur in dialysis patients. May have antipyretic effect through its anti-inflammatory and histamine release–blocking action Has been shown to reduce inflammation, free radicals, and leukotriene B 4 so could work in uremic pruritus Curcumin, a substance in turmeric, has an anti-inflammatory effect May act as an antagonist of calcium and prevents degranulation of mast cells
Monoclonal antibodies[18]	Dupilumab (Dupixent)	All origins	Is a human monoclonal antibody that blocks interleukin-4 and interleukin-13, therefore decreasing the sensation of itch
Antihistamine[18,21,22]	Hydroxyzine hydrochloride (Vistaril)	HIV origin	It helps treat itching by stopping the effects of a natural chemical in the body called histamine
Vasodilator/anti-inflammatory; phosphodiesterase inhibitor[18,21,22]	Pentoxifylline (Trental)	HIV origin	Improvement of red blood cell flexibility and platelet deaggregation contribute to the decrease in blood viscosity
Corticosteroid[18,21,22]	Triamcinolone (Kenalog)	HIV origin	Decreases inflammation
NSAID[18,21,22]	Indomethacin (Tivorbex)	HIV origin	Decreases inflammation
Opioid antagonist[18,23–25]	Naloxone (Narcan)	Opioid	Blocks the effect of the opioid
Opioid agonist-antagonist[18,23–25]	Nalbuphine (Nubain)	Opioid	Blocks the effect of the opioid

GI, gastrointestinal; NSAID, nonsteroidal anti-inflammatory drug.

has been shown to lower serum bilirubin levels and would limit the amount of pruritus in cholestatic cases.[20]

Naltrexone, an opioid antagonist, has indications based on evidence for the management of CP. A higher than usual dose may be indicated for better management; however, higher doses in a palliative care patient could bring about worsening pain, so its use would need to be individualized for each patient. There is limited support suggesting that the use of corticosteroids may have a potential benefit for CP. Research supports the use of ondansetron as a potentially effective management strategy for CP, but additional studies are needed to support this as a viable option.[19,20]

Pruritus of HIV: Origin and Pharmacologic Treatment

Pruritus in HIV patients can have varying and complicated underlying mechanisms. The prevalence of pruritus in this population can be as high as 45%. A significant percentage of pruritus in this population is cutaneous in nature.[21] Limited research, including studies that consist of small numbers of subjects, provides some support for medications in the pharmacological management of HIV-related pruritus (HIVP). Hydroxyzine HCl, an antihistamine, has demonstrated some effectiveness in the management of HIVP. The anti-inflammatory effect of pentoxifylline, indomethacin, and triamcinolone may have some impact on HIVP as well (Table 21.1).[21,22]

Opioid-Induced Pruritus: Origin and Pharmacologic Treatment

For patients who require opioids to manage pain or dyspnea, the risk of developing pruritus can be high. Although pruritus is common with opioid use, the intensity can range from mild to severe. In mild cases, patients may get relief with nonpharmacological treatment; but in more severe cases, pharmacological treatment may be indicated.[23] Pharmacologic treatments that have shown evidence to alleviate opioid-induced pruritus include naloxone and nalbuphine. The primary mediator of opioid-induced pruritus appears to be the central mu-opioid receptors. Therefore, these medications could decrease the prevalence and severity of pruritus from opioid treatment. Naloxone is an opioid antagonist and could therefore improve pruritus from opioid use but could also lead to worsening pain. The route of administration could also be a potential barrier to the use of naloxone as nasal spray must be maintained at room temperature to be effective; therefore, more evidence is needed regarding the benefits of naloxone. However, nalbuphine is a partial opioid antagonist and has been shown to treat opioid-induced pruritus more effectively than naloxone (Table 21.1).[24,25]

Fever

The underlying mechanism of fever can vary in individual patients, particularly in the palliative care population.[26,27] Fever can result in emergency department visits and hospitalization in patients receiving palliative care. Patients who exhibit an elevated temperature must be evaluated for the underlying source of the fever.[27] A fever of unknown origin (FUO) is generally defined as a clinically documented temperature of 101°F or higher on several occasions associated with an unrevealing diagnostic workup.[27] FUO can be broken down into five potential causative categories: infection, malignancies, noninfectious inflammatory disease, other miscellaneous causes, and undiagnosed illness.[28] The category of noninfectious inflammatory disease has been linked to potential causes such as vasculitis and autoimmune, rheumatic, and granulomatous disorders.

A complete history and physical exam are needed to identify the source of the fever. FUO in a patient with a malignant disease might be related to the malignancy or an underlying infection. Since not all patients are at the end of life, it is important to consider the stage of disease and the goals of care. Fever is a common occurrence during malignancy, especially during chemotherapy. There are times when the use of antibiotics would be of potential benefit for the patient receiving palliative care by relieving symptoms associated with other medical conditions, such as urinary tract infection. When this is the case, antibiotics could be offered to the patient as an option for palliation. This will help to reduce symptoms, improve the patient's QOL, and decrease hospitalization. In situations where the patient is actively dying, antibiotics would have no benefit and should be avoided except for patients who are neutropenic, immunocompromised, or critically ill.[27]

Consider the case of Jody, a 67-year-old with a diagnosis of stage IV non-small cell lung cancer; because of the advanced stage, Jody was not a candidate for surgery. Jody had received chemotherapy for the past 6 months, with the last treatment being a few days ago, yet recent scans revealed widespread metastases to bone, liver, and brain. Jody had been told by the oncologist that the treatment plan no longer includes chemotherapy. The patient was referred to hospice for home palliative care. Upon arrival at the home, the nurse found Jody's temperature to be 40°C. Jody was not experiencing chills and had no other complaints. The nurse's role in care of such patients, includes a thorough head-to-toe assessment and relaying of pertinent information concerning the patient's condition to the appropriate member of the healthcare team through collaboration.

Nursing Assessment and Diagnostic Evaluation of Fever

The nursing assessment in a patient with fever starts with the history of the fever, including history of travel, home and work environment, recent medication use including substance use, contact with animals or sick people, and family health history.[27] Collecting information such as when the fever started, how long it has been present, other related symptoms, and whether this has happened in the past could help with current and future management of the fever.[27] A physical assessment that includes auscultations of the lungs and heart, abdomen, lymph nodes, genitalia, skin assessment including any wounds, and assessment of edema and capillary refill could help the nurse to identify signs of infection or a source for the fever.[27] In collaborating with the healthcare team, the nurse reports, through situation, background, assessment and recommendation communication, pertinent details of the health history to the physician or advanced practice care provider and anticipates that diagnostic tests may be ordered. Potential diagnostic tests that might aid in identifying the source of the infection include complete blood count (CBC), erythrocyte sedimentation rate (ESR), C-reactive protein (CRP), tuberculin test, blood culture, antinuclear antibody (ANA), stool cultures, and spinal tap. If ESR or CRP levels are elevated and fever origin has not been identified, the clinician may consider fluorodeoxyglucose positron emission tomography scan. If these noninvasive tests do not reveal the source of the fever, then tissue biopsy may be considered due to the relatively high diagnostic yield.[27] As in the above-mentioned case of Jody, the patient's pain was managed by oral oxycodone/acetaminophen (Percocet) three or four tablets per day. The nurse reviewed the patient's past medical history and found diabetes, hypertension, and a smoking history of two packs per day for 50 years. Lab work demonstrated normal CBC, ANA, ESR, CRP, and blood cultures. In each individual case, the patient's overall status and goals of care should be considered before the more aggressive tests are planned. If FUO persists after initial workup, the clinician may consider referral to infectious disease, rheumatology, hematology or oncology.[27] The following question should be asked: Will the test change our plan for therapy?

Pharmacological Treatment Options for Fever

The use of an antipyretic medication such as acetaminophen, ibuprofen, or aspirin could be of benefit for the patient with a fever especially if the patient has comorbidities, such as coronary heart disease and respiratory disease.[29] In Jody's case, the nurse provided assessment data including updated lab work to the hospice medical director who was overseeing Jody's admission to hospice, noting that Jody had a chemo treatment a few days before. The patient confirmed sometimes having an elevated temperature after getting chemo. The patient was prescribed acetaminophen 500 mg every 6 hours for elevated temperature as needed. The nurse also asked the medical director to change the oxycodone/acetaminophen to oxycodone alone so as not to deliver doses of acetaminophen exceeding 2,000–3,000 mg/day. Jody took the acetaminophen for 24 hours, and the fever subsided.

Nonpharmacological Treatment Options for Fever

As stated above, the nurse's role in the care of a patient with fever includes assessing the patient, collaborating with the healthcare team, providing nursing interventions and patient education, and documenting within the electronic health record to ensure effective communication. When documenting, the nurse will also include the nonpharmacological interventions provided to the patient by the nurse. Nurses spend a lot of time providing care at the bedside and are essential in helping to normalize the patient's body temperature by providing appropriate nursing interventions, which include nonpharmacological interventions. Evidence for nonpharmacological management of fever goes back many years. Some of the evidence-based nonpharmacological treatments for fever I would like to see the active role of nurse in this nonpharm management come out a little stronger include fans, cool cloths to head and axilla, ice packs, drinking cool liquids, tepid water bath, changing clothes frequently, and other treatments including a cooling blanket.[30] Education of patients, family members, and caregivers concerning normal body temperature values, accompanying symptoms to be concerned about, and when to seek care should be performed by the nurse.[31]

Sweats

The human body contains between two and four million sweat glands that help to thermally regulate it.[32] These glands are subdivided into three different types: apocrine, eccrine, and apoeccrine.[33] Sweating results from thermal and emotional stimuli and physical exercise.[32] Thermoregulatory sweating is controlled by the sympathetic nervous system, cerebral cortex, and hypothalamus; and emotional sweating is controlled through the anterior cingulate cortex, hypothalamus, and limbic system.[33] Excessive sweating, referred to as "hyperhidrosis," can be generalized or focal.[33] When generalized, hyperhidrosis occurs in more than one location and can occur in any area where sweat glands are located. Focal hyperhidrosis is primarily seen in the face, palms, soles, and axillae.[34] In the palliative care population, sweating could be related to either an emotional cause or thermoregulation. Medications and/or medical conditions may cause sweating.[35] These causes may be seen in patients who are receiving palliative care. Since sweating often accompanies fever, many of the treatments for fever may also be used for patients who are experiencing sweating.[36]

Nursing Assessment of Sweats

The health history and nursing assessment of a patient who is experiencing sweating should focus on identifying the underlying cause.[35] Some data that should be collected during this health history include age at onset, distribution, frequency, temporal pattern, quantity, impact on daily activities, medical conditions, medications, family history, and related symptoms.[33,35] Understanding that there are both emotional and thermoregulatory factors involved can help the nurse to ask probing questions during the history. Because both the limbic system and the hypothalamus can be involved with sweating, there may be an underlying neurological issue that is leading to the sweating, which could mean the sweating is unrelated to any fever that the person may have. Some common neurological issues that often cause sweating include stroke, tumors, Parkinson's disease, neurologic lesions, psychiatric disorders, peripheral neuropathies, spinal cord injuries, and Arnold-Chiari malformations.[33,34] However, sweating could be linked to fever; therefore, when they are occurring together, the assessment should be made at the same time.[32] When the nurse is completing the physical assessment,[35] an assessment of the patient's comfort and QOL related to the sweating should also be evaluated.[35] Since sweat can create a moist environment and result in skin complications, such as infections, assessment of the skin and protection of the integrity of the skin are important and would be a nursing priority.[33]

Consider the case of Chris, a 43-year-old patient with a diagnosis of a malignant spinal cord lesion. The primary site of the malignancy had not been determined. The patient was being evaluated for symptom management by the acute care palliative care team. Chris complained of excess sweating of the palms and back of the neck for the past week. Chris stated it interfered with sleeping and verbalized feeling reluctant to leave the house because of the sweating. Chris reports trying to wear cool clothing and avoiding alcohol and spicy foods but with no relief from the sweating. On assessment, the patient had no fever and was alert, oriented, and ambulatory. The only other complaint was back pain around the lesion, which was controlled with oxycodone/acetaminophen.

Nonpharmacological Treatment Options for Sweating

For patients who are suffering with sweating, management should start with a conservative approach including modifications of lifestyle and behavior.[37] The nurse can provide patient education that wearing absorbent articles of clothing, such as undershirts, may improve QOL[35] and that sufficient hydration and ventilation, environmental temperature control, and loose articles of clothing made of cotton may provide some relief.[36] The nurse may also provide information regarding other nonpharmacological treatment options being offered to the patient and support the patient before, during, and/or after treatment. For example, the use of a technique called "iontophoresis" has patients immerse their hands and/or feet in water where a medical device is used to apply a low current of electricity.[35] The goal of this nonpharmacological treatment for sweating is to disrupt the ion transport in the secretory tangle of the sweat glands and is primarily effective for excessive sweating in the palms or feet. Acupuncture has also been shown to reduce sweating and improve overall feelings of well-being, anxiety, mood, and sleep.[38] Another potential treatment option is microwave therapy that targets and destroys sweat glands, providing a permanent reduction in sweating.[35] Sweating may also be reduced by fractionated microneedle radiofrequency in which radiofrequencies are applied to small needles placed under the skin.[34] More aggressive surgical options are available, such as an endoscopic thoracic sympathectomy, if the symptoms are distressing and altering the patient's QOL.[39] This procedure may result in the development of compensatory hyperhidrosis where sweating occurs in different areas of the body than prior to the procedure.[39] Surgical removal of the sweat glands in a focal region of excessive sweating is another aggressive treatment option, although this treatment has high rates of recurrence of sweating and complications.[34] Additional local surgical procedures may include curettage, liposuction, liposuction-curettage, limited skin excision, and laser therapy.[34,35] These procedures have high rates of recurrence of sweating, although they may reduce the sweating for several months.[34]

Pharmacological Treatment Options for Sweating

For patients who do not respond to nonpharmacological options, the use of medications may be of benefit. These medications vary in response rate and underlying reason for effectiveness. Topical antiperspirants containing aluminum salts, such as aluminum chloride, have been shown to be effective in focal areas of sweating through secretory cell destruction and sweat gland obstruction.[34] Nurses should educate patients using these prescription antiperspirants that they can dilute the solution if skin irritation occurs.[34] Clinical-strength over-the-counter antiperspirants have been shown to result in a decrease in sweating similar to that of prescription antiperspirants but with less irritation of the skin.[35] The injection of botulinum toxin has evidence to support its effectiveness in reducing focal sweating and improving QOL.[40] This inhibits the acetylcholine release from neurons innervating eccrine sweat glands, which will limit the secretory ability of these glands.[34] Patients should be informed that the results are temporary, usually lasting 6–9 months, and adverse effects may include bruising and pain at the site of injection and weakness of the muscles in the area of injection.[34] Oral or topical anticholinergic medications, including oral oxybutynin, oral methantheline bromide, and topical glycopyrrolate, have also been found to reduce sweating due to their drying effect.[40] However, due to this drying effect, the nurse should educate the patient that use of these medications may also result in a dry mouth, and additional possible adverse effects of these medications include sleepiness, tachycardia, blurred vision, urinary retention, constipation, and gastrointestinal symptoms.[34] When sweating is associated with fever, antipyretics such as paracetamol or nonsteroidal anti-inflammatory drugs may be used.[36] However, it should be noted that these medications can also cause sweating to worsen.[36] There is research that supports the use of antidepressants, such as amitriptyline and propantheline, and antipsychotics, such as olanzapine and thioridazine, for decreasing sweating in the palliative care patient.[36] Two additional medications, gabapentin and thalidomide, have been shown to be effective in reducing sweating.[36] Finally, in patients with cancer, some research has shown that cannabinoids, such as dronabinol, can decrease night sweats through cytokine activity modulation and hypothermia production, thereby improving QOL by reducing fatigue and anxiety, although the adverse effect of sedation may occur,[41] and palliative chemotherapy that results in tumor shrinking may reduce sweating.[41,42]

Consider again the case of Chris. The nurse's assessment findings were discussed with the palliative care team nurse practitioner to develop a treatment plan. Because of the lack of other related symptoms including fever, chills, signs of infection, or change in level of consciousness, the nurse practitioner felt the symptoms were neurologically linked. Since the sweating was focal in nature, the nurse practitioner prescribed a cream that included aluminum chloride 20%. The sweating lessened, and Chris returned to a regular routine with increased comfort leaving the house to walk in the neighborhood.

Conclusion

Patients who experience pruritus, fever, or sweating often report impaired QOL. For the patient receiving palliative care who may be approaching or currently is in the terminal phase of chronic illness, symptom management in a timely manner can be enhanced using evidence to guide practice. More research is needed to better understand the mechanisms of pruritus, fever, and sweating along with appropriate and effective interventions. This includes the need for improved research on the nonpharmacological interventions to treat these symptoms. The significance of these symptoms must not be underestimated in the patients who experience them. The nurse is the constant at the bedside no matter where that bedside may be. The nursing assessment is key in the success of a treatment plan for the patient. The nurse's role as manager and teacher cannot be stressed enough.

REFERENCES

1. National Coalition for Hospice and Palliative Care. National Consensus Project for Quality Palliative Care. 2020. https://www.nationalcoalitionhpc.org/ncp/.
2. Hospice and Palliative Nurses Association. 2022. https://advancingexpertcare.org/HPNA/HPNA/About_Us/About.aspx?hkey=63b4511d-eba6-4c88-b732-4685a5988b6d.
3. Chen S, Zhou F, Xiong Y. Prevalence and risk factors of senile pruritus: a systematic review and meta-analysis. *BMJ Open*. 2022;12(2):e051694. https://bmjopen.bmj.com/content/bmjopen/12/2/e051694.full.pd.
4. Agelopoulos K, Pereira MP, Wiegmann H, Ständer S. Cutaneous neuroimmune crosstalk in pruritus. *Trends Mol Med*. 2022;28(6):452–462. https://discovery.ebsco.com/linkprocessor/plink?id=bdb258af-eb09-3ebd-bbe1-ffd80a8e1351.

5. Kim D, Pollock C. Epidemiology and burden of chronic kidney disease–associated pruritus. *Clin Kidney J.* 2021;14:1–7. https://discovery.ebsco.com/linkprocessor/plink?id=8cf2839c-458c-360f-b10e-bdfe7ef95b66.
6. Sutaria N, Adawi W, Goldberg R, Roh YS, Choi J, Kwatra SG. Itch: pathogenesis and treatment. *J Am Acad Dermatol.* 2022;86(1):17–34. https://discovery.ebsco.com/linkprocessor/plink?id=9a07426a-d424-3f7f-92c4-11fe58b7a2ee.
7. Moosa AS, Leng NSY, Kum CL, Tan NC. A qualitative research study on the illness perception of chronic pruritus in older Asian adults based on the common-sense model of self-regulation. *Health Expect.* 2021;24(5):1801–1811. https://discovery.ebsco.com/linkprocessor/plink?id=44ace979-fa63-3533-86d1-d96f8112a918.
8. Cheng A-Y, Wong L-S. Uremic pruritus: from diagnosis to treatment. *Diagnostics.* 2022;12(5):1108. https://discovery.ebsco.com/linkprocessor/plink?id=c9c6f474-20ed-3dd6-8b02-546d90d11874.
9. Wu C-F, Hsiao Y-C, Ko P-C. The effects of nonpharmacological treatment on uremic pruritus patients: a systematic review. *Adv Nurs.* 2015;2015:1–9. https://discovery.ebsco.com/linkprocessor/plink?id=6946de21-c2b2-3dff-847e-5ba90f14a735.
10. Singh VS, V Vinayadev. Effectiveness of baby oil therapy for uremic pruritus in hemodialysis patients. *Saudi J Kidney Dis Transpl.* 2021;32(1):163–169. https://discovery.ebsco.com/linkprocessor/plink?id=8d11f14c-b72a-35d8-8ec4-f8298f7c3096.
11. Ragazzo J, Cesta A, Battistella M. Uremic pruritis. *CANNT J.* 2018;28(1):28–33. https://discovery.ebsco.com/linkprocessor/plink?id=ecfea52b-e2e0-356b-9ada-08c97636ddd2.
12. Visconti MJ, Haidari W, Feldman SR. Transcutaneous electrical nerve stimulation (TENS): a review of applications in dermatology. *J Dermatol Treat.* 2020;31(8):846–849. https://discovery.ebsco.com/linkprocessor/plink?id=0af78d62-d6a1-3cea-8095-ca3a8453d7a6.
13. Hercz D. Interventions for itch in people with advanced chronic kidney disease. *Cochrane Database Syst Rev.* 2020;12(12):CD011393. https://discovery.ebsco.com/linkprocessor/plink?id=3cb32c34-3a86-37d2-9e07-3be4b59e7254.
14. Ting S-W, Fan P-C, Lin Y S, et al. Uremic pruritus and long-term morbidities in the dialysis population. *PLoS One.* 2020;15(10):1–14. https://discovery.ebsco.com/linkprocessor/plink?id=69015880-7dbc-3571-8bf9-2a0e26e09faa.
15. Nakayama T, Morimoto K, Uchiyama K, et al. Serum thymus and activation-regulated chemokine level is associated with the severity of chronic kidney disease-associated pruritus in patients undergoing peritoneal dialysis. *Perit Dial Int.* 2022;42(4):415–424. https://discovery.ebsco.com/linkprocessor/plink?id=6c5a33fe-f5c5-3f13-98a5-6b4371b44bb7.
16. Verduzco HA, Shirazian S. CKD-associated pruritus: new insights into diagnosis, pathogenesis, and management. *Kidney Int Rep.* 2020;5(9):1387–1402. https://discovery.ebsco.com/linkprocessor/plink?id=158e115e-ab0f-3211-bcaf-9ed154f2853a.
17. Narita I, Tsubakihara Y, Uchiyama T, et al. Efficacy and safety of difelikefalin in Japanese patients with moderate to severe pruritus receiving hemodialysis a randomized clinical trial. *JAMA Netw Open.* 2022;5(5):e2210339. https://discovery.ebsco.com/linkprocessor/plink?id=919abfa2-6481-3e54-b1c7-7cca3fbe76b8.
18. Jeon J, Wang F, Badic A, Kim BS. Treatment of patients with chronic pruritus of unknown origin with dupilumab. *J Dermatol Treat.* 2022;33(3):1754–1757. https://discovery.ebsco.com/linkprocessor/plink?id=dabb42e6-c325-35bf-bddf-d5bcc382cc98.
19. Nietsche TR, Dotta G, Barcaui CB, Ferraz MLCG. Cholestatic pruritus: a knowledge update. *An Bras Dermatol.* 2022;97(3):332–337.
20. Patel SP, Vasavda C, Ho B, Meixiong J, Dong X, Kwatra SG. Cholestatic pruritus: emerging mechanisms and therapeutics. *J Am Acad Dermatol.* 2019;81(6):1371. https://doi.org/10.1016/j.jaad.2019.04.035.
21. le Dai D, van Anh Pham T, Bui TTH, et al. Symptom prevalence, burden and correlates among people living with HIV in Vietnam: a two-centre self-report study. *AIDS Care.* 2022;34(7):887–893. https://discovery.ebsco.com/linkprocessor/plink?id=1a783d2f-6882-3491-b6fd-e5c9c7ee4142.
22. Ozkoca D, Caf N, Atsu AN, Uzuncakmak TK, Kutlubay Z. The mucocutaneous manifestations in patients infected with the human immunodeficiency virus. *J Turk Acad Dermatol.* 2022;16(4):82–85. https://doi.org/10.4274/jtad.galenos.2022.83703.
23. Lipman ZM, Yosipovitch G. Substance use disorders and chronic itch. *J Am Acad Dermatol.* 2021;84(1):148–155. https://doi.org/10.1016/j.jaad.2020.08.117.
24. Kim BS, Inan S, Ständer S, Sciascia T, Szepietowski JC, Yosipovitch G. Role of kappa-opioid and mu-opioid receptors in pruritus: peripheral and central itch circuits. *Exp Dermatol.* 2022;31(12):1900–1907. https://doi.org/10.1111/exd.14669.
25. Buga S, Totoran AD. Itch, scratch, itch: the opioid-induced pruritus. *Oncol Hematol.* 2021;(56):27–30. https://doi.org/10.26416/onhe.56.3.2021.5647.
26. Fletcher T, Bleeker-Rovers C, Beeching N. Fever. *Acute Med II.* 2017;177–183.
27. David A, Quinlan JD. Fever of unknown origin in adults. *Am Fam Physician.* 2022;105(2):137–143. https://search-ebscohost-com.wvu.idm.oclc.org/login.aspx?direct=true&db=ccm&AN=155259008&site=ehost-live&scope=site.
28. Wright WF, Simner PJ, Carroll KC, Auwaerter PG. Progress report: next-generation sequencing, multiplex polymerase chain reaction, and broad-range molecular assays as diagnostic tools for fever of unknown origin investigations in adults. *Clin Infect Dis.* 2022;74(5):924–932. https://doi.org/10.1093/cid/ciab155.
29. Ludwig J, McWhinnie H. Antipyretic drugs in patients with fever and infection: literature review. *Br J Nurs.* 2019;28(10):610–618. https://doi.org/10.12968/bjon.2019.28.10.610.
30. Zhu Z, Yang F, Wang L, Zhao R. Non pharmacological fever management for persons living with HIV: a best practice implementation project. *JBI Database System Rev Implement Rep.* 2018;16(3):791–801. https://doi.org/10.11124/JBISRIR-2017-003347.
31. Ertem G, Hazar S. Symptom management and nursing care in palliative care of cervical cancer patients. *J Educ Res Nurs.* 2022;19(2):262–268. https://doi.org/10.5152/jern.2022.88886.
32. Kisielnicka A, Szczerkowska-Dobosz A, Purzycka-Bohdan D, Nowicki RJ. Hyperhidrosis: disease aetiology, classification and management in the light of modern treatment modalities. *Adv Dermatol Allergol.* 2022;39(2):251–257. https://doi.org/10.5114/ada.2022.115887.
33. Nawrocki S, Cha J. The etiology, diagnosis, and management of hyperhidrosis: a comprehensive review: etiology and clinical work-up. *J Am Acad Dermatol.* 2019;81(3):657–666. https://doi.org/10.1016/j.jaad.2018.12.071.
34. McConaghy JR, Fosselman D. Hyperhidrosis: management options. *Am Fam Physician.* 2018;97(11):729–734. https://search.ebscohost.com/login.aspx?direct=true&db=cmedm&AN=30215934&site=ehost-live&scope=site.
35. Zuzelo PR. Responding holistically to the person living with hyperhydrosis. *Holist Nurs Pract.* 2021;35(2):108–110. https://doi.org/10.1097/HNP.0000000000000437

36. O'Riordan J, Beatty S, Harnett I. Pharmacological management of paraneoplastic sweating in a palliative care setting. *Eur J Palliat Care.* 2016;23(1):6–9. https://search.ebscohost.com/login.aspx?direct=true&db=ccm&AN=112973683&site=ehost-live&scope=site.
37. Nawrocki S, Cha J. The etiology, diagnosis, and management of hyperhidrosis: a comprehensive review: therapeutic options. *J Am Acad Dermatol.* 2019;81(3):669–680. https://doi.org/10.1016/j.jaad.2018.11.066.
38. Ramasamy V. Acupuncture for the treatment of paraneoplastic night sweats. *J Acupunct Meridian Stud.* 2018;11(4):159–161. https://doi.org/10.1016/j.jams.2018.03.001.
39. Ho YL, Fauzi M, Sothee K, Basheer A. Diagnosis, impact and management of hyperhidrosis including endoscopic thoracic sympathectomy. *Med J Malaysia.* 2020;75(5):555–560. https://search.ebscohost.com/login.aspx?direct=true&db=cmedm&AN=32918426&site=ehost-live&scope=site.
40. Wade R, Llewellyn A, Jones-Diette J, et al. Interventional management of hyperhidrosis in secondary care: a systematic review. *Br J Dermatol.* 2018;179(3):599–608. https://doi.org/10.1111/bjd.16558.
41. Carr C, Vertelney H, Fronk J, Trieu S. Dronabinol for the treatment of paraneoplastic night sweats in cancer patients: a report of five cases. *J Palliat Med.* 2019;22(10):1221–1223. https://discovery.ebsco.com/linkprocessor/plink?id=14c21523-ad0e-36b5-85cc-3e3da3c37f79.
42. Strang P, Bergqvist J. Does palliative chemotherapy provide a palliative effect on symptoms in late palliative stages? An interview study with oncologists. *Acta Oncol.* 2017;56(10):1258–1264. https://doi.org/10.1080/0284186X.2017.1332426.

22

Neurological Disorders

Lauren Massimo and Brianna Morgan

Key Points

- Neurological disorders are common across healthcare settings, are often life-threatening, and significantly impact function and well-being.
- Palliative care nurses are an essential component of providing high-quality care to people living with neurological disorders and their caregivers from diagnosis through end of life.
- It is imperative for all palliative care nurses to understand the basic palliative care needs of people living with neurological disorders and be prepared to address these needs across all healthcare contexts.

Introduction

Nurses interact with people living with neurological disorders at every level of care. None of the neurological disorders included in this chapter—amyotrophic lateral sclerosis, Parkinson's disease, progressive supranuclear palsy, corticobasal syndrome, Huntington's disease, and multiple sclerosis—are curable with the treatments available today. Though some have disease-modifying treatments, all significantly impact the lives of people living with these disorders and their caregivers alike due to distressing symptoms and disability often requiring significant assistance. Most disorders carry a symptom burden greater than or equal to those caused by malignancies, yet few individuals living with these illnesses have access to palliative care. In addition, all the disorders discussed in this chapter can impact cognition, affecting autonomous decision-making; yet advance care planning is not commonplace. To that end, most people with these neurological disorders die in the hospital rather than at home with hospice.[1] While there has been a movement toward building a specialist palliative care workforce for persons with neurological disorders, there are not nearly enough specialists to meet the needs of this population.[2] Therefore, it is imperative for all nurses to understand the basic palliative care needs of this population and be prepared to address these needs in the settings where they encounter them. This chapter will provide an overview of six neurological disorders with high palliative care needs, outline common care needs that occur across these disorders, and review palliative interventions nurses can employ to reduce suffering and increase quality of life for people living with neurological disorders and their caregivers.

Neurological Disorders

Amyotrophic Lateral Sclerosis

Amyotrophic lateral sclerosis (ALS), also commonly known as Lou Gehrig's disease, is a progressive neurologic condition characterized by progressive muscle wasting from denervation (amyotrophy). ALS is the most common of all motor neuron diseases. It results from degeneration of both upper and lower motor neurons. Lower motor neuron signs include atrophy, weakness, and fasciculations, while upper motor neuron signs include spasticity, weakness, and hyperreflexia. ALS may also include cognitive impairment, such as impairment in executive function and behavior. Palliative nursing interventions for individuals living with ALS focus on symptom palliation and preserving functional ability.

The prognosis for ALS is 2–5 years, and life expectancy may be considerably shorter without medically administered nutritional or respiratory support. Therefore, serious illness communication early in the disease is essential. The care of a person with ALS is complex and requires an extensive multidisciplinary team including nurses, neurologists, pulmonologists, speech pathologists, physical and occupational therapists, and social workers. Physical and occupational therapy needs are immediate as patients with ALS may require assistive devices for muscle weakness at diagnosis. Therapy services can help individuals with ALS to maintain endurance and strength, promote functional independence, and limit complications such as pain from immobility.[3] Individuals with ALS are at high risk for malnutrition from dysphagia, sialorrhea, depression, cognitive impairment, difficulty with self-feeding, respiratory insufficiency, and fatigue with meals; therefore, speech–language pathology (SLP) and a nutritional assessment are helpful to evaluate swallowing and discuss feeding strategies.[4] Augmentative communication strategies will also become important as individuals with ALS develop speech difficulty. Both low-tech strategies such as alphabet boards and high-tech solutions like speech-generating devices can be helpful to enhance communication (Box 22.1). Table 22.1 outlines resources for individuals with ALS and their caregivers.

Box 22.1 Key Points for Optimizing Communication

- Provide the optimal setting for communication by ensuring there is adequate lighting and limit distractions in the environment.
- Ensure the patient is wearing eyeglasses and hearing aids, if appropriate.
- Avoid correcting grammatical mistakes or speaking for the individual with aphasia.
- Do not raise the volume of your voice unless the individual is hearing-impaired.
- Face the individual directly while communicating.
- Use facial expressions to emphasize spoken communication.
- Speak in context (e.g., discuss dinner plans in the kitchen).
- Simplify the message.
- Allow adequate time for comprehension and response.
- Consider augmentative and alternative communication devices such as communication boards, written communication, speech to text, and eye-gaze devices.

Table 22.1 Resources for people living with neurological disorders and their caregivers

Amyotrophic lateral sclerosis (ALS)
ALS Association https://www.als.org National Institute of Neurological Disorders and Stroke (NINDS) ALS Fact Sheet https://www.ninds.nih.gov/amyotrophic-lateral-sclerosis-als-fact-sheet
Parkinson's disease
Parkinson's Foundation www.parkinson.org Michael J. Fox Foundation for Parkinson's Research https://www.michaeljfox.org
Progressive supranuclear palsy (PSP)/corticobasal syndrome
The Association for Frontotemporal Degeneration https://www.theaftd.org Cure PSP https://www.psp.org NINDS PSP Fact Sheet https://www.ninds.nih.gov/progressive-supranuclear-palsy-fact-sheet
Huntington's disease
Huntington's Disease Society of America https://hdsa.org/ International Huntington Association https://huntington-disease.org/
Multiple sclerosis
National Multiple Sclerosis Society https://www.nationalmssociety.org/ Multiple Sclerosis Association of America https://mymsaa.org/ Multiple Sclerosis Foundation https://msfocus.org/
Symptoms
NINDS Motor Neuron Fact Sheet https://www.ninds.nih.gov/motor-neuron-diseases-fact-sheet NINDS Dystonia Fact Sheet https://catalog.ninds.nih.gov/publications/dystonia NINDS Myoclonus Fact Sheet https://www.ninds.nih.gov/myoclonus-fact-sheet American Speech–Language–Hearing Association https://www.asha.org/ National Aphasia Association https://www.aphasia.org/ Academy of Neurologic Communication Disorders Science http://www.ancds.org/
Neuropalliative care
International Neuropalliative Care Society https://www.inpcs.org/ Education in Palliative Care and End-of-Life Care Neurology www.EPEC.net

End of life with ALS is characterized by significant challenges, and symptoms are best managed by a hospice team.[5,6] Symptoms in late-stage ALS may include pain, loss of respiratory capacity, diminishing communicative ability, and increasing physical dependency. A remarkable responsibility thus falls to the family and caregivers. Due to progressive loss of diaphragmatic control, many individuals with ALS require mechanical ventilation to support respiratory function. Should the patient opt for long-term ventilatory support, the family and caregivers will require considerable teaching—from managing the tracheostomy wound to airway suctioning and maintaining equipment. Palliative sedation may be useful in select patients with ALS choosing to avoid or discontinue invasive ventilation.[7,8] Palliative sedation and physician-assisted suicide remain a topic of exploration and debate.[9]

Parkinson's Disease

Parkinson's disease (PD) is the second most common neurodegenerative disorder behind Alzheimer's disease. Characteristics of PD include resting tremor, postural instability, bradykinesia, and rigidity of the extremities or trunk. Non-motor symptoms may also occur in PD, including cognitive impairment, sleep disturbance, and mood symptoms such as apathy, depression, and anxiety. Motor symptoms such as tremor and bradykinesia are often treated with dopamine-based medications, such as dopaminergic therapies (e.g., carbidopa, levodopa) and dopamine agonists (e.g., pramipexole, ropinirole). For a select group of patients, surgical intervention may serve a role. Advanced surgical interventions include deep brain stimulator placement and ablative surgical techniques such as thalamotomy and pallidotomy. PD is a progressive disease, and over time motor and non-motor symptoms will worsen increasing dependence. People with PD typically live 7–14 years after their diagnosis.[10]

The palliative care nurse should initially focus on maximizing functional ability and reducing risk for falls. Medication education, home safety, physical and occupational therapy, and establishing a routine of exercise and rest are important initial goals of care. The pathogenesis of PD and side effects from dopamine-based medications (e.g., carbidopa, levodopa, pramipexole, ropinirole), which are used to treat motor symptoms, can result in a degree of autonomic instability (e.g., orthostatic hypotension, sexual dysfunction, exercise intolerance, increased or decreased diaphoresis); therefore, it is important for palliative care nurses to evaluate for life-threatening hypotensive episodes and symptoms impacting daily life. The speech therapist also has a role in the care of the patient with PD as dysphagia, dysarthria, sialorrhea, and aspiration are common. Fluctuating energy expenditure, medication–food interactions, impaired gastrointestinal motility, and impaired fluid balance leave people with PD at risk of nutritional deficiencies.[11,12] Therefore, a dietician may also be an important part of the palliative care team. Resources for individuals with PD and their caregivers are outlined in Table 22.1.

The end-of-life phase of PD is typically heralded by progressive loss of mobility, worsening dysphagia, and aspiration. PD-associated dementia can occur as well, which may include cognitive changes in one or more cognitive domain, such as memory and executive functioning. Unfortunately, dopaminergic medication in this phase may have limited efficacy; therefore, discussion of discontinuation may be warranted. Goals of nursing interventions in late-stage PD should include continence care, prevention of recurring infection such as urinary tract infections, preserving patient preferences, and education about symptoms at the end of life.

Progressive Supranuclear Palsy and Corticobasal Syndrome

Corticobasal syndrome (CBS) and progressive supranuclear palsy (PSP) are characterized by movement difficulty and cognitive impairment. Individuals with CBS can experience motor deficits such as limb rigidity, dystonia, and apraxia, while individuals with PSP present with early falls, akinesia, and axial rigidity. Additionally, people living with PSP will show a characteristic vertical supranuclear gaze palsy (i.e., slowing or restriction of vertical eye movements). Cognitive difficulties are also common in these conditions and may include impairment in executive function, visuospatial ability, and behavioral changes. Currently there are no curative treatments or medications that can be used to slow down the disease process. Patients with CBS and PSP will experience a gradual worsening of gait, speech, and swallowing with increasing dependence on others for their activities of daily living. Time from symptom onset until death is approximately 6 years.[13]

An early symptom of PSP and CBS is gait dysfunction, and falls are common. The palliative care nurse should evaluate gait and balance and spend time educating the patient and family about fall risk reduction (see "Gait Impairment and Falls"). Early intervention by physical therapy is often necessary for gait and balance therapy and may include recommendations for assistive devices such as walkers to assist with ambulation. Abnormal posturing of the limbs or dystonia may be associated with pain; therefore, pain is an important part of the assessment. Devices such as splints and braces and range-of-motion exercises may also be helpful in reducing pain associated with dystonia. Finally, botulinum toxin injections are an effective form of treatment for pain associated with focal dystonia or rigidity. Speech disorders are also common in CBS and PSP and may occur early and progress to mutism. Early intervention by SLP can help the patient and caregiver implement strategies and may suggest alternative communication, such as text-to-speech devices, to enhance communicative efficacy (Table 22.1 for resources, Box 22.1 for communication strategies).

Advanced CBS and PSP share similar disease trajectories, with severe stage disease marked by motor disability, swallowing impairment, falls, infection, and advancing cognitive impairment.[14] Identification of symptoms that increase risk for mortality is an important aspect of palliative care nursing. For example, aspiration pneumonia is a common cause of mortality; therefore, reinforcing strategies for a safe swallow is an important educational opportunity (see "Speech and Swallowing"). While there is growing recognition of palliative care for neurodegenerative disorders, there are several barriers to enrolling patients in palliative care. CBS and PSP are relatively rare conditions, and clinician discomfort with symptoms and disease trajectory often limit discussions around palliative care and hospice services.[14] Therefore, ongoing serious illness communication describing how palliative care and hospice services can support patient goals is important to enhance quality of life in persons with CBS and PSP.

Huntington's Disease

Huntington's disease (HD) is a life-threatening, progressive neurodegenerative disorder impacting multiple health domains, including motor function, cognition, and behavior. HD leads to functional decline and disability almost always requiring caregiver support. The health impacts of HD are overlapping and complex, requiring management by multidisciplinary health professionals across the healthcare system from hospital to home. Currently, there are no curative or disease-modifying treatments available, and people living with HD have significant symptom burden requiring highly skilled and complex management. Palliative nursing principles are well suited to meet the significant needs of people impacted by HD beginning at diagnosis.

HD is autosomal dominant, meaning that the disease occurs if an individual inherits one copy of the *HTT* gene from a parent. The age at onset can range from childhood to elderhood but is most common in midlife (40s–50s). Juvenile HD, or onset before age 20, occurs in 10% of cases. Time of onset and progression are impacted by the number of repeats, with more repeats leading to early onset and faster progression. Typical prognosis of HD is 10–20 years after symptom onset, though some individuals can live up to 40 years after symptom onset.

HD progression is characterized in three stages—early, middle, and late—which each have different symptom and function profiles (Table 22.2). Nursing care evolves across the illness trajectory

Table 22.2 Symptoms of Huntington's disease by stage

	Motor	Cognition	Behavior	Function	Other
Early stage	Minor chorea, tics,[a] myoclonus[a]	Mild difficulty with learning, slower processing speed, some impaired judgment and/or insight, mild executive dysfunction	Mild depression, irritability, apathy, anxiety, OCD, hallucinations, impulsivity	Independent in iADLs and bADLs	Illness understanding, emotional processing
Middle stage	Prominent chorea, tics,[a] myoclonus[a]	Moderate cognitive impairment including difficulty learning, slow processing, impaired judgment and/or insight, and executive dysfunction	Moderate to severe depression, irritability, apathy, anxiety, OCD, hallucinations, impulsivity, suicidality	Assistance with iADLs Independent/some assistance with bADLs	Dysphagia Imbalance Falls Weight loss Fatigue Sleep disorders Sexual disorders
Late stage	Significant chorea or rigidity, dystonia, and bradykinesia	Dementia-level cognitive impairment impacting daily function	More difficult to recognize	Dependent for all ADLs, often requiring assistive devices and/or durable medical equipment	Dysarthria Aspiration Incontinence

bADLs, basic activities of daily living; iADLs, independent activities of daily living; OCD, obsessive–compulsive disorder.
[a] Commonly seen in juvenile HD.

to meet these changing needs. Initially, in the early stage, palliative nursing care focuses on supporting the person with HD and their families with illness understanding, emotional support, genetic testing decision-making, resource-gathering, and advance care planning.[15,16] Given the typical age at onset and autosomal dominant nature of HD, many individuals with HD are navigating receiving a diagnosis while also worrying about the impact on their existing or future children. Blood relatives may consider predictive genetic testing in conjunction with specially trained Huntington's Disease Society of America (HDSA) genetic counselors, and persons with HD may consider reproductive support and prenatal testing.[16] Nurses and social workers play a vital role in connecting individuals with HD and their families with resources and information in a timely and individualized manner (Table 22.1). Finally, given the progressive nature of HD and the almost certain need for increasing level of dependence requiring assistive care, advance care planning is vital. However, only about one-third of people with HD have advance directives, and fewer than half have other end-of-life plans in place.[17,18] Nurses play an important role in facilitating early discussions about advance care planning that includes elicitation of goals and values, development of advance directives, and identifying family and surrogate decision makers.[19]

The middle stage of HD focuses on symptom management that maximizes function and quality of life. Motor symptoms are most common in HD, with choreiform movements, or involuntary irregular dance-like movements, as a hallmark sign. Pharmacological management of chorea by a neurologist with tetrabenazine is standard of care.[20] Cognitive dysfunction in HD is progressive and characterized by difficulty learning, slowed processing, impaired judgment and/or insight, and executive dysfunction.[20] No pharmacological agent has shown efficacy in delaying cognitive decline in HD, so nursing care focuses on augmenting a supportive environment to maintain as much independence as possible while ensuring safety. Appropriate referral for multidisciplinary supportive care such as occupational therapy, physical therapy, SLP, and nutritionists can support independence and function. Behavioral symptoms, such as emotional lability, irritability, depression, anxiety, hallucinations, suicidality, or homicidally, can be significant in HD. Treatments typically include off-label use of selective serotonin-reuptake inhibitors (SSRIs) for mild symptoms and antipsychotics for more severe symptoms like hallucinations and compulsions. Other symptoms may include dysphagia, imbalance, falls, weight loss, and fatigue, which are discussed later in the chapter.

Late-stage HD is characterized by near or total function dependence for most or all activities of daily living requiring 24-hour supervision and assistance. While some people with HD may live at home with 24-hour support, others prefer to reside in long-term care settings. Though HD progression has varying patterns, late-stage HD can persist for many years, even a decade or more; therefore, planning for this level of supervision is essential. HDSA social workers are specially trained to help with this decision-making and transition. Safety is a greater concern given risk for falls, aspiration pneumonia, and incontinence. At this point, ongoing serious illness communication will be a valuable resource, and many will consider hospice. Caregiver support during late-stage HD and into bereavement is also an important aspect of palliative nursing care.

Multiple Sclerosis

Multiple sclerosis (MS) is the most prevalent chronic neuroinflammatory disease, impacting nearly 1 million people in the United States. MS causes demyelination in the central nervous system (CNS), leading to neurologic symptoms and disability and is typically diagnosed in young to middle adulthood. While MS reduces the life span by an average of 7 years, most people will live with MS for several decades with disease-modifying therapies.[21] The main cause of death for people with severe MS is infection, such as urinary tract infection or pneumonia.[22] The pattern and course of MS vary. While 15% of people living with MS have a progressive course from the outset (primary progressive), 40% will develop progressive disease (secondary progressive) after 15 years with relapsing–remitting disease.[23] Palliative care can be beneficial for anyone with MS, but most guidelines and evidence focus on individuals with progressive MS.[24,25] Though people living with MS experience symptom burden similar to those with metastatic disease, there are many barriers to receiving palliative care. Therefore, palliative nursing, especially primary palliative care across all settings where these individuals receive care, is imperative to increasing access and improving quality of life.[26]

Palliative care guidelines for people living with progressive MS recommend advance care planning early and ongoing serious illness communication throughout the illness trajectory, symptom management, home-based palliative care, and caregiver support.[24,25] Early discussion of advance care planning that includes caregivers and decisions related to care preferences is recommended.[24] Symptom management should focus on common symptoms including spasticity, fatigue, pain, depression, sleeping problems, bladder problems, and mobility issues.[24,25] Palliative home-based care can reduce symptom burden and, in some cases, improve quality of life. Caregivers need education, training, and referral to resources (Table 22.1) that are tailored to their preferences and habits as well as emotional support.[24]

Common Neurologic Care Needs and Palliative Management Strategies

Advance Care Planning and Serious Illness Communication

There are several reasons why early advance care planning and ongoing serious illness communication including the person living with illness and selected surrogate decision makers are essential in neurological disorders. First, all the neurological disorders discussed in this chapter shorten life expectancy, though there is variability in prognosis. Second, all these neurological disorders increase the likelihood that a person will have one or more serious health events (e.g., falls, infections, respiratory emergencies) that will require in-the-moment decision-making about advanced interventions. Finally, almost all these neurological disorders (ALS, PD, PSP/CBS, HD) have the potential to impact cognition and therefore autonomous decision-making prior to end of life.

The approach to advance care planning and serious illness communication should be tailored to the unique needs of persons impacted by neurological disorders. First, while early communication about prognosis and decision-making is essential in all neurological disorders, expected prognosis should dictate the timing and content of communication. ALS has a short prognosis (2–5 years from symptom onset) and can present with immediate life-threatening circumstances (e.g., respiratory failure), which necessitates early serious illness communication about prognosis, goals, and care preferences to direct care decision-making. PD, CBS, and PSP have a middle-range prognosis (6–14 years after symptom onset), while individuals with MS and HD often live with the disease for a decade or more. Therefore, early conversations for individuals with these diagnoses should support awareness of prognosis and expected illness trajectory and elicit advance care planning preferences. Serious illness communication techniques should be used throughout the illness, especially at moments of disease progression or complications requiring increased care. Second, expected symptoms and complications for each neurological disorder should direct the content of serious illness communication. For example, ALS, HD, CBS/PSP, and PD often lead to significant disability requiring assistance for daily living. Therefore, serious illness communication should include preparation for assistance and preferences for living (e.g., home, assisted living facility). Finally, the need to designate a surrogate is essential in all neurological diagnoses but should be prioritized in diagnoses that carry an increased risk of cognitive impairment (e.g., ALS, PD, PSP/CBS, HD), which can threaten autonomous decision-making.

Mobility Symptom Cluster

Several symptoms occur in neurological disorders that impact mobility, including spasticity, myoclonus, and gait impairment. This section presents common symptoms and management strategies for palliative care nurses to consider. It also includes a case study that exemplifies these symptoms and will be discussed at the end of the section (Box 22.2).

Spasticity

Spasticity is an abnormal increase in muscle tone that can cause functional disability by interfering with movement and speech, exacerbating fatigue, or causing pain. Spasticity is typically caused by damage to the nerve pathways within the brain or spinal cord that control muscle movement (upper motor neurons). Spasticity occurs in many degenerative neurologic conditions and is commonly encountered with ALS, MS, PSP, CBS, and occasionally PD and HD, though it is more common in juvenile HD.

Box 22.2 Case Study: Mobility

Jack is a 47-year-old, self-identified male who was diagnosed with amyotrophic lateral sclerosis 1 year ago. He and his partner, Romeo, have been struggling to meet his functional needs at home, so he is now living in a nursing home. Romeo is concerned because Jack has fallen several times in the nursing home and had several episodes of urinary incontinence.

You are a palliative care nurse who is new to Jack's care. Upon further investigation, you find Jack uses a rolling walker at baseline, but he often leaves it behind because "it gets stuck on the rugs." There is no physical trauma from Jack's recent falls, but Jack notes that he is afraid to leave his room for fear of falling. You run a urine dipstick to rule out a new urinary tract infection, which is negative. You also note Jack is on several medications for spasticity, including baclofen, tizanidine, and dronabinol. Jack notes the nursing home physician has been increasing his medications for spasticity due to worsening pain, which is still unresolved, now 7 out of 10. Jack has been declining his physical therapy and occupational therapy appointments because he is "too tired."

Spasticity can occur in any muscle or muscle group, though it is common in antigravity muscles, such as the brachioradialis and hip flexors. The palliative care nurse should consider if the condition is new or established. In worsening, established spasticity, nurses should assess for secondary causes—infection, constipation, pain, or autonomic dysreflexia. If the spasticity is new, further investigation is required. Spasticity may signal disease progression in MS.

Many treatments are available for spasticity. The goal of pharmacological treatment for spasticity is to find a balance between reducing muscle tone to improve function while avoiding muscle laxity, which can impair gait and continence, and CNS depressant effects of medication (e.g., dizziness, drowsiness, and confusion), especially in older adults. Baclofen is the mainstay treatment due to its demonstrated efficacy, lower side effect profile (less hepatotoxicity), and low cost. Other commonly used oral antispasmodics include dantrolene, diazepam, and tizanidine. Medical marijuana and dronabinol, a synthetic tetrahydrocannabinol, show mixed efficacy at reducing spasticity and pain related to spasticity.[25] Phenol and botulinum toxin are injected for patients with persistent spasticity and torticollis, a condition that causes the neck to twist and the head to tilt. Surgical interventions are also available for the patient with medically intractable spasticity. Intrathecal administration of baclofen has become a mainstay of treatment for patients with persistent spasticity with significant side effects from oral baclofen.[27]

Nursing care for spasticity focuses on comfort and maximizing function. Physical and occupational therapy consultation are invaluable for prescribed stretching regimens and to determine appropriate durable medical equipment. Repositioning, application of heat, and strategies to improve functional abilities are helpful. Patient and family education are important to set realistic goals. Education also focuses on factors that worsen spasticity, prevention of pressure ulcers and contractures, fatigue, and psychosocial concerns. Early education is crucial to prevent complications and includes medication education.

Myoclonus

Myoclonus is a series of sudden and brief, lightning-like muscular contractions. The contractions are irregular in both amplitude and rhythm and denote a disturbance of the CNS. Neurological disorders impacting the basal ganglia can cause symptomatic myoclonus. Myoclonus occurs in roughly half of patients with CBS but is less common in PSP. Patients with juvenile-onset HD and a high number of repeats may develop myoclonus. PD, especially when Lewy bodies are present, can lead to myoclonus. MS can also lead to myoclonus depending on the location of neuroinflammation.[28]

Few medications have been shown to ease myoclonus associated with degenerative conditions. Anticonvulsants can be helpful in chronic myoclonus, although typically multidrug therapy is needed. Clonazepam is the most frequently used and most effective agent across all types of myoclonus.[28] Other drugs have been tested, including valproic acid, levetiracetam, zonisamide, acetazolamide, and sodium oxybate, although strong data for each of these medications is lacking.[29] Several non-antiepileptic drugs have been tried for myoclonus, including baclofen and dantrolene, also with varying success. In instances of peripherally mediated myoclonus, botulinum toxin injections may provide relief.[30,31] Importantly, palliative nurses should help to identify polypharmacy related to pharmacological management of myoclonus and discontinue medications that do not provide clinical benefit. Finally, it is also important to consider other factors that are common in palliative care settings that may cause or contribute to myoclonus. These causes include medications (e.g., opioids, antiseizure medications like lithium, and some cardiac medications like calcium channel blockers), infection (e.g., encephalitis, syphilis, Lyme disease), and other metabolic disturbances (e.g., hepatic failure, renal failure, hyponatremia, hypokalemia, etc.). In these instances, treatment focuses on reversing the underlying cause if possible. In the case of opioid-induced myoclonus, opioid rotation is indicated.

Nursing-specific care for myoclonus is multifaceted. Safety takes priority. Padded side rails and helmets may be necessary. For patients with severe myoclonus, ambulation may not be possible. Physical or occupational therapy assessment will determine whether durable medical equipment or assistive devices are needed. Offer strategies for safe transfers to families and caregivers. As with all palliative care measures, assessment for pain is necessary. Myoclonus is fatiguing and may even lead to weight loss. Teaching individuals with myoclonus and family members about energy conservation and non-stimulating environments (low light, minimizing noise) is important. Nutritional counseling and supplements may prevent weight loss.

Gait Impairment and Falls

One-third of community-dwelling older adults fall each year, increasing their risk of injury, institutionalization, and death.[32] All the neurological disorders discussed in this chapter can cause gait impairment and put individuals at an even higher risk for falls and fall-related injuries.[33] Gait impairment in neurological disorders can be caused by bradykinesia, spasticity, weakness, fatigue, sensory loss, visual loss, vestibular dysfunction, or executive dysfunction.

Nursing care for gait impairment and fall prevention should focus on a comprehensive gait assessment to understand the type of gait disturbance and appropriate interventions. Nurses should assess for and reduce risk factors that could increase falls including medications, environmental risks (e.g., poor lighting, lack of safety equipment, obstacles), and other contributing medical conditions (e.g., cardiac disease, musculoskeletal disease, visual or hearing disturbances). History of falls strongly predicts the likelihood of future falls.[34] All individuals with gait impairment should be assessed for appropriate assistive devices on an ongoing basis. Since many medications commonly used in this population can increase the risk for falls (e.g., SSRIs, neuroleptics, etc.), it is important for palliative nurses to create plans that balance function and safety based on the goals and values of each individual. Importantly, palliative nurses should include appropriate multidisciplinary team members, especially occupational therapy, physical therapy, and physical medicine and rehabilitation providers, to support function and safety. Exercise therapy has been shown to reduce falls in PD and other neurological conditions.[35,36] No evidence-based data supports the use of restraints to prevent falls.

Case Study: Mobility

As the palliative care nurse in Jack's case, you suspect the polypharmacy related to treating Jack's spasticity may be worsening his risk of falls, causing incontinence, and leaving his pain undertreated. You suggest this to the nursing home physician, who agrees. Jack says his goal is to have more control over his pain and still be able to get to the dining hall to have his meals with Romeo, who visits every evening. Together with Jack, Romeo, and the physician, you decide to slowly taper Jack's sedating medications, titrating to Jack's stated goal. You collaborate with physical and occupational therapy to evaluate Jack's environment and assistive equipment. You remove the rugs from his room and start heat, repositioning, and stretching recommended by physical therapy. A week later with no falls or incontinence, Jack's pain level has dropped to a 3 out of 10, and his energy level has improved. At your suggestion, he restarts physical and occupational therapy sessions. Later that week you see him sharing a meal with Romeo in the dining hall.

Speech and Swallowing

Neurological disorders can significantly impact speech and swallowing, which negatively impacts well-being and quality of life. Palliative care nurses can support individuals with neurological disorders experiencing these symptoms (Table 22.1 for resources). This section continues the case study from the previous section (Box 22.3).

Impaired Communication

Communication is at the heart of the human existence. Difficulty communicating is highly distressing to both the patient and care partner. Impairments in communication from neurological disorders can take the form of aphasia, mutism, deafness, agraphia, alexia, or dysarthria. Aphasia, or the inability to express speech or understand what is being spoken, is caused by any disease disturbing the cortex of the brain, responsible for language production or reception. Traditional neurologic teaching identifies the key cortical areas as Broca's area, Wernicke's area, and the supplemental motor area for speech production and comprehension. For most people, language production and comprehension occur in the left hemisphere of the brain.

Nursing care for individuals with disorders of speech or language focuses on strategizing alternative means of speech and maximizing comprehension. While there is currently no curative treatment or symptomatic pharmacological treatment available, several nonpharmacological strategies are important for the patient with aphasia (Box 22.1). SLPs are a wonderful resource for the palliative care nurse and can be immensely helpful to clarify specific

Box 22.3 Case Study Continued: Speech and Swallowing

Several weeks later, Romeo mentions to you that Jack has been having trouble during their nightly meals. He is coughing while eating and drooling, and sometimes Romeo finds food in Jack's mouth several hours after eating. Romeo notes that he is also having a harder time communicating with Jack as his speech declines. This is incredibly distressing to Romeo as good conversation has been a mainstay of their relationship.

communication deficiencies and strategize alternative communication methods.

Dysphagia

Dysphagia, or difficulty swallowing, is a common symptom in persons with neurological conditions and can increase risk for complications such as aspiration pneumonia that are associated with mortality. Nurses perform an essential role in the identification and treatment of dysphagia. The major goal of care for a person with dysphagia is to optimize a safe and effective swallow. Signs that a person is experiencing dysphagia include coughing during or after swallowing, a weakened voice, difficulty chewing, and getting food stuck in the back of the throat. Diagnosis of dysphagia starts with an evaluation of complaints about the timing of symptoms and consistency of foods that are problematic for the patient. Collaboration with SLPs is important to determine if special swallow studies such as a barium swallow are indicated.

Management of dysphagia is typically done in collaboration with SLP and may include strategies such as oral exercises to strengthen the tongue and lip, ensuring the patient is fully upright during meals, and limiting distraction during mealtime to ensure the patient can focus on swallowing. Dietary modification is an important strategy to improve swallowing and prevent aspiration. For patients who are unable to safely swallow liquids, food additives that can thicken liquids while retaining taste are commercially available without a prescription. Finally, for patients who are unable to tolerate oral nutrition, enteral nutrition may be indicated in some cases such as those with early-stage ALS. However, gastrostomy tubes may not be beneficial for those with advanced disease, especially in individuals with dementia. Therefore, it is important to have serious illness conversations early on to educate patients and families about dysphagia to determine their wishes for treatment.

Sialorrhea or excessive drooling is common in individuals with ALS and PD. Sialorrhea increases the risk for aspiration pneumonia and skin breakdown and may be a source of embarrassment for patients. Sialorrhea may occur due to overproduction of saliva or ineffective clearance of saliva.[37] Oral medications such as glycopyrrolate are often first-line treatment. Radiotherapy to the salivary or parotid gland and botulinum toxin injection may be helpful if oral medications are ineffective.[38] Nonpharmacological strategies which can be useful include oral suctioning and oral exercises to improve swallowing in patients with dysphagia.

Case Study: Jack's Speech and Swallowing Concerns

As the palliative care nurse, you suggest that the nursing home staff modify the consistency of his liquids with a thickener to prevent aspiration. You collaborate with the SLP, who performs a bedside evaluation and determines that Jack's chewing and tongue muscles are weak. You educate Jack and Romeo on strategies for a safe swallow, indicating the need for a quiet environment where Jack is sitting straight up. Next week Jack will begin regular speech therapy sessions for his dysarthria and dysphagia. You also discuss typical progression of speech and swallowing changes in ALS with Jack and Romeo. You discuss the risks and benefits of tube feeding, which Jack states he may consider when the time comes. You begin to discuss communication strategies, like communication boards and speech to text programs. Jack and Romeo are grateful for the recommendations, and Jack begins recording voice memos for Romeo to listen to later if he is no longer able to speak.

REFERENCES

1. Creutzfeldt CJ, Kluger B, Kelly AG, et al. Neuropalliative care: priorities to move the field forward. *Neurology*. 2018;91(5):217–226.
2. Boersma I, Miyasaki J, Kutner J, Kluger B. Palliative care and neurology: time for a paradigm shift. *Neurology*. 2014;83(6):561–567.
3. Burke T, Hardiman O, Pinto-Grau M, et al. Longitudinal predictors of caregiver burden in amyotrophic lateral sclerosis: a population-based cohort of patient-caregiver dyads. *J Neurol*. 2018;265(4):793–808.
4. Greenwood DI. Nutrition management of amyotrophic lateral sclerosis. *Nutr Clin Pract*. 2013;28(3):392–399.
5. Cheng HWB, Chan OMI, Chan CHR, Chan WH, Fung KS, Wong KY. End-of-life characteristics and palliative care provision for patients with motor neuron disease. *Am J Hosp Palliat Care*. 2018;35(6):847–851.
6. Ozanne A, Graneheim UH. Understanding the incomprehensible—patients' and spouses' experiences of comprehensibility before, at and after diagnosis of amyotrophic lateral sclerosis. *Scand J Caring Sci*. 2018;32(2):663–671.
7. Mitsumoto H, Rabkin JG. Palliative care for patients with amyotrophic lateral sclerosis: "prepare for the worst and hope for the best." *JAMA*. 2007;298(2):207–216.
8. Kettemann D, Funke A, Maier A, et al. Clinical characteristics and course of dying in patients with amyotrophic lateral sclerosis withdrawing from long-term ventilation. *Amyotroph Lateral Scler Frontotemporal Degener*. 2017;18(1–2):53–59.
9. Maessen M, Veldink JH, Onwuteaka-Philipsen BD, et al. Euthanasia and physician-assisted suicide in amyotrophic lateral sclerosis: a prospective study. *J Neurol*. 2014;261(10):1894–1901.
10. Macleod AD, Taylor KS, Counsell CE. Mortality in Parkinson's disease: a systematic review and meta-analysis. *Mov Disord*. 2014;29(13):1615–1622.
11. Sheard JM, Ash S, Mellick GD, Silburn PA, Kerr GK. Improved nutritional status is related to improved quality of life in Parkinson's disease. *BMC Neurol*. 2014;14:212.
12. Fereshtehnejad SM, Ghazi L, Sadeghi M, et al. Prevalence of malnutrition in patients with Parkinson's disease: a comparative study with healthy controls using Mini Nutritional Assessment (MNA) questionnaire. *J Parkinsons Dis*. 2014;4(3):473–481.
13. Stang CD, Turcano P, Mielke MM, et al. Incidence and trends of progressive supranuclear palsy and corticobasal syndrome: a population-based study. *J Parkinsons Dis*. 2020;10(1):179–184.
14. Akbar U, McQueen RB, Bemski J, et al. Prognostic predictors relevant to end-of-life palliative care in Parkinson's disease and related disorders: a systematic review. *J Neurol Neurosurg Psychiatry*. 2021;92(6):629–636.
15. El-Sourady M, Martin S, Wong HN, Carroll T. A scoping review of palliative care for adults with Huntington's disease: current practice and future directions. *J Palliat Med*. 2022;25(3):488–505.
16. Dawson S, Kristjanson LJ, Toye CM, Flett P. Living with Huntington's disease: need for supportive care. *Nurs Health Sci*. 2004;6(2):123–130.
17. Booij SJ, Rodig V, Engberts DP, Tibben A, Roos RA. Euthanasia and advance directives in Huntington's disease: qualitative analysis of interviews with patients. *J Huntingtons Dis*. 2013;2(3):323–330.

18. Kavanaugh MS, Noh H, Zhang L. Caregiving youth knowledge and perceptions of parental end-of-life wishes in Huntington's disease. *J Soc Work End Life Palliat Care*. 2016;12(4):348–365.
19. Bisson JI, Hampton V, Rosser A, Holm S. Developing a care pathway for advance decisions and powers of attorney: qualitative study. *Br J Psychiatry*. 2009;194(1):55–61.
20. Mestre TA, Shannon K. Huntington disease care: from the past to the present, to the future. *Parkinsonism Relat Disord.* 2017;44:114–118.
21. Scalfari A, Knappertz V, Cutter G, Goodin DS, Ashton R, Ebers GC. Mortality in patients with multiple sclerosis. *Neurology.* 2013;81(2):184–192.
22. Roberts M. End-of-life care in multiple sclerosis. *Br J Neurosci Nurs*. 2021;17(4):170.
23. Scalfari A, Neuhaus A, Daumer M, Muraro PA, Ebers GC. Onset of secondary progressive phase and long-term evolution of multiple sclerosis. *J Neurol Neurosurg Psychiatry*. 2014;85(1):67–75.
24. Solari A, Giordano A, Sastre-Garriga J, et al. EAN guideline on palliative care of people with severe, progressive multiple sclerosis. *Eur J Neurol*. 2020;27(8):1510–1529.
25. Wright S, Yadav V, Bever C Jr, et al. Summary of evidence-based guideline: complementary and alternative medicine in multiple sclerosis: report of the Guideline Development Subcommittee of the American Academy of Neurology. *Neurology.* 2014;83(16):1484–1486.
26. Cheong WL, Mohan D, Warren N, Reidpath DD. Accessing palliative care for multiple sclerosis: a qualitative study of a neglected neurological disease. *Mult Scler Relat Disord*. 2019;35:86–91.
27. Creamer M, Cloud G, Kossmehl P, et al. Intrathecal baclofen therapy versus conventional medical management for severe poststroke spasticity: results from a multicentre, randomised, controlled, open-label trial (SISTERS). *J Neurol Neurosurg Psychiatry.* 2018;89(6):642–650.
28. Kojovic M, Cordivari C, Bhatia K. Myoclonic disorders: a practical approach for diagnosis and treatment. *Ther Adv Neurol Disord.* 2011;4(1):47–62.
29. Stone P, Minton O. European Palliative Care Research Collaborative pain guidelines. Central side-effects management: what is the evidence to support best practice in the management of sedation, cognitive impairment and myoclonus? *Palliat Med.* 2011;25(5):431–441.
30. Valls-Sole J. Electrodiagnostic studies of the facial nerve in peripheral facial palsy and hemifacial spasm. *Muscle Nerve.* 2007;36(1):14–20.
31. Carnero-Pardo C, Sanchez-Alvarez JC, Gomez-Camello A, Minguez-Castellanos A, Hernandez-Ramos FJ, Garcia-Gomez T. Myoclonus associated with thoracodorsal neuropathy. *Mov Disord.* 1998;13(6):971–972.
32. Sattin RW. Falls among older persons: a public health perspective. *Annu Rev Public Health.* 1992;13:489–508.
33. Verghese J, Ambrose AF, Lipton RB, Wang C. Neurological gait abnormalities and risk of falls in older adults. *J Neurol.* 2010;257(3):392–398.
34. Thurman DJ, Stevens JA, Rao JK; Quality Standards Subcommittee of the American Academy of Neurology. Practice parameter: assessing patients in a neurology practice for risk of falls (an evidence-based review): report of the Quality Standards Subcommittee of the American Academy of Neurology. *Neurology*. 2008;70(6):473–479.
35. Axer H, Axer M, Sauer H, Witte OW, Hagemann G. Falls and gait disorders in geriatric neurology. *Clin Neurol Neurosurg.* 2010;112(4):265–274.
36. O'Malley N, Clifford AM, Conneely M, Casey B, Coote S. Effectiveness of interventions to prevent falls for people with multiple sclerosis, Parkinson's disease and stroke: an umbrella review. *BMC Neurol.* 2021;21(1):378.
37. Paine CC 2nd, Snider JW 3rd. When saliva becomes a problem: the challenges and palliative care for patients with sialorrhea. *Ann Palliat Med.* 2020;9(3):1333–1339.
38. Karam CY, Paganoni S, Joyce N, Carter GT, Bedlack R. Palliative care issues in amyotrophic lateral sclerosis: an evidenced-based review. *Am J Hosp Palliat Care*. 2016;33(1):84–92.

23

Acute Delirium

Shih-Yin Lin and Donna E. McCabe

Key Points

- This chapter discusses the symptoms, subtypes, risk factors, causes, assessment, and management of acute delirium.
- Acute delirium is common and associated with worse outcomes but can often be preventable or reversible.
- The diagnosis and classification of acute delirium in palliative care can be challenging.
- As part of an interprofessional team, nurses play a critical role in the identification of at-risk patient groups, as well as early recognition, assessment, and management of acute delirium.

Case Study

Mr. Lee is a 72-year-old man who has non-small cell lung cancer, hypertension, chronic obstructive pulmonary disease, benign prostatic hyperplasia, and untreated cataracts. He has been followed by the palliative care team for symptom management since his cancer diagnosis 2 years ago.

Mr. Lee lives with spouse Pat, who is also his primary care partner. Pat calls the palliative care clinic to speak with the nurse due to Mr. Lee's recent increase in fatigue and confusion. Mr. Lee asked Pat "Why are there children sitting at the table?" Pat also reports Mr. Lee has been sleeping more over the past 2 days and is "groggy" during the day. The nurse advises Pat to bring Mr. Lee into the clinic immediately. The nurse reminds Pat to bring all of Mr. Lee's medications.

Upon arrival to the clinic, Mr. Lee is assessed by the registered nurse. Vital signs are blood pressure 130/70, pulse 102, respiratory rate 22, O_2 saturation 95% on room air, and temperature 99°F. He is awake and anxious, yelling "Let me go home now, I didn't want to come here." Mr. Lee does not answer questions that are directed to him.

Recognizing a change in mental status, the nurse performs the Confusion Assessment Method (CAM), which yields a positive result due to the acute onset of symptoms, inattention, and presence of disorganized thinking.

On further physical exam, the nurse notes Mr. Lee's lower abdomen is firm and distended, consistent with a full urinary bladder. The nurse performs an in-and-out catheterization that yields 900 mL of urine. The nurse collects blood to evaluate a complete blood count and chemistry panel and a urine sample for urinalysis and culture and sensitivity.

Medications:

Metoprolol XL 100 mg taken daily
Fluticasone 45/salmeterol 21 inhalation aerosol
Acetaminophen 500 mg two pills taken twice a day
"Sleep Aid" doxylamine 25 mg

During the medication review the nurse learns that Mr. Lee developed difficulty sleeping due to worsening knee pain. His family member gave him the over-the-counter "Sleep Aid," doxylamine 25 mg, which he has taken for the past 4 nights. The clinic physician examines Mr. Lee, collaborates with the nurse, and reviews the lab results. Mr. Lee is found to have a urinary tract infection (UTI) and delirium. The team is also concerned Mr. Lee may develop sepsis. The decision is made to admit Mr. Lee to the inpatient unit to begin intravenous (IV) antibiotics and monitor.

What are Mr. Lee's risk factors for developing delirium?

What do you think the underlying cause of delirium may be for Mr. Lee?

Are there any medications which could have precipitated the development of Mr. Lee's symptoms?

Introduction

Delirium, sometimes referred to as "acute confusion," is a neurocognitive disorder characterized by an acute disturbance in attention and awareness combined with an additional disturbance in cognition; these disturbances often fluctuate in severity during the course of a day.[1] In this chapter, we use the term "delirium" to refer to "acute delirium" unless otherwise specified.

Prevalence

Delirium is common in palliative care settings[2]: the prevalence of delirium ranges from 6.6% to 73% at admission to inpatient palliative care and from 19% to 88% over the entire inpatient palliative care stay. At the initial inpatient palliative care consultation, the prevalence of delirium ranges from 9% to 57%; at the initial community palliative care assessment, 4% to 12%. Prior to death, the prevalence of delirium ranges from 42.5% to 44% in community settings and from 58% to 88% in inpatient settings.

Prognosis

Delirium is associated with worse outcomes in individuals receiving palliative care. For instance, a recent cohort study of 410 patients receiving palliative care showed that delirium is associated with prolonged hospitalization and increases in healthcare requirements/costs, institutionalization, and mortality.[3] Another study that followed 350 individuals with advanced cancer or major organ failure receiving inpatient or outpatient palliative care found that those who had delirium had significantly shorter median survival time (11 days in the delirium group vs. 62 days in the non-delirium group) and a lower survival rate (1.3% vs. 14.3%).[4] Given that delirium is predictive of death within days to weeks in individuals with serious illness, especially among those receiving hospice care or in a palliative care unit, if advance care planning has not been completed prior to the onset of delirium, it is often too late to do so.[5] Furthermore, delirium causes distress and burden in patients, their families, and clinicians.[6,7]

Diagnosis Criteria

The Diagnostic and Statistical Manual of Mental Disorders, fifth edition, Text Revision (DSM-5-TR)[1] offers five diagnostic criteria for delirium: (1) disturbances in attention and awareness to the environment; (2) an acute change (hours to a few days) in symptoms from baseline that often fluctuate in severity; (3) an additional disturbance in other cognitive functions such as memory deficit and disorientation; (4) disturbances in attention, awareness, and other cognitive functions that are not fully explained by another preexisting neurocognitive disorder or occur during a coma/severely reduced level of arousal; and (5) evidence from the history, physical examination, or laboratory findings that suggests a direct physiological consequence of another medical condition, substance intoxication/withdrawal, exposure to a toxin, or multiple etiologies.

Subtypes of Delirium

According to the DSM-5-TR, delirium can be further classified into subtypes by its duration, level of psychomotor activity, and etiology.[1] When delirium lasts from hours to days, it is termed "acute" delirium. When delirium lasts for weeks to months, it is termed "persistent" delirium. There are three psychomotor subtypes of delirium, namely, hyperactive, hypoactive, and mixed. Individuals with a *hyperactive* level of psychomotor activity (hyperactive delirium) tend to exhibit mood lability, agitation, and/or refusal to cooperate with medical care. Individuals with a *hypoactive* level of psychomotor activity (hypoactive delirium) tend to demonstrate sluggishness and lethargy that approaches stupor. Individuals with *mixed delirium*, in contrast, may demonstrate a normal level of psychomotor activity despite the disturbances in attention and awareness, or demonstrate fluctuating psychomotor activity levels.[1] In palliative care settings, hypoactive delirium is the most common psychomotor subtype, followed by mixed delirium.[2] The DSM-5-TR also provides specific diagnostic considerations and the *International Classification of Diseases* coding notes the following subtypes of delirium by etiology: substance intoxication delirium, substance withdrawal delirium, medication-induced delirium, delirium due to another medical condition, and delirium due to multiple etiologies.

Challenges in Delirium Diagnosis and Classification

The diagnosis and classification of delirium in palliative care can be challenging. Leonard and colleagues have outlined the following seven major challenges: (1) balancing the burden of investigation with the need for a thorough delirium assessment and management plan; (2) determining reversibility of delirium, considering the patient's proximity to death; (3) impaired capacity for communication and decision-making; (4) multimorbidity, cachexia, frailty, and fatigue; (5) polypharmacy and psychoactive drugs; (6) high possibility for misdiagnosis due to overlapping phenomenology between delirium, depression, dementia, and pain (e.g., hypoactive delirium tends to be misdiagnosed as depression); and (7) lack of clinical agreement regarding subsyndromal delirium.[8]

Pathophysiology

The exact pathophysiology of delirium is unclear. The syndrome of delirium has been described as "acute brain failure" to depict an understanding of the underlying brain dysfunction.[9] There are multiple complex pathways that are thought to be associated with the onset of delirium including inflammation, hypoxia, and oxidative stress.[9,10] The reticular activating system, the area of the brain that is responsible for a person's level of arousal, has been found to be altered in the presence of delirium.[9] Neurotransmitter dysfunction has also been identified as an alteration present with delirium, particularly a decrease in acetylcholine or an excess of dopamine.[10] The pathways to delirium often begin before symptoms are identified. Research is ongoing to understand the pathophysiology of delirium including identification of associated biomarkers.

Risk Factors

Risk factors for delirium can be broadly divided into predisposing factors and precipitating factors.[11] "Predisposing" refers to existing characteristics or conditions (e.g., age, cognitive impairment, or a chronic illness) that increase an individual's susceptibility/vulnerability to delirium. In contrast, "precipitating" factors are immediate events or assaults that trigger delirium (e.g., a new infection, a recent surgery, etc.). In older adults, common predisposing factors include advanced age, cognitive impairment/dementia, frailty, multimorbidity, sensory disorders, anemia, malnutrition, substance abuse, depression, and social isolation; common precipitating factors include surgery, anticholinergic drugs, psychoactive drugs, intensive care unit admission, acute blood loss, acute infection, electrolyte disturbances, hyponatremia or exsiccosis, sleep disturbances, immobility, physical restraints, substance withdrawal, urinary catheter, and foreign environment.[12]

It is important to note that some risk factors are modifiable (e.g., dehydration) while others (e.g., age) are not. Both modifiable and non-modifiable risk factors can inform clinical decision-making and be used to identify and prioritize high-risk patient groups.

Furthermore, through addressing modifiable risk factors and the underlying etiology, about 50% of the time, delirium is reversible even in persons facing a life-limiting serious illness.[13] According to a 2022 systematic review and meta-analysis,[14] potentially *modifiable* risk factors for delirium in adult patients receiving specialist palliative care include opioids, lower performance status, dehydration, hypoxemia, sleep disturbance, liver dysfunction, and infection; and *non-modifiable* risk factors include older age, male sex, primary brain cancer or brain metastases, and lung cancer.

Delirium Superimposed on Dementia

Due to population aging, dementia has become the top hospice principal diagnosis in the United States.[15] Both advanced age and dementia increase one's risk for delirium. When delirium occurs in persons living with existing dementia, it is termed "delirium superimposed on dementia" (DSD).[16] Compared to dementia alone, those with DSD have poorer prognosis, including accelerated cognitive and functional declines, lengthier hospital stays, and increased rates of rehospitalization, institutionalization, and death.[17] Due to overlapping symptoms between delirium and dementia, DSD is often undiagnosed or mistaken as worsening of existing dementia.[16] For instance, inattention is a diagnostic feature of delirium, but it can also occur in later stages of dementia. In contrast, an acute change in mental status from baseline and an altered level of consciousness are features unique to delirium and less common in dementia.[17] Thus, being vigilant about acute changes from baseline symptoms and levels of consciousness is essential to early detection of DSD and differential diagnosis between delirium, dementia, and DSD.

Etiology

The etiology of delirium is multifactorial. The model for delirium among older adults being the result of the relationship between the person's predisposing factors and precipitating factors can also be applied to a population of people dealing with serious illness.[18] The mnemonic DELIRIUMS (Table 23.1) can be used as a tool for the clinician to help identify the etiology of delirium. The mnemonic tool can also identify individuals at risk who will benefit from preventative care.

Table 23.1 DELIRIUMS mnemonic

DELIRIUMS mnemonic	
D	Drugs
E	Eyes, ears
L	Low O_2 states (myocardial infarction, stroke, pulmonary embolism)
I	Infection
R	Retention (of urine or stool)
I	Ictal (relating to after seizure or stroke)
U	Underhydration/undernutrition
M	Metabolic
S	Subdural hematoma

Assessment

Delirium is often unrecognized and undocumented by clinicians. Rates of unrecognized delirium, which is defined as the diagnosis of delirium after being unrecognized by a primary physician or nurse, is estimated to be about 60% of all cases.[17] This high rate of unrecognized delirium highlights the need for routine screening, while early recognition can improve outcomes for the person with acute delirium. The CAM[19] is considered the gold-standard tool for both screening for delirium and serving as an algorithm to diagnose delirium. The CAM has been proved as sensitive, specific, and reliable. The CAM tool is easy to use and intended for use by nurses and physicians. The CAM is available in a long form (10 items) or short form. The short-form CAM is the most commonly used in clinical practice. The clinician can assess for delirium by assessing for the presence or absence of four diagnostic features: (1) acute change or fluctuating course, (2) inattention, (3) disorganized thinking, and (4) altered level of consciousness. The diagnosis of delirium requires the presence of features (1) and (2) and either (3) or (4).[19] The CAM tool may be accessed for free after registration at https://help.agscocare.org/.

Other commonly used delirium assessment instruments in palliative care settings include the Memorial Delirium Assessment Scale,[20] the Nursing Delirium Screening Scale,[21] and the Delirium Observation Screening Scale.[22] For home hospice patients, the Buffalo Delirium Scale can be used to identify risk factors in the prodromal stage of delirium, help differentiate prodromal delirium from dementia, and identify individuals who may benefit from sleep interventions to delay the onset or reduce the occurrence of delirium.[23] Another two brief delirium assessment instruments recommended for nursing use are the 4 A's Test (4AT)[24–26] and the Richmond Agitation and Sedation Scale (RASS).[27,28] The 4AT is a rapid screening test that can be completed in 2 minutes. Although validation of the 4AT in palliative care settings is currently underway,[29] this instrument has been successfully implemented in an inpatient hospice quality improvement program and rated by the nursing staff as preferable to the short-form CAM.[24] Both the RASS and its modified version for serial administration[30] demonstrate moderate sensitivity and very high specificity for detecting DSD in older patients across clinical settings.[28] There is also a version of the RASS that is modified to assess level of sedation during palliative sedation therapy called the Richmond Agitation Sedation Scale—Palliative Version (RASS-PAL).[31] Table 23.2 provides a list of delirium assessment tools that have been validated in palliative care settings.

Informant-Based Delirium Assessments

Family and friends ("family care partners") of the patient may aid delirium assessment and early detection of delirium. There is an informant-based version of the CAM called Family Confusion Assessment Methods (FAM-CAM).[47,48] FAM-CAM is an 11-item instrument that can be administered to a care partner by a trained interviewer in person, on the telephone, or electronically or self-administered by the care partner. There are two other validated informant-administered assessments, the Informant Assessment of Geriatric Delirium[49] and Sour Seven.[50] However, these assessment instruments have not been validated in palliative care settings specifically.

Table 23.2 Delirium screening tools validated in palliative care settings

Instrument	Palliative care setting validated	Administration time
Bedside Confusion Scale[32]	Inpatient palliative care unit	2 minutes
Communication Capacity Scale - Item 4 (used as a single-item screener)[33]	Across inpatient and outpatient palliative care settings	<1 minute
Confusion Assessment Method (CAM)[34]	Specialist palliative care unit	5 minutes plus additional time to administer a cognitive testing test (To rate the CAM, a brief cognitive test such as the Short Portable Mental Status Questionnaire[35] or the Mini-Cog[36] and the digit span test should also be performed.)
Brief CAM[37]	Hospital palliative care services	2 minutes
Delirium Observational Screening Scale[38–40]	Inpatient palliative care unit, medical oncology ward, home hospice	5 minutes
Delirium Rating Scale—Revised 98[41,42]	Medical oncology wards and palliative care units	1-2 hours for gathering information (including family, staff interview, medical record review), and typically based on a 24-hour observation period.
Memorial Delirium Assessment Scale[20,43,44]	Acute palliative/supportive care units (advanced cancer patients)	≥10 minutes, plus additional time to establish rapport, review medical records, and speak to informants
Nursing Delirium Screening Scale[45]	Community hospice (advanced cancer patients within the final 7 days of life)	1–2 minutes
Single Question in Delirium[46]	Oncology inpatient service	<1 minute
Buffalo Delirium Scale[23]	Home hospice	Not reported

Additional Delirium Assessment Resources

For additional information and resources on delirium assessment instruments and how to choose among different tools, please visit the NIDUS website (https://deliriumnetwork.org/measurement/delirium-info-cards/). NIDUS stands for Network for Investigation of Delirium: Unifying Scientists. It is a collaborative, multidisciplinary network funded by the National Institute on Aging to advance scientific research on the causes, mechanisms, outcomes, diagnosis, prevention, and treatment of delirium in older adults.

Lab Results

A complete evaluation of a person with delirium may include laboratory data or other diagnostic tests to determine the possible etiologies and identify correctable issues. The specific tests will be determined by the provider, carefully considering the whole person including underlying medical issues and goals of care. The tests should be correlated to the common underlying causes of delirium. Common tests include serum analysis of electrolytes, complete blood count, blood urea nitrogen (BUN), creatinine, glucose, and urinalysis. Other diagnostic tests such as cardiac biomarkers, electrocardiogram, or imaging may also be considered by the interprofessional team and should be used in correlation with predisposing and precipitating factors.[51] Table 23.3 lists common laboratory and diagnostic tests possibly evaluated in the setting of delirium.

Table 23.3 Common laboratory and diagnostic tests to aid delirium assessment

Diagnostic evaluation	Indication
Complete blood count	Infection and anemia
Electrolytes	Electrolyte disorders particularly in sodium
Glucose	Hypoglycemia
Blood urea nitrogen and creatinine	Dehydration
Urinalysis, urine culture	Urinary tract infection
Thyroid function study	Hyper-/hypothyroidism
Electrocardiogram, cardiac biomarkers	Myocardial infarction
Chest X-ray	Pneumonia
Cerebral imaging (computed tomography, magnetic resonance imaging)	Suspicion for stroke or hemorrhage

Management

Early identification and treatment of delirium can improve outcomes for individuals. Delirium management requires an interprofessional, multifaceted approach. The treatment principles for delirium include identifying causes, treating those underlying causes as possible, and providing supportive care. The interprofessional team members involved in care may depend on the person's clinical setting but should always include family or care partners.

Nonpharmacological interventions to prevent delirium that can be implemented by the palliative care team and family care partners include optimize sleep–wake pattern; orient/reorient the patient to where they are, who they are, who you are, and what your role is; address sensory impairment and facilitate communication (using eyeglasses, hearing aids, and dentures where needed); encourage mobility; ensure adequate hydration and nutrition; monitor bladder and bowel function; and provide support and education.[18] Research shows that family care partners play a critical role in detection and prevention of delirium, symptom monitoring, and acting as advocates for their loved one with delirium.[52] To support these roles, family care partners would like to receive education and clear information on potential causes, progression, and treatment of delirium; how care partners can help to reduce the occurrence of delirium; and how to respond to their loved one with delirium. Family education and information should be provided early on or prior to the onset of delirium and may be provided in the format of information leaflets or booklets, along with routine discussion with a clinician.[53]

More specifically, nursing care for the individual experiencing delirium aims to reduce the distress associated with the syndrome, while the overall treatment for delirium includes treating the underlying cause or causes. Concurrent to treating the underlying etiology the nurse works with the older adult, interprofessional team, and care partners to provide supportive care aimed at reducing the length and severity of delirium.

Evidenced-based nonpharmacologic interventions to reduce delirium symptoms in general settings include promoting day/night routines, maintaining mobility, optimizing sensory function, optimizing nutrition, and providing reorientation as tolerated.[52,54] The palliative care nurse can tailor interventions to align with an individual's goals of care, as well as educate/engage family care partners in implementation of the tailored interventions. Table 23.4 describes interventions for each category.

Nurses are often the healthcare team members who spend the most time directly with patients and as such are key to delirium management. Evaluation of nurses' experiences with acute delirium management has found that, in addition to direct knowledge, nurses' perceptions and emotions, overall healthcare complexities, and team member influence can impact their delirium management. Interventions to address these related determinants of nurse delirium management include developing self-awareness of ageism, systems to facilitate effective teamwork and communication, and a supportive environment.[55]

Clinician training and education on delirium management that includes realistic clinical scenarios, interprofessional teams, and opportunities for nurses to practice clinical reasoning can improve delirium detection. Nurses found that the absence of delirium symptoms was more readily detectable than the presence of delirium symptoms. This was true particularly in the case of the hypoactive form of delirium in which delirium can present as a new onset of lethargy, inactivity, and slowed movement.[56]

There are no approved pharmacological treatments for delirium. The first pharmacological principle for treatment is to deprescribe the medications that may have precipitated the delirium. The nurse with the interprofessional team is alert to any medications that were recently added or changed. Anticholinergics, H_2-blockers, benzodiazepines, opioids, and antipsychotic medications are among the most common medications that may precipitate delirium.[57]

Existing evidence does not support the use of benzodiazepines to treat agitation in acute delirium. Benzodiazepines have proven efficacy only in treating delirium related to alcohol withdrawal. Benzodiazepines have been found to cause delirium particularly among older adults. Further, they have been found to extend the duration and severity of delirium when administered to those with delirium.[58]

There is growing evidence regarding antipsychotic use in the prevention and management of delirium. A meta-analysis conducted in 2019 found that evidence does not support the use of first-generation or second-generation antipsychotics for the routine treatment of delirium. Further, adverse events related to the use of antipsychotic medications include neurologic and cardiac issues, particularly QT prolongation and arrhythmias.[59]

Despite evidence for the lack of efficacy and the potential risks associated with antipsychotic medications in those with delirium, these medications may be indicated for individuals exhibiting certain symptoms. This subset of individuals includes those experiencing distressing hallucinations or delusions not amenable to nonpharmacological interventions and those with behavior that is dangerous to the person or others caring for the person. In these cases, antipsychotic medications with the best safety profile should be used judiciously in low doses for the least amount of time to avoid negative outcomes. The nurse and the interprofessional team members must continually monitor and reassess the patient for negative consequences, particularly the conversion of hyperactive delirium into hypoactive delirium due to the sedating properties of antipsychotics.[57] Furthermore, despite not being a prescriber, nurses play an important role in advocacy for appropriate medication use, given their knowledge of medications and delirium risk factors. The Beers Criteria is an evidenced-based list of potentially inappropriate medications (PIMs) among older adults.[60] This tool can assist the nurse in identifying PIMs to discuss with the older adult, family care partners, prescribers, and interprofessional team. The process of active deprescribing, stopping a potentially inappropriate medication before an adverse event occurs, is an important intervention for delirium prevention.[61]

Table 23.4 Nursing interventions to reduce delirium severity

Intervention domain	Strategy
Promote day/night routines	Provide activities during the day Limit daytime napping Daytime light exposure Sleep hygiene
Maintain mobility	Maintain activity and mobility Avoid prolonged bedrest Consider physical therapy referral
Optimize sensory function	Ensure sensory aids such as eyeglasses and hearing aids are used Provide adequate lighting Minimize extraneous noise
Optimizing nutrition	Provide hydration and nutrition Consider registered dietician referral
Reassurance and reorientation	Communicate with the person to reassure them frequently Include information to reorient and provide information Do not "force" reorientation as this can lead to agitation

Goal-Setting and Plan of Care

Delirium is a heterogenous syndrome; the severity of symptoms and likelihood of reversal of cognitive dysfunction will vary based on patient variables. Delirium is considered to be often preventable and reversible. Patient-centered and goal-concordant care plans that seek to treat the underlying factors can reduce the severity and length of symptoms. The duration and severity of symptoms vary greatly, dependent on the person's health status and the variable associated with the delirium development, including when it was identified. For some individuals, delirium may persist for months or longer and can be the initiating factor that leads to irreversible cognitive impairment (i.e., delirium reveals a new dementia diagnosis).[62]

Care plans or bundles that integrate evidence-based, interprofessional team–based interventions for delirium prevention and treatment have been found to improve outcomes. The Hospital Elder Life Program (HELP), a multicomponent intervention that began in 1993, used a treatment protocol that included daily visits, orientation, therapeutic activities, sleep enhancement, early mobilization, vision and hearing adaptation, fluid repletion, and feeding assistance.[63] This program has been proven effective to reduce delirium and associated negative outcomes such as falls in a variety of clinical settings including palliative care units.[64] Information regarding HELP can be found at https://help.agscocare.org/.

Another example of an integrated model of care is the ABCDEF or A2F bundle.[65] This group of interventions aims to improve outcomes for those with critical illness. Interventions in the bundle include awakening and breathing coordination, delirium monitoring/management, early exercise and mobility, and family engagement. A meta-analysis conducted in 2019 examined 15 interprofessional team–based, delirium preventive models of care and identified several models that had efficacy for reducing delirium or its duration.[66] However, there is a need for further research in models of care for both prevention and treatment of delirium across care settings.

Recap the Case Study

Mr. Lee was admitted to the inpatient palliative care unit and received intravenous antibiotics for the UTI. The over-the-counter sleeping aid medication doxylamine was deprescribed. Acetaminophen was changed to 625 mg every 6 hours to address the pain associated with the UTI as well as reduce fever. Significant lab results included sodium 152 mEq/L and BUN 42 mg/dL due to dehydration. He received IV fluids for 1 day and was encouraged to drink and eat with assistance.

Upon arrival to the inpatient unit, Mr. Lee was anxious and agitated. He was initially resistant to the placement of the IV, repeatedly yelling at the nursing staff to bring him home and attempting to get out of bed unassisted. The nursing staff implemented the delirium nursing care plan, which includes providing an environment with low stimuli and using calming and reassuring communication as well as reorientation as possible. Mr. Lee's attempts to walk unassisted were reduced after the nursing staff addressed his personal needs of hunger and use of the toilet.

The nursing staff continued to assess Mr. Lee using the CAM tool. His UTI symptoms as well as his attention and disorganized thinking improved over the 3 days he was hospitalized. As Mr. Lee transitioned home with his spouse the interprofessional team provided teaching and support including use of the FAM-CAM

Conclusion

Delirium is a serious and common syndrome in palliative care that can have poor outcomes. Nurses play an essential role as part of the interprofessional team in identifying those at risk, avoiding precipitating factors when possible, frequently assessing patients for signs and symptoms of delirium, and providing family and patient education on delirium. Nurses together with the healthcare team advocate for appropriate treatment to improve patient care outcomes and quality of life.

REFERENCES

1. American Psychiatric Association. *Diagnostic and Statistical Manual of Mental Disorders*. 5th ed., text rev. American Psychiatric Association ; 2022.
2. Watt CL, Momoli F, Ansari MT, et al. The incidence and prevalence of delirium across palliative care settings: a systematic review. *Palliat Med*. 2019;33(8):865–877. https://doi.org/10.1177/0269216319854944.
3. Seiler A, Schubert M, Hertler C, et al. Predisposing and precipitating risk factors for delirium in palliative care patients. *Palliat Support Care*. 2020;18(4):437–446. https://doi.org/10.1017/S1478951519000919.
4. Klankluang W, Tongsai S, Sriphirom C, Siriussawakul A, Chanthong P, Tayjasanant S. The prevalence, associated factors, clinical impact, and state of diagnosis of delirium in palliative care patients. *Support Care Cancer*. 2021;29(12):7949–7956. https://doi.org/10.1007/s00520-021-06367-7.
5. Bramati P, Bruera E. Delirium in palliative care. *Cancers*. 2021;13(23):5893. https://doi.org/10.3390/cancers13235893.
6. Featherstone I, Hosie A, Siddiqi N, et al. The experience of delirium in palliative care settings for patients, family, clinicians and volunteers: a qualitative systematic review and thematic synthesis. *Palliat Med*. 2021;35(6):988–1004. https://doi.org/10.1177/02692163211006313.
7. Schmitt EM, Gallagher J, Albuquerque A, et al. Perspectives on the delirium experience and its burden: common themes among older patients, their family caregivers, and nurses. *Gerontologist*. 2019;59(2):327–337. https://doi.org/10.1093/geront/gnx153.
8. Leonard MM, Agar M, Spiller JA, et al. Delirium diagnostic and classification challenges in palliative care: subsyndromal delirium, comorbid delirium-dementia, and psychomotor subtypes. *J Pain Symptom Manage*. 2014;48(2):199–214. https://doi.org/10.1016/j.jpainsymman.2014.03.012.
9. Maldonado JR. Delirium pathophysiology: an updated hypothesis of the etiology of acute brain failure. *Int J Geriatr Psychiatry*. 2018;33(11):1428–1457. https://doi.org/10.1002/gps.4823.
10. Thom RP, Levy-Carrick NC, Bui M, Silbersweig D. Delirium. *Am J Psychiatry*. 2019;176(10):785–793. https://doi.org/10.1176/appi.ajp.2018.18070893.
11. Bush SH, Lawlor PG, Ryan K, et al. Delirium in adult cancer patients: ESMO clinical practice guidelines. *Ann Oncol*. 2018;29:iv143–iv165. https://doi.org/10.1093/annonc/mdy147.
12. Iglseder B, Frühwald T, Jagsch C. Delirium in geriatric patients. *Wien Med Wochenschr 1946*. 2022;172(5–6):114–121. https://doi.org/10.1007/s10354-021-00904-z.
13. Leonard M, Raju B, Conroy M, et al. Reversibility of delirium in terminally ill patients and predictors of mortality. *Palliat Med*. 2008;22(7):848–854. https://doi.org/10.1177/0269216308094520.
14. Featherstone I, Sheldon T, Johnson M, et al. Risk factors for delirium in adult patients receiving specialist palliative care: a systematic review and meta-analysis. *Palliat Med*. 2022;36(2):254–267. https://doi.org/10.1177/02692163211065278.

15. National Hospice and Palliative Care Organization. *NHPCO Facts and Figures*. 2021 ed. National Hospice and Palliative Care Organization; 2021.
16. Apold S. Delirium superimposed on dementia. *J Nurse Pract*. 2018;14(3):183–189. https://doi.org/10.1016/j.nurpra.2017.12.010.
17. Oh ES, Fong TG, Hshieh TT, Inouye SK. Delirium in older persons: advances in diagnosis and treatment. *JAMA*. 2017;318(12):1161–1174. https://doi.org/10.1001/jama.2017.12067.
18. Bush SH, Tierney S, Lawlor PG. Clinical assessment and management of delirium in the palliative care setting. *Drugs*. 2017;77(15):1623–1643. https://doi.org/10.1007/s40265-017-0804-3.
19. Inouye SK, van Dyck CH, Alessi CA, Balkin S, Siegal AP, Horwitz RI. Clarifying confusion: the confusion assessment method. A new method for detection of delirium. *Ann Intern Med*. 1990;113(12):941–948. https://doi.org/10.7326/0003-4819-113-12-941.
20. Breitbart W, Rosenfeld B, Roth A, Smith MJ, Cohen K, Passik S. The Memorial Delirium Assessment Scale. *J Pain Symptom Manage*. 1997;13(3):128–137. https://doi.org/10.1016/s0885-3924(96)00316-8.
21. Gaudreau JD, Gagnon P, Harel F, Tremblay A, Roy MA. Fast, systematic, and continuous delirium assessment in hospitalized patients: the nursing delirium screening scale. *J Pain Symptom Manage*. 2005;29(4):368–375. https://doi.org/10.1016/j.jpainsymman.2004.07.009.
22. Schuurmans MJ, Shortridge-Baggett LM, Duursma SA. The Delirium Observation Screening Scale: a screening instrument for delirium. *Res Theory Nurs Pract*. 2003;17(1):31–50. https://doi.org/10.1891/rtnp.17.1.31.53169.
23. Breier JM, Meier ST, Kerr CW, Wright ST, Grant PC, Depner RM. Screening for delirium: development and validation of the Buffalo Delirium Scale for use in a home-based hospice setting. *Am J Hosp Palliat Med*. 2018;35(5):794–798. https://doi.org/10.1177/1049909117739386.
24. Baird L, Spiller JA. A quality improvement approach to cognitive assessment on hospice admission: could we use the 4AT or Short CAM? *BMJ Open Qual*. 2017;6(2). https://doi.org/10.1136/bmjoq-2017-000153.
25. Bellelli G, Morandi A, Davis DHJ, et al. Validation of the 4AT, a new instrument for rapid delirium screening: a study in 234 hospitalised older people. *Age Ageing*. 2014;43(4):496–502. https://doi.org/10.1093/ageing/afu021.
26. Bridwell RE, April MD, Long B. Is the 4AT score accurate in identifying delirium in older adults? *Ann Emerg Med*. 2021;77(6):628–630. https://doi.org/10.1016/j.annemergmed.2020.12.022.
27. Sessler CN, Gosnell MS, Grap MJ, et al. The Richmond Agitation–Sedation Scale: validity and reliability in adult intensive care unit patients. *Am J Respir Crit Care Med*. 2002;166(10):1338–1344. https://doi.org/10.1164/rccm.2107138.
28. Morandi A, Han JH, Meagher D, et al. Detecting delirium superimposed on dementia: evaluation of the diagnostic performance of the Richmond Agitation and Sedation Scale. *J Am Med Dir Assoc*. 2016;17(9):828–833. https://doi.org/10.1016/j.jamda.2016.05.010.
29. Arnold E, Finucane AM, Spiller JA, Tieges Z, MacLullich AMJ. Validation of the 4AT tool for delirium assessment in specialist palliative care settings: protocol of a prospective diagnostic test accuracy study. *AMRC Open Res*. 2021;3:16. https://doi.org/10.12688/amrcopenres.12973.1.
30. Chester JG, Harrington MB, Rudolph JL, Group on behalf of the VDW. Serial administration of a modified Richmond Agitation and Sedation Scale for delirium screening. *J Hosp Med*. 2012;7(5):450–453. https://doi.org/10.1002/jhm.1003.
31. Bush SH, Grassau PA, Yarmo MN, Zhang T, Zinkie SJ, Pereira JL. The Richmond Agitation–Sedation Scale modified for palliative care inpatients (RASS-PAL): a pilot study exploring validity and feasibility in clinical practice. *BMC Palliat Care*. 2014;13(1):17. https://doi.org/10.1186/1472-684X-13-17.
32. Stillman MJ, Rybicki LA. The Bedside Confusion Scale: development of a portable bedside test for confusion and its application to the palliative medicine population. *J Palliat Med*. 2000;3(4):449–456. https://doi.org/10.1089/jpm.2000.3.4.449.
33. Hamano J, Morita T, Ozawa T, et al. Validation of the Simplified Palliative Prognostic Index using a single item from the Communication Capacity Scale. *J Pain Symptom Manage*. 2015;50(4):542–547.e4. https://doi.org/10.1016/j.jpainsymman.2015.04.021.
34. Ryan K, Leonard M, Guerin S, Donnelly S, Conroy M, Meagher D. Validation of the Confusion Assessment Method in the palliative care setting. *Palliat Med*. 2009;23(1):40–45. https://doi.org/10.1177/0269216308099210.
35. Pfeiffer E. A short portable mental status questionnaire for the assessment of organic brain deficit in elderly patients. *J Am Geriatr Soc*. 1975;23(10):433–441. https://doi.org/10.1111/j.1532-5415.1975.tb00927.x.
36. Borson S, Scanlan J, Brush M, Vitaliano P, Dokmak A. The Mini-Cog: a cognitive "vital signs" measure for dementia screening in multi-lingual elderly. *Int J Geriatr Psychiatry*. 2000;15(11):1021–1027. https://doi.org/10.1002/1099-1166(200011)15:11<1021::aid-gps234>3.0.co;2-6.
37. Wilson JE, Boehm L, Samuels LR, et al. Use of the brief Confusion Assessment Method in a veteran palliative care population: a pilot validation study. *Palliat Support Care*. 2019;17(5):569–573. https://doi.org/10.1017/S1478951518001050.
38. Jorgensen S, Carnahan R, Nguyen C, Weckmann MT. Effectiveness of the Delirium Observation Screening Survey at identifying delirium in home hospice patients. *Am J Hosp Palliat Care*. 2017;34(8):744–747. https://doi.org/10.1177/1049909116658468.
39. Detroyer E, Clement PM, Baeten N, et al. Detection of delirium in palliative care unit patients: a prospective descriptive study of the Delirium Observation Screening Scale administered by bedside nurses. *Palliat Med*. 2014;28(1):79–86. https://doi.org/10.1177/0269216313492187.
40. Neefjes ECW, van der Vorst MJDL, Boddaert MSA, et al. Accuracy of the Delirium Observational Screening Scale (DOS) as a screening tool for delirium in patients with advanced cancer. *BMC Cancer*. 2019;19(1):160. https://doi.org/10.1186/s12885-019-5351-8.
41. Trzepacz PT, Baker RW, Greenhouse J. A symptom rating scale for delirium. *Psychiatry Res*. 1988;23(1):89–97. https://doi.org/10.1016/0165-1781(88)90037-6.
42. O'Sullivan R, Meagher D, Leonard M, et al. A comparison of the revised Delirium Rating Scale (DRS-R98) and the Memorial Delirium Assessment Scale (MDAS) in a palliative care cohort with DSM-IV delirium. *Palliat Support Care*. 2015;13(4):937–944. doi:10.1017/S1478951514000613.
43. Lawlor PG, Nekolaichuk C, Gagnon B, Mancini IL, Pereira JL, Bruera ED. Clinical utility, factor analysis, and further validation of the Memorial Delirium Assessment Scale in patients with advanced cancer: assessing delirium in advanced cancer. *Cancer*. 2000;88(12):2859–2867.

44. Mercadante S, Adile C, Ferrera P, Cortegiani A, Casuccio A. Delirium assessed by Memorial Delirium Assessment Scale in advanced cancer patients admitted to an acute palliative/supportive care unit. *Curr Med Res Opin*. 2017;33(7):1303–1308. https://doi.org/10.1080/03007995.2017.1315332.
45. de la Cruz M, Noguera A, San Miguel-Arregui MT, Williams J, Chisholm G, Bruera E. Delirium, agitation, and symptom distress within the final seven days of life among cancer patients receiving hospice care. *Palliat Support Care*. 2015;13(2):211–216. https://doi.org/10.1017/S1478951513001144.
46. Sands MB, Dantoc BP, Hartshorn A, Ryan CJ, Lujic S. Single Question in Delirium (SQiD): testing its efficacy against psychiatrist interview, the Confusion Assessment Method and the Memorial Delirium Assessment Scale. *Palliat Med*. 2010;24(6):561–565. https://doi.org/10.1177/0269216310371556.
47. Steis MR, Evans L, Hirschman KB, et al. Screening for delirium via family caregivers: convergent validity of the Family Confusion Assessment Method (FAM-CAM) and interviewer-rated CAM. *J Am Geriatr Soc*. 2012;60(11):2121–2126. https://doi.org/10.1111/j.1532-5415.2012.04200.x.
48. Inouye SK, Puelle MR, Saczynski JS, Steis MR. *The Family Confusion Assessment Method (FAM-CAM): Instrument and Training Manual*. Hospital Elder Life Program; 2012.
49. Rhodius-Meester HFM, van Campen JPCM, Fung W, Meagher DJ, van Munster BC, de Jonghe JFM. Development and validation of the Informant Assessment of Geriatric Delirium Scale (I-AGeD). Recognition of delirium in geriatric patients. *Eur Geriatr Med*. 2013;4(2):73–77. https://doi.org/10.1016/j.eurger.2012.11.006.
50. Shulman RW, Kalra S, Jiang JZ. Validation of the Sour Seven Questionnaire for screening delirium in hospitalized seniors by informal caregivers and untrained nurses. *BMC Geriatr*. 2016;16:44. https://doi.org/10.1186/s12877-016-0217-2.
51. Mattison MLP. Delirium. *Ann Intern Med*. 2020;173(7):ITC49–ITC64. https://doi.org/10.7326/AITC202010060.
52. Mulkey MA, Olson DM, Hardin SR. Top four evidence-based nursing interventions for delirium. *Medsurg Nurs*. 2019;28(6):357–362.
53. Finucane AM, Lugton J, Kennedy C, Spiller JA. The experiences of caregivers of patients with delirium, and their role in its management in palliative care settings: an integrative literature review. *Psychooncology*. 2017;26(3):291–300. https://doi.org/10.1002/pon.4140.
54. Harris C, Spiller J, Finucane A. Managing delirium in terminally ill patients: perspective of palliative care nurse specialists. *Br J Community Nurs*. 2020;25(7):346–352. https://doi.org/10.12968/bjcn.2020.25.7.346.
55. Lim XM, Lim ZHT, Ignacio J. Nurses' experiences in the management of delirium among older persons in acute care ward settings: a qualitative systematic review and meta-aggregation. *Int J Nurs Stud*. 2022;127:104157. https://doi.org/10.1016/j.ijnurstu.2021.104157.
56. Hoch J, Bauer JM, Bizer M, Arnold C, Benzinger P. Nurses' competence in recognition and management of delirium in older patients: development and piloting of a self-assessment tool. *BMC Geriatr*. 2022;22:879. https://doi.org/10.1186/s12877-022-03573-8.
57. Hollmann P. The American Geriatrics Society releases the 7th edition *Geriatric Nursing Review Syllabus*. *J Gerontol Nurs*. 2022;48(5):51–52. https://doi.org/10.3928/00989134-20220404-01.
58. Hui D. Benzodiazepines for agitation in patients with delirium: selecting the right patient, right time, and right indication. *Curr Opin Support Palliat Care*. 2018;12(4):489–494. https://doi.org/10.1097/SPC.0000000000000395.
59. Neufeld KJ, Needham DM, Oh ES, et al. *Antipsychotics for the Prevention and Treatment of Delirium*. Comparative Effectiveness Review No. 219. Agency for Healthcare Research and Quality; 2019. https://doi.org/10.23970/AHRQEPCCER219.
60. American Geriatrics Society Beers Criteria® Update Expert Panel. American Geriatrics Society 2019 updated AGS Beers Criteria® for potentially inappropriate medication use in older adults. *J Am Geriatr Soc*. 2019;67(4):674–694. https://doi.org/10.1111/jgs.15767.
61. Wright DJ, Scott S, Buck J, Bhattacharya D. Role of nurses in supporting proactive deprescribing. *Nurs Stand*. 2019;34(3):44–50. https://doi.org/10.7748/ns.2019.e11249.
62. Fong TG, Tulebaev SR, Inouye SK. Delirium in elderly adults: diagnosis, prevention and treatment. *Nat Rev Neurol*. 2009;5(4):210–220. https://doi.org/10.1038/nrneurol.2009.24.
63. Strijbos MJ, Steunenberg B, van der Mast RC, Inouye SK, Schuurmans MJ. Design and methods of the Hospital Elder Life Program (HELP), a multicomponent targeted intervention to prevent delirium in hospitalized older patients: efficacy and cost-effectiveness in Dutch health care. *BMC Geriatr*. 2013;13:78. https://doi.org/10.1186/1471-2318-13-78.
64. Hshieh TT, Yang T, Gartaganis SL, Yue J, Inouye SK. Hospital Elder Life Program: systematic review and meta-analysis of effectiveness. *Am J Geriatr Psychiatry*. 2018;26(10):1015–1033. https://doi.org/10.1016/j.jagp.2018.06.007.
65. Marra A, Ely EW, Pandharipande PP, Patel MB. The ABCDEF bundle in critical care. *Crit Care Clin*. 2017;33(2):225–243. https://doi.org/10.1016/j.ccc.2016.12.005.
66. Khan A, Boukrina O, Oh-Park M, Flanagan NA, Singh M, Oldham M. Preventing delirium takes a village: systematic review and meta-analysis of delirium preventive models of care. *J Hosp Med*. 2019;14:E1–E7. https://doi.org/10.12788/jhm.3212.

24

Anxiety and Depression

Katharine Adelstein and Elizabeth Archer-Nanda

Key Points

- Delineating normal adjustment to illness from psychiatric conditions can be challenging due to the presence of overlapping somatic symptomatology. Removing barriers to accurate diagnosis and intervention for psychiatric sequalae (depression and anxiety) in palliative care patients can be helpful for improving quality of life. Normalizing the importance of treatment of anxiety and depression in palliative care settings can be helpful for growing patient and family acceptance of care interventions.

Case Study

Sue is a 38-year-old woman diagnosed with advanced ovarian cancer. Sue is married and has three children, aged 21, 19, and 14. Her children have a good relationship with both her and her husband. They have long admired her independent spirit and wit. Sue has completed multiple rounds of chemotherapy without ability to achieve a sustained remission. Treatment sequelae have left Sue feeling fatigued, and she has limited appetite. Feelings of hopelessness have become overwhelming, with a growing belief she has let her family down. As a result of feeling ashamed, she has not been able to achieve a remission from her disease, she has begun isolating herself from friends and family, and she no longer finds enjoyment in spending time with her family or being with her horses.

Introduction

Psychiatric symptoms are common in patients with serious illnesses; among the most commonly diagnosed are anxiety and depression.[1] The Academy of Consultation-Liaison Psychiatry urges that good end-of-life care must also include attention to mental health disorders.[1] Adequate assessment and interventions are important for ameliorating emotional and psychological suffering.

Depression is the most common mental health condition arising in the context of advanced illness yet remains underdiagnosed and undertreated. Anxiety is also known to rise at diagnosis of serious illness for a panoply of reasons: fear, growing understanding of limitations to medical interventions, and co-occurring medical symptoms causing distress. Patients may exhibit emotional or behavioral symptoms arising from the onset of a stressor (advanced illness) with distress greater than expected and impairment in functioning consistent with a clinical adjustment disorder with either predominant anxious or depressed features. An understanding of common psychiatric conditions arising in palliative care is important for nursing staff to foster early intervention and the normalization of psychiatric intervention at the end of life.

Nurses are aptly positioned to aid in the elimination of barriers to timely mental health interventions. Among the most important nursing roles are patient advocate and extension of psychoeducation. Greater nursing understanding of the clinical significance of comorbid psychiatric conditions including anxiety and depression increases the likelihood that patients and families will gain access to appropriate interventions.

Prevalence and Scope

Symptoms of depression and anxiety are common in individuals receiving palliative care, yet they are still misunderstood, underdiagnosed, and undertreated.[2–6] Healthcare team members, including nurses, often fail to recognize the extent of a patient's mood symptoms until late in the course of the disease. The late diagnosis means treatment is often initiated too late for the patient to experience real relief.[3] Barriers to the recognition and appropriate treatment of depression and anxiety in patients with serious illness can include the belief that all patients facing the end of life are "depressed," the clinician's lack of knowledge or understanding related to the treatment of depression and other psychiatric disorders, fear of further upsetting the patient or family and disrupting them at a vulnerable time, the stigma associated with psychiatric diagnoses, concern about prescribing psychoactive medications and possible drug-drug interactions, and clinician feelings of helplessness and hopelessness when caring for patients across the palliative care trajectory.[7]

It is important to focus on psychological distress in patients nearing the end of life because it is one of the primary causes of suffering in this population.[8,9] Depression and anxiety are highly correlated with reduced health-related quality of life, decreased adherence to treatment, increased difficulty in managing the patient's primary treatment or course of illness, and earlier admission to hospice care.[2,10–15] Psychological symptoms also impair the patient's ability to experience joy, peace, pleasure, meaning, and connection as they attend to the tasks of the dying, the work of tying up loose ends, saying goodbyes, and separating from life.[16] This can make the dying process more difficult for the patient by increasing pain, both emotional and physical, and for the family, causing worry and intensifying the grief of losing a loved one.[17]

The estimated prevalence of depression in the palliative care population ranges from 24% to 70%.[18] Underdiagnosis,[19] lack of agreement regarding diagnostic criteria that are appropriate for the setting of advanced illness,[19] and difference in patient populations (e.g., demographics, disease type and stage),[20] and variation in assessment techniques[21] account for the large range in estimates of prevalence, though generally there is a higher rate of depression in patients experiencing greater levels of pain or disability.[22–24] The prevalence of depression in patients with cancer is estimated to range from 8% to 24%, with assessment technique, type of cancer, and treatment phase as significant influencers of the range.[25] Patients with other advanced medical illnesses also have elevated levels of depression. Depression was identified in end-stage kidney disease in approximately 27% of patients,[26,27] up to 40% of patients with Parkinson's disease,[28,29] approximately 35% of patients with advanced multiple sclerosis,[30] 46% of patients with advanced heart failure,[31] and 52% of patients with end-stage acquired immune deficiency syndrome.[32,33]

The prevalence of anxiety in palliative care settings may be even more difficult to estimate than depression due to varying assessment techniques and the overlay of medical factors mimicking anxious symptomatology and anxiety that rises to the level of a disorder, though all anxiety symptoms should be taken seriously and addressed by clinicians. Anxiety symptoms occur in up to 70% of patients with advanced illness.[11,34] Anxiety disorders, however, may occur in less than 10% of patients in palliative care, with younger age, female gender, and increased pain and disability as primary risk factors.[35]

Awareness of generalized risk factors for depression and anxiety in patients receiving palliative care can facilitate early diagnosis and interventions.[36]

- *Age and gender*: Several studies suggest that younger patients have higher rates of depression and anxiety and self-reported distress.[37–41] In the general population, women are twice as likely to receive a diagnosis of depression or anxiety; gender is not a consistently reported risk factor for depression or anxiety in patients with life-threatening illness.[42]
- *Prior history of mental illness*: A personal history of depression or anxiety is a major risk factor for depression and anxiety in palliative care patients.[4,43]
- *Uncontrolled symptoms*: The presence of uncontrolled symptoms, particularly pain, is a major risk factor for depression and suicidal thoughts in patients with serious illness.[44–46] Some studies suggest that depression may be amplified by pain, and others suggest that depression may lessen a patient's ability to tolerate pain; thus, the relationship between pain and anxiety may be bidirectional.[47–49] Symptoms such as dyspnea or air hunger are strongly correlated with anxiety in patients with late-stage lung disease.[50]
- *Type of illness and treatment-related factors*: In some cancers, depression or mood changes sometimes appear as a primary symptom of the disease. In patients with pancreatic cancer, psychiatric symptoms can precede the diagnosis by up to several months due to neuroendocrine changes associated with the tumor.[44,51,52] Tumors arising or metastasizing to the central nervous system can cause depression,[14,41,53,54] and tumors related to the production of increased cortisol can cause depression or anxiety due to increased levels of the hormone.[55,56] Patients with HIV are at additional risk of depression due to direct damage to the brain from virus and chronic stress related to the social ramifications of the illness.[57,58] Other cause of depression in patients with serious illness include autoimmune responses,[59] viral infection, nutritional deficiencies, and treatment-related factors such as treatment with steroid, certain anticonvulsant medications, some chemotherapies, and radiation to the head or brain.[60–66]
- *Existential concerns*: Facing mortality can bring to the surface many distressing existential concerns such as unfulfilled dreams or ambitions, unresolved relational conflicts, meaning in life and death, concerns related to dignity in dying, and spiritual questions related to what happens after death.[2] Existential suffering and personal emotional pain are some of the most distressing experiences that occur in the dying. [67] The relationship between existential suffering and depression or depressive symptoms in those with advanced illness is not well studied or understood; however, one study did show a higher correlation between depression and existential distress than physical symptoms, social isolation, or treatment-related factors.[40]

Screening

Sue presented to her palliative care team. She noted that she had been feeling down and hopeless recently, with less motivation to do what brings her joy, particularly walking with friends and spending time with her horse. Sue's nurse was also concerned about her reduced mood and increased fatigue, recognizing symptoms of possible depression. Sue's nurse screened her using the Patient Health Questionnaire (PHQ-9). Sue scored a 17 on the PHQ-9, and her nurse alerted the palliative care team to her depression symptoms and score on the PHQ-9.

A number of instruments have been studied regarding how to screen for depression and anxiety, with the Depression Cancer Consensus Group reporting validity studies involving at least 19 tools designed to help clinicians identify depression in the cancer setting.[68] The American Society of Clinical Oncology's guidelines recommend that all patients with cancer and cancer survivors be evaluated for symptoms of depression and anxiety at periodic times across the trajectory of care. Assessment should be performed using validated measures, such as the PHQ-9 and the Generalized Anxiety Disorder (GAD-7) for screening of depression and anxiety, respectively.[69] If moderate or severe symptomatology is detected through screening, individuals should have further diagnostic assessment to identify the nature and extent of the symptoms and the presence or absence of a mood or an anxiety disorder.[69]

There is no consensus on how to best screen for depression in patients receiving palliative care. Low completion rate due to patient frailty, refusal, or cognitive impairment is not uncommon. Shorter screening tools may be easier to use for both patients and providers. The sensitivity and specificity of different screening tools for depression in palliative care range from 0.72 to 1.0 and from 0.50 to 1.0, respectively.[70]

In a study by Chochinov et al. involving patients hospitalized and receiving palliative care, the sensitivity and specificity of a single question—"Have you felt depressed most of the day, nearly every day for two or more weeks?"—were both 1.0 and therefore diagnostic of depression.[71] In a small study within community patients receiving palliative care, the same single question had a high specificity of 0.85 and a low false-negative value of 0.94.[72] Thus, this single question seemed most helpful at screening out those patients who are not depressed and therefore do not more in-depth assessment of their mood. Due to low positive predictive value (0.57) in this study, it was determined that patients identified as possibly depressed by the single question need further assessment of their mood before they are started on treatment.

As far as screening for anxiety, the State-Trait Anxiety Inventory, the GAD-7, and the Fear of Disease Progression Scale have been reported as tools to be applied in cancer settings, although their acceptability is reported to be modest. The Hospital Anxiety and Depression Scale is a suitable tool for initial screening for both anxiety and depression, but it cannot be proposed as a diagnostic instrument.[73]

Diagnosis

Sue's score of 17 on the PHQ-9 represents a moderate to moderately severe depression. The palliative care team understood that this is, although common, not a normal part of serious illness and required the care of a mental health specialist. The palliative care team referred Sue to a psychiatric mental health nurse practitioner (PMHNP) within the cancer center for further diagnostic workup and treatment of her depression.

Even though depressive and anxious symptoms are common in patients receiving palliative care, these disorders are often misunderstood, underdiagnosed, and, hence, untreated. Studies indicate that up to 50%–60% of depression in patients with cancer is not properly recognized.[74]

There can be many barriers interfering with the recognition of clinically significant depression or anxiety. These may include:

- The clinician's own lack of knowledge or skill to diagnose and treat depression or anxiety
- Reluctance to bring up potentially upsetting topics (a very low proportion of patients discuss their low mood with their doctors or oncologists and choose to address somatic rather than affective and emotional symptoms)[75]
- Belief that depression is "normal" at the end of life
- Concerns about possible drug–drug interactions with antidepressants

The most widely used criteria to diagnose depression are those outlined in the *Diagnostic and Statistical Manual of Mental Disorders* (DSM-5, 2013).[76] If patients do not meet the full criteria for major depression or primary anxiety disorder, they can be classified as having "adjustment disorder" with depressive and/or anxiety features. A proposal to adopt a "substitutive" approach to diagnosis of depression has been debated for years. It suggests replacing somatic criteria (e.g., poor appetite, fatigue, impaired sleep) thought attributable to medical illness or its treatment with other substitutes, such as depressed appearance, social withdrawal, brooding/self-pity/pessimism, and lack of reactivity in situations that would normally be pleasurable.[77]

Table 24.1 Psychiatric disorders with depression as a predominant symptom

Adjustment disorder with depressed mood	Significant depressive symptoms in response to a life stressor causing undue distress and interference with daily functioning.
Major depressive disorder	Depression or anhedonia lasting for 2 weeks or more and present for most of the time. Associated symptoms include: weight loss, insomnia versus hypersomnia, psychomotor agitation or retardation, fatigue, feelings of worthlessness or inappropriate guilt, difficulty concentrating, and suicidal ideation.
Dysthymia	Depressed mood is present for most of the time for at least 2 years. Additional symptoms include changes in appetite and weight, fatigue, poor concentration, feelings of low self-esteem, and hopelessness.

However, most experts agree that, for clinical purposes, the use of an inclusive set of diagnostic criteria that incorporates both neuro-vegetative (somatic) and psychological symptoms of depression and emphasizes the presence of hopelessness, worthlessness, guilt, and suicidal ideation is most appropriate for the palliative care population.[78]

For this chapter, we will focus on major diagnostic categories for both depressive and anxiety disorders that are most likely to be identified in patients receiving palliative care (see Tables 24.1 and 24.2). A reader interested in more detailed diagnostic criteria is recommended to turn to two commonly used systems in nosology, the DSM-5 (2013) and the *International Classification of Diseases, 10th version*,[79] for further information.

Table 24.2 Psychiatric disorders with anxiety as a predominant symptom

Generalized anxiety disorder	Pervasive and excessive anxiety about a number of events/activities, occurring more days than not for at least 6 months. Additional symptoms include restlessness, easy fatigue, difficulty concentrating, irritability, muscle tension, and sleep disturbance.
Panic disorder	Recurrent unexpected panic attacks.
Adjustment disorder with anxiety	Occurs within 3 months of a major stressor and causes significant distress and functional impairments.
Phobias	Significant fear brought about by specific situations or objects (e.g., closed spaces, blood draws, needles). Often accompanied by avoidance of a feared stimulus.
Posttraumatic stress disorder	Follows a traumatic event. Presents with intrusion symptoms (e.g., memories), avoidance of stimuli associated with trauma, and negative alterations in cognition and mood. Increased arousal and reactivity are also present.

Depressive Disorders

At Sue's first appointment with her PMHNP, she provides a full history of her depression symptoms. She tells her nurse practitioner (NP) that for the last month or so she has been feeling down, with more crying than she is used to. She does not feel like getting out of the house for activities she used to enjoy and is instead staying in bed, using her illness as an excuse when friends or family ask to spend time with her. She is sleeping more but feeling more fatigued and notices that she is not interested in eating even when she is not struggling with nausea. She reports feeling hopeless about her illness and guilty that she has not had a response to treatment. She is worried about the effects of her illness and treatment on her husband and children and is concerned that she is a burden on them and that they wish she "just die already." Sue also notes that she has lost approximately 10 lb unintentionally over the last month.

Depressive syndromes are a common mental health problem in the palliative setting, but they are often unrecognized and undertreated. Clinicians often fail to appreciate the extent of a patient's depression until too late in the course of the disease.[3] Depressed mood, sadness, grief, and anticipatory feelings of loss are all appropriate responses to advanced disease and dying. However, feelings of hopelessness, helplessness, worthlessness, excessive guilt, lack of pleasure, and suicidal ideation (even passive) are among the best indicators of depressive syndromes in these patients.[79,80]

On the other hand, feelings of hopelessness, helplessness, and guilt must be considered in the context of the patient's illness. Hopelessness may be difficult to interpret in the setting of a disease where there is no hope for cure or recovery.[81] Almost all patients with advanced illness experience a certain degree of disengagement from areas of interest. However, a pervasive anhedonia that extends to loss of interest and pleasure in almost all activities warrants attention as an important indicator of clinically significant depression. Symptoms that seem out of proportion to the patient's actual situation should prompt concern for major depressive disorder. Major depression affects approximately 7% of the general population (8%–9% of women and 3%–4% of men), with data in oncology indicating a prevalence of 15%–40%, depending on several factors (e.g., type, stage of cancer, in-/outpatient, on/off treatment, type of diagnostic tool used).[82]

Important Factors for Consideration in the Diagnosis of Depression

During her initial appointment, her NP also took a complete medical and family history including a history of medications. Sue was an otherwise healthy 36-year-old woman when she began to experience abdominal bloating, constipation, and other vague gastrointestinal complaints. At the time of diagnosis, her medical history was not significant for any chronic illness, and she was only taking over-the-counter vitamins. She did not have a family history of cancer, heart disease, diabetes, or psychiatric illness including depression. Since her diagnosis she has been treated with surgery and the standard chemotherapeutic regimen for her ovarian cancer. At the present time she is not taking any medications thought to be contributors to depression, and her PMHNP was able to rule out any medical causes of depression symptoms including hypothyroid or hormonal alterations.

Depressive symptoms caused by medications or underlying medical conditions need to be taken into consideration. Some medications that are often given in advanced illness, for either therapeutic or palliative purposes, can have psychoactive effects that can mimic depression and anxiety. Additionally, circumstances related to medical illness itself can cause depression/anxiety or create symptoms that mimic depression and anxiety. When considering a diagnosis of depression or anxiety in a patient with advanced illness, it is important to include an examination of patient medications and a full medical workup. The following list of medications and medical considerations is not exhaustive and outlines only a few examples:

- *Medications*: corticosteroids, benzodiazepines, hormonal agents, amphotericin B, opioids
- *Chemotherapeutic agents*: vincristine, vinblastine, procarbazine, asparaginase, tamoxifen, interferon, interleukin-2
- *Medical factors*: electrolyte abnormalities (sodium, potassium, calcium), folate and/or vitamin B_{12} deficiencies, nutritional deficiencies, hypothyroidism, adrenal insufficiency, cognitive deficits, fatigue, pain, substance use concerns.[83]

Many of these medications or medical conditions can also contribute to delirium, which can present as confusion and/or agitation in its hyperactive form or withdrawal in its hypoactive form.[84] Patients with advanced illness may look depressed, withdrawn, apathetic, agitated, distressed, or unsettled; and the clinician should have a high level of suspicion for delirium if any of the medications or underlying medical abnormalities are present, prior to making a diagnosis of depression or anxiety.

Symptoms of depression should also be differentiated from normal grief reactions. During their end-of-life stage some patients go through a period of sadness or mourning while adjusting to loss and working through the existential issues that may arise. This "preparatory grief" process can be adaptive and appropriate. However, when a patient's grief becomes severe and lasting and includes pathological signs or symptoms such as persistent social withdrawal, pervasive hopelessness, or thoughts of suicide, they may be clinically depressed.[85] This distinction has clinical relevance for treatment as support for grieving patients may be different from support needed by those who are clinically depressed.[86]

Another important concept to consider as separate from major depression is demoralization or existential distress. Advanced illness and facing mortality can challenge a patient's fundamental assumptions about safety, personal control, and priorities in life.[87] This experience can lead to clinically relevant existential distress that is distinct from depression, though it is a risk factor for the development of depression.[87,88] Patients experiencing demoralization or existential distress as a result of the natural psychological tasks of dying may appear to have some symptoms of depression, but further investigation into the feelings underlying their symptoms will likely reveal a motivated desire for dignity and resolution of end-of-life conflicts. Patients in this situation crave a respect of their human autonomy, which strengthens their self-worth, acceptance, and hope and reinforces family connectedness.[89] Clinicians can provide dignity-conserving care that fosters coping strategies to control physical and psychosocial factors and alleviate suffering for these patients.[89]

Anxiety Disorders

Anxiety may be a natural response to suffering, uncertainty, disability, disfigurement, and impending death. While anxiety is often a normal response to terminal illness, clinical awareness of persistent symptoms and effective intervention can reduce undue suffering.[90] Somatic symptoms of anxiety including tachycardia, shortness of breath, diaphoresis, and gastrointestinal distress, are common, as are insomnia, hyperarousal, and irritability.[90]

Individuals approaching the end of life experience anxiety for a myriad of reasons. For many, illness is a disruptive event impacting individual roles, interpersonal relationships, capability to meet external demands, and future plans.[90] Anxiety can develop for many reasons and can increase as individuals become more aware of limitations to medical treatments.[90,91] Patients often experience gaps in understanding of medical terminology, further contributing anxiety in the context of fear arising from uncertainty. Characteristics associated with anxiety in the general population (female gender, younger age, and lower socioeconomic status) do not necessarily correlate to the development of anxiety in palliative care patients.[90] Anxiety affects an estimated 19.1% of the American population annually; approximately 31.1% of all US adults will experience anxiety across their lifetime.[92] A recent retrospective cross-sectional study including 351 cancer caregivers approximated 46.4% of patients to have experienced moderate to severe anxiety.[93]

Important Factors for Consideration in the Diagnosis of Anxiety

Similarly, to depressive symptoms, a clinician needs to take into consideration medications and underlying medical conditions when a patient with advanced illness presents with anxious symptoms. Many of the same medications, chemotherapeutic agents, and medical abnormalities can cause anxious symptoms as well as depressive symptoms, including the following:

- *Medications*: corticosteroids, dexamethasone, antiemetics (akathisia), bronchodilators, hormonal agents
- *Chemotherapeutic agents*: interferon, interleukin-2
- *Medical factors*: hypoxia, delirium, sepsis, bleeding, pulmonary embolus, arrhythmias, hypocalcemia, thyroid dysfunction, hypoglycemia
- *Substance-related*: intoxication and withdrawal

Many of these medications or medical conditions can also cause delirium, which may also present in a hyperactive form.[94] Patients may look agitated and hyperalert and could be experiencing hallucinations, delusions, or paranoia.[90]

Symptoms of anxiety should be delineated from medical factors creating anxious symptoms. Palliative care teams may consider obtaining laboratory studies to identify medical causes of anxiety and intervene as appropriate. Alcohol withdrawal should be managed as a medical emergency. Many patients approaching end of life have never seen a mental health practitioner.[90] Normalization of co-occurring anxiety and education related to the common role for mental health consultants in palliative care can ease additional anxiety related to the entry of an additional team member—the development of yet one more thing to "deal" with as a patient facing the end of life. Patients themselves may not identify as "anxious" and may prefer to use different terms, such as "concerned," "scared," or "worried."[95] Although it does not always reach a clinically significant level, it is important to recognize the presence of anxiety and its potential sources.[96]

Feelings of helplessness are common among individuals with advanced illness facing the end of life. It is important for nurses and other members of the team to help patients to manage practical concerns, rather than to attempt to change ineffective coping strategies.[90]

Treatment Considerations

Sue's PMHNP diagnosed her with major depressive disorder moderate to severe single episode as she had not had previous psychiatric illness. Sue's PMHNP consulted with her palliative registered nurse (RN) regarding Sue's symptoms of fatigue and loss of appetite. Sue's palliative RN advised her NP that her symptoms of fatigue and loss of appetite were unlikely to be related to her cancer or its treatment. Sue's NP recommended that Sue pursue psychotherapy with the licensed clinical social worker on the palliative care team and began a discussion about pharmacotherapy for depression with Sue.

When determining the best course of treatment for a patient suffering from anxiety and/or depression in the palliative care setting it is important to consider the degree of functional impairment and the severity and duration of the depressive symptoms.[97] Nurses are uniquely positioned to gain understanding of patient symptom experience and advocate for initiation of treatment. Before initiating treatment with psychotherapy or medication treatment for depressive or anxious symptoms it is crucial to treat uncontrolled physical symptoms such as pain, fatigue, or shortness of breath. Then further assessment of the patient's emotional symptoms, including the nature of the emotional distress; factors contributing to the symptoms, including psychosocial factors, demoralization, or existential distress; and comorbid symptoms such as pain and fatigue are important to determining what the most effective intervention may be.[98] Empirical evidence suggests that severe depression and anxiety are best treated with a combination of psychotherapy and pharmacotherapy.[98] Regardless of who undertakes the treatment of depression and anxiety symptoms pharmacologically (e.g., primary treating provider, palliative care provider, psychiatrist, psychiatric NP), a referral for psychotherapy or supportive counseling should be considered. Many palliative care teams also have the availability of a mental health professional such as a clinical psychologist or licensed clinical social worker (LCSW) or a chaplain trained to provide supportive counseling. Nurses are also able to use therapeutic communication to provide supportive care for patients in the palliative care setting.

Treatment Considerations: Psychotherapy

With the help of her palliative RN, Sue was able to schedule an appointment for counseling with the LCSW on her palliative care team. She worked with the LCSW on brief supportive therapy and engaged in therapeutic life review with meaning-centered psychotherapy woven throughout. She was also recommended some community resources including a support group for young people with cancer to help provide her with extra social support.

In non-palliative care settings, depression is usually treated with insight-oriented psychotherapy, which can be useful for patients in palliative care; however, for many patients, depressive symptoms are best managed with a combination of crisis intervention, brief supportive psychotherapy, and cognitive behavioral techniques.[99] Cognitive behavioral therapy focuses on understanding and controlling one's thoughts, which can change emotional and reactions and behaviors. This can be very helpful for intrusive thoughts about loss, life changes, or death and can help alleviate feelings of sadness, guilt, and worthlessness, thus reducing behaviors such as withdrawal and isolation.[99] Other goals of psychotherapy include enhancing coping skills, improving problem-solving skills, mobilizing support systems, reshaping negative or self-defeating thoughts, and directly reducing distress through a relationship with a knowledgeable and empathetic healthcare provider.[99,100] Disease-specific support groups can also be very helpful for patients as adjunctive therapies and have been shown to be effective at improving mood disturbance, promoting the use of positive coping strategies, and improving quality of life and have been linked to positive immune responses.[101,102] Resources for support groups can usually be found through disease foundations and through the social work, chaplaincy, or behavioral health departments at the hospital.

Existential psychotherapy may be particularly helpful in patients nearing the end of life. As patients in this situation grapple with changes in their sense of self, physical and psychological losses, challenges to their sense of wholeness and integrity, loss of control and independence (which together form the construct of dignity),[103] and challenges to self-determination and self-worth, psychotherapeutic approaches that are targeted at restoring these are extremely useful. Approaches such as dignity therapy,[103–107] meaning-centered psychotherapy,[108,109] and therapeutic review[110] are good choices for seriously ill patients who are struggling with questions about the meaning, purpose, and value of their lives. These therapeutic approaches can improve spiritual well-being, reduce sadness and depression, and promote or enhance a feeling of meaning, peace, and purpose at the end of life.

Treatment Considerations: Pharmacological

Depression

Once medical causes for depressive symptoms are ruled out and symptom burden is noted to interfere with functioning or enjoyment, a diagnosis of depression should be considered, and treatment should be initiated. It is important that psychopharmacological interventions are combined with psychotherapy for optimal patient benefit. Commonly used medications for the treatment of depression include selective serotonin reuptake inhibitors (SSRIs), serotonin norepinephrine reuptake inhibitors (SNRIs), atypical antidepressants, tricyclic antidepressants, psychostimulants, and wakefulness agents. Monoamine oxidase inhibitors are less commonly used due to adverse effects and interactions. Primary care providers are the largest group of prescribers of antidepressants, surpassing psychiatric prescribers, though this can lead to incomplete or ineffective treatment of depression.[91] Although 10% of the US adult population will fill one or more antidepressant prescriptions each year, many do not complete a full treatment course (9–12 months) and often do not understand that consistent use is needed to achieve benefit.[91] Astute understanding of the mechanisms of action, expectations for effectiveness, potential adverse effects, safety considerations, and potential contraindications and drug–drug interactions is important when prescribing antidepressants for patients on complex medication regimens. For a list of commonly used medications for depression and anxiety please see Table 24.3.

Anxiety

Once medication- and other medically related causes of anxious symptoms have been ruled out and anxiety is interfering with a patient's quality of life, nonpharmacological strategies (e.g., therapy, distraction, relaxation, breathing, or mindfulness exercises) should be considered first. If those interventions alone are not helpful at reducing symptoms, medications may be warranted.[91] Commonly prescribed medications for the treatment of anxiety include antidepressants (SSRIs, SNRIs), antipsychotics (generally second-generation atypical antipsychotics), antihistaminic medications, anticonvulsant medications (gabapentin or pregabalin), propranolol, and non-benzodiazepine anxiolytics. Benzodiazepines are best prescribed for short-term treatment of acute anxiety, such as during a test or procedure, and may also be used to treat acute alcohol or substance withdrawal. It is important to use benzodiazepines cautiously and for shorter periods of time (less than 2 weeks) due to increased risk for abuse, dependence, and diversion.

Medication Considerations

Sue's PMHNP elected to add citalopram at a dose of 20 mg by mouth daily, which was helpful in combination with the therapy delivered by her social worker and the added social interaction with her support group.

It can be helpful to consult with a clinical pharmacist when adding medications for patients approaching the end of life to ensure maximum benefit and minimize any adverse effects. With any medication, it is important to consider each patient's unique characteristics and weigh risk–benefit ratios and patient preference. Factors for consideration when prescribing medications include patient comorbidities, risk for drug interactions, capacity for adherence to medication regimens, route of administration, and absorption concerns. Additionally, prescribers must consider the pharmacokinetics of a medication to determine if patients will have time to enjoy the benefits of the medication or if a faster-acting option may be more useful.

*Delirium does not have any FDA approved medications, these are commonly used, however, off label.[89]

Considerations in Children

Due to challenges in diagnosing mental illness in a growing and developing brain, information about the incidence of depression and anxiety in children is limited. The Joint Commission on Mental Health of Children states that 1.4 million children under the age of 18 suffer from clinically significant depression or another similar disorder, and only one-third of these children receive help for their disorder.[99] A diagnosis of life-limiting or terminal disease

Table 24.3 Commonly prescribed medications for depression and anxiety psychiatric disorders with anxiety as a predominant symptom

Drug class (examples)	Indications	Considerations and potential adverse effects	Abuse potential
SSRIs (citalopram, escitalopram, fluoxetine, paroxetine, sertraline)	Depression Anxiety (may be used to help anxiety, OCD, panic, hot flashes)	Require daily use. May take 2–5 weeks to achieve benefit. Anxiety, restlessness, drowsiness, gastric upset.	None
SNRIs (venlafaxine, desvenlafaxine, duloxetine)	Depression Anxiety (may be used to help pain, hot flashes)	Require daily use. May take 2–5 weeks to achieve benefit. Anxiety, restlessness, drowsiness, gastric upset.	None
Other antidepressants (mirtazapine, bupropion)	Major depression (also used to help insomnia, poor appetite), depression, seasonal affective disorder, smoking cessation (may help attention, sexual dysfunction)	Require daily use. May take several weeks to achieve benefit. Less common to experience gastric upset, may help nausea. Requires daily use, may take weeks for benefit. Can be activating and contribute to agitation/ insomnia. Monitor for anorexia. May lower seizure threshold.	None None
Non-benzodiazepine anxiolytic (buspirone)	Generalized anxiety disorder (often used for other anxiety, can help air hunger)	Must be taken daily, may take several weeks to help. May not help those who have taken benzodiazepines in past. Rare for adverse effects.	None
Benzodiazepines (alprazolam, oxazepam, lorazepam, chlordiazepoxide, diazepam, chlorazepate, clonazepam, temazepam)	Anxiety withdrawal Anxiety-related insomnia IV forms to treat status epilepticus	Should be used for less than 2 weeks. Can increase risk for dependence, delirium, disinhibition. Limit use in individuals with hepatic dysfunction. Sedation, disinhibition, respiratory depression, impaired concentration, memory disturbance.	Moderate to high risk
Antihistamines (hydroxyzine, diphenhydramine)	Itching Anxiety (also used for sleep)	May contribute to sedation. Can cause anticholinergic side effects.	Low to no abuse potential
Atypical antipsychotics/ mood stabilizers (olanzapine, quetiapine, aripiprazole, haloperidol, ziprasidone, risperidone, lurasidone)	Mood and psychotic disorders (also used to treat agitation, severe anxiety, refractory depression, and delirium)	Many are used off-label in this population. Important to monitor for extrapyramidal symptoms. Olanzapine can be helpful for nausea/low appetite and insomnia. Quetiapine can be helpful for anxiety and insomnia. Aripiprazole may be more energy-producing. Important to have baseline electrocardiogram to ensure no presence of prolonged QTc. In addition to all being available orally, haloperidol is available IM/IV, ziprasidone is available IM, and olanzapine is available IM and in a zydis wafer. IM olanzapine and IV lorazepam should not be used concurrently due to black box warning.	Low to no abuse potential
Antiseizure medications (pregabalin, gabapentin)	Post-herpetic neuralgias, adjuvant seizure treatment, restless leg syndrome (often used off-label for anxiety, neuropathic pain [beyond diabetic], hot flashes)	May contribute to dizziness and sedation.	Growing concern for abuse potential Unclear
Wakefulness agents (modafinil, armodafinil)	Narcolepsy, sleep-work shift disorder, and obstructive sleep apnea (often used off-label in advanced illness for fatigue)	Generally well tolerated. May be difficult to achieve insurance coverage. Can improve energy, mood, and focus. Can contribute to nausea, anxiety, insomnia, and increased heart rate.	Moderate
Psychostimulants (methylphenidate, dexmethylphenidate, dextroamphetamine, mixed amphetamine salts)	Attention deficit hyperactivity disorder (used off-label for fatigue in advanced-state illness/end of life)	May be best reserved for patients approaching end of life. Can contribute to cardiac complications, agitation, anxiety, restlessness. Use caution in individuals with anorexia, however may increase activity and improve appetite. May help with attention and focus, may improve alertness.	High

IM, intramuscular; IV, intravenous; OCD, obsessive-compulsive disorder; SNRIs, serotonin norepinephrine reuptake inhibitors; SSRIs, selective serotonin reuptake inhibitors.

in childhood is a significant disruption for the entire family and can cause tremendous emotional upheaval. Most children, however, are able to cope with this upheaval and show evidence of adaptation and positive psychosocial growth and development.[111] However, some children do develop symptoms of emotional and psychological distress including symptoms of anxiety and depression, sleep disturbances, difficulties with interpersonal relationships, and noncompliance with treatment. Depression and anxiety may present differently in children than in adults. While in adults we look for a sad affect, social withdrawal, and depressed mood, in children long-term behavioral changes may be a clearer sign of depression. For example, if a child struggles with insomnia, irritability, changes in eating habits, changes in social adjustment or scholastic performance, lethargy, hyperactivity, somatization, or self-criticism when they previously did not struggle with these problems, and the duration is longer than a few weeks, it is prudent to seek help from a mental healthcare provider.[99] A trained mental healthcare provider will be able to distinguish these symptoms from behavioral responses to normal development. Assessment of depression in a child includes the family situation, level of emotional maturity, ability to cope with illness and treatment, age, level of development, and previous experience with illness.[99,112]

When attempting to diagnose depression and anxiety in children, it is important to have an understanding of childhood mental illness as a distinct entity from depression in adults because developmental tasks in childhood are distinctly different from those of adulthood, and that impacts both the development of mental illness and the manifestations.[113] Similarly, choosing a treatment modality for childhood depression, especially for children with life-limiting illness, is different than for adults. Individual, family, and group psychotherapy are first-line treatment and are directed at helping children problem-solve and manage emotions. Play therapy is commonly used in younger children to help explore the child's view of themself, the disease, and its treatment.[99,113] The conundrum of prescribing psychoactive medications for a developing brain has led to a hesitancy to prescribe for children; however, in recent years more research has suggested that, particularly for children with severe depression and anxiety, pharmacotherapy can be very helpful. SSRIs are used most frequently in low doses, and new research suggests that there may be a role for ketamine infusion in adolescents with severe refractory depression.[114,115]

End-of-Life Considerations

As individuals approach the end of life, nurses are well positioned to help patients achieve their goals around symptom management, participation in care, regaining a sense of control, and facilitation of important conversations, including legacy building. Nurses are among the most trusted professionals, invited in to care for patients at their most vulnerable moments. Nurses and other multidisciplinary team members and hospital staff bear witness to suffering and are afforded the opportunity to help patients and family members to create meaning and hope, especially at the end of life.

Depending on a patient's prognosis, willingness to accept limitations to curative treatments, and the availability of external supports, members of the patient care team may need to help facilitate understanding, shift to a more realistic hope, and re-establish a new set of care goals. Although some degree of distress is inevitable in the process of shifting to palliative treatment and end-of-life care, each patient can grow in acceptance of the unacceptable (impending death). The presence of co-occurring mental health sequelae can interfere with an individual's ability to set realistic care goals and place an individual at risk for impaired coping.

Assessment of patient psychosocial care concerns and engagement from multidisciplinary team members are of paramount importance to ease suffering at the end of life. Often, patients approaching the end of life have not interacted with mental health professionals previously. Normalizing the inclusion of multidisciplinary team members with psychosocial and mental health expertise is important.

Coping with life-threatening illness, treatment burden, changes to autonomy, and changes in family roles and functioning are enormous tasks for patients. Distressing uncertainty can be present from initial diagnosis, throughout treatment, and as patients transition to end-of-life care. But illness does not happen in a vacuum; concurrent stressors including work strain, financial stressors, interpersonal concerns, and barriers to receiving adequate psychosocial support can persist for many patients. Failure to recognize and treat comorbid psychiatric concerns, such as depression and anxiety, risks worsening quality of life and enhancing distress, feelings of hopelessness, and helplessness. Even as patients are stopping curative treatment and transitioning to comfort care or hospice, it is important for nurses and other members of the care team to regularly assess for depression, anxiety, and other mental health issues. Continued attention to psychological distress in patients near the end of life and swift intervention can reduce suffering for patients and their families and ease the inevitable grief following death.[116]

Suicide

Suicide is the 12th leading cause of death in the United States, and 45,979 individuals took their own life in 2020.[117] Desire for a hastened death or requests for assistance with dying among patients with serious illness remains a controversial topic in palliative care.[118] It is important to distinguish between suicide and physician-assisted death, with the primary distinction being that suicide occurs as a result of psychic suffering and physician-assisted death occurs after an in-depth assessment to ensure that the patient is not making the decision based on feelings of depression or hopelessness.[119] Feeling like a burden to others, loss of autonomy, hopelessness, fear, demoralization, and challenges to psychosocial support are associated with a desire for a hastened death, or suicidal thoughts, in patients with terminal illness.[118] Patients with a history of suicide attempts and those who expressed suicidal thoughts with intent are at particularly high risk and require additional screening and care; additional risk factors include substance use, comorbid psychiatric illness, poor social support, impulsivity, and access to lethal methods.[120]

Screening tools to further understand suicide risk include the PHQ-9, the Columbia Suicide Risk Assessment, the Beck Hopelessness Scale, and the Ask Suicide Screening Questions.[120]

In patients receiving palliative care, nursing assessment of patients at risk includes exploration of suicidal ideation (thoughts of suicide), presence of a plan for suicide ("Have you thought about how you would hurt yourself?"), and intent ("Do you intend at this time to carry out the plan?").[118]

Nurses can provide a safe space for patients to speak their feelings, consider individual risk factors, provide support around specific concerns, identify and promote sources of support, and advocate for the inclusion of mental health providers in a patient's care.[121] Nurses need to be aware of their own attitudes, beliefs, and responses to individuals at risk for suicide and above all demonstrate care and a positive regard for patient suffering.[81] The primary goal is to ensure patient safety and seek psychiatric evaluation when needed. Hospitalized patients expressing suicidal thoughts should be placed on one-to-one safety observation with employment of suicide safety measures. Ambulatory patients should be sent to the emergency room with a source of support; for individuals who will not seek emergency care, a home safety check may be done by law enforcement.[120] Staff may share the National Suicide Prevention Lifeline or Suicide Crisis Lifeline with patients (1-800-273 TALK [8225] or 988).

Integrative Therapies

Evidence-based interventions that have shown promise with patients with depression include integrative therapies such as acupressure, breathing exercises, guided imagery, relaxation, and emotive imagery in the management of symptoms of depression and anxiety in patients with cancer.[122] Massage therapy has also been shown to reduce patient-reported experiences of pain, anxiety, and depression symptoms. A systematic review of the effects of massage therapy on the alleviation of pain, anxiety, and depression yielded some promising results. Patients with limited social support and limited experience with physical contact and affection benefited most from the massage experience.[123]

Patient and Family Education

With Sue's permission, her palliative RN spoke with Sue's husband and children about her diagnosis of depression and helped them to understand that this is common in people with serious illness. Sue's palliative RN provided her family with educational materials regarding depression in serious illness, its treatment, and ways to help Sue to feel better. She also provided Sue's family with support for their own feelings about Sue's depression and some coping skills for managing their own feelings in addition to community mental health resources should they need further support.

Educated and empowered patients and families are better equipped and motivated to understand and manage their chronic illness. Effective patient education has been shown to improve adherence with patient instruction and reduce pain and anxiety.[124] Effective patient education is evidence-based and includes materials that reinforce understanding. In most facilities, nurses can partner with health educators who are skilled at developing patient-friendly, culturally sensitive, and health literacy–appropriate patient education. The goal of patient education is to increase patient/caregiver knowledge of health information and to assist patients who struggle to understand instructions. It seeks to engage, motivate, and empower patients with skills to self-manage their illness.[125]

In palliative care, patient education should focus on empowering patients to self-manage anxiety and depression.[126] Nurse-delivered, evidence-based, psychoeducational interventions focusing on problem-solving, coping techniques, and management of depression symptoms improve outcomes among depressed palliative care patients.[126] In a 2017 study, patients who received palliative care with education and coping skill building at the time of hematopoietic stem-cell transplant experienced "remarkable and sustained improvement" in depression and posttraumatic stress disorder symptoms 6 months posttransplant.[127]

Patient Empowerment and Self-Management

The Institute of Medicine defines self-management as "the systematic provision of education and supportive interventions to increase patient's skills/confidence in managing their health problems, including goal-setting and problem-solving support."[126,128(pE17)] The Chronic Care Model posits that patients with chronic illness need education and support to become effective managers of their own health condition.[129]

To increase patients' self-management and self-efficacy skills, the nurse must provide:

- Easy-to-digest information
- Tools for building self-management and problem-solving skills
- Ongoing support from care team, friends, and family

The nurse and patient/caregiver should set achievable, patient-centered goals and create a follow-up plan:

- Nurse assesses patient's skill, understanding, and confidence in managing symptoms.
- Patient identifies an action plan with specific goals/behaviors.[128]
- Nurse creates structured follow-up to review goals/progress via clinic visit, phone, or email.

Follow-Up for Patients with Chronic Conditions

Structured follow-up is an essential part of chronic care and self-management development and reinforcement.[130] The following are helpful tips in planning follow-up calls with patients and families:

- Schedule follow-up based on mutual goals developed with patients and families. Be flexible in allowing patients to determine the follow-up method.
- Include problem-solving techniques to help patients identify problems and create solutions in follow-up.
- Don't skip follow-up.
- Follow-up can be by phone, email, fax, home visit, clinic visit, or other. If possible, use trained, culturally competent laypeople for follow-up.

Returning to the case study, Sue's palliative care RN was the center of the interdisciplinary team, and her timely recognition and diligent follow-up helped Sue and her family to obtain the help they needed so that they could all enjoy quality time together.

Conclusion

Depression and anxiety are common in patients receiving palliative care, but clinically significant symptoms are often unrecognized and untreated, which can add to patients' suffering and undermine their quality of life. Active screening for depression and anxiety is recommended, and it should be combined with a systematic plan for appropriate intervention to be effective. Optimal treatment may involve the use of psychotropic medications, psychotherapy, and, in some cases, complementary treatment modalities. Clinicians should understand the difference between suicidality, wish for hastened death, and desire for physician-assisted death; actively screen for suicidal thoughts; and intervene as necessary. Patient and family education is indispensable in helping patients and their families to feel empowered by contributing to their care.

REFERENCES

1. Shuster JLH, Higginson I J Hospice and palliative care: a psychiatric perspective. In: Breitbart HMCW, ed. *Handbook of Psychiatry in Palliative Medicine*. 2nd ed. Oxford University Press; 2012:3–13.
2. Breitbart W, Bruera E, Chochinov H, Lynch M. Neuropsychiatric syndromes and psychological symptoms in patients with advanced cancer. *J Pain Symptom Manage*. 1995;10(2):131–141.
3. Lloyd-Williams M, Friedman T, Rudd N. A survey of antidepressant prescribing in the terminally ill. *Palliat Med*. 1999;13(3):243–248.
4. Meyer HA, Sinnott C, Seed PT. Depressive symptoms in advanced cancer. Part depression over time; the role of the palliative care professional. *Palliat Med*. 2003;17(7):604–607.
5. O'Mahony S, Goulet J, Kornblith A, et al. Desire for hastened death, cancer pain and depression: report of a longitudinal observational study. *J Pain Symptom Manage*. 2005;29(5):446–457.

6. Sharpe M, Strong V, Allen K, et al. Major depression in outpatients attending a regional cancer centre: screening and unmet treatment needs. *Br J Cancer*. 2004;90(2):314–320.
7. Passik SD, Dugan W, McDonald MV, Rosenfeld B, Theobald DE, Edgerton S. Oncologists' recognition of depression in their patients with cancer. *J Clin Oncol*. 1998;16(4):1594–1600.
8. Wilson KG, Chochinov HM, McPherson CJ, et al. Suffering with advanced cancer. *J Clin Oncol*. 2007;25(13):1691–1697.
9. Chochinov HM, Tataryn D, Clinch JJ, Dudgeon D. Will to live in the terminally ill. *Lancet*. 1999;354(9181):816–819.
10. Portenoy RK, Thaler HT, Kornblith AB, et al. Symptom prevalence, characteristics and distress in a cancer population. *Qual Life Res*. 1994;3(3):183–189.
11. Wilson KG, Chochinov HM, Skirko MG, et al. Depression and anxiety disorders in palliative cancer care. *J Pain Symptom Manage*. 2007;33(2):118–129.
12. Hinton J. Which patients with terminal cancer are admitted from home care? *Palliat Med*. 1994;8(3):197–210.
13. Christakis NA. Timing of referral of terminally ill patients to an outpatient hospice. *J Gen Intern Med*. 1994;9(6):314–320.
14. Pelletier G, Verhoef MJ, Khatri N, Hagen N. Quality of life in brain tumor patients: the relative contributions of depression, fatigue, emotional distress, and existential issues. *J Neurooncol*. 2002;57(1):41–49.
15. Jiang W, Alexander J, Christopher E, et al. Relationship of depression to increased risk of mortality and rehospitalization in patients with congestive heart failure. *Arch Intern Med*. 2001;161(15):1849–1856.
16. Rawlings D, Litster C, Miller-Lewis L, Tieman J, Swetenham K. The voices of death doulas about their role in end-of-life care. *Health Soc Care Community*. 2020;28(1):12–21.
17. Block SD. Assessing and managing depression in the terminally ill patient. ACP-ASIM End-of-Life Care Consensus Panel. American College of Physicians—American Society of Internal Medicine. *Ann Intern Med*. 2000;132(3):209–218.
18. Perusinghe M, Chen KY, McDermott B. Evidence-based management of depression in palliative care: a systematic review. *J Palliat Med*. 2021;24(5):767–781.
19. Rayner L, Loge JH, Wasteson E, Higginson IJ. The detection of depression in palliative care. *Curr Opin Support Palliat Care*. 2009;3(1):55–60.
20. Hayes RD, Lee W, Rayner L, et al. Gender differences in prevalence of depression among patients receiving palliative care: the role of dependency. *Palliat Med*. 2012;26(5):696–702.
21. Kelly B, McClement S, Chochinov HM. Measurement of psychological distress in palliative care. *Palliat Med*. 2006;20(8):779–789.
22. Mystakidou K, Rosenfeld B, Parpa E, et al. Desire for death near the end of life: the role of depression, anxiety and pain. *Gen Hosp Psychiatry*. 2005;27(4):258–262.
23. Julião M, Barbosa A. Depression in palliative care: prevalence and assessment. Article in Portuguese *Acta Med Port*. 2011;24(suppl 4):807–818.
24. Pham VA, Nguyen H, Krakauer EL, Harding R. "I wish I could die so I would not be in pain": a qualitative study of palliative care needs among people with cancer or HIV/AIDS in Vietnam and their caregivers. *J Pain Symptom Manage*. 2021;62(2):364–372.
25. Krebber AM, Buffart LM, Kleijn G, et al. Prevalence of depression in cancer patients: a meta-analysis of diagnostic interviews and self-report instruments. *Psychooncology*. 2014;23(2):121–130.
26. Murtagh FE, Addington-Hall J, Higginson IJ. The prevalence of symptoms in end-stage renal disease: a systematic review. *Adv Chronic Kidney Dis*. 2007;14(1):82–99.
27. Cohen LM, Dobscha SK, Hails KC, Pekow PS, Chochinov HM. Depression and suicidal ideation in patients who discontinue the life-support treatment of dialysis. *Psychosom Med*. 2002;64(6):889–896.
28. Lieberman A. Depression in Parkinson's disease—a review. *Acta Neurol Scand*. 2006;113(1):1–8.
29. Miyasaki JM, Shannon K, Voon V, et al. Practice parameter: evaluation and treatment of depression, psychosis, and dementia in Parkinson disease (an evidence-based review): report of the Quality Standards Subcommittee of the American Academy of Neurology. *Neurology*. 2006;66(7):996–1002.
30. Chwastiak L, Ehde DM, Gibbons LE, Sullivan M, Bowen JD, Kraft GH. Depressive symptoms and severity of illness in multiple sclerosis: epidemiologic study of a large community sample. *Am J Psychiatry*. 2002;159(11):1862–1868.
31. Rutledge T, Reis VA, Linke SE, Greenberg BH, Mills PJ. Depression in heart failure a meta-analytic review of prevalence, intervention effects, and associations with clinical outcomes. *J Am Coll Cardiol*. 2006;48(8):1527–1537.
32. Cook JA, Grey D, Burke J, et al. Depressive symptoms and AIDS-related mortality among a multisite cohort of HIV-positive women. *Am J Public Health*. 2004;94(7):1133–1140.
33. Selwyn PA, Rivard M, Kappell D, et al. Palliative care for AIDS at a large urban teaching hospital: program description and preliminary outcomes. *J Palliat Med*. 2003;6(3):461–474.
34. Roy-Byrne PP, Davidson KW, Kessler RC, et al. Anxiety disorders and comorbid medical illness. *Gen Hosp Psychiatry*. 2008;30(3):208–225.
35. Spencer R, Nilsson M, Wright A, Pirl W, Prigerson H. Anxiety disorders in advanced cancer patients: correlates and predictors of end-of-life outcomes. *Cancer* 2010;116(7):1810–1819.
36. Harrison J, Maguire P. Predictors of psychiatric morbidity in cancer patients. *Br J Psychiatry*. 1994;165(5):593–598.
37. Carroll BT, Kathol RG, Noyes R Jr, Wald TG, Clamon GH. Screening for depression and anxiety in cancer patients using the Hospital Anxiety and Depression Scale. *Gen Hosp Psychiatry*. 1993;15(2):69–74.
38. Kathol RG, Noyes R Jr, Williams J, Mutgi A, Carroll B, Perry P. Diagnosing depression in patients with medical illness. *Psychosomatics*. 1990;31(4):434–440.
39. Levine PM, Silberfarb PM, Lipowski ZJ. Mental disorders in cancer patients: a study of 100 psychiatric referrals. *Cancer*. 1978;42(3):1385–1391.
40. Noyes R Jr, Kathol RG, Debelius-Enemark P, et al. Distress associated with cancer as measured by the illness distress scale. *Psychosomatics*. 1990;31(3):321–330.
41. Walsh D, Donnelly S, Rybicki L. The symptoms of advanced cancer: relationship to age, gender, and performance status in 1,000 patients. *Support Care Cancer*. 2000;8(3):175–179.
42. Massie MJ. Prevalence of depression in patients with cancer. *J Natl Cancer Inst Monogr*. 2004(32):57–71.
43. Hughes JE. Depressive illness and lung cancer. I. Depression before diagnosis. *Eur J Surg Oncol*. 1985;11(1):15–20.
44. Kelsen DP, Portenoy RK, Thaler HT, et al. Pain and depression in patients with newly diagnosed pancreas cancer. *J Clin Oncol*. 1995;13(3):748–755.
45. Glover J, Dibble SL, Dodd MJ, Miaskowski C. Mood states of oncology outpatients: does pain make a difference? *J Pain Symptom Manage*. 1995;10(2):120–128.
46. Chochinov HM, Wilson KG. The euthanasia debate: attitudes, practices and psychiatric considerations. *Can J Psychiatry*. 1995;40(10):593–602.

47. Wilson KG, Chochinov HM. Physician-assisted suicide. *N Engl J Med*. 1996;335(7):518–519; author reply 519–520.
48. Spiegel D, Bloom JR. Pain in metastatic breast cancer. *Cancer*. 1983;52(2):341–345.
49. Spiegel D, Sands S, Koopman C. Pain and depression in patients with cancer. *Cancer*. 1994;74(9):2570–2578.
50. Baltaji S, Cheronis N, Bajwa O, Cheema T. The role of palliative care in COPD. *Crit Care Nurs Q*. 2021;44(1):113–120.
51. Boyd AD, Riba M. Depression and pancreatic cancer. *J Natl Compr Canc Netw*. 2007;5(1):113–116.
52. Shakin EJ, Holland J. Depression and pancreatic cancer. *J Pain Symptom Manage*. 1988;3(4):194–198.
53. Mainio A, Hakko H, Niemelä A, Koivukangas J, Räsänen P. Gender difference in relation to depression and quality of life among patients with a primary brain tumor. *Eur Psychiatry*. 2006;21(3):194–199.
54. Litofsky NS, Farace E, Anderson F Jr, Meyers CA, Huang W, Laws ER Jr. Depression in patients with high-grade glioma: results of the Glioma Outcomes Project. *Neurosurgery*. 2004;54(2):358–366; discussion 366–357.
55. Kelly WF, Checkley SA, Bender DA, Mashiter K. Cushing's syndrome and depression—a prospective study of 26 patients. *Br J Psychiatry*. 1983;142:16–19.
56. Weitzner MA, Kanfer S, Booth-Jones M. Apathy and pituitary disease: it has nothing to do with depression. *J Neuropsychiatry Clin Neurosci*. 2005;17(2):159–166.
57. Arseniou S, Arvaniti A, Samakouri M. HIV infection and depression. *Psychiatry Clin Neurosci*. 2014;68(2):96–109.
58. Cysique LA, Brew BJ. Comorbid depression and apathy in HIV-associated neurocognitive disorders in the era of chronic HIV infection. *Handb Clin Neurol*. 2019;165:71–82.
59. Brown JH, Paraskevas F. Cancer and depression: cancer presenting with depressive illness: an autoimmune disease? *Br J Psychiatry*. 1982;141:227–232.
60. Kelly C, Paleri V, Downs C, Shah R. Deterioration in quality of life and depressive symptoms during radiation therapy for head and neck cancer. *Otolaryngol Head Neck Surg*. 2007;136(1):108–111.
61. Sehlen S, Lenk M, Herschbach P, et al. Depressive symptoms during and after radiotherapy for head and neck cancer. *Head Neck*. 2003;25(12):1004–1018.
62. Kohda R, Otsubo T, Kuwakado Y, et al. Prospective studies on mental status and quality of life in patients with head and neck cancer treated by radiation. *Psychooncology*. 2005;14(4):331–336.
63. Armstrong CL, Gyato K, Awadalla AW, Lustig R, Tochner ZA. A critical review of the clinical effects of therapeutic irradiation damage to the brain: the roots of controversy. *Neuropsychol Rev*. 2004;14(1):65–86.
64. Patten SB, Barbui C. Drug-induced depression: a systematic review to inform clinical practice. *Psychother Psychosom*. 2004;73(4):207–215.
65. Devlen J, Maguire P, Phillips P, Crowther D, Chambers H. Psychological problems associated with diagnosis and treatment of lymphomas. I: Retrospective study. *Br Med J (Clin Res Ed)*. 1987;295(6604):953–954.
66. Stiefel FC, Breitbart WS, Holland JC. Corticosteroids in cancer: neuropsychiatric complications. *Cancer Invest*. 1989;7(5):479–491.
67. Boston P, Bruce A, Schreiber R. Existential suffering in the palliative care setting: an integrated literature review. *J Pain Symptom Manage*. 2011;41(3):604–618.
68. Mitchell AJ, Meader N, Davies E, et al. Meta-analysis of screening and case finding tools for depression in cancer: evidence based recommendations for clinical practice on behalf of the Depression in Cancer Care Consensus Group. *J Affect Disord*. 2012;140(2):149–160.
69. Andersen BL, DeRubeis RJ, Berman BS, et al. Screening, assessment, and care of anxiety and depressive symptoms in adults with cancer: an American Society of Clinical Oncology guideline adaptation. *J Clin Oncol*. 2014;32(15):1605–1619.
70. Lloyd-Williams M, Spiller J, Ward J. Which depression screening tools should be used in palliative care? *Palliat Med*. 2003;17(1):40–43.
71. Chochinov HM, Wilson KG, Enns M, Lander S. "Are you depressed?" Screening for depression in the terminally ill. *Am J Psychiatry*. 1997;154(5):674–676.
72. Taylor L, Lovell N, Ward J, Wood F, Hosker C. Diagnosis of depression in patients receiving specialist community palliative care: does using a single screening question identify depression otherwise diagnosed by clinical interview? *J Palliat Med*. 2013;16(9):1140–1142.
73. Grassi L, Caruso R, Sabato S, Massarenti S, Nanni MG; The UniFe Psychiatry Working Group Coauthors. Psychosocial screening and assessment in oncology and palliative care settings. *Front Psychol*. 2014;5:1485.
74. Caruso R, GiuliaNanni M, Riba MB, Sabato S, Grassi L. Depressive spectrum disorders in cancer: diagnostic issues and intervention. A critical review. *Curr Psychiatry Rep*. 2017;19(6):33.
75. Greenberg DB. Barriers to the treatment of depression in cancer patients. *J Natl Cancer Inst Monogr*. 2004(32):127–135.
76. American Psychiatric Association. *Diagnostic and Statistical Manual of Mental Disorders*. 5th ed. Washington DC; 2013.
77. Endicott J. Measurement of depression in patients with cancer. *Cancer*. 1984;53(10 suppl):2243–2249.
78. Block SD. Psychological issues in end-of-life care. *J Palliat Med*. 2006;9(3):751–772.
79. The ICD-10 Classifiction of Mental and Behavioural Disorders: Diagnostic Criteria for Research. Geneva: World Health Organization; 2015.
80. Breitbart W. Suicide in cancer patients. *Oncology (Williston Park)*. 1987;1(2):49–55.
81. Choy CH. Suicide in palliative care setting. *Ann Palliat Med*. 2017;6(suppl 2):S264–S265.
82. Abbey JG, Rosenfeld B, Pessin H, Breitbart W. Hopelessness at the end of life: the utility of the hopelessness scale with terminally ill cancer patients. *Br J Health Psychol*. 2006;11(pt 2):173–183.
83. Dauchy S, Dolbeault S, Reich M. Depression in cancer patients. *EJC Suppl*. 2013;11(2):205–215.
84. Marchington KL, Carrier L, Lawlor PG. Delirium masquerading as depression. *Palliat Support Care*. 2012;10(1):59–62.
85. Arantzamendi M, García-Rueda N, Carvajal A, Robinson CA. People with advanced cancer: the process of living well with awareness of dying. *Qual Health Res*. 2020;30(8):1143–1155.
86. McKee KY, Kelly A. Management of grief, depression, and suicidal thoughts in serious illness. *Med Clin North Am*. 2020;104(3):503–524.
87. Vehling S, Philipp R. Existential distress and meaning-focused interventions in cancer survivorship. *Curr Opin Support Palliat Care*. 2018;12(1):46–51.
88. An E, Lo C, Hales S, Zimmermann C, Rodin G. Demoralization and death anxiety in advanced cancer. *Psychooncology*. 2018;27(11):2566–2572.
89. Xiao J, Ng MSN, Yan T, Chow KM, Chan CWH. How patients with cancer experience dignity: an integrative review. *Psychooncology*. 2021;30(8):1220–1231.

90. Roth AJM, Massie MJ. Anxiety in palliative care. In: Breitbart HMCW, ed. *Handbook of Psychiatry in Palliative Medicine*. 2nd ed. Oxford university Press; 2012:69–80.
91. Roth A, Nelson C. *Psychopharmacology in Cancer Care: A Guide for Non-prescribers and Prescribers*. Oxford University Press; 2021.
92. National Institute of Mental Health: Any Anxiety Disorder. Accessed October 2, 2022. https://www.nimh.nih.gov/health.
93. Kozlov E, Phongtankuel V, Prigerson H, et al. Prevalence, severity, and correlates of symptoms of anxiety and depression at the very end of life. *J Pain Symptom Manage*. 2019;58(1):80–85.
94. Pralong A, Perrar KM, Kremeike K, Rosendahl C, Voltz R. Depression, anxiety, delirium and desire to die in palliative care: recommendations of the S3 guideline on palliative care for patients with incurable cancer. Article in German. *Nervenarzt*. 2020;91(5):391–397.
95. Anderson WG, Alexander SC, Rodriguez KL, et al. "What concerns me is …": expression of emotion by advanced cancer patients during outpatient visits. *Support Care Cancer*. 2008;16(7):803–811.
96. Stoklosa J, Patterson K, Rosielle D, Arnold RM. Anxiety in palliative care: causes and diagnosis #186. *J Palliat Med*. 2011;14(10):1173–1174.
97. Whooley MA, Simon GE. Managing depression in medical outpatients. *N Engl J Med*. 2000;343(26):1942–1950.
98. Hart SL, Hoyt MA, Diefenbach M, et al. Meta-analysis of efficacy of interventions for elevated depressive symptoms in adults diagnosed with cancer. *J Natl Cancer Inst*. 2012;104(13):990–1004.
99. National Cancer Institute. Depression PDQ-Health Professional Version. Updated 2022. Accessed September 30, 2022. https://www.cancer.gov/about-cancer/coping/feelings/depression-hp-pdq#_29.
100. Wilson KG, Lander M, Chochinov HM. Diagnosis and management of depression in palliative care. In: Breitbart HMCW, ed. *Handbook of Psychiatry in Palliative Medicine*. 2nd ed. Oxford University Press; 2012:39–68.
101. Montazeri A, Jarvandi S, Haghighat S, et al. Anxiety and depression in breast cancer patients before and after participation in a cancer support group. *Patient Educ Couns*. 2001;45(3):195–198.
102. Fawzy FI, Fawzy NW, Hyun CS, et al. Malignant melanoma. Effects of an early structured psychiatric intervention, coping, and affective state on recurrence and survival 6 years later. *Arch Gen Psychiatry*. 1993;50(9):681–689.
103. Chochinov HM, Hack T, Hassard T, Kristjanson LJ, McClement S, Harlos M. Dignity therapy: a novel psychotherapeutic intervention for patients near the end of life. *J Clin Oncol*. 2005;23(24):5520–5525.
104. Montross L, Winters KD, Irwin SA. Dignity therapy implementation in a community-based hospice setting. *J Palliat Med*. 2011;14(6):729–734.
105. Chochinov HM, Kristjanson LJ, Breitbart W, et al. Effect of dignity therapy on distress and end-of-life experience in terminally ill patients: a randomised controlled trial. *Lancet Oncol*. 2011;12(8):753–762.
106. Vuksanovic D, Green HJ, Dyck M, Morrissey SA. Dignity therapy and life review for palliative care patients: a randomized controlled trial. *J Pain Symptom Manage*. 2017;53(2):162–170.e161.
107. Martínez M, Arantzamendi M, Belar A, et al. "Dignity therapy," a promising intervention in palliative care: a comprehensive systematic literature review. *Palliat Med*. 2017;31(6):492–509.
108. Breitbart W, Rosenfeld B, Pessin H, Applebaum A, Kulikowski J, Lichtenthal WG. Meaning-centered group psychotherapy: an effective intervention for improving psychological well-being in patients with advanced cancer. *J Clin Oncol*. 2015;33(7):749–754.
109. Breitbart W, Pessin H, Rosenfeld B, et al. Individual meaning-centered psychotherapy for the treatment of psychological and existential distress: a randomized controlled trial in patients with advanced cancer. *Cancer*. 2018;124(15):3231–3239.
110. Keall RM, Clayton JM, Butow PN. Therapeutic life review in palliative care: a systematic review of quantitative evaluations. *J Pain Symptom Manage*. 2015;49(4):747–761.
111. Lockwood B, Humphrey L. Supporting children and families at a child's end of life: pediatric palliative care pearls of anticipatory guidance for families. *Child Adolesc Psychiatr Clin N Am*. 2018;27(4):527–537.
112. Erker C, Yan K, Zhang L, Bingen K, Flynn KE, Panepinto J. Impact of pediatric cancer on family relationships. *Cancer Med*. 2018;7(5):1680–1688.
113. Malhotra S, Das PP. Understanding childhood depression. *Indian J Med Res*. 2007;125(2):115–128.
114. Hazell P. Updates in treatment of depression in children and adolescents. *Curr Opin Psychiatry*. 2021;34(6):593–599.
115. Leichsenring F, Luyten P, Abbass A, Rabung S, Steinert C. Treatment of depression in children and adolescents. *Lancet Psychiatry*. 2021;8(2):96–97.
116. Ann-Yi S, Bruera E. Psychological aspects of care in cancer patients in the last weeks/days of life. *Cancer Res Treat*. 2022;54(3):651–660.
117. American Foundation for Suicide Prevention. Suicide Statistics. Updated February 17, 2022. Accessed October 4, 2022. https://afsp.org/suicide-statistics/
118 Olden M, Pessin H, Lichtenthal WG, Breitbart W. Suicide and desire for hastened death in the terminally ill. In: Breitbart HMCW, ed. *Handbook of Psychiatry in Palliative Medicine*. 2nd ed. Oxford University Press; 2012:101–113.
119. Pronk R, Willems DL, Van De Vathorst S. Do doctors differentiate between suicide and physician-assisted death? A qualitative study into the views of psychiatrists and general practitioners. *Cult Med Psychiatry*. 2021;45(2):268–281.
120. Fernandez-Robles CK, S. Psychiatric emergencies In: Rosenstein DA-N, E., ed. *American Psychosocial Oncology Society/Pfizer Psychosocial Pocket Guide*. American Psychosocial Oncology Society; 2022 (in press).
121. Washington KT, Albright DL, Parker Oliver D, Gage LA, Lewis A, Mooney MJ. Hospice and palliative social workers' experiences with clients at risk of suicide. *Palliat Support Care*. 2016;14(6):664–671.
122. Zeng YS, Wang C, Ward KE, Hume AL. Complementary and alternative medicine in hospice and palliative care: a systematic review. *J Pain Symptom Manage*. 2018;56(5):781–794.e784.
123. Candy B, Armstrong M, Flemming K, et al. The effectiveness of aromatherapy, massage and reflexology in people with palliative care needs: a systematic review. *Palliat Med*. 2020;34(2):179–194.
124. Thompson SL, Ward C, Galanos A, Bowers M. Impact of a palliative care education module in patients with heart failure. *Am J Hosp Palliat Care*. 2020;37(12):1016–1021.
125. Graul A, Haggerty A, Stickley C, et al. Effect of patient education on palliative care knowledge and acceptability of outpatient palliative care services among gynecologic oncology patients: a randomized controlled trial. *Gynecol Oncol*. 2020;156(2):482–487.
126. Schulman-Green D, Brody A, Gilbertson-White S, Whittemore R, McCorkle R. Supporting self-management in palliative care throughout the cancer care trajectory. *Curr Opin Support Palliat Care*. 2018;12(3):299–307.

127. El-Jawahri A, Traeger L, Greer JA, et al. Effect of inpatient palliative care during hematopoietic stem-cell transplant on psychological distress 6 months after transplant: results of a randomized clinical trial. *J Clin Oncol.* 2017;35(32):3714–3721.
128. Hoffman AJ. Enhancing self-efficacy for optimized patient outcomes through the theory of symptom self-management. *Cancer Nurs*. 2013;36(1):E16–E26.
129. Grady PA, Gough LL. Self-management: a comprehensive approach to management of chronic conditions. *Am J Public Health.* 2014;104(8):e25–e31.
130. Matcham F, Rayner L, Hutton J, Monk A, Steel C, Hotopf M. Self-help interventions for symptoms of depression, anxiety and psychological distress in patients with physical illnesses: a systematic review and meta-analysis. *Clin Psychol Rev*. 2014;34(2):141–157.

25

Fatigue

Stephanie Gilbertson-White and Nayung Youn

Key Points

- Fatigue is the most common chronic symptom associated with cancer and other chronic progressive diseases.
- Thorough assessment of all patient comorbidities and symptoms is critical to accurately diagnose and treat disease-related fatigue.
- Educational interventions in the management of fatigue for healthcare providers, patients, and families provide an important opportunity for consistent integration of current guidelines into practice.
- Ongoing research has provided evidence for improved patient outcomes through both pharmacological and nonpharmacological measures.

Introduction

Case Study Part 1

Kai Jefferson, a 67-year-old man, was diagnosed with stage IV lung cancer 6 months ago. Despite undergoing antineoplastic treatment regimens to limit tumor progression including chemotherapy and targeted therapy, his cancer has progressed, significantly impacting his quality of life (QOL). His primary complaint during recent palliative care visits has been a debilitating fatigue, one that does not improve with rest and that persists for most of the day. He is wondering if and how palliative care might provide some relief from his severe fatigue.

Fatigue is consistently noted to be one of the most prevalent, severe, and distressing symptoms in people with serious or life-threatening illnesses.[1] While there is no universally accepted definition of fatigue, it is often described as devastating tiredness regardless of the number of recent activities or rest.[2] Commonly, it is a symptom exhibited following a stressor, activity, disease, and or treatment. Physiologically, fatigue can be a natural and healthy response to physical or emotional stress, where symptoms are largely relieved following natural rest. However, in the context of cancer, chronic disease, or serious, life-threatening illness, fatigue is more prevalent and typically not relieved by rest.[1] In addition, fatigue frequently has a detrimental impact on QOL for patients as well as their families. The subjective nature of the experience and variability in presentation can result in significant management challenges for healthcare providers.

Fatigue is commonly associated with cancer as well as other chronic and/or serious, life-threatening illness such as chronic obstructive pulmonary disease (COPD),[3] irreversible cardiomyopathies,[4] chronic renal failure,[5] HIV/AIDS,[6] and multiple sclerosis.[7] The manifestation of fatigue in any disease process may differ across diagnoses and treatments. In the context of cancer, for example, people may perceive fatigue differently depending on when fatigue occurs in the disease trajectory.[8] Often, it is the development of fatigue that initiates pursuit of diagnosis or disease discovery and implementation of medical treatment.[8] In addition, fatigue may persist as a pervasive side effect even after disease-focused treatments are discontinued.[9]

Cancer-related fatigue is one of the most common, devastating, and multidimensional symptoms associated with cancer diagnosis and treatment. Fatigue associated with cancer or its treatments commonly occurs with groups of debilitating symptoms or side effects such as pain, depressed mood, and/or sleep disturbance.[10] These co-occurring symptoms are often referred to as a "symptom cluster."[10] Once diagnosed, a person with cancer may experience fatigue as a side effect of treatment, as well as the emotional consequence of a life-threatening diagnosis. Fatigue intensity and distress may vary with diagnosis, stage, and/or treatment severity. It can progressively interfere with common physical and/or social activity and potentially impact QOL and overall well-being.[1,8] Fatigue may have the greatest potential to interfere with quality at the end of life.[11]

People with chronic and/or serious, life-threatening illness often do not have the energy or forethought to communicate to healthcare professionals about their fatigue as they may perceive it to be a nonurgent symptom and do not want to be a bother.[2] Some people find it difficult to convey the extent of their fatigue to healthcare providers as a result of lack of understanding and a general attitude of acceptance that fatigue is part of the disease process, treatment, and side effects. Similarly, healthcare providers and other professional staff often consider fatigue or other symptoms as "expected side effects" of disease and treatment and are unaware of effective strategies to manage fatigue.[12] As such, unaddressed fatigue may have significant financial and psychosocial impacts for patients and their families as well as on clinical issues such as continuing with curative and/or various disease-focused treatments.[9]

Definitions of Fatigue

Fatigue is a complex phenomenon, one studied by many disciplines, yet it has no widely accepted definition.[3] Even within different nursing specialties there has been little agreement on a definition of fatigue. For example, cancer-related fatigue has been studied extensively and has been described as "*weariness, burnout, lassitude, malaise, apathy, impatience, and/or inability to perform daily activities*"[13(p131)] but also in terms of *lack of energy or exhaustion that interferes with normal activities and function* which may provide a useful person-centered definition that applies to other chronic and/or serious, life-threatening illnesses.[9] Similarly, the National Comprehensive Cancer Network (NCCN) Fatigue Practice Guidelines Panel, charged with synthesizing research on fatigue to develop recommendations for care, defines it as "a distressing, persistent, and subjective sense of physical, emotional, and/or cognitive tiredness, or exhaustion related to cancer or cancer treatment, that is not proportional to recent activity and interferes with usual functioning."[2(p3)] The American Cancer Society defines cancer-related fatigue as "feeling very weak, listless, drained, or washed out" and even "too tired to eat, walk to the bathroom, or even use the TV remote."[14] This definition is similar to that used by multiple sclerosis patients, who defined fatigue as one of the most frequent and most disabling symptoms—a subjective lack of physical and/or mental energy that interferes with usual and desired activities.[15] Sufferers of other nonmalignant diseases such as stroke and end-stage heart failure define fatigue as being "physically tired and mentally exhausted" and perceive it as one of their worst symptoms, yet one that often receives little attention.[16] The most frequent and problematic issue following an acute myocardial infarction is fatigue, which is often expressed in the same terminology used by those experiencing cancer-related fatigue.[17]

Descriptors of fatigue range from a single focus of tiredness to the broad, multifocal, and overwhelming multidimensional syndrome of exhaustion that differs from the anticipated feelings of tiredness that are often felt in healthy patients and are relieved by adequate rest. Fatigue is often perceived differently by those living the experience of disease, treatment, and recovery from those who observe the process, including healthcare providers and family. This difference in perception may continue to be observed differently throughout the course of disease or treatment.

People experiencing fatigue often use metaphorical language such as "I feel as if I have been run over by a truck." Differentiating the symptom of fatigue from feeling tired or sleepy and determining its impact on daily life and function are often difficult for the patients experiencing fatigue as well as healthcare providers, friends, and family.[18] Fatigue at the end of life may be experienced as the end of a very long struggle, a natural stage of the dying process; and it may protect against elements of suffering.[19]

Across these varied definitions of fatigue, two key elements are dominant: (1) a subjective perception with physical, emotional, and cognitive features and (2) interference with an ability to function, often negatively impacting QOL.[1]

Prevalence

Fatigue is currently reported to be one of the most common symptoms associated with cancer and other chronic diseases.[20,21] Estimates of prevalence are between 28% and 90% depending on the diagnosis, length of disease, course of treatment, complications, physical state, and various other psychosocial factors. In the context of palliative care in both community-based care and tertiary care settings, fatigue has been identified as the most common and distressing symptom.[20,21] Prevalence rates reported for fatigue are presented in Box 25.1, including cancer,[22] cardiac disease,[23] heart failure,[17]

Box 25.1 Prevalence of Fatigue and Populations at Risk

Cancer

Prevalence rates of cancer-related fatigue vary depending on cancer site and stage, as well as the measurement tool. Studies indicated that 62% of patients receiving treatment experience fatigue, as did up to 94% of incurable cancer patients.[22] Similarly, moderate/severe fatigue has been reported more often among those who have poorer performance. Fatigue is also the most common and distressing symptom experienced by pediatric cancer patients. Among older adults with cancer, the very old report lower levels of fatigue compared to younger patients.[25] In general, the prevalence of fatigue among patients under active treatment seems higher than that among patients who completed their treatments. However, we should note that in post-treatment cancer survivors, fatigue may persist months or even years after treatment, although the rate significantly decreases among survivors of more than 5 years except lung cancer patients.

Cardiac

Research suggests the widespread presence of fatigue in people with chronic heart failure and those who have gone through myocardial infarction. Prevalence rates range from 39% to 74% in people with heart failure.[16]

Chronic Obstructive Pulmonary Disease

Second only to breathlessness in its prevalence, fatigue is experienced by 96% of those with chronic obstructive pulmonary disease.[3]

Renal Disease

In renal disease, the prevalence of fatigue varies depending on the method of treatment employed.[24] Of those treated by hemodialysis, 82% report fatigue, notably physical fatigue and reduced activity. Fatigue prevalence in those treated by peritoneal dialysis was greater than 88%.[26]

HIV/AIDS

The diagnosis of HIV/AIDS is now more consistently addressed as a chronic disease rather than as a terminal illness as a result of antiviral therapy. However, as the disease becomes more chronic, fatigue is now recognized as an ongoing, chronic symptom and needs to be recognized and treated as such.[6]

The prevalence of fatigue in HIV-positive patients, according to one study, was 69%. While fatigue was not the most common symptom in AIDS patients, it was nonetheless widespread, affecting at least 42% of patients.

Multiple Sclerosis

Fatigue is the most prevalent and potentially debilitating symptom of multiple sclerosis. It is experienced by 75%–95% of multiple sclerosis patients, more than half of whom name fatigue as one of their most distressing symptoms.[7]

While symptoms rarely occur in isolation, there is growing evidence to support the occurrence of various *symptom clusters* as a significant contributor to symptom burden.[10] Fatigue has been found to be part of the psychoneuroimmune symptom cluster that also includes pain, sleep disturbance, and depressed mood. The underlying mechanism has not been fully identified, but there is compelling evidence supporting that the inflammatory response plays an important role in this cluster.

In addition, multimorbidity (i.e., having two or more chronic conditions) can have a significant impact on the development of fatigue. For example, when cancer co-occurs with rheumatoid arthritis, 60% of subjects reported fatigue.[27]

COPD,[3] renal disease,[24] HIV/AIDS,[6] and multiple sclerosis.[7] Despite the high prevalence, fatigue remains frequently underdiagnosed and undermanaged.

Fatigue has been more widely studied in people with cancer compared with other chronic or life-threatening illnesses. Fatigue has been identified as the most prevalent, disabling, and continuous phenomenon in patients receiving various treatments for cancer.[9] Fatigue cuts across all diagnoses, ages, genders, stages of disease, and treatment modalities.[11] Both chemotherapy and radiation therapy result in fatigue, while fatigue following combined chemoradiation therapy continues to be underestimated and profoundly affects QOL. Furthermore, "fatigue may persist for months or years" following completion of disease-modifying treatments.

Pathophysiology

Case Study Part 2

Understanding the pathophysiology of Kai's fatigue involves delving into the complex interplay of biological, physiological, and psychological elements. The presence of Kai's lung cancer has likely activated an immune response in his body, resulting in an increased release of inflammatory cytokines, which are implicated in fatigue. The chemotherapy and targeted therapy he underwent can compound this cytokine response and cause direct tissue damage, adding to his feelings of fatigue. Furthermore, his treatment could have affected his bone marrow function or caused blood loss, leading to anemia, a notable contributor to fatigue. His lung cancer may have also caused metabolic changes leading to muscle wasting (cachexia) and poor nutritional intake, thereby escalating his fatigue. Lastly, Kai's anxiety about his prognosis and the overall stress of living with a life-limiting diagnosis are significant psychological factors that can amplify his experience of fatigue.

Fatigue is also caused by medical/treatment-related factors including anemia, chemotherapy or other treatments, medications, and co-occurring symptoms such as pain, depression, and anxiety.[28] Anemia can result in severe fatigue and significantly impair QOL. It has a profound impact on patients, with additional complications that include dyspnea, palpitations, dizziness, and decreased cognitive function.[29] These symptoms can be common in patients with advanced disease or who are receiving aggressive, cure-focused therapies.

Some evidence suggests that dysregulation of pro-inflammatory cytokines may play a mechanistic role in the symptom of fatigue as a common biological mechanism across medical diagnoses.[14] Pro-inflammatory cytokines are released as part of the host response to infection, tumor, tissue damage from injury, or depletion of immune cells associated with treatments. These inflammatory stimuli can lead to signaling in the central nervous system, resulting in the perception of fatigue as well as changes in sleep, appetite, reproduction, mood, and social behavior.[13] A number of inflammatory biomarkers including interleukin 1 beta (IL-1β), tumor necrosis factor alpha (TNF-α), IL-6, IL-1 receptor antagonist, soluble TNF receptor, soluble IL-6 receptor, and C-reactive protein have been implicated for their role in development of fatigue.

Cachexia is believed to be a significant pathophysiologic cause of fatigue.[30] Decreased nutritional status and loss of muscle mass contribute to feeling lack of strength both in large muscle groups needed for ambulation and activities of daily living and in basic physiologic functions such as breathing and eating. In addition, research has shown that increased inflammation is associated with decreased transthyretin, subsequent poor muscle power, and increased fatigue.[31]

Factors Influencing Fatigue

Factors influencing the development of fatigue across various chronic and life-threatening illnesses have not been well studied. Fatigue, like pain, is not only explained by physiological mechanisms and must be understood as a multidimensional phenomenon that includes physical, psychological, social, and spiritual aspects. Demographic factors including age, gender, marital status, and income, as well as spiritual well-being and functional and emotional supports, can impact one's experience of fatigue. Box 25.2 provides a list of risk factors that are associated with fatigue.

Participants in a study exploring fatigue following acute myocardial infarction reported that fatigue interfered with daily functional status and described symptoms related to depression.[32] Similarly, patients with

Box 25.2 Risk Factors Associated with Fatigue

Personal Factors
- Age
- Marital status
- Menopausal status
- Income/insurance

Psychosocial Factors
- Mental and emotional state (depression, fear, anxiety, distress, conflicts)
- Culture/ethnicity
- Living situation

Care-Related Factors
- Number/cohesiveness of caregivers
- Responsiveness of healthcare providers

Disease-Related Factors
- Stage and extent of disease
- Comorbidities
- Anemia
- Pain
- Dyspnea
- Nutritional changes (weight loss, cachexia, and electrolyte imbalance)
- Continence
- Sleep patterns/interruptions

Treatment-Related Factors
- Any treatment-related effect from surgery, chemotherapy, or radiation (skin reaction, temporary altered energy level, urinary/bowel changes, pain)
- Medication issues (side effects, polypharmacy, taste changes, over-the-counter medications)
- Permanent physiological changes such as loss or damage to lung tissue that impairs gas exchange and loss of muscle mass from cachexia.

end-stage renal disease on chronic dialysis complain of high levels of pain and fatigue associated with other symptoms, including headaches, cramps, itching, dyspnea, nausea and vomiting, and sleep disruption, and often identify severe fatigue and symptom distress as significant.[26]

In one study, 100 patients with rheumatoid arthritis (RA) were asked to identify factors that contributed to their fatigue. Results indicated that the rheumatoid disease process itself was the primary cause of fatigue; joint pain was specifically mentioned.[27] Disturbed sleep was the second most frequent factor, and physical effort to accomplish daily tasks ranked third.[27] Patients with RA indicated that they had to exert twice the effort and energy to accomplish the same amount of work. In another study, women with RA reported more fatigue than men; the authors explained this variance as a result of female patients' higher degrees of pain and poor quality of sleep.[33]

Many characteristics that may predispose patients with other advanced diseases to develop similar fatigue syndromes have not been studied comprehensively. However, depression and fatigue are two related concepts often linked to cancer patients.[34] Fatigue is part of the diagnostic criteria for depression, and depression may develop as a result of being fatigued. While depression is reported less frequently, feelings of depression are common in patients with cancer. Research indicates that women who are fatigued score twice as high on the depression scale as those who were not fatigued and that depression is the strongest predictor of fatigue.[34]

Depression and fatigue may coexist with cancer without having a causal relationship since each can originate from the same cause.[34] Fatigue in people undergoing cancer treatment has been closely linked with other distressing symptoms, such as pain, dyspnea, anorexia, constipation, sleep disruption, depression, anxiety, and other mood states impacting patient QOL.[35]

Impact of Fatigue

Fatigue has been identified as a reason people miss clinic appointments. It is associated with decreased QOL in advanced cancer patients.[36] In pediatric cancer, fatigue was associated with distress related to other symptoms (anorexia, nausea, sleep disturbance, sadness, and irritability).[37] Fatigue is associated with increased caregiver burden across palliative care populations.[38] It is associated with overall suffering in hospitalized patients with cancer[39] and decreased performance status in people starting palliative radiation.[40]

For many people fatigue can be the most debilitating part of their diagnosis. People with fatigue experience worse sleep quality, disrupted circadian rhythms, decreased QOL, and lower activity levels. The management of fatigue is described as a common unmet need[41] and frequently identified by patients as a top priority.[42] Given the consequences and unmet needs, nurse clinicians and researchers should assess and address fatigue.

Assessment of Fatigue

Case Study Part 3

Kai met with the palliative care nurse to discuss options. The nurse's assessment provided important insights on Kai's fatigue and its impact on his life as well as possible options for management. His fatigue has severely limited Kai's daily activities, impairing his ability to perform even simple tasks such as eating or walking short distances. Kai also reports that he is not sleeping well at night due to discomfort from his illness and anxiety about his prognosis. Kai has always done the majority of the cooking for his family, and he especially loves hosting weekend family barbeques but finds he cannot handle all the prep work and standing that goes into making big family meals anymore. The combination of persistent fatigue and poor sleep has resulted in an exacerbation of his overall sense of physical weakness and psychological distress. Kai is especially distressed by the fact that he may not be able to host a family barbeque for his grandson's first birthday party next month due to his fatigue.

Assessment of the whole person, physical, psychosocial, and emotional, of the mind and spirit as well as the body, is essential in the recognition of fatigue. Fatigue, like all symptoms, is defined as a subjective experience that can best be identified by the person who is experiencing it. Caregiver or staff perceptions may differ from those articulated by the person experiencing fatigue. Unfortunately, up to 77% of professionals in palliative care report a lack of confidence in measuring and managing fatigue, and about half agree that fatigue is hard to control.[12] However, early and routine screening for fatigue has been shown to improve management for people receiving palliative care.[43] While there is evidence that muscle strength is positively correlated to fatigue severity, self-report is considered to be the gold standard for fatigue assessment.[44]

The NCCN guidelines[2] for cancer-related fatigue clearly delineate steps and processes to put the assessment and recognition of fatigue on the same level as pain and call for healthcare providers to assess patients at an initial visit; to follow up at regular intervals using an age-related severity scale; and, based on those findings, to implement a program of patient education and strategies to manage fatigue. The guidelines also include a step-by-step diagram from a "focused history" to specific interventions of nonpharmacological and pharmacological treatment, from the evaluation phase through active treatment, post-treatment, and the end of life. While these guidelines were developed for the assessment of fatigue in people with cancer, they provide a useful approach that can be implemented in any population of people with chronic or life-threatening illnesses in which fatigue is a concern.

There are numerous methods of assessing and diagnosing fatigue. Recognizing the importance of fatigue, the diagnosis has been proposed for inclusion in the *International Classification of Diseases* (Box 25.3). However, some researchers suggest that the diagnostic criteria are too restrictive, and the strict exclusion of those with possible "mood disorders" is of concern and may underestimate fatigue occurrence.

Fatigue, as with any symptom, is not static. Changes take place daily and sometimes hourly in the patient with an advanced illness. As such, adequate fatigue management requires frequent evaluation on the part of the healthcare team. An example of a thorough assessment of the symptom of fatigue is found in Box 25.3, which uses both a subjective and an objective framework to ascertain fatigue and possible underlying physiological events that may exacerbate the fatigue. Important areas to explore are patient and family beliefs and expectations related to the fatigue experience and awareness of

Box 25.3 Criteria for Diagnosing and Evaluating Fatigue

Criteria for diagnosing and evaluating fatigue include the presence, frequency (sporadic or constant), duration, and degree of interference with activities of daily living.

1. Complaints of generalized weakness or limb heaviness
2. Diminished concentration or attention
3. Decreased motivation or interest in engaging in usual activities
4. Insomnia or hypersomnia
5. Sleep is unrefreshing or nonrestorative
6. Perceived need to struggle to overcome inactivity
7. Marked emotional reactivity to feeling fatigued (sadness, frustration, irritability)
8. Difficulty in completing daily tasks attributed to feeling fatigued
9. Perceived problems with short-term memory
10. Post-exertional malaise lasting several hours

changes in energy levels, exacerbation and remission of symptoms, and what improves the level of fatigue.[28]

Many scales have been developed to measure fatigue in adults. Examples of fatigue measurement tools include the Multidimensional Assessment of Fatigue, the Symptom Distress Scale, the Fatigue Scale, the Fatigue Observation Checklist, and the Visual Analog Scale for Fatigue.[45] These scales are available for use in both research and clinical practice. A comprehensive review by Piper and colleagues[46] describes the advantages and disadvantages of the single-item as well as multi-item multidimensional fatigue measures currently in use. Single items are brief and especially useful for screening and tracking change over time, whereas multidimensional assessments provide a depth of understanding of the entire fatigue experience.

When fatigue is identified, healthcare providers must be aware of the presence of other clinically significant distresses or impairments in social, occupational, or other important areas of functioning and report these to the medical team. Other important considerations include evidence from the history, physical examination, or laboratory findings that symptoms are a consequence of disease-directed therapy or determination that symptoms are not primarily a consequence of a comorbid psychiatric disorder (e.g., major depression, somatization disorder, somatoform disorder, or delirium).

Fatigue can be quickly assessed using a single-item self-report scale, similar to the widely used 0–10 numeric rating scale commonly used to assess pain. A single-item assessment permits rapid quantification of fatigue, where 0 equals no fatigue and 10 equals severe fatigue that interferes with some function.[1] A single-item scale is particularly useful in monitoring change in fatigue within an individual over time. As with the use of any measurement tool, consistency of utilization is essential to understanding the symptom experience for both the patient and professional staff.

A practical approach nurses can take during an initial assessment of fatigue is to use a multidimensional assessment framework similar to ones used to assess pain. Assessments should include inquiring about severity, distress, and duration; exacerbating and relieving factors; related symptoms such as sleep, pain, and mood; and the impact on daily activities. Single-item fatigue assessments can be used to track progress once a plan of care has been implemented.

Management and Treatment of Fatigue

Case Study Part 4

The palliative care team implemented several nonpharmacological strategies to help manage Kai's fatigue. Firstly, he was introduced to a gentle, tailored exercise program overseen by a physiotherapist, designed to balance periods of activity with rest. Regular, short walks were encouraged to boost his energy levels and improve sleep quality. A registered dietitian was consulted to help Kai with his nutrition, focusing on energy-dense meals and snacks that are easy to consume and digest, along with sufficient hydration. Kai was taught various relaxation techniques, including mindfulness-based stress reduction and guided imagery, aimed at reducing his anxiety and promoting restful sleep. In addition, regular napping was recommended but with limited duration to avoid disruption to his nocturnal sleep cycle. Kai's bedroom was transformed into a conducive sleep environment—quiet, dark, and at a comfortable temperature—with a regular bedtime routine established. Lastly, the palliative care nurse worked closely with Kai to identify activities of importance to him, such as overseeing the grill for the barbeque, and activities he can give over to other people, such as grocery shopping and prepping all the side dishes. By respecting his preferences and taking a holistic approach in managing his fatigue the palliative care nurse was able to create a realistic and effective care plan for Kai.

Fatigue interventions can be grouped into two broad categories: pharmacological and nonpharmacological related to associated causes and symptoms. Treatment may include both of these modalities and should be adjusted to meet the changes in the patient's health status. The nurse plays an important role in developing a holistic plan of care to manage fatigue and providing personalized education to the patient and family to implement the fatigue management plan.

Within the context of palliative care, the management of fatigue can be extremely challenging. Palliative care can occur over a prolonged period ranging from early in the course of a disease when a person may be physically and socially active to a few weeks before death, when all activity may diminish considerably. With fatigue interventions, the wishes of the patient and family are paramount. Effective management takes into consideration the extent of the disease, other symptoms, whether and what disease-modifying treatments are being used, and the person's age, developmental and emotional status, and physical location.[47] Intervention and treatment for fatigue are suggested to occur at two levels: (1) management of symptoms that contribute to fatigue and (2) prevention of additional or secondary fatigue by maintaining a balance between restorative rest and restorative activity.

Fatigue can be treated more effectively when underlying factors such as anemia, deconditioning, depression, dehydration, hypoxia, metabolic and endocrine disorders, insomnia, pain, malnutrition, infection, or other comorbidities are effectively managed. Identifiable goals are to alleviate recognizable factors contributing to fatigue in general and provide support systems to develop or improve patients' and families' coping mechanisms. Often the acknowledgment of the potential of fatigue in any chronic or life-threatening illness assists with understanding of the experience.

It is beneficial for family members to understand the potential for feelings of fatigue and extreme exhaustion. In practice, it can be difficult to manage expectations around fatigue since patients and their family members are frequently under the impression that disease-focused treatments should also relieve disease-related side effects.[48] Helping patients and families to understand the interrelated factors that cause fatigue and to identify realistic goals is a critical component to fatigue management.

Pharmacological and Herbal Interventions

Pharmacological approaches to treat fatigue in patients with cancer or other chronic or life-threatening illnesses include both Food and Drug Administration–approved medications and herbal therapies. More frequently used pharmacological therapies include corticosteroids, psychostimulants, and, to a lesser degree, antidepressants, TNF-α, micronutrients, and various other classes of drugs.

Corticosteroids such as dexamethasone are commonly used to counteract fatigue, poor appetite, and nausea. However, side effects may include insomnia, mood swings, elevation of blood glucose, and increased occurrence of *Candida* infection.

Fatigue associated with anemia has been treated with erythropoietin in order to reduce the need for red blood cell transfusion; however, there is concern that it may "increase the risk of thromboembolic events."[29] Clinical trials of TNF-α (etanercept) have shown some effects on fatigue for patients experiencing RA with promising results.[49]

The addition of a central nervous system stimulant might counteract the somnolence of opioid use and, as a result, might enhance the effects of pain medication and increase patient activity levels. A large study was conducted with the psychostimulant methylphenidate to identify its effects on depression and cognition associated with cancer-related fatigue.[50] Analysis demonstrated limited evidence to support treatment and did identify some adverse events including vertigo, anxiety, anorexia, and nausea. The benefit of herbal psychostimulants has been demonstrated with a trial for treatment of cancer-related fatigue with the use of American ginseng 2,000 mg/day with no associated toxicities.[51] There continues to be mixed results of the effectiveness of psychostimulants in the management of fatigue across diagnoses.

Nurses play an important role in understanding the role of medications in the management of fatigue and providing patient education on the appropriate use of prescribed and over-the-counter medications including teaching about the dose and route, timing, interactions with food, and other medications and potential side effects.

Nonpharmacological Interventions

Historically, nurse clinicians and researchers have been the trailblazers in assessing and managing fatigue, with interventions encompassing several disciplines. Effective fatigue management strategies listed in Table 25.1 include identifying and managing disrupted sleep patterns, addressing nutritional deficits, and managing related symptoms such as pain, depressed mood, and/or appetite loss. In addition, interventions that calm the body and mind can have a significant positive impact on distress associated with fatigue. Bathing, specifically in a tub, was found to reduce distress associated with fatigue in people receiving hospice care.[52] Similarly music therapy has been found to be an effective intervention to decrease fatigue-related distress.[53] While the exact mechanism is unknown, the traditional Chinese medicine practices of acupuncture and acupressure may be effective interventions in the management of fatigue.[54]

A significant component of fatigue management is the role of pacing one's activities, choosing which activities to spend energy on, reframing expectations about what is a realistic amount of energy to individuals. Pacing and planning may not reduce the severity of fatigue but can significantly reduce the distress associated with fatigue. The nurse can play a critical role in working with the patient and family to identify how to plan and best implement strategies when in the context of limited energy.

Paradoxical to many people's expectations, fatigue severity and distress have been significantly improved with the implementation of exercise interventions. Strength training has been found to decrease fatigue in people with fibromyalgia.[55] Group exercise programs have been found to reduce physical fatigue in patients with incurable cancers receiving hospice care.[56] Exercise interventions have shown reduction in fatigue as well as related symptoms, including pain, insomnia, and shortness of breath, and improved functional capacities in people with advanced cancer.[57] Toward the end of life, the NCCN guidelines recommend general strategies for fatigue management that begin with energy conservation techniques, prioritizing activities, delegating, taking rest periods, and using labor-saving devices. They also recommend optimizing patient activity levels with the consideration of a referral to both physical and occupational therapies. Increased caution was emphasized for those with bone metastases and immunosuppression. Early research indicates that exercise may be an effective intervention for improving the severity of side effects of cognitive impairment, sleep problems, depression, pain, anxiety, and physical dysfunction. While exercise should be considered an important intervention to reduce fatigue in people with advanced cancer, there is a lack of evidence supporting its impact on other conditions.[58]

Nutritional consultation for patients has been shown to be key to managing physiological deficiencies from cachexia, nausea, and anorexia. Adequate hydration and the replacement of lost electrolytes enable the fatigue sufferer to have the best opportunity to control fatigue symptoms that are physiologically based. Vitamin D supplementation has been shown to decrease fatigue severity in randomized controlled trials of people in palliative care.[59]

Sleep disturbances are often reported together with fatigue. Sleep disruption is a common problem encountered by people with advanced chronic progressive disease and life-threatening illnesses. Sleep cycles may be negatively affected by multiple internal and external factors. The sleep disturbances may be actual or perceived, but both result in daytime fatigue and sleepiness. Common sleep disturbances resulting in fatigue include insomnia, breathing disorders, and movement disorders. Treating the underlying causes of sleep disturbance can have a significant impact on daytime fatigue. Perhaps through a related mechanism, light therapy has been found to decrease fatigue severity in a study of people with cancer.[60]

One of the identified barriers to fatigue management is lack of knowledge and understanding of the relationship between physical

Table 25.1 Nursing interventions to relieve fatigue

Problem	Intervention	Rationale
Lack of information or lack of preparation	Explain complex nature of fatigue and importance of communication of fatigue level with healthcare providers. Explain causes of fatigue in advanced cancer and chronic progressive diseases, and evaluate fatigue level with each visit. • Fatigue can increase in advanced disease. • Cancer cells can compete with body for essential nutrients. • Palliative treatments, infection, and fever increase the body's need for energy. • Anxiety, depression, and tension can contribute to fatigue. • Changes in daily schedules or interrupted sleep schedules contribute to fatigue development. Prepare patient for planned activities of daily living and other activities requiring significant energy (eating, moving, visitors, healthcare provider appointments).	Preparatory sensory information reduces anxiety and fatigue. Realistic expectations decrease distress and fatigue.
Disrupted rest/ sleep patterns	Evaluate/establish sleep routine: • Usual sleep pattern, length of uninterrupted sleep, temperature in room, activity prior to sleep. • Eating habits prior to sleep, medications, exercise. • Establish/continue regular, routine bedtime and awakening. • Obtain as long sleep sequences as possible, plan uninterrupted time. • Take short rest periods/naps that do not interfere with night sleep. • Use light sources to cue the body into a consistent sleep rhythm. • Pharmacologic management of insomnia should be used when behavioral and cognitive approaches have been exhausted.	Minimizing time in bed helps patients feel refreshed, avoids fragmented sleep, and strengthens circadian rhythm.
Deficient nutritional status	Recommend to patient: • High-protein, nutrient-dense food to "make every mouthful count." • Use protein supplements to augment diet. • Suggest small, frequent meals. • Coordinate time up in chair with meal arrival time. • Socialization may increase oral intake. • Encourage adequate intake of fluids, eight glasses/day or whatever is tolerated, unless contraindicated. • Consider requesting an appetite stimulant like medroxyprogesterone acetate (Megace).	Increased nutrition will raise energy level. Less energy is needed for digestion with small, frequent meals.
Multi-symptom occurrence	Assess and control symptoms contributing to or coexisting with fatigue such as pain, sleeplessness, depression, nausea, diarrhea, constipation, electrolyte imbalances, dyspnea, dehydration, infection. Assess for symptoms of anemia and evaluate for the possibility of pharmacologic intervention or transfusion.	Multiple distressing symptoms drain energy and will contribute to marked physical/ mental fatigue.
Decreased energy reserves	Plan/schedule activities: • Identify a person to be in charge (fielding questions, answering the phone, organizing meals). • Adjust method/pace of care and move slowly when providing care. • Prioritize and save energy for the most important events. • Eliminate or postpone noncritical activities. • Learn to listen to body; if fatigued, rest. Obtain physical therapy consult: • Mild physical therapy may help joint flexibility and prevent pain. • Engage in individually tailored, team-approved exercise/yoga program. Use distraction/restoration: • Encourage activities to restore energy: spending time in natural environment, gardening, listening to music, praying, meditating, engaging in hobbies (art, reading, journaling). • Spend time with family/friends, joining in passive activities (riding in car, watching meal preparation).	Energy conservation helps to reduce fatigue burden and efficiently use energy available. Pleasant activities may reduce/relieve mental (attentional) fatigue.

activity/inactivity as it relates to fatigue on the part of the patient and the family as well as the healthcare professionals. Education should include information on such topics as changes in disease status, progression, additional procedure or treatment needs, and medication side effects. Nurse-initiated and -planned educational sessions with the patient and family may provide a forum in which to respond to forgotten questions, reinforce nutritional information, and together manage symptoms to improve QOL.

As the practice guidelines and standards for fatigue management in palliative care continue to evolve, the NCCN fatigue guidelines provide a framework for adults, children, and adolescents suffering from fatigue.[2] It is recommended that quality management be ongoing and implemented as continuous quality improvement projects. Finally, the guidelines suggest that medical care contracts include reimbursement for fatigue-related treatments and that disability insurance addresses coverage for long-lasting fatigue.[1]

Conclusion

This chapter provides an overview of fatigue as it spans the illness trajectory and end-of-life experience for people with chronic progressive disease and life-threatening illnesses. While fatigue is a complex phenomenon that has been widely studied, it still has no universally accepted definition. Patients with cancer and many other chronic, progressive diseases continue to experience fatigue; and the costs associated with it—not only in the economic sense but also in its physical, emotional, and psychological impacts on life—need to be understood. Many factors, including age, psychological state, social support, access to care, disease type and status, pharmaceutical issues, cognitive impairment, and comorbid conditions, influence fatigue. Fatigue is a serious problem that interferes with physical, psychological, emotional, social, and economic functions. The need for healthcare providers to recognize and identify symptoms and explore management strategies is crucial to the lessening of human suffering. Professional nurses are in a unique position to recognize, identify, and explore the needs of patients who may prematurely decline further treatment as a consequence of their fatigue.

REFERENCES

1. Finsterer J, Mahjoub SZ. Fatigue in healthy and diseased individuals. *Am J Hosp Palliat Med*. 2014;31(5):562–575.
2. National Comprehensive Cancer Network. Cancer-Related Fatigue (Version 2). 2022. Accessed October 24, 2022, https://www.nccn.org/professionals/physician_gls/pdf/fatigue.pdf.
3. Chen Y-W, Camp PG, Coxson HO, et al. A comparison of pain, fatigue, dyspnea and their impact on quality of life in pulmonary rehabilitation participants with chronic obstructive pulmonary disease. *COPD*. 2018;15(1):65–72.
4. Williams BA. The clinical epidemiology of fatigue in newly diagnosed heart failure. *BMC Cardiovasc Disord*. 2017;17(1):1–10.
5. Ju A, Unruh ML, Davison SN, et al. Patient-reported outcome measures for fatigue in patients on hemodialysis: a systematic review. *Am J Kidney Dis*. 2018;71(3):327–343.
6. Barroso J, Leserman J, Harmon JL, Hammill B, Pence BW. Fatigue in HIV-infected people: a three-year observational study. *J Pain Symptom Manage*. 2015;50(1):69–79.
7. Khan F, Amatya B, Galea M. Management of fatigue in persons with multiple sclerosis. *Front Neurol*. 2014;5:177.
8. Bower JE. Cancer-related fatigue—mechanisms, risk factors, and treatments. *Nat Rev Clin Oncol*. 2014;11(10):597–609.
9. Whitehead LC, Unahi K, Burrell B, Crowe MT. The experience of fatigue across long-term conditions: a qualitative meta-synthesis. *J Pain Symptom Manage*. 2016;52(1):131–143. e1.
10. Dong ST, Costa DS, Butow PN, et al. Symptom clusters in advanced cancer patients: an empirical comparison of statistical methods and the impact on quality of life. *J Pain Symptom Manage*. 2016;51(1):88–98.
11. Charalambous A, Kouta C. Cancer related fatigue and quality of life in patients with advanced prostate cancer undergoing chemotherapy. *Biomed Res Int*. 2016;2016:3989286.
12. Ingham G, Urban K. How confident are we at assessing and managing fatigue in palliative care patients? A multicenter survey exploring the current attitudes of palliative care professionals. *Palliat Med Rep*. 2020;1(1):58–65. https://doi.org/10.1089/pmr.2020.0005.
13. Kolak A, Kamińska M, Wysokińska E, et al. The problem of fatigue in patients suffering from neoplastic disease. *Contemp Oncol (Pozn)*. 2017;21(2):131–135.
14. American Cancer Society. What Is Fatigue or Weakness? Updated February 1, 2020. Accessed October 24, 2022, https://www.cancer.org/treatment/treatments-and-side-effects/physical-side-effects/fatigue/what-is-cancer-related-fatigue.html.
15. Kratz AL, Murphy SL, Braley TJ. Pain, fatigue, and cognitive symptoms are temporally associated within but not across days in multiple sclerosis. *Arch Phys Med Rehabil*. 2017;98(11):2151–2159.
16. Eckhardt AL, DeVon HA, Piano MR, Ryan CJ, Zerwic JJ. Fatigue in the presence of coronary heart disease. *Nursing Res*. 2014;63(2):83–93.
17. Gandesbery B, Dobbie K, Gorodeski EZ. Outpatient palliative cardiology service embedded within a heart failure clinic: experiences with an emerging model of care. *Am J Hosp Palliat Care*. 2018;35(4):635–639. https://doi.org/10.1177/1049909117729478.
18. Mairesse O, Neu D. Tired of blunt tools? Sharpening the clinical assessment of fatigue and sleepiness. *Psychiatry Res*. 2016;238:100–108.
19. den Hartogh G. Suffering and dying well: on the proper aim of palliative care. *Med Health Care Philos*. 2017;20(3):413–424.
20. Dhingra L, Barrett M, Knotkova H, et al. Symptom distress among diverse patients referred for community-based palliative care: sociodemographic and medical correlates. *J Pain Symptom Manage*. 2018;55(2):290–296. https://doi.org/10.1016/j.jpainsymman.2017.08.015.
21. Bandeali S, des Ordons AR, Sinnarajah A. Comparing the physical, psychological, social, and spiritual needs of patients with non-cancer and cancer diagnoses in a tertiary palliative care setting. *Palliat Support Care*. 2020;18(5):513–518. https://doi.org/10.1017/s1478951519001020.
22. Delgado-Guay MO, Ferrer J, Ochoa J, et al. Characteristics and outcomes of advanced cancer patients who received palliative care at a public hospital compared with those at a comprehensive cancer center. *J Palliat Med*. 2018;21(5):678–685. https://doi.org/10.1089/jpm.2017.0236.
23. Fredriksson-Larsson U, Alsen P, Brink E. I've lost the person I used to be—experiences of the consequences of fatigue following myocardial infarction. *Int J Qual Stud Health Well-being*. 2013;8(1):20836.
24. Clark-Cutaia MN, Rivera E, Iroegbu C, Arneson G, Deng R, Anastasi JK. Exploring the evidence: symptom burden in chronic kidney disease. *Nephrol Nurs J*. 2022;49(3):227–255.
25. Pang L, de la Cruz M, Wu J, Liu D, Naqvi M, Bruera E. Symptom frequency and change of oldest old cancer patients. *Support Care Cancer*. 2019;27(11):4165–4170. https://doi.org/10.1007/s00520-019-04702-7.
26. Horigan AE, Schneider SM, Docherty S, Barroso J. The experience and self-management of fatigue in patients on hemodialysis. *Nephrol Nurs J*. 2013;40(2):113–122.
27. Hewlett S, Dures E, Almeida C. Measures of fatigue: Bristol Rheumatoid Arthritis Fatigue Multi-Dimensional Questionnaire (BRAF MDQ), Bristol Rheumatoid Arthritis Fatigue Numerical Rating Scales (BRAF NRS) for severity, effect, and coping, Chalder Fatigue Questionnaire (CFQ), Checklist Individual Strength (CIS20R and CIS8R), Fatigue Severity Scale (FSS), Functional Assessment Chronic Illness Therapy (Fatigue) (FACIT-F), Multi dimensional Assessment of Fatigue (MAF), Multi-dimensional Fatigue Inventory (MFI), Pediatric Quality of Life (PedsQL) Multi-dimensional Fatigue Scale, Profile of Fatigue (ProF), Short Form 36 Vitality Subscale (SF-36 VT), and visual analog scales (VAS). *Arthritis Care Res*. 2011;63(suppl 11):S263–S286.
28. Bower JE, Bak K, Berger A, et al. Screening, assessment, and management of fatigue in adult survivors of cancer: an American Society of Clinical oncology clinical practice guideline adaptation. *J Clin Oncol*. 2014;32(17):1840.
29. Bohlius J, Tonia T, Nüesch E, et al. Effects of erythropoiesis-stimulating agents on fatigue- and anaemia-related symptoms in cancer patients: systematic review and meta-analyses of published and unpublished data. *Br J Cancer*. 2014;111(1):33–45.

30. Flynn B, Barrett M, Sui J, Halpin C, Paz G, Walsh D. Nutritional status and interventions in hospice: physician assessment of cancer patients. *J Hum Nutr Diet*. 2018;31(6):781–784. https://doi.org/10.1111/jhn.12562.
31. Miura T, Amano K, Shirado A, et al. Low transthyretin levels predict poor prognosis in cancer patients in palliative care settings. *Nutr Cancer*. 2018;70(8):1283–1289. https://doi.org/10.1080/01635581.2018.1557213.
32. Robinson RL, Stephenson JJ, Dennehy EB, et al. The importance of unresolved fatigue in depression: costs and comorbidities. *Psychosomatics*. 2015;56(3):274–285.
33. Nikolaus S, Bode C, Taal E, van de Laar MA. Fatigue and factors related to fatigue in rheumatoid arthritis: a systematic review. *Arthritis Care Res*. 2013;65(7):1128–1146.
34. Ho S-Y, Rohan KJ, Parent J, Tager FA, McKinley PS. A longitudinal study of depression, fatigue, and sleep disturbances as a symptom cluster in women with breast cancer. *J Pain Symptom Manage*. 2015;49(4):707–715.
35. Deodhar JK, Noronha V, Muckaden MA, et al. A study to assess the feasibility of introducing early palliative care in ambulatory patients with advanced lung cancer. *Indian J Palliat Care*. 2017;23(3):261–267. https://doi.org/10.4103/ijpc.Ijpc_19_17.
36. Selina C, Bo Angela W, Pidduck W, et al. Symptoms predictive of overall quality of life using the Edmonton Symptom Assessment Scale in breast cancer patients receiving radiotherapy. *Clin Breast Cancer*. 2019;19(6):405–410. https://doi.org/10.1016/j.clbc.2019.05.007.
37. Ullrich CK, Dussel V, Orellana L, et al. Self-reported fatigue in children with advanced cancer: results of the PediQUEST study. *Cancer*. 2018;124(18):3776–3783. https://doi.org/10.1002/cncr.31639.
38. Celik E, Aslan MS, Sengul Samanci N, et al. The relationship between symptom severity and caregiver burden in cancer patients under palliative care: a cross-sectional study. *J Palliat Care*. 2022;37(1):48–54. https://doi.org/10.1177/08258597211045780.
39. Davis MP, Rybicki LA, Samala RV, Patel C, Parala-Metz A, Lagman R. Pain or fatigue: which correlates more with suffering in hospitalized cancer patients? *Support Care Cancer*. 2021;29(8):4535–4542. https://doi.org/10.1007/s00520-021-05996-2.
40. Nieder C, Kämpe TA. Symptom burden in patients with reduced performance status at the start of palliative radiotherapy. *In Vivo*. 2020;34(2):735–738. https://doi.org/10.21873/invivo.11832.
41. Simon H, Ganem G, Touboul C, Lhomel C, Morère JF. Patient perspectives on supportive care in cancer: results of the Calista 2 study. *Eur J Cancer Care*. 2020;29(6):1–11. https://doi.org/10.1111/ecc.13299.
42. Tometich DB, Mosher CE, Hirsh AT, et al. Metastatic breast cancer patients' expectations and priorities for symptom improvement. *Support Care Cancer*. 2018;26(11):3781–3788. https://doi.org/10.1007/s00520-018-4244-8
43. Vigstad S, Clancy A, Broderstad AR. Palliative patients get greater relief from early screening of symptoms and implementation of measures. Article in Norwegian. *Norwegian J Clin Nurs/Sykepleien Forskning*. 2019;13:e74591. https://doi.org/10.4220/Sykepleienf.2018.74591.
44. Schvartsman G, Park M, Liu DD, Yennu S, Bruera E, Hui D. Could objective tests be used to measure fatigue in patients with advanced cancer? *J Pain Symptom Manage*. 2017;54(2):237–244. https://doi.org/10.1016/j.jpainsymman.2016.12.343.
45. Aaronson LS, Teel CS, Cassmeyer V, et al. Defining and measuring fatigue. *Image*. 1999;31(1):45–50.
46. Borneman T, Piper BF, Sun VC-Y, Koczywas M, Uman G, Ferrell B. Implementing the fatigue guidelines at one NCCN member institution: process and outcomes. *J Natl Compr Canc Netw*. 2007;5(10):1092–1101.
47. Piper BF. Piper fatigue scale available for clinical testing. *Oncol Nurs Forum*. 1990;17(5):661–662.
48. Mohandas H, Jaganathan SK, Mani MP, Ayyar M, Thevi GR. Cancer-related fatigue treatment: an overview. *J Cancer Res Ther*. 2017;13(6):916.
49. Hunt L, Emery P. Etanercept in the treatment of rheumatoid arthritis. *Expert Opin Biol Ther*. 2013;13(10):1441–1450.
50. Gong S, Sheng P, Jin H, et al. Effect of methylphenidate in patients with cancer-related fatigue: a systematic review and meta-analysis. *PLoS One*. 2014;9(1):e84391.
51. Barton DL, Liu H, Dakhil SR, et al. Wisconsin ginseng (*Panax quinquefolius*) to improve cancer-related fatigue: a randomized, double-blind trial, N07C2. *J Natl Cancer Inst*. 2013;105(16):1230–1238.
52. Hayashi E, Aoyama M, Fukano F, Takano J, Shimizu Y, Miyashita M. Effects of bathing in a tub on physical and psychological symptoms of end-of-life cancer patients: an observational, controlled study. *J Hosp Palliat Nurs*. 2022;24(1):30–39. https://doi.org/10.1097/njh.0000000000000803.
53. Colwell CM, Fiore J. Feasibility of patient-created Orff chant as a music-based intervention in supportive cancer care. *J Music Ther*. 2020;57(4):e1–e31. https://doi.org/10.1093/jmt/thaa019.
54. Wong CHL, Wu IXY, Adams J, et al. Development of evidence-based Chinese medicine clinical service recommendations for cancer palliative care using Delphi approach based on the evidence to decision framework. *Integr Cancer Ther*. 2020;19:1–13. https://doi.org/10.1177/1534735420940418.
55. Andrade A, de Azevedo Klumb Steffens R, Sieczkowska SM, Peyré Tartaruga LA, Torres Vilarino G. A systematic review of the effects of strength training in patients with fibromyalgia: clinical outcomes and design considerations. *Adv Rheumatol*. 2018;58(1):36. https://doi.org/10.1186/s42358-018-0033-9.
56. Malcolm L, Mein G, Jones A, Talbot-Rice H, Maddocks M, Bristowe K. Strength in numbers: patient experiences of group exercise within hospice palliative care. *BMC Palliat Care*. 2016;15(1):1–8.
57. Bobrowski D, Bobrowski A, Lim F, et al. A review of the effect of exercise on patients with advanced cancer. *J Pain Manage*. 2018;11(3):267–285.
58. Mochamat, Cuhls H, Sellin J, Conrad R, Radbruch L, Mücke M. Fatigue in advanced disease associated with palliative care: a systematic review of non-pharmacological treatments. *Palliat Med*. 2021;35(4):697–709. https://doi.org/10.1177/02692163211000628.
59. Klasson C, Helde Frankling M, Warnqvist A, et al. Sex differences in the effect of vitamin D on fatigue in palliative cancer care—a post hoc analysis of the randomized, controlled trial "Palliative-D." *Cancers (Basel)*. Jan 31 2022;14(3):746. https://doi.org/10.3390/cancers14030746.
60. Çelik A, Usta Yeşilbalkan Ö. The effect of the bright white light application to cancer patients receiving palliative care on their fatigue level and sleep quality: a randomized control trial. *Omega (Westport)*. 2023;88(1):303–317. https://doi.org/10.1177/00302228221093462.

26

Insomnia

Patricia Carter

Key Points

- Insomnia is difficulty falling asleep, staying asleep, and awakening feeling unrefreshed.
- Comprehensive assessment is required to identify causative factors for insomnia. Management of insomnia in persons with serious illness is essential for quality of life.
- Patients and families should be included in developing the treatment plan for their insomnia as buy-in is essential for success.
- Cognitive behavioral therapy (single or multimodal) is the recommended first-line treatment for insomnia.
- Pharmacotherapy should be used in combination with behavioral therapies for the greatest effectiveness.
- Nurses need to be aware of over-the-counter remedies used by persons with serious illness.

Introduction

Insomnia disorder is commonly reported in the general population; however, the prevalence increases in those diagnosed with serious illness.[1] While the etiology of insomnia is still being debated, several contributing factors have been supported across numerous empirical studies.[2] One area that is well supported in the literature is the reciprocal relationship between serious illness and the development of insomnia disorder. Insomnia generally coexists with the following serious illnesses: cancers; HIV/AIDS; and gastrointestinal, cardiovascular, pulmonary, musculoskeletal, nephrological, endocrine, neurological, and psychiatric disorders.[3–6] To effectively manage insomnia in people with serious illness, it is critical to have a holistic approach to identify the unique contributing factors that each person is experiencing. This allows for a precision treatment to reduce or minimize those unique factors. This chapter provides a model for comprehensive assessment of insomnia disorder in persons with serious illness and describes the available evidence-based interventions that can be used to address insomnia symptoms.

Definition of Insomnia

According to the American Academy of Sleep Medicine, insomnia is defined as difficulty either falling or staying asleep despite adequate opportunity to sleep and results in daytime functional impairments.[7] A 30-minute rule helps to quantify insomnia; for example, taking more than 30 minutes to fall asleep, spending more than 30 minutes awake in the middle of the night, or waking up more than 30 minutes earlier than planned in the morning.[8] In 2014, the third edition of the *International Classification of Sleep Disorders*, the most widely used classification system for sleep disorders, revised how insomnia is defined.[9] It now subclassifies insomnia as short-term, chronic, or other. Short-term insomnia is if symptoms occur for less than 3 months, and chronic is if symptoms persist for 3 or more months. "Other" insomnia refers to temporary sleep disturbance that does not meet the full diagnostic criteria of insomnia disorder.[7]

Diagnosis

Diagnostic criteria for insomnia include difficulty falling asleep (long sleep onset latency), difficulty staying asleep (low sleep maintenance), and/or awakening feeling unrefreshed even with adequate opportunity to sleep.[9] Insomnia is often precipitated by a significant life stressor (e.g., acute pain, traumatic event). Insomnia symptoms may improve when the stressor resolves or the individual develops coping strategies to reduce the impact of the stressor, or they could become chronic. Chronic insomnia is a clinical diagnosis that relies on the individual's sleep history, medical and psychiatric conditions, and substance use.[10]

Prevalence and Impact

Insomnia symptoms are a nearly universal experience across patient populations with serious illness, with approximately 70% of all patients reporting these symptoms.[11] However, the prevalence within any specific patient population varies in the literature. For example, empirical reports suggest that up to 95% of persons with cancer, 70% of persons with Parkinson's disease, and 50% of persons with congestive heart failure (CHF) report insomnia symptoms.[12–14] It is important to note that these findings are from clinical research studies that frequently use differing assessment surveys and/or criteria for identifying insomnia, and this can contribute to the discrepancies. Furthermore, in clinically based evaluations, the numbers may be much higher; however, underreporting by both the patient and clinician is common.[15]

The impact of insomnia on physical, psychological, and social well-being is well established. Several epidemiological studies and meta-analyses associate persistent insomnia symptoms with increased incidence of hormonal disruption, inflammation, anxiety, depression, memory deficits, and impaired quality of life.[3–6] Persons with serious illness are at increased risk for many of these conditions; however, there is evidence that co-occurrence of chronic insomnia symptoms and other medical conditions can be mutually exacerbating,[8] further supporting the need for comprehensive assessment and treatment of all conditions to ensure optimal patient outcomes.

Case Study: A Patient with Insomnia

Mr. M. is a 60-year-old man, accompanied by his wife, who was seen in the clinic by his nurse practitioner (NP). This is a routine visit and medication refill. His major diagnosis is CHF. The nurse noticed that both he and his wife seemed more fatigued and irritable than usual. The NP asks about his sleep; this is the conversation:

Mr. M. "It's fine"

Ms. M. "He sleeps all day and roams the house at night. It is not fine."

The NP. "Mr. M. will you please describe what happens in the evening?"

Mr. M. "I just can't sleep at night, after I take my pills [including a beta-blocker and loop diuretic], I try to go to sleep, but I am up and down all night having to pee, my skin feels like it is crawling, and I just can't get comfortable. It is just easier to stay up and watch TV."

Ms. M. "I find him asleep in the recliner in the morning. Our whole schedule is out of whack."

The NP discovers Mr. M. takes his medications around 7 p.m. and tries to go to bed at 8 p.m. He lays in bed for 30–60 minutes and gets up to urinate and walks around the house to relieve the crawling sensation in his legs. This pattern repeats most of the night until he finally falls asleep in the recliner watching TV. When Ms. M wakes up at 5 a.m., she brings him coffee and wakes him up. Mr. M. is irritable and fatigued. Ms. M. is frustrated and fearful that they will never be on the same schedule again. She is also worried that these changes are predicting a worsening of his condition and that he may die soon.

This case presents many potential causes of insomnia, including physical, emotional, and treatment-related issues which could contribute to both Mr. and Ms. M's inability to sleep.

Pathophysiology

Insomnia is a complex interaction of psychological cognitive arousal and altered circadian and homeostatic mechanisms. Decreased function of the sleep–wake switch may also contribute to insomnia. During sleep, there is a slow transition through stages of non-rapid-eye movement (non-REM) sleep to cycles of REM sleep.[16] The American Academy of Sleep Medicine classifies sleep into five progressive stages[16]:

Stage W (wake)
Stage N1 (relaxed wake)
Stage N2 (light sleep)
Stage N3 (deep or slow-wave sleep)
Stage R (REM sleep)

Multiple areas of the brain work together to promote sleep or wakefulness. The sleep–wake cycle is a complex process in which wake and sleep are switched on and off by reciprocal systems in a feedback loop.[16] Circadian factors promote wakefulness on a roughly 24-hour biological clock, and homeostatic factors respond to accumulated sleep drive over periods of wakefulness.[16] A disruption to this delicately balanced and highly complex process results in insomnia.

The 3P behavioral model of insomnia helps to explain how acute insomnia becomes chronic and lays the groundwork for assessing insomnia in individual patients.[17] The 3Ps include factors that predispose an individual to insomnia, precipitate an acute episode of insomnia, and then perpetuate insomnia so that it moves from short-term (acute) to chronic.

Predisposing factors increase an individual's risk for developing insomnia and include genetics and personality traits that lead to physiologic and cognitive hyperarousal.[18] Precipitating factors are the trigger for insomnia and are typically distressing life events (e.g., health problems, family issues).[19]

Perpetuating factors allow insomnia to continue after the original trigger(s) has resolved.[19] Environmental stimuli such as light, noise, and temperature serve as frequent disruptors of sleep.[20] Additionally, dysfunctional thoughts and beliefs about sleep, such as "nothing can be done, I am a bad sleeper," contribute to catastrophizing and reduce motivation to try to improve sleep quality. Finally, maladaptive behaviors that are often used to cope with insomnia, such as excessive caffeine consumption, smoking or other tobacco use, alcohol, and use of electronic devices close to sleeping hours, all serve to disrupt sleep onset and contribute to fragmentation of sleep.[21]

Both predisposing and precipitating factors are generally non-modifiable and are thus not the target for treatment; however, perpetuating factors are prime treatment targets for behavioral therapies. The idea is not to minimize the traumatic event(s) that triggered the insomnia but to focus on the small behavioral changes that could help to reset the sleep–wake cycle balance. For persons with serious illness, there are additional illness- and treatment-related factors that can perpetuate insomnia symptoms[22]; therefore, it is critical to conduct a comprehensive assessment of all potential contributing factors.

Contributing Factors for Insomnia

Physical Factors

In the case of Mr. M. it is evident that there are physical factors that are likely contributing to his insomnia symptoms. Substantial evidence supports the coexistence of insomnia with nearly every serious illness.[23] Furthermore, persons with serious illness may experience physical symptoms that contribute to insomnia (e.g., pain, dyspnea, urinary frequency).[14] It stands to reason that poor symptom control may perpetuate insomnia symptoms. Additionally, the medications commonly prescribed to manage the primary medical condition, such as anti-inflammatories (steroids), anti-arrhythmics (quinidine), anti-parkinsonians (levodopa), bronchodilators (theophylline), anticonvulsants (phenytoin), antihypertensives (clonidine, methyldopa, propranolol), or diuretics (triamterene), have been shown to impede sleep onset, disrupt slow-wave (deep sleep), and contribute to daytime sleepiness.

Assessment for Physical Factors Contributing to Insomnia

Insomnia is primarily a self-reported condition. However, as has been described, there are perpetuating factors, many of which can be physical in nature, that cause insomnia. When assessing an individual with serious illness for physical causes of insomnia, a comprehensive approach is needed. It is important to gather information about the nature, frequency, evolution, and duration of symptoms, as well as the response to treatment(s) attempted. Using a sleep diary (e.g., the Consensus Sleep Diary) will provide detailed information that can assist in obtaining a sleep history.[24] A sleep diary will provide temporal information (time the person goes to bed, attempts to sleep, wake-up time, out of bed time), quantitative information (total sleep time, sleep onset latency, number and duration of awakenings), and qualitative information (satisfaction with sleep). The physical and medical history is necessary to identify general medical and psychological conditions that could be coexisting with insomnia and identify pharmacotherapies that may contribute to sleep–wake disturbances. Table 26.1 provides a list of areas to consider when taking a history about insomnia.

Nursing Intervention for Physical Factors Contributing to Insomnia

In the case study presented earlier, the nurse practitioner recognized that Mr. and Ms. M were showing signs of disturbed sleep (fatigue and irritability) and inquired about how the patient was sleeping. This allowed for a conversation about the quality of sleep and potential contributors to poor sleep. As was noted, there are several possible physical factors that may perpetuate insomnia in Mr. M. One factor is that the patient is taking medications that can contribute to restlessness and nocturia. The nurse can council the patient to take the medications earlier in the day, rather than right before bed. The nurse could also assess Mr. M.'s B_{12} and magnesium levels as they could be contributing to restless leg syndrome as he described the classic crawling feeling in his legs that is relieved with walking. Other instructions could include decreasing the amount of fluids in the hours prior to bedtime to reduce nocturia (Box 26.1).

Box 26.1 Physical Assessment of Contributing Factors to Insomnia

1. Physical assessment—to rule out other sleep disorders (e.g., restless leg syndrome, obstructive sleep apnea)
   a. Neurologic exam to include symptoms of restless leg syndrome
   b. Obesity
   c. Examine head and neck: neck circumference
   d. Crowded oropharynx
   e. Lab values
      i. Ferritin, magnesium, renal function, and vitamin B_{12}
2. Symptom assessment—to identify physical contributors to sleep-wake disruption
   a. Pain
   b. Cough
   c. Shortness of breath
   d. Urinary frequency
   e. Anxiety
3. Medication and substance assessment
   a. Evaluate medications which may contribute to insomnia
   b. Use of tobacco, caffeine, alcohol, or illicit drugs

Table 26.1 Taking a history about insomnia

Is the problem falling asleep, staying asleep, or getting back to sleep after awakening during the night? Is sleep disrupted, nonrestorative? Is the problem new (acute), intermittent, or chronic?	
If acute or intermittent • What stressors are they experiencing? • Travel across time zones • New medications or change in medications • New physical symptoms (e.g., dyspnea) affecting sleep • Change in medical or psychiatric condition • Change in substance use (caffeine, tobacco, alcohol) • Change in timing of sleep (bedtime, wake time) • Change in sleep environment (noise, light, temperature)	If chronic • Activities before sleep (caffeine, tobacco, alcohol, exercise, screen use, relaxation) • Over-the-counter medication use or prescription for sleep • Bedtime, wake up time, estimated sleep duration (current, past, ideal) • Time in bed versus sleep time • Sleep–wake schedule stability • Symptoms affecting sleep at bedtime (sleepiness, restless, anxiety, pain) • Symptoms affecting sleep during the night (snoring, choking dyspnea, hot flashes, nocturia) • Symptoms upon awakening (dry mouth, headache) • Habits when awakened at night (lying awake in bed, check clock, watch TV in bed) • Daytime impairment from insomnia (drowsiness or fatigue, irritability) • Daytime napping (when and for how long)

Cognitive and Emotional Factors Contributing to Insomnia

Acute insomnia can become chronic when perpetuating maladaptive cognitive (thoughts and beliefs) and emotional (stress-diathesis) are present. Persons with serious illness may experience sleep wake pattern disruptions as a result of physical symptoms and therapies for their illness (as described above). Maladaptive thoughts and beliefs about these sleep–wake pattern disruptions can lead to rumination and catastrophic thinking about sleep.[22] Once this pattern of thinking is engaged, it can lead to sleep reactivity.[25] Sleep reactivity is a physiological and emotional hyperarousal in response to stress that precipitates insomnia onset.[25] Additionally, persons with serious illness experience emotional responses to their diagnosis and illness state (depression, anxiety, fear) that have been linked to insomnia onset and perpetuation.[25] The more the individual worries, the more disrupted sleep becomes, and the more reactive the individual becomes to life stressors. This cyclic pattern can be disrupted and reset so that the person with serious illness can obtain quality sleep.

Assessment for Cognitive and Emotional Factors Contributing to Insomnia

Assessment for sleep reactivity and an individual's history of sleep disruption following stressful events will help to identify precipitating and perpetuating factors for insomnia. Individuals with a past history of insomnia are more likely to experience difficulties with falling asleep or maintaining sleep following a real or anticipated acute stressor. For this reason, it is important to ask patients about their sleep history. Use of a sleep diary (e.g., the consensus sleep diary) can help the patient to identify patterns of thoughts and emotions that contribute to sleep–wake disturbances. The sleep diary will also quantify actual sleep characteristics (sleep onset latency, nighttime awakenings, total sleep time). This information can be used to support cognitively reframing and resetting the catastrophic cascade of dysfunctional thoughts about sleep. The diary can also identify target behaviors to improve sleep habits (e.g., timing of exercise, caffeine intake, naps).[24] The following topics can be explored with patients to assess for cognitive and emotional factors that may precipitate and perpetuate insomnia.

Sleep patterns prior to illness—to establish a history of insomnia
Current or past stressors—to establish a precipitating event
Ongoing fears or concerns about sleep—to assess for dysfunctional thoughts or beliefs
Sleep–wake patterns—to assess for rumination and/or worry (sleep reactivity)

Nursing Intervention for Cognitive and Emotional Factors Contributing to Insomnia

In the case study, both Mr. and Ms. M. expressed cognitive and emotional responses that may precipitate and/or perpetuate insomnia. Specifically, Ms. M. is worried about Mr. M's health decline and how his poor sleep patterns may be signaling his further decline. While Ms. M. was not assessed for insomnia, it would be important for the nurse to engage both partners in the intervention to improve sleep quality and reverse or prevent insomnia. It will be important for the nurse to use supportive and therapeutic communication skills to explore the causes and potential interventions to reduce dysfunctional thoughts and beliefs as well as emotional responses. When addressing emotional issues surrounding insomnia, consider fears of being alone, life changes, and grief, which may increase nighttime sleep difficulties. The nurse should take time to listen to the concerns of the patient and the spouse and help them to identify personal and professional sources of support (e.g., family, church, social work, therapist). Cognitive behavioral therapy for insomnia (CBTi) is the preferred first-line treatment for insomnia and can be especially helpful with cognitive and emotional contributing factors for insomnia.

Environmental Factors Contributing to Insomnia

The environment that is most conducive to sleep is one that is quiet, dark, and cool. This may be a challenge if the person with serious illness also requires medical equipment to support them during the night. Ask the patient to go into their room with the lights off and look around, listen, and feel the temperature. Are there noises that can be silenced or removed? Are there light sources that can be blocked (e.g., blackout curtains for the street light outside)? Can the temperature of the room be changed to make it cool (not cold)?

Nursing Intervention for Environmental Factors Contributing to Insomnia

It is important to instruct people with serious illnesses and their families that the sleep environment needs to be relaxing, comfortable, and peaceful. Reducing light and noise and having a cool temperature will support melatonin release and facilitate rapid sleep onset and deep restorative sleep. Reserve the bed for sleep and sexual activities only. No reading, watching TV, eating, or other mentally stimulating activities. Use a small (red) night light in the bathroom at night. Use the overhead lights in the morning to stimulate wake.

In addition to creating a sleep environment that is conducive to sleep, it is important to establish a habitual pattern that will promote regularity in the sleep–wake cycle. These habits are often referred to as "sleep hygiene." Examples include the following:

- Get up at roughly the same time every day.
- Go to bed when sleepy.
- Establish a bedtime routine or sequence of activities that signal that bedtime is approaching. This may include making a list for the next day, brushing teeth, taking a bath, putting on night clothes, etc.
- If unable to fall asleep easily, get out of bed and go to another location and engage in non-stimulating activity (e.g., reading a paper book in low light). Return to bed when feel sleepy. This will reduce the association of the bed with wakefulness.

Treatment of Insomnia

The goals of insomnia treatment are to improve quantitative and qualitative aspects of sleep to reduce the distress and anxiety associated with poor sleep and to improve daytime function.[26] Persons with insomnia often try self-help strategies including reading, relaxation, sleep hygiene, over-the-counter remedies (e.g., antihistamines, herbal supplements), and/or alcohol to reduce insomnia symptoms. Rarely are these approaches fully effective, and in some cases, they may further perpetuate insomnia symptoms.

The first step in providing effective treatment for a person with serious illness who is experiencing insomnia is to identify and treat the comorbid medical and psychiatric conditions and therapies that may precipitate and/or perpetuate insomnia symptoms. Once these factors are addressed, treatment for insomnia may proceed to other interventions. Insomnia treatment includes two broad categories, nonpharmacological and pharmacological interventions. These treatments may be used individually or in combination, depending on the needs and preferences of the individual patient.

Cognitive Behavioral Interventions

Several nonpharmacological cognitive behavioral interventions have been used for the treatment of insomnia. The most commonly studied interventions in this category include both single-mode and multimodal interventions. Single-mode therapies include sleep hygiene education, stimulus control, sleep restriction therapy, relaxation training, and cognitive therapy. Multimodal therapies include CBTi and brief behavioral treatment of insomnia. See Table 26.2 for a description of these interventions.

CBTi

CBTi is the most widely studied multimodal nondrug treatment for insomnia and is recommended as a first-line treatment for insomnia.[27] The efficacy of CBTi has been demonstrated for chronic insomnia across the life span[27] and in individuals with serious illness.[28] The treatment effects are comparable with or

Table 26.2 Nonpharmacologic therapies for insomnia

Intervention	Description	Specific techniques
Sleep hygiene education	Recommendations promoting behaviors that promote sleep and discourage behaviors that disrupt sleep	Do not try to sleep Avoid stimulants (caffeine, nicotine) Limit alcohol intake Maintain a regular sleep schedule Avoid naps in the second half of the day Avoid strenuous exercise within 6 hours of bed Keep bedroom dark, cool, and quiet
Stimulus control	Based on operant and classical conditioning principles: non-sleep activities in the bedroom environment can serve as stimuli that interfere with sleep Treatment prescribes behaviors that strengthen associations between the environment and sleep	Go to bed only when sleepy Use the bed and bedroom for sleep and sexual activity only Avoid reading, watching TV, talking on the phone, or worry in the bedroom If unable to fall asleep within 15–20 minutes, leave the bed and bedroom Return to bed only when feeling sleepy again Set the alarm to wake up at a regular time each day Do not use the snooze button on the alarm If nap during the day, nap in bed
Sleep restriction therapy	Based on experimental evidence that sleep is regulated by circadian and homeostatic processes Treatment increased homeostatic sleep drive by reducing time in bed and maintaining a consistent wake time in the morning to reinforce circadian rhythms	Restrict time awake in bed by setting strict bedtime and rising schedules limited to the average number of hours of actual sleep reported in one night Keep a fixed wake-up time, regardless of actual sleep durations If after 10 days sleep efficiency is lower than 85%, further restrict bedtime by 15–30 minutes Increase time in bed by advancing bedtime by 15–30 minutes when the time spent asleep is >85% of time in bed
Relaxation training	Muscular tension and cognitive arousal prevent efficient sleep onset Relaxation decreases waking arousal and facilitates sleep onset and sleep maintenance	Specific techniques may include progressive muscle relaxation, guided imagery, paced breathing
Cognitive therapy	Identify, challenge, and replace dysfunctional thoughts and beliefs about sleep and insomnia These thoughts increase arousal and tension, which impede sleep onset and further reinforce the dysfunctional beliefs	Counseling to challenge unhelpful beliefs and fears about sleep such as: inaccurate expectations of required sleep duration, belief that sleep is not modifiable, fear that poor sleep will result in catastrophic Use of thought journaling to reduce rumination
Cognitive behavioral therapy for insomnia	Multimodal treatment combining elements of previously described techniques	Sleep hygiene education, stimulus control, sleep restriction, cognitive therapy, may include relaxation training
Brief behavioral treatment of insomnia	Core techniques from stimulus control, sleep restriction therapies	Limit time in bed to actual sleep time plus 30 minutes Establish regular wake time every day, regardless of prior night's sleep duration Do not go to bed until sleepy Do not stay in bed if awake

superior to those of hypnotic medications[29] and are maintained for up to 3 years of follow-up. Initial combination therapy (CBTi + pharmacotherapy) may be indicated for individuals with severe insomnia and/or multiple non-modifiable precipitating factors.[28] Individuals with complex serious illnesses may be best served with combination therapy. It is important for the nurse to include the patient and family in the plan of care for insomnia as several of the suggested behavioral therapies can be more successful with family support.

While CBTi is the first-line, gold-standard therapy for insomnia, it must be noted that CBTi is delivered by a highly trained therapist over a period of multiple weeks. The lack of availability and accessibility of these therapists is an ongoing issue across the nation. In response, brief behavioral therapies for insomnia have been developed and are being effectively delivered by nurses in clinic settings.[30,31] Additionally, evidence-based online applications are available for free to the general public (e.g., insomnia coach—https://mobile.va.gov/app/insomnia-coach) and provide accessible sleep hygiene information and a functional sleep diary that can be downloaded and shared with healthcare providers.

Pharmacological Interventions

There are several pharmacological options available for use in patients with insomnia. The pharmacological agents currently approved by the US Food and Drug Administration (FDA) are primarily classified as benzodiazepine sedatives, nonbenzodiazepine sedatives, melatonin receptor agonists, antidepressants, and orexin receptor antagonists. See Table 26.3 for a summary of pharmacologic therapies. The American Academy of Sleep Medicine has published clinical practice guidelines for pharmacological treatment of chronic insomnia.[10]

Caution should be taken when using pharmacological agents. For example, medication interactions, risk for falls, cognitive impairments, dependence, and adverse reactions should be thoroughly reviewed. Sedating medications should be carefully considered for each person based on indication for use, plan of care, and safety.

Table 26.3 Pharmacological interventions for insomnia

Medication by class	Common medication	Common doses	Onset/duration	Recommended use
Orexin receptor antagonist	Lemborexant	5, 10 mg	Slow/long	Sleep maintenance
	Suvorexant	10, 15, 20 mg	Slow/long	Sleep maintenance
Nonbenzodiazepine receptor agonists	Eszopiclone	1, 2, 3 mg	Rapid/intermediate	Sleep onset and sleep maintenance
	Zaleplon	5, 10 mg	Rapid/ultra-short	Sleep onset
	Zolpidem immediate-release sublingual tablet	1.75, 3.5 mg	Rapid/ultra-short	Nighttime awakening
	Zolpidem sublingual tablet	5, 10 mg	Rapid/short	Seep onset and sleep maintenance
	Zolpidem immediate-release oral tablet	5, 10 mg	Rapid/short	Seep onset and sleep maintenance
	Zolpidem controlled-release tablet	6.25, 12.5 mg	Rapid/short	Sleep onset and sleep maintenance
Benzodiazepines	Triazolam	0.125, 0.25 mg	Rapid/short	Sleep onset
	Temazepam	7.5, 15, 22.5, 30 mg	Slow/intermediate	Sleep onset and maintenance
Melatonin agonists	Ramelteon	8 mg	Rapid/short	Sleep onset
Tricyclic antidepressants	Doxepin	3, 6 mg	Slow/long	Sleep maintenance

Source: Adapted from Reference 10.

Over-the-Counter Preparations

Nurses need to stay informed about the over-the-counter remedies that their patients may use to treat their insomnia. Individuals with serious illness who are also experiencing insomnia are often quite distressed and will "try anything" to find relief. Several formulations are marked as sleep aids and are widely available over-the-counter in retail stores and online. However, the benefits of these formulations are often outweighed by the risks and/or negative side effects observed. For example, antihistamines such as diphenhydramine are added to "sleep medicines" for their sedative properties as well as for their anticholinergic properties. There is little to no evidence to support greater than a placebo effect on sleep onset over time. Additionally, the potential for negative effects observed in older persons' cognitive functioning and next-day drowsiness increases the risk profile of this common medication. In addition, several herbal supplements are currently marketed as having properties that will reduce insomnia symptoms (e.g., chamomile, lavender, St. John's wort, valerian, and melatonin). The studies evaluating the benefits of herbal therapies for managing insomnia have produced inconclusive or contradictory results. Although widely used in the general public, herbal supplements do not undergo rigorous regulation or clinical trials to determine efficacy and side effects and thus are not recommended by the FDA.

Returning to the case study, Mr. M's B_{12} and magnesium levels were tested and found to be slightly below normal; a supplement was prescribed. The nurse encouraged them to set a consistent evening routine that included moving night meds to the dinner hour and reducing fluid intake after dinner. Ms. M. was encouraged to speak with her minister regarding her fears. The nurse provided Ms. and Mr. M with a sleep diary to complete over the next 2 weeks and to return to a tele-med visit to discuss patterns that emerge.

During the tele-med visit 2 weeks later, both Ms. and Mr. M's sleep patterns had begun to improve. The sleep diary helped them to visualize the impact that their evening routine was having on their sleep quality. By changing the medication time and fluid intake along with the addition of sleep-promoting behaviors (sleep hygiene), both Mr. and Ms. M. are seeing improvements in their sleep, reduced daytime fatigue, and improved mood. They both verbalized that they will still have times when their sleep is disrupted, but now they know it is normal, not catastrophic. The nurse was instrumental in helping Mr. and Ms. M to learn about how sleep was impacting other areas of their life and to see that making small changes to their routine could positively impact their overall sleep–wake patterns.

Conclusion

In persons with serious illness, insomnia is one of the most common and distressing symptoms reported. Physical, emotional, and environmental factors serve to precipitate and perpetuate insomnia symptoms and increase the risk for acute insomnia to become chronic. A thorough assessment of these factors and the comorbid medical and psychiatric symptoms will help the nurse to identify effective treatment modalities. Nurses in palliative care are key investigators in helping analyze the causes of insomnia and providing interventions to assist in improving sleep.

The case study explored in this chapter illustrated the complex and multifactorial contributors to insomnia and the impact that it can have on both the patient and family. Interventions are focused on the precipitating and/or perpetuating factors that the nurse identifies through conversations and assessments with the patient and family. Insomnia is not an objective condition but instead is a deeply personal experience. The nurse must help the patient to create a plan to address the modifiable factors and to cognitively reframe the nonmodifiable ones. The goal for treatment of insomnia in persons with serious illness is to help them to have the best sleep possible within the context of the physical challenges they are experiencing.

Fortunately, evidence supports the effectiveness of nurses for providing brief behavioral sleep interventions for persons with serious illness. Therefore, nurses must integrate sleep education within the plan of care to promote healthy sleep patterns and advocate for appropriate multidisciplinary referrals.

REFERENCES

1. Perlis ML, Vargas I, Ellis JG, et al. The natural history of insomnia: the incidence of acute insomnia and subsequent progression to chronic insomnia or recovery in good sleeper subjects. *Sleep*. 2020;43(6):zsz299. https://doi.org/10.1093/sleep/zsz299.
2. Dopheide JA. Insomnia overview: epidemiology, pathophysiology, diagnosis and monitoring, and nonpharmacologic therapy. *Am J Manag Care*. 2020;26(4 suppl):S76–S84. https://doi.org/10.37765/ajmc.2020.42769.
3. Bayon V, Leger D, Gomez-Merino D, Vecchierini MF, Chennaoui M. Sleep debt and obesity. *Ann Med*. 2014;46(5):264–272. https://doi.org/10.3109/07853890.2014.931103.
4. Khurshid KA. Comorbid insomnia and psychiatric disorders: an update. *Innov Clin Neurosci*. 2018;15(3–4):28–32.
5. Ge L, Guyatt G, Tian J, et al. Insomnia and risk of mortality from all-cause, cardiovascular disease, and cancer: systematic review and meta-analysis of prospective cohort studies. *Sleep Med Rev*. 2019;48:101215. https://doi.org/10.1016/j.smrv.2019.101215.
6. Sadeghmousavi S, Eskian M, Rahmani F, Rezaei N. The effect of insomnia on development of Alzheimer's disease. *J Neuroinflammation*. 2020;17(1):289. https://doi.org/10.1186/s12974-020-01960-9.
7. Thorpy MJ. Classification of sleep disorders. *Neurotherapeutics*. 2012;9(4):687–701. https://doi.org/10.1007/s13311-012-0145-6.
8. Paul S, Vidusha K, Thilagar S, Lakshmanan DK, Ravichandran G, Arunachalam A. Advancement in the contemporary clinical diagnosis and treatment strategies of insomnia disorder. *Sleep Med*. 2022;91:124–140. https://doi.org/10.1016/j.sleep.2022.02.018.
9. Sateia MJ. International Classification of Sleep Disorders-third edition: highlights and modifications. *Chest*. 2014;146(5):1387–1394. https://doi.org/10.1378/chest.14-0970.
10. Sateia MJ, Buysse DJ, Krystal AD, Neubauer DN, Heald JL. Clinical practice guideline for the pharmacologic treatment of chronic insomnia in adults: an American Academy of Sleep Medicine Clinical Practice Guideline. *J Clin Sleep Med*. 2017;13(2):307–349. https://doi.org/10.5664/jcsm.6470.
11. Macedo PJOM, Oliveria RS, Foldvary-Schaefer N, Gomes M. Insomnia in people with epilepsy: a review of insomnia prevalence, risk factors and associations with epilepsy-related factors. *Epilepsy Res*. 2017;135:158–167.
12. Kwak A, Jacobs J, Haggett D, Jimenez R, Peppercorn J. Evaluation and management of insomnia in women with breast cancer. *Breast Cancer Res Treat*. 2020;181(2):269–277. https://doi.org/10.1007/s10549-020-05635-0.
13. Gharzeddine R, McCarthy MM, Yu G, Dickson VV. Insomnia and insomnia symptoms in persons with heart failure: an integrative review. *J Cardiovasc Nurs*. 2021;36(4):374–384. https://doi.org/10.1097/JCN.0000000000000719.
14. Patel D, Steinberg J, Patel P. Insomnia in the elderly: a review. *J Clin Sleep Med*. 2018;14(6):1017–1024. https://doi.org/10.5664/jcsm.7172.
15. Zhou ES, Partridge AH, Syrjala KL, Michaud AL, Recklitis CJ. Evaluation and treatment of insomnia in adult cancer survivorship programs. *J Cancer Surviv*. 2017;11(1):74–79. https://doi.org/10.1007/s11764-016-0564-1.
16. Berry RB, Budhiraja R, Gottlieb DJ, et al. Rules for scoring respiratory events in sleep: update of the 2007 AASM Manual for the Scoring of Sleep and Associated Events. Deliberations of the Sleep Apnea Definitions Task Force of the American Academy of Sleep Medicine. *J Clin Sleep Med*. 2012;8(5):597–619. https://doi.org/10.5664/jcsm.2172.
17. Spielman AJ, Caruso LS, Glovinsky PB. A behavioral perspective on insomnia treatment. *Psychiatr Clin North Am*. 1987;10(4):541–553.
18. Bethea TN, Zhou ES, Schernhammer ES, Castro-Webb N, Cozier YC, Rosenberg L. Perceived racial discrimination and risk of insomnia among middle-aged and elderly Black women. *Sleep*. 2020;43(1):zsz208. https://doi.org/10.1093/sleep/zsz208.
19. Rash JA, Kavanagh VAJ, Garland SN. A meta-analysis of mindfulness-based therapies for insomnia and sleep disturbance: moving towards processes of change. *Sleep Med Clin*. 2019;14(2):209–233. https://doi.org/10.1016/j.jsmc.2019.01.004.
20. Evandt J, Oftedal B, Hjertager Krog N, Nafstad P, Schwarze PE, Marit Aasvang G. A population-based study on nighttime road traffic noise and insomnia. *Sleep*. 2017;40(2):zsw055. https://doi.org/10.1093/sleep/zsw055.
21. Garland SN, Barg FK, Cakouros B, Gehrman P, DuHamel KN, Mao JJ. A qualitative examination of the factors related to the development and maintenance of insomnia in cancer survivors. *Palliat Support Care*. 2019;17(2):221–226. https://doi.org/10.1017/S1478951518000135.
22. Ellis JG, Perlis ML, Espie CA, et al. The natural history of insomnia: predisposing, precipitating, coping, and perpetuating factors over the early developmental course of insomnia. *Sleep*. 2021;44(9):zsab095. https://doi.org/10.1093/sleep/zsab095.
23. Bjorvatn B, Jernelöv S, Pallesen S. Insomnia—a heterogenic disorder often comorbid with psychological and somatic disorders and diseases: a narrative review with focus on diagnostic and treatment challenges. *Front Psychol*. 2021;12:639198. https://doi.org/10.3389/fpsyg.2021.639198.
24. Carney CE, Buysse DJ, Ancoli-Israel S, et al. The consensus sleep diary: standardizing prospective sleep self-monitoring. *Sleep*. 2012;35(2):287–302. https://doi.org/10.5665/sleep.1642.
25. Walker JL, Vargas I, Drake CL, Ellis JG, Muench A, Perlis ML. The natural history of insomnia: high sleep reactivity interacts with greater life stress to predict the onset of acute insomnia. *Sleep*. 2022;45(9):zsac149. https://doi.org/10.1093/sleep/zsac149.
26. Sutton EL. Insomnia. *Ann Intern Med*. 2021;174(3):ITC33–ITC48. https://doi.org/10.7326/AITC202103160.
27. Buysse DJ. Insomnia. *JAMA*. 2013;309(7):706–716.
28. Feng G, Han M, Li X, Geng L, Miao Y. The clinical effectiveness of cognitive behavioral therapy for patients with insomnia and depression: a systematic review and meta-analysis. *Evid Based Complement Alternat Med*. 2020;2020:8071821. https://doi.org/10.1155/2020/8071821.
29. Mitchell MD, Gehrman P, Perlis M, Umscheid CA. Comparative effectiveness of cognitive behavioral therapy for insomnia: a systematic review. *BMC Fam Pract*. 2012;13:40. https://doi.org/10.1186/1471-2296-13-40.
30. Troxel WM, Germain A, Buysse DJ. Clinical management of insomnia with brief behavioral treatment (BBTI). *Behav Sleep Med*. 2012;10(4):266–279. https://doi.org/10.1080/15402002.2011.607200.
31. Bramoweth AD, Lederer LG, Youk AO, Germain A, Chinman MJ. Brief behavioral treatment for insomnia vs. cognitive behavioral therapy for insomnia: results of a randomized noninferiority clinical trial among veterans. *Behav Ther*. 2020;51(4):535–547. https://doi.org/10.1016/j.beth.2020.02.002.

27

Complementary and Integrative Therapies in Palliative Care

Mary-Anne Meyer and Melinda Ring

Key Points

- Patients with chronic illness frequently use integrative medicine to help address symptoms and improve quality of life.
- Evidence of efficacy of specific therapies for common concerns such chronic pain, mood issues, and gastrointestinal symptoms is growing.
- The nursing profession plays a critical role in guiding patients and families in the safe and appropriate use of integrative medicine for palliative care.

Integrative Medicine and Palliative Care: The Critical Role of Nurses

Integrative medicine aims to provide whole-person care with a focus on healing and health rather than curing and disease, and thus it is inherently aligned with palliative care. Incorporating the broader toolbox of therapeutic practices, a social-spiritual emphasis, and a compassionate partnership between provider and patient (and family/support persons) can be of benefit at any time from diagnosis to end-of-life care. Earlier adoption is encouraged to allow for greater potential benefits. For many patients and families, beyond the actual relief of symptoms and management or reversal of disease processes, active engagement in an integrative approach provides a sense of empowerment over their disease; this paradigm shift can be healing in and of itself. Nurses on the front-line of caring for patients with chronic debilitating symptoms and end-of life care are ideally positioned to help patients understand their options and facilitate access to safe and appropriate resources. The nursing profession additionally has deep roots in the philosophical approach to holistic, relationship-centered healing. This chapter serves as an introduction to frequently encountered terminology, complementary and integrative medicine (CIM) practices, and current evidence for common concerns addressed via an integrative palliative care approach.

Current Prevalence of Complementary and Integrative Therapies in Palliative Care

In the United States, approximately 38% of adults (about 4 in 10) and approximately 12% of children (about 1 in 9) are using some form of CIM.[1] Previous studies have shown that individuals opt to use CIM to improve health and well-being, to relieve symptoms associated with chronic diseases, or to manage side effects of conventional medicine.[2] Palliation of chronic pain and management of symptoms and side effects related to oncology care are among the top conditions for which patients report using CIM.[3, 4]

In response to growing awareness in the medical community, integrative medicine services are increasingly available in academic and community health centers. The Academic Consortium for Integrative Medicine and Health membership increased from 9 North American academic institutions in 1999 to 69 in 2017.[5] The US military health system has been an early adopter of the use of integrative strategies for their stakeholders, especially in relation to its benefits for managing pain. In 2010, the Department of the Army Pain Management Task Force published its report with the recommendation for a comprehensive pain management strategy focused on an interdisciplinary, holistic, multimodal, patient-centered approach.[6] A survey of 14 Department of Defense medical treatment facilities found that 100% of the 14 facilities offered IM services, with 92% offering six or more modalities.[7] The research literature also documents a growing number of integrative oncology programs; at least 29 dedicated CIM oncology programs were noted, with many more integrative centers offering care to cancer populations.[8]

Hospice programs have also incorporated CIM options, with prevalence increasing over recent decades. In surveys from the early 2000s, 60–70% of responding hospice organizations offered CIM therapies.[9, 10] The most common services were massage therapy (83%), music therapy (50%), therapeutic touch (49%), pet therapy (48%), guided imagery (45%), Reiki (36%), aromatherapy (30%), harp music (23%), reflexology (20%), art therapy (20%), hypnotherapy (4%), yoga (3%), acupuncture (1%), and humor therapy (1%).[9] A recent survey of 108 Illinois-based organizations listed on the National Hospice and Palliative Care Organization website found that 90.3% of the responding organizations offered some type of CIM.[11] The top five most frequently offered options in this report were pet therapy (64.5%), music therapy (61.3%), massage therapy (54.8%), art therapy (29.0%), and energy therapies (25.8%). However, even in hospices and palliative care programs that offer these services, they are accessed by less than 25% of eligible patients.[10] Profit orientation and the number of patients served by hospices have been identified as significantly related to the probability that hospices will offer CIM.[12] Not-for-profit hospices were approximately four times more likely to offer CIM than for-profit hospices, and for every 100 patients served by the hospices, the odds of offering CIM increased by 13%. Constraints to providing and use of these services include lack of funding, lack of staff time, lack of qualified therapists, inadequate knowledge about these services, and patient and staff resistance to the services.[9] Preliminary research outcome data on CIM programs have been favorable, and Demmer and Sauer found that patients who received complementary therapies were more satisfied with their hospice services.[13, 14]

Patients may seek integrative medicine on their own or be referred by members of their healthcare team. A National Institute of Health (NIH)-funded study found that referrals to integrative medicine inpatient services at a tertiary hospital were often driven by nurses and mid-level providers.[15] In this survey, physicians and administrators indicated that nurses were better able to assess a need for CIM services, initiate discussions about them, and consequently recommend them to patients. In contrast, a survey about physician attitudes toward and knowledge about CIM reported that 76% had never referred a patient to a CIM practitioner, although 44% stated that they would refer a patient if a practitioner were available at their institution.[16] An online survey of professional members of the German Society for Palliative Care confirmed the stronger interest among nurses: among the 365 respondents (9.8% of all members), 85% of the physicians and 99% of the nurses claimed to be interested in CIM.[17] Combined, these findings highlight the important role of nurses in guiding patients to ensure safe and appropriate utilization of CIM services and therefore educating themselves on potential benefits versus risks for commonly seen conditions. The remainder of this article aims to provide an introduction for nurses to integrative health, with resources for additional learning and reference.

Terminology

It is helpful to have shared definitions when describing holistic system approaches to healthcare and the individual healing traditions and practices. The following basic terms are recommended by the National Institute for Health's National Center for Complementary and Integrative Health (NCCIH)[18]:

Complementary health approaches: Practices and products of non-mainstream origin

Integrative health: Incorporating complementary approaches into mainstream health care

A broader definition of integrative medicine as promoted by the Osher Collaborative, an international group of six academic centers funded by the Bernard Osher Foundation to study, teach, and practice integrative medicine follows.[19]

Integrative medicine:

Reaffirms the importance of the relationship between practitioner and patient, focuses on the whole person, is informed by evidence, and makes use of appropriate therapeutic approaches, healthcare professionals, and professions to achieve optimal health and healing.

Applies rigorous scientific research methods to evaluate physiological and therapeutic mechanisms, efficacy, and use of approaches in society as they affect health, resiliency, and well-being.

Educates practitioners, public, and policy to appreciate and address the full range of physical, emotional, mental, social, spiritual, and environmental influences that affect health.

Other descriptors of approaches to patient care that overlap with integrative medicine:

Alternative medicine refers to the much less common occurrence of a non-mainstream practice being used in place of conventional medicine.

Functional medicine, according to the Institute for Functional Medicine, determines how and why illness occurs and restores health by addressing the root causes of disease for each individual. It requires a "detailed understanding of each patient's genetic, biochemical, and lifestyle factors and leverages that data to direct personalized treatment plans that lead to improved patient outcomes."[20]

Holistic medicine, according to the American Holistic Health Association "is the art and science of healing that addresses the whole person—body, mind, and spirit. The practice of holistic medicine integrates conventional and alternative therapies to prevent and treat disease, and most importantly, to promote optimal health."[21]

Lifestyle medicine, per the American College of Lifestyle Medicine, "involves the use of evidence-based lifestyle therapeutic approaches, such as a predominantly whole food, plant-based diet, exercise, sleep, stress management, alcohol moderation and tobacco cessation, and other non-drug modalities, to prevent, treat, and, oftentimes, reverse the lifestyle-related, chronic disease that's all too prevalent."[22]

Complementary Health Approaches

There is overlap in the practice and proposed mechanism of different complementary health approaches; therefore, the NCCIH currently suggests considering them within two major subgroups: natural products or mind-body practices.[18]

Natural products include a diverse group of substances that includes vitamins, minerals, and probiotics, as well as compounds from diverse sources. Many natural products are produced from marine organisms, bacteria, fungi, and plants, herbs and botanicals.[23] Natural products can include complex extracts from whole plants or isolated compounds. In traditional herbalism, whole-plant extracts are often used due to purported positive synergistic interactions, while a more Westernized approach seeks to isolate the active compound.[24, 25] According to the 2012 National Health Interview Survey (NHIS), 17.7% of American adults had used a dietary supplement (not including vitamins and minerals) in the past year, making them the most popular form of complementary approaches in the survey.[2]

Mind-body practices include a large set of techniques ranging from meditation, yoga, and tai chi to acupuncture, massage, and chiropractic manipulation. These practices are often taught or provided by a trained teacher or practitioner, though self-use is also common.

A third category of *whole healing traditions* incorporates many aspects of both natural products and mind-body approaches. Examples of these include Ayurvedic medicine (the traditional medicine of India), traditional Chinese medicine, naturopathy, and traditional healers.

Applications in Palliative Care

Conventional medicine excels at treating emergency situations, acute conditions such as infection, and problems requiring a surgical intervention. However, many chronic conditions are not fully amenable to treatment with conventional medicine approaches, or the side effects and risks significantly impair a patient's quality of life (QOL). In these cases, an integrative strategy can often provide important relief. Here, we focus on three categories of frequently encountered issues with examples of current research behind potential therapeutic options: (1) chronic pain, (2) fatigue and mood disorders, and (3) gastrointestinal conditions.

Case Study: Integrative Medicine

Aurelia was a 55-year-old woman with a recent diagnosis of Stage 1B hormone-receptor-positive breast cancer who presented with insomnia, fatigue, and joint stiffness. She was diagnosed after an abnormal finding on her routine mammogram and subsequently underwent a lumpectomy with axillary node dissection, chemotherapy, and radiation therapy. She was started on the aromatase inhibitor letrozole 1 month ago. Prior to being diagnosed, her health history was unremarkable other than being overweight (body mass index 29). She had significant personal stressors in her life including the death of her father during cancer treatment and the end of her marriage of 20 years last year. She reported trouble both falling asleep and staying asleep. She was prescribed many medications but preferred to take nonpharmaceuticals. She presented to the integrative medicine team for "holistic treatment."

Integrative Medicine Plan and Response

The initial integrative medicine consult consisted of an in-depth discussion of Aurelia's view of her illness, goals for her health, and understanding of her current social, spiritual, emotional, and environmental aspects of well-being.

Psycho-social-spiritual: In discussion, it became clear that, in many ways, Aurelia had been compartmentalizing her feelings in order to focus on the demands of her healthcare during treatment. She noted a feeling of tightness or heaviness in her chest that she associates with her emotional and physical fatigue. She noted never having time to grieve the loss of her father due to her own illness, and additionally didn't fully process the grief of the loss of her marriage, and now the loss of her health as the one thing she saw as intact in her life. Her cardiac evaluation was normal, and she did work with a therapist in cognitive behavioral therapy (CBT) weekly for the past year.

Recommendation: The grief and emotional stressors were not the sole cause of fatigue, but could be significant contributors. Aurelia found CBT helpful as a support but didn't feel like it helped her fully process her emotions. Energy therapy with Reiki was suggested, with a discussion about how traumas sometimes benefit from a therapy that works at a different level and can help move "stuck" emotions and support healing. She was additionally taught a brief Loving Kindness Meditation (LKM), to send loving emotions to herself and to troubling situations. Aurelia had been exploring essential oils and chakra/energy readings, so this approach was very appealing to her. She saw an experienced Reiki practitioner at the Osher Center weekly for 8 weeks and did the LKM meditation twice daily. At her follow-up visit she noted that, in her first few treatments, she had deep releases where she was sobbing on the massage table. She said after this early session that she felt a bit drained, but also cleansed. At the end of 2 months, she noted no longer feeling any chest tightness; she felt lighter, and while she still struggled with feelings of loss they were more manageable. Her sleep was improved and more restorative. She planned to continue Reiki sessions monthly, continue the meditation practice, and still see her therapist twice monthly as she created her vision for what came next.

Musculoskeletal: The joint aching was clearly associated temporally with starting the aromatase inhibitor. She noted this was a barrier to her being physically active, as she knew the importance of both physical activity and weight management for reducing the risk of breast cancer recurrence. She was considering stopping the medication unless the symptoms could be controlled.

Recommendation: The data on acupuncture for her situation were reviewed with Aurelia. She had received acupuncture during her chemotherapy sessions in the infusion suites by Osher center acupuncturists, and she felt they helped minimize her symptoms. Given her positive experience, she was interested in exploring this option. She began acupuncture sessions in the Osher Center, and was also given Traditional Chinese Medicine (TCM) herbs based on her TCM diagnosis. At the 2-month follow-up she noted some improvement in the symptoms starting at the fourth session. Given the positive trend, she planned to continue to see if she could have complete resolution.

Prevention: Aurelia had already received basic nutrition and physical activity counseling through the Cancer Survivorship program. She was making positive changes but sought additional counseling and wondered if she should be taking any dietary supplements. A full dietary and physical activity history was taken, and while she had been making some positive changes, her prior diet was low in vegetables, fruits, and fibers and had daily added sugars and refined carbohydrates. Lab tests revealed vitamin D deficiency and low essential fatty acids. Vitamin D supplements and fish oil were recommended, along with a shift toward a whole-food plant-based diet. Given her prior sedentary lifestyle and joint discomfort, she started an exercise regimen that included longer daily walks at a higher intensity and twice-weekly restorative yoga classes. At 2-month follow-up she had lost 5 pounds and was ready to increase her program, so 30 minutes of high-intensity interval training was added twice a week.

Chronic Pain

Pain is a complex phenomenon involving physical, emotional, social, and spiritual aspects that all must be addressed. Depression, anxiety, and spiritual distress can all increase the perception of pain intensity, and addressing these components can reduce the need for pain medication.[26]

A comprehensive review of all effective integrative and complementary therapies for these concerns is impossible given the enormous diversity in this area. This chapter will share some of the most current data on mind-body approaches (e.g., movement, relaxation therapies, music, aromatherapy, massage, and acupuncture), and then review common dietary supplements for symptom management in serious illness or at end of life. Many modalities are quite effective for a number of symptoms in palliative care and have been studied in different populations.

Mind-Body Approaches for Pain

Physical Activity

Patients with cancer are often discouraged from engaging in exercise during cancer treatment, but the positive effects of continuing exercise on QOL, weakness, fatigue, and mood are documented in a number of studies.[27] A 10-year longitudinal study of post-treatment breast cancer patients showed that pain was significantly reduced in patients who maintained regular physical activity and an ideal body weight, as opposed to those women who had a weight gain of more than 5%, who were obese or overweight, and had a sedentary lifestyle.[26]

Massage Therapy

Massage therapy encompasses many different styles, but in patients with advanced chronic illness, gentler forms such as Swedish massage may be better tolerated. In a meta-analysis of studies involving massage for adult oncological patients receiving palliative care, 4 of 6 studies showed a statistically significant reduction in pain.[28] Other studies looking at the lasting benefits of massage on pain were less favorable, showing that the immediate benefits of massage seem to be higher than the longer term effects. Qualitative data from studies have also shown that interventions such as massage therapy seem to be effective if the patient is treated with empathy and if a relationship between the massage therapist and the patient had been formed beforehand.[29]

Aromatherapy

Aromatherapy—the therapeutic use of essential oils—is an increasingly popular option for use by nurses in inpatient and palliative care settings. The aromatic organic compounds are typically applied in one of three ways: (1) inhalation; (2) topically during baths, massage, or on a compress; or (3) through oral ingestion. A 2016 meta-analysis of 12 studies examined the use of aromatherapy for pain management.[30] It concluded that there was a significant positive effect of aromatherapy compared to controls (placebo or treatments as usual) in reducing pain reported on a visual analog scale, with stronger correlations found in nociceptive and acute pain versus inflammatory and chronic pain. Lavender was the most commonly studied essential oil, with others being orange, eucalyptus, clary sage, chamomile, rose, ginger, rosemary, peppermint, and lemongrass. Applications included hand massage, localized massage, acupressure, sitz baths, and vaporized, and the populations included children, pregnant women, and patients with chronic pain or in hospice. Many patients and healthcare providers are attracted to aromatherapy because of its low cost and minimal side effects.[31]

Acupuncture

Acupuncture involves the insertion of fine sterile disposable needles into specific body points along energy pathways known as *meridians* to address imbalances and thereby alleviate symptoms and prevent or treat disease. Traditional Chinese acupuncture is based on the health concept of Qi ("chee") or vital life force energy. Many studies and systematic reviews have been done but are generally not considered to be of sufficient quality to reach conclusions. However, a 2012 analysis of acupuncture for pain showed improved pain relief in patients who received acupuncture for back or neck pain, osteoarthritis, or chronic headache.[32] A 2016 meta-analysis of 20 randomized clinical trials (n = 892) reported that acupuncture alone was not superior to pharmacotherapy for cancer-related pain; but, of significance is that combination therapy may be more effective, resulting in quicker pain relief, longer pain remission, and improved QOL.[33] At the Sao Paulo Cancer Institute, 183 patients were enrolled in an acupuncture study that showed significant reductions in cancer pain, chemotoxicity, lumbar pain, and chronic postoperative pain.[34] Individual studies on acupuncture or electro-acupuncture for aromatase inhibitor-related arthralgias suggest reduced pain and stiffness in treatment groups versus placebo or sham acupuncture, though these results did not achieve significance in a meta-analysis.[35] In 2016, the National Cancer Institute held a symposium on Acupuncture for Symptom Management in Oncology with a call to action for additional research.[36]

Music/Music Therapy

Simple music that is relaxing can be provided by anyone—typically healthcare staff—in what has been termed "music medicine." In contrast, in "music therapy" patients work with a trained music therapist in a therapeutic relationship where music (prerecorded, live, and/or interactive) is individualized based on a professional assessment.[37] The interventions in this review are generally classified as either *music medicine* or *music therapy*. In music medicine interventions, patients listen to prerecorded music that is administered by healthcare staff and preselected by study investigators, who may or may not have any formal training in music therapy.[7,8] Because there are a wide variety of modalities of music therapy, it has been difficult to perform reviews that give strong recommendations. Music can raise endorphin levels in the brain and lower adrenaline levels.[38] Music therapy has been studied in intensive care unit settings: Zimbardo and Gerrig found that 30 minutes of classical music therapy equaled the relaxation effects of 10 mg of diazepam.[39] Two recent studies in inpatient palliative care units suggest music therapy in this setting is feasible, well-received, and associated with promotion of relaxation and well-being.[40,41]

Mindfulness

Mindfulness-based stress reduction (MBSR) is an 8-week program of teaching moment-to-moment awareness of mind-body interactions through practices such as meditation, Hatha yoga, breath awareness, and body scan meditation. A meta-analysis review of studies using MBSR was significantly correlated with reductions in the anxiety, chronic pain, stress, and depression often found in patients at the end of life.[42]

Guided Imagery

Guided imagery has been shown to reduce anxiety, pain, and stress and to promote relaxation in some small trials.[43] Through guided imagery techniques, patients can learn to control functions normally controlled by the autonomic nervous system such as heart rate, blood pressure, respiratory rate, and body temperature. Through guided imagery, the patient can create an image of pain and then transform it into something less powerful and frightening.

Natural Products for Pain

Polypharmacy with nutritional supplements is to be avoided, similar to polypharmacy with medications, as these can increase the burden on the patient and caregiver without significant benefit as well as increase risk of interactions. In most cases of patients imminently dying, almost all nutritional supplements can be discontinued except for those giving specific symptom relief.[44] Supplements and herbs often utilized in pain management include turmeric, capsaicin, arnica, polyunsaturated fatty acids, vitamin D, and medical cannabis.

Curcuma longa (turmeric) has a growing body of evidence for the treatment of pain associated with osteoarthritis. This is likely related to the laboratory evidence showing that curcumin functions as a selective cyclooxygenase-2 (COX-2) inhibitor. A head-to-head clinical trial of curcumin supplementation in comparison with ibuprofen in the treatment of knee osteoarthritis demonstrated a similar treatment effect of each medication, with less gastrointestinal adverse events associated with curcumin.[45]

Capsaicin has been used topically for pain. Numerous studies have shown safety and modest efficacy of low-concentration formulations. A single 60-minute application in patients with neuropathic pain produced effective pain relief for up to 12 weeks. Topical capsaicin acts in the skin to attenuate cutaneous hypersensitivity and reduce pain by a process best described as "defunctionalization" of nociceptor fibers.[46] Over-the-counter (OTC) strength capsaicin (.025% to.075%) has been available for a long time, and studies did not show benefit beyond placebo.[47] More recently an 8% capsaicin patch has been used with more positive results.[48] A single patch applied for 30–90 minutes showed significant relief in the treatment of postherpetic neuralgia. The patch is difficult to tolerate as it causes a severe burning sensation and must be premedicated with topical lidocaine and even oxycodone. Capsaicin has also been studied in other conditions. Although enrolling only small numbers, the work done by Bhaskar and colleagues in cancer-associated neuropathic pain showed that almost 71% of patients in this subgroup had 90% pain relief.[49]

Arnica gel is an OTC product that has promising benefit. In 2013, a Cochrane Database Systematic Review concluded that "arnica gel probably improves symptoms as effectively as a gel containing nonsteroidal anti-inflammatory drug.... Comfrey extract gel probably improves pain, and Capsicum extract gel probably will not improve pain or function at the doses examined in this review. Further high quality, fully powered studies are required to confirm the trends of effectiveness identified in studies so far."[50]

It is thought that *omega-3 fatty acid* supplementation may have an anti-inflammatory effect.[51] Ramsden and colleagues performed a randomized controlled trial (RCT) examining the impact of omega-3 fatty acid supplementation for the treatment of chronic headaches. There was a significant reduction in the measures of headache intensity pain, in addition to increased markers of anti-nociceptive lipid mediators.[52]

There have been significant efforts examining the role of *vitamin D* in pain processing that involve complex pathophysiologic pathways. Earlier studies have demonstrated that high rates of hypovitaminosis D are prevalent in subjects with fibromyalgia and chronic pain. Several review studies have concluded that, although there seems to be a trend toward vitamin D supplementation and decreased pain, there is a need for further RCTs.[53] Considering that much time in hospice and palliative care is spent indoors and away from the best source of vitamin D, the sun, this is a worthy consideration.

Cannabis can potentially help alleviate neuropathic pain. Cannabinoid receptors are located in the central and peripheral nervous system (CB1) and the immune system (CB2). Numerous studies have shown safety and efficacy for central and peripheral neuropathic pain, rheumatoid arthritis, and cancer pain.[54] Studies in chemotherapy-induced peripheral neuropathy have shown that the activation of CB1 and CB2 receptors suppresses the development of vincristine-induced peripheral neuropathy in rats.[55] Nabiximols is an oromucosal spray of a formulated extract of the *Cannabis sativa* plant that contains the principal cannabinoids delta-9-tetrahydrocannabinol (THC) and cannabidiol (CBD) in a 1:1 ratio. It is available in Canada and Europe for treatment of peripheral neuropathy. Studies in the United States were not found to be clinically significant but showed promise, and further study is warranted.[56]

THC has been shown to enhance the analgesic effect of narcotics. Abrams et al. performed a small study that showed significant decreases in overall pain scores after the addition of vaporized cannabis.[57] More study is needed, but this combination may lead to lower doses of opioid treatment with fewer side effects. Cannabis has been shown to be safe (no one has ever died from an overdose) and not likely to cause dependence (thought to be equally addictive as caffeine).[58]

Although CBD and THC are the most popular known cannabinoids, other cannabinoids within the whole plant also have significant therapeutic properties, including cannabigerol (antitumor), cannabichromene (analgesic, anti-inflammatory, and antibiotic), and tetrahydrocannabivarin (although psychoactive, contains antidiabetic and anti-obesity properties). CBD alone (the nonpsychoactive cannabinoid) has been shown to reduce nausea, pain, and inhibit cancer growth on its own. Because CBD can be derived from hemp and not the cannabis plant itself, individuals in states that do not license medical marijuana who wish to try this option may have access to hemp-derived CBD products.[59]

Mood and Sleep

Mind Body Approaches for Mood and Sleep

Physical Activity: Yoga

A meta-analysis of 13 randomized, controlled trials of yoga in cancer survivors documented significant reductions in distress, anxiety, and depression; moderate reductions in fatigue; moderate increases in social and emotional function and QOL; and a small increase in functional well-being.[27]

Aromatherapy

An RCT of 15 days of inhaled lavender essential oil in 60 patients in an intensive care unit showed statistically significant increased quality of sleep and reduced level of anxiety in patients with coronary artery disease based on the Pittsburgh Sleep Quality Index (PSQI) and the Beck Anxiety Inventory (BAI) scale.[60] Another RCT compared a 4-week trial of blended essential oil (*Lavendula angustifolia, Salvia sclarea*, and *Origanum majoranava*) versus lavender essential oil versus acupressure massage versus placebo in 132 career women.[61] All treatment groups showed significant improvements in PSQI and Short Form 36 Health Survey (QOL) ($p < 0.05$), with the greatest benefit in the blended essential oil treatment group.

A meta-analysis of mindfulness-based therapy suggests it is moderately effective for improving anxiety and mood symptoms from pre- to post-treatment in an overall sample totaling 1,140 participants in 39 studies.[62] Importantly, these effects were maintained over follow-up and were found in populations including those with cancer, generalized anxiety, and chronic pain disorders. Mindfulness-based therapies have also been developed to support caregivers of palliative care patients, with promising improvements in mental distress and life satisfaction.[63]

Energy Medicine

Biofield therapies are based on the premise that each person has an endogenous biofield, which affects physiologic processes.[64] Biofield or energy therapies are purported to improve the balance of the biofield through the practitioner's gentle laying on of hands, placement of hands within the biofield, or distance-based healing.

Healing Touch (HT) is a biofield therapy endorsed by the American Holistic Nurses Association and the Canadian Holistic Nurses Association.[65] HT has the most standardized training, with an independent certification after completing five levels of training. A pilot study of HT found it to have positive effects on stress, fatigue, pain, and mood of patients with cancer.[66]

Reiki is a system of natural healing considered an energy medicine practice. Reiki is administered by the gentle laying of hands on top of or above a clothed individual so the Reiki practitioner can act as a conduit for energy to flow to needed areas in the recipient. One small study showed benefit in well-being, relaxation, pain relief, sleep quality, and reduced anxiety.[67] More study is needed as most RCTs have yielded inconclusive results.

Therapeutic Touch is another energy therapy based on the restoration of balance using a technique in which the hands are used to direct energy for healing purposes, usually without any direct physical contact. A Therapeutic Touch Program was introduced to a geriatric palliative care unit with treatments provided by volunteer Therapeutic Touch Practitioners.[68] A retrospective chart review suggests that implementation is feasible and appears to be safe and well-tolerated, with patients achieving a state of relaxation or sleep after treatment.

Acupuncture

Several RCTs and meta-analyses support acupuncture as both a beneficial monotherapy and as adjunct treatment, though others did not find evidence of efficacy.[69] The Canadian Network for Mood and Anxiety Treatments 2016 Clinical Guidelines for the Management of Adults with Major Depressive Disorder (MDD) rate acupuncture as a third-line treatment for patients with MDD.[69] Two systematic reviews and meta-analyses of auricular acupuncture and acupuncture with moxibustion for primary insomnia had positive results; however, the findings are limited by studies of poor methodological quality, insufficient sample size, and possible publication bias.[70, 71]

Hypnosis

Hypnosis creates a state of "focused awareness and attention" during which the patient can be taught to undertake diversional thinking from unpleasant somatic experiences such as pain. One small study showed a select group of patients noted decreased anxiety and increased relaxation as a result of hypnosis.[72]

Natural Products for Mood and Sleep

Supplements and herbs commonly used for mood and sleep include S-adenosyl-L-methionine (SAMe), St. John's Wort, hydroxytryptophan (5HTP), and valerian.

SAMe

SAMe is a chemical found naturally in the body. SAMe is made in the body from methionine, an amino acid found in many proteins. It is known to help many of our cells function normally.[73] A meta-analysis of studies using SAMe in the treatment of depression showed favorable results.[74] SAMe also shows promise as an anti-inflammatory supplement used for pain relief in fibromyalgia.[75]

St. John's Wort

St. John's wort is a herb that is commonly used to treat depression. Many studies show that St. John's wort works as well as traditional antidepressants for the treatment of mild to moderate depression with fewer side effects. However, St. John's wort can react poorly with many medications and other supplements so drug–herb interactions should be checked before using.[76]

5HTP

5HTP is a serotonin precursor used to treat depression, fibromyalgia, migraines, insomnia, and tension headaches. While there is evidence that precursor loading may be of therapeutic value, particularly for the serotonin precursors 5-HTP and tryptophan, more studies of suitable design and size are needed for more conclusive results.[77]

Valerian Root

Valerian root is used primarily for insomnia, dyssomnia, and for anxiety-associated restlessness and sleeping disorders. It has also been used for many other conditions, but studies for these conditions are only preliminary in nature. A meta-analysis of 16 studies suggests that valerian might improve sleep quality without producing side effects.[78]

Melatonin

One well-known supplement used for sleep is melatonin. Orally, melatonin is used for jet lag, insomnia, shift-work disorder, circadian rhythm disorders in the blind, sleep–wake cycle disturbances, and nicotine and benzodiazepine withdrawal. Additionally, there are many studies using melatonin in combination with chemotherapeutic agents to promote cancer regression.[79]

Gastrointestinal Symptoms

Mind-Body Approaches for Gastrointestinal Symptoms

Acupuncture

The benefit of acupuncture for nausea and vomiting has been generally accepted for many years; the NIH Consensus Statement of 1997 supported acupuncture for adult postoperative and chemotherapy-related nausea and vomiting.[80] One point, the PC6 point (located 2½ to 3 fingerbreadths from the wrist crease up the arm), has the most convincing evidence, leading to FDA-approved wrist devices to provide acupressure at the PC6 point.[81, 82, 83] Acupuncture or acupressure that includes the PC6 point is a reasonable consideration for patients with persistent nausea and vomiting.

Hypnosis

Hypnosis is a psychotherapeutic technique performed by a trained clinician who uses therapeutic suggestions to produce changes in perception, cognition, affect, mood, behavior, and sensation that are mutually acceptable to the patient and provider.[84] Advanced practice nurses can receive training in hypnosis and can explore options through the Society for Clinical and Experimental Hypnosis and the American Society of Clinical Hypnosis. Hypnosis is a safe option for managing anticipatory nausea and vomiting for patients receiving chemotherapy. Patients can also be taught or can use audio versions of scripts for self-treatment.[85]

Progressive Muscle Relaxation and Guided Imagery

Progressive muscle relaxation (PMR) is a technique of alternately tensing and relaxing muscle groups in sequence throughout the body. Patients can do this on their own, but often will use a prerecorded script to guide the process. Guided imagery is often added to PMR to enhance mental visualization. The 2016 updated Multinational Association of Supportive Care in Cancer (MASCC)/ European Society for Medical Oncology (ESMO) consensus recommendations for anticipatory nausea and vomiting in children and adults receiving chemotherapy confirmed their prior recommendation of progressive muscle relaxation training as a valuable therapy.[86]

Natural Products for Gastrointestinal Symptoms

Supplements and herbs specific for gastrointestinal concerns include glutamine, ginger, magnesium, and calendula.

L-Glutamine

L-glutamine is an amino acid found in high levels in the body. Although glutamine is traditionally classified as a nonessential amino acid, it is essential for maintaining intestinal function, especially during times of severe stress. L-glutamine is used for many conditions including diarrhea, HIV wasting, chemotherapy-induced mucositis, and for protection of immune and gut barrier function in people with esophageal cancer undergoing radiochemotherapy. Taking glutamine orally seems to enhance intestinal absorption of nutrients, decrease intestinal permeability, and increase weight gain in people with HIV/AIDS.[87] Research findings in chemotherapy-induced diarrhea have been inconsistent.[88, 89]

Ginger

Ginger (*Zingiber officinale*) is a perennial plant grown in warmer climates. Its tuberous root is the source of the popular spice. Orally, ginger has been used for a host of conditions including motion sickness, diarrhea, dyspepsia, and anorexia, as well as nausea and vomiting. Topically, the fresh juice of ginger is used for treating thermal burns. The essential oil of ginger is used topically as an analgesic. Studies of ginger in treating antiretroviral-induced and chemotherapy-induced nausea and vomiting show promise.[90, 91]

Magnesium

Magnesium is a mineral that is involved in more than 300 biochemical functions in the body. Most magnesium comes from dietary sources. There is some evidence that magnesium supplementation may enhance opioid-induced analgesia without increasing side effects and may also help with constipation.[92]

Calendula

Calendula (*C. officinalis*) is commonly known as pot marigold. Orally, it is used as an antispasmodic, to reduce fever, and for treating inflammation of the oral and pharyngeal mucosa. Clinically, Calendula mouthwash ameliorated the severity of radiotherapy-induced oral mucositis in patients with head and neck cancer.[93] As with most supplements, more study is needed.

Resources

Resources for Natural Products, Evidence, and Safety

It would likely be impossible to have knowledge about all herbs and supplements patients might be using, so it is helpful to have access to resources that could help in the understanding of indications for use, overall and comparative effectiveness, and potential side-effect profiles (Table 27.1).

Resources for Natural Products and Quality

In the United States, herbal medicines and dietary supplements are not subject to strict oversight by the FDA. In response to concerns about supplement quality, several third-party organizations now perform independent quality-control testing of actual products, providing information on whether supplements contain the stated ingredients and are free of contaminants. Consumer Lab, Natural Products Association, NSF International, and United States Pharmacopeia (USP) are several of the most prominent and

Table 27.1 Resources: Natural products, evidence, and safety

Natural Medicines	https://naturalmedicines.therapeuticresearch.com/	Natural Medicines has several helpful point-of-care resources for the clinic setting including "Herb-Supplement Interaction," Medication Effectiveness," "Nutrient Depletion," and "Pregnancy-Lactation Checkers." The Clinical Management Series provides excellent diagnosis-based learning and monograph-based courses provide in-depth overviews of individual herbal medicines. Access to this resource is subscription-based: it is frequently included in hospital and health system libraries.
Memorial Sloan Kettering Cancer Center's About Herbs database	https://www.mskcc.org/cancer-care/diagnosis-treatment/symptom-management/integrative-medicine/herbs	A tool for the public as well as healthcare professionals with information on common herbs and other dietary supplements.

Table 27.2 Resources for deepening knowledge about integrative medicine and integrative nursing

Center for Spirituality & Healing: Integrative Nursing	https://www.csh.umn.edu/education/focus-areas/integrative-nursing	University of Minnesota offers the first Doctor of Nursing Practice (DNP) in Integrative Health and Healing and well as access to continuing education modules.
Center For Spirituality & Healing: Learning Modules	https://www.csh.umn.edu/education/online-modules-and-resources/learning-modules-healthcare-professionals	Online free modules offer an introduction to various topics in the field of complementary therapies. Each of the modules takes from 1 to 3.5 hours to complete and is organized into short sections. All modules feature content written by subject matter experts and reviewed by a faculty team from the schools of Nursing, Pharmacy and Medicine at the University of Minnesota.
American Holistic Nurses Association	http://www.ahna.org/	AHNA advocates for holistic nursing through continuing education, research, practice, networking, and advocacy.
Academy of Integrative Pain Management	https://integrativepainmanagement.site-ym.com/	AIPM mission: "To improve the lives of people with pain by advancing a person-centered, integrative model of pain care through evidence-guided education, credentialing, and advocacy that is now defined as 'best practice' in the National Pain Strategy published by NIH."
Osher Center for Integrative Medicine at Northwestern University	http://www.feinberg.northwestern.edu/sites/ocim/ http://ocim.nm.org/	The authors' location with websites highlighting clinical offerings, and an academic site with content for health professionals.
The Osher Collaborative for Integrative Medicine	https://www.oshercollaborative.org/	The Osher Collaborative for Integrative Medicine comprises an international group of six academic Centers at Harvard University, UCSF, Northwestern University, Vanderbilt University, University of Miami, and Karolinska Institute. The website provides links to resources from the programs.
National Center for Complementary and Integrative Health (NCCIH) is a National Institute of Health initiative	https://nccih.nih.gov/	NCCIH supports research and education in this evolving field. The website contains free online continuing medical education (CME), videocasts of the annual Distinguished Lecture Series, and databases for both clinical guidelines and systematic reviews.
Academic Consortium for Integrative Medicine & Health	https://www.imconsortium.org/	The mission of the Consortium is to advance integrative medicine and health through academic institutions and health systems. Many member institutions have clinical centers and education programs. Listings for members can be found on the site.
Academy of Integrative Health & Medicine	https://www.aihm.org/	An interprofessional association of integrative clinicians who embrace a person-centered, team-based approach to health care. AIHM provides transformational educational programs, connections to a global network, and resources and toolkits for our members.

commonly encountered organizations. Dietary supplements may have seals of approval from these organizations after successful testing. The website ConsumerLab.com is additionally an excellent resource available for a modest annual fee to help learn more about the supplements tested and recommended brands.

Resources for Deepening Knowledge about Integrative Medicine and Integrative Nursing

Learning about integrative nursing and health can be an enriching personal and professional experience. For many providers, it helps them reconnect to the reasons they pursued a career in healthcare in the first place. Learning can range from reading articles or online modules to conferences to degrees. Some examples of engaging courses are listed in Table 27.2.

Conclusion

CIM offers many more tools in the nurse's toolbox to deal with conditions and issues dealt with in palliative care. This chapter has only outlined in broad strokes some of the options available. Clinicians owe it to themselves and their patients to be aware, supportive, and even suggest some alternatives to conventional Western medicine. Embodying the principles of integrative nursing can bring connection and healing to the patient, the family, and, ultimately, to the caregiver.

REFERENCES

1. NCCIH. Statistics on complementary and integrative health approaches. https://nccih.nih.gov/research/statistics. Published December 21, 2011. Accessed January 16, 2018.
2. Clarke TC, Black LI, Stussman BJ, Barnes PM, Nahin RL. Trends in the use of complementary health approaches among adults: United States, 2002–2012. *Natl Health Stat Report*. 2015;(79):1–16.
3. NCCIH. Diseases/conditions for which CAM is most frequently used among adults—for 2007 and 2002. https://nccih.nih.gov/research/statistics/2007/diseases-conditions-for-which-cam-is-frequently-used-among-adults. Published March 22, 2016. Accessed January 16, 2018.
4. Horneber M, Bueschel G, Dennert G, Less D, Ritter E, Zwahlen M. How many cancer patients use complementary and alternative medicine: a systematic review and metaanalysis. *Integr Cancer Ther*. 2012;11(3):187–203.
5. History—Academic Consortium for Integrative Medicine & Health. https://www.imconsortium.org/about/history.cfm. Accessed January 16, 2018.
6. Thomas R. *Pain Management Task Force: Final Report*. Falls Church, VA: DIANE Publishing; 2011.

7. Petri RP Jr, Delgado RE. Integrative medicine experience in the US Department of Defense. *Med Acupunct*. 2015;27(5):328–334.
8. Seely DM, Weeks LC, Young S. A systematic review of integrative oncology programs. *Curr Oncol*. 2012;19(6):e436–e461.
9. Demmer C. A national survey of hospice bereavement services. *OMEGA*. 2003. http://journals.sagepub.com/doi/abs/10.2190/E2DY-42C7-7QP6-7052. Accessed January 16, 2018.
10. Running A, Shreffler-Grant J, Andrews W. A survey of hospices use of complementary therapy. *J Hosp Palliat Nurs*. 2008;10(5):304–312.
11. Van Hyfte GJ, Kozak LE, Lepore M. A survey of the use of complementary and alternative medicine in Illinois hospice and palliative care organizations. *Am J Hosp Palliat Care*. 2014;31(5):553–561.
12. Olotu BS, Brown CM, Barner JC, Lawson KA. Factors associated with hospices' provision of complementary and alternative medicine. *Am J Hosp Palliat Care*. 2014;31(4):385–391.
13. Demmer C, Sauer J. Assessing complementary therapy services in a hospice program. *Am J Hosp Palliat Care*. 2002;19(5):306–314.
14. Marchand L. Integrative and complementary therapies for patients with advanced cancer. *Ann Palliat Med*. 2014;3(3):160–171.
15. Griffin KH, Nate KC, Rivard RL, Christianson JB, Dusek JA. Referrals to integrative medicine in a tertiary hospital: findings from electronic health record data and qualitative interviews. *BMJ Open*. 2016;6(7):e012006.
16. Wahner-Roedler DL, Vincent A, Elkin PL, Loehrer LL, Cha SS, Bauer BA. Physicians' attitudes toward complementary and alternative medicine and their knowledge of specific therapies: a survey at an academic medical center. *Evid Based Complement Alternat Med*. 2006;3(4):495–501.
17. Muecke R, Paul M, Conrad C, et al. Complementary and alternative medicine in palliative care: a comparison of data from surveys among patients and professionals. *Integr Cancer Ther*. 2016;15(1):10–16.
18. Complementary, alternative, or integrative health: what's in a name? NCCIH Web site. https://nccih.nih.gov/health/integrative-health. Published November 11, 2011. Accessed January 16, 2018.
19. What Is Integrative Medicine? Osher Collaborative Web site. https://www.oshercollaborative.org/what-integrative-medicine. Accessed January 17, 2018.
20. Functional Medicine. The Institute for Functional Medicine Web site. https://www.ifm.org/functional-medicine/. Accessed January 17, 2018.
21. Principles of Holistic Medicine. American Holistic Health Association Web site. https://ahha.org/selfhelp-articles/principles-of-holistic-medicine/. Accessed January 17, 2018.
22. What is lifestyle medicine? American College of Lifestyle Medicine Web site. https://www.lifestylemedicine.org/What-is-Lifestyle-Medicine. Accessed January 17, 2018.
23. Natural products research—information for researchers. NCCIH Web site. https://nccih.nih.gov/grants/naturalproducts. Published June 26, 2012. Accessed January 17, 2018.
24. Dias DA, Urban S, Roessner U. A historical overview of natural products in drug discovery. *Metabolites*. 2012;2(2):303–336.
25. Bernardini S, Tiezzi A, Laghezza Masci V, Ovidi E. Natural products for human health: an historical overview of the drug discovery approaches. *Nat Prod Res*. 2017:1–25.
26. Forsythe LP, Alfano CM, George SM, et al. Pain in long-term breast cancer survivors: the role of body mass index, physical activity, and sedentary behavior. *Breast Cancer Res Treat*. 2013;137(2):617–630.
27. Buffart LM, van Uffelen JGZ, Riphagen II, et al. Physical and psychosocial benefits of yoga in cancer patients and survivors: a systematic review and meta-analysis of randomized controlled trials. *BMC Cancer*. 2012;12:559.
28. Falkensteiner M, Mantovan F, Müller I, Them C. The use of massage therapy for reducing pain, anxiety, and depression in oncological palliative care patients: a narrative review of the literature. *ISRN Nurs*. 2011;2011:929868.
29. Crawford C, Boyd C, Paat CF, et al. The impact of massage therapy on function in pain populations—A systematic review and meta-analysis of randomized controlled trials: Part I, Patients experiencing pain in the general population. *Pain Med*. 2016 Aug;17(8):1553–1568.
30. Lakhan SE, Sheafer H, Tepper D. The effectiveness of aromatherapy in reducing pain: a systematic review and meta-analysis. *Pain Res Treat*. 2016:8158693.
31. Louis M, Kowalski SD. Use of aromatherapy with hospice patients to decrease pain, anxiety, and depression and to promote an increased sense of well-being. *Am J Hosp Palliat Care*. 2002;19(6):381–386.
32. Vickers AJ, Cronin AM, Maschino AC, et al. Acupuncture for chronic pain: individual patient data meta-analysis. *Arch Intern Med*. 2012;172(19):1444–1453.
33. Hu C, Zhang H, Wu W, et al. Acupuncture for pain management in cancer: A systematic review and meta-analysis. *Evid Based Complement Alternat Med*. 2016; 2016:1–13.
34. Salmon J. Evaluation of an acupuncture service in oncology. *J Radiother Pract*. 2013;12(1):39–55.
35 Chien T-J, Liu C-Y, Chang Y-F, Fang C-J, Hsu C-H. Acupuncture for treating aromatase inhibitor-related arthralgia in breast cancer: a systematic review and meta-analysis. *J Altern Complement Med*. 2015;21(5):251–260.
36. Zia FZ, Olaku O, Bao T, et al. The National Cancer Institute's conference on acupuncture for symptom management in oncology: state of the science, evidence, and research gaps. *J Natl Cancer Inst Monogr*. 2017;2017(52). doi:10.1093/jncimonographs/lgx005.
37. Archie P, Bruera E, Cohen L. Music-based interventions in palliative cancer care: a review of quantitative studies and neurobiological literature. *Support Care Cancer*. 2013;21(9):2609–2624.
38. Koelsch S, Fuermetz J, Sack U, et al. Effects of music listening on cortisol levels and propofol consumption during spinal anesthesia. *Front Psychol*. 2011;2:58.
39. Gerrig RJ, Zimbardo PG, Campbell AJ, Cumming SR, Wilkes FJ. *Psychology and Life*. London: Pearson Higher Education AU; 2015.
40. Warth M, Keßler J, Hillecke TK, Bardenheuer HJ. Music therapy in palliative care. *Dtsch Arztebl Int*. 2015;112(46):788–794.
41. Kordovan S, Preissler P, Kamphausen A, Bokemeyer C, Oechsle K. Prospective study on music therapy in terminally ill cancer patients during specialized inpatient palliative care. *J Palliat Med*. 2016;19(4):394–399.
42. Khoury B, Sharma M, Rush SE, Fournier C. Mindfulness-based stress reduction for healthy individuals: a meta-analysis. *J Psychosom Res*. 2015;78(6):519–528.
43. Zech N, Hansen E, Bernardy K, Hauser W. Efficacy, acceptability and safety of guided imagery/hypnosis in fibromyalgia: A systematic review and meta-analysis of randomized controlled trials. *European Journal of Pain*. 2017. http://onlinelibrary.wiley.com/doi/10.1002/ejp.933/full. Accessed January 17, 2018.
44. Marchand LR. Palliative and end-of-life care. In: Rakel D, ed. *Integrative Medicine*. 4th ed. Buffalo Grove, IL: Elsevier; 2018:806–816.e4.
45. Kuptniratsaikul V, Dajpratham P. Efficacy and safety of curcuma domestica extracts compared with ibuprofen in patients with knee osteoarthritis: a multicenter study. *Clin Interv Aging*. 2014;9:451–458.

46. Anand P, Bley K. Topical capsaicin for pain management: therapeutic potential and mechanisms of action of the new high-concentration capsaicin 8% patch. *Br J Anaesth*. 2011;107(4):490–502.
47. Derry S, Moore RA. Topical capsaicin (low concentration) for chronic neuropathic pain in adults. *Cochrane Database Syst Rev*. 2012;(9):CD010111.
48. Derry S, Sven-Rice A, Cole P, Tan T, Moore RA. Topical capsaicin (high concentration) for chronic neuropathic pain in adults. *Cochrane Database Syst Rev*. 2013;(2):CD007393.
49. Bhaskar AK, England J, Lowe J. Management of neuropathic pain (NP) using the capsaicin 8% patch in patients with cancer. *Palliat Med*. 2012;26(4):658.
50. Cameron M, Chrubasik S. Topical herbal therapies for treating osteoarthritis. *Cochrane Database Syst Rev*. 2013;(5):CD010538.
51. Zhang MJ, Spite M. Resolvins: anti-inflammatory and proresolving mediators derived from omega-3 polyunsaturated fatty acids. *Annu Rev Nutr*. 2012;32:203–227.
52. Ramsden CE, Faurot KR, Zamora D, et al. Targeted alteration of dietary n-3 and n-6 fatty acids for the treatment of chronic headaches: a randomized trial. *Pain*. 2013;154(11):2441–2451.
53. Martin KR, Reid DM. Is there role for vitamin D in the treatment of chronic pain? *Ther Adv Musculoskelet Dis*. 2017;9(6):131–135.
54. Russo EB. Cannabinoids in the management of difficult to treat pain. *Ther Clin Risk Manag*. 2008;4(1):245–259.
55. Rahn EJ, Makriyannis A, Hohmann AG. Activation of cannabinoid CB1 and CB2 receptors suppresses neuropathic nociception evoked by the chemotherapeutic agent vincristine in rats. *Br J Pharmacol*. 2007;152(5):765–777.
56. Lynch ME, Cesar-Rittenberg P, Hohmann AG. A double-blind, placebo-controlled, crossover pilot trial with extension using an oral mucosal cannabinoid extract for treatment of chemotherapy-induced neuropathic pain. *J Pain Symptom Manage*. 2014;47(1):166–173.
57. Abrams DI, Couey P, Shade SB, Kelly ME, Benowitz NL. Cannabinoid-opioid interaction in chronic pain. *Clin Pharmacol Ther*. 2011;90(6):844–851.
58. Lachenmeier DW, Rehm J. Comparative risk assessment of alcohol, tobacco, cannabis and other illicit drugs using the margin of exposure approach. *Sci Rep*. 2015;5:8126.
59. Fulop JA, Grimone A, Victorson D. Restoring balance for people with cancer through integrative oncology. *Prim Care*. 2017;44(2):323–335.
60. Karadag E, Samancioglu S, Ozden D, Bakir E. Effects of aromatherapy on sleep quality and anxiety of patients. *Nurs Crit Care*. 2017;22(2):105–112.
61. Kao Y-H, Huang Y-C, Chung U-L, Hsu W-N, Tang Y-T, Liao Y-H. Comparisons for effectiveness of aromatherapy and acupressure massage on quality of life in career women: a randomized controlled trial. *J Altern Complement Med*. 2017;23(6):451–460.
62. Hofmann SG, Sawyer AT, Witt AA, Oh D. The effect of mindfulness-based therapy on anxiety and depression: a meta-analytic review. *J Consult Clin Psychol*. 2010;78(2):169–183.
63. Kögler M, Brandstätter M, Borasio GD, Fensterer V, Küchenhoff H, Fegg MJ. Mindfulness in informal caregivers of palliative patients. *Palliat Support Care*. 2015;13(1):11–18.
64. Henneghan AM, Schnyer RN. Biofield therapies for symptom management in palliative and end-of-life care. *Am J Hosp Palliat Care*. 2015;32(1):90–100.
65. Class/Program Information. Healing Touch Program Web site. https://www.healingtouchprogram.com/classes/class-program-information. Accessed January 19, 2018.
66. Danhauer SC, Tooze JA, Holder P, Miller C, Jesse MT. Healing touch as a supportive intervention for adult acute leukemia patients: a pilot investigation of effects on distress and symptoms. *J Soc Integr Oncol*. 2008;6(3):89–97.
67. Birocco N, Guillame C, Storto S, et al. The effects of Reiki therapy on pain and anxiety in patients attending a day oncology and infusion services unit. *Am J Hosp Palliat Care*. 2012;29(4):290–294.
68. Senderovich H, Ip ML, Berall A, et al. Therapeutic Touch in a geriatric palliative care unit: A retrospective review. *Complement Ther Clin Pract*. 2016;24:134–138.
69. Kennedy SH, Lam RW, McIntyre RS, et al. Canadian Network for Mood and Anxiety Treatments (CANMAT) 2016 clinical guidelines for the management of adults with major depressive disorder: section 3. pharmacological treatments. *The Can J Psychiatry*. 2016; 61(9):540–560.
70. Huang K-Y, Liang S, Grellet A, Zhang J-B. Acupuncture and moxibustion for primary insomnia: a systematic review and meta-analysis of randomized controlled trials. *Eur J Integr Med*. 2017;12:93–107.
71. Lan Y, Wu X, Tan H-J, et al. Auricular acupuncture with seed or pellet attachments for primary insomnia: a systematic review and meta-analysis. *BMC Complement Altern Med*. 2015;15:103.
72. Finlay IG, Jones OL. Hypnotherapy in palliative care. *J R Soc Med*. 1996;89(9):493–496.
73. S-Adenosyl-L-Methionine (SAMe): in depth. NCCIH Web site. https://nccih.nih.gov/health/supplements/SAMe/. Published October 11, 2012. Accessed January 18, 2018.
74. Bressa GM. S-adenosyl-l-methionine (SAMe) as antidepressant: meta-analysis of clinical studies. *Acta Neurol Scand Suppl*. 1994;154:7–14.
75. Jacobsen S, Danneskiold-Samsøe B, Andersen RB. Oral S-adenosylmethionine in primary fibromyalgia. Double-blind clinical evaluation. *Scand J Rheumatol*. 1991;20(4):294–302.
76. St. John's Wort. NCCIH Web site. https://nccih.nih.gov/health/stjohnswort/ataglance.htm. Published February 1, 2008. Accessed January 18, 2018.
77. Hinz M, Stein A, Uncini T. 5-HTP efficacy and contraindications. *Neuropsychiatr Dis Treat*. 2012;8:323–328.
78. Fernández-San-Martín MI, Masa-Font R, Palacios-Soler L, Sancho-Gómez P, Calbó-Caldentey C, Flores-Mateo G. Effectiveness of Valerian on insomnia: a meta-analysis of randomized placebo-controlled trials. *Sleep Med*. 2010;11(6):505–511.
79. Rondanelli M, Faliva MA, Perna S, Antoniello N. Update on the role of melatonin in the prevention of cancer tumorigenesis and in the management of cancer correlates, such as sleep-wake and mood disturbances: review and remarks. *Aging Clin Exp Res*. 2013;25(5):499–510.
80. The National Institutes of Health (NIH) Consensus Development Program: Acupuncture. https://consensus.nih.gov/1997/1997acupuncture107html.htm. Accessed January 19, 2018.
81. Cheong KB, Zhang J-P, Huang Y, Zhang Z-J. The effectiveness of acupuncture in prevention and treatment of postoperative nausea and vomiting: a systematic review and meta-analysis. *PLoS One*. 2013;8(12):e82474.
82. Van den Heuvel E, Goossens M, Vanderhaegen H, Sun HX, Buntinx F. Effect of acustimulation on nausea and vomiting and on hyperemesis in pregnancy: a systematic review of Western and Chinese literature. *BMC Complement Altern Med*. 2016;16:13.
83. Lee A, Chan SKC, Fan LTY. Stimulation of the wrist acupuncture point PC6 for preventing postoperative nausea and vomiting. *Cochrane Database Syst Rev*. 2015;(11):CD003281.
84. Kravits KG. Hypnosis for the management of anticipatory nausea and vomiting. *J Adv Pract Oncol*. 2015;6(3):225–229.

85. Non-drug treatments for nausea and vomiting. American Cancer Society Web site. https://www.cancer.org/treatment/treatments-and-side-effects/physical-side-effects/nausea-and-vomiting/other-treatments.html. Accessed January 19, 2018.
86. Dupuis LL, Roscoe JA, Olver I, Aapro M, Molassiotis A. 2016 updated MASCC/ESMO consensus recommendations: anticipatory nausea and vomiting in children and adults receiving chemotherapy. *Support Care Cancer*. 2017;25(1):317–321.
87. Noyer CM, Simon D, Borczuk A, Brandt LJ, Lee MJ, Nehra V. A double-blind placebo-controlled pilot study of glutamine therapy for abnormal intestinal permeability in patients with AIDS. *Am J Gastroenterol*. 1998;93(6):972–975.
88. Daniele B, Perrone F, Gallo C, et al. Oral glutamine in the prevention of fluorouracil induced intestinal toxicity: a double blind, placebo controlled, randomised trial. *Gut*. 2001;48(1):28–33.
89. Savarese D, Al-Zoubi A, Boucher J. Glutamine for irinotecan diarrhea. *J Clin Oncol*. 2000;18(2):450–451.
90. Dabaghzadeh F, Khalili H, Dashti-Khavidaki S, Abbasian L, Moeinifard A. Ginger for prevention of antiretroviral-induced nausea and vomiting: a randomized clinical trial. *Expert Opin Drug Saf*. 2014;13(7):859–866.
91. Lee J, Oh H. Ginger as an antiemetic modality for chemotherapy-induced nausea and vomiting: a systematic review and meta-analysis. *Oncol Nurs Forum*. 2013;40(2):163–170.
92. Bujalska-Zadrożny M, Tatarkiewicz J, Kulik K, Filip M, Naruszewicz M. Magnesium enhances opioid-induced analgesia—what we have learnt in the past decades? *Eur J Pharm Sci*. 2017;99:113–127.
93. Aghamohamamdi A, Hosseinimehr SJ. Natural products for management of oral mucositis induced by radiotherapy and chemotherapy. *Integr Cancer Ther*. 2016;15(1):60–68.

PART III
Psychosocial and Spiritual Care Across Lifespan

28

Cultural Considerations in Palliative Care

Carrie L. Cormack and Aminah Fraser-Rahim

Key Points

- The increasing diversity of the nation brings opportunities and challenges for interprofessional healthcare teams, healthcare systems, and policymakers to work together to create and deliver culturally competent services equitably for all suffering with serious illness and their families.
- The 21st century has heightened awareness of the value of assessing patient and family cultural values, practices, and beliefs as a vital component of palliative care.
- Individual and family culture is multidimensional including race, ethnicity, age, gender, languages, religion and spirituality, socioeconomic class, differing abilities, composition of family, and geographic environment.
- Cultural self-awareness is necessary if nurses are to better understand their own values, practices, and beliefs and the impact these may have on the care of others.

Culture Defined

Culture is "the integrated pattern of human knowledge, belief, and behavior that depends upon the capacity for learning and transmitting knowledge to succeeding generations."[1] Shaped over time, these beliefs, traits, values, and lifestyle patterns are designed to ensure well-being and guide one's worldview and decision-making.[2] The tendency for understanding culture is the assumption that beliefs and values are based on an individual's race, ethnicity, and religious affiliations. The definition of culture is much more multidimensional, encompassing such components as age, gender, languages, religion and spirituality, socioeconomic class, differing abilities, composition of family, and geographic environment.[3] Each cultural component plays a role in shaping individual responses throughout one's life span, from birth until time of death.[2,3] Included in components of this multidimensional definition of culture are the social determinants of health (SDOH). "SDOH" refers to "conditions in the environments where people are born, live, learn, work, play, worship, and age that affect a wide range of health, functioning, and quality-of-life outcomes and risks."[4] Understanding the multiple dimensions of culture and the impact of SDOH is essential in providing quality palliative care within a social justice lens.[5]

A broad definition of culture recognizes that various *subcultures* exist within the dominant cultures. These subcultures may further affect individuals' experiences and responses in any given situation, including dealing with trauma or serious illness and the end of life. It is essential that nurses consider the role that culture, or subcultures, may play in patient and family choice and decision-making during these more difficult times. The meaning of culture comes from the individual's perspective, not from guides or texts. In addition, the nurse must be aware that the culture of the healthcare system and the culture of the nursing profession, as well as their own personal beliefs, may shape the interactions with patients, families, and colleagues.

Culture as a Global Palliative Care Issue

Care of individuals and their families with serious illness and at the end of life is complex, with many patients coping with multiple chronic illnesses, age-related syndromes and needs, complicated medication regimens, and often a limited social support to help with care. Nurses around the world must acquire and maintain primary palliative care nursing knowledge and skills to address the unique needs of those coping with serious illness and their families. While variations in global nursing education and workforce challenges exist, attention to the cultural aspects of care, regardless of where one lives, is necessary to providing compassionate and skilled nursing care across disease states. In a global world, there is no "one size fits all," and no singular approach to palliative care is appropriate; there are, quite literally, infinite variations in cross-cultural dynamics.[6] Discussion of all cultural variations is beyond the scope of this chapter; however, the authors encourage readers to consider how to apply key concepts to their specific global setting.

On January 30, 2020, The World Health Organization (WHO) declared a global health emergency. This marked the sixth time in history where the WHO issued this level of public health emergency. The COVID-19 (coronavirus disease 2019) pandemic altered the delivery of and access to healthcare across the United States and the world. COVID-19 presented a global challenge unlike anything that the healthcare system has faced for generations in this country. The impacts of COVID have been widespread, but there is significant preliminary evidence of racial and socioeconomic disparities in the population affected by COVID-19 due to the reduction in, access to,

Box 28.1 Historically Excluded Groups with Neglected Access to Palliative Care

1. Those in low- and middle-income countries
2. People living in humanitarian crisis situations
3. Those who are incarcerated
4. People experiencing homelessness
5. Those who have contracted COVID-19
6. LGBTQ+ people
7. Frail older people
8. Those living with a physical or mental impairment
9. Those living with HIV and/or tuberculosis
10. Children and young people

Source: Reference 97.

Table 28.1 US ethnic group census estimates for 2021

Group	Percent
White alone	75.8%
White alone, non-Hispanic or Latino	59.3%
Hispanic or Latino alone	18.9%
Black or African American alone	13.6%
Asian alone	6.1%
American Indian/Alaska Native alone	1.3%
Native Hawaiian and Other Pacific Islanders	0.3%

Fact Notes
- Includes persons reporting only one race
- Hispanics may be of any race, so also are included in applicable race categories

Source: https://www.census.gov/quickfacts/fact/table/US/PST045221.

and utilization of healthcare services.[7] As a result, inadequate or inaccessible access to healthcare services has exacerbated the existing social advantages, stressing the system even more.[8]

Each year the world comes together to celebrate World Hospice and Palliative Care Day. The 2021 virtual celebration highlighted the fact that 88% of the worldwide need for palliative care is not being met and that palliative care is not part of universal health coverage or national health systems in most countries across the world.[9] Yet equity in access to care is a human right. See Box 28.1 for the 10 groups that historically lack equitable access to palliative care. Many of these groups lack access within the United States as well. This chapter will discuss how nurses and other members of the interprofessional palliative care team can support individuals who identify with many of these groups.

Cultural Perspectives

The complexity of culture and its impact on health outcomes is widely known and accepted and was magnified during the pandemic. It is essential that culture and cultural perceptions be considered in all aspects of healthcare. Cultural perceptions may affect the care provided to others, access to care, treatment provided, and fear of stigmatization.[10] It is important to assess the role of culture and avoid correlating disease with questionable cultural causations. This may lead to blaming specific populations for their high prevalence rate or stigmatizing of certain groups.[11] Cultural assessment is discussed throughout this chapter including components of an assessment and resources to assist with assessment.

Increasing Diversity in the United States

In a nation of increasing diversity, the growing range of treasured beliefs, shared teachings, norms, customs, and languages in the United States challenges the nurse to understand and respond to a wide variety of perspectives. The total US population in 2021 was estimated to be 331.89 million.[12] Population statistics from the US Census Bureau illustrate that the United States has become a more racially and ethnically diverse population in the last 10 years, with cultural diversity increasing among the five most common pan-ethnic groups. These groups are federally defined as American Indian, Alaska Native, Asian, Hawaiian and other Pacific Islander, Black or African American, Hispanic, and White (Table 28.1).[12]

With these changes in cultural diversity comes increasing diversity in the nursing workforce. Beliefs and attitudes about nursing's role and the status of the nurse may be underappreciated or not acknowledged in some parts of the world. Nurses must be aware of how their own cultural beliefs and norms shape their professional practice and differ from the beliefs and norms of the patients and families for whom they care.

Culture and Palliative Care

The essence of palliative care is to provide holistic supportive care for the patient and the family living with a serious illness. Palliative care is an interprofessional care delivery model designed to anticipate, prevent, and manage physical, psychological, social, and spiritual suffering to optimize quality of life (QOL) for patients, their families, and caregivers.[13,14] To meet these needs, nurses must recognize the vital role that culture has on one's experience of living and dying. The beliefs, norms, and practices of an individual's cultural heritage guide one's behavioral responses, decision-making, and actions.[3] Culture shapes how an individual makes meaning out of illness, suffering, and death.[15] Nurses, along with other members of the interprofessional team, partner with the patient and family to ensure that patient and family values, beliefs, and practices guide the plan of care.[13]

The National Consensus Project's *Clinical Practice Guidelines for Quality Palliative Care*[14] define the core concepts and structures for quality palliative care delivery. The guidelines comprise eight domains with corresponding criteria that reflect the depth and breadth of the specialty. Cultural Aspects of Care constitutes one of the eight domains, emphasizing the central role that culture plays in providing strength and meaning for patients and families facing serious illness.[14] This domain defines culture and outlines cultural competencies for interdisciplinary team members (Box 28.2).

Culture is a source of resilience for patients and families and plays an important role in the provision of palliative care. It is the responsibility of all members of the palliative care team to strive for cultural awareness to ensure that appropriate and relevant services are provided to patients and families. The following case illustrates the

Box 28.2 Clinical Practice Guidelines for Quality Palliative Care: Cultural Aspects of Care

Guideline 6.1 Global
The interdisciplinary team (IDT) delivers care that respects patient and family cultural beliefs, values, traditional practices, language, and communication preferences and builds upon the unique strengths of the patient and family. Members of the IDT work to increase awareness of their own biases and seek opportunities to learn about the provision of culturally sensitive care. The care team ensures that its environment, policies, procedures, and practices are culturally respectful.

Guideline 6.2 Communication and Language
The IDT ensures that patient and family preferred language and style of communication are supported and facilitated in all interactions.

Guideline 6.3 Screening and Assessment
The IDT uses evidence-based practices when screening and assessing patient and family cultural preferences regarding healthcare practices, customs, beliefs and values, level of health literacy, and preferred language.

Guideline 6.4 Treatment
A culturally sensitive plan of care is developed and discussed with the patient and/or family. This plan reflects the degree to which patients and families wish to be included as partners in decision-making regarding their care. When hosting meetings to discuss and develop the plan, the IDT ensures that patient and family linguistic needs are met.

Source: Reference 14.

challenges faced when caring for a patient and family with serious illness and importance of cultural considerations.

Case Study 1: Cultural Considerations of a Family

Lee, a 12-year-old girl, has a long medical history of end-stage renal disease. Lee is dialysis-dependent, withdrawn, soft-spoken, and fully dependent on others for all of her needs. She lives at home with her father, mother, brother, and grandmother. Her primary caretaker is her grandmother, Rosa, who is 65 years old. Rosa does not speak English. She came to the United States from China at 24 years of age, in hopes of a better life and better medical care for herself and her family. Lee and Rosa have a very close relationship. Lee's disease has progressed over the past few years, and unfortunately, she is not a candidate for a kidney transplant. Without a kidney transplant, the family is aware that Lee will not survive.

Lee's parents are the primary decision makers; but all medical information is shared in Rosa's presence, and her feedback and opinions are respected as she is an elder in their culture. An interpreter is needed for all family meetings since Rosa does not speak English. Medical team and parents want to transition Lee home with hospice services so that she can spend time with her family. Rosa is not in agreement. Rosa wants Lee to remain in the hospital and placed on a transplant list. She also wants all Chinese cultures and practices in place in case of an acute event and Lee passes away.

This complex case addresses several areas requiring cultural consideration and the need for comprehensive assessment of the values, practices, beliefs, and goals of the family.

Questions to Consider:

1. What cultural issues must be considered in this case, and how may these issues impact decision-making?
2. How may a palliative team be helpful to this family, and what resources may they access to assist with the cultural needs of this family?
3. What are some communication techniques that the nurse and other healthcare providers might use with this family?

Striving to Understand Culture: A Process

Striving to understand and respectfully engage with other cultures is a process. This next section defines the various terms used to describe this process and how they are applicable to palliative care.

Cultural Awareness

Healthcare team members should continually strive for cultural awareness especially when working with patients with serious illness and their families. Integrating cultural considerations into palliative care requires, first and foremost, awareness of how one's own values, practices, and beliefs influence care. Cultural awareness begins with an examination of one's own heritage, family's practices, experiences, and religious or spiritual beliefs.[16,17] Cultural awareness challenges the nurse to look beyond their own ethnocentric view of the world, asking the question, "How are my values, beliefs, and practices different from those of the patient and family?" rather than, "How is this patient and family different from me?"

Cultural Knowledge

Acquiring knowledge about different cultural groups is another component to striving for cultural awareness, but knowledge alone is insufficient in providing culturally appropriate care.[16] Having in-depth knowledge of all cultural variations of health and illness beliefs, values, and norms is an impossible task. A suggested strategy is to identify the most common ethnic groups/cultures living in one's community and to integrate a basic understanding of norms and practices impacting issues likely to arise in palliative and end-of-life (EOL) situations.

It is important to be aware that knowledge gained of a particular group should serve only as a guide to understanding the unique cultural needs of the patient and family, which comes through individualized assessments. Relying solely on culturally specific knowledge to guide practice, rather than individual assessment, is incongruent with culturally competent care. Resources may also be helpful to assist the nurse in acquiring knowledge about specific groups including cultural guides, literature, and web-based resources (examples listed in Box 28.3).[18]

Cultural Skill

Cultural skill is another important component of cultural awareness.[16] Skills in cultural assessment, cross-cultural communication, cultural interpretation, and appropriate intervention can be learned. Multiple tools are available to assess cultural behavior and beliefs. For the new nurse, key assessment questions, applicable in the palliative care setting, may be helpful in guiding the assessment (Box 28.4). These questions, although useful to guide a discussion, should not replace patient and family interaction. Listening to the stories of heritage/family history and asking about their cherished practices

Box 28.3 Web-Based Resources

Cross Cultural Health Care Program (CCHCP): www.xculture.org

- CCHCP addresses broad cultural issues that impact the health of individuals and families in ethnic minority communities. Its mission is to serve as a bridge between communities and healthcare institutions.

EthnoMed: http://ethnomed.org/

- The EthnoMed site contains information about cultural beliefs, medical issues, and other related issues pertinent to the healthcare of recent immigrants to the United States.

Palliative Care Network of Wisconsin: Home of Fast Facts and Fast Fact CME

- Fast Fact & Concept #78—Cultural Aspects of Pain Management: https://www.mypcnow.org/blank-a8lpj
- Fast Fact #216—Asking about Cultural Beliefs in Palliative Care: https://www.mypcnow.org/fast-fact/asking-about-cultural-beliefs-in-palliative-care/
- Fast Fact & Concept #435—End-of-Life Considerations for Muslim Patients: https://www.mypcnow.org/fast-fact/end-of-life-care-considerations-for-muslim-patients/
- Fast Fact & Concept #449—End-of-Life Considerations for the Pentecostal Patient: https://www.mypcnow.org/fast-fact/end-of-life-care-considerations-for-the-pentecostal-patient/

Office of Minority Health: https://minorityhealth.hhs.gov/

- This website has training tools for developing cultural competency.
- Transcultural Nursing Society: http://www.tcns.org
- The society (founded in 1974) serves as a forum to promote, advance, and disseminate transcultural nursing knowledge worldwide.

and beliefs is an invaluable way to learn more about the patient and family and build a trusting relationship.

Cultural Sensitivity

Being sensitive to other cultures is an underlying context in this process.[18,19] This is necessary in palliative care, as in any other clinical arena. Each new encounter should begin with an open mind, knowing that each individual and professional perspective is but one of many in the larger community being served. The goal of each provider should be to create a shared understanding.

Cultural Encounter

This next component encompasses the concept of cultural encounters.[16] The more opportunities for engaging with persons with differing values, practices, and beliefs, the more we learn about others and ourselves and the less likely we are to draw erroneous conclusions about each other. Active engagement with community leaders and use of learning tools such as case studies and role-play all help expose nurses to varied cultural experiences. Increasing exposure to cultural encounters may also improve confidence in one's ability to meet the needs of diverse populations.[16]

Cultural Desire

Cultural desire is the interest and openness with which the nurse strives to understand patients and families and the communities from which they come, with the motivation to "want to" engage in

Box 28.4 Key Cultural Assessment Questions

Formal cultural assessments are available for the nurse to use (see resources in **Box 28.3**). Remember that a checklist does not always instill trust. Listed here are some suggestions for ascertaining key cultural preferences from both patients and family caregivers.

Basic Assessment Questions

General

- Can you tell me a little bit about yourself (e.g., your family, your mother, father, siblings, etc.)?
- Where were you born and raised? (If an immigrant, "How long have you lived in this country?")
- What language would you prefer to speak?
- Is it easier to write things down, or do you have difficulty with reading and writing?
- To whom do you go for support (family friends, community, or religious or community leaders)?
- Is there anyone we should contact to come to be with you?
- I want to be sure I'm giving you all the information you need. What do you want to know about your condition? To whom should I speak about your care?
- Whom do you want to know about your condition?
- How are decisions about healthcare made in your family? Should I speak directly with you, or is there someone else with whom I should be discussing decisions?
- Addressed to patient or designated decision maker: Tell me about your understanding of what has been happening up to this point. What does the illness mean to you?
- We want to work with you to be sure you are getting the best care possible and that we are meeting all your needs. Is there anything we should know about any customs or practices that are important to include in your care?

Religion and Spirituality

- What are your religious or spiritual beliefs?
- Are you a part of a spiritual or religious community? If so, how does this group provide support?
- Are there any specific practices or restrictions you would like us to know about while we are providing care?

Gender

- We want to make sure we respect how you prefer to be addressed, including how we should act. Is there anything we should avoid? Is it appropriate for you to have male and female caregivers?
- Describe your gender identity. How has this changed at all throughout your life?

Race and Ethnicity

- Have you faced any challenges due to your race or ethnicity? If so, what were they?
- Where is your family originally from?
- Where were you born and raised?

Death Rituals and Practices

- Is there anything we should know about care of the body, about rituals, practices, or ceremonies that should be performed?
- What is your belief about what happens after death?
- Is there a way for us to plan for anything you might need, both at the time of death and afterward?
- Is there anything we should know about whether a man or a woman should be caring for the body after death?
- Should your family be involved in the care of the body?

Finances
- Do you have any concerns about how to pay for care, medications, or other services?

Other
- Do you feel safe?
- Do you have a dwelling to go home to?
- Does the dwelling have electricity, gas, appropriate heating/cooling?
- Do you have access to a food store?
- Do you have access to food and food storage?
- Are there any foods you would like or that you should avoid?
- Do you have access to transportation?
- Do you have access to a pharmacy?

Source: Reference 5 and Partners for Kids, Cultural Assessment Questions (https://partnersforkids.org/wp-content/uploads/2022/01/Cultural-Assessment-Questions.pdf).

the process of cultural awareness as opposed to being "forced to" participate in the process. The desire should be genuine and authentic. Such experiences lend opportunities for the nurse to grow both personally and professionally.[16]

Cultural Humility

Cultural humility is an approach that should be the goal for all healthcare professionals, which includes being open, self-aware, egoless, and supportive and incorporates self-reflection when interacting with diverse individuals, groups, or communities.[17,19] Self-reflection is essential for nurses in order to provide care that respects and honors others' culture. Cultural humility may be considered the epitome of commitment to cultural competence, when learners truly practice in a manner which represents dignity, compassion, caring, and empathy.[18,19]

Some researchers suggest that the term "cultural humility" is more acceptable than "cultural sensitivity" or "cultural competence" when trying to provide culturally appropriate care.[2,20] They have suggested that multiple generations of blended families and intercultural marriages have made it nearly impossible to know all about the healthcare practices of particular communities. These social scientists and writers recommend that nurses strive to mindfully respect each patient/family member as a unique individual rather than the components of culture (ethnicity, religion/spirituality, place of residence, etc.) that might label them.[17,19] Integrating the proposed model of cultural competence with cultural humility into clinical practice may strengthen nurses' and others' ability to respect and support patient and family wishes in palliative care settings.

Cultural Competence

"Cultural competence" refers to a dynamic, fluid, continuous process of awareness, knowledge, skill, sensitivity, interaction, desire, and humility.[17] While the term remains controversial, as some question whether true "cultural competence" can ever be achieved,[3] cultural competence along with cultural awareness remain important outcomes for nursing students[20] and essential for all nurses, as noted by nursing organizations worldwide.[21] Cultural competence can be employed as a strategy to reduce health disparities among minority groups and vulnerable populations.[22]Cultural Assessment

Self-Assessment

Exploring one's own beliefs by completing a personal self-assessment will help raise an awareness of differences that have the potential to foster prejudice and discrimination and limit the effectiveness of care.[23] Often identifying more similarities than differences, the nurse and patient can recognize universal aspects of life, family, trust, love, hope, understanding, and caring, which will enhance the quality of care. Exploring one's individual cultural competence will allow consideration of individual skills, knowledge, and awareness and how these may affect interactions with others, as well as recognition of what can be done to be more effective working and living in diverse environments.

Conducting a Cultural Assessment

In caring for diverse populations, nurses must understand and assess the essential components of culture as well as the SDOH. There are many guides and tools available to help with cultural assessment. These tools include the components of culture discussed throughout this chapter. Completing a cultural assessment involves asking questions that enhance the development of a trusting relationship. When meeting the patient and family early in the disease trajectory, the palliative care nurse has the advantage of time to establish such a relationship. Unfortunately, this luxury of time is not always available. The nurse must develop the skills of presence and active listening as these are often more beneficial than a standardized tool. Checklists do not necessarily build trust and can be burdensome. Asking the patient and/or the family member about themself and then listening to those narratives are powerful. Simple inquiries into patient and family practices and beliefs can assist the nurse in understanding needs and goals of care, and these stories often give clues that may trigger further questioning. Integrating assessment questions regarding SDOH within a cultural assessment ensures that the needs of those who are especially vulnerable because of serious illness and their SDOH are identified. Box 28.4 provides examples of trigger questions.

Components of Culture

Race

The commonly held misconception that "race" refers to biological and genetic differences and "ethnicity" refers to cultural variation is outmoded. Race exists not as a natural category but as a social construct.[24] Any discussion of race must include the harsh reality of racism issues and disparities that have plagued society and continue to exist even today. Recent studies have demonstrated discrimination against persons of certain races regarding healthcare practices, treatment options, and hospice utilization.[25] When viewed in relation to specific races, morbidity and mortality statistics point to serious gaps in access to quality care. Racial disparities are still evident worldwide, even after adjustments for socioeconomic status and other access-related factors are taken into account.[26]

There is often an underlying mistrust of the healthcare system. Memories of the Tuskegee syphilis study and segregated hospitals remain with older African Americans.[27] The combination of mistrust and numerous other complex variables influence palliative care issues such as medical decision-making and advance care planning.[28] Compounding the situation is the fact that healthcare providers often do not recognize existing biases within systems or themselves.[29]

Researchers have tried to identify causal mechanisms for healthcare disparities in psychosocial, cultural, and spiritual palliative care; however, the work is sparse and limited by methodological flaws. Evans and Ume[30] recommend using a conceptual framework such as that used in the *National Healthcare Disparities Report*[31] to explore causal mechanisms, which include access to care, receipt of care, and quality of care, as well as examination of barriers, usage, costs of care and effectiveness, safety, timeliness, and patient-centeredness.

Ethnicity

"Ethnicity" refers to "a group of people that share a common and distinctive racial, national, religious, linguistic, or cultural heritage."[31] The values, practices, and beliefs shared by members of the same ethnic group may influence behavior or response. Ethnicity has been identified as a significant predictor of EOL preferences and decision-making.[32] While the US Census recognizes only six ethnic categories in the United States (White, Black or African American, American Indian or Alaska Native, Asian, and Native Hawaiian or Other Pacific Islander),[12] individuals may self-identify with one of more than 100 ethnic groups nationwide.

Ethnicity has been shown to influence utilization of hospice and palliative care service. Ethnic minority groups are less likely to use hospice services when compared with non-Hispanic Whites. Furthermore, there has been little increase in hospice utilization in Black, Hispanic, or Asian populations in recent years.[32] Researchers have demonstrated an understanding of disparities in quality EOL care among ethnicities but have not yet identified why this is happening.[33,34] Further study into the multiple factors influencing utilization of these services is needed.[35]

Although an individual may belong to a particular ethnic group, they may not identify strongly with that group.[3,36] Members of the same family from the same ethnic group may have very different ideas about what is acceptable practice concerning important palliative care concepts such as communication with healthcare professionals, medical decision-making, and EOL rituals. In multigenerational families, some members may hold to the traditional beliefs and practices of their ethnic community of origin. Other family members may have a bicultural orientation, moving between the family culture of origin to the host society; and others may have left their cultural roots and identify with the host society. For example, in the United States, second- and third-generation members of immigrant families may be more assimilated into Western culture than first-generation members. This can lead to cultural conflicts within families around sensitive palliative care concepts.

The assumption that an individual will respond in a certain way because they are a member of an ethnic group contributes to stereotyping. The nurse should assess each individual's beliefs and practices rather than assuming that they hold the beliefs of a particular group. Note that many studies have demonstrated that regardless of race or ethnicity, all persons share common needs at the end of life: being comfortable, being cared for, sustaining or healing relationships, having hope, and honoring spiritual beliefs.[3,13,23,36,37]

Age and Developmental Stage

Age has its own identity and culture.[3] Each group has its own beliefs, attitudes, and practices, which are influenced by their developmental stage and by the society in which they live. The impact of a life-limiting illness on persons of differing age groups is often influenced by the loss of developmental tasks associated with that age group.[3]

Infant/Toddler

Although in modern society we expect that children will outlive their parents, in 2020 an estimated 5 million children from around the world under the age of five years died, mostly from preventable and treatable causes.[38] While many of the principles of adult palliative care can be applied to children, caring for an infant or toddler with a life-limiting condition or at the end of life brings new challenges to a nurse, which can be difficult to manage without experience or preparation.

Palliative care principles can be applied at time of diagnosis, which for some parents is during pregnancy. Compassionate care should be offered to the family during this time, and discussions should be facilitated to allow parents options regarding care and treatment.[39] The National Association of Neonatal Nurses,[39] the American Academy of Pediatrics,[40] and the National Hospice and Palliative Care Organization[41] have position statements outlining the values and recommendations for palliative care with newborns and their families. These recommendations include advocating for family-centered care throughout the illness trajectory and continuing to support following the death of a child because family members will continue to require support as they cope with their loss.[39,40,41]

School-Aged Children

Just as children develop and change as they grow, offering palliative care to children as they emerge from infancy and toddlerhood into the school-aged years requires another set of skills for the palliative care nurse. Depending on the developmental level of the child at the center of the care, the focus should be to assist the child to cope with the illness and offer support to the family. Typically developing children during the school-aged years have fears as well as vivid hopes and dreams, all which must be acknowledged during difficult times of illness. School-aged children strive for increased independence and autonomy and seek opportunity for control and responsibility,[42] traits often diminished by necessary medical procedures, clinical appointments, tests, and hospitalizations. Friends and a sense of belonging to groups of peers are important for this age group, and children with life-limiting illnesses are often excluded or forced into more solitary activities. This can be isolating and painful for the school-aged child, and recognition of this can help build trust between a patient and nurse. Family members also need support to consider the wishes of the child and help facilitate what may be important to them during this time.

Adolescence

Cultural considerations with adolescents coping with serious illness bring yet another set of concerns for caregivers. An increased sensitivity to their appearance[42] can be agonizing for teens going through bodily changes beyond their control. Peer groups and acceptance remain important, although adolescents strive to secure their own identities, including their own ethical and moral decisions. Adolescents should be involved in all decision-making regarding their care. Future goals and plans are often considered, and the impact that a serious illness may have on this trajectory can be distressing to both the teen and family. Providers must be sensitive to the self-preoccupation that teens have and the often critical self-image or low self-esteem that may be a factor during these difficult times. Spiritual development can be helpful and is often explored during this time. This may be an important implication for practice when caring for an adolescent with a life-limiting illness.[40]

Young and Middle-Aged Adulthood

Serious illness is less common in young and middle-aged adults than in older adults. The death-denying society of the United States does not expect young or middle-aged adults to have to face life-threatening illnesses or death. For young adults (aged 21–40) and middle-aged adults (aged 41–60), developmental tasks include finishing their education, starting and engaging in a work and career, finding a life partner, establishing a long-term relationship, and starting a family. A serious illness can interfere with being able to accomplish any or all of these tasks. Research has shown that patients with dependent children have more worry and anxiety over the uncertainty of the future and time away from family for treatment than those who do not have children at home.[43]

Older Adulthood

Census projections suggest that, by 2060, the combined minority groups that currently make up 37% of the US population will constitute the majority (57%). Globally, the population older than 60 is expected to more than double in the next several decades from 12% in 2015 to 22% in 2050, and the number of the "oldest old," the 85 and older age group, is expected to more than triple.[44]

As the population of young-old (60–69), middle-old (70–79), and very old (80 and older) adults rises, the importance of addressing the unique palliative care needs of the older adult becomes more evident.[44] Each group of older adults has specific developmental tasks that reflect cultural traditions and range from positive experiences (e.g., retirement, grandparenting) to losses associated with aging (e.g., loss of independence, death of those close to them, and physical and mental health changes).

Cultural considerations related to this aging population include the impact of serious illness on finances, home environment, caregiving needs and availability, medical decision-making abilities, management of complex medication regimens and comorbid conditions, availability of medications, and pain and symptom management disparities. Cognitive changes make decision-making and patient safety critical issues across the aging trajectory.

As the adult population lives longer, spousal caregivers, who may also be among the very old, often have their own medical issues that may impact their ability to provide care.[45] These trends will present significant challenges to health systems and interprofessional healthcare teams including nurses worldwide as they look to meeting the needs of older adults.

Gender

Gender Considerations

Cultural norms have guided specific roles for men and women regarding illness and EOL care. For some families, gender determines roles in decision-making and caregiving.

It is culturally sensitive to be aware of family dominance patterns in decision-making and determine which family member(s) holds that dominant role. In some families, decision-making may be the responsibility of the female head of the family, in others the male head of the family or eldest son. For example, those of Asian ethnicity who follow strict Confucian teaching believe that men have absolute authority and are responsible for family decision-making.[18] When caring for families who adhere to these norms, discussing prognosis and treatment with a female family member is likely to cause the patient and family distress and may result in significant clashes with the healthcare team and mistrust. It is critical to ask every person and family who should have the responsibility for decision-making and never assume how that family functions.[19]

In addition to decision-making, cultural expectations exist regarding the responsibilities of caregiving. In many families, women have traditionally been expected to take on the role of caregiver when someone in the family is facing a serious illness. This responsibility, in addition to responsibilities at work and for children, has been overwhelming for many women, affecting their physical and emotional well-being. Research has demonstrated that female caregivers tend to experience greater caregiver burden, anxiety, and depression than male caregivers.[46] Supportive interventions for family caregivers, regardless of gender, are an essential component of palliative care.[19,47]

Gender Identity

One of the most profound gender disparities in the delivery of quality palliative care involves those who are lesbian, gay, bisexual, transgender, or queer/questioning (LGBTQ).[45] It is recommended that the best way to address these disparities is by providing LGBTQ-inclusive palliative care rather than conceptualizing LGBTQ people as a "special population" that is separate from all others. Acquaviva[48] suggests that making subtle changes in the way palliative care is delivered will allow for inclusive, nonjudgmental hospice and palliative care for all persons.

There are some particular aspects of palliative care where the LGBTQ population may be at risk. Ethical and legal issues related to advance care planning, healthcare decision-making, disposition of the body after death, and property ownership are particularly important to address early in care.[49–51] Waiting until the end of life to have these discussions may be too late.

Risk for discrimination of LGBTQ older adults remains despite the mounting resources available for LGBT patients and their care providers to help navigate EOL issues together. There remains the need for improved research, clinical practice, provider education, and access to bereavement programs with the LGBT patient in mind.[50,51] Antidiscrimination policies and staff education should be mandatory for all care providers.

It is important to note that transgender individuals may have some unique health needs that can influence disease and symptom management in palliative care.[52] Some transgender persons have had medical or surgical interventions to help them achieve their gender identity,[48] and these interventions may have implications on morbidity and mortality. For example, cross-sex hormone therapy may have a negative effect on cardiovascular disease and diabetes in transgender men but may have important psychological benefits, thus requiring a benefit–burden conversation in palliative and EOL care. However, many healthcare professionals are not knowledgeable about the risks associated with medical or surgical interventions that should be monitored closely. Nurses should be aware of the benefits and burdens these individuals face across the life span in order to support them in treatment decision-making. To read more about delivery of palliative care for LGBTQIA+ individuals, please see Chapter 67, "Affirmative Palliative Care for LGTBQIA+ Patients and Their Families."

Language

It is essential to determine the dominant language and dialect spoken and the literacy level of both the patient and the family. If there is a language barrier, a professionally trained interpreter of the appropriate language should be contacted. This may include the use of a computerized interpreter service that offers secured services under the Health Insurance Portability and Accountability Act (HIPAA). If such services are not available, other health providers, ideally those trained in palliative care, may serve as interpreters. Family members should only act as interpreters in emergency situations and only if they agree to do so as family members placed in this role may feel uncomfortable should sensitive issues or questions arise.[3,14] Always determine what is culturally appropriate to disclose prior to discussion regardless of who is involved in the communication of medical information.[2] When using an interpreter, direct all verbal communication to the patient/family rather than the interpreter. Ongoing clarification that information is understood is critical.

Religion and Spirituality

Religion is the belief and practice of a faith tradition, a means of expressing spirituality. Spirituality, a much broader concept, is the life force that transcends our physical being and gives meaning and purpose.[53–55] Although religion and spirituality are complementary concepts, these terms are often mistakenly used interchangeably. It should be noted that an individual may be very spiritual but not practice a formal religion. In addition, those who identify themselves as belonging to a religion may not necessarily adhere to all the practices of that religion. As with ethnicity, it is important to determine how strongly the individual aligns with their identified faith and the significance of its practice rituals.

Chaplains or clergy from a patient's or family member's religious group—ideally their own community clergy—are key members of the interprofessional palliative care team. Those who turn to their faith-based communities for support may find the emotional, spiritual, and other tangible support they need when dealing with a life-limiting illness.[56] Keep in mind, however, that some individuals who are struggling with misconceptions of the tenets of their own faith may experience spiritual distress and need spiritual intervention from caring chaplains or spiritual care counselors. Also, be aware that many community clergy are not trained in EOL care and may need assistance from the palliative care team in order to support the patient's spiritual journey.

Spirituality is in the essence of every human being. It is what gives each person a sense of being, meaning, purpose, and direction.[56,57] It transcends the self to connect with others and with a higher power, independent of organized religion.[3,31,36,53] One's sense of spirituality is often the force that helps transcend loss and suffering.[35,53,54] Spiritual distress can cause pain and suffering if not identified and addressed. Assessing spiritual well-being and attending to spiritual needs, which may be very diverse, are essential to QOL for patients and families facing serious illness and confronting the end of life.[57] To read more about spirituality, please see Chapter 33, "Addressing Spiritual, Religious, and Existential Needs in Palliative Care."

SDOH

The National Academies of Sciences, Engineering, and Medicine report *The Future of Nursing 2020–2030: Charting a Path to Health Equity* (2021) identified the need to prepare nurses to address health equity, SDOH, systemic bias, and racism.[58] The components of SDOH make a cultural assessment more inclusive for all those who are considered "oppressed." These persons are not afforded equitable treatment, reflecting a societal structure that forces them into unjust conditions. Once referred to as marginalized populations, examples of those who are at risk for being oppressed include individuals who are Black, Latino, American Indian, Indigenous peoples, disabled, LGBTQ+, homeless, and incarcerated, as well as those with comorbid substance use disorder or serious psychiatric illness.[58] It is well known that these oppressed groups underutilize palliative and EOL care. Therefore, it is essential to include components of SDOH within a comprehensive cultural assessment.

Socioeconomic Status

One's socioeconomic status, which is usually measured as a combination of education, occupation, and income, is an important aspect of one's cultural identity, affecting physical and mental health and playing an important role in palliative care. Inequities in health distribution and resource availability are increasing in the United States and globally.[59] Individuals who are socioeconomically disadvantaged, with lower educational achievement, poverty, and poor health, face unique challenges when seeking healthcare and health insurance[59] and may struggle to navigate the healthcare system and to find information and support.

Financial costs, including those for medications, medical tests, and treatments not covered by limited insurance plans, transportation, and childcare, add further burdens. Regardless of financial status, an estimated 25% of families are financially devastated by a serious terminal illness.[3] Patients experiencing disease progression or in whom treatment side effects preclude the ability to work are forced to confront profound losses: loss of work and income, loss of identity, and loss of a network of colleagues.

While an exhaustive review of the impact of socioeconomic status and SDOH on health and health outcomes is beyond the scope of this chapter, we discuss some important aspects that the palliative care nurse should consider in the following paragraphs.

Health Literacy, Health Numeracy, and Financial Literacy

Individuals who are socioeconomically disadvantaged may experience additional difficulties when attempting to understand medical terms and basic body functions and when interpreting statistics and evaluating risks and benefits.[60] While no universal definition exists, most definitions identify *health literacy* as the degree to which an individual can obtain, process, and understand basic health information in order to make decisions related to health.[61,62] Even individuals with good literacy skills can have low health literacy, health numeracy, or financial literacy.[60,62]

Health numeracy is related to health literacy, referring to the degree to which individuals have the capacity to obtain, interpret, and process quantitative information for health behavior and decision.[62] Health numeracy includes four functional categories: basic numeracy skills (identify numbers and comprehend data), computational skills (ability to count, quantify, compute, and use simple manipulation of numbers or figures), analytical skills (e.g., inference, estimation, and proportions), and statistical numeracy skills (e.g., analytical skills plus the ability to critically analyze information and research findings and weigh risks and benefits).[62]

Financial literacy refers to an individual's ability to use knowledge and skills to manage financial resources effectively for lifelong financial well-being.[63] Individuals who lack the ability to consider health insurance options, calculate out-of-pocket expenses, and navigate other complex financial choices may have more difficulty in making important health decisions.[62,63]

Individuals facing serious illness need information in a format and language that are easily understood in order to make informed healthcare decisions.[64] For individuals who are socioeconomically disadvantaged, the challenges just described regarding health literacy, health numeracy, and financial literacy may be more significant. Nurses can assist patients and family by considering whether the information they receive reflects their socioeconomic status, age, cultural background, language, and literacy skills.

Place of Residence

Access to services is challenging for some individuals depending on their geographic location. For those living in rural areas, access to palliative care services is inadequate when compared to urban areas.[65] While access to and availability of specialty palliative care services have seen an increase in the past few years,[66,67] internationally, research suggests that lower socioeconomic status is associated with lower use of palliative care services.[68] Factors that affect poorer utilization include an inconsistent number of service providers in disadvantaged areas and increased travel time to specialist palliative care providers and facilities.[68] Hospice services are also lacking in rural counties, with discrepancies between needed and received hospice care.[69] Recent developments, including community support, academic partnerships, and telehealth initiatives, suggest that improvement in access for the seriously ill and dying may be feasible, even in the most remote areas.[70]

Individuals Who Are Homeless

People experiencing homelessness face significant mortality, comorbid conditions, and high disease burden compared to age- and sex-matched peers.[71] The last global survey of homelessness was completed by the United Nations in 2005 and estimated that 100 million people were homeless and that more than 1 billion people lacked adequate housing in both industrialized and developing nations.[72] In the United States, it is estimated that at least 500,000 persons are homeless and that nearly 1.5 million people use homeless shelters.[73]

Many of the health, numeracy, and financial literacy concerns mentioned earlier may be present for individuals who are homeless. Additionally, individuals may not have a trusted surrogate decision maker and may be estranged from family members.[74] Despite significant barriers to advance care planning with this population, research indicates that those who are homeless have the desire to complete advance directives when given the opportunity.[73–75]

Those struggling with homelessness with serious illness may have greater social challenges, mortality at a younger age, higher prevalence of physical symptoms associated with psychosocial distress, mistrust of the healthcare community, and a higher occurrence of psychological symptoms than the general population.[71,72,75] Individuals also experience a higher incidence of substance use, severe mental illness, and infectious diseases (e.g., HIV/AIDS, hepatitis C).[75]

Despite calls for improved palliative resources and access to services, those who are homeless continue to have limited access to quality palliative care services.[76] Access to transportation, stigmatization by healthcare providers, prioritizing basic needs of food and shelter, and ineligibility for health insurance may delay a person from accessing healthcare or obtaining adequate follow-up.[75,77] Healthcare professional attitudes (perceived or real negative stereotyping) and lack of experience may also contribute to existing barriers.[77]

Suggestions to improve palliative and hospice services for homeless persons include building trust and relationships, increasing collaboration between professionals, increasing flexibility within health services, and providing training and support for professionals working with people who are homeless.[77] Several examples of programs offer hope for homeless individuals facing serious illness, including shelter-based and street-based palliative care programs,[78] programs aimed at increasing advance care planning in the homeless population,[74] and increased education for health providers. With an increase in community-based palliative care, some of the access issues may begin to lessen; however, continuing financial concerns and adequate shelter and caregiving needs will require ongoing research and efforts in both rural and urban settings.

Prisons

Globally, the number of seriously ill and dying persons in prisons is growing. Most current literature focuses on US prison hospice programs or on identifying barriers to quality palliative and EOL care in prisons.[79] Examples of successful practices include the use of inmate volunteers alongside interdisciplinary teams and prison staff training and partnerships with local hospice organizations. Barriers to improved palliative care in prisons include mistrust between staff and prisoners, safety concerns, concerns regarding the use and potential misuse of opioids and other medications used to ameliorate symptoms, ethical dilemmas based on custody versus care, staff and public apathy toward rights to healthcare for this population, and debate over the use of compassionate release.[79]

Immigration Status

Immigrant populations face both cultural and logistical challenges when faced with serious illness and dying due to language differences, potential health literacy deficiencies, variations in family decision-making and role responsibilities, insurance barriers, and the possibility of lack of financial or social resources.[80] It is important to consider whether there are true disparities rather than differences in patient/family care preferences, as well as to consider professional bias toward perceived cultural differences when approaching goals-of-care discussions and assessments.[81] Over time, acculturation may decrease true variations in preferences; however, completing an in-depth cultural assessment is necessary to determine individual norms and preferences.

The number of undocumented immigrants varies worldwide. It is estimated that there were approximately 10.5 million undocumented immigrants in the United States in 2017, accounting for 3.2% of the nation's population,[82] many of whom are educationally and socioeconomically disadvantaged and living in rural areas without access to healthcare.[83] For undocumented immigrants, challenges to optimal healthcare include limited social support, geographic distance from family, language and cultural barriers, financial concerns, and fear of deportation. Most are not insured, and access relies on provisions for emergency medical treatment through the Emergency Medical Treatment and Labor Act and safety net clinics.[83–85] Disparities in hospice access for undocumented immigrants exist in areas where most hospice care is delivered by small, for-profit agencies.[86] Health insurance and healthcare access are limited. Undocumented individuals are excluded from federally funded insurance options (full Medicare and Medicaid). This lack of both insurance and access to needed health services negatively impacts patient and family care and support.

Disability Status

Individuals with physical disabilities or mental illness are at risk of receiving poorer-quality healthcare. Those with differing abilities constitute a cultural group in themselves and often feel stigmatized. This discrimination is evident in cultures where the healthy are more valued than the physically, emotionally, or intellectually challenged.[3] If patients are unable to communicate their needs, then pain and symptom management and EOL wishes are often not addressed. Additionally, this vulnerable population's losses may not be recognized or acknowledged, putting individuals at risk for complicated grief. Taking time to determine an individual's goals of care—regardless of differing abilities—and identifying resources and support to improve QOL is essential.

Essential Cultural Concepts in Palliative Care

Culture impacts all aspects of palliative care. This section focuses on key palliative care issues and concepts that are heavily influenced by patient and family values, practices, and beliefs. Communication, medical decision-making, pain and symptom assessment and management, nutrition, and EOL rituals are presented.

Case Study 2: The Impact of Culture on Palliative Care

Robert was a 74-year-old African American man, diagnosed six months ago with Stage IV pancreatic cancer, with metastases to the liver, lungs, and bones. The palliative care team of a large academic medical center was called to offer a consult during a recent hospitalization for uncontrolled upper back pain and dyspnea. He had previously received palliative radiation, which offered little relief from pain.

Since his diagnosis, he has been living with his daughter and her family (three children, ages 10, 14, and 17) in a small apartment in the inner city because he is unable to care for himself. He refused to take opioids for his back pain and dyspnea, stating "I don't want to become an addict like my brother." Robert's daughter did not want to have him living at her house taking opioids because her oldest daughter has been treated for substance use disorder and "I can't have those drugs in my house."

The oncology and palliative care team agreed that the patient had progression of his cancer, as evidenced by new bone metastases in his hips and new liver metastases. With his past medical history of Type 2 diabetes, hypertension, and renal insufficiency, no further cancer treatment was recommended. The oncologist met with the patient and his daughter and recommended hospice care. Robert was furious that "They are giving up on me," and his daughter states that "They are only suggesting this because they don't want to take care of Medicaid patients like my father at this hospital."

Questions to Consider:

1. What cultural considerations may have contributed to the challenges of pain and symptom management for Robert?
2. What cultural issues may have influenced Robert and his daughter in their mistrust of the healthcare system and his oncology care?
3. What communication strategies may have helped with the complexity of the patient's and daughter's fears and concerns?

Communication

Communication is the foundation for all encounters between nurses, patients, and family members.[87] When the nurse and the patient–family unit are from different cultural backgrounds, discussing news regarding serious illness or a poor prognosis can be challenging if the nurse is not aware of potential cultural conflicts. Communication disparities may lead to poorer outcomes and reduced patient and family satisfaction.[23,88] The establishment of a trusting relationship with the nurse, where the nurse seeks to understand the unique concerns of the patient and family, provides a foundation for all future communication and decision-making.[18]

Communication is an interactive, multidimensional process, often dictated by cultural norms; and it provides the mechanism for human interaction and connection. Given the complexities of communicating diagnosis, prognosis, and progression of a life-limiting disease, there is no common approach that works uniformly.[89] Cultural assessments, including cultural norms related to communication, should occur early in the initial assessment; and findings should be clearly documented and shared with all health providers involved in the care of the patient and family (Box 28.5).

Providing presence and active listening are the most important communication techniques for the nurse to master. Elicit patient and family concerns, customs, norms, beliefs, and values and take time to reflect back what is heard. Encourage patients and families to also reflect back what they have heard. Listening to words alone is not enough. Pay attention to nonverbal cues (e.g., gestures, posture, use or avoidance of eye contact). Nonverbal communication will give valuable information and insight into the emotional impact of what is being said and will help inform the clinician how to respond. The reader is referred to Chapter 5, "Palliative Nursing Communication," for further discussion on this subject.

Shared Decision-Making

Over the past 45 years in the United States, ethical and legal considerations of decision-making have focused on patient autonomy.[32,56] This focus replaced the more paternalistic approach—decision-making as solely the physician's responsibility—with an approach that emphasizes a model of shared responsibility with the patient's active involvement.[28] The Patient Self-Determination Act of 1991 sought to further clarify and to protect an individual's healthcare preferences with advance directives.[90] The principle of respect for

Box 28.5 Culturally Competent Communication Skills and Best Practices for Palliative Care

1. *Foster respect.* Baseline assessment and documentation should include primary language/dialect. Determine need for professional interpreter services. Determine how individuals prefer to be addressed and who should be involved in giving/receiving medical information and participating in decision-making, especially in regard to treatment options for serious illness.
2. *Engage in person-centered conversations through active and reflective listening.* Reflective listening involves hearing, understanding, retaining, analyzing, and evaluating information. Get to know the patient as an individual with values, beliefs, and hopes for the future. During conversations, be aware of cultural implications of nonverbal communication. Is eye contact or touch acceptable during active listening, or is it disrespectful?
3. *Provide presence.* This is the greatest gift nurses can give their patients and families. Listen to the stories, life goals achieved, and future goals. Pull up a chair for a few minutes and let the patient tell you what is important to them. Show empathy and compassion; be quiet/reflective during times of silence.
4. *Assess the patient's interpretation of what is important in life, what gives life meaning for them.* Understanding what is important to the individual and those closest to them will assist in individualizing the palliative care plan. Support the patient's strengths and encourage the patient to maintain hope. Life review can help identify what gives life meaning.
5. *Assess and address religious and spiritual preferences and concerns.* It is important to understand the role that a religious/faith community and spiritual beliefs and practice play in the patient's life. Consider including clergy and others that the individual/family identifies as key supports. Offer spiritual care (books, music, rituals, meditation, etc.) to enhance healing and peace.
6. *Demonstrate consideration of patient's privacy, decision-making strategies, and experience of loss and grief.* Early assessment of cultural issues related to beliefs about disclosure of diagnosis and decision-making preferences will ensure that care is given in ways that respect patient and family values. Observe for signs and symptoms of anticipatory or complicated grief and refer to appropriate interdisciplinary team members.
7. *Assess patient and family knowledge of disease trajectories, if culturally appropriate to discuss.* Assess and address distressing symptoms, side effects of treatment, and likely disease progression. Reaffirm goals of care and attempt the relief of symptoms and other concerns. Incorporate preferred healing practices and traditions. Discuss early access to hospice care to support goals as disease progresses.
8. *Anticipate times when communication will be difficult.* Dealing with serious illness is often stressful. Be proactive by anticipating situations when communication may be difficult (i.e., breaking bad news, holding family meetings, and helping patients and family members communicate last wishes at end of life). Utilize appropriate interdisciplinary team members to provide support to the patient and family during these difficult times.

Source: Reference 98.

patient autonomy points to a patient's right to participate in decisions about the care they receive. Associated with this is the right to be informed of diagnosis, prognosis, and the risks and benefits of treatment to make informed decisions. Inherent in the movement for patient autonomy is the underlying assumption that all patients want control over their healthcare decisions. Yet, in fact, for some individuals, patient autonomy may violate the very principles of dignity and integrity it proposes to uphold and may result in significant distress.[56]

This European–American model of patient autonomy has its origin in the current dominant culture, a predominantly White, middle-class perspective that does not consider diverse cultural perspectives.[3] In fact, in some cultures, patient autonomy may be viewed not as empowering but rather as isolating and burdensome for patients who are too sick to have to make difficult decisions.[56]

Emphasis on autonomy as the guiding principle assumes that the individual, rather than the family or other social group, is the appropriate decision maker.[28] However, in many non–European–American cultures, the concept of interdependence among family and community members is valued more than individual autonomy.[32,56] Cultures that practice family-centered decision-making, such as the Korean American and Mexican American cultures, may prefer that the family, or perhaps a particular family member, rather than the patient receives and processes information.[31,56] The traditional Chinese concept of "filial piety" requires that children, especially the eldest son, are obligated to respect, care for, and protect their parents.[18] Based on the values and beliefs of this culture, the son is obligated to protect the parent from the worry of a terminal prognosis.

Although full disclosure may not be appropriate, it is never appropriate to lie to the patient. If the patient does not wish to receive information and/or telling the patient violates the patient's and family's cultural norms, the healthcare provider may not be respecting the patient's right to autonomously decide not to receive the information. Some cultures believe that telling the patient they have a terminal illness strips away any and all hope, causes needless suffering, and may indeed hasten death.[56] For example, for those adhering to traditional Navajo values, imposing negative information, such as prognosis of a life-limiting illness, on the person who is ill is a dangerous violation of their values.[56]

The nurse must consider the harm that may occur when the health system or providers violate cultural beliefs and practices. Assessing and clarifying the patient's and family's perspectives, values, and practices may prevent a cultural conflict.[3,21] The nurse is in a key position to address these critical patient and family issues (see Box 28.4 for examples of questions to ask). By asking how decisions are made and whether the patient wishes to be involved in both being told information and participating in the decision-making process, nurses respect patient autonomy and honor individual beliefs and values.[21]

Pain and Symptom Assessment and Management

It is important to remember that the acknowledgment and expression of pain and symptoms are heavily influenced by culture. Assessment must be performed with a cultural lens. For some, even the word "pain" has a negative connotation, and some patients may not answer the assessment questions when those terms are used. For example, in certain cultures, it is unacceptable for a male to report pain; admission of pain is a sign of weakness.[3] These individuals may respond more openly to questions about "discomforts," "something hurting you" or "aching," rather than pain.

The same is true when assessing for symptoms. For example, depression, a common symptom in palliative care, may not be assessable simply using the standard assessment question "Are you depressed?" Patients who are unable to admit depression due to stigma or other cultural considerations may be open to discussing feelings of "sadness" or "having no energy" or "no interest in things that usually bring joy." An association between the report of symptoms and symptom distress has been reported. Individuals from Asian-speaking communities in the United States have reported low symptom distress because of their fatalistic beliefs regarding acknowledging symptoms and their meaning. Sensitivity to the language used in assessment of pain and symptoms is essential for an accurate assessment.

Managing pain and symptoms may also be culturally challenging. If a patient and family have relied on remedies commonly used in their culture to manage symptoms, insisting on more Western-style medications/interventions is inappropriate and can result in a cultural clash and an ethical dilemma. These dilemmas can be exacerbated in the current cultural climate surrounding the use of opioids and substance use disorder. It is important that the nurse work together with the patient and family and the team to identify safe, effective, and culturally respectful ways to address pain and symptoms associated with the serious illness.

Research has demonstrated that racial and ethnic differences continue to exist in pain assessment and pain management.[25] The unmet needs for good pain management in an African American population when compared to a Caucasian population at the time of a palliative care consult highlight this issue in the United States.[91] Western providers are reported to underestimate pain in 75% of African Americans and 64% of Hispanics experiencing pain.[92] It is important to be aware of these disparities in delivery of quality palliative care and work to ensure equal care for all.

Nutrition

One of the most central aspects of caring for each other in nearly every culture is feeding. Food and nutrition are essential human needs, and sharing food together is an essential social interaction for families and communities. When patients with serious illness no longer have the desire or ability to take food in, families often become distressed. Many mistakenly believe that providing food or fluids at the end of life will prolong survival.[93] Research has shown that the burdens associated with medically administered nutrition or hydration at the end of life usually outweigh the benefits.[34] Families need to be educated about the burdens and taught ways to provide care other than making food or feeding. For example, teaching them how to do good oral care for the patient, keeping the mucous membranes and lips moist, will allow them to provide comfort and physical caregiving. Encouraging them to offer small bites of favorite foods for pleasure and tasting can be enjoyable for the patient and family. This is especially important when certain cultural foods are essential for QOL.[11,37,93]

EOL Rituals

It is critical that the nurse explores what cultural rituals should be honored as death approaches, at the time of death, and immediately after death. These important rituals and practices should be known well in advance of the death, if possible. Rituals are important social aspects of care that can provide a means to express emotions, ease anxiety, and offer structure in times of distress.[94] However, if the patient and family are not given the opportunity to engage in valued rituals, needless suffering occurs, and the grieving process may be complicated. Memories of the loved one's death will stay with the family forever.

Examples of rituals prior to death that may be offered include, among others, having a priest administer the sacrament of the sick to practicing Catholics. Those who are practicing Hindi may prefer to die at home, lying on the floor close to Mother Earth.[55] Every effort should be made to get the patient home and honor that valued practice. Immediately after death, for those adhering to the Muslim faith, the body should be placed facing Mecca or the east. This should be known ahead of time and honored immediately following death. In the Orthodox Jewish tradition, as well in other cultures, care of the body after death is gender-dependent.[18] Therefore, it is important after death that a female nurse not clean a male body if the family is adhering to Orthodox practices.

Rituals that are spiritual and nondenominational can be a tremendous support to families after the death of their loved one. A bathing and honoring ritual, developed by hospice nurses at Cottage Hospice in California, has been shown to be a meaningful way to respect the patient's body, honoring the person-centeredness of that individual and comforting the family.[95] This ritual can be offered by nurses in acute care, hospice or home care, and long-term care.

Finally, rituals that honor the work that professionals have done in caring for the deceased patient and family are extremely important to our profession. Taking a moment at the time of death to honor the person who has died as "somebody's mother, somebody's daughter, somebody's loved one" is essential to healthy grieving for the healthcare team. A ritual called "The Pause," performed after death in the emergency room or in the intensive care unit, is appropriate in all healthcare settings and important in preventing compassion fatigue in healthcare workers.[96]

Conclusion

Given the changing population of the United States, nurses must advocate for the integration of cultural considerations in providing comprehensive palliative care. It is imperative that each of us move beyond our own ethnocentric view of the world to appreciate and respect the similarities and differences in each other. We are challenged to embrace a better understanding of various perspectives. Striving for this understanding first requires an awareness of how one's own cultural background impacts care. In addition, acquiring knowledge about cultures and developing skill in cultural assessment and communication are essential to improving palliative care for patients with life-limiting illnesses and their families. Most importantly, maintaining a sense of cultural humility, caring for each patient/family member as a unique human being with unique needs, and attending to those needs with dignity and respectfulness are the essence of providing culturally sensitive care.

This chapter encourages nurses to integrate cultural assessment and culturally appropriate interventions into palliative care. It is the hope of the authors that readers will enrich their practice by seeking new knowledge about different cultures through available resources and, most importantly, by respectfully interacting with the most valuable resources on cultural considerations we have—our patients and their families.

Acknowledgment

We would like to acknowledge Polly Mazanec and Joan Panke for their efforts and significant contributions in the previous edition of this chapter that laid the foundation for this version.

REFERENCES

1. Merriam-Webster. Culture. Accessed October 17, 2022. https://www.merriam-webster.com/dictionary/culture.
2. Purnell LD, Fenkl EA. Transcultural diversity and health care. In: *Handbook for Culturally Competent Care*. Springer International Publishing; 2019:1–6. https://doi.org/10.1007/978-3-030-21946-8_1.
3. American Association of Colleges of Nursing. End-of-Life Nursing Education Consortium. Updated 2022. Accessed October 13, 2022. http://www.aacnnursing.org/ELNEC.
4. US Department of Health and Human Services. Social Determinants of Health. 2022. Accessed October 20, 2022. https://health.gov/healthypeople/priority-areas/social-determinants-health.
5. Dahlin C, DePace N, Ford J, Maani-Fogelman P, Chow K. Promoting health equity: palliative nurses on the frontlines. *J Hosp Palliat Nurs*. 2022;24(4):218–224. https://doi.org/10.1097/NJH.0000000000000864.
6. Rosa WE, Krakauer EL, Farmer PE, et al. The global nursing workforce: realising universal palliative care. *Lancet Glob Health*. 2020;8(3):e327–e328. https://doi.org/10.1016/S2214-109X(19)30554-6.
7. Abedi V, Olulana O, Avula V, et al. Racial, economic, and health inequality and COVID-19 infection in the United States. *J Racial Ethn Health Disparities*. 2021;8(3):732–742. https://doi.org/10.1007/s40615-020-00833-4.
8. Núñez A, Sreeganga SD, Ramaprasad A. Access to healthcare during COVID-19. *Int J Environ Res Public Health*. 2021;18(6):2980. https://doi.org/10.3390/ijerph18062980.
9. Rosa WE, Pandey S, Epstein AS, et al. The 2nd annual US celebration of world hospice and palliative care day: a virtual coming together to support equity in palliative care access. *Palliat Support Care*. 2022;20(3):307–312. https://doi.org/10.1017/S147895152200013X.
10. Bruns DP, Kraguljac NV, Bruns TR. COVID-19: facts, cultural considerations, and risk of stigmatization. *J Transcult Nurs*. 2020;31(4):326–332. https://doi.org/10.1177/1043659620917724.
11. Sovran S. Understanding culture and HIV/AIDS in sub-Saharan Africa. *SAHARA J*. 2013;10(1):32–41. https://doi.org/10.1080/17290376.2013.807071.
12. US Census Bureau. QuickFacts United States. Accessed October 17, 2022. https://www.census.gov/quickfacts/fact/table/US/PST045216.
13. Ferrell, B. Introduction to palliative care. In: Ferrell BR, Paice JA, eds. *Oxford Textbook of Palliative Nursing*. 5th ed. Oxford University Press; 2019:3–4.
14. National Consensus Project for Quality Palliative Care. *Clinical Practice Guidelines for Quality Palliative Care*. 4th ed. National Consensus Project for Quality Palliative Care; 2018. https://www.nationalcoalitionhpc.org/ncp/.
15. Ferrell BR, ed. *Spiritual, Religious, and Cultural Aspects of Care*. Oxford University Press; 2016.
16. Campinha-Bacote J. A model and instrument for addressing cultural competence in health care. *J Nurs Educ*. 1999;38(5):203–207.
17. Foronda C, Porter A, Phitwong A. Psychometric testing of an instrument to measure cultural humility. *J Transcult Nurs*. 2021;32(4):399–404. https://doi.org/10.1177/1043659620950420.
18. Spector R. *Cultural Diversity in Health and Illness*. 9th ed. Pearson Education; 2016.
19. Neubauer K, Dixon W, Corona R, Bodurtha J. Cultural humility. In: Wittenberg E, Ferrell B, Goldsmith J, et al., eds. *Textbook of Palliative Care Communication*. Oxford University Press; 2015:79–89.
20. Gradellini C, Gómez-Cantarino S, Dominguez-Isabel P, Molina-Gallego B, Mecugni D, Ugarte-Gurrutxaga MI. Cultural competence and cultural sensitivity education in university nursing courses. A scoping review. *Front Psychol*. 2021;12:682920. https://doi.org/10.3389/fpsyg.2021.682920.
21. Sharifi N, Adib-Hajbaghery M, Najafi M. Cultural competence in nursing: a concept analysis. *Int J Nurs Stud*. 2019;99:103386. https://doi.org/10.1016/j.ijnurstu.2019.103386.
22. Abualhaija N. Clarifying cultural competence in nursing: a concept analysis approach. *J Cult Diversity*. 2021;28(1):3–14.
23. Foley H, Mazanec P. Culture and considerations in palliative care. In: Plakovic K, Bobb B, Coyne P, eds. *Conversations in palliative care: questions and answers with the experts*. Hospice and Palliative Nurses Association; 2017:189–198.
24. Koffman J, Calanzani N. Ethnic and cultural aspects of palliative care and end of life care. In: Cherny N, Fallon M, Kaasa S, Portenoy R, Currow D, eds. *Oxford Textbook of Palliative Medicine*. 6th ed. Oxford University Press; 2021:76–92.
25. Payne R. Racially associated disparities in hospice and palliative care access: acknowledging the facts while addressing the opportunities to improve. *J Palliat Med*. 2016;19(2):131–133.
26. Chen J, Vargas-Bustamante A, Mortensen K, Ortega AN. Racial and ethnic disparities in health care access and utilization under the Affordable Care Act. *Med Care*. 2016;54(2):140–146.
27. Brandon DT, Isaac LA, LaVeist TA. The legacy of Tuskegee and trust in medical care: is Tuskegee responsible for race differences in mistrust of medical care? *J Natl Med Assoc*. 2005;97(7):951–956.
28. Bullock K. The influence of culture on end-of-life decision making. *J Soc Work End Life Palliat Care*. 2011;7(1):83–98.
29. Callaghan KA, Fanning JB. Managing bias in palliative care: professional hazards in goals of care discussion at the end of life. *Am J Hosp Palliat Care*. 2018;35(2):355–363.
30. Evans BC, Ume E. Psychosocial, cultural, and spiritual health disparities in end-of-life and palliative care: where we are and where we need to go. *Nurs Outlook*. 2012;60(6):370–375.
31. Office of Minority Health. National Center on Minority Health and Health Disparities. Accessed October 17, 2022. http://www.nimhd.nih.gov/.
32. Portanova J, Ailshire J, Perez C, Rahman A, Engvidanos S. Ethnic differences in advance directive completion and care preferences: what has changed in a decade. *J Am Geriatr Soc*. 2017;68(6):1352–1357.
33. Teno JM, Plotzke M, Christian T, Gozalo P. Examining variation in hospice visits by professional staff in the last 2 days of life. *JAMA Intern Med*. 2016;176(3):364–370.
34. Abunafeesa H, Elsayem AF. Cultural diversity and barriers to high-quality end of life care. *Ann Palliat Med*. 2017;6(2):183–186.
35. Balboni TA, Fitchett G, Handzo GF, et al. State of the science of spirituality and palliative care research part II: screening, assessment, and interventions. *J Pain Symptom Manage*. 2017;54(3):441–453.
36. Leininger M. Quality of life from a transcultural nursing perspective. *Nurs Sci Q*. 1994;7(1):22–28.

37. Prince-Paul M, Daly BJ. Ethical considerations in palliative care. In: Ferrell B, Paice JA, eds. *Oxford Textbook of Palliative Nursing*. 5th ed. Oxford University Press; 2019:824–836.
38. World Health Organization. Child Mortality (under 5 Years). January 28, 2022. Accessed October 19, 2022. https://www.who.int/news-room/fact-sheets/detail/levels-and-trends-in-child-under-5-mortality-in-2020.
39. Catlin A, Brandon D, Wool C, Mendes J. Palliative and end-of-life care for newborns and infants: from the National Association of Neonatal Nurses. *Adv Neonatal Care*. 2015;15(4):239–240. https://doi.org/10.1097/ANC.0000000000000215.
40. Linebarger JS, Johnson V, Boss RD, et al. Guidance for pediatric end-of-life care. *Pediatrics (Evanston)*. 2022;149(5):e2022057011. https://doi.org/10.1542/peds.2022-057011.
41. National Hospice and Palliative Care Organization. *Standards of Practice for Pediatric Palliative Care: Quality Improvement Resource*. National Hospice and Palliative Care Organization; 2022. https://www.nhpco.org/wp-content/uploads/Pediatric_Standards.pdf.
42. Burns C, Dunn A, Brady M, Starr N, Blosser C. *Pediatric Primary Care*. 5th ed. Elsevier; 2013.
43. Mack JW, Cronin A, Fasciano K, Block SD, Keating NL. Cancer treatment decision-making among young adults with lung and colorectal cancer: a comparison with adults in middle age. *Psychooncology*. 2016;25(9):1085–1091.
44. World Health Organization. Ageing and Health. 2022. Accessed October 13, 2022. https://www.who.int/news-room/fact-sheets/detail/ageing-and-health.
45. Morgan T, Ann Williams L, Trussardi G, Gott M. Gender and family caregiving at the end-of-life in the context of old age: a systematic review. *Palliat Med*. 2016;30(7):616–624.
46. Kent E, Rowland J, Northouse L, et al. Caring for caregivers and patients: research and clinical priorities for informal cancer caregivers. *Cancer*. 2016; 122(3):1987–1995.
47. Ferrell B, Wittenberg E. A review of family caregiving intervention trials in oncology. *CA Cancer J Clin*. 2017;67(4):318–325.
48. Acquaviva K. *LGBTQ-Inclusive Hospice and Palliative Care*. Harrington Park Press; 2017.
49. National LGBT Cancer Network. LGBT Palliative Care. 2022. Accessed October 17, 2022. https://cancer-network.org/cancer-information/cancer-and-the-lgbt-community/lgbt-palliative-care/.
50. Cloyes KG, Hull W, Davis A. Palliative and end-of-life care for lesbian, gay, bisexual, and transgender (LGBT) cancer patients and their caregivers. *Semin Oncol Nurs*. 2018;34(1):60–71. https://doi.org/10.1016/j.soncn.2017.12.003.
51. Barrett N, Wholihan D. Providing palliative care to LGBTQ patients. *Nurs Clin North Am*. 2016;51(3):501–511.
52. Jacobson J. LGBT older adults in long-term care. *Am J Nurs*. 2017;117(8):18–20.
53. Taylor EJ. Spiritual assessment. In: Ferrell B, Coyle N, Paice J, eds. *Oxford Textbook of Palliative Nursing*. 5th ed. Oxford University Press; 2019:432–446.
54. Puchalski CM. Spirituality in geriatric palliative care. *Clin Geriatr Med*. 2019;31(2):245–252.
55. Shah M, Sorajjakool S. Hinduism. In: Sorajjakool S, Carr M, Bursey E, eds. *World Religions for Healthcare Professionals*. Routledge Taylor & Francis Group; 2017:32–48.
56. Johnstone MJ, Kanitsaki O. Ethics and advance care planning in a culturally diverse society. *J Transcult Nurs*. 2009;20(4):405–416.
57. Puchalski CM, Ferrell BR, O'Donnell EO. Spiritual issues in palliative care. In: Yennurajalingam S, Bruera E, eds. *Oxford American Handbook of Hospice and Palliative Medicine & Supportive Care*. 2nd ed. Oxford University Press; 2016:257–272.
58. National Academies of Sciences, Engineering, and Medicine; National Academy of Medicine; Committee on the Future of Nursing 2020–2030. In: Flaubert JL, Le Menestrel S, Williams DR, Wakefield MK, eds. *The Future of Nursing 2020–2030: Charting a Path to Achieve Health Equity*. Washington (DC): National Academies Press (US); May 11, 2021.
59. American Psychological Association. Education and Socioeconomic Status. 2017. Accessed October 17, 2022. http://www.apa.org/pi/ses/resources/publications/education.aspx.
60. Centers for Disease Control and Prevention. Understanding Health Literacy. September 13, 2022. Accessed October 17, 2022. https://www.cdc.gov/healthliteracy/learn/understanding.html.
61. Centers for Disease Control and Prevention. What Is Health Literacy? February 2, 2022. Accessed October 17, 2022. https://www.cdc.gov/healthliteracy/learn/index.html.
62. Centers for Disease Control and Prevention. Understanding Literacy and Numeracy. June 10, 2022. Accessed October 17, 2022. https://www.cdc.gov/healthliteracy/learn/UnderstandingLiteracy.html.
63. Bauhoff S, Carmann K, Wuppermann A. *Financial Literacy & Consumer Choice of Health Insurance: Evidence from Low-Income Populations in the US*. RAND Center for the Study of Aging, RAND Population Research Center; 2013.
64. Panke JT, Bayne S. Palliative care and hospice care for patients with cancer. In: Camp-Sorrell D, Hawkins R, eds. *In Practice Oncology Nursing*. 3rd ed. Burlington, MA: Jones & Bartlett Learning; 2017:287–303.
65. Lynch S. Hospice and palliative care access issues in rural areas. *Am J Hosp Palliat Care*. 2013;30(2):172–177.
66. Center to Advance Palliative Care. Growth of Palliative Care in US Hospitals: 2022 Snapshot (2000–2020). 2022. Accessed October 17, 2022. https://www.capc.org/documents/download/1031/.
67. Institute of Medicine. *Dying in America: Improving Quality and Honoring Individual Preferences Near the End of Life*. National Academies Press; 2014.
68. Currow DC, Allingham S, Bird S, et al. Referral patterns and proximity to palliative care inpatient services by level of socio-economic disadvantage. A national study using spatial analysis. *BMC Health Serv Res*. 2012;12:424.
69. Baernholdt M, Campbell CL, Hinton ID, Yan G, Lewis E. Quality of hospice care: comparison between rural and urban residents. *J Nurs Care Qual*. 2015;30(3):247–253.
70. Taylor R, Dionne-Odom N, Currie E, Stockdill M, Bakitas M. Rural palliative care. In: Ferrell B, Coyle N, eds. *Oxford Textbook of Palliative Nursing*. 5th ed. Oxford University Press; 2019:670–681.
71. Sumalinog R, Harrington K, Dosani N, Hwang SW. Advance care planning, palliative care, and end-of-life care interventions for homeless people: a systematic review. *Palliat Med*. 2017;31(2):109–119.
72. United Nations Commission on Human Rights. *Report of the Special Rapporteur on Adequate Housing as a Component of the Right to an Adequate Standard of Living*. February 25, 2005. Accessed October 17, 2022. http://www.un.org/womenwatch/ods/E-CN.4-2005-43-E.pdf.
73. Tobey M, Manasson J, Decarlo K, Ciraldo-Maryniuk K, Gaeta JM, Wilson E. Homeless individuals approaching the end of life: symptoms and attitudes. *J Pain Symptom Manage*. 2017;53(4):738–744.
74. Ko E, Nelson-Becker H. Does end-of-life decision making matter? Perspectives of older homeless adults. *Am J Hosp Palliat Med*. 2013;31(2):183–188.

75. McNeil R, Guirguis-Younger M, Dilley LB. Recommendations for improving the end-of-life care system for homeless populations: a qualitative study of the views of Canadian health and social services professionals. *BMC Palliat Care*. 2012;11:14.
76. Huynh L, Henry B, Dosani N. Minding the gap: access to palliative care and the homeless. *BMC Palliat Care*. 2015;14:62.
77. Hudson BF, Flemming K, Shulman C, Candy B. Challenges to access and provision of palliative care for people who are homeless: a systematic review of qualitative research. *BMC Palliat Care*. 2016;15(1):96.
78. Hughes A. Poor, homeless, and underserved populations. In: Coyle N, Ferrell BR, eds. *HPNA Palliative Nursing Manuals: Legal and Ethical Aspects of Care*. Oxford University Press; 2016:89–117.
79. Maschi T, Marmo S, Han J. Palliative and end-of-life care in prisons: a content analysis of the literature. *Int J Prison Health*. 2014;10(3):172–197.
80. Yarnell CJ, Fu L, Manuel D, et al. Association between immigrant status and end-of-life care in Ontario, Canada. *JAMA*. 2017;318(15): 1479–1488.
81. Harhay MO, Halpern SD. End-of-life care among immigrants: disparities or differences in preferences? *JAMA*. 2017;318(15):1448–1449.
82. Budiman A. Key Findings about US Immigrants. Pew Research Center. 2020. Accessed October 19, 2022. https://www.pewresearch.org/fact-tank/2020/08/20/key-findings-about-u-s-immigrants/.
83. Helft PR. To keep them from injustice: reflections on the care of unauthorized immigrants with cancer. *J Oncol Pract*. 2012;8(4):212–214.
84. Hastings Center. Undocumented Immigrants and Health Care Access in the United States. March 29, 2022. Accessed January 14, 2025. https://undocumented.thehastingscenter.org/executive-summary/.
85. Beck TL, Le TK, Henry-Okafor Q, Shah MK. Medical care for undocumented immigrants: national and international issues. *Prim Care*. 2017;44(1):e1–e13.
86. Gray NA, Boucher NA, Kuchibhatla M, Johnson KS. Hospice access for undocumented immigrants. *JAMA Int Med*. 2017:177(4):579–580.
87. Dahlin C, Wittenberg-Lyles E. Communication in palliative care: an essential competency for nurses. In: Ferrell B, Coyle N, Paice J, eds. *Oxford Textbook of Palliative* Nursing. 5th ed. Oxford University Press; 2022:55–78.
88. Butow P, Bell M, Goldstein D, et al. Grappling with cultural differences; communication between oncologists and immigrant cancer patients with and without interpreters. *Patient Educ Couns*. 2011;84(3):398–405.
89. Williams SW, Hanson LC, Boyd C, et al. Communication, decision making, and cancer: what African Americans want physicians to know. *J Palliat Med*. 2008;11(9):1221–1226.
90. US Congress. H.R.4449—Patient Self Determination Act of 1990. 101st Cong. (1989–1990). Accessed October 22, 2022. https://www.congress.gov/bill/101st-congress/house-bill/4449.
91. Kamal AH, Bull J, Wolf SP, Portman D, Strand J, Johnson KS. Unmet needs of African Americans and Whites at the time of palliative care consultation. *Am J Hosp Palliat Care*. 2017;34(5):461–465.
92. Brant J. Holistic total pain management in palliative care: cultural and global considerations. *Palliat Med Hosp Care Open J*. 2017;SE(1):S32–S38.
93. Lynch MT. Palliative care at the end of life. *Semin Oncol Nurs*. 2014;30(4):268–279.
94. Berry P, Griffie J. Planning for the actual death. In: Ferrell B, Coyle N, Paice J, eds. *Oxford Textbook of Palliative Nursing*. 4th ed. Oxford University Press; 2019:420–431.
95. Rodgers D, Calmes B, Grotts J. Nursing care at the time of death: a bathing and honoring practice. *Oncol Nurs Forum*. 2016;43(3):363–371.
96. ProvidenceSpokane. The Pause. Youtube. February 3, 2014. Accessed October 17, 2022. https://www.youtube.com/watch?v=_HVXM2YhZ2A&app=desktop.
97. Worldwide Hospice Palliative Care Alliance. Campaign Toolkit: Leave No One Behind. 2021. http://www.thewhpca.org/resources-2021/category/campaign-toolkit-leave-no-one-behind.
98. Long CO. Ten best practices to enhance culturally competent communication in palliative care. *J Pediatr Hematol Oncol*. 2011;33(suppl 2):S136–S139.

29

Supporting Families and Family Caregivers in Palliative Care

Tamryn F. Gray and J. Nicholas Odom

Key Points

- The diagnosis of a life-threatening illness affects not only the patient but individual family members, relatives, friends, and the entire family.
- Family members who provide care—family caregivers—require support from nurses and the healthcare system to sustain them in their caregiving role. The health and well-being of the family caregiver are just as important as those of the patient, regardless of the caregiver's age, racial and ethnic background, socioeconomic and immigrant status, health condition, health literacy, or location of residence.
- Family members look to nurses and other health professionals to provide quality care to the patient in palliative care but also expect nurses to meet their needs for information, emotional support, and assistance with care. For the vast majority of families, contributing to the care of their loved one is important. Individualizing care based on the needs of each family and its members is a key role for nurses who provide family-centered palliative care.

Introduction

When a family member is faced with a life-threatening illness, it affects the entire family. Anticipating the loss of a significant other not only causes disruptions to the family unit as a whole but can challenge individual family members to make sense of the impending loss. Many families show resilience and adaptation in the face of such stress,[1–4] and these experiences have the potential to create a deeper sense of meaning and connection among family members.[5] At the same time, research suggests a significant percentage of family members—18%–35%—experience some form of psychological morbidity,[6,7] and if family members are giving care—family caregiving—the physical and financial consequences can be substantial.[8,9]

Nurses working with people diagnosed with a serious illness are in a primary position to provide support to family members and families. Family-centered care is an important part of nursing practice, and, in the context of palliative care, the family as the unit of care has been central since the inception of the modern hospice and palliative care movement. The World Health Organization states that palliative care should improve the quality of life of patients and their families. A family's experience of having an ill member is best understood in the context of their relationships with each other, and this becomes even more so when a family member is ill and requires care.[10] Changing patterns of dependency, reciprocity, and the rewards and challenges that arise influence each family in different ways. As such, palliative care focuses on family as the unit of care,[11] experienced uniquely for each family and the individuals in it.

This chapter focuses on the family as the unit of care and places emphasis on family caregivers in palliative care. Family members who provide care to a relative or friend make substantial contributions to that individual's overall healthcare. Many families willingly assume the role of family caregiver for someone with life-limiting illness, often doing so out of a sense of love, compassion, or obligations to care. Providing such support can result in positive changes in family members and personal growth[12–14]; however, many families and family caregivers are not always fully prepared for the potential cost of caregiving to their physical, mental, and financial health, particularly when they are full low-income households.[15] Some family caregivers do not perceive themselves to be in need of support from healthcare professionals and the healthcare system, even when giving care and support to an ill member becomes overly burdensome.[16,17]

In recent years, family caregiving has become a more critical public health issue for several reasons. Improvements in treatments to control diseases mean that patients can often live an extended period of time with life-limiting illness. Depending on the illness, the decline toward death is sometimes precipitous, allowing little time for the family and the caregiver to adapt and acquire the necessary knowledge to support the person dying and themselves.[18] Additionally, many family caregivers are now asked to perform tasks and procedures in the home (and sometimes in the hospital)[19–21] that were once the exclusive domain of nursing care.[22] Family caregivers assist individuals with serious illness by meeting their basic needs (e.g., meals, shelter, transportation, essential daily personal care), providing social and emotional support, coordinating healthcare and appointments, participating in healthcare decision-making, managing medication, procuring and overseeing the use of medical equipment, performing medical/nursing tasks in the home, and acting as advocates and surrogates for legal and financial matters.[23] Fewer children per family and a more mobile society mean that there are usually fewer family members present to care for dying relatives and those with complex needs.[24] And, since we are living longer with more comorbidity, caregiving is more complex; spouse caregivers are older and often have their own serious illnesses as well.[24] Additionally, a growing older adult population, smaller family sizes, and greater geographic and social mobility place considerable demands on family caregivers whose contribution to the sustainability of health and social care systems is significant.[25,26]

As a basis for offering optimal support to families in palliative care, this chapter will discuss family-centered palliative care and the experience of family members in supporting their significant others. In addition to presenting research that will inform nursing interventions for families, this chapter will include what is involved in being a family caregiver and some of the challenges that family caregivers face. In keeping with a core focus in palliative care on quality of life, important elements in promoting family caregiver quality of life and the needs of caregivers will be outlined. Considerations in family caregiver assessment and how to support family caregivers in the home, in the hospital, and in intensive care, perioperative, and long-term care settings will also be highlighted, as will the family's role in decision-making and advance care planning, including providing resources that nurses can use to promote family-centered palliative care.

Family-Centered Palliative Care

Currently, an estimated 66 million Americans, or roughly 30% of the adult population, are caregivers, and nearly two thirds are women.[27] Recognizing the importance of a family focus necessitates clearly defining what is meant by "family" and "family caregiving." Most often, families in palliative care consist of patients, their partners, and their children. But, in today's world of divorce, repartnering, remarriage, and cohabitation,[28–30] step-relatives must also enter into the family portrait. In other instances, people unrelated by blood or marriage (also referred to as "families of origin" and "families of choice")[31,32] and families made up of lesbian, gay, bisexual, trans, and queer or questioning (LGBTQ) individuals mean that our definitions of families in palliative care must necessarily be broad and diverse.[29] Census definitions of family have tended to focus on defining family as people living in one household; but we know that not all family members live together, and how family is defined can vary from country to country.[33]

For the purposes of this chapter, family is defined as a group of individuals inextricably linked in ways that are constantly interactive and mutually reinforcing. Family can mean direct blood relatives, relationships through an emotional commitment, or the group or person with whom an individual feels most connected.[32] In its broadest sense, family is defined as whoever the person says their family is, including relatives, partners, neighbors, and friends.[32] Family caregivers in the palliative care context are defined as individuals who provide unpaid care and support to a family member, friend, neighbor, or significant other who has a physical or mental disability, is chronically ill or frail, and, in particular, is diagnosed with a disease where the likelihood of death is high.[33]

Palliative care programs are based on the principle that the family is the unit of care. In practice, the family is often viewed as a group of individuals who are sometimes perceived to be helpful or to resist efforts to deliver care. Regardless of the family situation and composition in palliative care, nurses and other health professionals must strive to understand the meaning of the palliative experience to the family as a whole, as well as to its individual members.[34] Some of the best outcomes are achieved when appropriate interventions are directed toward family members both individually and as a group.[34,35] If quality care is to be provided, nurses need to understand how all family members perceive their experience, how the relationships fit together, and that a multitude of factors interact to make families what they are.[35]

In the past 10–15 years, research has gone beyond focusing on the needs of dying patients for comfort and palliation to addressing issues relevant to other family members. Much of this research has focused on the family's perceptions of their needs,[36,37] experiences and challenges faced,[24] adaptation and coping skills required for home care,[38,39] the supportiveness of nursing behaviors[40,41] or physician behaviors,[42] and satisfaction with care.[41] Though research used to focus primarily on families of patients with cancer, palliative care extends the focus to other life-threatening illnesses. Reports for other diagnostic populations, such as Parkinson's disease,[43,44] heart disease,[45] motor neuron disease,[46] lung disease,[42,47] kidney disease,[48,49] and neurodegenerative diseases,[40,42] are becoming more available, as is research and clinical care focused on the care needs of people with dementia and their families.[49,50] Regardless of disease or condition, research makes it clear that family members look to nurses and other health professionals to provide quality care to the patient.[48] Family members expect health professionals to meet their needs for information, emotional support, and assistance with care.[41] Recent research suggests that one of the most effective ways to support families may be to help them be successful in their caregiving roles.[41] Providing care might not always be what families desire,[51] but, for the vast majority of families and their members, contributing to the care of their significant other is important. Individualizing care for each family and its members is a key role for nurses who provide family-centered palliative care.

Supporting Family Members and Family Caregivers from Historically Marginalized and Underrepresented Backgrounds

Racially Diverse Caregivers

Demographic shifts in the United States have led to an increased interest in research on racial and ethnic differences in caregiving.[52] Currently, nearly 40% of caregivers identify as Black/African American, Latino, and Native American/Indigenous.[53] In particular, Latino and Black/African American family caregivers experience higher burdens from caregiving and spend more time caregiving on average than their White or Asian American counterparts. On average, 57% of Black/African American family caregivers experience high caregiver burden and work 30 hours per week, compared to Hispanic family caregivers (45% and 30 hours per week), White caregivers (33% and 20 hours per week), and Asian American caregivers (30% and 16 hours per week).[53] Family caregivers from historically marginalized racial and ethnic backgrounds often provide more intensive caregiving, for longer, and have outcomes that are worse than those experienced by White caregivers.[54] Given the racial disparities that exist in palliative and end-of-life care, it is essential for clinicians to consider the unique needs of caregivers from racially marginalized backgrounds and understand how many of their concerns may be grounded in cultural, historical, and racial experiences. Systemic injustice, mistrust and stigmatizing behavior, and historical discrimination from clinicians and health systems play a role in caregiver access to and use of formal services for involvement in care, caregiver support and training, and respite care. Research has demonstrated that caregiver stress centers around key areas, including lack of family support, communication barriers with healthcare professionals, minority stress, caregiver burden, and lack of spiritual support.[55] Linking these caregivers with faith-based organizations, community-based organizations, culturally and linguistically competent educational materials, and support groups with other caregivers who have similar background and experiences is key to providing optimal care for these family caregivers.

Strategies to Support Racially Diverse Caregivers

National guidelines endorse cultural competence training as a strategy to advance health equity and reduce disparities in care.[56] With the growing racial and ethnic diversity of our caregiving population, it has become increasingly important for palliative care nurses to understand how caregivers' racial backgrounds and culture influence their role. Additionally, when palliative care nurses screen for and evaluate racially diverse caregiver needs, they must ensure that the assessment tools accurately measure variables that are culturally appropriate and culturally relevant to these caregivers, and they must ensure to adequately capture these caregivers' experiences.

LGBTQ Caregivers

There is a growing body of work addressing specific issues and concerns facing the LGBTQ community, but until recently the fields of palliative care and hospice have been largely silent on best practices regarding members of the community.[57] Due to long-standing historical events, members of the LGBTQ population have experienced multiple societal barriers to living life fully and safely as well as aging gracefully.[58] However, the number of individuals who identify as LGBTQ is expected to continue rising over the next 10 years, thus prompting the urgent need to address the inadequate, disrespectful, discriminatory, and abusive care that many patients and their chosen families receive.[59] At the level of the clinical encounter, sexual and gender minorities and their chosen families are at risk for implicit and explicit biases throughout the care continuum.[60] On an institutional/systemic level, the lack of sexual orientation and gender identity data collection stymies efforts to track relevant outcomes.[60]

Strategies to Support LGBTQ Caregivers

There are several strategies recommended to support LGBTQ caregivers of persons with serious illness. First, it is imperative that clinicians foster a welcoming environment to build trust and perceived safety with their patients and caregivers.[60] Palliative care nurses are well-positioned to provide supportive and competent care for LGBTQ family caregivers who provide care for individuals with serious illnesses. Learning and applying competent care are necessary to understand and address LGBTQ caregivers' social and historical structures of oppression (e.g., homophobia, transphobia, heteronormativity, lack of legal protection, institutionalized discrimination) and how these structures intersect with their need for holistic, patient- and family-centered palliative and end-of-life care.[57] Beyond individuals' behaviors and knowledge, palliative and hospice service providers must also pay attention to environmental and cultural factors that support inclusivity and continuity of care by allowing family members opportunities to be involved in care and decision-making, acknowledged by the care team, and able to disclose their sexual and gender orientation. Second, these family caregivers should be asked about their relationship status with the patient and receive support and grief services that are welcoming and affirming.[57] Palliative care nurses should inquire about the relationship with family members of origin and patients' preferences about their role in caregiving and surrogate decision-making as well as ask patients if they have discussed their care wishes with designated surrogates and clarified whether there is conflict between the family of origin and the chosen family caregivers if different.[60]

Summary

In summary, when engaging with caregivers from historically marginalized and underrepresented backgrounds, palliative care nurses have a responsibility to use a relationship-based approach as well as take the time to understand family relationship and attune communication and practice based on the individual caregiver. To mitigate bias and behaviors of oppression toward these caregivers, nurses must be trained in implicit bias education and held accountable for discriminatory behaviors. Additionally, there must be enhanced recruitment and retention efforts targeting nurses from racially and ethnically diverse backgrounds into palliative care as well as nurses who are sexual and gender minorities to mirror the nation's diverse population.[61] Figure 29.1 provides a figurative description of the diversity and heterogenous needs of family caregivers within the individual caregiver-, care recipient-, caregiving-, and caregiving-context levels.

Understanding the Experiences of Families in Palliative Care

The Transition of Fading Away

When a family member is faced with a life-threatening illness, the impending death presents a challenge to the entire family. Family members must try to find new balance during the illness and after their significant other has died. One of the most comprehensive research programs directed toward understanding the experiences of families in palliative care evolved from nurses' concerns about how to provide family-centered palliative care.[63] Steele and Davies[64] noted that nurses in a regional cancer center constantly had to attend to the needs of not only patients but also patients' families, particularly as they moved back and forth between hospital and home. In searching the literature for guidelines about family-centered care, Davies and her colleagues[63] found that many articles were about the needs of patients and family members, about levels of family members' satisfaction with care, and about family members' perceptions of nurses;

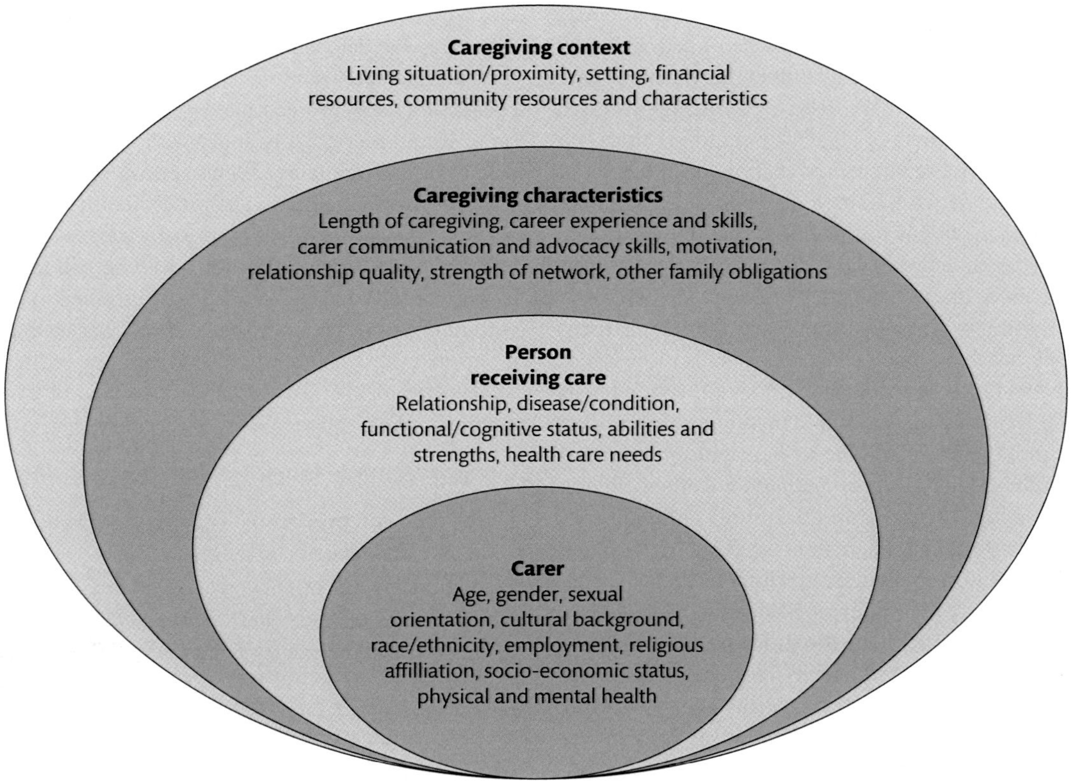

Figure 29.1 Family caregivers themselves are diverse and have heterogeneous needs that are shaped by a wide range of factors.
Source: Reference 62.

but nothing really described the families' experiences as they coped with the terminal illness of a beloved family member. Their research program, studying families of patients with advanced cancer and, later, families with AIDS, Alzheimer's disease, cardiac disease, and children with progressive, life-threatening illness resulted in a conceptualization—the *transition of fading away*—as a basis for thinking about the experiences of families in palliative care.[63]

The transition of fading away is characterized by seven dimensions: redefining, burdening, struggling with paradox, contending with change, searching for meaning, living day by day, and preparing for death. The dimensions do not occur in linear fashion; rather, they are interrelated and inextricably linked to one another. While transitions are often initiated by changes defined as the start of something new, many transitions are changes that begin with endings. This is true for families in palliative care. As Davies et al.[63] found, the transition of fading away begins with the ending of life as a person knows it. Family members come to realize that the ill family member is no longer living with a life-threatening illness but is now dying from it.

Despite the fact that family members have been told about the seriousness of the prognosis, often since the time of diagnosis, they experience the usual rewards and challenges associated with the illness trajectory; for many the "gut" realization that a patient's death is inevitable occurs suddenly: "It struck me hard—it hit me like a bolt. Dad is not going to get better!" The awareness is triggered when family members see, with "new eyes," a change in the patient's body or physical capacity, such as the patient's weight loss, extreme weakness, lack of mobility, or diminished mental capacity. Realizing that the patient will not recover, family members begin the transition of fading away. As one patient commented, "My body has shrunk so much—the other day, I tried on my favorite old blue dress and I could see then how much weight I have lost. I feel like a skeleton with skin! I am getting weaker.... I just can't eat much now, I don't want to. I can see that I am fading.... I am definitely fading away." To help further illustrate the transition of fading away, we use case exemplars loosely based on our clinical experiences and research.

Dimensions of the Transition of Fading Away

Redefining

Redefining involves a shift from "what used to be" to "what is now." It demands adjustment in how individuals see themselves and each other. Patients maintain their usual patterns for as long as possible and then begin to implement feasible alternatives once they realize that their capacities are seriously changing.

Case Study 1: Redefining in Different Ways

Shelly, a young woman diagnosed with metastatic colon cancer, redefined what she was capable of as her illness progressed. Once an avid tap dancer, she could no longer participate in dance competitions in her age group. As she became more fatigued, she gave up dancing altogether but was still able to help her dance group behind the scenes with costume changes and makeup. As her illness progressed, she became an audience member, cheering on her dance company. One day, Shelly realized that even that required more energy than she had. She was able to maintain connections with her dance community even toward the very end of her life, but those connections changed and were redefined; her family kept her updated about the dance group, posted pictures in her bedroom of her "dance friends," and made arrangements for friends to visit when Shelly felt well enough. Another patient, Fred, owned a landscaping business, and, as his chronic obstructive pulmonary disease (COPD) progressed and he became increasingly short of breath, he could no longer do the physical work required. Fred lamented that he loved being out in the garden, but as time went on, he took over bookkeeping duties while his son took over the family business. Eventually, he could no longer do that as his health deteriorated.

Both Shelly and Fred, like other patients, accepted their limitations with much sadness and a sense of great loss. Their focus narrowed, and they began to pay attention to details of everyday life that they had previously ignored or overlooked. While Shelly wanted to maintain connections to her dance community, over time, that became more difficult, and she set her sights on spending more time with family and her nieces and nephews. Both Shelly and Fred talked about feeling "the same on the inside," although they acknowledged the drastic changes in their physical appearance. Some patients, like Shelly, became more spiritual in their orientation to life and nature. Early in her illness, Shelly organized groups of friends to go to the ocean early in the morning for a "healing circle," where meditation, yoga, and prayer were practiced. When patients are able to redefine themselves as Shelly did, they make the best of their situation, differentiating what parts of them are still intact. While Fred could no longer continue working as a landscaper, he could still enjoy going into his own backyard and "puttering around" when he felt well enough. His son, Jeremy, even built a backyard gazebo where Fred took up bird watching; he replaced one joy in life with another as a way to continue to connect with the outdoors.

Caregiver Questions to Consider:

1. How might the family and friend caregivers of Shelly and Fred also redefine their activities and identities differently?
2. What set of questions could you ask the caregivers of Shelly and Fred to help them further reflect on how they and the patient are going through the process of redefinition?
3. What additional resources might you provide to caregivers to help them navigate how they might redefine themselves?

Patients who are unable to redefine themselves in this way often attempt to maintain their regular patterns despite the obvious changes in their capacity to do so. Sometimes patients end up frustrated, angry, and feeling worthless. These reactions distance them from others, resulting in the patient feeling alone and, at times, abandoned.

Case Study 2: Resistance to Letting Go

Lisa worked in a law office as a paralegal. Even though her health was deteriorating, she was unable to recognize that she could no longer work to full capacity. The demands of her job were high, often with tight timelines and occasions when she had to work overtime. While her workplace and employer were respectful of her need to contribute and maintain her work identity, Lisa had difficulty giving up responsibility. As the work piled up, it became clear that she could no longer complete assigned duties. Her co-workers began helping Lisa with her work, often working overtime themselves. At first, they were happy to help, but, as the months went by and Lisa's health further deteriorated, some co-workers started to feel resentful. Lisa became increasingly frustrated with her inability to complete work on time and increasingly angry with her boss who she felt was too demanding. Eventually, Lisa was encouraged to take time off work, with pay, to enable her to look after herself. Her husband, Dan, remarked that not being able to work was devastating to Lisa, who had previously enjoyed her job and who still felt that she was able to work at full capacity. While Lisa continued to have a relationship with her co-workers once she left work, her husband remarked that it was awkward and strained at times. According to Dan, her co-workers began visiting less and less, leaving Lisa feeling abandoned and misunderstood.

Caregiver Questions to Consider:

1. What do you think Dan's experience has been like through all of Lisa's work-related challenges?
2. What questions might you ask Dan to assess how he is coping?
3. How could you help support Dan as he reflects on preparing for the future and knowing what to expect?

For the most part, we have found that partners take the patient's physical changes in stride. They attribute the changes to the disease, not to the patient personally and, as a result, are able to empathize with the patient. Patients' redefining tends to focus on themselves, the changes in their physical status and intrapersonal aspects; partners' redefining centers on their relationship with the patient. Partners did their best to "continue on as normal," primarily for the sake of the patient. In doing so, they consider alternatives and reorganize their priorities.

Sometimes family members experience the "reciprocity of suffering" that results from the physical and emotional distress that is rooted in their anguish of dealing with the impending death of a loved one and in their attempt to fill new roles as family caregivers. It appears that the degree to which family members experience reciprocal suffering relates to how patients redefine themselves. When patients are able to redefine themselves, partners have an easier time. Such patients accepted partners' offers of support; patients and partners were able to talk about the changes that were occurring. Partners felt satisfied in the care that they provided. But when patients were less able to redefine, partners' offers of support were rejected or unappreciated. For example, Louis was the main trumpet player in a military band. He loved to perform, and when he could no longer keep up with band members, his wife Donna encouraged him to quit, telling Louis that it was unfair to his band members. Louis got angry with Donna, telling her that "you don't know anything, I'm fine." Louis continued to play with the band, having Donna drive him to twice-weekly performances. One night at a performance, Louis collapsed and was taken to the hospital. Donna was frustrated that her concerns had not been heard by Louis, and Louis in turn was upset that Donna did not understand his need to continue performing. Their relationship became strained as Louis struggled to redefine life after his cancer diagnosis, and Donna struggled to know how to best help Louis.

In such situations, partners often avoid talking about or doing anything that will remind the patient of the changes they are experiencing but not acknowledging. This often causes strain in relationships. Rather than feeling satisfied with their care, partners become frustrated and angry, although often they remain silent and simply "endure" the situation. The ill person contributes significantly to the caregiver's ability to cope. In their systematic review of factors that influence family caregiving of persons with advanced cancer, Li and Loke[65] found that the spousal relationship contributed significantly to the capacity of the partners to adjust their caregiving role and expectations in order to provide care despite their experience of overwhelming emotional and physical strain. Caregivers drew strength from the dying person when the ill person accepted the impending death, had an understanding of the caregivers' needs, and had attitudes, values, and beliefs that sustained their caregiving.[65]

Adult children also redefine the ill family member; they redefine their ill parent from someone who was strong and competent to someone who is increasingly frail. As Davies and colleagues report,[39] children perceive that the changes in their ill parent are the result of disease and not intentional. Younger children are particularly sensitive to keeping the situation private, claiming they want to protect the dignity of the patient; but they seemed to want to protect their own sense of propriety. Adolescents in particular had a difficult time redefining the situation. They preferred to continue as if nothing was wrong and to shield themselves against any information that would force them to see the situation realistically. This is consistent research with adolescents who have a dying family member.[66]

Case Study 3: The Difficulty of Witnessing Changes in a Patient's Health

When Jeremy took over his father's landscaping business, he expressed disbelief at watching his father's strong body wither away. He had always viewed his father as a "strong man," and it was difficult to see him in a weakened state. Jeremy felt vulnerable in ways he had not previously experienced. For example, Jeremy, a young man in his early 20s, was "devastated" when his father's urinary bag dragged behind him as he left the living room when his friends were visiting. It was difficult for Jeremy to accept such manifestations of his parent's illness.

Questions to Consider:

1. What emotions do you think Jeremy might be experiencing as he witnesses his father's change in health?
2. How do you think child–parent relationships might change when the parent experiences a life-limiting illness?
3. What challenges might you expect in situations where caregivers have difficulty accepting their loved one's serious illness?

When a patient is able to redefine, children are also better able to accept that dying is a natural part of life. Often, children (and others) recommit to their own health when they have a family member who is dying, and the experience causes them to reflect on their own life and the changes that they want to make. Fred's son David, for example, was estranged from his own children as a result of a long history of substance use. Though he had been alcohol-free for 5 years, he had been afraid to reach out to his now teenage children. Fred and his wife had not spent much time with their grandchildren. When David realized that his father was dying, it prompted him to get in touch with his ex-wife, which resulted in a meeting with his children. Fred's illness, while challenging for the family, prompted David to reconnect with his children and allowed Fred the opportunity to spend time with his grandchildren before he died. In contrast, when a dying person is unable to redefine, it can also affect their adult children. Dealing with the patient's angry emotions sometimes makes the relationship difficult. Valerie and her mother had experienced conflict in their relationship when Valerie was growing up. When her mom was diagnosed with metastatic cancer and her health began to deteriorate, Valerie began spending more time with her mother than she had in the past; but her mother was not overly receptive. After her mother had died, Valerie expressed regrets and wished that her mother had been able to accept her offers of help. Valerie said that she had spent many hours in bereavement counseling trying to reconcile her feelings about the relationship with her mother, suggesting that her mother's inability to redefine their relationship had affected her personal life in profound ways.

Burdening

One of the most common feelings that people who are dying express is a desire to not be a burden to their family.[67] If patients see themselves as purposeless, dependent, and immobile, they have a greater sense of burdening their loved ones. The more realistically that patients redefine themselves as their capacities diminish, the more accurate they tend to be in their perceptions of burdening.[63] They acknowledge other family members' efforts, appreciate those efforts, and encourage family members to rest and take time to care for themselves. According to Steele and Davies,[64] patients who are less able to redefine themselves do not tend to see that they are a burden on other family members in any way. Frances, a retired nurse, retold the story of her husband Bernie and how he did not seem to realize that she needed a break. Frances explained that when Bernie became ill and was no longer able to attend their weekly bridge group, he insisted that she also stay home to be with him. Frances arranged to have home help for Bernie so that she could continue her weekly outing as she found it a great source of support. When Bernie refused the help, Frances felt she had no choice but to give up her weekly game. She commented that Bernie "just didn't seem to have a clue that I needed to get out.... It wasn't about him, it was just that I needed the break."

Most partners acknowledge that providing care and support to a loved one is hard work, and it can be overwhelming. While some partners do feel overburdened, most often partners feel a deep desire to provide care to their loved one out of a sense of love and obligation.[16] Partners often do not focus on their own difficulties and, in fact, often put their own needs aside. Stories of loneliness and helplessness often surface during the experience, but caring for a loved one can also bring couples closer together as they revisit their relationship and deepen their love and respect for one another. Partners of patients who are able to redefine often feel proud of their caregiving efforts and appreciated for their contributions to their partner's life and dying process. Partners who are not able to redefine can feel unappreciated and exhausted, and some have even confessed to "waiting for the patient to die."

Steele and Davies[64] suggest that children, too, experience burdening, but the source stems from the additional responsibilities of helping to care for a dying parent, superimposed on their work responsibilities, career development, and their own families. As a result, adult children of all ages feel a mixture of satisfaction and exhaustion. Debbie's mother was diagnosed with metastatic lung cancer just as she was graduating from university and starting a new job in another city. While Debbie was reluctant to move, her father encouraged her to do so; but, over time, Debbie began to feel the strain of living at a distance. As her mother's disease progressed, Debbie, an only child, would fly home on weekends to help her father but often felt pulled between her work responsibilities and her responsibilities to her family. Both of Debbie's parents were understanding and recognized that Debbie was doing all she could to support them; they appreciated her efforts and were thankful when she was home. Adult children are influenced by the ill parent's redefining—if the ill parent acknowledges their efforts, they are more likely to feel satisfaction. Children's sense of feeling burdened is also influenced by the state of health of the well parent. If that parent is also ill or debilitated, the burden on children is compounded. Children who are able to prioritize their responsibilities while also attending to their own needs do tend to feel less burdened, according to Steele and Davies.[64] As such, nurses can play an important role in coaching adult children toward self-care and balance so that they do not feel burdened by the multiple responsibilities that they can incur when a parent is dying.

Struggling with Paradox

Struggling with paradox stems from the fact that the patient is both living and dying. For patients, the struggle focuses on wanting to believe they will survive and knowing that they will not. Steele and Davies[64] write that on "good days," patients felt optimistic about the outcome; on other days, they succumbed to the inevitability of their approaching demise. Often, patients did not want to "give up" but at the same time were "tired of fighting." They wanted to "continue on" for the sake of their families but also wanted "it to end soon" so their families could "get on with their lives." Patients coped by hoping for miracles, fighting for the sake of their families, and focusing on the good days. Rose, a young woman diagnosed with advanced cancer, rarely talked about dying. Although she had been a palliative care volunteer, had journeyed with many dying people, and was told what the eventual outcome of her diagnosis would be, she focused exclusively on her cancer treatment, on living, and praying for a cure. As her functional status changed, her mobility declined, and she developed pain, it was difficult for Rose to ignore that the disease was progressing. Some days she talked about being healed, and on others she doubted that this would happen. It was not until 2 days before she died that Rose agreed to register with the palliative care program.

Caregivers also struggle with paradox. They want to care for and spend time with the patient, and they also wanted a "normal" life. Frances desperately wanted to continue with her bridge playing for the social outing but also because the social support that the group provided helped her cope with caring for Bernie. Because Bernie feared being left alone but would refuse help, Frances felt that she had to put her life on hold and soon became exhausted herself. Eventually, Frances decided to invite the bridge group to her home. Even though this created more work for her as she prepared for their arrival, and it was not the complete break that she desired, it did provide her with a welcome distraction and created some normalcy in her life. Steele and Davies[64] report that partners who manage to find ways of tending to their own needs usually are less exhausted and report fewer health problems than partners who neglect their own needs.

Children struggle with hanging on and letting go to a greater extent than their parents. They want to spend time with their ill parent and to "get on with their own lives." Feeling the pressure of dual loyalties (to their parents and to their own young families), the demands of both compound the struggle that children face.

Contending with Change

Those facing life-limiting illness in a family member experience changes in every realm of daily life—relationships, roles, socialization, and work patterns. The focus of the changes differs among family members. Patients face changes in their relationships with everyone they know.[64] They realize that the greatest change of their life is under way and that life as they knew it will soon be gone. Patients tend to break down tasks into manageable pieces, and, increasingly, they focus inward. The greatest change that partners faced was in their relationship with the patient. They cope by attempting to keep everything as normal as possible. Children contend with changes that are more all-encompassing; they cannot withdraw as their ill parent did, nor can they prioritize their lives to the degree that their well parent could.[64] They easily become exhausted. As Debbie explained, it was hard to fly home every weekend to help her mother and father. She had just started a new job in a new city, and she wanted to begin building her professional career; but she felt "the pull" to be at home. She felt guilty for not being there to help her father with the everyday demands but also stressed at learning her new job and wanting to impress her employer. She contemplated moving home and quitting her job several times but, in the end, continued to travel back and forth for several months, up until her mother died and she helped her father after her mother's death.

Searching for Meaning

Searching for meaning has to do with seeking answers to help in understanding the situation. Patients tend to journey inward, to reflect on spiritual aspects and deepen their most important connections. Partners and others close to the dying person often look toward their own personal growth and reconciling issues from the past. Gail and Nancy had been close childhood friends. They spent most of their summers together up until they each got married and moved to different parts of the country. Over time, their relationship became distant, but when Gail was diagnosed with bladder cancer, Nancy was the first person she called. Nancy visited Gail and her husband several times over the 2 years before she died. They reminisced about their childhood and young adult days and tried to understand why their friendship had diminished. They sought experiences that reminded them of their earlier times together—going to the beach, fishing, and staying at lakeside cottages. After Gail died, Nancy remarked that spending time with Gail had caused her to reflect and re-evaluate her own life. The experience helped her "put things in perspective," and she described becoming less concerned about bolstering her career and more concerned about spending time with family and friends. Children also tend to reflect on and re-evaluate aspects of their lives when a parent dies.[64] One son said that his father had worked hard his whole life trying to provide for his children as they were growing up. He often worked late, traveled for work, and missed family celebrations. While he was appreciative of his father's efforts, he vowed to make changes in his own life so that he could spend more time with his children.

Living Day to Day

Living day to day is characterized by a focus on the present, on the "here and now," and trying to make the most of a challenging situation. When patients are able to find meaning in their experiences, they are more able to take one day at a time and often experience less turmoil.[63] Catherine approached her cancer diagnosis pragmatically. She had always been organized, a strong planner, and, when diagnosed with cancer, decided to not dwell too much in "what could have been" but rather focused on "the here and now." Once she could no longer work, she turned her attention to learning new skills that she could handle and that would keep her busy. She began knitting hats and blankets for her family, and, when she tired, she would put that aside and rest. She was not discouraged but rather decided on adopting an attitude of living each day to the fullest that she could. Not all patients are able to live day to day. For patients who are unable to find meaning in their situations, they tend to focus on persevering through difficult times and "getting through it."[63]

Partners who are able to find meaning in the situation are better able to live day to day. They cherished the time that they had with their partner and made the best of things. Fred's wife Betty even suggested that Fred's diagnosis meant that they could spend time in their own garden together after years of Fred landscaping the yards of others. Although they could no longer make their yearly trip to Arizona, Betty said she "didn't mind" as she wanted to make the best of the time that she and Fred had left. Other partners simply endure the situation without paying much attention to philosophizing about the experience. Steele and Davies[64] comment that children often have difficulty concentrating on living day to day because they are unable to defer their obligations and therefore worry about what else needs to be done. Other children cope differently and are able to "live for the day."

Preparing for Death

In preparing for death, patients, partners, and children come to terms with the practical aspects of dying. Patients often have their family's needs uppermost in their minds and work hard to teach or guide family members with regard to various tasks and activities that the patient will no longer be around to do. Bea spent many months teaching her husband Harold how to cook and do laundry as he had not been responsible for those tasks in their married life together. Even though it was hard for both of them, Bea was determined that Harold be prepared. Many patients are also committed to leaving legacies for their loved ones, not only as a means of being remembered but also as a way of comforting loved ones in their grief. Gail learning to knit blankets and hats for those she loved enabled her to leave something special behind. She also created multiple memory books for her friends and family.

Caregivers tend to concentrate on meeting the patient's wishes. They attend to practical details and anticipate their future in practical ways. Children offer considerable help to their parents with legal and financial matters. They also prepare their own children for what is to come. A central aspect of preparing is reassuring the dying parent that they would take care of the surviving parent.[63] Children also prepare for the death by envisioning their future without their parent.

In summary, the transition of fading away and its related dimensions provide a comprehensive picture of the families' experience in palliative care, how life-threatening illness can affect the family as a whole and its individual members. This conceptualization provides nurses with guidance for interventions with families. Table 29.1 summarizes key strategies that nurses caring for families can use in their everyday practice to promote family-centered palliative care.

Family Caregiving in Palliative Care

The primary goal of palliative care is to improve the quality of life and quality of death of dying people and their families through provision of excellent care. Families share most intimately the experience of living with and dying from a life-threatening illness. They are strongly affected, both positively and negatively. Many also wish to provide care, and, in these cases, nurses and other healthcare professionals play a key role in supporting them so that they do not endanger their own health.

Family caregiving in palliative care involves many things, but, at its core, family caregivers provide most of the physical and emotional care for the individual who is dying.[68] Family caregivers manage medications, symptoms, and other aspects of patient care,[69] and, as the person who is dying functionally declines and is less able to get out and socialize with others, family caregivers provide social support.[68] Providing the person who is dying with practical support for activities of daily living, such as bathing and eating, as well as other household tasks, is a common role for family caregivers, including taking on new roles that were previously those of the person who is dying. Family caregivers act as the spokesperson, advocate, and proxy decision maker for their significant other; and they assume primary responsibility for coordinating the care of the patient.[69] There are many challenges for family caregivers. For example:

- The physical demands of providing care can be extremely difficult for family caregivers.[70] Many family caregivers are older and have health concerns of their own, which can make caregiving particularly challenging.[24]
- Developing assessment and caregiving skills may be challenging for family caregivers. They often report that they do not feel prepared for their caregiving role, especially in regard to medication management.[71]
- Family caregivers who look for information to help them prepare for caregiving often feel overwhelmed by the complexity and amount of information needed to fulfill their caregiving role, adding to their stress.[72]
- Caregiving responsibilities, carrying out multiple roles, facing loneliness and social isolation, and often being unable to leave the patient alone result in significant disruptions in family caregivers' regular routines and restrictions on their time and ability to participate in social and health-related activities that they value.[73–75] Younger caregivers, women, and those who are a child of the person who is dying often find disruptions to their own schedules especially difficult,[76] likely due to the stress of competing demands from work and family life.[72]

Family caregivers may also experience financial stressors associated with caring for a dying person at home.[77] Many family caregivers quit their job, lose work hours, or use special leave or holiday time

Table 29.1 Dimensions of fading away: Nursing interventions for family members

Dimension	Nursing interventions
Redefining	Ensure effective symptom management to allow patients and family members to focus more outside the illness. Appreciate that relinquishing old and comfortable views of themselves occurs over time and does not necessarily occur simultaneously with physical changes in the patient. Tailor interventions according to the various abilities of family members to assimilate the changes.
Contending with change	Reassure family members that a range of responses and coping strategies is to be expected within and among family members. Create an environment in which family members can explore and manage their own concerns and feelings. Encourage dialogue about family members' beliefs, feelings, hopes, fears, and dilemmas so they can determine their own course of action. Provide opportunities for patients to talk about the illness, the enforced changes in their lives, and the ways in which they have adapted; for partners to talk about how changes in the patient affect their marital relationship; and for children to talk about their own feelings of vulnerability and the degree to which they want to be open or private about the situation. Recognize that families communicate in well-entrenched patterns and their ability to communicate openly and honestly differs. Normalize the experience of family members and explain that such feelings do not negate the positive feelings of concern and affection. Reinforce normal patterns of living for as long as possible and as appropriate. When patterns are no longer viable, consider adjustments or alternatives. Provide information so families can explore the available resources, their options, and the pros and cons of the various options. Provide information in writing as well as verbally. Focus on the patient's attributes that remain intact, and acknowledge that roles and responsibilities may be expressed differently. Consider adjustments or alternatives when former patterns are no longer feasible. Explain the wide-ranging nature of the changes that occur within the patient's immediate and extended family.
Searching for meaning	Help family members consider how they might reorganize life priorities and consider resources to help them search for meaning during this time. Appreciate that the search for meaning involves examination of the self, of relationships with other family members, and of spiritual domains. Help patients appreciate their family members from another perspective, such as in recalling favorite stories or identifying ways to leave lasting legacies. Realize that talking about the current situation and their recollections of past illness and losses is part of making sense of the situation.
Burdening	Provide opportunities for patients and family members to talk about fears and anxieties about dying and death and to consider with whom to share their concerns. Encourage life reviews and reminiscing of past memories. Listen to the life stories that family members tell. Help patients stay involved for as long as possible as a way of sustaining self-esteem and a sense of control. Suggest approaches for reflective practices and self-examination such as journal writing and digital storytelling and approaches for facilitating interactions between family members such as writing letters. Assist family members to take on tasks appropriate to their comfort level and skill and share tasks among themselves.
Living day to day	Support family members' reassurances to patient that they are not a burden. Explain that when patients reaffirm family members for their efforts, this contributes to their feeling appreciated and lessens the potential for feeling burdened. Listen carefully for the subtle shifts in orientation to living with a dying relative and gauge family members' readiness for a new orientation. Ensure effective control of symptoms so that the patient can make the most of the time available. Assess the need for aids. Explain the importance of breaks for family members. Encourage others to take over for patients on a regular basis so family members can take a break. Without minimizing their losses and concerns, affirm their ability to appreciate and make the most of the time left. Facilitate conversations with patients and family members related to exploring gratitude and positive psychology after the diagnosis. Assist patients and family members with redefining hope that includes more than "being cured." Acknowledge the reorganization of priorities and the considerable adjustment in family routines and extra demands placed on family members. Acknowledge the "work" of caring for all family members. Review resources that would free family members to spend more time with the patient.
Preparing for death	Assess your own comfort level in talking about the inevitability of death, describing the dying process, and helping families make plans for wills and funerals. Assess and mitigate your own individual biases regarding different cultural practices and beliefs surrounding the death and dying process. Realize that family members will vary in their ability to assimilate the changes and that a range of reactions and coping strategies is normal. Provide information about the dying process. Recognize and address spiritual and existential distress in patients and their family members during impending death. Collaborate with other members of the interdisciplinary clinical team to assist in the provision of quality spiritual care, particularly chaplains, social workers, psychologists, palliative care clinicians, etc.
Struggling with paradox	Discuss patients' preferences about the circumstances of their death. Encourage patients to discuss these issues with their family. Acknowledge how difficult such discussions can be. Appreciate that you, as a nurse, cannot completely alleviate the psychosocial–spiritual pain inherent in the family's struggle. Assess your own comfort level in working with people facing paradoxical situations and ambivalent feelings. Encourage patients to do important "last things," such as completing a project as a legacy for their family. Provide adequate time and opportunities for family members to mourn the loss of their hopes, plans, and the future they once envisioned. Do not minimize these losses; help them modify their previous hopes and plans and consider new ones. Provide opportunities for partners and children to express their concerns about their future without the patient. Provide them with opportunities to reminisce about their life together. Acknowledge that such remembrances will have a bittersweet quality. Listen to their expressions of ambivalence, and be prepared for the ups and downs of opinions.

Source: Reference 63.

in order to fulfill caregiving responsibilities.[78–80] Loss of income and out-of-pocket costs incurred for items such as prescription and over-the-counter medications, home care, and equipment and home modifications result in many family caregivers having some type of financial difficulty due to home-based caregiving.[81]

These challenges often leave family caregivers feeling burdened by the demands of care. The literature provides a comprehensive description of the multidimensional nature of the burden experienced by family caregivers. Caregiver burden, commonly experienced by partners, has been described in terms of physical burden, which includes fatigue and physical exhaustion, sleeplessness, and deterioration of health.[50] Social burdens encompass limited time for self and social stress related to isolation.[46] Financial burdens, reported as the costs of caring for a person at the end of life, are substantial.[55] Despite the burdens and challenges reported by many family caregivers, research shows that many caregivers continue to want to provide palliative care even when the experience becomes burdensome and overwhelming for them.[82]

Family Caregiver Quality of Life

Family caregivers identify that they are better able to cope with their caregiving roles when their quality of life concerns are addressed and their needs are attended to. Family caregivers are diverse, and what is important to quality of life at an individual level will vary greatly from person to person and even for the same person over time. Research shows, however, that there are some commonalities in what family caregivers say is important to their quality of life. Cohen and colleagues[83] identified seven dimensions that family caregivers identify as important to their quality of life:

1. *The state of the family caregiver*: Physical well-being, mental health, being able to think clearly and think of something other than the patient's illness and a sense of feeling in control.
2. *Their family member's condition*: When the patient has a good day, the family caregiver also has a good day.
3. *Their environment*: When family caregivers believe that their significant other is in the best place, be that at home, the hospital, or other facility, and having privacy when they want it.
4. *The family caregiver's outlook on life*: When life has meaning, when faith and spirituality is comforting, and when providing care to their significant other is rewarding.
5. *Healthcare*. The family caregiver is comfortable with the way that decisions are made for their family member and is satisfied with the care their family member receives and how they are both treated by the healthcare team.
6. *Relationships*: That they have a relationship with the person they are caring for and with other people who are important to them.
7. *Financial concerns are addressed and not negatively affecting their life.*

Family caregiver quality of life is associated with the extent to which family caregivers perceive that their and the patient's needs are met.[84] Family caregivers have many needs related to both their own well-being and that of the patient. It is important that they focus on meeting both types of need. If they focus only on meeting their needs related to caring for the patient and neglect to take care of themselves, then they are likely to become unable to continue providing care, because they either become ill themselves or become overwhelmed.[85] Their own health and well-being is just as important as that of the patient. Some common needs found in studies of family caregivers are summarized in Table 29.2. Though they may not apply to all family caregivers in palliative care, it is important that these needs are taken into consideration when conducting family caregiver assessment.

Family Caregiver Assessment in Palliative Care

In both practice and research, palliative care has had the majority of its focus centered on families affected by cancer.[5,6,9,22,87] Yet in the past several years, a number of organizational reports, research priority papers, organizational statements, and reviews of the literature have synthesized and catalogued the state of the science of family caregiving generally[24,29,32] and within the context of serious noncancer illnesses, including dementia and Alzheimer's disease,[50,88] heart failure and stroke,[89–91] kidney disease,[48,49] lung disease/COPD,[42,47] and pediatric serious illness.[92,93] There can be several differences in the caregiving experience that are attributed to these specific illnesses. These differences can include the duration and intensity of caregiving (e.g., cancer caregiving tends to be of relatively short duration but very intense),[7] the types of treatment decisions faced (e.g., heart failure caregivers often assist with decisions about mechanical circulatory support device placement or pacemaker deactivation),[89] and special challenges due to a care recipient's cognitive impairment (e.g., dementia caregivers dealing with their care recipient's deteriorating sense of self). Hence, palliative care nurses are encouraged to review these cited resources for their respective areas of practices.

Despite these and other differences in the caregiving experience that may be characteristic of specific serious illnesses, there are common elements of assessment that the palliative care nurse should consider. Family caregiver assessment is important because research has found that nurses tend to focus on the patient, tend not to undertake comprehensive screening of family caregivers, and may be reluctant to openly do so in the patient's presence.[94] Without having a comprehensive understanding of the support needs of family caregivers, nurses' capacity to provide assistance is limited. The following points summarize these elements and are based on published guidelines and other texts.[24]

An initial comprehensive assessment should be initiated when a patient is first diagnosed with serious, potentially incurable illness, even if disease-modifying and curative therapies remain the focus of medical treatment.

Caregiver assessment should be tailored to an institution's resources, setting, and culture and yet result in a plan of care that is determined collaboratively with the family and that has measurable objectives of success.

The purpose of caregiving assessment should ideally include (but not be limited to): (1) identifying the primary caregiver and other family members who assist with caregiving tasks, (2) assessing caregivers' physical and psychological health, (3) understanding the demands that the patient's illness is likely to place on the family, and (4) determining the capacity of the family to meet these demands.

Assessment might also include what caregivers understand about how their patient's illness and its progression may impact their lives in the future. What have they discussed with the patient

Table 29.2 The needs of family caregivers in palliative care

Maintaining a balance	
Family caregivers' own needs 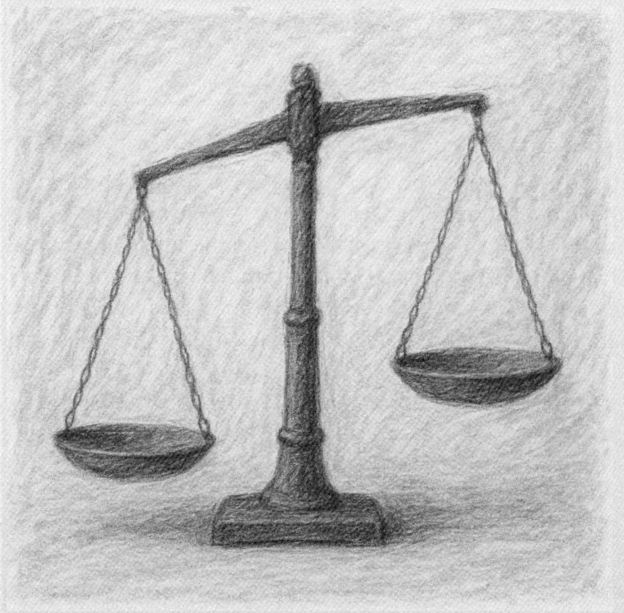	Needs to be able to provide care for the patient
Physical Maintain physical health Strength to provide care Respite care Sleep Rest ***Psychological*** Cope with strong and difficult emotions Maintain mental health Manage anxiety Avoid depression Be supported emotionally Maintain self-esteem Recognition of their anticipatory grief ***Cognitive*** Maintain cognitive functioning Get a mental break from caregiving and the illness Have privacy ***Existential/spiritual*** Retain hope Feel in control Find meaning in their new situation Strength from spirituality/faith Feel reward from caregiving Prevent isolation ***Social*** Financial security Learn new roles Be helped with other roles Cultural needs/differences to be respected	***Information*** Obtain and understand information about patient's condition Feel prepared to provide care ***Healthcare*** Healthcare team to be competent Healthcare team to be available Access to assistive devices Be comfortable with the way they are involved in decisions for the patient's care ***Relationships*** Appreciation of their caregiving Have a good and trusting relationship with the patient Have a good and trusting relationship with the healthcare team ***Environment*** Have modifications made to the home Have a safe environment ***Psychological*** Feel confidence in their caregiving ability/role ***Taught how to and/or help with*** Administer medications through numerous routes (i.e., injections, suppositories, oxygen masks, etc.) Move and position the patient Be able to safely toilet, feed, and transfer the patient from one position to another Monitor/assess Emotionally support patient Household tasks (they are increased) Coordinate and navigate care Organize Ask others for help Access available financial benefits Transport the patient and themselves if patient is not living at home Plan for death

Source: Reference 86.

concerning advance care planning? Have they talked about surrogate decision-making?

The history of the caregiver–care recipient relationship can be a significant determinant of how family members cope with the caregiver role. Not all family members will take on a caregiving role willingly, and hence this should be assessed.

Assessment findings should be used to provide caregivers with educational materials relevant to immediate priorities and expressed concerns and to link caregivers to existing resources and community services. Family carers with assessment findings indicating clinically significant physical or mental health changes due to caregiving should be referred to a specialized professional or service.

Caregivers should be reassessed at regular intervals, including any time there is an acute change in the care recipient's health status, a care recipient transition in living situation or care setting, and prior to major treatment decisions (e.g., heart transplant, continue or discontinue dialysis).

Caregiver assessment should be driven by a conceptual framework.

Tools to assist in the assessment of family caregiver support needs exist in the literature.[95,96] One recent example is the Carer Support Needs Assessment Tool (CSNAT) developed by researchers in the United Kingdom.[40] The CSNAT consists of 14 questions and can be used by nurses as a screen to identify family caregivers' key support needs that require further assessment. The tool is designed both to help legitimize family caregiver needs for support to family caregivers themselves and to make such needs visible and explicit to nurses and other health professionals. It focuses on support domains that enable the family caregiver to care for the patient ("Do you need more support with ... Understanding your relative's illness? Managing your relative's symptoms, including providing medicines? Providing personal care for your relative? Knowing who to contact if you are concerned about your relative? Equipment to help care for your relative? Talking with your relative about their illness? Knowing what to expect in the future when caring for your relative?") and on more direct support domains for family caregivers themselves (i.e., "Do you need more support with ... Having time for yourself in the day? Your financial, legal, or work issues? Dealing with your feelings and worries? Looking after your own health (physical problems)? Your beliefs or spiritual concerns? Practical help in the home? Getting a break from caregiving overnight?"). In addition to the 14 questions assessing family caregivers' needs for support, the tool includes one optional question to capture anything that might not have been addressed.

Supporting Family Caregivers in Different Settings

While the majority of care families provide is in the home, there are many different settings where family caregivers play a critical role. Notably, as the delivery of palliative care services moves increasingly to community and/or primary care,[97] there is a growing expectation that families and family caregivers will become even more involved in the delivery of palliative care and operate as extensions to formal services.[98,99]

The following sections describe the roles that caregivers can play in different settings, and general guidance is provided for the palliative care nurse on how to best prepare and support family members in these different settings.

In the Home and Community

Family members of patients with advanced illnesses have been reported to provide support an average of 8 hours per day for community-dwelling relatives in the home.[100] The tasks that are performed include routine tasks such as meal preparation, housework and lawn maintenance, managerial and financial tasks, transportation, and care for other family members. While some of these routine tasks may have already been part of the family member's normal daily routine, others may have been formerly managed by the patient until they became too sick to assume these tasks. Other tasks involve medical/nursing and hands-on patient care. These tasks might include healthcare and medical appointment coordination, emotional and spiritual support, medication management and administration, wound and medical device care, symptom monitoring and management, assistance with instrumental and other activities of daily living, promotion of care recipient self-care (e.g., physical activity), and healthcare decision-making. A large survey conducted in the United States found that just 14% of family members had received some kind of training to perform these medical/nursing tasks.[87]

The fundamental challenge that the palliative care nurse can help families with as they care for relatives with serious illness in the home is how to balance the additional demands of caregiving, their paid work, family life, and their own needs. This can be facilitated by helping caregivers make lists of their tasks and responsibilities and identify which tasks are absolutely necessary to accomplish and maintain. The next step is to help the family member estimate how much time each task takes. The family member then has three options to accomplish these tasks: (1) do the task(s) themselves, (2) ask and organize help from other family members and friends, or (3) hire outside assistance. If the caregiver decides to do the task themselves, assess how competent they are in doing the task and encourage them to acquire additional training if needed. For employed caregivers, there may be opportunities for leave, both paid and unpaid. A second option is to rally the assistance of family and friends. It can be difficult for caregivers to ask for volunteer assistance, so it should be emphasized to caregivers that most family members and friends appreciate the opportunity to be helpful. The palliative care nurse can help caregivers make a list of the family and friends who could offer assistance and urge them to ask for help with specific tasks. A third option for families with the financial means is to hire someone or an agency to assist with tasks in the home. Different ways to find services to meet specific needs include referrals through the patient's provider or social worker, contacting a hospital's patient services department, searching the internet, and asking family, friends, and community groups for recommendations.

Another particular issue of family caregiving for the palliative care nurse to be aware of are the preferences and special considerations for caregivers providing in-home care at the end of life. Home has surpassed the hospital as the most common place of death in the United States for the first time since the early 20th century.[101] Deciding to provide home care for relatives at the end of life can have a profound effect on family caregivers. Many caregivers believe that providing home care for their loved one is the only option. Some make uninformed decisions, giving little consideration to the implications of their decision. Such decisions are often made early in the patient's disease trajectory or when the patient is imminently dying and may be influenced by the unrealistic portrayal in the media about dying at home. The patient's needs and wishes often drive decisions, with caregivers paying little attention to their own needs. Negotiated decisions for home care typically occur if caregivers and patients are able to talk openly about dying and have done so throughout the disease trajectory. For some families, a home death can bring additional burdens, worries, and responsibilities, so it is important that open discussion be facilitated. Large variations exist in the provision of home-based palliative and end-of-life care, although the development of hospice home services has enabled increasing numbers of seriously ill patients to experience care at home. Indeed, dying at home has been cited as the preference of the majority of patients, and research on quality of life at the end of life has shown home deaths to be associated with higher-quality death and dying.[102] However, dying at home can present special challenges for family members. Clinicians must recognize the emotional impact of providing palliative care at home and must be sensitive to the potentially overwhelming task that caring for a dying relative imposes on family members. Care should be provided within a team context so that families understand that they are not alone in supporting the care recipient at the end of life in the home and have access to a range of services from the palliative and hospice care team when needed. Furthermore, clinicians must work with the dying patients, with family caregivers, and with each other as equal partners in the caregiving process. Importantly, ongoing attention should be paid to improving hospital end-of-life care so that families feel they have a meaningful alternative to home care.

In the Hospital

Family caregivers play critical roles when their care recipients with advanced illness are admitted as inpatients into the hospital. They function as the patient's primary advocate, often having a close relationship to the patient that affords them an enhanced understanding of the patient's interests and values. Family caregivers are often present with patients over their illness trajectories and across settings. Hence, they are prime historians and "experts" in the patient's past and ongoing treatments and will often be a co-spokesperson with the patient in their encounters with different healthcare professionals. Though typically relieved of providing medical and nursing tasks while patients are in the hospital, family caregivers will often continue to provide essential companionship and emotional and spiritual support to patients. When appropriate, families may also provide hands-on patient care assistance such as bathing, dressing, hygiene, and feeding. And, finally, caregivers play an essential role in the discharge and transition-of-care process. To ensure patients continue to receive high-quality care after leaving the hospital, it is critical that families are prepared to assume and coordinate duties that patients cannot do for themselves but are made necessary by their medical condition and functional status.

For palliative care nurses interacting with families in the hospital, there are a few general principles to offering support that promotes their resiliency in the face of what can be a very intimidating and stressful event for them. First and foremost, and unless otherwise directed by the patient, include family caregivers in all discussions with the patient about their condition, treatments, and tests. Treat them as partners in the patient's care. Clinicians should be aware that their own attitudes about the involvement of families in the care of patients is critical; if families feel they are a "nuisance" to healthcare providers, they will often become less cooperative with and more resentful of the healthcare system (which may ultimately negatively impact the patient). Second, help orient caregivers to what the different roles are of the different healthcare professionals. Many families may never have heard of palliative care or may associate it with hospice care or death and dying. It is important to convey that palliative care is not terminal illness care but instead serious illness care that is focused on providing an extra layer of support by offering relief from symptoms, pain, and the stress of serious illness. Finally, encourage caregivers to keep a small notebook whenever they talk with a member of the palliative care team. Family members should be reassured that nothing is trivial. All questions are important, and all observations are valuable. They should be encouraged to say when they do not understand something and to ask for information to be repeated as necessary. Palliative care professionals can help by spelling words that family members do not understand or by jotting down explanations. They should reassure family members that asking for help is not a sign of failure but rather a sign of good common sense. Following such simple guidelines helps keep families from feeling overwhelmed.

In the Intensive Care Unit

Many family caregivers will experience seeing their care recipients in the intensive care unit (ICU), where the most invasive and aggressive medical treatments are performed. What caregivers do in the ICU is similar to what they might be seen doing in the hospital setting, and yet there are differences of relevance for the palliative care clinician. Studies report that family members in the ICU can be under marked psychological duress due to seeing their critically ill relative unconscious and connected to machines, having limited visitation with the patient, witnessing invasive procedures, experiencing distressing uncertainty, and being physically exhausted.[103] Being under such duress can challenge the ability of family members to cognitively process information,[104] and yet they are often asked to speak on behalf of patients' interests, participate in family meetings, and perform as surrogate decision makers. A palliative care priority in interacting with family members in the ICU is the delivery of honest, easily understandable, and timely information as poor communication has been reported by families as the most frequent complaint in the ICU.[105] Families need to have their emotions and feelings acknowledged by clinicians, reassurance that everything is being done to help the patient, and as liberal access to the patient's bedside as is possible; and they most generally want to know the patient's prognosis.[106] Palliative care nurses interacting with families in the ICU should become familiar with resources that further elaborate best practices for ICU communication skills,[107] conducting family meetings,[108] delivering prognosis,[109] and dealing with family emotions.[110,111]

In the Perioperative Setting

Regardless of whether a patient's surgery is planned or emergent, the perioperative experience for family caregivers can be physically and psychologically exhausting and manifest a range of intense emotions, including uncertainty, fear, and anxiety.[112] A prospective cohort study by Juarez et al.[112] of family caregivers of patients undergoing palliative surgery identified a number of ways that nurses can support families. These included (1) identifying any physical or psychological limitations of family members caring for patients after discharge, (2) educating families on patient postoperative symptom management, (3) ascertaining the caregiver's prior experiences with supporting the patient, (4) initiating referral for suspected psychosocial issues (e.g., depression, financial strain) or spiritual needs, (5) discussing anticipated out-of-pocket costs, (6) communicating patient needs after discharge that will require assistance from the caregiver, and (7) discussing distance and access to care for return visits and urgent care. Prospectively addressing caregiver distress related to uncertainty may be helped by informing families as early as possible about exactly what to expect before, during, and after surgery.[113] Offering support to family members by palliative care–trained nurses may be especially important in situations where the surgery was unexpected or emergent; the surgery is potentially futile or inappropriate; if there are complicated family dynamics;

if family members are functionally debilitated, burned out, distressed, or depressed; if there are actual or foreseen ethical dilemmas; if there is expected to be complicated postoperative home care requiring intense symptom and medication management; and any time it would be unsurprising if the patient died within a year despite surgery.[114]

In the Long-Term Care Setting

Unpaid caregivers provide the majority of long-term services and support (LTSS), in part because long-term services are expensive and not covered by Medicare.[115] LTSS are covered by Medicaid but only for those who are income-eligible; and with many ineligible or unable to afford formal LTSS, the burden falls to unpaid family and other caregivers to provide care.[116]

Long-term care (LTC) is provided in many settings, including nursing homes, assisted living facilities, group homes, and personal residences,[117] and is defined as the health and supportive services provided to people unable to practice self-care, usually over months or years.[118] LTC includes personal care, social services, room and board, transportation, and medical and rehabilitative care.[118] Unlike care in the community, where family members often provide intensive care assistance unilaterally, a distinct shift occurs when a relative is placed in an LTC setting.[119] Within LTC, family caregivers account for up to 30% of care including feeding, washing, toileting, social, emotional and memory support, and mobilization. While they are often unseen and underrecognized by the care team, they are key partners in LTC but inconsistently included as part of the circle of care and care planning.[120] Communication and relationship-building between family members and LTC clinicians, including direct care nursing staff, have the potential to reduce costly avoidable hospitalizations as well as timely and proactive education of family members on availability of on-call clinical teams and the ability of the LTC workforce to manage medical needs and the risk of hospitalizations and engage family members in decisions that are congruent with the resident's wishes.[121] Palliative care for people living in LTC settings is complex and involves responding to physical, psychological, social, and spiritual needs; discussing wishes and care preferences; updating families to reduce distress, confusion, and miscommunication; as well as supporting families before and after bereavement.[122] Additionally, both families and LTC providers suggest that more staff–family communication is significantly related to better family perception of resident quality of life,[123] but more research is needed to explore the role of palliative care clinicians in providing support for families of LTC residents.

The conceptual model shown in Figure 29.2, developed by Gaugler,[124] illustrates opportunities for family involvement in residential LTC, their antecedents (e.g., aspects of the residential setting, sociodemographic context of family and resident, resident functional status), and potential outcomes among an array of stakeholders (i.e., family, staff, residents, and facilities). This model can help to guide palliative care interventions, particularly driven by the nursing workforce, to aid in the support of LTC residents and their families across the continuum from pre-placement to post-placement.

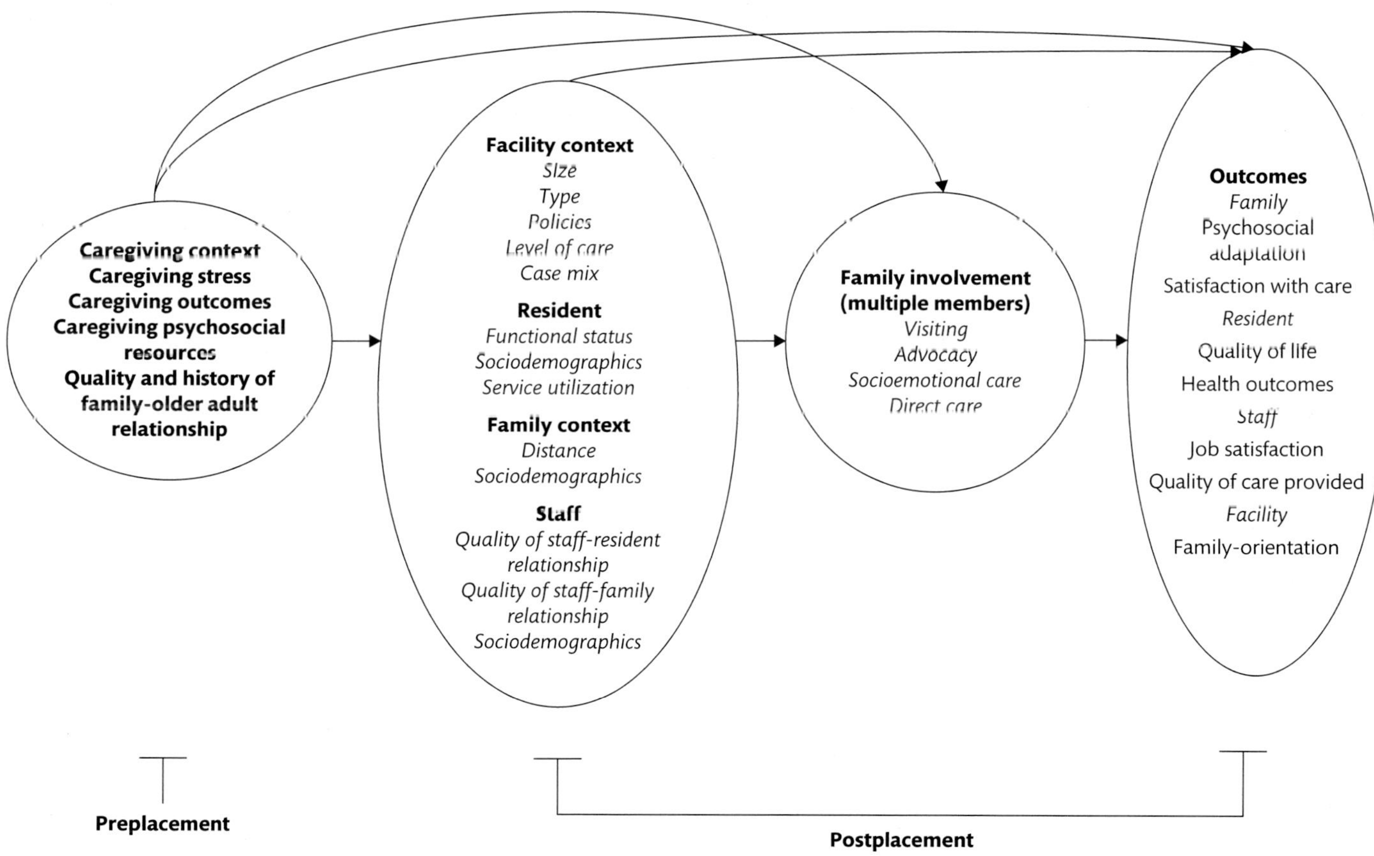

Figure 29.2 Conceptual model of family involvement in residential long-term care.
Source: Reference 124.

The Caregiver's Role in Decision-Making and Advance Care Planning

The effects of serious illness on the day-to-day lives of patients and their families inevitably give rise to new problems and challenges where choices have to be made about the best course of action. Some of these decisions are treatment-related, such as deciding about whether or not to pursue an investigational new chemotherapy or whether to pursue a heart transplant. Others are wellness-related, such as deciding to engage in an exercise program or to change one's diet to reduce symptoms. Other decisions have little to do with health per se but are imposed upon patients and families by the serious illness, such as whether to hire outside help to assist in the home, whether to sell a business to pay for medical expenses, whether to relocate the patient to a different care setting (e.g., home to assisted living or patient's home or caregiver's home), and even whether to give away a pet because the patient has become too ill to care for it.

In all these decisions, family caregivers play two key roles. First, they act as decision partners with patients who still have the ability to make decisions for themselves.[125] In some cases, patients even regard their family members and sometimes even community members (e.g., pastors) as co–decision makers along with them. For decisions about medical treatments, studies have reported that family members often help patients comprehend their medical situation, prognosis, and treatment options; are key communicators and coordinators with providers during office visits where treatment decisions are made; and trigger help-seeking decisions when symptoms worsen.[126] For both healthcare and non-healthcare decisions, family caregivers are information gatherers and holders who often seek out and gather information about available options and the pros and cons of a decision. This can give family caregivers a great deal of influence because they are able to selectively seek out and relay information that consciously or unconsciously favors their own values and preferences. Family caregivers are also the individuals most proximally impacted by the consequences of patient decisions and, in this sense, have a vested stake in the choice selected and the outcome incurred. Evidence suggests that patients themselves are sensitive to this and often weigh decisions about palliative care and life-sustaining treatments based on how much they feel they are burdening family caregivers with their healthcare decisions and care.[127,128]

The second key role that caregivers play in the decision-making of patients is as a surrogate decision maker when patients become unable to make decisions for themselves, often at the end of life. Whether care is provided in the hospital or by families in the home or at a distance, patients at the end of life may not be able to make decisions about their own care. Family members, therefore, are often asked to make those decisions on the patient's behalf according to ethical standards of *concordance*, which require that decisions approximate as closely as possible those choices the patient would have made if they had been able.[129] These decisions are often about (though not limited to) the withdrawal or withholding of life-sustaining treatments such as mechanical ventilation, dialysis, and vasopressor support. A few challenges have been noted for family members in this role, including that the role itself can be extraordinarily burdensome and is often associated with negative psychological aftereffects that may persist for months to years after the death of a patient.[130] These psychological aftereffects can include depression, anxiety, and guilt about whether or not the "right" decision was made. Surrogates have also been repeatedly shown to be poor predictors of patients' treatment preferences.[131]

Many of the difficulties encountered in surrogate decision-making are related to family members not knowing what the patient would want. The palliative care clinician is thus urged to involve family members and their patients as early as possible in advance care planning. *Advance care planning* is a process that allows the patient's preferences to be made known to the family and to healthcare professionals. It involves discussions between the patient and their family and friends, as well as written instructions in the event that a patient can no longer express their choices verbally. Advance care planning is best begun while family members are healthy but, when someone is ill, as early as possible in the illness experience and revisited as needed because preferences can change over time. However, even in the less than 30% of cases when an adult has an advance directive, it may be neither specific enough nor available when needed. Clinicians should ask if advance directives are available, and they might invite family discussion regardless of whether or not such directives are in place. It is important for clinicians to be familiar with a patient's advance directive and to advocate for the patient if needed.

Recognizing the family caregiver's involvement in decision-making is critical to helping patients achieve their goals and receive care that is reflective of their values. When family members are involved in the advance care planning and decision-making process, they are more likely to work toward helping the patient achieve their preferences. Clinicians should be available to families, offering anticipatory guidance and support through the caregiving experience. Healthcare professionals must assist family members as they traverse the maze of treatment and care decisions, ranging from whether to give particular "as-needed" medications or what food to make for the patient to eat to whether or not to seek hospice care, to sign "do-not-resuscitate" documents, or to terminate treatment. It is critical that palliative care professionals continually engage with caregivers in forward planning, interpretation, and monitoring of the inevitable decline and dying process of the ill person to facilitate the feeling in caregivers that they are secure and supported in their physically and emotionally exhaustive work. Families need to know whom to call and when and how to reach them. Table 29.3 provides information on various resources available for family caregivers; palliative care nurses can supplement this table with local resources and service agencies.

Conclusion

Family members and family caregivers are strongly affected by the diagnosis of a serious illness, both positively and negatively. As a result, an overarching goal of palliative care is to improve the quality of life and quality of death in individuals facing serious illness and their families through provision of excellent care. Many also wish to provide care for their loved one, but they require support from nurses and others on the healthcare team to do so without being overburdened and endangering their own health and well-being. Family caregivers need greater recognition, information, and meaningful support to help them care for older relatives or friends and to maintain their own health, financial

Table 29.3 Family caregiver resources for palliative care nurses

Advance care planning/decision-making/planning for the future	
Advance Care Planning Australia	https://www.advancecareplanning.org.au/
Five Wishes	https://www.fivewishes.org/
Get Your Stuff Together	www.gyst.com
Gold Standards Framework: Advance Care Planning	http://www.goldstandardsframework.org.uk/advance-care-planning
Patient Decision Aids	Patient Decision Aids | Center for Collaborative Care Decisions | Washington University in St. Louis
Planning Ahead for the End of Life	https://www.nhs.uk/Planners/end-of-life-care/Pages/planning-ahead.aspx.
PREPARE for your care	www.prepareforyourcare.org
Speak Up: Advance Care Planning	Advance Care Planning Canada: A CHPCA Initiative
The Conversation Project	www.theconversation.org
Family caregiver resources	
AARP (American Association of Retired Persons): Caregiving	https://www.aarp.org/caregiving/
American Psychological Association—Caregiver Briefcase	http://www.apa.org/pi/about/publications/caregivers/
Caregiver Action Network	www.caregiveraction.org
Carers Australia	http://www.carersaustralia.com.au/
Carers Canada	http://www.carerscanada.ca/
Carers UK	www.carersuk.org
Caring.com	www.caring.com
Family Caregiver Alliance	https://www.caregiver.org/
Global Sickle Cell Disease Family Network	https://www.globalscd.org/global-sickle-cell-disease-family-network/
HealthWell Foundation	https://www.healthwellfoundation.org/
Lotsa Helping Hands	www.lotsahelpinghands.com
National Alliance for Caregiving	www.caregiving.org
Next Step in Care	www.nextstepincare.org
Sickle Cell Family Support Network Inc.	https://www.onescdvoice.com/place/sickle-cell-family-support-network-inc/
Palliative and hospice care	
Get Palliative Care	https://getpalliativecare.org/
Hospice UK	https://www.hospiceuk.org/
National Hospice and Palliative Care Organization	www.caringinfo.org
Palliative Care Australia	http://palliativecare.org.au/im-a-carer/
The National Council for Palliative Care	http://www.ncpc.org.uk/
Virtual Hospice	http://www.virtualhospice.ca/
Grief and bereavement support	
AARP: Caregiving Grief & Loss	Dealing With Grief, Loss and End of Life Planning
CarersUK—Bereavement	When caring ends or changes | Carers UK
Dying Matters	http://www.dyingmatters.org/
Family Caregiver Alliance—Grief and Loss	https://www.caregiver.org/grief-and-loss
National Cancer Institute—Grief, Bereavement, and Coping with Loss	https://www.cancer.gov/about-cancer/advanced-cancer/caregivers/planning/bereavement-pdq
Virtual Hospice—My grief	http://www.mygrief.ca/
Information on specific illnesses	
ALS Association	http://www.alsa.org/als-care/caregivers/for-caregivers.html
Alzheimer's Association	https://www.alz.org/care/
American Association for the Study of Liver Diseases	https://www.aasld.org/
American Heart Association	http://www.heart.org/HEARTORG/Support/Support_UCM_001103_SubHomePage.jsp
Be The Match	NMDP (Formerly Be The Match) Global Nonprofit in Cell Therapy | NMDP
MS Society of Canada	https://mssociety.ca/support-services/caregivers/information-and-resources
National Cancer Institute	https://www.cancer.gov/about-cancer/coping/caregiver-support
National Kidney Foundation	https://www.kidney.org/patients/resources_Caregiver

security, and well-being.[24] Nurses play a key role in helping families to navigate uncharted territory, in identifying the family's needs for support, and in assessing and personalizing a plan of care not only for the patient but for the family as a whole and its individual members. While not all families generate positive benefits from the experience of losing a loved one, many families and family caregivers derive significant meaning from the experience of supporting another in the palliative phases of care. Tailored palliative care interventions are critical to supporting family members and family caregivers of people with serious illnesses. In addition, practice changes and research priorities should respond to the heterogeneous needs of caregivers from diverse populations and historically marginalized backgrounds.

Acknowledgments

The authors are very grateful for the original work on this chapter completed by Betty Davies, PhD, and Rose Steele, RN, PhD, and previous revisions by Dr. Kelli I. Stajduhar, RN, PhD, FCAHS, FCAN. The contributions they have made to the field of palliative care nursing cannot be overstated.

REFERENCES

1. van Roij J, Brom L, Sommeijer D, van de Poll-Franse L, Raijmakers N. Self-care, resilience, and caregiver burden in relatives of patients with advanced cancer: results from the eQuiPe study. *Support Care Cancer*. 2021;29(12):7975–7984. https://doi.org/10.1007/s00520-021-06365-9.
2. Palacio GC, Krikorian A, Gómez-Romero MJ, Limonero JT. Resilience in caregivers: a systematic review. *Am J Hosp Palliat Med*. 2020;37(8):648–658. https://doi.org/10.1177/1049909119893977.
3. Opsomer S, Lauwerier E, De Lepeleire J, Pype P. Resilience in advanced cancer caregiving. A systematic review and meta-synthesis. *Palliat Med*. 2022;36(1):44–58. https://doi.org/10.1177/02692163211057749.
4. Dionne-Odom JN, Azuero A, Taylor RA, et al. Resilience, preparedness, and distress among family caregivers of patients with advanced cancer. *Support Care Cancer*. 2021;29(11):6913–6920. https://doi.org/10.1007/s00520-021-06265-y.
5. Ferrell B, Wittenberg E. A review of family caregiving intervention trials in oncology. *CA Cancer J Clin*. 2017;67(4):318–325. https://doi.org/10.3322/caac.21396.
6. Ferrell BR, Temel JS, Temin S, et al. Integration of palliative care into standard oncology care: American Society of Clinical Oncology clinical practice guideline update. *J Clin Oncol*. 2017;35(1):96–112. https://doi.org/10.1200/JCO.2016.70.1474.
7. Griffin J, Meis L, Greer N, et al. *Effectiveness of Family and Caregiver Interventions on Patient Outcomes among Adults with Cancer or Memory-Related Disorders: A Systematic Review*. Department of Veterans Affairs; 2013. https://www.ncbi.nlm.nih.gov/books/NBK148475/.
8. Lee J, Cagle JG. Measures of financial burden for families dealing with serious illness: a systematic review and analysis. *Palliat Med*. 2021;35(2):280–294. https://doi.org/10.1177/0269216320973161.
9. Kent EE, Rowland JH, Northouse L, et al. Caring for caregivers and patients: research and clinical priorities for informal cancer caregiving. *Cancer*. 2016;122(13):1987–1995. https://doi.org/10.1002/cncr.29939.
10. Schulz R, Eden J. *Families Caring for an Aging America*. National Academies Press; 2016. https://nap.nationalacademies.org/catalog/23606/families-caring-for-an-aging-america.
11. Oliveira C, Fonseca G, Areia N, Sotero L, Relvas A. Caring for people who take care: what is already done? *Palliat Support Care*. 2022;20(5):720–730.
12. Harvey J, Berndt M. Cancer caregiver reports of post-traumatic growth following spousal hematopoietic stem cell transplant. *Anxiety Stress Coping*. 2021;34(4):397–410. https://doi.org/10.1080/10615806.2020.1845432.
13. Borstelmann N, Gray T, Gelber S, et al. Psychosocial issues and quality of life of parenting partners of young women with breast cancer. *Support Care Cancer*. 2022;30(5):4265–4274.
14. Autio T, Rissanen S. Positive emotions in caring for a spouse: a literature review. *Scand J Caring Sci*. 2018;32(1):45–55. https://doi.org/10.1111/scs.12452.
15. Bradley CJ, Kitchen S, Owsley KM. Working, low income, and cancer caregiving: financial and mental health impacts. *Journal of Clinical Oncology*. 2023;41(16):2939–2948. doi:10.1200/JCO.22.02537.
16. Dionne-Odom J, Applebaum A, Ornstein K, et al. Participation and interest in support services among family caregivers of older adults with cancer. *Psychooncology*. 2018;27(3):969–976. https://doi.org/10.1002/pon.4603.
17. Wolff J, Spillman B, Freedman V, Kasper J. A national profile of family and unpaid caregivers who assist older adults with health care activities. *JAMA Intern Med*. 2016;176(3):372–379. https://doi.org/10.1001/jamainternmed.2015.7664.
18. Hoefman R, Al-Janabi H, McCaffrey N, Currow D, Ratcliffe J. Measuring caregiver outcomes in palliative care: a construct validation study of two instruments for use in economic evaluations. *Qual Life Res*. 2015;24(5):1255–1273.
19. Salifu Y, Almack K, Caswell G. "My wife is my doctor at home": a qualitative study exploring the challenges of home-based palliative care in a resource-poor setting. *Palliat Med*. 2021;35(1):97–108. https://doi.org/10.1177/0269216320951107.
20. Reckrey J, Federman A, Bollens-Lund E, Morrison R, Ornstein K. Homebound status and the critical role of caregiving support. *J Aging Soc Policy*. 2020;32(6):590–603.
21. Ambrosi E, Biavati C, Guarnier A, et al. Factors affecting in-hospital informal caregiving as decided by families: findings from a longitudinal study conducted in acute medical units. *Scand J Caring Sci*. 2016;31(1):85–95.
22. Li Q, Loke A. The positive aspects of caregiving for cancer patients: a critical review of the literature and directions for future research. *Psychooncology*. 2013;22(11):2399–2407.
23. Bell J, Whitney R, Young H. Family caregiving in serious illness in the United States: recommendations to support an invisible workforce. *J Am Geriatr Soc*. 2019;67(S2):S451–S456. https://doi.org/10.1111/jgs.15820.
24. Schulz R, Eden J, eds. *Families Caring for an Aging America*. National Academies Press; 2016.
25. Zarzycki M, Seddon D, Bei E, Dekel R, Morrison V. How culture shapes informal caregiver motivations: a meta-ethnographic review. *Qual Health Res*. 2022;32(10):1574–1589. https://doi.org/10.1177/10497323221110356
26. Bei E, Zarzycki M, Morrison V, Vilchinsky N. Motivations and willingness to provide care from a geographical distance, and the impact of distance care on caregivers' mental and physical health: a mixed-method systematic review protocol. *BMJ Open*. 2021;11(7):e045660. https://doi.org/10.1136/bmjopen-2020-045660.

27. Hudson P, Morrison R, Schulz R, et al. Improving support for family caregivers of people with a serious illness in the United States: strategic agenda and call to action. *Palliat Med Rep.* 2020;1(1):6–17. https://doi.org/10.1089/pmr.2020.0004.
28. Guzzo K. Shifts in higher-order unions and stepfamilies among currently cohabiting and married women of childbearing age. *J Fam Issues.* 2017;38(12):1775–1799.
29. Brennan-Ing M, Seidel L, Larson B, Karpiak S. Social care networks and older LGBT adults: challenges for the future. *J Homosex.* 2014;61(1):21–52.
30. Gillis L, Aronson J, Pierre M, Brotman S, MacDonnell J, Daley A. Providing health and social services to older LGBT adults. *Annu Rev Gerontol Geriatr.* 2017;37(1):143–160.
31. Baernholdt M, Campbell C, Hinton I, Yan G, Lewis E. Quality of hospice care: comparison between rural and urban residents. *J Nurs Care Qual.* 2015;30(3):247–253.
32. Roberto K, Blieszner R. Diverse family structures and the care of older persons. *Can J Aging.* 2015;34(3):305–320.
33. Williams AM, Wang L, Kitchen P. Differential impacts of caregiving across three caregiver groups in Canada: end-of-life care, long-term care and short-term care. *Health Soc Care Community.* 2014;22(2):187–196. https://doi.org/10.1111/hsc.12075.
34. Shin DW, Cho J, Kim SY, et al. Discordance among patient preferences, caregiver preferences, and caregiver predictions of patient preferences regarding disclosure of terminal status and end-of-life choices. *Psychooncology.* 2015;24(2):212–219. https://doi.org/10.1002/pon.3631.
35. Hudson P, Trauer T, Kelly B, et al. Reducing the psychological distress of family caregivers of home based palliative care patients: longer term effects from a randomised controlled trial. *Psychooncology.* 2015;24(1):19–24. https://doi.org/10.1002/pon.3610.
36. Angelo J, Egan R. Family caregivers voice their needs: a photovoice study. *Palliat Support Care.* 2015;13(3):701–712.
37. Gallagher R, Krawczyk M. Family members' perceptions of end-of-life care across diverse locations of care. *BMC Palliat Care.* 2013;12(1):25.
38. Holm M, Henriksson A, Carlander I, Wengström Y, Öhlen J. Preparing for family caregiving in specialized palliative home care: an ongoing process. *Palliat Support Care.* 2015;13(3):767–775.
39. Davies B, Reimer JC, Brown P, Martens N. *Fading Away: The Experience of Transition in Families with Terminal Illness.* Routledge; 2020.
40. Aoun S, Grande G, Howting D, et al. The impact of the Carer Support Needs Assessment Tool (CSNAT) in community palliative care using a stepped wedge cluster trial. *PLoS One.* 2015;10(4):e0123012. https://doi.org/10.1371/journal.pone.0123012.
41. Jack B, Mitchell T, Cope L, O'Brien M. Supporting older people with cancer and life-limiting conditions dying at home: a qualitative study of patient and family caregiver experiences of Hospice at Home care. *J Adv Nurs.* 2016;72(9):2162–2172. https://doi.org/10.1111/jan.12983.
42. Aasbø G, Rugkåsa J, Solbrække K, Werner A. Negotiating the care-giving role: family members' experience during critical exacerbation of COPD in Norway. *Health Soc Care Community.* 2017;25(2):612–620.
43. Theed R, Eccles F, Simpson J. Experiences of caring for a family member with Parkinson's disease: a meta-analysis. *Aging Ment Health.* 2017;21(10):1007–1016.
44. Greenwell K, Gray W, van Wersch A, van Schaik P, Walker R. Predictors of the psychosocial impact of being a carer of people living with Parkinson's disease: a systematic review. *Parkinsonism Relat Disord.* 2015;21(1):1–11.
45. Van den Heuvel L, Hoving C, Schols J, Spruit M, Wouters E, Janssen D. Barriers and facilitators to end-of-life communication in advanced chronic organ failure. *Int J Palliat Nurs.* 2016;22(5):222–229.
46. Weisser F, Bristowe K, Jackson D. Experiences of burden, needs, rewards and resilience in family caregivers of people living with motor neurone disease/amyotrophic lateral sclerosis: a secondary thematic analysis of qualitative interviews. *Palliat Med.* 2015;29(8):717–745.
47. Aslakson R, Reinke L, Cox C, Kross E, Benzo P, Curtis J. Developing a research agenda for integrating palliative care into critical care and pulmonary practice to improve patient and family outcomes. *J Palliat Med.* 2017;20(4):329–343.
48. Axelsson L, Klang B, Hagelin C, Jacobson S, Gleissman S. Meanings of being a close relative of a family member treated with haemodialysis approaching end of life. *J Clin Nurs.* 2015;24(3–4):447–456.
49. Tong A, Cheung K, Nair S, Tamura M, Craig J, Winkelmayer W. Thematic synthesis of qualitative studies on patient and caregiver perspectives on end-of-life care in CKD. *Am J Kidney Dis.* 2014;63(6):913–927.
50. McCabe M, You E, Tatangelo G. Hearing their voice: a systematic review of dementia family caregivers' needs. *Gerontologist.* 2016;56(5):e70-e88. https://doi.org/10.1093/geront/gnw078.
51. Stajduhar K, Nichel D, Martin W, Funk L. Situated/being situated: client and co-worker roles of family caregivers in hospice palliative care. *Soc Sci Med.* 2008;67(11):1789–1797.
52. National Alliance for Caregiving. *Caregiving in a Diverse America: Beginning to Understand the Systemic Challenges Facing Family Caregivers.* National Alliance for Caregiving; 2021. https://www.caregiving.org/wp-content/uploads/2021/12/NAC_AmgenDiverseCaregiversReport_FinalDigital-112121.pdf.
53. National Alliance for Caregiving. *Caregiving in the United States 2015.* National Alliance for Caregiving; 2015. https://www.aarp.org/ppi/info-2015/caregiving-in-the-united-states-2015.html.
54. Recognize, Assist, Include, Support, and Engage (RAISE) Act Family Caregiving Advisory Council, Advisory Council to Support Grandparents Raising Grandchildren. *First Principles: Cross-Cutting Considerations for Family Caregiver Support.* Advisory Councils; 2022. Accessed February 12, 2022. https://acl.gov/sites/default/files/RAISE_SGRG/NatlStrategyFamCaregivers_FirstPrinciples.pdf.
55. Kayser K, DeMarco R, Stokes C, DeSanto-Madeya S, Higgins P. Delivering palliative care to patients and caregivers in inner-city communities: challenges and opportunities. *Palliat Support Care.* 2014;12(5):369–378.
56. Boucher NA, Johnson KS. Cultivating cultural competence: how are hospice staff being educated to engage racially and ethnically diverse patients? *Am J Hosp Palliat Med.* 2021;38(2):169–174. https://doi.org/10.1177/1049909120946729.
57. Cloyes K, Hull W, Davis A. Palliative and end-of-life care for lesbian, gay, bisexual, and transgender (LGBT) cancer patients and their caregivers. *Semin Oncol Nurs.* 2018;34(1):60–71. https://doi.org/10.1016/j.soncn.2017.12.003.
58. Javier N. Palliative care needs, concerns, and affirmative strategies for the LGBTQ population. *Palliat Care Soc Pract.* 2021;15:26323524211039230.
59. Stein G, Berkman C, O'Mahony S, Godfrey D, Javier N, Maingi S. Experiences of lesbian, gay, bisexual, and transgender patients and families in hospice and palliative care: perspectives of the palliative care team. *J Palliat Med.* 2020;23(6):817–824.

60. Rosa WE, Banerjee SC, Maingi S. Family caregiver inclusion is not a level playing field: toward equity for the chosen families of sexual and gender minority patients. *Palliat Care Soc Pract.* 2022;16(10):1–5. https://doi.org/10.1177/26323524221092459.
61. National Academies of Science, Engineering and Medicine. *The Future of Nursing 2020–2030: Charting a Path to Achieve Health Equity*. National Academies Press; 2021. https://nap.nationalacademies.org/catalog/25982/the-future-of-nursing-2020-2030-charting-a-path-to.
62. Young H, Bell J, Whitney R, et al. Social determinants of health: underreported heterogeneity in systematic reviews of caregiver interventions. *Gerontologist.* 2020;60(suppl 1):S14–S28. https://doi.org/10.1093/geront/gnz148
63. Davies B, Reimer J, Brown P, Martens N. *Fading Away: The Experience of Transition in Families with Terminal Illness.* Baywood Publishing; 1995.
64. Steele R, Davies B. Supporting families in palliative care. In: Ferrell B, Coyle N, Paice J, eds. *Oxford Textbook of Palliative Nursing.* 4th ed. Oxford University Press; 2015:500–514.
65. Li Q, Loke A. A literature review on the mutual impact of the spousal caregiver–cancer patients dyads: "communication", "reciprocal influence", and "caregiver–patient congruence." *Eur J Oncol Nurs.* 2014;18(1):58–65. https://doi.org/10.1016/j.ejon.2013.09.003.
66. Huizinga G, Visser A, Van Der Graaf W, Hoekstra H, Stewart R, Hoekstra-Weebers J. Family-oriented multilevel study on the psychological functioning of adolescent children having a mother with cancer. *Psychooncology.* 2011;20(7):730–737. https://doi.org/10.1002/pon.1779.
67. Tang S, Hsieh C, Chiang M, et al. Impact of high self-perceived burden to others with preferences for end-of-life care and its determinants for terminally ill cancer patients: a prospective cohort study. *Psychooncology.* 2017;26(1):102–108.
68. Morris S, King C, Turner M, Payne S. Family carers providing support to a person dying in the home setting: a narrative literature review. *Palliat Med.* 2015;29(6):487–495.
69. Given B, Reinhard S. Caregiving at the end of life: the challenges of family caregivers. *Generations.* 2017;41(1):50–57.
70. Roth D, Fredman L, Haley W. Informal caregiving and its impact on health: a reappraisal from population-based studies. *Gerontologist.* 2015;55(2):309–319.
71. Sexson K, Lindauer A, Harvath T. Discharge planning and teaching. *Am J Nurs.* 2017;117(5):522–524.
72. DePasquale N, Polenick C, Davis K, Moen P, Hammer L, Almeida D. The psychosocial implications of managing work and family caregiving roles: gender differences among information technology professionals. *J Fam Issues.* 2017;38(11):1495–1519.
73. Hajek A, Kretzler B, König H. Informal caregiving, loneliness and social isolation: a systematic review. *Int J Environ Res Public Health.* 2021;18(22):12101. https://doi.org/10.3390/ijerph182212101.
74. Gray TF, Azizoddin DR, Nersesian PV. Loneliness among cancer caregivers: a narrative review. *Palliat Support Care.* 2020;18(3):359–367. https://doi.org/10.1017/S1478951519000804.
75. Li L, Wister A, Mitchell B. Social isolation among spousal and adult-child caregivers. *J Gerontol B Psychol Sci Soc Sci.* 2021;76(7):1415–1429.
76. Clendon J, Walker L. Nurses as family caregivers—barriers and enablers facing nurses caring for children, parents or both. *J Nurs Manag.* 25(2):93–101.
77. Gardiner C, Brereton L, Frey R, Wilkinson-Meyers L, Gott M. Approaches to capturing the financial cost of family care-giving within a palliative care context: a systematic review. *Health Soc Care Community.* 2016;24(5):519–531. https://doi.org/10.1111/hsc.12253.
78. Schulz R. The intersection of family caregiving and work: labor force participation, productivity, and caregiver well-being. In: Czaja S, Sharit J, James J, eds. *Current and Emerging Trends in Aging and Work.* Springer; 2020:399–413. https://doi.org/10.1007/978-3-030-24135-3_20.
79. Simard-Duplain G. Heterogeneity in informal care intensity and its impact on employment. *J Health Econ.* 2022;86:102647.
80. Nadash P, Alberth A, Tell E, Jansen T. Policies to sustain employment among samily caregivers: the family caregiver perspective. *J Appl Gerontol.* 2023;42(1):3–11. https://doi.org/10.1177/07334648221125635.
81. Shooshtari S, Duncan K, Roger K, Fast J, Han J. Care-related out-of-pocket spending and caregiving consequences: results from a Canadian population-based study. *J Fam Econ Issues.* 2017;38(3):405–420.
82. Young J, Snowden A. A systematic review on the factors associated with positive experience in carers of someone with cancer. *Eur J Cancer Care (Engl).* 2017;26(3):12544.
83. Cohen R, Leis A, Kuhl D, Charbonneau C, Ritvo P, Ashbury F. QOLLTI-F: measuring family carer quality of life. *Palliat Med.* 2006;20(8):755–767.
84. Kim H, Myungsun Y. Unmet needs and quality of life of family caregivers of cancer patients in South Korea. *Asia Pacific J Oncol Nurs.* 2015;2(3):152–159.
85. Wu M, Huang S, Tsao L. The life experiences among primary family caregivers of home-based palliative care. *Am J Hosp Palliat Med.* 2020;37(10):816–822.
86. Alam S, Hannon B, Zimmerman C. Palliative care for family caregivers. *J Clin Oncol.* 2020;38(9):926–936.
87. National Alliance for Caregiving. *Cancer Caregiving in the US: An Intense, Episodic, and Challenging Care Experience.* National Alliance for Caregiving; 2016. https://www.caregiving.org/wp-content/uploads/2020/05/CancerCaregivingReport_FINAL_June-17-2016.pdf.
88. Murphy E, Froggartt K, Connolly S, et al. Palliative care interventions in advanced dementia. *Cochrane Database Syst Rev.* 2016;12(12):CD011513. https://doi.org/10.1002/14651858.CD011513.pub2.
89. Dionne-Odom J, Hooker S, Bekelman D, et al. Family caregiving for persons with heart failure at the intersection of heart failure and palliative care: a state-of-the-science review. *Heart Fail Rev.* 2017;22(5):543–557. https://doi.org/10.1007/s10741-017-9597-4.
90. Pollock A, St George B, Fenton M, Firkins L. Top 10 research priorities relating to life after stroke—consensus from stroke survivors, caregivers, and health professionals. *Int J Stroke.* 2014;9(3):313–320.
91. Doherty L, Fitzsimons D, McIlfatrick S. Carers' needs in advanced heart failure: a systematic narrative review. *Eur J Cardiovasc Nurs.* 2016;15(4):203–212.
92. Weaver M, Heinze K, Bell C, et al. Establishing psychosocial palliative care standards for children and adolescents with cancer and their families: an integrative review. *Palliat Med.* 2016;30(3):212–223. https://doi.org/10.1177/0269216315583446.
93. Weaver M, Heinze K, Kelly K, et al. Palliative care as a standard of care in pediatric oncology. *Pediatr Blood Cancer.* 2015;62(suppl 5):S829–S833. https://doi.org/10.1002/pbc.25695.
94. Kirch R, Reaman G, Feudtner C, et al. Advancing a comprehensive cancer care agenda for children and their families: Institute of Medicine Workshop highlights and next steps. *CA Cancer J Clin.* 2016;66(5):398–407. https://doi.org/10.3322/caac.21347.

95. Tanco K, Park J, Cerana A, Sisson A, Sobti N, Bruera E. A systematic review of instruments assessing dimensions of distress among caregivers of adult and pediatric cancer patients. *Palliat Support Care.* 2017;15(1):110–124. https://doi.org/10.1017/S1478951516000079.
96. Whittingham K, Barnes S, Gardiner C. Tools to measure quality of life and carer burden in informal carers of heart failure patients: a narrative review. *Palliat Med.* 2013;27(7):596–607.
97. Murray S, Firth A, Schneider N, et al. Promoting palliative care in the community: production of the primary palliative care toolkit by the European Association of Palliative Care Taskforce in primary palliative care. *Palliat Med.* 2015;29(2):101–111.
98. Finucane A, Bone A, Evans C, et al. The impact of population ageing on end-of-life care in Scotland: population-based projections of place of death and recommendations for future service provision. *BMC Palliat Care.* 2019;18(1):112. https://doi.org/10.1186/s12904-019-0490-x.
99. McCauley R, McQuillan R, Ryan K, Foley G. Mutual support between patients and family caregivers in palliative care: a systematic review and narrative synthesis. *Palliat Med.* 2021;35(5):875–885.
100. Ornstein K, Kelley A, Bollens-Lund E, Wolff J. A national profile of end-of-life caregiving in the United States. *Health Aff (Millwood).* 2017;36(7):1184–1192.
101. Cross S, Warraich H. Changes in the place of death in the United States. *N Engl J Med.* 2019;381:2369–2370. https://doi.org/10.1056/NEJMc1911892.
102. Liu W, Koerner J, Lam L, et al. Improved quality of death and dying in care homes: a palliative care stepped wedge randomized control trial in Australia. *J Am Geriatr Soc.* 2020;68(2):305–312.
103. Dionne-Odom J, Willis D, Bakitas M, Crandall B, Grace P. Conceptualizing surrogate decision making at end of life in the intensive care unit using cognitive task analysis. *Nurs Outlook.* 2015;63(3):331–340.
104. Starcke K, Brand M. Decision making under stress: a selective review. *Neurosci Biobehav Rev.* 2012;36(4):1228–1248.
105. Hinkle L, Bosslet G, Torke A. Factors associated with family satisfaction with end-of-life care in the ICU: a systematic review. *Chest.* 2015;147(1):82–93.
106. Al-Mutair A, Plummer V, O'Brien A, Clerehan R. Family needs and involvement in the intensive care unit: a literature review. *J Clin Nurs.* 2013;22(13–14):1805–1817. https://doi.org/10.1111/jocn.12065.
107. Back A, Arnold R, Tulsky J. *Mastering Communication with Seriously Ill Patients: Balancing Honesty with Empathy and Hope.* Cambridge University Press; 2009.
108. Singer A, Ash T, Ochotorena C, et al. A systematic review of family meeting tools in palliative and intensive care settings. *Am J Hosp Palliat Care.* 2016;33(8):797–806. https://doi.org/10.1177/1049909115594353.
109. Fakhreddine M, Galvan E, Pawlowski J, Jones W. Communicating effectively with elderly cancer patients. *Int J Radiat Oncol Biol Phys.* 2017;98(4):741–742.
110. Back A, Arnold R. "Isn't there anything more you can do?": when empathic statements work, and when they don't. *J Palliat Med.* 2013;16(11):1429–1432.
111. Back A, Arnold R. "Yes it's sad, but what should I do?" Moving from empathy to action in discussing goals of care. *J Palliat Med.* 2014;17(2):141–144.
112. Juarez G, Ferrell B, Uman G, Podnos Y, Wagman L. Distress and quality of life concerns of family caregivers of patients undergoing palliative surgery. *Cancer Nurs.* 2008;31(1):2–10. https://doi.org/10.1097/01.NCC.0000305682.13766.c2.
113. Sun V, Krouse R. Palliative surgery: incidence and outcomes. *Semin Oncol Nurs.* 2014;30(4):234–241.
114. Sipples R, Taylor R, Kirk-Walker D, Bagcivan G, Dionne-Odom J, Bakitas M. Perioperative palliative care considerations for surgical oncology nurse. *Semin Oncol Nurs.* 2017;33(1):9–22.
115. Doty P, Spillman B. Help for family caregivers available from government programs and policies. In: *Family Caregiving in the New Normal.* Academic Press; 2015:153–190.
116. Reyes AM, Thunell J, Zissimopoulos J. Addressing the diverse needs of unpaid caregivers through new health-care policy opportunities. *Public Policy Aging Rep.* 2020;31(1):19–23. https://doi.org/10.1093/ppar/praa039;
117. Ersek M, Carpenter J. Geriatric palliative care in long-term care settings with a focus on nursing homes. *J Palliat Med.* 2013;16(10):1180–1187.
118. Huskamp H, Kaufmann C, Stevenson D. The intersection of long-term care and end-of-life care. *Med Care Res Rev.* 2012;69(1):3–44.
119. Gaugler J, Mitchell L. Reimagining family involvement in residential long-term care. *J Am Med Dir Assoc.* 2022;23(2):235–240.
120. Tupper S, Ward H, Parmar J. Family presence in long-term care during the COVID-19 pandemic: call to action for policy, practice, and research. *Can Geriatr J.* 2020;23(4):335–339.
121. Abrahamson K, Bernard B, Magnabosco L, Nazir A, Unroe K. The experiences of family members in the nursing home to hospital transfer decision. *BMC Geriatr.* 2016;16(1):184.
122. Bolt S, van der Steen J, Mujezinović I, et al. Practical nursing recommendations for palliative care for people with dementia living in long-term care facilities during the COVID-19 pandemic: a rapid scoping review. *Int J Nurs Stud.* 2021;113(2021):103781.
123. Roberts A, Ishler K. Family involvement in the nursing home and perceived resident quality of life. *Gerontologist.* 2018;58(6):1033–1043.
124. Gaugler J. Family involvement in residential long-term care: a synthesis and critical review. *Aging Ment Health.* 2005;9(2):105–118. https://doi.org/10.1080/13607860412331310245.
125. Gray TF, Nolan MT, Clayman ML, Wenzel JA. The decision partner in healthcare decision-making: a concept analysis. *Int J Nurs Stud.* 2019;92:79–89. https://doi.org/10.1016/j.ijnurstu.2019.01.006.
126. Lamore K, Montalescot L, Untas A. Treatment decision-making in chronic diseases: what are the family members' roles, needs and attitudes? A systematic review. *Patient Educ Couns.* 2017;100(12):2172–2181.
127. Lee J, Shin D, Cho J, et al. Caregiver burden, patients' self perceived burden, and preference for palliative care among cancer patients and caregivers. *Psychooncology.* 2015;24(11):1545–1551.
128. Tang S, Chen J, Chou W, et al. Prevalence of severe depressive symptoms increases as death approaches and is associated with disease burden, tangible social support, and high self-perceived burden to others. *Support Care Cancer.* 2016;24(1):83–91. https://doi.org/10.1007/s00520-015-2747-0.
129. Beauchamp T, Childress J. *Principles of Biomedical Ethics.* 7th ed. Oxford University Press; 2012.
130. Torke A, Sachs G, Helft P, et al. Scope and outcomes of surrogate decision making among hospitalized older adults. *JAMA Intern Med.* 2014;174(3):370–377. https://doi.org/10.1001/jamainternmed.2013.13315.
131. Moorman S, Inoue M. Predicting a partner's end-of-life preferences, or substituting one's own?. *J Marriage Fam.* 2013;75(3):734–745.

30

Hope and Meaning in Illness

Anessa M. Foxwell and Darcy Alimenti

Key Points

- Those living with serious illness may question, reassess, or search for meaning within their experience of serious illness; supporting patients and their families through this process is an integral responsibility of the palliative care nurse.
- Hope, meaning, and purpose are central concepts in the psychological and spiritual holistic care of patients with serious illness and their families.
- Distress—psychological, spiritual, and existential—as well as grief occur commonly in serious illness; palliative nurses are in a unique position to support patients and their families through their distress and grieving process.
- Assessing patients' hope, meaning, and purpose through skilled communication is integral to holistic palliative nursing.

Introduction

As a nurse who cares for patients with serious illness, it is important to bring a holistic perspective, that is, to care for patients and families as whole persons with physical, emotional, psychological, spiritual, and existential dimensions. Those living with serious illness may question, reassess, or search for meaning within their experience of serious illness; supporting patients and their families through this process is an integral responsibility of the palliative care nurse. This can often occur at serious illness diagnosis, any loss or change in condition—exacerbation, decline in functional status, starting or stopping a new treatment—or any failure of treatment. Each person has a unique definition for hope, meaning, and purpose; often, meaning and purpose are not even the same within a patient and caregiver dyad.

Similarly, hope(s) during illness and for the future is unique to each individual. Hopes during illness and wishes for the future are one of the ways persons and their families cope with illness and make sense of the insensible. Thus, to understand one's meaning, purpose, and hope is an intimate and reflective process. Indeed, when meaning, purpose, and hope are ill-defined or misaligned, a patient may experience psychological, spiritual, and/or existential distress.

The purpose of this chapter is to (i) explore the concepts of meaning, purpose, and hope; (ii) differentiate the types of psychological, spiritual, and existential distress and grief due to loss; (iii) define the role of nurses in supporting patients in their search for meaning, purpose, and/or hope; and (iv) provide nurses with assessment and intervention strategies to guide patients and families in redefining meaning. To get started, the case of Ms. R (see Case Study 1) explores meaning in the early stages of cancer diagnosis.

Case Study 1: Ms. R

Ms. R, a 71-year-old woman, was diagnosed with non-metastatic left breast cancer earlier this year and is recovering from a left mastectomy. She lives with her husband of 45 years, with whom she has four children and seven grandchildren. Since diagnosis she has experienced increased anxiety as she processes this whirlwind diagnosis and treatment. After her treatment, she has struggled with loss of identity and finding meaning in her life. She is not used to feeling so unsettled due to uncertainty about her future, grappling with questions such as "Should I have reconstructive surgery?" and "Will I need additional chemotherapy and radiation?" She has experienced grief about a variety of losses—the loss of her breasts, a loss of meaning and purpose, loss of healthiness, and loss of life as she knew it. She worries about her relationship with her husband and getting back to the love and intimacy they enjoyed. Her anxiety and worry cause her mind to race in circles. She tries to see the light in life but notes that at times life feels "dark."

Questions to Consider:

1. What statements/questions indicate that Ms. R is struggling to process her illness?
2. What type(s) of distress is Ms. R experiencing?
3. Identify three losses Ms. R has named.

Meaning and Purpose

Each of us has our own unique meaning and purpose that define, shape, and motivate our lives. Meaning and purpose are complementary concepts. Meaning can be defined as what and how people subjectively experience meaningfulness.[1] Purpose is defined as "a sense of core goals, aims and direction in life."[1(p534)] One's meaning and purpose are not stagnant but rather can evolve throughout the course of our lives, whether in the spur of the moment, because of a major life change, or due to an anticipated pivot. For many, a serious illness often forces a reappraisal of meaning and purpose in life.

It is important to separate meaning in life as a psychological question, as opposed to the search for the meaning of life, which is a philosophical question.[1] Meaning in life is a subjective experience, whereas meaning of life can be viewed as a more collective question of existence. The psychotherapist Viktor Frankl popularized meaning in his book *Man's Search for Meaning*, chronicling his Holocaust survival through an ability to find meaning and purpose in life.[2,3] Frankl was the founder of "logotherapy," a psychotherapeutic approach to the analysis of one's meaning and guidance to find meaning and purpose in life.[3] In trauma or crisis, the ability to make meaning can be likened to one's ability to make sense of the insensible or to redeem the unredeemable.[3]

Everything is assigned meaning based on our judgments of its significance and value.[4] Each person comes to new situations with unique life experiences and the meanings gained from them. This is true when confronted with a serious illness. While living with a serious illness, it is normal for people to experience a plethora of emotions—both positive and negative emotions. For instance, a person with end-stage renal disease feels gratitude and love while at the same time feeling anger and fear. On the positive side, they experience gratitude that dialysis is available to them and love for their family who has created a schedule for their dialysis treatments. Simultaneously, they experience the negative emotions of anger that their body is failing them and fear that something will go wrong. The simultaneous experience of both positive and negative emotions is part of living with serious illness. In those with cancer, the concept of existential experience has been described as a balance of dialectical coping between existential health and existential suffering.[5] Thus, patients swing between these extremes and live in the gray of the experience, rather than being categorized into a binary of health or suffering.

Despite one's illness, a strong sense of meaning has been correlated with self-awareness, self-acceptance, and feelings of peace and control of their environment.[6–8] Meaning in serious illness can be derived from religion, an educational purpose, a sense of connection, or a service mission. For instance, cancer patients enrolled in clinical trials find meaning when they give back to society through participation in trials that may benefit future generations.[9,10] An individual with serious illness may have one meaning and purpose, while caregivers or loved ones may have a different meaning. Because different roles and relationships exist, diagnosis and loss will create different meanings for each person involved.

A patient's journey through serious illness implores the nurse to go beyond assessment, diagnosis, intervention, and evaluation. In order to reach shared connectedness, nurses must be willing to match a patient's vulnerability within the therapeutic nurse–patient relationship. Skilled communication is integral to support a patient's interpretation of meaning while living with serious illness. Nurses can be a catalyst for helping the patient and family find meaning in the illness and in the process. Specific communication techniques and nursing interventions are described in more depth in the later section "Nursing Assessment of Meaning in Illness and Role of the Nurse."

Loss of Meaning and Purpose

When a person loses their sense of meaning and purpose, they may feel listless, hopeless, demoralized, or sad. During serious illness, a person may reassess or reappraise their meaning and purpose and feel a sense of meaninglessness or purposelessness. This can show up as depression, anxiety, listlessness, insomnia, anger, or uncertainty. It can impact relationships, career, motivations, and almost all aspects of life. When a person with a serious illness loses their sense of meaning and purpose, it is commonly due to the losses associated with their illness. In the case of Ms. R (see Case Study 1), her meaning was derived from her identity as a mother, grandmother, wife, and caregiver. Her cancer diagnosis and loss of her breast have caused her to question her identity and meaning moving forward.

A loss of meaning and purpose can lead to distress—whether mild or severe. Often, when someone has a loss of meaning and purpose, there is a sense of separation or disconnectedness. In other words, while they remain the same person, they also become permanently different from others. They may fear that no one can possibly understand or appreciate what they are going through. When meaning is threatened by a serious diagnosis, people may fear the loss of who they are as functioning, productive, relatable, and relational human beings.

Case Study 2: Mr. M

Mr. M. is a 44-year-old successful engineer at a pharmaceutical company, devoted husband, and father of two young children. His ability to solve challenging problems at work earned him the nickname "Fix." His identity as a "fixer" meant providing for his family gave him meaning and purpose. Then, in 2017, he was diagnosed with amyotrophic lateral sclerosis (ALS) after months of clinic visits trying to diagnose his symptoms—stumbling more, slurred speech, and frequently dropping things. By the time he was diagnosed he was categorized as middle-stage ALS. This was a shock for both him and his family. He was immediately worried about "suffering a slow death" due to the progressive nature of ALS. Over time, he became paralyzed and dependent on a feeding tube for all nutrition. His anxiety about his future and his family is heightened. He feels his situation is "futile" and perseverates on a fear of suffering. As he becomes weaker, Mr. M shares that witnessing his "own decline disturbs" him. When he sees a reflection of himself in the mirror, he thinks "Why is this happening to me?" He continues to worry about his family, especially his young children. Although Mr. M. tries to draw strength from his family and faith, he struggles with the uncertainty. His inability to "fix" his health, his situation, his decline is devastating. Given his prognosis, he questions the merit of life-sustaining treatment, such as feeding tubes and tracheostomies, if he is going to die "anyway." At the same time, he expresses a desperate desire to live for his wife and children. He feels very isolated in his distress, and the process of living with his serious illness is "dehumanizing."

Questions to Consider:

1. How has Mr. M's illness impacted his identity and meaning and purpose?

2. What type of distress does Mr. M display when he states, "Why is this happening to me?"
3. What continues to give Mr. M strength as he copes with his diagnosis?

Types of Distress

Distress can be broadly defined as "pain or suffering affecting the body, a bodily part, or the mind."[11] Distress surfaces in many forms—physical, emotional, psychological, spiritual, existential, moral, or ethical. The National Comprehensive Cancer Network defines distress as "a multifactorial unpleasant experience of psychological (i.e., cognitive, behavior, emotional), social, spiritual, and/or physical nature that may interfere with one's ability to cope effectively"[12(pDIS-1)] with serious illness. In the field of oncology, there has been much research to explore distress in its many forms while patients are dealing with the serious illness of cancer. Psychological or emotional assessment and treatment is an important component of palliative and serious illness care.[13–16] Moreover, in a retrospective study of bereaved caregivers, almost half felt the decedent experienced some form of psychological distress at the end of life.[17] A meta-analysis found that the prevalence of mood disorders in hospitalized patients with cancer was 30%–40% of cases.[18] Further, depressive symptoms have been associated with poor quality of life and greater burden of associated symptoms.[19,20]

Suffering is a related concept to distress. Sociologist Martha Beck describes suffering as what remains after the physical experience of pain—physical, emotion, or psychological—is gone.[21] Thus, people experience suffering on a spectrum of absence. Cassell goes further in linking suffering and distress: "Suffering is a state of severe distress induced by the loss of the intactness of a person, or by a threat that the person believes will result in the loss of his or her intactness."[4 (p. 63)] Suffering is an individual and private experience and will be greatly influenced by the personality and character of the person; for example, the patient who has needed control during times of wellness will find the out-of-control experience of illness as suffering.[4] Healthcare clinicians can contribute to suffering when making patients feel objectified or by providing fragmented care.[22]

The following sections will describe the most common types of distress associated with meaning in serious illness. Experiences of distress and suffering can be discrete or multifactorial or have overlapping qualities depending on how a patient feels at that particular time.

Psychological Distress

Psychological distress has to do with an unpleasant emotional, behavioral, or cognitive state. Psychological distress can be situational, as in demoralization or hopelessness, or broad, as when a patient confronts mortality. Psychological distress manifests in one or more of the following emotions: anxiety, guilt, fear, worry, shame, regret, despair, etc. In serious illness, patients and family members may talk about persuasive guilt, fear of burden, fear of resentment, or unresolved traumas that resurface (i.e., the need to be forgiven for previous wrongdoings).

It is important for the palliative nurse to collaborate with colleagues (especially palliative care social workers, therapists, and psychologists as applicable) to differentiate psychological distress from clinical depression, anxiety disorder, or other mental health diagnoses. Psychological distress is difficult to recognize as symptoms vary and do not typically qualify for psychiatric diagnoses (i.e., depression and anxiety). Nonetheless, psychological and emotional distress, if unaddressed, may lead to more severe depression, anxiety, suicidal ideation, or other psychiatric comorbidities.[23,24]

If a person experiences psychological distress related to the desire to be forgiven, then the nurse can help explore these desires and facilitate conversations. Sometimes, patients need guidance to forgive themselves for past action or inaction; other times, patients seek reconciliation with others. Reconciliation during serious illness can be powerful and healing for the patient and family. Forgiveness allows both physical and emotional energy to be used to create and enjoy the time left to live. In fact, those who practice self-acceptance and self-forgiveness have transformative experiences of living with illness, according to a qualitative meta-synthesis,[25] and perhaps less psychological distress.

Spiritual Distress

Spiritual distress can broadly be defined as the loss of, or questioning of, previously held beliefs. Spirituality can be associated with religiosity or can be a separate experience. Spirituality is a central component of hope.[26–28] Hopefulness is consistently associated with spiritual well-being,[25–27,29] and studies have shown that spirituality and spiritual practices provide a context in which to define hope and articulate hope-fostering activities.[26,29] Patients have unique spiritual needs and concerns depending on their views and experiences of spiritual care; globally patients and caregivers want staff competence in spiritual care to support unique needs.[30] For many, spirituality helps transcend losses and find ways to maintain connections—whether it is the belief that one's love, work, or creativity will remain after the physical separation or the belief that one's spirit goes on to an afterlife. Although spirituality is almost always viewed as a hope-fostering influence, serious illness and suffering can challenge one's religious belief and trust in a benevolent deity or be viewed as punishment from God; either interpretation of suffering can result in hopelessness. Meaning in life is a potential mediator of the relationship between religiousness and psychological well-being.[31–33]

Existential Distress

Existential distress is similar to spiritual distress; however, a key distinction is that there is always a loss of meaning and/or purpose. Existentiality is associated with what is beyond the human body; therefore, existential distress may be due to a dread of "what comes next" after one dies. Existential distress can be recognized by the unanswerable questions that one may pose (see Table 30.1). If a person's meaning and purpose are connected to their spirituality, then they may also experience spiritual distress. For those believing in life after death, the questions may focus on the uncertainty of eternal life or

Table 30.1 Example of existential questions

Existential questions	Why me? What have I done to deserve this? What happens when I die? Is there really a God? How could my God do this to me?

the possibility of this being a "test" of faith. No matter what the belief system, existential questions are frequently asked in serious illness.[5]

When faced with uncertainty, many may reach out for a connection to something beyond the self (i.e., God, nature, etc.) to obtain some sense of security and stability. Persons with serious illness may grapple with existential questions that they are afraid to ask aloud. It is important for the palliative care nurse to be trained to hear these questions and intervene with additional support, such as referral to a spiritual care provider or social worker trained in palliative care. In the case of Mr. M (see Case Study 2), he experiences existential distress as he has lost his sense of meaning and purpose—that of a fixer, that of a provider—and he is asking the red flag question "Why me?" For additional reading on spiritual and existential distress, please see Chapter 33, "Addressing Spiritual, Religious, and Existential Needs in Palliative Care."

Grief

For many, being diagnosed with a serious illness is a loss of their future as they once knew it. Grief refers to the subjective feelings that accompany an anticipated or realized loss. Loss is an expansive concept that can be associated with dying, change, or anticipation of a loss. Persons with serious illness experience grief at diagnosis because they will never be the same person. They also experience loss of a future as they had imagined it. The patient may miss events while hospitalized or have to cancel trips, leave work and go on disability, and give up certain responsibilities at home. Each of these losses deserves time and space to grieve.

Caregivers too can experience grief as they care for a loved one with serious illness. These losses may be similar or different. They may grieve the loss of the way they used to imagine life and how it would have been with that person. It is also the loss of an image of oneself, the abandonment of plans for the future and what might have been.[34,35] For a child and the surviving parent, those losses of dreams will be played out on important days—birthdays, milestones, anniversaries, weddings, etc. For additional reading on grief, please see Chapter 58, "Grief and Bereavement."

Distress in Serious Illness

As described, distress in serious illness can be related to psychological issues, spiritual concerns, existential struggles, and/or grief. To return to the case of Ms. R, she experienced psychological distress as well as grief due to loss—loss of identity, loss of self, loss of the future as she imagined it.

Case Study Revisited: Ms. R

After her mastectomy, Ms. R is referred to a wound care nurse who is also a certified hospice and palliative nurse through the Hospice & Palliative Nurses Association. Ms. R laments that having her wounds tended to by the nurse is the most intimate she has been with anyone besides her husband. They quickly develop a therapeutic relationship based on trust, care, and connection. The nurse recognizes Ms. R's anxiety and psychological distress on the first visit and holds space for Ms. R to process her emotions and her situation. Over time, Ms. R's psychological distress lessens. She feels more in control of her anxiety as she plans for the future. She makes plans with her husband for a date night, schedules time with her grandkids, and asks friends to stop by. She remains unsure what her future with cancer will look like but is clear that minimizing stress is a priority.

As her surgical wound heals, the nurse prepares to discharge Ms. R from home care. Ms. R reflects that the process of living with cancer is humbling. Previously, her motto was to "power through" life. She now understands that healing and recovery take time. Cancer has been the most complicated struggle she has gone through and has taught her how fragile life is.

Questions to Consider:

1. What strategies did the palliative care nurse use to help support Ms. R?
2. What tools has Ms. R utilized to cope with her serious illness and distress?
3. What signs indicate that Ms. R has less distress after interventions from the palliative care nurse?

The palliative care certified wound care nurse supports Ms. R and helps her to reframe her distress and grief. When a patient experiences distress in serious illness, it is rare that they reach a state of transcendence and remain there through the illness process. Instead, for most, it is a process in which there are moments when they reach a sense of expansion that supports them to face the uncertainty of the future.

Hope in the Context of Serious Illness

Hope is central to the human experience of living and dying, and it is integrally entwined with spiritual and psychosocial well-being. Although serious illness can challenge and even temporarily diminish hope, the dying process does not inevitably bring despair. The human spirit manifests its creativity and resiliency to forge new and deeper hopes at the end of life. Palliative care nurses play important roles to support patients and families with this process through expert physical, psychosocial, and spiritual care. Sensitive, skillful attention to maintaining hope can enhance quality of life and contribute significantly to a "good death" as defined by the patient and family. Fostering hope is a primary means by which palliative care nurses accompany patients and families on the journey through serious illness.

Hope influences health and adaptation to illness. Empirical evidence indicates that diminished hope is associated with poorer quality of life[36] and persistence of suicidal ideation.[37] Hopelessness also increases the likelihood that people will consider medical aid in dying as an option for themselves.[38]

Despite these somber realities and the inevitable suffering, many people do maintain hope within the context of serious illness, and families recover and find hope even within the experience of loss. This can partially be attributed to the nature of hope itself—its resiliency and capacity to coexist with suffering. For instance, relationships with significant others are another important dimension of hope. Interconnectedness with others is continually cited as a source of hope, and physical and psychological isolation from others is a frequent threat to hope.[39–41] In addition to family members and friends, nurses offer patients a unique and independent source of support for hope.[42,43] As witnesses to suffering and hope, palliative care nurses must understand these complexities and be confident and sensitive in their efforts to address hope and hopelessness in the people for whom they care.

Another strategy is to help the patient and family identify goals, which can motivate and energize people and thereby increase hope.[44,45] To identify goals, people assess what they desire and value within a context of what is realistically possible.[46] They appraise the resources necessary to accomplish their goals against the resources that are available to them. They then take action to secure the resources or meet the goals, and they decide on a reasonable time frame in which to accomplish the goals.[47] Active involvement in one's situation and attainment of goals increase the sense of personal control and self-efficacy, which, in turn, increases hope.[46] If a person repeatedly fails to attain valued goals, then hopelessness and negative emotions, such as anxiety, depression, or anger, can result.[44] People also adopt specific strategies to foster hope at the end of life.[48,49]

Many people with serious illness turn to activities and coping strategies that cultivate generalized hope rather than an emphasis on achievement and control. These strategies reflect a sense of peace and acceptance of death and center on "being" rather than "doing."[48] These strategies are described in Box 30.1. On the other hand, Olsson and colleagues found that patients preserved their hope using two goal-oriented or problem-solving processes: (1) maintaining life and (2) preparing for death.[50] The patients tried to maintain life in several ways: continue their day-to-day tasks and hobbies; communicate with others about practical matters and emotional feelings; involve other people such as family, friends, or professionals; and actively search elsewhere for something to give them hope.

Although hope tends to change in people with serious illness, the delicate balance between acceptance of death and hope for a cure often remains an important task up until the time of death, even when people acknowledge that cure is virtually impossible.[49,50] The dying person also needs to envision future moments of happiness, fulfillment, and connection.[48,51]

Although some people continue to search for a cure after receiving a serious or life-threatening diagnosis, hoping for a cure can coexist with awareness of mortality and engagement with life's activities.[48] Most people eventually accept their prognosis and mourn the loss of their original goals. At this point, they need to develop and pursue alternative goals that are possible in light of their diminished physical function, end-of-life symptoms, and loss of energy. These different approaches to maintaining hope are important to describe and understand because they assist the palliative care nurse to design effective strategies to foster and reframe hope. See Case Study 3 to review the case of Mx. S where the palliative care advanced practice registered nurse (APRN) supports Mx. S to reframe hopes for their future.

Box 30.1 Sources of Hope/Hope-Fostering Strategies in Seriously Ill Adults

Love of family and friends
Spirituality/having faith
Setting goals and maintaining independence
Positive relationships with professional carers
Humor
Personal characteristics
Uplifting memories

Source: Reference 49.

Case Study 3: Mx. S

Mx. S is a 56-year-old queer person who was diagnosed with chronic obstructive pulmonary disease (COPD) 5 years ago due to a 40-year smoking history. They are single, live alone, have no children, and recently went on long-term disability from a career at FedEx. They have two supportive brothers who live within 2 hours. They have experienced progressive disease, with six hospitalizations for COPD exacerbations in the last year. Mx. S has high prognostic awareness and understands their time is limited and could be as short as months to years. They especially hate taking steroids for exacerbations as they become hyperactive and insomniac on steroids; more recently they have begun to notice Cushingoid features, which have been troubling. They worry about the future, especially suffering at the end of life, and question what happens after death. They worry about losing their independence and becoming a burden to their brothers. Mx. S converted to Buddhism decades ago and values an interconnectedness to a greater being and finds calm in meditation.

During a palliative care consultation, Mx. S speaks with the palliative care APRN and acknowledges that they are no longer the person they once were. Living with a serious illness has allowed them to reprioritize their life and focus on what they can control. They work with the palliative care ARPN to complete an advance directive and estate will to decrease burden on family. After this is complete, Mx. S talks about their hope to travel solo. They have always wanted to ride the train cross-country. They yearn to see national parks across America and Canada. They look forward to time alone on the train, immersed in the beauty of the world, and hope to be reminded there is something bigger and better beyond their illness.

Questions to Consider:

1. Identify three losses Mx. S has experienced due to COPD.
2. What types of distress is Mx. S experiencing?
3. The palliative care APRN helped Mx. S reframe hope. What goals was Mx. S then able to name?

Reframing Hope

Acceptance, comfort, contentedness, or peace is an individual experience for each person. Another important nursing intervention is to help patients reframe hope. Reframing hope can be as simple as the nurse recalibrating assessment questions from long-term to short-term. Instead of "What are your hopes for the future?" the nurse can ask "What are your hopes for today [or the next week]?" Or if time is a triggering concept, the nurse can ask about hopes for specific events, such as "How do you hope this visit with your loved one will go?" Reframing hope to more concrete, achievable goals help patients focus on the present. There are also psychotherapy interventions. For instance, inspired by Viktor Frankl,[2] there are meaning-centered psychotherapy interventions that show that if the patient could manipulate or reframe their sense of meaning, they would have positively impacted the foundational elements of despair at the end of life.[52] When patients are able to reframe their sense of meaning and purpose, their hopefulness may be sustained.

There is a role for the nurse to assist families with reframing hope. Often, when friends and family try to encourage or help the patient find meaning, they may unintentionally minimize the loss and pain by comparing losses; they can deny the patient the freedom to be angry or by immediately focusing on the time left to live. Ultimately, the goal is not to merely arrive at a single meaning within the patient–family dyad but, rather, encourage them to share their individual meanings so that all can learn and relationships can be deepened and strengthened.[26,30,53]

Nursing Assessment of Meaning in Illness and Role of the Nurse

Nurses help patients diagnosed with a serious illness process complex emotions related to meaning and purpose. Armed with both the skills and tools, nurses are precisely situated to support patients in coping with their ever-changing reality. Ethically, nurses have a responsibility to provide the care and support needed. The American Nurses Association's *Code of Ethics for Nurses* asserts that nurses are obligated to address the alleviation of suffering and provide supportive care to individuals with serious illness: "Optimal nursing care enables the patient to live with as much physical, emotional, social, and spiritual well-being as possible and reflects the patient's own values."[54 (p. 2)] In order to best support patients during this time, nurses must draw on their knowledge of the nursing process. A comprehensive assessment must be performed prior to an appropriate intervention. Ultimately, with time the nurse functions as a key support of the patient with serious illness and their caregivers as they seek to redefine hope and reappraise their meaning and purpose.

Nursing Assessment

Thorough assessment of physical, psychosocial, and spiritual/existential factors must precede a thoughtful plan and implementation of therapeutic strategies. Therefore, consistent and comprehensive evaluations of hope, meaning, and purpose should be included in the palliative care nursing assessment. Assessment should focus on patients' self-reports as the elements of hope and meaning and purpose are highly subjective and individualized experiences. Open-ended questions offer an opportunity for patients to express their emotions, look inward as they contemplate their distress, and guide the conversation. Table 30.2 provides examples of questions a palliative care nurse can use to assess hope and meaning and purpose. Oftentimes patients will need time and space to express their feelings. This may be the first time they are being asked these questions, and they may not know the answers immediately. Patients may feel uncomfortable divulging their deepest emotions, thoughts, and worries. If a patient responds with a one-worded answer, the nurse can further explore the patient's thoughts with statements like, "Tell me more." The goal of the assessment is to have a better sense of the patient's character and how the illness has impacted their core being.

Nurses also utilize their astute assessment skills to discern more about the patient's emotional state. The nurse can learn more about the patient's internal state of mind when they pay attention to the patient's behavior and physical presentation. Behavioral cues often provide insight into a person's internal state. Hopelessness is a central feature of depression; therefore, behaviors such as social withdrawal, flat affect, alcohol and substance use, insomnia, lethargy, loss of appetite, and passivity may be indicative of hopelessness. Loss of meaning and purpose may come across as anger, anxiety, depression, insomnia, restlessness, tearfulness, and flat affect. Ultimately, when a patient with serious illness has new physical complaints or altered behavior patterns the nurse uses these signals to gather more data about how they are doing emotionally, mentally, and spiritually.

Table 30.2 Examples of language for nursing assessment of hope and meaning

Assessing hope	What are you hoping for? What is most important to you when you think about the future? What are you looking forward to? In the past, what have been sources of strength? What sustains you and keeps you going? What do you hold onto during difficult times?
Assessing meaning	Tell me about your life and who you were before your illness. How has your illness impacted your life? How has your illness changed who you were before your illness? How has your illness impacted your ability to do the things that are most important to you? How do you make sense of your illness? What typically brings you meaning and purpose in life? What gives you joy and pleasure in life?

In light of holistic care, the hope, meaning, and purpose of the patient's family, loved ones, caregivers, and support people should be also assessed. A serious illness affects the patient–caregiver dyad in a bidirectional manner. Changes to the patient's hope, meaning, purpose, and distress will impact their caregivers. Caregivers have their own distress and worry as they struggle to know how best to support the patient. Caregivers may express feelings of helplessness and fear as they bear witness to changes in the patient's being. They do not want to say or do things that may result in further distress to the patient. Meanwhile they internalize their own worry that when mixed with the demands of caregiving can result in caregiver burnout. Similarly, patients with serious illness often struggle with fear of burdening their loved ones. Often, patients harbor their emotions and choose not to share their deep worries, which causes them to feel isolated. The nurse can assess the patient–caregiver dyad together or separately. Some patient–caregiver dyads may prefer to communicate openly with the nurse present as a guide and mediator. Others prefer to speak to the nurse separately as they continue to process the impacts of a serious illness. In assessing patient and caregiver distress levels, the nurse is already having an impact. Assessment provides space for the patient and caregiver to be heard and demonstrates that the nurse cares about their well-being.

When the palliative care nurse physically assesses the patient and caregiver, it is important to evaluate for psychological, spiritual, and existential distress. If a psychological, spiritual, or existential crisis is noted, then the nurse should call upon their interdisciplinary palliative care team or place a referral to spiritual care providers and other professionals with expertise in psychological, spiritual, or existential counseling.

Assessing Diversity

Much of the research pertaining to hope and meaning and purpose in illness does not adequately reflect the experience of people from non-European cultures. Several known cultural differences limit the applicability of current conceptualizations of hope, meaning, and purpose, especially within the palliative care context. Three issues that theoretically could have a major impact on multicultural views of hope, meaning, and purpose are time orientation, truth-telling, and one's beliefs about control.

Time orientation is identified as a cultural phenomenon that varies among cultural groups. Some cultural groups, usually highly individualistic ones, are future-oriented. Within these groups, people prefer to look ahead, make short- and long-term plans, and organize their schedules to meet goals.[55] Because hope is defined as being future-oriented, with hopeful people more likely to identify and take action to meet goals, members of these future-oriented cultures may possibly appear more hopeful than people who are predominantly present-focused. When confronted with a serious illness, people who are future-oriented tend to have greater fears and worries about the future as they grapple with uncertainty and their mortality. On the other hand, people who are more focused on the present and are guided by meaning may be better able to sustain hope while seriously ill, given that their ability to create long-term goals is hindered by the uncertainty surrounding a life-threatening diagnosis. People who do not focus on the what-ifs and worst-case situations and are more focused in the present tend to not have fears and worries about the future with their serious illness. Additional research is needed to clarify these relationships.

The value of truth-telling in Western healthcare systems also may affect hope, meaning, and purpose. Current ethical and legal standards require full disclosure of all relevant healthcare information to patients.[56] Informed consent and patient autonomy in medical decision-making, two eminent values in US healthcare, are impossible without this disclosure.[56] Although few would advocate that clinicians should lie to patients, truth-telling is not universally viewed as helpful or desirable.[57–59] In some cultures, it is believed that patients should be protected from burdensome information that could threaten hope. Truthful, but blunt, communication may also be seen as rude and disrespectful in some cultures and can have a negative impact on hope. In addition to the threats to hope that frank discussion is believed to engender, people who prefer nondisclosure of threatening information may be seen as clinging to unrealistic hopes and refusing to listen to discouraging facts about their condition.

A third cultural concept that may affect hope, meaning, and purpose is one's feeling of being in control. Control is a core attribute in many conceptualizations of hope. Although control can be relinquished to others, including healthcare providers or a transcendent power, personal control often is central to hope and meaning-making. In Euro-American cultures, it is natural and desirable for patients to direct their will and energy to alter the course of an illness or the dying process. Advance directives are one culturally sanctioned way in which members of these societies exert control over the dying process.[60] However, this desire for and belief in personal control is not a common feature in many other cultures. In cultures where death is viewed as part of the inherent harmony of life, attempts to exert any influence over the dying process may seem unnatural or inappropriate.[60] People from diverse cultures who take a more passive role in their healthcare or who do not espouse a desire to control their illness or the dying process may be viewed as less hopeful than people who manifest a "fighting spirit" and active stance. Every person and caregiver has individual needs when living and dying with a serious illness. The palliative nurse should assess and acknowledge individual losses. For certain patient populations there are unique needs that the nurse should be aware of. For example, in the LGBTQIA+ community there are unique psychological stressors of serious illness and advanced care planning, such as surrogate designation and memorialization in their chosen name.[61] For additional reading specific to care of LGBTQIA+ individuals, please see Chapter 67, "Affirmative Palliative Care for LGBTQIA+ Patients and Their Families."

These, among other reasons, provide evidence that an individual's values and preferences are impacted by cultural and societal constructs. How much stock one places on the value of time, the importance of truth-telling, and the need for control of self and environment is subjective. Thus, cultural values associated with hope, meaning, and purpose should be situated within the palliative nursing assessment. In the same vein, when the nurse understands a patient's cultural and ethnic background this does not presume insight alone. The palliative nurse must be curious about how culture shapes the individual's values and how their illness impacts their personal experience of hope, meaning, and purpose. For additional reading regarding culture, diversity, and inequalities, please see Chapter 28, "Cultural Considerations in Palliative Care," and/or Chapter 66, "Addressing Health Inequities, Social Determinants of Health, and Underrepresented Individuals in Palliative Care."

Nursing Role

The palliative care nurse has a dynamic role in supporting patients with serious illness. The patient's ability to cope, emotions, psychosocial distress, and physical state will change over time. The nurse–patient relationship will also evolve as trust is built. There are many skills the nurse utilizes to tend to patient suffering and distress; these skills are outlined below. Of note, there is no one algorithm for this type of work. Rather, each patient–nurse relationship and each interaction is unique, thus requiring the nurse to draw upon a variety of skills. Patient experiences are all individualized; thus, the palliative care nurse must meet the patients where they are and utilize the appropriate techniques. See the Case Study Revisited: Mr. M for an example of the nurse's role within the interdisciplinary team to support Mr. M in his existential distress.

Case Study Revisited: Mr. M

In order to support Mr. M to live with the diagnosis of ALS, neurology recommends consultation with home palliative care. The interdisciplinary palliative care team includes a nurse, social worker, and chaplain. Each of the interdisciplinary team members addresses Mr. M's existential distress in unique, but complementary, ways. The nurse employs communication skills to actively listen to Mr. M's sources of distress with silence and presence. They build a therapeutic relationship where Mr. M feels a sense of connection and empathy. The nurse provides initial education on assistive devices (i.e., eye-gaze device and other technologies) should Mr. M need assistance in the future. This gives Mr. M a restored sense of autonomy and control of some aspects of his uncertain future. The social worker works with him to set some new goals of getting his affairs in order and legacy work. Through the creation of an advance directive and living will, he is now less worried about burdening his wife with the responsibilities after his death. As a part of legacy work, he writes letters for his children in celebration of future milestones. Finally, Mr. M and the spiritual call provider spend time delving into his existential despair. This allowed him to find a new sense of meaning and purpose as a devoted husband and father. He comes to accept he cannot fix the ALS and the uncertainty associated with it and focuses his time and energy on cuddling his children as his wife reads bedtime stories.

Questions to Consider:

1. What strategies does the nurse use to support Mr. M?
2. Culturally, what is something the nurse should be mindful of when considering advanced care planning?
3. What should the nurse assess for before assisting a patient with legacy work?

Patients will present with their own coping strategies as they seek to maintain hope and redefine meaning and purpose in the face of serious illness. For example, some people pray; others distract themselves with television watching, conversation, or other activities; and many patients use cognitive strategies, such as minimizing negative thoughts, identifying personal strengths, and focusing on the positive. For many patients and families, careful observation and active support of an individual's established strategies to maintain hope and reframe meaning and purpose will be most successful. Family caregivers and other support people should be included in these approaches. Ample evidence demonstrates that patients and people within their support systems reciprocally influence one another's hope. In addition, family and significant others are always incorporated into the palliative care plan and considered part of the unit of care. Maintenance of hope also is a goal after death, in that hope-restoring and hope-maintaining strategies must be an integral part of bereavement counseling.[62,63]

Nursing Interventions

Therapeutic Presence

It is the duty of all who care for patients to alleviate suffering and not just treat the physical dimensions of the illness. This is no small task as professionals must first be free from denial and the need to self-protect in order to see the suffering of another. Then, they must be able to attend to it without trying to fix it or simplify it. Suffering needs to be witnessed; amid suffering, presence and compassion become the balm and hope for its relief. The skill of presence provides patients with confirmation, nurturing, and compassion as space is given for the patient to express their thoughts. The act of listening is more than the collection of data; it is therapeutic in providing the environment for the narrative to take place.[64–66] The skill of holding space, being with, and presence ultimately serves as an essential transcendent act. To master the skill, respect is the starting point—respect for the individual's experience with suffering and attempts to make sense of the illness. Finally, therapeutic presence allows for a safe environment and time for telling.[67,68]

Nonverbal Communication Skills

Communication starts before a sound leaves the nurse's mouth. Nonverbal communication skills allow the nurse to express compassion and demonstrate presence. Examples of nonverbal communication skills include sitting, leaning in, eye contact, open body language, facial expressions, and touch. When the nurse sits down to be with the patient, it signals to the patient the nurse is committed to being present with the patient. Through leaning in, the nurse indicates they are engaged in the patient's story and paying attention. Eye contact allows the nurse to convey respect and interest. With open body language the nurse demonstrates they are approachable and receptive to the patient's narrative. Facial expressions allow the nurse to communicate emotions and engage with the patient. Touch is a way of connection that allows the nurse to demonstrate a level of humanness. Touch has also been shown to reduce anxiety, pain, and fatigue in adults as well as children.[69–71]

Silence

Silence is a powerful skill employed by the palliative care nurse. In allowing for silence, the nurse demonstrates their pivotal role as the listener, giving the patient their voice. For many patients, it takes courage to share their thoughts. Silence gives them time to open up and begin processing the emotions. Through expression, a patient with serious illness has the opportunity to redefine hope and reappraise meaning and purpose. Important life themes are shared, and the unanswerable questions are asked. As a relative stranger, the nurse develops intimacy and trust with the patient, and meaning takes hold.

Acknowledging Emotion

Nurses have a wonderful opportunity to verbally acknowledge and name the emotions being expressed by patients and their caregivers. A serious illness will provoke an array of emotions—sadness, anger, worry, fear, loneliness, confusion, uncertainty, and hopelessness. By taking time to name the emotion expressed, the nurse allows the patient and caregiver to further examine the subtext below the flurry of questions or statements. Once the emotion is exposed, further work and exploration can take place. Oftentimes the patient will repeat the named emotion in statements such as "Yes, I'm angry." Coupled with silence and therapeutic presence, the patient may feel comfortable divulging the underlying thoughts behind the emotion. Additionally, the simple act of acknowledging the emotion allows the patient to feel heard and understood.

Reframing

Reframing is a technique employed by palliative care nurses to encourage patients and their caregivers to find meaning in the loss. Through reframing the nurse can assist the patient in altering their perspective and shifting the locus of control from the serious illness and back to the patient. For example, by adjusting the statement of "dying well" to "living well" nurses can help patients refocus their time and energy on how to live the days they have to the fullest. Reframing allows the patient to take back some control that was lost at diagnosis. This technique can also be utilized with the concept of hope. A common statement in palliative care is "Our hope is to allow you more days without pain, so that you can live your life fully." There is a cognitive shift in reframing that moves from a negative, catastrophizing narrative to a more neutral and possibly positive framework.

Listening for Hope

Hope is a very important coping skill. It is common to hear clinicians questioning the feasibility of a patient's or caregivers' hope and labeling it as "unrealistic" or noting that the patient remains in denial. However, true denial is very rare. Researchers and psychologists question whether denial and "unrealistic" hope are maladaptive. Instead, they argue that to believe these patients' professions of hope are unrealistic is to challenge or negate the legitimacy of the dominant depiction of the promise and potential cure provided by medical science.[48,51] Clinicians should not be concerned whether hope is real or unreal, true or false, present or not; rather, they should view hope as an attempt to articulate, share, and value with others those things that connect the patient to what give their lives meaning and, ultimately, to life.[51] In addition to the nurses role to promote positive outcomes, "unrealistic" hopes need to be assessed within the context of uncertainty. For instance, people frequently respond to dire prognostic news with the observation that they can always "beat the odds." Given that no one can predict the future with absolute certainty, it is impossible to predict which individuals with a small chance of remission or recovery will actually be cured. So, if a person hopes for something in the future that appears highly unlikely, can it be known for certain that it will not occur? It may be psychologically easier for patients and families to live in this uncertainty than to remind themselves of the more dire, pending mortality. Research supports the idea that patients' and families' hopes and goals are effective coping strategies, even when the likelihood of obtaining them seems remote.[48,72]

Reappraisal of Meaning, Purpose, and Hope

Reappraisal is a cognitive technique, often employed by older adults, that allows them to alter the meaning and impact of a serious illness in order to change the emotional impact. For example in a meta-synthesis of qualitative research, hope was described as an important psychological resource that helped older adults deal with chronic illness.[73] Older adults used two interrelated processes to help deal with their experience: (1) transcendence, a process of reaching inwardly and outwardly, and finding meaning and purpose, and (2) positive reappraisal, a recognition and acknowledgment that their situation had changed and they could see positive possibilities for the future.[73] For example, an older, married woman with advanced breast cancer may comment that, despite the seriousness of her disease, she feels luckier than another woman with the same disease who is younger or without social support. She takes solace in recognizing that "things could be worse" when she compares herself to others less fortunate. This act of comparison allows the older adult to change the meaning of their situation without changing it objectively.

Symptom Management

The mind and body are intimately connected. Unattended physical distress will result in emotional distress. Uncontrolled symptoms, such as pain, fatigue, dyspnea, and anxiety, cause suffering and challenge patients' and caregivers' hopefulness and meaning in illness. When patients suffer physically, it impacts their overall quality of life and perspective. They begin to question their meaning and purpose and can experience hopelessness. Timely and adept symptom prevention and management are central to maintain hope and optimize quality of life. Palliative care nurses, across settings, teach patients and families the knowledge and skills to manage symptoms confidently and competently.

Distraction

Other ways to help people find hope in suffering is to provide them a cognitive reprieve from their situation. One powerful strategy to achieve this temporary suspension is through humor. Humor helps put things in perspective and frees the self, at least momentarily, from the onerous burden of illness and suffering. Making light of a grim situation brings a sense of control over one's response to the situation, even when one has little influence over it. Of course, the use of humor with patients and families requires sensitivity as well as a sense of timing. The nurse should take cues from the patient and family, observe how they use humor to dispel stress, and let them take the lead in joking about threatening information and events. In general, humor should be focused on events outside the immediate concerns of the patient and family.

Positive Self-Talk

Another strategy the palliative care nurse can draw upon is to support patients or caregivers in their own positive self-talk. Often people naturally cope with stress by identifying attributes of personal strength that help them find hope.[45,49] Similarly, patients maintain hope when they focus on particular talents or previous accomplishments that indicate an ability to cope with illness. Patients cite their high level of motivation as a reason to feel hopeful about the future. They may also discuss prior experiences with adversity or describe their personal growth as sources of strength in the face of a serious illness. Acknowledgment and validation of these attributes support hope and affirm self-worth for patients and families.

Supporting Spirituality

Palliative care nurses can encourage and support a patient's spirituality as a way to cope with an illness. This strategy allows the nurse to provide opportunities for the patient to express spiritual beliefs and arrange for involvement in religious rituals and spiritual practices across palliative care settings. Another useful approach is when the nurse assists patients and families to explore and make meaning of their trials and suffering. The nurse can encourage patients and families to keep a journal of thoughts and feelings to help process their experiences. Another strategy is to suggest books, films, or art that focus on religious or existential understanding and transcendence of suffering to help people make sense of illness and death. Finally, the nurse can support a patient spiritually when they place a referral for a palliative spiritual care provider or hospital chaplain.

Interdisciplinary Legacy Work

Leaving a legacy may be one of the most concrete ways for patients to find meaning in the final stage of their lives.[74–76] It most often requires the patient to master the existential challenge—where the person with serious illness recognizes that death is near—and to choose the direction of their end-of-life course, how they will be remembered, and what they leave behind. Some patients will design their funeral or memorial service and use rituals, readings, and songs that reveal their values and messages for others. Others will create videos, write letters, or distribute their assets in meaningful ways.

Dignity therapy, life review, and legacy documents are interventions that have been utilized successfully with patients with serious illness.[77,78] Another effective tool to decrease isolation and increase a sense of connection is blogging—by writing or video recording. "Cypercoping" has been used by patients and family members to record their experiences and also leaves a permanent imprint of their lives on the internet.[79–83] It becomes a diary of the illness and has been shown to increase a sense of purpose and meaning as the patient shares with others.[79,84–86] Vlogging—video blogging—is another way for patients to share their cancer experiences as well as a means for leaving a legacy.[87,88]

Self-Care for the Nurse

Self-care is essential for the palliative care nurse to remain resilient in their care of those with a serious illness. Nurses should seek a mentor as they face their own complex emotions that accompany their witness to suffering and their first patient death, as well as navigating work–life boundaries. Scheduled time for formal debriefing with an interdisciplinary team helps the nurse grow as a clinician and serves as a safe space to process. Many palliative care teams have formal interdisciplinary team meetings to allow for this self-care work to take place. The element of suffering is a focal point for a small-group process that unburdens cumulative effects of the work and teaches skills and rituals on how to cope with work demands. In addition, it is important that the nurse learn clear boundaries between their professional and personal lives. Some traditional self-care strategies, such as journaling, meditation, exercise, adequate nutrition and hydration, and relaxation and breathing techniques, can be helpful as the nurse copes with the work.

Palliative care nurses will experience grief as the patients they care for die. The nurse can honor those who have died to establish a sense of closure. There are a variety of ways to honor and acknowledge those who have died and allow for the staff to grieve. For example, an interdisciplinary team may read the names of all of those who have died in the past week with an opportunity for sharing short stories about the patient, followed by a moment of silence and poetry reading. Other teams send personal cards to caregivers; bereaved families are often touched by these notes and feel a connection to the care team after their loved one has died.[89] Some teams create mosaics, with a new stone for each patient who has died. Regardless of the act, the sentiment remains, and a safe space is created to allow the nurse to process their grief individually and within the context of their interdisciplinary team members. For more strategies of self-care, see Chapter 73, "Occupational Stress, Burnout, and Self-Care in Palliative Nursing."

Self-Appraisal for the Nurse

To nurture psychosocial and spiritual skills, nurses should continually reflect on and evaluate their own hopes, beliefs, and biases and identify how these factors influence their care. It is important the nurse has insight into themselves to avoid projection of their biases onto the patients and their caregivers. Self-appraisal is not a one-time act; rather, it is an iterative process that will continue throughout the nurse's career as their own personal life evolves. When nurses acknowledge their own biases, they become more conscientious in their care of patients and their caregivers and avoid misleading circumstances. Questions like "What would you recommend" and "What would you do if this was your mother/brother/father/loved one" are frequently heard in palliative care. If the nurse responds directly to these questions, they are doing a disservice as these questions stem from a place of overwhelm as the patient and caregivers struggle to make a decision. There is no right answer to these questions as every patient and situation is unique. The nurse should not reply with a response that is about their own hopes, beliefs, and biases but rather use their astute assessment tools to dig deeper and better understand the emotion and distress that drive the questions.

Conclusion: Fostering a Therapeutic Relationship between Nurse-Patient-Family in Serious Illness Care

To foster a person's sense of meaning, purpose, and maximal hope, nurses should establish and maintain an open relationship with patients and members of their support network. The palliative care nurse must take the time to learn what their priorities and needs are and then address those needs in timely, effective ways. The demonstration of respect, genuine interest with the use of therapeutic presence, and skills of silence to listen and be with people—that is, affirming each person's worth—are essential. Connectedness among the patient, family, and friends can be fostered and sustained with time for uninterrupted interactions, which is especially important in institutional settings. Nurses can foster hope, meaning, and purpose when they enlist help from others—including caregivers, family, friends, other clinicians, and palliative care specialists—to help achieve goals.

Acknowledgments

Dr. Foxwell and Ms. Alimenti would like to acknowledge Tami Borneman, MSN, RN, CNS, FPCN; Katherine Brown-Saltzman, MA, RN; Dr. Valerie T. Cotter; and Dr. Mary Ersek for their contributions to the previous editions of this chapter.

REFERENCES

1. Martela F, Steger MF. The three meanings of meaning in life: distinguishing coherence, purpose, and significance. *J Positive Psychol.* 2016;11(5):531–545. https://doi.org/10.1080/17439760.2015.1137623.
2. Frankl VE. *Man's search for meaning: an introduction to logotherapy.* Beacon; 1959.
3. Pytell TE. Redeeming the unredeemable: Auschwitz and *Man's search for meaning. Holocaust Genocide Stud.* 2003;17(1):89–113. https://doi.org/10.1093/hgs/17.1.89.
4. Cassell EJ. The relationship between pain and suffering. *Adv Pain Res Ther.* 1989;11:61–70.
5. Tarbi EC, Meghani SH. A concept analysis of the existential experience of adults with advanced cancer. *Nurs Outlook.* 2019;67(5):540–557. https://doi.org/10.1016/j.outlook.2019.03.006.

6. Steger MF, Kashdan TB, Sullivan BA, Lorentz D. Understanding the search for meaning in life: personality, cognitive style, and the dynamic between seeking and experiencing meaning. *J Pers*. 2008;76(2):199–228. https://doi.org/10.1111/j.1467-6494.2007.00484.x.
7. Zhang J, Peng J, Gao P, et al. Relationship between meaning in life and death anxiety in the elderly: self-esteem as a mediator. *BMC Geriatr*. 2019;19(1):308. https://doi.org/10.1186/s12877-019-1316-7.
8. Merluzzi TV, Salamanca-Balen N, Philip EJ, Salsman JM. "Letting go"—relinquishing control of illness outcomes to God and quality of life: meaning/peace as a mediating mechanism in religious coping with cancer. *Soc Sci Med*. 2023;317:115597. https://doi.org/10.1016/j.socscimed.2022.115597.
9. Ulrich CM, Knafl KA, Ratcliffe SJ, et al. Developing a model of the benefits and burdens of research participation in cancer clinical trials. *AJOB Prim Res*. 2012;3(2):10–23. https://doi.org/10.1080/21507716.2011.653472.
10. Ulrich CM, Ratcliffe SJ, Wallen GR, Zhou Q, Knafl K, Grady C. Cancer clinical trial participants' assessment of risk and benefit. *AJOB Empir Bioeth*. 2016;7(1):8–16. https://doi.org/10.1080/23294515.2015.1034381.
11. Merriam-Webster Dictionary. Distress. Accessed December 7, 2019. https://www.merriam-webster.com/dictionary/distress.
12. National Comprehensive Cancer Network. *Clinical Practice Guidelines in Oncology: Distress Management*. Version 1.2025. 2025. Accessed January 9, 2025. https://www.nccn.org/professionals/physician_gls/pdf/distress.pdf
13. McKee KY, Kelly A. Management of grief, depression, and suicidal thoughts in serious illness. *Med Clin North Am*. 2020;104(3):503–524. https://doi.org/10.1016/j.mcna.2020.01.003.
14. Graham-Wisener L, Dempster M, Sadler A, McCann L, McCorry NK. Validation of the Distress Thermometer in patients with advanced cancer receiving specialist palliative care in a hospice setting. *Palliat Med*. 2021;35(1):120–129. https://doi.org/10.1177/0269216320954339.
15. Fava GA, Guidi J, Porcelli P, et al. A cluster analysis-derived classification of psychological distress and illness behavior in the medically ill. *Psychol Med*. 2012;42(2):401–407. https://doi.org/10.1017/S0033291711001231.
16. Bradley N, Lloyd-Williams M, Dowrick C. Effectiveness of palliative care interventions offering social support to people with life-limiting illness—a systematic review. *Eur J Cancer Care*. 2018;27(3):e12837. https://doi.org/10.1111/ecc.12837.
17. Kozlov E, Phongtankuel V, Prigerson H, et al. Prevalence, severity, and correlates of symptoms of anxiety and depression at the very end of life. *J Pain Symptom Manage*. 2019;58(1):80–85. https://doi.org/10.1016/j.jpainsymman.2019.04.012.
18. Mitchell AJ, Chan M, Bhatti H, et al. Prevalence of depression, anxiety, and adjustment disorder in oncological, haematological, and palliative-care settings: a meta-analysis of 94 interview-based studies. *Lancet Oncol*. 2011;12(2):160–174. https://doi.org/10.1016/s1470-2045(11)70002-x.
19. Grotmol KS, Lie HC, Hjermstad MJ, et al. Depression—a major contributor to poor quality of life in patients with advanced cancer. *J Pain Symptom Manage*. 2017;54(6):889–897. https://doi.org/10.1016/j.jpainsymman.2017.04.010.
20. Grotmol KS, Lie HC, Loge JH, et al. Patients with advanced cancer and depression report a significantly higher symptom burden than non-depressed patients. *Palliat Support Care*. 2019;17(2):143–149. https://doi.org/10.1017/s1478951517001183.
21. Beck M. Victory by Surrender. *Martha's Blog* (blog). October 1, 2022. https://marthabeck.com/2011/09/victory-by-surrender/.
22. Berglund M, Westin L, Svanstrom R, Sundler AJ. Suffering caused by care—patients' experiences from hospital settings. *Int J Qual Stud Health Well-being*. 2012;7:18688. https://doi.org/10.3402/qhw.v7i0.18688.
23. Bobevski I, Kissane DW, Vehling S, McKenzie DP, Glaesmer H, Mehnert A. Latent class analysis differentiation of adjustment disorder and demoralization, more severe depressive and anxiety disorders, and somatic symptoms in patients with cancer. *Psychooncology*. 2018;27(11):2623–2630. https://doi.org/10.1002/pon.4761.
24. Zhong B-L, Li S-H, Lv S-Y, et al. Suicidal ideation among Chinese cancer inpatients of general hospitals: prevalence and correlates. *Oncotarget*. 2017;8(15):25141–25150. https://doi.org/10.18632/oncotarget.15350.
25. Hayden L, Byrne E, Deegan A, Dunne S, Gallagher P. A qualitative meta-synthesis examining spirituality as experienced by individuals living with terminal cancer. *Health Psychol Open*. 2022;9(2):20551029221121526. https://doi.org/10.1177/20551029221121526.
26. Ripamonti CI, Giuntoli F, Gonella S, Miccinesi G. Spiritual care in cancer patients: a need or an option? *Curr Opin Oncol*. 2018;30(4):212–218. https://doi.org/10.1097/cco.0000000000000454.
27. Laranjeira C, Baptista Peixoto Befecadu F, Da Rocha Rodrigues MG, et al. Exercising hope in palliative care is celebrating spirituality: lessons and challenges in times of pandemic. *Front Psychol*. 2022;13:933767. https://doi.org/10.3389/fpsyg.2022.933767.
28. Olsman E, Leget C, Onwuteaka-Philipsen B, Willems D. Should palliative care patients' hope be truthful, helpful or valuable? An interpretative synthesis of literature describing healthcare professionals' perspectives on hope of palliative care patients. *Palliat Med*. 2014;28(1):59–70. https://doi.org/10.1177/0269216313482172.
29. Olsman E, Duggleby W, Nekolaichuk C, et al. Improving communication on hope in palliative care. a qualitative study of palliative care professionals' metaphors of hope: grip, source, tune, and vision. *J Pain Symptom Manage*. 2014;48(5):831–838.e2. https://doi.org/10.1016/j.jpainsymman.2014.02.008.
30. Selman LE, Brighton LJ, Sinclair S, et al. Patients' and caregivers' needs, experiences, preferences and research priorities in spiritual care: a focus group study across nine countries. *Palliat Med*. 2018;32(1):216–230. https://doi.org/10.1177/0269216317734954.
31. Aglozo EY, Akotia CS, Osei-Tutu A, Annor F. Spirituality and subjective well-being among Ghanaian older adults: optimism and meaning in life as mediators. *Aging Ment Health*. 2021;25(2):306–315. https://doi.org/10.1080/13607863.2019.1697203.
32. Arslan G, Yıldırım M. Meaning-based coping and spirituality during the covid-19 pandemic: mediating effects on subjective well-being. *Front Psychol*. 2021;12:646572. https://doi.org/10.3389/fpsyg.2021.646572.
33. Krok D. The role of meaning in life within the relations of religious coping and psychological well-being. *J Relig Health*. 2015;54(6):2292–2308. https://doi.org/10.1007/s10943-014-9983-3.
34. Tarbi EC, Gramling R, Bradway C, Broden EG, Meghani SH. "I had a lot more planned": the existential dimensions of prognosis communication with adults with advanced cancer. *J Palliat Med*. 2021;24(10):1443–1454. https://doi.org/10.1089/jpm.2020.0696.
35. Asgeirsdottir GH, Sigurbjörnsson E, Traustadottir R, Sigurdardottir V, Gunnarsdottir S, Kelly E. In the shadow of

death: existential and spiritual concerns among persons receiving palliative care. *J Pastoral Care Counsel.* 2014;68(1–2):4. https://doi.org/10.1177/154230501406800104.
36. Rustoen T, Cooper BA, Miaskowski C. The importance of hope as a mediator of psychological distress and life satisfaction in a community sample of cancer patients. *Cancer Nurs.* 2010;33(4):258–267. https://doi.org/10.1097/NCC.0b013e3181d6fb61.
37. Zhang Y, Law CK, Yip PS. Psychological factors associated with the incidence and persistence of suicidal ideation. *J Affect Disord.* 2011;133(3):584–590. https://doi.org/10.1016/j.jad.2011.05.003.
38. Dees MK, Vernooij-Dassen MJ, Dekkers WJ, Vissers KC, van Weel C. "Unbearable suffering": a qualitative study on the perspectives of patients who request assistance in dying. *J Med Ethics.* 2011;37(12):727–734. https://doi.org/10.1136/jme.2011.045492.
39. Kavradim ST, Ozer ZC, Bozcuk H. Hope in people with cancer: a multivariate analysis from Turkey. *J Adv Nurs.* 2013;69(5):1183–1196. https://doi.org/10.1111/j.1365-2648.2012.06110.x.
40. Øgård-Repål A, Berg RC, Fossum M. A scoping review of the empirical literature on peer support for people living with HIV. *J Int Assoc Provid AIDS Care.* 2021;20:232595822110664. https://doi.org/10.1177/23259582211066401.
41. Piccinelli C, Clerici CA, Veneroni L, Ferrari A, Proserpio T. Hope in severe disease: a review of the literature on the construct and the tools for assessing hope in the psycho-oncologic setting. *Tumori J.* 2015;101(5):491–500. https://doi.org/10.5301/tj.5000349.
42. Reinke LF, Shannon SE, Engelberg RA, Young JP, Curtis JR. Supporting hope and prognostic information: nurses' perspectives on their role when patients have life-limiting prognoses. *J Pain Symptom Manage.* 2010;39(6):982–992. https://doi.org/10.1016/j.jpainsymman.2009.11.315.
43. Haugan G. Nurse–patient interaction is a resource for hope, meaning in life and self-transcendence in nursing home patients. *Scand J Caring Sci.* 2014;28(1):74–88. https://doi.org/10.1111/scs.12028.
44. Weis R, Speridakos EC. A meta-analysis of hope enhancement strategies in clinical and community settings. *Psychol Well-Being.* 2011;1(1):5. https://doi.org/10.1186/2211-1522-1-5.
45. Harris GE, Larsen D. HIV peer counseling and the development of hope: perspectives from peer counselors and peer counseling recipients. *AIDS Patient Care STDS.* 2007;21(11):843–60. https://doi.org/10.1089/apc.2006.0207.
46. Kylmä J, Duggleby W, Cooper D, Molander G. Hope in palliative care: an integrative review. *Palliat Support Care.* 2009;7(3):365–377. https://doi.org/10.1017/S1478951509990307.
47. Rustoen T, Cooper BA, Miaskowski C. A longitudinal study of the effects of a hope intervention on levels of hope and psychological distress in a community based sample of oncology patients. *Eur J Oncol Nurs.* 2011;15(4):351–357. https://doi.org/10.1016/j.ejon.2010.09.001.
48. Eliott JA, Olver IN. Hope, life, and death: a qualitative analysis of dying cancer patients' talk about hope. *Death Stud.* 2009;33(7):609–638. https://doi.org/10.1080/07481180903011982.
49. Buckley J, Herth K. Fostering hope in terminally ill patients. *Nurs Stand.* 2004;19(10):33–41. https://doi.org/10.7748/ns2004.11.19.10.33.c3759.
50. Olsson L, Ostlund G, Strang P, Jeppsson Grassman E, Friedrichsen M. Maintaining hope when close to death: insight from cancer patients in palliative home care. *Int J Palliat Nurs.* 2010;16(12):607–612. https://doi.org/10.12968/ijpn.2010.16.12.607.
51. Eliott JA, Olver IN. Hope and hoping in the talk of dying cancer patients. *Soc Sci Med.* 2007;64(1):138–149. https://doi.org/10.1016/j.socscimed.2006.08.029.
52. Rosenfeld B, Saracino R, Tobias K, et al. Adapting meaning-centered psychotherapy for the palliative care setting: results of a pilot study. *Palliat Med.* 2017;31(2):140–146. https://doi.org/10.1177/0269216316651570.
53. Carolan CM, Smith A, Forbat L. Conceptualising psychological distress in families in palliative care: findings from a systematic review. *Palliat Med.* 2015;29(7):605–632. https://doi.org/10.1177/0269216315575680.
54. American Nurses Association. *American Nurses Association Code of Ethics for Nurses with Interpretive Statements.* American Nurses Association; 2015.
55. Purnell LD. Transcultural health care: a culturally competent approach. In: Purnell LD, ed. *The Purnell Model for Cultural Competence.* 4th ed. F. A. Davis; 2013:15–44.
56. Beauchamp TL, Childress JF. *Principles of Biomedical Ethics.* 7th ed. Oxford University Press; 2013.
57. Tang W-R, Hong J-H, Rau K-M, et al. Truth telling in Taiwanese cancer care: patients' and families' preferences and their experiences of doctors' practices. *Psychooncology.* 2017;26(7):999–1005. https://doi.org/10.1002/pon.4257.
58. Alsirafy SA, Abdel-Aziz HI, Abdel-Aal HH, El-Sherief WA, Farag DE. Not telling patients their cancer diagnosis in egypt: is it associated with less anxiety and depression and better quality of life? *JCO Glob Oncol.* 2022;(8):e2200080. https://doi.org/10.1200/go.22.00080.
59. Testoni I, Wieser MA, Kapelis D, Pompele S, Bonaventura M, Crupi R. Lack of truth-telling in palliative care and its effects among nurses and nursing students. *Behav Sci.* 2020;10(5):88. https://doi.org/10.3390/bs10050088.
60. Giger JN, Davidhizar RE, Fordham P. Multi-cultural and multi-ethnic considerations and advanced directives: developing cultural competency. *J Cult Divers.* 2006;13(1):3–9.
61. Bajwah S, Wilcock A, Towers R, et al. Managing the supportive care needs of those affected by COVID-19. *Eur Respir J.* 2020;55:2000815. https://doi.org/10.1183/13993003.00815-2020.
62. Holtslander L, Duggleby W. An inner struggle for hope: insights from the diaries of bereaved family caregivers. *Int J Palliat Nurs.* 2008;14(10):478–484. https://doi.org/10.12968/ijpn.2008.14.10.31491.
63. Holtslander LF. Caring for bereaved family caregivers: analyzing the context of care. *Clin J Oncol Nurs.* 2008;12(3):501–506. https://doi.org/10.1188/08.CJON.501-506.
64. Alicea-Planas J. Listening to the narratives of our patients as part of holistic nursing care. *J Holist Nurs.* 2016;34(2):162–166. https://doi.org/10.1177/0898010115591396
65. Lima DWDC, Vieira AN, Silveira LC. Therapeutic listening in clinical mental health care nursing. *Texto Contexto Enfermagem.* 2015;24(1):154–160. https://doi.org/10.1590/0104-07072015002450013.
66. Kornhaber R, Walsh K, Duff J, Walker K. Enhancing adult therapeutic interpersonal relationships in the acute health care setting: an integrative review. *J Multidiscip Healthc.* 2016;9:537–546. https://doi.org/10.2147/JMDH.S116957.
67. Carlson LE, Zelinski E, Toivonen K, et al. Mind–body therapies in cancer: what is the latest evidence? *Curr Oncol Rep.* 2017;19(10):67. https://doi.org/10.1007/s11912-017-0626-1.
68. Prince-Paul M, Kelley C. Mindful communication: being present. *Semin Oncol Nurs.* 2017;33(5):475–482. https://doi.org/10.1016/j.soncn.2017.09.004.
69. Goldberg DR, Wardell DW, Kilgarriff N, Williams B, Eichler D, Thomlinson P. An initial study using healing touch for women

undergoing a breast biopsy. *J Holist Nurs*. 2016;34(2):123–134. https://doi.org/10.1177/0898010115585414.
70. Lu DF, Hart LK, Lutgendorf SK, Oh H, Silverman M. Effects of healing touch and relaxation therapy on adult patients undergoing hematopoietic stem cell transplant: a feasibility pilot study. *Cancer Nurs*. 2016;39(3):E1–E11. https://doi.org/10.1097/NCC.0000000000000272.
71. Wong J, Ghiasuddin A, Kimata C, Patelesio B, Siu A. The impact of healing touch on pediatric oncology patients. *Integr Cancer Ther*. 2013;12(1):25–30. https://doi.org/10.1177/1534735412446864.
72. Duggleby WD, Swindle J, Peacock S, Ghosh S. A mixed methods study of hope, transitions, and quality of life in family caregivers of persons with Alzheimer's disease. *BMC Geriatr*. 2011;11:88. https://doi.org/10.1186/1471-2318-11-88.
73. Duggleby W, Hicks D, Nekolaichuk C, et al. Hope, older adults, and chronic illness: a metasynthesis of qualitative research. *J Adv Nurs*. 2012;68(6):1211–1223. https://doi.org/10.1111/j.1365-2648.2011.05919.x.
74. Keall R, Clayton JM, Butow P. How do Australian palliative care nurses address existential and spiritual concerns? Facilitators, barriers and strategies. *J Clin Nurs*. 2014;23(21–22):3197–3205. https://doi.org/10.1111/jocn.12566.
75. Korte J, Bohlmeijer ET, Cappeliez P, Smit F, Westerhof GJ. Life review therapy for older adults with moderate depressive symptomatology: a pragmatic randomized controlled trial. *Psychol Med*. 2012;42(6):1163–1173. https://doi.org/10.1017/S0033291711002042.
76. Xiao H, Kwong E, Pang S, Mok E. Perceptions of a life review programme among Chinese patients with advanced cancer. *J Clin Nurs*. 2012;21(3–4):564–572. https://doi.org/10.1111/j.1365-2702.2011.03842.x.
77. Martinez M, Arantzamendi M, Belar A, et al. "Dignity therapy," a promising intervention in palliative care: a comprehensive systematic literature review. *Palliat Med*. 2017;31(6):492–509. https://doi.org/10.1177/0269216316665562.
78. Vuksanovic D, Green HJ, Dyck M, Morrissey SA. Dignity therapy and life review for palliative care patients: a randomized controlled trial. *J Pain Symptom Manage*. 2017;53(2):162–170.e1. https://doi.org/10.1016/j.jpainsymman.2016.09.005.
79. Ressler PK, Bradshaw YS, Gualtieri L, Chui KK. Communicating the experience of chronic pain and illness through blogging. *J Med Internet Res*. 2012;14(5):e143. https://doi.org/10.2196/jmir.2002.
80. Kim JN, Lee S. Communication and cybercoping: coping with chronic illness through communicative action in online support networks. *J Health Commun*. 2014;19(7):775–794. https://doi.org/10.1080/10810730.2013.864724.
81. Lagerkvist A, Andersson Y. The grand interruption: death online and mediated lifelines of shared vulnerability. *Feminist Media Stud*. 2017;17(4):550–564. https://doi.org/10.1080/14680777.2017.1326554.
82. Taylor J, Pagliari C. #Deathbedlive: the end-of-life trajectory, reflected in a cancer patient's tweets. *BMC Palliat Care*. 2018;17(1):17. https://doi.org/10.1186/s12904-018-0273-9.
83. Zanchetta MS, Cognet M, Lam-Kin-Teng MR, Dumitriu ME, Renaud L, Rheaume J. From early detection to rehabilitation in the community: reading beyond the blog testimonies of survivors' quality of life and prostate cancer representation. *Health Qual Life Outcomes*. 2016;14(1):171. https://doi.org/10.1186/s12955-016-0568-6.
84. Donovan EE, Nelson EC, Scheinfeld E. Cyberframing cancer: an exploratory investigation of valenced cybercoping on cancer blogs. *Health Commun*. 2017;32(1):1–10. https://doi.org/10.1080/10410236.2015.1089467.
85. Keim-Malpass J, Steeves RH. Talking with death at a diner: young women's online narratives of cancer. *Oncol Nurs Forum*. 2012;39(4):373–378. https://doi.org/10.1188/12.ONF.373-378.
86. Keating DM, Rains SA. Health blogging and social support: a 3-year panel study. *J Health Commun*. 2015;20(12):1449–1457. https://doi.org/10.1080/10810730.2015.1033119.
87. Huh J, Liu LS, Neogi T, Inkpen K, Pratt W. Health vlogs as social support for chronic illness management. *ACM Trans Comput Hum Interact*. 2014;21(4):23. https://doi.org/10.1145/2630067.
88. Lee JL, Frey M, Frey P, Hollin IL, Wu AW. Seeing is engaging: vlogs as a tool for patient engagement. *Patient*. 2017;10(3):267–270. https://doi.org/10.1007/s40271-017-0215-2.
89. Morris SE, Nayak MM, Block SD. Insights from bereaved family members about end-of-life care and bereavement. *J Palliat Med*. 2020;23(8):1030–1037. https://doi.org/10.1089/jpm.2019.0467.

31

Sexuality and Sexual Function in Serious Illness

Christina M. Wilson and Marloe V. Esch

Key Points

- There are differences between sexual health, sexual function, and sexuality.
- Physical and psychosocial changes can occur related to serious illnesses.
- Patients with serious illnesses desire guidance regarding sexual issues and want clinicians to ask about sexuality and sexual health.
- Palliative care clinicians should recognize and integrate a person's sexual health into their care.

As universal elements of the human experience across the life span, sexuality and sexual function continue to carry significance and importance for individuals facing serious illness. Palliative care clinicians are adept at communicating about sensitive issues, and these skills can be translated to discussions addressing sexuality and sexual health with this population.[1,2] A sex-positive paradigm which endorses sexuality as a natural part of humanity and acknowledges the diversity of sexual expression and experience fits well within the patient centered philosophy of palliative care.[2–4] Providing compassionate and holistic palliative care requires the recognition that sexual health is influenced by myriad physical and psychosocial elements over time. Chronic illnesses can influence any or all of these dimensions and result in reduced sexual well-being and quality of life. This chapter will detail some of the physical and psychosocial changes that can occur in relation to a chronic illness, as well as the clinician's role in assessing and providing sexual healthcare to these patients.

An Overview of Sexual Health Concepts

To provide comprehensive, high-quality sexual healthcare, clinicians must understand the basic terminology comprising sexual health and be able to integrate these aspects of care into their practice. Sexual health is a broad concept, defined by the World Health Organization as "a state of physical, emotional, mental, and social well-being in relation to sexuality, not merely the absence of disease, dysfunction, or infirmity, [and] a positive and respective approach to sexuality, sexual relationships, as well as the possibility of having pleasurable and safe sexual experiences."[5(p3)] As a component of sexual health, sexuality "encompasses sex, gender identities and roles, sexual orientation, eroticism, pleasure, intimacy and reproduction. [It] is experienced and expressed in thoughts, fantasies, desires, beliefs, attitudes, values, behaviours, practices, roles, and relationships."[5(p3)] Understanding the concept of sexuality requires clarity on the differing definitions for the terms "sex" and "gender." Colloquially, "sex" is often used as a term to denote sexual activity. Scientifically, however, sex describes differences in biology and/or physiology, including hormones, chromosomes, and reproductive organs.[6] In contrast, "gender" refers to how an individual identifies themselves and is a socially constructed phenomenon with historical and cultural implications.[6] Lastly, the term "sexual function" specifically pertains to the ability to engage in sexual activities. Sexual function has both neurologic and physiologic components that occur within the sexual response cycle.[7] Sexual dysfunction typically occurs when there are alterations within one of these aspects leading to a change that is distressing to the individual.[8]

Physical Impact of Serious Illness on Sexuality and Sexual Function

Changes to physical appearance, function, and sensation resulting from a serious illness or its treatment can significantly impact sexuality and may be related to both direct and indirect effects of the illness or treatment on one's reproductive or sexual organs. However, physiological alterations disrupting sexual function and sexuality are not limited to the reproductive system as numerous systems play a role in optimal sexual health and functioning. Some of the common serious illnesses and their subsequent physical changes that impact sexual function and sexuality are described below.

Case Study, Part 1: The Impact of a Serious Illness on Sexual Health

Kelsey is a 32-year-old female recently diagnosed with invasive breast cancer. She is being seen in the interdisciplinary breast clinic, and options for surgery, radiation, chemotherapy, and endocrine therapy are being discussed. Of note, she is currently in a long-term relationship with her partner Kevin.

Questions to Consider:

1. When helping Kelsey make informed decisions about her care, what sexual side effects are important to share for each treatment modality?
2. What special considerations are important to keep in mind regarding this patient's age and life stage?
3. When and how might nurses involve the partners of patients in sexual health conservations?

Cancer

Both cancer and its treatments can have a detrimental effect on sexual function. The ability to engage in sexual activity may be directly impacted by the presence of cancer or the tumor itself, especially diagnoses affecting reproductive organs or those within the pelvic cavity (e.g., gynecologic, prostate, bladder, colorectal). Cancers that do not directly affect reproductive organs may still lead to changes in sexual function if they play a role in the sexual response cycle or are stimulated during sexual activity (e.g., brain, breast). In addition to the cancer itself, cancer treatments including surgery, radiation, chemotherapy, and endocrine therapies can impact sexual function. Surgical procedures within the abdomen may affect pelvic nerves responsible for sensation, arousal, and orgasm and can lead to scarring and pelvic pain or pain with intercourse. Radiation to the pelvic region can also lead to changes in satisfaction, arousal, or orgasm or cause erectile dysfunction and painful intercourse in individuals.[9–12]

Cardiac Illnesses

Cardiovascular disease, including hypertension and atherosclerosis, have been shown to cause sexual dysfunction in both men and women.[13,14] Erectile dysfunction, specifically, has been found to be related to heart disease, atrial fibrillation, and congestive heart failure.[14,15] Female sexual dysfunction, including difficulties with desire, arousal, lubrication, and pain, have been commonly reported in cardiac conditions.[13,14] Cardiac illnesses that result in reduced blood flow can decrease arousal and orgasm in women and contribute to erectile dysfunction in men,[13] and the side effects of medications used to treat them can also produce sexual dysfunction.

Endocrine Illnesses

Illnesses affecting the hypothalamus–pituitary–adrenal axis, such as Cushing's disease, Addison's disease, and tumors of the pituitary and adrenal glands, may lead to significant impairments in sexual function, including erectile dysfunction and decreased desire, arousal, and lubrication.[16–18] Thyroid conditions are also culprits of sexual dysfunction. Hyperthyroidism has been shown to potentially decrease libido in both men and women, whereas hypothyroidism has been shown to have significant negative effects on desire, arousal, lubrication, and orgasm in women.[19] Diabetes mellitus has a strong association with sexual dysfunction in both men and women. Erectile dysfunction, pain, and changes in desire, arousal, and lubrication have all been shown to be impacted by diabetes and its complications.[20]

Neurologic Illnesses

Spinal cord injuries have been noted to impair sensation and orgasm, lubrication, ejaculation, the ability to achieve/maintain an erection, as well as genital arousal engorgement.[21,22] These impairments may vary based on where the injury to the spinal cord originates. Individuals who have had strokes may have similar issues, but libido and erectile dysfunction have been noted to markedly change within this population.[23] Parkinson's disease can also affect sexual function in both men and women, with substantial effects on erectile function due to the role of the dopaminergic system and subsequently higher incidence rates of dysfunction in men.[24]

Autoimmune Illnesses

Sexual dysfunction has been reported in both men and women with Crohn's disease and ulcerative colitis, two autoimmune diseases that affect the digestive tract.[25] Common types of sexual dysfunction include decreased sexual satisfaction, infrequent sexual activity (due to symptoms), dyspareunia, and lubrication difficulties.[25] Autoimmune rheumatologic diseases, specifically Sjogren's syndrome and systemic sclerosis, can also significantly impair sexual dysfunction.[26,27]

Other Considerations

Comorbid illnesses may have unfortunate culminating effects on worsening sexual dysfunction. While the illness itself can lead to complications with sexual functioning and sexuality, symptoms such as fatigue, pain, shortness of breath, neuropathies, and sleep disturbances can all have negative consequences as well. Moreover, medications used to treat the illness or its symptoms (outlined in Table 31.1) may further impair sexual function in various ways.

Table 31.1 Common medications and impacts on sexual function[a]

Common classes of medications	Common subclasses with sexual side effects	Common impacts on sexual function
Antihypertensive	Beta blockers Thiazide diuretics	Erectile dysfunction, decreased libido[28]
Antidepressants	Selective serotonin reuptake inhibitors	Orgasm difficulties, decreased libido, impotence[29]
Analgesics	Opioids	Erectile dysfunction, decreased libido, decreased arousal, orgasm difficulties[30]
Hormonal agents	Aromatase inhibitors Antiandrogens	Dyspareunia, erectile dysfunction, decreased libido[31]
Anxiolytics	Benzodiazepines	Decreased libido, erectile dysfunction[32]
Corticosteroids	Glucocorticoids	Decreased libido, erectile dysfunction[29]

[a] Note: This is not a comprehensive list but rather a list of common offenders. There are many other medications that can impact sexual function.

Case Study, Part 2: Utilizing Anticipatory Guidance to Address Sexual Concerns in Serious Illness

At her consultation, Kelsey learns that she will need surgery, chemotherapy, a hormonal blocking agent, and possibly radiation. In considering her options, Kelsey asks about some of the physical effects that might occur with these treatments. You are happy to provide some anticipatory guidance regarding what Kelsey can expect with her planned treatments. You explain that a lumpectomy surgery conserves the majority of the breast tissue but may lead to scarring and an indentation in the breast, while a mastectomy removes as much breast tissue as possible and will result in scarring as well as loss of the nipple and substantial changes to breast sensation. Removal of any axillary lymph nodes with surgery will put Kelsey at risk for developing lymphedema as well. Long-term effects of breast radiation can include skin changes in texture and color. You also explain that chemotherapy will require a chest port-a-cath to be placed and that she will experience hair loss with her chemo regimen. You describe that chemotherapy and endocrine agents can suppress ovarian function, affecting fertility and causing menopausal symptoms. Lastly, you describe some of the sexual side effects of treatment-induced estrogen loss, including vulvovaginal dryness, decreased libido, and dyspareunia.

Questions to Consider:

1. Why is it important to include body image and sexual side effects in a conversation about the physical effects of treatments for serious illness?
2. How might you also provide anticipatory guidance on possible changes to a couple's relationship after diagnosis of a serious illness?
3. What management options could be offered to help mitigate or minimize the impact of some of these common sexual side effects?

Psychosocial Impact of Serious Illness on Sexuality and Sexual Function

In addition to the physiological challenges that a diagnosis of a serious illness brings, psychosocial ramifications occur. These include the influence of sexual changes on one's sexual self-concept, body image, and the dynamic of one's relationships.

Sexual Self-Concept and Body Image

Alterations in body integrity may not only make it difficult to participate in sexual activity from a functional standpoint but also interfere with how individuals view themselves as sexual beings and their willingness to be physically intimate with others. Visible signs of illness or treatment can reduce an individual's feelings of desirability and lead to embarrassment, loss of sexual self-confidence, and poor body image. For example, things like the presence of a colostomy, tracheostomy, feeding tube, drainage tubes, wounds, and bladder or bowel incontinence can contribute to self-consciousness and avoidance of sexual activity.

Functional changes in sexual performance such as erectile difficulties, the loss of breast sensation with mastectomy surgery, or the inability to participate in vaginal intercourse due to shortened vaginal canal or dyspareunia can also threaten a person's sense of self and sexual vitality. The physical effects of hormonal alterations with treatments like androgen deprivation therapy, anti-estrogen therapy, and bilateral oophorectomy may lead individuals to mourn the lost sense of their previous (pre-illness) sexual self-identity. Young people with serious illness may experience anticipatory grieving as they recognize that some of their expected future life experiences, including establishing romantic relationships, engaging in partnered sex, and the ability to have biological children, may not be achievable.[2] Clinicians can validate these experiences and help individuals navigate this emotional territory with strategies that promote exploring and reflecting on the meaning of such losses and by focusing on resilience and the reframing of goals and abilities.[2]

Interpersonal Relationships

How individuals relate to others is deeply influenced by their personal cognitions and emotional responses, and the diagnosis of an illness can disrupt a couple's relationship dynamics and patterns of intimacy and create interpersonal distress.[1,33–35] Couples may struggle to adjust to the loss of sexual spontaneity and potentially altered sexual and intimacy needs, which may no longer align.[34] Persons with serious illness and their partners may find it difficult to communicate openly about sexual concerns, and feelings of guilt, sadness, and rejection may occur as couples attempt to maneuver these emotionally charged changes.[2,34] However, facing obstacles together also provides an opportunity for shared growth and resilience. Couples have reported strengthened relationships in the face of serious illness and identify sexual expression as a way to cultivate these connections, provide a sense of normalcy, and find mutual joy and pleasure.[1,34,36] Clinicians can support couples by facilitating conversations and providing strategies for discussing these sensitive issues as effective sexual communication has been shown to improve sexual and relationship satisfaction.[37]

Case Study, Part 3: Weaving Sexual Health Conversations into Routine Care

Kelsey chose to have a mastectomy with reconstruction in order to avoid radiation treatment. Her mastectomy surgery went well, although she developed some postsurgical complications that have delayed her plans for breast reconstruction. She is halfway through her chemotherapy regimen and arrives at the breast clinic for a surgical follow-up appointment. You recognize that sexual health is an important component of supportive care, and you bring up this topic with each of your patients receiving treatment. Today, you broach the subject with Kelsey by asking "Is there anything regarding how your illness and its treatment has impacted your sexuality or intimacy that you'd like to discuss today?" Kelsey appears relieved to be asked this question and responds "Well, Kevin has been really supportive, but we haven't really been intimate since everything started, and I'm concerned about him seeing and touching me with the scarring and without reconstruction." She also describes that since losing her hair with chemotherapy, "I just don't feel like myself anymore. I don't feel pretty or attractive at all."

Questions to Consider:

1. List the various biopsychosocial factors that may be contributing to Kelsey's concerns.
2. How might you respond in a way that acknowledges and normalizes Kelsey's experiences?
3. What additional details would be important to know regarding her concerns that would help inform a plan of care?

Sexuality and Sexual Function across the Life Span

An individual's sexuality and sexual relationships evolve over time. Clinicians must be aware of and sensitive to the individualized nature of sexuality, as well as the capacity for a person's sexual and relationships needs, attitudes, behaviors, priorities, and goals to change with life circumstances, aging, and illness.[38] A person-centered approach to understanding and supporting the needs of individuals with serious illnesses and their partners allows clinicians to help them realistically achieve sexual well-being throughout their lives, however they define it.

Early Adulthood

Adolescence and young adulthood, defined as individuals aged 15–39, is a time of multiple complex sexual and romantic relationship developmental milestones. In this phase of life, individuals are gaining independence, expanding their social networks and peer groups, developing a sexual identity, participating in sexual exploration and experimentation, establishing romantic relationships, and planning for their futures.[12] Whether diagnosed in childhood or in early adulthood, the presence of serious illness at this phase of life does not take away the importance of fulfilling psychosexual milestones. Rather, it adds a layer of complexity to these already challenging tasks and can significantly alter an individual's trajectory of psychosexual development. Despite challenges, young adults living with chronic illnesses do establish sexual relationships, engage in sexual activities, and rate sexual health as an important component of their care.[39,40] Thus, clinicians must be sensitive to the sexual health needs in this population, including discussions addressing safer sex and contraception.[40]

Middle Adulthood

Middle adulthood spans the ages of 40–65, and individuals in this phase of life may find themselves in the familiar routines of managing established long-term romantic relationships, families, and careers. As they enter retirement and children leave home, couples may find freedom in the renewed time to spend on one another and their relationship.[35] Conversely, others may be experiencing the loss of a partner through separation or widowhood.[12] Dating and finding new sexual partners may become an important goal for these individuals.

At this phase of life, individuals may begin to notice the progressive age-related physiological changes that impact sexual functioning. Men may experience changes in arousal response and erectile function.[41] Women will experience the menopausal transition, with hormonal fluctuations contributing to perimenopausal symptoms such as increasingly irregular menstrual cycles, vasomotor symptoms, mood changes, sleep disturbances, and vulvovaginal symptoms.[42] Menopause is defined by a woman's final menstrual period, which is retrospectively determined following 12 months of amenorrhea and occurs at an average age of 51.[42] Postmenopausal status has been found to be significantly associated with sexual problems, including lack of desire, vaginal dryness, and pain.[35,41,43] For middle-aged adults newly diagnosed or living with a serious illness, generalized and pervasive illness symptoms such as pain, fatigue, shortness of breath, mobility issues, and impaired immunity may impact the ability of a couple to engage in their normative sexual routines.[1,33] In palliative settings, something as simple as newly necessary medical equipment or a lack of privacy can interfere with intimacy or sexual activity.[1,3,33,34]

Older Adulthood

Sexual functioning in older adulthood continues to be impacted by the aging process. Older men and women may notice genital changes, including atrophy and reduced sensation, as well as diminished sensitivity to touch and decreased arousal and engorgement.[35,43] Difficulties achieving orgasm can occur, and sexual desire may decrease.[35,43] For women, genitourinary symptoms of menopause may worsen, and men may experience more progressive difficulties with erectile function. Additionally, the absence of a partner or having a partner in poor health or with sexual dysfunction is a common barrier to engaging in sexual activity for this population.[43] However, older adults can and do find ways to express themselves sexually and derive pleasure through non-partnered experiences such as fantasy, reminiscing, and self-touch.[38,44]

Although the prevalence and frequency of engaging in sexual activities decline with advancing age, sexuality and sexual relationships continue to be an important part of overall quality of life and well-being in older adulthood and for older individuals experiencing serious illness.[36,43] Individuals and couples are often able to adjust their sexual routines and expand their definitions and expectations of what it means to be sexual in order to accommodate sexual limitations related to aging and illness.[1,35,36,38] The frequency of sexual activity and the physical ability to perform specific sexual acts may become less important to one's sense of sexual wellness.[1,38] Instead, a wider continuum of sexual and sensual shared experiences are explored that provide opportunities to continue to fulfill this important aspect of their lives and relationships.[38] The role of non-genital sensual touch, such as massage, hand-holding, kissing, and cuddling, also gains increasing significance as a way for older couples to build and maintain emotional intimacy and connection in the face of illness.[3,33,35]

Considerations for LGBTQIA+ Individuals

Although people of any age receiving palliative care who identify as LGBTQIA+ have many of the same needs as heterosexual and cisgender individuals and couples, the unique circumstances of sexual and gender-minority populations place them at greater risk for receiving inferior-quality healthcare.[45] Both a pervasive sociocultural stigma and the historical pathologizing of non-heteronormative and gender-minority identities by the medical community contribute to the ongoing negative healthcare experiences of persons who identify as LGBTQIA+. They report both covert and overt discrimination and disrespect, as well as subjection to ignorant, inappropriate, and misinformed care practices. Cultivating a safe and inviting context within palliative settings begins by validating patients' lived experiences and engaging in individualized supportive care for LGBTQIA+ people and their families throughout the life span. For additional reading on the palliative care for persons who identify at LGBTQIA+, see Chapter 67, "Affirmative Palliative Care for LGBTQIA+ Patients and Their Families."

Nursing Approach to Sexual Health in the Palliative Care Setting

Open communication that centers sexual health within the context of overall well-being and quality of life during serious illness provides an opportunity for clinicians to normalize and validate patient experiences, provide emotional support, offer patient education and anticipatory guidance regarding possible changes, and implement individualized management strategies for specific concerns. Unfortunately, sexuality and sexual dysfunction remain inadequately addressed in the palliative care setting.[1–3,33,34,36] Identified barriers include a lack of knowledge and training; inadequate time or privacy; clinician discomfort with the topic or concerns about embarrassing or upsetting patients; a failure to view sexual health as relevant to medical care; and making false assumptions about patient priorities based on characteristics such as age, gender, partner status, disease process, or phase of care.[1,3,34,36]

There is a significant discrepancy between clinician perceptions and patient priorities. While clinicians tend to underestimate the significance of sexuality for patients facing serious illness, patients receiving palliative care and their partners report that sexuality and intimacy continue to be an important component of their lives.[36] Further, clinicians often believe that patients will raise the topic if they are having concerns or questions or if it is important to them, but this is rarely the case.[36] Instead, patients expect and prefer that sexual health discussions are initiated by their health team. This disconnect results in a gap in care and contributes to psychosocial distress for patients.[34]

Integrating Sexual Health into Nursing Practice

The most recent guidelines developed by the National Consensus Project for Quality Palliative Care stipulate that psychosocial assessments should include "the effect of illness or injury on intimacy and sexual expression . . . "[4(p27)] As members of the interdisciplinary palliative care team, nurses are in an ideal position to engage patients and their partners in meaningful discussions that explore how illness has impacted sexual expression and intimacy in their relationships. Holistic nursing practice provides a framework for recognizing and addressing sexual health challenges though a biopsychosocial lens.[1,36] Guided by the nursing process, nurses can assess the multiple and interconnected physiological, cognitive, emotional, and interpersonal contributing factors to sexual problems identified by patients; assist in goal-setting and identifying patient priorities; facilitate plans of care that aim to maximize adaptation, pleasure, and connection for patients and couples; and evaluate patient outcomes to ensure that needs within this domain of health are being met.

Incorporating questions about sexuality and intimacy into routine nursing practice helps ensure that opportunities to address this issue with patients are not overlooked.[1,33,36] Clinicians may include a simple, open-ended question into a standardized review of systems,[1] such as "How has your illness impacted your sexuality?"[2] Doing so signals to patients that sexuality is a legitimate and important aspect of their care and that the clinician is comfortable and willing to discuss the topic.[1,36] Based on a patient's response, a more comprehensive assessment and sexual history may be performed to further delineate patient needs and provide opportunities for management and nursing intervention.[12,46]

It is important to recognize that clinicians do not need to have expertise in sexual healthcare to be able to identify patient needs, provide education and reassurance, and create plans of care to manage patient concerns. Several models have been developed and proposed as a way to adopt a standardized method for initiating and addressing patient concerns about sexuality and sexual functioning (see Table 31.2). Some models serve to guide clinicians through the assessment of various domains of sexual health, such as the ALARM and PLEASURE frameworks.[46] Others outline the process of addressing sexual health through a series of steps, including the 5 A's, BETTER, PLISSIT, and Ex-PLISSIT frameworks.[37,46] Each of these latter models proposes a way to initiate a discussion on the topic; assess patient needs and concerns; provide education and management strategies within the clinicians' scope of practice, comfort level, and knowledge base; and offer referrals to interdisciplinary care for more complex patient needs. Adopting any of the models into routine nursing practice can facilitate patient–clinician communication on this topic with all individuals and their partners.

Intervention Strategies for Sexual Health Concerns

A biopsychosocial approach is also necessary to the successful management of any identified patient sexual health concerns, including consideration for effective pharmacologic and nonpharmacologic interventions. Physical challenges such as erectile difficulties may be improved with either prescription or mechanical erectile aids. Over-the-counter vaginal moisturizers and personal lubricants may relieve symptoms of vulvovaginal dryness or pain with sexual activity. Topical hormonal preparations for genitourinary symptoms may be appropriate for some patients. Adequate control of symptoms such as pain, fatigue, or nausea should be encouraged. Nurses can offer practical suggestions such as planning time for intimacy when individuals have the most energy (e.g., in the mornings, after a nap) and after the administration of medications or strategies for pain control (e.g., warm baths, analgesics). Creativity with positioning and the use of sexual aids may alleviate discomfort and provide adequate stimulation. Couples can be encouraged to explore non-penetrative activities.

In the inpatient palliative care setting, clinicians can facilitate sexual and sensual intimacy between partners.[3] This may include encouraging affectionate physical contact between partners such as lying next to one another, holding hands, massage, and physical caresses.[3] Clinicians can also ensure privacy through the closing of doors, planning and providing uninterrupted alone time, and knocking prior to entering a room.[3] Clinicians should be knowledgeable on the various professional resources and clinical practice guidelines available that detail evidence-based strategies for approaching and managing sexual challenges in illness and can be utilized when creating plans of care. Collaboration with interdisciplinary care and referrals to specialty services, including sexual

Table 31.2 Sexual health communication frameworks

Communication framework	Framework components
5 A's[37]	• Ask • Assess • Advise • Assist • Arrange follow-up
PLEASURE[46]	• Partner • Lovemaking • Emotions • Attitudes • Symptoms • Understanding • Reproduction • Energy
ALARM[46]	• Activity • Libido • Arousal • Resolution • Medical information
BETTER[37]	• Bring up the topic • Explain sexuality as a normal part of quality of life • Tell patients about available resources • Timing of discussions should be tailored to patient needs • Educate about possible changes to sexual functioning or sexuality • Record the process in the patient's documentation record
PLISSIT[37]	• Permission • Limited information • Specific suggestions • Intensive therapy
Ex-PLISSIT[37]	Expansion of the original PLISSIT model to include: • The opportunity for clinicians to reflect on their own attitudes and beliefs throughout each stage in an effort to provide nonjudgmental care free of bias • The recommendation that permission should be sought at each of the stages, as should a review for patient understanding • The understanding that referrals may take place at any stage of the PLISSIT framework

counseling or therapy, can be considered for complex needs or for issues outside a clinician's scope of practice.

Conclusion

By its very nature, a sex-positive, person-centered approach to palliative care is innately inclusive of the unique circumstances of all genders, sexual orientations, and ages. Incorporating a routine sexual health assessment into palliative practice builds the foundation for welcoming spaces that affirm the humanity and dignity of all individuals. In order to achieve the goal of improving well-being and quality of life in serious illness, palliative nurses must work to actively overcome their own personal, contextual, and sociocultural biases and barriers related to sexuality. Sexual health is a human right and a relevant component to comprehensive nursing care across the illness trajectory.

Case Study, Part 4: Guiding Care with a Communication Framework

You have just provided permission (P) to Kelsey to discuss sexual health, and she has shared her concerns about her physical changes, sexuality, and body image. You decide to proceed with the next steps of the PLISSIT (Permission, Limited Information, Specific Suggestions, Intensive Therapy) communication framework to address her concerns. You choose to validate her feelings and provide some limited information (LI) by stating, "A lot of people who have gone through surgery and chemotherapy for breast cancer feel differently about their bodies and have worries about how their romantic relationships may be impacted by some of the physical changes that occur with treatment. The good news is that many women find that they and their partners are able to successfully adjust to these changes and resume a satisfying sexual relationship." You then provide several specific suggestions (SS), including informational patient resources on intimacy after cancer. You offer for her to consider bringing Kevin with her to her next appointment, and you remind her that counseling services through your clinic's quality-of-life center are available if she would like additional support regarding accepting some of the body changes she has endured (intensive therapy [IT]). Kelsey expresses appreciation for the information and states she is looking forward to reviewing some of the material with Kevin when she gets home. She states, "Thank you for helping me feel normal, I feel much more hopeful that Kevin and I can figure this out together!"

Questions to Consider:

1. How and when would you plan to follow-up with this patient regarding her concerns and to evaluate the outcomes of your recommendations?

2. When you meet Kelsey's partner at a future appointment, how might you guide a conversation around sexual health using a couple-centered approach?
3. What findings might indicate that Kelsey and/or her relationship could benefit from additional sexual health counseling or therapy?

REFERENCES

1. Leung MW, Goldfarb S, Dizon DS. Communication about sexuality in advanced illness aligns with a palliative care approach to patient-centered care. *Curr Oncol Rep*. 2016;18(2):11. https://doi.org/10.1007/s11912-015-0497-2.
2. Chando SC, Haley EM, Moore CM, Neault M. Introduction to sex-positive palliative care: best practices and interventions. *J Palliat Med*. 2021;24(7):1111–1116. https://doi.org/10.1089/jpm.2020.0262.
3. Benoot C, Enzlin P, Peremans L, Bilsen J. Addressing sexual issues in palliative care: a qualitative study on nurses' attitudes, roles and experiences. *J Adv Nurs*. 2018;74(7):1583–1594. https://doi.org/10.1111/jan.13572
4. National Consensus Project for Quality Palliative Care. *Clinical Practice Guidelines for Quality Palliative Care*. 4th ed. National Coalition for Hospice and Palliative Care; 2018. https://www.nationalcoalitionhpc.org/wp-content/uploads/2020/07/NCHPC-NCPGuidelines_4thED_web_FINAL.pdf.
5. World Health Organization. *Sexual Health and Its Linkages to Reproductive Health: An Operational Approach*. World Health Organization; 2017. Accessed July 20, 2022. https://apps.who.int/iris/handle/10665/258738.
6. National Institutes of Health, Office of Research on Women's Health. Sex & Gender. Accessed September 5, 2022. https://orwh.od.nih.gov/sex-gender.
7. Bancroft J. Biological factors in human sexuality. *J Sex Res*. 2002;39(1):15–21. https://doi.org/10.1080/00224490209552114.
8. American Psychiatric Association. *Diagnostic and Statistical Manual of Mental Disorders*. 5th ed. American Psychiatric Association; 2013. https://doi.org/10.1176/appi.books.9780890425596.
9. Gao H, Xiao M, Bai H, Zhang Z. Sexual function and quality of life among patients with endometrial cancer after surgery. *Int J Gynecol Cancer*. 2017;27(3):608–612. https://doi.org/10.1097/IGC.0000000000000905.
10. Lane JA, Donovan JL, Young GJ, et al. Functional and quality of life outcomes of localised prostate cancer treatments (Prostate Testing for Cancer and Treatment [ProtecT] study). *BJU Int*. 2022;130(3):370–380. https://doi.org/10.1111/BJU.15739.
11. Damast S, Alektiar KM, Goldfarb S, et al. Sexual functioning among endometrial cancer patients treated with adjuvant high-dose-rate intra-vaginal radiation therapy. *Int J Radiat Oncol Biol Phys*. 2012;84(2):e187–e193. https://doi.org/10.1016/j.ijrobp.2012.03.030.
12. Katz A. *Breaking the Silence on Cancer and Sexuality: A Handbook for Healthcare Providers*. 2nd ed. Oncology Nursing Society; 2018.
13. Rosman L, Cahill JM, McCammon SL, Sears SF. Sexual health concerns in patients with cardiovascular disease. *Circulation*. 2014;129(5):e313–e316. https://doi.org/10.1161/CIRCULATIONAHA.113.004846.
14. Jaarsma T. Sexual function of patients with heart failure: facts and numbers. *ESC Heart Fail*. 2017;4(1):3. https://doi.org/10.1002/EHF2.12108.
15. Platek AE, Hrynkiewicz-Szymanska A, Kotkowski M, et al. Prevalence of erectile dysfunction in atrial fibrillation patients: a cross-sectional, epidemiological study. *Pacing Clin Electrophysiol*. 2016;39(1):28–35. https://doi.org/10.1111/PACE.12753.
16. Krysiak R, Drosdzol-Cop A, Skrzypulec-Plinta V, Okopien B. Sexual function and depressive symptoms in young women with elevated macroprolactin content: a pilot study. *Endocrine*. 2016;53(1):291–298. https://doi.org/10.1007/S12020-016-0898-5.
17. Salvio G, Martino M, Giancola G, Arnaldi G, Balercia G. Hypothalamic–pituitary diseases and erectile dysfunction. *J Clin Med*. 2021;10(12):2551. https://doi.org/10.3390/JCM10122551.
18. Zamponi V, Lardo P, Maggio R, et al. Female sexual dysfunction in primary adrenal insufficiency. *J Clin Med*. 2021;10(13):2767. https://doi.org/10.3390/JCM10132767.
19. Gabrielson AT, Sartor RA, Hellstrom WJG. The impact of thyroid disease on sexual dysfunction in men and women. 2019;7(1):57–70. https://doi.org/10.1016/J.SXMR.2018.05.002.
20. Maiorino MI, Bellastella G, Esposito K. Diabetes and sexual dysfunction: current perspectives. *Diabetes Metab Syndr Obes*. 2014;7:95–105. https://doi.org/10.2147/DMSO.S36455.
21. Aikman K, Oliffe JL, Kelly MT, McCuaig F. Sexual health in men with traumatic spinal cord injuries: a review and recommendations for primary health-care providers. *Am J Mens Health*. 2018;12(6):2044–2054. https://doi.org/10.1177/1557988318790883.
22. Piatt JA, Simic Stanojevic I, Stanojevic C, Zahl ML, Richmond MA, Herbenick D. Sexual health and women living with spinal cord injury: the unheard voice. *Front Rehabil Sci*. 2022;3:74. https://doi.org/10.3389/FRESC.2022.853647.
23. Rosenbaum T, Vadas D, Kalichman L. Sexual function in post-stroke patients: considerations for rehabilitation. *J Sex Med*. 2014;11(1):15–21. https://doi.org/10.1111/JSM.12343.
24. Ng YF, Chen CYT, Chia GTH, Tan BBJW, Chan LL, Tan EK. The association between Parkinson's disease and sexual dysfunction: clinical correlation and therapeutic implications. *Ageing Res Rev*. 2022;79:101665. https://doi.org/10.1016/J.ARR.2022.101665.
25. de Arce EP, Quera R, Barros JR, Sassaki LY. Sexual dysfunction in inflammatory bowel disease: what the specialist should know and ask. *Int J Gen Med*. 2021;14:2003. https://doi.org/10.2147/IJGM.S308214.
26. Minopoulou I, Pyrgidis N, Tishukov M, et al. Sexual dysfunction in women with systemic autoimmune rheumatic disorders: a systematic review and meta-analysis. *Rheumatology (Oxford)*. 2023;62(3):1021–1030. https://doi.org/10.1093/RHEUMATOLOGY/KEAC457.
27. Al-Ezzi M, Tappuni AR, Khan KS. The impact of Sjögren's syndrome on the quality of sexual life of female patients in the UK: a controlled analysis. *Rheumatol Int*. 2022;42(8):1423–1429. https://doi.org/10.1007/S00296-021-04830-6.
28. Imprialos KP, Stavropoulos K, Doumas M, Tziomalos K, Karagiannis A, Athyros VG. Sexual dysfunction, cardiovascular risk and effects of pharmacotherapy. *Curr Vasc Pharmacol*. 2018;16(2):130–142. https://doi.org/10.2174/1570161115666170609101502.
29. Conaglen HM, Conaglen J V. Drug-induced sexual dysfunction in men and women. *Aust Prescr*. 2013;36(2):42–46. https://doi.org/10.18773/AUSTPRESCR.2013.021.

30. Salata B, Kluczna A, Dzierżanowski T. Opioid-induced sexual dysfunction in cancer patients. *Cancers (Basel)*. 2022;14(16):4046. https://doi.org/10.3390/CANCERS14164046.
31. Zhou ES, Frederick NN, Bober SL. Hormonal changes and sexual dysfunction. *Med Clin North Am*. 2017;101(6):1135–1150. https://doi.org/10.1016/J.MCNA.2017.06.008.
32. Hosseinzadeh Zoroufchi B, Doustmohammadi H, Mokhtari T, Abdollahpour A. Benzodiazepines related sexual dysfunctions: a critical review on pharmacology and mechanism of action. *Rev Int Androl.* 2021;19(1):62–68. https://doi.org/10.1016/J.ANDROL.2019.08.003.
33. Kelemen A, Cagle J, Chung J, Groninger H. Assessing the impact of serious illness on patient intimacy and sexuality in palliative care. *J Pain Symptom Manage*. 2019;58(2):282–288. https://doi.org/10.1016/j.jpainsymman.2019.04.015.
34. Hjalmarsson E, Lindroth M. "To live until you die could actually include being intimate and having sex": a focus group study on nurses' experiences of their work with sexuality in palliative care. *J Clin Nurs*. 2020;29(15–16):2979–2990. https://doi.org/10.1111/jocn.15303.
35. Ricoy-Cano AJ, Obrero-Gaitán E, Caravaca-Sánchez F, de la Fuente-Robles YM. Factors conditioning sexual behavior in older adults: a systematic review of qualitative studies. *J Clin Med*. 2020;9(6):1716. https://doi.org/10.3390/jcm9061716.
36. Wang K, Ariello K, Choi M, et al. Sexual healthcare for cancer patients receiving palliative care: a narrative review. *Ann Palliat Med*. 2018;7(2):256–264. https://doi.org/10.21037/apm.2017.10.05.
37. Katz A. *Sexuality and Illness: A Guidebook for Health Professionals*. Routledge; 2022.
38. Syme ML, Cohn TJ, Stoffregen S, Kaempfe H, Schippers D. "At my age …": defining sexual wellness in mid- and later life. *J Sex Res*. 2019;56(7):832–842. https://doi.org/10.1080/00224499.2018.1456510.
39. Kazmerski TM, Prushinskaya O V, Hill K, et al. Sexual and reproductive health of young women with cystic fibrosis: a concept mapping study. *Acad Pediatr*. 2019;19(3):307–314. https://doi.org/10.1016/j.acap.2018.08.011.
40. National Comprehensive Cancer Network. (2024). NCCN Guidelines: Adolescent and Young Adult (AYA) Oncology. Version 2.2025. Accessed January 12, 2025. https://www.nccn.org/professionals/physician_gls/pdf/aya.pdf
41. Quinn-Nilas C, Milhausen RR, McKay A, Holzapfel S. Prevalence and predictors of sexual problems among midlife canadian adults: results from a national survey. *J Sex Med*. 2018;15(6):873–879. https://doi.org/10.1016/j.jsxm.2018.03.086.
42. Kelly L. The menopause transition. In: Schadewald DM, Pritham UA, Youngkin EQ, Davis MS, Juve C, eds. *Women's Health: A Primary Care Clinical Guide*. 5th ed. Pearson Education; 2020:410–443.
43. Træen B, Hald GM, Graham CA, et al. Sexuality in older adults (65+)—an overview of the literature, part 1: sexual function and its difficulties. *Int J Sex Heal.* 2017;29(1):1–10. https://doi.org/10.1080/19317611.2016.1224286.
44. Lindau ST, Schumm LP, Laumann EO, Levinson W, O'Muircheartaigh CA, Waite LJ. A study of sexuality and health among older adults in the United States. *N Engl J Med*. 2007;357(8):762–774. https://doi.org/10.1056/NEJMoa067423.
45. Higgins A, Hynes G. Meeting the needs of people who identify as lesbian, gay, bisexual, transgender, and queer in palliative care settings. *J Hosp Palliat Nurs*. 2019;21(4):286–290. https://doi.org/10.1097/NJH.0000000000000525.
46. Ayaz S. Sexuality and nursing process: a literature review. *Sex Disabil.* 2013;31(1):3–12. https://doi.org/10.1007/S11195-012-9280-6.

32

Ethical Considerations in Palliative Care

Phyllis B. Whitehead and Mark G. Swope

Key Points

- Effective palliative care that rests on a sound ethical foundation requires ongoing discussions about patient and family values and preferences and medically beneficial interventions.
- Decisions regarding ethical dilemmas and the choices that are necessary require thoughtful discussion and critical communication skills.
- The ethical duties of all healthcare providers include the obligation to respect diversity in the views of colleagues as well as patients.
- All healthcare professionals have the right to maintain and responsibility for maintaining their own ethical integrity.

Ethics and Moral Reasoning

Ethics or morality poses questions about how we ought to act and how we should live. It is an inquiry into the justification or actions. Are these actions right or wrong?

"Ethics," broadly defined, is the branch of philosophy that is concerned with the study of human conduct, with the rational analysis of how human beings ought to behave and the methods by which we can identify good and evil, right and wrong.[1,2] In contrast, the term "morality" is conventionally used to refer to accepted and rational codes of conduct governing behavior, aimed to promote good and minimize evil.[2–4] As can be seen, these terms are closely related and are often used interchangeably.

Much of this text is concerned with the practical sense of nursing—that is, the application of natural and behavioral sciences in designing and implementing effective processes of care. The focus will be on the most common issues faced by nurses in palliative care. Our objective is to prepare the nurse for identifying, addressing, and resolving the complex questions that arise in caring for individuals and families facing life-limiting illnesses.

In confronting ethical questions, nurses may experience varying levels of moral quandaries. Given the complexity of the healthcare system and individual patient situations, nurses often are uncertain about the right or most ethically sound action. *Moral uncertainty* can produce discomfort, but it is the hallmark of a morally sensitive agent. It signals doubt or confusion about values or rules, but it can usually be resolved with careful analysis, as we will illustrate with case studies. In contrast to uncertainty, *moral dilemmas* are more troublesome and occur when nurses find themselves in a situation with conflicting demands or one in which every possible action seems to involve violating an ethical duty. Dilemmas may be associated with significant stress and anxiety; resolution may require assistance of others to sort through the conflicts involved. *Moral distress* is the most damaging state and occurs when the nurse perceives a moral duty but is unable, often because of external constraints, to fulfill that duty. Persistent moral distress can lead to disillusionment, moral apathy, and eventual resignation.[5–7]

Dealing with ethical questions before moral distress occurs requires knowledge and skill in ethical reasoning. While thorough exploration of ethical theories is beyond the scope of this chapter, a brief review of the major theories that are the basis for the commonly accepted principles of autonomy, beneficence, nonmaleficence, and justice will be helpful. Following this review, specific issues that the palliative care nurse is likely to face will be explored, with particular attention paid to analysis of the problems (see Box 32.1).[1,2,8,9]

Moral Reasoning

As mentioned, ethics as a discipline has its roots in philosophy. There are many ethical theories that have been developed over the years, each with its own justification. The best known of these are deontological theories and consequentialist theories. *Consequentialist theories* evaluate the justification for actions by examining consequences. The action that produces the best consequences for the greatest number is the preferred or "right" action. *Deontological theories*, in contrast, argue that actions are right or wrong according to their adherence to duties and obligations, not by virtue of the consequences of the actions. Both types of theories generate principles, such as autonomy (the right of self-determination), beneficence (the duty to promote good), and nonmaleficence (the duty to do no harm). From principles, in turn, more specific moral rules can be derived. For example, the general duty to respect autonomy and the right of self-determination is the basis of the specific rule that we obtain informed consent before interventions.[8–10]

Both deontological and consequentialist theories are forms of a *principlist approach* to ethics. Principlist approaches, although they may rest on differing theoretical premises, all use general and relatively universal principles as the central tool for ethical analysis. Universal

Box 32.1 Ethical Framework

Focus on the Ethical Dimensions of Care

1. What ought we to do? (Not just can we do.)
2. Which obligation is primary? (There will be multiple obligations.)
3. What are the goals of care? (Based upon what is medically indicated)
4. Have they changed?
5. Do they need to change?

What Would a Reasonable Person in This Patient's Circumstance Consider?

- Balance between benefit and burden
  - For example, morphine is believed to decrease the burdens of life (terminal illness).
  - For example, the benefit is decreased pain severity, so a reasonable person would not refuse, even if the treatment has some sedation or lowered blood pressure.

Box 32.2 Steps of Ethical Problem-Solving

1. Define the problem/issue
   Differentiate clinical problems, such as uncertainty or disagreement about prognosis, from ethical problems, such as determining how to balance duties to provide benefit and duties to respect autonomy. Assure that everyone identifies the same issue for consistency in messaging to the patient and/or family members.
2. Clarify facts and assumptions
   Differentiate known facts from assumptions about the situation, such as presumed motives of family members; assure that all parties have access to the same facts.
3. Develop a list of all options
   Delineate what are the medical standards of care and clarify with all medical and surgical teams their medical recommendations.
4. Evaluate all options
   Consider relevant laws, policies, and ethical principles; address rights, duties, and interests of all involved.
5. Choose the optimal option and implement

principles play a key role in developing mature ethical agency, provide reliable rules of thumb for responding quickly in real-life dilemmas, and reflect the considered wisdom of decades of philosophical analysis. Nevertheless, abstract and somewhat rigid principles can be insensitive to the nuances of specific clinical situations and conflict with the deep intuitions of experienced clinicians. More recently, appreciation for the importance of context has grown.[9,10]

Feminist ethics, an *ethic of care*, and *narrative ethics* are relatively new approaches to ethical analysis. The development of feminist ethics, an outgrowth of the feminist movement, was encouraged by the work of Carol Gilligan, who studied moral reasoning in children and found that boys typically relied on a rule-oriented, justice-based approach, while girls tended to analyze situations in terms of relationships and context, seeking resolution in the details of the story or narrative. Consistent with Gilligan's work, caring as a basis for ethics rests on the assumption that morality is rooted in human relationships and feelings. Nel Nodding, recognized as the originator of this theory, argues that morality must stem from the caring instinct and that the ethical ideal is located in the reciprocal caring relationship between and among persons.[8,11,12]

Narrative ethics uses the stories of patients and health professionals as the unit of analysis. In seeking understanding of ethical dilemmas from a narrative perspective, the elements of the situation are viewed as components of the story, and aspects such as the relation among participants, predominant voices, intentions of the actors, and consideration of whose voices are heard and not heard are central to developing an understanding of the ethical dimensions.[9,12] As with the ethic of care and feminist ethics, understanding the relationships among all participants, the meaning of what is stated and unstated, and the motives of all involved is key to the evaluation of how best to respond in ethical dilemmas. Sara Fry has argued that the traditional approach to medical ethics, which centers on application of objective principles and simply evaluating which principle takes priority, is no longer adequate as a foundation for nursing ethics.[12] She points out that caring, as an ideal, is a more comprehensive basis for the traditional values of autonomy and doing good for patients. Rather than relying on moral theory, Fry suggests that nursing ethics rests on a moral view of persons. Thus, in the discussion that follows, we will evaluate ethical issues and use illustrative cases with reference to the usual moral principles. In addition, we will consider the moral obligations that may stem from the caring relationship that nurses have with their patients.[1]

Regardless of the theoretical underpinnings of ethical analysis, the nurse who identifies ethical issues or questions will need to use a systematic process to examine the situation and reach a decision about what action to take. There are many suggested models for analyzing ethical dilemmas, and any thoughtful, deliberative process can be helpful. One approach that is similar to the problem-solving steps most nurses have learned is illustrated in Box 32.2. The process begins with identifying the issue or question; this step helps to focus the ethical issue, clarify what aspect of a complex patient care situation is raising concerns, and differentiate the ethical dilemma from clinical problems. The second step, a review of facts and assumptions, directs the nurse to be clear about relevant data and to be sensitive to assumptions that may not be based on adequate data. The third step, to list all options, is intended to prompt the nurse to think carefully about all possible actions, rather than fall into the temptation to dichotomize the possible answers (e.g., withdraw all treatment or continue all treatment, accept the patient's decision or do not accept it, etc.). The fourth step is the point at which the nurse must bring to bear considerations related to ethical principles, relevant professional norms, laws, policies, and personal values. In this step, each option is evaluated against these touchstones or criteria. Finally, having evaluated each option, the final decision is made as the fifth step. Most ethical dilemmas are multifaceted, with conflicting demands. The case studies that follow in this chapter will demonstrate the complexity of these challenges, the need to address them in a methodical and logical process, and the essential caring role of the nurse in responding to such dilemmas.[1,2,8,9,13]

Common Ethical Dilemmas

Case Study 1: Determining Decisional Capacity

A 55-year-old woman with an 8-year history of coronary artery disease, hypertension, diabetes, and chronic obstructive pulmonary disease entered the hospital after an aneurysm that has left her partially aphasic and hemiparetic, and she now is aspirating food and liquids. Seven days after external ventricular drain placement, her mentation fluctuates, leading to a question of whether she has medical decisional capacity. At times she can answer "yes" and "no," although the responses are inconsistent. The attending physician is convinced that the patient lacks decision-making capacity, while two family members (her daughter and younger sister) are equally convinced that she has decisional capacity. The patient does not have an advance directive. The patient's husband states that they never had any specific or detailed conversations about preferences for life-sustaining treatment. Until her aneurysm, she had been active and enjoyed gardening. He believes that she would not want to live in a condition that would not allow her to function as fully as she was prior to the aneurysm, but he is ambivalent about the placement of a feeding tube. Other members of the patient's family (daughter and sister) insist that a feeding tube be placed because not doing so would be "killing her." The attending physician and the rest of the interdisciplinary healthcare team do not recommend placing the feeding tube as they are worried that the patient will not have a meaningful medical recovery. Several nurses and physicians during this hospitalization state that the patient indicated to them that she would not want to be sustained by artificial means. The neurological consultant verifies that, at this point, further significant recovery would be unlikely due to dense damage to the cerebral cortex. The registered nurse is concerned about whether the patient would have wanted the feeding tube and whether medically administered nutrition would serve her best interests in the long term. The nurse needs help to resolve this conflict.

Questions to Consider:

1. Does the patient understand the benefits and risks of a feeding tube and medically administered nutrition?
2. What are the alternatives to a feeding tube and medically administered nutrition including not having it? Can she communicate her wishes?

Palliative care and end-of-life (EOL) patients with serious illness, their families, and healthcare clinicians may encounter a variety of ethical dilemmas and subsequent choices. Although moral questions can arise about any aspect of nursing practice, from ensuring informed consent to duties to colleagues, many issues are encountered in palliative care around EOL decisions. These situations include withholding or withdrawing treatment (e.g., mechanical ventilation, hemodialysis, cardiopulmonary resuscitation, and cardiac assist devices), concerns about use of medically administered nutrition and hydration (MANH), requests for hastened death, surrogate refusal of basic pain and symptom management, and palliative sedation. In order to properly address these challenges, it is important to have an understanding of the legislation that has led to the current healthcare environment.[2,14–17]

It has been more than three decades since the Patient Self-Determination Act was made law in 1990. The Patient Self Determination Act of 1990—Amended titles XVIII (Medicare) and XIX (Medicaid) of the Social Security Act required hospitals, skilled nursing facilities, home health agencies, hospice programs, and health maintenance organizations to: (1) inform patients of their rights under state law to make decisions concerning their medical care; (2) periodically inquire as to whether a patient executed an advance directive and document the patient's wishes regarding their medical care; (3) not discriminate against persons who have executed an advance directive; (4) ensure that legally valid advance directives and documented medical care wishes are implemented to the extent permitted by state law; and (5) provide educational programs for staff, patients, and the community on ethical issues concerning patient self-determination and advance directives.[2]

Since 1990, healthcare has shifted from a "paternalism" approach to medical decision-making to consumerism. Paternalism is defined as when a physician or other healthcare professional makes decisions for a patient without the explicit consent of the patient. The physician believes the decisions are in the patient's best interests. Whereas healthcare consumerism is where patients take more control of their own health benefits and healthcare decisions. The intent is for patient empowerment, allowing patients to be conscious of the benefits and the risks of their choices.[3]

Unfortunately, what has occurred over the last several decades is a loss of the balance between the ethical principles of autonomy, beneficence, and nonmaleficence. Patients and surrogates are asked "what do you want" rather than being offered a discussion on the benefits, risks, and expected outcomes. Healthcare clinicians have a moral and ethical obligation to properly inform patients of the intended and unintended consequences of recommended interventions and to make medical recommendations so that patients can make informed decisions. At the end of life, these conversations are most crucial but incredibly challenging for clinicians.[2]

Family meetings help establish goals of care for patients. How we communicate during these meetings/discussions and especially the words we choose are important. One word that should be avoided is "want": "What would mom want or have wanted?" Unfortunately, asking about "wants" can lead to less information and more of a desire that "she wants to live." Focusing on "wants" encourages the family to reflect on unfeasible hopes rather than the patient's preferences. The intention of asking a patient's wants is to initiate a conversation about the patient's values. Rather, asking what a patient would "want" only directs surrogates to think about what a patient would choose. Instead of asking "what mom would want," one would ask the surrogate "What would your mom say about her serious illness?" or "Has your mom ever discussed or experienced with other family members serious illness?"[2]

The real question is not if we can offer a medical intervention but, rather, should we, based upon the expected outcome and patient's preferences. Are the treatments being considered the medical standards of care? If not, then they should not be offered. There should be limits to what patients can request, and it is important to clearly articulate what interventions are under consideration and those that are not with applicable rationales.

Based on the principles of beneficence and nonmaleficence, providers are not bound to offer treatments which do not have a reasonable chance of benefiting their patients. Support for this comes from the American Medical Association's (AMA's) Council on Ethical and Judicial Affairs: "Physicians are not ethically obligated to deliver care that, in their best professional judgment, will not have a reasonable chance of benefiting their patients." Further, many states have regulations that support this position. For example, the Virginia Health Care Decisions Act (54.1-2990) states, "Nothing in this article shall be construed to require a physician to prescribe or render medical treatment to a patient that the physician determines to be medically or ethically inappropriate." Clinicians should be familiar with their statutes as they vary state to state.

As with all interventions, the conventional and accepted process of shared decision-making (including informed consent, consultation of relevant specialists, and meeting with the patient and/or family/representative to elicit and understand their values and expressed goals of care) should be carried out.

When determining interventions the clinician should consider whether the proposed intervention is medically nonbeneficial, defined as treatment which[2]

1. Will be ineffective for producing the physiological effect that the patient or legally authorized decision maker desires or expects of the medical treatment
2. Will produce no effects that can reasonably be expected to be experienced by the patient as furthering the patient's expressed and medically obtainable goals
3. Will cause harm to the patient significantly disproportionate to the benefit
4. Has no realistic chance of securing patient survival outside of an acute care hospital
5. Qualifies exclusively as "life-prolonging"

For the most part, ethical analyses of these issues are grounded in three aspects[2]:

1. Medical indications
2. Preferences of patients
3. Quality of life (QOL) as defined by the patient

However, there are many important social, cultural, professional, and legal influences that have made these choices complex. The continual expansion of technological options and biomedical interventions, particularly over the past few decades, has enabled medical treatments that can prolong life through sophisticated interventions while appropriate ethical norms have not been clearly established.

Beneficence and nonmaleficence are the driving ethical principles when determining medical recommendations for treatment.[2] Consequently, it is imperative for clinicians to understand whether the intervention under consideration is indicated or not for their specific patient at hand.[2] The facts about the patient's physical and psychological condition provide the reasonable foundation for the clinical judgment, so the clinician can formulate the overall goals of the treatment. Every discussion of an ethical problem should begin with a statement of the medical indications for treatments and their clinical recommendations.

Respect for autonomy is the guiding ethical principle for eliciting patient preferences. When there are medical indications for treatment, the clinician should propose a treatment plan that a patient may accept or reject. Shared decision-making is an important aspect. After being presented with the medically reasonable options, patients may choose to receive or not receive the recommended treatment. Clinicians should honor the patient's preferences, and respect for autonomy does not require a clinician to accede to a patient's request for medically nonbeneficial treatments.[2]

Both autonomy and beneficence are the primary ethical principles for ascertaining QOL.[18–20] QOL refers to the degree of a person's satisfaction with the experience of living based on their current condition of their serious illness and/or anticipated functionality and mental engagement for their future. It is imperative that this determination be based upon the patient's beliefs, values, and preferences and not the clinician's view of QOL.

Clearly, this approach requires careful and repeated discussions with clinicians, patients, and their families. As can be seen in Case Study 1, it would have been much more helpful to know the patient's feelings and attitudes about what states or conditions would have been acceptable to her rather than general statements about use of "artificial means." Our words matter, and many times we get caught up using medical jargon that confuses patients and families. Taking the time to understand who our patients are beyond their diagnoses and problems is key to aligning treatment to our patient's preferences and avoiding ethical dilemmas.

Advance Care Planning

With the high pace and demands of healthcare today, it is even more important to encourage patients to inform their healthcare team who they would like to make medical decisions on their behalf and how they would like to be treated in the future if they were unable to participate in their care decisions.[2,17,21–23]

Because of the many difficult decisions that will be faced by most people as they age and experience serious illnesses, having thoughtful discussions before serious illness occurs can be quite helpful in preventing later uncertainties and dilemmas (see Case Study 1). *Advance care planning* is a process of communication and documentation to identify patients' preferences about goals of care and to identify an authorized proxy who can provide competent, confident, and informed representation for choices when the patient is unable to express wishes. *Advance directives* are written instructions to healthcare providers that are established before the need for medical intervention. Advance directives have three major purposes: to provide a mechanism to enable providers to respect patient autonomy in situations in which the patient cannot express their wishes, to provide guidance to healthcare professionals and family members regarding how to proceed with decision-making about life-sustaining interventions, and to provide immunity for professionals from civil and criminal liabilities when certain stated conditions are met.[24]

A *living will* is a form of advance directive which is often accompanied by a *durable power of attorney for healthcare* (DPAHC) or *healthcare proxy*. Living wills are used to declare wishes to refuse, limit, or withhold life-sustaining treatment under such circumstances that the individual is incapacitated or unable to communicate or that death is imminent (very close) and medical treatment will not help the patient recover, while the DPAHC authorizes the agent or proxy to make all healthcare decisions, presumably acting as the patient would have. A living will, as the patient's own treatment preference, takes precedence over the DPAHC if there are conflicts. However, in many states, the living will statute specifies that this document is only in effect when death is imminent, as determined by a physician, and thus it may not be helpful in situations such as major cerebrovascular accident, significant dementia, coma, or other serious illnesses where the patient may eventually succumb to the disease but death is not imminent. Unfortunately, because predicting and outlining all possible choices regarding healthcare scenarios are difficult, advance directives are rarely specified as precisely as needed, especially when a disease progresses and the context of the situation changes. Additionally, states have varying procedures for making advance directives. For example, some states require advance directives to be notarized, while others require two witnesses. It is important to understand these requirements and advocate for your patients and families. Despite their shortcomings, advance directives are the best instruments we have to ensure that an individual's goals and preferences for care are met.[25]

Other forms of advance directives include *do-not-attempt-resuscitation* (DNAR) orders and the *Five Wishes*, a detailed guide for discussions of preferences for EOL care. The Five Wishes document helps individuals who are seriously ill and unable to speak for themselves express how they want to be treated from medical, personal, emotional, and spiritual perspectives. The Five Wishes document is especially useful when caring for children and their families. This unique document helps patients discuss their wishes with family and the healthcare team prior to loss of capacity and can be used in all 50 states and in all countries around the world (available in 30 languages); however, it meets the legal requirements for an advance directive in only 46 states and the District of Columbia. In the other states, the Five Wishes document can be included with the state's required form.[25,26]

Healthcare advance directives differ widely in format and content, making the already complex issues that palliative care nurses face even more difficult. Additional barriers exist when patients transfer from one care facility to another, and the requirements change, or the previously existing document is not incorporated or honored. In addition, some advance directives are not sufficient to direct care in many healthcare institutions until a physician's order is written in the medical record. These barriers have led to an attempt to remedy these problems through the creation of other methods such as *Physician Orders for Life-Sustaining Treatment/Portable Medical Orders* (POLST) and *Medical Orders for Life-Sustaining Treatment* (MOLST). The overall aim of these forms of advance directives is to improve the communication of personal wishes about life-sustaining treatments, resulting in higher-quality medical care that is consistent with patient choice.[27]

The POLST Paradigm, as the concept is called, was originally developed in Oregon to improve EOL care by overcoming many of the shortcomings and pitfalls of advance directives. Because the POLST document is designed to translate shared decision-making into actionable medical orders and to be long-lasting and portable across treatment settings, it can be posted on the patient's refrigerator or on the front of the patient's medical record, where it can be easily located by emergency medical personnel and other healthcare providers. The POLST form provides specific treatment orders for mechanical ventilation, antibiotics, cardiopulmonary resuscitation, and MANH and is recommended for persons who have a life-limiting disease, who might die in the next year, or who want to further define their preferences for care and treatment to help prevent initiation of unwanted, disproportionately burdensome, and extraordinary treatment.[27]

Other states have adopted similar programs with different names, although all share the same core elements with similar forms (e.g., medical orders on scope of treatment, physician's orders on scope of treatment, and transportable physician orders for patient preferences). The National Consensus Project for Quality Palliative Care's fourth edition of the *Clinical Practice Guidelines for Quality Palliative Care* recommends that the POLST model be adopted nationwide because it more accurately reflects treatment goals and ensures that the information is transferable and applicable across all healthcare settings. Unfortunately, many state statutes require modification before this goal can be reached. Evidence, however, continues to support the implementation of POLST form completion and its relationship with preference concordance for less life-sustaining treatment. If a patient is unable to communicate their preferences about care, then other individuals, known as "surrogates," are allowed to do so. If the patient has not formally appointed a surrogate, then next of kin are considered national surrogates. It is important to familiarize oneself with the statutes and regulations that govern your state or states of practice as there may be some variability.[27]

Nursing responsibilities related to advance care planning include initiating conversations about patient overall goals and specific wishes related to hospitalization, use of cardiopulmonary resuscitation (CPR), and other forms of advanced life support. These discussions will be most helpful if they focus on values rather than specific treatments. Patients and families should be asked about the existence of advance directives and be educated about the formal documents, their completion, and the process of advance care planning.

DNAR

As noted, decisions about the level and type of interventions to be used must stem from consensus and understanding of the indication for the recommended interventions while integrating the goals of care for the patient and/or surrogate decision maker. For patients in acute care settings and those who have not yet elected to focus on comfort rather than cure, the specific issue of resuscitation status is a frequent source of distress for clinicians as well as for patients and families. In addition to discomfort and inexperience with the topic, there continues to be widespread misunderstanding about the efficacy of CPR efforts and the meaning of decisions to withhold CPR in the event of an arrest.[25]

Although survival rates following in-hospital cardiac arrest have improved over the past decade, currently, approximately half of all adult patients achieve return of spontaneous circulation following an in-hospital cardiac arrest, and less than 20% survive to hospital discharge. This success rate has changed little in the 50 years since the technique of CPR was first developed. The relative ineffectiveness of CPR reflects the inappropriate widespread use of resuscitation efforts in situations in which multiple preexisting chronic illnesses have led to an irreversible state and death is inevitable. Unfortunately, the public has very little understanding of what occurs in CPR, the limited benefit except in situations of single-organ disease and immediate intervention, and the potential for cognitive impairment if circulation is restored.[25]

Once a DNAR order is obtained, for many there is a misperception that the patient's care needs diminish with clinicians. Ethically, this is inappropriate for several reasons. First, more than 50% of patients with a DNAR survive to discharge; and, second, there may not be medically beneficial interventions directed toward cure, but there are always beneficial interventions focused on comfort and symptom management, such as palliative care and hospice care. The following medical proverb comes to mind: cure sometimes, provide relief often and comfort always.[25]

Clinicians, too, may inadvertently contribute to misunderstandings about this issue in several ways. In addition to the tendency to

Table 32.1 Phrases to avoid and consider

Avoid	Consider
"What do you want us to do if your loved one's heart stops?"	"We need to talk about where we go from here if your loved one's condition continues to worsen."
"Would you want us to do CPR if your loved one's heart stops?"	"There are many things we can do, but it's very important that we talk together about what your loved one would want done in this situation. Have you and they ever known anyone who was this ill ... did they say anything about what they would tell us to do in a situation like this?"
"We need your permission to do a (tracheostomy, PEG, angiogram, etc.)."	"Given what we've discussed about your loved one's situation and the most likely benefits and burdens of the procedure, we need your help in determining what they would tell us to do (tracheostomy, PEG, angiogram, etc.)."
"We'll do whatever you want us to ... it's your decision ... we'll support whatever you decide." "We need to withdraw care."	"We have to make some decisions about where to go from here. It's our job to give you information about the medical facts and our recommendations, and we need you to help us know what would be important to your loved one now. Then, we need to talk and come up with a plan together." "We recommend stopping the dialysis based on your husband's goals of care. We will not abandon you or your husband and will still use everything we can to make sure he is comfortable."

CPR, cardiopulmonary resuscitation; PEG, percutaneous endoscopic gastrostomy.

avoid discussions of goals of care, too often the topic of resuscitation status is raised in the form of a question to patients, or more commonly to families, such as "What do you want us to do if his heart stops?" (Table 32.1). This approach reflects a well-intentioned but misguided attempt to identify patient and family preferences. It is misguided in that it places full responsibility for decision-making on the shoulders of family members and implies that it is possible to restore circulation through CPR. It is important for clinicians to provide medical recommendations for CPR based upon the medical standards of care and the patient's goals of care.[7,28,29]

As part of improving the standard of care in any institution, nurses can encourage providers to adopt the newer acronym "DNAR." The American Heart Association, the recognized experts in emergency cardiac care, converted to the acronym "DNAR" (do not attempt resuscitation), rather than the former "DNR" (do not resuscitate) in their 2005 standards, signaling recognition that CPR, with its current wide application, more accurately is an *attempt* to restore cardiac function. This attempt is most often unsuccessful, and this change in language will hopefully facilitate recognition that a DNAR order does not entail a decision to allow a preventable death to occur. Rather, a DNAR order indicates a decision to withhold a very invasive and aggressive intervention that has little chance in promoting survival to hospital discharge.[30]

Clarification of resuscitation status is best done as part of overall care planning. Nurses can play a key role in raising this topic, encouraging sensitive but straightforward communication, and facilitating discussion. Because the intention to use CPR in the event of an arrest is the default in virtually all healthcare settings today, resuscitation status must be addressed in every situation of serious illness. This is particularly important when patients change care settings or begin care with new providers, such as with admission to a long-term care facility, home healthcare, or home hospice.

Although use of DNAR orders is the standard method to indicate to healthcare personnel that CPR is not to be used, these orders are only effective within the facility in which they are issued. The need to have portable orders and valid indicators of DNAR status for patients moving between facilities or patients being cared for at home has led to the creation of out-of-hospital forms and identifiers. In some cases, these have been specific clauses in the living will; and, in other cases, a specific out-of-hospital standard order form has been developed. Unlike most advance directives, the out-of-hospital DNAR document is a valid physician order that takes effect as soon as it is signed; it is not limited by the patient's diagnosis or terminal status. When available, these forms should be initiated when the decision is made to forgo CPR, and patients should be encouraged to carry them with them as they go between facilities and services.[1,26]

A frequent challenge nurses face is how to manage situations in which they perceive the patient's condition is deteriorating and no one has addressed the issue of resuscitation status with the patient or family. Common concerns are that initiating such a discussion is outside the scope of nursing practice, that physicians will be angry if the nurse raises the topic, or that patients or families will be upset. It is important for nurses to recognize that it is within our scope of practice and is part of our professional responsibilities to identify the need to develop consensus as to goals of care and treatment plans and to facilitate discussions surrounding difficult decision-making.

Proxy Decision-Making

Because patients with serious illness frequently lack cognitive capacity at some point during the illness, professionals must rely on surrogates, family, or friends to represent their wishes and participate in decision-making. This creates several possible areas of conflict and uncertainty, including the need to make careful assessments of capacity, questions about the moral authority of family and friends to make decisions for patients, and, in some cases, the need to manage conflicts among and between families and the care team, as occurred in Case Study 1.

"Incompetency" refers to a status that is conferred by a court, establishing the inability of an individual to act as an autonomous and legally responsible person. Only the court can make a determination of *competence*; clinicians provide evidence to the court regarding the *capacity* of the individual, including data about diagnosis, cognitive and functional ability, and likelihood of recovery.[2] The elements of a clinical determination of decisional capacity include the patient's ability to understand what decision is being made; to understand the alternative to the proposed intervention; to understand the relevant risks, benefits, and uncertainties related to each alternative; to maintain consistent reasoning; and to clearly communicate the desired decision. An individual who has been deemed "incompetent" loses the right to make all decisions, including healthcare decisions, and must have a guardian appointed by the court to manage all affairs. Clinicians, therefore, cannot establish competency but instead do have an ongoing responsibility to assess the capacity of the patient to participate in decision-making.[17,31–36]

When patients are not able to express their wishes or make decisions and do not have a designated healthcare agent, family members are asked to act as proxies. Although this is common practice, states vary in the extent to which this is authorized by law and the precise specification of which family members have priority in decision-making. The moral basis for allowing one adult to make decisions for another is the assumption that family members are committed to furthering the best interests of the patient and that family members who share background, experiences, religion, and culture with the patient are well-equipped to represent the preferences and values of the patient. Substituted judgment is when a surrogate relies upon the known preferences of the patient to make a decision about medical treatment. These assumptions are usually quite valid, but there are situations in which nurses question the ability of the family member to act as a valid proxy for the patient. These situations are difficult, and nurses must be prepared to seek guidance from the hospital ethics committee or hospital legal counsel, as well as collaborate with physicians and social workers on the care team.[37,38]

Proxy decision-making, even under the best of circumstances, can be very burdensome to families already stressed by the realization of the seriousness of their loved one's illness. Several studies have demonstrated that family members are not able to consistently identify the preferences of their ill relative even when an advance directive is in place. As mentioned earlier, this is related to reluctance to discuss EOL issues before a crisis and, when discussion does occur, the likelihood that the discussion was of a general nature and does not necessarily apply to the very specific decisions that have to be made in situations of prognostic uncertainty. An additional common occurrence is lack of consensus among family members about specific decisions, such as limiting treatment, DNAR status, or a transition to a focus of comfort.[2]

In the absence of formal advance directives, intrafamily conflict, as exemplified in Case Study 1, is not uncommon. In that case, the patient's husband seemed to be leaning against use of MANH, but the patient's daughter and sister felt compelled to provide MANH. Even if the patient had completed an advance directive that established the husband's authority as a decision maker, the nurse can provide significant assistance to the family, as a unit, in providing education, as discussed in the next section, and helping the family come to consensus.[39–42]

There are several steps the nurse can take to prevent or minimize concerns related to proxy decision-making. First, all patients who have a serious illness and do not have an advance directive should be asked to identify a proxy to make decisions if they should become unable and for the appropriate documentation to be completed. This can be done on admission to the hospital or any other healthcare delivery system in a nonthreatening manner, simply pointing out that sometimes patients become too ill or too sleepy due to medication. This will enable the team to know, if there are disagreements later, who has the strongest claim to the decision maker role.[39,43]

Second, the time to obtain information about the patient's lifestyle, values, and preferences is before specific decisions about pursuing invasive diagnostic tests or procedures are needed. Talking with family members about what the patient was like, what they enjoyed, and what was important can be helpful in later discussions. Third, when it is necessary to ask a family proxy to provide input into the plan of care, it is essential to address the task as one of helping the clinicians to know what the patient would tell us if they understood the medical situation. This can be done by referring back to earlier discussions about what was most important to the patient. One approach is to consider the best interests of the patient, while it is important to promote the patient's welfare such as relief of suffering, restoration of functionality, and promotion of QOL. The goals here are twofold: to minimize the burden of responsibility the family member might feel and to remain focused on the ethical mandate to act according to the patient's wishes, not the family members' wishes. In addition to Table 32.1, which provides some examples of ways to phrase questions that are not helpful and some ways that can be more useful in supporting family decision-making, there are a number of more detailed communication suggestions that have been published.[39,42–45]

Refusal of Pain and Symptom Management

Pain and symptom management are vitally important parts of good healthcare and quality care for patients at the end of life. Several studies have shown that pain and symptom management are core domains for quality EOL care. However, family members sometimes will refuse these medications on a patient's behalf. This request rightfully raises an ethics red flag for any healthcare provider because of the strong moral duty to prevent harm and suffering. Patients can refuse medications, but family members should not be allowed to refuse them.[29,46–50]

The evaluation and treatment of severe pain remain ongoing problems despite educational efforts and quality improvement measures. Physician factors, patient and family concerns, and institutional and regulatory constraints have all been cited as barriers to effective pain and symptom management. The elderly and patients without capacity are particularly vulnerable and at high risk of having their pain and symptoms undertreated. Pain and palliative care clinicians often need to educate patients and family members who may be reluctant to use strong opioids for moderate or severe pain, as often occurs with advanced cancer or HIV.[29,47]

Studies have shown that family caregivers share many of the same attitudinal biases against analgesic use as patients, yet little guidance is available for clinicians when surrogates or family members attempt to refuse adequate analgesia for patients without capacity. Concerns about side effects can be addressed by educating family members about the different classes of medication and what the real risks are of addiction or decreased level of consciousness. In some cases, their concerns are unjustified with respect to the particular medication being used. If the risk of addiction is a legitimate consequence of the medication, it can be explained to family members that the risk of addiction is the lesser of two evils (compared to dying in pain) for patients near the end of life. When engaged in a discussion about this, most family members will come to agree that the most important thing is to keep the patient comfortable. Sometimes denial is a factor as their concern about addiction may stem from a belief that the patient is going to recover and will then have to deal with the addiction.[48,51]

The concern about decreased level of consciousness is a bit more complicated because the interaction between patients and family members is often of great importance not only to the patient's QOL but also to the family. Anecdotally, this is probably the number one reason why patients themselves will refuse pain medications near the end of life; many patients would be willing to accept a certain amount of pain and suffering if it allows them to remain alert enough to interact with people important to them.[7,29]

Fear of hastening death with certain pain medications is common not only among family members of patients but also among healthcare professionals, and this fear has been shown to contribute to the undertreatment of pain. The fear usually applies to opioids, which were long thought to carry an increased risk of respiratory depression. However, numerous clinical studies have shown no significant association among opioid use, respiratory depression, and shortened survival. The consensus among many professional organizations, such as the Hospice and Palliative Nurses Association in the United States, is that the risk of hastening death is minimal if opioids are used responsibly within established guidelines.[29,52]

A competent adult has an indisputable and absolute right to refuse medical treatment. This reflects the importance the law places on respecting people's right to determine what happens to their own body. However, complex situations arise in clinical practice when it may be difficult for nurses to respect a patient's decision to refuse treatment, for example, where their decision could cause them serious harm or if there is doubt over their capacity to make autonomous choices. An understanding of ethics and law is therefore important to guide decision-making. Ultimately this can help to uphold patients' rights and protect vulnerable people from harm.[4,7,23]

MANH

Per the American Nurses Association (ANA), adults with decision-making capacity, and surrogate decision makers for patients who lack capacity, are in the best position to weigh the risks, benefits, and burdens of nutrition and hydration at the end of life, in collaboration with the healthcare team. The acceptance or refusal of clinically appropriate food and fluids, whether delivered by oral or artificial means, must be respected, provided the decision is based on accurate information and represents patient preferences. If a patient chooses food, even if that intake may cause harm (e.g., oral feedings in people who are at risk of aspirating), the nurse is responsible for minimizing risk (i.e., using both positional changes and slow, assisted feedings). This is consistent with the ANA's values and goals of respect for autonomy, relief of suffering, and expert care at the end of life.[39,41–45,53]

The decision to voluntarily stop eating and drinking, referred to here as VSED, with the intention of hastening death can be made only by those patients with decision-making capacity, not by surrogates. A patient's decision regarding VSED remains binding, even if the patient subsequently loses capacity. A fundamental caregiving task is to provide food and fluids. The provision of nutrition and hydration symbolizes the essence of care and compassion, and eating serves as a symbol of health. In most societies, celebrations involve eating, and through these traditional social events we communicate sharing and well-being. Clearly, human life is represented as social and communal through the provision of food. When a loved one has an advanced illness, these opportunities wane; and when one is dying, they are often lost.[39,40,43,44]

However, providing MANH is not synonymous with eating or feeding another person. In health, people eat in a socially acceptable form, with others, in a social setting. MANH does not share these social characteristics. The technology of feeding tubes was developed to address specific temporary medical problems (e.g., postsurgical gastric motility issues, swallowing impairment following a stroke in a patient expected to recover). However, the use of feeding tubes and medically provided nutrition and hydration has become widespread in patients with very poor prognoses and for those with little likelihood of regaining functional abilities. Few decisions are more value-laden than those to withhold or withdraw a medical intervention that is thought to be able to prolong life. As with all decisions about the use of any medical device or treatment, this decision should be based on the patient's goals of care, the medical need, and the burdens and benefits of the treatment.[40,41,44,53,54]

In general, patients (or their surrogates) have the right to withhold or withdraw MANH if they believe that the burden or risks outweigh the benefits. There is widespread agreement in ethics and law that patients or their surrogates have a right to choose or refuse MANH. All decisions about nutrition and hydration should be made considering a patient's goals and outcomes of care. These goals of care may change as the disease progresses and the patient's cognitive and physical functioning decline. Consequently, nurses should create opportunities for discussion and negotiation of goals and priorities of care with the patient and family/surrogate on an ongoing basis.[42,44,45]

MANH requires the placement of a temporary or permanent feeding tube or the initiation of intravenous access. These interventions are associated with risks, including bleeding, tube displacement, and infection, as well as the potential need for repositioning and replacement. In patients with impaired renal function, intravenous fluids may promote peripheral or pulmonary edema and increase the need for suctioning. Tube feedings do not appear to prevent aspiration pneumonia and may increase the risk as compared to those patients who do not take anything by mouth. Other potential side effects of tube feeding include diarrhea, nausea, and vomiting. Hospitalized nursing home residents who received a percutaneous endoscopic gastrostomy (PEG) tube were 2.7 times more likely to develop a new pressure ulcer, and those with a pressure ulcer were less likely to show healing of the ulcer when they had a PEG tube inserted. Similarly, there is particularly strong evidence confirming the failure of PEGs and tube feeding to prolong survival in states of advanced dementia.[40,54]

Many patients and family members have deep concerns about the issue of "hunger" and "starvation." Contrary to what many believe, a patient with a terminal disease, who is often anorexic from the effects of the disease, is unlikely to be bothered by hunger. In fact, many patients in whom the disease is progressing tend to report a complete lack of hunger and enter into a state of fasting. Evidence suggests that natural physiological processes that accompany the cessation of food and fluid intake naturally suppress both hunger and thirst. In addition, there is strong consensus among palliative care clinicians and oncology professionals that use of parenteral hydration in terminally ill patients is most often associated with unpleasant symptoms of fluid retention and overload. Nursing interventions that can assist with the palliation of symptoms associated with dry mouth or thirst include small sips of oral intake, ice chips, meticulous mouth care, and lubrication of the lips. Involving caregivers, family members, and loved ones in this activity may replace the family's desire and need to feed with another caregiving activity that can provide the family with the opportunity to provide physical comfort.[41]

Some hospice programs cover the cost of MANH based on the individual plan of care and the goals of care, but others do not. Some extended-care facilities (i.e., nursing homes) mandate MANH when a person stops eating and/or drinking, often related to misunderstanding and concern about state regulations or to philosophical and religious missions. One approach involves bolus feedings when the patient is hungry for pleasure. Consequently, discussions with families about decisions to use MANH, as in Case Study 1, should include consideration of these factors. In Case Study 1, the nurse would have several responsibilities, including clarifying the facts about the patient's previously stated wishes, educating all family members regarding the likely benefits and risks of tube feedings, and focusing discussions with physicians and family members on what was known about the patient's values and preferences.

Despite the lack of proven benefit in states of irreversible and advanced illness, MANH will remain an emotionally laden topic and one of the most difficult decisions to make. There is a persistent widespread belief that healthcare professionals have a moral duty to feed all patients and that the benefits of MANH always outweigh the burdens. This misunderstanding, in combination with concerns about causing suffering, is a significant barrier to careful ethical evaluation of the decision to use or withhold MANH. Assuring informed decision-making about this aspect of the care plan often must begin with addressing the concerns of the care team and providing the necessary education about this issue. A valuable resource for families includes Improving Decision-Making about Feeding Options in Dementia, available at https://www.med.unc.edu/pcare/resources/feedingoptions/, provided by the University of North Carolina Palliative Care Program.

Case Study 2: Withdrawal of Life Support in the Intensive Care Unit

Ms. Smith is a 40-year-old, divorced Caucasian woman who had been diagnosed with metastatic colorectal adenocarcinoma 2 years ago. She had undergone three cycles of adjuvant chemotherapy and radiation to reduce tumor burden and had successfully survived a colorectal resection with ileostomy placement. Over the past 2 years, she described her QOL as meaningful due to her relationship with her two college-aged children. Unfortunately, her liver metastasis progressed, and the last imaging revealed widespread lung metastasis with mediastinal involvement. While at home over a break, her sons found her having difficulty breathing and called 911. Upon arrival to the emergency department, additional imaging revealed the thoracic lesion was now compressing her bronchus, and she was taken to the operating room for stent placement as a palliative measure. This was able to be done, and she was transferred to the intensive care unit (ICU), intubated, and placed on mechanical ventilation. Several attempts, over the course of the next 2 weeks, were made to extubate her; but she was unable to maintain a patent airway without the positive pressure of the ventilator. Each time the ventilator support was reduced, Ms. Smith was unable to protect her airway. She was awake and alert, was able to write notes, and wanted to see her sons. On rounds, the ICU physician mentioned to the team that it was time to consider performing a tracheostomy since Ms. Smith could not remain intubated indefinitely, and, after all, she was young. Her nurse Camille was concerned that this would just subject Ms. Smith to another procedure that would not change the eventual outcome. Camille was also uncertain whether anyone on the healthcare team had discussed Ms. Smith's condition with her and her sons and the high probability that she would never be able to leave the ICU.

Questions to Consider:

1. What is Ms. Smith's prognosis?
2. Should a tracheostomy be offered based upon Ms. Smith's condition and prognosis? (Just because a tracheostomy can be done should it be done?)
3. Should a palliative care team consult be requested to coordinate a patient and family meeting to communicate the prognosis and recommendations for helpful interventions?

Hastening Death

A central issue in decision-making in states of serious illness is the moral acceptability of actions that can be seen as hastening death. As has been noted throughout this chapter, it is well established in Western bioethics that competent patients have an almost unlimited right to accept or refuse medical interventions, regardless of the established efficacy of the intervention or its necessity for survival. Supporting and advocating for this right is a critical function of the nurse and one which has been identified as a frequent source of ethical distress.[55–60]

The recognized right of the individual to elect to stop life-sustaining technology, such as mechanical ventilation or hemodialysis, has been used by some as the basis for arguing that there is no difference between this act and acts that intentionally hasten death, including medical aid in dying (MAID).[57] Arguments that there is a difference usually rely on the distinction between allowing a death caused by disease (allowing natural death to occur) as occurs when removing unwanted or ineffective life-prolonging therapies such as mechanical ventilators and dialysis, and killing, which entails being the direct cause of death (see Case Studies 1 and 2). There is ongoing debate in the bioethics community about whether this is a morally relevant distinction, and each nurse who cares for patients with a serious disease will have to carefully identify their own beliefs.

Euthanasia is defined as an intentional act performed for the purpose of causing the death of another for reasons of mercy, whereas MAID is the provision of assistance in some form (e.g., supplying lethal medications or instructions) to an individual who then acts to take their own life.[57] Euthanasia in all forms is illegal in the United States and is condoned by none of the professional associations (see Box 32.3). However, MAID has been legalized in Oregon since 1997. Given that MAID is legally sanctioned in several states and that legislation in additional states is anticipated, guidelines to assist palliative and hospice nurses on how to respond when hastened death is requested are germane to the delivery of comprehensive hospice and palliative care. At this time, professional nursing organizations do not condone nurses actively participating in MAID (Box 32.3). In 2017, the Hospice and Palliative Nurses Association developed guidelines for the role of the registered nurse and advanced practice registered nurse when hastened death is requested.[7,61]

As of 2022, 11 jurisdictions in the United States—Oregon, Washington, Montana, Vermont, California, Colorado, Hawaii, New Jersey, Maine, New Mexico, and the District of Columbia—have authorized physicians to prescribe a lethal dose of medication

Box 32.3 Position Statements from Recognized Professional Organizations

Medically Administered Hydration and Nutrition

1. Hospice and Palliative Nurses Association (HPNA). *Position Statement: Medically Administered Nutrition and Hydration*. Hospice and Palliative Nurses Association; 2020.
2. National Hospice and Palliative Care Organization (NHPCO). *Position Statement: Artificial Nutrition and Hydration Narrative and Statement*. National Hospice and Palliative Care Organization; 2010.
3. American Nurses Association Position Statement (ANA). *Position Statement: Nutrition and Hydration at the End of Life*. American Nurses Association; 2017.
4. American Academy of Hospice and Palliative Medicine (AAHPM). *Position Statement: Artificial Nutrition and Hydration Near the End of Life*. American Academy of Hospice and Palliative Medicine; 2013.

Medical Aid in Dying

1. Hospice and Palliative Nurses Association (HPNA). *Position Statement: Physician Assisted Death/Physician Assisted Suicide*. Hospice and Palliative Nurses Association; 2017.
2. American Nurses Association Position Statement (ANA). *Position Statement: The Nurse's Role When a Patient Requests Medical Aid in Dying*. American Nurses Association; 2019
3. National Hospice and Palliative Care Organization (NHPCO). *Statement on Medical Aid in Dying*. National Hospice and Palliative Care Organization; 2021.
4. American Academy of Hospice and Palliative Medicine (AAHPM). *Position Statement: Physician Assisted Dying*. American Academy of Hospice and Palliative Medicine; 2016.
5. International Association for Hospice and Palliative Care. *Position Statement: Euthanasia and Physician-Assisted Suicide*. International Association for Hospice and Palliative Care; 2016

Palliative Sedation

1. Hospice and Palliative Nurses Association (HPNA). *Position Statement: Palliative Sedation*. Hospice and Palliative Nurses Association; 2016.
2. American Academy of Hospice and Palliative Medicine (AAHPM). *Position Statement: Palliative Sedation*. American Academy of Hospice and Palliative Medicine; 2014.
3. National Hospice and Palliative Care Organization. *Position Statement: Use of Palliative Sedation in Imminently Dying Terminally Ill Patients*. National Hospice and Palliative Care Organization; 2010.
4. National Hospice and Palliative Care Organization. *Position Statement: Palliative Sedation in Hospice and Palliative Care*. National Hospice and Palliative Care Organization; 2012.

to a terminally ill patient for the purpose of hastening death. The legal status of MAID has been in a state of rapid change across the country over the last several decades. Before 2008, MAID was legal only in Oregon. MAID is currently being discussed in many additional states. There are widespread and ongoing legislative and judicial efforts to legalize MAID in more than 30 other states. The expanded legislation of MAID seems inevitable. Surveys consistently show that more than 70% of the American public supports MAID. But the battle will be fought by bill in each state.[1,9,15]

The current statutes that make MAID legal allow physicians to prescribe, but not administer, a lethal drug for a competently requesting patient who is terminally ill. A 2-week waiting period is required. The physician must be confident that the patient is making a competent and informed request. If the physician suspects that the patient suffers from mental illness, then a psychiatric consultation is required. Most states have similar conditions regarding patient eligibility, the role of physicians, and the role of the patient. The patient must: (1) be an adult (aged 18 or older), (2) have decision-making capacity, (3) be able to self-ingest the medication, and (4) be terminally ill, with a prognosis of 6 months or less.[23,62]

A patient's request for hastened death is a complex phenomenon that is motivated by different aspects of the patient's situation. One systematic review identified four factors that contributed to a request to hasten one's death: (1) those pertaining to physical function (i.e., loss of physical function, pain, other distressing symptoms), (2) psychological and emotional conditions (i.e., fear and hopelessness), (3) social interactions (i.e., not wanting to be dependent or a burden on others, causing loved ones to suffer), and (4) a loss of the sense of self (i.e., loss of self-worth, dignity, and identity). However, it is important to recognize that factors such as these may add up to a request for hastened death that does not necessarily reflect a true desire for death.[37,63,64]

Recent data reports that typical patients who seek MAID are older, white, and well-educated and have cancer; most of these patients state that impending loss of autonomy is the primary motivation for requesting MAID.[13,65] Since the law passed in Oregon in 1997, a total of 3,280 people have received prescriptions under the Death with Dignity Act (DWDA) and 2,159 people (66%) have died from ingesting the medications. During 2021, DWDA deaths accounted for an estimated 0.59% of total deaths in Oregon.[37,66] In 2016, most patients seeking MAID were enrolled in hospice care. In Oregon, 133 died ingesting medication (88% enrolled in hospice); in Washington, 192 died (77% enrolled in hospice). Although no healthcare professional is obligated to engage in MAID, all members of the interdisciplinary healthcare team will need to determine how to balance patients' rights with personal values and professional obligations.[67,68]

Given the legal status of specific actions related to MAID, ethical conflicts can arise among those individuals who support the actions permitted in the statute and those who may hold a different moral position. To improve professional tolerance around such discussions, healthcare providers should not lose sight of serving the good of the patient, including patient preferences and religious and cultural values. These situations require very careful attention from the nurse, awareness of legal and ethical considerations, and a well-developed and collaborative plan for responding.[66]

The first, and perhaps most important, responsibility of the nurse is clarification and assessment. The expression of thoughts of hastening death may be an accurate report of a serious intention; it may be a relatively off-hand comment, an expression of distress prompted by unrelieved symptoms, or intended as a test of the nurse's views about hastening death. In addition to clarifying the meaning of the patient's statements, the desire for hastened death should always prompt a thorough evaluation of the adequacy of symptom management, reassurance about commitment to address future problems, advance care planning, and hospice. There are several guidelines developed by professional associations and groups to assist the clinician in responding to requests for hastened death (see Box 32.3). Reassessing and focusing on palliative care efforts to relieve distress are essential. Assessment of the emotional state of the person is necessary when the request for hastened death is affected by depression, anxiety, or delirium.

Cardiovascular Implantable Electronic Devices, Palliative Sedation, "Nonbeneficial Interventions," VSED, and Left Ventricular Assistive Devices

There are some specific issues that present particularly challenging questions in palliative care. These are the acceptability and methods of withdrawing life-sustaining interventions that consist of cardiac assistive devices (pacemakers, automatic internal cardiac defibrillators [AICD], left ventricular assistive devices [LVAD]), concerns about requests for potentially inappropriate treatments or nonbeneficial interventions (formerly known as "futility"), palliative sedation, and VSED.[2,11,31,35,69]

Cardiovascular Implantable Electronic Devices

One of the most concrete examples of the complexities created by advancing technologies is the situation of patients who have elected to forego continued use of cardio-assistive devices in order to allow a peaceful death. There are several implantable mechanical assistive devices intended to either support or replace normal cardiac electrical and mechanical function, including LVADs, right ventricular assistive devices, total implantable hearts, internal AICDs, and pacemakers. Each of these raises unique issues.[35,69]

Internal automatic cardiac defibrillators are very commonly used in the United States as treatment of recurrent ventricular fibrillation. Pacemakers have been a long-standing therapy for bradyarrhythmias, and combined AICD-pacemakers are recommended for some forms of heart failure. Hundreds of thousands of patients in the United States have cardiovascular implantable electronic devices, primarily due to the nearly 800,000 individuals who have end-stage refractory heart failure. It is therefore very likely that palliative care nurses will find themselves caring for patients with either or both devices. In most cases, both AICDs and pacemakers are on-demand therapy; that is, they are programmed to deliver therapy only on demand (when heart rate decreases or a lethal arrhythmia develops). Therefore, their function should be disabled when the plan of care is based on a goal of allowing a peaceful death with no further intervention. AICDs should be turned off so that they will not deliver a shock as the heart rate falls or ventricular arrhythmias occur, and a magnet should be placed over the device until it can be deactivated. Demand pacemakers can have the rate and sensitivity decreased so that they do not prolong the dying process. Cardiologists or cardiac technicians usually must be called and requested to make these changes.[69]

When cardiac function is dependent on active device operation, as is the case with some pacemakers and most cardiac assistive devices, there are more difficult challenges and unresolved questions. Some argue that discontinuing a cardiac assistive device, with the expectation that death will follow, is no different, morally, than discontinuing mechanical ventilation for a patient who has elected (or family has elected) to have life-sustaining therapy discontinued. However, others believe that the act of deactivation constitutes euthanasia. The crucial difference lies in the primary intention: termination of a life versus termination of a therapy. Thus, death that follows withdrawal of LVAD support occurs from the underlying heart failure. As the burden of these devices may outweigh benefits when patients' goals and preferences change, patients have the right to request deactivation. This right is well-accepted and supported by the American College of Cardiology Foundation and the American Heart Association. In fact, the Heart Rhythm Society issued a consensus statement that asserts that "withdrawal of a treatment is a personal right of the patient" and is ethically and legally permissible.[35,69]

Since 2002, LVADs have been considered "destination therapy" for patients who are ineligible for transplant or for those patients whose estimated 1-year mortality is greater than 50% with medical therapy. LVADs will alter EOL trajectories. Although intended to prolong survival related to heart failure, LVADs have the potential to decrease the overall QOL of these patients because of serious infections, neurological complications, and device malfunction. Numerous research studies have shed light on the importance of the ethical obligations clinicians hold to provide significant emotional support to these patients and their families and have a palliative care consult prior to device placement.[35,69]

When caring for the patient with an implanted cardiac device, the nurse has several responsibilities. First, the exact status of the device's operation has to be determined. As with all components of the palliative care plan, the plan for adjusting the device should stem from a clear understanding of the patient's goals of care and treatment indications. If, for example, the goal is to make the most of whatever time is left and there is hope for more time, all cardiac devices should remain active and in place. On the other hand, if the patient is actively dying or has expressed an informed desire to remove any therapy that could interfere with the dying process (whenever that might occur), the devices should be inactivated (or turned to an inactive setting). Each of these decisions, of course, must be made in collaboration with the care team. If there is consensus about discontinuing a device on which cardiac function is entirely dependent, extra care must be taken to assure that the patient, family members, and the entire care team agree. The timing of the discontinuation must be carefully considered and a plan to address likely symptoms put in place.[35,69]

Palliative Sedation

There are a few situations at the end of life in which patient symptoms cannot be adequately relieved despite multiple pharmacologic and nonpharmacologic regimens. Despite the provision of evidence-based, state-of-the-art palliative care, some patients will continue to experience protracted, intractable, intense suffering toward the end of life. In these cases, the option of palliative sedation is sometimes raised. "Palliative sedation" refers to the use of medications to induce sedation, either intermittently or continuously, for the purpose of providing relief of intractable symptoms and suffering. The intention is not to cause death but to provide symptom relief via sedation for a dying patient when all other efforts have failed.[2,11,48,70]

To clarify the different types of palliative sedation and how each may be used, three definitions of sedation have surfaced: ordinary, proportionate palliative sedation (PPS), and palliative sedation to unconsciousness (PSU). Although these definitions have helped to clarify the types of sedation, there remains great fear that access to these practices may become too easy. However, in a systematic review of the literature regarding palliative sedation and survival, Barathi and colleagues[71] found no evidence to suggest that palliative sedation has any detrimental effect on survival of patients with advanced cancer. In fact, they suggested that it is a medical intervention that should be included in the list of interventions to relieve suffering and must involve informed consent as with any other intervention.[11,48,70]

Despite these views and data, the wide variation in the reported use of palliative sedation and limited research evidence about best practice are likely reflections of ambivalence and uncertainty about the ethical acceptability of the practice. Perhaps the most common objection to palliative sedation is the belief that PPS and PSU will directly hasten death. Nevertheless, use of PPS and PSU does require also addressing other interventions, such as the continuation of oral medications and the administration of food and fluids. In general, these other decisions should be made separately and before palliative sedation is begun. If there are adequate reasons to stop food, fluids, and other medications (i.e., if the patient is in the final stages of dying, has been refusing food and fluids, and other medications are not needed for promotion of comfort), there is no reason to insist they be used when palliative sedation begins. On the other hand, if nutrition and hydration were indicated before sedation, there may be good reason to continue their use, or sedation should be stopped or lightened intermittently to offer food and fluid.[71]

Palliative sedation is morally permissible and supported by the *principle of double effect*. This principle, well established in bioethics, asserts that an act that is intended to achieve a "good" effect (in this case, respecting autonomy and preventing suffering) is permissible even if the act also carries with it an unintended "bad" effect (hastened death). In addition to intending only the good effect, this principle requires that the good not be achieved by means of the bad (i.e., the relief of suffering is achieved by the sedation, not by causing death), and the weight of the good achieved must be greater than the bad effect.[52]

Although many professional organizations (see Box 32.3) support the use of palliative sedation in carefully selected situations, all emphasize the importance of clarity in the intended objective (relief of suffering) and the need for thorough discussion and *informed consent* from the patient. In addition, all healthcare institutions providing palliative and EOL care should have a written policy about palliative sedation and the types of sedation that will be offered to patients if requested. This policy should be provided to patients or their proxies who ask about the possibility of having PSU in the future or request it when other interventions have failed to relieve intractable suffering. Moreover, if the healthcare institution offers PSU but an individual physician objects to its provision, the providers must make alternative arrangements for the care to be transferred to another provider or institution.[2,52]

Given the importance of communication in the final stages of life, use of palliative sedation should be reserved for those few situations in which all other interventions have been ineffective, and the patient finds continued consciousness to be intolerable. Clinicians have an obligation to describe as clearly as possible the likely scenarios for a patient who is considering palliative sedation and should work with patients, families, and the interdisciplinary team to establish a clear plan of care before sedation is initiated. This should include discussion about what life-sustaining treatments will be continued or withdrawn after the patient has been sedated.[52]

Medically Inappropriate and Nonbeneficial Treatments (Futility) and Alternative Terminology

The task of medicine is to care even when we cannot cure. Physicians and their patients must continually evaluate the use of technology at their disposal. Despite the attempts of many physicians, bioethicists, and organizations to define futility, it is apparent that no one definition covers all the clinical situations. However, the moral obligation to furnish treatment diminishes as medical effectiveness decreases. Disputes arise when a patient or surrogate decision maker requests, rather than refuses, an intervention which the physician believes to be medically inappropriate. Some people are unreasonably hopeful, insisting on aggressive therapy for their loved one even when such treatment would cause additional suffering with little or no chance of success. Communication is an essential part of dealing with unreasonable hope. The goal is not to deprive people of hope but to transform it into something that is valuable and reality-anchored.[2,6,72]

The concept of futility is one of the most controversial issues in contemporary medical practice. The dilemmas that surround the topic began to intensify in the early part of 1990s. At that time physicians sought objective standards for determining when the provision of continued medical treatment should be considered futile. The following classic cases served as catalysts for prompting the pursuit of accepted standards: Karen Ann Quinlan (1975), Paul Brophy (1975), Baby Doe (1982), Nancy Cruzan (1983), and Terri Schiavo (2005).[2,72]

Medical futility is among the most ambiguous issues in medicine. Modern medical technology has made it possible to prolong the lives of people with irreversible illness. When the question arises whether to withhold or withdraw life-sustaining treatment from an individual, people are confronted with a confusing myriad of legal, ethical, and clinical issues. The lack of consensus on the use of the term "futile" and the need for a clear definition of the concept as well as the diverse opinions regarding when and when not to continue life support create immense complexity for clinicians, patients' families, and policymakers.[6]

In all its complexity, there is a growing affirmation in a physician's clinical ability to determine when continuing medical treatment is futile. Scholars continue to make arguments against the allocation of limited resources in cases of futility and in favor of professional integrity and expertise of clinical judgment. The importance of process in decision-making including the attending physician, specialist, and nurses is essential to each case. A process approach when determining futility or EOL decisions is less subject to the accusations of mistrust that unilateral decision-making invites. Despite the unilateral decision that treatment is futile, mistrust can be a factor of the patient's family not trusting the clinical judgment.

"Futility" is a term that refers to a medical effort to provide a benefit to a patient which reason and experience suggest is highly likely to fail and whose rare exceptions cannot be systematically produced.[2] There are many definitions in the literature regarding the term "futility," but because there is no consensus about an accepted definition, the preferred term is "nonbeneficial." Nonbeneficial treatments include situations where treatments are highly likely to be medically ineffective as well as those treatments that may be physiologically effective but where the patient will not receive any significant benefit due to the critical nature of their clinical condition.[6,72]

Good communication is a basic and necessary component for a successful process of decision-making. Candid and timely communication aids in preventing distrust, strengthens relationships, and avoids unnecessary stress. Members of the healthcare team collaborate with patients and/or their authorized surrogate decision maker to develop goals of care that respect patient preferences. Physicians should only recommend and provide interventions that are medically appropriate. Physicians are not required to offer or provide interventions that in their best medical judgment cannot reasonably be expected to yield an intended clinical benefit. Respecting patient autonomy does not mean that patients should receive interventions simply because they or their surrogates request them.[73–76]

Patient and family demands for the initiation or continuation of nonbeneficial treatment continue to be a major issue. Inappropriate intervention disputes occur frequently with patients with advanced illness and their families and are one of the primary reasons for hospital ethics consultation. Differences of opinion between clinicians and families about what are medically appropriate interventions are often highly straining on the entire medical team. It is important to recognize the moral and emotional distress experienced by all the parties involved. The right of a patient to accept or refuse medical treatment offered to them has been long established in both medical ethics and law. This acceptance or refusal is considered under the principle of autonomy and patient rights. Equally valid is the physician's right to refuse to provide medical interventions that they determine to be medically and ethically inappropriate. This is also well established in both medical ethics and law.[13,73–77]

Even when complete and open discussions have occurred, disagreement may continue. For cases in which the patient and or surrogate refuses a medical intervention, proper informed consent or refusal processes apply. For cases in which the patient and/or surrogate requests or demands treatments or procedures that the healthcare team determines are medically inappropriate, it is essential to have an alternate means of assessing the appropriateness of the treatment plan and how it affects the patient.

An example of a potentially inappropriate treatment is prolonged use of mechanical ventilation in a patient who has widely metastatic and incurable cancer (see Case Study 2). Over the past decade, clinicians have increasingly encountered situations in which patients and families request or demand therapies that the clinician believes have no meaningful chance of prolonging life or improving well-being. Over the years, there has been a growing consensus that the right of patients and families to accept or refuse therapies does not entail the right to demand therapies which the physician does not believe are medically justified. This stems from the principle of autonomy, which establishes the duty to refrain from interfering in the life choices of competent persons.[16,76]

The gradual move away from the paternalism of the past and a commitment to supporting patient autonomy has unfortunately led to a tendency to shift the responsibility for decision making entirely to patients and families. This is sometimes seen in the reluctance of clinicians to advise or guide patients and families in decisions and, instead, to present options in a completely impartial fashion. Not infrequently, families will express the wish to have "everything" done for their loved one. When this is said, the nurse or physician should respond by assuring the patient and family that they are heard and that their wish to receive all therapies that have any meaningful chance of maintaining or improving the patient's condition will be used. The use of shared decision-making should be emphasized from the start. As the condition of the patient deteriorates and it becomes apparent that continued interventions will not be helpful, it is best to set the stage for later decisions by affirming that the clinicians will provide honest and direct information and will identify when there are no further curative options, with assurances that the plan of care will always be discussed before changes are made. When the situation is such that CPR or other interventions are no longer indicated, this should be stated; patients or families should not be asked to give permission to withhold an ineffective intervention. If consensus appears to be unreachable, other resources, such as clergy or ethics consultants, should be utilized. Although seeking guidance from the court may be required in intractable disputes, in general this should be viewed as a last resort; and thoughtful, interdisciplinary procedural approaches are preferable.[76]

In Case Study 2, the nurse, Camille, may have believed that performing a tracheostomy on Ms. Smith would indeed be futile. Although the procedure could be safely performed, it would not save the patient's life or even allow her to recover enough to leave the ICU—she would always require mechanical ventilation. To address this issue, Camille would need to first validate her assumption about the location of Ms. Smith's tumor and the ineffectiveness of a tracheostomy to relieve the obstruction. Next, a care conference with the entire multidisciplinary team would have to be arranged to develop consensus about the best approach. If the team reaches agreement about the lack of any effective treatment options for the cancer, a plan will have to be developed, including who would talk with Ms. Smith and her sons, what recommendation would be offered, what options would be acceptable, and how to manage her symptoms when she was ready to discontinue mechanical ventilation.

Although it is becoming increasingly recognized that clinicians have not only the right but the professional duty to refrain from interventions that are harmful, it is essential to be cautious in judging interventions as "futile" or medically inappropriate. There are many treatments or therapies that offer neither cure nor improvement in patient condition but which are effective in supporting survival, such as mechanical ventilation following anoxic brain injuries. Today, the claim of "futility" should not be used to justify withholding therapies in situations in which the clinician believes that the proposed therapy would accomplish its intended purpose but that the resulting QOL would be undesirable. Judgments such as this reflect the subjective opinions and values of clinicians and are not a valid basis for withholding therapy against the wishes of patients and families. Decisions based on treatments used must be guided by what is medically indicated and what is beneficial. Treatments must be based on evidence-based medicine. Nonbeneficial treatment is considered any treatment procedure for patients who are naturally dying that will not make any difference in their survival, will probably impair their remaining QOL, can potentially cause them pain or prolonged suffering, or leave them in a worse state of health than they were before admission. Nonbeneficial treatment/therapy by its very definition cannot be helpful, and indeed can be harmful, to patients and hence cannot be justified no matter what the source or kind of reasons used to support its use.[2,13,16,31,73,76]

VSED

Voluntary refusal of food and fluids is another option to hasten death and anecdotally seems to have increasing prevalence, specifically in states where MAID has not been legalized. Persons with a terminal illness who retain decisional capacity may elect to stop eating and drinking; it is both legally and morally permissible. In contrast to MAID, VSED requires no action by a physician and requires no physical action by the patient. Persons who elect this approach usually die within 7–21 days. In contrast, VSED in a non–terminally ill patient is usually considered a form of suicide and must be evaluated as such. The ANA recently published a favorable position statement regarding VSED (see Box 32.3), yet almost no medical association, either in the United States or in Europe, has formally supported or taken a neutral position on the subject. Institutions should have established policies in place that address VSED and include educational offerings for the staff and family, safeguards for the patient (e.g., psychiatric evaluation), and ethics committee consultation when requested.[39–45]

Nursing Issues, Moral Distress, and Compassion Fatigue

Decisions regarding ethical dilemmas and the choices that are necessary require thoughtful discussion and critical communication skills. Stemming from the priority of the principle of autonomy or self-determination, decisions about care should be made in accordance with patients' preferences for care, beliefs, and values and aligned to the medical standards of practice and the ethical principles of beneficence and nonmaleficence. With increased medical technology, the advances in science, and conflicting interests of patients and families, nurses stand in a pivotal position to lead the way in ensuring patient access to quality palliative care. This charge does not come without the risk of the nurse feeling like they are "in the middle," trying to provide the best possible care to the patient and supporting the family members while preserving personal values.[5,78–83]

Nurses and other members of the interdisciplinary healthcare team daily face ethical and legal issues in decision-making related to EOL care in clinical practice. These dilemmas have a strong potential to provoke conflict among those involved in patient care, sometimes between professionals and sometimes between patients, families, and professionals. The ANA Code of Ethics states that nurses have the right to withdraw from providing care to patients when their own values conflict with those of patients so long as the patient's care can safely be transferred to another care provider. The ANA goes on to discuss the importance of "preservation of integrity." Specifically, Provisions 5 and 6 of the ANA Code of Ethics discuss moral self-respect and the influence of the environment on ethical obligations, moral virtues, and values. According to these provisions, nurses have a duty to remain consistent with both their personal and professional values and to possess character strengths such as compassion and patience. Although simply stated, these behaviors may be challenged when faced with ethical and moral dilemmas.[80,82,84–88]

Close, personal relationships are often formed with patients and their families as palliative care nurses care for them over a prolonged period. Moral and ethical dilemmas, often associated with patient/family situations and healthcare environments, may leave the hospice and palliative care nurse feeling physically, emotionally, and spiritually drained. As nurses continue to be exposed to patients with greater healthcare needs, staff shortages, heavy and intense workloads, an aging workforce, and a lack of resources to work effectively, the opportunity to develop moral distress, moral fatigue, burnout, and compassion fatigue is a real possibility.[23,61,74,89–93]

"Compassion fatigue" is a term used to describe a stress response in a healthcare provider; it has been widely studied and is pervasive within the nursing profession. Compassion fatigue is a state in which the compassionate energy that is expended by nurses outweighs the restorative processes, and the ability to recover has been lost; it is the negative aspect of helping that can be related to the actual provision of care, the environment, colleagues, and/or beliefs about self. "Burnout," on the other hand, relates to work-related hopelessness; it is the inability to cope with job stress that produces feelings of inefficacy.

"Moral distress" is a phenomenon in which an individual perceives they know the right action to take but is constrained from taking it. Moral distress arises when one must act in a way that contradicts personal values and beliefs, resulting in the compromise of their moral integrity; "moral fatigue" is the consequence of continued moral distress. For example, nurses might act in a way that is contrary to personal and professional values or be unable to translate moral choices into action. This creates anguish, and the consequences can be profound and have lasting effects. Although nearly all healthcare professionals experience some moral distress during their tenure in caring for those who are ill, nurses seem to be at a higher risk. Nurses who appear to be at a higher risk for compassion fatigue include those who are younger, who have a history of personal trauma and have not worked through issues related to that trauma, who are working with large caseloads and/or long hours, who are already experiencing professional burnout, who have inadequate training in effective communication or are less competent in communication, and who are without adequate collegiate and personal support systems.[5,82]

According to Potter [52] and colleagues, the risk and incidence of compassion fatigue among nurses could largely be decreased with education regarding its existence, prevention, and institutional interventions that foster better work–life balance. One of the most crucial elements in dealing with moral distress is knowing *what* support is available and *how* to navigate the system in place. Ethics committees are one source of support and serve to assist in resolving complicated ethical problems that affect the care and treatment of patients within healthcare organizations. Just as preventive ethics should be used before an ethical dilemma arises, so should they be used to guide nursing practice before a crisis occurs. Moral distress consult services are another important resource for nurses to be aware of. Moral distress consultation is an organization-wide mechanism for addressing moral distress. Consultation does not resolve moral distress but helps staff identify strategies to improve the situation.[82]

Allocation of Scarce Resources

Public health emergencies occur with unpredictable frequency and scale. If sufficiently severe, they may create scarcity of medical resources, including healthcare staff and equipment. Public health emergencies occur with unpredictable frequency and scale. The COVID-19 pandemic strained healthcare systems throughout the world. For some, available medical resources could not meet the increased demand, and rationing was ultimately required. As the coronavirus pandemic intensified, many communities in the United States experienced shortages of ventilators, intensive care beds, medical supplies, and treatments. Currently there is no single national response to provide guidance on allocation of scarce resources. Accordingly, states have formulated various "triage protocols" to prioritize those who will receive care and those who may not.[94–97]

Rationing healthcare and treatments has always carried negative connotations, and until the current coronavirus, its mention would have raised some eyebrows. However, the need to restrict the allocation of healthcare resources in the face of COVID-19 has been widely accepted as a required response to the pandemic.[94,98] The COVID-19 pandemic spread rapidly across the globe and caught most healthcare systems unprepared. There was a lack of readiness in many healthcare systems. Many items that were needed to fight the pandemic were items that became quickly scarce. The scarcity of protection equipment triggered protests in many countries. Dialysis and ICU beds were some of the most agonizing to patient providers as rapid life-and-death decisions at bedside were being made. Other ethical dilemmas faced by front-line workers included withdrawal of life support and denying families in-person access to dying relatives.[8,68,94,99,100]

The COVID-19 pandemic generated considerable reflection and debate in the medical community, the public arena, as well as among ethicists regarding the rationing of scarce healthcare resources. There is ongoing debate on how to fairly allocate scarce resources to patients with COVID-19. The debate revolves around two views: that priority for scarce resources should primarily aim at saving the most lives or at saving the most life-years. And many states, although not all, have responded by publishing crisis standards of care (CSCs). In March 2020, the governors of Arizona, Florida, California, Georgia, and New York declared a state of emergency based on the coronavirus. By March 17, 2020, 48 states had followed suit. Following the emergency declarations, states drafted new or prepared CSC guidelines, which provide in part the method to ration healthcare services when patient demand exceeds medical services supply.[13] Many of the states use the prognostic tool the Sequential Organ Failure Assessment (SOFA) to allocate resources, with the goal of maximizing the overall number of lives saved. While saving as many people as possible during a healthcare crisis is laudable, this utilitarian ethics approach is questionable in leaving many questions about what is "fair" unanswered.[68,96,101]

During the COVID-19 pandemic, equity and transparency helped shape guidelines created for allocating resources like ventilators and dialysis machines. The anticipation was where the availability of the interventions would be limited or less than the number of patients in need. Some state guideline proposals urged giving precedence to healthcare workers and pregnant women. Criticisms leveled against various CSCs that discriminated by race, disability, and age occurred.[96,98,101] No rationing tool is perfect, which is why responsiveness, accountability, transparency, and fairness are crucial. Multiple stakeholders are needed to ensure that equity is protected and that any triage process used is fair and transparent. The heavy decisions of life and death should never be placed on or decided by any one clinician.

Conclusion

There will always be new ethical dilemmas that require decision-making, and the answers to those dilemmas will not always be obvious or easily identified. It is often in states of uncertainty that serious wrongs occur. As partners in the care of patients and families with advanced illness who must make difficult decisions, nurses must be empowered to facilitate discussion and to be heard by all parties involved. The challenge today is to ensure that all nurses acquire attributes of leadership, excellent communication skills, and self-reflection that enable them to fulfill the crucial role of nursing.

REFERENCES

1. Dzeng E, Bein T, Curtis JR. The role of policy and law in shaping the ethics and quality of end-of-life care in intensive care. *Intensive Care Med.* 2022;48(3):352–354. https://doi.org/10.1007/s00134-022-06623-2.
2. Jonsen AR, Siegler M, Winslade WJ. *Clinical Ethics: A Practical Approach to Ethical Decisions in Clinical Medicine.* 9th ed. McGraw-Hill; 2022.
3. Latimer T, Roscamp J, Papanikitas A. Patient-centredness and consumerism in healthcare: an ideological mess. *J R Soc Med.* 2017;110(11):425–427. https://doi.org/10.1177/0141076817731905.
4. Lim A, Kim S. Nurses' ethical decision-making during end of life care in South Korea: a cross-sectional descriptive survey. *BMC Med Ethics.* 2021;22(1):94. https://doi.org/10.1186/s12910-021-00665-9.
5. Epstein EG, Whitehead PB, Prompahakul C, Thacker LR, Hamric AB. Enhancing understanding of moral distress: the measure of moral distress for health care professionals. *AJOB Empir Bioeth.* 2019;10(2):113–124. https://doi.org/10.1080/23294515.2019.1586008.
6. Morata L. An evolutionary concept analysis of futility in health care. *J Adv Nurs.* 2018;74(6):1289–1300. https://doi.org/10.1111/jan.13526.
7. Nnate DA. Treatment withdrawal of the patient on end of life: an analysis of values, ethics and guidelines in palliative care. *Nurs Open.* 2021;8(3):1023–1029. https://doi.org/10.1002/nop2.777.
8. Wangi KYW. Ethno-ethics lens for palliative care decision making in COVID-19. *Int J Community Based Nurs Midwifery.* 2021;9(3):265–266. https://doi.org/10.30476/ijcbnm.2021.89239.1718.
9. Weaver MS, Boss RD, Christopher MJ, et al. Top ten tips palliative care clinicians should know about their work's intersection with clinical ethics. *J Palliat Med.* 2022;25(4):656–661. https://doi.org/10.1089/jpm.2021.0521.
10. Dzeng E, Bein T, Curtis JR. The role of policy and law in shaping the ethics and quality of end-of-life care in intensive care. *Intensive Care Med.* 2022;48(3):352–354. https://doi.org/10.1007/s00134-022-06623-2.
11. Pesut B, Wright DK, Thorne S, et al. What's suffering got to do with it? A qualitative study of suffering in the context of medical assistance in dying (MAID). *BMC Palliat Care.* 2021;20(1):174. https://doi.org/10.1186/s12904-021-00869-1.
12. Wright DK, Chan LS, Fishman JR, Macdonald ME. "Reflection and soul searching": negotiating nursing identity at the fault lines of palliative care and medical assistance in dying. *Soc Sci Med.* 2021;289:114366. https://doi.org/10.1016/j.socscimed.2021.114366;
13. Chang T, Darshani S, Manikavasagam P, Arambepola C. Knowledge and attitudes about end-of-life decisions, good death and principles of medical ethics among doctors in tertiary care hospitals in Sri Lanka: a cross-sectional study. *BMC Med Ethics.* 2021;22(1):66. https://doi.org/10.1186/s12910-021-00631-5.

14. Courtright KR, Benoit DD, Curtis JR. Focus on ethics and palliative care in the intensive care unit. *Intensive Care Med.* 2019;45:885–886. https://doi.org/10.1007/s00134-019-05602-4.
15. Hatefimoadab N, Cheraghi MA, Benton DC, Pashaeypoor S. Ethical advocacy in the end-of-life nursing care: a concept analysis. *Nurs Forum.* 2022;57(1):127–135. https://doi.org/10.1111/nuf.12656.
16. De Panfilis L, Di Leo S, Peruselli C, Ghirotto L, Tanzi S. "I go into crisis when …": ethics of care and moral dilemmas in palliative care. *BMC Palliat Care.* 2019;18(1):70. https://doi.org/10.1186/s12904-019-0453-2.
17. Sellars M, Morton R, Clayton J, et al. Case-control study of end-of-life treatment preferences and costs following advance care planning for adults with end-stage kidney disease. *Nephrology.* 2019;24:148–154.
18. Hanson LC, Kistler CE, Lavin K, et al. Triggered palliative care for late-stage dementia: a pilot randomized trial. *J Pain Symptom Manage.* 2019;57(1):10–19.
19. Ernecoff NC, Lin FC, Wessell KL, Hanson LC. Quality of life with late-stage dementia: exploring opportunities to intervene. *J Am Geriatr Soc.* 2019;67:1189–1196.
20. Ernecoff NC, Wessell KL, Hanson LC, et al. Does receipt of recommended elements of palliative care precede in-hospital death or hospice referral? *J Pain Symptom Manage.* 2020;59(4):778–786.
21. Ernecoff NC, Zimmerman S, Mitchell SL, et al. Concordance between goals of care and treatment decisions for persons with dementia. *J Palliat Med.* 2018;21(10):1442–1447. https://doi.org/10.1089/jpm.2018.0103.
22. Foglia MB, Lowery J, Sharpe VA, Tompkins P, Fox E. A comprehensive approach to eliciting, documenting, and honoring patient wishes for care near the end of life: the Veterans Health Administration's life-sustaining treatment decisions initiative. *Jt Comm J Qual Patient Saf.* 2019;45(1):47–56. https://doi.org/10.1016/j.jcjq.2018.04.007.
23. Schofield G, Dittborn M, Huxtable R, Brangan E, Selman LE. Real-world ethics in palliative care: a systematic review of the ethical challenges reported by specialist palliative care practitioners in their clinical practice. *Palliat Med.* 2021;35(2):315–334. https://doi.org/10.1177/0269216320974277.
24. Skeath P, Berger A. "Living in the moment" among cancer survivors who report life-transforming change. *Ann Palliat Med.* 2017;6(3):227–236. https://doi.org/10.21037/apm.2017.06.22.
25. Abdul-Razzak A, Heyland DK, Simon J, Ghosh S, Day AG, You JJ. Patient–family agreement on values and preferences for life-sustaining treatment: results of a multicentre observational study. *BMJ Support Palliat Care.* 2019;9(1):e20. https://doi.org/10.1136/bmjspcare-2016-001284.
26. Five Wishes. Accessed August 26, 2022. https://www.fivewishes.org/for-myself/.
27. Torke AM, Hickman SE, Hammes B, et al. POLST facilitation in complex care management: a feasibility study. *Am J Hosp Palliat Med.* 2019;36(1):5–12. https://doi.org/10.1177/1049909118797077.
28. Akdeniz M, Yardımcı B, Kavukcu E. Ethical considerations at the end-of-life care. *SAGE Open Med.* 2021;9:205031212110009. https://doi.org/10.1177/20503121211000918.
29. Takla A, Savulescu J, Wilkinson DJC. A conscious choice: is it ethical to aim for unconsciousness at the end of life? *Bioethics.* 2021;35(3):284–291. https://doi.org/10.1111/bioe.12838.
30. Rong J. End of life care in the ICU: the ethics of sedation. *Nurs Crit Care.* 2020;15(5):7–8. https://doi.org/10.1097/01.CCN.0000694104.93935.d6.
31. Mo L, Geng Y, Chang YK, Philip J, Collins A, Hui D. Referral criteria to specialist palliative care for patients with dementia: a systematic review. *J Am Geriatr Soc.* 2021;69(6):1659–1669. https://doi.org/10.1111/jgs.17070.
32. Hernández-Marrero P, Fradique E, Pereira SM. Palliative care nursing involvement in end-of-life decision-making: qualitative secondary analysis. *Nurs Ethics.* 2019;26(6):1680–1695. https://doi.org/10.1177/0969733018774610.
33. Kang KA, Han SJ, Lim YS, Kim SJ. Meaning-centered interventions for patients with advanced or terminal cancer: a meta-analysis. *Cancer Nurs.* 2019;42(4):332–340. https://doi.org/10.1097/NCC.0000000000000628.
34. Moynihan KM, Dorste A, Siegel BD, Rabinowitz EJ, McReynolds A, October TW. Decision-making, ethics, and end-of-life care in pediatric extracorporeal membrane oxygenation: a comprehensive narrative review. *Pediatr Crit Care Med.* 2021;22(9):806–812. https://doi.org/10.1097/PCC.0000000000002766.
35. Shaw M, Shaw J, Simon J. Listening to patients' own goals: a key to goals to care decisions in cardiac care. *Can J Cardiol.* 2020;36:1135–1138.
36. Wong A, Billett A, Milne D. Balancing the hype with reality: what do patients with advanced melanoma consider when making the decision to have immunotherapy? *Oncologist.* 2019;24(11):e1190–e1196. https://doi.org/10.1634/theoncologist.2018-0820.
37. Burns RB, Waikar SS, Wachterman MW, et al. Trends in hospital-based specialty palliative care in the United States from 2013 to 2017. *J Pain Symptom Manage.* 2018;10(1):774–780. https://doi.org/10.1111/jocn.13925.
38. Hum A, Tay RY, Wong YKY, et al. Advanced dementia: an integrated homecare programme. *BMJ Support Palliat Care.* 2019;10(4):e40. https://doi.org/10.1136/bmjspcare-2019-001798.
39. Cardenas D. Ethical issues and dilemmas in artificial nutrition and hydration. *Clin Nutr ESPEN.* 2021;41(2021):23–29. https://doi.org/10.1016/j.clnesp.2020.12.010.
40. Mayers T, Kashiwagi S, Mathis BJ, et al. International review of national-level guidelines on end-of-life care with focus on the withholding and withdrawing of artificial nutrition and hydration. *Geriatr Gerontol Int.* 2019;19(9):847–853. https://doi.org/10.1111/ggi.13741.
41. Newcomer KF, Fine RL, Newman AF. Food as love: ethical and moral dilemmas in withdrawal of artificial nutrition and hydration in the minimally conscious state. *J Palliat Care.* 2023;38(4):407–411. https://doi.org/10.1177/08258597211014359.
42. Schwartz DB, Barrocas A, Annetta MG, et al. Ethical aspects of artificially administered nutrition and hydration: an ASPEN position paper. *Nutr Clin Pract.* 2021;36(2):254–267. https://doi.org/10.1002/ncp.10633.
43. Marcolini EG, Putnam AT, Aydin A. History and perspectives on nutrition and hydration at the end of life. *Yale J Biol Med.* 2018;91(2):173–176.
44. American Nurses Association. *Position Statement: Nutrition and Hydration at the End of Life.* American Nurses Association; 2017.
45. Rochford A. Ethics of providing clinically assisted nutrition and hydration: current issues. *Frontline Gastroenterol.* 2021;12(2):128–132. https://doi.org/10.1136/flgastro-2019-101230.
46. Compton P, Blacher S. Nursing education in the midst of the opioid crisis. *Pain Manag Nurs.* 2020;21:35–42.
47. Fogger S, Dobbs G. Treating pain while mindful of opioid risks. *Am Nurse J.* 2020;15(10):20–26.
48. Herr K, Coyne PJ, Ely E, Gélinas C, Manworren RCB. ASPMN 2019 position statement: pain assessment in the patient unable to

self-report. *Pain Manag Nurs.* 2019;20:402–403. https://doi.org/10.1016/j.pmn.2019.07.007.
49. Jerpseth H, Dahl V, Nortvedt P, Halvorsen K. Older patients with late-stage COPD: their illness experiences and involvement in decision-making regarding mechanical ventilation and noninvasive ventilation. *J Clin Nurs.* 2018;27(3–4):582–592. https://doi.org/10.1111/jocn.13925.
50. Wilkinson D, Truog R, Savulescu J. In favour of medical dissensus: why we should agree to disagree about end-of-life decisions. *Bioethics.* 2016;30(2):109–118. https://doi.org/10.1111/bioe.12162.
51. Von Heymann-Horan AB, Puggaard LB, Nissen KG, et al. Dyadic psychological intervention for patients with cancer and caregivers in home-based specialized palliative care: the Domus model. *Palliat Support Care.* 2018;16(2):189–197. https://doi.org/10.1017/S1478951517000141.
52. Potter J, Shields S, Breen R. Palliative sedation, compassionate extubation, and the principle of double effect: an ethical analysis. *Am J Hosp Palliat Med.* 2021;38(12):1536–1540. https://doi.org/10.1177/1049909121998630.
53. Albanesi B, Piredda M, Marchetti A, et al. Oncology and palliative care nurses' knowledge and attitudes toward artificial nutrition and hydration for patients at end of life in Italy: a cross-sectional survey. *Cancer Nurs.* 2021;44(2):E99–E107. https://doi.org/10.1097/NCC.0000000000000803.
54. Pengo V, Zurlo A, Voci A, et al. Advanced dementia: opinions of physicians and nurses about antibiotic therapy, artificial hydration and nutrition in patients with different life expectancies. *Geriatr Gerontol Int.* 2017;17(3):487–493. https://doi.org/10.1111/ggi.12746.
55. Brassfield ER, Buchbinder M. Clinicians' perspectives on the duty to inform patients about medical aid-in-dying. *AJOB Empir Bioeth.* 2020;11(1):53–62. https://doi.org/10.1080/23294515.2019.1695016.
56. Endsley S, Main R. Palliative care in advanced dementia. *Am Fam Physician.* 2019;99(7):456–458.
57. Escher M, Nendaz MR, Cullati S, Hudelson P. Physicians' perspective on potentially non-beneficial treatment when assessing patients with advanced disease for ICU admission: a qualitative study. *BMJ Open.* 2021;11(5):e046268. https://doi.org/10.1136/bmjopen-2020-046268.
58. Johnson SB, Butow PN, Kerridge I, Tattersall MHN. Patient autonomy and advance care planning: a qualitative study of oncologist and palliative care physicians' perspectives. *Support Care Cancer.* 2018;26(2):565–574. https://doi.org/10.1007/s00520-017-3867-5.
59. Koh S-J, Kim S, Kim J, et al. Experiences and opinions related to end-of-life discussion: from oncologists' and resident physicians' perspectives. *Cancer Res Treat.* 2018;50(2):614–623. https://doi.org/10.4143/crt.2016.446.
60. Quill TE, Back AL, Block SD. Responding to patients requesting physician-assisted death: physician involvement at the very end of life. *JAMA.* 2016;315(3):245–246. https://doi.org/10.1001/jama.2015.16210.
61. Walling AM, Ahluwalia SC, Wenger NS, et al. Palliative care quality indicators for patients with end-stage liver disease due to cirrhosis. *Dig Dis Sci.* 2017;62(1):84–92. https://doi.org/10.1007/s10620-016-4339-3.
62. Bolt S, van der Steen J, Schols J, Zwakhalen S, Meijers J. What do relatives value most in end-of-life care for people with dementia? *Int J Palliat Nurs.* 2019;25(9):432–442.
63. Rodríguez-Prat A, Balaguer A, Booth A, Monforte-Royo C. Understanding patients' experiences of the wish to hasten death: an updated and expanded systematic review and meta-ethnography. *BMJ Open.* 2017;7(9):e016659. https://doi.org/10.1136/bmjopen-2017-016659.
64. Zertuche-Maldonado T, Tellez-Villarreal R, Pascual A, et al. Palliative care needs in an acute internal medicine ward in Mexico. *J Palliat Med.* 2018;21(2):163–168.
65. Elbaum A. Black lives in a pandemic: implications of systemic injustice for end-of-life care. *Hastings Cent Rep.* 2020;50(3):58–60. https://doi.org/10.1002/hast.1135.
66. Chua KZY, Quah ELY, Lim YX, et al. A systematic scoping review on patients' perceptions of dignity. *BMC Palliat Care.* 2022;21(1):118. https://doi.org/10.1186/s12904-022-01004-4.
67. National Coalition for Quality Palliative Care. *Clinical Practice Guidelines for Quality Palliative Care.* 4th ed. National Coalition for Hospice and Palliative Care; 2018. https://www.nationalcoalitionhpc.org/ncp.
68. Mohsin A, Sume A, Hussain M. Analysis of the causes of moral injury in the outbreak of COVID-19. *Psychol Trauma.* 2020;12(suppl 1):S162–S164. https://doi.org/10.1037/tra0000720.
69. Hutchison K, Sparrow R. Ethics and the cardiac pacemaker: more than just end-of-life issues. *Europace.* 2018;20(5):739–746. https://doi.org/10.1093/europace/eux019.
70. Ashkenazy S, DeKeyser Ganz F. The differentiation between pain and discomfort: a concept analysis of discomfort. *Pain Manag Nurs.* 2019;20(6):556–562. https://doi.org/10.1016/j.pmn.2019.05.003.
71. Barathi B, Chandra PS. Palliative sedation in advanced cancer patients: does it Shorten Survival Time?—A Systematic Review. *Indian J Palliat Care.* 2013 Jan;19(1):40–47. doi:10.4103/0973-1075.110236. PMID: 23766594; PMCID: PMC3680838.
72. Schwarzkopf D, Ruddel H, Thomas-Ruddel D, et al. Perceived nonbeneficial treatment of patients, burnout, and intention to leave the job among ICU nurses and junior and senior physicians. *Crit Care Med.* 2017;45(3):265–273. https://doi.org/10.1097/CCM.0000000000002081.
73. Cohen KR, Loewy ZG, Rumore MM. End of-life care: law, ethical principles, and Jewish medical ethics. *Ann Long-Term Care.* 2018;26(4):25–31.
74. Emmerich N. Leadership in palliative medicine: moral, ethical and educational. *BMC Med Ethics.* 2018;19(1):55. https://doi.org/10.1186/s12910-018-0296-z.
75. Gómez-Vírseda C, De Maeseneer Y, Gastmans C. Relational autonomy: what does it mean and how is it used in end-of-life care? A systematic review of argument-based ethics literature. *BMC Med Ethics.* 2019;20(1):76. https://doi.org/10.1186/s12910-019-0417-3.
76. Gómez-Vírseda C, De Maeseneer Y, Gastmans C. Relational autonomy in end-of-life care ethics: a contextualized approach to real-life complexities. *BMC Med Ethics.* 2020;21(1):50. https://doi.org/10.1186/s12910-020-00495-1.
77. De Panfilis L, Tanzi S, Perin M, Turola E, Artioli G. "Teach for ethics in palliative care": a mixed-method evaluation of a medical ethics training programme. *BMC Palliat Care.* 2020;19(1):149. https://doi.org/10.1186/s12904-020-00653-7.
78. Chan P, Spertus J, Kennedy K, Nallamothu B, Starks M, Girotra S. In-hospital cardiac arrest survival in the United States during and after the initial novel coronavirus disease 2019 pandemic surge. *Circ Cardiovasc Qual Outcomes.* 2022;15(2):e008420. https://doi.org/10.1161/CIRCOUTCOMES.121.008420.

79. Hamric A, Epstein E. A health system-wide moral distress consultation service: development and evaluation. *HEC Forum.* 2017;29(2):127–143. https://doi.org/10.1007/s10730-016-9315-y.
80. Epstein EG, Hurst AR. Looking at the positive side of moral distress: why it's a problem. *J Clin Ethics.* 2017;28(1):37–41. http://www.ncbi.nlm.nih.gov/pubmed/28436927.
81. Litam S, Balkin R. Moral injury in health-care workers during COVID-19 pandemic. *Traumatology.* 2021;27(1):14–19. https://doi.org/10.1037/trm0000290.
82. Ma K, Wright DK, Vanderspank-Wright B, Peterson WE, Carnevale FA. Nurses' moral experiences of ethically meaningful end-of-life care: distress, resilience, responsibility, and care. *Res Theory Nurs Pract.* 2020;34(3):269–285. https://doi.org/10.1891/RTNP-D-19-00114.
83. Meeker MA, White D. Transition to comfort-focused care: moral agency of acute care nurses. *Nurs Ethics.* 2021;28(4):529–542. https://doi.org/10.1177/0969733020952128.
84. McCarthy J, Monteverde S. The standard account of moral distress and why we should keep it. *HEC Forum.* 2018;30(4):319–328. https://doi.org/10.1007/s10730-018-9349-4.
85. Prestia AS, Sherman RO, Demezier C. Chief nursing officers' experiences with moral distress. *J Nurs Adm.* 2017;47(2):101–107. https://doi.org/10.1097/NNA.0000000000000447.
86. Sajjadi S, Norena M, Wong H, Dodek P. Moral distress and burnout in internal medicine residents. *Can Med Educ J.* 2017;8(1):e36–e43. https://doi.org/10.1016/j.jcrc.2015.10.011.
87. Balboni TA, Fitchett G, Handzo GF, et al. State of the science of spirituality and palliative care research part II: screening, assessment, and interventions. *J Pain Symptom Manage.* 2017;54(3):441–453. https://doi.org/10.1016/j.jpainsymman.2017.07.029.
88. Sinclair S, Hack TF, Raffin-Bouchal S, et al. What are healthcare providers' understandings and experiences of compassion? The healthcare compassion model: a grounded theory study of healthcare providers in Canada. *BMJ Open.* 2018;8(3):e019701. https://doi.org/10.1136/bmjopen-2017-019701.
89. Casey D. Hospice and palliative care: what's the difference? *MEDSURG Nurs.* 2019;28(3):196–197.
90. Coyne PJ, Bobb B, Plakovic K, eds. *Conversations in Palliative Care: Questions and Answers with the Experts.* 4th ed. Hospice and Palliative Nurses Association; 2017.
91. Erel M, Marcus EL, Dekeyser-Ganz F. Barriers to palliative care for advanced dementia: a scoping review. *Ann Palliat Med.* 2017;6(4):365–379.
92. Philip J, Russell B, Collins A, et al. The ethics of prioritizing access to palliative care: a qualitative study. *Am J Hosp Palliat Med.* 2019;36(7):577–582. https://doi.org/10.1177/1049909119833333.
93. Sullivan NM, Blake LE, George M, Mears SC. Palliative care in the hip fracture patient. *Geriatr Orthop Surg Rehabil.* 2019;10:2151459319849801. https://doi.org/10.1177/2151459319849801.
94. Makhoul AT, Drolet BC. Reserve system implementation during the COVID-19 pandemic. *Chest.* 2021;160(6):2005–2006. https://doi.org/10.1016/j.chest.2021.08.067.
95. Persad G, Peek ME, Shah SK. Fair allocation of scarce therapies for coronavirus disease 2019 (COVID-19). *Clin Infect Dis.* 2022;75(1):e529–e533. https://doi.org/10.1093/cid/ciab1039.
96. Rubin E, Dryden-Peterson SL, Hammond SP, et al. A novel approach to equitable distribution of scarce therapeutics: institutional experience implementing a reserve system for allocation of COVID-19 monoclonal antibodies. *Chest.* 2021;160(6):2324–2331. https://doi.org/10.1016/j.chest.2021.08.003.
97. Wolfe ID, Patel SJ. SARS-CoV-2 monoclonal antibodies in children: ethical considerations. *Clin Ther.* 2021;43(6):e157–e162. https://doi.org/10.1016/j.clinthera.2021.04.008.
98. Elsner AM. After COVID-19: the way we die from now on. *Camb Q Healthc Ethics.* 2020;30(1):69–72. https://doi.org/10.1017/S0963180120000572.
99. Haller M, Norman S, Davis B, Capone C, Browne K, Allard C. A model for treating COVID-19 related guilt, shame, and moral injury. *Psychol Trauma.* 2020;12(suppl 1):S174–S176. https://doi.org/10.1037/tra0000742.
100. Sheahan L, Brennan F. What matters? Palliative care, ethics, and the COVID-19 pandemic. *J Bioeth Inq.* 2020;17:793–796. https://doi.org/10.1007/s11673-020-10046-3.
101. Ho CWL, Lin CC. How the COVID-19 pandemic could reshape palliative care into high-tech and high-touch care: an ethics of care perspective. *Cancer Nurs.* 2020;43(6):429–430. https://doi.org/10.1097/NCC.0000000000000883.

33

Addressing Spiritual, Religious, and Existential Needs in Palliative Care

Elizabeth Johnston Taylor and William E. Rosa

Key Points

- Spiritual, religious, and/or existential (S/R/E) needs are prevalent and salient among persons living with a serious illness. These needs manifest in many ways, such as a need for meaning, forgiveness, hope, peace, and self-worth, among others.
- Numerous psychometrically evaluated tools and scales exist for screening for spiritual distress and for a more in-depth, multifaceted understanding of one's S/R/E needs (i.e., for obtaining a history).
- There are several S/R/E interventions nurses can use to promote personhood and dignity for those with serious illness, requiring continued self-development, competency building, and application of various modalities, including therapeutic presence.

Addressing Spiritual, Religious, and Existential Needs in Palliative Care

The biomedical model, the predominant model adopted by most Western health systems, is based on a physiological understanding of health and illness. Through a biomedical lens, good health is defined as the absence of illness; the body is assessed and treated as machinery exhibiting varying amounts of function. This reductionist view of health and illness considers only the individual, whose health and illness are uninformed by environmental determinants of health. Nurses working in such a model often fall prey to a system that rarely supports authentic person-centeredness rooted in caring for the person as a whole, never mind as a person who has meaningful relationships. Rather, nurses steeped in the biomedical model sometimes define their work in terms of the interventions rendered rather than the quality of time spent, healing facilitated, and personhood preserved.

Palliative nursing employs an inherently holistic approach that accounts for biopsychosocial considerations, as well as the spiritual, religious, and existential (S/R/E) needs that arise in the context of serious illness, end of life, and bereavement. The practice of palliative nursing relies on evidence-based science to improve outcomes and ensure the highest standards of care. It also involves addressing S/R/E experiences of patients, their loved ones, and their communities; this core component of palliative nursing merges science and art and has clear opportunities to enhance a dignity and meaning for all involved, including the nurse. Beyond the clinical obligations to address S/R/E needs and ensure responsible, respectful, and inclusive S/R/E care, this domain invites the nurse to experience sacred ground with those in their care—a domain which may not always have words, definitions, or explanations. Thus, the Case Study 1 can illustrate and provide a matrix for further exploration.

Case Study 1: Navigating Disbelief and Divine Abandonment

Lee is a widowed 67-year-old accountant recently diagnosed with a life-limiting illness that causes considerable physical pain and fatigue. Given his circumstances, a palliative care consult is ordered. During the initial assessment, when Lee is asked about what he understands of his illness and prognosis, he makes the following comments: "Why would this happen to me? It's such a shocker! I've eaten my spinach, never smoked, volunteered in the community, and went to church every Sunday. I just always assumed God would take care of me, but now I feel like he dumped me."

Questions for Reflection:

1. What might be the scope of Lee's S/R/E needs, given their social background that includes being a widower, active in a church and the community, and nearing 70?
2. What feelings do you have when a patient asks you "why" about their illness or condition?
3. Given this exchange occurs during initial consultation, what might be the key elements of your palliative nursing plan of care as you build a relationship with Lee?

Lee's case provides a peek into how patients receiving palliative care could respond in ways that reflect an S/R/E dimension. Indeed, serious illness and facing one's mortality inherently conjure S/R/E needs. For some—at least 10%–22%—these needs are distressing.[1,2] Even if not distressing, spiritual care needs are often reported among persons with advanced illness (e.g., 62% in an Australian palliative care sample[3]). Thus, one of the eight domains identified by the National Coalition for Hospice and Palliative Care is that of caring for S/R/E aspects.[4] Therefore, this chapter will provide an overview of how palliative nurses can address these needs. Specifically, this chapter presents guidance on how to screen for and more deeply assess S/R/E needs and provide care that can promote S/R/E well-being.

What Are S/R/E Needs?

Most people around the world are religious; if they are not religious, they often self-describe as spiritual.[5] The very few who deny being religious or spiritual typically accept that they do have the existential need to make sense of their world and their life, including their death. Furthermore, as Allie's story in Case Study 2 illustrates, for many of those who are religious "nones" or "dones," their religious upbringing or culture can still influence them.

Case Study 2: Being Spiritual while "None and Done"

Allie is a 44-year-old partnered woman who cooked for a living. After years of living with a chronic and increasingly debilitating illness, her physician tells her she has less than 6 months to live and that it is "time to get her life in order." She accepts the offer to receive hospice care. During the intake assessment, the nurse learns that although Allie rejected the religion of her childhood, she considers herself "sort of spiritual." Allie suspects a chaplain visit is unnecessary and counters with: "I'm not sure there really is a God to make peace with. Besides, if there is a heaven and the people there are like the religious people here, I don't want to go there!"

Questions for Reflection:

1. What new or changing S/R/E needs, if any, do you typically observe as patients transition to hospice care?
2. Suppose Allie's rejection of her childhood religion is related to painful memories. What is your comfort level attending to a patient's religious or spiritual injury?
3. What skills and actions can you take so as to remain fully present with Allie as she sits in her spiritual uncertainty?

Numerous analyses of the concept of spirituality have identified key aspects of this ethereal and intangible phenomenon. Nursing conceptualizations of spirituality often include the following as aspects of spirituality: the need for purpose and meaning, forgiveness, love and relatedness (or connectedness to self, others, and nature), peace and harmony, self-transcendence.[6] Many nurses distinguish religion from spirituality; they view religion as the beliefs (e.g., stories, theologies) and practices (e.g., rituals, lifestyle) that are shared within a collective or organization. Religious beliefs and practices support and allow expression of one's spirituality. Thus, religious needs can involve the need to worship within one's faith community, find comfort from religious practices, or make decisions according to one's beliefs.[7] Existential needs are fundamentally about needing to know one's existence is meaningful, purposeful, and of worth.[8]

These components of S/R/E are found in the widely accepted definition for spirituality developed by consensus among international palliative care experts.[9] This definition states:

> Spirituality is a dynamic and intrinsic aspect of humanity through which persons seek ultimate meaning, purpose, and transcendence, and experience relationship to self, family, others, community, society, nature, and the significant or sacred. Spirituality is expressed through beliefs, values, traditions, and practices.[9 (p. 646)]

Given it is a most essential, inherent, and vitalizing aspect of humans, it is unsurprising that it comes to the fore as one faces one's mortality.

How Do S/R/E Needs Manifest?

To understand how to address S/R/E needs, the palliative nurse must know how they may present. Although many descriptive studies have identified spiritual needs of patients and their loved ones facing the end of life, systematic reviews that synthesize what are S/R/E needs provide stronger evidence.[10–13] Whereas any listing of S/R/E needs would be incomplete, Table 33.1 provides an overview.

Although the terminology S/R/E "need" may unintentionally and inappropriately suggest a problem or spiritual pathology, spiritual needs can also be of a positive nature. The following examples illustrate:

- need to express their joy about sensing closeness to others
- need to pursue activities that allow expression of creative impulses (e.g., artwork, music-making, writing)
- need to develop, foster, and express gratitude (e.g., "I wish I didn't need to rely on others so much, but I am so thankful for how people do help me.")
- need to experience awe (e.g., need to sit under the stars and transcend self)
- need to serve others or return love outwardly (e.g., "I want to pay it forward")
- need to tell their story and share their experiential wisdom (e.g., legacy-building)

Indeed, it must be remembered that even though an S/R/E need may manifest with discomforting emotions such as anger or grief, these "negative" emotions can prompt continued inner S/R/E growth. The S/R/E journey involves awakening to how one's misaligned ego, inner irrationalities, or shadow self can better align with one's truest or best self (also known as "God's will")—or with what is most loving, truthful, beautiful, ethical, of virtue.[14]

S/R/E Assessment

A three-tiered approach to assessing patient spirituality is advocated by experts.[15] That is, the process of assessment of S/R/E can potentially include: screening, history-taking, and a more in-depth assessment. Because it is unlikely that nurses, as spiritual care generalists (rather than specialists), would conduct an in-depth S/R/E

Table 33.1 Spiritual/religious/existential needs of persons receiving palliative care

S/R/E needs	Examples
Need for meaning and purpose (in life, in suffering, in death)	"Why do I have to suffer on the way to death? Why couldn't I just go to my death in my sleep?" "I feel like I never really did anything important in life, and now it's too late." "I am going to leave a legacy; my imprint on the world will be my children and the values and good I transmit through them."
Need for hope	"I just want to give up; it is not worth it anymore." (despair) "I have nothing to live for."
Need to resolve inner religious struggle	"Sometimes it is hard to believe there is a loving God upstairs that has my best interests in mind." "I used to believe . . . but now how could it? The world is just so capricious and life is unfair."
Need to forgive self or others	"I think my cancer is a punishment for something I did when I was young." (guilt) "I'm mortified that I'd get cancer in my private area." (shame)
Need to sense self-worth and dignity	"Look and smell this body! It's so embarrassing . . . it's not me anymore." "I'm such a burden now."
Need to sense being loved	"Everyone is so busy . . . too busy to take care of me."
Need to resolve anger at God/others/faith community	"Why would a loving God allow this to happen to me?" "Why did that corporation pollute the water where we lived for so long?" "The folks from church have stopped coming to visit; I guess I've been sick too long and they are tired of me."
Need to understand a "dark night of the soul" (e.g., feeling abandonment by God)	"I feel like my prayers aren't being answered . . . where is God?"
Need for reconciliation	Desire to be reunited with estranged family members
Need to mourn losses	"I feel a deep sadness about not being able to be there for my kids and grandkids when they need my comfort and wisdom." Spiritual issues often accompany the various losses persons mourn when living with a terminal illness, such as the loss of independence, social roles and vocation, body image, and function.
Need to feel autonomous or "in control"	"I wish I could control my body and my life! I can't even control my own schedule, when doctors and nurses keep coming in unannounced." "I'm ready to go . . . but it's not happening."
Need to "come to terms" with one's death	"I wish I could say 'I'm at peace' about dying, but I can't. It's hard to accept that soon I'll just decay into nothing." "Death is just so final; I know my friends will eventually move on, and I'll have been like a blip on the monitor."

assessment, only approaches to conducting a spiritual screening or history are presented.

S/R/E Screening

One purpose of a spiritual screening is to determine if the patient presents with any spiritual distress and if they wish for the healthcare specialist or team to provide spiritual support. This screening can be conducted by anyone who has received training to do so.[15] Thus, a screening should involve only one or very few questions. For this review, only screeners with fewer than four or five questions are presented.

Several stand-alone screening questions have been empirically evaluated. Particularly noteworthy is the work of Bahraini et al., who compared the psychometric evidence available for 24 S/R/E screening measures.[16] Although there are many screening approaches, those with the greatest empirical support (e.g., highest specificity and sensitivity) are presented in Table 33.2.

Whereas all of these approaches to screening assess how important spirituality is to the patient or how much spiritual distress or well-being they experience, for some settings it will be important to screen the preferences of the patient with regard to receiving spiritual support.

S/R/E History

An expert panel recommended that the spiritual history be obtained by the primary care provider.[15] In palliative care, it is typically the patient's primary nurse who is responsible for coordinating care and should complete this level of assessment. Compared to screening, the history provides a brief but more comprehensive understanding of what types of spiritual needs and resources might exist.

Many tools for spiritual screening or assessment published in the literature are quantitative measures of S/R/E that may have originally been designed for use in research. Systematic reviews and evaluation of these tools for use with life-threatening illness are available.[13,16,22–25] These may be useful for learning about a patient's S/R/E history. Likewise, some of the longer tools proposed for screening may also be helpful for the history. Table 33.3 presents a selection of tools or measures that are most likely to hold promise for palliative care patient spiritual history-taking. These questionnaires were selected for their brevity, validity, and/or clinical relevance to palliative care.

Whereas these tools and measures allow a quick, written quantification of various types of S/R/E needs without much clinician engagement, assessing one's S/R/E history will be woefully lacking if there is not also a more qualitative and personal approach. That is, to allow assessment to provide a foundation for S/R/E care, the relationship between the primary provider and patient is paramount. Although a history is not to require the time or expertise of an in-depth assessment interview, simply asking one or two open questions when collecting the history data will benefit. For example, if the patient completed a measure independently, the nurse can follow this up with something like the following: "Thank you for answering these questions about your spirituality. I'm just wondering if they prompted some additional thoughts or feelings that you'd like to share?" Or "I'm curious about what you thought of these questions?"

Table 33.2 Spiritual, religious, and existential screening questions with empirical support

Questions	Empirical support
1. (How much) Do you have pain deep in your soul (being) that is not physical?	An adaptation of this screener evaluated in an Israeli sample was given a top ranking by Bahraini et al., who observed it to have both high specificity and sensitivity.[16] Fashioned after the Edmonton Symptom Distress Scale, this item is accompanied by response options from 0 (best) to 10 (worst) spiritual pain.[17]
1. Do you struggle with the loss of meaning and joy in your life? 2. Do you currently have what you would describe as spiritual or religious struggles?	These screeners demonstrate high specificity and sensitivity.[16,18]
1. Are you at peace?	Although Bahraini et al. ranked this item eighth (of 24 S/R screeners), it is worth presenting here given its brevity and evidence for its support.[16] Responses to this screener, identified by Steinhauser et al., were found to correlate highly with spiritual and emotional well-being in a large study of terminally ill patients.[19]
1. Associated with your health, do you suffer due to feeling punished/fearful/shame/guilty/angry with God/no meaning in life/disconnected/other issues? 2. Has suffering limited you from doing what you need to do for >14 days over the last 30 days? 3. Do you seek additional professional help for these concerns?	As part of a general screening for suffering appropriate for use with seriously ill patients in low- and middle-income countries, Vallath et al. included an item for S/R/E.[20] This item includes possible sources of distress (question 1). If the patient agrees, then question 2 can be asked, followed by question 3.
1. Is religion or spirituality important to you as you cope with your illness? 2. Has there ever been a time when S/R was important to you? 3. How much strength/comfort do you get from your S/R right now?	Chaplain Fitchett's research team has developed and evaluated the Rush Spiritual Screening Protocol over several years.[2] Based on the patient response to question 1, the clinician follows up. If the patient responds with no to question 1, then follow up with question 2. If the patient responds with yes to question 1, then move to question 3. If the patient indicates either that S/R used to be a resource or that it is failing to provide adequate strength/comfort now, then a referral to a chaplain is advised.[2] When comparing various S/R screeners, Bahraini et al. observed that this protocol had the highest specificity (as high as 90% in one study).[16]
1. Instructions for thermometer: Please circle the number (0–10) that best describes how much distress you have been experiencing in the past week including today. 2. Problem list: Please indicate if any of the following has been a problem for you in the past week including today (includes options for S/R concerns).	The National Comprehensive Cancer Network offers a Distress Thermometer for S/R concerns. The thermometer indicates responses can range from no distress to extreme distress. Handzo et al. observed that nurses at a comprehensive cancer center did not accept this screening tool as well as the Fitchett protocol.[21]

S/R, spiritual/religious; S/R/E, spiritual/religious/existential.

Or "Do you think these questions covered what you think is important?" Allow time for the patient to gather their thoughts and speak; verbalizing one's innermost experience can be difficult and requires effort. It also requires a relationship that is safe. Table 33.4 provides additional prompts for encouraging spiritual discourse, as well as patients' responses that can indicate need for referral to a chaplain.

S/R/E Screenings and Histories: Putting Them into Practice

The nurse participating in the initial palliative care consult for Lee, the newly diagnosed patient spontaneously complaining that he feels God "dumped" him, can assume Lee is experiencing S/R/E distress. His comment indicates an affirmative response to many of the screening items recommended (e.g., Do you have pain deep in your soul [being] that is not physical? Do you suffer due to feeling punished/fearful/shame/guilty/angry with God?). Indeed, this spontaneous comment may be more reliable than the likelihood of a patient confessing yes to not "being at peace" or "currently having what they would describe as spiritual or religious struggles"—extraordinarily painful admissions. Such admissions require not only an awareness of great inner pain but vulnerability and a sense of safety with the clinician receiving the confession. Thus, the next step for Lee's nurse will be to assess resources and how the palliative care team can provide support. If the primary care coordinator, this nurse will follow up to obtain an S/R/E history so as to better understand Lee's distress and plan care.

The nurse conducting the intake assessment of Allie, the new hospice patient who rejects the religiosity of her childhood, will benefit from conducting a screening and history. If her hospice has selected a standardized scale or tool that quantifies S/R/E distress, this can be given to Allie to complete. Regardless of whether the screening tool indicates distress requiring immediate attention, a history should be obtained to provide person-centered care. When the nurse receives the completed screening and/or history survey, they would do well to ask an open question to prompt further insight and rapport. Indeed, not only will the narrative assessment allow the nurse to understand Allie's worldview and preferences for care at the end of life; it will also give Allie an opportunity to gain self-awareness. The process of assessing S/R/E inherently involves providing caring.

Interventions for Attending to the S/R/E Domain

Human-centered S/R/E care requires the nurse to be clear on intention and *how* they are entering into relationship with the other. Caring for the S/R/E needs of another person calls for the nurse to be quite grounded and attuned to their innate strengths, challenges, and wisdom. Some find benefit in adopting nursing theories to assist in giving language to the less tangible elements of their practice and substantiate their unique contributions to providing comfort and alleviating suffering. For instance, Watson's human caring science provides a moral-ethical framework known as the Ten Caritas

Table 33.3 Tools and measures for a spiritual/religious/existential (S/R/E) history

Name	Description	Illustrative items
FICA[26]	Structured interview that inquires about faith, import, community, address (FICA). Widely cited. Has been validated as feasible within a hospital palliative care service.	F = What faith, if any, nurtures you? I = How important is it to you? C = How do you participate in your faith community? A = How would you like your healthcare team to support your S/R/E?
Spiritual Pain Assessment Sheet[27]	When screening determines there is spiritual pain, a structured interview with 14 questions is conducted by trained nurses. It allows inquiry about: (a) relationships, (b) autonomy, and (c) temporality. Evaluated in Japanese patients with advanced cancer.	Relationships: worries about family; being a burden Autonomy: loss of purpose; loss of control Temporality: regrets; absurdity of life
Existential Distress Scale[8]	10 items with response options from *never* (1) to *all the time* (4).	I don't matter. No one cares about me. My life is empty. I have nothing to live for.
Spiritual Care Checklist[3]	17-item checklist with items evaluated in a sample of palliative care patients in Australia. Evidence exists for structural and concurrent validity and reliability.	Fear of dying process Fear of losing control Guilt over past behaviors Prayers being unheard
Spiritual Needs Questionnaire[28]	The 20-item version of this scale measures the follow factors: religious needs (6 items), need for inner peace (5 items), existential/meaning (5 items), and actively given of oneself (3 items). A 10-item "screener" version for palliative care patients eliminates last factor as it addresses "generativity." Response options (4-point) allow measurement of agreement/disagreement. Developed in Germany, so wording may not be fitting for North American patients. Evidence for strong psychometric properties.	Inner peace: To talk with others about your fears and worries? Existential need: To talk with someone about the question of meaning in life? Religious need: To turn to a higher power?
Spiritual/Religious Struggles Scale—Short Form (RSSS-SF)[29]	The RSSS includes six subscales (in 14 items) that measure supernatural (i.e., divine and demonic), interpersonal, and intrapersonal (moral, ultimate meaning, doubt) struggles. The RSSS-SF was rigorously developed and evaluated. The 5-point response options include *never* and *does not a apply*.	Questioned whether my life will really make any difference in the world. Felt troubled by doubts or questions about religion or spirituality. Felt as though God had abandoned me.
Spiritual Injury Scale[24]	This 8-item scale developed in Israel is a top-ranked tool for predicting spiritual distress.[16] Response options allow measurement of frequency (*never* to *very often*).	Does anger or resentment block your peace of mind? Do you feel that God/life has treated you unfairly?

Table 33.4 Useful prompts and responses indicating need for a chaplain referral

Spiritual care questions from nurse to patient	Questions/statements by the patient requiring chaplain referral
• How is your spirit doing today? • Are you scared? • What are you most afraid of? • What are you most worried about? • What makes life worth living? • Is there anything you haven't done that you need to do? • What do you hope for? • What is your deeper hope? • Is there anything worse than death? • What are you most proud of in your life? • Do you have regrets? • Do you need to forgive anyone? • Do you need to ask forgiveness from anyone? • What will your legacy be? • What do you love most about your life? • Are you at peace?	• What have I done to deserve this? • I pray, but I am still sick. • I used to believe in God, but now I'm not so sure. • I feel like all hope is gone. • No one has ever accepted me because I'm different • How will my family get along without me? • What did my life mean? • What is there left to care about? • No one understands. • I'm scared.

Source: Reference 35.

Processes* that can be used as a personal compass for guiding S/R/E-oriented palliative nursing.[30] These include: embracing altruistic values and practicing loving-kindness; honoring others while instilling faith and hope; showing sensitivity to others by attending to one's own beliefs and practices; developing relationships that are helping, trusting, and caring; promoting and accepting the full range of positive and negative feelings while listening to another; using creative scientific problem-solving approaches; adapting teaching and learning to the individual; creating a healing environment that prioritizes the protection, promotion, and preservation of human dignity; assisting with the basic physical, emotional, and S/R/E needs; and opening to the possibility of mystery and miracles.

These processes can directly inform palliative nursing practices. For instance, when hearing Lee feels abandoned by God, the nurse can invite the full depth of disappointment and sadness (so-called negative emotions) that are driving his experience. By responding with love and kindness, the palliative nurse forges an authentic relationship that offers help, facilitates trust, and demonstrates caring at a time when Lee may feel quite isolated. As the nurse prioritizes Lee's most basic needs at the physical, emotional, and S/R/E levels, Lee feels cared for and cared about; this experience of safety creates a healing environment where his dignity is maintained even amid substantial internal instability.

Quinn sounds the call for nurses to become an instrument for healing by developing several competencies that are iterative and require lifelong development.[31] Examples include:

- Embarking on spiritual self-knowledge to promote comfort and ease when engaging in S/R/E/ questions with others
- Committing to spiritual self-care and personal wholeness to ensure the nurse remains spiritually vital and healthy

- Developing the ability to center oneself, to know stillness, and to create healing environments "from the inside out"
- Learning to let go of tasks, agendas, plans, and objectives to remain authentically present with the needs arising in this moment with this person in this sacred encounter
- Listening deeply while using all ways of knowing, allowing heart and intuition to support the science of nursing practice
- Staying connected to the nature of compassion while allowing self to nurture and be nurtured by the relationships with those in our care
- Reflecting and remaining self-aware of thoughts, emotions, and physical responses while being with another
- Remaining open-minded and open-hearted, identifying and releasing judgment and bias, creating opportunities for full self-expression and freedom of being
- Dwelling in the space of uncertainty and "not knowing" and surrendering the role of "expert" to reconnect with the human condition of vulnerability without the need to fix, change, or alter

These competencies may require great commitment from the nurse to remain emotionally grounded in their work in the context of busy health settings and overtaxed teams. This type of fortitude is more easily described than accomplished. Yet S/R/E interventions detached from this authenticity may be potentially harmful and lack the individualized attention required to respectfully attend to the distress that often accompanies serious illness.

Consider the nurse responding to Allie, a woman likely to have a history of traumatic spiritual injury. To assess and plan care for her S/R/E will require that a nurse remain present to S/R/E pain and struggle. As Allie shares the hurts that have led to her current perspective, the nurse can choose to stay present for Allie, to get still, to self-assess S/R/E discomfort, and to remain nonjudgmental. When Allie experiences the nurse's compassion, she will likely be able to share openly (perhaps for the first time) how her S/R/E history is influencing her responses to serious illness. New possibilities are created for Allie in the face of an open-minded and open-hearted nurse, someone who is truly there for the betterment of Allie.

Integrative healing modalities become vehicles for tending to the S/R/E needs of someone with serious illness. Quinn[31] categorized modalities that tend to S/R/E needs into four main groups:

- Approaches to tending the spirit through the individual, inner experience (e.g., spiritual practices from one's religion, meditation aligned with one's beliefs, cultivating self-awareness, forgiveness practices, reflective journaling)
- Approaches to tending the spirit through the body (e.g., ritual, yoga, mindful eating, sacred dance, making or listening to music, walking meditation, viewing or making art)
- Approaches to tending the spirit through the shared inner experience with other people (e.g., group prayer or meditation, pastoral care/counseling, support groups, time spent with loving friends or family, seeking healing of broken relationships, spiritually oriented therapy)
- Approaches to tending the spirit through natural, social, cultural, and institutional environments (e.g., being in nature, being with pets/animals, gardening, working for positive social change, participating in community or charity initiatives and celebrations, caring for the environment)

Palliative nurses should remember that the modality is simply one part of the intervention; the nurse as the healing instrument of care is the other and most essential part.[32] In other words, the modality itself may be powerful, but *how* the modality is offered is offered with compassion is of essential concern.

Lee may find connection and regain his confidence in faith through support groups for widowed persons and spiritually oriented therapy that integrates his religious uncertainty into a care plan. His palliative nurse may be able to facilitate such experiences by listening to reflections from Lee's journaling and ensuring access to the music that calms and centers him. Allie might regain and nourish her sense of safety through time spent in the hospice garden and through sharing a few moments of mindful breathing with her nurse. Her access to the pet therapy program has potential to reawaken joy and connection even in her moments of worry.

Conclusion

This chapter, the synthesis of two more in-depth chapters on the topics of spiritual assessment[33] and therapeutics,[34] advances the promotion of S/R/E well-being as a pillar of palliative care. To do so, a major cultural shift within healthcare is required. We posit that to sustainably prioritize the S/R/E experience of patients, S/R/E literacy must be embedded into clinical training and research. This training needs to teach clinicians to foster self-awareness and self-development.[35]

The palliative nurse attending to S/R/E needs is never expected to fix, change, or alter "what is"; rather, the nurse is called to "be with," witness, and holistically support the recipient of palliative care. Being fully available to those who are suffering in the S/R/E domain requires self-knowledge and a staunch commitment to the delivery of dignified nursing care. Such care also requires an alignment with the highest moral standards and practices to facilitate healing and wholeness, not least of which is love.

REFERENCES

1. Robinson KL, Connelly CD, Georges JM. Pain and spiritual distress at end of life: a correlational study. *J Palliat Care*. 2022;37(4):526–534. https://doi.org/10.1177/08258597221090482.
2. Fitchett G, Murphy P, King SDW. Examining the validity of the Rush Protocol to screen for religious/spiritual struggle. *J Health Care Chaplain*. 2017;23(3):98–112. https://doi.org/10.1080/08854726.2017.1294861.
3. Michael NG, Bobevski I, Georgousopoulou E, et al. Unmet spiritual needs in palliative care: psychometrics of a screening checklist. *BMJ Support Palliat Care*. 2020;13(e1):e170–e176. https://doi.org/10.1136/bmjspcare-2020-002636.
4. National Coalition for Hospice and Palliative Care. *Clinical Practice Guidelines for Quality Palliative Care*. 4th ed. National Coalition for Hospice and Palliative Care; 2018.
5. Association of Religion Data Archives. http://www.thearda.com.
6. Murgia C, Notarnicola I, Rocco G, Stievano A. Spirituality in nursing: A concept analysis. *Nurs Ethics*. Aug 2020;27(5):1327–1343. https://doi.org/10.1177/0969733020909534.
7. Taylor EJ. *Fast Facts about Religion: Implications for Nursing*. Springer; 2019.

8. Lo C, Panday T, Zeppieri J, et al. Preliminary psychometrics of the Existential Distress Scale in patients with advanced cancer. *Eur J Cancer Care (Engl)*. 2017;26(6):12597. https://doi.org/10.1111/ecc.12597.
9. Puchalski CM, Vitillo R, Hull SK, Reller N. Improving the spiritual dimension of whole person care: reaching national and international consensus. *J Palliat Med*. 2014;17(6):642–656. https://doi.org/10.1089/jpm.2014.9427.
10. Mesquita AC, Chaves ECL, Barros GAM. Spiritual needs of patients with cancer in palliative care: an integrative review. *Curr Opin Support Palliat Care*. 2017;11(4):334–340. https://doi.org/10.1097/spc.0000000000000308.
11. Lormans T, de Graaf E, van de Geer J, van der Baan F, Leget C, Teunissen S. Toward a socio-spiritual approach? A mixed-methods systematic review on the social and spiritual needs of patients in the palliative phase of their illness. *Palliat Med*. 2021;35(6):1071–1098. https://doi.org/10.1177/02692163211010384.
12. Benites AC, Rodin G, Leite A, Nascimento LC, Dos Santos MA. The experience of spirituality in family caregivers of adult and elderly cancer patients receiving palliative care: a meta-synthesis. *Eur J Cancer Care (Engl)*. 2021;30(4):e13424. https://doi.org/10.1111/ecc.13424.
13. Daly L, Fahey-McCarthy E, Timmins F. The experience of spirituality from the perspective of people living with dementia: a systematic review and meta-synthesis. *Dementia (London)*. 2019;18(2):448–470. https://doi.org/10.1177/1471301216680425.
14. Edinger E. *Ego and Archetype: Individuation and the Religious Function of the Psyche*. Shambala; 1992.
15. Puchalski C, Ferrell B, Virani R, et al. Improving the quality of spiritual care as a dimension of palliative care: the report of the consensus conference. *J Palliat Med*. 2009;12(10):885–904. https://doi.org/10.1089/jpm.2009.0142.
16. Bahraini S, Gifford W, Graham ID, et al. The accuracy of measures in screening adults for spiritual suffering in health care settings: a systematic review. *Palliat Support Care*. 2020;18(1):89–102. https://doi.org/10.1017/s1478951519000506.
17. Delgado-Guay MO, Chisholm G, Williams J, Frisbee-Hume S, Ferguson AO, Bruera E. Frequency, intensity, and correlates of spiritual pain in advanced cancer patients assessed in a supportive/palliative care clinic. *Palliat Support Care*. 2016;14(4):341–348. https://doi.org/10.1017/s147895151500108x.
18. King SD, Fitchett G, Murphy PE, Pargament KI, Harrison DA, Loggers ET. Determining best methods to screen for religious/spiritual distress. *Support Care Cancer*. 2017;25(2):471–479. https://doi.org/10.1007/s00520-016-3425-6.
19. Steinhauser KE, Voils CI, Clipp EC, Bosworth HB, Christakis NA, Tulsky JA. "Are you at peace?": one item to probe spiritual concerns at the end of life. *Arch Intern Med*. 2006;166(1):101–105. https://doi.org/10.1001/archinte.166.1.101.
20. Vallath N, Salins N, Ghoshal A, et al. Developing a screening tool for serious health-related suffering for low- and middle-income countries - phase-1: domain identification and item generation. *Indian J Palliat Care*. 2022;28(1):51–63. https://doi.org/10.25259/ijpc_25_2021.
21. Handzo G, Bowden JM, King S. The evolution of spiritual care in the NCCN distress management guidelines. *J Natl Compr Canc Netw*. 2019;17(10):1257–1261. https://doi.org/10.6004/jnccn.2019.7352.
22. Nissen RD, Falkø E, Stripp TK, Hvidt NC. Spiritual needs assessment in post-secular contexts: an integrative review of questionnaires. *Int J Environ Res Public Health*. 2021;18(24):12898. https://doi.org/10.3390/ijerph182412898.
23. Cosentino C, Harrad RA, Sulla F, Bertuol M, Sarli L, Artioli G. Nursing spiritual assessment instruments in adult patients: a narrative literature review. *Acta Biomed*. 2020;91(12-s):e2020015. https://doi.org/10.23750/abm.v91i12-S.10998.
24. Schultz M, Meged-Book T, Mashiach T, Bar-Sela G. Distinguishing between spiritual distress, general distress, spiritual well-being, and spiritual pain among cancer patients during oncology treatment. *J Pain Symptom Manage*. 2017;54(1):66–73. https://doi.org/10.1016/j.jpainsymman.2017.03.018.
25. Perry KR, King HA, Parker R, Steinhauser KE. Coordinating assessment of spiritual needs: a cross-walk of narrative and psychometric assessment tools used in palliative care. *J Health Care Chaplain*. 2022;28(3):365–377. https://doi.org/10.1080/08854726.2021.1904653.
26. Gomez-Castillo BJ, Hirsch R, Groninger H, et al. Increasing the number of outpatients receiving spiritual assessment: a pain and palliative care service quality improvement project. *J Pain Symptom Manage*. Nov 2015;50(5):724–729. https://doi.org/10.1016/j.jpainsymman.2015.05.012.
27. Ichihara K, Ouchi S, Okayama S, et al. Effectiveness of spiritual care using spiritual pain assessment sheet for advanced cancer patients: a pilot non-randomized controlled trial. *Palliat Support Care*. 2019;17(1):46–53. https://doi.org/10.1017/s1478951518000901.
28. Büssing A. The Spiritual Needs Questionnaire in research and clinical application: a summary of findings. *J Relig Health*. 2021;60(5):3732–3748. https://doi.org/10.1007/s10943-021-01421-4.
29. Exline JJ, Pargament KI, Wilt JA, Grubbs JB, Yali AM. The RSS-14: development and preliminary validation of a 14-item form of the Religious and Spiritual Struggles Scale. *Psycholog Relig Spiritual*. 2023;15(4):592–604. https://doi.org/10.1037/rel0000472.
30. Watson J. *Unitary Caring Science: Philosophy and Praxis of Nursing*. University Press of Colorado; 2018.
31. Quinn JF. Integrative nursing and care of the human spirit. In: Kreitzer MJ, Koithan M, ed. *Integrative Nursing*. 2nd ed. Oxford University Press; 2019:82–99.
32. Rosa W, Estes T. What end-of-life care needs now: an emerging praxis of the sacred and subtle. *Adv Nurs Sci*. 2016;39(4):333–345. https://doi.org/10.1097/ANS.0000000000000136.
33. Taylor EJ. Spiritual screening, history, and assessment. In Ferrell BR, Paice JA, eds. *Textbook of Palliative Nursing Care*. 5th ed. Oxford University Press; 2019:432–446
34. Rosa W. Spiritual care intervention. In Ferrell BR, Paice JA, eds. *Textbook of Palliative Nursing Care*. 5th ed. Oxford University Press; 2019:447–455.

PART IV
Pediatric Palliative Care

34

Pain Management in Pediatric Palliative Care

Juliana H. O'Brien and Gina Santucci

Key Points

- Infants and children experience pain.
- Pediatric pain assessment is specific to age and developmental level and includes both observational and self-reporting tools and strategies.
- Pain management plans are individualized based on the pain source and physiology (acute vs. chronic, somatic vs. neuropathic), the patient's history (past pain experience), and the patient's goals for pain management.
- Children and their families should be engaged in assessment and management of pain.
- Pediatric medication dosing is based on the child's age, body weight, and potentially hepatic or renal function.

Introduction

Infants and children, like adults, experience pain as a serious complication of disease and injury. Until the 1980s, it was thought that neonates were unable to perceive pain due to their immature neuro logic system.[1] Clinicians now know that not only do neonates feel pain but pain is associated with worse neurodevelopmental out comes for neonates.[2,3] For older children, untreated pain can lead to anxiety, decreased school functioning, social isolation, sleep disorders, and mood changes.[3,4] Pain prevention and pain management for this pediatric patients are imperative for their overall physical and mental growth and well-being.

Pain assessment and management in infants and children require that palliative care nurses understand the developmental stages of childhood. A child's response to pain may differ based on their developmental stage. Careful attention should be paid to eliciting both the child's and family's perspectives about pain, including past pain experiences, cultural and social perspectives on pain, and individual behaviors around pain. Children and families should be engaged as a part of the healthcare team, with their input being important in the management of pain. The pediatric pain experience can be influenced by emotional, psychological, and existential distress, just as in adults.

Pediatric Pain Assessment

Taking a Pain History and Self-Reporting Pain Scales

Self-report of pain is an integral part of the pediatric pain assessment whenever it is developmentally and clinically feasible. At the same time, self-report is not the only aspect of the pain assessment; it is considered along with behavioral observations, caregiver report, and clinical data.[5]

Children can affirm or deny pain at a young age. The ability to describe pain will correlate with the child's expressive language and vocabulary. The interviewer should be mindful to use a word for pain that the child is familiar with, such as "hurt," "owie," or "ouchie." Toddlers can begin to either communicate pain location with words or by pointing but may not always be consistent or reliable. A preschool-aged child (>3 years) begins to be more reliable and can utilize a self-reporting pain scale such as the Faces Pain Scale—Revised: six cartoon faces that depict varying levels of pain severity. The child is asked to "point to the face that shows how much you hurt right now."[6] A school-aged child (>8 years old) may be able to provide a more detailed pain history, and the interviewer can use similar questions to those utilized in obtaining a pain history from an adult (Box 34.1). School-aged children with numerical processing skills (about age 8) can make use of the numeric rating scale. See Table 34.1 for examples of pediatric self-reporting pain scales. If a child's self-report when using a validated scale does not correlate with the clinical observation and/or pain behaviors exhibited, the nurse should clarify the child's understanding of the pain scale and potentially utilize a different scale. This is an opportunity for "teach back," having the child explain the pain scale to the nurse. It is important for the interviewer to be mindful of the motivations to underreport or over report pain (see Table 34.2 for examples). The nurse could also use reflective listening to clarify their understanding of the child's report: "I hear you say that you are not having

Box 34.1 OLDCARTS Mnemonic for Obtaining Pain History

O: Onset: When and/or how did your pain start? Did it happen all of a sudden?
L: Location: Where is your pain? Can you point to where you hurt on the stuffed animal?
D: Duration: How long does your pain last? All day versus comes and goes?
C: Characteristics: How would you describe your pain? What does it feel like?
A: Aggravating factors: What makes your pain worse? What makes it hurt more?
R: Relieving factors: What makes your pain better? What takes the "ouch" away?
T: Treatments: What treatments have you tried to help make it better? Play, movement, being held by caregiver?
S: Severity: Rate your pain using a given pain scale. How much is your pain affecting your life (mood, sleep, daily functioning)? Can you play/sleep/eat/move with the pain?

any pain, but then again you are not wanting to get out of bed or move around. What do you feel in your body?"

Physical Exam and Observational Assessment of Pain Intensity

For children who cannot self-report either due to age (infants and toddlers), developmental disability, or medical intervention (i.e., intubation), the caregiver must rely on observational signs of pain and caregiver report. Examples of age-appropriate observational pain scales are listed in Table 34.3.[7–9] For those children who can self-report pain, it is still important for the examiner to also observe the child's behavior for signs of pain as part of their physical exam. Examples are listed in Table 34.4. The nurse should note congruence between the self-report of pain and presence of pain behaviors. If there is a positive self-report of pain *and* pain behaviors are observed, this congruence supports the child's pain experience. Incongruence between self-report and behavior does not invalidate the pain report; for example, a child may report no pain on the numeric scale but have limits to function and grimacing during activities of daily living. The examiner should first ensure that the child understands the self-reporting pain scale to avoid misinterpretation and then, once again, be mindful of motivations to underreport pain. Conversely, children who suffer from chronic pain, such as with rheumatoid arthritis, sickle cell disease, or chronic pancreatitis, may report a significant amount of pain but may not exhibit pain behaviors. For these children, assessment of daily functioning may better indicate their level of impairment from pain.

Just as in adults, some children can articulate what are acceptable or intolerable levels of pain and what are acceptable or intolerable side effects from pain treatments. When children decline pain treatment, caregivers and clinicians should seek to better understand their reasoning. Children may misunderstand the purpose, effects, or risks of the treatment or medication. If children do not like the

Table 34.1 Pediatric self-reporting pain scales

Age	Scale	Parameters	Comments
4–12 years old	Faces Pain Scale–Revised	Uses six cartoon faces showing increasing signs of pain/distress	Complete instructions and translations may be downloaded at https://www.iasp-pain.org/resources/faces-pain-scale-revised/
>8 years old	Numeric Rating Scale (NRS)	Uses a 0–10 scale, where 0 denotes no pain and 10 signifies the worst pain. *Hint*: It is helpful to note what the child considers to be "the worst pain imaginable." The "anchor effect" may lead to misinterpretation or skewed pain report (e.g., whether a "10" to an individual child is a stubbed toe vs. multiple broken bones)	Requires language skills and numerical processing. To reduce failure rates, consider use of a visual analogue scale (a 10-cm visual scale) or Faces Pain Scale–Revised in children 8–12 years of age who do not seem to understand the NRS

Table 34.2 Children's motivations for underreporting and overreporting of pain

Underreporting	Overreporting
Fear of being admitted to the hospital or having to stay in the hospital longer Desire for healthcare provider to leave the room Fear of needles or procedures that might come if pain is reported Fear of what admitting pain means (e.g., cancer returning, disease progression, becoming sicker) Social construct (e.g., boys/big kids don't cry) Lacking language to articulate pain Feelings that providers do not believe reports of pain	School avoidance Not wanting to be discharged from hospital Liking the way pain medicine makes one feel Getting more attention from caregiver Not wanting caregiver to leave bedside Fear of future pain

Table 34.3 Observational pain scales for infants, toddlers, and children

Age	Scale	Parameters	Comments
Infants (0–6 months)	CRIES	Assess crying, required oxygen, increased vital signs, expression (facial), and sleepiness. A score of 0–2 is given for each parameter based on changes in the patient's baseline.	Score out of 10
Infants and toddlers	FLACC	Assesses *face*, *legs*, *activity*, *crying*, and *consolability*.	Score out of 10
Developmentally delayed/cognitively impaired	Revised-FLACC	Uses same parameters as FLACC but allows for the addition of individualized pain behaviors.	Score out of 10 Engage caregivers to help individualize this scale.

Table 34.4 Observed pain behaviors

Age	Pain behaviors
Infant (0–12 months)	High-pitch crying Facial grimacing Furrowed eyebrows Difficulty sucking Frequent hiccupping Frequent yawning Avoidance of eye contact or inability to console Change in level of activity Irritability/restlessness
Toddlers (12 months–4 years)	Facial grimacing Furrowed eyebrows Sleep difficulties Guarding area of discomfort Crying/moaning Decreased interest in play Irritability/restlessness Loss of appetite Needs to be held more than normal
School-aged and adolescent (5–17 years)	Facial grimace Furrowed eyebrows Difficulty sleeping Crying Guarding area of discomfort Decreased activity level Withdrawn Irritability Anger Change in eating habits Breath holding

taste or side effects of a given treatment, other therapies or medications can be trialed. Children and adolescents may prefer to tolerate pain as opposed to feeling lethargic or impaired from pain medications. This can become distressing for caregivers and clinicians caring for children and adolescents, particularly for those at the end of life. Care should be respectful and honor the wishes and values of the child or adolescent with respect to pain management. Consider further assessment of cultural or religious beliefs around the experience or presence of pain.

Case Study: A Pediatric Patient with Pain

Brian was an 8-year-old boy with end-stage metastatic rhabdomyosarcoma who was receiving oral palliative chemotherapy. He reported generalized body pain (3–5 out of 10 on numeric scale, sore with deep aching feeling) and described it as tolerable (reports that tolerable is up to 6/10 on numeric scale). He was using heat packs, gentle massage, and distraction with movies, as well as scheduled acetaminophen and ibuprofen for pain management. Brian described "the worst pain imaginable" was after he had a thoracotomy to resect pulmonary lesions, which was several months ago. On your assessment, Brian was observed to be cachectic and weak, moving gingerly and wincing when turning over in bed; he preferred to be carried in and out of clinic by his dad as opposed to using a wheelchair. The oncology team wanted to trial long-acting opioids in the hopes of improving his pain control, but Brian refused, stating he did not like the way opioids "made him feel in his head," that they made him sleepy and not himself. Brian had trialed oral oxycodone, oral morphine, oral hydromorphone, and methadone, each one with a similar intolerable side-effect profile. While oncology and palliative care teams continued to work with Brian and his family to find alternative methods of improving pain control, they respected Brian's desire to avoid sleepiness to maximize time awake with family and friends. Brian was discharged to home with recommendations for continued use of nonpharmacologic and non-opioid therapies, as well as a prescription for an as-needed oral opioid should pain progress to more than tolerable.

Assessment of Pain in Child with Severe Neurologic Impairment

Children with severe neurologic impairment who are nonverbal are at risk for the underrecognition and undertreatment of pain.[10] A child may be severely neurologically impaired from an anoxic or traumatic brain injury or from a specific disease, such as a congenital anomaly, brain malformation, or metabolic disorder. The revised FLACC is a pain scale to aid in the assessment of the nonverbal, neurologically impaired child.[9,10] When pain behaviors are observed, common sources of acute pain in the severely neurologically impaired child such as spasticity, dental caries, constipation, fracture, subluxation, feeding intolerance, corneal abrasion, and urinary retention should be considered and addressed.[10] If pain behaviors persist without any findings of tissue injury or inflammation indicating an acute pain source, then some experts propose that it may be reasonable to trial neuropathic pain agents, arguing for the empiric treatment of a central neuropathic pain syndrome in this population.[10]

Procedural Pain Management

Procedural pain is the most commonly experienced pain event of hospitalized children.[11] Hospitalized children experience painful procedures including, but not limited to, venipuncture, intramuscular injections, lumbar puncture, stabilizing fractures, heel lancet, subcutaneous port access, urinary catheterization, feeding tube placement, wound dressing change, chest tube placement, and minor surgical procedures (e.g., sutures). Children who experience unrelieved or severe pain from procedures may in the future have a worse pain response to the same procedure or be avoidant of medical care altogether.[12]

In infants, procedural pain management includes caregiver education and preparation for the procedure (anticipated duration, steps prior to painful part of intervention, how to position infant, anticipated infant response), skin-to-skin contact with caregiver in position of comfort, and preemptive analgesia with sucrose and non-nutritive sucking or breastfeeding.[13]

In children, developmentally appropriate procedural preparation is important to help reduce pain perception. This includes counseling caregivers on how to respond to their child in pain and how to support their child's positioning and coping during the procedure. Children should be offered guidance on what to expect from the procedure, with attention to how the child will be supported and what role the child will have in the procedure (i.e., counting, taking deep breaths, holding caregiver's hand, staying still). Children may benefit from medical play prior to the procedure to destigmatize the tools and environment (i.e., water play with needleless syringes, tour of casting room or lab draw station prior to procedure time). Child life specialists may be helpful in supporting the child's coping in a developmentally appropriate manner.

Children should be allowed to help with determining their positioning for the procedure in a way that supports comfort and safety. For toddlers, a hug position with arms and legs wrapped around caregivers may allow one arm free for intramuscular injection or phlebotomy procedure. School-aged children may prefer to sit on a caregiver's lap or in a chair facing away from the affected body part. For procedures around the eyes or face, children may prefer their head supported by a caregiver. Children should be allowed to hold a support object (stuffed animal or blanket) if desired and safe. When possible, avoid painful procedures in the child's hospital bed to allow this to be a safe space. Procedure rooms and sitting outside of the bed are alternative settings.

Children may benefit from visual stimuli such as pictures or moving lights. Distraction techniques include video games, having children identify objects in a book, singing a song, or listening to music. Hypnosis techniques may also reduce children's perception of pain.[14] Application of cold and vibration stimulus have also been shown to reduce pain during intravenous line starts.[14]

Preemptive analgesia is appropriate for procedures when pain is expected. This may include topical analgesia (lidocaine-based creams EMLA, LMX-4) or a needleless injection of lidocaine (J-Tip). Pharmacologic therapies are similar to those used in acute pain management, noting that onset and duration of action are important to match with the expected duration of the procedure and resulting pain.

Table 34.5 Nonpharmacologic interventions for pain management

Age	Nonpharmacologic interventions
Infant (0–12 months)	Cuddle/swaddle infant Skin-to-skin care Massage Dim lights Lower voices/noise Non-nutritive sucking (pacifier, bottle) Music Breastfeeding Physical therapy
Toddlers (12 months–4 years)	Positioning for comfort and control Distraction (storytelling, reading favorite book, games, play with toys) Art and music therapy Massage Guided imagery/visualization Physical therapy Relaxation through deep breathing (using bubbles or pinwheel) Heat or cold therapy
School-aged and adolescent (5–17 years)	Positioning for comfort and control Environmental changes to promote safety Dim lights Procedural preparation Relaxation through deep breathing Guided imagery/visualization Distraction (television, reading a book, video games, board games) Art and music therapy Acupuncture (>8 years) Massage Hypnosis Aromatherapy Heat or cold therapy Physical therapy Biofeedback Transcutaneous electrical nerve stimulation (TENS unit)

Acute Pain

Acute pain typically lasts less than 30 days and is associated with tissue injury, with improvement of pain as the tissue heals. Pain persisting more than 3 months and after the complete healing of tissue damage is considered chronic pain. Examples of acute pain include postoperative pain, pain resulting from injury, chemotherapy-induced mucositis pain, and sickle cell vaso-occlusive pain crisis.

Acute pain management includes nonpharmacologic and pharmacologic approaches. Medications should be used in addition to nonpharmacologic interventions—not instead of them. See Table 34.5 for examples of age-appropriate nonpharmacologic interventions for pain management. Updated in 2020, the World Health Organization (WHO) guidelines provide clinicians the basic tenets for the use of analgesics for pediatric pain management.[15,16]

1. Use a stepwise strategy for pain medications, also referred to as "by the ladder."
2. Dose medications at regular intervals: "by the clock" and have available "as needed" medication for breakthrough pain.
3. Use the least invasive, most convenient route of administration: "by the mouth," when possible. Oral route includes nasogastric or gastrostomy tube.
4. Tailor the treatment to the individual child: "by the individual," adapting to their needs and response

Using a Two-Step Strategy

The pediatric two-step strategy replaces the three-step analgesic ladder introduced by the WHO in 1986. Like the three-step ladder, the two-step strategy outlines medications to be used based on the child's pain severity but no longer recommends the use of weak opioids (e.g., codeine) for moderate pain. For mild pain, Step 1 treatments are non-opioids including acetaminophen and/or ibuprofen (or an alternative nonsteroidal anti-inflammatory drug [NSAID]); see Table 34.6 for Step 1 medications and dose recommendations. If the child has moderate to severe acute pain related to tissue injury, then Step 2 treatments are strong opioids, and these should be used in conjunction with Step 1 treatments.[17] See Table 34.7 for Step 2 medications and dose recommendations. (Providers should confirm doses using their institutional formulary, guidelines, and/or Lexi comp™.[18])

Opioids with Limited or No Use in Pediatrics

Medications that have limited uses in pediatrics include nalbuphine (Nubain), a mixed opioid agonist–antagonist. Nalbuphine can be helpful for an opioid-naive, postoperative patient whose acute pain is expected to get better quickly or to treat opioid-induced itching.[19] It can also be used as a premedication prior to procedures if sedation is needed. It does not cause pruritus, nausea, vomiting, or urinary retention like other opioids; however, nalbuphine is not recommended for patients with pain that is expected to get worse (i.e., cancer pain). Nalbuphine reverses the adverse reactions (pruritus,

Table 34.6 Treatment of acute pain Step 1: Mild pain, non-opioids

Medication	Route	Term neonate–6 months	6 months–12 years	>12 years	Maximum daily dose	Comments
Acetaminophen	PO, IV, PR	10–15 mg/kg/dose q 4–6 h	10–15 mg/kg/dose q 4–6 h	650–1,000 mg q 4–6 h	75 mg/kg/day or 3,000 mg	Avoid use in hepatic impairment; requires dose adjustment in renal impairment
Ibuprofen	PO		5–10 mg/kg/dose q 6–8 h	400–800 mg q 6–8 h	40 mg/kg/day or 2,400 mg/day, whichever is less	Chronic use increases risk of thrombotic events, GI bleed, and renal impairment; may impair platelet aggregation
Naproxen	PO		5–7 mg/kg/dose q 8–12 h	200–400 mg q 12 h	600 mg/day	Chronic use increases risk of cardiovascular thrombotic events, GI bleed, and renal impairment
Ketorolac	IV		0.5 mg/kg q 6–8 h	15–30 mg q 6 h	120 mg/day	Increases risk of bleeding, stroke, GI bleed, cardiovascular events, and renal impairment Maximum duration of use 5 days
Celecoxib	PO		10–25 kg: 50 mg q 12 h	100–200 mg/day	400 mg/day, may be used short-term	Chronic use increases risk of cardiovascular thrombotic events, GI bleed, and renal impairment

GI, gastrointestinal; IV, intravenous; PO, orally (per os); PR, per rectum; q, every.

urinary retention) of other opioids and can be given to oppose those symptoms without significantly decreasing the analgesic properties of opioids.[20] It is an option for treating limited postoperative pain in children.

Combined opioid and acetaminophen products should only be used with caution in children given the risk of dosing errors with both opioid and acetaminophen contents[21] and risk of hepatotoxicity with acetaminophen overdose. In pediatrics, it is preferred that the medication components be dosed and administered separately, even in acute surgical pain. For some children, surgical pain may be well controlled with acetaminophen taken together with an NSAID. Others may benefit from having an opioid available as a separate third-line agent for breakthrough pain. This depends on the anticipated pain severity and recovery time. For children with disease-related pain that is expected to worsen over time, fixed opioid and acetaminophen combination products limit the flexibility for opioid titration since the dose is limited by the recommended daily acetaminophen maximum. If the opioid and acetaminophen are separated, the patient can take the same opioid scheduled around the clock and as needed for breakthrough pain.

The US Food and Drug Administration recommends against the use of codeine and tramadol in children and adolescents given the risk of oversedation with associated respiratory depression and potential death.[22] Both codeine and tramadol are prodrugs, which means they must be metabolized by the body into their active metabolite to produce analgesia. There is genetic variability in metabolism. Those persons who are ultra-rapid metabolizers will have too much of the active metabolite in their body too quickly and potentially suffer the side effects of opioid-induced respiratory depression.

Dosing at Regular Intervals

When pain is constantly present, analgesics should be administered at regular intervals, not simply on an as-needed basis. With as-needed dosing alone, the risk is undertreatment and uncontrolled pain. The addition of an as-needed or "rescue dose" to scheduled analgesia is appropriate for management of breakthrough pain.[23] This can be achieved by using one or more routes of medication administration.

Case Study: A Patient in Pain Crisis

Molly is a 12-year-old admitted to the hospital for acute vaso-occlusive pain crisis secondary to sickle cell disease. For the 48 hours prior to admission, she had been taking oxycodone 7.5 mg orally every 4 hours, with an additional oxycodone 5 mg orally every 1 hour as needed for breakthrough pain. She typically began this regimen at the onset of acute pain crisis symptoms. On admission, Molly and her father reported that she had taken 17.5 mg of oxycodone in the prior 4 hours with only minimal pain relief. She received heat packs to apply to painful sites, distraction with movies, intravenous hydration, and scheduled intravenous ketorolac and was started on a patient-controlled analgesia (PCA) pump (morphine 1 mg/h plus a 1-mg demand dose every 10-minute lockout) since she was complaining of upset stomach and was unable to tolerate any more oral medications. After several hours, she had improved pain control and was using her demand dose on average once per hour.

By the Appropriate Route

Analgesics should be administered by the simplest, most effective, least painful route, making oral analgesics preferred, if possible. The intramuscular route is to be avoided given its painful administration. Alternative routes of administration, including buccal, intravenous, intranasal, subcutaneous, rectal, or transdermal, should be used when the oral route is not available or based on clinical judgment and patient preference.

Case Study: Varying the Route of Medication Delivery

Heather is an 8-year-old with spinal muscular atrophy who was preparing for hospital discharge following spinal fusion surgery. She had been hospitalized for 4 weeks and required high-dose opioids for pain control during her intensive care stay. The critical care unit had been reducing her intravenous hydromorphone doses over time to avoid withdrawal symptoms, without need for breakthrough dosing. Heather had severe gastroparesis at baseline and was dependent on total caregiver nutrition. She had a

Table 34.7 Treatment of acute pain Step 2: Moderate to severe pain, opioids

Medication	Route	Pediatric starting dose	Adult starting dose	Comments
Fentanyl	IV	0.5–2 mcg/kg IV bolus q 5 min–1 h, 0.5–3 mcg/kg/h continuous infusion	25–50 mcg/dose IV bolus q 5 min–1 h, 25–200 mcg/h continuous infusion	Skeletal muscle and chest-wall rigidity can be seen with rapid IV dosing Has no active metabolites and is considered relatively safe to use in patients with renal failure
	Intranasal	1.5 mcg/kg once (maximum: 100 mcg/dose); may repeat 0.5 mcg/kg q 5 min to a max of 3 mcg/kg	100 mcg/dose	Use IV preparation
	Transdermal patch			Not intended for opioid-naive patients Half-life 20–27 h, steady state reached after 2 sequential 72-h patch applications Refer to Duragesic patch package insert for dose recommendations when converting from another opioid to a fentanyl patch
	Transmucosal (i.e., sublingual, buccal)	Not approved for use in children, could consider for adolescents receiving end-of-life care	100–200 mcg	Available as a lozenge, dissolving tablet, buccal film, sublingual spray. Onset of action 5–15 min
Hydromorphone	Oral	0.03–0.08 mg/kg/dose q 3–4 h as needed	1–4 mg/dose q 3–4 h as needed	Use with caution in renal impairment (inactive metabolite accumulation can lead to neurotoxicity)
	IV	0.01 mg/kg/dose q 3–6 h as needed Continuous IV infusion: 0.003–0.005 mg/kg/h	0.2–1 mg q 2–3 h as needed	Titrate dose to effectiveness
Methadone	Oral	0.1 mg/kg/dose q 4 h for 2–3 doses, then q 6–12 h	Initial 5–10 mg; dosing interval may range 4–12 h during initial therapy; decrease in dose or frequency may be required (~2–5 days after initiation of therapy or dosage increase) due to accumulation with repeated doses	Not recommended for opioid-naive patients Long and unpredictable half-life of 5–100 h Used in management of opioid dependence and weaning
	IV	0.1 mg/kg/dose q 4 h for 2–3 doses, then q 6–12 h as needed; maximum dose: 10 mg/dose	2.5–10 mg q 8–12 h; titrate slowly to effect	Helpful in treatment of neuropathic pain given its NMDA receptor activity and has some inhibitory effect on the reuptake of serotonin and norepinephrine Use with caution in hepatic impairment, metabolized primarily by liver QTc prolonging drug, consider checking EKG prior to initiation and with dose titration
Morphine	Oral	0.15–0.3 mg/kg/dose q 3–4 h as needed	5–15 mg q 4 h as needed	Use with caution in renal impairment (inactive metabolite accumulation can lead to neurotoxicity) Titrate dose to effectiveness
	IV	0.05–0.1 mg/kg/dose q 2–4 h as needed; continuous infusion: 0.01–0.04 mg/kg/h	2–5 mg q 2–4 h as needed; continuous infusion: 1 mg/h	
Oxycodone	Oral	0.1–0.2 mg/kg/dose q 4–6 h as needed	5–15 mg/dose q 4–6 h as needed	

EKG, electrocardiogram; IV, intravenous; q, every; NMDA, *N*-methyl-D-aspartate.

gastrostomy tube, but her mother reported that medications appeared to "just come right back out" when her gastrostomy tube was vented. The team decided to transition her from her intravenous hydromorphone to buccal concentrated morphine for home use and expected her to continue her opioid wean as an outpatient.

Treatment for the Individual Child

Consideration should be given to other sources of non-opioid-responsive pain and distress (emotional, existential, and spiritual) and non-pain symptoms that children may report as pain (constipation, spasticity, gastrointestinal upset). Analgesic regimens should be multimodal, including both nonpharmacologic and pharmacologic strategies; combination therapy of non-opioids, opioids when necessary, and adjuvant medications for neuropathic pain may be utilized.[15] Analgesic regimens should target the primary source and pathophysiology of the individual child's pain. The child's age and ability to metabolize medications should also be considered. Opioid regimens should be tailored and titrated on an individual basis, taking into consideration a child's previous opioid exposure and response. There is no absolute maximum dose of opioids; the appropriate dose achieves desired pain relief with side effects tolerable to the patient and caregivers.

Neuropathic Pain

Neuropathic pain occurs when there is damage to a nerve either by chemical damage, nerve compression, or prolonged excitation. On physical exam, there may be autonomic changes to the affected area including changes in skin color, skin temperature, or edema. There may be sensory abnormalities (Box 34.2) and motor function changes (as evidenced by decreased strength or diminished reflexes). A child may describe a burning sensation, "prickling," numbness, tingling, "pins and needles," shock waves, or shooting pain. Some children may not have the vocabulary to describe neuropathic pain characteristics. Neuropathic pain can be constant or intermittent. Common causes of peripheral neuropathic pain in pediatrics include medications (i.e., chemotherapy), metabolic conditions, tumor compression of the nerve root, post-amputation pain, and nerve compression caused by musculoskeletal abnormalities such as scoliosis in neuromuscular disease. Recent surgery can be a risk factor for peripheral neuropathic pain. Central pain syndromes can occur as a result of a malformation or damage to the central nervous system. Children with severe neurologic impairment are at risk for neuropathic pain.[10] Severe neurologic impairment may result from injury (severe anoxic brain injury), congenital brain malformation (schizencephaly or lissencephaly), or metabolic disorders (mitochondrial cytopathy, Leigh's syndrome).

Neuropathic pain treatment is focused on decreasing the firing of the ascending pathways and increasing the descending or inhibitory pathways of the peripheral and central nervous systems.[25,26] Gabapentin is most used in pediatrics as it is available in liquid formulation and has a limited side-effect profile. In pediatric orthopedic surgery patients, gabapentin has been shown to decrease postoperative opioid use, decrease hospital length of stay, and improve functioning postoperatively.[27] Serotonin norepinephrine reuptake inhibitors may be helpful for patients with neuropathic pain and comorbid depression. Methadone and ketamine (oral or intravenous) may be indicated for severe neuropathic pain.[28] Table 34.8 details medications used to treat neuropathic pain; medications are listed in what would be a stepwise approach. The medications used to treat peripheral neuropathic pain and central neuropathic pain syndromes are the same. Concurrent treatment with physical and occupational therapy supports improved functioning and reduction in pain over time.[29]

Box 34.2 Sensory Abnormalities Seen in Neuropathic Pain Syndromes

Paresthesia: An abnormal (not unpleasant) sensation, whether spontaneous or evoked

Dysesthesia: An unpleasant abnormal sensation, whether spontaneous or evoked

Allodynia: Pain due to a stimulus that does not normally provoke pain

Hyperalgesia: Increased pain from a stimulus that normally provokes pain

Hypoalgesia: Diminished sensation of pain form normally painful stimulus

Source: Reference 24.

Case Study: A Pediatric Patient with Peripheral Neuropathy

Brittany was a 17-year-old girl with leukemia who was hospitalized for continued chemotherapy. She had severe chemotherapy-induced peripheral neuropathy in her hands and feet. She cried when her hands or feet were lightly touched by her bed sheets. On exam, she was sedated, her hand grasp was extremely weak, and she was unable to stand due to pain and lethargy. She was receiving hydromorphone PCA of 1.5 mg/hour plus a 2-mg demand dose with every 20-minute lockout. Brittany was engaging in a function-focused rehabilitation plan with desensitization through physical and occupational therapy. Meditation, animal-assisted therapy, and art therapy supported her coping with pain. She was receiving scheduled acetaminophen, oral gabapentin 1,200 mg three times a day, and clonidine 0.3 mg/24 hours by transdermal patch. She had pancytopenia following chemotherapy and was thus unable to take NSAIDs. She was started on a ketamine infusion and achieved improved pain control within 24 hours. Over the course of the next week, the hydromorphone PCA could be weaned with continued pain control, less sedation, and improved functioning. She was eventually transitioned off her hydromorphone and ketamine infusions and onto scheduled oral methadone, which was continued after hospital discharge and then slowly weaned over the next 3 months as her neuropathy resolved. She continued outpatient physical therapy and psychotherapy for support of her symptoms.

Chronic Pain

Pain is considered chronic if present for more than 3 months; in children it is often underidentified and undertreated.[31] It is often divided into two subcategories: cancer pain and chronic nonmalignant pain. Examples of chronic nonmalignant pain conditions seen in pediatric patients include avascular necrosis, musculoskeletal pain secondary to neuromuscular deformities, and abdominal pain in patients with inflammatory bowel disease. In chronic nonmalignant pain, pain persists even after the tissue injury has healed.

Treatment of chronic pain in children should use a multimodal approach, including interventions to address the physical and emotional impacts of chronic pain, such as pharmacotherapy, physical therapy, and psychotherapy.[32] The goals of treatment are primarily to improve function and coping because pain frequency may not change.[33] Improvement in daily functioning, mood, and sleep may occur over weeks to months with adherence to medication, exercise, and psychotherapy.

Opioids are appropriate for chronic use in cancer patients who have clear tissue injury or malignant disease. Opioids are not indicated for use in nonmalignant chronic pain and should be avoided given their limited benefit long-term, risk of side effects, and risk of abuse.[34] In nonmalignant chronic pain, pharmacologic treatment should target neuropathic etiologies[32] (refer to Table 34.8 for recommended medications). Children should be empowered to continue daily functioning despite pain and encouraged to maintain a healthy lifestyle with good sleep hygiene, daily exercise, and good nutrition. Appropriate referrals to physical therapy, occupational therapy, psychotherapy, and psychiatry should be made as needed. Comorbid depression and anxiety are commonly seen in patients who experience

Table 34.8 Medications used in the treatment of neuropathic pain and chronic pain syndromes

Medication or drug class	Route	Dose	Titrations	Comments
Gabapentin (Neurontin)	PO	Start 2–5 mg/kg/dose q HS	Titrate every 1–4 days by 5 mg/kg/day until effective analgesia Minimum effective dose for children <5 years 40–60 mg/kg/day; children >5 years 30 mg/kg/day Maximum dose 50–75 mg/kg/day (2,400–3,600 mg/day) divided TID Children with severe neurologic impairment may require higher doses	Monitor for side effects: nystagmus, sedation, tremors, ataxia, swelling May see increased fatigue/sleepiness when initiating or titrating May give 50% of total dose in evening if symptoms occur mostly overnight *Dose-adjust for altered kidney function
Pregabalin (Lyrica)	PO	Start 0.3 mg/kg q HS[31] Adults: 150 mg divided BID–TID	Titrate every 3 days to 1.5 mg/kg/dose BID (max 6 mg/kg/dose) Adults: titrate in 1 week to 300 mg divided BID–TID, max daily dose 600 mg	*Dose-adjust for altered kidney function
Clonidine	PO, TD	Day 1–3: 0.002 mg/kg q HS	Day 4–6: 0.002 mg/kg bid Day 7–9: 0.002 mg/kg TID	PO and TD daily dosing is equivalent, but TD patch takes 2–3 days to reach full effect Monitor blood pressure
Tricyclic antidepressant	PO	Nortriptyline: Start 0.1 mg/kg q HS, titrate up to 0.5 mg/kg, max 1 mg/kg		Nortriptyline has less anticholinergic effect than amitriptyline Given at night can help with sleep
		Amitriptyline: Start 0.1 mg/kg q HS, titrate up to 0.5 mg/kg, max 1–2 mg/kg		
Serotonin norepinephrine reuptake inhibitors	PO	Duloxetine: 20 mg q HS, titrate up to 60 mg QD, max 60 mg BID, cannot be crushed		
		Venlafaxine: 12.5–37.5 mg daily ×1 week, then BID, then increase by 12.5–37.5 mg every week, max 225 mg/day; immediate-release tabs can be crushed		
Methadone	PO, IV	0.1 mg/kg/dose q 6–12 h		Strong opioid with NMDA receptor channel blocker Long and variable half-life, 3–60 h, requires prescriber to be skilled in methadone use Determine QTc within normal limits before use, discuss risk benefit before prescribing
Ketamine	PO, IV	PO: 0.2–0.5 mg/kg/dose TID–QID[19] IV: 0.06–0.3 mg/kg/h	PO: can titrate to 1 mg/kg/dose	NMDA receptor channel blocker Ketamine may reduce opioid tolerance allowing for opioid dose reduction
Cannabinoids	PO	Dronabinol (Marinol) 2.5 mg PO BID, max 20 mg/day		In some states, medical marijuana has been approved for use in pediatric patients

BID, twice a day; HS, hour of sleep; IV, intravenous; NMDA, *N*-methyl-D-aspartate; PO, orally (per os); q, every; QD, every day; QID, four times a day; TD, transdermal; TID, three times a day.
Sources: References 10 and 31.

chronic pain and should be treated accordingly. Psychotherapy can be especially helpful for patients to learn and practice coping techniques such as guided imagery, self-hypnosis, cognitive behavioral reframing, and progressive muscle relaxation. Grief support may be helpful if children have experienced a loss or an anticipated loss due to illness (e.g., loss of independence or functioning, amputation of limb, loss of normal childhood experiences, death).

Case Study: A Pediatric Patient with Chronic Pain

Alice was a 15-year-old girl (45 kg) with Charcot-Marie-Tooth disease and subsequent scoliosis and muscle weakness. She complained of several months of constant pain in her low back and right hip (sore, with shooting and tingling) and an intermittent shooting pain down her right leg. She took oral gabapentin 600 mg three times a day and diazepam at bedtime because pain limited her restful sleep. She also took oral oxycodone 5 mg every 4 hours as needed and as prescribed by her orthopedist; she used on average one dose per day. Alice was referred to outpatient physical and occupational therapy, massage therapy, and a psychologist for support in coping with her chronic illness and chronic pain. She was also started on oral amitriptyline 25 mg at bedtime to help with chronic neuropathic pain secondary to scoliosis, and the team hoped the anticholinergic effects of amitriptyline would also help Alice sleep. She was seen a month later in follow-up and stated that she saw an improvement in her sleep with the first dose and that her pain improved over the next few weeks in alignment with functional improvements brought on by concurrent physical therapy. She continued to take her gabapentin in addition to her amitriptyline but had not needed to use any diazepam or oxycodone in the past month.

Medical Marijuana in Pediatrics

Many states have adopted laws legalizing the use of medical marijuana, but the laws differ from state to state. Prescribers should become familiar with the regulations in the state in which they practice. The use of medical marijuana in pediatrics is growing, and its use for children with certain types of epilepsy and other neurological disorders in particular is expanding. Medical marijuana for children became popularized by case reports of its benefit in the treatment of epilepsy.[35] The outcomes are mixed, but there is emerging evidence that medical marijuana can provide relief beyond epilepsy, including easing nausea/vomiting, improving appetite, and reducing inflammation.[36] The use of medical marijuana for the management of pain is uncertain, and there is insufficient data to strongly support or refute its use for pain.[37] Caregivers whose children are suffering from refractory symptoms such as pain, muscle spasms, and seizures may be open to trying anything that may help. The nurse should know the status of the medical marijuana laws in their state, eligibility criteria, and the process to obtain medical marijuana. Currently, the American Academy of Pediatrics opposes medical marijuana outside the regulatory process of the US Food and Drug Administration given data supporting that marijuana use can negatively affect brain development in children and adolescents.[38] The patient and the family may want to consider consultation with a pain or palliative care specialist to discuss the potential risks/benefits of trialing medical marijuana for their child.[39] Nurses have an ethical responsibility to remain open to the conversation with caregivers and families as more is understood about the use of medical marijuana.[40]

Polypharmacy

The concurrent use of multiple medications to treat a single condition is more widely recognized in adults; however, children with chronic and serious illness are also at risk. While some conditions may require more than one medication, it is important to review if the medication continues to improve the child's quality of life and not put them at risk for adverse drug interactions. The nurse is key in monitoring whether prescribed medications are beneficial or causing harmful unwanted side effects[41] and in identifying medications that may no longer be helpful and can be removed from a child's medication regimen.

Conclusion

The plan of care for assessment and management of pain in children should be individualized, with an understanding of developmental and behavioral norms taken into consideration. Children and families facing serious illness desire to be engaged and empowered in their care, and the palliative care clinician should include them in determining a plan to best manage the child's pain. A child's developmental age and cognitive understanding of pain and its impact on quality of life and optimizing or maintaining functionality whenever possible can help the provider determine the best approach to pain management. The ramifications of untreated pain can be multifactorial, affecting one's physical, emotional, and spiritual well-being. Although opioids have been considered the foundation of acute pain, their role in managing chronic pain is less effective and often does not improve function. Employing an interprofessional approach, incorporating pharmacological and nonpharmacological interventions, (i.e., physical therapy, music therapy, guided imagery, acupuncture) based on the readiness of the child, may not only treat pain but also reduce dependence on opioids. Although the common conditions seen in pediatric palliative care are different from those in the adult population, children still experience the same types of pain and sequelae of untreated pain, and their pain must be addressed.

REFERENCES

1. Agakidou E, Tsoni K, Stathopoulou T, et al. Changes in physicians' perceptions and practices on neonatal pain management over the past 20 years. A survey conducted at two time-points. *Front Pediatr.* 2021;9:667806. https://doi.org/10.3389/fped.2021.667806.
2. Giordano V, Deindl P, Gal E, et al. Pain and neurodevelopmental outcomes of infants born very preterm. *Dev Med Child Neurol.* 2023;65(8):1043–1052. https://doi.org/10.1111/dmcn.15505.
3. Connolly ME, Bills SE, Hardy SJ. Neurocognitive and psychological effects of persistent pain in pediatric sickle cell disease. *Pediatr Blood Cancer.* 2019;66:e27823. https://doi.org/10.1002/pbc.27823.
4. Noel M, Rosenbloom B, Pavlova M, et al. Remembering the pain of surgery 1 year later: a longitudinal examination of anxiety in children's pain memory development. *Pain.* 2019;160(8):1729–1739. https://doi.org/10.1097/j.pain.0000000000001582.
5. Cohen LL, Donati MR, Shih S, Sil S. Topical review: state of the field of child self-report of acute pain. *J Pediatr Psychol.* 2020;45(3):239–246. https://doi.org/10.1093/jpepsy/jsz078.
6. Birnie K, Hundert A, Lalloo C, et al. Recommendations for selection of self-report pain intensity measures in children and adolescents—a systematic review and quality assessment of measurement properties. *Pain.* 2019;160(1):5–18. https://doi.org/10.1097/j.pain.0000000000001377.
7. Popowicz H, Kwiecień-Jaguś K, Olszewska J, Mędrzycka-Dąbrowska WA. Pain scales in neonates receiving mechanical ventilation in neonatal intensive care units—systematic review. *J Pain Res.* 2020;13:1883–1897. https://doi.org/10.2147/JPR.S248042.
8. Crellin D, Harrison D, Santamaria N, et al. Comparison of the psychometric properties of the FLACC Scale, the MBPS and the observer applied visual analogue scale used to assess procedural pain. *J Pain Res.* 2021;14:881–892. https://doi.org/10.2147/JPR.S267839.
9. Chan AYL, Ge M, Wong ICK, et al. Pain assessment tools in paediatric palliative care: a systematic review of psychometric properties and recommendations for clinical practice. *Palliat Med.* 2022;36(1):30–43. https://doi.org/10.1177/02692163211049309.
10. Hauer J, Houtrow AJ. AAP section on hospice and palliative medicine, council on children with significant impairment of the central nervous system. *Pediatrics.* 2017;139(6):e20171002.
11. Friedrichsdorf SJ, Postier A, Eull D, et al. Pain outcomes in a US children's hospital: a prospective cross-sectional survey. *Hosp Pediatr.* 2015;5(1):18–26.
12. Susam V, Friedel M, Basile P, Ferri P, Bonetti L. Efficacy of the Buzzy System for pain relief during venipuncture in children: a randomized controlled trial. *Acta Biomed.* 2018;89(6 suppl):6–16. https://doi.org/10.23750/abm.v89i6-S.7378.
13. Bresesti I, Vanzù G, Redaelli F, et al. New perspective for pain control in neonates: a comparative effectiveness research. *J Perinatol.* 2021;41(9):2298–2303. https://doi.org/10.1038/s41372-021-01025-6.
14. Geagea D, Tyack Z, Kimble R, et al. Clinical hypnosis for procedural pain and distress in children: a scoping review. *Pain Med.* 2023;24(6):661–702. https://doi.org/10.1093/pm/pnac186.
15. World Health Organization. *Guidelines on the Management of Chronic Pain in Children.* World Health Organization; 2020. https://www.who.int/publications/i/item/9789240017870.
16. Anekar AA, Cascella M. WHO analgesic ladder. In: StatPearls. Stat Pearls Publishing; 2022. https://www.ncbi.nlm.nih.gov/books/NBK554435/.

17. Bramati PS, Bruera E. The end of the second step of the World Health Organization analgesic ladder? *Ann Oncol.* 2022;33(12):1212–1213. https://doi.org/10.1016/j.annonc.2022.08.085.
18. Lexidrug. Update December 26, 2022. https://online.lexi.com/lco/action/home/tox?langCode=de.
19. Tubog TD, Harenberg JL, Buszta K. Use of nalbuphine for treatment of neuraxial opioid-induced pruritus: a systematic review and meta-analysis. *AANA J.* 2019;87(3):222–230.
20. Reiter PD, Clevenger AC. Nalbuphine reduces opioid-associated urinary retention in pediatric patients. *Pediatr Crit Care Med.* 2019;20(5):e240–e244. https://doi.org/10.1097/PCC.0000000000001920.
21. Caruso TJ, Trivedi S, Chadwick W, et al. A quality improvement project to reduce combination acetaminophen–opioid prescriptions to pediatric orthopedic patients. *Pediatr Qual Saf.* 2020;5(3):e291. https://doi.org/10.1097/pq9.0000000000000291.
22. Fortenberry M, Crowder J, So TY. The use of codeine and tramadol in the pediatric population-what is the verdict now? *J Pediatr Health Care.* 2019;33(1):117–123. https://doi.org/10.1016/j.pedhc.2018.04.016.
23. Moody K, Baig M, Carullo V. Alleviating terminal pediatric cancer pain. *Children (Basel).* 2021;8(3):239. https://doi.org/10.3390/children8030239.
24. International Association for the Study of Pain. Terminology. Accessed December 23, 2022. https://www.iasp-pain.org/resources/terminology/.
25. Jääskeläinen S. Differential diagnosis of chronic neuropathic orofacial pain: role of clinical neurophysiology. *J Clin Neurophysiol.* 2019;36(6):422–429. https://doi.org/10.1097/WNP.0000000000000583.
26. Colloca L, Ludman T, Bouhassira D, et al. Neuropathic pain. *Nat Rev Dis Primers.* 2017;3:17002. https://doi.org/10.1038/nrdp.2017.2.
27. Reed LA, Patel M, Luque K, Theiss SM. Opioid sparing analgesics in spine surgery. *Adv Orthop.* 2022;2022:1026547. https://doi.org/10.1155/2022/1026547.
28. Anghelescu DL, Tesney JM. Neuropathic pain in pediatric oncology: a clinical decision algorithm. *Paediatr Drugs.* 2019;21(2):59–70. https://doi.org/10.1007/s40272-018-00324-4.
29. Harrison LE, Pate JW, Richardson PA, Ickmans K, Wicksell RK, Simons LE. Best-evidence for the rehabilitation of chronic pain part 1: pediatric pain. *J Clin Med.* 2019;8(9):1267. https://doi.org/10.3390/jcm8091267.
30. Friedrichsdorf SJ, Goubert L. Pediatric pain treatment and prevention for hospitalized children. *Pain Rep.* 2019;5(1):e804. https://doi.org/10.1097/PR9.0000000000000804.
31. Friedrichsdorf SJ, Giordano J, Desai Dakoji K, Warmuth A, Daughtry C, Schulz CA. Chronic pain in children and adolescents: diagnosis and treatment of primary pain disorders in head, abdomen, muscles and joints. *Children (Basel).* 2016;3(4):42. https://doi.org/10.3390/children3040042.
32. Collins AB. Chronic pain in children: interdisciplinary management. *Pediatr Clin North Am.* 2023;70(3):575–588. https://doi.org/10.1016/j.pcl.2023.01.010.
33. Lynch-Jordan AM, Soumitri S, Peugh J, Cunningham N, Kashikar-Zuck S, Goldschneider K. Differential changes in functional disability and pain intensity over the course of psychological treatment for children with chronic pain. *Pain.* 2014;155(10):1955–1961.
34. Knipper E, Banta-Green CJ, Jimenez N. Opioid use disorder and misuse: a review of the epidemiology and medical implications for pediatric anesthesiologists. *Paediatr Anaesth.* 2017;27:1070–1076.
35. Moreira GA, Moraes Neto R, Ribeiro RG, Crippa ACS. Cannabidiol for the treatment of refractory epilepsy in children: a critical review of the literature. *Rev Paul Pediatr.* 2022;41:e2021197. https://doi.org/10.1590/1984-0462/2023/41/2021197.
36. Patel AD. Medical marijuana in pediatric neurological disorders. *J Child Neurol.* 2015;31(3):388–391. https://doi.org/10.1177/0883073815589761.
37. Fisher E, Moore RA, Fogarty AE, et al. Cannabinoids, cannabis, and cannabis-based medicine for pain management: a systematic review of randomized controlled trials. *Pain.* 2021;162(suppl 1):S45–S66. https://doi.org/10.1097/j.pain.0000000000001929.
38. Ammerman SD, Ryan SA, Adelman WP, et al.; Committee on Substance Abuse, Committee on Adolescence. The impact of marijuana policies on youth: clinical, research, and legal update. *Pediatrics.* 2015;135(3):584–587. https://publications.aap.org/pediatrics/article/135/3/584/75419/The-Impact-of-Marijuana-Policies-on-Youth-Clinical.
39. Campbell CT, Phillips MS, Manasco K. Cannabinoids in pediatrics. *J Pediatr Pharmacol Ther.* 2017;22(3):176–185. https://doi.org/10.5863/1551-6776-22.3.176.
40. Ryan JE, McCabe SE, Boyd CJ. Medicinal cannabis: policy, patients, and providers. *Policy Polit Nurs Pract.* 2021;22(2):126–133. https://doi.org/10.1177/1527154421989609.
41. Fraser LK, Gibson-Smith D, Jarvis S, et al. Polypharmacy in children and young people with life-limiting conditions from 2000 to 2015: a repeated cross-sectional study in England. *J Pain Symptom Manage.* 2022;64(3):213–221.e1. https://doi.org/10.1016/j.jpainsymman.2022.05.020.

35

Symptom Management in Pediatric Palliative Care

Camara van Breemen and Nadine Lusney

Key Points

- Distressing symptoms in seriously ill and dying children should be recognized and treated promptly. Symptom assessment and management should always incorporate input from the child/caregiver, the fragility of a child's health condition, the setting of care (what is possible and clinically responsible), the caregivers' understanding of the illness/symptom, and the overall goals and preferences the caregiver and their child have based on clinical guidance.
- All symptom management plans that provide a guide for caregivers should be modified when symptoms change or the overall condition of the child changes. The care plan should consider the current symptoms along with symptoms that are likely to arise based on the diagnosis and trajectory of the condition or illness. Also essential is to incorporate pharmacological, physical, and psychological interventions (3 P approach) into each individualized care plan.
- Good communication and shared decision-making with the child, caregivers, and other team members are essential. Emotional, spiritual, and psychosocial issues (total pain) can affect the child's symptoms and their management and must be taken into consideration.

Introduction

Pediatric palliative care promotes comfort for children with life-threatening conditions (serious illnesses) and their families through a holistic approach addressing physical, emotional, social, and spiritual needs.[1–3] Pediatric palliative care is collaborative, person- and family-centered care delivered using a team-based, developmental approach throughout the continuum of care across all ages and stages of illness, including bereavement.[2,3] It values choice and honest and compassionate communication.[2–4]

Assessing and managing symptoms in seriously ill and dying children should be approached collaboratively in a manner that fosters respectful, compassionate, culturally appropriate/safe, and competent care that is responsive to the needs, values, beliefs, and preferences of the child and family/caregivers.[3,4] In this chapter, "family" refers to the child's identified caregivers and guardians of care. Palliative care in the pediatric setting has some notable challenges compared to adult palliative care. Many seriously ill children are nonverbal due to their age or their condition, making it more difficult to identify the cause of distress. Typically, more than one subspecialist is involved; thus, symptom assessment and care coordination are more complex. An altered central nervous system may be the source of a symptom, complicating symptom assessment.[5,6] Moreover, it is more common to have a surrogate decision maker for a pediatric palliative patient. Thus, incorporating the whole family, including siblings, as part of the care team can be helpful.[3,5] Family members are the most familiar with the child's reactions and methods of communicating.[3,5,7] Ideally, the nurse will develop a trusting relationship with the family while remaining objective in assessing and treating the symptoms.

Comprehensive symptom management must start early in the disease trajectory[2,3]—at diagnosis of a life-threatening condition—and continue in conjunction with curative and/or life-prolonging treatments[1–3] for as long as needed. If symptoms are not managed along the trajectory of the illness, caregivers and children can experience distress that healthcare providers may fail to recognize.[8] The child and family may fear the unknown future and worry that increasing symptoms signal disease progression and decline.[9]

Symptoms arise from physical, emotional, social, and spiritual domains. This chapter focuses on physical symptoms, apart from pain (described in other chapters), commonly found in children with palliative care needs,[3,10–12] including some respiratory, gastrointestinal, and neurological symptoms.[8,9,12,13] All physical symptom assessment should be accompanied by a comfort/pain assessment to address suffering and distress. Emotional and spiritual suffering will be discussed briefly and addressed more completely in other chapters. A resource list is provided (Box 35.1) so that each symptom can be explored in depth through other resources.

Box 35.1 Useful Websites

1. Together for Short Lives (www.togetherforshortlives.org.uk) is a UK-based organization working to improve care and services for children with life-threatening or terminal conditions and their families. They have a list-serve and other resources, such as Basic Symptom Control in Paediatric Palliative Care (https://www.togetherforshortlives.org.uk/resource/basic-symptom-control-paediatric-palliative-care).
2. EPEC: Education in Palliative and End of Life Care–Pediatrics (https://www.bioethics.northwestern.edu/programs/epec/curricula/pediatrics.html) is a comprehensive adaptation of the EPEC curriculum designed to address the needs of children, their families, and pediatric oncology providers and other pediatric clinicians.
3. The National Pediatric Hypnosis Training Institute (http://www.nphti.org/) provides training in ongoing clinical hypnosis skill development for advanced practice pediatric clinicians to assist children and teens in developing self-regulation, optimizing resilience related to medical and mental health issues and stressful experiences, and maximizing well-being and peak performance.
4. The Initiative for Pediatric Palliative Care (https://icpcn.org/) is a comprehensive website with curricula and resources, including videotapes and other helpful educational resources.
5. The National Hospice Palliative Care Organization (www.nhpco.org) hosts the ChiPPS Curriculum, a collaboration between the Children's International Project on Palliative/Hospice Services and the National Hospice and Palliative Care Organization; visit https://www.nhpco.org/pediatrics/#:~:text=Pediatric%20palliative%20and%20hospice%20care%20focuses%20on%20enhancing%20quality%20of,for%20personal%20and%20spiritual%20growth.
6. The End of Life/Palliative Education Resource Center—Fast-Facts offers downloadable resources relating to education about end-of-life care (not specific to but includes pediatrics), oriented for physicians and applicable to other health professionals. This resource will now be housed in the American Academy of Hospice and Palliative Medicine at https://aahpm.org/
7. The Canadian Virtual Hospice (www.virtualhospice.ca) is for patients of all ages, their families and friends, healthcare professionals, and healthcare volunteers. It provides information about physical symptoms of illness and deals with some of the emotional reactions and spiritual questions often experienced by patients and their families. It has excellent learning modules, such as www.kidsgrief.ca that outlines supporting a child with death and dying.
8. The Centre for Pediatric-Pain Research (http://pediatric-pain.ca) is an international internet forum for informal discussion of any topic related to pain in children.
9. The Ian Anderson Continuing Education Program in End-of-Life (www.cme.utoronto.ca/endoflife) is an accredited national continuing education program tailored to the needs of both family physicians and specialists.
10. The goal of the Courageous Parents Network (https://courageousparentsnetwork.org) is to empower parents caring for children with serious illness through video, shared community, professional guidance, and palliative care.
11. The *Dana Farber Pediatric Pain and Symptom Management Guidelines 2020* https://pinkbook.dfci.org/assets/docs/blueBookv2.pdf) booklet is a guide to symptom management in children and a tool for identifying areas for self-study. Pharmacologic options for pain and other distressing symptoms are provided. (Use of medications requires adequate knowledge of side effects and drug–drug interactions. These suggestions cannot replace medical consultation.)
12. The Canuck Place Children's Hospice, Vancouver, Canada (www.canuckplace.org) is a caring, innovative children's hospice and community-based service that fully embraces the life of each child and family. It provides leadership in improving pediatric palliative care regionally, nationally, and internationally through collaboration, education, and research.
13. The International Children's Palliative Care Network (http://www.icpcn.org/) works to raise awareness of children's palliative care, lobbying for the global development of children's palliative care services and sharing expertise, skills, and knowledge.
14. Davies B, Steele R, Baird J. *Pediatric Palliative Care: A Model for Exemplary Practice*. Routledge; 2021. This incredible resource provides essential and timely suggestions for practitioners seeking to improve and build their relational skills with children and families.

Overview of Symptom Assessment and Factors

Distressing symptoms should be recognized and treated promptly in all seriously ill and dying children. The focus of the assessment is on understanding the whole child within the context of their family and community of care.[3,4] In particular, a comprehensive assessment through a pediatric palliative care lens considers the goals of care, the fragility of a child's health condition, anticipated illness trajectory, current care location of the child, child's developmental age/capacity, cultural and language considerations, and possible role of a pediatric palliative care subspecialty team.[3]

The comprehensive assessment includes a physical head-to-toe assessment along with a more detailed assessment of the symptom of concern, child's health history, recent investigations, and current medications and treatments.[3] Consider Case Study 1. A child's history can serve as an overarching guide to anticipating symptoms along the illness trajectory by providing context to the extent of disease, prognosis, and anticipated disease progression. The fragility of the child's health condition indicates how at risk a child is for deterioration and thus the possibility of needing more detailed anticipatory plans and parallel planning to mobilize appropriate healthcare services/resources.[2,3]

Case Study 1: Trevor

Trevor was diagnosed at 16 years of age with alveolar rhabdomyosarcoma of the prostate and adjacent lymph nodes. Initial chemotherapy was initiated along with radiation and brachytherapy. Sixteen months later his end treatment demonstrated no residual disease. Unfortunately, Trevor's disease relapsed 7 months later, presenting as new-onset back pain, with positron emission tomography–computed tomography (PET-CT) demonstrating bilateral pulmonary, nodal, and mediastinal metastases. Relapse chemotherapy and thoracic radiation therapy were initiated along with several other supportive treatments. Scans showed partial response of disease, but following treatment, scans revealed progressive diffuse disease in the lungs.

Trevor reports occasional back pain, treated well with ibuprofen, but overall reports feeling well. He also had occasional shortness of breath, typically when anxious or when sleeping at night, for which

Ativan was effective. The oncology team consulted the pediatric palliative care team when Trevor began experiencing increasing pain and intermittent shortness of breath. Trevor has an older sister, Madeline, and lives with both his parents. Prior to his diagnosis, he spent his time playing sports, hanging out with his friends, and walking his dog, Ralph.

All symptom assessments include a comfort assessment, with a focus on the level of distress/suffering the symptom is causing, along with the use of validated pain scales. The child's developmental stage, verbal ability, and cultural factors must be considered when engaging a child and family meaningfully in the assessment process. For a child who is nonverbal, caregiver input is especially essential.[3,5,7,8] The family's distress, connections between child distress and family distress, and family capacity and coping ability should also inform management plans. A comprehensive assessment may not always be appropriate/possible due to the urgency of symptoms (i.e., palliative symptom emergencies).

Frameworks for Assessment

Symptoms can be better understood if symptom-specific assessment tools are used. In general, a comprehensive assessment of any symptom should include OPQRSTUV[14] (Table 35.1); a rating component; review of systems; observation of child; input from child, when appropriate, and caregiver and other team members; and, if possible, a physical exam. There are several validated pain tools but fewer tools for other symptoms. The pediatric Memorial Symptom Assessment Scale[15] is validated and can be used to assess symptom burden or severity in children.

Nurses must have a dynamic process of assessing, treating, evaluating, documenting, communicating, and collaborating with the child, parents, and interdisciplinary team members through an equity, trauma-informed, and person-centered lens. Attention to relationship-building and attunement to healthcare conversations with families can affect parents' perception of care as well as long-term outcomes.[4] Communication with a child/family should always include principles of permission and an exploration of understanding and reciprocal/attuned responses (verbal/nonverbal); in pediatric palliative care, the care and communication are relational in nature, and human-to-human connection should be emphasized as central to the relationship.[3,4,16–18]

Table 35.1 OPQRSTUV mnemonic

O Onset	When did it begin? How long does it last? How often does it occur?
P Provoking/ palliating	What brings it on? What makes it better? What does that feel like in your body? What makes it worse? What does that feel like in your body?
Q Quality	What does it feel like? Can you describe it?
R Region/ radiation	Where is it? Does it spread anywhere?
S Severity	What is the intensity of this symptom (on a scale of 0 to 10 with 0 being none and 10 being worst possible)? Can use validated tools here. Right now? At best? At worst? On average? How bothered are you by this symptom? Are there any other symptom(s) that accompany this symptom?
T Treatment	What medications and treatments are you currently using? How effective are these? Do you have any side effects from the medications and treatments? What medications and treatments have you used in the past?
U Understanding/ impact on you	What do you believe is causing this symptom? How is this symptom affecting you and/or your family? Meaning of the pain/symptom to the sufferer, "total pain."
V Values	Goals and expectations of management for this symptom. What is your goal for this symptom? What is your comfort goal or acceptable level for this symptom (on a scale of 0 to 10 with 0 being none and 10 being worst possible)? Are there any other views or feelings about this symptom that are important to you or your family?

Creating a Treatment/Management Plan

Considerations for Treatment/Management Plans

A child's treatment plan should consider the child's illness (extent of disease, prognosis, and fragility), the child/family experience (symptom intensity, impact, suffering/distress), and the child as a person (goals, hopes, culture, plans). Realistic goals and expectations for symptom alleviation with estimated timelines or reassessment points should be set in collaboration with the child/family.[3,7] In pediatric palliative care, the expectation may be not to eliminate symptoms but to decrease/alleviate symptoms and promote function and well-being in the child.[3]

Parents value interactive patterns where the healthcare provider gives information and the context of its impact on their child's health while also consistently attending to questions and emotional responses of the child and family.[4] The centrality of authentic interactions with children and families is essential to build relationships grounded in actions of attunement, connection, and empowerment, while also taking into consideration worldviews and influencing factors.[4]

Treat Underlying Causes and Consider Additional Medical Tests/Specialist Referrals

Before any investigation or test is ordered, the burdens and benefits should be weighed (risk:benefit assessment). Where is the investigation or test available? Will it require care coordination or travel or undue expense for the family? How long will any associated treatment last? If an intervention/investigation seems reasonable for the child/family, then options should be shared with the child/family in a supportive manner, as described in the continuation of Case Study 1. Healthcare providers should strive to ensure the family understands the stage of the child's illness.[16,17] Although disease prognostication is fraught with many inaccuracies, especially in pediatric illness, children and families deserve context so that they can better adapt to their child's illness.[16,17]

Case Study 1 Continued: Trevor

Trevor had an X-ray and was found to have a significant pleural effusion of the right side. The team felt that draining it would be helpful. They knew from Trevor that he wanted to be at home as much as possible and that any medical procedure was a burden to him—especially if he had to stay in hospital. Interventional radiology suggested an indwelling catheter that could be intermittently drained. An indwelling catheter would mean he would have to have home visits and/or outpatient clinic visits regularly. In exploring the benefits and burdens, the nurse voiced her hope that draining the lung would relieve symptoms—at least for some time—but that she worried that the indwelling would be a burden and would stop Trevor's plans of going to the lake with his friends this weekend. The nurse explored with Trevor what he feels is most important for him right now. Trevor chose to go home to talk about this with his family before coming to a decision.

Tensions may arise between different members of the healthcare team and even between family members in terms of how aggressively to pursue treatments or interventions. Some may see the benefits outweighing the burdens, while others may feel the benefits are too onerous. Palliative care teams are experts in helping to navigate these types of situations and journeying alongside families. Questions to consider when weighing benefit versus burden of treatments or investigations can be found in Box 35.2.

Support Shared Decision-Making in Symptom Management

Informed recommendations provided by pediatric palliative care clinicians can help families make the best decisions for the child in terms of location of care, intensity of treatment, goals of care, and support regarding advance care planning. For example, twice-weekly blood transfusions for a child with a good quality of life (QOL) would likely be worth the burden, whereas an increase in fluids for a child showing signs of deterioration or end of life likely would not. However, each situation is unique, and the team and family together should make the best choice for the child. With any new or ongoing symptoms, nurses need to be keenly aware of the pathophysiologic factors that may be causing or contributing to the symptom.

Box 35.2 Questions to Consider

Questions to Consider (Weighing Benefit versus Burden):

- Do I need to know the underlying cause, or can I manage the symptom effectively without confirming the cause?
- Is the underlying cause likely to be treatable? Are the investigations of the underlying cause appropriate?
- Will treating the underlying cause improve prognosis or quality of remaining life?
- How effective could any potential treatment be? What are the potential negative outcomes?
- Will the child have to move to another location for the investigation and/or treatment? Will this be possible? Will they be willing to do this?
- Would treatment be congruent with the wishes and goals of the child and family?
- Is the intervention appropriate for the developmental age of the child?

Source: Reference 30.

Box 35.3 Wish, Worry, Wonder Framework from Serious Illness Conversation Guide for Pediatrics, Adapted by Canuck Place from Ariadne Labs.

I Wish, I Worry, I Wonder Framework

"I wish" allows for alignment with the parents' and child's hopes.
"I worry" allows for being truthful while sensitive.
"I wonder" is a subtle way to make a recommendation.

Align with Parents' and Child's Hopes, Acknowledge Concerns, Then Propose a Way to Move Forward

"*I wish* we could slow down or stop your child's cancer/disease, and I promise that I will continue to look for options that could work for them."
"*But I worry* that you and your child won't be prepared if things don't go as we hope. I wonder if we can discuss a Plan B today."

The wish, worry, wonder framework[16–18] (Box 35.3) can be extremely helpful in discussing what may be ahead if a certain active treatment or investigation is pursued. The nurse can utilize this approach to not only respectfully share their concerns based on their clinical knowledge but also invite discussion with the child or parents about their beliefs, hopes, and worries for a patient centred approach.[19]

Symptom Management

A stepwise approach is often used, whereby interventions are escalated in response to the nature and severity of the symptoms.[20] This reduces the potential of overwhelming the family with too many choices at once. Once symptoms are brought under control, the interventions can be tapered to determine which ones are most effective. The healthcare team should be aware of any integrative interventions the family or child may be pursuing that may adversely interact with medications and treatment protocols. Exchanging information in a nonjudgmental manner allows for clinicians and parents to hear about the potential benefits and burdens of any given treatment.[16,17] Biologically based integrative modalities include herbs, supplements, and related nutritional therapies. "Natural" does not guarantee safety; supplements can interact with other medications, have adverse effects, or even cause toxicity. A trusting relationship between the nurse and parents allows honest sharing to discuss the burdens, cost, and potentially unrealistic hope for cure.

The management plan of care will incorporate a 3 Ps (pharmacological, psychological, physical) approach, as seen in Figure 35.1, to co-create symptom management interventions using a biopsychosocial, spiritual, and integrative approach.

Pharmacologic Interventions

Generally, the medications utilized for symptom management in pediatric palliative care are the same as those for adult palliative care, albeit with specific dosing recommendations.[21] Medication doses and compatibilities are not included in this chapter. Having access to a hospital formulary, online resources, and a pharmacist with expertise in palliative care is valuable.

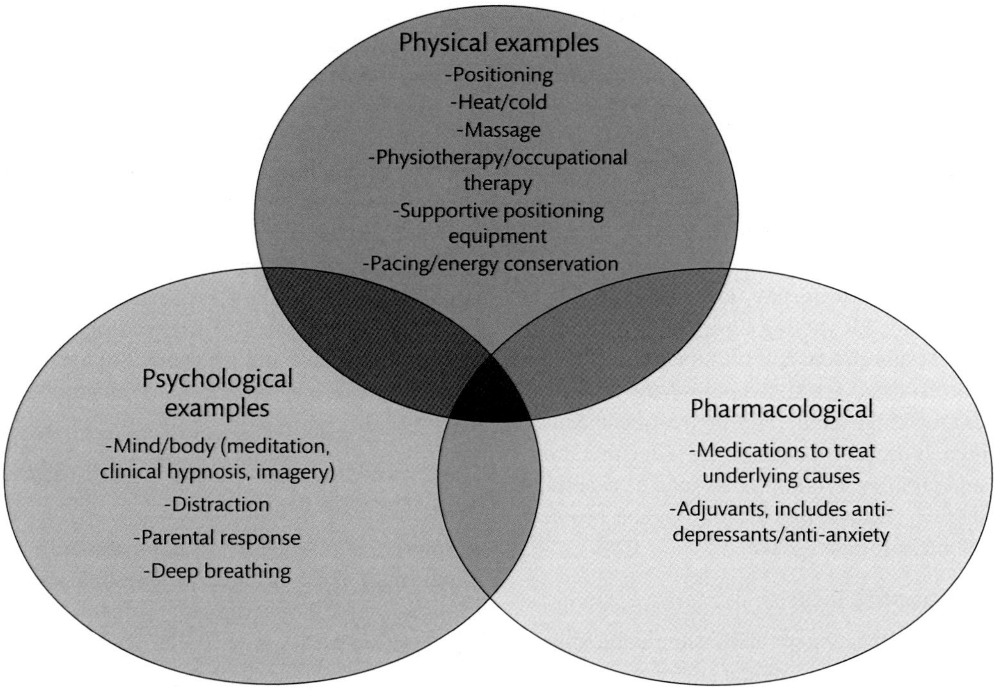

Figure 35.1 Examples of a 3 P approach to be integrated to support symptom management.

Nurses also need to consider which route of administration is most appropriate for the child, taking into account the symptom, the onset/duration of medication, compatibility with other medications, adverse effects, and the possible harms. The oral/enteral route is safest and often preferred but may not be possible as the child deteriorates. Rectal administration (use caution in neutropenia), especially for younger or less conscious children, may be a good alternative route; and staff at specialized pharmacies are able to compound appropriate products. When possible, subcutaneous in situ catheters or sublingual routes offer faster medication delivery and do not rely on an adequate swallow. Using central lines offers an effective route but entails more technical care. The intramuscular route should be avoided as it is too painful. Anticipating medication adverse effects and adverse reactions should be incorporated into management plans.

Psychological Interventions

Mind–body modalities rely on the body's ability to self-regulate. Integrating effective psychological interventions into treatment plans may serve to empower the child and family as it can demonstrate their agency in symptom control. Common practices include prayer, hypnosis, biofeedback, mental imagery, deep breathing, distraction, and music therapy.

Clinical hypnosis has proven useful for pain and symptom management, including nausea, in pediatric palliative care as well as for painful procedures such as lumbar punctures and blood draws.[22] Hypnosis is best understood as an alternative state of awareness,[22] one of concentration and intense focus. Children have active imaginations that help them enter a world of "make believe."[23] Hypnosis also highlights the importance of language to optimize comfort and invite engagement in the child.[24] For example, the pain/symptom/distress the child is exhibiting should be acknowleged.[24] The value of listening to the child's/family's experience of the symptom can often be a powerful intervention, the concept of feeling heard and seen.[24] When possible, pace conversations and assessments at a rhythm that works for the child/family to convey respect and support shared power in exchange.[24] The work of healthcare providers when supporting a family is through active coaching, guiding, and teaching to work with the discomfort alongside the support of the healthcare team and caregivers.[24]

Another psychological intervention is music, which can bring both comfort and distraction. Many parents/caregivers sing songs or recite rhymes for young children, while older children may listen to music on headphones. Music therapists offer insight into deepening the effectiveness of this intervention.[25]

Aromatherapy generally involves diluted topical application or inhalation of an essential oil. Essential oils can also be a way to invoke memories or to distract from noxious smells. Inhaled aromatherapy can be delivered via an infuser or simply by taping a cotton ball saturated with the oil to a pillowcase or article of clothing. Lavender is typically used for relaxation and has been shown to be supportive for pediatric acute care settings.[26] Although aromatherapy is not well researched, it is easy to use, has few adverse effects, and has shown usefulness in palliative care.[27] The child should be monitored for any allergic reactions.

Physical Interventions

Physical and occupational therapies can augment symptom assessment and management through appropriate exercises, physical equipment, rehabilitation, and functional improvements. If possible, refer the child to a therapist who has pediatric training and may provide specific treatment such as manipulation, acupressure, massage, or exercise/stretching.[28] Physiotherapists and occupational therapists will recommend the best equipment to support the child's activities of daily living. Nurses can follow care plans outlined by occupational or physical therapists that may include specific positioning and equipment. Nurses can also work with the family to determine the usefulness of hot/cold compresses, supportive positioning, mobility aids, and transfer methods.

Energy therapies include esoteric arts, such as reiki, healing touch, craniosacral therapy, and chi gong. Families may seek these treatments out for their child on their own or may ask for guidance around the benefit or potential harms.

Reassessment and Monitoring

All symptom management plans need integrated reassessment or follow-up plans by supporting healthcare teams. Reassessment and monitoring should include identifying signs and symptoms of increasing severity, medical side effects, and imminent dying. Often goals of care need to be revisited when symptoms are worsening causing excessive stress for child/family and/or treatment benefit versus burden has shifted. If time for the child's life is deemed short, healthcare providers and families should discuss specific aspects of care planning including such things as best location (home, hospital, hospice) and escalate comfort-focused goals.

Documentation and Support Tools

Symptom assessment and management plans should be shared and communicated among healthcare providers determined by the child and family as involved in and supporting care. Co-creation of documentation and support tools for families should take into consideration the family's literacy level, language, and individualized barriers/access to care. For example, a symptom support tool might be created to be more visual (e.g., drawing out the clock times) or to include words from other languages. Symptom management tools can include individualized care plans, symptom algorithms, summary letters for emergency room guidance, and communication plans for team members. Care plans need to be individualized to include the physical and psychological support interventions each child identifies as helpful to their comfort. Communication plans support a child/family, and healthcare teams know when, why, and how best to communicate with each other. For example, the family physician may call the family weekly, but the home care nurse might visit the family twice weekly and report to the family physician after the visit. Setting up routine communication patterns collectively decided between teams and families allows everyone to set expectations surrounding minimum communication, methods, and updates. Symptom management algorithms serve as roadmaps for families to know when to use what medication and support integration of physical and psychological measures when under stress. An example of a symptom management algorithm can be seen in Figure 35.2.

Communication and Care Coordination to Support Symptom Management

Communication with a child/family should always include principles of permission, exploring understanding, and reciprocal/attuned responses (verbal/nonverbal).[16–18] Consider the use and adaptation of conversation guides, such as The Serious Illness Conversation guide for pediatrics,[16,18] which provides a framework for exploring how the child and family understand specific symptoms. Exploring a family's understanding of the child's symptoms can provide insight to their overall perception of the illness and why they are experiencing distress and suffering. For example, increasing shortness of breath in a child with neuroblastoma may be interpreted by the child/family as a viral cold that will improve versus understanding that the symptom is the consequence of further metastasis of the cancer to the lung.[17]

Nurses should determine with parents how much their child understands about their symptoms and illness and how much

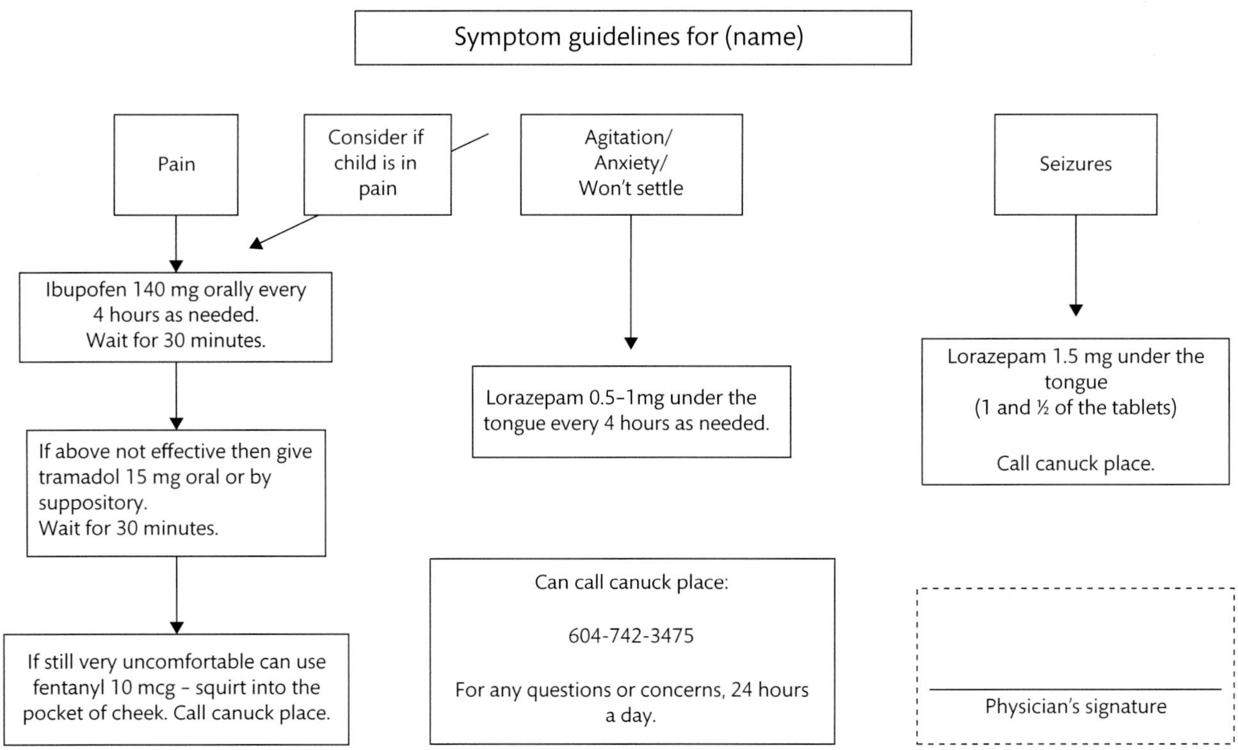

Figure 35.2 Symptom guidelines. Example of a symptom algorithm from Canuck Place, Canada.

information they feel their child is ready to receive.[17,18] When appropriate, the child can be asked how much they want to know about the cause of their symptoms, what is happening with their body, and what the plan is to support them.

Although often hope is seen to be contradictory in the context of a life-threatening illness, the child's symptoms and distress can often be framed within the concept of hope rather than doom.[22] A clinician should be cautious not to placate or falsely assure the child/family and maintain honest and clear information surrounding symptoms and management.[17] It can be helpful to respond by recognizing the child/caregiver experience and the ongoing commitment, support, and collaboration of the healthcare team to manage symptoms as partners. When appropriate, nurses should focus on function or symptom easement to subtly inspire strength and sustain hope.[22] The child should be supported to live as fully as possible (e.g., legacy-making, create special memories, pursue bucket-list items).

Education of the Child and Family

The goal of education is to empower a child and their family to understand the current and potential symptoms, services available to them, and their capacity to respond to symptoms. It is helpful to explore with a family or caregiver how they best learn and what supports them in their learning. Some people might be more visual learners, while others prefer written form or learning through discussion. With all education, nurses need to affirm understanding or enact different levels of teaching (i.e., teach back).

Families can be introduced to simple symptom assessment techniques and learn to recognize common triggers for some symptoms. For instance, a child with dyspnea may experience increased symptoms with the daily shower or other movement. Guidance can be provided on how to identify symptoms and support the child (e.g., pacing, use of equipment to decrease effort, pre-medicate with an opioid, and use of a fan). Adverse effects of medications should be anticipated and managed (e.g., start a laxative when an opioid is started to prevent constipation). Finally, the child/family should know when and how to contact a clinician when symptom management plans are no longer working or new symptoms arise. Families should have access to a clinician in a timely manner so that visits to emergency departments can be minimized.

Dyspnea/Respiratory Distress

Respiratory distress in a previously well child requires an urgent response, and the cause of the distress must be identified and managed. However, for seriously ill children receiving palliative care, the cause may be well known or expected. In the circumstance of increasing respiratory distress or dyspnea—the subjective feeling of being short of breath—the clinician and family need to review the course of action based on reversibility of cause, the level of distress the child is experiencing (from both dyspnea and possible treatments), and the goals of any treatment (see Case Study 2).

Case Study 2: A Pediatric Patient with Dyspnea and Panic

Rachel is a 17-year-old with metastatic osteosarcoma and extensive lung disease. Recently, she has experienced increasing work of breathing with activity. She was having difficulty getting to class using her crutches, and showers were exhausting. She was more comfortable when sitting and found a handheld fan helpful for dyspnea. She had a mild cough but no secretions, fever, or nasal congestion. Her hope was to continue to attend school. Rachel started on 5 mg of immediate-release morphine to be taken hourly as needed. A salbutamol inhaler every 4 hours as needed decreased her cough. After a few days, her morphine was converted to a short-acting formulation, then finally to a long-acting formulation of 30 mg every 12 hours (she had used an average of 12 breakthrough doses/day) with a breakthrough dose of 3 mg every hour as needed. This provided much better control of her dyspnea.

Rachel's dyspnea continued to worsen over several weeks, especially at night when prone. She was struggling to rise, shower, and get to class. The breakthrough doses helped but left her drowsy and unable to pay attention in class. Rachel was getting weaker. She found that the short-acting opioid fentanyl 25 mcg sublingually prior to exertion reduced her dyspnea without making her "zoned-out." A fan at her bedside was helpful, while oxygen was not. She agreed to try lorazepam 1 mg as needed along with mind–body (imagery and meditation) skills she had gained while working with a counselor.

As the dyspnea got more severe, her panic increased. She identified that it was not only the sensation of feeling breathless but also her sadness and fear of knowing she was dying. She said talking helped sometimes. Other times, she just wanted her mom to hold her hand and look at old photos. The lorazepam helped control the overwhelming fear. Meditating to a safer place, which she identified as a beach setting with a cool breeze, was also helpful for her. By having a number of interventions to use, Rachel was able to control her dyspnea, improve her comfort, and feel some control over her increasing symptoms.

Dyspnea can be assessed by asking the person to rate how short of breath they feel. If the child is unable to articulate this, respiratory distress can be observed by others as a symptom that includes increased work of breathing and decreased ability to exert oneself, along with signs of distress, panic, or agitation. In babies, retraction of the ribs and head bobbing are often observed alongside signs of distress/discomfort. Dyspneic symptoms can present at any age and with a variety of conditions. Anticipation of dyspnea is essential in care planning to enable quick and prepared responses. When appropriate, the underlying cause should be explored to better understand other treatment options.

Nurses must ensure that the parents/caregivers can assess respiratory distress, treat with physical and psychological interventions (e.g., fan, cool room, positioning, physical supportive presence), and escalate medications safely and confidently when needed. Opioids are first-line and benzodiazepines secondary options for managing dyspnea.[29] These medications are often used together to treat a child's experience of the symptom and their anxiety/emotional distress surrounding the symptom. Different agents have different pharmacokinetic profiles and are therefore suitable for certain situations. Care planning should focus on anticipating temporary dyspneic episodes as well as longer dyspneic events. For breathlessness that occurs with increases in activity (such as during a shower), fentanyl, a highly lipid-soluble opioid, can be given transmucosally[30] (buccal, sublingual, or nasal) as its onset of action is within 5–10 minutes and the duration is approximately 30 minutes. For a child who is requiring breakthrough medications for breathlessness, the background opioid should be increased, and administering a benzodiazepine regularly may be trialed to try to lessen the overall symptom burden.

Excessive Secretions

Excessive secretions can be problematic at different times across the child's journey and do not need to be treated unless causing distress or discomfort. Increased salivation is very common in children with neuromuscular disorders, such as cerebral palsy (see Case Study 3). At times, a dry bib will suffice, but drooling/excessive secretions can cause perioral dermatitis, dental problems, dehydration, respiratory distress, and aspiration pneumonia.[31] Thick secretions may be hard to mobilize and cause respiratory issues; increased humidity or nebulized saline can be helpful.

Case Study 3: A Patient with Excessive Secretions

At age 3 years, Ali was diagnosed with a neurodegenerative condition. He slowly lost his ability to swallow. A gastrostomy tube was inserted for nutrition. His increased secretions irritated his face and neck, requiring frequent clothing changes. Barrier creams and bibs helped for a short time, but frequent aspiration pneumonia and chronic sores in the folds of his neck became serious complications. Oral glycopyrrolate was prescribed, and later in his disease course sublingual atropine and Botox injections to his salivary glands were employed but did not resolve the issue. The family chose no other aggressive interventions. As Ali's disease progressed, the secretions increased, requiring suctioning every 10–15 minutes, while his gastrostomy feeds continued at the same rate. Palliative care staff talked with the family about the burdens of overhydration causing increased secretions at the end of life. Ali's mother said she would allow Ali to "tell her" when he had too much by the amount of secretion he was experiencing. With the technique of "feed to comfort," his comfort level improved.

As with other symptoms, the team should assess whether any of the current treatments or medications are exacerbating the problem. Excessive medical hydration can cause increased oral secretions.[31] Physical measures to treat excessive secretions include adjusting fluid intake and positioning in a drainage position. It is crucial to assess secretions in children who are being fed enterally. Often, reducing the volume or concentration of feed can improve the child's overall comfort. The medical order may offer a range of feed volume so that if the child is experiencing more respiratory symptoms on a particular day, the volume can be reduced. On other days, the child may be able to tolerate more. This balance requires frequent reassessment, especially as the child becomes closer to end-of-life care.

Chronic and problematic secretions can often be managed with oral anticholinergic agents such as glycopyrrolate[31] or hyoscine or by administering atropine 1% eye drops orally. However, adverse effects, such as thick secretions and urinary retention, can occur. In some children, injection of Botulinum toxin (Botox) into the salivary gland can be helpful to reduce secretions.[32]

At the end of life, secretions can collect in the back of the throat in children whose swallowing muscles have become too weak to function well. The associated gurgling noise can be very distressing for family members. The nurse can help family members recognize signs of distress in the child's face, provide education to normalize these sounds, and know which comfort medications can be helpful.

Gastrointestinal Symptoms

Nausea/Vomiting

Nausea is a complex symptom with a wide variety of causes.[33] Nausea can be caused by chemicals such as drugs or toxins, central nervous system abnormalities, vestibular changes, and multiple issues in the gastrointestinal tract including constipation.[33] Identifying the underlying cause will determine the most effective intervention.

Psychosocial and emotional aspects play a significant role in gastrointestinal symptoms, and managing anxiety, anger, and other stressful emotions can provide relief of these symptoms. Conducting a very careful history and assessment, involving the parent and, if possible, the child, along with observational assessment skills and trending of symptoms can provide insight. Understanding the frequency, duration, and timing of nausea/retching or vomiting can help delineate contributing factors, but further investigation may be needed. The emotional element is illustrated in Case Study 4.

Case Study 4: A Patient with Nausea

Olivia was a 6-year-old with a brain tumor. She had symptoms of nausea at the time of her radiation treatment and was on regular ondansetron, which seemed to control the vomiting. When her tumor relapsed and the intracranial pressure increased, her parents noted that she started to have a morning vomit and an increase in headaches. It was decided to trial a pulse (5 days) of dexamethasone to see if that would be advantageous.

After 3 days, Olivia was feeling better with no morning headache or nausea. Teaching and support were given to parents that another pulse could be tried in the future but that there were other agents that could be used if the dexamethasone did not have the same result.

Reducing intestinal distention can relieve nausea, retching, or vomiting. Regular bowel movements are key. For some children, this may mean multiple bowel movements in a day. Children who receive their nutrition orally often have control over their intake, while those who are "tube-fed" often do not. The volume and rate of the feeding should be adjusted individually and venting offered when appropriate. Children with severe neurological impairment often have lower energy requirements than healthy children, and overfeeding may cause abdominal distention and discomfort.[34] Working alongside families/caregivers to adjust the rate and concentration of feed when the goals are comfort and not weight gain might be beneficial.

Clinical hypnosis, music therapy, mind–body therapy, and aromatherapy can be tried. Peppermint, chamomile, fennel, ginger, or other mild teas may settle an upset stomach. Chicken soup, tea and toast, or family remedies, although not scientifically proven, may be helpful. The placebo effect is real.

Establishing the cause of the nausea, if possible, will determine the medications used. Some common medications used for nausea and vomiting include dimenhydrinate, 5HT-3-receptor antagonists (e.g., ondansetron), corticosteroids (e.g., dexamethasone), benzodiazepines (e.g., lorazepam), and prokinetics (e.g., domperidone). The best route for medications is the one that is simplest and most acceptable for the child and family.

Constipation

Children with complex medical conditions frequently have difficulty with bowel movements; thus, diet (type, amount, fiber, fluid, etc.), frequency and consistency of stool, and what agents or routines the families have found particularly helpful should be assessed with every visit. Constipation commonly occurs secondary to medications, neurological disorders, and disease processes. Fruit laxative recipes may be a medication-free way to support softer and bulkier stools.[35] When constipation is more severe or long-standing, medications are needed to both soften the stool and help move the stool through the gut. Polyethylene glycol powder, stimulant laxatives such as senna or bisacodyl, and lactulose can be used to accomplish the softening and promote resulting push action.[31] Consider the formulation and the route carefully and with the child's and family's input (see Case Study 5). Sodium phosphate enemas and glycerin or stimulant suppositories may need to be used occasionally to clear lower bowel impaction when there is no known obstruction. In cases of severe opioid-induced constipation, intravenous methylnaltrexone can be effective.[36]

Case Study 5: A Patient with Constipation

Jennifer was a single mother of Tyler (3 years), who had encephalopathy secondary to birth asphyxia. He was fed by gastrostomy tube. During one home visit with the nurse, Jennifer mentioned that Tyler has started vomiting after his feeds. On further discussion, she reported he had not had a bowel movement for 1 week. Polyethylene glycol 5 g was being given once daily, and though it seemed to work when they were in hospital, it was not working now. The nurse did an assessment and noted that the abdomen was firm with bowel sounds in all four quadrants. She did note hard stool when she did a digital exam. A pediatric enema was given with good effect, and the dose of polyethylene glycol was increased to twice daily with an extra dose to be given if Tyler did not have a bowel movement after 2 days. In a follow-up 1 week later, Jennifer reported that Tyler had a moderate-volume, soft bowel movement every 1 to 2 days, and there was no further feeding intolerance.

Feeding Difficulties/Appetite Issues

Diet and feeding are essential aspects of care, and there are multiple ways that illness, environment, symptoms, and circumstances affect a child's ability to enjoy, tolerate, or metabolize food. Across all ages and cultures, food is symbolic of love, nurturing, and interconnectedness. When disease or treatments decrease the child's appetite, families are distressed, even if the child is not. Medications, nutritional history, physical condition, and disease process must be carefully assessed. This may reveal treatable issues such as poor oral hygiene, mouth sores, or dental issues that can contribute to nutritional problems. Finances may prevent families from accessing nutritious food, but they may hesitate to mention this. Social workers can help navigate these situations.

Assessment should also include the family's understanding of why the child is unable to tolerate or has a reduced appetite. It is also helpful to explore families' goals in terms of diet and what their worries are if their child was to continue to lose weight. If the cause of low appetite is reversible or time-limited, small, frequent snacks may be more palatable for the child or foods in other forms, such as popsicles. If it is painful to eat or there is underlying nausea, this must be treated. Tracking diet and intake should not be obsessive but should include the overall goals of the child's wellness. This may include weight gain or a certain calorie/day plan, or it may focus on time with family at the dinner table or celebration without the expectation of certain intake measures.

In children whose condition is close to the end of life, weight loss is part of the natural dying process. Parents are often focused on growth and development up to this point, so having conversations about the changing needs of the child and how to monitor comfort may look different than counting the calories or doing weekly/monthly weights. For children who can direct their oral nutrition, parents/caregivers must recognize the child's agency in this aspect and that a decrease in appetite/intake enables the child to have fewer symptoms.

Children who receive long-term artificial nutrition and hydration (ANH) via medical interventions (e.g., gastrostomy, jejunostomy, or parenteral infusions) do not have control over their body's intake. At the end of life, ANH can be more burdensome than beneficial. This may be present as increased edema, vomiting, and increased secretions.[37] At this point, the team needs to help the family re-examine their goals of care and determine what actions would be most effective. The family can learn to adapt the interventions to meet those goals. Often, this is a long process as families and the team adjust the rate, frequency, amount, and type of formula to find what other forms of nutrition the child can benefit from before accepting the child's change in condition (see Case Study 6). At times a "feed to comfort" medical order may be needed to relieve the child of the suffering from an inability to process ANH. This type of order allows for feeding flexibility to adjust to the child's comfort, even if that means decreasing or stopping feeds. This is a sensitive and particularly difficult time as feeding is seen as an inherent part of providing care and nurturing. The team's understanding, patience, and ongoing support for the family are essential at this time; it may be an issue that takes time or several trials to resolve. A spiritual care provider working in collaboration with the team can be of great support, particularly at the end of life when a child refuses to eat or cannot tolerate ANH.

Case Study 6: A Patient with Multiple Symptoms

Mya was born with a fatal genetic disorder and irreparable cardiac condition; she was expected to live only weeks to months after birth. The parents wanted comfort care only and were eager to go home.

They were happy to have her home but struggled to cope with her long periods of crying. No curable causes for the crying could be found. The team was concerned that this was neuro-irritability, also known as "central neuropathy." Physical and psychological interventions along with an over-the-counter medication were tried. These helped but did not resolve the problem.

There was parental resistance to consistent medication use; however, with further supportive discussions they decided to "listen" to what Mya's body was "saying" she needed. Gabapentin was helpful during the day, and lorazepam at night allowed everyone to sleep.

While initially the parents did not want any tubes, they now feared she was hungry and requested a nasogastric tube be placed for extra feeds. A nasogastric tube was trialed, with the focus being on comfort versus growth. The palliative care team taught the parents how to place the tube and had the family use a reliable YouTube video as an additional guide.

The extra feeds increased Mya's oral secretions, requiring frequent suctioning; and she began to vomit with feeds. None of the medications or adjustments prevented this. The relational care of the team supported conversations around focusing on what Mya's body was telling us about what she needed or did not need for her comfort. This was a difficult time for the family, but the family, in collaboration with the team, decided to remove the tube and only feed her orally if she was showing signs of hunger. The parents provided excellent mouth care to Mya to keep her comfortable and satiate their need to nurture her through food. Mya was more comfortable and died peacefully.

At the end of life, when a child's body is no longer able to tolerate nutrition or hydration, natural changes occur in the body. Though body changes can be difficult for family members to witness—dry skin, weight loss, seeing ribs and cheekbones more prominently—these changes do signal to the parents/caregivers that time is short. This emotional and psychological connection to "what is" can be helpful in years to come as death will not be remembered as something that "came out of the blue." Acknowledging the physical symptoms gently and providing context for the family about the body's process in relation to comfort can be extremely helpful. For some parents, this may include discussing how the body slows down and may be more comfortable when metabolic needs are reduced and when it is not stressed from trying to process food and fluids. Nurses can highlight that the dying process is due to the underlying condition and not because the child is not eating; in fact, the child is not eating (or not tolerating feeds) because they are dying. Although the physical body may be shutting down at this time, the connection spiritually and psychologically to the child can remain intact.

The "phase" of imminent dying can be very protracted. Providing certainty around an anticipated time of death is generally not helpful for parents/caregivers as it sets expectations that cannot be guaranteed. Nurses need to be prepared and assess symptoms while also supporting parents living each moment and day with uncertainty, following the child's lead.

Neurological Symptoms

Children with serious neurological impairment, with or without an underlying progressive condition, typically experience a complicated disease course, with times of stability interrupted by acute health decline and recovery, followed by a new baseline with an uncertain trajectory.[2] Seizures, increased tone or spasticity, and irritability wreak havoc on the QOL of the child and the family. The wide range of specialist teams involved can make sharing information a challenge.

Box 35.4 Neuro-irritability Assessment

A child may have neuro-irritability if:

1. Actions known not to be painful (wearing socks, touching) seem to cause pain or distress
2. Child fusses or cries for no apparent reason
3. Child's crying is difficult to control or is prolonged
4. Parent cannot tell the difference between the child's cries for attention and cries due to pain/discomfort
5. Child's pain/discomfort cannot be localized

Physical and Psychological Measures for Inconsolability

1. Environment: Quiet, dim lighting; rested parents
2. Swaddling
3. Music therapy
4. Aromatherapy: Lavender oil diffuser or drop on a cotton ball on the pillow
5. Massage
6. Prayer
7. Rocking: Infant swing, rocking chair, held rocking
8. Therapeutic touch or Reiki

Source: Reference 34.

A comfort log is an individualized tool for determining the extent or severity of the symptoms and the helpfulness of an intervention. These tools are easy to design and can be used during a hospital stay or at home. They can include descriptions of the symptom, duration, severity, helpful interventions (pharmacological, physical, and psychological), and effect of interventions. This enables clinicians and family members to get an overview, perhaps notice trends or triggers, and assess the effectiveness of interventions. See the neuro-irritability assessment in Box 35.4. In assessing a child for neuro-irritability, any signs of allodynia and hyperalgesia should be noted.[13] Benzodiazepines, gabapentin or pregabalin, neuroleptics, and adrenergic agonists and antagonists are the medications most often used to manage neuro-irritability symptoms.[37]

Children who have increasing frequency of seizures or a potential to have a seizure (e.g., brain tumor) require a stepwise approach to management involving regular antiseizure medications (e.g., levetiracetam) and rescue medications (e.g., diazepam). An individualized algorithm that incorporates interventions and next steps is helpful. When there is potential for life-threatening seizures, clinicians have an obligation to discuss this with the family so that direction of care can be considered. For example, a child with a progressive brain tumor may need treatment for a seizure within the context of their dying. Part of the algorithm may explicitly state that the parent's role is to not only medicate the seizure but also to hold and comfort the dying child. For children who are otherwise stable, the plan may include responding to the symptom with medication and then engaging emergency services for further treatment.

Severe Bleeds

Bleeds in children can occur due to a variety of reasons. Certain diseases and treatments may place a child at a higher risk for a bleed (such as advanced leukemia). Management plans need to align with goals of care, stage of disease progression, type of bleed, and likely cause.[31] Symptoms are often dependent on the rate and duration of the bleed.[14] Bleeds can be visible or invisible depending on the location and can range from small to life-ending. Bleeding that is visual to the parents, even if the amount is small, can be distressing to parents or even the child. If blood from mucous membranes, coughing, from a wound, or per rectum is seen or anticipated, an individualized plan should be made for that child. It is helpful to prepare children and families for what is happening or what could happen and to inform them that there are supports in place for how to manage. Physical interventions can be dependent on the exit site of the bleed. If the child is vomiting, then a drainage position might be helpful. Low platelets might cause bleeding out of small cuts or a child's mouth. Using dark towels for bleeds can decrease the visual impact for the caregivers; however, the focus should be on integrating psychological interventions such as maintaining the physical presence of a loved one with the child, staying calm, and supportive pharmacologic interventions, such as tranexamic acid.[31] Caregivers can be reassured that in the circumstance of a catastrophic bleed (internal or external), it is often not painful for the child as they do lose consciousness quickly. Post-management includes support for debriefing and ongoing support.[31]

Emotional and Existential Distress

It is beyond the scope of this chapter to critically explore anxiety and depression from emotional and existential distress in children with palliative conditions. Children of any age may experience suffering during the dying process that goes beyond the physical. Moreover, parents and children are connected in ways that are not like other relationships, with each influenced by the other in the face of ultimate physical separation.

Children of any age should be assessed from a developmental framework regarding their emotional and spiritual health. Are they experiencing joy and times of pleasure and having opportunities to play and express themselves? What is it like to spend months in neonatal intensive care or receive chemotherapy? How are they adjusting to the changes in friendships and activities? What gives them hope and purpose?

Families and children have different capacities to communicate, find meaning, and adjust to the multitude of changes that serious illness brings. An interdisciplinary palliative care team can be instrumental in supporting the family unit and the child in these tasks. If physical symptoms can be controlled, the child and the family may be better able to process the symptoms of emotional and spiritual distress. Often, families need coaching and modeling in how to listen to their children's questions about the changes in their body and how to respond with both honesty and hope. Children and parents/caregivers may need different and separate confidants to share their questions, worries, and fears as a way of protecting each other.

When existential distress and emotional suffering do not seem to be responding to multiple attempts from family, community, healthcare providers, counseling professionals, spiritual support, and other therapy, medications such as antidepressants, benzodiazepines, antipsychotics, or stimulants may be helpful in the short or medium term.

Refractory Symptoms

In rare circumstances, difficult-to-manage symptoms may become refractory—all possible treatments available have either failed or no reasonable methods are available for palliation within a tolerable time frame for the child.[38] Lack of availability of interventions/resources can contribute to determining that a symptom is refractory.

Labeling a symptom refractory requires excellent assessment and communication skills and a thorough evaluation of the symptom through a multidisciplinary team approach, including the child's and family's input, experience, and insights, when possible. Palliative sedation is an extraordinary intervention to intentionally lower a child's level of consciousness when symptoms are extremely difficult to manage. Framing these discussions with families often entails significant expertise and should be done by a pediatric palliative care clinician. Palliative sedation can be trialed as a "respite" from the symptom for several days with a plan to then lighten the sedation to determine if it continues to be needed. Parents desire engagement with their child and grieve intensely as that engagement lessens in the dying process. When palliative sedation is required, psychosocial support and guidance to parents and siblings is essential. Nurses who work in pediatric palliative care need to be informed about and familiar with the policy of palliative sedation at their institution.[38]

Conclusion

Although many of the symptoms commonly seen in dying children are similar to those in adult palliative patients, children are often less able to describe and localize their symptoms. Nurses must therefore be careful listeners, imaginative problem-solvers, and evidenced-based professionals. They need to be able to draw on a broad skill set, including excellent assessment, critical thinking, communication, and relational skills, as well as flexibility/adaptability. The family must be closely integrated with the palliative care team as care planning and decision-making are shared. If this collaboration is not present, managing distressing symptoms may be difficult. Building trusting relationships is vital to ensure excellent care of the child, the designated "family" of the child, the interdisciplinary care team, and community resources.

Physical and psychological interventions, medication dosages, and routes of administration must be tailored to the child and family. Understanding of the care and the chosen goals can be influenced by culture, religion, past experiences/traumas, and the child's stage of development. Evidence-based clinical guidelines and pediatric-specific communications tools can be helpful as a starting point for developing individualized care plans.

REFERENCES

1. World Health Organization. *Integrating Palliative Care and Symptom Relief into Paediatrics*. World Health Organization; 2018. Accessed September 23, 2022. https://www.who.int/publications/i/item/integrating-palliative-care-and-symptom-relief-into-paediatrics.
2. Together for Short Lives. What Is Children's Palliative Care. 2021. Accessed September 23, 2022. https://www.togetherforshortlives.org.uk/changing-lives/supporting-care-professionals/introduction-childrens-palliative-care/.

3. Benini F, Papadatou D, Bernada M, et al. International standards for pediatric palliative care: from IMPaCCT to GO-PPaCS. *J Pain Symptom Manage.* 2022;63(5):529–543.
4. Davies B, Steele R, Baird J. *Pediatric Palliative Care: A Model for Exemplary Practice.* Routledge; 2021.
5. Bogetz J, Lemmon M. Pediatric palliative care for children with severe neurological impairment and their families. *J Pain Symptom Manage.* 2021;62(3):662–667.
6. Hauer J. Feeding intolerance in children with severe impairment of the central nervous system: strategies for treatment and prevention. *Children (Basel).* 2018;5(1):1–11.
7. Bogetz J, Trowbridge A, Lewis H, et al. Parents are the experts: a qualitative study of the experiences of parents of children with severe neurological impairment during decision-making. *J Pain Symptom Manage.* 2021;62(6):1117–1125.
8. Hauer J, Wolfe J. Supportive and palliative care of children with metabolic and neurological diseases. *Curr Opin Support Palliat Care.* 2014;8(3):296–302.
9. McHugh M, Buschman P. Communication at the time of death. In: Ferrell B, ed. *Advanced Practice Palliative Nursing.* Oxford University Press; 2016:395–404.
10. Siden H. Pediatric palliative care for children with progressive non-malignant diseases. *Children (Basel).* 2018;5(2):28. https://doi.org/10.3390/children5020028.
11. Hoell J, Weber H, Warfsmann J, et al. Facing the large variety of life-limiting conditions in children. *Eur J Pediatr.* 2019;178:1893–1902.
12. Steel R, Siden H, Cadell S, et al. Charting the territory: symptoms and functional assessment in children with progressive non-curable conditions. *Arch Dis Child.* 2014;99:754–762.
13. Sisk B, Widger K, Feudtner C. The new and changing landscape of children receiving pediatric palliative care in the US: an evidence base emerges. In: Wolfe J, ed. *Interdisciplinary Pediatric Palliative Care.* 2nd ed. Oxford University Press; 2021:10–25.
14. BC Centre for Palliative Care. Symptom Management Guidelines. Accessed September 29, 2022. https://www.bc-cpc.ca/publications/symptom-management-guidelines/.
15. Collins JJ, Devine TD, Dick GS, et al. The measurement of symptoms in young children with cancer: the validation of the Memorial Symptom Assessment Scale in children aged 7–12. *J Pain Symptom Manage.* 2002;23(1):10–16.
16. Ariadne Labs. Serious Illness Conversation Guide. 2017. https://www.ariadnelabs.org/wp-content/uploads/2018/04/Serious-Illness-Conversation-Guide.2017-04-18CC2pg.pdf.
17. van Breemen C, Johnston J, Carwana M, Louie P. Serious illness conversations in pediatrics: a case review. *Children (Basel).* 2020;7(8):102. https://doi.org/10.3390/children7080102.
18. van Breemen C. Adapting the serious illness conversation guide for use in pediatrics. *J Palliat Med.* 2018;21(12):1683. https://doi.org/10.1089/jpm.2018.0515.
19. Institute for Patient and Family Centered Care. Patient and Family-Centered Care Defined. Accessed March 3, 2023. https://www.ipfcc.org/bestpractices/sustainable-partnerships/background/pfcc-defined.html.
20. Brock K, Wolf J, Ullrich C. From the child's word to clinical intervention: novel, new, and innovative approaches to symptoms in pediatric palliative care. *Children (Basel).* 2018;5(4):45.
21. Association of Paediatric Palliative Medicine. *The Association of Paediatric Palliative Medicine Master Formulary.* 5th ed. Together for Short Lives. 2020. Accessed March 25, 2023. https://www.togetherforshortlives.org.uk/app/uploads/2018/03/APPM-Master-Formulary-2020-protected.pdf.
22. Friedrichsdorf S, Kohen D. Integration of hypnosis into pediatric palliative care. *Ann Palliat Med.* 2018;7(1):136–150. https://doi.org/10.21037/apm.2017.05.02.
23. Kuttner L. Pediatric hypnosis: treatment that adds and rarely subtracts. *Int J Clin Exp Hypn.* 2020;68(10):16–28.
24. Kuttner L. Chapter 5 Psychological Methods to Relieve Pain. In *A Child in Pain: What Health Professionals Can Do to Help.* Crown House Publishing; 2010:147–153.
25. You H, Ross S. The impact of music therapy in paediatric palliative care in residential hospice. *J Pain Symptom Manage.* 2018;56(6):e75.
26. Czarnecki M, Michlig J, Norton A, Stelter A, Hainsworth K. Use of aromatherapy for pediatric surgical patients. *Pain Manag Nursing.* 2022;23(6):703–710.
27. Weaver M, Robinson J, Wichman C. Aromatherapy improves nausea, pain and mood for patients receiving pediatric palliative care symptom-based consults: a pilot design study. *Palliat Support Care.* 2019;18(2):158–163.
28. Weekly T, Riley B, Wichman C, Weaver M. Impact of massage therapy intervention for pediatric palliative care patients and their family caregivers. *J Palliat Care.* 2019;34(3):164–167.
29. Friedrichsdorf SJ. From tramadol to methadone: opioids in the treatment of pain and dyspnea in pediatric palliative care. *Clin J Pain.* 2019;35(6):501–508.
30. Chang A, Roeland EJ, Atayee RS, Revta C, Ma JD. Transmucosal immediate-release fentanyl for breakthrough cancer pain: opportunities and challenges for use in palliative care. *J Pain Palliat Care Pharmacother.* 2015;29(3):247–260.
31. Together for Short Lives. Basic Symptom Control in Paediatric Palliative Care. June 14, 2022. Accessed September 29, 2022. https://www.togetherforshortlives.org.uk/resource/basic-symptom-control-paediatric-palliative-care/.
32. Gok G, Cox N, Bajwa J, Christoudoulou D, Moody A, Howett D. Ultrasound-guided injection of botulinum toxin A into the submandibular gland in children and young adults with sialorrhoea. *Br J Oral Maxillofac Surg.* 2013;51:231–233.
33. Russel AC, Stone AL, Waker LS. Functional nausea in children: a review of literature and the need for diagnostic criteria. *Children (Basel).* 2016;3(1):5.
34. Gale R, Namestnic J, Singer P, Kagan I. Caloric requirements of patients with brain impairment and cerebral palsy who are dependent on chronic ventilation. *J Parenter Enteral Nutr.* 2017;41(8):1366–1370.
35. Provincial Health Services Authority British Columbia Cancer. Oncology Nutrition. October 2018. Accessed March 15, 2023. http://www.bccancer.bc.ca/nutrition-site/Documents/Patient%20Education/Fruit-lax-recipes.pdf.
36. Yoemanson D, Chohan O, Mayer A. Paediatric palliative care: intravenous methylnaltrexone relieves constipation. *BMJ Support Palliat Care.* 2013;3:103–105.
37. Hauer J. Pediatric Palliative Care. UpToDate. July 2017. Accessed March 25, 2023. https://www.uptodate.com/contents/pediatric-palliative-care.
38. Cuviello A, Ang N, Morgan K, Baker J, Anghelescu D. Palliative sedation therapy practice comparison—a survey of pediatric palliative care and pain management specialists. *Am J Hosp Palliat Care.* 2022;40(9):977–986.

36

Values and Perspectives Influencing Goals of Care and Decision-Making in Pediatric Palliative Care

Christina McDaniel and Jordan M. Desai

Key Points

- End-of-life goals-of-care conversations require effective communication, empathy, and active listening.
- It is critical to understand the values of the patient and family to enable decision-making that centers on what they consider important.
- Quality care, as a metric used to help guide the decision-making of pediatric palliative care patients and their families, is bound in and to the culture of the individual family.
- Understanding parent and family perspectives is essential not only for providing care during the illness trajectory but also in assisting families through bereavement.
- Guiding conversations around goals addressing physical, emotional, spiritual, and social needs is necessary to ensure holistic care is delivered.

Introduction

> I suddenly realize that my own pregnancy, the status of being in good hope, no longer exists. There are just black clouds, there is just the feeling, oh my god, perhaps I am carrying a curious being, disfigured and malformed and ill and disabled.[1]

From the moment a family is faced with the life-threatening illness of a child, they are thrust into a stressful, perhaps devastating, new world. This world often communicates with a medical culture and language that are unfamiliar to most families. From an ethnographic perspective, the language and culture of medicine require clinicians' fluency and essentially demand that ill children and their families learn at least some level of competency. The palliative care clinician must serve as a kind of bicultural figure and must have a keen understanding of both worlds.[2] The pediatric care clinician must consistently find ways to bridge the gap between the culture of medicine and the culture of the individual families served.

When asked to reflect on his rotation with a local hospice, a general pediatrics resident noted, "I had no idea his life [the patient] had *quality*. Every time I've seen this patient in the hospital, he looks miserable and never interacts with anyone. Here at home, he was smiling, he was laughing; that was an entirely different kid." Any clinician who has had the privilege of being invited into the sacred ground of a pediatric hospice patient's home can appreciate this assessment.

Quality, as a metric used to help guide the decision-making of pediatric palliative care patients and their families, is bound in and to the culture of the individual family. It is also tied into setting; quality of life (QOL) defined by the bed-bound patient residing in the intensive care unit (ICU) might look very different from quality as defined by the newly diagnosed asymptomatic patient. The suggestion then becomes that quality must be a fluid metric that is influenced by values and goals established by the patient and family. However, it is possible that clinicians interacting with families have an entirely different definition of quality and subsequent outcomes. Understanding the need for early palliative care integration is perhaps best demonstrated by the following case example.

Case Study: A Patient's QOL

Upon Landry's birth, she was diagnosed with trisomy 13, exhibiting characteristics such as a ventricular septal defect, rocker bottom feet, low-set ears, microcephaly, and clenched hands, posing a high risk for aspiration. Transferred to the neonatal ICU (NICU), she spent her initial 4 weeks there. The family sought palliative care consultation to navigate the challenging decisions ahead. Landry's mother, overwhelmed, expressed a desire for her daughter's recovery, while Landry's father struggled with the complexities of medical choices.

Following family meetings, Landry's parents opted to bring her home with a nasogastric tube and safety medications, deferring decisions on surgical interventions. Landry's mother spoke optimistically about a nursery awaiting Landry at home. Discharged with hospice care, Landry's parents aimed to keep her comfortable, adjusting her code status for a natural death. However, the strain on the parents became evident during a social work hospice visit, with Landry's mother expressing a sense of waiting for her daughter to die.

Introducing home health support and with Landry gaining weight, the parents regained hope after 2 months of home hospice. Yet, as Landry's condition improved, her mother reconsidered the goals of care, seeking potential surgical interventions. Engaging with a supportive online community of mothers with similar experiences, she felt empowered to advocate for Landry. The family transitioned from hospice to palliative care, celebrating Landry's progress with a "hospice graduation" party.

Under the outpatient palliative care team's guidance, Landry underwent successful ventricular septal defect closure and received a button G-tube. Regular appointments with specialists followed, and after a year under palliative care, Landry's mother confidently stated that they were doing well and questioned the ongoing need for support. Surpassing life expectancy expectations, Landry thrived until shortly after her third birthday when seizures and increased hospitalizations surfaced.

Reintroducing palliative care, Landry's mother sensed a significant change, describing it as "the big one." Landry's interactivity diminished, raising concerns about neurological delays. After a substantial ICU stay, Landry's parents opted for hospice care at home, where she peacefully passed away surrounded by family and cherished stuffed animals. Reflecting on Landry's strength, her mother remarked, "Landry never had it easy, but she always did things her own way and was the strongest person I know."

Outcome Considerations and the Power of Social Networking

The experiences described in Landry's case study illustrate the challenges families face when navigating goals of care. In the case of trisomy 13 and 18, many families have reported experiencing bias by clinicians due to their child's diagnostic label.[3] While Landry's parents were not aware of her diagnosis until birth, the research suggests that when trisomy 13 and 18 are discovered in utero, families are often counseled toward termination.[4] Remarkably, despite feeling the pressure to terminate, the majority of parents elect to continue their pregnancy. In a survey of parents facing prenatal diagnosis of trisomy 13 and/or 18, parents chose to ignore recommendations toward termination based on their own reported moral beliefs (68%), child-centered reasons (64%), religious beliefs (48%), parent-centered reasons (28%), and practical reasons (6%).[5] This research demonstrates the disconnect that can exist between clinicians and parents when determining treatment courses for their medically fragile children.

A retrospective cohort study found that among children born with trisomy 13 or 18 in Ontario, Canada, early mortality was the most common outcome; however, 10%–13% of children survived for 10 years, and, among children who underwent surgical interventions, 1-year survival was actually high.[6] So how should palliative care clinicians approach assisting families with decision-making in the face of such prognostic ambiguity and potential clinician bias?

The palliative care clinician should not only attune themself to what families might be hearing from their primary medical providers but also consider what families might be learning in their own examination of the diagnosis. In the example of trisomy 13 and 18, clinicians relied on the multitude of resources that suggested this diagnosis will mean extreme suffering and shortened life span. Meanwhile, families researching the condition on the internet were introduced to an alternative narrative, one that suggested that patients who do survive experienced meaningful lives and QOL.

Parents, like Landry's mother, who engage with parental support groups online may discover an alternative positive description about children with trisomy 13 and 18.[5] A quick internet search reveals shockingly different results when the words "trisomy 13 and 18" are used alone versus "trisomy 13 and 18 support." While the diagnosis-alone internet search yields a clinical, medically complex, and seemingly negative perspective, the diagnosis and support search results in a multitude of support groups such as the Support Organization for Trisomy,[7] which presents smiling children and relatable language. Understanding that families might hold the clinical perspective and the support perspective in equal regard will help the palliative care clinician assist families in navigating decision-making through uncertain outcomes.

Guiding with Uncertainty

The sometimes dichotomous relationship between the perspective of the clinician and the patient and family is no more evident than when considered through the lens of prognostication in pediatric life-threatening illness. In the case of cancer, which remains one of the leading causes of nonaccidental death in childhood, one study reports that children who die of cancer experience significant suffering and inadequate palliation in the last month of life.[8,9] The team investigating these parent-reported outcomes suggested that unrealistic prognostic expectations, by both physicians and parents, may be leading to inappropriate treatment goals. A survey of parents of children who died of cancer between 1990 and 1997, along with 42 pediatric oncologists, confirmed that parents first recognized that the child had no realistic chance for cure a mean of 109 days before the child's death, while physician recognition occurred earlier at 206 days before death,[10] furthering the idea that palliative care often acts as a bridge between medical understanding and family understanding.

Considerable delay exists in parental recognition that children have no realistic chance for cure, but earlier recognition of this prognosis by both providers and families is associated with a stronger emphasis on treatment directed at lessening suffering and greater integration of palliative care.

Case Study: A Patient Undergoing Hematopoietic Stem Cell Transplantation

Ravi, a 17-year-old boy of Indian descent, lived at home with his parents and younger sister. Born with a severe primary immunodeficiency, Ravi faced recurring, long-lasting infections throughout his life, resulting in extended stays in the ICU for treatment. Despite these challenges, Ravi excelled academically, graduating a semester early by frontloading his classes. Following the advice of his medical team, Ravi and his family decided to pursue hematopoietic stem cell transplant through bone marrow transplant.

In adherence to hospital protocol, the pediatric palliative care team was called upon to meet Ravi and his family at the time of the transplant. During the initial consultation, Ravi described his choice in timing for the transplant, stating, "I'd rather take a year off now, finish up my last semester, and go into college without having to worry about this." When questioned about concerns regarding the transplant, he remarked, "I mean, I guess I'm worried it won't work, but I don't want to spend the rest of my life in and out of hospitals, so it's worth it." Actively participating in the decision-making process, Ravi's parents remained hopeful and confident in their choice to proceed with transplantation.

Throughout the engraftment period, Ravi and his family engaged easily with care team providers. Like many of his peers, he loved discussing sports and technology with all providers who visited him. Discharged from the hematology/oncology unit after 30 days of engraftment, Ravi looked forward to returning home, playing video games, and catching up with his friends as he continued the recovery process. Unfortunately, a week after discharge, he returned to the unit with low counts and fever, causing understandable discouragement and worry for his family. Ravi had lost almost all his hair and had severe nausea. This was especially challenging for his family as his mother identified feeding Ravi as a primary exhibition of her love and care.

Ravi would always be the first to tell staff that he loved food, and any restrictions on his eating habits felt like a major setback. Ravi had grown close to his primary nurses, palliative care social worker, and child life specialist, routinely requesting visits to "check in" and report on new technology or projects he was working on. He arranged a special Super Bowl viewing party in his room on the floor and invited all staff and his friends to attend. While Ravi remained upbeat in his interactions with his teams, his condition worsened.

Ravi developed graft-versus-host disease, which presented with skin sloughing and progressive gastrointestinal involvement. Ravi was acutely aware of his decline, and, during one visit with his palliative care social worker, when asked if there were things he was worried about, he tearfully replied, "I'm worried I won't get to do the things I want to do with my life." Ravi was a very imaginative young man and was able to explore some of these "bucket list" items through guided imagery. All the teams involved in Ravi's care had grown close to Ravi and his family. In a preconference to a care team meeting, each of his specialists had begun speaking about the aspect of Ravi's disease process that they were responsible for when the palliative care physician interjected, "No one is acknowledging the reality here; Ravi is dying."

While each clinician cognitively understood this clinical reality, the team was challenged with how to communicate this to a family who had been such strong advocates for hoping against hope. When the change in Ravi's prognosis was presented to his parents, they explained that they needed to maintain hope and that there were forces outside those of medicine that might intervene. They both felt that the care team had become "like family" and reported that Ravi would want to be on the unit in the event he should die. When asked what they felt brought their son comfort, Ravi's parents reported that he loved listening to his favorite book read aloud. During the last 3 days of Ravi's life, he remained unresponsive while members of the care team and Ravi's parents took turns reading Ravi's favorite book aloud to him.

Parent Outlook and Understanding

While hematopoietic stem cell transplantation presents the potential for cure for patients like Ravi, it remains an intensive therapy that presents many risks for complications and lasting health effects.[11] Can families truly understand what the transplantation process could look like? Understanding patient and family perspectives on proposed interventions is essential to facilitating goals-of-care conversations. In the case of bone marrow transplantation, one qualitative study found that parents reported being either incapable or unwilling to think about the potential for negative outcomes. Some parents refused to acknowledge the possibility that their child might die, in order to move forward with transplantation.[12]

In Ravi's case, this was certainly true for his parents. He had spent his life dealing with infections that had the potential for significant harm, so a path without transplantation still presented significant risk to Ravi's life. If they elected not to move forward with transplantation, they could imagine a future decline. However, transplantation presented the possibility of a different future, a future that was *potentially* symptom-free and curative. At one point Ravi's mother even remarked, "If it doesn't work, he will be sick, and he's always been sick." What they repeatedly reported not "being ready for" was the way things like graft-versus-host would present. They had read that this was possible, but they had not imagined what it would be like to see Ravi experience significant pain with the slightest touch. They had not imagined seeing Ravi's skin break down to the point of bleeding or that he would become too weak to walk the short distance to his bathroom.

Fortunately, palliative care consultation began early for Ravi, and continued conversations about his parents' outlook and concerns throughout the transplantation course were possible. This type of communication can greatly assist parents with coping during this uncertain process.[13] Research centered on parent outlook in hematopoietic stem cell transplantation helps make the case for early and frequent goals-of-care conversations. The team concluded that, "understanding parent outlook is a cornerstone of clear and compassionate communication throughout the course of hematopoietic stem cell transplantation, allowing mutual understanding of hopes, fears, expectations, and goals of care."[12] In Ravi's case, this meant continued readjustment of goals of care as his disease progressed. The trust necessary to hold both hope and prognosis was well established through continued open and honest communication.

Clinician Impact on Bereavement Course

Understanding parent and family perspectives is essential not only for providing care during the illness trajectory but also in assisting families through their bereavement. Communication and continuity of care are two of the most important aspects of the parent-reported grief experience that the clinician can impact.[14] Many families will want to reconvene their care team to ask, "Did I make the right decision?" or "What could I have done differently?" These meetings can be an important opportunity to revisit family decision-making and reiterate that parents have made the most loving decisions possible with the information they had available.

These bereavement care team meetings can have significant impact for families. Four major meaning-making processes have been identified in qualifying the impact of these meetings. These processes include sense-making, benefit-finding, continuing bonds, and identity reconstruction.[15] See Tables 36.1, 36.2, 36.3 and 36.4 for detailed descriptions of the four processes and examples of parental response. While the extent to which meaning-making during bereavement meetings affects parental health outcomes remains unknown, the research in the pediatric ICU (PICU) setting suggests that bereaved parents are at a high risk for complicated grief and that meaning-making is associated with a reduction in the severity of these symptoms.[15]

Consideration should also be given to the bereaved sibling. The death of a sibling can have significant impact on the life course of the surviving sibling. In Ravi's case, his sister, Madison spent most of her afternoons doing homework in Ravi's hospital room. If she wanted her parents present for something in her life, Ravi's illness always had to be considered. Many of the same challenges in meaning-making exist in the bereavement course of a sibling. How a sibling experiences the death of a child could impact their long-term psychosocial well-being. Sibling-directed communication and concurrent supportive care during the illness experience and the immediate bereavement course may mitigate poor long-term outcomes.[16]

Communication throughout the Trajectory

When caring for children with complex life-threatening illnesses, communication needs change rapidly and sometimes unexpectedly. Given the uncertainty of prognostication, effective communication surrounding goals of care is essential. Guiding conversations around goals to address physical, emotional, spiritual, and social needs is necessary to ensure holistic care is delivered. Communication is the basis for all decision-making, and, throughout an illness trajectory, decision-making hinges on effective communication.[17] Providers

Table 36.1 Sense-making processes observed during follow-up meetings (*N* = 35)

Sense-making process	Example (follow-up meeting number)	*n* (%)*a*
Biomedical explanations	Do you think there's anything we should be asking as far as from a medical perspective that maybe we're just not—any information that we should know that we might not already know? (#21)	34 (97)
Details of illness	What about the high blood sugar? ... And did his weight have anything to do with it? (#4)	32 (91)
Course of illness	My question was how things happened chronologically. For me it was a blur. (#28)	27 (77)
Counterfactuals	I just have the "what-ifs," like what if we waited one day and they would have done surgery. (#23)	23 (66)
Cause of death	Do you know what her cause of death is? Is it blunt force trauma to her head? (#8)	20 (57)
Autopsy	So, was there anything in the autopsy that was surprising or significant? (#25)	13 (37)
Parents' prior decisions	You're always going to have that question whether or not you made the right decision. (#21)	24 (69)
End-of-life care	One of B's main concerns is that we didn't pull the plug too soon or gave up on her too soon. (#23)	17 (49)
Treatment	The feeding tube, we understand we want to try to feed him.... But was it worth it? (#15)	14 (40)
Blame	What happens is a lot of times when you try to get all the answers you're trying to find somebody to blame. (#30)	18 (51)
For child's death	You can tell me when my pizza's going to be here. But you can't tell me when they're going to be here to pick up a child who's dying? It's just unacceptable. (#41)	9 (26)
For parents' experience	Why did it take 4 hours for the nurse to call us? If they're telling us everything started around 9 p.m., we didn't we get a call until 1:15 a.m., and we're a half an hour away. (#16)	16 (46)
Blessings	And every day he lived was a blessing. Every day was better than anybody had ever told me. (#29)	18 (51)
Inevitability of death	Even though he had his ups and downs, he was on a downward cycle. (#25)	18 (51)
Parents' role in the death	Has smoking ever been connected to any kind of heart problem in pregnancy? I smoked when I was pregnant. (#32)	15 (43)
Downward comparisons	There's been a couple sudden deaths in our area.... In some ways that would be even harder. (#13)	14 (40)
God's will	Maybe that was her day to be with the Lord. (#11)	13 (37)
Did everything	I do believe you all did everything you could to save my daughter. (#20)	11 (31)
No longer suffering	He's in a good place. He's not suffering anymore. (#3)	7 (20)
Exceeded expected age	I had 9 months. Nine months that technically I never should have had. (#10)	7 (20)
Child's will	He [child] told Dr. S, "I'm not having no more surgery." He said, "This is my last one." (#22)	4 (11)
Why me?	It's unfair, but it's my life, you know. This is what I was dealt. (#2)	3 (9)
Parent not capable	I know I can't handle a sick baby.... I wouldn't be able to take care of a sick child forever. (#2)	2 (6)
No sense made	When we got the results back, basically we were told they didn't find anything wrong. So, we're still left without an answer.... It's like getting handed a blank piece of paper. It's like, why? Why did we go through what we went through for no answer? (#16)	9 (26)
No need to make sense	I believe this stuff happens and that's just how it was supposed to happen, you know. Left your house an hour early, got in a car accident, that's just what was supposed to happen. (#2)	9 (26)

a n (%) = number and percentage of follow-up meetings demonstrating each meaning-making process.

Table 36.2 Benefit-finding processes observed during follow-up meetings (*N* = 35)

Benefit-finding process	Example (follow-up meeting number)	*n* (%)*a*
Ways to help others	We're trying to get to the point where we can help, instead of them helping us. (#13)	29 (83)
Feedback	It's a lot easier to have repetitive nurses than to keep having new ones take care of your child.... To ask the parents if they would rather have that would be nice for other parents. (#3)	15 (43)
Donations	I was lucky that we had this equipment sitting around to donate to them. (#22)	8 (23)
Research	I just didn't want to not participate in the research to help other families. (#21)	8 (23)
Volunteerism	And as far as any sort of parent outreach or anything that you need I would feel—I would always be open and available to helping any way I can. (#33)	5 (14)
New medical knowledge	I know that he was sent here for a reason and, like I said, now these doctors know what they need to do for the next baby. (#10)	6 (17)
Organ donation	It comforts us knowing that she would be able to live on through other people. (#17)	2 (6)
Change in others for the better	Even in his slow motion, he helped them slow down and smell the roses and think better of what they were doing. (#7)	90 (26)
Change in parents for the better	I feel like she helped me get to a different appreciation and respect things on many different levels way different than I did before. (#21)	7 (20)

a n (%) = number and percentage of follow-up meetings demonstrating each meaning-making process.

Table 36.3 Continuing bond manifestations observed during follow-up meetings (*N* = 35)

Continuing bond	Example (follow-up meeting number)	*n* (%)*a*
Parents' inner lives	Every time I hear a bird I think of him. (#9)	33 (94)
Child attributes	She had a strong personality, that one. She had the biggest, biggest brown eyes ever. She was so beautiful. (#4)	28 (80)
Child life events	He played baseball, he played soccer. He'd drive the power chair around the bases on his own, stealing bases and everything. (#1)	21 (60)
Personal rituals	We wanted to take our little girl home with us in our way instead of having her sitting in some cold place. (#31)	21 (60)
Photos	Just have a family picture here of all of us. (#5)	18 (51)
Linking objects	So, you know it's still sitting there. His diaper pail is, gross as it is, we haven't emptied it. (#15)	17 (49)
Angel	My friend's grandpa was having surgery for cancer ... the first thing I did was I looked up and I was like, "[deceased child], can you look out for grandpa?" (#8)	8 (23)
Imagine	I can only imagine what she would have said if she was still living. (#13)	3 (9)
Parents' social world	I just have to talk about her. (#20)	26 (74)
Community	The funeral director said he had never seen so many people come out for a baby. They ran out of flags for the cars; that's how many people came out. (#16)	19 (54)
Health professionals	It really meant a lot to me how good they were with R and how much they treated her like a child and not a series of medical events. (#18)	15 (43)
Siblings	They talk about her a lot. If I say, "C, who's my favorite daughter?" she's like, "Your favorite daughter on earth is me; your favorite daughter in heaven is her." (#5)	7 (20)

a n (%) = number and percentage of follow-up meetings demonstrating each meaning-making process.

Table 36.4 Identity reconstruction process observed during follow-up meetings (*N* = 35)

Identity reconstruction	Example (follow-up meeting number)	*n* (%)*a*
Good parent	I have no doubt that I did a really good job caring for him. (#6)	23 (66)
Life changes	I have to figure out what my purpose is now. (#18)	22 (63)
Relationships	I had another baby. Yeah, L, and everything's well with him. And that's kept me going. (#4)	18 (51)
Work	I am getting ready to go back to school and hopefully going to be up here working soon. (#10)	9 (26)
Environment	She said, "We have to sell the house." We have another house on the river. We bought it a few years ago for investment.... So, he said, "Fix that up and we're going to go." (#34)	5 (14)
Travel	We're going on a cruise ... getting away, just the two of us ... we met on a cruise 22 years ago. (#1)	2 (6)
Hobbies	I'm back to the choir now ... I got to do something I like, and he liked, and so I'll do it in his honor and move on. (#1)	1 (3)
Number of children	There's always that question, how many kids do you have? I hate that question. I have four kids, but ... (#2)	2 (6)

a n (%) = number and percentage of follow-up meetings demonstrating each meaning-making process.

must understand how to meet a family where they are in order to foster open communication around the issues that are most important to the patient and the family.

When families are faced with having to make hard healthcare decisions for their children, open and effective communication impacts how information is received. The necessary communication skills that the provider must possess include marrying effective general communication with complex medical topics and patient-centered decisions.[18] Training medical professionals how to effectively communicate with their patients builds confidence in the provider. This confidence then facilitates a trusting relationship in which difficult conversations are more productive.[19]

Preparation for the conversation is key for the provider and the family. Understanding the goals of the communication and the topics that will be covered allows the participants to feel more at ease with the expectations. Giving space for the concerns of the family and how they will best be supported in having difficult conversations is essential to ensuring productivity. This facilitation fosters trust and opens the door to effective communication regardless of how difficult the topic. Conversations that help align family perspectives and values with anticipated medical outcomes will be more accepted if the communication is trusted and facilitated appropriately. This rapport allows for trust during the times when communication is occurring with medical uncertainty and the communication is rapidly changing. Parents consider communication to be a key component of their QOL.[20]

Communication surrounding goals of care across the illness trajectory empowers the patient and family to make informed decisions in the face of uncertainty. An interdisciplinary approach to goals-of-care communication ensures that all aspects of the patient's care are being addressed. Cohesive goal conversations hinge largely on care providers being consistent in their messaging and collaboration as a healthcare interdisciplinary team. When planning communication, whether there is a need to revisit goals or have an initial meeting, making sure that all disciplines are involved will ensure that the patient's needs are effectively and globally addressed.

Case Study: A Patient with a Congenital Heart Defect and Hydrocephalus

Matthew was diagnosed at birth with a congenital heart defect and hydrocephalus, requiring shunt placement. His challenging journey involved spending 9 months in the NICU/PICU. Upon discharge, he went home with private duty nursing services and the necessary durable medical equipment for in-home care. Over a 3-day period, his mother received education and training, attending approximately six care team meetings during his hospitalization.

After just a week at home, Matthew had to be readmitted to the hospital due to a code event. Further investigation revealed a malfunction in his shunt, necessitating replacement. Unfortunately, he experienced a cardiac arrest during surgery but was successfully resuscitated. Due to infection, his shunt was externalized, and he was placed in the PICU on ventilator support. Another 4 weeks passed before a palliative care consult took place, prompted by yet another code event and unsuccessful conversations regarding Matthew's code status and prognosis with his mother.

Following the palliative care consult, a comprehensive care team meeting was scheduled, involving the PICU physician, PICU nurse, neurosurgeon, cardiologist, social worker, palliative care physician and nurse, and the child life specialist for the PICU. The palliative care team nurse met with Matthew's mother beforehand to discuss his trajectory and care goals. She admitted that, prior to the consult, she had not fully grasped the severity of Matthew's condition, despite previous code events and discussions about the futility of treatment. Realizing the need for decisions on limiting interventions due to his fragile state and recent health decline, she acknowledged the importance of the upcoming care team meeting.

On the morning of the meeting, the palliative care nurse once again met with Matthew's mother, clarifying the goals and attendees. Preliminary questions were addressed to ensure a productive meeting. During the session, Matthew's mother actively engaged, asking relevant questions. Care goals were thoroughly discussed, and she sought more information on a tailored resuscitation plan instead of signing a do-not-resuscitate form. Post-meeting, the care team collectively agreed that this was the most productive care goal discussion since Matthew's PICU admission. The palliative care nurse also met with Matthew's mother afterward to confirm the consistency of the message conveyed during the meeting. Overall satisfaction among the team and Matthew's mom improved significantly following this enhanced level of communication.

Communication and Impact on Outcomes

Matthew's case illustrates how patient outcomes are directly impacted by the way communication is handled. Parental reports of dissatisfaction can stem from the way in which communication was handled during the critical times of their child's illness trajectory. Similar to Matthew's case, families report that they are not confident in the medical knowledge provided; they feel there is a lack of emotional consideration, a continued emphasis on a cure without realistic conversations surrounding refocusing care goals, a delay in this realistic communication, and a lack of privacy during these delicate conversations.[18]

Even though the intention of the care team was to provide Matthew's mother with education and guidance regarding his diagnosis and prognosis, the tenuous environment of the PICU challenged Matthew's mother's communication needs. The rapport necessary to foster the trusting relationship needed for these difficult conversations effectively must be established early in the trajectory.[21]

Families express that the information they find most critical during early diagnostic discussions is regarding symptom management, what to expect from the diagnosis, and what testing is necessary.[18] Parents who report good communication experiences with their healthcare providers include such contributing factors as communication skills that included open and sympathetic dialogue and direct communication regarding the diagnosis in private with adequate time to absorb and clarify the information provided.[18] Parents like Matthew's mom express the inherent desire to have their needs valued and heard.

Value-Based Decision-Making

Just as parents want their children's needs communicated and valued, they also want to know that the decisions they are making regarding the care of their children are based on the values that are important to them. The child's value and significance are important to the family, and how care goals are handled by providers has a reflection on this value. Engaging conversations around goals of care not only to include what medical needs may be present but also understanding the importance of the family's values will guide these goals regardless of the medical trajectory. Quality of life is defined by the World Health Organization as an individual's view of their role in life, shaped by the cultural and value systems they are part of, and influenced by their goals, expectations, standards, and concerns.[22] Promoting an environment where QOL and personal values are at the forefront when discussing goals of care will foster collaboration and cohesiveness.[23]

Preparing Families for Uncertainty

Patients and families report realistic expectations about the possibility for decline when faced with life-threatening illnesses, but uncertainty around when or how this decline will occur.[24] The complexity of the illness and making value-based decisions for their child's health management can be complicated by this unknown. Parents confronted with the fact that their child's health had declined over time talked about *when* the child would die in contrast to parents faced with the immediate threat of acute changes who talked about *whether* the child would die.[25]

Pediatric palliative care is designed to support families through this uncertainty with a collaborative team approach that changes as the patient's and/or family's needs change.[26] Understanding the changing landscape of the illness trajectory is both crucial and difficult for healthcare providers and parents alike. Parents do not expect that healthcare providers have all of the answers but instead seek honest and caring providers who are available to answer their questions.[21] Uncertainty throughout the illness trajectory is not an unexpected difficulty; however, the challenge comes with preparing families and patients to anticipate changing care goals. Palliative care should be delivered in a way that anticipates these unique and changing needs. This care should be delivered in a flexible and collaborative manner while anticipating the needs of the patient and family.[26]

The timing of palliative care involvement plays an important part in establishing care goals that transcend the initial diagnosis. Integrating the palliative care team as part of the primary care team will foster the trust necessary when uncertainty and difficult conversations present themselves. Timely involvement of the palliative care team can positively impact outcomes, for both children and adults, including pain and symptom management; effective patient–provider communication; support for decision-making; coordination of care; spiritual, emotional, and psychological care; and bereavement.[27]

Whether the child has been chronically or acutely ill, changing trajectories and uncertain outcomes are stress-inducing for the family. Fear and anticipation of the next hospitalization or setback are constant when caring for a child with a life-threatening illness. The decline may have been seen over a longer period, or it may be a more rapid illness that prompts the hospitalization that could mean the change in the current trajectory. Provider support for both the physical and emotional needs during this critical time is invaluable. Palliative care has often been considered when having end-of-life conversations, when, in reality, palliative care is most supportive when utilized across the illness trajectory to ensure the anticipation of changes in the patient's goals of care.[28]

Case Study: A Patient with an Evolving Trajectory of Care

Upon birth, Payton was diagnosed with a rare genetic disorder impacting her overall health. Her early life was marked by complications such as cataracts, hip dysplasia, a heart murmur, and hearing loss. By her first birthday, Payton had undergone eight surgeries, initiating a prolonged and intricate medical journey characterized by persistent uncertainty. Despite enduring numerous surgeries and hospitalizations over 6 years, Payton's mental capacity remained limited, never progressing beyond a 9-month-old level. She lacked the ability to sit, crawl, or talk. The trajectory of her health was consistently challenged by new medical complexities, resulting in 20 surgeries and countless hospital stays. Each hospitalization introduced fresh concerns and necessitated goal adjustments, with what was considered a return to baseline at the end of each hospital stay. In retrospect, her mother noted a gradual and subtle decline in Payton's overall baseline, which, as her primary caregiver, was not immediately apparent.

At the age of 6, Payton was admitted to the hospital with suspected feeding intolerance. During this hospitalization, her parents engaged in daily rounds with the medical team, learning about her evolving health status and the uncertainty surrounding her condition. This uncertainty was not unfamiliar, given the rarity of Payton's case. However, this hospitalization brought a new level of uncertainty—not about what was acutely happening but about whether she would recover from this setback. With no pediatric palliative care team available, the general pediatric team managed her care and consulted specialists to address the complex health needs faced by Payton and her family.

After 2 weeks in the hospital, it became evident that this was not a typical admission. Payton's lab values could not be normalized, and her body seemed to be in decline. On the 17th day, an external pediatric hospice team was consulted to assess the possibility of providing care at home. During the meeting with Payton's mother, it became clear that returning to her baseline health status was unlikely. The family expressed their desire to shift the focus to symptom management, discontinuing exhaustive testing that had characterized previous attempts to understand Payton's decline. The primary pediatrician documented the family's wishes, establishing an order for allowing natural death and discontinuing enteral feeds due to their symptom burden.

Given the complexity of Payton's care and the presence of a sibling at home, a follow-up meeting was scheduled. The pediatrician, hospice nurse, social worker, and child life specialist collaborated with the family to answer questions and plan for the end of Payton's life. Considering the circumstances, it was decided that Payton would remain in the hospital under the care of the hospice team, working in tandem with the hospital care team. The family was offered memory-making and legacy-building opportunities, and a hospice care plan was devised to provide comprehensive support. On the 40th day of her hospitalization, Payton passed away with her family by her side. The family received bereavement support for 2 years after her death.

Reflecting on the experience, Payton's mother emphasized the increasing complexity of medical issues and the realization that no treatment could remedy her condition. Involving the appropriate hospice team provided concurrent support, helping the family navigate their daughter's life-threatening illness with compassion and empathy. The decision to incorporate hospice care aimed to ensure a compassionate support system during the last 40 days of Payton's life, facilitating a smoother transition from illness to loss and grief. The hospice care team proved to be an invaluable resource for the entire family during this challenging time.

Clinician Challenges when Leading through Uncertainty

As illustrated in Payton's case, uncertainty is a constant when caring for patients with life-threatening illnesses. Supporting families through rapidly changing health status and goals of care is challenging at best. Understanding the delicate balance between hope and realistic expectations is essential to the well-being of the patient, family, and clinician. Clinician support is often overlooked in the pursuit to care for the patient and family. The severe illness and death of a child is out of the "natural order" of things. Bearing witness to the isolation or suffering of children is distressing for families and providers alike.[29]

Clinicians need support while guiding families through uncertainty. Without proper support, clinicians can become ineffective in the care they are able to provide, which will further complicate the course. Promoting a professional environment that validates the providers' needs throughout the time they are caring for a complex patient will foster healthy discussion and support.[28] Understanding their own grief is paramount, given how this grief can impact the care the clinician is able to provide. Clinicians may have been providing care for this patient throughout the illness trajectory, and an acute change in the patient's health status or the patient entering a terminal phase is emotionally distressing.[30]

Families express effective communication as a consistent theme when discussing their satisfaction with the delivery of care for their children living with complex health needs. For clinicians to be effective communicators, they must first understand their personal comfort level with having these conversations and supporting families through uncertainty. To avoid their discomfort being misconstrued as insensitivity, the clinician must fully grasp this concept. Self-awareness is crucial.[31] Providers are faced with identifying their own emotions surrounding their mortality and grief processes. Continuously providing care to critically ill children, where the focus needs to shift from curative to more palliative care, is emotionally taxing. Having a grasp of how each clinician handles this emotion is essential to ensure quality care for the patient and sustainability for the clinician.[32]

Conclusion

In conclusion, the journey through the challenging terrain of pediatric palliative care illuminates the profound disparities in understanding and defining the QOL for children facing life-threatening illnesses. As families navigate the intricate intersection between the medical culture and their own, the role of the palliative care clinician emerges as pivotal—a bicultural figure tasked with facilitating comprehension and bridging the gap between two worlds. QOL, viewed through the lens of young patients and their families, becomes a dynamic and context-dependent metric, intimately entwined with individual values and goals. The bed-bound child in the ICU perceives quality differently from the newly diagnosed asymptomatic patient, emphasizing the need for a flexible and personalized approach. The understanding that clinicians may harbor distinct perspectives on quality and outcomes further underscores the imperative for early integration of palliative care, including eliciting values and perspectives that influence goals of care and decision-making. In essence, the journey of pediatric palliative care patients reveals a spectrum of life that defies conventional expectations, challenging clinicians to broaden their understanding and embrace the unique narratives embedded in each family's cultural and personal context.

REFERENCES

1. Flaig F, Lotz JD, Knochel K, Borasio GD, Führer M, Hein K. Perinatal palliative care: a qualitative study evaluating the perspectives of pregnancy counselors. *Palliat Med.* 2019;33(6):704–711. https://doi.org/10.1177/0269216319834225.
2. Brouwer MA, Maeckelberghe ELM, van der Heide A, Hein IM, Verhagen EAAE. Breaking bad news: what parents would like you to know. *Arch Dis Child.* 2021;106(3):276–281. https://doi.org/10.1136/archdischild-2019-318398.
3. Kawasaki H, Yamada T, Takahashi Y, Nakayama T, Wada T, Kosugi S; Neonatal Research Network of Japan. The short-term mortality and morbidity of very low birth weight infants with trisomy 18 or trisomy 13 in Japan. *J Hum Genet.* 2021;66(3):273–285. https://doi.org/10.1038/s10038-020-00825-6.
4. Buskmiller C, Ho S, Chen M, Gants S, Crowe E, Lopez S. Patient-centered perinatal palliative care: family birth plans, outcomes, and resource utilization in a diverse cohort. *Am J Obstet Gynecol.* 2022;4(6):100725. https://doi.org/10.1016/j.ajogmf.2022.100725.
5. Janvier A, Farlow B, Barrington KJ, Bourque CJ, Brazg T, Wilfond B. Building trust and improving communication with parents of children with trisomy 13 and 18: a mixed-methods study. *Palliat Med.* 2020;34(3):262–271. https://doi.org/10.1177/0269216319860662.
6. Nelson KE, Rosella LC, Mahant S, Guttmann A. Survival and surgical interventions for children with trisomy 13 and 18. *JAMA.* 2016;316(4):420–428.
7. Soft. Support Organization for Trisomy. September 22, 2022. Accessed December 18, 2023. https://trisomy.org/.
8. Cuviello A, Pasli M, Hurley C, Bhatia S, Anghelescu DL, Baker JN. Compassionate de-escalation of life-sustaining treatments in pediatric oncology: an opportunity for palliative care and intensive care collaboration. *Front Oncol.* 2022;12:1017272. https://doi.org/10.3389/fonc.2022.1017272.
9. Rosenberg AR, Wolfe J. Approaching the third decade of pediatric palliative oncology investigation: historical progress and future directions. *Lancet Child Adolesc Health.* 2017;1(1):56–67.
10. Srivastava R, Srivastava S. Parental perspective in paediatric palliative care: a systematic review of literature using the PRISMA method. Indian Journal of Palliative Care. 2022;28:199–215. https://doi.org/10.25259/IJPC_37_2021.

11. Klages KL, Chardon ML, Drake SN, Myers KC, Morrison CF, Pai ALH. Pain, depressive symptoms, and health-related quality of life among survivors of pediatric hematopoietic stem cell transplant. *Pediatr Blood Cancer*. 2022;69(10):e29846. https://doi.org/10.1002/pbc.29846.
12. Ullrich CK, Rodday AM, Bingen K, et al. Parent outlook: how parents view the road ahead as they embark on hematopoietic stem cell transplantation for their child. *Biol Blood Marrow Transplant*. 2016;22(1):104–111.
13. Gunter MD, Duke G. Social support to reduce uncertainty in childhood cancer in south Texas: a case study. *J Pediatr Oncol Nurs*. 2019;36(3):207–218. https://doi.org/10.1177/1043454219835450.
14. Bronsema A, Theißen T, Oechsle K, et al. Looking back: identifying supportive care and unmet needs of parents of children receiving specialist paediatric palliative care from the bereavement perspective. *BMC Palliat Care*. 2022;21(1):87. https://doi.org/10.1186/s12904-022-00971-y.
15. Meert KL, Eggly S, Kavanaugh K, et al.; for Eunice Kennedy Shriver National Institute of Child Health and Human Development Collaborative Pediatric Critical Care Research Network. Meaning making during parent–physician bereavement meetings after a child's death. *Health Psychol*. 2015;34(4):453–461.
16. Rasouli O, Moksnes UK, Reinfjell T, Hjemdal O, Eilertsen MEB. Impact of resilience and social support on long-term grief in cancer-bereaved siblings: an exploratory study. *BMC Palliat Care*. 2022;21(1):93. https://doi.org/10.1186/s12904-022-00978-5.
17. Buang SNH, Loh SW, Mok YH, Lee JH, Chan YH. Palliative and critical care: their convergence in the pediatric intensive care unit. *Front Pediatr*. 2022;10:907268. https://doi.org/10.3389/fped.2022.907268.
18. Fratantoni K, Livingston J, Schellinger SE, Aoun SM, Lyon ME. Family-centered advance care planning: what matters most for parents of children with rare diseases. *Children (Basel)*. 2022;9(3):445. https://doi.org/10.3390/children9030445.
19. James C, Styres C, Palombo S, Morvant A. Impact of pediatric palliative care intensive educational session on resident confidence in caring for children and families with serious illness (QI727). *J Pain Symptom Manage*. 2021;61(3):666.
20. Zhukovsky D, Herzog C, Kaur G, Palmer J, Bruera E. The impact of palliative care consultation on symptom assessment, communication needs, and palliative interventions in pediatric patients with cancer. *J Palliat Med*. 2009;12(4):343–349. https://doi.org/10.1089/jpm.2008.0152.
21. Lewis-Newby M, Sellers DE, Meyer EC, Solomon MZ, Zurakowski D, Truog RD. Location of clinician–family communication at the end of life in the pediatric intensive care unit and clinician perception of communication quality. *J Palliat Med*. 2020;23(8):152–159. https://doi.org/10.1089/jpm.2019.0511.
22. Rasalingam A, Brekke I, Stenberg U, Haaland-Øverby M, Helseth S. "Struggling to participate in everyday life": emerging adults' experiences of living with long-term health challenges. *BMC Public Health*. 2023;23(1):1368. https://doi.org/10.1186/s12889-023-16291-6.
23. World Health Organization. The World Health Organization quality of life assessment (WHOQOL): position paper from the World Health Organization. *Soc Sci Med*. 1995;46:1569–1585.
24. Coombes L, Braybrook D, Roach A, et al. Achieving child-centred care for children and young people with life-limiting and life-threatening conditions—a qualitative interview study. *Eur J Pediatr*. 2022;181(10):3739–3752. https://doi.org/10.1007/s00431-022-04566-w.
25. Kline C, Reineke A, Auger J, Willert J, Roberts W, Schiff D. Effects of a unique pediatric hematology–oncology palliative care program on medical decision-making and communication between healthcare providers and families: results of a supportive care survey. *Prog Palliat Care*. 2012;20(1):13–18.
26. Lovell T, Mitchell M, Powell M, et al. Dying in intensive care: an analysis of the perspectives of families and clinicians on end-of-life care. *Aust Crit Care*. 2023;36(4):595–603. https://doi.org/10.1016/j.aucc.2022.07.004.
27. Green DJ, Bennett E, Olson LM, et al. Timing of pediatric palliative care consults in hospitalized patients with heart disease. *J Pediatr Intens Care*. 2023;12(1):63–70. https://doi.org/10.1055/s-0041-1730916.
28. Davis JAM, Bass A, Humphrey L, Texter K, Garee A. Early integration of palliative care in families of children with single ventricle congenital heart defects: a quality improvement project to enhance family support. *Pediatr Cardiol*. 2020;41(1):114–122. https://doi.org/10.1007/s00246-019-02231-y.
29. Jonas D, Bogetz J. Identifying the deliberate prevention and intervention strategies of pediatric palliative care teams supporting providers during times of staff distress. *J Palliat Med*. 2016;19(6):679–683.
30. Shorey S, Chua C. Nurses and nursing students' experiences on pediatric end-of-life care and death: a qualitative systematic review. *Nurse Educ Today*. 2022;112:105332. https://doi.org/10.1016/j.nedt.2022.105332.
31. Beckstrand RL, Willmore EE, Macintosh JLB, Luthy KE. Critical care nurses' qualitative reports of experiences with physician behaviors, nursing issues, and other obstacles in end-of-life care. *Dimens Crit Care Nurs*. 2021;40(4):237–247. https://doi.org/10.1097/DCC.0000000000000479.
32. Stayer D. Living with dying in the pediatric intensive care unit: a nursing perspective. *Am J Crit Care*. 2016;25(4):350–356.

37

Communication Components for Determining Goals of Care and Advance Care Planning in Pediatric Palliative Care

Deborah Lafond and Kathy Perko

Key Points

- Effective communication between children, their families, and their healthcare team is an integral part of pediatric palliative care, and assessing and identifying what is most important to the child and family are crucial to guide care.
- Understanding the values of children and their families is critical to enable decision-making that respects their perspective on what they consider most important.
- Children may have a desire to be involved in making decisions. Each child should be assessed in terms of their cognitive development, interest, and understanding to help determine their competence in assisting with decision-making.
- Nurses have a professional responsibility to facilitate communication and informed child and family decision-making.

Case Study

Aniya is a 12-year-old Black female diagnosed with a malignant brain tumor. The treatment plan includes surgery, radiation, and chemotherapy. Her blended family actively practices a deep Christian faith. Aniya is in the sixth grade and an honor student. She hopes to be an engineer when she grows up. Her parents divorced when Aniya was 3 years old. Her mother remarried and has two other children (ages 4 years and 8 years) with her new husband. Aniya's father is single and is very involved in Aniya's life. Maternal and paternal grandparents are also actively involved and are a great support to Aniya and her parents. Aniya's mother, stepfather, and father work full time. She attends an afterschool program at her school. She enjoys reading, cheerleading, and playing with her siblings and friends.

Introduction

What is most important to Aniya and her family guides best care practices. Effective communication between children, families, and the healthcare team is an integral part of pediatric palliative care (PPC), and assessing and identifying what is most important to the child and family are crucial. Goals of care include medical and non-medical hopes and expectations.[1] Goals of care are established at diagnosis, and discussions continue throughout the trajectory of the illness.[2] They involve a broad range of elements, including joining a family event, planning an adventure or a trip, attending school or other important activities, or completing a milestone. These goals represent their hopes of a future and may not rely on an understanding of the seriousness of their current illness. It is not uncommon for an adolescent to plan for a future even with a clear understanding of their terminal disease.

Advance care planning evolves from goals-of-care conversations. Advance care planning discussions and documentation capture the child's voice and wishes, ideally prior to the child losing the ability to express their wishes. Many children are unable to fully participate in advance care planning discussions due to age, developmental abilities, or child or family preference. At these times, advance care planning often becomes less about documenting preferences before capacity is lost and more about helping surrogate decision makers, typically parents, think and plan for decisions that need to be made at the time and in the future.[3] While the previous chapter focuses on understanding the values and perspectives that influence patients' and families' goals of care and the decision-making process, this chapter will describe the essential components of communicating with children and their families around goals of care and decision-making through the trajectory of serious illness. A case example will illustrate the use of talking maps as one way to structure and navigate these challenging conversations.

Background

While pediatric deaths are relatively rare compared to adult deaths, these lives represent the loss of the future of society.[4] These lives also represent significant impact on families and friends. There is also impact on the workforce through loss of caregivers to care for the ill child or delay in return to work following the death of a child.

Decisions such as goals of care driven by child and family values, advance care planning, and those at the end of life, and how they are made, may impact parent grief and bereavement as well. Many parents indicate that feeling that they have been good parents, doing everything possible, and having their wishes for their child's care respected are priorities in making decisions at the end of life.[5]

Decision-Making

Shared decision-making (SDM) is the cornerstone of child- and family-centered care and imperative in eliciting goals of care. SDM has been described as a process by which children, families, and clinicians work together to make optimal healthcare decisions that align with what matters most to the child.[6] The SDM process is especially challenging in pediatric care as it includes the wishes of the child, the legal authority of the parents, and the expertise of the healthcare team in an ever-evolving relationship as the child's developmental level and understanding may be changing. What is essential to facilitate effective SDM with families is accurate and honest communication between the healthcare team and the family, as shown in Table 37.1.

In a systematic review of studies from 2000 to 2016, Sisk et al.[7] noted that parents also need to understand the diagnosis and prognosis. Communication of prognosis is essential to parents' understanding and will allow them to make decisions regarding their children's treatment that best align with their values and preferences. Assessing the children's and families' preferences in receiving information will provide the healthcare team with essential data in conveying this sensitive and valuable information. Uncertainty will always exist in prognostication. Clinicians must be mindful that family preferences about how and how much information to receive regarding diagnosis and prognosis are variable, not only between differing backgrounds but between any given individual within any culture, race, ethnicity, or religion.[8] This is further complicated by the fact that accurate prognostication is difficult for even the very

Table 37.1 Essential core functions of clinician–child/parent communication defined for pediatrics

Core function	Definition	Examples
Foster healing relationships	Providing emotional supports and anticipatory guidance to inform understanding of the child's underlying illness and treatment options.	The primary medical team relays information from the time of diagnosis in an honest, clear, and compassionate way, which facilitates trust throughout the trajectory of the child's illness.
Exchanging information	The child, parents, and healthcare team share information about their understanding of the diagnosis, treatment options, prognosis, and anticipated adverse events.	The parents provide the primary medical team with information they have found on the internet about a promising treatment and seek the healthcare team's guidance on beginning this treatment. The healthcare team provides information about any results in previous studies, risks and benefits of this treatment, and how it may help or hinder the child's prognosis.
Responding to emotions	From the time of diagnosis throughout the trajectory of the child's illness, parents and the child may experience a variety of emotions, such as anger, denial, sadness, worry, anxiety, depression, etc. The healthcare team acknowledges these emotions and actively seeks to provide appropriate resources to support the child and parents, clarifying their emotional state, communicating understanding, and responding in an empathetic manner.	The mother of a child with a serious illness is noted to be crying in the radiology waiting room while her child is undergoing testing. The social worker acknowledges that she can see that the mother is upset and asks her to explain why she is in distress. The social worker listens actively to the mother's expressed worries and fears that her child's illness is worsening because she has seen physical signs and symptoms that are similar to those seen at diagnosis. The social worker validates that she understands why the mother may be worried and reassures her that she will stay with her until the test is completed, then let the primary medical team know her worries so that they can communicate the results of testing as soon as possible.
Managing uncertainty	There are many periods of uncertainty during the trajectory of childhood cancer, for example, prognosis, unanticipated adverse events, survivorship, late effects of treatment, options for treatment, etc. In managing uncertainty, the healthcare team provides as much information as known to anticipate periods of uncertainty and dispel uncertainty when answers are known.	A child with a progressive serious illness is entering the active dying phase. The family asks when to anticipate death. The advanced practice nurse provides anticipatory guidance of the signs and symptoms of the dying process and how the family can comfort their dying child during this time.
Making decisions	Accurate and timely information on the diagnosis, prognosis, treatment options, anticipated side effects, and alternatives to treatment is essential to making decisions. Communication of this information must be clear, honest, and given in a developmentally appropriate way. The family's values, preferences, and style of decision-making must be assessed carefully.	The physician, nurse, and social worker meet with the family of a child with a newly diagnosed serious, potentially life-limiting, illness. The team assesses the family's understanding of the diagnosis and their values, preferences, and fears. Options for disease-directed care and palliative care are discussed with the family. The physician discusses the risks/benefits, anticipated side effects, and required testing with the family.
Enabling child and family health-seeking behaviors	The healthcare team carefully assesses the family's past history with medical care and decision-making, the child's current medical condition with anticipated treatments, and other variables which may affect the child's and family's ability to cope effectively. By acknowledging the role of the child, the family, and the healthcare team, better health-seeking behaviors can lead to improved coping skills throughout treatment and beyond into survivorship or a peaceful death, if that is the ultimate outcome.	The social worker performs a thorough psychosocial assessment of the child and family to identify strengths and areas for needed supports. These are communicated to the healthcare team so that a comprehensive plan of care can be developed to address physical, emotional, spiritual, and environmental needs.

Source: Reference 6.

experienced clinician. Conversations can be unclear, leading to ambiguity for families in weighing their decisions. In some cases, parents may not be offered all treatment options due to the unconscious biases of clinicians.

Utilizing the skill of "best case, worse case, most likely case" may help in providing reasonable expectations without focusing on an exact timeline. This skill involves the use of clinical data and scenarios to illustrate the best and worst potential outcomes. Families may define their "best" case or "worst" case differently based upon their values and preferences, which may or may not align with outcomes defined by the healthcare team. The clinician adds a most likely outcome based on the expertise of the clinical teams involved. This intervention may alleviate mistrust that happens when the prognostication does not match the child's condition. Clinicians should use clear language when prognosticating. Some families are not ready to make decisions to limit non-beneficial life-prolonging interventions, despite skilled conversations about late goals of care. In this case, proposing a trial of an intervention for a reasonable time to evaluate benefits and burdens may be appropriate. Be sure to discuss the length of the trial, what parameters will be assessed for benefit, and the next steps.

Back et al.[9] convey the importance of using the words "death" and "dying" and to avoid the temptation to provide reassurance about the actual prognosis and confuse the message. The process of decision-making is complex. Families may request a recommendation from the healthcare team. Linebarger et al.[10] share that families appreciate a recommendation that is consistent with their own shared values and goals. A recommendation from the team helps families feel the decision-making process is a truly shared one.[11] It is important to remember that a child and family have a right to accept the recommendation or not.

Hinds and colleagues identified important reasons that influence parent end-of-life (EOL) treatment decision-making. In interviews with more than 100 parents of children with incurable cancers across several studies, the majority of parents (approximately 80% within each study) identified their definition of being a good parent as influencing their EOL decision-making on behalf of their very ill child.[12] Key characteristics of their definition of being a good parent to a seriously ill child are listed in Box 37.1 These characteristics did not differ by type of EOL decision made or by diagnosis.[13] Parents also identified clinician behaviors that helped them to achieve their definition of being a good parent before their child died. This research has been replicated in the pediatric intensive care unit (PICU), documenting the most common factors in being a good parent to their seriously ill child included prioritizing their child's QOL, advocating with the healthcarel team for their child's needs, and focusing on their child's needs over their own.[14,15] Engaging parents in a discussion of what it uniquely means to them to be a good parent to their child may illuminate things that matter most to the child and family.

Ethical and Legal Considerations in Goals of Care and Advance Directive Conversations

Ethical issues and decision-making in PPC are different than for adults, who are largely considered competent and able to make their own decisions. Macauley[16] shares that the unique diagnoses and illness trajectories and the societal expectation that "children aren't supposed to die" often lead to more aggressive treatment and delays in palliative care consultations. Another important distinction is that the decision maker is rarely the child, and the best-interest standard is more often used than in the adult model of autonomy. Please see Chapter 38, "Ethical Considerations in Pediatric Palliative Care," for more information.

Communication Pearls in Pediatric Goals of Care and Advance Care Planning

What is said and how it is said are crucial in providing child- and family-centered care for children with serious illness and their families. One size does not fit all, and while tools exist to enhance communication in pediatric serious illness, conversations must be tailored to each unique child, each unique family, and each unique clinical situation. This section will provide examples of tools and skills that may assist nurses at all levels of practice in developing the skills needed to be compassionate in crucial conversations with children with serious illness, their families, and other members of the healthcare team.

Box 37.1 Parent Themes from Their Definition of Being a Good Parent to Their Seriously Ill Child[12]

Parent themes	Clinician strategies
Doing right by my child	All that can be done is being done
Being there for my child	Staff respect me and my decisions
Conveying love to my child	Staff continue to comfort my child and me
Being a good life example	Staff know our special needs
Being an advocate for my child	Staff like our child
Letting the Lord lead	Staff are pleasant
Not allowing suffering	Staff coordinate care
Making my child healthy	Staff ask about our faith
Making sure I have all the information I need	Give us the facts
Feeling valued	Staff tell us we are good parents
Not feeling abandoned	Do not quit on us

Goals-of-Care Conversations

Goals-of-care conversations are essential to PPC. Ideally, goals-of-care conversations should occur at diagnosis of any serious illness and continue throughout the trajectory of the disease.[17]

Initiating these conversations during less stressful times is ideal; however, there are times when conversations need to happen during a crisis. Especially at those times, the human aspect of communication is crucial, and families must be provided as much time and empathy as possible. Creating these connections allows for trust and an environment to discuss values, hopes, and worries for the child and family.

Conversations around goals of care begin with asking about families' beliefs, values, and experiences. It is only after their preferences are shared that the healthcare team can begin an honest and realistic discussion of care. The child and family make decisions based on understanding the information they have received, trust in their healthcare providers, and individual preferences in care. The American Academy of Pediatrics Policy Statement on Pediatric Palliative and Hospice Care Commitments, Guidelines and Recommendations, emphasize the importance of goals-of-care conversations occurring over time and being revisited when requested by the child or family, with significant change in prognosis, and at least yearly for children with chronic disease.[18] A goals-of-care conversation is often part of a family care conference. Careful preparation for family meetings will allow thoughtful and fruitful conversations for both families and clinicians and assures that the healthcare team will provide a united conversation. Please see Chapter 9, "Enhancing Team Effectiveness," for more information.

Approaching a family meeting in a stepwise fashion may be helpful.[19]

Pre-meet to ask for each member of the healthcare team's view and propose an agenda for the meeting. This is done prior to meeting with the child (if present) and the family.

Introduce each person at the meeting, including their role or social connection to the family. It is advised to ask the family if there is anyone they would like included in the care conference, which could be additional family members or members of the healthcare team. Beginning with the family members, offer respect for their time and commitment to their child. Thank each person for coming, ask the family for any specific information they would like to discuss, add that to the proposed agenda, and explain the purpose of the meeting.

Assess what the family knows. It is important not to ask the family what they "understand" as that may sound like a test. Another way to assess knowledge would be to ask what their medical team has shared about their child during their last visit or phone call.

Update the medical condition before moving on to decisions. Provide important updates, and to assure their understanding, you can ask "Was I clear in explaining this?"

Empathize with each person to show that you are fully engaged. Acknowledging emotion creates psychological safety and shows you care. A short, clear statement is most helpful: "I can see you care so much about your child."

Prioritize the child's values (if present) while also asking about family values.

Align with the families' values and offer matching treatments. Reflecting back values shows the family you are listening. It might be helpful to say "This is what I am hearing is important to you and your child. Did I get that right?"

It is important to include the psychosocial members of the team at a goals-of-care discussion. Care conferences are often full of tense moments and big emotions. They offer an additional opportunity to respond to emotion and check the room for possible questions or misunderstandings. They also offer someone to be in tune with the child or adolescent if they attend the conference. Disclosed information should be tailored to the child's developmental stage and desire.[20] If they become overwhelmed or disengaged and the parents wish to continue, the psychosocial team member may accompany them out and offer support.

Successful family meetings involving goals-of-care discussions are often perceived as "high-stakes" conversations and are challenging for all involved. Taking time to prepare prior to engaging with the family is a necessary step to assure a clear and united conversation. This should include who will begin the conversation. Parents differ in who should initiate the conversation but desire it be done with kindness and sensitivity with appropriate involvement of their child.[21] Clinician training and experience with these discussions are often limited, which may increase the complexity of the discussion. These factors increase the importance of the team approach to these discussions. This allows each healthcare team member to participate in areas they are most comfortable with while providing personal and requested support for the child and family.

Responding to Emotion

Providing support to the child and family is paramount to successful goals-of-care conversations. Communicating serious news is one of the most challenging aspects of healthcare. Research suggests that many clinicians feel ill-prepared in communication techniques.[22] Managing heightened emotions during intense conversations may provoke anxiety. The key to addressing this anxiety is recognizing the emotion and responding to it with empathy. The mnemonic NURSE(S) provides six different ways to respond empathetically to emotion. They are not meant to be prescriptive or to be used all at once or in any specific order. It is a guide for supportive language when responding empathetically to an emotion cue.[23]

N = Name: Put the emotion into words to acknowledge it.
U = Understand: Explain how you see it from their perspective.
R = Respect: Admire what you genuinely see and feel good about.
S = Support: Offer caring, expertise, and presence.
E = Explore: Ask for more data or information.
S = Silence: Allow silence to encourage conversation from the child or family.

Case Study Continued

Aniya's parents are talking with Aniya's primary nurse prior to their first meeting with the palliative care team. Both parents have questions about palliative care and why they are meeting with them now. Aniya's mom shares that she already has "too much going on" and does not need "one more team" to help with Aniya and her disease when they are trying to cure her. "It is enough that we have oncology, neurology, and rehab services. Enough is enough!" The nurse recognizes that mom's emotion is high and uses NURSE(S) statements to support her with empathy.

Name: "This situation must feel overwhelming."
Understand: "I can only imagine how challenging it is to meet so many different teams."
Respect: "You are such an incredible advocate for Aniya."
Support: "As Aniya's primary nurse, I will continue to support all of you through her treatment."
Explore: "Can you tell me a bit more about what you are thinking?"

Aniya's mom sighs and shares "It is just all too much. She's been through so much already . . . we just want her to get better." The nurse allows silence, and Aniya's mom continues tearfully, "Of course we always want what is best for Aniya, and if you think they could be helpful, we can meet them."

NURSE(S) statements help de-escalate the emotion of Aniya's mother, allowing her to process the information more fully. Using one NURSE statement and allowing silence is a good starting point. It is not appropriate to use the NURSE statements back to back, without allowing silence and time for the person to respond.

Talking Maps for Goals of Care Discussions

Goals-of-care conversations may be awkward, even for the very experienced clinician. Several helpful tools, or talking maps, have been developed that aid in structuring these conversations. They can serve as algorithms for conversation planning and are not meant to be step-by-step prescriptions that replace the human connection in these meaningful conversations.[24] These talking maps, or guides, are simply a way to provide structure to the conversation; one size does not fit all. Clinicians should find a talking map, or combination of talking maps, that resonates with their professional communication style. Practice using them to become familiar with the structure of the talking map so that when used in conversations with children and families, it is natural and seamless. The talking maps discussed below are by no means an exhaustive review. There are many talking maps to choose from. These were chosen as examples that have been useful in PPC practice. In any conversation, it is imperative to assess the readiness of the child and family for these important conversations.[25] PPC brings additional challenges to consider as children age and mature over time, and some parents change their priorities over time.[5] Conversations will need to be revisited as clinical and developmental changes occur, which may change goals of care.

The GUIDE Talking Map

The GUIDE talking map developed by Vital Talk™ communication training[26] is helpful in framing conversation in serious illness for all ages. It is similar to the SPIKES model,[27] which includes *S*etting, *P*erception, *I*nvitation, *K*nowledge, *E*motion, and *S*trategy or *S*ummary. The GUIDE talking map reframes the "Invitation" section because some view the "Invitation" as irrelevant as no one ever will be "ready" for serious news.[28] The GUIDE Talking Map (Table 37.2) has similar steps: *G*et ready, *U*nderstand, *I*nformation, *D*eepen, and *E*quip. Know the current clinical, emotional, social, and cultural situation. Review the chart carefully and talk with the pertinent members of the medical teams in advance to establish what information is to be shared. Expect and respond to emotions; one's own, those of the child and/or family, and those of other members of the various medical teams and various disciplines. The GUIDE talking map can be used at any time in the trajectory of illness.

Case Study Continued

The palliative care team is meeting with the family for the first time. After introducing the team, using the GUIDE talking map is helpful in discussing difficult news at diagnosis. In this case, the GUIDE talking map may include:

G = Thorough review of the medical record and discussion with the neurologist, neurosurgeon, and oncologist to learn more about the diagnosis, prognosis, and plan of treatment. Other team members who may be essential to this case initially may include the social worker, chaplain, child life specialist, or other psychosocial clinicians. Discussion with these team members about the appropriateness of including Aniya in the initial conversations is key. One approach may be to first have a conversation with her parents and ask their thoughts on when and how to include Aniya.

U = Asking Aniya and/or her parents to share what the other medical teams have told them about the diagnosis and next steps. Avoid asking them to tell you what they "understand" as this may seem like a test of their knowledge.

I = Share what you know and understand about the diagnosis, prognosis, and treatment plan, including that you have reviewed the medical record and spoken with the pertinent medical teams.

D = Aniya and/or her family may respond with a variety of emotions, including sadness, anger, defeat, criticism, etc. Use NURSE(S) statements to respond appropriately to these emotions. This will help the clinician align with the family and begin to develop a relationship based on mutual respect and trust.

E = Share how the palliative care team can be helpful to Aniya and her family. Using language such as the 4 Ws (Table 37.2) can be helpful to let the family know you share their worries and you wish the situation was different, the ways quality of life and quality of time can be optimized, and what the next steps will be with the palliative care team. Equip them with the tools, support, and resources they most need.

The PAUSE Talking Map for Early Goals of Care

The PAUSE talking map[29] is helpful to frame discussions of goals of care earlier in the trajectory of serious illness. Evidence has shown that discussions of goals of care before a crisis allow the child and/or family to thoughtfully consider the things that matter most to them so that when the crisis occurs, they have already had discussions with the important people involved in decision-making. Decision-making in pediatric serious illness is never easy, and even early discussions of goals of care will not mitigate all potential issues. The most common barrier to these discussions is time. Being intentional to make time early in the trajectory of illness facilitates mutual respect and trust and uncovers what is meaningful to the child and

Table 37.2 The GUIDE Talking Map

	Meaning	Sample language	Pediatric considerations
G = Get Ready	• Get ready before the conversation. Know the clinical, social, emotional, and cultural situation through chart review and talking with key players in the child's care. • Choose and prepare the setting, considering privacy and a quiet location. • Invite the essential people to the conversation, keeping in mind not to overwhelm the child and/or family.		• Who are the legal decision makers? • Who are the important people to that child and/or family? • Is the child cognitively able to participate in the discussion and is it appropriate? • Children often have multiple medical teams involved. Who is essential to be at the meeting, and who will lead the discussion? Decide this in advance.
U = Understand	• Find out what the family and/or child already knows. • DO NOT ask them "What do you understand about you/your child's illness as this may cause them to feel they are being tested or their opinions are being challenged.	"What have the other doctors (teams) shared with you about your child's illness?" "We have reviewed your/your child's medical record and talked with the various teams about the current situation. Please share with us your thoughts and questions so that we can plan together what makes sense for the next steps."	• While decision-making usually defaults to the parents or legal guardian, children often have strong opinions on what is best for them. Grandparents and members from blended families may also have strong opinions that inform decision-making.
I = Inform	• Use a one- or two-sentence headline to deliver the key information.	• "The biopsy showed the cancer is back." • "The results of the genetic testing showed your child has muscular dystrophy."	• Keep language simple, and do not go into deeper explanations. • Use terms the child and/or family have used to describe the illness.
D = Deepen	• Respond to emotions to deepen the connection with the child and/or family.	• "I can only imagine how difficult this is to hear." • "This must be very difficult to hear. We were all hoping for different news."	• Use NURSE(S) statements. • If you are nervous or anxious, acknowledge that to yourself and ask yourself why you might be feeling this way. • If what you say does not come out quite right, acknowledge it and ask permission to try again.
E = Equip	• Equip the child and/or family with what the next steps are.	• The 4 Ws: "I wish . . ." "I worry . . ." "I wonder . . ." "I will . . ." • "Tell me what you will tell your family when you get home about this news." • "This has been a difficult conversation for us today. I wonder if meeting again this afternoon or tomorrow would be helpful so that you have time to think about all that we have talked about?"	• Summarize the information. • Explain the next steps. • Use a teach-back approach, as appropriate.

Source: Reference 26.

family. The PAUSE talking map (Table 37.3) includes the following steps: *P*ause, *A*sk permission, *U*ncover values, *S*uggest a surrogate, and *E*xpect emotion.

Case Study Continued

Aniya has completed 6 weeks of radiation therapy (XRT) and is due to have her first post-XRT magnetic resonance imaging (MRI) next week. The family anticipates talking with the medical team about chemotherapy options for the next steps in treatment. The palliative care team is seeing Aniya in a routine outpatient clinic appointment. They have conferred with the neuro-oncology team, and most of the team members agree to begin goals-of-care discussions. They have asked the palliative care team to lead this discussion with the family. The PAUSE talking map may be a helpful tool to structure this conversation.

P = Let the family know before the scheduled appointment that goals of care will be a topic of conversation. Be intentional about scheduling time for this discussion. Assessing readiness is essential. While this conversation may be on the team's agenda, it may not be the best timing for the family; however, many families avoid this conversation. Preparing the family that these types of conversations are held with all families of children with serious illness will normalize the experience and not portray that there has been news held back from the family that urgently needs discussion now. An analogy may be that automobile insurance is for support if one has a car accident. No one plans to have a car accident, and planning for what to do just in case is helpful.

A = Ask permission if now is a reasonable time to talk about some important things that are helpful for the team to know in planning the best possible care for Aniya. Frame this in terms of the family as experts in Aniya and what is important to her and the rest of the family. Sincerely offer that you value their opinion as part of the team.

U = Ask the family to tell you about Aniya as a person, especially since diagnosis and the early phases of treatment. Get to know them

Table 37.3 The PAUSE Talking Map

	Meaning	Sample language	Pediatric considerations
P = Pause	• Pause to make time for this discussion early in the child's illness.	"I would like to take some time to discuss the things that are most important to you/your child/your family."	• Be intentional in planning for goals-of-care conversations. • It is a series of conversations over time. • Keep in mind developmental changes over time as discussions will need to be revisited as the child matures.[3] • Who are the legal decision makers, and who are the caretakers who would be involved in carrying out these decisions? They may or may not be the same.
A = Ask Permission	Ask permission as you begin the conversation to indicate the importance of the discussion.	"You know your child better than anyone else. Sometimes a child gets sick suddenly, and we don't have time to ask them about the things that are most important to them." "I would like your opinion . . ." "Could we talk about an extreme situation that is very different from where we are now?"	• The most common barrier is time. • Avoid using personal attributions, such as "your child" and try more neutral terms such as "a child" or "other children," which distances the conversation a bit to make it a safer place to talk about the "what ifs."
U = Uncover Values	Find out what is most important to the child and family.	"What do I need to know about your child and you as people to give the best care possible?" "If the illness were to get very serious and it may take your child's life, what are the things that are most important to you/your child/your family?" "What are you hoping for?" "What would reaching that hope mean?"	• Do not start with a discussion of code status. • Establish mutual respect and trust. • Asking about an extreme situation is a way to rehearse what decisions may need to be made. • It is possible to hold two or more hopes at the same time. Hope for cure and hope for quality of life.
S = Suggest a Surrogate	Who will make decisions if the child is unable to speak for themselves.	"If you/your child were too sick to speak for yourself/themself, who should help us make those decisions?" "The best surrogate is someone who knows you well and will help us decide what you would want, if you could tell us."	• Many children want to protect their parents from these difficult decisions. • Children want to be involved in decision-making and have opinions on what is most important to them.
E = Expect Emotion	Expect emotion, and respond using NURSE(S) statements as appropriate.	"This is hard to even think about. Knowing what is most important to you/your child will help us take better care of you/your child." "You are such a good mother/father/parent/family member. We talked about a lot today. Thank you for sharing your thoughts with me. You have made such thoughtful decisions, and I really value your opinion."	• Make it about the medical team. Relate past experiences in similar situations where knowing what was important to a family was helpful. • Praise is a powerful tool that supports.

Source: Reference 29.

as more than the diagnosis so that you can uncover what matters most to them. Talk about decision-making in the third person, for example, "Some children may get sick quickly, and we have not had time to find out what matters most to them. Knowing what is important to you and Aniya will help us give better care."

S = Discuss who will make decisions, legally, culturally, and spiritually. Often the discussion of a surrogate is a great first step to introduce potential issues in decision-making. Children may be protective of parents and prefer an older sibling, grandparent, or other trusted adult to participate in decision-making. Given that Aniya's family has a strong faith, consider the role of their spiritual advisors.

E = Expect and acknowledge emotion when goals of care are discussed. Once might respond with something like "I can imagine this is hard to think about. It is important to know what is most important to you and Aniya so that we can take the very best care of her.". Make the focus on the medical team by being curious and open to doing better based on past experiences. "I want to take better care of Aniya by learning more about what is important to her and you."

The REMAP Talking Map for Later Goals-of-Care Discussions

People and situations change over time. Even with careful planning and early discussions of values and goals of care, decisions still need to be made late in the trajectory of serious illness. Reframing the current clinical situation is imperative to facilitate understanding. The REMAP talking map[30,31] is a tool that is helpful in these conversations. The REMAP talking map (Table 37.4) includes the following steps: *R*eframe, *E*xpect emotion, *M*ap values, *A*lign, and *P*lan. It is easy to get stuck in open-ended questions, and while they are very helpful, they can detract from the message that the underlying illness has no or very limited options for treatment. Reframing the current situation is key as children may have been in serious conditions before, yet they have improved. What makes this time different? As in any serious conversation, expect emotion. This is an indication that the news you have shared has been heard. Respond empathetically to continue to build trust. Empathy leads to uncovering values. Avoid discussion of code status early in the conversation as this may lead the family to feel the medical teams have "given up." Discuss next steps by aligning reasonable interventions with the child's and family's values. Using one or more of the 4 Ws—"I wish . . . ," "I worry . . . ," "I wonder . . . ," and "I will . . . "—allows next steps to be framed as what

Table 37.4 The REMAP Talking Map[30,31]

	Meaning	Sample language	Pediatric considerations
R = Reframe	Why is the current situation different? Why is what has been working no longer working?	"We are in a different place now." "Given this news, I think it is time to talk about what makes sense to do next."	• Children with serious illness may have had "brink of death" experiences multiple times and improved.
E = Expect Emotion	Expect emotion, and respond using NURSE(S) statements as appropriate.	"Tell me what you are thinking right now." "I can imagine this is very hard to hear."	• Emotional responses often reflect that the family did hear the message you wanted them to hear.
M = Map Values	Find out what is most important to the child and family.	"Tell me more about your child and your family as people. Knowing more about what is most important to you helps us plan the best care."	• Discussing interventions before understanding the values of the child and family may lead to getting stuck in technical details.
A = Align	Aligning with the child's and family's values shows that you heard them and care about them as people, not just a diagnosis.	"What I hear you say is that being at home with family is important. Let's talk about how we might be able to make that happen." "I wish we had different news to share. I remember (your child) shared that they most wanted to be at home. Can we talk about how we might be able to make that happen?"	• Reflect back the values to show that you are listening and their input is important.
P = Plan	Plan interventions that align with the child's and family's values.	"You said being at home was important to you. We want to help you do more of that." "I worry that (this intervention) will not help your child and will only cause more pain and suffering." "I hope with you for that miracle, and as we are waiting, let's talk about how we can help your child to have the best life possible."	• Talk in terms of what can be done, not what cannot be done. • If the family says something like "Do everything," probe to find out what they mean by this statement. Do not assume it means a full code. • Consider time-limited trials.

Sources: References 30 and 31.

can and should be done versus what cannot be done. Plan interventions that promote comfort and align with values.

What If a Family Wants to "Do Everything"

Even with the most skilled communication, a family may say "do everything." Do not assume that "do everything" means full code interventions. The family may be sad and feeling desperate. They never wanted to be in this situation. Respond with empathy. Probe to find out what "do everything" means to them. Avoid pushing decisions for limitations of life-prolonging interventions too soon. This may result in a "fight-or-flight" response. Discuss benefits and burdens in terms of the child's and family's values and what is reasonable given the change in clinical status. Keep in mind the cognitive, emotional, cultural, and spiritual factors that may impact decision-making. Involving trusted cultural or spiritual advisors may be helpful to frame the conversation. Expect and respond to emotion appropriately using NURSE(S) statements. Clinicians need to check their emotions as well. Many clinicians report feeling they did not do their best when a family says something like "There must be something more you can do." Using "I wish . . . " statements aligns the clinician with the family and conveys empathy for their situation. Use "and" and not "but" when responding to an unrealistic statement by a family. Using "but" discounts their hopes. Try responding by indicating the clinician "wish" that their hope could be realized "and" "worry" or "wonder" to frame why that hope may not be possible. Some examples of the 4 W statements are highlighted when the case study is revisited below.

Regoaling

In most pediatric illness, initial goals include cure or stabilization. Regoaling occurs when cure or stabilization is not possible, and the focus turns more toward optimizing quality of life and quality of time. Regoaling occurs for clinicians as well as the child with serious illness and their family. Walter et al.[32] note barriers to regoaling for clinicians may include challenges related to hierarchy in or between medical teams, avoiding criticism of colleagues, communication challenges, focus remaining on cure or remission, confusion in whose responsibility it is to have goals-of-care discussions with families, and need to avoid expressions of sorrow, lack of support, labeling, and conflict. They conclude that facilitators for clinician regoaling include building a shared mental model, mutual respect, and trust between clinicians and teams; anticipating conflict and moving into conflict resolution; processes for re-evaluation of goals; communication of serious news as a team; and flexibility in and between medical teams.

Children and families most often share the initial goals of cure or stabilization and may persist in these hopes even when they understand the serious nature of the underlying illness and clinical condition. It is possible to hold two or more hopes simultaneously: hopes for clinical stabilization and hopes for optimal quality of life. Hill et al.[33] describe regoaling for families as disengaging from initial goals of cure/remission to accept that they are no longer possible or desirable and re-engaging in new hopes that align with realistic goals. In order to achieve successful regoaling, clinicians must give clear and consistent information about the child's clinical condition.[34] Responding to the emotional cues of the child and family, as well as praising them for the thoughtful decisions they have made along the way, will also support regoaling.[33]

Case Study Continued

Aniya completed treatment 15 months ago and has been followed closely with serial MRI scans and neurological exams. She presents to the neuro-oncology clinic with worsening ataxia, diplopia, and headache. An MRI scan reveals recurrence of the tumor and spread to the spine. The neuro-oncology team shares there are limited treatment options; however, there are potential experimental therapies that may improve her symptoms for a while. The neuro-oncology and palliative care teams are meeting with the family to discuss these findings. Aniya's clinical condition is deteriorating, and time is limited. She had multiple ICU stays in the past, requiring intubation and extensive medical support, yet eventually improved and was able to go home. Using the REMAP talking map will aid in reframing goals from cure to optimizing quality of life and promotion of comfort. An example of how REMAP might be used in this scenario follows:

R = Review the current clinical situation and why this time things are different. Aniya has been extremely ill in the past with aggressive medical interventions. Sharing with the family that in those situations the cause of her symptoms and deterioration was due to surgery and/or complications of prior therapies, such as increased intercranial pressure following surgery or sepsis with chemotherapy. Using language such as "We are in a different place now. Given what we know now, there are no reasonable treatment options." Pause after that statement to allow the family time to process it.

E = Expect the family to be emotional. This is usually a broad indicator that they heard the information that was shared. Every family, and even different family members, may respond with different emotions. How they have responded to serious news in the past gives clues and is not always indicative of how they will respond to this news. Use NURSE(S) statements to respond to emotion.

M = Find out what is most important to the family. The neuro-oncology and palliative care teams likely have a respected and trusted relationship with Aniya and her family. Reflect on what they may have shared in other encounters: "I remember early on, when we first met, you shared with us that Aniya is most happy at home. I wonder if it would be helpful to talk about how we might be able to make that happen."

A = Hope is essential to human existence. It is possible to hold multiple hopes at the same time. For example, Aniya's family may still be hoping that the new experimental treatment will slow disease progression and give her more time. At the same time, they want whatever time she has left to live to be as joyful as possible and for her to be able to be as pain-free as possible. They may even refer to hoping for a miracle. Using "I wish . . . " statements can help to align with these multiple hopes and support the family, such as "I wish things were different. Aniya and you have been so strong through all of this. We hope for that miracle with you. I wonder if talking about what we can do to support Aniya while we are waiting for that miracle would be helpful?"

P = Make a plan together with all the medical teams, Aniya, and her family. It is imperative that all be on the same page to avoid confusing messages to the family. If there is disagreement about the experimental treatment, for example, suggesting a time-limited trial may be useful. Be honest and open in communication of what can be done, rather than what cannot be done. Avoid promising things that cannot be delivered. For example, most home hospice agencies do not provide 24/7 private duty nursing, and many insurance plans have limited coverage for home healthcare.

Talking maps are simply guides. Practice these conversations with trusted colleagues, attend communication training, jump into role plays for difficult conversations, and observe other skilled communicators at work in sharing difficult news with children and their families. No one is perfect 100% of the time. Some days clinicians are skilled communicators, and other days things may not come out the way they were intended. Do not be afraid to ask for a "do over" with a family or another colleague. For example, using a phrase like "That didn't come out quite the way I meant it. May I try again?" may be helpful. The key is to be truthful, open to listening, responsive to emotion, and compassionate.

Advance Care Planning in Pediatric Serious Illness

Advance care planning is a discussion of values and preferences in care to inform decision-making in pediatric serious illness. It should be distinguished from an *advance directive*, which is a legal document for children 18 years of age and older that typically names a surrogate decision maker if the child is unable to make informed decisions themselves, with preferences for cardiopulmonary resuscitation (CPR) and life-sustaining supports.[35] Advance care planning should be a series of conversations regarding care preferences, often revisited over time as the clinical condition changes, and may or may not result in completion of a written advance directive.

The pediatric population is unique in that most children are below the legal age of consent and may also have developmental challenges that impact decision-making. Legally, decision-making falls to the parents or legal guardian, that is, a surrogate decision maker (see Chapter 6, "Advance Care Planning"). In the case where a child is in state foster care, the child may be appointed a guardian ad litem, who facilitates discussion, and the court makes the final healthcare decisions. Regardless of who the legal decision maker is, these conversations are challenging as the parent or legal guardian (referred to as "parents" henceforth) must make decisions on the best interests of their child. See Chapter 38, "Ethical Considerations in Pediatric Palliative Care," for more information on the best-interest standard. The situation may be clouded by many factors, some of which include blended families, mature minors, grandparents, friends, and spiritual advisors, all of whom may have opinions on what should be done. Knowing the players in the child's family is imperative so that accurate information can be shared with the people the family chooses, knowing final decisions most often rest with parents.

Healthcare providers are often uncomfortable with facilitating advance care planning conversations, and parents struggle with initiating these conversations with older children and adolescents/young adults (AYAs). Lyon et al.[36–38] have consistently demonstrated that facilitated conversations by specially trained personnel do not cause undue harm and are desired by parents and AYAs. This facilitator can be the physician or another trusted member of the healthcare team. Trained facilitators who are not part of the AYA's care team may have fewer unconscious biases which could influence the discussion.[39] Parents and AYAs should be asked for their preferences regarding who is best to facilitate advance care planning discussions for them.

Table 37.5 Sample tools for advance care planning in pediatrics

Name	Information
My Wishes—Useful for younger children to help children express what is most important to them. Utilizes drawing and storytelling to help children express what is most important to them. Available in English and Spanish. Not a legal document.	https://agingwithdignity.org/shop/product-details/pediatric-my-wishes
Voicing My Choices—Useful for older children, adolescents, and young adults. Based upon the Five Wishes document and guided by young adults living with serious illness. Written in easier-to-understand language. Available in English and Spanish. Not a legal document.	https://agingwithdignity.org/shop/product-details/voicing-my-choices
Five Wishes—A legal advance directive document in many states. Most useful for adults over the age of 18 years. Available in paper and digital formats. Available in multiple languages.	https://www.agingwithdignity.org/shop/product-details/five-wishes
Shop Talk—A board game designed for children (ages 7–16) with cancer and other serious illnesses to facilitate conversations about the emotional issues faced during illness. Questions written in English and Spanish.	https://ccr.cancer.gov/Pediatric-Oncology-Branch/psychosocial/education
Pediatric Go Wish Together—A card-sorting game designed for children, adolescents, young adults, and families to facilitate conversations about serious illness and what matters most. Available in English only.	Pediatric GoWish Together—Coda Alliance https://codaalliance.org/pediatric-gowish/

There is no roadmap or algorithm for parents in making decisions for their child. There are several helpful tools to guide conversations, which are discussed later in this chapter (Table 37.5). Medical providers often miss opportunities to engage with families in advance care planning for a variety of factors, including lack of time, lack of comfort/skill in having the advance care planning conversation, feeling ill-equipped to manage emotions in the moment, and confusion over which medical team or even which provider should lead these discussions with a family.[40] Multiple studies have shown that, although difficult, families want to engage in advance care planning discussions, which actually support their feelings of being a good parent.[37,38,41] Fratantoni et al.[37] found that parents of children with rare diseases value most having their child be able to get out and move freely even if wheelchair-dependent, human connection, feeling included and being engaged, symptom management, coordination of care between multiple providers, managing the daily cares and burdens of care, and planning for the future. These things that matter most to parents are key aspects of advance care planning discussions. Parents often focus on the short-term or near-future goals for their child. Fahner et al.[42] note that, even with a near focus, parents do think about what may happen in the future. Initially parents may focus on immediate needs and treatment. It is incumbent on the healthcare team to also frame discussions toward the future. As noted in the section above, being intentional and preparing for advance care planning discussions are key to uncovering the child's and family's values and planning care that honors those values.

Pediatric advance care planning is complex, and what is known from advance care planning with adults is not directly applicable to pediatrics.[43] The goal is to provide accurate and honest information for families to inform their decision-making and guide them appropriately in what makes sense. No one can plan for all possible scenarios, yet using knowledge, skills, and experience with other children with serious illness will allow families to have time to reflect on what is most important to them. Crisis decision-making is to be avoided when possible. Assessing readiness to begin these conversations requires skill and empathy. No one is ever ready to discuss the possibility of their child's death.[24] Framing the discussion as part of a normal part of care planning is helpful in early discussions of advance care planning and goals of care.[29] If later in the trajectory of illness, frame the discussion on changes in the clinical condition and why things are different now.

Hein et al.[43] note that key components in pediatric advance care planning include mutual respect and trust, ongoing discussions over time taking into account the individual child and family's needs, including medical and psychosocial specialists in these discussions, documentation of the discussions and sharing with other team members to ensure consistency, sharing of the documents with all pertinent medical teams including the child's community-based pediatrician, and acknowledging that there is no "right time" for goals-of-care and advance care planning conversations. They also note that healthcare professionals often made assumptions that the family was not willing to have goals-of-care and advance care planning discussions, when in fact parents desired these discussions but were reluctant to bring up the topic themselves. In this study, parents also noted they wanted documentation of not only the decisions for life-sustaining treatments but also documentation of the decision-making process. Barriers to the process included providers feeling increased moral distress when there were disagreements between the medical teams and the family, where parents experienced distress when they felt their decisions were being challenged. Emergency personnel noted feeling powerless as they perceived "do not resuscitate" as "do nothing." Medical providers needed support as they guided families through these difficult conversations and when the time of death approached. Medical providers feared parents would change their minds and often required validation of choices, which in turn caused the family to feel their decisions were being challenged. Another barrier was lack of access to documented advance care planning decisions across care settings.[43]

Tools for Pediatric Advance Care Planning

Several helpful tools exist that are helpful in starting goals-of-care and advance care planning conversations. As with talking maps, one size does not fit all. Use the tool that best suits the child and family. Examples of advance care planning conversation tools can be found in Table 37.5. One resource that is helpful is the Courageous Parents Network (CPN; https://courageousparentsnetwork.org/). CPN is a nonprofit organization with educational tools for families and clinicians that reflect the experiences of children with serious illness and their families, as well as the clinicians who care for them. CPN has a vast library of videos, podcasts, printable guides, and blogs that highlight the child and family voice in communication and decision-making throughout the trajectory of serious illness.[44]

Documentation of Goals of Care and Advance Care Planning

Discussions with the child and family to elicit values, clarify goals of care, and plan for future care in the event of changing health status are critical to providing high-quality palliative care. However, having the discussion is not enough. The conversation and outcomes must be documented in the medical record in a clear and concise manner. Advance care planning documents may or may not be legal documents depending upon the child's age and the state recognition of these forms. Medical Orders for Life-Sustaining Therapies or Physician Orders for Life-Sustaining Therapies (MOLST/POLST) forms are medical orders for specific interventions to be done in the event of a cardiopulmonary arrest. The exact title of the form may vary from state to state. Most states have a form which can be found at https://www.everplans.com/articles/state-by-state-polst-forms. There is a national POLST form which has been adopted by many states and is portable across state lines (https://polst.org/state-polst-programs/). Most states require the child's (if of legal age), the parent's or legal guardian's, and physician's or advance practice provider's signatures.

Most state advanced directive forms are paper-based. An institution may choose to develop a summary document of these paper forms in the electronic medical record for ease of use or to scan the paper document into the electronic medical record so that all members of the child's healthcare team are aware of it. This includes all hospital-based providers, the community-based pediatrician, home health agencies, home hospice agencies, and any other pertinent providers. The family should also have copies of any documents such as the MOLST/POLST forms or written advanced directives, such as Voicing My Choices™ or Five Wishes™. The originals of these forms should be provided to the family and copies placed in the medical record with each agency or provider's office.

These documents should be reviewed regularly for changes. That does not mean that a full discussion of goals of care and advance care planning should be done every time. The conversation for review of these plans will depend upon the child's clinical condition, any changes in developmental understanding, and if the family has any changes they wish to make. While some providers feel that an in-depth discussion must occur at specific frequencies, the child and parent may feel it is distressing to have such a difficult discussion again. If the child's clinical or developmental status has changed or the parents have indicated changes in their goals, then a full goals-of-care and advance care planning conversation may be warranted.

The Role of the Nurse in Goals of Care and Advance Care Planning in Pediatric Serious Illness

Nurses are in a unique position to provide education and anticipatory guidance for the decisions that children and their families face throughout the trajectory of serious illnesses (Table 37.6).[35] Nurses develop trusting relationships with children and families at the bedside, which creates an environment that empowers parents to make informed decisions and helps the child and family to transcend the experience of end of life with a peaceful death.[45,46] Accurate family education about side effects and interventions is essential to clarifying realistic expectations. Nurses provide support for children and families at all stages of the illness experience, from diagnosis through survivorship, end of life, and into bereavement.

Providing empathetic listening, presence, and supportive care enhances the trusted relationship. Allowing children and families time to express their feelings and providing empathy for the family's point of view will aid the family in processing the information about the child's condition and in making immediate, as well as future, decisions. Nurses also provide realistic information about prognosis based on the clinical evidence, as well as their experience, to gently inform the family that a child is unlikely to survive. Hearing this information from a trusted member of the healthcare team may support the family's decision to forgo more aggressive medical and life-sustaining interventions. The expertise of nurses in facilitating and advocating in decision-making conversations is helpful to elicit the child's and parents' voices in goals of care. The impact of nursing involvement in goals-of-care and advance care planning conversations with children and families may help families realize the child is dying and make informed decisions regarding realistic next steps.

Table 37.6 Nurses' role in advance care planning

Clinical practice
• Advance care planning is essential to family-centered, person-centered care. • Children and their families have the same rights as adults to have their values and preferences in care honored. • Nurses should advocate for the child's and family's voices to be heard, valued, respected, and included in care. • Nurses should honor the child's and/or family's decision not to engage in advance care planning.
Education
• Nurses should be educated on the tenets and processes of advance care planning for children with serious illness and their families at any stage of illness. • Nurses should be provided with opportunities for training in the skills to facilitate advance care planning discussions with children and their families. • Nurses must respect and attend to preferences for advance care planning discussions related to culture, ethnicity, spirituality/religion, and other factors unique to each individual child and family.
Institutional policies
• Institutions must incorporate advance care planning as a key initiative in quality care for all children with serious illness. • Policies and standards for implementing advance care planning as a standard of care should be developed for all adolescents and young adults 18 years of age and older and should be thoughtfully considered for younger children with capacity, as well as for certain high-risk medical conditions or procedures with high risks of morbidity and/or mortality (i.e., bone marrow transplant, heart failure, etc.).

Support of Professional Nursing Organizations of the Nurse's Role in Decision-Making

The American Nurses Association (ANA) Code of Ethics[47] supports the nurse in advocating for the rights, health, and safety of all children and families. Guidelines to support members of the healthcare team may be helpful to frame discussions with families and among the healthcare team (Box 37.2). The ANA has published position statements to guide nurses in participating in end-of-life decision-making, including *Nursing Care and Do Not Resuscitate (DNR) Decisions*[48] and *Nurses' Roles and Responsibilities in Providing Care and Support at the End of Life.*[49] These statements are not specific to pediatrics; however, they do endorse developing an adequate skill set to facilitate discussions and encourage children and families to actively participate in decision-making. The Hospice and Palliative Nurses Association (HPNA)[35] advocates for a dynamic process in a series of conversations with families over time, beginning before anticipated health crises. The ANA and HPNA Palliative and Hospice Nurses Professional Issues Panel endorses the role of the nurse in facilitating informed decision-making for all children with serious illness.[50] Advocating, supporting, and facilitating decision-making for children with cancer

Box 37.2 Guidelines for the Healthcare Team to Use in Assisting Parents with End-of-Life Decision-Making

1. At the time of diagnosis and throughout treatment, actively seek opportunities to provide information to the parent about treatment and the child's response to treatment.
2. At the time of diagnosis and throughout treatment, involve the parent in treatment-related discussions and decision-making. Be available to discuss and rediscuss decisions and related concerns.
3. Ask parents if they would like to talk with parents of other children with similar conditions.
4. Verbally and nonverbally reassure the parents that they are "good" parents who are committed to the well-being of their child and that they have made good decisions for the child all throughout the child's treatment.
5. Provide assurances that everything that can be done to help the child is being done and being done well.
6. As the child's disease progresses, provide clear verbal (and written, if desired by the parent) explanations of the child's status. Provide visual sources of evidence such as actual scans, with appropriate interpretations.
7. Inform parents of treatment options as they become available in the treating institution or elsewhere.
8. At each treatment juncture, ask the parents what they are hoping for and anticipate that they will have more than one hope.
9. Include more than one healthcare team member in end-of-life discussions with the parents.
10. When discussing end-of-life options with parents:
    a. Strongly emphasize the team's commitment to the child's comfort and to providing expert care at all times.
    b. Offer professional recommendations.
    c. Describe how their child is likely to respond to each option (the child's physical appearance, ability to communicate, etc.).
    d. Give information about other support resources (ethics committees, social services, other healthcare professionals, etc.).
11. When discussing end-of-life options with parents, anticipate:
    a. Parents' vacillation between certainty and uncertainty about the decision.
    b. Parents' need for clarification and additional information to resolve their uncertainties.
    c. Parents' need for practical information about ways to explain the end-of-life decision to other family members.
    d. Being asked to give personal advice (i.e., what you would do if this was your child?).
12. Allow parents private time to consider the options.
13. Maintain sensitivity to any specific ethnic, cultural, or religious preferences during end-of-life care.
14. Convey respect for the parents' right to change decisions when clinically feasible.
15. Consider seeking an ethics consultation for the family and/or the healthcare team as a whole.
16. Consider seeking consultation from palliative care experts.
17. Demonstrate commitment to maintaining the child's comfort and dignity and to affirming the parents' role.
18. Do not question the parents' decision after it has been made.
19. Carefully document the end-of-life treatment or care decision once it is made so that all clinicians can be fully informed of this decision.

Box 37.3 Guidelines for the Healthcare Team to Use in Assisting Each Other with End-of-Life Decision-Making

1. Know the guidelines offered by specific disciplines regarding roles in end-of-life decision-making (i.e., the American Nurses Association's official statements on what the nurse is expected to do to help parents and children make decisions) because it is possible that the guidelines differ from expectations held by others outside the discipline.
2. Before initiating end-of-life discussions with children and parents, all members of the healthcare team should discuss and agree on:
    a. The need for such a discussion.
    b. Which options are appropriate and available.
    c. Whether outside consultants, such as an ethics committee, palliative care specialists, or an external oncology expert, are needed to identify which options are in the best interest of the child.
    d. Which other team members will participate in the discussion with the parents and child.
    e. The time of the discussion and specific staff members who will participate.
    f. Which staff member will document the discussions in the medical record.
    g. Availability of the appropriate staff time and resources to address any questions parents and children may have. Communicate to the team members who were not present at the child-and-parent discussion what specific language was used to provide support to the parents and child in making this decision.
3. Be available to team members and to the child and parents to discuss and rediscuss decisions and related concerns. When considering whether the child should be present during such discussions, evaluate the developmental stage of the child and the severity of illness and symptoms at the time of the discussion.
4. Explore with the team all appropriate options to ensure that all that can be done is being done and being done well.
5. Consider consulting an ethics and/or palliative care expert on behalf of the entire team.
6. Inform other team members if feedback from or assessment of the child, parents, or both indicates that any decision needs clarification or reconsideration.
7. Directly approach other team members regarding aspects of decision-making rather than seek such information from the parents.
8. Make certain that decision-making is fully documented in the healthcare record and accessible for all members of the team.

and their families is not only a professional obligation supported by key nursing organizations but also ethically our responsibility in providing high-quality child- and family-centered care (Box 37.3).

Conclusion

Decision-making in pediatric serious illness is complex and dynamic, from the time of diagnosis throughout the trajectory of disease to survivorship or death and into bereavement. Children and families should be actively engaged in conversations that elicit their unique values and preferences. Key components of communication include responding to emotions evoked by these conversations and the use of talking maps to guide decision-making. Healthcare providers must provide accurate and timely information to elicit goals of care and inform decision-making in a developmentally appropriate manner. This information should be reviewed frequently, framed in terms of the child's stable or changing clinical condition, the child's changing developmental level, and respect for the values of families as experts on their child. The child and family should be provided with opportunities for advance care planning, beginning before health crises. Nurses are key to advocating, initiating, and facilitating discussions with family that educate, inform, and elicit goals of care that honor the values and preferences of the child and family.

REFERENCES

1. Myers J, Simon J. Advance care planning and goals of care discussions. In: MacDonald S, Herx L, Boyle A, eds. *Palliative Medicine: A Case-Based Manual.* 4th ed. Oxford University Press; 2021. https://doi.org/10.1093/oso/9780198837008.003.0001
2. Grier K, Koch A, Docherty S. Pediatric goals of care communication: a socioecological model to guide conversations. *J Hosp Palliat Nurs.* 2023;25(1):E24–E30.
3. Lusney N, van Breemen C, Lim E, Pawliuk C, Hussein Z. Pediatric advance care planning: a scoping review. *Children (Basel).* 2023;10(7):1179.
4. National Hospice and Palliative Care Organization. *Pediatric Facts and Figures.* National Hospice and Palliative Care Organization; 2023.
5. Hill DL, Faeber JA, Li Y, et al. Changes over time in good-parent beliefs among parents of children with serious illness: a two-year cohort study. *J Pain Symptom Manage.* 2019;58:190–197.
6. Kon AA, Morrison W. Shared decision-making in pediatric practice: a broad view. *Pediatrics.* 2018;142(suppl_3):S129–S132. https://doi.org/10.1542/peds.2018-0516B.
7. Sisk BA, Mack JW, Ashworth R, DuBois J. Communication in pediatric oncology: state of the field and research agenda. *Pediatr Blood Cancer.* 2018;65(1):10.1002/pbc.26727.
8. Mack JW, Joffe S. Communicating about prognosis: ethical responsibilities of pediatricians and parents. *Pediatrics.* 2014;133(suppl 1): S24–S30.
9. Back AL, Arnold RM, Baile WF, Tulsky JA, Fryer-Edwards K. Approaching difficult communication tasks in oncology. *CA Cancer J Clin.* 2005;55(3):164–177.
10. Linebarger S, Johnson V, Boss RD. Guidance for pediatric end-of-life care. *Pediatrics.* 2022;149(5):e2022057011. https://doi.org/10.1542/peds.2022-057011.
11. Eaton S, Clark JD, Cummings CL, et al. Pediatric shared decision-making for simple and complex decisions: findings from a Delphi panel. *Pediatrics.* 2022;150(5):e2022057978. https://doi.org/10.1542/peds.2022-057978.
12. Weaver MS, October T, Feudtner C, Hinds PS. "Good-parent beliefs": research, concept, and clinical practice. *Pediatrics.* 2020;145(6):e20194018.
13. Weaver MS, Neumann ML, Lord B, Wiener L, Lee J, Hinds PS. Honoring the good parent intentions of courageous parents: a thematic summary from a US-based national survey. *Children (Basel).* 2020;7(12):265.
14. October T, Fisher K, Feudtner C, Hinds P. The parent perspective: "being a good parent" when making critical decisions in the PICU. *Pediatr Crit Care Med.* 2014;15(4):291–298.
15. Wool J, Irving SY, Meghani SH, Ulrich CM. Parental decision-making in the pediatric intensive care unit: an integrative review. *J Fam Nurs.* 2021;27(2):154–167.
16. Macauley RC. *Ethics in Palliative Care: A Complete Guide.* Oxford University Press; 2018. https://doi.org/10.1093/med/9780199313945.001.0001.
17. Feudtner C, Beight LJ, Boyden JY, et al. Goals of care among parents of children receiving palliative care. *JAMA Pediatr.* 2023;177(8):800–807.
18. Linebarger S, Johnson V, Boss RD. Guidance for pediatric end-of-life care. *Pediatrics.* 2022;149(5):e2022057011. https://doi.org/10.1542/peds.2022-057011.
19. Vital Talk. Family Conference. 2019. Accessed October 15, 2022. https://www.vitaltalk.org/guides/family-conference/.
20. Stein A, Dalton L, Rapa E, et al. Communication with children and adolescents about the diagnosis of their own life-threatening condition. *Lancet.* 2019;393(10176):1150–1163.
21. Thompkins JD, Needle J, Baker JN, et al. Pediatric advance care planning and families' positive caregiving appraisals: an RCT. *Pediatrics.* 2021;147(6):e2020029330.
22. Ekberg S, Parry R, Land V, et al. Communicating with patients and families about illness progression and end of life: a review of studies using direct observation of clinical practice. *BMC Palliat Care.* 2021;20:186.
23. Vital Talk. Responding to Emotion: Articulating Empathy Using NURSE Statements. 2019. Accessed November 14, 2023. https://www.vitaltalk.org/guides/responding-to-emotion-respecting/.
24. Madrigal VN, Kelly KP. Supporting family decision-making for a child who is seriously ill: creating synchrony and connection. *Pediatrics.* 2018;142 (suppl 3):s170–s177.
25. Wiener L, Bell CJ, Spruit JL, Weaver MS, Thompson AL. The road to readiness: guiding families of children and adolescents with serious illness towards meaningful advance care planning discussions. *NAM Perspectives.* 2021;2021:10.31478/202108a.
26. Vital Talk. Serious News: Breaking Bad News Using the GUIDE Tool. 2019. Accessed October 7, 2022. https://www.vitaltalk.org/guides/serious-news/.
27. Kaplan M. SPIKES: a framework for breaking bad news to childs with cancer. *J Oncol Nurs.* 2010;14(4):514–516.
28. Porsensky EK, Carpenter BD. Breaking bad news: effect of forecasting diagnosis and framing prognosis. *Child Educ Couns.* 2016;99(1):68–76.
29. Vital Talk. PAUSE Talking Map. 2019. Accessed October 7, 2022. https://www.vitaltalk.org/guides/pause-talking-map/.
30. Vital Talk. Addressing Goals of Care: Using the REMAP tool. 2019. Accessed October 8, 2022. https://www.vitaltalk.org/guides/transitionsgoals-of-care/.
31. Childers JW, Back AL, Tulsky JA, Arnold RM. *REMAP:* A framework for goals of care conversations. *J Oncol Pract.* 2017;13(10):e844–e850.

32. Walter JK, Hill DL, DiDomenico C, Parikh S, Feudtner C. A conceptual model of barriers and facilitators to primary clinical teams requesting pediatric palliative care consultation based upon a narrative review. *BMC Palliat Care*. 2019;18(1):116–124.
33. Hill DL, Miller V, Walter JK, et al. Regoaling: a conceptual model of how parents of children with serious illness change medical care goals. *BMC Palliat Care*. 2014;13(1):9–16.
34. Mack JW, Cronin AM, Uno H, et al. Unrealistic parental expectations for cure in poor-prognosis childhood cancer. *Cancer*. 2020;126(2):416–424.
35. Hospice and Palliative Nurses Association. HPNA Position Statement: Advance Care Planning. 2017. Accessed October 15, 2022. https://advancingexpertcare.org/acp.
36. Lin CJ, Cheng YI, Garvie PA, D'Angelo LJ, Wang J, Lyon ME; Adolescent Palliative Care Consortium. The effect of family-centered (FACE®) pediatric advanced care planning intervention on family anxiety: a randomized controlled clinical trial for adolescents with HIV and their families. *J Fam Nurs*. 2020;26(4):315–326.
37. Fratantoni K, Livingston J, Schellinger SE, Aoun SM, Lyon ME. Family-centered advance care planning: what matters most for parents of children with rare diseases. *Children (Basel)*. 2022;9(3):445–455.
38. Thompson JD, Needle J, Baker JN, et al. Pediatric advance care planning and families' positive caregiving appraisals: an RCT. *Pediatrics*. 2021;147(6):e20200293309330. https://doi.org/10.1542/peds.2020-029330.
39. Dupont-Thibodeau A, Hindie J, Bourque CJ, Janvier A. Provider perspectives regarding resuscitation decisions for neonates and other vulnerable childs. *J Pediatr*. 2017;188:142–147.e3.
40. Johnson KA. Advance care planning in pediatric serious illness: centering the family experience. *Pediatrics*. 2021;147(6):e2020048660. https://doi.org/10.1542/peds.2020-048660.
41. Carr K, Hasson F, McIlfatrick S, Downing J. Parents' experiences of initiation of paediatric advance care planning. *Eur J Pediatr*. 2022;181:1185–1196.
42. Fahner JC, Tholking TW, Rietjens JAC, van der Heide A, van Deiden JJM, Kars MC. Towards advance care planning in pediatrics: a qualitative study on envisioning the future as parents of a seriously ill child. *Eur J Pediatr*. 2020;179:1461–1486.
43. Hein K, Knochel K, Zaimovic V, et al. Identifying key elements for paediatric advance care planning with parents, healthcare providers and stakeholders: a qualitative study. *Palliat Med*. 2020;34(3):300–308.
44. Courageous Parents Network. 2023. Accessed November 5, 2023. https://courageousparentsnetwork.org/.
45. Head BA, Song MK, Wiencek C, Nevidjon B, Fraser D, Mazanec P. Palliative nursing summit: nurses leading change and transforming care: the nurse's role in communication and advance care planning. *J Hosp Palliat Nurs*. 2018;20(1):23–29.
46. Fliedner M, Halfens RJG, King CR, Eychmueller S, Lohrmann C, Schols JMGA. Roles and responsibilities of nurses in advance care planning in palliative care in the acute care setting: a scoping review. *J Hosp Palliat Nurs*. 2021;23(1):59–68.
47. American Nurses Association. *Code of Ethics for Nurses: With Interpretive Statements*. Amerian Nurses Association; 2015.
48. ANA Center for Ethics and Human Rights. *Nursing Care and Do-Not-Resuscitate (DNR) Decisions*. American Nurses Association; 2020.
49. American Nurses Association. *Nurses' Roles and Responsibilities in Providing Care and Support at the End of Life*. American Nurses Association; 2016.
50. ANA Professional Issues Panel. *Call for Action: Nurses Lead and Transform Palliative Care*. American Nurses Association; 2017.

38

Ethical Considerations in Pediatric Palliative Care

Hilary Carroll McGuire and Nicole Fernandez

Key Points

- Nurses working in pediatric palliative care may face unique ethical dilemmas related to difficulty in prognostication, questions of autonomy, and multiple involved stakeholders including children, parent(s), and medical teams.
- Children should be involved in ethical discussions and decision-making as appropriate based on their developmental stage.
- Nurses may rely on specific techniques to minimize moral distress while engaging in a systematic process to navigate pediatric ethical dilemmas.

Introduction

Given the complexities involved in caring for children with serious illnesses and advancement in medical technologies with now more interventions than ever before, it seems natural for ethical issues to arise. How, though, are these issues different from those experienced by adult patients, their families, and the nurses who care for them? Children are not merely small adults. They have unique developmental stages that impact understanding of medical information and ability to participate in decision-making and care. Pediatric patients, who for the purpose of this chapter are those less than 18 years old, experience changing needs from birth through adolescence into young adulthood as well as a growing capacity to take on more ownership of self.

Parents/caregivers of pediatric patients are surrogate decision makers, meaning they act in the best interest of their children. The authors use the term "parent" in this chapter to denote a parent in any capacity, guardian, or legally appointed representative who has the responsibility to care for and make decisions on behalf of a child. This differs from substitute decision makers for adults, whose responsibility is to put the wishes of the patient into action irrespective of their own beliefs.[1] Additionally, some children live with and are cared for by individuals other than their biological or adoptive parents, such as those in foster care, which adds a layer of complexity to decision-making.

Determination of best interest is further complicated in pediatrics as there can be difficulty in prognostication. Babies born prematurely might experience complications whose effects can span into adolescence and young adulthood.[2,3] Furthermore, it is appropriate to engage children of certain developmental stages in conversations about their care and offer opportunities to assent to their treatment; at times, their preferences may differ from their parents. Additionally, there are circumstances when a healthcare team may determine that further life-prolonging treatment may be clinically ineffective or offer limited benefit to quality of life. This may result in conflict between the medical team and family unit.[2] Who holds the ethical responsibility to make the final decision in these situations? How should nurses navigate these emotionally charged situations while relying on ethical principles as a guide? This chapter will outline some of the frequently encountered ethical dilemmas in pediatric palliative care and offer a framework to support navigating these complex issues while offering a better understanding of ethical principles as they apply to pediatric patients. This chapter should encourage nurses to think critically as ethical questions arise in practice and increase their confidence and competence to care for patients while upholding their own moral values.

Case Study

The pediatric oncology team was caring for a 15-year-old female with myelodysplastic syndrome which had progressed to high-risk acute myelogenous leukemia. Her disease was refractory to standard chemotherapy, and unfortunately, she relapsed 50 days after allogeneic hematopoietic stem cell transplant. Her leukemia course was notable for multiple prolonged admissions, some over 100 days, due to complications including antibiotic-resistant infections, grade 4 graft versus host disease of the gut, severe pneumatosis intestinalis with resultant ileostomy placement, a subdural hematoma, COVID-19 infection, mild restrictive lung disease, anxiety related to treatment, and refractory nausea.

This patient had a close relationship with the palliative care team and inpatient nurses from prior admissions. When she received the information that her disease had relapsed, she shared her worry that there would be no further treatment for her disease and that her path forward was uncertain. Despite an incredibly complex and difficult medical course, she felt prepared to trial any offered treatment as she had already endured so much. She requested to be included in conversations about her chances of survival and felt her anxiety was exacerbated when medical conversations occurred out of her earshot with just her parents.

After relapse, her blast count continued to rise. She hoped to receive chimeric antigen receptor T-cell therapy at another hospital but was found to be ineligible and therefore was offered a phase 1 clinical trial of oral medication. The medical team, though offering a clinical trial, still felt her prognosis was grave; they did not believe the trial would offer her a cure and felt unsure whether it would provide benefit. The patient expressed ambivalence about further treatment; however, she was incredibly distressed about taking oral medications and potential symptoms associated with the trial. She felt her life had become difficult, often used the word "suffering," and expressed that she did not feel her family would allow her to decline treatment even if she did not want it. She acknowledged that her leukemia would worsen without treatment and that she may die, though felt unsure if she would die even with more treatment. The nurses caring for her felt distressed regarding her enrollment in a phase 1 clinical trial given that she, at times, told those she trusted that she did not want this treatment. The nurses caring for her contemplated what to do next.

Table 38.1 Steps to analyze ethically challenging situations

Steps
1. Review the overall situation—identify what is going on in this case.
2. Identify the ethical dilemma(s).
3. Gather all relevant facts about the patient and the contextual situation including:
a. significant medical and social history
b. involved family
c. decision-making capacity
d. existence of advance directives—written, appointed, or verbal—and any pertinent institutional policies
e. surrogate or healthcare agent if decision-making capacity is absent
4. Identify the parties or stakeholders involved in the situation, including those who will be affected by the decision(s).
5. Identify relevant legal data, including both state and federal laws.
6. Identify religious or cultural issues.
7. Identify specific conflicts of ethical principles or values. Identify and consider nursing guidelines and the profession's code and position statements.
8. Identify possible options, their purpose, and their probable consequences to the welfare of the patient. Identify and make use of interdisciplinary and institutional resources, including ethics committees, social workers, chaplains, and other experienced colleagues.
9. Identify practical constraints to decision-making, including institutional, legal, organizational, and economic.
10. Review and evaluate the situation after action has been taken—debrief and support the staff.

Source: Reference 7.

Pediatric Nursing Competencies in Ethical Reasoning

Providing nursing care for children with serious illnesses may raise unique ethical challenges including providing medical interventions which may cause pain,[4] infringing on autonomy, and invoking conflicting perspectives of the interdisciplinary team.[5] In navigating these challenges, pediatric nurses are especially susceptible to moral uncertainty, dilemmas, and distress[6] (see Chapter 32 for discussion of moral distress). Utilizing a systematic process to evaluate ethical dilemmas and reach decisions about what action to take may lead to resolutions of ethical dilemmas and reduce moral distress. This will be referred to as the "ethical process." Table 38.1 illustrates the steps of this process.

Utilizing a Stepwise Approach to Analyze Ethical Concerns

When encountering an ethically challenging situation, the ethical process (Table 38.1) may be used to evaluate the dilemma and decide what action to take. The first steps in this process are to obtain information and identify the ethical dilemma.[7] Nurses caring for pediatric patients and their families are in the unique position to be privy to the narratives of many key stakeholders including child, parent(s), and medical team. Nurses may rely on their palliative communication skills of eliciting child/family values and preferences to explore these narratives (see Chapter 27, 37). Individuals vary in their lived experiences and interpretations of ethical dilemmas; thus, factors such as religious, social, and cultural considerations must also be considered (see Chapter 28-29, 39). The nurse may be the first to recognize conflicting narratives, ineffective communication patterns, and ethical concerns, as was evident in the case described above. If an ethical concern is raised, the American Nurses Association (ANA) *Code of Ethics* states that there is an inherent responsibility for nurses to "bring forward difficult issues related to patient care and/or institutional constraints upon ethical practice for discussion and review."[8]

In the next steps of the ethical process, gathering relevant facts and identifying stakeholders, the pediatric nurse must rely on the interdisciplinary team, including both palliative care and ethics consulting teams when available, as well as pediatric-specific roles such as social workers and child life specialists. While the roles and responsibilities of palliative care consultants and ethics consultants may overlap, clinical ethics teams are specifically adept at identifying the ethical issues at hand, debriefing how child and/or parent goals of care and preferences were or were not met, and addressing systemic factors that may have influenced care.[9] The support offered by these ethics consultants may help address and mitigate moral distress. In the case example, ethics consultants provided strategies for staff involved to rely on when experiencing moral distress while participating in the patient's care.

Cultivating a Reflective Practice

Just as evaluation is a crucial step in the nursing process, it also is a critical step in processing an ethical dilemma. Multiple studies have shown that pediatric nurses desire formal and informal opportunities to reflect and deliberate on ethical concerns and that doing so may lessen the moral burden of care.[4,5] Prioritizing time to reflect may also contribute to personal and professional growth and improve future practice. Evaluation may involve self-reflection, in which pediatric nurses consider how their own biases and emotions have impacted their nursing care, as well as reflection-on-practice, which is a way to process the ethical dilemma and outcomes in a team setting where the nuances of a case are discussed. This can be especially important for nurses in pediatric settings given the complexity of interests and concerns between the child, family, and medical teams.[2]

Fostering a Positive Ethical Climate

Situations may arise in pediatric palliative care that are emotionally distressing without necessarily being morally distressing. Or a nurse may feel moral distress without encountering a specific ethical dilemma, such as experiencing time constraints or inadequate staffing levels.[4] One protective factor of moral distress in pediatric settings is the presence of a positive ethical climate.[4,10] "Ethical climate" refers to an individual's perception of how ethical issues are handled within an organization, including practices, procedures, policies, and organizational culture.[11] Pediatric nurses who perceive their organization as having a positive ethical climate report less frequent and less intense moral distress.[4,10] According to provision 6 of the ANA *Code of Ethics*, a nurse "establishes, maintains, and improves the ethical environment of the work setting"[8]; thus, pediatric nurses, and especially their nurse leaders, must be prepared to contribute to a positive ethical climate through respectful colleague interactions, peer support, identification of organizational barriers to care, and efforts to address concerns.[4,8]

Coping Skills and Duty to Self

Nurses have a duty to maintain their own health and well-being, understanding that compassion fatigue may negatively affect their nursing care and ability to navigate ethical dilemmas.[8] A nurse's own morality and definition of quality of life may not align with a family's or the direction of medical care, and they have a right and responsibility to uphold their ethical and moral integrity. If a nurse or team member disagrees with the consensus and believes they are unable to act impartially, they should be supported to have another staff member fill their role.[12]

Ethical Reasoning in Pediatrics

"Morality" and "ethics" are closely related terms, though not interchangeable. Morality concerns personal values, character, and behaviors of an individual or group and is often influenced by personal experiences, upbringing, and religion.[8] Ethics concerns the study of morality and applying principles of right and wrong to a societal or professional context.[8] Exploring overarching ethical theory is beyond the scope of this chapter (see Chapter 32 for brief review of major theories). However, there are specific situations that may arise in pediatric palliative care in which an understanding of underpinning ethical theory may be helpful for the nurse to identify and evaluate the ethical dilemma.

Autonomy in Pediatric Palliative Care

The ethical principle of *autonomy*, the right to self-determination, is at the center of many ethical dilemmas encountered in pediatric palliative care. Autonomy is a basic principle of bioethics which underpins moral rules, such as the duty to respect autonomy, which is the foundation for medical law and procedures such as informed consent. Autonomy is a central principle in ethical dilemmas arising in caring for pediatric patients in two primary ways: nurse concerns regarding infringing on autonomy and autonomy in decision-making.[4,5]

Autonomy Infringement

The concern of violating a child's autonomy is one of the most frequent experiences of moral distress encountered by pediatric nurses.[4] A nurse may perceive that they are inflicting suffering (e.g., causing pain to children in forced procedures, such as a blood draw) or engaging in limiting truth-telling (e.g., the child is questioning their diagnosis or prognosis, but the nurse is prevented from answering the child's question truthfully).[5,13] In the case study, nurses expressed distress administering a trial medication that the patient, at times, voiced concern over. While the ethical process (Table 38.1) may lead to resolution of dilemmas, the pediatric nurse may also consider other measures to lessen the moral distress associated with these dilemmas.

Preparing children in developmentally appropriate ways for planned procedures with information about what sensations to expect and potential coping mechanisms may help lessen anxiety, fear, and negative feelings.[14] Though a child may not provide *consent* (legal agreement to a procedure), having a nurse that seeks and obtains *assent* (agreement to take part in a procedure) may also lessen anxiety in the child, promote trust between the nurse and child, and acknowledge the child's growing autonomy.[15] One example of this would be to ask a child where to receive an injection instead of whether to receive it.

Regarding truth-telling, a nuanced approach to information sharing is now widely accepted: inform children in developmentally appropriate ways according to their assessed communication needs.[16] In navigating this dilemma regarding parents' preference to limit information to their child, nurses or other members of the interdisciplinary team may find that it can be helpful to validate parents' inclination to protect their child while assisting them to understand that intentional deception may do the opposite.[2,17]

Autonomy in Pediatric Medical Decision-Making

With the exception of emancipated minors, children under the age of 18 are not considered legally competent to make their own medical decisions in most states.[18] Instead, parents make substituted judgment decisions via parental autonomy.[2] Relational autonomy is another model of autonomy based upon a shared decision-making process in which the child's and family's values and beliefs are guided by the medical expertise of the interdisciplinary healthcare team to determine the best course of action.[9] This supports the family's decision-making process while accounting for the expertise of the medical team.[9,16] Though children under age 18 may not be legally competent to make medical decisions, children may still have the capacity, or the ability to understand, reason, and express a choice, at younger ages depending on their developmental abilities.[16] In general, a school-aged to adolescent child may be able to express preferences and values which should be considered. Involvement of the child in medical decision-making conversations should be based on the child's level of cognitive and emotional development.[2]

Studies show that most parents reflected positively upon engaging their children in these conversations when supported and prepared in doing so.[17]

Supporting Parental Decision-Making

The responsibility to make medical decisions for a child is an immense one, and there are differing ethical and legal principles to consider. In the *Substituted Judgment* standard, parents are asked to try to make the decision the child would have made for themselves. However, flaws to this approach include that many children have never expressed treatment preferences and that preferences may change over time.[19] An alternative framework is the *Best Interests Standard*, defined as maximizing benefits while minimizing harm "in the context of the child's/family's known values, beliefs, familial relationships, and cultural norms." Choices must meet a minimum acceptable threshold, defined as the *Reasonable Person Standard*.[15] Use of this framework can be complicated as it relies on a nuanced understanding of the medical question and potential outcomes. The interests of pediatric patients and their parents are often intertwined; thus, parents may need support from the interdisciplinary team including social work or pastoral care to make these decisions.[2] The *Zone of Parental Discretion* postulates that parents should be able to make decisions for their children "even if the decisions are considered, by some, to be suboptimal."[16,20] The limitation to this exists when a parent makes a choice that deviates from the range of options offered by the medical team and/or exposes a child to a risk of excess harm, defined as the *Harm Principle*.[16,20] In situations such as these, legal and regulatory authorities may become involved.[9]

Ethical Dilemmas Encountered in Pediatric Palliative Care

In the following section, we will discuss ethical dilemmas that nurses may encounter when caring for pediatric patients. Winter et al.[18] describes that formal ethics consultations are uncommon in pediatric medical care, though they are more prevalent when children have advanced or refractory disease.[21] They postulate that low incidence of consultation is not due to a lack of ethical issues when caring for pediatric patients but that there may be a myriad of supportive services available to help medical teams and parents through difficult situations. While unable to provide an exhaustive list of ethical issues in pediatric palliative care, the aim here is to highlight considerations which may provide guidance in navigating these often-complex scenarios when experienced in practice.

Information Sharing

As previously discussed, it can be distressing and complicated to determine what information to share and when to share it with pediatric patients. In contrast to adult patients where the dyad of decision-making includes the competent patient or surrogate and their medical provider, pediatric care involves three parties—the medical provider, the patient, and the family.[1,18] Parents may express worry that diagnostic information will produce distress or that their child will not comprehend.[2,17] There are developmental stages that occur as children progress from neonate through the age of majority, 18, when they legally transition to an adult status with decision-making responsibility if they have the capacity to do so. These stages impact the ability to receive, understand, and participate in medical conversations and are influenced by biologic, psychological, and social factors.[22] The International Society of Pediatric Oncology working committee on psychosocial issues in pediatric oncology recognizes a child's right to participate in their medical decision-making in accordance with their developmental level.[22]

While there is ongoing debate about at what age a child may offer informed consent, it is hypothesized that children aged 14 and older can be assessed for assent to medical interventions that qualify as research and that children aged 12 and older can have decision-making competence.[23,24] Even within this definition, however, there will be variability among children based on their development and experience.[25] The American Academy of Pediatrics outlines that assent includes four elements: assisting the patient to have a developmentally appropriate understanding of their condition, clarifying expectations of treatment or procedures, assessing the child's understanding and what influences their response, and inquiring about willingness to undergo the proposed care.[26] Some feel that assent should only be solicited when there is a choice to be made. Others argue that a child's preference should always be sought as it bears moral weight even when it will not be ultimately authoritative.[25] Irrespective of age, if a child is going to be included in medical decisions, the medical team must foster a supportive environment that respects their developing autonomy.[27]

The patient in the case was an adolescent (aged 15–18) who not only had expressed her preference to be involved in medical conversations but had a remarkable understanding of her illness and likely death if she did not receive further treatment. Her preference for inclusion is not uncommon among patients her age and should be supported as exclusion can produce anxiety and feelings of isolation.[2,16] Honoring patients' wishes can be difficult when they conflict with their parents' wishes. In the case, the patient felt unsure about participation in a clinical trial, though her parents wanted to afford her a potential life-prolonging opportunity. Her parents agreed to discuss medical care, prognosis, and preferences with her as they felt their daughter was developmentally able to participate. When a disagreement occurred, ethics consultants were able to facilitate discussions and bridge the parents' and patient's goals. In determining the patient's and parents' influences on decision-making (the patient's worry about side effects of treatment and the parents' worry that without treatment their daughter would certainly die), they were able to reach an agreement. It was established that if the patient felt there were intolerable side effects, her participation in the trial would be reconsidered.

Complications of Prematurity

This section discusses events that may arise as a complication of prematurity, though these situations are also experienced outside of the neonatal intensive care unit and newborn stage.

It remains difficult for medical providers to deduce which babies born prematurely will go on to live with limited to no disability and who will have significant impairment.[2] There will be times when discussions occur about ongoing benefit of care in relation to expected outcome or quality of life.[2] When a child has a life-limiting, irreversible condition, a healthcare team and family may make the collaborative decision to limit care that lacks clear benefit.[28,29] In such circumstances the discontinuation of life-sustaining ventilator support, with the understanding that natural death will occur, may be pursued.[30,31] This discontinuation is radically different from an intervention to hasten death despite the same outcome. The difference stems from the intent behind discontinuation or withdrawal of life-sustaining therapies, which is to reduce suffering and promote the greatest quality of life while allowing for the natural course of disease progression.[32,33] When these decisions are made, it is critically important for nursing and medical providers to offer support for parents. The parents will carry the story of their child with them throughout their lives, and they deserve the necessary support to feel confident that they have made the best possible decisions for their child's well-being.[33–35] Supporting a family through shared decision-making can alter bereavement as it has been reported that when parents feel the decision was strictly theirs, they are at risk for experiencing grief throughout their lifetime.[36]

Initiating Extracorporeal Membrane Oxygenation

Initiation of extracorporeal membrane oxygenation (ECMO), an advanced life support technology supporting heart and lungs, might be considered for a myriad of conditions such as congenital diaphragmatic hernia, congenital heart conditions, or persistent pulmonary hypertension in newborns. This intervention is typically initiated urgently or emergently, therefore complicating the ability to obtain truly informed consent.[37,38] When offering ECMO, it is typically a bridge to therapy to allow a patient to recover or allow for clarification of prognosis and associated decision-making or potentially as a bridge to organ transplant.[29] Not every center treating pediatric patients can offer such advanced technology, and it is an incredibly resource-intensive intervention; therefore, providers must have criteria for which children are suitable candidates and how long this support will be maintained.[29,37] As with ventilatory support, ECMO too can be discontinued and decannulation pursued when no further benefit is expected or this support is no longer in line with the family's goals.[29]

Declining Treatment

As previously discussed, the discontinuation of life-sustaining therapy is acceptable within the medical community when there is thought to be an irreversibility of condition and the burden of treatment is believed to outweigh potential benefit.[12] Parents, however, do not have the ability to refuse treatments that offer clear benefit to their child as this could infringe on the child's right to an open future.[39,40] The Child Abuse Prevention and Treatment Act of 1974 was amended to include conditions that would allow declining treatment and not consider this act neglect.[41] Exceptions include when the infant is chronically and irreversibly comatose, when treatment prolongs the dying process and will not correct all life-threatening conditions, and when treatment is futile or inhumane.[12] The interpretation of therapeutic futility, however, varies widely among medical providers.[2,22,42,43] Understanding parents' beliefs and values can aid in navigation of complex decision-making that often occurs in palliative care.[2,36] When curative options are no longer present for a child, it is imperative for medical providers to solicit from the family and child, if able to participate, what promotes quality within their lives and cater discussions related to future interventions around this. These interventions can include, but are not limited to, use of antibiotics, blood products, noninvasive respiratory support, disease-directed therapy, and artificial nutrition or hydration. When the burden of any of these interventions might outweigh the benefit, there is ethical precedent that supports forgoing or discontinuation.[1,12,44]

Case Conclusion

The patient in the case did begin the phase 1 clinical trial with agreement to rediscuss her participation if she felt her symptom burden became too significant. When the patient made statements of doubt, staff were encouraged to probe deeper into the motivation behind the statement. An example of this is when she shared that she "did not want to take the drug." Her nurse gracefully navigated this, inquiring what her worry with taking the medication was. It was deduced that she had an aversion to oral medications due to taste and ongoing nausea rather than a desire to discontinue treatment indefinitely. Ultimately, she participated in 1 month of the trial prior to experiencing a disease complication that resulted in her death. Even during her dying process, her parents voiced that they would be able to rest knowing they did everything they could to help their daughter.

Conclusion

Nurses caring for children with serious illnesses may face unique ethical dilemmas; these dilemmas may continue to evolve as both medical technologies advance and legal landscapes shift. Additionally, it would be remiss not to mention that caring for seriously ill children can be challenging in many ways. Children are supposed to outlive their parents and be afforded a chance to blossom into their own person. When this pathway is disrupted, it impacts all involved in their care—family, friends, and nurses—in different ways. Nurses, in partnership with both the patient and family and as an integral part of the broader medical team, must be prepared to use their communication skills and a systematic process to navigate these ethical dilemmas while mitigating and coping with the moral distress that may arise.

REFERENCES

1. Wolfe J, Hinds P, Sourkes B. *Interdisciplinary Pediatric Palliative Care*. 2nd ed. Oxford University Press; 2022.
2. Grace P, Milliken A, Uveges M. Neonatal and pediatric acute and palliative care. In: *Clinical Ethics Handbook for Nurses*. Vol. 93. The International Library of Bioethics. Springer; 2022.
3. Crump C. An overview of adult health outcomes after preterm birth. *Early Hum Dev*. 2020;150:105187. https://doi.org/10.1016/j.earlhumdev.2020.105187.
4. Ventovaara P, af Sandeberg M, Räsänen J, Pergert P. Ethical climate and moral distress in paediatric oncology nursing. *Nurs Ethics*. 2021;28(6):1061–1072. https://doi.org/10.1177/0969733021994169.
5. Bartholdson C, Lützén K, Blomgren K, Pergert P. Experiences of ethical issues when caring for children with cancer. *Cancer Nurs*.

2015;38(2):125–132. https://doi.org/10.1097/NCC.0000000000000130.

6. Bong HE. Understanding moral distress: how to decrease turnover rates of new graduate pediatric nurses. *Pediatr Nurs.* 2019;45(3):109–114.
7. Coyle N. Palliative care, hospice care, and bioethics a natural fit. *J Hosp Palliat Nurs.* 2014;16(1):6–12. https://doi.org/10.1097/NJH.0000000000000032.
8. American Nurses Association. *Code of Ethics for Nurses with Interpretive Statements.* American Nurses Association; 2015. https://www.nursingworld.org/coe-view-only.
9. Weaver MS, Boss RD, Christopher MJ, et al. Top ten tips palliative care clinicians should know about their work's intersection with clinical ethics. *J Palliat Med.* 2021;25(4):656–661. https://doi.org/10.1089/jpm.2021.0521.
10. Pergert P, Bartholdson C, Blomgren K, af Sandeberg M. Moral distress in paediatric oncology: contributing factors and group differences. *Nurs Ethics.* 2019;26(7–8):2351–2363. https://doi.org/10.1177/0969733018809806.
11. Koskenvuori J, Numminen O, Suhonen R. Ethical climate in nursing environment: a scoping review. *Nurs Ethics.* 2019;26(2):327–345. https://doi.org/10.1177/0969733017712081.
12. Sacco J, Virata R. Baby O and the withdrawal of life-sustaining medical treatment in the devastated neonate: a review of clinical, ethical, and legal issues. *Am J Hosp Palliat Med.* 2017;34(10):925–930. https://doi.org/10.1177/1049909116672177.
13. af Sandeberg M, Bartholdson C, Pergert P. Important situations that capture moral distress in paediatric oncology. *BMC Med Ethics.* 2020;21(1):6. https://doi.org/10.1186/s12910-020-0447-x.
14. Bray L, Appleton V, Sharpe A. The information needs of children having clinical procedures in hospital: Will it hurt? Will I feel scared? What can I do to stay calm? *Child Care Health Dev.* 2019;45(5):737–743. https://doi.org/10.1111/cch.12692.
15. Coughlin KW. Medical decision-making in paediatrics: infancy to adolescence. *Paediatr Child Health.* 2018;23(2):138–146. https://doi.org/10.1093/pch/pxx127.
16. Sisk BA, Canavera K, Sharma A, Baker JN, Johnson L. Ethical issues in the care of adolescent and young adult oncology patients. *Pediatr Blood Cancer.* 2019;66(5):e27608. https://doi.org/10.1002/pbc.27608.
17. van der Geest IMM, van den Heuvel-Eibrink MM, van Vliet LM, et al. Talking about death with children with incurable cancer: perspectives from parents. *J Pediatr.* 2015;167(6):1320–1326. https://doi.org/10.1016/j.jpeds.2015.08.066.
18. Winter MC, Friedman DN, McCabe MS, Voigt LP. Content review of pediatric ethics consultations at a cancer center. *Pediatr Blood Cancer.* 2019;66(5):e27617. https://doi.org/10.1002/pbc.27617.
19. Torke AM, Alexander GC, Lantos J. Substituted judgment: the limitations of autonomy in surrogate decision making. *J Gen Intern Med.* 2008;23(9):1514–1517. https://doi.org/10.1007/s11606-008-0688-8.
20. Gillam L. The zone of parental discretion: an ethical tool for dealing with disagreement between parents and doctors about medical treatment for a child. *Clin Ethics.* 2016;11(1):1–8. https://doi.org/10.1177/1477750915622033.
21. Johnson LM, Church CL, Metzger M, Baker JN. Ethics consultation in pediatrics: long-term experience from a pediatric oncology center. *Am J Bioeth.* 2015;15(5):3–17. https://doi.org/10.1080/15265161.2015.1021965.
22. Juárez-Villegas LE, Altamirano-Bustamante MM, Zapata-Tarrés MM. Decision-making at end-of-life for children with cancer: a systematic review and meta-bioethical analysis. *Front Oncol.* 2021;11:739092. https://doi.org/10.3389/fonc.2021.739092.
23. Wendler D, Shah S. Should children decide whether they are enrolled in nonbeneficial research? *Am J Bioeth.* 2003;3(4):1–7.
24. Grootens-Wiegers P, Hein I, van den Broek J, de Vries M. Medical decision-making in children and adolescents: developmental and neuroscientific aspects. *BMC Pediatr.* 17(1):120. https://doi.org/10.1186/s12887-017-0869-x.
25. Navin M, Wasserman J. Capacity for preferences and pediatric assent implications for pediatric practice. *Hastings Cent Rep.* 2019;49(1):43–51. https://doi.org/10.1002/hast.980.
26. American Academy of Pediatrics. Informed consent in decision-making in pediatric practice—policy statement. *Pediatrics.* 2016;138(2). https://doi.org/10.1542/peds.2016-1484.
27. Hopkins KA, Ott MA, Salih Z, Bosslet GT, Lantos J. When adolescent and parents disagree on medical plan, who gets to decide? *Pediatrics.* 2019;144(2):e20190291. https://doi.org/10.1542/peds.2019-0291.
28. Dryden-Palmer K, Garros D, Meyer E, Farrell C, Parshuram C. Care for dying children and their families in PICU: promoting clinician education, support, and resilience. *Pediatr Crit Care Med J.* 2018;18(suppl 8):S79–S85. https://doi.org/10.1097/PCC.0000000000001594.
29. Kirsch RE, Munson D. Ethical and end of life considerations for neonates requiring ECMO support. *Semin Perinatol.* 2018;42:129–137.
30. de Araújo Affonseca C, Andrade de Carvalho L, de Pinho Barroso Quinet R, da Cunha Guimarães M, Cury V, Rotta A. Palliative extubation: five-year experience in a pediatric hospital. *J Pediatr (Rio J).* 2019;96(5):652–659.
31. Donoho K, Dabagh S, Caliboso M, Lotstein D, Nair S. Compassionate extubation protocol to improve team communication and support in the neonatal intensive care unit. *J Perinatol.* 2021;41(9):2355–2362.
32. Kirsch RE, Balit CR, Carnevale FA, Latour JM, Larcher V. Ethical, cultural, social, and individual considerations prior to transition to limitation or withdrawal of life-sustaining therapies. *Pediatr Crit Care Med.* 2018;19(suppl 8):S10–S18. https://doi.org/10.1097/PCC.0000000000001488.
33. Gibson JA, Boerstler JJ, Chase J, Smith C. Withdrawing life-sustaining treatments v. euthanasia: the ethical difference. *Nursing (Lond).* 2022;52(7):59–61. https://doi.org/10.1097/01.NURSE.0000832380.26717.3d.
34. Efstathiou N, Vanderspank-Wright B, Vandyk A, et al. Terminal withdrawal of mechanical ventilation in adult intensive care units: a systematic review and narrative synthesis of perceptions, experiences and practices. *Palliat Med.* 2020;34(9):1140–1164.
35. Kreicbergs U, Valdimarsdottir U, Onelov E, Bjork O, Steineck G, Henter JI. Care-related distress: a nationwide study of parents who lost their child to cancer. *J Clin Oncol.* 2005;23(36):9162–9171.
36. Eden LM, Callister LC. Parent involvement in end-of-life care and decision making in the newborn intensive care unit: an integrative review. *J Perinat Educ.* 2010;19(1):29–39. https://doi.org/10.1624/105812410X481546.
37. Moynihan KM, Dorste A, Siegel BD, Rabinowitz EJ, McReynolds A, October TW. Decision-making, ethics, and end-of-life care in pediatric extracorporeal membrane oxygenation: a comprehensive narrative review. *Pediatr Crit Care Med.* 2021;22(9):806–812. https://doi.org/10.1097/PCC.0000000000002766.
38. Friedman M, Hobson M. Extracorporeal membrane oxygenation for acute pediatric respiratory failure. In: Mastropietro CW, Valentine

KM, eds. *Pediatric Critical Care*. Springer International Publishing; 2019:17–41. https://doi.org/10.1007/978-3-319-96499-7_2.
39. Millum J. The foundation of the child's right to an open future. *J Soc Philos*. 2014;45(4):522–538. https://doi.org/10.1111/josp.12076.
40. Garrett JR, Lantos JD, Biesecker LG, et al. Rethinking the "open future" argument against predictive genetic testing of children. *Genet Med*. 2019;21(10):2190–2198. https://doi.org/10.1038/s41436-019-0483-4.
41. Child Welfare Information Gateway. (2019). About CAPTA: A legislative history. Washington, DC: U.S. Department of Health and Human Services, Children's Bureau.
42. Marron JM, Jones E, Wolfe J. Is there ever a role for the unilateral do not attempt resuscitation order in pediatric care? *J Pain Symptom Manage*. 2018;55(1):164–171. https://doi.org/10.1016/j.jpainsymman.2017.09.006.
43. Leeuwenburgh-Pronk WG, Miller-Smith L, Forman V, Lantos JD, Tibboel D, Buysse C. Are we allowed to discontinue medical treatment in this child? *Pediatrics*. 2015;135(3):545–549. https://doi.org/10.1542/peds.2014-0548.
44. Diekema D, Botkin J. Forgoing medically provided nutrition and hydration in children. *Pediatrics*. 2009;124(2):813–822.

39

Pediatric Spiritual Assessment and Care

Dianne Richoux and Judy Zeringue

Key Points

- Pediatric spiritual assessment is an essential component of palliative care as it provides significant information to be incorporated into the plan of care.
- A family's spiritual, religious, and/or cultural beliefs may influence decision-making and coping skills.
- Understanding the spiritual and developmental level of each child is an important factor in meeting their specific needs.
- Some barriers to obtaining a spiritual assessment include trauma situations, unanticipated deaths, and limited chaplain coverage.
- Hope can create space for coping and healing, irrespective of whether the goal is cure or comfort.
- Regardless of religion, faith, or culture, it is important to treat all patients and families with dignity and respect regarding end-of-life decisions.

Introduction

Understanding a child's spirituality is essential to caring for the whole child. Of note, throughout this chapter the terms "child" and "children" will represent neonates through adolescents.

The spiritual domain is, and has always been, integral to palliative care. The World Health Organization emphasizes that spiritual care is vital for enhancing quality of life and should be included in caring for patients and their families.[1] This insight of spiritual needs was first identified by Dame Cicely Saunders, the founder of modern palliative care, when she identified the multidimensional spiritual suffering at the end of life (EoL) which came to be known as "Total Pain."[1] The goals of palliative care include improving a patient's quality of life by assessing physical, psychosocial, and spiritual needs.[2] Research has also shown that spiritual needs are often not adequately assessed. Communication skills are essential in assessing the spiritual dimensions of patients and families. Attention to spiritual needs may positively impact a patient's quality of life; however, clinicians continue to report a lack of confidence in addressing a patient's spiritual distress.[3]

Definition of Spirituality

The National Consensus Project guidelines define spirituality as "a dynamic and intrinsic aspect of humanity through which persons seek ultimate meaning, purpose, transcendence, and experience relationship to self, family, others, community, society, nature, and the significant or sacred."[4 (p. 1687)] Spirituality is expressed through beliefs, values, traditions, and practices. As noted in this very collaborative definition, spirituality may encompass many aspects for everyone.[5] For some, spirituality is a part of transcendence and finding meaning in their life. Some find this through a particular community of faith or beliefs or values; others may not share any religious affiliation or beliefs. Some individuals may identify more with the strength and meaning found in the beauty of nature. Regardless of an individual, family, or caregiver's sources of strength, palliative care clinicians seek with humble curiosity to best determine how patients may be supported on their unique journeys.

As with religion, the heart of spirituality is the quest for meaning in human existence, especially in the presence of suffering and death.[6] The role of palliative care clinicians is to meet the patient/family/caregiver and support the holistic individual. Spirituality is an essential component to consider as a potential source of strength. Through humble curiosity, the clinician leans in, listens, and learns what is most important to this person. Spirituality is the aspect of humanity that refers to the way individuals seek and express meaning and purpose and the way they experience their connectedness to the moment, to self, to others, to nature, and to the significant or sacred.[1]

The expression of beliefs may be reflected through cultural beliefs and practices, traditions, and an individual's values. Members of a palliative interdisciplinary team (IDT) strive to incorporate this vital information into spiritual assessments. Religious beliefs or nonbeliefs may impact decisions regarding goals of care and EoL decisions. It is imperative to practice cultural humility and have humble curiosity to gain better insights into beliefs and values which are most important for a patient/family/caregiver. Recognizing where families are in their journeys at the initial consultation is essential to building relationships and trust. Emphasis on reassessing spiritual needs and providing support that individuals/families may or may not desire should be based on their unique journeys. An important component of holistic care is inclusion of a spiritual care assessment to identify important aspects to include in the care of a child and family.[7]

Definition of Spiritual Care

Compassionate Presence

Spiritual care begins with compassionate relationships. Compassion helps the nurse establish therapeutic communication with patients and facilitates their ability to understand patients, recognize their emotions and needs, and meet their spiritual needs.[8] Spiritual care is considered a component of relationship-centered compassionate care, with all members of the IDT having a unique role.[9] The term "bearing witness" entails compassionate presence, deep listening, watching, observing, and being with.[10] Presence offers time and space to build connections and help alleviate suffering.[11]

Empathetic Listening

Sitting in silence with a patient/family/caregiver is an important expression of spiritual care. Actions or nonverbal responses may speak louder than words. Empathetic listening and support offer an outlet to express emotions. Beginning with an open mind, listening with a sensitive heart, and acknowledging and validating feelings may help bring a sense of peace and hope to a difficult situation.[11] It is important that clinicians bring sincerity to each encounter. Spiritual care can be assessed through an open conversation, leaning in, and listening attentively to learn how to best support a particular patient, family, or caregiver. Regardless of a person's spiritual or religious belief or nonbelief, it is essential to engage in a way that builds trust and support.

Providing Prayer and Support

Whether meeting someone face to face or having a virtual visit or a phone conversation, clinicians must be mindful of expressing dignity and respect for every individual. Sharing in prayer, for those who find faith in prayer, is a way to instill hope.[12] Families with children who experience chronic illness and may be dying have shared remarkable insights based on the support of their faith. Providing space for presence and empathetic listening, nurses may encounter shared sacred thoughts during the illness journey.[13]

Spiritual Assessment

Spiritual assessment is an ongoing extensive process of evaluating a patient's spiritual needs and resources and should be explored by nurses or any member of the team.[14] Chaplains or spiritual care providers must cultivate cultural and spiritual humility as the true intent of spiritual assessment is to enter another person's spiritual world with reverence and compassionate curiosity.[1] This may reveal how spiritual aspects possibly impact healthcare decisions, goals-of-care discussions, and EoL desires, rituals, or limitations.

Spiritual Screening Tools

Asking about sources of strength for families can assist in spiritual screening. A brief screening tool may involve questions such as "Are you at peace?" or "What gives you strength?" Another question may be "Do you have a particular religious or spiritual belief?" This screening can be done by any nurse or any member of the IDT. Responses may elicit basic preferences of spiritual needs and identify the need for additional support. A table of three screening tools are listed below. Each provides guiding questions to assist in a spiritual assessment. These tools may be incorporated into nursing care and assessment.

Spiritual History

It is essential that palliative care nurses know how to assess spirituality. Additional spiritual care training courses may be necessary if not included in formal nursing education for nurses to feel more proficient in providing spiritual care to patients.[15] A spiritual history includes interviewing patients, from children to adults, in order to come to a better understanding of their spiritual needs and resources.[16] If patients and families identify with a specific faith, clinicians can ask if there are any religious or spiritual needs and how they may assist with them.[17] It may also be helpful to ask how families can be best supported during their hospitalizations. Addressing spiritual needs for a family who identify as finding strength in faith can be as important as identifying and addressing any other needs, such as pain or psychological support.[7] Engaging beliefs, values, experiences, and practices especially in the context of coping during illness can be a source of strength.[18]

Comparison of Models

In obtaining a spiritual history, some useful tools include the models outlined in Table 39.1. These models are grounded in the fundamental need to honor the dignity of all people and to provide compassionate presence to all patients and families.[16]

Table 39.1 Spiritual history models

FICA model	SPIRIT model	HOPE model
F (faith, belief, meaning)	**S** (spiritual belief system)	**H** (sources of hope)
I (importance or influence)	**P** (personal spirituality)	**O** (organized religion)
C (community)	**I** (integration with a spiritual community)	**P** (personal spirituality or spiritual practices)
A (address in care)	**R** (ritualized practices and restrictions)	**E** (effects on medical care and/or end-of-life issues)
	I (implications for medical care)	
	T (terminal events planning)	

Source: Reference 32.

Spirituality in Children

Childhood spirituality and faith can be a complex mixture, often making it difficult to distinguish one from the other.[19] Understanding the spiritual and faith development of children at each developmental stage is an important component of meeting the needs of each child.[19]

Spiritual conversations between nurses and children reveal that children may question God and the reason for their illnesses and want to talk and share descriptions of an afterlife as a way of understanding their limited life span.[20] This reinforces the need for nurses to be present and engage in spiritual communication with children.[12]

Spiritual Development by Age

Spiritual and religious experiences have implications for many aspects of development across the life span, including early childhood.[21] Spirituality may help some children deal with illnesses, especially those that are life-threatening. A child's spiritual dimension may not be directly related to their stage of cognitive development.[19] Childhood development may occur before faith development. Developmental psychology looks at the relationship between what children know and how they think.[19] Researchers such as Piaget explained the different stages in the structure of children's thinking.[19] Goldman and others explored how this affects thoughts about a child's faith. Based on these suggestions, there are three phases of childhood spiritual thinking, beginning with the preschooler and moving toward the adolescent.[19] Table 39.2 compares these phases in the development of theory and faith.

James Fowler's life-span "stages of faith" model was influenced by the work of many notable theorists, including Lawrence Kohlberg's work on moral development, Erik Erikson's understanding of psychosocial development, and Jean Piaget's understanding of the typical stages in a child's intellectual development.[19] Table 39.3 describes Fowler's life-span stages of faith.

Parental Influence

Emerging technology has extended children's lives, creating challenges for decision-making.[22] Religion and/or spirituality are important values for many parents; however, how religion and/or spirituality influence treatments options for their child, or how they respond to significant events during their child's illness treatment, remains unclear.[23] Understanding parental spiritual and religious beliefs may be important in the decision-making process. Incorporation of the expertise of spiritual care providers may provide the optimal context for enhanced collaboration with the IDT in the care of children at the EoL.[20]

When a child faces a serious illness, it has a profound effect on a family's physical, psychological, and spiritual health. When a family struggles with a child's serious illness, there are four spiritual themes that emerge: anger with God, blame/regret, forgiveness, and ritual/cultural traditions.[20] Blaming God for letting their children get sick, and sometimes anger at God, may cause families to abandon their faith. Many families find new meaning through spirituality as anger about illness results in spiritual distress and the need for support. Some families need to express blame or regret, especially at the end of a child's life. Some parents and siblings blame themselves, questioning whether something they had done caused the child's illness or, perhaps, why a cure was not found. Parents and families often seek forgiveness from their dying child or children from their parents at the EoL.[20]

Table 39.2 Development of theory and faith

Stage	Scripture	God image	Prayer	Religious identity
Stage 1 Intuitive religious thinking Age 2–5	Magical explanations of religious events.	A magical power.	A wishful magical activity.	Automatic, unquestioned.
Stage 2 Literal religious thinking Age 5–11	Engrossed by narrative but cannot extract meaning.	Anthropomorphic (e.g., a man with a beard).	Instrumental; bargaining to get things I like.	Literal logic.
Stage 3 Abstract religious thinking Age 11+	Can use symbolic, metaphorical levels of meaning to make sense; deeper concepts are possible.	Can be abstract, multifaceted.	Exploration of oneself before God; communicative.	Outcome of making a personal choice.

Source: Reference 19.

Table 39.3 Fowler's life-span stages of faith

Stage	Type	Definition
Stage 0 Infants up to 3 years	Primal or undifferentiated	Faith emerges as a sense of trust.
Stage 1 Age 3–6 years	Intuitive-projective	Faith is led by imagination and feelings.
Stage 2 Age 6–12	Mythical-literal	Faith begins to be simple thinking.
Stage 3 Adolescents	Synthetic-conventional	Faith becomes a form of loyalty.

Source: Reference 19.

Preserving Hope

Hope is a uniquely powerful mechanism that enables coping and promotes resilience among children experiencing serious illness. Hope is described as a life-sustaining factor, one that impacts decision-making.[24] Hope can help create space for coping and healing, irrespective of whether the goal is cure or comfort and may change over time. Faith or spiritual beliefs may align with one's hopes. Families with children who experience serious illness will often strive to keep that hope throughout the journey of the child's illness.[24]

Rituals/Cultural Traditions

Rituals may include presentation to the congregation; communion; anointing of the sick; prayer; scripture reading, chanting, or singing; or saying the rosary.[25] Focusing on what may be most meaningful to support families, nurses may identify the need to provide sacred space to support the family's beliefs and means of finding strength. Rituals are not always religious in nature and are often created in the moment to honor a loved one, event, or circumstance.[10] A time to honor a loved one with words from the heart can be a beautiful and spontaneous ritual to bring connection and soothe the soul. The gathering of those near and dear is a sacred time to cherish and express support for someone's beloved child. The recognition of the influence of culture and religious or spiritual practices can also have a meaningful influence on how families process grief and bereavement.[6] Family religious faith traditions may include dedication, prayers, chanting/singing/music, or a rosary. A sacred space for a family may be the patient's room, a significant location, or the hospital's chapel.

Rituals

It is human nature to acknowledge when significant experiences or transitions occur in our lives. Rituals are used to give honor and provide connection and order to such events.[13] Significant experiences in the lives of people are often honored with rituals to acknowledge an event or transition.[16] An important aspect to consider and assess is a patient/family's need for meaning and memory-making, within the context of their unique health journey. Some families employ religious rituals such as prayer, baptism, reading of sacred texts, singing of sacred music, and blessings; others may desire hospital visits and emotional and spiritual support from a local faith leader, clergy person, or hospital chaplain. Many families practice their spiritual beliefs at the bedside by providing a peaceful presence and offering tender, loving care to their loved one.[26]

Case Study: Honoring Religious Beliefs with Cultural Humility

A beautiful baby boy came into this world and was part of a family who loved him dearly. Ezra was born with multiple complex congenital anomalies which presented challenges in his journey. Meeting this family in consultation, it was important to learn about the patient, his family, and other factors which influenced and impacted their life and decisions and their coping strategies. This was a family who found strength in their faith. They identified as members of the Coptic Orthodox Church which included a supportive faith community. To honor their religious beliefs, the family invited their priest to come to the hospital and perform a beautiful sacred baptism. When the family realized that time was short, they made the most of every day. Sibling visits were important for making lifetime memories by allowing precious time for Ezra's siblings to bond with him. The child life specialist worked with the siblings to prepare them for visits based on their developmental level. Photos were taken to capture these sacred memories. These special moments helped to develop and enrich family bonding and brought great comfort to the family.

Through spiritual assessment and open communication, the palliative care team, nurses, and primary team members began a relationship built on trust, honoring the wishes and desires of this loving family. As members of the Coptic (Egyptian) Orthodox religion the family found great support in their community of faith. These are Christians who practice their faith away from their unique homeland of Ethiopia. There were some family members who lived near and other extended family support in Ethiopia. With the focus being on the family's values and beliefs, all decisions and discussions were directed toward the family's goals of care and included any specific rituals. Nurses caring for Ezra provided a level of comfort by compassionately caring for him when the family could not be present.

At the time of Ezra's death, his loving family and extended family members gathered in his room. They prayed with him, lovingly took turns holding him, and shared this sacred time as a family. It was beautiful to witness the incredible outpouring of love for this beloved child. This sacred time that Ezra and his family were able to experience at the end of his life is one that made a lasting impression and provided great comfort to the family. Nurses also shared in the experience by granting the family the time they needed together and inviting them to participate in postmortem care. As the hospital chaplain visited this family to express his condolences, they invited him to share in prayer. This prayer was concluded by Ezra's father in his native language.

Support for Patients/Families

As a family/caregiver experiences the suffering of a beloved child, they seek support for strength and hope. Spirituality often provides this needed strength and support to lean on in the most difficult time.[26] Assessment of spiritual or religious needs is an important aspect of caring for the whole person, especially in pediatrics. Identification of the family's strengths and support is important to include in the spiritual assessment and should be approached with humble curiosity and presence.[6] Utilizing a practice of sincere cultural humility, we are open to inquiring about the special needs and beliefs of those entrusted to our care.[6] Nurses have a unique vantage point to incorporate spiritual questions with humble curiosity, great compassion, and respect to elicit spiritual beliefs and support which may be beneficial in the care of patients, families, and caregivers. By simply altering one's approach from one of an expert to that of an attentive learner, most patients/families/caregivers will be more open and honest regarding their beliefs.[27] Spirituality is an extremely valued dimension for those who receive palliative nursing care. It is essential that nurses know how to assess spirituality since it is an ongoing process. Spiritual assessment and integration of this information into a patient care plan are important to provide holistic care.[27] Nurses must be attentive to recognizing their own spiritual and emotional needs. This knowledge can be important in reaching the people nurses care for and in finding rich meaning in care and support.[26] Treatment decisions, care planning, direct services, and all roles of the palliative care team revolve around the meaning of life for a particular patient and family. By their own definition and prioritization, the family's hopes and needs are the aspects which will make life most meaningful during the remaining days, weeks, months, or years of the child's life.[27]

Chaplains

Chaplains are identified leaders who have acquired an extended education in pastoral care. They may be ordained, commissioned, or otherwise based in their religious-tradition community.[8] Chaplains can assist families to locate or connect with local clergy and may help children explore their spirituality and ability to wonder, providing children with a safe space to engage in their spirituality.[22] A key value of pediatric chaplaincy is to offer supportive care even if it may not align with the religious beliefs of patients and families.[10] Chaplains and spiritual care providers should be open to all in need. Providing a ministry of presence, attentive listening, and hospitality is important in building relationships and developing trust. Nurses often struggle with time constraints and available resources to provide necessary spiritual care. By performing a spiritual assessment, the need for a chaplain may be identified. Chaplains are a source of expertise in areas of specific rituals, spiritual distress, or a desire for greater focus on discussions on spiritual needs and support. Chaplains and other members of the healthcare team, including nurses, can impact the experience of a patient/family/caregiver by allowing space to share their inner thoughts and being fully present with an open mind and compassionate heart.[11]

Barriers to Obtaining a Spiritual Assessment

Trauma/Unanticipated Deaths

When pediatric deaths occur within minutes to days of the cause (unintentional injury, extremely preterm birth, catastrophic illness), it becomes a challenge to meet the spiritual needs of patients and families as the focus may be more on the patient's physical needs than the spiritual needs of the patient and family.[28] To address the spiritual and psychological needs of patients and families facing unexpected death or in the critical care areas, it is essential that nurses perform a spiritual assessment and provide spiritual care as needed. The awareness that spirituality is an essential component of quality of life has led to the recognition of the need for further development of complementary and effective spiritual care in the critical care areas to relieve the distress of patients and their families.[29]

Limited Chaplain Coverage

One growing approach has been to utilize the generalist/specialist model in providing spiritual care in the hospital setting. While most healthcare givers appreciate the importance of spirituality in patient-centered care, few have received adequate training to undertake it skillfully.[30] Some focused spiritual education is provided through the Interprofessional Spiritual Care Education Curriculum for Pediatrics (ISPEC-Peds). ISPEC provides a systematic way to address spirituality and assessment as the important aspect of care is caring for the whole patient.[30] When needing greater spiritual expertise, a consultation with the chaplain should be started. If chaplain coverage is limited, utilization of resources within an IDT such as nurses, doctors, social workers, and child life specialist can provide support.

EoL Decisions

Postmortem Care

Religious beliefs and traditions may impact postmortem care. Table 39.4 shows some specific examples regarding postmortem care based on religion. It is essential to clarify what is most important to each family regarding their specific beliefs and desires. Regardless of religion, faith, or culture, it is important to treat all with dignity and respect. For the Islamic tradition, a same-sex Muslim must wash the body, and it is essential to keep the body covered. In Judaism, it is important for nurses to assess and respect the tradition that individuals outside of the family handle the body as little as possible. In Hinduism, prayers and meditation in a quiet environment may be important. In Sikhism beliefs, the family often desires to wash the body.[31]

Burial

Time of burial and/or cremation may be significantly impacted based on one's religion. Please refer to Table 39.4 for some examples.[31] It is important to keep in mind that these examples may or may not apply to all people within a certain religion. It is not appropriate to assume, but express humble curiosity and ask the family for their specific desires and wishes related to death. Death preference location is another important aspect for thoughtful consideration if time and condition permit. Please see Table 39.4, which lists the most prevalent religions and provides an overview of traditions.

Spiritual Distress

The idea of spiritual distress is so closely aligned with the idea of existential suffering that they are often indistinguishable.[6] As nurses, we should never underestimate the profoundness of a child's spiritual experience, especially dying children.[10] Spiritual care of the child begins by building trust and respect. Allowing a dying child to share their thoughts through words, art, or play minimizes spiritual distress. Clinicians should always be mindful of a child's sacred space.

IDT

Each member of the IDT may contribute to including spiritual assessment within the initial palliative care consult. Nurses are trained to have compassion and to serve those in need, meeting all aspects of care dimensions when providing a holistic-care approach. Nurses

Table 39.4 Religious considerations as death is near and care after death, burial, and bereavement

Religion	Faith leader	Rituals in anticipation of death	Postmortem	Religious traditions for burial	Bereavement traditions based on religion
Christianity	Chaplain Priest Minister Reverend	Anointing with oil, prayer, communion, repentance	Treat the body with respect and dignity.	Burial or cremation permitted.	No official mourning practices.
Islam	Imam	Family may wish patient to face Mecca (southeast)	Same-sex Muslims must wash the body. Body must be kept covered. It is important to ask permission to touch the body.	Timely burial is essential, within 24 hours facing Mecca. (southeast)	Tradition of mourning period of 40 days. Food is provided by family.
Judaism	Rabbi	Prayer and confession on deathbed.	Shema is recited. (declaration of death). Body is not left alone after death until time of burial. Individuals outside of the family handle the body as little as possible.	Burial as soon as possible, within 24 hours. Some non-orthodox permit cremation.	Mourners sit shiva at home.
Buddhism	Monk	Provide a peaceful environment for meditation.	Prayers and meditation may take place. Buddhists believe that reincarnation of the soul takes place after death.	The body is cremated after the service. Burial up to 1 week after death.	Ask the family as practices vary. There is often a funeral service with an altar for the deceased person.
Hinduism	Hindu priest	Prayers and hymns from Hindu holy books. Water from the Ganges is sacred.	Do not remove jewelry, straighten limbs. Family may want to wash the body.	Children under 3 years old are buried. Older children and adults are kept in the family home until cremated within 24 hours.	Mourners walk around the coffin. Hindu priest chants from scripture, and eldest performs rituals. Mourning period 10–16 days.
Sikhism	Guru	Hymns from the Sikh holy book.	Family members may wash the body. Do not trim hair. Plain white cloth to cover the body. Name of God (Waheguru) recited. Holy water (Amrit).	Cremation as soon as possible. They believe that cremation will let the soul detach from the body and reunite with God or Waheguru.	Up to 10 days of reading from scriptures. The eldest son is given a turban as a sign that he is now head of the family.

Source: Reference 31.

may assess these spiritual needs longitudinally as the illness progresses. For some healthcare professionals, spiritual care may be intuitive, but most will need to develop the knowledge and skills for providing high-quality and competent spiritual care.[1] Spiritual care providers may offer emotional support for those who find strength in faith, religion, or spirituality.[8] Nurses have a strong voice and unique lens to assess and address those important spiritual needs which may be identified as they share in care. As spirituality becomes an integral part of the medical structure, it is important to help caregivers identify spiritual themes and needs.[9] Nurses often report feeling ill-equipped to care for these children and their families and, in particular, a lack of self-confidence in discussing suffering, death, spirituality, hope, or EoL care with families.[22] In order to provide compassionate care, nurses must practice good self-care. This will allow nurses to be at their best when leaning in and supporting those in need. One source of strength may be in a routine awareness of strengthening spiritual beliefs and practices.

Spiritual Care Education to Support the Development of Spiritual Care

Opportunities for further training are emerging, such as ISPEC, which is now being adapted into the pediatric-specific ISPEC-Peds.[18] This interdisciplinary approach to providing spiritual care offers a much broader perspective in assessing the spiritual needs of those we serve. Ongoing education and support of the interprofessional healthcare team will be critical elements in the sustainability of the change in practice for attending to patients' spiritual needs.[27]

Conclusion

Understanding pediatric patients' and families' spiritual, religious, and cultural beliefs is an essential component of pediatric palliative care. Because spiritual or religious beliefs may influence decision-making and coping efforts, it is necessary that a spiritual assessment is part of the patient's history. It is also important to understand the spiritual developmental level of each child to better create more meaningful relationships with children and their families. There may be barriers to obtaining a spiritual assessment including traumatic situations, unanticipated deaths, and limited chaplain coverage. Families of children with life-threatening illness may have diverse cultural and ethnic beliefs, customs, practices, or rituals surrounding illness and/or death. A thorough spiritual assessment ensures that this significant information is incorporated into the patient's plan of care. Spiritual support and care may be provided by nurses in various ways and are vital in providing quality care.

REFERENCES

1. Puchalski CM. *Making Health Care Whole: Integrating Spirituality into Health Care*. New Age Books; 2012.

2. Wierstra IR, Liefbroer AI, Post L, Tromp T, Körver J. Addressing spiritual needs in palliative care: proposal for a narrative and interfaith spiritual care intervention for chaplaincy. *J Health Care Chaplain*. 2023;29(1):64–77. https://doi.org/10.1080/08854726.2021.2015055.
3. Ferrell BR, Buller H, Paice JA, Glajchen M, Haythorn T. Interprofessional communication training to address spiritual aspects of cancer care. *J Health Care Chaplain*. 2023;29(4):381–393. https://doi.org/10.1080/08854726.2022.2097781.
4. Ferrell BR, Twaddle ML, Melnick A, Meier DE. National Consensus Project clinical practice guidelines for quality palliative care guidelines, 4th edition. *J Palliat Med*. 2018;21(12):1684–1689. https://doi.org/10.1089/jpm.2018.0431.
5. Puchalski CM. *A Time for Listening and Caring: Spirituality and the Care of the Chronically Ill and Dying*. Oxford University Press; 2006.
6. Wolfe J, Hinds PS, Sourkes BM. *Interdisciplinary Pediatric Palliative Care*. Oxford University Press; 2021.
7. Smith C, Lakin T. Effects of an interprofessional spiritual care education project. *J Hosp Palliat Nurs*. 2022;24(1):78–83. https://doi.org/10.1097/NJH.0000000000000819.
8. Türkben Polat H, Özdemir AA. Relationship between compassion and spiritual care among nurses in Turkey. *J Relig Health*. 2022;61(3):1894–1905. https://doi.org/10.1007/s10943-021-01287-6.
9. Falkenburg JL, van Dijk M, Tibboel D, Ganzevoort RR. The fragile spirituality of parents whose children died in the pediatric intensive care unit. *J Health Care Chaplain*. 2019;26(3):117–130. https://doi.org/10.1080/08854726.2019.1670538.
10. Ferrell BR. *Spiritual, Religious, and Cultural Aspects of Care*. Oxford University Press; 2015. https://doi.org/10.1093/med/9780190244231.001.0001.
11. Bartel M, Nash S, Nash P. *Paediatric Chaplaincy: Principles, Practices and Skills*. Jessica Kingsley Publishers; 2018.
12. Ferrell B, Wittenberg E, Battista V, Walker G. Nurses' experiences of spiritual communication with seriously Ill children. *J Palliat Med*. 2016;19(11):1166–1170.
13. Carter BS, Levetown M, Friebert SE. *Palliative Care for Infants, Children, and Adolescents: A Practical Handbook*. 2nd ed. Johns Hopkins University Press; 2011.
14. Muehlhausen BL, Foster T, Smith AH, Fitchett G. Patients' and loved ones' expectations of chaplain services. *J Health Care Chaplain*. 2022;28(3):350–364. https://doi.org/10.1080/08854726.2021.1903734.
15. Lukovsky J, McGrath E, Sun C, Frankl D, Beauchesne MA. A survey of hospice and palliative care nurses' and holistic nurses' perceptions of spirituality and spiritual care. *J Hosp Palliat Nurs*. 2021;23(1):28–37. https://doi.org/10.1097/NJH.0000000000000711.
16. Taylor EJ. Initial spiritual screening and assessment: five things to remember. *J Hosp Palliat Care*. 2020;23(1):1–4. https://doi.org/10.14475/kjhpc.2020.23.1.1.
17. Kim K, Bauck A, Monroe A, Mallory M, Aslakson R. Critical care nurses' perceptions of and experiences with chaplains. *J Hosp Palliat Nurs*. 2017;19(1):41–48. https://doi.org/10.1097/NJH.0000000000000303.
18. Taylor EJ, Trippon M. What chaplains wish nurses knew. *Holist Nurs Pract*. 2020;34(5):266–273. https://doi.org/10.1097/HNP.0000000000000401.
19. Nye R. Child spirituality and faith development. In: Bartel M, Nash S, Nash P, eds. *Paediatric Chaplaincy*, Jessica Kingsley Publishers; 2018:23–36.
20. Arutyunyan T, Odetola F, Swieringa R, Niedner M. Religion and spiritual care in pediatric intensive care unit: parental attitudes regarding physician spiritual and religious inquiry. *Am J Hosp Palliat Med*. 2018;35(1):28–33. https://doi.org/10.1177/1049909116682016.
21. Abo-Zena MM, Midgette A. Developmental implications of children's early religious and spiritual experiences in context: a sociocultural perspective. *Religions*. 2019;10(11):631. https://doi.org/10.3390/rel10110631.
22. Superdock AK, Barfield RC, Brandon DH, Docherty SL. Exploring the vagueness of religion & spirituality in complex pediatric decision-making: a qualitative study. *BMC Palliat Care*. 2018;17(1):107. https://doi.org/10.1186/s12904-018-0360-y.
23. Uveges MK, Hamilton JB, DePriest K, Boss R, Hinds PS, Nolan MT. The influence of parents' religiosity or spirituality on decision making for their critically ill child: an integrative review. *J Palliat Med*. 2019;22(11):1455–1467. https://doi.org/10.1089/jpm.2019.0154.
24. Kaye EC, Kiefer A, Blazin L, et al. Bereaved parents, hope, and realism. *Pediatrics*. 2020;145(5):e20192771.
25. Hall EJ, Hughes BP, Handzo GH. Spiritual care: what it means, why it matters in health care. *Health Chaplain Netw*. 2016;(October):1–16.
26. Limbo R, Wool C, Carter BS. *Handbook of Perinatal and Neonatal Palliative Care: A Guide for Nurses, Physicians, and Other Health Professionals*. Springer Publishing; 2020.
27. Denney-Koelsch EM, Côté-Arsenault D, eds. *Perinatal Palliative Care: A Clinical Guide*. Springer International Publishing; 2020. https://doi.org/10.1007/978-3-030-34751-2.
28. Pierce A, Hoffer M, Marcinkowski B, Manfredi RA, Pourmand A. Emergency department approach to spirituality care in the era of COVID-19. *Am J Emerg Med*. 2021;46:765–768. https://doi.org/10.1016/J.AJEM.2020.09.026.
29. Willemse S, Smeets W, van Leeuwen E, Nielen-Rosier T, Janssen L, Foudraine N. Spiritual care in the intensive care unit: an integrative literature research. *J Crit Care*. 2020;57:55–78. https://doi.org/10.1016/J.JCRC.2020.01.026.
30. Szilagyi C, Lion AH, Varner Perez SE, et al. Interprofessional spiritual care education in pediatric hematology-oncology: a pilot study. *Pediatr Blood Cancer*. 2022;69(3):e29515. https://doi.org/10.1002/pbc.29515.
31. Santucci G, ed. *Core Curriculum for the Pediatric Hospice and Palliative Nurse*. Hospice and Palliative Nurses Association; 2017.
32. Taylor E. Spiritual screening, history, and assessment. In: Ferrell BR, Paice JA, eds. *Oxford Textbook of Palliative Nursing*. 5th ed. Oxford University Press; 2019:432–446.

40

Palliative Care in the Perinatal Setting: Neonatal Intensive Care Unit and Labor and Delivery Unit

Cheryl Ann Thaxton, Kathleen Ellis, and Andrea Biondi

Key Points

- Care for an infant, either prenatally or postnatally, with a life-limiting or life-threatening condition is one of the most intimate times that a nurse can share with a family.
- Palliative care incorporates comfort care in addition to pain and symptom management for the infant. It also includes emotional, psychosocial, and spiritual support for the infant and family members.
- Palliative care involves a dynamic exchange of information between the interdisciplinary team and the family; the nurse has a compelling role in prenatal and neonatal palliative and end-of-life care.[1,2]

Introduction

According to the American College of Obstetricians and Gynecologists (ACOG), "perinatal palliative care refers to a coordinated care strategy that comprises options for obstetric and newborn care that include a focus on maximizing quality of life and comfort for newborns with a variety of conditions considered to be life-limiting in early infancy... with a dual focus on ameliorating suffering and honoring patient values, perinatal palliative care can be provided concurrently with life-prolonging treatment."[3(pe84)] Due to technological advances in the past 30 years in diagnosing fetal anomalies and genetic disorders during the prenatal period, parents may face months of anguish and uncertainty as they prepare for the birth of an infant with a life-limiting, life-threatening, or lethal condition.[4,5] The sudden delivery of a prematurely born infant also may pose existential stress within the family unit. In 2020, the infant mortality rate in the United States was 5.4 deaths per 1,000 live births; the 10 leading causes of infant death were congenital malformations, low birth weight, sudden infant death syndrome, unintentional injuries, maternal complications, cord and placental complications, bacterial sepsis of newborn, respiratory distress of newborn, diseases of the circulatory system, and neonatal hemorrhage.[1]

Care of the family as a unit is vital to implementing the highest-quality palliative care. "A dedicated multidisciplinary team that is comprehensive of all the specialists involved in the perinatal care path should continually reassess all the needs (of the body, mind, and spirit) of the newborn and family while trying to give timely and concrete answers to each of them."[6(p2)] As the time draws near for the birth of the baby, each family member will individually transition through thoughts that pose more questions than answers as they come to understand the long-term consequences of the infant's underlying condition, poor prognosis, and/or poor quality of life.[7] The nurse is in a key position to provide support and bring the needed aspects of care together during this challenging time. In addition to the nurse and social work leaders, neonatologists, nurses, social workers, pastoral care, and child life specialists are the frontline providers for end-of-life care.[8]

After delivery, the baby may receive care in the neonatal intensive care unit (NICU) or remain in the labor and delivery (L&D) unit for post-delivery care. When palliative care is initiated early in a disease process, even absent the likelihood of death, the focus may shift to decision-making, setting value-based goals, and building relationships between clinicians and families.[9] Nurses should recognize the sensitive nature of this subject and use language to promote a culturally sensitive, patient- and family-centered approach to the care of the infant during this difficult time for the family. Several evidence-based communication strategies can be utilized to facilitate this process of communication. Vague communication can lead to confusion and frustration about the specific prognosis of a fetus or infant.[10] Providing a seamless transition into palliative care requires an interdisciplinary effort and the support of the entire healthcare team. Implementing a palliative care protocol involves tremendous individual planning that supports a variety of choices, which may include various aspects of active life-sustaining measures up until the end of the infant's life. A medical interpreter must be utilized whenever the provider and the family do not share the same primary language.[11] The nurse has a vital role in ensuring that communication with the family is not fragmented and that parents are reassured that the best effort will be made to support their wishes throughout the uncertainty of the journey. The dignity of the infant and family should be maintained at all costs.

Patient- and family-centered care measures seek to ensure that the final hours of a dying infant are spent in a peaceful environment and in the presence of the family. This chapter presents the core values of perinatal and neonatal palliative care nursing within the context of providing culturally appropriate, compassionate, individualized, family-centered developmental care (IFDC) and patient-focused care for infants receiving care in the L&D and in the NICU environment. Core components of IFDC include parent engagement, cue-based care, and the provision of a supportive environment.[12] To illustrate the use of palliative care with the neonatal population, the following case study will provide a unique scenario for reflection.

Case Study: A Broken Heart: Coco's Story

Coco was born at 29 weeks' gestation after the onset of preterm labor, prolonged rupture of membranes, and subsequent womb infection called "chorioamnionitis." At age 39 the pregnancy was "a miracle" after years of failed infertility services. Coco's mother, Greta, was classified as "advanced maternal age and high risk." She married late in life to a busy enlisted officer, John, a widower and single parent to two young, busy teenage girls. Greta's parents had died, and her sister lived on the opposite side of the country. For Greta, it was tough and lonely at times being a military wife and stepmom, but this was not unusual on the Army base where the family lived. The stress of failed conception attempts and John's frequent deployments put physical and emotional distance between them. The surprise pregnancy seemed to bring back the joy in their lives, if only briefly.

They decided not to do some of the typical prenatal tests that could detect birth defects, nor did they want to know the gender of the infant. The 14-week fetal ultrasound showed a heart with four chambers and possible trisomy. This was a shock to the parents, and John would not discuss it with the high-risk obstetric physician, explaining to the physician that he and Greta expected everything to be "normal" and that the tests were "not always right." He was resolute and stoic when any mention of the baby came up in conversation. They planned to deliver at the military hospital nearby that had a Level II nursery. Greta continued her prenatal visits, and John deployed, leaving preparations at home for the baby to her alone. Greta had been on and off antidepressants for the past few years but decided not to take any medications other than her prenatal vitamins during the pregnancy. The joy of finally being pregnant seemed to carry her through each day.

Greta eventually went into preterm labor, and Baby Coco was born by emergency C-section at 30 weeks and 1 day, weighing 900 g. Coco did not cry at first, and her skin was a color between blue and gray. Swiftly acting NICU staff placed an endotracheal tube to help her breathe and wheeled the transporter nearby. Greta held Coco's tiny hand that was tightly clenched and noticed her unusual facial features. Greta knew there was something different about her right away.

Coco was whisked to the NICU, and several hours later, Greta could visit her. NICU staff was around her incubator, doing all sorts of tasks and discussing her vital signs and lab results. Greta could tell some were seasoned nurses. There were also younger nurses in training nervously performing tasks while medical students observed attending physicians and neonatal nurse practitioners in charge of Coco's care. Some staff made eye contact with Greta, some did not, and she could hear whispers from other parents through thin hanging curtains in the unit about "a sick baby" just admitted. She could see parents holding their babies, some touching their preemies through incubator portals, and even moms breastfeeding some healthier infants. Greta felt as if her world was spinning. An older nurse with kind eyes approached her and gently touched her arm. Her name was Sherry, and she would be Coco's primary nurse. That meant she would care for her each shift she was at work. Sherry told Greta her baby was beautiful and explained she would do everything she could to help make Coco comfortable and to ensure Greta understood everything the team was doing to stabilize her child. Greta felt her confidence, making her feel stronger and less alone.

The neonatologist explained that Coco had a very loud murmur, and her oxygen was low despite supplementation. A pediatric cardiologist was on the way to examine her, but they suspected she might have a heart defect. Greta stood by her incubator, exhausted, as the cardiologist performed the echocardiogram and shared the devastating news of Coco's congenital heart defect. It was operable, but with her diagnosis of trisomy 18, it would be unlikely that a pediatric cardiothoracic surgeon would be willing to do the extensive repairs to help her survive. The left side of Coco's heart was underdeveloped, and her chances of surviving due to genetics and low birth weight were slim. She also was diagnosed with a large atrioventricular defect. The cardiologist hand-drew a heart diagram to make it more understandable. It was too much to take in all at once, and Greta was left feeling hopeless. The NICU staff were supportive and kind and told her they would keep Coco stable until a decision was made to transport her to a hospital over 2 hours away or make plans for "comfort care." The neonatal nurse practitioner (NNP) ordered an intravenous (IV) drip medication called prostaglandin, which would keep her patent ductus arteriosus open and allow blood to flow better to her extremities. It was going "to buy Coco time" until John, Greta's husband, could return, and they could make decisions together about her care. The Red Cross was contacted to help bring John back from deployment.

Coco required mechanical ventilation for 3 days and could wean to continuous positive airway pressure (CPAP). Her lungs were immature, but she was able to breathe on her own with this respiratory support device. Genetic tests were sent, and Greta was forced to confront a flurry of confusing medical jargon, tests, tubes, wires, pumps, and machinery, all to keep Coco stable. The NICU team was certain Coco would be diagnosed with trisomy 18.

Sherry showed Greta how to touch Coco to calm her and encouraged "skin-to-skin" holding once she was on CPAP. Sherry was always encouraging and told her how well she did with Coco's sponge bath and how peaceful Coco looked in her arms. She swabbed Coco's tiny mouth with pumped breast milk, which was slowly increasing in volume each day, and showed her how to change her diaper without interfering with the IV and monitor wires. Greta was pumping every three hours, but it was only drops of milk, which became frustrating. The staff offered donor breast milk to supplement maternal expressed milk, but Greta knew her husband would disapprove. They used a preterm formula to feed her and slowly increased the amount given every 12 hours.

Finally, the Red Cross was able to arrange the return of John from deployment, and he arrived at the hospital on Coco's sixth day of life. He was distant and quiet and wanted to meet with the NICU providers and cardiologist right away. He was a soldier who was accustomed to being in control and wanted to hear all the options for Coco's care. Without any discussion with Greta, he explained to the care team that "we" wanted everything done for Coco to survive and giving up was not an option. He needed sleep from his long flight home and left the hospital with plans to return the next morning.

Days passed, and no hospital with a pediatric cardiothoracic surgeon was willing to accept care for Coco. In their expert opinions, the low survival odds combined with her trisomy 18 and very low birth weight excluded her from the surgery she needed to repair her "broken" heart. The NICU team was gently helping Greta accept the inevitable outcome, but her husband insisted that Coco have heart surgery.

Coco's vital signs were not stable one night. She began to have apneic events, and her oxygen saturation dropped periodically. The NICU NNP increased her caffeine dose and intubated her, placing her back on mechanical ventilation to help her rest her lungs. Her blood gasses showed metabolic acidosis, and an X-ray of her lungs showed excess fluid. Her belly became full and firm in the early morning hours, and her feedings of Greta's precious drops of breastmilk were stopped as she was made NPO. Greta sat at her bedside again, only to receive more bad news that Coco's intestines showed inflammation and that air had been seen in the intestinal walls in a process called pneumatosis. Bacteria had caused this as well as the bloody stool the nurses had reported being found in her tiny diaper overnight. Coco had necrotizing enterocolitis (NEC).

Three types of antibiotics were given to Coco, and a pediatric surgeon was consulted to look at her abdominal X-ray. It was a poor prognosis based on the amount of bowel that was involved in addition to her confirmed diagnosis of trisomy 18 and a complex heart defect. Greta called her husband and explained that he needed to come back to the hospital right away. Coco's blood pressure was dropping, and the skin on her abdomen looked tight and uncomfortable. The neonatologist explained that she would likely die in the next 24 hours and staff would do their best to make her comfortable. Greta felt overwhelmed and alone.

Greta got to know the nurses by name in just a few days. Some of the younger nurses she noticed would not make eye contact but continued to assist Coco's primary nurse. She could tell they did not know what to say, but Greta felt confident they were skilled at Coco's physical care. The primary nurse, Sherry, was there on the last day; and she was the one who gently placed Coco's tiny, frail body in Greta's arms, knowing she was leaving them soon and wanting her to have as much time holding Coco as possible. In just a few days, Sherry seemed to understand so much about the family and knew compassion and calmness were what Greta needed the most. John finally arrived. He sat beside Greta as the neonatologist explained that Coco's heart and lungs were failing as her intestinal infection spread. He refused to hold Coco but sat with Greta as the nurses carefully removed her umbilical lines and the complicated tangle of wires and tubes. John and Greta asked if Coco could be given pain medication since Sherry had mentioned her abdomen was likely very tender. They saw her little face relax as she was medicated, and soon after, once her heart rate became very slow and irregular, the respiratory therapist removed the breathing tube and tape from her face. She slipped away peacefully. John disappeared from the room, stoic, leaving Greta with her baby girl, who had suffered so much in her short life. Greta could see many of the NICU staff standing quietly by. Some made eye contact, while others kept busy with bedside tasks. She felt that gentle hand again on her arm, and Sherry explained she would not leave Greta's side. Sherry would move Coco and Greta to a more private area of the NICU. Greta was grateful Sherry was such a confident, kind, and empathic nurse who seemed to intuitively know what needed to be done.

Sherry helped Greta bathe Coco and put her in a tiny, white preemie dress with ribbons and a ruffled hat. Sherry printed Coco's feet onto a beautiful card and put her name band, umbilical clamp, crib card, and a lock of hair into a tiny treasure box. Greta held her for hours in the privacy of a quiet, softly lit NICU annex in a large, cushioned chair. Greta heard the door open gently and felt a hand on her shoulder. John stood over her, tears running down his face, and he knelt to wrap his arms around Greta and Coco. Greta nodded at Sherry, and she silently retreated from the annex. Greta told John it was okay to let Coco go peacefully and without pain. He could not speak, but he was there; and Greta understood him enough to know this was how he began to grieve. Greta didn't know if they could heal from this, but she had so much gratitude for the support Sherry and the NICU team gave and had even tried to offer John. The time Greta had to bond with her baby and the reassurance from the care team about letting Coco go would be something she would carry with her forever.

Before they left the hospital, Sherry explained she was a lead nurse on the bereavement team and asked if it would be okay to keep in contact. Greta agreed but was not sure it would help and might even make it harder to get over the loss of her baby. About a month later, a notecard came in the mail, handwritten by Sherry, and signed by the nurse, NNPs, and neonatologists who cared for Coco. They wanted Greta to know that she and her family were not forgotten and how special Coco was. A tiny silver angel medallion was enclosed as well as a contact for the bereavement counselor and a monthly support group at the Army base hospital. It was a simple compassionate gesture that helped Greta begin her journey to closure over the loss of Coco. Greta wrapped her hand around the medallion and took a deep breath.

Summary of Coco's Case

The NICU nurse must be present at the most difficult time for the family, be fully attentive to the infant and family, and separate personal values regarding birth, life, and death. Nurses must adapt and individualize their care to help families cope emotionally with the unexpected loss of an infant. Coco's primary nurse communicated appropriately and shared her compassion with this family while advocating for their privacy, addressing Coco's pain, and keeping them informed of what the medical team was doing. She helped Coco's mother to build her confidence in simple tasks that promoted bonding as well.

The Integration of Palliative Care Principles within the Neonatal Setting

The care of the neonatal palliative care patient is not setting-specific. Care can be provided within the L&D unit, NICU, a newborn special care unit, or through a perinatal home hospice program.[4] Integration of perinatal and neonatal palliative care services in tertiary care centers is increasing in the United States and other developed countries. For example, premature infants with multiple comorbidities are potential candidates for early and consistent perinatal or neonatal palliative care. The nurse is instrumental in providing goal-directed support through care that integrates potential curative therapies with palliative measures.

Role of the Neonatal Nurse in Palliative Care

Nurses usually spend more time with families, hear the parents' perceptions, and learn of their wishes for the baby's care in addition to serving as the conduit between the family and other health professionals and acting as an advocate for their wishes.[13] Nurses work with the interdisciplinary team (IDT) to ensure that the patient and family have all needs addressed. The nurse often leads communication with the family and should participate in palliative care discussions as part of the palliative care team because the nurse spends the most time with the infant and family. Neonatal nurses have the challenging role of caring for critically ill infants and integrating care that must maintain multiple modes of communication with the IDT. Neonatal nurses participate in weekly IDT meetings and parent care conferences; they are sometimes asked to serve as primary care nurses for specific infants within the NICU. Serving as strong advocates to help facilitate the infant's care plan is an imperative role of the neonatal nurse. The nurse interprets data with the medical team, listens to the family's concerns, and offers suggestions to members of the healthcare team, thus allowing the nurse to form a holistic view of the baby's strengths and needs; the result is highly individualized, expert plans of care.[14]

The neonatal nurse also serves as a translator between the high-tech medical world and the fears and concerns of the family. This includes answering questions, giving descriptions, and providing anticipatory guidance of the sights, sounds, and experiences that they will have as their infant grows closer to death. Parents who are surprised by their infants' changes tend to believe that their infants suffered more and tend to experience more difficulties in their grief process.[15] Furthermore, ensuring that referrals to other specialty team members are completed aligns with the role of the neonatal nurse. When parents and caregivers have sudden changes in their ability to spend time with the critically ill infant, it is the neonatal nurse who helps to keep the connection in place by providing regular updates about the infant's status. Neonatal nurses partner with L& D nurses in instances in which a newly delivered infant needs to remain in the L&D unit for comfort care; there are variations of how the dual support is provided to families, which need to be worked out ahead of the delivery. In summary, the role of the neonatal nurse in palliative care is dynamic (see Table 40.1).

Role of the L&D Nurse in Palliative Care

The role of the L&D nurse in palliative care has become more established in recent years. Perinatal loss encompasses loss during pregnancy through the neonatal period. Intrauterine fetal demise (IUFD) is commonly called a "stillbirth," although the birth of an infant at 20 weeks' or greater gestation is considered a neonatal death in the L&D setting.[16] Perinatal death, although not always fitting the traditional palliative care referral criteria, results in grief and bereavement unique in human relationships. Regardless of the circumstances surrounding the loss, parents are often devastated and heartbroken.[10] For families with a perinatal life-limiting condition or those going through unexpected loss, the L&D unit becomes a palliative care unit. The goals of care in these circumstances are to help families face the diagnosis, listen to and discuss options as the family is ready, and facilitate communication with providers and other ancillary team members, as well as being present while the family experiences a situation like no other.[17] The parent may learn of the life-limiting condition at a prenatal visit and have months to plan and anticipate the baby's birth. In the months leading up to birth, time can be spent deciding on wishes for the pregnancy and birth. Birth plans can be developed, outlining specific wishes related to L&D care (both antepartum and postpartum) and for photography.

Perinatal palliative care involves caring for the mother, her unborn child, and the family during the antepartum, intrapartum, and postpartum periods and actively participating in bereavement care planning before and after birth.[10] Flexibility is needed when working with families experiencing perinatal loss because parental decisions can change. Nurses are on the front line and are with the parents at the time of diagnosis and delivery, as well as providing bereavement care. Specifically, L&D nurses work with the IDT to ensure as seamless a communication process following the delivery as possible. They also partner with the neonatal nurse to care for both the mother and the baby during the most precious moments of delivering palliative care. The IDT, including medical residents, fellows, neonatal nurse practitioners, social workers, chaplains, lactation consultants, and others, must maintain contact with the L&D nurse to support the family in the palliative care setting.

It is the L&D nurse's role to help the mother through labor and to remain present when the parents face the challenge of saying

Table 40.1 Role of the neonatal nurse and the labor and delivery (L&D) nurse in palliative care

Role of the neonatal nurse in palliative care	Role of the L&D nurse in palliative care
• Supports the infant and family • Collaborates with the interdisciplinary team (IDT) • Arranges family care conferences • Provides clinical support to infant in the neonatal intensive care unit and/or the L&D unit • Communicates status of the infant to the family • Actively involved in end-of-life care for infant • Consults social worker, chaplain, child life specialist, and/or others to ensure adequate support for infant and family • Integrates pharmacologic and nonpharmacologic therapies for the infant • Liaison to bereavement support	• Supports the infant and family in addition to dual role of caring for birth mother • Collaborates with the IDT • Arranges family care conferences • Provides clinical support to infant in the L&D unit • Communicates status of infant and mother to the family • Actively involved in end-of-life care for infant in collaboration with the neonatal team • Consults social worker, chaplain, child life specialist, and/or others to ensure adequate support for infant and family • May have early involvement with birth plan discussions in collaboration with the palliative care team and high-risk obstetrics team • Integrates pharmacologic and nonpharmacologic therapies for the infant in collaboration with the neonatal team • Provides continuum of care to mother of the infant • Liaison to bereavement support

goodbye to the newborn. For those patients with previous knowledge of life-limiting conditions, an L&D plan is created with an interdisciplinary team.[10] Patient teaching and perinatal palliative and bereavement care begin with admission and continue through discharge and beyond. Answering questions about the labor and birth process and what the baby will look like becomes the focus during labor. During labor, patients who have a fetus with a deformity or IUFD are often waiting anxiously and have fears about the appearance of the baby. Nurses should create a supportive and open environment for questions, concerns, and fears. After delivery, the teaching focuses on self-care, family grief, community resources, and infant disposition.[18]

L&D nurses should be honest and compassionate when explaining what caregivers should anticipate. A fetus with IUFD, for example, may have peeling skin and pale skin tones. Blankets and clothing can cover any area of the skin that may not be intact. Deformities and congenital syndromes often have characteristic traits that can be described to prepare the parents and family for the baby's appearance. Before delivery, the patient and family should discuss their expectations about social media posts, photographs on cell phones, videos, cultural rituals, or desires with their caregivers, family, and friends (40). The focus of the L&D nurse includes medical care such as induction medication management, pain control, and comfort measures, as well as encouragement and reassurance.

After members of the delivery team have completed the delivery process, a plan is in place to allow the family privacy. It is the L& D nurse who remains with the patient and family, giving care to the dying or deceased infant and the mother. Interdisciplinary support is vital to support the patient and family. Family presence is at the discretion of the parent(s). Parents may weep quietly and hold their baby, or they may not appear sad at all; while looking at the baby, they may talk about any familial features of the baby while enjoying their moments together.

The L&D nurse must help the patient and the family navigate this time while displaying compassion, understanding, presence, and patience. It is common for families to ask the same questions repeatedly. The L&D nurse becomes the mediator, giving families privacy, having side conversations (with permission) with the extended family, answering questions, listening, and being present. Care should emphasize the importance of the baby. If agreed to by the parents, the L&D nurse will collect and create mementos such as a lock of hair, pictures, footprints, and molds of the hands or feet and allow the parents to take as much time as they desire.[19] This can be completed in collaboration with the neonatal team if there is a neonatal nurse assigned to support the family. Perinatal loss resources should be given to the patient and family that allow connection to others experiencing the same loss.[18] In summary, the role of the L&D nurse in palliative care is dynamic.

Cultural Influences on the Integration of Neonatal Palliative Care Practices

For culturally competent care to reflect the complexity of care that is much broader than ethnicity, the nurse must be sensitive to cultural, ethnic, and religious values. Importantly, parents must be asked whether they have personal, cultural, or religious preferences for the goals of care for their child. The concept of "suffering" may have differing interpretations between members of the care team and the family, creating a potential for conflict.[20] In some cultures, suffering can relate to a test of faith or can be seen as an unavoidable part of life.[21] For families who belong to groups that have been historically marginalized, communication is of particular importance. Previous experiences with healthcare discrimination or concerns about being discriminated against may lead families to be guarded, lack trust, and/or feel that they are not receiving the full scope of information about their child's condition.[22]

In a stressful situation, such as anticipating the loss of a child, communication may become difficult for people whose first language does not match that of the dominant culture of the hospital. Even families who have spent many years speaking the dominant language may feel more comfortable and better understand when information is presented in their native tongue. Additionally, one parent may have more experience with the dominant language than the other, potentially leading to an unequal experience of understanding discussions with the care team. An experienced medical interpreter can be valuable in this context.[23]

The nurse should not assume that because the family is of a particular race, ethnicity, or religious sect their reactions or requests are reflective of all individuals of that race, ethnicity, or religious sect.[4] For example, bereavement interventions such as mementos (i.e., hand- and footprints; a lock of hair) or photographs of the deceased infant may not be acceptable in all cultures. In an example of a nurse working with a Native American family, the nurse must consider combining healing ceremonies from tribal rituals, if that is what the family desires, with Western medicine to alleviate suffering. In this instance, ethnic and religious beliefs are intertwined. But, in other instances, religious and ethnic values must be differentiated and incorporated into individualized care. It is important to remember that not every family that identifies with an organized religion strictly adheres to all principles of that faith. Families who do not ascribe to a formal religious tradition also have spiritual needs that should be recognized. These include making meaning out of important life transitions, recognizing the impact of this infant's life, and creating practices to honor their memory.[21]

Thus, individualized nursing care must include considerations of cultural assimilation, healthcare literacy and language barriers, educational attainment, health insurance status, and socioeconomic factors. The principles of diversity, equity, and inclusion should also be integrated into the care of the infant and family. Evidence demonstrates that, due to misunderstandings, lack of communication, and healthcare provider bias, racial and ethnic minorities (Asians, African Americans, Latinos) may have a delay in the initiation of palliative care services and pain alleviation as compared to White patients.[18] This delay or underutilization of palliative care measures may increase the infant's and family's pain and emotional suffering. The nurse needs to examine their own beliefs and biases because these personal constructs will influence the delivery of culturally sensitive palliative care.[17]

Neonatal Palliative Care Guidelines

In 2016, the National Association of Neonatal Nurses published position statement no. 3015 entitled "NICU Nurse Involvement in Ethical Decisions, Treatment of Critically Ill Newborns.[41]" This position statement reiterates the importance of the contribution of the neonatal nurse to the palliative care team. In addition, the American Academy of Pediatrics published its recommendations in a guideline for the care of infants, children, and adolescents in need of pediatric palliative care (PPC) and hospice care.[42] The guideline emphasizes the goals of PPC and the importance of collaboration among the IDT. Standards of care for patients in the NICU must be followed, and evidence-based practices should guide protocols for implementing palliative care. According to ACOG recommendations and conclusions, the perinatal palliative care team should prepare families for the possibility that there may be differences of opinion between family members before and after the delivery of the infant and that there may be differences between parents and the neonatal care providers about appropriate postnatal therapies, especially if the postnatal diagnosis and prognosis differ substantially from antenatal predictions.[3] The opportunity for palliative care following the birth can be helpful to families who choose not to terminate the pregnancy for religious beliefs, who wish to meet the child and say goodbye, and who may not be convinced of the extent of their child's diagnosis.[24]

In 2022, ACOG joined by 24 medical organizations submitted an amicus brief to the US Supreme Court in the case of *Dobbs v. Jackson Women's Health Organization*, a case challenging the Mississippi law imposing a ban on the provision of abortion after 15 weeks of pregnancy for most individuals.[25] It is important for neonatal and L&D nurses to remember that patients and families have their thoughts and opinions about the *Dobbs v. Jackson* decision; respect for each family's perspective is imperative and necessary to provide the highest quality of care and support.

Bereavement Support Services

Working alongside neonatologists, social workers, medical photographers, and other staff members, nurses are often the team members who introduce the idea of photography to families as part of the transition to end-of-life care and take photos for families during their stay.[26] In some areas, bereavement photography specialists can assist with providing compassionately developed photographs of the deceased infant, such as the Now I Lay Me Down to Sleep organization (https://www.nowilaymedowntosleep.org). Nurses can serve as advocates to ensure that comprehensive support is being offered to the family. The benefit of providing these bereavement support services should be of utmost consideration. Healthcare providers, especially nurses, are in the unique position of facilitating the bereavement process for parents, beginning when the infant's life-limiting condition is diagnosed and continuing until after the infant's death.[27] The neonatal nurse and L&D nurse have roles in ensuring that the bereavement support measures are optimized. Asking parents or caregivers if they want to have their community spiritual support or emotional support team members engaged in the process will provide a clear path for aligning support. Some palliative care teams have additional bereavement support members such as chaplains, child life specialists, bereavement specialists, and others. In addition to bereavement photography, a memory box is an important part of the process, with items such as the infant's ID band, hospital cap, lock of hair, baptism gown, hand or foot molds, or any other items the family desires to keep. Other bereavement keepsake checklist items can be found in Figure 40.1. The use of cooling devices (such as pads or special bassinets) has been introduced to facilitate keeping the infant with the parents or caregivers after the infant has died. The cooling process slows the normal decomposition process, allowing the infant to stay with the family for visitation.[10]

Perinatal Palliative Care Resources for Education, Training, and/or Advocacy

More institutions are interested in neonatal-specific content to start their palliative care teams. Despite support from the American Academy of Pediatrics and the World Health Organization for the provision of palliative care, there are still many barriers. One of the greatest ways to build upon knowledge in neonatal palliative care nursing is to attend formal training sessions. The End-of-Life Nursing Education Consortium (ELNEC) project

> is a national and international education initiative to improve palliative care, and it is a collaboration between the City of Hope, Duarte, CA, and the American Association of Colleges of Nursing, Washington, DC; the project, administered by City of Hope, provides undergraduate and graduate nursing faculty, CE providers, staff development educators, specialty nurses in pediatrics, oncology, critical care and geriatrics, and other nurses with training in palliative care so they can teach this essential information to nursing students, practicing nurses and other healthcare professionals.

The ability of the nurse to deliver care to the dying newborn is impacted by many barriers to access in addition to the ongoing need for educational support to help novice nurses gain the confidence and skill set needed to provide competent care. Educational initiatives such as ELNEC provide an avenue for neonatal and L&D nurses to gain a baseline foundation in knowledge of the principles of palliative care; the curriculum contains perinatal and neonatal modules. For more information, see https://www.aacnnursing.org/ELNEC.([28])

There are additional educational resources, training sessions, and neonatal advocacy support networks available, as listed in Table 40.2.

Promoting Comfort for Neonatal Palliative Care Patients

Neonatal comfort should be promoted at all times. Parents and caregivers expect clear communication from the IDT about the plan for promoting comfort. At most, explanations should include simple language, avoiding medical jargon. There can be general apprehension about medication utilization for pain and symptom management. It is important to dispel myths and provide direct answers to parental and family concerns about pharmacologic and nonpharmacologic measures utilized to promote comfort (Table 40.3).

Pharmacologic Measures to Promote Comfort in the Neonatal Palliative Care Setting

The perinatal palliative care team should ensure that a thorough pain assessment has been conducted. For newborns with minutes to hours to live, the plan for comfort should involve an overview

Bereavement Keepsake Checklist

- __Use supportive communication and offer choices
- __Ask for assistance from experienced bereavement team members and interdisciplinary team (social work, chaplain, child life specialist)
- __Request music therapist to provide soft music, if comforting to family
- __Sign Consent Form (parent) for permission to prepare keepsakes
- __Offer bath, skin-to-skin, family members' help with keepsakes
- __Offer music therapist recording of baby's heartbeat to music
- __Provide the following, per family members' choice:
  - __Hand-painted keepsake boxes and/or quilted bag
  - __Bereavement information folder
  - __Certificate of Life
  - __Beaded name bracelet
  - __Memory stone
  - __Ink handprints and footprints
  - __Foam impressions – baby's hands & feet, parents' & siblings' hand(s) with baby's
  - __Alginate impressions – hands, feet, face
  - __Locket of hair (2 x 2 baggie, no tape); strip of baby's heartbeat
  - __Seashell used for baptism
  - __Bereavement gown and/or gown crafted from donated wedding dress
  - __Photos (with outfit chosen by parents) – printed photos and DVD
  - __Donated journal, photo album, blanket, books on grief
- __Prepare the following items for siblings:
  - __Keepsake box
  - __Children's storybooks
  - __Stuffed animal(s)
  - __Memory stone
  - __Ink handprints and footprints
  - __Impressions – siblings' hand(s) with baby's
- __Give as many of the belongings/photos as possible to family before they leave
- __Escort parents and siblings to car or make sure extended family member does
- __Chart on Bereavement Form
- __Place sympathy card for family at charge desk
- __Place support/appreciation card for staff at charge desk
- __Call parents when remaining keepsakes are ready – offer pick up or mailing
  - __If mailing, verify address and describe contents in detail to prepare them
  - __If parents express they are not ready, give them contact information and store keepsakes

Figure 40.1 Bereavement keepsake checklist.
Source: Reference 8.

of possible medication options and should be supported by a neonatologist, neonatal pharmacist, and/or NNP. In terms of opioids, fentanyl and morphine are the two most commonly prescribed opiates in the NICU and have both similar and distinctive side effects; when compared to morphine, fentanyl, with its shorter half-life, is more potent and possesses a more rapid onset of action.[29] Opioids are often utilized for pain and/or dyspnea. The role of the neonatal and L&D nurse includes ensuring that open discussions are held between the family and medical teams involved in administering comfort medications. Intranasal fentanyl provides an additional route of administration for neonates who do not have established IV access.[29] Titration of opioids in neonates is a delicate process and requires the expertise of the neonatologist and/or NNP. The benefits of treatment versus the burden of symptoms should be transparently discussed. There are other opioids utilized in the neonatal palliative care setting. Hibo et al. conducted a study reviewing the use of gabapentin in the NICUs across the United States and found that neonates with chronic genetic, neurologic, and gastrointestinal diagnoses were more likely to receive gabapentin.[30]

Neonatal anxiety must be addressed. Parents and family members witnessing anxious neonates also have the risk of experiencing anxiety. Lorazepam or midazolam is utilized as a sedative or as an adjunct to the analgesic effects of opioids both in everyday care and, more specifically, at the end of life in many newborns.[30] Diazepam

Table 40.2 Perinatal palliative care resources for education, training, and/or advocacy

Name of resource	Mission and vision/description	Website
Courageous Parents Network	Mission: To empower, support, and equip families and providers caring for children with serious illness. Vision: Families have confidence in their ability to be the best caregivers they can possibly be, resulting in minimal regret and maximal healing. Pediatric medical providers feel increased efficacy in delivering family-centered care.	https://courageousparentsnetwork.org/about/what-we-do
National Association of Neonatal Nurses (NANN)	Mission: Is the professional voice that shapes neonatal nursing through excellence in practice, education, research, and professional development. Description: NANN is an inclusive, diverse community of registered nursing professionals at all stages of their careers who care for newborn infants born with a variety of health challenges, including prematurity, birth defects, infection, cardiac malformations, and surgical problems.	http://nann.org/about/national-association-of-neonatal-nurses
Neonatal Comfort Care Program	Mission: The Neonatal Comfort Care Program honors babies' lives with life-limiting conditions by creating a safe and loving space for bonding, attachment, comfort, and joy for them and their families. They journey with families from diagnosis through birth and beyond, offer them guidance and support, and provide a unique medical plan that follows the natural course of each baby's life. The Neonatal Comfort Care Program offers a service of perinatal/neonatal palliative care, and its specialized approach encompasses the following: • Individualized medical evaluation and plan, including alleviation of pain • Comfort measures, such as holding, skin-to-skin contact, and feeding • Memory-making activities, such as handprints + footprints, photographs, and personalized keepsakes • Emotional, psychological, and spiritual care, including both short- and long-term bereavement support The Neonatal Comfort Care Program is also committed to teaching and research, to inspire and guide professionals in the perinatal field to develop similar programs. Vision: Because each baby's life is precious, the Neonatal Comfort Care Program is devoted to providing the best interdisciplinary care, teaching, and research so that our specialized approach will become the standard of care around the world for any baby born with life-limiting conditions.	http://www.neonatalcomfortcare.com/home-page
Pediatric Division, formerly known as the Pediatric Palliative Care Task Force	Mission: Activate interdisciplinary collaborations and create real-world solutions to continuously improve access to pediatric palliative care. Vision: Equitable access to high-quality pediatric palliative care for everyone.	https://www.nationalcoalitionhpc.org/pediatric/
Perinatal Hospice & Palliative Care	Description: Perinatalhospice.org is a clearinghouse of information about perinatal hospice and palliative care, including many resources for parents and caregivers as well as an international list of more than 300 programs.	https://www.perinatalhospice.org/about
Perinatal Loss and Infant Death Alliance (PLIDA)	Mission: PLIDA's mission is to promote the highest quality of consistent, evidence-based perinatal bereavement care for all families who experience the death of a baby. We express this mission through continuing professional education, the establishment of position statements and practice guidelines, unified responses to issues in the media or legislation, and by creating a network for professionals to share questions, resources, insight, and support. PLIDA strives to create position statements that promote the highest standard of supportive care for bereaved parents. PLIDA position statements advocate for parents' emotional needs and the provision of compassionate, relationship-based care. Available to all members, these position statements can be used to increase awareness, educate others, inform policy, sustain supportive programs, or encourage change. Vision: PLIDA's overriding goal is to support those whose work supports bereaved families. We are committed to serving as leaders in perinatal and neonatal bereavement care by offering the most up-to-date resources available to our members	https://www.plida.org/

Table 40.3 Pharmacologic and nonpharmacologic measures to promote comfort in the neonatal palliative care setting

Pharmacologic measures to promote comfort	Nonpharmacologic measures to promote comfort
• Pain: acetaminophen, morphine, fentanyl, methadone (some opioids can be utilized for chronic pain) • Anxiety and/or agitation: lorazepam, midazolam, diazepam; agitation and/or feeding intolerance: neurontin • Excessive secretions: glycopyrrolate • Constipation: glycerin suppository, osmotic laxatives, if needed methylnaltrexone subcutaneous	• Skin-to-skin care • Swaddling/facilitated tucking • Non-nutritive sucking • Oral sucrose • Breastfeeding • Management of oral secretions • Ocular care • Oral care

is a long-acting benzodiazepine that can be utilized in the setting of chronic symptoms. Untreated anxiety impacts the ability of the family to hold the infant comfortably; end-of-life care is geared toward fewer restrictions on physical touch and as much time as desired for the infant and family to remain in close contact. Effective management requires anticipation of the disease manifestations as well as the severity of symptoms for each patient; this can vary greatly and is often related in part to the underlying diagnoses and conditions leading to death.[31]

The side effects of opioids can lead to constipation, which is typically addressed with glycerin suppositories, osmotic laxatives, and, if needed, methylnaltrexone subcutaneously.[32] The goal is to alleviate distressing abdominal pain, bloating, and constipation by starting with the least invasive method possible. This can help to promote comfort and relax the patient enough for cuddling with the family when permitted. In addition, oral secretions which can cause audible frightening sounds for the neonate should be addressed with glycopyrrolate at the end of life, oral suctioning may lead to distress, but oral care should be considered and discussed with the family.

Nonpharmacologic Measures to Promote Comfort in the Neonatal Palliative Care Setting

Due to the immaturity of the renal and hepatic systems, neonatal care already uses many nonpharmacologic methods to decrease pain and agitation. NICU nurses can independently implement these options, but their use varies by infant acuity, practitioner preference, NICU policies, and availability of resources. It is also important to pay close attention to the milieu of the NICU setting. Protecting the infant from excess light, noise, noxious touch, and cold contributes to the success of both pharmacologic and nonpharmacologic management of pain and discomfort.[33] The use of multiple simultaneous nonpharmacologic methods is encouraged as these techniques have synergistic effects.[33]

Skin-to-skin care (also called "kangaroo care") is a common therapy used in the NICU. Typically, the infant is placed prone directly on the chest of a parent. Its use is dependent on the physiological stability of the infant, the presence or absence of specific treatments (such as mechanical ventilation or umbilical catheters), and individual unit policies and procedures.[34] For infants whose care has moved from curative to palliative, their prior health status may have precluded parents from holding their infant or from providing skin-to-skin care. Skin-to-skin care provides several benefits for infant health and has been shown to promote attachment as well as decrease stress in parents.[35]

Positioning of the neonate is important to maintain comfort, decrease stress, and improve sleep. Older, healthy infants will naturally place themselves into the fetal position—slightly curved spine with flexed limbs contained close to the body. Infants born ill and/or premature often lack the strength and muscular control to move themselves into this soothing position. Instead, nurses can use the process of facilitated tucking—using blankets or special positioning helps infants maintain a soothing position while lying supine, prone, or on their side.[36] If the infant can maintain their temperature, swaddling produces the same effects and facilitates parent holding.

Non-nutritive sucking begins early in gestation, but the infant's ability to use this self-calming mechanism relates to the strength of their oral muscles and the energy available to expend. In the ill or preterm infant, non-nutritive sucking is typically facilitated by a pacifier. Specialty pacifiers are available in various sizes and shapes, accommodating the smallest infants. Non-nutritive sucking has been shown to ease pain and provide comfort with and without the addition of oral sucrose. The addition of oral sucrose typically increases the pain relief associated with non-nutritive sucking.[37]

Breastfeeding can be maintained for comfort for both the mother and the infant. Palliative care can also bring an opportunity for a mother to put an infant to breast who has not previously been able to attempt breastfeeding. This can be an important component of closure for the mother; some mothers may wish to continue pumping to donate to a milk bank or to help decrease engorgement by slowing down pumping before ceasing. Nurses should provide support for the mother's choice and should share lactation resources with them.[38]

As the dying infant develops less control over their bodily functions, it becomes imperative for the nurse to manage oral and ocular care more carefully. This is a comfort measure for infants as well as a method of alleviating distress in parents. As the infant loses control of basic bodily functions, whether due to imminent death or the effects of medications, two main areas of concern are the management of oral secretions and ocular care. Oral secretions may be increased related to the infant's decreased ability to swallow. This can result in excess noise breathing, which can be disturbing to family members. The infant may or may not be able to perceive discomfort related to the excess secretions. The nurse can maintain oral care using gentle oral suction and application of moisture (water) to the lips and mouth. Ocular care may become necessary if infants cannot fully close their eyes. This can be distressing to the family and uncomfortable to the infant as the partial opening of the eyes does not allow for full ocular lubrication. The nurse can assist by the application of artificial tears and/or ointment to the eyes.[39]

Conclusion

Neonates and their families can greatly benefit from timely interdisciplinary palliative care services. Families with an infant diagnosed with a life-limiting diagnosis are often unprepared for the news and need guidance from healthcare professionals. The emotional burden for families is complex—feelings of grief, fear, disbelief, and guilt are common. It is important for healthcare professionals to answer questions, help the parents make plans, and honor the needs of a family whose future is uncertain. Clear, honest communication is vital to building trust.

Interdisciplinary planning should start as soon as palliative care is selected. During pregnancy, birth plans can help provide direction as to who will be included in the delivery room, plans for resuscitation (if any), and spiritual or cultural aspects that are important to the family. With some diagnoses, it is not uncommon for a family to initially choose resuscitation to see how well the infant will adapt to extrauterine life. Infants who receive palliative care consultations in the NICU often endure painful procedures when the focus is on life-saving care. The infant's illness trajectory can be unpredictable, which can impact the transition to palliative care as families hold out hope that another treatment could help save their child's life.

Nursing care of the infant needs to focus on excellent pain and symptom management while promoting supportive developmental care. Nursing care for the family includes a holistic approach to emotional, psychological, spiritual, and cultural needs. Families and healthcare professionals can work together with a common goal of providing comfort and dignity while accepting that the infant may not live a long time.

Some infants will be able to go home with their parents. Community resources are vital—the palliative care team can help to plan the transition home and can arrange for home assistance. A comprehensive plan must include all necessary equipment, emergency plans, and plans for when the infant dies. Bereavement care needs to include resources for the family after the death. These can include counselors, support groups, memorial services for the infant, and memorial events for families who have lost a child.

Experiencing the death of a child is incredibly difficult. Palliative care offers the opportunity to support families, honor the wishes of the parents, ease the pain of the infant, and create memories of the infant's short life. Healthcare providers should recognize the emotional toll that an infant loss creates in the workplace as well. Senior staff members should support those who are experiencing their first infant death. A debrief after death can help answer questions and reassure staff of the roles that they played in supporting the family.

REFERENCES

1. Centers for Disease Control and Prevention. Infant Mortality. Accessed September 8, 2022. https://www.cdc.gov/reproductivehealth/maternalinfanthealth/infantmortality.htm.
2. Institute of Medicine. *Dying in America: Improving Quality and Honoring Individual Preferences Near the End of Life*. National Academies Press; 2015.
3. American College of Obstetricians and Gynecologists. Perinatal Palliative Care. Accessed September 25, 2022. https://www.acog.org/clinical/clinical-guidance/committee-opinion/articles/2019/09/perinatal-palliative-care?utm_source=redirect&utm_medium=web&utm_campaign=otn.
4. Kenner C, Press J, Ryan D. Recommendations for palliative and bereavement care in the NICU: a family-centered integrative approach. *J Perinatol*. 2015;35:S19–S23.
5. Marty CM, Carter BS. Ethics and palliative care in the perinatal world. *Semin Fetal Neonatal Med*. 2018; 23(1):35–38. https://doi.org/10.1016/j.siny.2017.09.001.
6. Lago P, Cavicchiolo ME, Rusalen F, Benini, F. Summary of the key concepts on how to develop a perinatal palliative care program. *Front Pediatr*. 2020;8:596744 https://doi.org/10.3389/fped.2020.596744.
7. Bidegain M, Younge N. Comfort care vs palliative care: is there a difference in neonates? *NeoReviews*. 2015;16:333–339.
8. Levick J, Fannon J, Bodemann J, Munch S. NICU bereavement care and follow-up support for families and staff. *Adv Neonatal Care*. 2017;17(6):451–460. https://doi.org/10.1097/ANC.0000000000000435.
9. Quinn M, Weiss A, Crist, J. Early for everyone. *Adv Neonatal Care*. 2020;20(2):109–117. https://doi.org/10.1097/ANC.0000000000000707.
10. Mendes J, Wool J, Wool C. Ethical considerations in perinatal palliative care. *J Obstet Gynecol Neonatal Nurs*. 2017;46(3):367–377. https://doi.org/10.1016/j.jogn.2017.01.011.
11. Sieg SE, Bradshaw WT, Blake S. The best interests of infants and families during palliative care at the end of life: a review of the literature. *Adv Neonatal Care*. 2019;19(2):E9–E14. https://doi.org/10.1097/anc.0000000000000567.
12. Lisanti A, Vittner D, Medoff-Cooper B, Fogel J, Wernovsky G, Butler S. Individualized family-centered developmental care. *J Cardiovasc Nurs*. 2019;34(1):85–93. https://doi.org/10.1097/JCN.0000000000000546.
13. Kenner C. The role of neonatal nurses in palliative care. *Newborn Infant Nurs Rev*. 2016;16(2):74–77. https://doi.org/10.1053/j.nainr.2016.03.009.
14. Welborn AC. Supporting the neonatal nurse in the role of final comforter. *J Neonatal Nurs*. 2017;23(2):58–64. https://doi.org/10.1016/j.jnn.2016.09.005.
15. Cortezzo DE, Meyer M. Neonatal end-of-life management. *Front Pediatr*. 2020;8:574121.
16. Beresford S. Response to placenta in intrauterine fetal demise (IUFD): a comprehensive study from a tertiary care hospital. *J Matern Fetal Neonatal Med*. 2020;33(21):3723. https://doi.org/10.1080/14767058.2019.1580261.
17. Wool C. Clinician perspectives of barriers in perinatal palliative care. *MCN: Am J Maternal Child Nurs*. 2015;40(1):44–50.
18. Ryan A, Bernhard H, Fahlberg B. Best practices for perinatal palliative care. *Nursing*. 2015;45(10):14–15.
19. Homer CSE, Malata A, Hoope-Bender P. Supporting women, families, and care providers after stillbirths. *Lancet*. 2016;387:516–517.
20. Tate T. Pediatric suffering and the burden of proof. *Pediatrics*. 2020;146(suppl. 1):S70–S74.
21. Kain VJ. Perinatal palliative care: cultural, spiritual, and religious considerations for parents—what clinicians need to know. *Front Pediatr*. 2021;9:597519. https://doi.org/10.3389/fped.2021.597519.
22. Sample E, Mikulic C, Christian-Brandt A. Unheard voices: underrepresented families' perspectives of pediatric palliative care. *Clin Pract Pediatr Psychol*. 2021;9(3):318–322.
23. Dreier LA, Zernikow B, Wager J. Quantifying the language barrier: a total survey of parents' spoken languages and local language skills as perceived by different professions in pediatric palliative care. *Children*. 2020;7(9):118.
24. Hasegawa SL, Fry JT. Moving toward a shared process: the impact of parent experiences on perinatal palliative care. *Semin Perinatol*. 2017;41:95–100.

25. American Medical Association. Leading Medical Groups File Amicus Brief in Dobbs v. Jackson. September 21, 2021. Accessed October 3, 2022. https://www.ama-assn.org/press-center/press-releases/leading-medical-groups-file-amicus-brief-dobbs-v-jackson.
26. Furingsten L, Sjogren R, Forsner M. Ethical challenges when caring for dying children. *Nurs Ethics*. 2015;22(2):176–187.
27. Martel S, Ives-Baine L. Nurses' experiences of end-of-life photography in NICU bereavement support. *J Pediatr Nurs*. 2018;42:e38–e44. https://doi.org/10.1016/j.pedn.2018.05.011.
28. End-of-Life Nursing Consortium. FAQs about ELNEC. Accessed October 7, 2022. https://www.aacnnursing.org/ELNEC/ELNEC/FAQs.
29. Carter BS, Brunkhorst J. Neonatal pain management. *Semin Perinatol.* 2017;41(2):111–116. https://doi.org/10.1053/j.semperi.2016.11.001.
30. Abdi HH, Maitre NL, Benninger KL, Hester ME, Slaughter JL. Gabapentin use for hospitalized neonates. *Pediatr Neurol.* 2019;97:64–70. https://doi.org/10.1016/j.pediatrneurol.2019.02.012.
31. Cortezzo DE, Meyer M. Neonatal end-of-life management. *Front Pediatr*. 2020;8:574121. https://doi.org/10.3389/fped.2020.574121.
32. Haug S, Dye A, Durrani S. End-of life care for neonates: assessing and addressing pain and distressing symptoms. *Front Pediatr*. 2020;8:574180. https://doi.org/10.3389/fped.2020.574180.
33. Garten S, Buhrer C. Pain and distress management in palliative neonatal care. *Semin Fetal Neonatal Med*. 2019;24(4):101008.
34. Fluharty M, Nemeth LS, Logan A, Nichols M. What do neonatal intensive care unit policies tell us about kangaroo care implementation? *Adv Neonatal Care*. 2020;21(4):E76–E85.
35. Garnica-Torres Z, Gouveia A, da Silva Pedroso J. Attachment between father and premature baby in kangaroo care in a neonatal unit of a public hospital. *J Neonatal Nurs*. 2020;27(5):334–340.
36. Lavalee A, De Clifford-Faugere G, Garcia C, Fernandez Oviedo AN, Heon M, Aita, M. Part 1: narrative overview of developmental care interventions for the preterm newborn. *J Neonatal Nurs*. 2019;25(1):3–8.
37. Gai H, Li M, Gao H, et al. Effect of non-nutritive sucking and sucrose alone and in combination for repeated procedural pain in preterm infants: a randomized controlled trial. *Int J Nurs Stud*. 2018;83:25–33.
38. Marc-Aurele KL. Decisions parents make when faced with potentially life-limiting fetal diagnoses and the importance of perinatal palliative care. *Front Pediatr*. 2020;8:574556. https://doi.org/10.3389/fped.2020.574556.
39. Haug S, Dye A, Durrani S. End-of life care for neonates: assessing and addressing pain and distressing symptoms. *Front Pediatr*. 2020;8:574180. https://doi.org/10.3389/fped.2020.574180.

41

Considerations for Adolescents in Pediatric Palliative Care

Lauren Greco and Faith Kinnear

Key Points

- Pediatric palliative care is family-centered care that focuses on a child's and family's quality of life through the prevention and relief of suffering along a physical, psychological, emotional, spiritual, and social continuum.
- The adolescent and young adult (AYA) population can be especially vulnerable when faced with chronic or serious illness and benefit from support with decision-making, medical therapy adherence, coping strategies, and advance care planning or legacy-building.
- Pediatric palliative care providers play a key role in guiding AYAs through serious illness to support their autonomy while acknowledging their unique needs.
- Pediatric palliative care nurses and providers are knowledgeable in communication, symptom management, advance care planning, legacy-building, coping strategies, and recognition of distress—spiritual, physical, emotional, and social.
- Special considerations should be given to the AYA population that is not neurotypical.

Case Study

Bill is a 13-year-old who was diagnosed with Emery-Dreifuss muscular dystrophy after a prolonged hospital stay. He was discharged home with nighttime bidirectional positive airway pressure (BiPAP) support, cough assist, and vest therapy for airway clearance; a gastric tube for feeding; and multiple specialty follow-ups including neurology, pulmonology, nutrition, genetics, cardiology, and palliative care (PC). The PC team met Bill and his parents during his admission with plans to follow up in the outpatient clinic for longitudinal support.

Introduction and Timing of PC

Adolescence and young adulthood is often an exciting, transitional time as individuals in this stage are trying to establish independence, autonomy, confidence, and social status as they transition into adulthood. Developing identities separate from their parents and fostering social and intimate relationships are prioritized.[1] For adolescents and young adults (AYAs) living with a life-threatening diagnosis, this period is compounded by increased distress around achieving milestones, social isolation, body image and self-esteem, intimacy, fertility, potential employment, and financial independence.[2]

Unfortunately, AYAs as a group have been historically neglected by both the pediatric and adult world.[2] Too old for services geared toward children and not yet old enough for adult services, this group has long "fallen through the cracks." It is now widely accepted that this is a distinct population with unique needs and challenges.[2] AYAs represent a large percentage of uninsured or underinsured individuals. Insurance status and/or feelings of immortality often result in delayed care.[1]

Clinicians must honor patients' desires to become more independent and make decisions, while also responsibly caring for, in many cases, minors. Compounding this is the discomfort many clinicians feel about having conversations around decision-making and advance care planning (ACP). The American Academy of Pediatrics acknowledges healthcare communication as a "critical but generally neglected component of pediatric and pediatric subspecialty practice and training."[3(p7)] Thus, it is important to advocate for both generalist PC training for clinicians and early specialist PC integration to provide an additional layer of support in addressing pain, symptom management, and communication needs.

Early PC integration and high-quality prognostic communication have been associated with improved symptom control and increased trust, hope, peace of mind, and satisfaction with medical care.[1,4] Evidence suggests that PC for AYAs living with life-threatening illness as part of routine care results in improved quality of life and should be a professional standard.[3] In the case of Bill, it is recommended that PC be introduced during his initial admission and continue in the outpatient setting to provide longitudinal support. Unfortunately, the involvement of PC is inconsistent and often late in the disease trajectory.[4] This delay is frequently the result of the continued misconception about the role of a PC team, limited access to PC, or time constraints and communication barriers.[4] Improved education, enhanced interdisciplinary communication, standardized screening tools, and referral practices could help mitigate the delay in introduction and integration of PC into the care for AYA patients and their families.

One of the ways a PC team can be most beneficial is by providing additional support around conversations—be it prognosticating, decision-making, or ACP. AYAs benefit from opportunities to have truthful, developmentally appropriate conversations based on what they would find most helpful and including whomever they would like to participate. In an attempt to protect, family members can often act as "gate keepers"—delaying or preventing conversations in an effort to avoid distress.[5] This actually has the opposite effect as a lack of communication or information often results in increased fear, distrust, and internalization for the patient. Clinicians should encourage honest communication based on cognitive maturity and experience rather than age, allowing AYAs to hope for the best, while discussing or planning for the worst.[5,6]

Allowing AYAs a sense of control in how information is provided to them may better prepare them to participate in future conversations, and many AYAs prefer that ACP conversations are initiated by their providers.[7] AYAs should first be asked if they want to participate in conversations and, if so, how they would like to receive information. They should also be offered the opportunity to speak with a clinician privately and re-evaluate their level of participation at any time.[7] In the case of Bill, it should be made clear that there are opportunities to have visits as a family, that Bill can meet alone with members of the PC team, and that there are times when Bill can opt out of a visit or conversation and allow his parents to meet with his team. (See Table 41.1 for example conversation phrases.) For additional information regarding questions to ask or strategies to address "hopes and worries," please refer to the Chapter 37 on communication.

In addition to communicating with providers, AYAs may need to communicate with extended family, friends, school, and people with whom they work. Knowing what to say can be difficult, and AYAs should be reassured that they are not required to disclose any more information than what they are comfortable with. In fact, as many AYAs emphasize their desire to "try and be normal," reminding them that setting boundaries and choosing not to always discuss their illness is healthy and appropriate. Members of the PC team could support Bill and his family by providing a developmentally appropriate description of his diagnosis to share with friends, a letter to the school sharing an update and outlining necessary supports so that they do not have to constantly repeat the story, and resources for siblings.

Symptom Management

AYAs may experience pain, fatigue, depression, and anxiety due to their diagnosis or treatment and side effects. These symptoms may require a multimodal approach including pharmacologic, nonpharmacologic, spiritual, and/or psychosocial interventions.[7] Please see Chapter 35 on symptom management for details.

Disease Implications

Quality PC interventions should address the physical, emotional, mental, and social well-being of patients through education, resources, and support. This support is not limited to issues related to a life-threatening illness but includes any issue that impacts the whole person. Physical changes are not just a perceived concern. A change in appearance or functional status can have far-reaching social, emotional, and physical implications. Children as young as first grade have been shown to indicate preferential reactions in favor of children without physical limitations over physically limited peers.[8] Preparing AYAs for changes such as variation in habitus, implanted devices, or potential amputation is essential. Thoughtful interventions to address physical changes, such as therapeutic conversations, preoperative photos or videos, medical device or prosthetic manipulation, hypnosis, or peer-modeling, have significant physical and emotional benefits including decreased anxiety, better coping and adjustment, decreased use of pain medication, and shorter hospital stays.[8] Studies indicate there is benefit in first sharing difficult news, especially around permanent physical changes, with parents or caregivers to allow them to process their initial emotions in a safe, separate space; and these conversations are best facilitated by an interdisciplinary team. In instances where there is a potential permanent change such as the support of a tracheostomy or amputation, it is often helpful to invite parents or caregivers to see their AYA in the operating room prior to reversing anesthesia.[8]

Adolescence and young adulthood are marked by increased awareness of one's peers' physical attributes, constant exposure to social media, and societal pressure.[9] In addition to permanent physical changes, AYAs are often distressed by reversible changes, such as port placements, gastrostomy tubes, hair thinning or loss, weight and muscle fluctuation, facial swelling, and dermatological changes. While physical changes present a clear impact to quality of life for AYA patients, there are many invisible wounds that are equally distressing and should be addressed by clinicians. Acceptance by peers, ability to establish or continue intimate relationships, reliance on family members, and concern about caring for young children, if an AYA is a parent, all require attention. In the case example, a member of the PC team should speak with Bill about how he is feeling and offer to make a referral to a mental health clinician for him or members of his family.

Fertility

A diagnosis where fertility may be impacted is a significant source of stress for both males and females as they have most of their reproductive years ahead of them. This is especially true for patients diagnosed with cancer where the 5-year survival is greater than 80% but where alkylating chemotherapy, radiation, and hematopoietic stem cell transplant are significant risk factors for infertility.[10] Even for those for whom parenthood is far off, counseling around fertility preservation such as oocyte cyropreservation, ovarian tissue preservation, and sperm cryopreservation should be considered standard of care.[10] Additional counseling should be provided for AYAs who are undergoing immunotherapy such as chimeric antigen receptor T-cell treatment. The hope is that fertility will be preserved as advances in immunotherapy reduce exposure to gonadotoxic therapies; however, more research is needed.[10]

Coping and Well-Being

A serious illness is associated with negative psychosocial outcomes including impaired quality of life, poor mental health, social isolation,

Table 41.1 Methods and example phrases for engaging adolescent and young adult (AYA) patients in conversations around prognosis and advance care planning and decision-making in advanced cancer

Element of conversation Element of Conversation is how it is written on the guide we requested permission to use	Example phrases Example Phrases is how it is written in the original text
Offer the opportunity for the AYA to be involved in the conversation	We have some new findings about your disease. Would you like to be a part of this conversation right now? Or are there things you would rather we talk to your parents about first?
Determine the preferred way the AYA patient would like to receive information	How much information would you like us to share with you? The phrasing from the guide is: How much information do you want us to share with you?
	Do you prefer written materials that you can read on your own? The phrasing from the guide is: Do you do better with written materials that you can read on your own?
Offer the opportunity to speak privately with AYA and/or the patient's parent or guardian Or guardian is not part of the table text.	Are there things you would like to speak privately to me about? (or conversely is part of the table text)
	How do you feel about giving your parent(s) the opportunity to speak privately with me?
Offer AYA the choice to be involved and explore their preferred Offer the AYA the choice to be involved and explore the preferred level of involvement at every meeting level of involvement in every meeting	I know in the past you have not wanted to be a part of some of the discussions that I have had with your parents. We are going to talk again about what is going on with your cancer and what the next steps might be. Would you like to be a part of this conversation today? I know if the past you have not wanted to be a part of some of the discussions that I have had with your parents. We are going to talk again about what is going on with your cancer and what the next steps might be. Would you like to be a part of this conversation today?
Elicit goals of care and preferences	Although we have other options for continuing treatment, we want to make sure we hear what is important to you. For example, when thinking of next steps, would you like us to focus more on you having the best quality of life, such as being away from hospital as much as possible, or on treatments that might control your cancer, but may require you to be in the hospital for a period of time? Although we have other options for continuing treatment, we just want to make sure we are considering what you want. For example, when thinking of next steps, would you like us to focus more on you having the best quality of life, such as being away from the hospital as much as possible, or on treatments that might control your cancer but may require you to be in the hospital for a period of time?
	Can you share with us what is most important and/or most concerning to you? Can you tell us what is most important or concerning to you at this moment?
In patients with relapsed or progressive disease, reframe conversation around current disease state	We are at a place now where we no longer have any treatments that can stop your cancer from progressing.
	Your cancer will continue to worsen, and you are at risk for (e.g., pain, trouble breathing, spinal cord compression and death). We want to know how you would like us to treat you if this happens. Would you like to talk about some decisions we might be able to make together? Your cancer will likely continue to grow, and you are at risk for (e.g., continued disease progression, spinal cord compression). We want to make sure that we know how you would like us to treat you if this happens. Would you like us to talk with you about what we know and about some decisions we might be able to make together?
Discuss spirituality and/or spiritual support or distress	Some people find comfort in their spiritual beliefs or specific traditions in their faith or religion. Do you? Some AYAs find great comfort in their spiritual beliefs or traditions in their faith or religion. Do you ?
	It sounds like you are really struggling with your spiritual beliefs right now There are no right or wrong ways to be spiritually or emotionally comforted.
Introduce advance care planning principles and/or guides	We wanted you. We thought you might like to know that there is a guide that was created by and for persons your age who had concerns about what would happen if they got sicker. Too sick to speak for themselves. It allows you to make decisions about things that may be important or meaningful to you, such as how you want to be treated if you are in pain, if there are certain friends you would like around, if you would want doctors in the future to learn about your cancer from your cells or tumour, or how much time you want to spend in the hospital. If you would like, we can show you the guide.

Source: Wolters Kluwer Health, Inc. Reference 7.

and limited educational or professional attainment.[11] This is true for not only the individual living with the illness but the family as well. When an AYA has a serious illness, the family and community are impacted in ways not seen in the adult world. Those closest to the AYA can experience significant distress. A life-threatening illness forces families to manage long periods of separation, disruptions to family routines, absences from work, shifts in roles, and increased marital dissatisfaction.[12] AYAs and their caregivers should receive psychosocial assessments examining prior and current family structure and functioning, family dysfunction, and the presence of other psychosocial stressors such as financial hardship.[7] At the same time, AYAs and their families learn to cope well and exhibit resilience.[13]

Targeted social support, clinical intervention, and education can facilitate growth during the time they are living with a serious illness.[13] Additionally, encouraging AYAs and their families to rely on the support of family, friends, and faith community is imperative as it often results in a sense of peace, connection, comfort, and purpose.[12]

Clinicians should encourage peer relationships in the form of maintaining previous relationships or fostering new ones with peers who have shared experiences. Peer support and social media groups can have a powerful impact. This is especially true of groups facilitated by skilled psychosocial professionals through the AYA's home institution. In addition to relationships, there are many local and national organizations which can provide guidance on school and career concerns and may offer limited one-time financial support. AYAs who are parents themselves face a unique set of challenges. They are often torn between their hopes as an individual and the narrative they want to leave for their child or children. This often results in a desire to "do everything" for more time or exhausting all possible interventions so that their child/children know they "fought to the end" for them.[14]

Adolescence and young adulthood are a time for significant reflection and evaluation with regard to religious and spiritual beliefs and practice. This time is marked by the exploration of meaning and morality and beginning to form personal faiths and beliefs.[15] This population is burdened by determining the meaning of life, "while placing their diagnosis within the context of a meaningful life."[15(p271)] A hallmark of the AYA period is moving from an inherited system of beliefs to considering the abstract and forming a personal theology based on lived experience.[15] Living with a serious illness alters the lens through which AYAs view the nature of suffering and fairness and see the world as a safe, caring, and just space.[15] AYAs with serious illness no longer have the luxury of time in pondering these questions, and they often do not have a peer, parent, or teacher who has the spiritual maturity or comfort in wrestling with these questions along with them. As such, special attention needs to be given to the spiritual needs of this population as spiritual pain may manifest as physical pain just as physical pain may result in spiritual pain.[15]

Spirituality is often overlooked unless an AYA expresses an affiliation in a faith-based community. Spiritual struggles and distress are associated with poorer health outcomes and impaired quality of life.[16] The majority of AYAs want their providers to address their spiritual and existential questions or concerns, and the desire for these conversations increases with disease acuity.[16] Even asking something as simple as "Do you feel peace?" is a nonthreatening way to approach a larger conversation.[16] Intervention from a hospital chaplain is often only initiated when an AYA expresses a religious affiliation. However, it is often those who do not express a specific affiliation and want to explore their spirituality who can benefit most from a chaplain. In addition to spiritual or existential distress, there are religious implications to treatment. For more specific information, please refer to Chapter 39 on spiritual Assessment and Care.

Intimate and potentially risky health behaviors are common in this population. The majority of AYA patients are sexually active, and in multiple studies, fewer than half reported consistent condom use or birth control.[11] AYAs who identify as LGBTQ+ are more likely to have engaged in sexual activity than their peers who identify as heterosexual or unsure.[17] As such, it is important that clinicians ask about sexual activity in an inclusive way, to provide the most comprehensive education. While engaging in sexual activity is normative, and in some cases indicates the AYA is coping well, it can have seriously unintended outcomes such as interfering with treatment, exacerbating health problems, and increasing the risk for late effects.[18] In order to facilitate affirming, candid conversations, taking steps such as displaying inclusive images like flags, pronoun pins, and inclusive terms on forms is helpful. There is still significant concern around discussions of sexual or gender identity as fears around safety and acceptance are legitimate. AYAs should be assured that conversations are confidential, and discussions with parents/family members should be approached by keeping a family's individual and cultural beliefs in mind.[17] Alcohol and illicit substance use is common.[11] These behaviors should be normalized and inquired about regardless of whether the need is expressed by the AYA.

Difficulty coping with caring for an AYA with a life-limiting illness is not confined to families and caregivers. Some clinicians see themselves in their patient or associate them with their own child. While this often fosters early connection and relatability, it can result in clinicians experiencing significant distress in caring for this population.[19] Many clinicians cite a greater sense of tragedy in caring for a young person, which can result in emotional agony, helplessness, and feelings of failure.[19] It is important for clinicians to check in with colleagues, participate in debriefings, and seek peer supervision depending on discipline.

Implications on the Family Unit

When an AYA is facing a life-threatening illness, the entire family is impacted. Siblings play an important role in providing comfort, distraction, and a sense of normalcy. While siblings often experience feelings of love and gratitude toward their ill sibling, it is normal and expected that they may experience feelings of grief, loss, guilt, and resentment. Parents may be less available for major events, and other family members, or friends, might step in to manage day-to-day needs. In addition to the disruption to family life, a significant impact for siblings is the medicalization of their home.[20] Family members are forced to cope with new equipment and people in what was once a private space. It is not uncommon to see siblings mature quickly and try not to draw any attention to themselves or act out in hopes of drawing the attention of their parents. Special attention should be provided to the well-being of siblings including encouraging use of psychosocial supports in the hospital and community setting—and emphasizing participation in school and extracurricular activities. School is often a sanctuary, in addition to a place for learning, leisure, and friendship, for the siblings of seriously ill AYAs.[20]

Parents of AYAs with life-limiting illness report increased marital dissatisfaction, anxiety, depression, and posttraumatic stress symptoms.[12] While this is often most acute in the time period surrounding diagnosis, many parents present as clinically distressed for years.[12] As such, it is imperative that psychosocial needs be evaluated at regular intervals.

ACP

Decision-making for the AYA can be challenging as decisions often involve risks and benefits with multiple paths forward. The timing for discussing ACP is often delayed due to provider discomfort and fear of causing stress for the patient and family. Providers fear taking away hope by discussing "what ifs," potential side effects, or negative outcomes; but one study showed a decrease in AYA anxiety around ACP and better communication with their family members using the *Voicing My Choices* document as a tool to discuss ACP.[21] One strategy may be to ask Bill during a routine outpatient visit "Can I ask you a difficult question?" This provides a warning shot that the conversation may be uncomfortable or difficult and elicits permission from the patient. "Have you thought about who may know what you would want if you got too sick to speak for yourself?" can initiate the ACP conversation. Healthcare providers can ask patients 18 years and older if there is an adult family member they would trust to make decisions on their behalf, known as a "medical power of attorney" (MPOA), as another way to introduce and normalize ACP. One could further the discussion by asking the AYA how they would want to communicate their desires to their MPOA—verbally versus written or both. Some individuals may prefer to discuss ACP at home, and others may welcome the support of a trusted interdisciplinary team member. A few communication tools and guides exist that may be helpful to explore ACP with the AYA including *Voicing my Choices* and *Five Wishes*.[22] It is important to remember that AYAs may have different wishes and worries than their loved ones and could benefit from their PC provider facilitating communication among their specialty teams and family members to support the AYA's autonomy in decision-making.[23] For additional details on ACP, please refer to Chapter 6.

Living with Chronic Illness and/or Long-Term Effects of Treatment

Several chronic complex illnesses, such as congenital heart disease, cystic fibrosis, pulmonary hypertension, muscular dystrophies, epilepsy, pain, autoimmune diseases, and cerebral palsy, may have fluctuating disease trajectories, with periods of stability followed by more acute illness or complications followed by convalescence or new baselines. Other illnesses, like cancer, organ transplant, and traumatic injuries, may have long-term consequences or secondary injury related to the original treatment including medication side effects, radiation, surgery, etc.[24] This may be a time the AYA is most vulnerable as they try to anticipate what is going to happen next, and healthcare providers may be uncomfortable with prognostication or addressing uncertainty.[25] Providers should provide anticipatory guidance about illness trajectory and disease progression in a clear, compassionate, and timely way. Telling Bill, for example, that he may have to wear his BiPAP longer with respiratory illnesses while recommending preventative health maintenance such as compliance with airway clearance and receiving annual flu vaccines would be helpful guidance. It is imperative to provide AYAs with ongoing evaluation and care of not only their underlying disease process but their entire social, emotional, spiritual, and sexual being.

AYAs may rely heavily on support outside of their medical teams and families. The PC provider should be aware of local and national support groups, social media groups, camps, online forums, and school accommodations. The AYA population benefits from peer and social support and often finds comfort in realizing they are not alone.[26] There will likely be a time to discuss with Bill and his family the transition to adult medicine, and this should be broached thoughtfully by the medical team. It is important to identify which specialties will transition to adult medicine and which may remain with their current team, if any, and to begin communicating this to Bill and his family 12–24 months in advance, if possible. Bill and family may find comfort in being given a provider's name and contact information for transition in addition to anticipatory guidance on general differences between adult and pediatric medicine.[27] In some cases an AYA may feel that they are burdening their family or loved ones, and they may request to reside in a long-term care facility. Healthcare providers should partner with their interdisciplinary team and adult colleagues to provide accurate information to patients and families and to maintain honest and accurate communication on this sensitive subject.

Crisis Management

Healthcare providers recognize that in addition to the chronic phase of illness, there will be acute illnesses or crises for many AYA patients. The potential for these crises should be discussed with patients and families, especially during outpatient visits in a controlled setting. For example, when seeing Bill in clinic, it may be helpful to mention that he may notice that he is more easily fatigued or is waking up fatigued as a sign of progressive muscle weakness. This provides Bill anticipatory guidance about potential symptoms and allows exploration of management strategies that may be offered such as inpatient admission, increased airway clearance modalities, and longer noninvasive ventilation use. The goal is to help Bill and his family understand potential signs of disease progression and what options may be available to alleviate or improve symptoms and prolong quality of life in line with their goals.[28] These times of disease progression or acute on chronic illness offer the opportunity for the PC team to help Bill reexamine wishes and worries, to provide medical decision-making support about medical management or added technology, and to continue longitudinal support.

Hospice

Hospice is an insurance benefit for patients with a life expectancy of 6 months or less and is different in pediatric versus adult medicine.[29] AYA patients aged 21 or younger qualify for concurrent benefits, allowing them to seek illness-directed therapies such as chemotherapy, surgery, and infusions, while also receiving hospice support at home. Patients older than 21 do not qualify for concurrent care and must choose between hospice support and further illness-directed therapies.[29] It is important to understand each patient's hospice benefit as AYA patients like Bill need accurate and honest information from their care teams about how hospice can impact their care. Often hospice is an additional layer of support at home that can provide specialized physical and emotional assessment, management and treatment of symptoms, and support in the home and is not intended to replace subspecialty care teams.[29] It should also be explained what medications, therapies, and equipment hospice may cover in addition to services already being provided by home nursing or equipment companies. Bill may ask if the team is out of options or is giving up on him, and the PC provider should be experienced in addressing this concern. One strategy may be to share with Bill and his mom what the team worries about for Bill and how they hope hospice could enhance his care while acknowledging it is his decision which will be respected. For additional information about hospice, please see Chapter 42.

End-of-Life Care

If AYAs and their families do not have discussions about ACP, they are more likely to experience an intensive care stay at the end of their lives.[29] Sensitive, honest, timely, and open communication and support will benefit Bill, his family, and care teams and should not be delayed. ACP should be a part of routine visits to address Bill's wishes, worries, wants, and needs as his disease progresses. A potential benefit of discussing a provider's fear about Bill getting sicker and nearing the end of life is affording Bill the opportunity to do some legacy-building.[30] This may be letters, videos, TikToks, drawings, or songs to express how he is feeling to those most important to him. It may allow Bill the chance to make something meaningful out of a shortened life.[30] Some AYAs may want to allocate belongings or prized possessions, and others may want to be a part of their funeral or celebration of life planning.[31] Bill may express wanting to achieve or experience certain milestones: graduation, prom, having a job, going on a date, or being in a relationship. He may want to experience something new, repeat an experience, or seek physical intimacy with a partner. Legacy-building may improve communication around the end of life between Bill and his family by allowing exploration of wishes and worries while painting, making a video, or recording a song.[30] Not all AYAs will want to discuss their end of life, and some may need permission to not have to share everything. Attempts should be compassionately made to elicit their fears and where they would prefer to die to provide them with dignity and respect at their end of life. Many patients will have been supported by their family throughout their illness journey, and it is important to acknowledge and offer these family members support as well. For detailed information, please refer to Chapter 43 on end-of-life care and Chapter 44 on grief and bereavement.

Special Population Considerations

As advances in pediatric medicine continue and children live longer with chronic or life-threatening conditions, there is a growing population of AYAs who are neurologically and or developmentally impaired. A large portion of these patients will not be able to make decisions for themselves, and therefore all the subjects mentioned above will likely be directed to their parents or guardians. Currently, there is not a tool available for guardians making decisions on behalf of their adult children. The PC provider may be helpful to guardians by discussing guardianship, which varies by state, and transition from pediatric medicine to adult medicine. It is imperative to continue to discuss symptom burden, wishes and worries, legacy-building, and advance directives with the guardians as well. The PC provider and primary physician should coordinate who will be leading these discussions to provide consistency and continuity.

Summary

The AYA population living with chronic, serious, and life-threatening illness deserves the skills of an integrated pediatric PC team to foster and support independence and healthcare autonomy. Skilled clinicians should be able to introduce PC, guide difficult conversations, address wishes and worries, provide symptom relief, and respect desires for treatment and the end of life. Additionally, the healthcare provider can provide longitudinal support for the AYA and family unit to learn strategies for coping with serious illness or death, encourage legacy-building, and provide exceptional end-of-life care that respects the AYA's desires when necessary.

REFERENCES

1. Sisk BA, Canavera K, Sharma A, Baker JN, Johnson LM. Ethical issues in the care of adolescent and young adult oncology patients. *Pediatr Blood Cancer*. 2019;66(5):e27608. https://doi.org/10.1002/pbc.27608.
2. Burgers VWG, van der Graaf WTA, van der Meer DJ, et al. Adolescents and young adults living with an uncertain or poor cancer prognosis: the "new" lost tribe. *J Natl Compr Canc Netw*. 2021;19(3):240–246. https://doi.org/10.6004/jnccn.2020.7696.
3. Cuviello A, Raisanen JC, Donohue PK, Wiener L, Boss RD. Defining the boundaries of palliative care in pediatric oncology. *J Pain Symptom Manage*. 2020;59(5):1033–1042.e1. https://doi.org/10.1016/j.jpainsymman.2019.11.022.
4. Cuviello A, Raisanen JC, Donohue PK, Wiener L, Boss RD. Initiating palliative care referrals in pediatric oncology. *J Pain Symptom Manage*. 2021;61(1):81–89.e1. https://doi.org/10.1016/j.jpainsymman.2020.07.008.
5. Kenney AE, Bedoya SZ, Gerhardt CA, Young-Saleme T, Wiener L. End of life communication among caregivers of children with cancer: a qualitative approach to understanding support desired by families. *Palliat Support Care*. 2021;19(6):715–722. https://doi.org/10.1017/S1478951521000067.
6. Friebert S, Grossoehme DH, Baker JN, et al. Congruence gaps between adolescents with cancer and their families regarding values, goals, and beliefs about end-of-life care. *JAMA Netw Open*. 2020;3(5):e205424. https://doi.org/10.1001/jamanetworkopen.2020.5424.
7. Snaman J, McCarthy S, Wiener L, Wolfe J. Pediatric palliative care in oncology. *J Clin Oncol*. 2020;38(9):954–962. https://doi.org/10.1200/JCO.18.02331.
8. Loucas CA, Brand SR, Bedoya SZ, Muriel AC, Wiener L. Preparing youth with cancer for amputation: a systematic review. *J Psychosoc Oncol*. 2017;35(4):483–493. https://doi.org/10.1080/07347332.2017.1307894.
9. Brierley ME, Sansom-Daly UM, Baenziger J, McGill B, Wakefield CE. Impact of physical appearance changes reported by adolescent and young adult cancer survivors: a qualitative analysis. *Eur J Cancer Care (Engl)*. 2019;28(4):e13052. https://doi.org/10.1111/ecc.13052.
10. Ligon JA, Fry A, Maher JY, et al. Fertility and CAR T-cells: current practice and future directions. *Transplant Cell Ther*. 2022;28(9):605.e1–605.e8. https://doi.org/10.1016/j.jtct.2022.06.002.
11. Rosenberg AR, Bona K, Ketterl T, Wharton CM, Wolfe J, Baker KS. Intimacy, substance use, and communication needs during cancer therapy: a report from the "Resilience in adolescents and

young adults" study. *J Adolesc Health*. 2017;60(1):93–99. https://doi.org/10.1016/j.jadohealth.2016.08.017.

12. Arruda-Colli MNF, Bedoya SZ, Muriel A, Pelletier W, Wiener L. In good times and in bad: what strengthens or challenges a parental relationship during a child's cancer trajectory? *J Psychosoc Oncol*. 2018;36(5):635–648. https://doi.org/10.1080/07347332.2018.1485813.
13. Wiener L, Bluebond-Langner M. Commentary: treating the pediatric cancer patient: insights that have stood the test of time. *J Pediatr Psychol*. 2019;44(7):764–767. https://doi.org/10.1093/jpepsy/jsz022.
14. Buxton D. Child and adolescent psychiatry and palliative care. *J Am Acad Child Adolesc Psychiatry*. 2015;54(10):791–792. https://doi.org/10.1016/j.jaac.2015.05.017.
15. Weaver MS, Wratchford D. Spirituality in adolescent patients. *Ann Palliat Med*. 2017;6(3):270–278. https://doi.org/10.21037/apm.2017.05.09.
16. Grossoehme DH, Friebert S, Baker JN, et al. Association of religious and spiritual factors with patient-reported outcomes of anxiety, depressive symptoms, fatigue, and pain interference among adolescents and young adults with cancer. *JAMA Netw Open*. 2020;3(6):e206696. https://doi.org/10.1001/jamanetworkopen.2020.6696.
17. Bright Futures: Guidelines for Health Supervision of Infants, Children, and Adolescents, 4th Edition. Last updated: July 2022 Downloaded from: https://www.aap.org/brightfutures.
18. Fladeboe KM, Scott S, Bradford MC, Ketterl TG, Yi-Frazier JP, Rosenberg AR. Sexual activity and substance use among adolescents and young adults receiving cancer treatment: a report from the PRISM randomized controlled trial. *J Adolesc Young Adult Oncol*. 2020;9(5):594–600. https://doi.org/10.1089/jayao.2020.0001.
19. Avery J, Geist A, D'Agostino NM, et al. "It's more difficult . . .": clinicians' experience providing palliative care to adolescents and young adults diagnosed with advanced cancer. *JCO Oncol Pract*. 2020;16(1):e100–e108. https://doi.org/10.1200/JOP.19.00313.
20. Lyon ME, Wiener L. Special issue: psychosocial considerations for children and adolescents living with a rare disease. *Children (Basel)*. 2022;9(7):1099. https://doi.org/10.3390/children9071099.
21. Wiener L, Bedoya S, Battles H, et al. Voicing their choices: advance care planning with adolescents and young adults with cancer and other serious conditions. *Palliat Support Care*. 2022;20(4):462–470. https://doi.org/10.1017/S1478951521001462.
22. Aging with Dignity. Five Wishes: https://www.fivewishes.org/. Accessed September 21, 2022. https://store.fivewishes.org/ShopLocal/en/p/VC-MASTER-000/voicing-my-choices.
23. Needle JS, Peden-McAlpine C, Liaschenko J, et al. "Can you tell me why you made that choice?": a qualitative study of the influences on treatment decisions in advance care planning among adolescents and young adults undergoing bone marrow transplant. *Palliat Med*. 2020;34(3):281–290. https://doi.org/10.1177/0269216319883977.
24. Suh E, Stratton KL, Leisenring WM, et al. Late mortality and chronic health conditions in long-term survivors of early-adolescent and young adult cancers: a retrospective cohort analysis from the Childhood Cancer Survivor Study. *Lancet Oncol*. 2020;21(3):421–435. https://doi.org/10.1016/S1470-2045(19)30800-9.
25. Burgers VWG, van den Bent MJ, Darlington AE, et al. A qualitative study on the challenges health care professionals face when caring for adolescents and young adults with an uncertain and/or poor cancer prognosis. *ESMO Open*. 2022;7(3):100476. https://doi.org/10.1016/j.esmoop.2022.100476.
26. LeBeau K, Collins S, Zori G, et al. Evaluating a novel hospital-based online health community to address palliative and psychosocial care factors for chronically ill adolescent and young adult patients. *Palliat Support Care*. 2024;22(3):432–443. https://doi.org/10.1017/S1478951523000147.
27. Coyne I, Sheehan A, Heery E, While AE. Healthcare transition for adolescents and young adults with long-term conditions: qualitative study of patients, parents and healthcare professionals' experiences. *J Clin Nurs*. 2019;28(21–22):4062–4076. https://doi.org/10.1111/jocn.15006.
28. Friebert S, Grossoehme DH, Baker JN, et al. Congruence gaps between adolescents with cancer and their families regarding values, goals, and beliefs about end-of-life care. *JAMA Netw Open*. 2020;3(5):e205424. https://doi.org/10.1001/jamanetworkopen.2020.5424.
29. Pyke-Grimm KA, Fisher B, Haskamp A, Bell CJ, Newman AR. Providing palliative and hospice care to children, adolescents and young adults with cancer. *Semin Oncol Nurs*. 2021;37(3):151166. https://doi.org/10.1016/j.soncn.2021.151166.
30. Cahalan L, Smith A, Sandoval M, Parks G, Gresham Z. Collaborative legacy building to alleviate emotional pain and suffering in pediatric cancer patients: a case review. *Children (Basel)*. 2022;9(1):33. https://doi.org/10.3390/children9010033.
31. Wiener L, Zadeh S, Battles H, et al. Allowing adolescents and young adults to plan their end-of-life care. *Pediatrics*. 2012;130(5):897–905. https://doi.org/10.1542/peds.2012-0663.

42

Pediatric Hospice Perspectives

Alice Bass and Rebecca Turner

Key Points

- Pediatric palliative and hospice care is a rapidly growing field providing multifaceted care that focuses on a child's and family's well-being along a physical, psychological, emotional, spiritual, and social continuum.
- Pediatric hospice should be considered a necessary part of comprehensive palliative care. Concurrent care is aimed at improving access to hospice, an invaluable service for pediatric patients.
- Initial and ongoing education and care delivered by an interdisciplinary team of healthcare professionals is essential in addressing the complex physical, emotional, spiritual, and practical needs and concerns of children and their families.
- Relieving suffering and improving quality of life, for even a brief life, can benefit not only the child but all those affected by the illness or death of the child, including siblings, parents, grandparents, other relatives, teachers, school friends, faith community, and neighbors, as well as the healthcare professionals involved in their care.
- Nurses who care for dying children and their families need a significant personal and professional support system and opportunities for renewal, personal growth, and ongoing education.

Case Study

Taylor is a 3-year-old with a chromosomal deletion syndrome that has led to significant cardiac defects, chronic kidney disease, global developmental delay, and severe laryngomalacia. The inpatient pediatric palliative care (PPC) team was consulted for Taylor and her family on day of life 4. Taylor's parents were receptive to services, and goals were aimed at interventions that would prolong Taylor's quality and length of life as their hope was that Taylor would be given every opportunity to live as normal of a life as was possible alongside her three older siblings. As such, she received a tracheostomy in the first month of life, was ventilator-dependent, and received enteral nutrition via gastrostomy tube.

Overview of Pediatric Hospice and Palliative Care

Universally, children symbolize the "future," representing their parents' hopes and dreams. The experience of serious illness or the death of an infant, child, or adolescent therefore generates a legitimate threat to such hopes. Bearing witness and walking alongside children and their families motivates clinicians to do their best to prevent children's suffering. This chapter provides an overview of pediatric palliative and hospice care (PPHC) and the impact of nurses who are called on to provide this unique type of care.

Definition of PPC

The World Health Organization developed one of the earliest and most widely accepted definitions of PPC, describing it as the active total care of the child's body, mind, and spirit and involving an evaluation of a child's psychological, physical, and social distress.[1] PPC is provided by an interdisciplinary team (IDT) of professionals from medicine; nursing; social work; spiritual care; child life; art, music, and massage therapy; and other areas of healthcare. These clinicians and providers receive specialized training to offer expertise on the impact of disease processes on pediatric development, pain and symptom prevention and management, family-centered care, and maximizing quality of life. Together, they can provide comprehensive care for children and serve as good resources for other allied professionals (including psychiatrists, psychologists, representatives from other consulting services, primary care providers, other therapists [physical, occupational, speech, and respiratory], as well as community representatives [teachers, coaches, religious leaders, hospice team members]) who are also part of a child's care team. PPHC serves as the foundation for collaborative decision-making regarding goals of care while aiming to preserve the integrity of the family throughout disease progression, addresses anticipatory grief, and includes bereavement support following death.

Comparing PPHC

The terms "palliative care" and "hospice care" are often used interchangeably (as in this chapter) because of their similar core values and philosophical approaches to care. However, it is important to appreciate and understand their distinctive features. Primarily, palliative care can be provided at any time during the course of the disease (including the time of diagnosis), whereas hospice care focuses more around true end-of-life (EOL) care.[2] PPHC provision is unique because children go through developmental stages while having more complex, lifelong chronic conditions, thereby complicating the identification of treatment plans, trajectories, and ethical issues around legal decision-making, all while dealing with larger community involvement, inadequate palliative and hospice care resources, and more complicated grief.

Concurrent Care

When first developed, state and federal hospice regulations and standards governing hospice care and the clinical guidelines for ongoing appropriateness (Medicare and Medicaid) did not address pediatrics. Determining the required 6-months-or-less prognosis is extremely difficult for pediatricians because of the wide variability of prognoses in children, often varying from days to weeks or from months to years. Referral to hospice care by pediatric providers made them feel as though they were "giving up."

In addition, there was a question as to what, if any, treatments might be acceptable under hospice admission guidelines. Programs varied on whether blood products, antibiotics, infusions, lab tests, and more were considered "too aggressive" an approach to care, expecting parents to surrender all means of therapies before enrollment in hospice. These interventions were also a great financial burden or unfeasible for many programs without substantial foundational support. The option of forgoing treatment for their child to receive palliative or hospice care was simply too difficult a decision for parents to make, and the rigidity of these strict choices has been identified as a barrier to enrollment in pediatric hospice services at the end of life.

On March 23, 2010, the US government responded to these challenges with the enactment of the provision "Concurrent Care for Children" in Section 2302 of the Patient Protection and Affordable Healthcare Act.[3] This legislation allows patients under the age of 21 with state Medicaid or Children's Health Insurance Program to receive hospice support while still pursuing disease-directed or curative therapies. Its ratification was a step toward healthcare systems and the government acknowledging that the needs of children with life-threatening illnesses/conditions are distinctly different from those of adults. Hospices could now accept pediatric patients up to age 21 who had interventions not traditionally covered under the hospice benefit such as tracheostomies, ventilators, chemotherapy, frequent hospitalizations, and expensive medications. Hospice could still be reimbursed the daily per diem rate, and qualifying insurers would cover these patients' non-hospice-covered needs separately.

To better understand and interpret this new act, in 2012, a pediatric-focused Continuum Briefing titled "Pediatric Concurrent Care" was composed at the Mary J. Labyak Institute for Innovation at the National Center for Care at the End of Life. This briefing identified some barriers to the provision: (1) a physician still needs to certify that the child is expected to die in less than 6 months, (2) every state has different Medicaid-covered services/resources, and (3) the provision itself does not specify what treatments/services are deemed curative.[4] The District of Columbia Pediatric Palliative Care Collaborative and the National Hospice and Palliative Care Organization also recognized these barriers, as well as the effort involved for individual states to acclimate to and utilize concurrent care. In response, they developed the Concurrent Care for Children Implementation Toolkit, designed to guide providers and interested parties in understanding the effect that concurrent care could have on their individual state Medicaid programs. It describes how each state has its own amendment and waiver options and encourages learning from other states' experiences to help facilitate a statewide collaborative approach in adapting and implementing effective and efficient concurrent PPC services.[5]

In "Concurrent Care for the Medically Complex Child: Lessons of Implementation," Miller et al.[6] discussed some general issues they identified in coordinating concurrent care for medically complex children. They found that, when adding hospice services to care, existing providers (some who cared for the patient for many years) needed much education and support regarding the concept and the clinical interventions/treatment. They also discovered a high level of complexity in coordinating and integrating hospice care with the current services and providers already in place. Lastly, there were challenges and complexities in determining whether the current durable equipment company or hospice agency was responsible for providing equipment and what services were still covered under the primary commercial insurance (if applicable).

Case Study Continued

Taylor developed worsening pulmonary hypertension during her hospitalization, and in the context of Taylor's many medically complex needs, her cardiology team shared their worry that Taylor would not be a good candidate for future disease-directed cardiac surgeries due to extremely high risk of mortality. The palliative care team continued to discuss her mother's hopes in light of this new information. Taylor's parents ultimately shared that their hopes were still to get Taylor home to be with family for as much time as possible while hoping to have the opportunity to discuss benefits and burdens of recommended procedures or interventions due to worry for suffering that would not necessarily promote better time at home. If a complication could be treated or reversed (e.g., pneumonia), the parents felt it important to try, though recognized that Taylor would ultimately succumb to heart failure over time. Taylor's parents expressed that their most important wish would be that Taylor die at home surrounded by her immediate family.

Progress and Challenges

The advancement of palliative care as a model for care in the United States has reached unprecedented levels in many types of settings. There is a surge of robust development and integration for PPHC programs and services from prenatal diagnosis, throughout childhood, to adolescents on the brink of adulthood. Growth has been evidenced on many fronts: legislative action, research, hospital based palliative care, community-based hospice teams/programs, and specialty areas of palliative care. As a government-based coverage provider, Tricare has adopted concurrent care coverage as well, allowing military families to receive the extra support they need to care for their ill children.[7] While private insurance companies are not required to cover hospice with concurrent care, several will on a case-by-case basis. Despite this, many challenges to delivering optimal PPC and improving the quality of life (QOL) of children and families still exist. Much work remains regarding understanding the differences between palliative care and hospice, clearly defining the population being served, better understanding the needs of children with life-threatening conditions and of their families, developing an approach that will be appropriate across different communities, and providing timely care that responds adequately to suffering.[8] Changing the pervasive stigma of how PPC and hospice are often perceived as synonymous with "giving up," "there's nothing more that can be done," or "death must be near" is a long-term goal.

The ongoing painful dilemmas and struggles for families with children who are facing life-threatening illness and the end of life remain hidden from society's view, yet the demands and challenges of caring for a dying child are being addressed continually within hospitals and homes. The landmark report from the Institute of Medicine *When Children Die: Improving Palliative and End-of-Life Care of Children and Their Families*[9] became the catalyst for a cascade of national initiatives, research, funding, and heightened awareness that continues to evolve today. In addition, the National Consensus Project's *Guidelines for Quality Palliative Care*, originally published in 2004, provide clinical practice guidelines to foster consistent and high standards in palliative care and to encourage continuity of care across settings for both children and adults living with life-threatening illness.[10] Concurrent care exists to help optimize the child's QOL for as long as possible and in a manner that is most in line with the family's goals. Despite the development of toolkits and resources to guide implementation of concurrent care among states, research shows significant variability in how concurrent care is carried out across the country.[11]

The Settings Where PPC Occurs

"Hospice and palliative care can be provided in almost any setting as long as those providing the care are willing to enter the patient's world and honor their setting of choice."[12 (p. 310)] Figure 42.1 and its associated Event Key provide a glimpse into various opportunities where PPC may be introduced during a child's illness trajectory. Irrespective of the setting, PPC should be patient-/family-centered, interdisciplinary, and collaborative with optimal and ongoing communication among all caregivers.[13] The American Academy of Pediatrics recommends that large healthcare organizations should have interdisciplinary PPC teams with expertise and experience to effectively manage and coordinate the complex and intricate

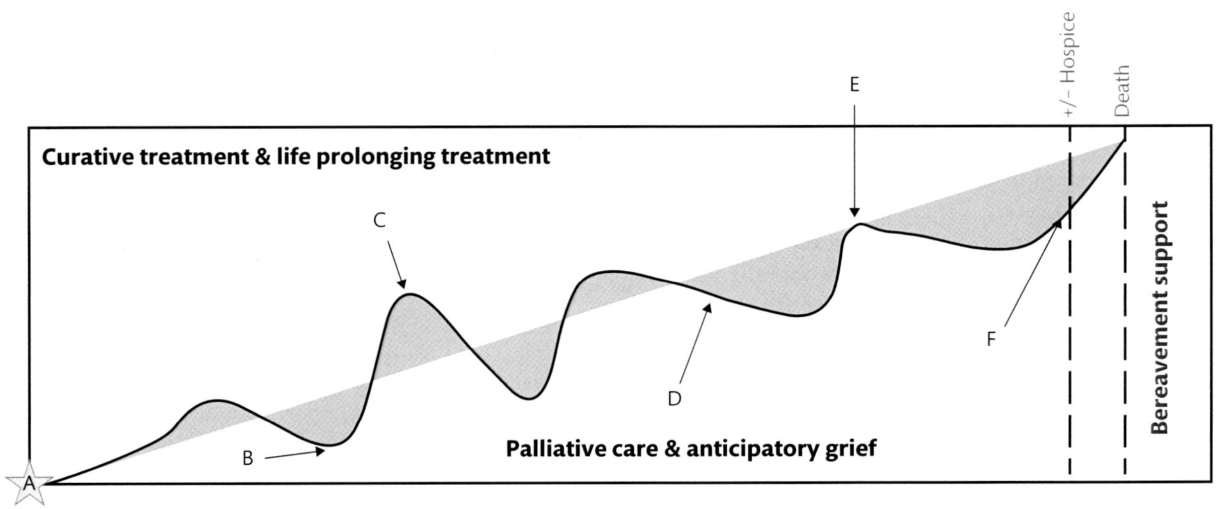

Figure 42.1 "The rollercoaster." A general visualization of the extent of pediatric palliative care (PPC) involvement for a child diagnosed with a potentially life-limiting illness. PPC integration may occur at any time along a child's illness trajectory, with multiple cases that can occur in the inpatient, clinic, or home setting. The associated event key lists examples of PPC introduced along many points in a child's illness trajectory—from diagnosis to near end of life. Multiple opportunities exist along the continuum, in a variety of possible care settings, for PPC services to partner with primary providers in support of family goals and to enhance quality of life for the child and family.

Event key	Sample description of events surrounding introduction of pediatric palliative care (PPC) services
A	At the time of diagnosis—the recommended ideal time to introduce PPC[15]—even with curative options available and driving a family's journey, PPC can initially play a small role getting to know the family and their unique values and goals.
B	Following a particularly challenging or unexpected acute episode/hospitalization to establish rapport, provide support around grief themes and explore goals of care (GOC)—the child may be medically stable, but family could benefit from initial conversations around pediatric advanced care planning (pACP)
C	In the midst of a period where symptom management is a priority alongside curative or life-prolonging interventions where PPC may assist not only with goal-setting but also with pain or other signs of physical distress, discussing how the patient/family wishes to prioritize time at home, including use of available home-based resources.
D	PPC is sometimes introduced during a prolonged hospitalization where it may be important to address GOC/pACP, assist with symptoms, facilitate communication, or coordinate care to ensure medical decisions remain in line with family goals.
E	As curative or life-prolonging treatment options begin to fail or the child endures repeated life-threatening events, there is a clinic visit with news of relapse or progression, or there is concern that future options may negatively impact quality of life, PPC may be introduced to discuss advance care planning around the "what ifs," including family's critical illness treatment preferences.
F	Parents and family elect to redirect goals toward aggressive comfort measures, or child begins showing signs of active decline despite interventions, and PPC is introduced to facilitate goals, discussing family's desire to maximize time at home, including available hospice options, and involvement is heavy from the start.

arrangements in transitioning pediatric patients between healthcare and/or home settings while maintaining the highest quality of care possible.[14] Recommendations also include that these PPC teams stay involved and fully engaged across all settings to ensure continuity of care and appropriate treatment and interventions which align with the patient's and family's goals of care at all times.[15]

PPC and Hospice Service Availability

In assessing the landscape of outpatient PPC and hospice agencies dedicated to nurturing children, the National Hospice and Palliative Care Organization (NHPCO) published its 2023 edition of *Pediatric Facts and Figures*. This report showed that within the United States, home-based services are available across only 895 counties for hospice and 591 for palliative care. Delving deeper, the statistics revealed that PPHC accessibility was limited to 21.8% (hospice) and 12.3% (palliative) of non-metro counties, in contrast to the 39.8% (hospice) and 29.8% (palliative) of metro counties.[16] A clear disparity emerges regarding access to these life-affirming pediatric services in regions beyond metropolitan thresholds.

As the field of home-based hospice and palliative care continues to grow and expand across the United States, NHPCO reported that 71.5% (hospice) and 81.2% (palliative care) of counties remain void of pediatric home-based hospice or palliative care services.[16] Despite fewer resources arising for pediatric applications than their adult counterparts, there is a growing interest in and number of resources to help care for children requiring PPC. The collective aspiration is to steadily grow the quality and available resources for this vulnerable patient population.

Barriers to Accessing PPHC

Barriers to providing hospice or palliative care services for pediatric patients differ from those for adult patients. In general, society's belief that "children shouldn't die," along with denial of the process, make EOL care for this population a difficult and often misunderstood concept. Within the healthcare profession, a profound silence of discomfort and denial exists regarding babies and children dying. Clinical expertise in advanced illness or EOL care should be available for families who may transition their focus of care from a strictly curative mode to one of comfort and QOL.

In PPC, ethical issues, law, and policy are sensitive and complex and therefore create additional barriers that may intimidate providers regarding palliative and EOL care. Healthcare providers, as well as the public, need to be aware of local and state laws, especially about adolescents having a say in their medical decision-making and goals/limitations of care.[2] Patients over the age of 18 treated at a pediatric institution who do not have decision-making capacity should have guardianship verified by care teams, and their IDTs should ensure the patient's best interests are kept in mind at all times when making care plans.[2]

Children with complex chronic conditions often have frequent life-threatening events and acute illnesses. Technological advances and treatments have helped children survive these events, making care, decision-making, and instituting limitations more difficult for both providers and patients/families. Common thought becomes, "If the child survived the last life-threatening event, they would survive the next." As a result, another barrier has emerged over the years: death is seen as a failure of the healthcare system and not a natural process of the illness/disease.[17] Advocates for PPC recognize that advanced technology/treatment saves lives but fear it may cloud decision-making and prolong suffering.

Pain and symptom management also have become more complex and challenging. Children with complex conditions often end up on multiple medications and/or treatment modalities, making it harder to cross-check interactions and determine doses and effectiveness. Feudtner et al. found that 73.3% of parents receiving PPC across the United States perceived that their child experienced polysymptomatology (identified as having five or more symptoms), which further highlights just how critical PPC can be in appropriately assessing and managing this patient population.[18] Hospice agencies tend to feel their expertise in EOL care is insufficient in caring for the complex pediatric patient. Provider education and ongoing support from palliative care colleagues help diffuse some anxiety in caring for these children and thus should remain an integral part of caring for children and families within the context of PPC.

Lastly, the cost of caring for children with chronic life-limiting illnesses/conditions has been a barrier to pursuing pediatric hospice. Pediatric hospice or palliative care typically requires longer, more frequent home visits; longer time for family meetings and decision-making; more coordination of care with multiple physicians, other providers, and insurance companies; and hiring or access to pediatric experienced nurses, social workers, and child life specialists and aides. Ongoing therapies for palliation of distressing symptoms, including blood transfusions, antibiotics, chemotherapy, and enteral and gavage feedings, typically continue longer for children than for adults. The cost and responsibility for covering these therapies may be an additional factor for home-based providers in deciding whether to serve children. Now with concurrent care and Medicaid waiver programs, this barrier is being addressed and will hopefully become less of an issue as implementation becomes more uniform and consistent across healthcare settings.

Nursing Considerations

Nurses providing PPC and EOL care often experience emotional pain and suffering themselves related to their young patients' declining conditions and poor prognosis. In programs where nurses are not clinically trained or emotionally prepared to manage pediatric patients, many issues can emerge because of their anguish. Previous losses of a similar nature, unresolved grief issues, conflicting beliefs regarding "supportive care-only" interventions, and insecurities and self-doubt are all common, even within the hospice setting. Nurses who are trained properly report feeling honored and privileged to help patients and families during one of their most painful, private, and intimate experiences. Therefore, the better prepared, supported, and educated nurses are, the better chance they will help influence a more positive and less traumatizing experience for all involved.[19,20]

Parents as Advocates

Nurses can support parents and families in the hospital and at home by identifying their concerns and fears regarding things such as routine care in the hospital, life outside the security of the hospital, what to expect at home, how to handle emergencies, and knowing when to call for help. Nurses have an important role in preparing families for care in different situations, making sure they have appropriate medications, resources, and contacts in place when needed. In the home setting, it may be helpful to think of parents as "first responders," and, as such, they require access to what is needed to respond best to their child's issue when it arises. For example, having an "emergency kit" with a few medications in one or two doses for common crisis situations can prevent needless fear and suffering until a home care nurse arrives. Educating parents as thoroughly as possible for transitions in care and settings will reduce anxiety and unnecessary problems faced at home. PPC places special demands on healthcare providers, not the least of which is an obligation to nurture relationships that can hold both vulnerability and suffering within their embrace.[21]

Case Study Continued

After four long months in the hospital's neonatal intensive care unit (NICU) and cardiothoracic ICU, Taylor was discharged home with a local hospice program that had cared for many pediatric patients in the past but none quite as complex as Taylor. The hospice wanted to find ways to best support Taylor but was unsure how to do this given the parents' goals. The PPC team provided just-in-time training, and resources were provided to better assist the hospice in understanding some of the nuances of concurrent care coverage. The hospice agreed to enroll Taylor in services and began developing a relationship with the family, gaining better insight into parents' experiences in the hospital and desire to be the best parents they can be to Taylor for whatever time she may have remaining.

General Considerations for PPHC

The philosophy of palliative care for children is similar to that for adults; however, the practical elements of PPC differ in many ways. Clinicians providing PPC must not only learn the nuances inherent to care focused on comfort and QOL but also pay particular attention to the specific needs of children and families as they assist them through their experience of the child's illness and death. The essential elements of PPC (Figure 42.2)[22] need to be woven into every aspect of nursing care, with consideration given to how each component of care will affect the child's and family member's daily life and over time. Hospice and palliative healthcare providers are specifically skilled at providing high-quality and family-centered dialogue

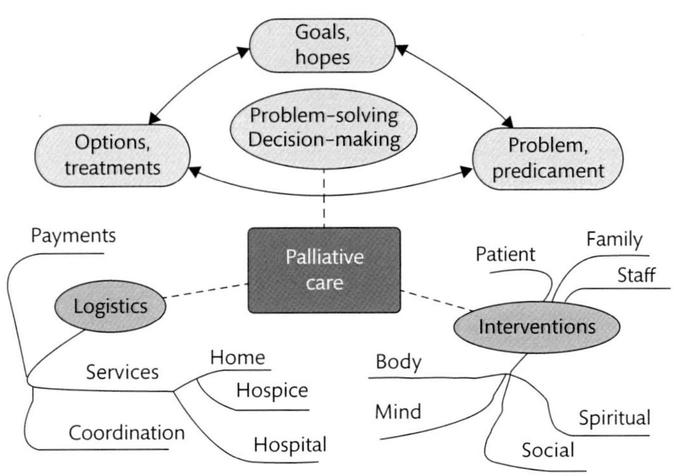

Figure 42.2 Essential elements in pediatric palliative care.
Source: Reference 22.

and education around their child's condition changes. This ability fosters trust and provides families with the information they need to make the right decisions to meet their definition of QOL for the patient and their entire family.

One must consider the reality of the burdens placed on families when caring for children with life-threatening illnesses and how their entire existence can center on details of medication schedules, treatment plans, medical appointments, and trips to the hospital, as well as the minutiae of providing constant care, leaving little time or energy for anyone or anything else. Taking these elements into consideration, it is the responsibility of interdisciplinary PPC providers to create individualized plans of care that are consistent with the goal of maintaining "normalcy" as much as possible while simultaneously adjusting to the "new normal" that families are often challenged to embrace. In these situations, one must consider the support and guidance that families will need when the focus of care changes as the end of life draws near. Nurses have a crucial role in supporting families through their fears and frustrations along with normalizing the full range of feelings that may ebb and flow throughout the course of a child's illness and death. Collectively, it is the role of the IDT to accompany the child and family throughout illness, death, and bereavement and to support families in coping with the challenges of living with a life-limiting illness and the suffering that may come along with it (Figure 42.2).[22]

Family-Centered Care

In essence, palliative care considers the patient and family as a unique entity whose members all require care.[2] When a child is diagnosed with a life-threatening condition, the entire family, whomever that may include, is affected on both an individual and a collective level.[22] Special attention should be paid to the role of each person in the family and to how those roles may change throughout the course of a child's illness; thus, understanding existing and evolving relationships among family members is extremely important. Understanding the meaning of the illness and/or death experience must also be considered within the historical, cultural, spiritual, and environmental contexts of each family.[23] See Table 42.1[24] for guidelines for children's developmental understanding of death.

Support for Parents/Guardians

Families often describe their experiences of living with a child with a life-threatening illness as "being on a roller coaster." From the first time a parent senses something is wrong until the time of death, parents are faced with stressors associated with daily life/providing care, making difficult decisions, and often feelings of anger, sadness, disbelief, and withdrawal.[23] Parents may feel as if they are losing control over several aspects of their lives, and it is therefore helpful for nurses and other members of the IDT to find ways to continually allow parents to remain in control, for example, by involving them in planning the child's daily routine, allowing them to participate in care, and asking if there is a certain way they would like things done. Nurses can assist parents with methods to help themselves and their child feel in control regarding aspects of their experience. Things such as establishing a daily routine; having children participate in conversations about care, when appropriate; and knowing what side effects to anticipate from medications, treatments, and therapies are empowering and foster an environment of mutual trust and respect.

Table 42.1 Developmental stages and perceptions of death

Age	Basic conflict	View of death	Suggestions
Birth–18 months	Trust versus mistrust	No sense of finality; death is viewed as continuous with life, child is reactive to the stress.	Use simple physical communication and provide comforting and nurturing care.
Early childhood: 2–3 years	Autonomy versus shame and doubt	Death is seen as reversible and not final; the child may feel that death is a punishment. Children may feel that they are responsible for death.	Expect regression, clinging, or aggressive behavior. Encourage expression as the child may be concerned about family function after a member dies. Use honest and clear language to explain death and dying.
Preschool: 3–5 years	Initiative versus guilt	Death continues to be understood as temporary. The child may have a literal understanding of death and will respond with curiosity and questioning.	Open communication with clear language should continue to be utilized. The child should be encouraged to ask questions about death and dying.
School age: 6–11 years	Industry versus inferiority	Death is understood as permanent, and the child understands that the body does not function (no breathing, heart stops beating). The child may also feel responsible and guilty for the illness. The child may have spiritual ideas about afterlife. The child may not want to discuss feelings.	Reassure the child that death is not their fault. Aim to maintain as normal a structure as possible. Include the child in afterlife plans (funeral planning, last wishes).
Adolescence: 12–18 years	Identity versus role confusion	Adolescents understand the finality of death and may develop a mature understanding of death. They may try to take responsibility for adult concerns within the family (such as finances and caretaking). Feelings of anger may be present.	Allow time for the child to reflect. Listen to concerns and questions. Support efforts for autonomy and control.

Source: Reference 24.

Support for Siblings

Along with parents' needs, siblings' unique needs must also be considered when caring for a child and family living with life-threatening illness. Parents may find it difficult to provide support for both their sick child and their other children due to the controlling nature of the needs of a child with a serious or life-threatening illness. For this reason, caregivers and healthcare providers must pay close attention to the siblings for signs and symptoms of emotional distress and then identify strategies and resources to support their needs accordingly.[2] Available hospice team members can be utilized to support parents to care for siblings, help to explain condition changes and interventions, and help to create moments of special attention. In addition to the medical care provided to the child, all team members can support siblings. Nursing, chaplains, and social workers are always a supportive presence for a hospice team. There can also be a wide range of available resources such as music therapy, art therapy, child life specialist, hospice volunteer, etc. reminding families to allow space for some level of normalcy.[25]

Strategies for engaging with siblings may be as simple as including them during visits (e.g., greeting a sibling by name when entering a room), asking about their favorite toys or interests, or participating in a small activity together during a home visit. It is important to repeatedly evaluate the sibling's level of understanding about the child's condition. Family meetings are also a good setting in which to discuss how everyone is doing (including sick and well siblings), how they each perceive the situation, how their needs are/are not being met, and how their fears and concerns can be addressed. Hospice and hospital volunteers, art therapists, and child life specialists are also extremely helpful for activities specifically with siblings such as picnics, outside play, reading stories, or memory-making activities including handprints/molds, "memory boxes" to store keepsakes, memory beads, and/or picture collages. The goal for siblings of terminally ill children is to enhance their feelings of involvement from the time of diagnosis to the greatest degree possible to facilitate a healthy adjustment and eventual grieving process.

Interaction with Schools

In addition to family members, multiple professionals are involved in the care of children living with life-threatening illnesses and are committed to maintaining their QOL. Children living with complex chronic and/or life-threatening illnesses may also have an IDT of caretakers at school, including teachers, healthcare providers, and a range of therapists (e.g., occupational, speech and language, physical). Because children spend significant time at school, it can serve as a sanctuary of normalcy for the patient or their siblings. School personnel are intimately involved in helping meet their various educational, therapeutic, medical, and basic care needs (i.e., feeding, toileting, hygiene) and play a fundamental role in advocating for them. Families often develop supportive relationships with members of their children's school-based care teams and rely on them for support and guidance as they face different care choices throughout their children's lives, as well as for responsible execution of care plans to meet children's individual needs. The hospice team can act as a resource to the school as well, with the family's permission. While any of the care team can assist, social workers can be especially helpful to provide education, support, and resources to members of the school team, as well as to children's classmates and/or their family members, whenever possible.

Case Study Continued

Over time, Taylor's home looked more and more like an ICU—ventilators, monitors, equipment, private duty nursing, and multiple medications filled her room. Each time the parents were concerned for an acute issue, they called the hospice team, who supported the parents in their decision whether or not to seek hospitalization or treatments such as antibiotics, cardiac catheterizations, intravenous diuretics, etc. The palliative care inpatient team continued to follow whenever Taylor was admitted for continuity and assistance with goals-of-care discussions.

Components of Care

This section will address some of the essential components of effective pediatric hospice care. Each section is meant to give a brief overview and explain why the topic is important or relative to comprehensive PPHC. Because these topics will be reviewed in greater detail in other chapters of this text, the following sections are not meant to provide an exhaustive explanation or to be all-inclusive regarding all aspects of how to provide such care.

Communication

Effective communication considers everyone's needs, including all family members and children, and it involves the use of verbal and nonverbal cues. Thus, it is important to pay attention to subtle cues that may be offered by both children and adult family members. In pediatrics, it is important to ask families whether and how they would like to include their child in discussions, and it is also essential to consider the child's chronological and developmental age. Effective communication is a skill that must be learned and can be developed over time by all healthcare team members so that all hospice or palliative interactions with children, families, and other healthcare team members facilitate the development of trust and allow children and families the opportunity to ask questions and engage in a healthy, honest dialogue with their healthcare team.[26] Please see Chapter 37 for more information on the essential components of communication that apply across hospice and palliative care.

Pain and Symptom Management

Pain and symptom management are other essential components of comprehensive and effective PPHC as no parent or healthcare provider wishes for children to suffer unnecessarily. Assessment and management of pain and other symptoms are domains that parents value most regarding PPHC in the home setting.[27] It is also important to recognize that there is often reluctance to manage pain aggressively in children based on myths and societal, cultural, religious, and familial beliefs that may make parents/guardians leery of opioid use to treat pain, such as the fear of "giving up" on their children, along with the notion that opioids may be "too strong" or that their children will become addicted. Healthcare providers' reluctance may stem from significant gaps in the existing evidence base; lack of sufficient education regarding pain management[28]; and misconceptions about opioids, such as frequency and severity of side effects, shortened life expectancy, and increased tolerance leading to difficulty managing pain at the end of life. Being aware of these hesitations is helpful so that fears can be addressed, and healthcare team members and family members can be educated about the realities of pain management in children with life-threatening illness and at the end of life.

Aside from pain, other symptoms commonly identified in children receiving palliative care include dyspnea, sleep disturbance, gastrointestinal disturbances, fatigue, mood concerns, delirium/agitation, hematological concerns, and seizures.[29] Adequate symptom control is a necessary part of effective PPHC, and assessment should consider developmental needs with treatment done in a manner that considers the most gentle, appropriate route for delivery that minimizes further distress and/or suffering.[26]

Many excellent resources are available to nurses for gaining competence in pain and symptom management for children, and nurses who care for children over time will become adept at recognizing when children are in pain or are uncomfortable. In addition, families require practical help, information, explanations, and support. Attention must be paid to the practical issues of preparing for pediatric-appropriate supplies, medications, formulas, feeding tubes, medical equipment, documentation, and teaching tools for parents and children. Ongoing support and education for children and families is an essential part of delivering effective PPHC.

Psychological, Emotional, Social, Religious, Spiritual, and Cultural Care

PPHC is best delivered by an IDT, including individuals who can provide psychological, social, emotional, and spiritual support, such as psychiatrists, psychologists, social workers, and chaplains; however, it is important to recognize that all members of the team are also an integral part of providing this type of support to families. Careful assessment should be conducted regarding the child's and family's developmental level and ability to complete developmental tasks; the experience of emotional symptoms; practical factors such as financial status, living situation, and social support; and religious or spiritual/existential background, preferences, beliefs, rituals, and practices.[2,26] See Table 42.2 for examples of open-ended questions that may be helpful when assessing psychosocial concerns and strengths in children receiving PPHC and in their families.[10,29–31]

Psychological Symptoms and Suffering

It is essential to recognize that the experience of caring for a child with a life-threatening illness may cause increased psychological and emotional distress for family members as the illness progresses and the level of care needed increases. Parents may experience heightened psychological distress, anxiety, or depression as a result.[32] The IDT must assess and recognize the stresses that families endure and talk with them about this routinely. It is also important to be aware that while worry and sadness are natural in the context of having or caring for a child with a serious illness, increasing frequency of these symptoms and significant impairment in functioning are signs that the individual and/or family should be evaluated by a mental health clinician.[26] Thus, it is appropriate for families and children to be offered early psychological and psychiatric referrals to assess the intensity of potential emotional distress, especially given that the symptoms of anxiety and depression are common, treatable, and associated with distress and morbidity yet are often unrecognized and undertreated in this population.[33] Also, it is essential to offer resources for coping (via social workers, chaplains, psychologists, etc.) in an attempt to support the best functioning possible for the child and family members.[2] Doing so may facilitate open discussions, relationship-building, and survival strategies that may help to offset the emotional distress experienced by family members. Also, strategies offered by healthcare providers may enable family members to

Table 42.2 Open-ended questions to help assess psychosocial factors impacting children receiving palliative care and their families

Assessment area	Examples of open-ended questions for the child or family
Developmental appropriateness and understanding	Tell me about what you understand about your/your child's diagnosis. What has your team shared with you? What have the past few weeks or months been like? What are you anticipating? What questions do you have that you have been too shy/too scared to ask?
Beliefs surrounding pain	What do you think is happening now that is making you hurt? What about your pain are you most worried about? What do you like (or not like) about using your pain medications? What concerns do you have about using your pain medication(s)? Can you tell me more about your pain?
Emotional needs	How are you feeling? What are you hoping for most? What else? What worries you most? Can you tell me more? What have been the most significant changes in your life? What is most important to you right now? How have you coped with difficult situations in the past?
Communication	Sometimes it's hard to talk about some things. Who can you usually talk to about difficult/challenging/hard things? How do you and your family best receive information? Is it best to start with big picture information or details? What things would you like to talk or hear about? What opportunities are people offering you to talk, and how does it work if you tell them you don't feel like talking?
Social context	How have the extra medical expenses and any lost income you may have experienced affected your family? How do you get to the hospital for visits? What meals do you eat when here? Who is caring for members of the family still at home? Who lives at home with you? Who helps care for your child when they are not in the hospital? What space is available in your home for hospital equipment, if needed? Sometimes nurses can come out to your home to provide certain skills or help with caretaking for your child. What would it be like for your family to have nursing in your home?
Spiritual considerations	What religious group or faith tradition, if any, do you belong to? How do your personal spiritual beliefs help you? What traditions or rituals does your family practice when someone is sick or dying? What support from the hospital would be most helpful to you regarding your faith or spirituality?

Source(s): References 10, 29, 30, and 31.

plan effectively for the future when the child's prognosis is unclear and if the child's life span may be limited.[13,26]

Social Aspects

Practical factors in a child's and family's life can have a direct impact on physical as well as psychological symptoms and treatment. Things such as family constellation, financial resources and constraints, employment status, healthcare benefits, childcare, transportation, and the ability to manage the myriad practical demands of living with and caring for a child with a life-threatening illness should be considered.[30] The impact of a child's illness is significant on the family, often requiring significant time away from work and attention being pulled away from siblings and self-care, and this can lead to strain on relationships. The hospice IDT should assess and provide support around the many social factors that play a role in a child's care using all available resources (social workers, child life, psychiatry, psychology, music therapy, etc.).

Religious/Spiritual and Cultural Considerations

Another integral part of providing PPHC is an understanding of children's and families' spiritual, religious, and cultural beliefs and how these beliefs influence the decisions that they make[29,30]; and addressing the spiritual needs of children and families is an important component of palliative care nursing. Chaplains serve to address spiritual suffering, improve family–team communication, and provide rituals that families may request,[10] such as ceremonies or sacraments. Although matters of faith are often discussed with chaplains, any member of the hospice IDT should have some level of comfort in giving families the space they need to talk about religious and spiritual beliefs, practices, and values.[10] It is important for PPHC teams to be open to such discussions and to be aware of and utilize available hospital- and community-based pastoral care services.[30] Please see Chapter 39 for more information on spirituality in palliative and hospice care.

The PPHC IDT needs to talk to families about their cultural and ethnic beliefs, customs, and practices, which may or may not be tied into their religious or spiritual beliefs. Of note, using a certified interpreter may be necessary and should not be overlooked when children and families have limited English proficiency, even if they say they understand what is being said. Various cultures approach children with life-threatening illnesses differently and have different beliefs and practices or rituals surrounding illness and/or death. It may be unacceptable to speak about illness or death or to discuss medical information in front of children. Nurses and other members of the healthcare team cannot be expected to be familiar with customs from every cultural background. Likewise, it should also not be assumed that just because someone comes from a particular cultural or ethnic background they subscribe to the particular beliefs and practices from that group; thus, it is always important to ask children and families about their personal preferences.

Preserving Hope

It is a common myth that families must choose between "fighting" or "giving up hope," when in reality one can choose to continue disease-directed therapy despite realizing cure may not be attainable. Similarly, families may choose to forgo disease-focused treatment while continuing to maintain hope.[34] A common characteristic of children living with life-threatening illness and their families is a prevailing and powerful experience of hope, evidenced in their language and decision-making. No matter how grim the situation, one should always strive to deal with matters in a positive, yet realistic, manner, taking the lead from the child and family. The focus of hope may change over time; for example, from hope for cure to hope for a longer remission than previously to hope that the child can continue to be cared for at home or to hope that the child will die without pain. Hope may also be centered on a child-specific wish, such as to return to school once more, to celebrate an important birthday, or to reach a significant milestone or rite of passage. Other expressions of hope include planning a trip or visits from extended family and close friends.[34] The IDT can help provide support to let children know that their loved ones will survive and be "OK" after they die. Hope offers opportunities for growth for the child and family, yet it can also be challenging to balance remaining hopeful with realistic expectations. Thus, it is important to openly discuss hopes and fears with children and family members, as well as with other members of the IDT.

Case Study Continued

About 18 months later, Taylor began struggling with her response to enteral diuretics at home—her kidney function continued to decline, electrolyte derangement became a growing concern, and it seemed as though every time Taylor was hospitalized, the days at home in between grew shorter and shorter. Her parents met with their hospice team at home and lovingly discussed what symptom management would look like at home if they chose to focus solely on comfort and avoid further hospitalizations. Their hospice nurse, social worker, and chaplain had developed great rapport with family and with siblings over the past year and were well poised to support Taylor and her family as they worked hard to maintain some level of normalcy at home while grieving the idea of limited time with Taylor. Taylor's siblings participated in memory-making, and a referral to psychology was made to help her eldest sibling work through concerns for depression.

Ethical Considerations

A large part of PPHC involves helping families with decision-making. Clinical ethical dilemmas are inherent to issues surrounding palliative and EOL care, and it will often be the role of the nurse and/or advanced practice registered nurse (APRN) to anticipate, recognize, define, examine, and manage ethically problematic situations that arise in the care of patients and families, particularly during times of serious illness and/or at the end of life. Ethical dilemmas abound when providing such a wide array of care surrounding topics that are deeply rooted in personal, cultural, religious, and social values. Although nurses and other members of the PPHC IDT are not expected to be ethicists, it is helpful to be mindful of the potential ethical dilemmas that will arise when working with families in these circumstances and to be aware of when to consult with their organization's ethics committee, if available, when additional support is needed. It is, therefore, also the role of the nurse/APRN to recognize, contemplate, and use appropriate resources to guide such discussions and decision-making processes with patients and families.[10]

Resources are available to help guide the decision-making process and to help children, adolescents, and adults express how they want to be treated throughout their illness and at the time of death from a medical, personal, emotional, and spiritual perspective.[26,35] Some helpful documents include *My Wishes* (for young children), *Voicing My Choices* (for adolescents), and *Five Wishes* (for adults) published by Aging with Dignity and available at www.agingwithdignity.org.[35] This section serves not to provide an all-inclusive discussion of ethics in PPHC but rather to highlight some of the dilemmas nurses may face. Please see other chapters in this text for a more thorough discussion of ethical considerations and EOL decision-making, such as Chapter 38.

Perinatal Palliative Care

Perinatal palliative and hospice care is an innovative and compassionate model of support that can be offered to parents who learn during pregnancy that their baby has a fatal condition, an unfortunate situation that occurs with increasing frequency as prenatal testing advances. This unique group of parents faces the daunting challenge of anticipating and preparing for the birth *and* the possibility of death of their baby simultaneously. For families who choose to continue their pregnancies, even if the baby may die shortly after birth, perinatal hospice helps them embrace whatever life their baby might have, before and after birth. Perinatal hospice support begins at the time of diagnosis, even before the child is born. It can be thought of as "hospice in the womb," including birth planning and preliminary medical decision-making prior to birth, as well as more traditional hospice care after birth, depending on how long the child survives.

Nurses play a unique and vital role in assisting and supporting families in creating palliative care plans for pregnancy and/or birth.[36] With the support of perinatal palliative care, families with a fetal diagnosis associated with shortened life expectancy, uncertain prognosis, or other medically complex trajectory are given the opportunity to coordinate obstetrical and neonatal care in a manner guided by family values and desired outcomes, whether this means neonatal comfort care following birth or trial of interventions aimed at prolonging life.[37] It provides families the opportunity to honor their baby in a way that is meaningful to them and helps families participate in memory-making experiences.

Perinatal hospice is not a place. Ideally, it is a comprehensive team approach that includes obstetricians, perinatologists, labor and delivery nurses, neonatologists, NICU staff, chaplains/pastors, and social workers as well as genetic counselors, therapists, and traditional hospice professionals. Perinatal hospice is a beautiful and practical response to some of the most heartbreaking challenges of prenatal testing.[38] Some programs exist within a hospital setting, such as the labor and delivery unit, NICU, and maternal and child areas. Other times, it presides within community settings. Perinatal palliative care may naturally extend into neonatal palliative care as some infants will live anywhere from days to months to years after birth. Please see Chapter 40 for more information on the essential components of neonatal palliative care.

Care at the Time of Death

Nothing can fully prepare families for the final moments of their loved ones' lives, yet there is much that can be done to help families anticipate what to expect so as to avoid unnecessary surprises when the time comes. The education provided and conversations about such a sensitive topic may feel difficult to initiate. The skilled clinicians who care for these patients know that parents are often worrying about these things and are often afraid to ask. Thus, after taking the time to build trust and rapport, experienced PPC practitioners must delicately initiate the conversation and provide education that may help to address their concerns. Families should be reminded that PPC clinicians cannot predict exactly when and how death will occur as it can be different for everyone, but parents and family members should be prepared for the possible range of changes that can happen.

Families should be prepared for when they might expect such changes and what things may look like, feel like, sound like, smell like, and so forth. Consider all the senses for both the adults and any other children who will be present. Parents also may appreciate written handouts in language that is not too clinical or frightening so that they have them to review at a time when they feel ready to do so. Having such knowledge may also prepare parents to talk with each other, other children, and family members. Families may have memories from previous experiences of death of other family members and may conjure images or memories from that time that may or may not be helpful, depending on what the particular experience was like for them.

Children and family members will likely have fears associated with death and the dying process. This may include fears about what dramatic events can unfold, fear of being alone at time of death, fear of a loved one missing the death, and fear of being unprepared for an unexpected emergency. Understanding the physical progression of events and the nearing-death awareness that is common among children and adolescents may be reassuring for both members of the team and the family. It is essential to review goals for the time of death well before the time comes so that families feel as in control of the situation as possible. For example, children and families likely will have an idea of where they would like for the final hours or days of life to occur, and, when possible, nurses and other members of the IDT can try to align the proper resources to allow this to happen. If families desire to remain in the hospital, they should be given a private space or room to be together as a family. Several children's hospitals allocate a specific room or space, often called a "comfort corner," where children may be moved to spend their final hours together with their family. Typically, changing locations close to the end of life is not desired; however, for some families, it may be very important to make it home from the hospital or to get to the hospital in the event of an emergency before death.

It is also crucial to consider whom a family may want to be present. In most instances, family members will be called to visit as the time of death nears, and the child's bedside, whether in the hospital or at home, can become the gravitational force for loved ones to gather. Families may also have particular wishes about who should be present at the actual moment of death as sometimes parents want to be alone with their child, with or without other children being present. Other times, families may choose to get in bed with their child. The tenderness and intimacy of these final moments is beyond description, and being present at this time with a family is a very precious privilege for everyone involved in the child's care, especially nurses who often spend the most time at the bedside.

Creating a Sacred Space

When a child is dying, regardless of their age, the very space becomes sacred ground; and it is important to maintain the purity of that space immediately following death. This also allows for a brief pause to honor the nurse's role in maintaining the dignity of a child and their family surrounding death before moving on to the next task. Some programs place a special sign on the door or an image of a dove, butterfly, flower, or leaf to subtly designate this sacred space and to minimize interruptions in and out of the room during this time. Honoring and respecting the space also model to staff that it is not just "business as usual."

When a child dies at home, if a hospice nurse is not already present, the family will call for postmortem care. The nurse is able to complete the assessment that the hospice providers will use to call the official time of death. While there can be exceptions, the nurse will stay with the family until their child leaves their home, often with chaplain and/or social work support. Some families may choose to have the child remain in their bed for a short time before having the body removed. Other families may desire the prompt removal of their child's body, which is a personal decision that should also be respected.[13] Cultural and religious practices may guide what happens at time of death and immediately following, but generally time is allowed for bathing, dressing, holding or rocking the child, offering prayers, obtaining handprints (if not obtained before), cutting a lock of hair,[13] and gathering the clothing items that may have the child's scent on them (to be preserved in a timely manner in a zipper bag). Families may or may not choose to partake in these activities. Some families may wish to accompany their child's body to the morgue, if the child dies in the hospital and hospital policy allows for this to happen, or out of the house if the child dies at home. Siblings and parents or others may choose to send along a note or a little something with the child's body as a symbolic way to remain connected while apart, and sometimes children may have previously stated their wishes about what objects they would like to keep with them.

It is also important to recognize that some families may choose to consider organ donation or autopsy, which ideally should be discussed with families before the time of death. Hospitals usually have programs that require that the option for organ donation be presented to families, and procedures are in place for representatives from the appropriate organizations to be notified near or at the time of death to have these discussions with families. If families elect to donate organs or have an autopsy performed, timing will be of the essence, and members of the team and the nurse should be aware of what needs to happen within what time frame to ensure that a family's wishes are met appropriately.

Self-Care

Providing PPHC puts nurses and other providers at particularly high risk for burnout,[39] and pressure around only having "one chance to get it right" may add to nurses' sense of stress and duty. It is important to recognize that the team members caring for the child and family will need support before, during, and following the time of death. The nurses present with the family will likely have other tasks to move on to, but it is very important to have support available to allow for at least a brief respite, break, or time away from the immediate setting. In some instances, nurses may be given a lighter caseload or, when possible, have time to debrief with another colleague, chaplain, or member of the PPHC IDT both immediately following and/or at a period after the death has occurred.[13] Great wisdom can be shared, burdens lessened, and insights and renewal gained from the time spent debriefing clinically as well as through other efforts to support colleagues.[13] In addition to opportunities to debrief, creation and maintenance of a self-care supportive work environment and clinical nursing supervision may be beneficial in helping to mitigate moral distress, compassion fatigue, as well as death anxiety.[40] It takes a lot of energy to care for seriously ill children and members of their family physically as well as emotionally and psychologically. Preserving the meaning of and sustaining this type of work require self-discipline and intentionality to tend to one's own centering practices and methods of self-care, whether physical, spiritual, or emotional. One review found that self-compassion in healthcare professionals, including hospice nurses, can be associated with greater capacity for self-care, mindfulness, and professional quality of life while decreasing burnout risk and secondary traumatic stress.[41] Some coping strategies may be personally beneficial, such as self-reflection and self-care, even for a few minutes throughout the day, along with building in time for ongoing renewal and reflection outside of work. Also important is professional support as many team members find relationships with colleagues in PPC to be especially supportive because no one else quite understands the emotional stressors of the work. The burden and grief experienced from caring for children with life-threatening illness and their families can be intense and serious and require formal and informal support to prevent burnout and to cope effectively with the challenges of this work.[17]

Anticipatory Grief and Bereavement

Chapter 44 is devoted entirely to grief and bereavement in PPC; however, it is essential to highlight the importance of anticipatory grief, grief surrounding death, and bereavement in PPC. Children and families will often begin the process of anticipatory grief at the time of diagnosis, and it is helpful for PPC team members to talk with children and families continually about the ongoing losses they are experiencing. Grief continues through and beyond the time of death, and families, community members, and team members who cared for the child and family will need ongoing bereavement support. Many hospitals have at least annual ceremonial remembrance services that families and team members find helpful for honoring and remembering the children who have died.

Case Study Continued

At about 2 years of age, Taylor developed worsening respiratory distress on home vent settings due to worsening cardiac function—her hospice nurse was present at the home, providing frequent and thorough assessment and management of symptoms, including the use of enteral morphine for dyspnea. Taylor's extended family members were able to visit and spend time with her in the weeks prior as her symptoms started to progress. She ultimately died in her mother's arms, surrounded by her father and siblings. Taylor's family received bereavement support through the hospice for about 13 months following Taylor's death, which included periodic phone calls, home visits from the hospice social work and chaplain, as well as grief resources.

Overview of Nursing Care Issues for PPHC

As evident, the responsibilities of caring for children living with life-threatening illnesses and their families are extensive and require an understanding of the interconnectedness of the myriad aspects of illness and suffering: physical, emotional/psychological, spiritual, and social. Nurses and members of the PPHC IDT must assess for imbalances and indications of suffering in each of these areas to appropriately intervene and provide comprehensive and effective PPC. They must ensure that families are well supported while also supporting each other and not allowing all of the burden to fall on one member of the team.[38] PPHC nurses and other professionals may also experience suffering in the form of moral distress, and thus self-care, adequate support, and ongoing education and professional training are also essential components of delivering effective PPHC.[40]

Education and Training

Healthcare professionals face many obstacles and challenges while providing intense and unique care to seriously ill children and their families, including lack of professional education and training.[42] A 2018 survey of hospice nurses noted that a majority of nurses received no formal training in PPHC and that half had no experience caring for this population.[42] Nurses specifically have reported perceived lack of skill in providing PPHC, including inadequate knowledge and expertise in areas such as psychosocial assessment, symptom assessment and management, communication, and medication use, among others.[42] Many educational programs exist to train nurses and other healthcare professionals in various aspects of PPHC. Interdisciplinary case discussions, "lunch-and-learn" sessions, journal clubs, and/or regularly scheduled community-based educational seminars can result in a commitment from nursing and other team members to work together and support each other. Of note, PPC has been integrated into national nursing professional practice guidelines and standards, such as those of the Society of Pediatric Nursing.[43]

There is an increasing number of educational offerings and opportunities for nurses and other healthcare professionals to expand their knowledge of PPHC. In recognizing that hospice and palliative nursing care has become a specialized area of nursing, there is a growing number of professional organizations and nationally recognized training options available. The Hospice and Palliative Nurses Association was established in 1986. This membership organization relies on evidence-based research and data to assist members in delivering quality nursing care, symptom management, grief and bereavement support, guidance with difficult conversations, education, certification options, and encouragement in leadership and mentoring efforts.[44] The End-of-Life Nursing Education Consortium (ELNEC) is a well-established and respected "train the trainer" initiative to teach nurses at all levels how to provide effective PPC, as well as how to teach this information to other nursing students and colleagues.[45] The Center to Advance Palliative Care provides healthcare professionals with the tools, training, and technical assistance necessary to start and sustain palliative care programs in hospitals and other settings and includes an extensive listing of other trainings that are available on its website: http://www.capc.org. The Initiative for Pediatric Palliative Care, sponsored by the Educational Development Center, is an interdisciplinary model of case-based experiential training offering PPC-specific training events.[46] The NHPCO also has pediatric curriculum options to address the ongoing demand for training for adult hospice programs to be prepared to care for children.[2]

In addition to national educational resources, training can be effective at the local and regional levels. Seeking partnership with specialized PPC teams may be of benefit to hospices hoping to expand their pediatric services. PPHC coalitions exist in multiple states including California, Illinois, Massachusetts, Michigan, Ohio, and Pennsylvania and are often composed of PPHC clinicians, clinical therapists, community advocates, and healthcare organizations with a breadth of hospice and palliative care experience. These alliances may additionally serve to offer education, training, and networking opportunities to hospice nurses in their respective areas; as robust community resources, there may be greater opportunity to provide nursing education around parent/caregiver psychosocial support, communication, and management of symptoms.[47] While an undoubtedly useful starting point, singular seminars, general written material, and shadowing experiences may not be enough to help hospice nurses gain the expertise and skills needed to feel confident in their role caring for pediatric patients and their families. Ongoing identification of knowledge gaps may help drive focused continuing education and creation of improved policies and resources for training hospice nurses in the community.

The Future Unfolding for PPHC

PPHC continues to grow rapidly with an increasing number of individual providers specializing in this type of care, growth of new and existing IDTs, and the expansion of available community resources. Each step toward increasing awareness about PPC is a step forward on behalf of the children who are dying without access to all of the resources that should be available to them and their loved ones.[48] The future of PPC is aimed at improved recognition and increased utilization of PPHC services and better reimbursement for palliative care providers. Nurses who choose to care for seriously ill and dying children, and their families, need a significant support system both professionally and personally, to maintain the tenuous task of balance and longevity in this field.[39] While challenging, this type of work is also humbling and rewarding as those caring for children with life-threatening illnesses have the privilege of being a part of families' most intimate and powerful experiences, both throughout children's lives and during the time of their death.

REFERENCES

1. World Health Organization. WHO Definition of Pediatric Palliative Care. 1998. Accessed October 23, 2022. http://www.who.int/cancer/palliatve/definition/en/.
2. National Hospice and Palliative Care Organization. *Standards of Practice for Pediatric Palliative Care: Quality Improvement Resource*. National Hospice and Palliative Care Organization; 2022.
3. Office of the Legislative Counsel. Compilation of Patient Protection and Affordable Care Act. 2010. Accessed November 1, 2022. https://housedocs.house.gov/energycommerce/ppacacon.pdf.
4. Mary J. Labyak Institute for Innovation. Pediatric Concurrent Care. National Hospice and Palliative Care Organization. December 2012. Accessed November 1, 2022. https://www.nhpco.org/wp-content/uploads/2019/04/Continuum_Briefing-2013.pdf.
5. National Hospice and Palliative Care Organization. Concurrent Care Implementation Tool Kit: Section 2302 of the Patient Protection and Affordable Care Act. Accessed March 16, 2023. https://www.nhpco.org/wp-content/uploads/2019/06/CCCR_Tool kit.pdf.
6. Miller EG, LaRagione G, Kang TI, Feudtner C. Concurrent care for the medically complex child: lessons of implementation. *J Palliat Med*. 2012;15(11):1281–1283.
7. Lotstein DS, Lindley LC. Improving home hospice and palliative care policies. *Pediatrics*. 2019;144(2):e20183287. https://doi.org/10.1542/peds.2018-3287.
8. Battista V, Thaxton C. Pediatric palliative care. In: Coyne PJ, Bobb B, Plakovic K, eds. *Conversations in Palliative Care: Questions and Answers with Experts*. 4th ed. Hospice and Palliative Nurses Association; 2017:359–371.
9. Field MJ, Behrman RE. *When Children Die: Improving Palliative and End-of-Life Care for Children and Their Families*. Report of the Institute of Medicine Task Force. National Academies Press; 2003.
10. Ferrell BR, Twaddle ML, Melnick A, Meier DE. National Consensus Project Clinical practice guidelines for quality palliative care guidelines, 4th edition. *J Palliat Med*. 2018;21(12):1684–1689. https://doi.org/10.1089/jpm.2018.0431.
11. Laird J, Cozad MJ, Keim-Malpass J, Mack JW, Lindley LC. Variation in state Medicaid implementation of the ACA: the case of concurrent care for children. *Health Aff (Millwood)*. 2020;39(10):1770–1775. https://doi.org/10.1377/hlthaff.2020.01192.
12. Lyckholm L, Slycord S. Improving palliative care across settings. In: Coyne PJ, Bobb B, Plakovic K, eds. *Conversations in Palliative Care: Questions and Answers with Experts*. 4th ed. Hospice and Palliative Nurses Association, 2017:307–314.
13. Linebarger JS, Johnson V, Boss RD, et al. Guidance for pediatric end-of-life care. *Pediatrics*. 2022;149(5):e2022057011. https://doi.org/10.1542/peds.2022-057011
14. American Academy of Pediatrics. Pediatric palliative care and hospice care commitments, guidelines and recommendations. *Pediatrics*. 2013;132(5):966–972. Policy reaffirmed 2019. https://doi.org/10.1542/peds.2013-2731.
15. Weaver MS, Rosenberg AR, Tager J, Wichman CS, Wiener L. A summary of pediatric palliative care team structure and services as reported by centers caring for children with cancer. *J Palliat Med*. 2018;21(4):452–462. https://doi.org/10.1089/jpm.2017.0405.
16. National Hospice and Palliative Care Organization. *NHPCO Pediatric Fact and Figures*. National Hospice and Palliative Care Organization; 2023. Accessed November 18, 2023. https://www.nhpco.org/wp-content/uploads/NHPCO_Pediatric_Facts_Figures_2023.pdf.

17. Himelstein BP, Hilden JM, Boldt AM, Weissman D. Pediatric palliative care. *N Engl J Med*. 2004;350:1752–1762.
18. Feudtner C, Nye R, Hill DL, et al. Polysymptomatology in pediatric patients receiving palliative care based on parent-reported data. *JAMA Netw Open*. 2021;4(8):e2119730. https://doi.org/10.1001/jamanetworkopen.2021.19730.
19. Mesquita Garcia AC, Domingues Silva B, Oliveira da Silva LC, Mills J. Self-compassion in hospice and palliative care: a systematic integrative review. *J Hosp Palliat Nurs*. 2021;23(2):145–154. https://doi.org/10.1097/NJH.0000000000000727.
20. Hussain FA. Psychological challenges for nurses working in palliative care and recommendations for self-care. *Br J Nurs*. 2021;30(8):484–489.https://doi.org/10.12968/bjon.2021.30.8.484.
21. Akard TF, Hendricks-Ferguson VL, Gilmer MJ. Pediatric palliative care nursing. *Ann Palliat Med*. 2019;8(suppl 1):S39–S48. https://doi.org/10.21037/apm.2018.06.01.
22. Feudtner C. Collaborative communication in pediatric palliative care: a foundation for problem-solving and decision-making. *Pediatr Clin North Am*. 2007;54(5):583–608.
23. Dombrowski D. Care of the patient and family. In: Santucci G, ed. *Core Curriculum for the Pediatric Hospice and Palliative Nurse*. 2nd ed. Hospice and Palliative Nurses Association; 2017:109–122.
24. Mandac C, Battista, V. Contributions of palliative care to pediatric patient care. *Semin Oncol Nurs*. 2014:30(4):212–226. https://doi.org/10.1016/j.soncn.2014.08.003.
25. Kreicbergs U, Nilsson S, Jenholt Nolbris M, Lövgren M. Using communication tools to explore young siblings' experiences of having a brother or sister with pediatric palliative care needs. *Children (Basel)*. 2022;9(5):641. https://doi.org/10.3390/children9050641.
26. Norris S, Minkowitz S, Scharbach K. Pediatric palliative care. *Prim Care*. 2019;46(3):461–473. https://doi.org/10.1016/j.pop.2019.05.010.
27. Boyden JY, Ersek M, Deatrick JA, et al. What do parents value regarding pediatric palliative and hospice care in the home setting? *J Pain Symptom Manage*. 2021;61(1):12–23. https://doi.org/10.1016/j.jpainsymman.2020.07.024.
28. City of Hope, American Association of Colleges of Nursing. End-of-Life Nursing Education Consortium (ELNEC): Pain Management in Pediatric Palliative Care. End-of-Life Nursing Education Consortium; 2003; revised 2021.
29. Hauer J. Pediatric Palliative Care. UpToDate. 2023. Accessed March 16, 2023. https://www.uptodate.com/contents/pediatric-palliative-care.
30. McSherry M, Kehoe K, Carroll JM, Kang TI, Rourke, MT. Psychosocial and spiritual needs of children living with a life-limiting illness. *Pediatr Clin North Am*. 2007;54(5):609–630.
31. Jackson VA, Jacobsen JC. The Initial Interview in Palliative Care Consultation. UpToDate. 2023. Accessed November 20, 2023. https://www.uptodate.com/contents/the-initial-interview-in-palliative-care-consultation?topicRef=6252&source=see_link.
32. Boyden JY, Hill DL, Nye RT, et al. Pediatric palliative care parents' distress, financial difficulty, and child symptoms. *J Pain Symptom Manage*. 2022;63(2):271–282. https://doi.org/10.1016/j.jpainsymman.2021.08.004.
33. Mullaney EK, Santucci, G. Symptom management in pediatric palliative care. In: Santucci G, ed. *Core Curriculum for the Pediatric Hospice and Palliative Nurse*. 2nd ed. Hospice and Palliative Nurses Association; 2017:73–107.
34. Friedrichsdorf SJ, Bruera E. Delivering pediatric palliative care: from denial, palliphobia, pallilalia to palliactive. *Children (Basel)*. 2018;5(9):120. https://doi.org/10.3390/children5090120.
35. Aging with Dignity. My Wishes, Voicing My Choices, and Five Wishes. 2017. Accessed October 24, 2022. http://www.agingwithdignity.org/index.php.
36. Tatterton MJ, Fisher MJ, Storton H, Walker C. The role of children's hospices in perinatal palliative care and advance care planning: the results of a national British survey. *J Nurs Scholarsh*. 2023;55(4):864–873. https://doi.org/10.1111/jnu.12866.
37. Buskmiller C, Ho S, Chen M, Gants S, Crowe E, Lopez S. Patient-centered perinatal palliative care: family birth plans, outcomes, and resource utilization in a diverse cohort. *Am J Obstet Gynecol MFM*. 2022;4(6):100725. https://doi.org/10.1016/j.ajogmf.2022.100725.
38. Perinatal Hospice & Palliative Care. A Gift of Time. 2016. Accessed October 31, 2022. http://www.perinatalhospice.org/.
39. Horn DJ, Johnston CB. Burnout and self care for palliative care practitioners. *Med Clin North Am*. 2020;104(3):561–572. https://doi.org/10.1016/j.mcna.2019.12.007.
40. Hussain FA. Psychological challenges for nurses working in palliative care and recommendations for self-care. *Br J Nurs*. 2021;30(8):484–489.https://doi.org/10.12968/bjon.2021.30.8.484.
41. Mesquita Garcia AC, Domingues Silva B, Oliveira da Silva LC, Mills J. Self-compassion in hospice and palliative care: a systematic integrative review. *J Hosp Palliat Nurs*. 2021;23(2):145–154. https://doi.org/10.1097/NJH.0000000000000727.
42. Kaye EC, Applegarth J, Gattas M, et al. Hospice nurses request paediatric-specific educational resources and training programs to improve care for children and families in the community: qualitative data analysis from a population-level survey. *Palliat Med*. 2020;34(3):403–412. https://doi.org/10.1177/0269216319866576.
43. American Nurses Association of Pediatric Nurse Practitioners, Society of Pediatric Nursing. Pediatric Nursing: Scope and Standards of Practice. 2017. Accessed October 31, 2022. http://www.nursingworld.org/scopeandstandardsofpractice.
44. Hospice and Palliative Nursing Association. Accessed October 31, 2022. https://advancingexpertcare.org.
45. American Association of Colleges of Nursing. End-of-Life Nursing Education Consortium (ELNEC). 2017. Accessed October 31, 2022. https://www.aacnnursing.org/ELNEC.
46. Education Development Center. Initiative for Pediatric Palliative Care (IPPC). 2014. Accessed October 31, 2022. https://www.ipfcc.org/bestpractices/ipe/ippc.html#:~:text=Spearheaded%20by%20the%20Education%20Development%20Center%2C%20Inc.%20%28EDC%29%2C,family-centered%20care%20for%20children%20living%20with%20life-threatening%20conditions.
47. Bogetz JF, Anderson A, Holland M, Macauley R. Pediatric hospice and palliative care services and needs across the northwest United States. *J Pain Symptom Manage*. 2022;64(1):e7–e14. https://doi.org/10.1016/j.jpainsymman.2022.02.015.
48. Pyke-Grimm KA, Fisher B, Haskamp A, Bell CJ, Newman AR. Providing palliative and hospice care to children, adolescents and young adults with cancer. *Semin Oncol Nurs*. 2021;37(3):151166. https://doi.org/10.1016/j.soncn.2021.151166.

43

Nursing Care for the Pediatric Patient at the End of Life

Jenna Freitas and Chelsea Heneghan

Key Points

- Nurses should be integrated into team and family discussions surrounding goals of care and advanced care planning to provide effective end-of-life care to the pediatric patient and family.
- The end-of-life period is unpredictable; and anticipatory guidance should be provided around expected symptoms, and management should be both interprofessional and tailored to the patient.
- Caring for a child at the end of life can come with intense grief; the nurse should be prepared to respond to patient and family emotions throug.h utilization of communication strategies.

Introduction

The purpose of this chapter is to outline nursing care for the pediatric patient at the end of life. As is true in other pediatric specialties, when addressing the end of life, it is important to recognize that children are resilient and that the ability to prognosticate the end of life experience can be challenging. Ensuring patients and families have a shared understanding with their healthcare team about the road ahead will help them identify what matters most, otherwise known as "goals of care." For more information, please refer to Chapters 36 and 37, which highlight communicating with patients and families, including delivering prognosis and understanding and delineating goals. Additionally, it is important to highlight the holistic nature of palliative care nursing when considering how to provide care at the end of a child's life.[1] Ensuring the physical, spiritual, emotional, and social needs are understood and met is imperative.[2] As each patient and family is unique, care at the end-of-life period must be tailored to individual needs and values, including location of care, communication preferences, and symptom management. Finally, the terms "family" and "caregiver" will be used interchangeably throughout this chapter, recognizing there is no one definition of family.

Case Study: Introduction

When the pediatric palliative care team first met Malik and his family, Malik was a sophomore in high school. He was a social young man with an extensive peer group. His greatest love was playing basketball; he had just made the varsity team. Malik was the eldest of three children. He had plans to go to college, study anthropology, and play basketball.

At initial presentation, Malik was healthy without any significant medical history aside from three febrile seizures in infancy and childhood. A few months prior to consultation, Malik's parents noticed some things were "not quite right." Malik was missing shots on the basketball court that had previously been easy for him to make and described him as overall seeming clumsier. They also noticed that Malik's grades were slipping as he went from a straight-A student to getting all Cs. Given their observations and concerns, Malik was seen by a neurologist for testing. Malik was diagnosed with a progressive neurologic disorder associated with both functional and cognitive decline as well as progressive, refractory seizures leading to early mortality. Although clinical trials are on the horizon, there is no cure for Malik's underlying disorder.

At the time of diagnosis, pediatric palliative care was consulted to support decision-making and symptom management in the setting of medical complexities and Malik's progressive disease.

Location of Care

Just as pediatric palliative care spans diagnoses and settings, end-of-life care for the pediatric patient is not confined to a specific location.[3] Children with serious illness, like most children, spend their lives between locations, living well at home, participating in school, engaging in the community, and being cared for, as needed, in the hospital. A hospital death may be expected for children who have experienced an acute event, such as a trauma, and are in the intensive care unit (ICU) or for critically ill infants in the perinatal care setting.[4] However, for children with a progressive disease, or for families caring for a child with a complex chronic condition, preferences around location of death are unique to the child/family, culture, and clinical circumstances. While most pediatric deaths occur in the hospital,[5] other settings for end-of-life care include home, with or without hospice support, and, less often, in a hospice house. Please see Chapter 42 for further detail on the pediatric hospice perspective, including hospice houses. For neonatal and pediatric patients nearing the end of life in an ICU, some institutions have the infrastructure to consider palliative transports home should home death be preferred.

Communicating Prognosis

Early and ongoing conversations around clinical trajectory and prognosis are important to ensure transparency and build trust. As delineated in Chapter 36 on communication, when assessing how much information might be helpful to provide, a good starting place is assessing a patient's and family's understanding of prognosis. This provides assurance that the provider and patient and/or family have a shared understanding of the clinical situation to make informed decisions moving forward. While the nurse will not be delivering the prognosis, it is important for the nurse to be present during these conversations to continue to deliver consistent messaging. The nurse is often the first team member to hear the hopes, worries, and concerns of families. Identifying when further discussions may be beneficial to support a patient's/family's understanding of prognosis and the decision-making process is an integral role of the nurse at the end of life. Collaboration with the interprofessional team during this time is key.[6]

Oftentimes providers hesitate to deliver serious news to families, worrying it could diminish patients' and families' hopes. However, research has shown honest and transparent communication may alleviate uncertainty and allows caregivers to make the best decisions for their children.[7,8] There are many techniques that can be utilized by practitioners to deliver serious news; see Chapter 37 for more information surrounding communication skills.

Defining the End-of-Life Period

While prognostication at any age is never precise, pediatrics poses specific challenges to predictions surrounding end-of-life timing.[9] Oftentimes pediatric patients receive disease-directed therapies, in addition to other life-sustaining interventions, until their death. Although certain interventions may alter life expectancy, in general the end-of-life period is considered *the time when there is no expectation of cure.*[10] This period may vary considerably based on the clinical scenario, and therefore it is often easiest and most accurate to think about time in ranges: weeks to months, days to weeks, hours to days, and/or moments to hours.[11] As the nurse caring for a child during the end-of-life period, it is helpful to understand where the child may be in the clinical trajectory during any given hospitalization.[12]

When the child's prognosis has changed, the healthcare team should provide this update to the family and patient (when developmentally appropriate) (see Chapters 36 and 37 for communication in palliative care). A change in prognosis or readmission to the hospital may offer an opportunity to address concerns about the future and advance care planning.[13,14] It provides the team a space to share changes they anticipate over time (both acute and chronic) and make goal-concordant recommendations for resuscitative efforts.

End-of-Life Period: Weeks to Months

A child in the advanced stages of an incurable disease may have weeks to months to live. This will present differently depending on the diagnosis; however, it may include progression of cancer or an underlying neurologic, cardiac, or pulmonary disease. At this stage the child is likely living at home and may be able to participate in usual activities with some adjustments (i.e., shortened school days, short outings, activities with assistance, etc.), while coming into the hospital as needed for more intensive support. Progression may be related to the natural course of the underlying disease or triggered by intercurrent illness. If goal-concordant, introduction of concurrent hospice care should be considered during this time (see Chapter 42, "Pediatric Hospice Perspectives").

Case Study Continued

Malik has been going back and forth from home to hospital for the past 2 years, often for electroencephalogram monitoring and adjustment of his antiepileptic medications. Over this time the nursing staff has come to know Malik well, understanding that he deeply values his independence, particularly in the face of a rapidly progressing disease. While he can no longer ambulate independently and has trouble feeding himself without support, Malik is determined to take care of himself. He loves to watch basketball and maintains hope that he will graduate from high school and attend college away from home. Malik is now admitted for intravenous antibiotics and supplemental oxygen support in the setting of aspiration pneumonia. While Malik continues to engage with visitors, his verbal responses are delayed, and he is frequently confused about why he is in the hospital. Malik's parents have been asked to consider whether gastrostomy placement for artificial nutrition/hydration would align with their goals for Malik.

Nursing Role

As the nurse caring for a child who has a prognosis of weeks to months, ensuring that the patient and family are receiving information in a way that works best for them to make decisions is paramount. At this point in the illness trajectory, the child may continue to live mostly out of the hospital; therefore, it is important for the nurse to assess for symptoms that could be negatively impacting the child's quality of life both in the hospital and at home. If distressing symptoms are present, the nurse is often the first care team member to recognize this and raise concerns to the larger interprofessional team for additional support. Being present and providing a listening ear for the patient and family continue to be cornerstones of nursing practice.[15] While gaining an understanding of what is most important for a child and family, the nurse may recommend interventions and opportunities to optimize the quality of life for the child while in the hospital. When the child goes home, if enrolled in hospice, the nurse should collaborate with the hospice nurse to coordinate care and communication across settings.[16,17]

End-of-Life Period: Days to Weeks

Weeks to months may turn to days to weeks for the child with advanced illness, whose disease has continued to progress to the point where current therapies to maintain clinical stability and comfort are no longer effective. At this time in the illness trajectory, the child may come to the hospital more frequently with increased length of hospital admissions.[18] During this time the child and family may feel the impact of the disease progression, and they often adjust their typical routines to accommodate increased care needs.[2]

Case Study Continued

Despite placement of a gastrostomy tube for artificial nutritional support and medication administration, Malik has been coming into the hospital more frequently. His admissions have included transfers to the ICU for intensive support during episodes of status epilepticus as well as multiple courses of antibiotics for separate bouts of pneumonia. The neurology team has shared their concern that Malik's condition is worsening, and antiepileptic medication options are limited. The palliative care team has engaged with Malik's family around decision-making and advance care planning. Based on their goals to allow Malik to live as long and as well as possible, while also minimizing suffering, the team provides a medical recommendation that if Malik's heart were to stop, chest compressions would not change the course of his underlying progressive disease and would signify the end of his natural life. Given this, Malik's parents accept the team's recommendation to protect Malik from attempts at cardiac resuscitation should his heart stop while expressing their desire to continue to provide full respiratory support should he experience respiratory insufficiency. Malik's parents want "to leave no stone left unturned" in their search for a clinical trial, in an attempt to continue allowing Malik to live as long and as well as possible.

Nursing Role

As the nurse caring for a child who has a prognosis of days to weeks, recognizing how disease progression impacts a child and family is imperative. It is at this stage, when a child may be coming to the hospital more often and staying longer, that identifying a continuity nursing team is most helpful. Some units have this in place already, while others may need to think with leadership about how to best establish continuity among providers. As a continuity nursing team, coordinating services such as child life therapy, social work, chaplaincy, etc., can enhance the support for the patient, family, and clinical care team. Performing frequent symptom assessments, being a listening ear, and ensuring the child's/family's voice is heard remain constant and central to the nursing role. Nurses may also be the ones to hear seemingly contradictory statements as the family integrates new prognostic information into their hopes for their child. Families can hold many priorities at the same time.[19] It is important that the nurse continues to listen, remains objective, and takes a nonjudgmental approach while caring for the child and family.

End-of-Life Period: Hours to Days

As an underlying disease progresses, it is likely that children will exhibit physiologic changes or worsening symptoms that alert families and providers to a clinical change. At this time families may work with the care team to consider discontinuing interventions or treatments, such as chemotherapy or total parenteral nutrition, that provide little benefit and may cause increased symptom burden.[20] Elective admission to an inpatient unit for physical, emotional, and spiritual support at the end of life should be considered. Alternatively, families may elect to stay at home, in which case continuous nursing care through hospice may be put into place (see Chapter 42, "Pediatric Hospice Perspectives").

Case Study Continued

Malik has been out of the hospital for many weeks, during which time his parents describe that he has been mostly somnolent with only a few hours each day of alertness. He has shown little interest in eating by mouth and is receiving all nutrition via gastrostomy tube. He is having multiple seizures each day despite being on numerous antiepileptic medications and is receiving rescue seizure medications daily. While he has been mostly comfortable, Malik's parents worry about the ability to control his seizures at home. They recognize time is short. Their goals have shifted to prioritizing comfort in an environment that feels supportive. They have made the decision to return to the hospital to focus intensely on comfort at the end of Malik's life. After discussion with the palliative care team and the neurology team, limitations have been placed on attempts at cardiac and respiratory resuscitation. Together with the team, a care plan is made for Malik to remain on the floor without plans to return to the ICU unless needed for comfort. Given his increased somnolence, waning interest in eating by mouth, and concern for increased secretions, Malik's family has also made the loving decision to discontinue artificial nutrition and hydration through the gastrostomy tube.

Nursing Role

As the nurse caring for a child who has a prognosis of hours to days, sharing the assessment that death is imminent will help the family prepare for what to expect. Ensuring the family has their basic needs met to be fully present with the child is key. While many support services may already be in place, as the bedside provider the nurse is often the first to know of ancillary stressors that could be weighing on the family. Given this trusted role, nurses are typically in the best position to coordinate clinician efforts to holistically support a patient and family. Frequent assessment and reassessment of symptoms is necessary during this stage, while also being flexible around changing interventions to support comfort as needed.[21] Finally, the nurse provides essential anticipatory guidance to families and caregivers regarding physiologic changes at the end of life.

End-of-Life Period: Moments to Hours

There are specific clinical scenarios during which death within moments to hours is most likely. For instance, a child in an ICU supported by maximal ventilator settings whose family has made the loving decision to discontinue ventilatory support to allow natural death will likely have moments to hours to live once the ventilator is discontinued.[22] For the child with advanced illness not supported by technology at baseline, this period may be less predictable. As the nurse caring for a patient, there are physiologic changes that will alert you that death may be imminent such as somnolence, labored breathing, decreased urine output, mottling and cooling of extremities, and weak pulses.

Case Study Continued

Malik has been inpatient for 4 days. Over the last 24 hours he has become more somnolent and is difficult to arouse. His breathing pattern has changed, with longer pauses between breaths, and his skin tone appears dusky. Extended family and close friends have come to visit. Malik is surrounded by his immediate family, including his parents and two younger siblings. Malik continues to receive medications for comfort and seizure control via gastrostomy tube; no additional fluids have been administered. Overnight his parents express worry about Malik's experience of breathlessness. The nurse provides education regarding expected changes in breathing at the end of life, while also engaging the advanced practice clinician regarding his parents' concern. In conjunction with a fan to support breathlessness, opioid medications are titrated as needed in response to Malik's symptoms. Malik appears calmer and more comfortable with these changes. Malik dies in the early hours of the morning surrounded by his loving family.

Nursing Role

As the nurse caring for a child who has a prognosis of moments to hours, it is essential to first be aware of one's own emotions. There is a balance that each nurse should strike between being present and giving space; one should always monitor for avoidance.[23] While every family is unique in what they find most helpful, direct communication to understand their wishes can provide clarity.[24] When a child is imminently dying, the nurse may want to encourage family members to stay present and continue to provide the child with familiar voices, sounds, and touch that will be comforting. At the same time, the nurse should encourage those at the bedside to maintain self-care and allow for breaks as needed. Working with unit leadership to find a private space outside the patient room for family members to take breaks is important.

Anticipatory Guidance

Caring for the Dying Child

While the body goes through many physiologic changes near the end of life (discussed later in this chapter), families may benefit from guidance on how to care for and be present with their child throughout the dying process.[25] It is the role of the nurse to guide patients and their loved ones during this time.

While recognizing familial and cultural beliefs around death and dying are unique to the individual, many loved ones find it difficult to know their role at the bedside. The nurse should provide reassuring guidance that being present is enough. At the same time, family members may find it difficult to be at the bedside during the end of life. Providing a listening ear and giving space for family members to share their experiences and concerns will help the nurse best support a patient and family. The nurse is often looked to for guidance around timing of family, sibling, and/or friend visitation.[26] While at times it can be overwhelming for the child and family to host visitors, the nurse can support enforcement of resting hours and space as needed. During visits, caregivers may benefit from the nurse modeling honest and developmentally appropriate communication about the changes they are seeing in the patient. Ongoing collaboration with social work and child life colleagues is particularly important to support children and their families during this time.[27]

There is inherent uncertainty in the dying process, which can be challenging for families and staff. It is important for interprofessional team members to work together to help set clear expectations as the end-of-life process is emotionally, physically, and spiritually challenging.[28] Avoiding promises and assuring families the team will do their best to ensure their child is as comfortable as possible is honest, transparent, and supportive. These times of uncertainty may provide an opportunity to optimize quality-of-life experiences, for example, going outside/on walks, having visitors present (as mentioned above), and finding opportunities for legacy- and memory-making.

Another aspect of caring for the family during this time may include offering space to think about what happens after the death of a child. While some families are unable to engage in these conversations ahead of time, it is often something on their minds. Consider the following question: "Are there important cultural or familial traditions for us to consider when your child dies?" This question provides an opportunity for the family member to share what they have been thinking about. Funeral and burial expenses may be a concern they have yet to voice to others. Additionally, there may be time constraints around burial or cultural considerations about aftercare they would like to share with someone.

Nursing Communication at the End of Life

Nurses are best situated to be part of intimate discussions with a patient and family. The nurse may be asked difficult questions or overhear challenging conversations.[29] The nurse should expect hard questions but should not be expected to have all the answers (see Table 43.1). The nurse should enter every clinical situation with a spirit of curiosity, never assuming they know exactly what a patient/family is most worried about. To best prepare for responding to the needs of a patient, family, or colleague, it is recommended to practice communication skills which attend to emotion. One tool that many find helpful is following the NURSE acronym to respond to a patient's needs[30]:

Name
Understand
Respect
Support
Explore

The nurse may also support patients and families in thinking and planning ahead (see Chapter 37 for more information regarding communication in pediatric palliative care, including more about using NURSE as well as tools to supplement advanced care planning conversations).

Physiologic Changes at the End of Life

The physiologic changes that may occur during the end-of-life process can be scary for both patients and their family if unexpected. A vital role of the nurse caring for a patient nearing the end of life is

Table 43.1 10 difficult questions the nurse is asked

Example difficult questions	
1. Can we just end this? Can't you just give her something to stop her suffering? 2. How do I go on ... after? 3. How will I know if they are suffering? 4. How much time do they have left? Should my family come to visit? 5. Can they hear me?	6. Do you think they're hungry? 7. Will opioids hasten their death? 8. Am I/my child dying? How will I know? 9. What happens when you die? 10. Have we done everything?
Guidelines for responding	
Expect difficult statements or questions during times of immense grief; do not expect to have all the answers. Below is a framework for how to respond to any number of difficult questions.	
Make empathetic statements: • I can only imagine what you are going through at this time. • This is so hard; this situation is so difficult. • I wish things were different. • I can only imagine how challenging this uncertainty has been. • You have such incredible advocates; you've made such loving decisions.	
Ask open-ended questions to ensure you understand worries of patient and family and to clarify questions: • Can you tell me more about what you are worried about ... ? • What do you think about ... ? • I want to make sure I understand, can you tell me what you mean by ... ? • What are you most hopeful for?	
As for permission: • Would it be okay if I shared my thoughts on that?	
Provide objective information and reassurance: • Opioids are medications commonly used to provide relief to distressing symptoms. When titrated appropriately to a patient's symptoms, they do not hasten death. We will continue to assess and reassess the effectiveness of each intervention we initiate. • While I cannot be certain of X's experience, the following clinical signs are telling me ... ; we will continue to assess and respond to any changes we are seeing. • As the nurse, offer to connect with the primary clinical team to support family member in accessing more information.	

providing anticipatory guidance. This begins with an assessment of how much and what type of information is most helpful to the patient and/or family. As the patient's prognosis moves from months to weeks and more imminently from weeks to days, the nurse should share expected physiologic changes and offer guidance in how the caregiver may take part in caring for the child.

As the child nears the end of life, they may have decreased or little interest in food/drink. Throughout the dying process, the body requires less caloric intake; in fact, excess food and/or fluids may even be distressing and cause discomfort.[31] It is also important to acknowledge food is connected to culture, protection, love, and care. Find ways to maintain the child's physical comfort by supportively educating families on the body's caloric requirements at the end of life.[6] The nurse may encourage caregivers to use oral swabs for lip moistening or ice chips for taste.

Given decreases in intake and changes in organ function at the end of life, the child will experience decreased urinary output. They may even become incontinent. Normalizing that this is something family members may expect to see will help them anticipate changes that do occur. Consider the use of additional disposable chucks or extra sheets to keep bedding clean.

Sleep patterns and level of alertness may change during this period. Increased sleep and decreased arousal are part of the dying process. The nurse should encourage patients and families to enjoy time together while awake and alert, supporting the delicate balance of stimulation and rest. While their child/patient is sleeping, families can continue to speak with them softly, play quiet or favorite music, snuggle, and create an environment that they would enjoy.

Near the end of life, the child may become agitated/delirious/confused. The nurse's role is pivotal in providing anticipatory guidance about agitation, confusion, delirium, and differentiating between anxiety and delirium. A helpful way to distinguish anxiety versus delirium with families is to wonder whether the child seems like themself. They may be disoriented to time/place/loved ones. Reassuring patients that they are "safe, loved, and well cared for" is calming and models supportive presence for caregivers at the bedside. Orienting a patient to time and place is often helpful and may have to be repeated frequently during this period. If the child/patient becomes anxious, the nurse can initiate calming techniques that have worked in the past. Many children are reassured by a light massage to their forehead, holding their hand, reading, or playing music for them.

As the child nears the end of life, breathing patterns change. Additionally, breathing may sound noisy or gurgly or may rattle. These are signs and sounds of upper airway secretions and are not bothersome to the child/patient. The nurse should reassure family members the sounds are most distressing to those listening.[32] A rolled towel behind the neck to prop up the chin can help open the airway, while turning the child to their side allows pooled secretions to drain. If the child/patient appears dyspneic, defined as the patient's perception of breathlessness, a handheld fan pointed toward their face stimulates the trigeminal nerve and may provide relief.[33] The nurse may consider nonpharmacologic techniques, for example, distraction using the child's favorite movie and encouraging family members that they can also implement these interventions.

Additional changes may occur at the end of life. Skin may change in color (blotchy, blue) this is called "mottling." It can also feel damp and cool. The nurse can provide guidance to family members, sharing with them that this is part of the end-of-life process. Offer that they can use extra blankets for warmth and hold the child's hands and feet. Dry eyes may also occur. Lubricant and artificial tears may be helpful in preventing dry eyes.

Ongoing collaboration with multidisciplinary team members including child life, social work, psychiatry/psychology, and chaplaincy will ensure holistic support as families navigate the changes at the end of life. For inpatient nurses, close collaboration with on-service physicians fosters teamwork during emotionally challenging times.

Interventions at the End of Life

The translation of a family's and/or child's goals of care to direct nursing care at the end of life is specific to each patient.[34] Providers may become overwhelmed with decision-making regarding what interventions to continue or discontinue. When a child is nearing the end of life, recommendations surrounding interventions should be made based on the big picture of what is most important to the child and family. Questions often arise surrounding what to do about vital sign monitoring, lab evaluation, transfusions, nonessential medications, etc. There is no one way to approach these interventions at the end of life; rather, decisions should be made in conjunction with the family based on balancing the benefits and burdens of each intervention. Questions to ask oneself to guide decision-making may include: Will this intervention enhance the quality of the child's life in the short time they have left?[35] What burdens could this intervention pose on the child's and/or family's experience? Will this intervention provide valuable information that could change/enhance the end-of-life period for the child?

End-of-Life Symptom Management

Inherent to both palliative care and nursing practice is the desire to alleviate suffering.[36] Suffering is multidimensional and therefore requires a multidimensional approach to treatment.[37] While salient themes may emerge in defining suffering, suffering is unique to every child and family. In addition to physical discomfort/pain, individuals may experience emotional, psychosocial, and spiritual suffering. See Chapter 39 for further information on psychosocial and spiritual suffering.

What about Opioids?

Physical distress is an aspect of suffering nurses may encounter while caring for a child at the end of life.[38] Studies have shown that children at the end of life can have a high symptom burden, which contributes to patient and family distress.[39,40] While nurses aim to alleviate suffering, there can be hesitation around administration of medications, specifically opioids, at the end of life.[41] This hesitation is often attributed to misconceptions surrounding opioids and approaches to symptom management. Opioids, when prescribed appropriately, do NOT hasten death but rather provide much needed relief to the pediatric patient experiencing symptoms related to disease progression at the end of life.[42] It is important that nurses feel confident in the therapies being provided and therefore should advocate to be part of larger healthcare team discussions to be well-informed and share their knowledge of the patient and family.[43–45]

End-of-Life Huddle

Given evolving symptoms and the potential for rotating providers, an end-of-life team huddle can be a nurse-led interprofessional care coordination intervention in various settings. See Figure 43.1 for an example of an end-of-life discussion tool.[46] This example outlines important team members to include in the huddle and topics to discuss to ensure providers are aligned in the care plan.

Acute Symptom Management at the End of Life

It is important to understand the disease process to best anticipate and manage acute symptoms at the end of life. Titrating medications to meet symptoms is the most effective and strategic approach.[47] Table 43.2 summarizes the common nonpharmacologic and pharmacologic interventions utilized for symptom management at the end of life.

Pain is complex and outlined in more detail in Chapter 34. The etiology of pain may vary and could include malignancy, infection, trauma, etc. A stepwise approach to pain management is helpful.[48] The nurse often has the most up-to-date understanding of how nonpharmacologic and pharmacologic interventions have benefited the patient. Frequent assessment and reassessment, in addition to close collaboration with the team, will ensure timely and effective pain management. Ensure comfort strategies such as changing position, venting gastrostomy tube, and removing painful stimuli are being considered in conjunction with pharmacologic management.[49]

Children may experience difficulty breathing for a variety of different reasons during the end-of-life period.[32,50] Dyspnea, the sense of breathlessness, can be distressing to the child and those around them. A low-dose opioid and calming techniques can help a lot. A fan to blow air directly onto the child's face is often even more beneficial than supplemental oxygen.[51,52] Consider providing increased oxygen support if the child already has oxygen supplementation.

Secretions can be challenging to manage and cause noisy breathing. As the muscles in the body relax toward the end of life, pooling of secretions can be common. Support nonpharmacologic interventions, such as repositioning and gently wiping the child's mouth and nose. Typically suctioning is not recommended and can worsen secretions. Atropine and glycopyrrolate are common medications that may be considered during this time.[53]

Anxiety is common in children and their family members at the end of life. Providing space and exploring what may be contributing to the child's anxiety are important. Allowing the opportunity for the child to ask questions or share their concerns can alleviate many worries. When available, collaboration with psychosocial colleagues (e.g., social work, psychology, psychiatry) can provide additional benefits. Given their short-acting nature and quick onset, benzodiazepines are a common pharmacologic intervention for anxiety during the end-of-life period.[54]

Confusion, disorientation, and agitation, commonly referred to as "delirium," can be seen in a child as their body goes through changes at the end of life. Ongoing reorientation, promotion of the sleep–wake cycle, and a calming presence in conjunction with antipsychotic therapy such as haloperidol or olanzapine are shown to be

EOL Huddle Discussion Tool ___/___/___ **Time** __

An end-of-life team huddle is recommended as needed, particularly with an anticipated change in providers, change in symptoms/escalation, prior to the weekend/holiday, etc.

- ***Charge or Bedside RN to facilitate EOL Huddle***

Patient discussed ____________________

Team members (recommended)

- Nurse ____________
- Charge/ Resource Nurse ____________
- Clinical Coordinator(s) ____________
- Primary team (Attending, Fellow, NP, Resident, RT, etc.) ____________
- Child Life Specialist (CLS) ____________
- Palliative Care Team ____________
- Pain Service ____________
- Pharmacy ____________
- Social Work ____________
- Other ____________

____

*Team member's/ contact information if they would like to be notified of patient's death: ____________

____

Topics to Discuss

Advance Care Planning

- Family goals discussed
- Resuscitation status documented
- Guidance in how the caregiver may take part in caring for the child.

Emotional/Social/Spiritual Care

- CLS and Music Therapy involved, and legacy making discussed, if appropriate
- Spiritual Care Team and/or Interpreter Services involved, if appropriate
- Any questions around funeral planning addressed (this does not need to be done prior to patient's death/discharge from hospital)

Contingency Planning

- Discuss next steps for symptom escalation
- Do next steps require a potential change in concentration of Patient Controlled Analgesia (PCA) if applicable?
- Consideration of additional drips (if applicable)? (Discuss additional teams to consult)
- Discuss acute symptoms management plans, if appropriate
  - **Risk** for seizure? Seizure PRN medication ordered
  - **Risk** for bleed? Sedation medication ordered
- Signs and symptoms of imminently dying discussed with family (changes in vital signs, respiration, skin, neurological response)
- Additional information: ____________________

Figure 43.1 End-of-life team huddle discussion tool.
Source: Edson J, Heneghan C. EOL Huddle Discussion Tool. Boston Children's Hospital; 2022.

Table 43.2 Summary table of end-of-life symptom management

Symptom	Typical nonmedication strategies	Typical medications	Helpful pearls
Agitation/delirium	Gentle reorientation to person, time, and place Ensuring lights on/windows open during the day Prioritizing lights off/darkness at night	Antipsychotics (haloperidol, olanzapine)	Benzodiazepines may worsen agitation/delirium
Bleeding	Use of dark towels Pressure Anticipatory guidance	Antifibrinolytic agents (topical aminocaproic acid, tranexamic acid)	Pre-planning is key
Dyspnea	Fan/cool air Limit fluids/hydration Calming/reorientation techniques	Low-dose opioids Benzodiazepines	Supplemental oxygen may not be needed
Pain	Positioning Adjust/vent gastrostomy tube Hot packs/cold packs Integrative therapies (reiki, massage, aromatherapy)	Analgesics (acetaminophen, NSAIDs, opioids)	Layer a multimodal approach to target different pain types and receptors
Secretions/noisy breathing	Reposition Wipe secretions Limit fluids/hydration	Anticholinergics (glycopyrrolate, atropine, hyoscyamine)	Noisy breathing is often more distressing to families than to patients; refocus on patient's calm face
Seizures	Anticipatory guidance Emergency action plan	Antiseizure agents (benzodiazepines, barbiturates)	Pre-planning is key

CLS, child life specialist; EOL, end of life; NP, nurse practitioner; NSAID, nonsteroidal anti-inflammatory drug; PRN, as needed; RN, registered nurse; RT, respiratory therapist.

most effective.[55] If possible, avoiding benzodiazepines, which could contribute to worsening delirium, is preferred.[56]

Bleeding may be an anticipated acute symptom at the end of life, particularly in some leukemic malignancies. Providing anticipatory guidance that this may be expected and creating a plan with the interdisciplinary team can alleviate concerns. Blood can be particularly distressing to patients and families. While scary to see, bleeding is not painful. Providing dark towels and sheets can help alleviate some of the shock of seeing blood on white linens. Consider the use of topical aminocaproic acid on mucous membranes to slow nose and gum bleeding.[57]

Seizures may be an expected acute symptom that occurs during the end-of-life period. While some institutions may recommend seizure prophylaxis, others may not.[58,59] Ensuring the team engages with the family in a conversation about expected or anticipated symptoms and management can help the family, nurse, and team to consider an antiepileptic action plan.

Though not discussed in detail in this chapter, palliative sedation, or sedation to unconsciousness, may be indicated when a patient experiences refractory symptoms that cannot be captured through appropriate titration of symptom-relieving medications.[60,61] Given the complexity at the end of life in pediatric patients, palliative sedation therapy is complicated and nuanced. A general approach to palliative sedation therapy in adults is discussed in Chapter 11.

Chronic Symptom Management at the End of Life

In addition to acute symptoms during the end-of-life period, children with medical complexities often live with chronic symptoms that continue to be present at the end of life. It is important to think through the risks and benefits of continuing to treat these symptoms. When the goal is to prioritize comfort, careful consideration should be taken surrounding how interventions/medications could improve or worsen the symptom burden. Constipation and pressure ulcers are two examples of long-standing symptoms that may require a different management approach at end of life.[62]

Medical Emergencies at the End of Life

In rare circumstances, the child may experience a sudden change in symptoms related to an emergency during the end-of-life period. When a known possibility, offering anticipatory guidance that this type of emergency may occur can help prepare patients, families, and teams to formulate an effective treatment plan. Interventions for these emergencies during the end-of-life period may align with the patient's and family's goals, or they may not. For example, consider a tension pneumothorax, which may develop in the setting of pulmonary metastases in which the child may experience sudden gasping. While needle thoracotomy would be the typical management, this may be more distressing to the child and family.[63] Regardless of intervention, management should involve anxiolytics and rapid initiation of opioids for the patient at bedside.

A patient with sudden bowel obstruction may similarly benefit from intervention (i.e., placement of nasogastric suction). At the same time, placement of a nasogastric tube with suction may be more distressing to the patient and family. In such a case, collaboration with the clinician in the escalation of opioids and anxiolytics should occur. Like a pneumothorax and bowel obstruction, upper airway obstruction, from disease or infection, can be anxiety-provoking for patients, families, and teams. Ensuring a clear plan is communicated about this potential and facilitating ongoing discussions on how to respond to an airway obstruction are important. Function can be assessed by asking questions about difficulty with chewing, swallowing, and/or breathing. Steroids can be helpful at reducing swelling, in conjunction with opioids and anxiolytics that can relieve pain and anxiety, respectively. Regardless of the type of medical emergency, planning ahead ensures the response is symptom-focused and goal-concordant.[64]

Care at and after Death

Patient Assessment

The nurse provides care at time of death and is looked to by members of the team as the expert in that care. While every institution may have unique policies regarding procedures at the end of life, there are common measures taken by nurses across institutions. When death is imminent, ongoing communication with the team and frequent assessment of patient comfort are imperative. During this time, some families may require intensive support from nursing, while others may prefer a more intimate environment. Continue to ensure family needs (as discussed above) are met, while gauging the level of physical presence that is necessary. When the nurse or the family notices the patient has not taken a breath in some time, the nurse should auscultate for a heartbeat for one minute. The nurse must continue to maintain a calm, respectful, and competent presence. If no heartbeat is heard, the nurse may step outside the room and call the on-service provider to confirm the child has died. All clinicians can assess a heartbeat and declare time of death in a clear and compassionate manner. An important role during this time is ensuring social work and chaplaincy (if indicated) are notified.

There are hospital policies for nursing and provider steps to follow once a patient has been declared deceased. Common tasks for advanced practice clinicians during this time include contacting the medical examiner, contacting the organ donation organization, completing the death certificate, and completing appropriate documentation in the medical record. Common tasks for nurses include aftercare (see next section for details) as well as documentation in the medical record.

Aftercare

Caring for the body of a child who has died is an intimate nursing task. The nurse should never feel alone in this process and should be encouraged to have a co-worker present to assist with the care. While some families may choose to participate in aftercare of their child, such as bathing and dressing, others may choose to step away prior to this care. Regardless of family preference for involvement, always offer time and a supportive presence once a child has died. The nurse should recognize the magnitude of this moment and be flexible to allow families the time they need.

While planning how to approach aftercare, be aware that muscle rigidity, known as "rigor mortis," sets in within hours after death and can be distressing for families to witness.[65] If possible, encourage bathing the child prior to rigor mortis setting in. Remove all stickers and clean up any bodily fluid. Prior to removing any hardware (central line, port-a-cath, tracheostomy, etc.), ensure a conversation is had with the provider about policies, cultural/familial considerations, or whether this patient will have an autopsy.

After the child has been bathed, and the family has been given the time they need at the bedside, the nurse can share with them what will happen next. Typically, the nurse is responsible for transportation of the body to the morgue. Families may find it comforting to hear that their child's body will not be left alone. Institution depending, if there is a special item such as an outfit, blanket, or stuffed animal they want to stay with the child, that can typically be arranged. Social work colleagues can help to ensure the family has a place to stay and/or safe transportation home. Many families benefit from being ushered out of the hospital by familiar staff as this is an incredibly overwhelming time.

End-of-Life Considerations

While the death of a child always comes with immense sadness, children and families have a remarkable way of thinking ahead toward the future. Many people find solace in legacy-making or thinking of ways for the child to have lasting impact after death.[66] Child life therapists, music therapists, and art therapists are common collaborators in pediatric settings to initiate legacy work.[67] Major decisions to consider at the end of life to support legacy include (1) organ donation and (2) autopsy. The provider is responsible for discussing organ donation and autopsy with patients and families prior to and after a child dies. The nurse should be present during these conversations and included in the family's decision-making around these topics when possible. Decisions surrounding organ donation and autopsy may influence nursing care after the death as there may be specific timing requirements for the nurse to follow.

Organ/Tissue Donation

Organ/tissue donation, the procurement of organs/tissues with intent to transplant, is a common decision point at the end of life.[68] While many families hope for their child's organs to be donated, there are strict clinical criteria that must be met for a patient to be eligible. Equitable distribution standards are set forth by the Organ Procurement and Transplantation Network.[69] For patients who are not eligible to donate organs for transplantation, research organizations may offer a family another avenue to support their child's legacy.

Autopsy

Autopsy, postmortem examination of the body, is an important consideration after the death of a child.[70] The scope of an autopsy may vary based on family preference and clinical indication. Autopsies may yield new information or provide confirmation for a family regarding their child's diagnosis.[71] Review of information gathered from a postmortem examination may also provide a venue for families to ask outstanding questions. Families should be guided through autopsy review by longitudinal providers.

Staff Commemoration and Expressing Condolences

The illness experience encompasses care of the child from time of diagnosis through the end-of-life period and into bereavement. Caring for a family after a child dies is one of the many roles of the nurse. Research shows that hearing from clinicians following the death of a child is helpful to support caregiver grief.[72–74] Unfortunately, ways for nurses to connect with families after the death of a child are typically not formalized. Small gestures can often go a long way in helping a family process the death of a child, such as letter writing, a card, or making a follow-up phone call.[72]

Part of caring for a child at the end of their life is also being attuned to the needs of the providers. Recognizing the importance for staff to have an opportunity to express their experiences in caring for that patient and family is paramount. Many units and programs offer staff-led debriefings for nurses to commemorate the patient and the care they received.[75] To care for themselves and allow for longevity within the field, nurses must acknowledge that this work is both emotionally and physically taxing.[76–78] In addition to staff-led interventions, it is important to consider and develop individual coping strategies to process caring for children and their families at the end of life.

Case Conclusion

After months of caring for Malik and his family through multiple hospitalizations, the nursing staff felt the loss after his death. Recognizing the hard work that many staff members participated in, and the impact Malik's death had, the nurse manager worked together with interprofessional colleagues to organize a unit debrief and celebration of life. It was a space for nurses and others (certified nursing assistants, social work, and child life specialist) to share their experiences, memories, and lessons learned from caring for Malik. The unit sent a bereavement card to Malik's family, who were extremely grateful. Malik's family returned to the unit months after his death to share their appreciation of the care they all received during Malik's life and expressed their immense gratitude for the support and guidance they received from staff during the most difficult time of their lives.

Conclusion

The nurse plays an essential role in caring for a child at the end of life. The nurse ushers the patient and family through the end-of-life experience with compassion and confidence. Inclusion in medical discussions and family meetings can help with consistent messaging and care planning. Providing anticipatory guidance to patients and families helps set expectations and gives families the opportunity to think ahead and ask questions. Ongoing assessment and reassessment are key in ensuring emotional, physical, and spiritual needs are met. Collaboration with interdisciplinary colleagues can ease this difficult process for all parties involved. Finally, the opportunity to reflect on one's experience caring for a child at the end of life may help build both internal and external resources to support sustainability within the field of nursing.

REFERENCES

1. American Nurses Association. Nurses' Role and Responsibilities in Providing Care and Support at the End of Life. Position Statement. 2016. Accessed June 19, 2016. https://www.nursingworld.org/~4af078/globalassets/docs/ana/ethics/endoflife-positionstatement.pdf.
2. Linebarger JS, Johnson V, Boss RD, et al. Guidance for pediatric end-of-life care. *Pediatrics*. 2022;149(5):e2022057011. https://doi.org/10.1542/peds.2022-057011.
3. Johnston EE, Martinez I, Currie E, Brock KE, Wolfe J. Hospital or home? Where should children die and how do we make that a reality? *J Pain Symptom Manage*. 2020;60(1):106–115. https://doi.org/10.1016/j.jpainsymman.2019.12.370.
4. Trowbridge A, Walter JK, McConathey E, Morrison W, Feudtner C. Modes of death within a children's hospital. *Pediatrics*. 2018;142(4):e20174182. https://doi.org/10.1542/peds.2017-4182.
5. Gibson-Smith D, Jarvis SW, Fraser LK. Place of death of children and young adults with a life-limiting condition in England: a retrospective cohort study. *Arch Dis Child*. 2021;106:780–785. https://doi.org/10.1136/archdischild-2020-319700.
6. Jordan M, Keefer PM, Lee YA, et al. Top ten tips palliative care clinicians should know about caring for children. *J Palliat Med*. 2018;21(12):1783–1789. https://doi.org/10.1089/jpm.2018.0482.
7. Wiener L, Tager J, Mack J, Battles H, Bedoya SZ, Gerhardt CA. Helping parents prepare for their child's end of life: a retrospective survey of cancer-bereaved parents. *Pediatr Blood Cancer*. 2020;67(2):e27993. https://doi.org/10.1002/pbc.27993.
8. Sedig LK, Spruit JL, Paul TK, et al. Supporting pediatric patients and their families at the end of life: perspectives from bereaved parents. *Am J Hosp Palliat Care*. 2020;37(12):1009–1015. https://doi.org/10.1177/1049909120922973.
9. Bergstraesser E, Thienprayoon R, Brook LA, et al. Top ten tips palliative care clinicians should know about prognostication in children. *J Palliat Med*. 2021;24(11):1725–1731. https://doi.org/10.1089/jpm.2021.0439.
10. Hui D, Nooruddin Z, Didwaniya N, et al. Concepts and definitions for "actively dying," "end of life," "terminally ill," "terminal care," and "transition of care": a systematic review. *J Pain Symptom Manage*. 2014;47(1):77–89. https://doi.org/10.1016/j.jpainsymman.2013.02.021.
11. Hui D, Paiva CE, Del Fabbro EG, et al. Prognostication in advanced cancer: update and directions for future research. *Support Care Cancer*. 2019;27(6):1973–1984. https://doi.org/10.1007/s00520-019-04727-y.
12. Newman AR, Callahan MF, Lerret SM, Oswald DL, Weiss ME. Pediatric oncology nurses' experiences with prognosis-related communication. *Oncol Nurs Forum*. 2018;45(3):327–337. https://doi.org/10.1188/18.ONF.327-337.
13. Rosa WE, Izumi S, Sullivan DR, et al. Advance care planning in serious illness: a narrative review. *J Pain Symptom Manage*. 2023;65(1):e63–e78. https://doi.org/10.1016/j.jpainsymman.2022.08.012.
14. Rosenberg AR, Popp B, Dizon DS, El-Jawahri A, Spence R. Now, more than ever, is the time for early and frequent advance care planning. *J Clin Oncol*. 2020;38(26):2956–2959. https://doi.org/10.1200/JCO.20.01080.
15. American Nurses Association. ANA Code of Ethics Revision. Accessed June 22, 2023. https://www.nursingworld.org/practice-policy/nursing-excellence/ethics/code-of-ethics-for-nurses/.
16. Brock KE. Urgent appeal from hospice nurses for pediatric palliative care training and community. *JAMA Netw Open*. 2021;4(10):e2127958. https://doi.org/10.1001/jamanetworkopen.2021.27958.
17. Porter AS, Zalud K, Applegarth J, et al. Community hospice nurses' perspectives on needs, preferences, and challenges related to caring for children with serious illness. *JAMA Netw Open*. 2021;4(10):e2127457. https://doi.org/10.1001/jamanetworkopen.2021.27457.
18. Blazin LJ, Cecchini C, Habashy C, Kaye EC, Baker JN. Communicating effectively in pediatric cancer care: translating evidence into practice. *Children (Basel)*. 2018;5(3):40. https://doi.org/10.3390/children5030040.
19. Jackson VA, Jacobsen J, Greer JA, Pirl WF, Temel JS, Back AL. The cultivation of prognostic awareness through the provision of early palliative care in the ambulatory setting: a communication

guide. *J Palliat Med*. 2013;16(8):894–900. https://doi.org/10.1089/jpm.2012.0547.

20. Diekema DS, Botkin JR, Committee on Bioethics. Clinical report—forgoing medically provided nutrition and hydration in children. *Pediatrics*. 2009;124(2):813–822. https://doi.org/10.1542/peds.2009-1299.
21. Mack JW, Currie ER, Martello V, et al. Barriers to optimal end-of-life care for adolescents and young adults with cancer: bereaved caregiver perspectives. *J Natl Compr Canc Netw*. 2021;19(5):528–533. https://doi.org/10.6004/jnccn.2020.7645.
22. Postier A, Catrine K, Remke S. Interdisciplinary pediatric palliative care team involvement in compassionate extubation at home: from shared decision-making to bereavement. *Children (Basel)*. 2018;5(3):37. https://doi.org/10.3390/children5030037.
23. Gibson K, Hofmeyer A, Warland J. Nurses providing end-of-life care for infants and their families in the NICU: a review of the literature. *Adv Neonatal Care*. 2018;18(6):471–479. https://doi.org/10.1097/ANC.0000000000000533.
24. Bogetz JF, Revette A, Rosenberg AR, DeCourcey D. "I could never prepare for something like the death of my own child": parental perspectives on preparedness at end of life for children with complex chronic conditions. *J Pain Symptom Manage*. 2020;60(6):1154–1162.e1. https://doi.org/10.1016/j.jpainsymman.2020.06.035.
25. Sansom-Daly UM, Wakefield CE, Patterson P, et al. End-of-life communication needs for adolescents and young adults with cancer: recommendations for research and practice. *J Adolesc Young Adult Oncol*. 2020;9(2):157–165. https://doi.org/10.1089/jayao.2019.0084.
26. Long KA, Lehmann V, Gerhardt CA, Carpenter AL, Marsland AL, Alderfer MA. Psychosocial functioning and risk factors among siblings of children with cancer: an updated systematic review. *Psychooncology*. 2018;27(6):1467–1479. https://doi.org/10.1002/pon.4669.
27. Michelson KN, Arenson M, Charleston E, et al. Parental views of social worker and chaplain involvement in care and decision making for critically ill children with cancer. *Children (Basel)*. 2022;9(9):1287. https://doi.org/10.3390/children9091287.
28. Greenfield K, Holley S, Schoth DE, et al. A mixed-methods systematic review and meta-analysis of barriers and facilitators to paediatric symptom management at end of life. *Palliat Med*. 2020;34(6):689–707. https://doi.org/10.1177/0269216320907065.
29. Montgomery KE, Sawin KJ, Hendricks-Ferguson V. Communication during palliative care and end of life: perceptions of experienced pediatric oncology nurses. *Cancer Nurs*. 2017;40(2):E47–E57. https://doi.org/10.1097/NCC.0000000000000363.
30. VitalTalk. Responding to Emotion: Respecting. 2019. Accessed October 18, 2022. https://www.vitaltalk.org/guides/responding-to-emotion-respecting/.
31. Lazzara A, Boss RD. Observation of child experience during discontinuing of medically provided nutrition and hydration. *J Pain Symptom Manage*. 2023;65(3):155–161. https://doi.org/10.1016/j.jpainsymman.2022.12.008.
32. Campbell ML, Donesky D, Sarkozy A, Reinke LF. Treatment of dyspnea in advanced disease and at the end of life. *J Hosp Palliat Nurs*. 2021;23(5):406–420. https://doi.org/10.1097/NJH.0000000000000766.
33. Luckett T, Phillips J, Johnson MJ, et al. Contributions of a hand-held fan to self-management of chronic breathlessness. *Eur Respir J*. 2017;50(2):1700262. https://doi.org/10.1183/13993003.00262-2017.
34. Lichtenthal WG, Roberts KE, Catarozoli C, et al. Regret and unfinished business in parents bereaved by cancer: a mixed methods study. *Palliat Med*. 2020;34(3):367–377. https://doi.org/10.1177/0269216319900301.
35. Bogetz JF, Rosenberg AR. Adults are just big children: what we can learn about quality end-of-life care from pediatrics. *Cancer*. 2021;127(14):2393–2396. https://doi.org/10.1002/cncr.33548.
36. Sekse RJT, Hunskar I, Ellingsen S. The nurse's role in palliative care: a qualitative meta-synthesis. *J Clin Nurs*. 2018;27(1-2):e21–e38. https://doi.org/10.1111/jocn.13912.
37. Sisk BA, Feudtner C, Bluebond-Langner M, Sourkes B, Hinds PS, Wolfe J. Response to suffering of the seriously ill child: a history of palliative care for children. *Pediatrics*. 2020;145(1):e20191741. https://doi.org/10.1542/peds.2019-1741.
38. Snaman J, McCarthy S, Wiener L, Wolfe J. Pediatric palliative care in oncology. *J Clin Oncol*. 2020;38(9):954–962. https://doi.org/10.1200/JCO.18.02331.
39. Broden EG, Hinds PS, Werner-Lin AV, Curley MAQ, Investigators RS. "I didn't want my baby to pass, but i didn't want him suffering either": comparing bereaved parents' narratives with nursing end-of-life assessments in the pediatric intensive care unit. *J Hosp Palliat Nurs*. 2022;24(5):271–280. https://doi.org/10.1097/NJH.0000000000000884.
40. Wolfe J. Suffering in children at the end of life: recognizing an ethical duty to palliate. *J Clin Ethics*. 2000;11(2):157–163.
41. Garten L, Daehmlow S, Reindl T, Wendt A, Munch A, Buhrer C. End-of-life opioid administration on neonatal and pediatric intensive care units: nurses' attitudes and practice. *Eur J Pain*. 2011;15(9):958–965. https://doi.org/10.1016/j.ejpain.2011.03.009.
42. National Institute on Aging. Providing Care and Comfort at the End of Life. October 18, 2022. https://www.nia.nih.gov/health/providing-comfort-end-life.
43. Zaal-Schuller IH, Willems DI, Ewals F, van Goudoever JB, de Vos MA. Involvement of nurses in end-of-life discussions for severely disabled children. *J Intellect Disabil Res*. 2018;62(4):330–338. https://doi.org/10.1111/jir.12473.
44. Cole MA, Foito K. Pediatric end-of-life simulation: preparing the future nurse to care for the needs of the child and family. *J Pediatr Nurs*. 2019;44:e9–e12. https://doi.org/10.1016/j.pedn.2018.09.005.
45. De Brasi EL, Giannetta N, Ercolani S, et al. Nurses' moral distress in end-of-life care: a qualitative study. *Nurs Ethics*. 2021;28(5):614–627. https://doi.org/10.1177/0969733020964859.
46. Edson J, Heneghan C. *EOL Huddle Discussion Toll*. Boston Children's Hospital; 2022.
47. Drake R, Frost J, Collins JJ. The symptoms of dying children. *J Pain Symptom Manage*. 2003;26(1):594–603. https://doi.org/10.1016/s0885-3924(03)00202 1.
48. Berde C, Wolfe J. Pain, anxiety, distress, and suffering: interrelated, but not interchangeable. *J Pediatr*. 2003;142(4):361–363. https://doi.org/10.1067/mpd.2003.194.
49. Snaman JM, Baker JN, Ehrentraut JH, Anghelescu DL. Pediatric oncology: managing pain at the end of life. *Paediatr Drugs*. 2016;18(3):161–180. https://doi.org/10.1007/s40272-016-0168-2.
50. Pieper L, Zernikow B, Drake R, Frosch M, Printz M, Wager J. Dyspnea in children with life-threatening and life-limiting complex chronic conditions. *J Palliat Med*. 2018;21(4):552–564. https://doi.org/10.1089/jpm.2017.0240.
51. Qian Y, Wu Y, Rozman de Moraes A, et al. Fan therapy for the treatment of dyspnea in adults: a systematic review. *J Pain Symptom Manage*. 2019;58(3):481–486. https://doi.org/10.1016/j.jpainsymman.2019.04.011.
52. Pan CX, Palathra BC, Leo-To WF. Management of respiratory symptoms in those with serious illness. *Med Clin*

North Am. 2020;104(3):455–470. https://doi.org/10.1016/j.mcna.2019.12.004.
53. Arcuri JF, Abarshi E, Preston NJ, Brine J, Pires Di Lorenzo VA. Benefits of interventions for respiratory secretion management in adult palliative care patients—a systematic review. *BMC Palliat Care.* 2016;15:74. https://doi.org/10.1186/s12904-016-0147-y.
54. Kamell A, Smith LK. Attitudes toward use of benzodiazepines among U.S. hospice clinicians: survey and review of the literature. *J Palliat Med.* 2016;19(5):516–522. https://doi.org/10.1089/jpm.2015.0376.
55. Tran PM, Moss J, Koh E, Ort K, Shaw RJ, Goldsmith M. Pediatric delirium in the palliative care setting. In: Wolfe J, Sourkes BM, eds. *Interdisciplinary Pediatric Palliative Care.* Oxford University Press; 2022:264–281.
56. Mody K, Kaur S, Mauer EA, et al. Benzodiazepines and development of delirium in critically ill children: estimating the causal effect. *Crit Care Med.* 2018;46(9):1486–1491. https://doi.org/10.1097/CCM.0000000000003194.
57. Prommer E. Management of bleeding in the terminally ill patient. *Hematology.* 2005;10(3):167–175. https://doi.org/10.1080/10245330500093237.
58. Krouwer HG, Pallagi JL, Graves NM. Management of seizures in brain tumor patients at the end of life. *J Palliat Med.* 2000;3(4):465–475. https://doi.org/10.1089/jpm.2000.3.4.465.
59. Baenziger PH, Moody K. Palliative care for children with central nervous system malignancies. *Bioengineering (Basel).* 2018;5(4):85. https://doi.org/10.3390/bioengineering5040085.
60. Cuviello A, Ang N, Morgan K, Baker JN, Anghelescu DL. Palliative sedation therapy practice comparison—a survey of pediatric palliative care and pain management specialists. *Am J Hosp Palliat Care.* 2023;40(9):977–986. https://doi.org/10.1177/10499091221138298.
61. Cuviello A, Johnson LM, Morgan KJ, Anghelescu DL, Baker JN. Palliative sedation therapy in pediatrics: an algorithm and clinical practice update. *Children (Basel).* 2022;9(12):1887. https://doi.org/10.3390/children9121887.
62. Raepsaet C, Blomberg K, Falk-Brynhildsen K, Gethin G, Beeckman D. Promoting and maintaining skin integrity in end-of-life care: a systematic review. *Adv Skin Wound Care.* 2022;35(11):617–631. https://doi.org/10.1097/01.ASW.0000833616.40632.40.
63. Sahota RJ, Sayad E. Tension pneumothorax. In: *StatPearls.* StatPearls Publishing; 2022.
64. Skoch BM, Sinclair CT. Management of urgent medical conditions at the end of life. *Med Clin North Am.* 2020;104(3):525–538. https://doi.org/10.1016/j.mcna.2019.12.006.
65. Shedge R, Krishan K, Warrier V, Kanchan T. Postmortem changes. In: *StatPearls.* StatPearls Publishing; 2022.
66. Love A, Greer K, Woods C, Clark L, Baker JN, Kaye EC. Bereaved parent perspectives and recommendations on best practices for legacy interventions. *J Pain Symptom Manage.* 2022;63(6):1022–1030.e3. https://doi.org/10.1016/j.jpainsymman.2022.02.003.
67. Schaefer MR, Wagoner ST, Young ME, Madan-Swain A, Barnett M, Gray WN. Healing the hearts of bereaved parents: impact of legacy artwork on grief in pediatric oncology. *J Pain Symptom Manage.* 2020;60(4):790–800. https://doi.org/10.1016/j.jpainsymman.2020.04.018.
68. Nakagawa TA, Shemie SD, Dryden-Palmer K, Parshuram CS, Brierley J. Organ donation following neurologic and circulatory determination of death. *Pediatr Crit Care Med.* 2018;19(8 suppl 2):S26–S32. https://doi.org/10.1097/PCC.0000000000001518.
69. Organ Procurement and Transplantation Network. Accessed October 18, 2022. https://optn.transplant.hrsa.gov/.
70. Feinstein JA, Ernst LM, Ganesh J, Feudtner C. What new information pediatric autopsies can provide: a retrospective evaluation of 100 consecutive autopsies using family-centered criteria. *Arch Pediatr Adolesc Med.* 2007;161(12):1190–1196. https://doi.org/10.1001/archpedi.161.12.1190.
71. Raghuram N, Alodan K, Bartels U, et al. Diagnostic discrepancies between antemortem clinical diagnosis and autopsy findings in pediatric cancer patients. *Virchows Arch.* 2021;478(6):1179–1185. https://doi.org/10.1007/s00428-020-03002-4.
72. Weaver MS, Lichtenthal WG, Larson K, Wiener L. How I approach expressing condolences and longitudinal remembering to a family after the death of a child. *Pediatr Blood Cancer.* 2019;66(2):e27489. https://doi.org/10.1002/pbc.27489.
73. Snaman JM, Kaye EC, Torres C, Gibson DV, Baker JN. Helping parents live with the hole in their heart: the role of health care providers and institutions in the bereaved parents' grief journeys. *Cancer.* 2016;122(17):2757–2765. https://doi.org/10.1002/cncr.30087.
74. Kaye EC, Kiefer A, Blazin L, et al. Bereaved parents, hope, and realism. *Pediatrics.* 2020;145(5):e20192771. https://doi.org/10.1542/peds.2019-2771.
75. Holbert E, Dellasega C. De-stressing from distress: preliminary evaluation of a nurse-led brief debriefing program. *Crit Care Nurs Q.* 2021;44(2):230–234. https://doi.org/10.1097/CNQ.0000000000000356.
76. Morgan D. Caring for dying children: assessing the needs of the pediatric palliative care nurse. *Pediatr Nurs.* 2009;35(2):86–90.
77. Pattison N, Droney J, Gruber P. Burnout: caring for critically ill and end-of-life patients with cancer. *Nurs Crit Care.* 2020;25(2):93–101. https://doi.org/10.1111/nicc.12460.
78. Whiting L, O'Grady M, Whiting M, Petty J. Factors influencing nurse retention within children's palliative care. *J Child Health Care.* 2021;25(4):587–602. https://doi.org/10.1177/1367493520971426.

44

Grief and Bereavement in Perinatal and Pediatric Palliative Care

Kathie Kobler, Rana Limbo, and Betty Davies

Key Points

- Bereavement care for all family members, including children of all ages, is an integral component of pediatric palliative care.
- Grief assessment begins at the time of diagnosis of a child's serious illness, applies to all family members, and continues into the bereavement period following the child's death.
- Grieving after a death is a normal process because grief is experienced from the loss or alteration of a close relationship; however, some grief reactions are complicated, and nurses must assess for factors that put family members at risk for such reactions.
- Nurses have the responsibility to create supportive relationships in which family members feel free to express their grief.
- Caring for children at the end of life requires nurses to attend to their own personal professional responses to death, dying, and bereavement as a basis for providing optimal care to families.

To best capture the many facets of supporting grieving parents, children, and healthcare professionals, brief exemplars and a case study are incorporated throughout this chapter.

Grief and Bereavement Overview

Guidelines and standards outlined by national neonatal, pediatric, and palliative care organizations emphasize the importance of providing compassionate interdisciplinary bereavement support to families of children with life-threatening conditions from diagnosis through death and bereavement.[1–5] Regardless of the cause, the death of a child is an incomparable life event impacting family members, friends, and their community. A child's death also affects the healthcare professionals who provide care for the child and family.

The purpose of this chapter is to discuss grief as a lifelong, relational process. Grief can arise at any point in care for all connected in relationship with the child, even well before death occurs. The trajectory of grief reflects how survivors of loving relationships maintain closeness and connection, cherishing dear ones who are no longer physically present. The progression of such care has been summed up this way: "Grief flows from relationship. Relationship forms a bridge from suffering to hope. Hope transforms."[6(p1)] The authors highlight practical strategies for grief assessment and supporting bereaved parents and children. Also included are the experiences of healthcare professionals as they maintain relationships with the child, the family, and team members and are affected by loss. The authors recognize the impact of social determinants of health on marginalized communities and their influence on the experience of grief. The ideas promoted in this chapter are intended for all, to support the highest-quality perinatal and pediatric palliative care. No matter the differences between clinician and patient(s), the power of relationship, a true understanding of the one cared for, creates connection and protection.

Grief as a Process

Death is a part of each individual life, something faced when contemplating our own mortality. Children are expected to outlive their parents; the death of one's child is outside of that hoped-for pattern. The grief associated with a child's serious illness can begin at diagnosis as parents and family members consider the possibility of no cure, while also simultaneously hoping for a good outcome.[7] The integrative model of curing and healing[8] in Figure 44.1 shows bereavement and hope as intertwining experiences throughout a serious illness, accompanying the moments that make up each day. As a serious illness progresses, a realignment of goals occurs—a result of shifting hopes and preferences in response to a child's deteriorating condition.[9]

When a child transitions to dying, grief responses intensify, and family members' grief continues long past the child's death. Parents may resume daily activities, adjust to life without their child's presence, and find new pleasures in life; but most parents feel vulnerable and that they are not the same people they were before the child's death. The death of a child, or any beloved person, is not something one gets over; rather, as time unfolds, one learns to integrate the loss into one's life. Indeed, grief is a process that is not always orderly and predictable; an individual's unique experience of loss is manifested in diverse ways.

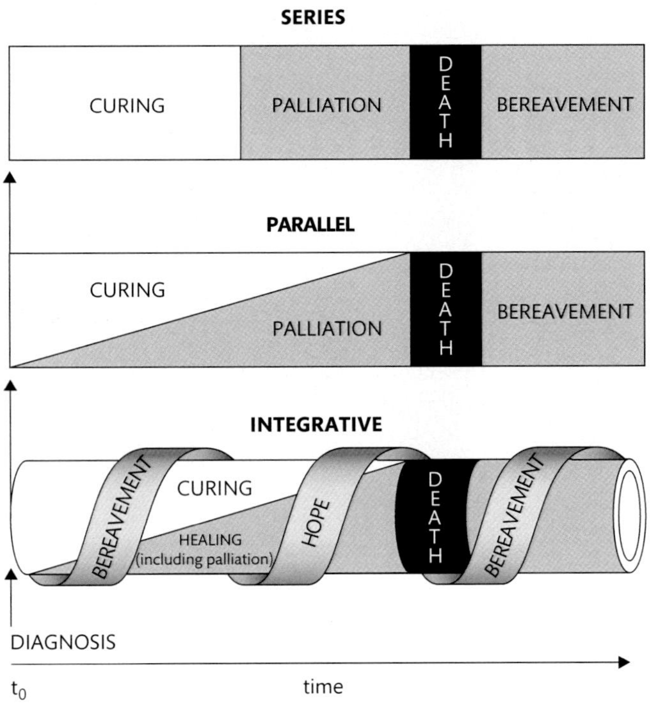

Figure 44.1 Integrative model of curing and healing (with bereavement and hope).
Source: Reference 8.

Grief, Bereavement, and Mourning

The term "grief" is used to refer to the emotional response to a loss.[10] But grief is much more than emotion. Grief is the personalized feeling and response that an individual makes to real, perceived, or anticipated loss or death. Grief encompasses every domain of human life: physical, emotional, psychological, social, and spiritual. Sadness, anger, numbness, sleep and eating disturbances, inability to concentrate, fatigue, existential angst, and tension in interpersonal interactions are among the responses to a loved one's death.

"Disenfranchised grief" arises when an individual's grief is not acknowledged in a social context due to socially stigmatized circumstances of the death, such as suicide, termination of pregnancy, or an early pregnancy loss (miscarriage). Young children, those with cognitive challenges, or even healthcare professionals may also experience disenfranchised grief if they are not expected, and therefore not allowed, to grieve.[11]

"Complicated" or "prolonged grief" refers to a response to loss that is more intense and longer in duration than usual and may include prolonged searching and yearning. Prolonged grief disorder (PGD) is a new diagnostic category that consists of persistent yearning for a year or more, creating suffering, such as meaninglessness, despair, and withdrawal from one's social network.[12] There is some evidence that bereaved parents are slightly more apt to experience PGD[13]; however, the research is insufficient to make a conclusive case.[14]

"Traumatic grief" depends on individual perceptions and experiences; however, these types of death are generally more traumatic than others: death of a child (at any age), homicide and other violence, suicide, severe accident, or disaster-related deaths. Research findings show that traumatic deaths resulted in different ways of finding meaning and making sense of the death and the world than did deaths for which one could prepare.[15]

Grief occurs when an individual experiences a loss deemed personally significant. To a certain degree, who or what we consider to be personally significant is culturally defined. For example, in the contemporary United States, the death of one's child is expected to result in profound grief.[16] Parents suffering from the traumatic loss of a child may be diagnosed with posttraumatic stress disorder (PTSD) by showing symptoms of intrusion, avoidance, negative alterations in cognitions, mood, arousal, and reactivity for at least 1 month.[17] To summarize the epidemiological literature, there is some evidence of an elevated risk of bereaved parents developing mental disorders; however, the research is still insufficient. New data was recently published about PGD and other mental health concerns (complicated grief, depression, PTSD), with one finding showed the birthing parent more at risk for all three conditions.[18]

The term "bereavement" refers to the state of being bereaved or deprived of something. The word derives from the Old English word "reave," which means to plunder, spoil, or rob.[10] This meaning implies the lost object is a valued one. This definition is especially apt for bereaved parents, who often report feeling as though a part of them has been torn away or is missing. As the bereaved mother of a 22-month-old who died sighed, "When my son died, it was as if my heart had been stolen from my breast, and my arms that held him ripped from their sockets."

"Mourning" refers to the outward, social expression of grief—often through ritual—and sometimes to the psychological process of adapting to loss.[19,20] Expression of loss is dictated by cultural norms, customs, and practices, including rituals and traditions. Religious and cultural beliefs and customs may also dictate how long one mourns and how one behaves during the bereavement period; outward expression of loss may be influenced by the individual's personality and life experiences.[21]

For parents of seriously ill children, grief often begins at the time of diagnosis, continues in waves throughout their child's serious illness, and continues long after their child's death. Parents appreciate nurses who understand the many dimensions of grief and support them as they face the challenges of living with grief.

Grief Models

The historical significance of Kübler-Ross (1969)[22] is acknowledged along with her role in opening doors to discussions about dying and death; however, Corr's (2021)[23] conclusions are supported that the Kübler-Ross five-stages model[22] describes the *reactions* and *responses* to a diagnosis of life-threatening illness, not the experience of loss, grief, or bereavement. Her five stages are only a few of the many possible responses that are affected by social, cultural, and situational factors specific to an individual death. The Kübler-Ross descriptive model[22] has mistakenly become widely prescriptive, implying that all grief is the same for everyone. In fact, empirical and scholarly literature does not support the concept of linear stages but rather focuses on grief as an individual's unique and personal process.

Thus, the field has seen a shift from stage models[24] to models that when used *descriptively* (C. M. Parkes, MD, oral communication, June 2007) provide a framework for understanding grief and

Table 44.1 Models of Grief

Stage model	Based on her work as a psychiatrist with hospitalized dying patients, Kübler-Ross (1969)[22] identified five stages of grief: denial, anger, bargaining, depression, and acceptance. Subsequent stage model research with grief after death identified these five stages: despair, yearning, anger, depression, and acceptance.[28]
Work of grief	Effort is put forth in grieving, described as "grief work."[20]
Phases model	Early work in acute grief based on survivors of those who died in the Cocoanut Grove fire in Boston, Lindemann (1944)[24] identified these symptoms: somatic disturbance (e.g., tightness in the throat, shortness of breath or choking), preoccupation with the image of the deceased, guilt (e.g., reviewing behavior that occurred before the death for evidence of negligence and/or failure), feelings of hostility or anger, and difficulty carrying out everyday routines. Grief occurs in *overlapping* phases, which highlights the process of grief as dynamic: numbing, including demonstrating outbursts of anger; searching and yearning; disorganization and despair; and reorganization, a reconstructing of self within the context of loss.[25,29] When the phase model, derived from attachment theory, is used *descriptively*, it provides a framework for understanding grief and bereavement (C. M. Parkes, MD, oral communication, June 2007).
Two-track model	Focuses on both biopsychosocial functioning and relational aspects of grief.[26] Authors recommend the model for helping an individual to rebalance from traumatic grief.
Meaning-making	Constructivist paradigm that emphasizes the role of meaning-making throughout the grieving process.[27]
Dual-process model (DPM)	Entails a duality of coping with alternating restoration and loss orientations.[19] Partner-oriented self-regulation—holding grief in to protect one's partner—brings the DPM into the context of the relationship and family.[30]
Model of relearning the world	Central challenge of grief is relearning and re-establishing all aspects of one's life.[31] Particularly suited to nursing's focus on attending to people's responses to the situation in which they find themselves.[32] Parents are constantly actively involved in regoaling[9] or actively relearning their world.

bereavement,[25] to the two- track model that considers both functioning and relational aspects of grief,[26] to a more constructivist paradigm that emphasizes the role of meaning-making throughout the grieving process,[27] and the duality of coping with alternating restoration and loss orientations.[19] It is important for nurses to understand how various terms, concepts, models, and theories pertaining to grief have progressed over time to conceptualize and make use of the most current knowledge in the field. See Table 44.1 for further explanations.

Grief in the Context of Relationship

Without relationship, there would be no grief; parents, grandparents, siblings, healthcare professionals, and all who cared about the child are affected when death occurs. These next sections reflect the ways relationship influences and is influenced by grief.

Child and Parent

Parent–child relationships are sacred, unique, and complex. The connectedness between parent and child has its roots in the biological and emotional bonds that precede birth. It grows as the parent begins to know and care for the child. Watching a child become sick and die is a crisis of meaning for families, and it is through their cultural understandings and practices that families make sense of this experience.[33] Gender, culture, temperament, and a variety of other factors influence grieving styles. Many parents whose child is receiving palliative care are likely having their first experience with illness, hospitals, medical technology, dying, and death. Consequently, they may have few practiced skills for dealing with significant loss.

A parent's grief can be all-consuming, affecting every aspect of their existence; no two people grieve a shared loss in the same way. Nurses should assess each parent individually to determine how they make sense of their experience and grief. Parents often struggle with guilt throughout their child's illness and following death because of deep-rooted feelings of responsibility for their child's welfare. Parents are responsible for protecting and sustaining their children[34] and shielding them from all danger; many parents feel they should have protected their child from illness and death. When children die from an inherited disease, such as cystic fibrosis or sickle cell anemia, parents know that their child's condition results from their unknowingly passing on the genetic material.[35]

Bereaved parents may cling to guilt because it is often easier to accept blame, with its fantasy of control, than it is to accept the total loss of control with their child's death. For example, one young mother's intense guilt was rooted in her belief that her baby's premature birth and eventual death were caused by her eating too many spicy foods early in pregnancy. Parents may also blame someone else for their child's death. Sometimes this guilt is targeted toward a partner or spouse or another child or family member. Nurses should be aware of these dynamics and help parents find an appropriate place for their anger and blame.[34]

Professionals who support bereaved parents are attuned to parents' own descriptions of being different after their child died. Gilmer and colleagues[36] found that changes in bereaved parents occurred primarily in two realms: in their personal lives (e.g., emotions, beliefs, work habits) and in relationships. Parents themselves reported changes in priorities, while their surviving children noted the intensity of their parents' sadness.[36] Davies and Limbo[37 (p.78)] share the story of one mother who asked her college-age son, "Did I change?" Her son was in grade school when his brother—and, a year later, his sister—were stillborn. Her son was flabbergasted that she was not aware of how different she was from the way she had been before the loss of her babies. He responded, "You were never happy, you stopped being a room mother or participating with any of our sports teams. You cried all the time."

The death of a child can affect the parents' relationship with each other. Odds of divorce are higher after miscarriage or stillbirth,[38] and the rate of relationship dissolution after such a loss increases for both married and cohabiting partners.[39] Some bereaved parents experience unique interpersonal dynamics when attempting to hold in their own grief in order to spare their partner, increasing their own and their partner's grief over time, a phenomenon termed "partner-oriented self-regulation."[30(p395)] Nurses who work with bereaved parents may hear one parent say, "I feel like I need to be strong for her" or "If he sees how I'm hurting, I don't think he can deal with it." Listening for such expressions provides nurses with insight into couple dynamics and can inform follow-up supportive interventions.

Nurses must also be cognizant of the special needs of those bereaved parents who cope with additional stressors in their everyday lives. Single parents or same-sex parents may not have as many options for support as married parents in a heterosexual relationship. Black and Fields[40] provide several clinical practice guidelines for nurses and others caring for lesbian couples who experience perinatal loss, including recognizing the complexity of always needing a third party to get pregnant; understanding the financial, legal, and social ramifications of achieving the pregnancy; and considering that the couple may feel disenfranchised in their bereavement by those who judge their lifestyle choices. Same-sex couples whose baby dies appreciate being treated as any bereaved couple, not considered different or unusual as they navigate factors associated with their pregnancy and subsequent loss.[40]

Child and Grandparents

The grief of grandparents is twofold: they grieve the loss of their grandchild, and they must also bear witness to the grief of their own child, the parent of the ill child. Grandparents also experience pain from their own past losses, along with pain common to all grief, and witnessing negative changes in their child, termed a "cumulative pain."[41] Grandparents identified two factors highly relevant to nursing care that helped them with their grief: having their loss acknowledged and being considered a part of the bereaved family.[41] Nurses should hold in mind that grandparents have their own unique needs in the moments surrounding their grandchild's end-of-life care, especially if they experienced the death of one of their own children or siblings many years prior.

Impact of Family Dynamics on Relationship

Families have characteristic ways of being in the world, of solving problems, of managing crises, of interacting with one another, and of relating to those outside the family. When a child is seriously ill and dies, families respond in the ways that are typical of how they manage other life events. Past experiences with death and the learned response to loss also affect how each family member will grieve a child's death. Other deaths of a similar nature may have occurred in the family, such as when more than one child suffers from the same life-threatening genetic disorder or when grandparents experienced the death of their own baby years ago.

Researchers of families with adults[42] and with children who had serious illness[43] documented eight dimensions of family functioning: communicating openly, dealing with feelings, defining roles, solving problems, using resources, incorporating changes, considering others, and confronting beliefs. These dimensions occur along a continuum of functionality so that family interactions tend to vary along the continuum rather than being positive–negative or good–bad.[43] Family members are better able to manage their grief and support one another in families where thoughts and opinions are expressed freely without fear of recrimination, where a wide range of feelings is expressed and differences are tolerated, where roles are flexible and problem-solving instead of blaming is the pattern for dealing with challenges, where families are able to ask for and receive assistance from others, and where beliefs and values are confronted and examined. Through establishing relationships with a child and family, nurses bear witness to the family's functioning in both happy and difficult moments, which in turn provides important insight into supportive measures that would best honor their grief and bereavement.

Child and Siblings

Siblings often develop special bonds that are unlike any other. The closer two siblings are to one another before death, the more behavior problems the surviving sibling may have following the death.[43] Siblings may be forgotten as grievers; even teenagers may feel overlooked. Parents are often so overcome with grief they may have little energy for the needs of their surviving children. The impact of a child's death on surviving siblings is manifested in four general responses, best characterized in the words of the children themselves: "I hurt inside," "I don't understand," "I don't belong," and "I'm not enough."[43,44] Not all bereaved siblings experience all four responses, but most demonstrate all responses to varying degrees.

"I hurt inside." This first response includes all the emotions typically associated with grief—sadness, anger, frustration, loneliness, fear, guilt, restlessness, and a host of other emotions. Unlike adults, who talk about their grief, children manifest their responses in various behaviors, such as withdrawing, seeking attention, acting out, arguing, fear of going to bed at night, overeating, or undereating. In response to children who are hurting inside, nurses need to allow, and even encourage, the expression of the hurt the children are feeling. Nurses can share their own feelings to let children know that they are not alone in this situation. If adults do not allow for or facilitate expression of feelings, children learn that there is something wrong with such feelings and may suppress what is on their minds and in their hearts.

"I don't understand." Children's difficulty in understanding death is greatly influenced by their level of cognitive development. However, once children know about death, their cognitive worlds are forever altered. Without guidance from adults in helping them to understand the death in clear, simple, and age-appropriate ways, children make up their own explanations, which usually involve taking responsibility for their sibling's death and their parents' distress. Without explanations, they can become more frightened and insecure. Nurses working with siblings should have a solid grasp of children's cognitive development, provide appropriate explanations for events that happen, and be open to supporting the family as questions from siblings arise.

"I don't belong." A death in the family disrupts the usual day-to-day activities and patterns of living. Surviving children are overwhelmed with the flurry of activity and the depth of emotion surrounding them after the death. They often feel uncertain about what to do; they may want to help, but they do not know how, or, if they try, their efforts are often not acknowledged by grieving family members. Bereaved siblings may feel as if they are in the way or as if they are not a part of what is happening. They feel different from their peers as well and begin to feel that they do not belong anymore. During a sibling's illness, nurses play a critical role in encouraging parents to include siblings in care-related events, such as holding their sibling's hand or blowing bubbles together for distraction during procedures. After death, the nurse can help the parents by modeling or guiding exploration of what to say to the surviving siblings.

"I'm not enough." Assuming that they are somehow responsible for their parents' distress, surviving siblings may feel as if they are not enough to make their parents happy ever again. They may feel their deceased sibling was the favorite child and that they should have been the ones to die instead. Some siblings respond by striving to be as good as they can be, trying to prove that they are worthy. Moreover, surviving siblings may not want to burden their parents with their own feelings and may keep the depth of their grief private. Bereaved siblings benefit from feeling accepted just for being themselves and not from being compared with their deceased brother or sister. Nurses can assist siblings to feel special by asking questions about their lives and acknowledging their unique characteristics or abilities.

Children and Adolescents at the End of Life

Assessing and responding to a child's experience of serious illness are the very essence of palliative care provision. Children experience their own disease progression and impending death within their cognitive and emotional capabilities, and they communicate such feelings to others as they are able.[45] They live and die as children but often with much apparent wisdom, sometimes seeming to surpass that of their adult caregivers. Researchers found that very ill children are indeed aware of death and are more anxious than children hospitalized for nonserious illnesses or nonhospitalized children.[46] Adolescents with a terminal disease are sensitive to their parents' reactions and have a strong desire to maintain relationships with their friends, regardless of their illness status: "I couldn't say anything with my Mom. She pretends to smile to me, but I know how she feels so sad whenever looking at me. I want to come out and share my emotions with my friends at least. But now there is nobody around me."

Children and teens with terminal illness often wish to please their parents, and parents may want their child to maintain hope and not give up, resulting in barriers to honest communication.[47] In such cases, nurses can honor the feelings of all involved while helping family members to open to the possibility of truthfully sharing perspectives, hopes, and grief.

Child and the Healthcare Team

Professionals who care for children with serious illness are constantly reminded of the frailty and preciousness of life. From the very beginning moments of awareness that a child will not survive, healthcare professionals hold much in mind and heart as they guide the family in the early phases of end-of-life decision-making.[48] When a child dies, healthcare professionals experience their own grief and miss the relationship once shared through daily communication with the child and family.[49] In one study of nurses' experiences following the death of a child,[50] participants described two types of distress: (1) *moral distress* resulted when the nurses knew the child's death was imminent and were required to carry out painful treatments they perceived as unnecessary and (2) *grief distress* occurred in response to the child's death. Both types of distress resulted from lack of open communication within the care team and lack of consideration of the nurses' viewpoints.[50]

Working with children at the end of life can also trigger nurses' awareness of their own personal losses and fears about their own death, the death of their own children, and mortality in general.[48] The process is complicated by cumulative loss—that is, a succession of losses experienced by nurses who work with patients with life-threatening illness and their families, often on a daily basis.[50] Nurses who work in settings where death occurs frequently seldom have time to grieve one child before the next death occurs on their unit.

Papadatou[51] describes how healthcare professionals manage grief, as they fluctuate between both experiencing and avoiding intense emotions. She notes that professionals are profoundly affected by what is required of them in working with children and bereaved parents, and, as such, they learn to regulate their grief in clinical settings.[51] For example, a nurse may cry at a child's bedside and be fully present to a father who has just watched the removal of his child's ventilator. Later that day, the same nurse may avoid the intensity of the emotions garnered from the child's death to engage in a dinner out with her family.

Understanding the normalcy of the grief responses provides healthcare professionals with an awareness of how they can simultaneously support families and themselves. Papadatou proposes that meanings are attributed to death and dying through grieving, that grief complications occur when there is no fluctuation, and that grief provides opportunities for personal growth.[51] Other researchers have found that caring for children at the end of life provides opportunities for such growth and transformation as healthcare professionals report finding meaning and enhanced life views through their work.[52]

Assessing Grief throughout the Trajectory of Care

Bereavement care is interdisciplinary in nature, with all team members collaborating to understand the experiences of each individual's grief, as well as those of the family as a whole. Grief assessment begins when the child is diagnosed with serious illness and continues throughout disease progression, transition to end of life, death, and aftercare. Five questions serve as a simple way for pediatric palliative teams to learn more about parents' perception of their child's needs and key issues: Who is your child as a person? What is your understanding of your child's illness (or condition today)? What are your hopes? What are your worries? What sustains you or gives you strength?[53,54]

These questions, followed by respectful probes such as "What are the most important things we should address for you and your child right now?" or "What do you think should happen next?"[54] can help to elicit what is weighing heaviest on parents' minds and serve as a bridge to learning more about their feelings. In addition, statements such as "This feels so difficult" or "Other parents/children have told me ... it sounds like this is similar to you" can aid in acknowledging experiences and open a way for eventual sharing of tender feelings.

During such interactions, nurses should also be mindful of periods of extended silence because there may be much that the child or parent is holding deep inside that cannot yet be spoken aloud.[45] Honoring silence in a compassionate manner offers the child or parent the opportunity to focus on these private thoughts or grief that may eventually be spoken aloud and shared with a trusted healthcare professional.[45,55] Nurses can introduce deliberate quiet spaces during caring conversations while allowing the child/family the opportunity to lead out of the silence as they are ready.[55]

Family Assessment

The nurse's role is to assess each family's way of functioning and to realize that some families are more challenging to assess and work with than others. For example, some families may not wish to share information in the presence of their children, others do not wish to discuss matters with any relatives in the room, while other families include everyone in most discussions. Thus, it is important for the nurse to gather information over time and to talk with more than one family member to appreciate the varied perspectives. As trusted relationships are established with the child and family, the nurse can assess family functioning with questions such as "What have you done in the past when you had a difficult decision to make?" or "Can you help me to know how your family found their way through previous losses (or deaths)."[54] Responses to such questions can help the nurse identify strategies that will honor and facilitate the family's grief work.

Factors Affecting the Grief Experience

In assessing grief, the healthcare team should keep in mind the range of factors that affect the grief of family members while noting those factors that put individuals and families at risk for disenfranchised or complicated grief. The passage of time is not a useful consideration in assessing grief responses; instead, one should assess the degree of grief's intrusiveness into each family member's life and the extent to which they can carry out their usual activities.

Decisions made at the end of life may have left parents second-guessing or wondering afterward about their choices. Lasting images or smells may be comforting or concerning to families, depending on their associations. In fact, pain or other distressing symptoms the child might have experienced provide powerful material for families to process during their grief.[13] Death following years of treatment is experienced very differently from a death that happens quickly. Where or when a child died can also impact the family's grief. Ideally, the location (home or hospital) of a child's death is based on the family's specific needs and requests, but circumstances (insurance issues, nursing shortages, transportation issues) may preclude achieving this goal. Long-term outcomes for bereaved parents and siblings suggest an early pattern of differential adjustment in favor of home-care deaths.[56]

When families convey less functional capacity, practitioners may choose to explore their experiences and offer potential resources one at a time, with considerable attention paid to the possible disruption that would result from each suggestion. In more functional families, a list of possible options can be presented and considered all at once. Most families value the opportunity to tell their story. Thus, listening becomes a central aspect of assessing and caring for all grieving families.

Interventions and Supporting the Bereaved

Nurses play a central role in a family's initial bereavement experience, holding in mind the family's sense of loss while pursuing with interdisciplinary team members (e.g., social workers, chaplains) care that addresses the bereaved family's well-being. Most children's deaths still occur in the hospital; nurses are most often present at the time of death. The nurse's words and actions at that time leave indelible imprints upon family members. The next section explores models of practice and strategies for supporting bereaved individuals as they grieve the loss of a beloved baby or child.

Perinatal and Pediatric Palliative Care—A Model of Exemplary Practice

Parents in perinatal or pediatric palliative care are deeply affected not only by what nurses say but also by what they do and how they convey a sense of connection with, caring about, and compassion for individual parents and their seriously ill or deceased baby or child.[57] Supportive interaction is especially important for non-English-speaking and socially and economically disadvantaged parents. Insensitive interactions with caregivers threaten parents' well-being during the entire course of their child's illness and death, into bereavement.

Relatively little attention has been directed to helping nurses focus on optimal interaction. Davies and colleagues'[57] research identified what makes it possible for some nurses more than others, despite facing the same constraints, to engage in excellent or exemplary interactions with parents of children with life-threatening conditions. Research participants included nurses as well as providers from several disciplines; exemplary care was evident across disciplines, but in this chapter, we refer specifically to how the resulting model of exemplary practice can help nurses practice perinatal/pediatric palliative care in a way that ensures parents are supported as human beings and helps nurses feel that they are doing what they entered their profession to do.

Davies and her colleagues[57] use a metaphorical prairie windmill to represent their findings (see Figure 44.2). The windmill model[57] shows how the many components of exemplary practice fit together, are interrelated and of equal importance, and result in optimal outcomes and how each component is essential but insufficient in and of itself to achieve optimal interaction. For example, nurses can be adept at carrying out one or more components of practice (such as skill completing certain procedures or showing empathy for grieving parents), thus being seen as providing very good care; but it is only when nurses carry out all components of the model that they are perceived to be exemplary.

The Windmill Model

The wind puts windmill blades into action; similarly, nurses' encounters with parents initiate an interaction. A rudder turns the blades in the direction of the wind to optimally capture the wind's energy. Likewise, optimal engagement with parents is guided by

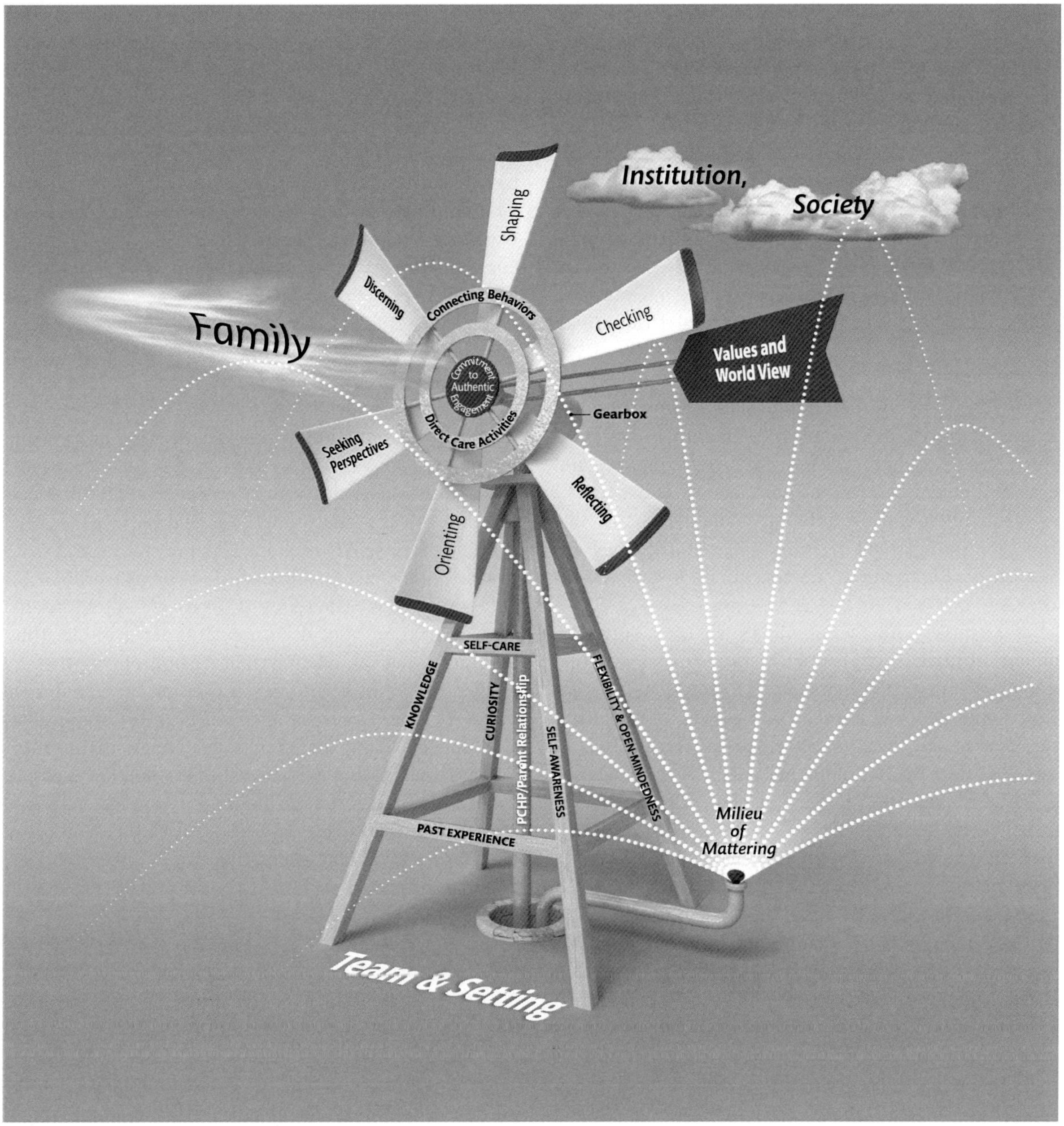

Figure 44.2 Exemplary practice in pediatric palliative care model.
Source: Reference 57.

nurses' expansive *worldview* whereby they perceive the many facets of the human condition as interconnected and interrelated and applying to all persons; as one nurse described, "If I think of what grounds me in my work, it's my worldview ... knowing that there will always be life and death, distress and joy—both are part of what all life is."[57] Inherent in this worldview are *values* of respect for the worth of all persons, diversity, social justice, family-centered care, and personal and professional integrity. A windmill's hub is the central point where all moving parts come together to ensure the viability of the windmill. Likewise, for exemplary interaction to occur, nurses' *commitment to authentic engagement* means they aim to know parents as people, not just as parents, and to collaborate with them as partners in the child's care and support them in their grief. The blades are central to a windmill's function; similarly, exemplary interaction requires that nurses *attune to the particularities of the situation in the moment* (via orienting, seeking parents' perspectives, discerning, sharing, checking, and reflecting), that is, responding to parents according to their individual situation and what matters most to them at the time.

Stabilizing bands ensure the stability of windmill blades. For exemplary interaction, an inner stabilizing band represents the direct care activities that all healthcare providers are obligated to carry out as part of their professional role. These activities include *doing for* parents what they cannot do for themselves (e.g., carrying out procedures) and *empowering* behaviors (teaching, sharing information, navigating, supporting) that enable parents to do what they want and need to do for themselves. The second stabilizing band represents *connecting behaviors* (e.g., listening, empathizing, showing kindness) that permeate every aspect of nurse–parent encounters; each is necessary but not sufficient on its own for optimal attuning.

Legs and struts provide a supporting framework. Exemplary interactions are supported by *personal influencing factors* (depth and breadth of nurses' knowledge, curiosity, flexibility/open mindedness, and self-awareness) as well as by their past experiences and self-care. Additionally, a windmill is subject to the climatic conditions that surround it. Likewise, nurses are influenced by the context in which they practice: the setting, their team's functioning and institutional leadership, and societal factors, such as societal attitudes toward death. Exemplary palliative care nurses recognize and operate from seeing that attachment, love, loss, and grief are integral to the human condition.

The windmill's conversion of the wind's energy into mechanical energy results in pumping the groundwater that sustains life. Similarly, the energy formed by exemplary interaction is expressed in a professional and meaningful relationship between nurses and parents. The coming together of all the components of exemplary interaction creates a milieu (or social climate) of mattering that, like the nourishing water pumped out by a windmill, optimally sustains parents during times of extreme duress and nurses in their exemplary practice.

The model of exemplary interaction shows what is involved in producing milieus of mattering.[57] It teaches nurses to ask not only "What is the matter?" but also "What matters to you?" "What matters to you in this moment?" In a milieu of mattering, parents and exemplary nurses alike feel that they and their concerns matter to each other and that they are not alone in facing the challenges of caring for the child at the end of life and of supporting parents in grief following their child's death. Parents feel that they and their family members are treated with respect and human dignity.

Similarly, exemplary nurses feel that they are valued and respected by parents. Both perceive a sense of cohesion, of belonging, and that they are in it together. Parents feel that exemplary nurses relate to them as fellow human beings, as companions in dealing with one of life's most challenging experiences. Importantly, in this milieu parents freely express their appreciation to exemplary nurses who, in turn feel valued by the parents. Both exemplary nurses and parents feel that they are making a difference in the lives of one another, an important illustration of societal mattering. Further, while working within their team to make a difference in the lives of families, exemplary nurses engage in exemplary interactions with their colleagues and contribute to team members feeling that they too belong and matter to each other.

Model of Exemplary Practice: Reflection and Self-Awareness for Nurses

The windmill model[57] offers guidance about how to achieve exemplary practice by optimally interacting with others. The model directs nurses to ask of those in their care what matters to them, but it also emphasizes that nurses are persons and professionals, thus encouraging nurses to ask, What matters to me? In thinking about this question, three components of the model come into play: reflecting, worldview/values, and self-awareness.

Reflecting is a vital component of the process of attuning where exemplary nurses purposefully step back and think about what they are doing: What happened here? What can I learn from this situation? But reflecting also is inherent in examination of nurses' own worldview/values and the focus of their commitment by asking multiple questions of themselves: How did I come to be who I am today? What positive or negative childhood experiences about death or grief do I carry with me, and how do they affect my worldview? Do I see myself as being interrelated to all other human beings, and how does that perception relate to how I support grieving parents? What have I learned about life, living, and dying from contact with people who are different than I am? How is it that I ended up doing the work that I do now? What is my level of commitment to authentic engagement with others? Have I even considered that concept before now?[57]

Reflecting is also closely related to self-awareness, which involves acknowledging one's own internal signals (thoughts, feelings, or bodily sensations) that something is out of line and needs attention. It is clear from the model that nurses need to understand themselves and their own strengths and weaknesses so that they can continually self-monitor for potential biases and act as needed to correct such biases, asking questions such as: Do I ever pause and think about the feelings and thoughts that arise in me as a child is dying? Or when caring for grieving parents? When I think about my life or my work, do I feel joy or sadness, anxiety? Do I find meaning in my work?[57]

In their book, Davies et al.[57] provide questions to guide personal reflection about all components of the model, thus facilitating learning about the relational dimension of care that is inherent in self-learning and is integral to exemplary neonatal and pediatric palliative care. As such, the model is useful in teaching nurses and all clinicians about the interconnectedness that predisposes to the feelings of mattering that are at the very heart of exemplary practice. Indeed, the model reflects something that has been inferred in the literature but not made explicit—that is, the components of exemplary provider/parent interaction *can* be identified, described, and taught and learned.

Middle-Range Theory: Guided Participation for Clinical Practice

Guided participation for clinical practice (GP) is a middle-range theory of teaching and learning designed for all levels of clinical practice and applicable when providing grief and bereavement care.[58,59] GP fosters caring for diverse families in an inclusive way as the teacher/guide (the nurse) focuses on identifying the learner's (child or parent's) unique needs and then applies GP strategies to achieve a mutually decided upon goal. GP fosters relationship-focused care and is a dynamic method for adapting to changes in a child's or parent's supportive or learning needs as goals are set and reset during caring interactions.[59]

There are three components in the GP model: processes, competencies, and issues.[58] Figure 44.3 provides a visual depiction of how GP components work together, along with descriptions for each. Nurses using GP can begin with any one of the three GP components (i.e., starting at any point of the triangle in Figure 44.3). For example, the teacher/guide may first identify an issue in the child's care (e.g., the nurse assessing a family's preferences for being with their child who is dying), the need for a competency (e.g., the parent articulating end-of-life care choices that would be meaningful), or the focus for a process (e.g., joining attention between the teacher/guide [nurse] and learner [parent] to discuss the issues at hand together). From there, the nurse can choose the next point in the GP triangle to build caring interactions.

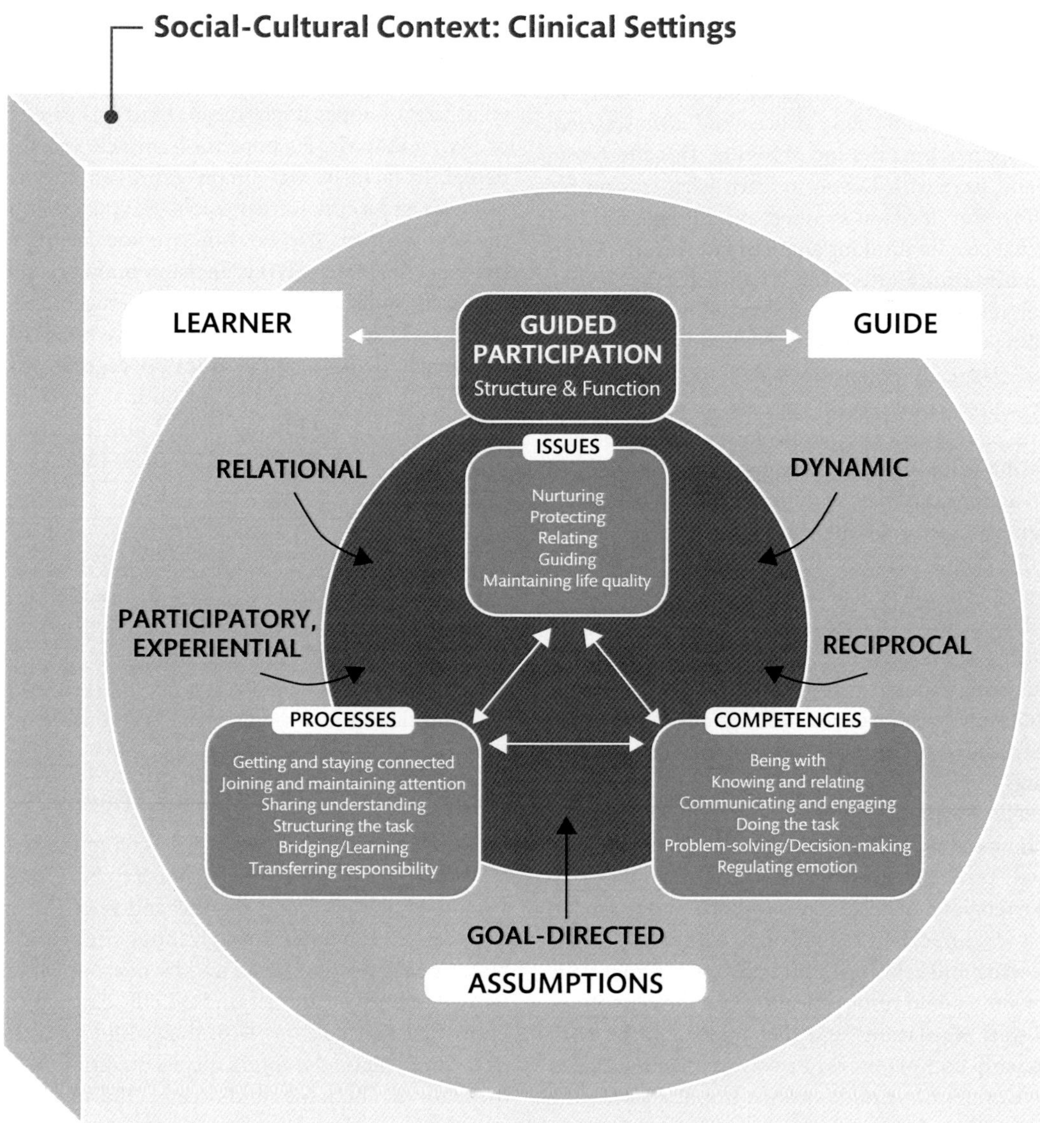

Figure 44.3 Guided participation issues, processes, and competencies triangle. Reproduced with permission from Limbo R. et al.
Source: Reference 59.

When first meeting a grieving child or family, it is helpful for healthcare professionals to begin by mindfully assessing all that is going on. The GP process of *getting and staying connected* works well to help establish relationship with the family and to foster the GP competencies of *being with and knowing* and *relating to the other* (see Figure 44.3). For example, when a young boy with terminal cancer shared quietly that his Lego superhero figure could "probably fly up all the way to heaven, too," his palliative nurse used this interest in his toy figures to establish rapport that eventually led to the boy disclosing how he would miss his family and toys when he died.

GP depends on sustaining a relationship, and such relationships are strengthened through holding another in mind, that is, being thought about in one's absence. A nurse can convey holding a child or family in mind by simply sharing, "I've thought about what you asked me yesterday before I left" or "I smiled this morning as I was getting ready for work, thinking of Jeremy's smile." Being in relationship may also mean sitting together quietly in the child's room, with both parents and the healthcare professional realizing that gaining trust and being with can also occur in moments of silence, when words are difficult to utter aloud.

The GP process of *joining and maintaining attention*, also referred to as "joint attention," requires that guide and learner understand whatever the issue is in a like manner—that is, that they share understanding.[59] Numerous potential issues could result in lack of shared understanding, such as navigating the complex needs that arise for the grieving family as a child's condition significantly deteriorates. In such moments, both the family and the child's team will experience a shift from familiar interactions to new, more uncertain situations.[60] The relationships that support a GP approach to teaching and learning can result in a shared understanding between family and team that results in meaningful actions, such as those in the following case study: the processes, competencies, and issues of GP and their application to a nurse guide, an adolescent, and the adolescent's grandparent and primary parent. GP processes, competencies, and issues are highlighted in bold.

Case Study

Adolescent palliative care nurse Brad had cared for 16-year-old Devon for several days. Devon's bone cancer had metastasized; Devon knew he was approaching the end of his life. This afternoon, Brad wanted to spend time with Devon to learn what was on his mind. Brad saw that Devon's face was strained, even though he rated his pain as a "3." "What are you thinking about today, Devon?" (**process: joining and maintaining attention**). "I wish Nana (Devon's primary caregiver all his childhood) would stop talking about miracles. She keeps telling me not to give up hope, that God performs miracles all the time" (**issue: divergent views on hope**).

Through further conversation, Brad engaged as a guide with Devon to explore his values, the expectations he had about the end of his life, and what he would like to see happen with his beloved Nana. "I want her to understand that I'm dying and it's OK" (**competency: emotion regulation through identifying his goal**).

Brad knew Devon's Nana (aka Ms. B.) was coming to visit in about an hour. He arranged his patient care responsibilities so that he could visit with Devon and Ms. B. together. Brad's GP processes would focus on joining attention and a shared understanding between Devon and his Nana about how hope could still be relevant for both. "Could you talk to your Nana about your goals?" Brad asked Devon (**process: structuring the task; competency: communicating and engaging**).

Brad remembered how experts write about the cultural aspects of hope,[61] describing how often clinicians incorrectly use the stigmatizing term "in denial," especially for African American families who possess deeply held religious beliefs linked to hope and miracles. Brad believed that it was important for Devon to witness his Nana's **competence** in **knowing and relating** to him during this final stage of his life. This discussion could result in feeling that their emotions were in sync (**emotion regulation**) and that they could **be with each other** (**relationship competency**) in a way that demonstrated shared goals about Devon's impending death without abandoning hope. Developing these shared goals was the centerpiece of the identified issue as Brad reflected on his conversation with Devon. He saw his role as guide to engage Devon and his Nana about what their mutual hopes might be.

(The following are *excerpts* of the conversation among Devon, his Nana, and Brad that highlight GP. They are not intended to represent the entire conversation.) Brad saw Ms. B. approach Devon's room and wanted them to have some private time. When Brad came into the room, the three talked about what Devon's Nana had done in the past days and how Devon was feeling. Devon's Nana then reminded him that the prayer circle at their church was praying for a miracle, and she was sure their prayers would be answered. Brad took this as a door opening to a conversation about hope and miracles. "Ms. B (Nana), what do you think a miracle would look like for Devon?" (**process: bridging**). "Well, I hope it means that he would be cured." Brad brought both Devon and his Nana into the conversation by **transferring responsibility** to Devon by asking, "Devon, if the miracle of a cure doesn't happen, what else might you be hoping for?" (**process: sharing understanding; structuring the task**). "That I'd do OK with my pain." "Ms. B., I think you and Devon might be able to figure out a set of hopes, in other words, how would it be if the two of you could agree that you might have more than one hope?" (**process: joining and maintaining attention; extending sharing understanding**). The room was quiet. Brad recognized that the three of them were sharing in a meaningful moment of silence that likely meant that Ms. B. and Devon had **joint attention**, considering what a set of hopes might mean. Brad was careful to avoid thinking or saying that Ms. B.'s hope for a miracle was the same as being in denial. In fact, she was simply expressing her religious belief that miracles and a cure were possible. Having other hopes did not erase the one she had. "Devon, how are you feeling right now?" (**competency: problem solving/decision making; emotion regulation**). "I'm glad Nana and I could talk to you together. I love you so much, Nana, and I am happy we can each have hope" (**issue: maintaining life quality; competency: emotion regulation**). "Ms. B., do you think your prayers could be for both a cure and pain relief?" Brad asked (**competency: being with, knowing and relating, decision making**). "I'll think about that. I know I want to do the best for my Devon."

As exemplified in this case study, GP processes and competencies provide a dynamic framework to address the issues faced by children and families in palliative care settings. Readers are encouraged to refer to Figure 44.3 showing the GP model and reflect on how they may incorporate aspects of GP into their daily practice when initiating and maintaining relationship with the families in their care.

Being Present for the Bereaved Family

Healthcare professionals may fear saying the wrong thing to a bereaved family member or may worry about not knowing what to say amid such profound sadness and grief. A compassionate presence can be conveyed through thoughtful words acknowledging a family's love for their child and by bearing witness to their experience. A nurse can sit or stand quietly, close to the family, let them know that they can stay with their child for as long as they would like, comment on the child's special qualities, and acknowledge their own sadness about the child's death. Offering to help in practical and concrete ways also conveys a caring presence.

Most family members have a need to share their story, telling and retelling anecdotes about the child and the events of their living and dying. For some families, reviewing what happened during their child's end-of-life care with the healthcare team is critical. Bereaved parents report that parent–physician bereavement meetings following their child's death helped them to understand the biomedical reasons for the death and to review their decision-making, resulting in making sense, finding benefit, staying connected with their child, and reconstructing their parental identity.[62]

Follow-up telephone calls or visits with the team members who cared for the child are much appreciated by families. This is especially true for those parents who, over the many years of their child's care, developed close relationships with their child's team members. Such families worry that the team will forget their deceased child; some families want to maintain an ongoing connection with those who cared for their child.[63] Thus, during the transition after the child's death, families and staff must navigate the changing relationship.

Preparing Bereaved Parents for Their Grief Experience

Many parents who are unaware of the normal manifestations of grief can find some comfort in knowing that their experience is normal. Providing either written or virtual resources about the common facts of grief can be helpful. Understanding that each person's grief experience is unique helps parents understand that there is no single right way to grieve. It also helps them realize that it is okay if they do not express their grief in the same ways that other family members do. Team members should identify any need for additional assistance and make referrals as necessary to those interdisciplinary professionals who can assist with ongoing grief support in the community.

Supporting Bereaved Grandparents

Grandparents, like their adult children, benefit from compassionate bereavement support that honors their life experiences. Healthcare professionals should be especially attentive to those grandparents who were actively involved in their grandchild's daily care. In one study, researchers found that grandparents who provided childcare for their grandchild experienced more intense symptoms of grief, depression, and PTSD than grandparents who were not directly involved in caregiving.[64] Grandparents report valuing the opportunity to participate in intergenerational perinatal bereavement programs, receiving support with the entire family following a perinatal death.[65]

Grief Support for Children and Teens

Bereaved siblings may harbor lingering questions and concerns along with the normal manifestations of grief; they can be at risk for negative long-term outcomes of a brother's or sister's death. How adults and other providers respond to children's and adolescents' grief has the potential to intensify the risk of problem behaviors or, conversely, to promote healing and health. Adults' ability to optimally support grieving siblings depends in large part on their understanding of the typical or normal reactions that characterize siblings' grief and siblings' reactions as an attempt to make sense of the death and to act out their distress.

Like adults, children feel denial, anger, sadness, guilt, and longing in response to the loss of a loved one. They may experience lack of sleep, lack of appetite, and difficulty concentrating and maintaining usual patterns of interaction with others. However, most children have limited ability to verbalize and describe their feelings; they also have limited capacity to tolerate the emotional pain generated by open recognition of their loss.[66] Moreover, children's cognitive developmental levels interfere with their ability to understand the irreversibility, universality, and inevitability of death and to understand the reactions of their parents. They also deeply fear being different in any way from their peers and, therefore, are often unable to find comfort, as adults do, in sharing their discomfort with their friends.

Play is the work and the language of childhood, so children are often able to express their feelings through their play, as well as through music and art. Bereaved children will benefit from spending time with art therapists, music therapists, or child life specialists who can foster creative avenues for children to process their experiences and grief.[67] During an art therapy session with clay, a young girl carefully and quietly made a creation, then smashed it flat. After observing her repeat this action, the art therapist inquired what she was thinking about. Following more silence, the girl eventually confided that she heard when someone dies, they get a new body, so she was trying to figure out what her new body would look like. This confession was the first time she expressed an understanding of her terminal condition and opened the door for honest communication among the child, her parents, and team.

Self-help support groups for teens, either in person or online, often prove valuable to grieving adolescents. Adolescents are often open to writing, art, or music when working through their grief. Adults should take care to follow the adolescents' lead, respecting confidentiality and permitting them to interpret the significance of their grief work in their own way.

Bereavement Support Groups for Siblings

The goal of bereavement support groups is to normalize children's grief experiences. Programs do vary in structure and format (depending on the setting, resources, and intent), with some being time-limited and others ongoing, and with some being curriculum-based and others nondirective. Efforts are directed toward providing a safe, contained environment in which bereaved children can share their experiences and can ably chart their own course through grief, rather than simply accommodating the wishes of others.[68] The National Alliance of Grieving Children, formed in 2004, provides resources and education on the many children's bereavement programs and models (www.nacg.org).

Bereavement support groups provide children with opportunities to express their emotions, including the hurt, sadness, and pain associated with grief. Art supplies, musical instruments, outdoor and indoor play equipment, quiet corners, rituals—all serve this purpose. Being with others in similar circumstances, children can listen to and learn from them about their experiences with death and grief. From the adult leaders, siblings also can learn such things as the facts about various illnesses, treatments, or dying and death, thus helping to clarify any misunderstandings they might have. Groups are not for everyone. Depending on their individual preference, preexisting mental health, behavior, or family system challenges, some grieving siblings and/or their families might benefit more from individual or family therapy. Thus, orientation sessions about support groups must be conducted prior to children joining a peer support group to assess the fit between each child and the program.[68]

Supporting Grieving Healthcare Professionals

Caring for dying children requires nurses to explore, experience, and express their personal feelings regarding death. Reflection is a key process for pediatric palliative care nurses in being with the child and family before, during, and after death.[48,57] The PRAM model can be helpful for nurses in their daily practice; PRAM incorporates reflection and self-awareness as one *P*auses, *R*eflects on what is happening, *A*cknowledges one's feelings and thoughts, and is *M*indful when starting a patient care encounter.[6] The model for exemplary practice[57] offers numerous questions that nurses can use to reflect on their interactions with children and families.

Knowing oneself is a lifelong process essential to personal and professional well-being through mindful reflection on personal beliefs, preferences, strengths, and challenges.[69] Self-awareness about one's own history of loss and one's own beliefs about death, dying, and the afterlife is essential to ensure that our personal preferences do not interfere with the experience of the family. Personal death-awareness activities and exercises, discussion of belief systems about death/afterlife with friends and colleagues, self-exploration, and reflection may promote an understanding and acceptance of death as part of life.

Nurses have responsibilities for acknowledging their own personal and professional limitations, seeking assistance, and engaging in self-care activities.[69] They must give themselves permission, space, and time to process feelings when a beloved patient dies and to regulate when and how to become connected in relationship again with the next child and family.[69] Free-writing, journaling, poetry, music, art, ritual—all have a place in processing professional experiences of grief.[69] Nurses also benefit from processing the impact of shared patient losses with their team members. When the death of a child resonates throughout the child's entire team, opportunities for group reflection can be helpful, especially if the death occurred unexpectedly or was traumatic to the team.[70] In such situations, facilitation of team processing should be offered using differing strategies over time to meet the unique needs of each grieving healthcare professional.[69,70]

Hospital Bereavement Programs

Development of interdisciplinary perinatal and pediatric bereavement programs in healthcare institutions has increased notably despite budget and resource concerns.[71,72] A bereavement program within a pediatric palliative care program or as part of an agency or system-wide initiative can be of considerable service to both families and staff. These services typically include staff with specific training in bereavement care and a follow-up component.[8] An interdisciplinary bereavement team ensures that all families are educated on and supported in their grief and are made aware of available services, such as support groups, memorial services, or grief workshops. Bereavement program leaders facilitate family referral to grief therapists as needed and may also help bereaved families to be with one another as a source of support. Parents report feeling supported by staff through hospital bereavement programs and value the opportunities offered by such programs to grieve and stay connected with their deceased child.[71,72] In addition to helping bereaved families, institutional bereavement programs serve the needs of staff. Programs can be structured to offer help in debriefing after a death, validating staff feelings, offering support groups, and encouraging informal support through the one-on-one sharing of experiences with co-workers, peers, or pastoral care workers.[69,70]

Ritual and Meaning-Making

Ritual is used by people across all time and cultures to mark or acknowledge significant life events, providing opportunities for meaning-making and transformation.[6,69,73]

Ritual creates a bridge from suffering to hope and reminds all involved of the importance of moments in the care of bereaved families.[6] Ritual can also play an important role in helping healthcare professionals process their experiences and reconnect to the purpose in their work.[69,70,73]

Nurses can aid in co-creating ritual with both families and interdisciplinary team members.[73] Discussions about ritual often begin when a nurse notices a parent letting out a deep sigh or sharing a poignant memory. In such moments, a nurse can inquire, "What is most important to you right now?" or "Holding in mind what you are thinking and feeling right now, what would be meaningful to do next?"[6,69] Answers can provide insight into ways that a ritual could honor all that is unfolding. For a mother whose baby was dying in the neonatal intensive care unit, the idea of holding her baby over her heart was very important. Together, the mother and nurse decided to pause in silence, with the nurse letting the mother decide when and how to lift and snuggle her baby close. The mother later shared how important it was to decide when and how she was ready for the ritual; for the nurse, this moment became a treasured reminder of trusting parents as experts in their children's care and in discerning their own grief support needs.

Box 44.1 Creating Ritual: Ideas to Share with Families

Ritual is something we use to fill the deep need to acknowledge, make sense, and find meaning when hard things happen, including when someone we love dies. It is a way to pause with intent, then act and reflect what is most important to you.

Creating Your Ritual

The following questions may be helpful as you plan your ritual:

- What is most important for me to do right now to remember my child?
- Are there others who would like to share this experience of ritual with me?
- Will this time of remembering and honoring be in my home or outside in nature?
- How will the ritual begin?
- What actions, words, or music could be shared?
- What real things can I use to help honor my child?
- How will the ritual close or end?

Ideas to Consider

- Grieving together and sharing ritual with others can happen in person or connecting by phone or the internet.
- Ritual can be as simple as telling stories and sharing memories of your pregnancy/child.
- Using items that belonged to your child can help you feel connected in a special way.
- Sacred text, poems, prayer, written passages, or letters may contain words that could be shared.
- Adding an action may be meaningful, such as lighting a candle, planting a seed, holding a special object or photo to your heart, or folding your hands during a time of quiet thought.
- Using favorite music or a song or adding sounds like a bell chiming can be helpful at the beginning, middle, or ending of the ritual.
- Be open to what meets you during the ritual, especially if things do not go exactly as planned. The most meaningful moments often unfold as you take in the experience and adjust what is happening as needed.

Children are intuitively drawn to ritual and are adept at co-creating ritual when invited to participate.[6] One young boy, standing at his sister's gravesite burial ceremony, noticed all the flowers nearby. When the chaplain finished speaking, the boy asked aloud what would become of the flowers. The chaplain wisely asked the little boy to share more what he was thinking about, which led the boy to declare that he wanted to give his sister one last flower. With his parents' tearful permission, the boy carefully took out a single white rose from a nearby arrangement, knelt before the open grave, and reverently tossed the flower in. Without spoken word, his parents followed their son's action, and eventually all chose a flower and knelt to honor the boy's sister one last time—a ritual that arose out of the moment and connected all participants together in a meaningful way. Box 44.1 offers choices for families to consider when creating ritual.

Conclusion

Nurses bear witness to the impact of a child's serious illness and death on all who love and care for the child. Providing compassionate bereavement care when a baby or child dies begins with honoring the relationship and requires a willingness to be present, to listen carefully, and to offer individualized strategies to support those who grieve. Through the children and their families, nurses are reminded of the fragility of life and that hope and love are everlasting.

REFERENCES

1. National Consensus Project for Quality Palliative Care. *Clinical Practice Guidelines for Quality Palliative Care*. 4th ed. National Consensus Project for Quality Palliative Care; 2018.
2. American Academy of Pediatrics Section on Hospice and Palliative Medicine and Committee on Hospital Care. Pediatric palliative care and hospice care commitments, guidelines, and recommendations. *Pediatrics*. 2013;132(5):966–972; reaffirmed April 2019.
3. Feudtner C, Zhong, W, Faerber J, Dai D, Feinstein J. Appendix F: Pediatric end-of-life and palliative care: epidemiology and health service use. In: *Dying in America: Improving Quality and Honoring Individual Preferences Near the End of Life*. National Academies Press; 2015:533–572.
4. National Association of Neonatal Nurses Board of Directors. *Palliative and End-of-Life Care for Newborns and Infants*. Position Statement #3063. National Association of Neonatal Nurses; 2015. http://nann.org/uploads/About/PositionPDFS/1.4.5_Palliative%20and%20End%20of%20Life%20Care%20for%20Newborns%20and%20Infants.pdf.
5. Resolve Through Sharing. *Perinatal Palliative Care: A Resolve Through Sharing Position Statement*. 3rd ed. Gundersen Lutheran Medical Foundation; 2022.
6. Limbo R, Kobler K. *Meaningful Moments: Ritual and Reflection When a Child Dies*. Gundersen Medical Foundation; 2013.
7. Hill DL, Feudtner C. Hope, hopefulness, and pediatric palliative care. In: Black B, Wright PM, Limbo R, eds. *Perinatal and Pediatric Bereavement in Nursing and Other Health Professions*. Springer Publishing; 2016:223–247.
8. Kobler K, Limbo R. Making a case: creating a perinatal palliative care service using a perinatal bereavement program model. *J Perinat Neonatal Nurs*. 2011;25(1):32–41.
9. Hill DL, Boyden JY, Feudtner C, Munson DA. Perinatal regoaling in the face of serious illness: hopeful thinking, good-parent belief, and uncertainty. In: Limbo R, Wool C, Carter BS. *Perinatal and Neonatal Palliative Care: A Guide for Nurses, Physicians, and Other Health Care Professionals*. Springer Publishing; 2020:201–215.
10. Merriam-Webster Dictionary. Grief. Anticipatory. Reave. Accessed October 8, 2022.
11. Lathrop D. Disenfranchised grief and physician burnout. *Ann Fam Med*. 2017;15(4):375–378.
12. Prigerson HG, Kakarala S, Gang J, Macjejewski PK. History and status of prolonged grief disorders as a psychiatric diagnosis. *Annu Rev Clin Psychol*. 2021;17:109–126.
13. Pohlkamp L, Krecicbergs U, Sveen J. Factors during a child's illness are associated with levels of prolonged grief symptoms in bereaved mothers and fathers. *J Clin Oncol*. 2020;38(2):137–144.
14. Kochen EI, Jenken F, Boelen PA, et al. When a child dies: a systematic review of well-defined parent-focused bereavement interventions and their alignment with grief and loss theories. *BMC Palliat Care*. 2020;19(1):28.
15. Lichtenthal WG, Corner GW, Sweeney C, Roberts KE. Grieving the traumatic death of a child. In: Black B, Wright PM, Limbo R, eds. *Perinatal and Pediatric Bereavement in Nursing and Other Health Professions*. Springer Publishing; 2016:249–286.
16. Cacciatore J. *Bearing the Unbearable: Love Loss, and the Heartbreaking Path of Grief*. Wisdom Publications; 2017.
17. American Psychiatric Association. Trauma and stressor-related disorders. In *Diagnostic and Statistical Manual of Mental Disorders*. 5th ed. American Psychiatric Association; 2013:265–290.
18. Baumann I, Künzel J, Goldbeck L, Tutus D, Niemitz M. Prolonged grief, posttraumatic stress, and depression among bereaved parents: prevalence and response to an intervention program. *Omega (Westport)*. 2022;84(3):837–855.
19. Stroebe MS, Schut H. The dual process model of coping with bereavement: rationale and description. *Death Stud*. 1999;23:197–224.
20. Worden JW. *Grief Counseling and Grief Therapy: A Handbook for the Mental Health Practitioner*. 5th ed. Springer Publishing; 2018.
21. Johnson KA. A mother's tears: contemplating Black grief. *Ann Fam Med*. 2022;20(4):381–382.
22. Kübler-Ross E. *On Death and Dying*. Macmillan Company; 1969.
23. Corr CA. Should we incorporate the work of Elisabeth Kübler-Ross in our current teaching and practice and, if so, how? *Omega (Westport)*. 2021;83(4):706–728.
24. Lindemann E. Symptomatology and management of acute grief. *Am J Psychol*. 1944;101:141–148.
25. Bowlby J. *Loss: Sadness and Depression*. Basic Books; 1980.
26. Rubin SS, Malkinson R, Witztum E. Traumatic bereavements: rebalancing the relation to the deceased and the death story using the two track model of bereavement. *Front Psychiatry*. 2020;11:537596.
27. Neimeyer RA, Klass D, Dennis MF. A social constructionist account of grief: loss and the narration of meaning. *Death Stud*. 2014;38(6–10):485–498.
28. Maciejewski PK, Zhang B, Block SD, Prigerson HG. An empirical examination of the stage theory of grief. *JAMA*. 2007;292:716–723.
29. Parkes CM. The first year of bereavement. *Psychiatry*. 1970;33(4):444–467.
30. Stroebe M, Finkenauer C, Wijngaaards-de Meij L, Schut H, van den Bout J, Stroebe W. Partner-oriented self-regulation among bereaved parents: the costs of holding in grief for the partners' sake. *Psychol Sci*. 2013;24(4):395–402.
31. Attig T. *How We Grieve: Relearning the World*. Oxford University Press; 2010.
32. American Nurses Association. *Nursing, A Social Policy Statement*. 3rd ed. American Nurses Association; 2015.
33. Gillies J, Neimeyer RA, Milman E. The meaning of loss codebook: construction of a system for analyzing meanings made in bereavement. *Death Stud*. 2014;38(4):207–216.
34. Duncan C, Cacciatore J. A systematic review of the peer-reviewed literature on self-blame, guilt, and shame. *Omega (Westport)*. 2015;71(4):312–342.
35. Bonanno L, Bennett M, Pitt, A. The experience of parents of newborns diagnosed with a congenital anomaly at birth: a systematic review protocol. *JBI Database System Rev Implement Rep*. 2013;11(11):100–111.
36. Gilmer MJ, Foster TL, Vannatta K, et al. Changes in parents after the death of a child from cancer. *J Pain Symptom Manage*. 2012;44(4):572–582.
37. Davies B, Limbo R. The grief of siblings. In: Webb NB, ed. *Helping Bereaved Children: A Handbook for Practitioners*. 3rd ed. Guilford Press; 2010:69–90.
38. Shreffler K, Hill T, Cacciatore J. The impact of infertility, miscarriage, stillbirth, and child death on marital dissolution. *J Divorce Remarriage*. 2012;53(2):91–107.
39. Gold KJ, Sen A, Hayward RA. Marriage and cohabitation outcomes after pregnancy loss. *Pediatrics*. 2010;125:1202–1207.

40. Black BP, Fields WS. Contexts of reproductive loss in lesbian couples. *MCN Am J Matern Child Nurs*. 2014;39(3):157–162.
41. Gilrane-McGarry U, O'Grady T. Forgotten grievers: an exploration of the grief experiences of bereaved grandparents (part 2). *Int J Palliat Nurs*. 2012;18(4):179–187.
42. Davies B. *Fading Away: The Experience of Transition in Families with Terminal Illness*. Baywood Publishing; 1995.
43. Davies B. *Shadows in the Sun: The Experiences of Sibling Bereavement in Childhood*. Brunner/Mazel; 1999.
44. Davies B, van Breemen C, Poitras S, Stephanson E. Bereavement in young children with siblings in pediatric palliative care. In: Black BP, Wright PM, Limbo R, eds. *Perinatal and Pediatric Bereavement in Nursing and Other Health Professions*. Springer Publishing; 2016:307–326.
45. Duncan J, Kobler K. Communication in pediatrics. In: Dahlin C, Coyne PJ, Ferrell BR, eds. *Textbook in Advanced Practice Palliative Nursing*. Oxford University Press; 2016:597–608.
46. Waechter EH. Children's awareness of fatal illness. *Am J Nurs*. 1971;7(6):1168–1172.
47. Bluebond-Langner M, Belasco JB, Wander MD. "I want to live, until I don't want to live anymore": involving children with life-threatening and life-shortening illnesses in decision making about care and treatment. *Nurs Clin North Am*. 2010;45(3):329–343.
48. Kobler K, Bell C, Kavanaugh K, Gallo AM, Corte C, Vincent C. Health care professionals' awareness of a child's impending death. *Qual Health Res*. 2020;30(9):1314–1325.
49. Jankowski JB. Professional boundary issues in pediatric palliative care. *Am J Hosp Palliat Care*. 2014;31(2):161–165.
50. Davies B, Clarke D, Connaughty S, et al. Caring for dying children: nurses' experiences. *Pediatr Nurs*. 1996;22(6):500–507.
51. Papadatou D. *In the Face of Death*. Springer Publishing; 2009.
52. Beaune L, Muskat B, Anthony SJ. The emergence of personal growth amongst health care professionals who care for dying children. *Palliat Support Care*. 2018;16(3):298–307.
53. Waldman E, Wolfe J. Palliative care for children with cancer. *Nat Rev Clin Oncol*. 2013;10:100–107.
54. Limbo R, Kavanaugh K, Kobler K. Honoring relationship and hope. In: Kobler K, Limbo R, eds. *Conversations in Perinatal, Neonatal, and Pediatric Palliative Care*. Hospice and Palliative Nurses Association; 2017:35–47.
55. Kaye E, Rockwell SL, Lemmon ME, Baker JN, Mack JW. The art of saying nothing. *Pediatrics*. 2022;149(6):e2022056862.
56. Mulhern RK, Lauer ME, Hoffmann RG. Death of a child at home or in the hospital: subsequent psychological adjustment of the family. *Pediatrics*. 1983;71(5):743–747.
57. Davies B, Steele R, Baird J. *Pediatric Palliative Care: A Model for Exemplary Practice*. Routledge; 2022.
58. Pridham KF, Limbo R. Guided participation for clinical practice: a middle-range theory of teaching and learning. *ANS Adv Nurs Sci*. 2023;46(3):306–321.
59. Limbo, R, Pridham KF. Applying the theory of guided participation to clinical practice. *ANS Adv Nurs Sci*. 2024;47(2):E41–E57.
60. Kobler K. Relationship-based approach to caring for children with serious illness. In: Pridham K, Limbo R, Schroeder M, eds. *Guided Participation for Pediatric Nursing Practice: Relationship-Based Teaching and Learning with Parents, Children, and Adolescents*. Springer Publishing; 2018:21–32.
61. Hill DL, Boyden JY, Feudtner C. Hope in the context of life-threatening illness and the end of life. *Curr Opin Psychol*. 2023;49:101513.
62. Meert KL, Eggly S, Kavanaugh K, Berg RA, Wessel DL. Meaning making during parent–physician bereavement meetings after a child's death. *Health Psychol*. 2015;34(4):453–461.
63. Melin-Johannson C, Axelsson I, Grundberg MJ, Hallqvist F. When a child dies: parents' experiences of palliative care—an integrative literature review. *J Pediatr Nurs*. 2014;29:660–669.
64. Younblut JM, Brooten D, Blais K, Kilgore C, Yoo C. Health and functioning in grandparents after a young grandchild's death. *J Community Health*. 2015;40(50):956–966.
65. Roose RE, Blanford CR. Perinatal grief and support spans the generations: parents' and grandparents' evaluations of an intergenerational perinatal bereavement program. *J Perinat Neonatal Nurse*. 2011;25(1):77–85.
66. Webb NB. *Helping Bereaved Children: A Handbook for Practitioners*. Guilford Press; 2002.
67. Wood DD, Lancto Near R. Using expressive arts when counseling bereaved children. In: Balk D, Corr C, eds. *Children's Encounters with Death, Bereavement and Coping*. Springer Publishing; 2010:373–393.
68. Schuurman DL, DeCristofaro J. Principles and practices of peer support groups and camp-based interventions for grieving children. In: Balk D, Coor C, eds. *Children's Encounters with Death, Bereavement and Coping*. Springer Publishing; 2010:1–47.
69. Kobler K. Strategies to honor professional well-being in perinatal and neonatal palliative care. In: Limbo R, Wool C, Carter BS, eds. *Perinatal and Neonatal Palliative Care: A Guide for Nurses, Physicians, and Other Health Care Professionals*. Springer Publishing; 2020:385–400.
70. Kobler K. Leaning in and holding on: team support with unexpected death. *MCN Am J Matern Child Nurs*. 2014;39(3):148–154.
71. Morris SE, Dole OR, Joselow M, Duncan J, Renaud K, Branowicki P. The development of a hospital-wide bereavement program: ensuring bereavement care for all families of pediatric patients. *J Pediatr Health Care*. 2017;31(1):88–95.
72. Snamen JM, Kaye EC, Torres, C, Gibson DV, Baker JN. Helping parents live with the hole in their heart: the role of health care providers and institutions in the bereaved parents' grief journeys. *Cancer*. 2016;122(17):2757–2765.
73. Kobler K, Limbo R, Kavanaugh K. Meaningful moments: the use of ritual in perinatal and pediatric death. *MCN Am J Matern Child Nurs*. 2007;32(5):288–295.

PART V

Issues in Populations of the Seriously Ill

45

Pulmonary-Palliative Care

Patricia A. Maani-Fogelman and Jennifer Wescoe-Singley

Key Points

- Rationale for early integration of palliative care for the advancing/chronic lung disease patient, in accordance with the American Thoracic Society Clinical Policy Statement on Palliative Care for Patients with Respiratory Diseases and Critical Illness.
- There are available triggers to use to identify patients in need of referral to a pulmonary-palliative medicine clinic.
- Regardless of prognosis, much can be done to optimize management of the advanced pulmonary patient.

Introduction

Persons living with advanced/terminal lung disease require early collaboration with palliative care to assure a comprehensive approach through the trajectory of their chronic, progressive illness which may often have prognostic variation and unexpected declines.[1] Advanced lung disease patients have physical, psychological, social, and spiritual issues that reduce their quality of life (QOL). In these patients, it may be difficult to diagnose depression[2,3]; however, diagnosis and treatment are essential. These emotional dimensions of chronic conditions are often overlooked when medical care is considered, and their impact on both patients and their caregivers cannot be overemphasized. In addition to patient care delivery, there is ample need demonstrated in the realm of caregiver needs.[2] The impact of chronic disease–related health costs can be seen from reviewing US healthcare spending, which rose by nearly 10%, $4.1 trillion, in 2020, much faster than the 4.3% of 2019, which is wholly attributed to the COVID-19 pandemic. Simultaneously, the gross domestic product deteriorated 2.2%, with allocation of total healthcare spending reaching a high of nearly 20%.[4] Patients with advancing, chronic medical illness do not have comprehensive advanced care planning discussions, and in the United States, our high healthcare expenditures do not translate to outcomes better than in other high-income countries.[4] Today's healthcare providers are well-equipped for the biomedical aspects of care but not for the challenges of understanding the psychological, social, and cultural dimensions of illness and health. Nurses on every level can play an important part in helping their patients to develop and maintain healthy coping skills.[5]

One of those prevalent, progressive lung diseases is chronic obstructive pulmonary disease (COPD). In the *Global Strategy for the Diagnosis, Management, and Prevention of Chronic Obstructive Pulmonary Disease* (GOLD) 2020 Report, it is noted that in the United States the estimated direct costs of COPD are $32 billion and the indirect costs $20.4 billion, with exacerbations as the largest cost of COPD burden on the healthcare system. Additionally, the costs of COPD rise exponentially as disease progresses (i.e., hospital admissions, supplemental oxygen, home health, etc.). Perhaps the greatest irony in advanced lung disease care, as noted in GOLD 2020: "Any estimate of direct medical expenditure for home-based care underrepresents the true cost of home-based care to society, because it ignores the economic value of the care provided by family members to people with COPD."[6(p7)] In addition, the mortality of COPD should be highlighted; more people die every day from COPD than from diabetes or breast cancer: 377 per day from COPD versus 193 per day from diabetes or 112 per day from breast cancer.[6,7] In a very similar pattern, advanced lung diseases all begin to have high-frequency exacerbations and mounting expenses as the disease worsens.

Most people nearing their end of life (EOL) exhibit a preference for care focused on alleviating pain and suffering.[5] Advanced lung disease patients may begin to experience some impairment in their information processing as their illness worsens, due to the gross nature of hypercapnic and hypoxemic respiratory failure. Nurses play a vital role in helping to drive the focus toward addressing goals of care early and in an ongoing manner, over the course of continued visits, to ensure person-centered care is best provided to this population who can develop substantial physical and, at times, cognitive impairment as they approach the EOL. Frequent nurse–patient conversations about EOL care values, goals, and preferences are necessary to avoid unwanted treatment. Incentives, quality standards, and system support are needed to promote improved communication skills and more frequent conversations.

Recommendations from the American Thoracic Society (ATS),[8] Institute of Medicine,[2,3] National Consensus Project (NCP) *Clinical Guidelines*,[9] and the American Society of Clinical Oncology[10] provide support for the framework of this comprehensive care plan. Much of the data stems from cancer-based research. However, the 2013 NCP report analyzed patients of any age with multiple comorbid/chronic conditions, with the intent

Box 45.1 Common Lung Diseases

Chronic obstructive pulmonary disease (COPD): emphysema, asthma, chronic bronchitis
Interstitial lung diseases: idiopathic pulmonary fibrosis, acute interstitial pneumonitis, hypersensitive pneumonitis, nonspecific interstitial pneumonitis, sarcoidosis, asbestosis
Pulmonary hypertension: idiopathic, heritable, and drug/toxin-induced
Cystic fibrosis/bronchiectasis
Pulmonary cancers
Alpha-1 anti-trypsin deficiency
COVID-associated respiratory disease

Box 45.2 Dyspnea Empathy Exercise

While seated, take a normal resting breath but only exhale partially.
Wait a few seconds and take another resting breath and only exhale partially.
Wait a few seconds and repeat.
After a few more seconds, breathe normally.
After this simple exercise, ask yourself these questions:
What was your experience? How did you feel? Were you a little anxious? Did you feel some stress? Was it unpleasant?
This exercise causes a 4–5 mm Hg elevation in CO2 from your baseline, with an associated dyspnea and affective (fear/anxiety) response. While this is a temporary, controlled exercise that can be stopped at any time, it does effectively reflect minor dyspnea. Now take a moment to imagine if this feeling was dramatically amplified, as it is with advanced lung disease patients who have no recourse or relief from the severity of their lung disease.
Source: Reference 38.

to offer the focus of palliative care interventions for the most seriously ill. The NCP integrates central quality assessment and improvement initiatives into palliative care, and it describes the comprehensive care necessary for patients at the EOL. These clinical guidelines emphasize the patient- and family-centered focus of palliative care, promoting access to palliative care across all patient populations and all health settings. In addition, there is expansion of the composition and necessary education of the intradisciplinary team beyond chaplaincy, medicine, nursing, pharmacy, and social work to include rehabilitation therapists, respiratory care, and other therapies.[8–10]

In September 2022, the ATS issued its Official ATS Policy Statement "Palliative Care Early in the Care Continuum among Patients with Respiratory Disease," which delineates the obligations of pulmonary providers to the patients we serve. The ATS acknowledges that pulmonary providers routinely care for patients with chronic or advanced respiratory diseases and critical illnesses (see common lung diseases, Box 45.1).[8] In this continuum of chronic disease management, the vitality of implementing palliative care into standard clinical management, whether it is curative or restorative, is an essential element of assuring comprehensive care (which has also been demonstrated in cancer care.) The ATS recognizes the growing importance and complexity of palliative care for patients with life-threatening and life-limiting diseases and disorders and the need for improving professional competence and teamwork in providing such care. The policy statement strongly endorses the concept that palliative care should be available to patients at all stages of illness and should be individualized based on the needs and preferences of the patient and the patient's family. Finally, the ATS believes that clinicians should consult with palliative care specialists as appropriate for managing palliative care situations beyond the clinician's level of competence.[8] This chapter will review primary distress symptoms of advanced lung disease, how to ameliorate them, and the steps nurses can take to assure comprehensive palliative care delivery for this vulnerable population.

Dyspnea: Why Is It Important?

Before reading this section, please see the Dyspnea Empathy Exercise in Box 45.2 developed by Dr. Betty Ferrell. Dying patients fear dyspnea and pain; therefore, symptom control is one cornerstone of pulmonary-palliative care. Dyspnea is a prominent symptom of the patient with advanced respiratory disease of any cause: Nearly all patients with COPD experience severe dyspnea during the last 3 days of their lives.[11,12] Breathing is a primal need. When the ease of breathing is dysregulated by advancing respiratory disease, there is a building fear. And although there has been progress in dyspnea mechanisms research, there remains a scarcity regarding its treatment.[13] In spite of many advances in the therapy of cardiopulmonary disorders, millions of persons living with advanced lung disease remain severely disabled by breathlessness because it is efforts to cure a disease which generate biomedical research and tend to grab the public's attention. However, the duty to alleviate suffering must remain a top priority. The ATS concludes: "Patients with serious respiratory illness and their caregivers suffer from significant physical, emotional, spiritual, and financial burdens and are in need of early palliative care to help guide treatment planning."[8] To learn more about treating the symptom of dyspnea, cough, and other respiratory symptoms, see Chapter 12, "Dyspnea and Cough." Patients with serious respiratory illness and their caregivers suffer from significant physical, emotional, spiritual, and financial burdens and are in need of early palliative care to help guide treatment planning

Pulmonary-Palliative Clinic: A New Construct

Although those with advanced lung disease may receive "palliative" or life-prolonging treatment, this usually does not address their physical, psychological, social, or spiritual issues—and may worsen them. During Dr. Maani-Fogelman's time at Geisinger Medical Center, she established a dedicated pulmonary-palliative clinic, assuring that advanced lung disease patients had access to providers who had the experience, training, and time to address these issues for both patients and their families, in an outpatient clinic setting where a continued dialogue could be sustained and evolved over time. There is substantial evidence demonstrating how earlier involvement of palliative care leads to improved QOL for patients and families, as well as a more efficient utilization of medical resources in a more appropriate, even cost-saving, manner[14,15] and higher patient satisfaction when the "unknown" is no longer a dark, scary mystery. The intention of the pulmonary-palliative medicine clinic is to encourage these discussions earlier in the trajectory of chronic, progressive illness; and it is through the dynamic process of ongoing education, close-interval follow-up, and relationship-building that palliative registered nurses (RNs) have the opportunities to deeply impact patient care: frequent reassessment of QOL changes, activity level changes, weight loss, mood, and relationships with others are key elements to how patients identify their self-worth. In keeping with the tenets of palliative care, the RN advocates for earlier referral and integration of palliative care services into the management of advanced disease, with the goal of ultimately improving QOL and patient and family satisfaction.[16] Pulmonary-palliative practice is a shared and collaborative effort, carried out by members of a multidisciplinary team with nurses, providers, and respiratory therapy partners. With these efforts must come the understanding that there are different levels of training among providers of palliative care:

Specialist: Professionals with advanced palliative care training/certification who specialize in providing symptom management and support to those with serious medical illness in parallel with their treatment as well as at EOL. The palliative care specialist is adept at managing complex and refractory symptoms that may occur with disease progression as well as being an experienced navigator of the psychosocial challenges and family dynamics which accompany these circumstances.

Generalist: Professionals from other specialties with training in basic palliative care concepts/content who identify the need for and initiate advance care planning, symptom management, and QOL support for their patients. Ideally all providers should be familiar with providing basic palliative care and then refer to and collaborate with palliative specialists as needed.

The goal is to improve education and outreach to be able to arrive at an equipoise where all professionals provide basic palliative care to most patients but will refer to palliative care specialists when higher intensity/higher levels of palliative care are required to optimize patient care.[17] Pulmonary-palliative nurses have the opportunity to initiate early engagement and evolve a highly specialized role in their clinic with the delivery of early and consistent primary palliative care. Please see Chapter 61, "Palliative Care Nursing in the Outpatient Setting," for more information on nursing's role in this setting.

Palliative Care for People with Advanced Lung Disease

Palliative care encourages and supports family involvement in planning and providing care to the extent desired by the patient. This is because chronic or advanced respiratory diseases and critical illnesses impact both patients and their families. All patients with symptomatic or life-threatening diseases, particularly those with chronic or advanced respiratory diseases or critical illnesses, regardless of age or social circumstances, should have access to palliative care. Perhaps more importantly, healthcare providers should have an appropriate level of competence in palliative care, where training and educational experiences equip the pulmonary provider with the core competencies necessary to provide compassionate and individualized palliative care.[18,19] The ATS supports efforts at public education about the availability and value of incorporating palliative care in the care of persons living with chronic or advanced respiratory diseases or critical illnesses, including advocacy for research and professional education to improve the quality and availability of palliative care services.[8]

Table 45.1 Decedent advanced lung disease demographics

Gender:	Race:	Diagnosis:
51.6% Female	92.4% White	COPD 88.9%
		ILD 10.8.%
		CF 0.3%

CF, cystic fibrosis; COPD, chronic obstructive pulmonary disease; ILD, interstitial lung disease.

Cross et al.[20] reviewed the trends for EOL care in advanced lung disease patients. Table 45.1 shows the 2003 to 2017 breakdown of over 2.2 million deaths attributed to chronic lung disease.

They note that while hospital and nursing facility deaths reduced from 44.4% to 19.7%, home and hospice facility deaths increased from 23.3% to 34.7%. Of interest was the finding that being male, being married, and having moderate collegiate education came with a higher prevalence of home-based deaths, though patients with interstitial lung disease (ILD) and cystic fibrosis (CF) remain in the higher rates of in-hospital or facility deaths. These findings reaffirm the need for earlier integration of palliative care, especially for the higher-intensity and higher-mortality lung diseases such as ILD and CF.

Advanced Lung Disease and Unique Circumstances

Historically, palliative care has focused on persons living with malignant cancers. In more recent years, the awareness of COPD-associated mortality and morbidity has led to a growing recognition of the need for similar services for persons living with respiratory conditions. This includes other nonmalignant end-stage pulmonary diseases such as CF, ILD, pulmonary arterial hypertension, sarcoidosis, and occupational lung disease. Often, these conditions are treated without a concomitant palliative component, until there is a sudden change in the trajectory of the illness or a decline, necessitating a sort of crisis approach to their needs.[20,21] Symptom management should address air hunger, exertional dyspnea, chest tightness, anxiety/panic, increased work of breathing as evidenced by increased accessory muscle use, increased oxygen needs, spiritual or existential distress, and grief. For clinically addressing specific symptoms, please see the corresponding chapter for each symptom.

Uncertainty in Prognosis and Disease Trajectory

Prognostication in lung disease is not straightforward. These diseases are, by definition, chronic. They will chronically progress over time, with declines in functionality that will be variable for patients: there may be fast versus slow/subtle decline for COPD, CF, or pulmonary hypertension, whereas another layer of complexity is added when caring for ILD patients, for whom a diagnosis may take 3 years or more, with patients seeing three providers or more before receiving a definitive diagnosis. This impacts their trajectory, delaying advanced therapies developed to slow disease progression. Conversations about advance illness planning are accelerated in the setting of late-stage diagnoses.[21-23]

The disease trajectories for lung diseases such as pulmonary hypertension or lung transplant recipients differ depending on the cause of the disease, comorbid conditions, complications related to therapy, response to treatment, or surgery. These are changing with the advent of newer therapies and experienced centers for treatment.[24]

Advanced therapies to slow the progression of illness present special challenges at EOL. Patients may not understand that these are not curative, which may be a factor of the communication and education they receive about these medications at the beginning. When medications are offered, they are often not offered with a statement about how they are not curative but will help buy some time *if they work*. These therapies are expensive, and, with current regulations, the patient must often choose between continuing therapy and hospice.

Of special note is idiopathic pulmonary fibrosis (IPF), a progressive disease with median survival of 2 to 7 years. IPF now has therapies available which do not reverse damage but have been shown to slow the decline in the loss of lung function as measured by forced vital capacity (FVC) on the pulmonary function test. Again, we highlight the importance of early and ongoing discussions with patients and their caregivers/families about the incurability of the disease and the aim of the drugs is to help buy time but that they will not cure/reverse the illness. As research into this disease continues, it is reasonable to hope for future drugs which may be of more efficacy. It is worth noting that these medications may have varied side effects which will also impact QOL, leaving patients with unintended compromise of accepting drug-related symptoms for a hopefully longer life span.

Early Integration of Palliative Care in Advanced Pulmonary Disease

Despite recommendations for early integration of palliative care, few studies are available on EOL recommendations for this population. Patients may continue to have a significant symptom burden, most commonly dyspnea and cough. Their oxygen need increases over time. According to a recent study, IPF has a major impact on daily living and family relationships.[24] This slowing rather than reversal or stopping of progression may be difficult for patients and families to understand. It is important when initiating these therapies that their efficacy be clearly explained and that this information be reviewed periodically. Early referral to a lung transplant center, if applicable and if the patient agrees, is recommended.

More than 100 types of ILDs have been identified, and, for most of these patients, lung transplant is not an option.[22] Therapy varies depending on etiology, and, for some, no therapy is available. Most of these patients die in a hospital setting with ongoing life-prolonging procedures until death. Often EOL decisions are still made very late. Early integrated palliative care with advance care planning could improve their EOL care. Further studies on the care received and ways to improve EOL for this population are needed.[22,25]

Nurses are not only patient advocates but also the champions of building a therapeutic rapport of trust that helps initiate conversations early in their care concerning when to expect to stop or reduce therapy, which should then be integrated into advance directive decisions. Nurses have the opportunity when assessing patients to inquire about changes, functional decline, and mood issues, as well as inquiring to caregivers about patient status. When patients affirm decline, it is the nurse's opportunity to further explore patient needs and desires. Patients and families may find it difficult to stop therapy even in the face of a decline in functional status. In the face of irreversible functional decline, the focus should be to continue treating comorbidities and be directed toward aggressive symptom management. Pulmonary rehabilitation can be considered an attempt to improve functional status and QOL.[21]

Medication Dilemmas

Pulmonary medications have a special challenge because their efficacy often is limited, and continual use may contribute to functional decline. For diseases such as pulmonary hypertension, many of them are titrated or combined to maximize efficacy and carry the risk of rebound if abruptly stopped.[24] Patients also note improvement when they are started, so they may be reluctant to reduce or stop them for fear of becoming symptomatic. COPD patients may feel "instant" relief with as-needed albuterol, which fixates their conviction that inhalers must always be continued, though the long-acting therapies may begin to lose efficacy as disease worsens. Nurses have an opportunity to be the patient's navigator through these changes, revisiting the goals of care and bringing to provider attention when medications may be more harmful than helpful. As the disease progresses beyond the ability of medications to control it and the patient experiences a functional decline or a dying process for another reason, the cessation of certain medications may become necessary. As with other EOL planning, nurses along with pulmonary medicine providers should meet and collaborate with the patient and family on the timing of tapering medications down. The plan should include aggressive measures to manage common EOL symptoms for advanced lung disease patients such as dyspnea, anxiety, hypertension, edema, or related symptoms. When it comes to medication de-escalation, this may begin with reducing the number of tablets or frequency stepwise over time. For pulmonary hypertension patients specifically, these meds may be infused, therefore requiring a gradual stepping down of rate of infusion, which may take days to a week or more to mediate symptoms. When possible, consider tapering off inhaled or intravenous therapy but continue phosphodiesterase 5 inhibitors or another oral pulmonary hypertension medication. Diuretics in pulmonary hypertension should be continued as possible and as tolerated for management of edema and breathlessness.[24] These medications have been the patient's lifeline, many times for years, so patients may approach the process of tapering or stopping them with fear and with questions about hastening their demise despite indications of loss of clinical efficacy and functional decline.

Advanced Ventilatory Technology

Noninvasive ventilation (NIV), bimodal positive airway pressure (BiPAP) therapy, and nocturnal ventilation via tracheotomy are becoming increasingly common therapies. In the later stages of disease and at EOL, home NIV may provide symptom relief and rest periods to offset the increased work of breathing.[25,26] In an acute situation, it may provide time for decision-making or family interaction. Patients and providers may elect noninvasive support to treat a possibly reversible comorbidity such as infection. It should be combined with aggressive management of dyspnea for patient comfort but also to facilitate the patient's ability to remove the device for communication with family and pleasure feeds. Nurses should advocate for patients to have continued symptom relief and provide ongoing supportive care for the families; medications such as opioids and anxiolytics should be requested for patients to have optimal symptom control.[27] Like other advanced therapies, an early conversation about this being a temporizing therapy and when to discontinue it should occur before initiating therapy. Patients and families should be encouraged to participate in this decision as it may involve waiting for a distant member to arrive or meeting or avoiding a special date or milestone.[26]

Forecasting

Identifying which individual with an advanced pulmonary disease will have a rapid versus more indolent progression of their illness remains the challenge. Efforts are underway to broaden our understanding. Diffusion capacity of the lungs for carbon monoxide (DLCO) is a measure done as part of a full pulmonary function test; it measures the transfer of gas from air in the lung to the red blood cells in lung blood vessels. A DLCO of less than 40% predicted, desaturation with exercise, and concomitant pulmonary hypertension are poor prognostic signs. The prognosis of combined pulmonary fibrosis and emphysema is worse than either disease alone. For ILDs, worsening fibrotic changes on radiology, decline in diffusion capacity, increasing oxygen need and dyspnea, decline in distance on 6-minute walk test, and decline in FVC are longitudinal indicators. Unintentional weight loss, repeated hospital admissions, and progressive decline in functional status are general clinical indicators.[25]

With pulmonary arterial hypertension, accepted guidelines use N-terminal pro b-type natriuretic peptide and renal function as markers of disease severity. Other inflammatory markers such as interleukin 6, growth differentiation factor 15, and red cell distribution width are useful but not commonly available. Research is underway to find other markers, for example, a nine-protein panel that will provide information on prognosis and response or lack of response to therapy. These could be beneficial in guiding therapy as well as in decision-making.[28]

When assessing readiness or suitability for pulmonary-palliative intervention, there are various triggers we use embedded within our daily pulmonary medicine practice:

1. The *BODE index* (*b*ody mass index, airflow *o*bstruction, *d*yspnea, and *e*xercise) is a scored index used to assess patients with COPD to predict long-term outcomes for them.[29] The degree of airflow obstruction is determined by the forced expiratory volume percentage predicted after using a bronchodilator to open airways from the pulmonary function test, the dyspnea is as reported by the patient, and the exercise component is measured using a 6-minute walk test distance. While it should not be used alone to guide treatment, the BODE score is a helpful adjunct to promote early conversations about advancing lung disease, allowing a focused conversation on the reality of their prognosis using clinical evidence. In general, patients with a higher BODE are at increased risk of mortality and often have increased frequency of COPD exacerbations and hospitalizations. This score can be calculated with an online calculator: https://www.mdcalc.com/bode-index-copd-survival#creator-insights.
2. The *GAP index* is a risk assessment system used for clinical prediction of prognosis in patients with IPF[30]. Using the frequently measured clinical and physiologic variables of gender (*G*), age (*A*), and two lung physiology variables (*P*; FVC and DLCO, described earlier), the GAP index provides an estimation of individual risk of mortality. This score can be easily determined using an online calculator: https://www.acponline.org/journals/annals/extras/gap/.

Tools like BODE and GAP assist in shaping prognostic conversations, but nurses and providers alike are encouraged to remember that end-stage lung disease patients, especially those with COPD, remain a notoriously difficult population to predict. Patients can lose ground with a viral illness and never regain it, or they can plateau and remain there for months, even years. Clinically, we also look at severity of lung function, frequency of exacerbations, need for oxygen, and declining functional status. Early identification and intervention is key because the symptom burden in severe COPD can be as high as in patients with lung cancer, but COPD patients may have a longer survival.[31] We continue usual management of dyspnea with opioids, inhaled medications, and oxygen. Even for those with respiratory derangement, doses of opioid are safe and effective. Other considerations include anxiety (a result of and contributor to breathlessness), deconditioning, depression, fatigue, and pain[32-34]. Patients with end-stage lung disease have significantly impaired QOL and emotional well-being. Those with end-stage COPD have broader needs to optimize well-being which may include rehabilitation, psychosocial support and ongoing medical management which can be complex and requiring multiple specialists. These needs that are not as well met as patients with lung cancer, and, at times, their survival is shorter.[12,19,20,26,32-35]

The majority of patients seen in this clinic are those with COPD or ILD, a statistic that correlates with the national prevalence of COPD as the leading lung disease and ILD as a more fatal, though less frequently occurring, lung disease.[31] This clinic initiated a change in practice based on the rising national recognition of palliative care, access to palliative care for all chronic illness patients,[36] and, most specifically, the needs of advanced lung disease patients and their families.[8] It is the commitment of the providers to assure that all lung disease patients have access to high-quality palliative care earlier in their advancing disease trajectory. The projected outcome is to provide a more comprehensive paradigm of care for advanced lung patients. In essence, this clinic epitomizes a new construct, built to provide palliative care in conjunction with best practice guidelines for the care of advanced lung disease patients. We recognize that this new construct/model has broad application potential for other chronic disease management clinics—as seen with similar models of palliative care delivery and the evidence established in oncology patient management.[9-12]

Toll of Serious Illness on Persons and Their Families/Caregivers

Like many persons living with advanced illness, those with advanced lung disease fear they will be a physical and financial burden.[29,30] Studies have demonstrated that caregivers of persons living with advanced lung disease report needing/desiring support with physical care and education/information about advanced illness and EOL processes, as well as the all too important but all too often underacknowledged need for emotional and spiritual support.[30] Persons and their families often worry about if "nothing more can be done," will the healthcare team abandon them? They are often consumed with worries about how their families and caregivers adjust to role changes: many drain life savings or go bankrupt to cover medical costs.[29] Approximately 40% of all persons living with COPD are affected by severe depressive symptoms or clinical depression, with the prevalence of depression as high as 57%; and this can often be a challenge to diagnose because of overlapping symptoms between COPD and depression.[6,8,12,29,30] As a result, persons living with advanced lung disease often feel helplessness or powerlessness due to their loss of mobility and freedom and their growing weakness. They report tense relationships with friends and family, often develop panic attacks with episodes of uncontrolled dyspnea, and increasing social isolation as they interact less and less with their world. This can often lead to more depression, anxiety, insomnia, or sleep disturbance.[6,12,27,30]

Medicare data confirms that many older adults may be cared for by an aging, also chronically ill spouse; additionally, older children caring for a parent may have acute or chronic illnesses.[31] This creates a situation where you have one chronically ill person(s) caring for another. The potential for either individual to have a rapid decline or complication from their medical issue may be higher. Nurses can assist patients to empower themselves to gain strength and optimize conditioning by educating and assisting patients to begin regular exercise (which can often be "jump-started" by enrollment in pulmonary rehabilitation for qualified patients); cognitive behavioral therapy; support groups, such as the Better Breathers Club; keeping oneself emotionally open to those seeking to assist and care for them; and the positive reinforcement felt by engaging in activities which promote happiness such as time with friends and family, hobbies that bring personal joy, or meditation.[32]

Assuring Equity Requires Patient, Caregiver, and Provider Advocacy

A variety of education options abound for advanced lung disease patients. As outlined in the earlier discussion, lung disease patients and their caregivers struggle with isolation and decreased socialization. It is in this space where the opportunity to build connections, improve resilience, and provide support, the most fundamentally vital impacts, can be made.

Wescoe Foundation for Pulmonary Fibrosis

The Wescoe Foundation for Pulmonary Fibrosis is a 501(c)3 nonprofit organization based in Pennsylvania which provides support, advocacy, and resources for people with IPF and their families to sustain the highest possible QOL. Their offerings include pulmonary fibrosis support groups embedded at regional advanced lung disease clinics, fundraising and awareness campaigns, connecting patients to clinical trials, and other educational materials including their *IPF Carebook* to help patients easily navigate IPF. The *Carebook* is available free to anyone on the website or can be sent in hardcopy form by request by visiting www.wescoe.org.

Managing Advanced Lung Disease Requires Attention to the Importance of Supportive Care for Patients and Families/Caregivers

As part of the pulmonary-palliative care construct, the benefits of connecting patients and families/caregivers to supportive care are essential for better compliance to treatment. As far back as 1995, the SUPPORT study indicated that a remarkable disparity between patient and provider communication led to inadequate understanding of their disease process.[11] Not only does this encourage providers to acknowledge the importance of this approach, but it emphasizes the necessity of the multidisciplinary team to integrate supportive care to improve overall patient care and QOL.

Upon initial diagnosis of advanced lung disease, a patient can often feel overwhelmed, which can lead to isolation, depression, and/or anxiety. It affects not only the patient but also the dynamics of the family system. The integration of patient advocacy organizations, such as the Wescoe Foundation for Pulmonary Fibrosis, is paramount to significantly increase the opportunity for patients and families/caregivers to get connected with supportive care. This mindset unites the community, including healthcare providers, in understanding the importance of another part of the care team and putting it into practice. Ultimately, this collaborative effort helps patients manage their disease as well as fulfill the void of the supportive care that many times healthcare providers do not always have the time to address.

The Wescoe Foundation for Pulmonary Fibrosis provides education, support, and resources for patients living with IPF, their caregivers, and healthcare providers. The mission is deeply woven into the fabric of the organization as Executive Director Jennifer Wescoe Singley's father succumbed to IPF in October 2004. At that time, there was very little to no support for families managing this insidious disease, and Jennifer made it her life's mission to connect the pulmonary fibrosis community with supportive care.

The Wescoe Foundation for Pulmonary Fibrosis exemplifies the effectiveness of a patient advocacy organization for better overall patient care. Jennifer has firsthand experience working with patients initially diagnosed and their caregivers and seeing the transition from being overwhelmed to being empowered and advocating for their own healthcare.

In unifying the pulmonary fibrosis community, the Wescoe Foundation created the only statewide support network in the United States, called the PA-IPF Support Network. It is a program that connects patients and caregivers to supportive care through effective, practical resources and educational programming. The Wescoe Foundation's work expands to other states, such as New Jersey and Delaware.

The support groups have been developed to meet the needs of the patients/families; they include IPF journey, lung transplantation, caregiver, veterans, and grief groups. Patients and caregivers not only learn about their disease, but they learn from and support each other. Some examples of practical resources are provider/patient checklists, pulmonary fibrosis podcasts, and the only web app in the United States connecting the pulmonary fibrosis community at one's fingertips. The educational programming prioritizes the interactive nature with providers and patients. It is a much more active model to engage, teach, and empower.

Learn more about The Wescoe Foundation for Pulmonary Fibrosis by visiting the website at www.wescoe.org and www.paipfsupportnetwork.org for more information.

Pulmonary-Palliative Care: We Be-LUNG Together: ATS Breathe Easy Series

This podcast provides informative dialogue about issues surrounding advanced lung disease patients and their needs. Topics include advanced illness planning, early communication about prognosis, symptom management, and pandemic planning. Additional information can be found at https://www.thoracic.org/about/ats-podcasts/.

End-of-Life Nurse Education Consortium

The End-of-Life Nurse Education Consortium (ELNEC; https://www.aacnnursing.org/ELNEC) project is a national and international education initiative using a "train-the-trainer" format to improve palliative care through education for nurses of all levels. ELNEC offers specialized and general palliative care tracks so that nurses may enroll in the coursework most relevant to their practice settings such as intensive care units or oncology. The education can then be brought back to the nurses' organization for ongoing education.

Four Seasons Consulting Group Palliative Care Immersion Course

Four Seasons Consulting (https://fourseasonsconsultinggroup.com/) is a national organization offering a renowned immersion course in palliative care that is accessible for all levels of palliative care: novice to expert, social work, nursing, providers, and administrators. The highly developed curriculum develops strong competencies and a knowledge base in palliative care across disease entities and healthcare settings.

The Pulmonary-Palliative Medicine Clinic at Geisinger Medical Center

At Geisinger Medical Center, a Level 1 shock-trauma academic medical center located in rural north-central Pennsylvania, a shared modality clinic was initiated and developed by nurse practitioners (NPs) with the goal of providing advanced lung disease patients with palliative and pulmonary care. This clinic allows patients and their families the opportunity to integrate ongoing management of lung disease with advanced illness planning and symptom management. Preliminary research found no previous existence of such a clinic; therefore, the need to build this from inception using evidence-based medicine became a necessity. The Geisinger Medical Center's Pulmonary-Palliative Medicine Clinic is a dedicated clinic with the time and trained staff to address the multifaceted issues of advancing lung disease in a safe forum for patients and their families to pursue an ongoing dialogue across the continuum of clinical care.

This enterprise began in 2008, with the Geisinger Medical Center's Divisions of Pulmonary and Palliative Medicine. This clinic was started by Patricia Maani-Fogelman, DNP, with the leadership support of the respective division directors Paul Simonelli, MD (Pulmonary-Critical Care), and Neil Ellison, MD (Palliative). In this setting, patients with advanced lung disease are seen by a pulmonary-palliative care NP (the author of this chapter) with extensive pulmonary, critical care, and palliative care backgrounds. Specific attention is given to the management of advanced lung disease symptoms, especially dyspnea, anxiety, depression, and fatigue, as well as to initiating discussions to establish goals of care, advance directives, code status, and more. When appropriate, hospice discussions and referrals are initiated with these patients, subsequently managed by the pulmonary-palliative NPs through the course of their progressive lung failure. The guidelines for the clinic's practice mission came from the ATS policy and consensus statements as well as from the NCP, which issued clinical practice guidelines (updated in 2018) for the delivery of quality palliative care for patients with advanced disease. These guidelines were not cancer-specific and included patients of any age living with progressive chronic conditions as well as those who are seriously and terminally ill. These are patients for whom intensive palliative care is the predominant focus for the remainder of their lives.[8,9,12,13,15–17]

The prognostication dilemma is managed through this specialty clinic by integrating palliative care early in the trajectory of advanced lung disease. Ongoing discussions are embedded into routine care, which normalizes the discussion and avoids creating a space for negative perceptions of "bad news." When providers are able to provide follow-up and continued dialogue across the continuum of the patient's disease trajectory, the long-held barrier that impeded the delivery of palliative care is lifted; and, as advocated by the ATS, it becomes a truly integrated, fundamental component of comprehensive pulmonary care.[1,6,8]

There is a need for education and training for healthcare and social care professions to plan and provide high-quality EOL care, and this is intensified in pulmonary medicine where patients have incurable, progressive illness with relatively high mortality and morbidity as disease advances.[6,8,9] Pulmonary-palliative care consults and ongoing care emphasize patient dignity, autonomy, and comfort. The first focus is to determine the patient/family understanding and goals. Part of this process is often early discussion and intervention for advanced illness planning in hopes of avoiding inappropriate medical interventions in favor of those that will not prolong a process of dying but serve to prolong a process of living.[33,34]

If indicated, the pulmonary-palliative NPs arrange aggressive, state-of-the-art medical care for patients with advanced illness, which may include measures such as high-flow nasal cannula, NIV, and continuous positive airway pressure or BiPAP therapy. Underlying this is ongoing medical management and psychosocial support for patient, family, and caregivers. All too often, there is the need to dispel myths concerning mechanical ventilation as most think death is swift and sudden or that they will be unconscious if on life support.

Nurses have the opportunity to be part of developing a clinic like this at their organization, with focused education, training, and multidisciplinary partnerships. The experience of this clinic has beautifully demonstrated that human beings are adaptable—because patients control their breathlessness by decreasing what they do on a daily basis, they are surprised when told they have a life-limiting illness and should consider palliative care.

Case Study: A Patient with COPD and Secondary Pulmonary Hypertension

Mr. B is a 74-year-old man seen in a clinic following admission for severe oxygen-dependent COPD, He is a former heavy smoker who currently smokes approximately half a pack of cigarettes daily. His recent admission for severe dyspnea, weakness, and cough included an echocardiogram which demonstrated significant increases in right heart pressures with an estimated pulmonary artery systolic pressure of 50 mm Hg. After further cardiologic investigation, it was concluded this was not cardiac in origin and determined to be World Health Organization Group III right heart disease, pulmonary hypertension attributed to chronic lung disease. Past medical history includes hypertension, diet-controlled diabetes, and a prior basal cell carcinoma lesion removed from his temple. At this visit, he reports dyspnea at rest. Pulmonary function testing indicated lung function of 26% predicted. He has been repeatedly referred to pulmonary rehabilitation and additional smoking cessation programs and counseling, which he declined. He needs help with most activities of daily living, cannot walk more than 3–5 feet without stopping, and is reliant on supplemental oxygen by nasal cannula around the clock. His nebulizers are not helping as much as they once did, and you determine his progressive shortness of breath and frequent exacerbations are not ameliorated with best-practice efforts and medical maximization. Due to continued decline in functional state, he was referred to the pulmonary-palliative clinic. At the initial visit, he reports the above symptoms. The nurse reviews this with the respiratory therapist and pulmonary-palliative NP. Together, they agree to add daily airway clearance with a flutter device and continued nebulizer therapies. The nurse advises providers not to increase nebulizer frequency because the patient shared with her how difficult and time-consuming this was for him. The nurse initiated advance illness planning discussions across multiple clinic visits, which included a multidisciplinary meeting about prognosis, discussion of advance directives, code status, EOL care, and hospice education. Both the patient and his significant other expressed great relief at being able to begin this discussion. With continued visits, hospice was discussed further, and code status was addressed: the patient verbalized satisfaction and happiness that he could be in control of his EOL decisions. Mr. B was a retired military officer who then went on to a second career in landscaping. He enjoyed working with his hands and creating beauty for his customers' property. He is also proud of his work as a soldier, noting that he was an active duty officer deployed in two wars and a proud patriot. His sense of duty, obligation, fidelity, and commitment run deep. He shares that he has some legal and financial matters he wants to get in order so that his spouse will always be cared for after he has died. The nurse provided ongoing support through this time, connecting Mr. B to a social worker. In partnership with the patient's pulmonary-palliative NP, they offered him the addition of hospice at home, which, after a few weeks, he accepted and which they arranged in conjunction with Mr. B's primary care office. During follow-up visits at the pulmonary-palliative clinic, Mr. B repeatedly expressed his gratitude for the focused care provided because the attention to learning about and developing a plan of care that was aligned with his wishes and preferences allowed him to make the arrangements he needed for his family and brought him tremendous peace of mind. His military career, devotion to family, and creative work were also acknowledged and validated, which brought him extraordinary pride and joy. There was a reinforcement of his dignity with this—it was important that he was known as a person, from the time before he was a "patient." With several months of attentive, ongoing palliative care and the support of visiting nurses from home-based hospice, he died at home, in peace and comfort, with his family by his side.

Conclusion

The person living with advanced lung disease suffers from multifaceted symptoms which, in combination, contribute to a loss in QOL, emotional distress, and, perhaps the most egregious loss of all, their functional independence. A commitment to whole-person care begins with the awareness of how this illness is more than just the single patient entity and extends to those in the patient's life, from family members to caregivers, perhaps even beyond—such as work groups and civic organizations. As advancing lung disease ensures, patients begin to lose more facets of their self-identity, may have to stop working, and become the one needing caregiving versus having been the traditional breadwinner. They need support, ongoing care, and open dialogue about the illness, what to expect, how to adjust/manage/cope; and we have evidence from around the world that affirms how patients and their families/caregivers value transparent and compassionate communication in an ongoing, organic manner regarding their prognoses and options for terminal stages of lung disease.[37] Preserving and promoting the dignity of the person living with advanced lung disease vis-à-vis early palliative care engagement, advocacy for strong symptom management, and comprehensive management of their global needs will best assure a goal of true optimization in both patient care and well-being. The foundation of strong nursing care begins with assuring clear, honest dialogues with patients, which is an ongoing process of education, discussion, and engagement with available supportive resources to assure we do our very best to deliver goal-concordant care. Pulmonary-palliative care is a construct whose time has long since arrived. They Be-LUNG together.

REFERENCES

1. Phongtankuel V, Meador L, Adelman RD, et al. Multicomponent palliative care interventions in advanced chronic diseases: a systematic review. *Am J Hosp Palliat Care*. 2018; 35(1):173–183.
2. Sullivan R, Peppercorn J, Sikora K, et al. Delivering affordable cancer care in high-income countries. *Lancet Oncol*. 2011;12(10):933–980. https://doi.org/10.1016/S1470-2045(11)70141-3.
3. Johnson T, McMurry-Heath M, Okon T, Rubin D, Carlson RW. NCCN policy summit: innovative solutions to drive down healthcare costs: implications for access to high-quality cancer care. *J Natl Compr Canc Netw*. 2021;19(9):1021–1026. https://doi.org/10.6004/jnccn.2021.7084.
4. Hartman M, Martin AB, Washington B, Catlin A; National Health Expenditure Accounts Team. National health care spending in 2020: growth driven by federal spending in response to the COVID-19 pandemic. *Health Aff (Millwood)*. 2022;41(1):13–25. https://doi.org/10.1377/hlthaff.2021.01763.
5. Institute of Medicine of the National Academies. *Dying in America: Improving Quality and Honoring Individual Preferences*

Near the End of Life. National Academies Press; 2014. Accessed October 25, 2022. http://www.nationalacademies.org/hmd/Reports/2014/Dying-In-America-Improving-Quality-and-Honoring-Individual-Preferences-Near-the-End-of-Life.aspx.

6. Halpin DMG, Criner GJ, Papi A, et al. Global initiative for the diagnosis, management, and prevention of chronic obstructive lung disease. The 2020 GOLD Science Committee Report on COVID-19 and Chronic Obstructive Pulmonary Disease. *Am J Respir Crit Care Med*. 2021;203(1):24–36. https://doi.org/10.1164/rccm.202009-3533SO.
7. Qaseem A, Wilt TJ, Weinberger SE, et al.; for the American College of Physicians, the American College of Chest Physicians, the American Thoracic Society, and the European Respiratory Society. Diagnosis and management of stable chronic obstructive pulmonary disease: a clinical practice guideline update from the American College of Physicians, American College of Chest Physicians, American Thoracic Society, and European Respiratory Society. *Ann Intern Med*. 2011;155:179–191.
8. Sullivan DR, Iyer AS, Enguidanos S, et al. Palliative care early in the care continuum among patients with serious respiratory illness: an official ATS/AAHPM/HPNA/SWHPN policy statement. *Am J Respir Crit Care Med*. 2022;206(6):e44–e69. https://doi.org/10.1164/rccm.202207-1262ST.
9. Ferrell BR, Twaddle ML, Melnick A, Meier DE. National Consensus Project Clinical Practice Guidelines for Quality Palliative Care Guidelines, 4th edition. *J Palliat Med*. 2018;21(12):1684–1689. https://doi.org/10.1089/jpm.2018.0431.
10. Ferrell BR, Temel JS, Temin S, et al. Integration of palliative care into standard oncology care: American Society of Clinical Oncology clinical practice guideline update. *J Clin Oncol*. 2017;35(1):96–112.
11. SUPPORT Principal Investigators. A controlled trial to improve care for seriously ill hospitalized patients. The study to understand prognoses and preferences for outcomes and risks of treatments (SUPPORT). *JAMA*. 1995;274(20):1591–1598.
12. Claessens MT, Lynn J, Zhong Z, et al. Dying with lung cancer or chronic obstructive pulmonary disease: insights from SUPPORT. *J Am Geriatr Soc*. 2000;48:S146–S153.
13. Mooren K, Wester D, Kerstjens H, Bergkamp F, Spathis A, Engels Y. Filling the gap: a feasibility study of a COPD-specific breathlessness service. *COPD*. 2022;19(1):324–329. https://doi.org/10.1080/15412555.2022.2099821.
14. Bakitas MA, Dionne-Odom JN, Ejem DB, et al. Effect of an early palliative care telehealth intervention vs usual care on patients with heart failure: the ENABLE CHF-PC randomized clinical trial. *JAMA Intern Med*. 2020;180(9):1203–1213. https://doi.org/10.1001/jamainternmed.2020.2861.
15. Dalal S, Bruera E. End-of-life care matters: palliative cancer care results in better care and lower costs. *Oncologist* 2017;22(4):361–368.
16. Kelley AS, Covinsky KE, Gorges RJ, et al. Identifying older adults with serious illness: a critical step toward improving the value of health care. *Health Serv Res*. 2017;52(1):113–131. https://doi.org/10.1111/1475-6773.12479.
17. Quill TE, Abernethy AP. Generalist plus specialist palliative care—creating a more sustainable model. *N Engl J Med*. 2009;368(13):1173–1175.
18. Knauft E, Nielsen EL, Engelberg RA, Patrick DL, Curtis JR. Barriers and facilitators to end-of-life care communication for patients with COPD. *Chest*. 2005;127:2188–2196.
19. Au DH, Udris EM, Fihn SD, McDonell MB, Curtis JR. Differences in health care utilization at the end of life among patients with chronic obstructive pulmonary disease and patients with lung cancer. *Arch Intern Med*. 2006;166:326–331.
20. Cross SH, Ely EW, Kavalieratos D, Tulsky JA, Warraich HJ. Place of death for individuals with chronic lung disease: trends and associated factors from 2003 to 2017 in the United States. *Chest*. 2020;158(2):670–680. https://doi.org/10.1016/j.chest.2020.02.062.
21. Kalluri M, Orenstein S, Archibald N, Pooler C. Advance care planning needs in idiopathic pulmonary fibrosis: a qualitative study. *Am J Hosp Palliat Care*. 2022;39(6):641–651. https://doi.org/10.1177/10499091211041724.
22. Wijsenbeek M, Suzuki A, Maher TM. Interstitial lung diseases. *Lancet*. 2022;400(10354):769–786. https://doi.org/10.1016/S0140-6736(22)01052-2.
23. Celli BR, Singh D, Vogelmeier C, Agusti A. New perspectives on chronic obstructive pulmonary disease. *Int J Chron Obstruct Pulmon Dis*. 2022;17:2127–2136. https://doi.org/10.2147/COPD.S365771.
24. Hendriks PM, Staal DP, van de Groep LD, et al. The evolution of survival of pulmonary arterial hypertension over 15 years. *Pulm Circ*. 2022;12(4):e12137. https://doi.org/10.1002/pul2.12137.
25. Gersten RA, Seth B, Arellano L, et al. Provider perspectives on and access to palliative care for patients with interstitial lung disease. *Chest*. 2022;162(2):375–384. https://doi.org/10.1016/j.chest.2022.03.009.
26. Owusuaa C, Dijkland SA, Nieboer D, van der Rijt CCD, van der Heide A. Predictors of mortality in chronic obstructive pulmonary disease: a systematic review and meta-analysis. *BMC Pulm Med*. 2022;22(1):125. https://doi.org/10.1186/s12890-022-01911-5.
27. Maddocks M, Lovell N, Booth S, Man WD, Higginson IJ. Palliative care and management of troublesome symptoms for people with chronic obstructive pulmonary disease. *Lancet*. 2017;390(10098):988–1002. https://doi.org/10.1016/S0140-6736(17)32127-X.
28. Rhodes JR, Wharton J, Ghataorhe P, et al. Plasma proteome analysis in patients with pulmonary arterial hypertension: an observational cohort study. *Lancet Respir Med*. 2017;5:717–726.
29. Dal Negro RW, Celli BR. Patient Related Outcomes-BODE (PRO-BODE): a composite index incorporating health utilization resources predicts mortality and economic cost of COPD in real life. *Respir Med*. 2017;131:175–178.
30. Raghu G, Remy-Jardin M, Myers JL, et al. Diagnosis of Idiopathic Pulmonary Fibrosis. An Official ATS/ERS/JRS/ALAT Clinical Practice Guideline. *Am J Respir Crit Care Med*. 2018;198(5):e44–e68. doi:10.1164/rccm.201807-1255ST
31. Ferrera MC, Labaki WW, Han MK. Advances in chronic obstructive pulmonary disease. *Annu Rev Med*. 2021;72:119–134. doi:https://doi.org/10.1146/annurev-med-080919-112707.
32. Gordon CS, Waller JW, Cook RM, Cavalera SL, Lim WT, Osadnik CR. Effect of pulmonary rehabilitation on symptoms of anxiety and depression in COPD: a systematic review and meta-analysis. *Chest*. 2019;156(1):80–91. doi:https://doi.org/10.1016/j.chest.2019.04.009.
33. Sohanpal R, Pinnock H, Steed L, et al. Tailored, psychological intervention for anxiety or depression in people with chronic obstructive pulmonary disease (COPD), TANDEM (Tailored intervention for ANxiety and DEpression Management in COPD): protocol for a randomised controlled trial. *Trials*. 2020;21(1):18. Published 2020 Jan 6. doi:https://doi.org/10.1186/s13063-019-3800-y.
34. Brien SB, Lewith GT, Thomas M. Patient coping strategies in COPD across disease severity and quality of life: a qualitative study. *NPJ Primary Care Respiratory Medicine*. 2016;26;16051.

35. Kasdorf A, Dust G, Hamacher S, et al. The last year of life for patients dying from cancer vs. non-cancer causes: a retrospective cross-sectional survey of bereaved relatives. *Support Care Cancer.* 2022;30(6):4971–4979. doi:https://doi.org/10.1007/s00520-022-06908-8.
36. Koh MYH, Hum AYM, Khoo HS, et al. Burnout and resilience after a decade in palliative care: what survivors have to teach us. A qualitative study of palliative care clinicians with more than 10 years of experience. *J Pain Symptom Manage.* 2020;59(1):105–115. https://doi.org/10.1016/j.jpainsymman.2019.08.008.
37. Owusuaa C, van Lent LGG, van't Spijker A, van der Rijt CCD, van der Heide A. Discussing prognosis and the end of life with patients with advanced cancer or COPD: A qualitative study. *PLoS One.* 2022;17(9):e0274201. https://doi.org/10.1371/journal.pone.0274201.
38. American Association of Colleges of Nursing and City of Hope. Dyspnea empathy exercise. In: *ELNEC-Critical Care Curriculum.* Module 3—Symptom Management, Supplemental Teaching Materials section. American Association of Colleges of Nursing; 2017.

46

Palliative Care in Heart Failure

Rachel D. Wells, Avery C. Bechthold, Keith M. Swetz, and J. Nicholas Odom

Key Points

- The heart failure disease trajectory is progressive, although highly unpredictable, with periods of high function interspersed with sudden life-threatening exacerbations leading to emergent hospitalizations and often rapid deterioration and death.
- The focus of palliative, supportive care is on symptom management, particularly shortness of breath, fatigue, and leg swelling, and promoting positive health behaviors (diet, exercise, and smoking cessation).
- Management of advanced heart failure includes medications and devices to sustain adequate circulation and prevent life-threatening arrhythmias.

Introduction

Heart failure is a complex syndrome resulting from any functional or structural disorder of the heart that lowers the ability of the heart to pump blood and/or leads to systemic or pulmonary congestion.[1] Heart failure is not a disease but a syndrome, and hence diagnosis relies on a myriad of clinical indicators and functional ability assessment.[2] Since the 1970s, heart failure in the United States has been described as an epidemic as newer therapies have increased survival.[3,4] Heart failure can be a slowly developing condition that results from coronary artery disease, hypertension, diabetes, and valvular disease or one that develops precipitously after a myocardial infarction.[1,5] Those living with symptomatic heart failure experience lower quality of life (QOL) and high morbidity and mortality; however, advances in therapies including angiotensin-converting enzyme (ACE) inhibitors, beta-blockers, coronary revascularization, implantable cardioverter-defibrillators, and cardiac resynchronization have substantially improved outcomes.[2]

An estimated 6 million Americans and 64.3 million individuals worldwide are affected by heart failure.[1,6] While the incidence of heart failure has decreased, the rate of heart failure in older adults has increased[1] and accelerated in the post-Covid era.[7] In the United States, there are over 900,000 new cases of heart failure each year and nearly 400,000 heart failure–related deaths.[1,8] By 2030, it is estimated that the number of Americans with heart failure will increase to 8 million.[9] African Americans have the highest incidence of heart failure, followed by Hispanic Americans, White Americans, and Asian Americans, with many of these differences mediated by differences in hypertension, diabetes, and low socioeconomic status.[1] Comorbidities are common in adults living with advanced heart failure, the most prevalent of which include chronic kidney disease, anemia, diabetes, and chronic obstructive pulmonary disease (COPD).[5,10]

The toll of heart failure on economic and healthcare utilization resources is considerable.[11] Worldwide, the economic cost of heart failure has been estimated at $346.7 billion per year.[11] In the United States, medical costs directly related to heart failure amounted to $22.3 billion in 2016,[12] with estimates predicting an increase to $69.8 billion in 2030.[9] These costs drastically increase in the last months of life, mostly due to increased number and length of hospitalizations.[13,14] Indeed, periodic exacerbations of heart failure require intensive treatments that nearly always require hospitalization. Close to 1 million hospitalizations occur each year due to heart failure, and it is one of the leading causes of hospitalization for individuals 65 years of age and older in both the United States and Europe.[15,16]

To help persons and families affected by heart failure manage the high symptom burden, complex decision-making, and ever-present risk of exacerbation and death, the early integration of palliative care is critical and has been recommended in numerous organizational statements in both the United States and worldwide.[5,17–21] Palliative care in the setting of heart failure seeks to mitigate complex symptoms and maximize function; promote positive coping, psychological health, and spiritual behaviors; enhance communication and decision-making; facilitate prognostic understanding and advance care planning (ACP); and coordinate care, including transitions to hospice care when appropriate.[1–4] To describe the role of palliative care further, this chapter provides an overview of the palliative care aspects of heart failure care.

Heart Failure Pathogenesis

Cardiac output is the primary indicator of cardiac performance. It equates to the product of the number of beats per minute (heart rate) and how much blood the heart pumps with each beat (stroke volume). *Heart rate* increases through sympathetic nervous system activation that speeds up the heart and is decreased by the parasympathetic nervous system. *Stroke volume* is determined by preload, afterload, and myocardial contractility. *Preload*, also called *end-diastolic volume*, is the amount of blood present in the ventricle at the end of diastole just prior to the heart pumping (or systole). As preload increases, myocardial muscle fibers stretch and eject with a proportionate force according to the Frank-Starling mechanism. The fraction of blood ejected by the ventricle relative to the preload is called *ejection fraction* and is the most commonly used metric for assessing heart failure. *Afterload* is the amount of resistance against which the ventricles must contract to eject blood and is a function of systemic vascular resistance and ventricular wall tension. The higher the systemic vascular resistance, the more forceful the systolic contraction must be to push blood out of the ventricle. *Contractility*, or *inotropy*, is the ability of the heart muscle fibers to contract against a load in the atria and ventricles. Myocardial contractility is governed at the cellular level by calcium ions (Ca^{++}) and the sodium–Ca^{++} exchange pump; hence, many drugs for heart failure target these cellular mechanisms.

Heart Failure with Reduced versus Preserved Ejection Fraction

Based on measurement of the left ventricular ejection fraction (LVEF), heart failure is most commonly characterized as having reduced (≤40%), mildly reduced (41%–49%), improved (prior ≤40% with a subsequent >40%), or preserved LVEF (≥50%) (see Table 46.1). In *heart failure with reduced LVEF* (HFrEF; also referred to as "systolic dysfunction"), myocardial contractility has been weakened, resulting in a lower ejection fraction (EF) and cardiac output. Common co-occurring conditions are supraventricular tachycardias (e.g., atrial fibrillation), ventricular arrhythmias, bradycardia, venous thromboembolism, anemia, and sleep disruption. For some individuals, their EF may improve to >40%. With *heart failure with improved LVEF* (HFimpEF), individuals may still have symptomatic heart failure or abnormal biomarkers. Improvement in LVEF may be due to reversible/resolving cause of heart failure (e.g., stress cardiomyopathy) or treatment.

In 2021, all international professional cardiology organizations issued a consensus statement proposing a universal classification of heart failure, thereby codifying the use of the term *heart failure with mildly reduced LVEF* (HFmrEF), to characterize a new heart failure phenotype when individuals present with heart failure signs and symptoms (e.g., elevated natriuretic peptides) or diastolic dysfunction with only a slight reduction in LVEF.[22] Given that those with mildly reduced EF are often in transition to either improving from or deteriorating to HFrEF, the etiology of HFmrEF is similar to that of heart failure with reduced EF though clinical presentation can be varied.[23]

In contrast, and increasing in incidence,[5] *heart failure with preserved LVEF* (HFpEF; also called "diastolic dysfunction") retains a normal EF (50%–65%), but the ventricles are stiff, less compliant, and unable to stretch normally. Consequently, venous blood returning from the systemic circulation is unable to adequately fill the ventricles, thereby compromising preload and reducing stroke volume. As heart rate increases, diastolic filling time decreases, and hence HFpEF worsens with tachycardia. Resultant co-occurring conditions mirror that of HFrEF.

Right versus Left Ventricular Dysfunction

Heart failure can be classified according to whether the right or left ventricle is primarily affected (although both ventricles are typically affected over the long term). Right ventricular heart failure is the inability of the right ventricle to move deoxygenated venous blood from the systemic circulation into the pulmonary circulation. Major effects include dependent peripheral edema, reduced left ventricular cardiac output, and hepatomegaly due to blood backing up into the hepatic veins. If hepatic circulation remains congested for a prolonged period, blood will begin engorging the spleen and the gastrointestinal tract, resulting in decreased hepatocellular function, ascites, altered nutritional uptake, and gastrointestinal discomfort. The most common cause of right ventricular heart failure is left ventricular heart failure. Other causes include chronic pulmonary hypertension (also called "cor pulmonale") due to thromboembolic disease or structural lung disease, tricuspid or pulmonic valve stenosis or regurgitation, right ventricular infarction, cardiomyopathy, and congenital heart defects (e.g., tetralogy of Fallot, ventricular septal defect).

Left ventricular heart failure occurs when oxygenated blood from the pulmonary circulation is not effectively pumped into the

Table 46.1 Heart failure type

Heart failure type	Criteria	Common causes
HF with reduced EF (HFrEF)	• LVEF ≤40%	• Coronary artery disease • Hypertension • Ischemic heart disease • Valvular disease (e.g., aortic stenosis)
HF with improved EF (HFimpEF)	• Prior LVEF ≤40% *and* follow-up measurement of LVEF >40%	• Dilated cardiomyopathy • Hypertension
HF with mildly reduced EF (HFmrEF)	• LVEF 41%–49% *and* spontaneous/provokable ↑ LV filling pressures	• Ischemic heart disease • Hypertension (systolic elevation) • Valvular disease (e.g., aortic stenosis) • Coronary artery disease
HF with preserved EF (HFpEF)	• LVEF ≥50% *and* spontaneous/provokable ↑ LV filling pressures	• Pericardial effusion • Constrictive pericarditis • Hypertrophic cardiomyopathy • Ischemic heart disease

HF, Heart failure; EF, ejection fraction; LV, left ventricle; LVEF, left ventricular ejection fraction.
Source: Reference 5.

systemic circulation. This lower cardiac output results in blood backing up into the left ventricle, left atrium, and pulmonary circulation. Consequently, pulmonary capillary pressures increase and, if high enough, cause intravascular fluid to infiltrate the lung interstitium, resulting in impaired gas exchange (i.e., hypoxia) and pulmonary edema. The most common causes of left ventricular heart failure are hypertension and myocardial infarction. Aortic or mitral valve stenosis or regurgitation may also cause this type of heart failure.

Disease Trajectory and Prognosis

Illness Trajectory

The heart failure disease trajectory is progressive yet highly unpredictable, with periods of high function interspersed with sudden life-threatening exacerbations leading to emergent hospitalizations and sometimes rapid deterioration and death.[24] For many, heart failure begins with an emergent presentation to the emergency department with severe breathlessness and chest pain or discomfort (e.g., acute myocardial infarction); for others, the onset is gradual with increasing breathlessness and fluid retention that might be first evaluated by a primary care clinician. Depending on the severity of the initial insult, medications combined with lifestyle modifications (e.g., low-sodium diet, increased physical activity, weight loss) and fluid management can effectively ameliorate nearly all symptoms, helping persons living with advanced heart failure reach a state of near-baseline functioning that can potentially last several years. However, as heart failure progresses, symptoms begin to reoccur, and management requirements exceed oral medication therapy and include consideration of intravenous inotropes and implantable cardiac devices, such as pacemakers and ventricular assist devices. Cause of death among individuals with heart failure varies considerably.[4] For some, a spontaneous cardiac event, such as a lethal arrhythmia, can occur unexpectedly and result in rapid deterioration and sudden death. For others, the dying phase is prolonged due to progressive pump failure marked with episodes of acute decompensation and severe symptoms.

Classification

Two classification systems are most commonly used to grade the severity of heart failure: the American College of Cardiology/American Heart Association (ACC/AHA) stages and the New York Heart Association (NYHA) classes (see Table 46.2).[5] Of note, the 2021 universal classification consensus statement also included a guide for universal staging that closely aligns with the ACC/AHA stages.[22]

The two classification systems have some similarities; however, the ACC/AHA system includes criteria for both physical symptoms and structural abnormalities of the heart, whereas the NYHA system only includes physical symptom criteria. An individual's NYHA class can fluctuate based on clinical status, but their ACC/AHA stage progresses unidirectionally; hence, one's stage and class are not direct corollaries of one another.

Estimating and Communicating Prognosis

Estimating and communicating prognosis in heart failure are critical to help persons living with advanced heart failure and their families plan and make decisions about treatment. However, accurate prognosticating is extremely difficult due to the interactions of frailty, polypharmacy,[26] and comorbidities,[27] discerning treatment-responsive from treatment-nonresponsive situations, and wide variations in end-of-life events.[28] After a period of improvement through the year 2000, survival trends have plateaued,[29,30] with approximately 25% of US adults newly diagnosed with heart failure dying within 1 year and 50% within 5 years.[1,31] However, these rates vary by geographic location,[29] age, and type of heart failure. Further, individuals 80 years of age or older and those with HFrEF experience the highest mortality rates.[32] It is also important to note that about half of heart failure deaths are due to complications of comorbidities, particularly respiratory conditions and cancer.[10,27]

Despite the challenges in accurate prognostication, recommendations in the current literature suggest using a combination of objective risk models[33,34] and clinical gestalt.[35] The Seattle Heart Failure Model (https://depts.washington.edu/shfm/) and the Meta-Analysis Global Group in Chronic Heart Failure (http://www.heartfailurerisk.org) risk calculators are well-validated multivariable models and available online. While predicting death in heart failure using these models is imperfect, predicting *nonsurvival* outcomes of importance to patients and families—such as QOL, symptom burden, and rehospitalizations—using prognostic models is even poorer.[36,37]

Despite the many challenges to accurate prognosis, prognostic assessments are recommended yearly and subsequent to hospitalization and stabilization after major health changes and events.[38–40] Such events represent "inflection points" that warrant reappraisal of goals of care, patient and family preferences, and treatment modalities. Approaches to "serious illness," "bad news," and "prognosis" conversations are covered in greater depth elsewhere[41,42]; and the palliative care nurse clinician is encouraged to continually enhance skills and prepare in advance for these conversations.

Overview of Assessment and Medical Management in Stage D Heart Failure

A number of major guidelines and consensus papers are published and regularly updated for the treatment of advanced Stage D heart failure, including the 2022 ACC/AHA/Heart Failure Society of America guideline,[5] the 2021 European Society of Cardiology guidelines,[17] and the National Institute for Health and Care Excellence chronic heart failure guideline (available at https://www.nice.org.uk/guidance/cg187 and https://www.nice.org.uk/guidance/ng106).[21] The following overview of heart failure clinical assessment and treatment is consistent with these guidelines.

Health History

Important health history information to collect during assessment includes:

- History of present illness including heart failure progression history and precipitating factors for most recent episode
- Heart failure risk factors and preventive behaviors (e.g., exercise, weight loss)
- Exacerbation episodes and hospitalizations
- Current and past treatments, therapy response, and compliance

Table 46.2 Classification systems for heart failure and typical treatments

ACC/AHA heart failure stages		NYHA heart failure classes		Typical treatments
Stage A (at risk)	No limitations or symptoms of HF. No structural heart abnormalities. Often presence of hypertension, diabetes, coronary artery disease, and metabolic syndrome.	No comparable class.		Lifestyle changes including regular exercise, smoking cessation. ACE inhibitor or ARB if confirmed coronary artery disease, diabetes, and hypertension. Beta-blockers if post-MI or hypertension.
Stage B (pre-HF; asymptomatic)	No limitations or symptoms of HF. Structural heart abnormalities present (e.g., left ventricular hypertrophy or other evidence of remodeling). Decreased ejection fraction. Often follows MI, valvular disease, and/or cardiomyopathy.	Class I	No limitations of physical activity. Ordinary physical activity does not cause fatigue, dyspnea, or palpitation.	ACE inhibitor or ARB. Beta-blockers if post-MI. Aldosterone inhibitor if the symptoms continue while taking beta-blockers and ACE/ARB medications. Surgery for coronary artery repair and valve repair or replacement. Implantable cardiac defibrillator-EF <30%, >40 days post-MI.
Stage C (symptomatic)	Shortness of breath, fatigue, and activity intolerance with activities of daily living. Structural heart abnormalities present.	Class II	Slight limitation of physical activity. Comfortable at rest. Ordinary physical activity causes fatigue, dyspnea, and/or palpitation.	ACE inhibitors and beta-blockers. Aldosterone inhibitor if symptoms severe and other medications have been initiated.
		Class III	Marked limitation of physical activity. Comfortable at rest. Less than ordinary activity causes fatigue, dyspnea, and/or palpitation (e.g., walking distances of 20–100 meters).	ARBs and neprilysin inhibitors. Mineralocorticoid receptor antagonists. SGLT2is[25] in the setting of chronic HFrEF. Hydralazine/nitrate combination if symptoms persist. Diuretics and digoxin if symptoms persist. Biventricular pacemaker. Implantable cardiac defibrillator.
Stage D (end stage)	Presence of progressive and/or persistent severe signs and symptoms of HF driven primarily by the HF syndrome itself despite optimal medical, surgical, and device management. Frequent hospitalization, severely limited exertional tolerance, and poor-quality of life are typically present.	Class IV	Physical activity not possible without discomfort. HF symptoms at rest.	Strict fluid and sodium restriction. Surgery (e.g., valve replacement). Heart transplantation. Ventricular assist devices. Continuous intravenous inotropic support.

ACC, American College of Cardiology; ACE, angiotensin-converting enzyme; AHA, American Heart Association; ARB, angiotensin II receptor blocker; EF, ejection fraction; HF, heart failure; HFrEF, HF with reduced EF; MI, myocardial infarction; NYHA, New York Heart Association; SGLT2i, sodium-glucose cotransporter 2 inhibitor.
Sources: References 5, 17, and 24.

- History of physical (e.g., diabetes, COPD, dyslipidemia) and psychosocial (e.g., anxiety, depression) comorbid conditions
- Symptom assessment, particularly dyspnea, fatigue, pain, edema, anorexia and cachexia, depression, and anxiety, focusing on exacerbating and relieving factors (see below, "Management of Symptoms in Stage D Heart Failure")
- Patient's and family's understanding of the illness and prognosis, to date, as well as current goals for care and treatment preferences
- Spiritual and faith-based practices and beliefs that may impact care

Physical Exam

The physical exam should begin with assessment of vital signs, height and weight, overall appearance, and mood/affect. In general, physical exam findings in heart failure lack sensitivity; however, a head-to-toe assessment may be remarkable for several of the following findings[31,43–45]:

- *Blood pressure and heart rate*: Tachycardia and systolic blood pressure less than 90–100 mm Hg are common if treatment is suboptimal. Presence of a weak, thready pulse and/or pulsus alternans (alternating strong and weak pulse) may indicate decreased cardiac output.
- *Jugular venous distension*: Assessed with the patient supine at a 45-degree angle. A distance of more than 3 cm between the sternal angle and the top of the internal jugular venous pulsation is a specific but not sensitive sign of elevated left ventricular filling.
- *Point of maximal impulse*: Assessed with finger palpation, the point of maximal impulse is typically located at the midclavicular line at the fifth intercostal space. Presence of cardiomegaly will shift this point laterally and downward.
- *Third and fourth heart sounds*: One or both of these heart sounds are present in nearly all cases of heart failure.

- *Pulmonary assessment*: Auscultation often reveals rales and/or wheezing. In some cases, increased lymphatic drainage compensates for increased pulmonary congestion over time.
- *Liver size and hepatojugular reflux*: Hepatomegaly may present in right-sided heart failure and can be assessed using the hepatojugular reflux. With the patient supine at a 45-degree angle and instructed to keep the mouth open (to prevent Valsalva maneuver), moderate pressure is applied to the middle of the abdomen for 30–60 seconds. Hepatojugular reflux is present if the height of the neck veins increases by 3 cm or more and remains increased during compression of the abdomen.
- *Lower extremity edema*: Usually detectable when the extracellular volume exceeds 5 L. The edema may be accompanied by stasis dermatitis, a chronic, eczema-like condition characterized by edema, hyperpigmentation, and sometimes ulceration.

Laboratory Data and Diagnostic Tests

Laboratory data and diagnostic tests are often performed prior to palliative care evaluation. Relevant tests and data to assess in relevance to heart failure include:

- *Hypokalemia*: Possibly due to thiazide diuretics.
- *Hyperkalemia*: Possibly due to potassium-sparing diuretics and ACE inhibitors.
- *Elevated blood urea nitrogen and creatinine*: Consider prerenal azotemia related to pump failure and decreased renal perfusion.
- *Elevated liver enzymes, including serum transaminase and bilirubin*: Potentially hepatic congestion from right-sided (or left-sided) heart failure. Jaundice may be present. In cases of chronic hepatomegaly, cardiac cirrhosis may occur, signaled by hypoalbuminemia, hypoglycemia, and increased prothrombin time.
- *Decreased hemoglobin*: May indicate (1) normocytic anemia secondary to decreased production of erythropoietin (and thus decreased red blood cell production) due to chronic kidney disease (comorbid kidney disease is present in 20%–40% of persons living with heart failure) and/or (2) anemia secondary to hemodilution through plasma volume expansion triggered by the renin–angiotensin system.
- *Elevated cardiac biomarkers including B-type natriuretic peptide (BNP) and N-terminal pro-B-type natriuretic peptide (NT-proBNP)*. Abnormally high levels typically indicate presence of acute and/or chronic heart failure and can be used to assist in diagnosis or exclusion of heart failure as a cause of symptoms (e.g., dyspnea, weight gain), inform prognosis, and estimate the likelihood of hospital readmission. Utility may be limited with concurrent renal failure.
- *Electrocardiogram (ECG)*: Abnormalities in advanced heart failure are typically present and may indicate atrial and ventricular arrhythmias, heart block and other conduction problems due to electrolyte disturbances, ischemia (new and old infarctions), and cardiac remodeling.
- *Echocardiography*: Used to assess left ventricular size, mass, and function; valve function; regional wall motion; and ACC/AHA heart failure staging. Also allows for the estimation of EF.
- *Chest radiograph*: Can be used to evaluate heart size, pulmonary edema, and pleural effusions.
- *Cardiac catheterization*: Assesses coronary artery occlusion and pressure gradients across heart valves. Can also be used as a platform for stent placement of occluded vessels. Right-sided catheterizations can assess pressures on the right side of the heart and pulmonary pressures.
- *Stress test*: Used to assess cardiac function in response to external stress induced through either physical exertion (e.g., walking on a treadmill, pedaling on an exercise bicycle) or intravenous medications (e.g., adenosine).

Treatment

Pharmacologic Treatment

Table 46.3 lists commonly used medications in the management of advanced heart failure by class.[5,17,46,47] The primary goals of pharmacologic management are to improve cardiac function and reduce symptoms. While pharmacologic therapies can improve the clinical status and symptoms of a person living with advanced heart failure, underlying cardiac structure and function are not restored to normal states. As heart failure worsens, the person's condition may become refractory to maximal doses of medications, prompting consideration of surgery, mechanical circulatory support devices, and heart transplant options.

Lifestyle Recommendations

While evidence for the impact of lifestyle modifications on morbidity and mortality in advanced heart failure is limited, patients with advanced heart failure should be generally encouraged to (1) quit smoking, (2) limit or abstain from alcohol intake and illicit drug use, (3) lose weight if obese, and (4) monitor daily weight to track fluid retention and overload. For patients with symptomatic congestion (1) sodium restriction to 2,300 mg/day[48] and (2) fluid restriction to 1.5–2 L/day may improve symptoms and QOL[49–51]; however, any dietary restriction should include careful monitoring for hyponatremia and malnutrition.

Implantable Cardioverter-Defibrillators

Implantable cardioverter defibrillators (ICDs) are medical devices implanted inside the body that perform cardioversion and/or defibrillation upon detection of a lethal arrhythmia (e.g., ventricular fibrillation, ventricular tachycardia). The benefits of ICDs are most frequently observed in terms of prolonged survival in patients who have HFrEF and are at risk for sudden cardiac death.[5] The devices alone do not improve cardiac function and are not recommended for patients with diastolic dysfunction or for patients with poor functional status and a prognosis of less than 1 year. ICDs are also not recommended for NYHA Class IV patients with medication-refractory congestive heart failure who are not candidates for heart transplantation. Patients should be informed *prior to ICD placement* about the option to deactivate the device as they approach the end of life.[52–55]

Mechanical Circulatory Support

For patients with HFrEF who are symptomatic despite optimal pharmacological management, mechanical circulatory support devices (MCSDs), including left ventricular assist devices (LVADs) and total artificial hearts (TAHs), may be viable options to partially or completely replace the function of the heart. MCS is considered

Table 46.3 Common medications in heart failure

Medications	Dose routes and ranges	Side effects	Special considerations
Angiotensin-converting enzyme inhibitors (ACE inhibitor)			
Captopril	6.5–50 mg three times a day PO	**Hyperkalemia**; **dizziness**; cough; less frequent: pruritus, skin rash, taste loss (dose-related and reversible); agranulocytosis, renal impairment, angioedema	Frequent urinary/blood analysis needed. Monitor liver enzymes. Do not use in patients with history of angioedema or patients taking aliskiren with diabetes, lithium, gold, or mTOR inhibitors (sirolimus). Caution with patients with renal insufficiency. Dose adjustment required for hemodialysis.
Enalapril	2.5–20 mg twice a day PO		
Lisinopril	2.5–40 mg daily PO; 2.5 mg starting dose with hyponatremia or creatinine clearance <30 mL/min		
Angiotensin II receptor blockers (ARBs)			
Losartan	25–150 mg daily PO; recommended hepatic initial dose: 25 mg PO daily	**Cough**; **dizziness**; **muscle ache**; hypotension; renal insufficiency; hyperkalemia	Caution with patients with low systemic blood pressure. Caution with concomitant use of potassium-sparing diuretics or NSAIDs. Do not use in diabetic patients taking aliskiren. Caution with patients on lithium—monitor serum lithium levels.
Valsartan	20–160 mg twice daily PO		
Angiotensin receptor-nephrolysin inhibitor			
Sacubitril/valsartan	49/51–97/103 mg twice daily PO; 24/26 mg starting dose for patients ACE inhibitor/ARB-naive, creatinine clearance <30 mL/min, or moderate hepatic impairment	**Hypotension**; **hyperkalemia**; dizziness; renal insufficiency; angioedema	Not all doses tested in HF trial. 36-hour wait period switch to/from ACE inhibitor. Risk of angioedema. High cost due to lack of generic availability—might not be covered by some insurances. Do not use in diabetic patients taking aliskiren.
Loop diuretics			
Furosemide	20–80 mg daily PO	**Hypotension**; **dry mouth**; muscle pain/cramps; hyperglycemia; dermatitis; tinnitus; systemic vasculitis; pancreatitis	Do not use in patients with anuria or those taking aminoglycoside antibiotics or ethacrynic acid (ototoxicity). Caution with patients with sulfonamide allergy. Caution with patients with hepatic cirrhosis, ascites. Caution with digitalis—may exaggerate hypokalemic metabolic effect.
Bumetanide	0.5–10 mg daily PO	**Muscle cramps**; **dizziness**; hypotension; hypokalemia; ototoxicity; pruritus; EKG changes; thrombocytopenia	Do not use in patients taking indomethacin. Caution in patients with hepatic impairment or allergic to sulfonamides. Caution with patients on lithium—monitor serum lithium levels.
Thiazide diuretics			
Metolazone	2.5–20 mg daily PO	**Dizziness**; **hypotension**; **fatigue**; **electrolyte disturbances**; agranulocytosis; hepatitis; necrotizing vasculitis; seizures	Do not use in patients with anuria. Caution in patients with hyperglycemia or taking NSAIDs, digitalis glycosides, lithium.
Chlorothiazide	250–500 mg twice daily PO	**Photosensitivity**; **hyperglycemia**; **gastrointestinal distress**; **dizziness**; agranulocytosis; pancreatitis; hepatic impairment; renal failure	Do not use in patients with anuria. Caution in patients with hyperglycemia or taking NSAIDs, digitalis glycosides, lithium.
Hydrochlorothiazide	25 mg once or twice daily PO	**Hypotension**; **dizziness**; **phototoxicity**; hyperglycemia; electrolyte disturbances; pancreatitis; glaucoma; renal impairment	Do not use in patients with anuria or taking dofetilide (risk of QT prolongation). Caution in patients with hyperglycemia or taking methotrexate, cyclophosphamide, NSAIDs, digitalis glycosides, lithium.
Chlorthalidone	12.5–100 mg once daily PO	**Hyperuricemia**; cardiac arrhythmias; pancreatitis; pulmonary edema	Do not use in patients with anuria. Caution in patients with hyperglycemia or taking NSAIDs, digitalis glycosides, lithium.
Mineralocorticoid receptor antagonists			
Spironolactone	25–50 mg daily PO; starting dose of 12.5 mg/day for patients with creatinine clearance 30–50 mL/min	**Hyperkalemia**; **dizziness**; hypotension; gynecomastia; renal dysfunction; leukopenia	Do not use in patients with anuria, Addison's disease, hyperkalemia, or taking other potassium-sparing diuretics. Caution in patients with hepatic impairment, or taking NSAIDs, cholestyramine, heparin, lithium, trimethoprim.
Eplerenone	25–50 mg daily PO	**Hyperkalemia**; **renal dysfunction**; angina; myocardial infarction	Do not use in patients with hyperkalemia or taking other potassium-sparing diuretics. Caution in patients taking strong CYP3A4 inhibitors (clarithromycin, itraconazole, ketoconazole).
Cardiac glycosides			
Digoxin	0.25 mg daily PO or IV; 0.0625–0.125 mg daily for patients with renal impairment; use with caution in age >70 years	**Bradycardia**; **gastrointestinal distress**; headache; yellow vision	Use with caution in patients taking amiodarone, cholestyramine, cyclosporine, erythromycin, loop diuretics, metoclopramide, methotrexate, oral aminoglycosides, thiazide diuretics, thyroid hormone, or verapamil.

Table 46.3 Continued

Medications	Dose routes and ranges	Side effects	Special considerations
Beta-blockers			
Metoprolol succinate extended release	12.5–25 mg daily PO	**Dizziness**; **bradycardia**; **fatigue**; bronchospasm; exercise intolerance; gastrointestinal distress; laryngospasm; paresthesia; hypoglycemia unawareness	Do not use in patients with second- or third-degree AV block, severe sinus bradycardia. Taper to discontinue. Caution in patients with renal impairment or patients taking cimetidine, clonidine, epinephrine, hydralazine, lidocaine, NSAIDs, prazosin, rifampin, verapamil.
Carvedilol (also has alpha-blocker properties)	3.125–50 mg twice daily PO for 2 weeks; may adjust starting dose with patients with hepatic impairment	**Bradycardia**; bronchospasm; hepatic injury; tinnitus; constipation; fatigue; headache; hypoglycemia unawareness	Do not use in patients with second- or third-degree AV block, severe sinus bradycardia. Taper to discontinue. Frequently monitor serum glucose level in diabetic patients. Caution in patients taking amiodarone, clonidine, cyclosporine, digoxin, diltiazem, rifampin, verapamil.
Bisoprolol	1.25–10 mg daily PO	**Bradycardia**; rhinitis; gastrointestinal distress; fatigue; headache; hypoglycemia unawareness	Do not use in patients with second- or third-degree AV block, severe sinus bradycardia. Taper to discontinue. Frequently monitor glucose level in diabetic patients. Caution in patients taking anticholinergics, hormonal contraceptives, insulin, NSAIDs, prazosin, aspirin.
Vasodilators (combination hydralazine + isosorbide dinitrate indicated for HF)			
Isosorbide dinitrate	25–50 mg four times daily PO	**Headache**; dizziness; hypotension; rebound hypertension; tachycardia; weakness	Need to be taken with hydralazine for heart failure. Not for acute angina episodes. Headache common upon discontinuation. Potential for nitrate tolerance. Do not use in patients taking phosphodiesterase inhibitors (Viagra, etc.) or soluble guanylate cyclase (riociguat). Caution in patients taking calcium channel blockers.
Hydralazine	20–30 mg four times daily PO	**Tachycardia**; **palpitations**; anorexia; headache; back, arm, or chest pain; shortness of breath; blood dyscrasias	Need to be taken with isosorbide dinitrate for HF. Not for acute angina episodes. Caution in patients with renal insufficiency or lupus or patients taking adrenergic blockers.
Sodium-glucose cotransporter 2 inhibitor			
Dapagliflozin	10 mg daily PO	**Change in appetite/thirst**; **dizziness**; **thrush**; **genitourinary infections**; changes in urinary frequency; anxiety; back pain; hypoglycemia	Not to be taken if patient taking gymnema. Do not use in patients with Type 1 diabetes or advanced kidney disease or at risk for bone fractures or dehydration. Caution in patients with a history of ketoacidosis or infections of the bladder or perineum.
Empagliflozin	10 mg daily PO	**Change in appetite/thirst**; **dizziness; thrush**; **genitorurinary infections**; changes in urinary frequency; anxiety; back pain; hypoglycemia	Not to be taken if patient taking gymnema. Do not use in patients with Type 1 diabetes or advanced kidney disease or at risk for bone fractures or dehydration. Caution in patients with a history of ketoacidosis or infections of the bladder or perineum.

Bolded side effects are most common; common medications as indicated in reference 5. Typical dose ranges provided: dosing for patients is dependent on individual health status, comorbidities, and institutional recommendations. Consultation with pharmacy is recommended. AV, atrioventricular; CYP3A4, cytochrome P450 3A4; EKG, electrocardiogram; HF, heart failure; IV, intravenous; mTOR, mammalian target of rapamycin; NSAID, nonsteroidal anti-inflammatory drug; PO, orally (per os).

Sources: References 5, 17, 46, and 47.

an approach that can bridge a patient to recovery, heart transplantation ("bridge to transplant"), and medical stabilization so that optimal decision-making can occur ("bridge to decision"). LVADs are also used as a *destination therapy*, where the device's goal is to improve functional status and QOL for those who will not be considered for heart transplantation. Considerations for placement of a MCSD include (but are not limited to) type and severity of heart failure, likelihood of potential complications, presence of significant comorbidities, ability to tolerate long-term anticoagulation, adequate psychosocial and family caregiver support, and feasibility of future heart transplantation.[5] Several guidelines,[5,17,56,57] including the seminal set of recommendations published by the International Society of Heart and Lung Transplantation,[58] recommend palliative care consultation for any patient being considered for an MCSD with follow-up as needed from implantation through deactivation. Furthermore, the US Joint Commission now requires that a palliative care specialist be part of accredited LVAD destination therapy programs.[59,60] Palliative care nurses working frequently with the MCSD population should consult the most recent clinical guidelines as well as seek more detailed guidance in working with patients and families considering and living with MCSDs.[39,57,61–64]

Heart Transplantation

Patients receiving heart transplantations have a median survival of 12 years and typically experience marked improvement in functional capacity.[5] While heart transplantation may be a viable option for eligible patients with advanced heart failure, this option is constrained by the relatively limited number of donor hearts,[65] the contraindications in patients with comorbidities, and the risk of posttransplant complications.[66] Patients considering transplantation should be made aware of the trade-offs involved, including the risks of organ rejection and side effects of immunosuppression, the details of which can be found in the most recent clinical guidelines.[67]

Intravenous Inotrope Therapy

Intravenous inotrope therapy, using medications such as dobutamine and milrinone, is initiated in the inpatient setting to stabilize heart failure patients with decompensation not improving to decongestive treatment with diuretics. While many patients can be weaned off these mediations, others become dependent and must consider either chronic intravenous inotrope therapy that is managed in the community setting or another destination therapy (e.g., heart transplantation, LVAD). Before decisions are made to receive chronic continuous infusions for symptom relief, patients' and families' treatment and prognostic understanding should be assessed (including risk of arrhythmia), and they should be guided in goals-of-care discussion. Nearly all patients on home inotrope therapy die within 1 year.[68,69]

Renal Replacement Therapies

For heart failure patients with symptomatic fluid overload that is refractory to diuretic therapy, hemofiltration or hemodialysis can provide relief of symptoms. Generally, this occurs when patients have concurrent renal failure and require intermittent hemodialysis for clearance of nitrogenous toxins, maintenance of electrolyte status, and management of volume status. However, in severe cases of volume overload, hemofiltration is used to manage excess volume even if glomerular filtration and electrolyte balance remain preserved.[70]

Management of Symptoms in Stage D Heart Failure

Patients with Stage D heart failure often experience multiple symptoms that can compromise function and reduce QOL.[71,72] In the following sections, palliative care considerations in managing some of the most commonly encountered symptoms in advanced heart failure are summarized; however, nurses are encouraged to refer to cited and other material for further clinical guidance.

Dyspnea

When the heart is unable to effectively pump blood forward into the systemic circulation, the lung vasculature can become congested, impairing gas exchange and making breathing difficult.[35] This makes dyspnea one of the most common symptoms experienced in heart failure,[73] and it has been reported that patients increasingly experience dyspnea in the days preceding the end of life.[74] Dyspnea management focuses on reducing fluid overload through prudent diuretic use and optimization of cardiac performance.[46] For HFrEF, ACE inhibitors, angiotensin II receptor blockers, and mineralocorticoid antagonists can be considered for optimizing volume status chronically. Digoxin and intravenous inotropic agents (e.g., milrinone, dobutamine) are also commonly initiated and titrated to relieve symptoms. First-line adjunctive therapies include low-dose opioids (e.g., morphine, hydromorphone, oxycodone) that can be used safely with careful monitoring. Hydromorphone or oxycodone are safer short-acting agents than morphine or codeine for patients with compromised kidney function, given that the risk of accumulating toxic metabolites is less. For chronic use, transdermal fentanyl and oral methadone should be considered with appropriate monitoring for side effects. Oxygen should be administered only if patients become hypoxemic (oxygen saturation less than 88%), and benzodiazepines are considered if patients experience dyspnea-related anxiety.

Fatigue

Reduced cardiac output results in diversion of blood away from skeletal muscles, interference in waste product removal, deconditioning and cachexia, poor sleep, depression, and decreased red blood cell production.[75] For all these reasons and others, fatigue is one of the most common symptoms in heart failure, and yet it is one of the most underassessed and undertreated. Treatment should be focused on optimizing cardiac performance, exercise (as tolerated), energy conservation, sleep hygiene, nutritional support, and identifying concurrent comorbid contributors such as hypothyroidism.[76] Corticosteroids (e.g., dexamethasone 2–8 mg/day) may be considered for short-term relief (i.e., 4–6 weeks), but caution is warranted due to potential for fluid overload; it may be of limited benefit in patients with longer prognoses.[75] There is scant evidence regarding the benefits and risks of modafinil and methylphenidate in heart failure–related fatigue, but they may be beneficial and considered with caution due to cardiac side effects.

Pain

Pain attributable to underlying heart failure includes pressure from edema (especially in the legs below the knees), anginal pain, and musculoskeletal pain from decreased perfusion, immobility, and deconditioning.[75,77] Approaches to pain should generally follow the World Health Organization's analgesic ladder.[78] Given the high prevalence of comorbidities in heart failure patients, non–heart failure–related causes of pain should also be assessed, such as arthritis and diabetic neuropathy. Nonsteroidal anti-inflammatory drugs, whether nonselective or cyclooxygenase-2-specific, are generally contraindicated in heart failure due to risk of renal failure, worsening of sodium and water retention, and increased risk of stroke and myocardial infarction.[79] Opioids are appropriate for moderate to severe pain; however, careful monitoring of opioid-induced hypotension (particularly when patients are intravascularly hypovolemic) is prudent, especially if co-administered with benzodiazepines.[80] Methadone and buprenorphine may prolong QTc, and thus ECG monitoring at baseline and following dose titration is warranted.[80]

Edema

Edema is a nearly universal sign in heart failure. The site of edema can vary depending on the type of heart failure. In right-sided failure, fluid accumulates in the lower extremities and often produces ascites. In left-sided failure, pulmonary edema and pleural effusions may result, potentially causing dyspnea and respiratory distress. Adding to the obstructive effects of underperforming ventricles, edema may result from underperfused tissues that activate the sympathetic and renin–angiotensin systems, thereby promoting sodium and water retention and plasma volume expansion. Therapeutic approaches include optimizing cardiac performance, diuresing excess fluid, and restricting sodium and fluid intake.[75] Nonpharmacologic interventions include lower extremity elevation, use of compression stockings, and paracentesis and thoracentesis for relief of refractory ascites and pleural effusions, respectively.

Cachexia

Cachexia is a poor prognostic indicator in heart failure and is defined as a 6% or greater loss in nonedematous total body weight over a 6-month period.[81] The mechanisms of cardiac cachexia are not fully understood but appear to be multifactorial and mediated by changes in endocrine function, insulin uptake, nutritional malabsorption in the gut, catecholamines, cortisol, natriuretic peptides, and pro-inflammatory cytokines.[81,82] Management includes optimizing nutrition and exercise as tolerated. There are no approved medications for cardiac cachexia; however, there may be some protective benefit of ACE inhibitors and beta-blockers; more information can be found in cited reviews.[81,82]

Depression

While estimates vary, approximately 40% of patients with advanced heart failure experience depression,[83] which has been associated with poorer medication adherence and other outcomes in this population,[84–87] including higher mortality.[88] Treatment approaches include cognitive behavioral therapy, spiritual support, and medications. First-line medications include low-dose selective serotonin reuptake inhibitors (e.g., sertraline); however, these drugs can result in fluid retention and hyponatremia and may prolong the QTc interval Other medication options include selective serotonin–norepinephrine reuptake inhibitors and psychostimulants (e.g., methylphenidate), but tricyclic antidepressants are rarely utilized due to adverse cardiac events.[46]

Primary Palliative Care in Heart Failure and Indications for Specialty and Hospice Referral

Due to the difficulties of prognostication in heart failure, it has been recommended that palliative care approaches and specialty referral be symptom-centered rather than prognosis-driven.[89] In a recent consensus study, an expert panel identified 25 major criteria for referral to specialty palliative care, including (1) disease-related triggers like disease progression, inability to tolerate guideline-directed medical therapy, comorbidities, and two or more hospitalizations in the last 3 months; (2) needs-related triggers like significant symptom burden or patient/care partner concerns; and (3) a time-based trigger of ≤6 months' life expectancy.[90]

In the United States, hospice services are eligible under Medicare funding and most private insurer coverage if a patient with heart failure is deemed by two physicians or one physician and one nurse practitioner to have an estimated prognosis of 6 months or less, and the patient is willing to forego curative-intent therapies. Guidelines stipulate that patients have NYHA Class IV heart failure and are either (1) optimally treated with medications or (2) experiencing angina at rest despite nitrate therapy and have been deemed ineligible or have opted out of invasive cardiac procedures. Other supporting indications for hospice include LVEF of 20% or less, treatment-resistant symptomatic arrhythmias, concomitant acquired immunodeficiency syndrome, and histories of cardiac syncope, embolism, and resuscitation.

End-of-Life Care

Advance Care Planning

ACP is a process aimed at supporting shared understanding of patients' values, goals, and preferences for care.[5] The process includes eliciting patient values[5]; discussing disease trajectory and prognosis, interventions and procedures, life-sustaining treatments, and general attitudes toward care[91,92]; documenting plans for medical treatments[5]; and designating a surrogate decision maker.[5,92] Despite mixed evidence on ACP and alignment of care with goals and utilization,[93] ACP has been found to decrease anxiety, grief, posttraumatic stress, and burden for surrogate decision makers.[91,94–97] However, many clinicians remain hesitant to engage in ACP,[98] and few patients have formally documented their care goals and designated a surrogate.[5] ACP has been most effective when initiated by a trusted provider over multiple visits,[92] introduced at key milestones in the disease trajectory,[91] treated as a continuous process rather than a one-time event,[91] and it considers cultural preferences and includes family members.[91] Thus, discussions of patients' values and goals for care should occur between the patient, the healthcare team, and other relevant individuals identified by the patient. Conversations should occur across the disease trajectory to promote concordance between the care plan and what is most important to the patient. Documented care preferences in written form (e.g., advance directives or living wills)[99] in addition to surrogate understanding of what matters most to the patient helps to guide care decisions once the patient loses the capacity to express their wishes.[94] Advance directives have been criticized for low completion rates and not being able to account for all possible health scenarios[99]; however, in recent years, ACP has been recognized as engagement in high-quality discussions with patients and families, rather than a one-time checkbox.[94] Written directives may serve as a useful tool for initiating conversations about the patient's values and goals between the patient, family, and healthcare team and documenting treatment preferences and preferred place of death.[5] Given the progressive and unpredictable trajectory of heart failure, marked by exacerbations and recoveries,[91,100] and the potential for complex devices and life-sustaining therapies (e.g., ICDs,[101] pacemakers,[102] LVADs,[103] or TAH[104]),[5] patients' values and wishes should be elicited proactively.

Withdrawal of Life-Sustaining Therapies

Advancements in medical technology have led to various cardiac devices (e.g., pacemakers, ICDs, MCSDs) that may be used to sustain life processes.[105] Patients may opt for life-sustaining devices with the hope of achieving specific values and life goals, whereas other patients (or their surrogates, if applicable) may opt out after weighing their (or the patient's) personal benefits and risks, even if such a refusal results in death. The patient's unique goals, beliefs, and circumstances should be discussed and documented (i.e., advance directives, patient's chart) prior to implantation, and iteratively as goals of care evolve, to ensure ongoing consistency with the patient's values, goals, and preferences.[5,105] A specialist palliative care consultation should also be initiated.[1] Discontinuing treatments found to no longer be effective is legally and ethically acceptable and does not constitute physician aid in dying, manslaughter, or suicide.[106] Patients eventually succumb to the underlying disease process (i.e., advanced heart failure), regardless of whether the treatment was

Box 46.1 Important Steps and Pointers for Left Ventricular Assist Device Deactivation

Prior to Deactivation

1. Inform key members of the healthcare team, including (but not limited to): physician of record, cardiologist, cardiothoracic surgeon, left ventricular assist device (LVAD) coordinator, bedside nurse, unit nurse manager, palliative care consultant, social worker, chaplain, and ethics consultant (if needed).
2. Confirm and document the presence of advance directives, do-not-resuscitate orders, and designated healthcare proxy or durable power of attorney for healthcare.
3. Confirm and document the treatment plan goals and the content of any family meetings.
4. Discuss with patients and families, noting (1) any ethical concerns; (2) the process for deactivation, including the unpredictable timing of death after deactivation (minutes to short days); (3) who would like to be present at the time of deactivation; (4) what religious preferences or rites the patient or family would like to have recognized and/or performed; and (5) decisions that may need to be made after death such as organ donation, autopsy, and funeral arrangements.
5. After eliciting patient's and family's values and goals of care, make direct recommendations about other treatments besides the LVAD that should be stopped (e.g., mechanical ventilation, defibrillator) to align with those values and goals.
6. Discuss goals of comfort during and after LVAD deactivation and what treatments will be offered to meet those goals. Reassure the patient and family that patients can be kept comfortable without life-sustaining treatment.
7. Set the date and time for LVAD deactivation, assuring appropriate resources are present.

During Deactivation

1. LVAD deactivation is similar in many respects to mechanical ventilator withdrawal. Clinicians should be prepared to treat the rapid onset of dyspnea/labored respirations, agitation, and other signs of discomfort.
2. Verify the presence of appropriate healthcare staff and all family members who expressed a desire to be at the bedside during deactivation.
3. Discontinue all monitoring that is not symptom-directed.
4. There are many different LVAD models with different steps to deactivation. Be familiar and review the specific steps to deactivate the device before performing the task in front of patients and families (especially alarm silencing, which can be distressing to patients and families). Consult your institution's LVAD coordinator as needed.
5. Once the LVAD is deactivated, cardiovascular circulation may greatly diminish. Thus, it is strongly encouraged to bolus with appropriate medications such as morphine for pain and dyspnea, lorazepam for agitation, and glycopyrrolate for secretions *prior* to deactivation and prior to withdrawal of other life-sustaining therapies. Have additional medication drawn up and ready to administer after deactivation if needed.
6. Once any post-LVAD deactivation symptoms have been appropriately managed, proceed with withdrawal of other life-sustaining treatments.
7. Monitor carefully for any signs of distress or discomfort, treat accordingly, and educate those present as needed regarding signs and symptoms observed.

After Deactivation and Death

1. Spend time with the family to discuss any concerns or questions.
2. After death occurs, encourage the family to spend as much time at the bedside as they desire.
3. Provide acute grief support and follow-up bereavement support.

Sources: References 39, 64, and 107–109.

never started or started and discontinued. However, discontinuation may be perceived as more psychologically and ethically difficult for patients, surrogates, and members of the healthcare team.[105,106] Clinicians whose moral or ethical beliefs oppose deactivating a device should promptly transfer care to another clinician who is able to carry out the patient's wishes.[105] Box 46.1 describes steps clinicians should be aware of when deactivating LVADs.

Case Study: A Patient with Heart Failure

Patricia Sterett is a 71-year-old woman who presented through the hospital emergency department with progressive dyspnea, orthopnea, and edema. She has been treated for acute heart failure decompensation with reduced EF, which was previously stable until her current admission. She has a medical history pertinent for coronary artery disease, diabetes mellitus Type 2 requiring insulin therapy, obesity, dyslipidemia, hypertension, chronic kidney disease, and depression. Three-vessel coronary artery bypass surgery was successfully completed 6 years ago. She states that she "is usually on top of all her medications," though she recently lost her husband of 46 years and may have missed a few days. Her A1C is presently 8.2, her glomerular filtration rate is 34, and her depression is well-controlled.

Presently, her cardiology team is counseling her on options for ongoing treatment. Her echocardiogram features worsening dilated cardiomyopathy now with an LVEF of approximately 15% with global hypokinesis and negative for severe valvular disease. All electrolyte abnormalities have been addressed and corrected, her renal function is near baseline, and there have been no new arrhythmias noted on telemetry during her stay in the hospital. A left heart catheterization shows that her bypass grafts are stable and patent. She remains dependent upon large doses of diuretics and inotropes to remain comfortable.

She expresses no suicidal ideation and has good insight into her present situation. She frequently tells her nurse that she enjoys just being able to talk and be around people. Her closest child lives about 4 hours away and visits a few times a year. This daughter will be arriving tonight to visit her mom. Given her inotrope dependency, the care team discussed some potential next steps including evaluation for LVAD implantation or home inotropes. The palliative care team has been involved with Ms. Sterett since her admission to the cardiac intensive care unit. Initially, she was steadfastly against any surgery and says "If I have more time on the Earth, then that's alright; but I'm ready to go. I have lived a long time and I'm ready to join my husband." She stated that she is disinterested in a long hospital stay and desires to sleep in her own bed and see her dog. But now that her daughter is arriving and talking about staying for a few months, Ms. Sterett asked to know more about her options.

The next day, the palliative care nurse practitioner visits Ms. Sterett and her daughter and queries about how she is doing and her preferences regarding the home inotropes and other therapies. They discuss other potential treatments for her heart failure. Guided by the nurse practitioner, Ms. Sterett expresses some goals of care, including grief counseling and a time trial of home inotropes. Plans are made to discuss possible home milrinone with Ms. Sterett's cardiologist, and Ms. Sterett is connected to the bereavement support group sponsored by the local hospital.

Conclusion

The initiation of palliative care for patients with heart failure may be at the time of diagnosis concurrent with traditional treatment and continue along the illness trajectory with periods of increased palliative care utilization during acute exacerbations. Given the high prevalence of comorbidities in heart failure patients as well as the rise in first-time heart failure diagnosis in the elderly population, the focus of palliative care in heart failure is improved QOL, self-care, symptom management, care coordination, prognosis understanding, and decision-making. Despite poor functional status and significant symptom burden, including frequent emotional symptoms (of anxiety and depression), patients with advanced heart failure are often referred to palliative care services late or are resistant to palliative approaches due to optimal treatment response during exacerbations and an unpredictable disease trajectory. Yet the burden of heart failure is ripe for palliative approaches by informed nurses guided by recent evidence-based practice guidelines. Relying on symptoms and progression, not prognosis, may promote greater uptake of specialty palliative services, especially in the outpatient setting. While pharmacological and nonpharmacological therapies may be used to address common symptoms of breathlessness, pain, fatigue, and depression, goals-of-care discussions support the patient and their caregivers (or support persons) during medical decisions such as heart transplantation, mechanical circulatory support devices, or home inotrope infusion considerations. Palliative care addresses the multifaceted disease burden experienced by those living with advanced heart failure, and nurses are at the forefront of incorporating palliative care to improve QOL and alleviate suffering.

REFERENCES

1. Tsao CW, Aday AW, Almarzooq ZI, et al. Heart disease and stroke statistics—2022 update: a report from the American Heart Association. *Circulation*. 2022;145(8):e153–e639.
2. Truby LK, Rogers JG. Advanced heart failure: epidemiology, diagnosis, and therapeutic approaches. *JACC Heart Fail*. 2020;8(7):523–536.
3. Roger VL. Epidemiology of heart failure: a contemporary perspective. *Circ Res*. 2021;128(10):1421–1434.
4. Warraich HJ, Hernandez AF, Allen LA. How medicine has changed the end of life for patients with cardiovascular disease. *J Am Coll Cardiol*. 2017;70(10):1276–1289.
5. Heidenreich PA, Bozkurt B, Aguilar D, et al. 2022 AHA/ACC/HFSA guideline for the management of heart failure: a report of the American College of Cardiology/American Heart Association Joint Committee on Clinical Practice Guidelines. *Circulation*. 2022;145(18):e895–e1032.
6. Emmons-Bell S, Johnson C, Roth G. Prevalence, incidence and survival of heart failure: a systematic review. *Heart*. 2022;108(17):1351–1360.
7. Salah HM, Fudim M, O'Neil ST, et al. Post-recovery COVID-19 and incident heart failure in the National COVID Cohort Collaborative (N3C) study. *Nat Commun*. 2022;13(1):4117.
8. Benjamin EJ, Blaha MJ, Chiuve SE, et al. Heart disease and stroke statistics—2017 update: a report from the American Heart Association. *Circulation*. 2017;135(10):e146–e603.
9. Heidenreich PA, Albert NM, Allen LA, et al. Forecasting the impact of heart failure in the United States: a policy statement from the American Heart Association. *Circ Heart Fail*. 2013;6(3):606–619.
10. Screever EM, van der Wal MHL, van Veldhuisen DJ, et al. Comorbidities complicating heart failure: changes over the last 15 years. *Clin Res Cardiol*. 2023;112(1):123–133.
11. Lippi G, Sanchis-Gomar F. Global epidemiology and future trends of heart failure. *AME Med J*. 2020;5:15.
12. Bhatnagar R, Fonarow GC, Heidenreich PA, et al. Expenditure on heart failure in the United States: the Medical Expenditure Panel survey 2009–2018. *JACC Heart Fail*. 2022;10(8):571–580.
13. Obi EN, Swindle JP, Turner SJ, et al. Healthcare costs among patients with heart failure: a comparison of costs between matched decedent and survivor cohorts. *Adv Ther*. 2017;34(1):261–276.
14. Obi EN, Swindle JP, Turner SJ, et al. Health care costs for patients with heart failure escalate nearly 3-fold in final months of life. *J Manag Care Spec Pharm*. 2016;22(12):1446–1456.
15. Jackson SL, Tong X, King RJ, et al. National burden of heart failure events in the United States, 2006 to 2014. *Circ Heart Fail*. 2018;11(12):e004873.
16. Bragazzi NL, Zhong W, Shu J, et al. Burden of heart failure and underlying causes in 195 countries and territories from 1990 to 2017. *Eur J Prev Cardiol*. 2021;28(15):1682–1690.
17. McDonagh TA, Metra M, Adamo M, et al. 2021 ESC guidelines for the diagnosis and treatment of acute and chronic heart failure: developed by the task force for the diagnosis and treatment of acute and chronic heart failure of the European Society of Cardiology (ESC). With the special contribution of the Heart Failure Association (HFA) of the ESC. *Eur J Heart Fail*. 2022;24(1):4–131.
18. Antonione R, Sinagra G, Moroni M, et al. Palliative care in the cardiac setting: a consensus document of the Italian Society of Cardiology/Italian Society of Palliative Care (SIC/SICP). Article in Italian. *G Ital Cardiol (Rome)*. 2019;20(1):46–61.
19. García Pinilla JM, Díez-Villanueva P, Bover Freire R, et al. Consensus document and recommendations on palliative care in heart failure of the Heart Failure and Geriatric Cardiology Working Groups of the Spanish Society of Cardiology. *Rev Esp Cardiol (Engl Ed)*. 2020;73(1):69–77.
20. Sobanski PZ, Alt-Epping B, Currow DC, et al. Palliative care for people living with heart failure: European Association for Palliative Care Task Force expert position statement. *Cardiovasc Res*. 2020;116(1):12–27.
21. National Guideline Committee. *National Institute for Health and Care Excellence: Guidelines. Chronic Heart Failure in Adults: Diagnosis and Management*. National Institute for Health and Care Excellence; 2018.
22. Bozkurt B, Coats AJS, Tsutsui H, et al. Universal definition and classification of heart failure: a report of the Heart Failure Society of America, Heart Failure Association of the European Society of Cardiology, Japanese Heart Failure Society and Writing Committee of the Universal Definition of Heart Failure: endorsed by the Canadian Heart Failure Society, Heart Failure Association of

India, Cardiac Society of Australia and New Zealand, and Chinese Heart Failure Association. *Eur J Heart Fail.* 2021;23(3):352–380.
23. Zhou Q, Li P, Zhao H, et al. Heart failure with mid-range ejection fraction: a distinctive subtype or a transitional stage? *Front Cardiovasc Med.* 2021;8:678121.
24. Kheirbek RE, Alemi F, Citron BA, et al. Trajectory of illness for patients with congestive heart failure. *J Palliat Med.* 2013;16(5):478–484.
25. Shah KS, Fang JC. Sodium–glucose cotransporter 2 inhibitors in heart failure. *Annu Rev Pharmacol Toxicol.* 2022;62:109–120.
26. Beezer J, Al Hatrushi M, Husband A, et al. Polypharmacy definition and prevalence in heart failure: a systematic review. *Heart Fail Rev.* 2022;27(2):465–492.
27. Rashid M, Kwok CS, Gale CP, et al. Impact of co-morbid burden on mortality in patients with coronary heart disease, heart failure, and cerebrovascular accident: a systematic review and meta-analysis. *Eur Heart J Qual Care Clin Outcomes.* 2017;3(1):20–36.
28. Uszko-Lencer N, Frankenstein L, Spruit MA, et al. Predicting hospitalization and mortality in patients with heart failure: the BARDICHE-index. *Int J Cardiol.* 2017;227:901–907.
29. Glynn PA, Molsberry R, Harrington K, et al. Geographic variation in trends and disparities in heart failure mortality in the United States, 1999 to 2017. *J Am Heart Assoc.* 2021;10(9):e020541.
30. Glynn P, Lloyd-Jones DM, Feinstein MJ, et al. Disparities in cardiovascular mortality related to heart failure in the United States. *J Am Coll Cardiol.* 2019;73(18):2354–2355.
31. Groenewegen A, Rutten FH, Mosterd A, et al. Epidemiology of heart failure. *Eur J Heart Fail.* 2020;22(8):1342–1356.
32. Dharmarajan K, Rich MW. Epidemiology, pathophysiology, and prognosis of heart failure in older adults. *Heart Fail Clin.* 2017;13(3):417–426.
33. Corrà U, Magini A, Paolillo S, et al. Comparison among different multiparametric scores for risk stratification in heart failure patients with reduced ejection fraction. *Eur J Prev Cardiol.* 2020;27(2_suppl):12–18.
34. Codina P, Lupón J, Borrellas A, et al. Head-to-head comparison of contemporary heart failure risk scores. *Eur J Heart Fail.* 2021;23(12):2035–2044.
35. Blum M, Gelfman LP, McKendrick K, et al. Enhancing palliative care for patients with advanced heart failure through simple prognostication tools: a comparison of the surprise question, the number of previous heart failure hospitalizations, and the Seattle heart failure model for predicting 1-year survival. *Front Cardiovasc Med.* 2022;9:836237.
36. Rahimi K, Bennett D, Conrad N, et al. Risk prediction in patients with heart failure. *JACC Heart Fail.* 2014;2(5):440–446.
37. Ouwerkerk W, Voors AA, Zwinderman AH. Factors influencing the predictive power of models for predicting mortality and/or heart failure hospitalization in patients with heart failure. *JACC Heart Fail.* 2014;2(5):429–436.
38. Allen LA, Stevenson LW, Grady KL, et al. Decision making in advanced heart failure: a scientific statement from the American Heart Association. *Circulation.* 2012;125(15):1928–1952.
39. Warraich HJ, Maurer MS, Patel CB, et al. Top ten tips palliative care clinicians should know about caring for patients with left ventricular assist devices. *J Palliat Med.* 2019;22(4):437–441.
40. Cavanagh CE, Rosman L, Spatz ES, et al. Dying to know: prognosis communication in heart failure. *ESC Heart Fail.* 2020;7(6):3452–3463.
41. Back A, Arnold R, Tulsky J. *Mastering Communication with Seriously Ill Patients: Balancing Honesty with Empathy and Hope.* Cambridge University Press; 2009.
42. Dunlay SM, Strand JJ. How to discuss goals of care with patients. *Trends Cardiovasc Med.* 2016;26(1):36–43.
43. Elder A, Japp A, Verghese A. How valuable is physical examination of the cardiovascular system? *BMJ.* 2016;354:i3309.
44. Selvaraj S, Claggett B, Shah SJ, et al. Utility of the cardiovascular physical examination and impact of spironolactone in heart failure with preserved ejection fraction. *Circ Heart Fail.* 2019;12(7):e006125.
45. Selvaraj S, Claggett B, Pozzi A, et al. Prognostic implications of congestion on physical examination among contemporary patients with heart failure and reduced ejection fraction: PARADIGM-HF. *Circulation.* 2019;140(17):1369–1379.
46. McGuinty C, Leong D, Weiss A, et al. Heart failure: a palliative medicine review of disease, therapies, and medications with a focus on symptoms, function, and quality of life. *J Pain Symptom Manage.* 2020;59(5):1127–1146.e1.
47. Ferrari F, Martins VM, Scheffel RS, et al. The role of sodium–glucose cotransporter-2 inhibitors in patients with heart failure, regardless of diabetes status: focus on cardiovascular disease. *Ann Pharmacother.* 2021;55(10):1267–1275.
48. Van Horn L, Carson JAS, Appel LJ, et al. Recommended dietary pattern to achieve adherence to the American Heart Association/American College of Cardiology (AHA/ACC) guidelines: a scientific statement from the American Heart Association. *Circulation.* 2016;134(22):e505–e529.
49. Yancy CW. The uncertainty of sodium restriction in heart failure: we can do better than this. *J Am Coll Cardiol.* 2016;4(1):39–41.
50. Yancy CW. Sodium restriction in heart failure: too much uncertainty—do the trials. *JAMA Intern Med.* 2018;178(12):1700–1701.
51. Mahtani KR, Heneghan C, Onakpoya I, et al. Reduced salt intake for heart failure: a systematic review. *JAMA Intern Med.* 2018;178(12):1693–1700.
52. Herman M, Horner K, Ly J, et al. Deactivation of implantable cardioverter-defibrillators in heart failure: a systematic review. *J Hosp Palliat Nurs.* 2018;20(1):63–71.
53. Padeletti L, Arnar DO, Boncinelli L, et al. EHRA expert consensus statement on the management of cardiovascular implantable electronic devices in patients nearing end of life or requesting withdrawal of therapy. *Europace.* 2010;12(10):1480–1489.
54. Lampert R, Hayes DL, Annas GJ, et al. HRS expert consensus statement on the management of cardiovascular implantable electronic devices (CIEDs) in patients nearing end of life or requesting withdrawal of therapy. *Heart Rhythm.* 2010;7(7):1008–1026.
55. Tracy CM, Epstein AE, Darbar D, et al. 2012 ACCF/AHA/HRS focused update of the 2008 guidelines for device-based therapy of cardiac rhythm abnormalities: a report of the American College of Cardiology Foundation/American Heart Association Task Force on Practice Guidelines. *J Thorac Cardiovasc Surg.* 2012;144(6):e127–e145.
56. Centers for Medicare & Medicaid Services. Decision Memo for Ventricular Assist Devices for Bridge-to-Transplant and Destination Therapy (CAG-00432R). October 30, 2013. Accessed November 20, 2019. https://www.cms.gov/medicare-coverage-database/details/nca-decision-memo.aspx?NCAId=268.
57. Cook JL, Colvin M, Francis GS, et al. Recommendations for the use of mechanical circulatory support: ambulatory and community patient care: a scientific statement from the American Heart Association. *Circulation.* 2017;135(25):e1145–e1158.
58. Feldman D, Pamboukian SV, Teuteberg JJ, et al. The 2013 International Society for Heart and Lung Transplantation guidelines for mechanical circulatory support: executive summary. *J Heart Lung Transplant.* 2013;32(2):157–187.

59. Centers for Medicare & Medicaid Services. Proposed Decision Memo for Ventricular Assist Devices for Bridge-to-Transplant and Destination Therapy (CAG-00432R). August 1, 2013. http://www.cms.gov/medicare-coverage-database/details/nca-proposed-decision-memo.aspx?NCAId=268.
60. Salomon S, Frankel H, Chuang E, et al. Implementing routine palliative care consultation before LVAD implantation: a single center experience. J Pain Symptom Manage. 2018;55(5):1350–1355.
61. Swetz KM, Kamal AH, Matlock DD, et al. Preparedness planning before mechanical circulatory support: a "how-to" guide for palliative medicine clinicians. *J Pain Symptom Manage.* 2014;47(5):926–935.e6.
62. Wordingham SE, McIlvennan CK, Dionne-Odom JN, et al. Complex care options for patients with advanced heart failure approaching end of life. *Curr Heart Fail Rep.* 2016;13(1):20–29.
63. Thompson JS, Matlock DD, McIlvennan CK, et al. Development of a decision aid for patients with advanced heart failure considering a destination therapy left ventricular assist device. *JACC Heart Fail.* 2015;3(12):965–976.
64. Wordingham SE, McIlvennan CK, Fendler TJ, et al. Palliative care clinicians caring for patients before and after continuous flow-left ventricular assist device. *J Pain Symptom Manage.* 2017;54(4):601–608.
65. Goff RR, Uccellini K, Lindblad K, et al. A change of heart: preliminary results of the US 2018 adult heart allocation revision. *Am J Transplant.* 2020;20(10):2781–2790.
66. Mehra MR, Canter CE, Hannan MM, et al. The 2016 International Society for Heart Lung Transplantation listing criteria for heart transplantation: a 10-year update. *J Heart Lung Transplant.* 2016;35(1):1–23.
67. Costanzo MR, Costanzo MR, Dipchand A, et al. The International Society of Heart and Lung Transplantation guidelines for the care of heart transplant recipients. *J Heart Lung Transplant.* 2010;29(8):914–956.
68. Hashim T, Sanam K, Revilla-Martinez M, et al. Clinical characteristics and outcomes of intravenous inotropic therapy in advanced heart failure. *Circ Heart Fail.* 2015;8(5):880–886.
69. Nizamic T, Murad MH, Allen LA, et al. Ambulatory inotrope infusions in advanced heart failure: a systematic review and meta-analysis. *JACC Heart Fail.* 2018;6(9):757–767.
70. Schaubroeck HA, Gevaert S, Bagshaw SM, et al. Acute cardiorenal syndrome in acute heart failure: focus on renal replacement therapy. *Eur Heart J Acute Cardiovasc Care.* 2020;9(7):802–811.
71. Alpert CM, Smith MA, Hummel SL, et al. Symptom burden in heart failure: assessment, impact on outcomes, and management. *Heart Fail Rev.* 2017;22(1):25–39.
72. Parshall MB, Schwartzstein RM, Adams L, et al. An official American Thoracic Society statement: update on the mechanisms, assessment, and management of dyspnea. *Am J Respir Crit Care Med.* 2012;185(4):435–452.
73. Filippatos G, Angermann CE, Cleland JGF, et al. Global differences in characteristics, precipitants, and initial management of patients presenting with acute heart failure. *JAMA Cardiol.* 2020;5(4):401–410.
74. Campbell ML, Kiernan JM, Strandmark J, et al. Trajectory of dyspnea and respiratory distress among patients in the last month of life. *J Palliat Med.* 2018;21(2):194–199.
75. Stewart D, McPherson ML. Symptom management challenges in heart failure: pharmacotherapy considerations. *Heart Fail Rev.* 2017;22(5):525–534.
76. Mücke M, Mochamat M, Cuhls H, et al. Pharmacological treatments for fatigue associated with palliative care. *Cochrane Database Syst Rev.* 2015;2015(5):CD006788.
77. Kang Y, Sheng X, Stehlik J, et al. Identifying targets to improve heart failure outcomes for patients receiving home healthcare services: the relationship of functional status and pain. *Home Healthc Now.* 2020;38(1):24–30.
78. Kida K, Doi S, Suzuki N. Palliative care in patients with advanced heart failure. *Heart Fail Clin.* 2020;16(2):243–254.
79. Curseen KA, Taj J, Grant Q. Pain management in patients with serious illness. *Med Clin North Am.* 2020;104(3):415–438.
80. Chen A, Ashburn MA. Cardiac effects of opioid therapy. *Pain Med.* 2015;16(suppl 1):S27–S31.
81. von Haehling S, Ebner N, dos Santos MR, et al. Muscle wasting and cachexia in heart failure: mechanisms and therapies. *Nat Rev Cardiol.* 2017;14(6):323–341.
82. Saitoh M, Ishida J, Doehner W, et al. Sarcopenia, cachexia, and muscle performance in heart failure: review update 2016. *Int J Cardiol.* 2017;238:5–11.
83. Moradi M, Doostkami M, Behnamfar N, et al. Global prevalence of depression among heart failure patients: a systematic review and meta-analysis. *Curr Probl Cardiol.* 2022;47(6):100848.
84. Sheffler JL, Schmiege SJ, Sussman J, et al. A longitudinal analysis of the relationships between depression, fatigue, and pain in patients with heart failure. *Aging Ment Health.* 2021;25(12):2272–2278.
85. Haedtke CA, Moser DK, Pressler SJ, et al. Influence of depression and gender on symptom burden among patients with advanced heart failure: insight from the pain assessment, incidence and nature in heart failure study. *Heart Lung.* 2019;48(3):201–207.
86. Haedtke C, Smith M, VanBuren J, et al. The characteristics of pain in patients diagnosed with depression and heart failure. *Pain Manag Nurs.* 2017;18(6):353–362.
87. Haedtke C, Smith M, VanBuren J, et al. The relationships among pain, depression, and physical activity in patients with heart failure. *J Cardiovasc Nurs.* 2017;32(5):E21–E25.
88. Correll CU, Solmi M, Veronese N, et al. Prevalence, incidence and mortality from cardiovascular disease in patients with pooled and specific severe mental illness: a large-scale meta-analysis of 3,211,768 patients and 113,383,368 controls. *World Psychiatry.* 2017;16(2):163–180.
89. Hogg KJ, Jenkins SMM. Prognostication or identification of palliative needs in advanced heart failure: where should the focus lie? *Heart.* 2012;98(7):523–524.
90. Chang YK, Allen LA, McClung JA, et al. Criteria for referral of patients with advanced heart failure for specialized palliative care. *J Am Coll Cardiol.* 2022;80(4):332–344.
91. Schichtel M, Wee B, Perera R, et al. The effect of advance care planning on heart failure: a systematic review and meta-analysis. *J Gen Intern Med.* 2020;35(3):874–884.
92. Thammana RV, Goodlin SJ. Telecommunication for advance care planning in heart failure. *Card Fail Rev.* 2022;8:e11.
93. McMahan RD, Tellez I, Sudore RL. Deconstructing the complexities of advance care planning outcomes: what do we know and where do we go? A scoping review. *J Am Geriatr Soc.* 2021;69(1):234–244.
94. Sudore RL, Hickman SE, Walling AM. Controversies about advance care planning. *JAMA.* 2022;327(7):685.
95. Morrison RS, Meier DE, Arnold RM. Controversies about advance care planning—reply. *JAMA.* 2022;327(7):686.
96. Myers J, Steinberg L, Seow H. Controversies about advance care planning. *JAMA.* 2022;327(7):684–685.
97. Kernick LA, Hogg KJ, Millerick Y, et al. Does advance care planning in addition to usual care reduce hospitalisation for patients with advanced heart failure: a systematic review and narrative synthesis. *Palliat Med.* 2018;32(10):1539–1551.

98. Schichtel M, Wee B, Perera R, et al. Effect of behavior change techniques targeting clinicians to improve advance care planning in heart failure: a systematic review and meta-analysis. *Ann Behav Med*. 2021;55(5):383–398.
99. Yadav KN, Gabler NB, Cooney E, et al. Approximately one in three US adults completes any type of advance directive for end-of-life care. *Health Aff (Millwood)*. 2017;36(7):1244–1251.
100. Nishikawa Y, Hiroyama N, Fukahori H, et al. Advance care planning for adults with heart failure. *Cochrane Database Syst Rev*. 2020;2(2):CD013022.
101. Merchant FM, Binney Z, Patel A, et al. Prevalence, predictors, and outcomes of advance directives in implantable cardioverter-defibrillator recipients. *Heart Rhythm*. 2017;14(6):830–836.
102. Pasalic D, Tajouri TH, Ottenberg AL, et al. The prevalence and contents of advance directives in patients with pacemakers: advance directives in pacemaker patients. *Pacing Clin Electrophysiol*. 2014;37(4):473–480.
103. Verdoorn BP, Luckhardt AJ, Wordingham SE, et al. Palliative medicine and preparedness planning for patients receiving left ventricular assist device as destination therapy—challenges to measuring impact and change in institutional culture. *J Pain Symptom Manage*. 2017;54(2):231–236.
104. DeMartino ES, Wordingham SE, Stulak JM, et al. Ethical analysis of withdrawing total artificial heart support. *Mayo Clin Proc*. 2017;92(5):719–725.
105. Jericho BG. Withdrawal of life-sustaining therapy. *Curr Opin Anaesthesiol*. 2018;31(2):179–184.
106. McIlvennan CK, Wordingham SE, Allen LA, et al. Deactivation of left ventricular assist devices: differing perspectives of cardiology and hospice/palliative medicine clinicians. *J Card Fail*. 2017;23(9):708–712.
107. Makdisi T, Makdisi G. Ethical challenges and terminal deactivation of left ventricular assist device. *Ann Transl Med*. 2017;5(16):331.
108. Woodburn JL, Staley LL, Wordingham SE, et al. Destination therapy: standardizing the role of palliative medicine and delineating the DT-LVAD journey. *J Pain Symptom Manage*. 2019;57(2):330–340.e4.
109. Gafford E, Luckhardt AJ, Swetz KM. FF #269 Deactivation of a Left Ventricular Assist Device at the End-of-Life. PCNow: Palliative Care Network of Wisconsin. 2019. FF #269 Deactivation of A Left Ventricular Assist Device at the End-of-Life | Palliative Care Network of Wisconsin

47

Palliative Care for People Living with HIV

Jacquelyn Slomka

Key Points

- Over more than three decades, HIV has evolved from a terminal illness to a manageable chronic illness.
- People living with HIV (PLWH), especially those who are developing additional chronic diseases as they age, can benefit from early palliative care.
- In assessing PLWH for palliative care services, clinicians should be aware of the association of HIV with mental health issues and substance use.
- Perceptions of stigma associated with HIV/AIDS and marginalized lifestyles may interfere with effective care of PLWH.
- PLWH may be wary of advance care planning discussions because of the historic association of palliative care, hospice, and death prior to the extraordinary advances in treatment for HIV.

Introduction

People living with human immunodeficiency virus (HIV) present unique challenges for the provision of palliative care due, in part, to the nature of HIV infection and its medical and social history. Since the virus was identified more than three decades ago, the world has witnessed a remarkable evolution of a (then) newly emerged disease condition and its eventual clinical control. At its onset, HIV was a mysterious infection, associated first with gay men and not amenable to treatment with traditional antibiotics.[1, 2] Individuals who contracted HIV in this early period most often experienced progression to acquired immunodeficiency syndrome (AIDS), with inevitable death. The spread of HIV and its progression to AIDS created a pandemic affecting people of all ages.[1, 2]

Scientists learned that HIV infection was caused by a type of virus called a "retrovirus" which attacked the body's immune system, causing a deficiency of CD4 (T) cells that allowed opportunistic infections and certain cancers to occur.[1, 2] AIDS is generally defined as severe progression of HIV infection or as the presence of a CD4 count of less than 250.[1, 2] The virus is spread through certain body fluids; risk of transmission was higher with certain activities such as sexual behaviors and injection drug use.[2] Over time, little progress was made in producing a vaccine to prevent HIV. But advances in drug treatments were made, and the deadly epidemic was transformed into a manageable chronic disease. Still without an effective vaccine, prevention efforts in recent years have focused on the use of pharmacological agents for pre- and postexposure prophylaxis.[3] As further evidence of the evolution of this once-deadly infection into a controllable chronic condition, the Center for Disease Control and Prevention (CDC) reported that studies now show viral suppression (i.e., reducing the levels of HIV in the blood and body to a very low or undetectable level) is the best way for PLWH to maintain health and prevent HIV transmission.[3, 4, 5]

HIV may not evoke the fear that it once did in the past, but it still remains a significant public health threat. The CDC estimates that 1.1 million people in the United States are living with HIV and that 1 in 7 individuals are not aware they are infected.[6, 7] Although the CDC estimated that the number of HIV diagnoses decreased by 12% between 2018 and 2022, a reported 31,800 individuals were newly diagnosed in 2022.[6] According to the CDC, the largest number of diagnoses were among gay and bisexual men (21,400, 67%), varying by ethnicity: Hispanic/Latino (9,374), Black/African. Twenty-two percent (7,000) of diagnoses were due to heterosexual contact, 15% (4,900) of women received diagnoses, and injection drug use (2,300, 7%). Disparities in HIV prevalence and treatment exist, with African American populations bearing a disproportionate HIV disease burden relative to Hispanic/Latino and white populations.[6]

HIV affects all organs of the body, and PLWH still die from HIV/AIDS. However, we know that today, with increasing survival rates, PLWH are more likely to die from non–AIDS-defining conditions (i.e., non-HIV/AIDS illness) than from HIV/AIDS. Although any chronic, potentially life-threatening illness is challenging for the individual, HIV may lead to additional stresses due to its social stigma. HIV infection has no social, economic, ethnic, or class boundaries, but perceived associations with marginalized or low-income life styles and fears of a potentially life-threatening condition may add stigma and additional stressors for the patient with HIV.

As with other chronic conditions, palliative care provides comprehensive treatment of the physical, psychological, and spiritual aspects of illness and management of symptoms. Ideally, palliative care begins at diagnosis of a chronic illness and continues throughout the trajectory of the disease.[8] This chapter identifies directions for the provision of palliative care for PLWH, beginning with identification of the need for palliative care, followed by potential interventions in various phases of coping with HIV. The focus will be limited to palliative care needs within the psychosocial context of HIV. Information on current medical treatment and prevention of HIV is constantly being updated as new research findings become available. Palliative care nurses who plan to work with PLWH are encouraged to enhance their familiarity with HIV and its clinical aspects, history, and current therapies through a variety of resources available to professionals and the public

The Need for Palliative Care in HIV

In the early epidemic, the trajectory of HIV/AIDS most often ended in palliative care, hospice, and death. By the early to mid-1990s, major developments in antiretroviral therapy (ART) had begun the transformation of HIV/AIDS into a controllable medical condition.[1] Pharmaceutical developments did not occur in isolation but were affected by patient activism leading to changes in the conduct of clinical trials to speed drug development.[9] PLWH who may have experienced and survived the terrors and uncertainties of the early HIV/AIDS epidemic may find themselves today facing other chronic diseases of aging.[10, 11, 12]

Among the current challenges of HIV is its chronicity and association with other comorbidities resulting in higher risk of mortality and increased symptom burden.[7] Studies have shown that, even with effective medical treatment, PLWH continue to experience both physical and psychological symptoms.[13, 14] PLWH may benefit greatly from palliative care from initial diagnosis and throughout disease progression. In a review article focused on identifying palliative care needs from the beginning of recognized HIV illness, Simms and colleagues[15] evaluated and reviewed 34 studies of individuals diagnosed within their first 6 months. The authors chose this time period because of its common usage in research studies that support clinically observed differences between newly diagnosed and those diagnosed longer than 6 months ago.[15] Although studies varied in design, aims, sample size, world geographic area, income level of country, and quality of methodology, these authors were able to identify commonalities in palliative care needs in the early HIV diagnosis period. Key findings were that symptoms were prevalent at initial diagnosis in all dimensions of palliative care needs, including psychological and emotional distress, spiritual well-being, and physical symptoms such as pain, fatigue, itching, and weight loss.[15] These authors concluded that palliative care needs are present and manageable beginning with the diagnosis of HIV but may be overlooked by clinicians. They recommended patient-centered, multidimensional assessment, with early referral to palliative care specialists.[15]

A number of observational studies in a variety of settings in the United States and Canada have documented the needs of PLWH at mid- and late stages of disease, and these show a similarity to the needs of individuals at an early stage of illness. At one large HIV outpatient clinic, researchers noted that patients usually were referred to palliative care when the primary clinician could no longer manage the patients' symptoms.[16] Multidrug-resistant AIDS infection, AIDS-related dementia, progressive loss of function, and uncontrolled symptoms were major reasons for referral, leading the authors to conclude that better integration of primary care, palliative care, and mental health and substance abuse services could improve the care of PLWH.[16] These study findings document the complex needs of PLWH and support a growing advocacy for referral of PLWH to palliative care earlier in the disease trajectory.[16, 17]

Others also have noted the greater need for multidisciplinary care and the higher illness burden sustained by PLWH as they reach the later stage of chronicity. Data from one study showed that physical, social, and mental health functioning were important to PLWH but were impacted by disease burden.[18] As PLWH grow older, a greater disease burden leads to lower quality of life (QOL) for individuals.[18, 19] Caring for PLWH throughout the disease trajectory involves an understanding of complex interactions of physical and mental health, including cognitive disorders and substance use, as well as social factors (e.g., housing instability resulting from unresolved psychological issues) associated with HIV.[20] Furthermore, the high association of HIV, substance use, and mental health disorders, the so-called *triple diagnosis*, has been well-recognized in the literature.[21] Assessment of substance use and mental health should be a part of the complete assessment of PLWH.

While palliative care nurses alone cannot address all of the complex issues involved in caring for PLWH, they can serve as valuable members of the interdisciplinary team, primarily in the area of symptom management. Palliative care expertise is especially valuable in the management of chronic pain because primary care physicians may be reluctant to treat pain adequately in individuals with a psychiatric or substance use history.[22] In their description of an HIV palliative care clinic embedded within an HIV primary care clinic, Perry and colleagues noted that of 124 first-time admissions to the HIV palliative care clinic, 91% were referred for chronic pain, more than one-third had depression or anxiety, and more than one-half had a history of substance abuse.[22] A history of substance abuse is a risk factor in PLWH for unrelieved pain.[23] Pain is a frequently reported symptom among PLWH, and better systematic assessment and treatment of pain by clinicians is needed.[24] All clinicians should become familiar with the latest guidelines for management of chronic pain in PLWH.[25] These guidelines provide evidence-based recommendations for treatment of chronic pain in PLWH in a variety of patient situations (see Table 47.1).

Another important type of symptom cluster prevalent in PLWH is that of HIV-associated neurocognitive disorders, also referred to as "HAND." A pathological feature of HIV infection is the potential for cognitive impairment. Tedaldi and colleagues[26] reviewed the relationships among HIV infection, cognitive impairment, and physical and social comorbidities. They noted that cognitive impairment in PLWH can be due to many overlapping causes, both physical and psychosocial. Examples of physical effects on impairment include the HIV disease process, effects of medications, cardiovascular disease, hepatitis C virus (HCV) coinfection, sleep disorders, illicit drug use, depression and other mental illness, and the aging process.[26] The authors also describe possible systemic inflammation, biomarker, and cellular level factors that may be associated with HIV cognitive impairment. They note that social factors related to the physical assessment of HAND may include poverty and low literacy if the individual comes from a disadvantaged educational background. Having a low-income or marginalized lifestyle and exposure to trauma often related to poverty may lessen an individual's resilience and add to physically adverse effects on cognition.[26] The palliative care nurse should be aware of the potential for cognitive

Table 47.1 Management of chronic pain in people with HIV: Summary of content of guidelines

Screening, initial assessment, general approaches to management, and management approaches at end of life (I, II, III)
Nonpharmacological treatments (IV)
Pharmacological treatments for chronic neuropathic and non-neuropathic pain (V)
Opioid treatment for chronic non-neuropathic pain; assessing potential negative consequences; safeguards, and minimizing adverse effects of opioids (VI, VII, VIII, IX)
Prescribing controlled substances in the presence of a history of substance abuse; management of individuals undergoing pharmacological treatments for opioid use disorder (X, XI, XII)
Instruments for mental health screening (XIII)

Source: From Bruce RD, Merlin J, Lum PJ, et al. 2017 HIVMA of IDSA clinical practice guideline for the management of chronic pain in patients living with HIV. *Clin Infect Dis.* 2017;65(10):e1–e37. (Roman numerals denote number of guideline.)

disorders in PLWH and their impact on the comprehensive care needs of the patient.

Multimorbidity and Aging with HIV

As length of survival with HIV increases, PLWH experience a more rapid physical aging process due to long-term effects of ART and cellular-level changes of inflammation and immune system damage.[11] In the ART-era literature, 50 years was generally considered the age of an "older" adult with HIV.[27] But many PLWH are living beyond age 50 and are likely to experience significant impacts on their health as HIV-related pathologies and the aging processes coincide.[28]

One of the greatest challenges of caring for the older patient with HIV is managing the chronic illness burden of multimorbidity, with many individuals having two or more chronic conditions. PLWH older than 50 years are likely to have one or more health problems in addition to HIV.[18] Types of comorbid conditions reported by PLWH commonly include hypertension, chronic pain, hepatitis, arthritis, diabetes, neurocognitive impairment syndrome, malignancy, cardiovascular disease, renal failure, bone disease and fractures, liver disease and frailty.[10, 11, 18, 19]

Like other aging individuals, older PLWH are at risk for the development of geriatric syndromes. Rather than focus on a single disease, geriatric syndromes focus on the impact of multimorbidity on outcomes related to the ability to function in activities of daily life and to maintain independence and QOL.[10] Such syndromes are associated with multiple physical, psychosocial, and environmental factors and include function-related impairments such as frailty, sensory and/or cognitive deficits, falls, urinary incontinence, and depression.[12] In a study of geriatric syndromes in 155 older PLWH, the most frequent geriatric syndromes found were pre-frailty, difficulty in activities of daily living, cognitive impairment, and depression.[12] Managing geriatric syndromes is important to decrease age-related complications. Treatment and prevention of comorbid conditions and exercise and diet to control and maximize function and reduce inflammatory influences on aging have been recommended to decrease adverse effects of aging and geriatric syndromes in older PLWH.[10, 29, 30, 31, 32]

Living and Coping with HIV

A diagnosis of HIV can be devastating for an individual. Even if a person suspects HIV infection, the confirmation may come as shock. Newly diagnosed individuals may have difficulty accepting the diagnosis and delay initiation of treatment. Or they may have difficulty with adhering to a medication regimen or dealing with the emotional and psychological struggles of having HIV.[30, 31] In contrast to situations of the newly diagnosed, many long-term HIV survivors have come to terms with their life-long HIV infection. Knowledge of how PLWH have positively coped with HIV over the long term may provide examples of coping strategies for other patients who must deal with the burdens of HIV infection.

A qualitative, in-depth interview study of 16 long-term survivors of HIV/AIDS described how these individuals coped and what positive traits and characteristics were helpful to their survival.[31] Time from diagnosis ranged from 8 to 26 years, with a mean of 17 years; age ranged from 38 to 67 years, with a median of 50 years. Thirteen (81%) were male. Based on this study, three categories of positive coping strategies (disease coping, practical coping, and emotional coping) and a context of social support were elicited from individual patient interviews.[31] Elaboration on the dimensions of coping and social support and their key representative qualities (Table 47.2) provides a framework for assessing and addressing the palliative care needs of older adults living with HIV.

These dimensions of positive coping have been experienced or utilized by PLWH at various times throughout the illness trajectory. However, each person has a unique life history. The most effective

Table 47.2 Dimensions of positive coping identified by long-term survivors of HIV

Disease coping	Practical coping	Emotional coping	Social support
Clinician–PLWH communication	Reasons for living	Resilience	Family/friends/pets
Medication challenges	Managing disclosure	Religion/spirituality	Support from professionals
Self-management of health	Giving back to others	Manage negative emotions	Peer support, individual and group

Source: From Reference 31.

ways to address patient needs will depend on individual factors: age, health status related to HIV and comorbidities, socioeconomic level, geographic location, and the like.[32] For example, a 67-year-old man with diabetes, hypertension, chronic obstructive pulmonary disease (COPD), and arthritis; on ART for many years; and living on Social Security in a depressed rural area will have different needs than someone living in an urban area where access to medical and social supports is easier to obtain.[32, 33] Listening carefully to the patient's story and allowing it to unfold over time will enable the nurse to see the broader landscape of the individual's coping challenges.

Disease Coping

Disease coping involves the ability to deal with the medical and physiological aspects of HIV.[31] For a person newly diagnosed with HIV, addressing the psychological and emotional trauma of diagnosis may be the first hurdle for the patient. Developing a therapeutic relationship with primary care clinicians may help the patient move toward taking a greater role in his or her own healthcare.[34] For long-term survivors of HIV, having good physician–patient relationships, dealing with their multiple medications, and taking charge of their own health was important.[31] As older PLWH develop other chronic conditions, their diagnosis of HIV may become less prominent for them as they find themselves facing new diagnoses, medications, and treatments.[32, 35, 36] For patients with HIV and multimorbidity, additional medications are likely to accompany new diagnoses. Sorting out drug names, their target diseases, their dosages, timings, adverse effects, and interactions with other medications may be a significant challenge for PLWH and adds to the complexity of their healthcare.[32, 35]

The palliative care nurse's role in disease coping will include support for the patient by communicating effectively and facilitating communication between the patient and multidisciplinary team members. The palliative care nurse may be the first to assess new symptoms or to identify inaccurate usage and other problems with medications. The role of patient educator is especially important but requires humility on the part of the palliative care nurse. Many PLWH who have lived with HIV long term and have successfully coped with the complexities of HIV infection are very knowledgeable about their condition. Learning from patients, as well as educating them, is an important aspect of patient-centered care of PLWH.

Practical Coping

Practical coping means the ability of long-term survivors to deal not only with the demands of everyday life with a chronic condition, but with the unique condition of HIV.[31] Individuals who successfully coped were able to find reasons to continue their everyday existence. PLWH identified children, grandchildren, pets, and meaningful employment as reasons to go on.[31] Ability to manage disclosure of one's HIV status or the outcomes of involuntary disclosure[37] also demonstrated practical coping. Research has shown that PLWH who voluntarily or involuntarily have their HIV status disclosed may risk stigmatization by some but gain social support from others.[37] Some patients choose to remain private to the extent that even closest family members may not know they have HIV, but they may risk accidental exposure during an illness or accident in which their medical history is evident.[38] Other PLWH choose partial disclosure, selecting the individuals to whom they wish to disclose and the timing of disclosure.[31, 38]

The term "giving back" was often heard among PLWH and was seen as a component of practical coping.[31] This theme has been noted elsewhere as a component of resilience in aging with HIV.[39] Individuals who had overcome significant barriers in their struggle to survive HIV/AIDS often did so with help from many sources. They often expressed a desire to give back some of the help they received by volunteering to teach, counsel, or help others affected by HIV.[31, 39]

The notion of practical coping by PLWH has implications for palliative care nursing. Important to the assessment of mental health of PLWH is understanding what is meaningful for them in their lives. Nurses may need to work closely with HIV social workers to address certain needs. For example, if having a job provides meaning, but the person is unable to find employment or lacks purpose in life, a social worker may be able to provide referrals to agencies or organizations that provide help targeted specifically for PLWH.

Understanding and maintaining confidentiality is essential for all patients but is especially important in regard to disclosure of HIV status due to the potential for stigmatization and discrimination. At the onset of care, the palliative care nurse should discuss with the patient which individuals know his or her status and with whom the nurse is able to discuss, or not discuss, the patient's healthcare. The nurse should take care to prevent an accidental breach of confidentiality that may occur by linking the patient to HIV-associated entities (e.g., a research study recruiting PLWH), leaving phone messages that may unintentionally disclose private information, or using unsecured social media to communicate with other healthcare providers. Furthermore, the palliative care nurse should become familiar with state laws regulating HIV confidentiality and sexual partner notification.

Emotional Coping

Emotional coping was viewed broadly as encompassing resilience, management of negative emotions, and spiritual/religious support.[31] Long-term HIV survivors often described an ability to take in stride setbacks in their health or social situation and continue with their lives. In a different interpretation of similar themes, Emlet and colleagues[39] characterized a concept of resilience in HIV as encompassing themes of self-acceptance, optimism (similar to "managing negative emotions"), a will to live ("reasons for living"), generativity ("giving back"), self-management ("taking charge of one's health"), relational living ("social support"), and independence. Consistency in some of the themes across the two studies, in spite of the difference in geographic locations (Midwest and Western United States), suggests reliability of these findings for older PLWH.

Although Emlet et al.[39] did not identify spirituality/religious support as part of resilience, Slomka et al.[31] found it to be a recurrent theme of positive coping with HIV for some study participants. Influences of spirituality/religious support on health-related outcomes have been addressed frequently in the HIV literature. In a review of 15 studies examining relationships between spirituality/religion and HIV outcomes, researchers identified 10 studies that showed positive outcomes such as increased CD4 count, undetectable viral load, and an association with increased survival.[40] Other studies in the review showed negative effects, no effect, or a mixed effect on HIV outcomes. According to the authors, some study results may have been affected by inadequately clarified concepts such as the meaning of "spiritual struggle" and views of God as either benevolent or harsh.[40] Findings from other studies showed that PLWH who had religious support after divorce or death of a spouse had slower increases in viral loads.[41] Contact with a spiritual advisor was associated with an absence of major depression, and spirituality/religion was beneficial in promoting medication adherence.[42] In another study focused on adherence and actual spiritual/religious practices, researchers associated praying once a day with 90% HIV medication adherence rate.[43] All authors agreed on the need to further clarify relationships between spirituality/religion and HIV outcomes. At this stage of research, say Doolittle et al.,[40] clinicians should neither encourage nor discourage spirituality/religion for PLWH, but try to understand its role in patients' lives.

Discussing spiritual/religious needs of the patient is part of the role of the palliative care nurse. PLWH may have strong spiritual beliefs but may have rejected or feel rejected by formal religion, especially if a religious institution stigmatizes HIV because of associations with illicit drug use or homosexuality. Spirituality/religion assessment by the nurse can help to clarify this aspect of care. In addition to support for spiritual/religious aspects of care, the palliative care nurse can further promote emotional coping by reinforcing patients' attitudes and behaviors that lead to resiliency. The nurse can also help the patient manage negative thoughts by suggesting ways to reframe them into more positive attitudes.

Social Support

PLWH described the importance of having supportive relationships in their lives, with family, friends, healthcare providers, HIV peer support groups, jobs, community-based social organizations, and even pets as part of their social networks.[31, 39] In a more nuanced study of social support and HIV, Oetzel and colleagues[44] examined both social support and social undermining and its relation to health-related QOL (HRQOL). They found that social support positively related to QOL and that it was more important for PLWH to avoid negative interactions that undermined perceptions of support (e.g., low-paying jobs, disapproval by family, perceived stigmatization) than to have positive interactions. They also noted that work status was the strongest correlate of socioeconomic status in HRQOL, a finding that could have potential policy implications for funding such services as job training programs.[44] These authors suggest that healthcare providers, through positive, supportive interactions with patients, can help to mitigate some of the effects of social undermining that PLWH may experience.

That support from health providers may counteract some of the effects of undermining of social supports for PLWH is an important finding. Health professionals who work with PLWH may have an enormous impact on how the individual sees himself and his illness. The perception of stigma by PLWH is common and is one of a constellation of factors that can impede access to care.[45, 46, 47] While stigmatizing social context may be difficult for individual clinicians to change, it is within the role of nurses to educate themselves and engage in civic action to improve social determinants of health.[48] One area of social action might be to examine laws that may be inappropriately harsh and stigmatizing toward PLWH who, because of past drug use and/or felony convictions, may be prevented from obtaining jobs, voting, or otherwise engaging in society as active citizens.

Advance Care Planning and Advance Directives

Although advance care planning (ACP) and advance directives (ADs) are not part of the coping framework just provided, they are part of palliative care and the healthcare provider role. The engagement of PLWH in ACP and/or formal execution of ADs varies. Researchers who studied AD completion rates in a US inner-city hospital learned that 92% of PLWH did not have an AD upon admission, and this number only decreased to 86.3% during admission.[49] Others reported AD completion rates among PLWH at 8.7%,[50] 23%,[51] and 47%[52] compared to the overall US population rate reported as 23.3%.[53]

Hansen and colleagues[54] studied relationships among rates of occurrence of ACP discussions with physicians and PLWH and their association with drug use, experience of pain, and family and physician communication. Discussions of ACP were more likely to occur when patients had good relationships with their physicians, higher rates of chronic pain, family arguments about end-of-life (EOL) issues, and comfort with discussing problems with one's family.[54] These authors note the importance for clinicians to assess patient–family relationships and communications. Patients who have chronic pain and/or conflicts with families over EOL care may be more amenable to ACP discussions with clinicians.[54]

Instead of EOL issues driving the need for ACP as in the early days of the epidemic, peace of mind and documentation of decision preferences now support ACP for PLWH.[55] With relatively low numbers of PLWH engaging in ACP, perceptions of palliative care, hospice, and ACP were elicited by researchers[56] as part of a larger study on palliative care. Twenty-two PLWH who had at least one other chronic condition participated in four focus groups. Findings indicated that individuals were not familiar with the term "palliative care" or the relevance of palliative care to chronic illness. Those who were familiar with palliative care tended to conflate it with hospice care, which was associated with end of life and viewed negatively by a number of participants. Participants also misunderstood the meaning of ACP. When palliative care and its role in chronic illness management and ACP were explained to participants, they expressed acceptance of the concept.[56]

Although healthcare professionals and the general public may equate palliative care with hospice, PLWH (and HIV clinicians) may do so because of the history of HIV/AIDS.[56] Older PLWH and HIV clinicians may have had first hand experience with the early AIDS epidemic, when medical treatments had not yet been developed, and palliation, hospice, and death was the inevitable endpoint of HIV/AIDS. Palliative care nurses should be aware that wariness in the acceptance of palliative care by PLWH may result from a collective memory of the history of HIV. Additionally, conversations with patients over time may reveal that some may have had conversations with family or friends about EOL care and may have chosen not to execute a formal AD. Nurses should be familiar with the AD laws in their state and encourage patients to reflect on who they would want to make healthcare decisions for them if they became incapacitated.

Case Example: A Patient Recently Diagnosed with AIDS

Ms. R is a 35-year-old, African American, divorced, single mother of a 7-year-old daughter. Ms. R has an MBA and had a well-paying job until she lost it as a result of postsurgery narcotic dependence that led to cocaine addiction. She contracted HIV from a sexual relationship with a male friend, a cocaine user who introduced her to the drug and who was unaware he was HIV-infected. Ms. R had been in drug treatment and sober for 10 months and was otherwise physically healthy. She was working two different jobs, trying hard to stabilize her life in order to regain custody of her daughter, who was under the care of grandparents (Ms. R's mother and father). Ms. R was diagnosed with HIV only 10 months ago, at the time she began drug treatment. Her HIV was under fairly good control with adequate CD4 count and viral suppression. She was having some trouble with adherence to ART due to some adverse medication effects and a fluctuating work schedule. She was dealing with her parents' anger and disappointment in her and with her own anger at herself and her ex-partner who infected her. Although her parents offered some emotional support, her social network deteriorated when she became addicted, and job and family stresses resulted in occasional episodes of depression. Ms. R felt she was young enough to rebuild her social and family life for her daughter. But she wondered whether she could have a "normal" life with HIV: Would anyone want to "date" her? Would she be able to remarry or become pregnant again? Would she live long enough to see her daughter grow up?

Comment

Ms. R was under an enormous amount of stress in dealing with a recent (<1 year) HIV diagnosis, HIV medication challenges, drug treatment, loss of her daughter, possible alienation from her parents, working two jobs, possible social isolation, and concerns about the future. Palliative care assessment and follow-up would involve coordination and collaboration with other health providers. Her current plan might include:

- Assessment of disclosure issues
- Medication review with patient, communication with primary HIV physician, diagnosis and assistance with adherence issues
- Symptom management for stress, anger; an HIV social worker may be able to advise regarding availability of individual counseling
- Assessment for clinical depression; encourage exercise; yoga
- Dealing with concern about future: ensure patient is linked to HIV resources online and in the community (e.g., AIDS Taskforce), peer counseling
- Assessment of family communication; need for counseling of child, grandparents
- Reinforce coping skills (e.g., daughter as "reason for living"), demonstrated resilience in seeking employment; self-management of health with goal of healthy, extended life; assistance in reframing negative thoughts; assess social isolation—suggest decreasing isolation by identifying a monthly group activity (participation in church or peer-support group) if job does not provide social support

Case Study: A Long-Term Survivor of AIDS

Mr. G was a 66-year-old, retired, white, homosexual male, diagnosed with HIV 25 years ago. He had been having an extramarital affair at the time with another man when he became gravely ill with Pneumocystis pneumonia (PCP) and AIDS. With intensive care and ART, he survived. His wife divorced him and gained custody of their two young children, a son and a daughter. His wife prevented him from seeing his children for a time, but as the children grew older he was able to re-establish a relationship with them. Mr. G had endured multiple other losses in his past, mainly a number of very close friends who contracted AIDS during the early years of the epidemic and did not survive. He considered himself lucky to be alive, having lived through a time when an HIV diagnosis meant an individual had no future. His life had not been very easy, but he was resilient. He had had to endure rejection from some family members who, lacking knowledge about HIV transmission, were afraid to associate with him, but he had had a good relationship with other family members. He experienced great anxiety in deciding to tell his children that he was gay and HIV-infected, but they now accepted his diagnosis and lifestyle. He remained physically and mentally active. He visited with grandchildren often and volunteered twice a week at a homeless shelter because he wanted to "give back" some of the help that people had given him over the past years. His HIV had been very stable, but in the past year his doctor had noted higher than normal fluctuations in his blood pressure. He also had chronic osteoarthritis pain, especially in his back and shoulders, that often kept him awake at night. He was unable to take nonsteroidal anti-inflammatory drugs (NSAIDs) due to gastric problems. Because Mr. G had a short history of illicit drug use more than 20 years ago, his physician still was reluctant to prescribe any medication that had the potential to become habit-forming.

Comment

In contrast to Ms. R, Mr. G has had many years to adjust to his HIV diagnosis and to cope with the challenges of living with HIV long term. He appeared to have stable and supportive social relationships and enjoyed meaningful activities. He was beginning to experience some of the comorbidities of aging and could benefit from symptom management. Pain management was complicated, but nonpharmacological therapies such as exercise might be helpful. He might also be at risk for comorbidities associated with HIV and with long-term ART use, as well as depression as a result of the losses in his life. The palliative care nurse would want to collaborate with the HIV team in monitoring Mr. G's symptoms, pain management, and depression risk.

Case Study: A Patient with AIDS and Multimorbidities

Mr. W was a 56-year-old African American diagnosed with HIV 15 years ago. He did not complete high school, dropping out at tenth grade. He had a former cocaine addiction and occasionally used marijuana. He had hypertension, diabetes, chronic kidney disease, anxiety, depression, and dental caries. He had a detectable viral load, but an acceptable CD4 count. He took a number of medications in addition to his HIV drugs. He sometimes skipped his drugs for anxiety and depression because he disliked how he felt when taking them. He also occasionally missed other medications when he ran out of them and could not afford to refill the prescriptions. Mr. W's only income was from disability and occasional odd jobs. He was incarcerated for a time for an offense related to his drug use. He lived in a poor neighborhood of the city and did not like to go out much because of the high crime rate. He did not rent or own a home or car, but had managed to keep off the streets because he stayed with friends or family, moving frequently so as not to burden those who took him in. He occasionally missed his clinic appointments because he had to take several buses to get to the clinic, depending on the time of day, and he sometimes did not have money for the fare. Sometimes he could get a friend to drive him, but his friends often cannot afford the extra gasoline necessary to transport him.

Comment

Mr. W. had a number of difficult problems related primarily to his poverty. His HIV needed to be controlled; he needed access to medicines and the ability to keep clinic appointments, but transportation and drug costs were problematic. His unstable housing situation and possible social isolation put him at risk for disease progression. His dental caries and possible food insecurity put him at risk for poor nutrition, infection, and other pathologies. The nurse could assess whether the patient had a therapeutic relationship with his physician and help him to establish one if lacking. The nurse may be able to provide continuity of care through home visits if the patient is unable to get to a clinic appointment. The team social worker should review Mr. W's situation to see if he is eligible for services to pay for food or medicine, a free dental clinic, or volunteers to help with transportation or to provide activities to decrease social isolation. Because Mr. W had a detectable viral load, he should be advised about condom use to prevent HIV transmission. Once the immediate "disease coping" challenges were addressed, the palliative care nurse/team can continue to assist the patient with other dimensions of coping.

Conclusion

The provision of early palliative care to PLWH is essential to manage symptoms and improve well-being for this challenging population. The palliative care nurse who chooses to work with PLWH can enhance his or her knowledge about the medical, psychosocial, economic, and historical aspects of this complex illness in several ways. Familiarity with clinical guidelines for HIV and chronic pain management[25] will enable provision of evidence-based care for a symptom that is often difficult to manage in this population. Professional HIV/AIDS literature is extensive and offers up-to-date clinical information. Organizations such as AIDS Taskforces can provide information on services for PLWH. Multiple websites, sponsored by government and private foundations, are publicly accessible with current information. Care should be taken to critically evaluate online information because disinformation based on "AIDS conspiracy" theories or denial of scientific therapies also abounds. Literature and films can offer historical views and insight into the "human" side of HIV infection. Numerous books and articles in the popular press, both fiction and nonfiction, are available about special groups such as ethnic and LGBT populations and about the experiences of drug users (Table 47.3). Such documents, films, and literature are not only informative, but also can help the palliative care nurse more fully understand the experiences of PLWH in the promotion of compassionate care.

Table 47.3 Selected resources

The science and global impact of HIV/AIDS
Center for Disease Control and Prevention (CDC): https://www.cdc.gov/hiv/
National Institutes of Health (NIH) – National Institute of Allergy and Infectious Diseases; https://www.niaid.nih.gov/diseases-conditions/hivaids
World Health Organization: www.who.int/hiv/en/
The human side of the early epidemic
Films:
Philadelphia, 1993 (drama)
How to Survive a Plague, 2012 (documentary film)
Dallas Buyers Club, 2013 (drama)
Books:
And the Band Played On. Politics, People, and the AIDS Epidemic by Randy Shilts, 1987 (also a 1993 film)
My Own Country. A Doctor's Story of a Town and Its People in the Age of AIDS by Abraham Verghese, 1994.

REFERENCES

1. Chu C, Selwyn PA. An epidemic in evolution: the need for new models of HIV care in the chronic disease era. *J Urban Health.* 2011;88:556–566.
2. A timeline of HIV and AIDS. https://www.hiv.gov/hiv-basics/overview/history/hiv-and-aids-timeline Accessed May 13, 2025
3. About HIV. https://www.cdc.gov/hiv/about/index.html Accessed may 13, 2025
4. Allen MA, Liang TS, La Salvia T, Tjugum B, Gulakowski RJ, Murguia M. Assessing the attitudes, knowledge, and awareness of HIV vaccine research among adults in the United States. *J Acquir Immune Defic Syndr*. 2005;40(5):617–624.
5. HIV treatment as prevention. Center for Disease Control and Prevention Web site. https://www.cdc.gov/hivpartners/php/hiv-treatment/index.html Accessed May 13, 2025 Updated November 3, 2017. Accessed November 13, 2017.
6. Hiv Diagnoses, Deaths, and Prevalence. https://www.cdc.gov/hiv-data/nhss/hiv-diagnoses-deaths-prevalence.html Accessed May 13, 2025.
7. Fausto JA, Selwyn PA. Palliative care in the management of advanced HIV/AIDS. *Prim Care Clin Office Pract.* 2011;38:311–326.
8. WHO definition of palliative care. World Health Organization Web site. http://www.who.int/cancer/palliative/definition/en/. Published 2017. Accessed November 5, 2017.
9. Epstein S. The construction of lay expertise: AIDS activism and the forging of credibility in the reform of clinical trials. *Sci Technol Human Values.* 1995;20(4):408–437.
10. Chirch LM, Hasham M, Kuchel GA. HIV and aging: a clinical journey from Koch's postulate to the chronic disease model and the contribution of geriatric syndromes. *Curr Opin HIV AIDS.* 2014;9(4):405–411.

11. Calcagno A, Nozza S, Muss C, et al. Ageing with HIV: a multidisciplinary review. *Infection*. 2015;43(5):509–522.
12. Greene M, Covinsky KE, Valcour V, et al. Geriatric syndromes in older HIV-infected adults. *J Acquir Immune Defic Syndr*. 2015;69(2): 161–167.
13. Karus D, Raveis VH, Alexander C, Hanna B, Selwyn P, et al. Patient reports of symptoms and their treatment at three palliative care projects servicing individuals with HIV/AIDS. *J Pain Symptom Manage*. 2005;30:408–417.
14. Harding R, Lampe FC, Norwood S, Date HL, Clucas C, et al. Symptoms are highly prevalent among HIV outpatients and associated with poor adherence and unprotected sexual intercourse. *Sex Transm Infect*. 2010;86:520–524.
15. Simms VM, Higginson IJ, Harding R. What palliative care-related problems do patients experience at HIV diagnosis? A systematic review of the evidence. *J Pain Symptom Manage*. 2011;42:734–753.
16. Ruiz M, Cefalu C. Palliative care program for human immunodeficiency virus-infected patients: rebuilding of an academic urban program. *Am J Hosp Palliat Care*. 2011;28:16–21.
17. Lofgren S, Friedman R, Ghermay R, et al. Integrating early palliative care for patients with HIV: provider and patient perceptions of symptoms and need for services. *Am J Hosp Palliat Care*. 2015;32(8): 829–834.
18. Balderson B, Grothaus L, Harrison RG, Mccoy K, Mahoney C, et al. Chronic illness burden and quality of life in an aging HIV population. *AIDS Care*. 2013;25(451–458):451–458.
19. Rodriguez-Penney AT, Iudicello JE, Riggs PK, et al. Co-morbidities in persons infected with HIV: increased burden with older age and negative effects on health-related quality of life. *AIDS Patient Care STDS*. 2013;27(1):5–16.
20. Halman M, Carusone SC, Stranks S, Schaefer-McDaniel N, Stewart A. Complex care needs of patients with late-stage HIV disease: a retrospective study. *AIDS Care*. 2014;26:320–325.
21. Durvasula R, Miller TR. Substance abuse treatment in persons with HIV/AIDS: challenges in managing triple diagnosis. *Behav Med*. 2014;40(2):43–52.
22. Perry BA, Westfall AO, Molony E, et al. Characteristics of an ambulatory palliative care clinic for HIV-infected patients. *J Palliat Med*. 2013;16(8):934–937.
23. Knowlton AR, Nguyen TQ, Robinson AC, Harrell PT, Mitchell MM. Pain symptoms associated with opioid use among vulnerable persons with HIV: an exploratory study with implications for palliative care and opioid abuse prevention. *J Palliat Care*. 2015;31(4):228–233.
24. Merlin JS, Cen L, Praestgaard A, Turner M, Obando A, et al. Pain and physical and psychological symptoms in ambulatory HIV patients in the current treatment era. *J Pain Symptom Manage*. 2012;43:638–645.
25. Bruce RD, Merlin J, Lum PJ, et al. 2017 HIV Medicine Association of Infectious Diseases Society of American clinical practice guideline for the management of chronic pain in patients living with human immunodeficiency virus. *Clin Infect Dis*. 2017; 65(10): 1601–1606.
26. Tedaldi EM, Minniti NL, Fischer T. HIV-associated neurocognitive disorders: the relationship of HIV infection with physical and social comorbidities. *Biomed Res Int*. 2015;2015:641913.
27. Aging with HIV. U.S. Department of Health and Human Services. https://www.hiv.gov/hiv-basics/living-well-with-hiv/taking-care-of-yourself/aging-with-hiv. Updated Updated August 20, 2024. Accessed May 14, 2025
28. Chambers LA, Wilson MG, Rueda S, et al. Evidence informing the intersection of HIV, aging and health: a scoping review. *AIDS Behav*. 2014;18(4):661–675.
29. Fortin M, Stewart M, Poitras ME, Almirall J, Maddocks H. A systematic review of prevalence studies on multimorbidity: toward a more uniform methodology. *Ann Fam Med*. 2012;10(2):142–151.
30. Graham JL, Grimes RM, Slomka J, Ross M, Hwang LY, Giordano TP. The role of trust in delayed HIV diagnosis in a diverse, urban population. *AIDS Behav*. 2013;17(1):266–273.
31. Slomka J, Lim JW, Gripshover B, Daly B. How have long-term survivors coped with living with HIV? *J Assoc Nurses AIDS Care*. 2013;24(5):449–459.
32. Justice AC, Braithwaite RS. Lessons learned from the first wave of aging with HIV. *AIDS*. 2012;26(suppl 1):S11–18.
33. Quinn K, Sanders C, Petroll AE. "HIV is not going to kill me, old age is!" The intersection of aging and HIV for older HIV-infected adults in rural communities. *AIDS Educ Prev*. 2017;29(1):62–76.
34. Chen WT, Wantland D, Reid P, et al. Engagement with health care providers affects self-efficacy, self-esteem, medication adherence and quality of life in people living with HIV. *J AIDS Clin Res*. 2013;4(11):256.
35. Slomka J, Prince-Paul M, Webel A, Daly BJ. Multimorbidity with HIV: views of community-based people living with HIV and other chronic conditions. *J Assoc Nurses AIDS Care*. 2017;28(4):603–611.
36. Warren-Jeanpiere L, Dillaway H, Hamilton P, Young M, Goparaju L. Taking it one day at a time: African American women aging with HIV and co-morbidities. *AIDS Patient Care STDS*. 2014;28(7):372–380.
37. Fletcher F, Ingram LA, Kerr J, Buchberg M, Bogdan-Lovis L, Philpott-Jones S. "She told them, oh that bitch got AIDS": experiences of multilevel HIV/AIDS-related stigma among African American women living with HIV/AIDS in the south. *AIDS Patient Care STDS*. 2016;30(7):349–356.
38. Emlet CA. Truth and consequences: a qualitative exploration of HIV disclosure in older adults. *AIDS Care*. 2008;20(6):710–717.
39. Emlet CA, Tozay S, Raveis VH. "I'm not going to die from the AIDS": resilience in aging with HIV disease. *Gerontologist*. 2011;51(1):101–111.
40. Doolittle BR, Justice AC, Fiellin DA. Religion, spirituality, and HIV clinical outcomes: a systematic review of the literature. *AIDS Behav*. 2018 June;22(6):1792–1801. doi: 10.1007/s10461-016-1`651-z.
41. Ironson G, Henry SM, Gonzalez BD. Impact of stressful death or divorce in people with HIV: a prospective examination and the buffering effects of religious coping and social support. *J Health Psychol*. 2017:1359105317726151.
42. Oji VU, Hung LC, Abbasgholizadeh R, Terrell Hamilton F, Essien EJ, Nwulia E. Spiritual care may impact mental health and medication adherence in HIV+ populations. *HIV AIDS (Auckl)*. 2017;9:101–109.
43. Dalmida SG, McCoy K, Koenig HG, et al. Examination of the role of religious and psychosocial factors in HIV medication adherence rates. *J Relig Health*. 2017;56(6):2144–2161.
44. Oetzel J, Wilcox B, Archiopoli A, et al. Social support and social undermining as explanatory factors for health-related quality of life in people living with HIV/AIDS. *J Health Commun*. 2014;19(6):660–675.
45. Sayles JN, Wong MD, Kinsler JJ, Martins D, Cunningham WE. The association of stigma with self-reported access to medical care and antiretroviral therapy adherence in persons living with HIV/AIDS. *J Gen Intern Med*. 2009;24(10):1101–1108.

46. Smit PJ, Brady M, Carter M, et al. HIV-related stigma within communities of gay men: a literature review. *AIDS Care*. 2012;24(4):405–412.
47. Toth M, Messer LC, Quinlivan EB. Barriers to HIV care for women of color living in the southeastern US are associated with physical symptoms, social environment, and self-determination. *AIDS Patient Care STDS*. 2013;27(11):613–620.
48. American Nurses Association. *Code of Ethics for Nurses with Interpretive Statements*. Silver Springs, MD: American Nurses Association, 2015.
49. deCaprariis PJ, Carballo-Dieguez A, Thompson S, et al. Advance directives and HIV: a current trend in the inner city. *J Community Health*. 2013;38:409–413.
50. Rhodes RL, Nazir F, Lopez S, et al. Use and predictors of end-of-life care among HIV patients in a safety net health system. *J Pain Symptom Manage*. 2016;51(1):120–125.
51. Barcoas JA, Erlandson KM, Belzer BK, Hess T, Sosman J. Advance directives among people living with HIV: room for improvement. *AIDS Care*. 2015;27:370–377.
52. Erlandson KM, Allshouse AA, Duong S, MaWhinney S, Kohrt WM, et al. HIV, aging and advance care planning: are we successfully planning for the future? *J Palliat Med*. 2012;15:1124–1129.
53. Rao JK, Anderson LA, Lin FC, Laux JP. Completion of advance directives among US consumers. *Am J Prev Med*. 2014;46:65–70.
54. Hansen ED, Mitchell MM, Smith T, Hutton N, Keruly J, Knowlton AR. Chronic pain, patient-physician engagement, and family communication associated with drug-using HIV patients' discussing advanced care planning with their physicians. *J Pain Symptom Manage*. 2017;54(4):508–513.
55. Martin CA. Promoting advance directives and ethical will with the HIV-aging cohort by first assessing clinician knowledge and comfort level. *J Assoc Nurses AIDS Care*. 2015;26:208–214.
56. Slomka J, Prince-Paul M, Webel A, Daly BJ. Palliative care, hospice, and advance care planning: views of people living with HIV and other chronic conditions. *J Assoc Nurses AIDS Care*. 2016;27(4):476–484.

48 Palliative Approaches to Dementia Care

Tatiana Sadak and Soo Borson

Key Points

Understanding Dementia

- Progressive cognitive decline sufficient to impair everyday functioning. Distinct from normal aging.
- Common types: Alzheimer's, vascular, Lewy body, and frontotemporal dementia.
- Early stages can affect just one cognitive ability; advanced stages result in global deterioration.

Palliative Care Principles

- Focus on whole-person care with specific goals.
- Prioritize quality of life, support for patient and loved ones, using team-based approaches.
- Address physical, psychosocial, and spiritual well-being.

The Six Domains of Health Framework

- Provides a practical clinical approach to identifying and addressing complexity.
- Starts with collecting information across key domains of health associated with clinical outcomes.
- Identifies current needs for action and what to track over time to ensure comprehensive care.

Nurse Roles

- Perform cognitive, functional, and caregiver assessments.
- Work as part of a clinical team to create and communicate personalized care plans.
- Educate and support caregivers.
- Advocate for systemic quality improvement.

Stages of Dementia Care

- Early Stage: Foster engagement in care planning and lifestyle adjustments to support health and quality of life.
- Moderate Stage: Manage behavioral symptoms, simplify routines, and ensure safety for patients and caregivers.
- Late Stage: Focus on comfort, address symptoms, and plan end-of-life care; support caregivers.
- End-of-Life: Offer hospice services and a peaceful, supportive environment.

Serious Illness Conversations

- Initiate conversations about personal and family goals of care, advance directives, and end-of-life preferences.
- Emphasize empathetic and skilled communication.

Healthcare System Needs

- Action to implement dementia-capable care processes at scale.
- Multi-level workforce training to fill care gaps and disseminate palliative competencies.

Call to Action for Nurses

- Nurses can and should lead in transforming dementia care using the Six Domains of Health framework.
- Advocate for patient-centered, comprehensive, and innovative system-wide care.

Introduction

Dementias are classified as major neurocognitive disorders, an umbrella term describing a group of conditions acquired in adulthood that cause a decline from an individual's prior level of cognition sufficient to interfere with everyday functioning. Not all dementias are characterized by prominent memory loss (an early feature of Alzheimer's disease). Deficits in intellectual ability, reasoning, social skills, behaviors, emotional reactions, problem-solving, and judgment occur in various combinations across different diagnostic subtypes of progressive dementias. The most common types are Alzheimer's disease and vascular, Lewy body, and frontotemporal dementias, defined by their clinical and neuropathological characteristics (Table 48.1). The general recommendations provided here are based on the most common cause of late-life dementia—Alzheimer's disease—but are broadly applicable to other dementia subtypes. These illnesses can disrupt lives, isolate individuals and families, drain financial resources, and eventually disable the affected individual. At the same time, they offer an opportunity to practice unconditional compassion, acceptance, appreciation of simple things and joys, and respect for our shared humanity. Although the future is promising for both public health and clinical interventions that may delay or mitigate the risk and outcomes of dementias, as of 2022, there is no cure or effective disease-modifying intervention for most dementias.[1] They remain incurable serious illnesses with profound effects beyond the individual, permanently altering roles, relationships, and life patterns. Most affected individuals live in the community and are cared for by their family members and

Table 48.1 Diagnostic criteria for common major neurocognitive disorders

Diagnosis	Hallmark symptoms	Implications for registered nurses	General references
Alzheimer	Cognitive difficulties that represent a decline from a previous level of functioning; interfere with usual activities; are not due to delirium; with objective evidence of impairment documented by screening or neuropsychological testing in two or more of the following areas: memory, reasoning, visuospatial ability, language, personality, and behavior. Impaired memory is the most commonly recognized cognitive change in early Alzheimer's disease, but in rare cases, difficulty with visual processing may predominate; in very rare cases, behavioral changes occur early and resemble frontotemporal dementia (below).	Gradual progression and slowly worsening cognitive abilities allow a person to maintain engagement in care planning during early and moderate stages. Behavioral symptoms are prevalent and are most common during moderate and more severe stages. The end stage can be prolonged and difficult to prognosticate. Most people with Alzheimer's disease die before they reach end-stage dementia.	McKhann et al.[47]
Vascular	Cognitive decline from a previously higher level of functioning manifested by impairment of memory and of two or more cognitive domains (orientation, attention, language, visuospatial functions, executive functions, motor control, and praxis); deficits interfere with activities of daily living and are not due to physical effects of stroke alone; there is evidence of cerebrovascular disease, including the presence of focal signs on neurologic examination (e.g., hemiparesis, lower facial weakness, Babinski sign, sensory deficit, hemianopia, and dysarthria) and neuroimaging consistent with stroke or significant cerebrovascular disease; and onset occurs within 3 months of a stroke or with abrupt deterioration or stepwise progression of cognitive deficits.	Reduction of vascular risk factors and overall physical and brain health–focused efforts may help slow progression and improve quality of life. Counseling care partners about the stepwise progression of cognitive impairment, without anticipated return to prior baseline, can help with estimating anticipating caregiving demands. When a person living with dementia is incapacitated due to a stroke, it is important to provide appropriate care partner coaching and teaching about performing medical/nursing tasks at home. It is important to monitor changes in gate and, when needed, institute fall precautions.	NINDS-AIREN Criteria for the Diagnosis of Vascular Dementia[48]
Lewy body	Progressive decline in cognitive function that interferes with normal functioning, causing prominent memory impairment and deficits in tests of attention, executive function, visuospatial ability, and fluctuating attention. Visual hallucinations are common and typically well-formed and detailed, and parkinsonian motor features occur. Other suggestive features include rapid eye movement (REM) sleep behavior disorder, severe neuroleptic sensitivity, and autonomic dysfunction.	Cognition is impaired but may be relatively stable during early stages and can fluctuate rapidly from confusion to moments of clarity during middle to late stages. Nurses should counsel care partners about the risks of harm to self or others caused by nighttime REM sleep behavior disorder when present. They should also guide care partners in identifying strategies for addressing vivid visual hallucinations and ensuring safety. It is important to carefully monitor the potential side effects of neuroleptics and to institute fall precautions.	McKeith et al.[49]
Frontotemporal	Selective degeneration of the frontal and temporal cortices and progressive deficits in behavior, executive dysfunction, or language, with three recognized clinical variants. The behavioral variant is characterized by early behavioral and personality changes, disinhibition, apathy, and executive dysfunction. The nonfluent variant is characterized by primary progressive aphasia and deficits in language production and comprehension. The semantic variant is characterized by aphasia and progressive deficits in knowledge and naming. For all variants, generalized memory decline symptoms usually appear after the primary behavioral or language/comprehension symptoms.	For these dementias, cognitive deficits may not present until later in the disease progression, and misdiagnosis of a primary psychiatric or personality disorder is common. Nurses should counsel care partners to recognize the signs of executive dysfunction, even in the absence of cognitive decline. Care partners should be helped to understand the involuntary nature of personality and behavioral changes and coached to monitor safety and to note, report, and mitigate difficult behaviors that can begin early in the disease course.	Bang et al.[50]

friends—the care partners.[1] With progression to moderate and severe stages, demands on care partners increase in parallel with the care recipient's declining ability to interact autonomously and intentionally with the world.[1,2] Taking on the role of care partner means becoming an interpreter, advocate, external memory, and safety surveillance system, in addition to helping navigate everyday tasks and managing health and illness. For nurses, dementia care is also inherently relational, involving the person living with dementia, one or more care partners, and a clinical team. Nurses' ability to understand and foster lasting partnerships with persons living with dementia and their support networks has decisive benefits for the quality of care, quality of life, and ultimate outcomes.

The critical components of dementia palliative care are listed in Box 48.1.[2–10] Early and consistent integration of palliative approaches, either embedded in or closely aligned with primary care, is an aspirational standard and a defining feature of dementia-capable health systems.[2–9] Despite the rising prevalence of dementia [2], and the

Box 48.1 Principles of Palliative Care in Dementia

Whole-person, trustworthy, transparent, proactive, equitable
Triadic: patient, care partner, clinical team
Flexible, relevant, specific, goal-directed
Optimized for quality of life
Responsive to psychosocial and spiritual needs
Continuous, coordinated, accountable, team-based
Supported by a responsive healthcare infrastructure

Box 48.2 Six Domains of Health

Domain 1. Cognitive Health and Function
Encompasses overall cognitive status and treatments. Cognition includes remembering, learning, thinking, making decisions, being aware of and responding appropriately to social cues, planning ahead, and completing everyday activities needed to live independently. Changes may be acute or chronic, stable or progressive. When progressive, dementia becomes an organizing principle of care: clinical decisions about all aspects of health must consider the impact of cognitive impairment on treatment choices.

Domain 2. Emotional, Behavioral, and Spiritual Health
Addresses mental health symptoms (e.g., loss of motivation, anxiety, depression, hallucinations, delusions), altered behavior (e.g., sleep, emotional reactivity, disinhibition, aggressive outbursts), and their treatment and management. It also focuses on identifying and meeting the overall emotional and spiritual needs of a person living with dementia.

Domain 3. Physical Health and Function
Includes general medical conditions and treatments; physical functioning and vulnerabilities; as well as frailty; mobility and fall risk; nutritional status; and sensory impairments (hearing, vision).

Domain 4. Care Partner Capacity and Needs
Focuses on building partnerships with care partners and how they can best integrate care demands into their everyday lives (e.g., manage stress, care for themselves, learn what they need to know about being a care partner, and activating additional supports as needed).

Domain 5. Health-Related Social Needs
Evaluates and intervenes to improve life conditions that affect well-being, health, social connection, and access to supportive care and services.

Domain 6. Care Delivery Framework
This domain specifies the attributes of dementia-capable healthcare systems and aspirational goals for universal, equitable access to high-quality care.

Registered Nurse Role Summary

- Administer and score cognitive and behavioral screens.
- Report results to the provider. The provider will follow up and may ask the registered nurse to do additional assessment.
- If impairment is identified, explore inclusion of a care partner, such as a family member or friend, in the diagnosis disclosure conversation.
- Engage in ongoing conversations about dementia diagnosis and impacts on everyday life, function, and safety.
- Obtain the recent history and functional status, identify any new or unresolved problems, check for needed prescriptions.
- Offer referrals to psychosocial and community services, provide focused person/family-centered teaching.
- Engage in ongoing comprehensive care planning, serious illness conversations, dementia staging, and care management.
- Iteratively assess care partner's capacity/needs and offer coaching and resources. Provide comprehensive care management.
- Evaluate health-related social needs and ensure culturally appropriate care delivery.
- Understand strengths and limitations of the health system and advocate for optimizing care delivery to become dementia-capable.

growing demand for primary palliative care, many providers remain uncomfortable diagnosing dementia, offering dementia-specific care, or addressing related questions.[10] Nurses are also reluctant to lead palliative and dementia care conversations due to a lack of role clarity and perceived knowledge and skills.[11] Consequently, fewer than a third of persons living with dementia/care partner dyads recall ever discussing the prognosis of dementia with a clinician, and many have no documented dementia-specific care plans.[12] Care teams need practical solutions to help simplify, organize, and track the inherent multi-complexity associated with dementia care over time. We present this solution as the Six Domains of Health framework (Box 48.2), which incorporates the critical components of dementia palliative care across stages of decline and can guide teams and health systems toward delivering high-quality dementia care across different settings. In this chapter, we outline the roles of nurses in providing dementia palliative care and issue the call to action for nurses to lead the transformation of dementia care to include palliative best practices and to expand the scope of nursing practice as leaders in comprehensive dementia care. Nursing roles and the application of the Six Domains of Health framework are illustrated in the case study.

Case Study

Ted C. was a 74-year-old retired terrorism/homeland security expert with well-controlled, uncomplicated, mild diabetes whose wife of 55 years called their primary care provider because "he didn't seem like himself," but she could not provide any concrete observations. She spoke to the practice registered nurse (RN), who asked a few screening questions and recommended that they schedule an evaluation visit. During this initial appointment Ted was diagnosed with mild Alzheimer's disease and was prescribed a trial of cognition-enhancing medication. Mr. and Ms. C. were sad and overwhelmed, and left the clinic quickly. Noticing their obvious upset, the RN called the couple the next day to invite them in for several follow-up visits that included medication reconciliation, functional and safety screening, evaluation of Ms. C's needs for support with caregiving tasks, and referrals to psychosocial and community services. Though grateful for this support, Ted and his wife declined to discuss advance directives: it felt "much too soon." Childhood sweethearts, both had experienced major early losses and been each other's primary confidant since their late teens. They could not imagine life without each other. During follow-up visits, Ms. C related that initiation of donepezil treatment perked Ted up: he was more engaged but still easily confused and becoming more reliant on her day by day. She clearly felt overwhelmed with her new caregiving responsibilities but refused to engage their children and other family members: she "did not want to burden them." The RN talked through with Ms. C how she could plan a program of regular self-care and coached her about the value of regular "time off." Sharing supportive resources eventually made Ms. C realize that she was not alone and that help with caregiving was good for both of them. Over the next several years, Ted's dementia care was managed by his primary care team, with regular assessment and stage-appropriate changes in the care plan. After 5 years, his dementia had reached the moderate stage, and his gait was mildly impaired. He remained at home in a close and loving relationship with his wife and could still warmly recognize his primary care nurse, and a paid caregiver was now visiting twice a week for a few hours. In separate conversations with Ms. C, the risks associated with advancing dementia (e.g., deteriorating behavioral control, physical risks of falling and injury, excessive care partner burden) were gently probed from time to time, with renewed encouragement to discuss advance care planning. His wife demurred: "It's in God's hands; what will be will be." By 7 years, his behavior was too disruptive for home management, prompting worried calls from Ms. C. to the primary care nurse. After a discussion with the primary care team, Ted moved into a memory care unit with a home-like environment, where he did well until the last months of his life. This new living environment offered structured, simplified routines, skillful nursing care, low-stimulation activities, and on-site church services that he and his wife could attend together. Low-dose medications helped to regulate sleep and alleviate his overall distress. In the tenth year of his decline, he was nonverbal and frail and stopped walking even with support. Suddenly, his wife called with an urgent message—he had fallen out of bed and was in transit by ambulance to the emergency room, as required by his residential community in the absence of a documented order to care for him on site. After discovery of a hip fracture, the orthopedic surgeon requested a palliative care team consultation with Ted's wife to help her understand and weigh the benefits and risks of surgery. During this conversation, they discussed whether hip surgery fit with Ted's goals of care and goals of life, and ultimately Ms. C. declined to proceed. Ted returned to his residential care community. After learning that Ted met hospice enrollment criteria (anticipated death from end-stage dementia within 6 months), Ms. C. agreed to initiate hospice services. Ted died peacefully 3 weeks later. His wife sought comfort in her church community and closure in conversation with the primary care nurse who had followed them together throughout the years.

Recognizing and Staging Dementia

Cognitive impairment can be detected during any healthcare encounter. For example, the Medicare annual wellness visit, a prevention-focused health service, offers an important opportunity for regular screening of cognition in older adults. Nurses can play an essential role in supporting this service by conducting initial steps to detect cognitive impairment (e.g., by administering brief, validated cognitive screening tests such as the Mini-Cog, which can be reliably administered by nonspecialists in under 5 minutes[13] and is included among widely recommended tools for this purpose). Care partners can provide important insight into the symptoms and course of cognitive decline; one useful tool nurses can use to elicit their report is the Informant Interview to Differentiate Aging and Dementia (AD-8).[14] The Kickstart, Assess, Evaluate, Refer (KAER model) is a detailed resource that nurses can use to guide follow-up conversations about brain health, cognition, and the next steps and to link persons living with dementia and their families to additional clinical and/or community-based services. It includes practical approaches, educational materials, and validated clinical tools.[15]

"Staging dementia" refers to establishing its severity and impact at a given point in time. Staging is essential for explaining the dementia process, communicating prognosis, anticipating care needs, identifying care partners' roles, and optimizing care planning. While different types of dementia vary in presenting symptoms and trajectories, stages of progression share certain features across subtypes. Different methods and instruments for staging dementia generally recognize at least three main stages. Staging is most efficiently conducted by integrating clinical cognition, behavior, and function measures, including information obtained from care partners. Simple clinical tools such as the Quick Dementia Rating System (QDRS)[16] can be integrated into the everyday nursing workflow. The key recommendations for all dementia stages are summarized in Table 48.2.

Discussing Dementia Diagnosis and Creating Care Plans

Although the initial determination and disclosure of the diagnosis are performed by a provider (e.g., nurse practitioner, physician assistant, or physician), diagnosis-related conversations are an ongoing process that requires the engagement of an interdisciplinary team.[3,6–9,17] Discussing the dementia diagnosis is challenging for many nurses, but this specialized, focused communication can be learned and practiced. Strategies and best practices for dementia-related communication can be adapted from approaches developed for discussing other difficult diagnoses. For example, the SPIKES model[18] and the NURSE mnemonic for guiding empathic communication[19] have successfully transferred to dementia.

In some situations, disclosing the diagnosis by a provider elicits feelings, fear, and questions that will be the only focus for the rest of the visit. Developing a care plan can be deferred to follow-up visits that a prepared nurse may conduct. Such conversations may include the discussion of common adjustment concerns, eliciting potential safety issues (e.g., around driving, financial management, and ability to handle firearms), and identifying needs across the six domains of care depicted in Table 48.2. Other aspects of care planning include discussing, assessing the need for, and referring to psychosocial and community services (e.g., counseling, early-stage support groups, the Alzheimer's Association 24/7 hotline) and encouraging healthy-brain activities (e.g., social and spiritual connection, cognitive stimulation, exercise, and a healthy diet). Nurses should frame the concept of living well with dementia as an attainable goal, taking positive action where possible, adapting to what cannot be changed, embracing preventive health and self-care strategies, cultivating what brings joy, and growing a network of meaningful support. Follow-up visits with providers may include decisions about prescribing cognition-enhancing medications, reviewing the appropriateness of prescribed and other medications, and strategies for managing multimorbidity.

Serious Illness Conversations in Dementia

The person and care partners need time to process the diagnosis, assess available resources and treatment options, and understand the initial care plan. Dementia qualifies as a serious illness: it has prognostic implications, impacts everyday life, and brings new responsibilities for family and friends that can have profound effects on their own futures. Serious illness conversations should take place shortly after dementia diagnosis is established but are best introduced in a follow-up appointment, such as part of a comprehensive care planning visit. The goals of these conversations are to support the person living with dementia in communicating their priorities now and understanding and communicating their values and preferences

Table 48.2 Key domains and palliative approaches in supporting people living with dementia (PLWD) and their care partners (CPs) across dementia stages

Dementia stages	Cognitive Health and Function	Emotional, Behavioral, and Spiritual Health	Physical Health and Function	CP Capacity and Needs	Health-Related Social Needs	Care Delivery Framework
Focus: optimizing quality of life—early/mild and middle/moderate dementia stages						
			Apply to all dementia stages			
	Recognize and plan	Anticipate, prevent, and manage	Reduce risks and acute care crises	Establish and maintain partnerships	Recognize and respond	Activate dementia capable age-friendly health system

Early/mild symptoms may include:
 	
forgetfulness; other mild cognitive, language, and judgment difficulties; IADL deficits.
 	
Cognitive impairment is a comorbidity. Consider its influence on treatment plans for other conditions.
	• Detect impairment early
	• Consider patient's and CPs' preferences when creating an evaluation plan
	• Disclose diagnosis
	• Explain dementia as a process and what to expect next
	• Initiate comprehensive care planning
	• Complete advanced directives and serious illness conversations
	• Evaluate safety (e.g., driving and guns)
	• Consider pharmacological options
	• Encourage engaging with early-stage support group
	• Encourage healthy-brain activities (e.g., social and spiritual connection, cognitive stimulation, exercise, diet)
	• Consider options for research participation
		• Detect psychological, behavioral, stress-related, and emotional changes (especially depression and anxiety)
		• Consider nonpharmacological options:
		  • Counseling, community support services
		  • Predictable routines
		  • Meaningful, pleasant experiences
		  • Physical and social activity
		• Consider pharmacological options
		• Address spiritual needs: a sense of value and belonging in the face of existential worries
		• Focus on adaptive strengths for high quality of life with dementia
		• Anticipate emergence of changes in behavior over time
			• Plan individualized preventive and follow-up visit schedule
			• Focus on crisis prevention (e.g., avoidable acute care episodes)
			• Consolidate clinical care and emphasize continuity
			• Identify and compensate for sensory deficits (hearing, vision)
			• Assess mobility, fall risk; consider physical therapy, exercise programs, supportive equipment
			• Screen, detect, and manage chronic conditions; reassess short and long-term goals
			• Explain rationale for all treatments and teach how to carry out plans at home
			• Anticipate and mitigate potential medical complications (e.g., recognize over- or undertreatment of hypertension or diabetes)
			• Examine all medications:
			  • assure accurate records
			  • limit polypharmacy including OTC
			  • ensure appropriate dosing
			  • eliminate low-value medications
			  • Teach home medication administration
				• Goals for CP:
				  • Understand PLWD diagnosis, prognosis, and health management needs
				  • Engage in care planning
				  • Accept CP role in evolving care needs
				  • Carry out recommended treatments at home; alert healthcare team when needed
				  • Ask questions, voice opinions and concerns
				  • Seek help for self when needed
				• Goals for healthcare team:
				  • Actively identify and track CP needs (knowledge, skills, resources)
				  • Actively encourage CP self-care: mental, emotional, physical, social, spiritual
				  • Observe CP for signs of stress, burnout, functional decline, cognitive impairment, family conflict, financial strain
				  • Offer rapid access to consultation, triage for acute needs
				  • Ensure continuity of care
				  • Link to community support services as needed
				  • Anticipate care transitions
					• Goals for PLWD/CP: Address needs through resource referrals as needed:
					  • Housing instability
					  • Food insecurity
					  • Transportation problems
					  • Utility help needs
					  • Interpersonal safety
					  • Physical safety
					  • Financial strain
					  • Family and community support
					  • Physical activity
					  • Substance use
						• Provides dementia and basic palliative care training to all staff
						• Identifies CPs in EHR
						• Facilitates systematic PLWD/CP evaluation using EHR tools, templates, and tracking of simple, relevant measures
						• Provides flexible scheduling options to accommodate the complexity
						• Offers care navigation, coordination, transitional, telemedicine, and home-based primary care services
						• Ensures that POLST and other advanced care planning documents are in the EHR
						• Ensures that pain/discomfort assessment and management tools are in the EHR
						• Promotes transparency about services covered by patient's insurance plan used to optimize affordability
						• Incorporates all relevant covered services into routine workflow (e.g., Medicare annual wellness visit, cognitive assessment and care planning, care management; advanced care planning; integrated behavioral health)
						• Offers acute medical care at home when feasible and delivers cognitively protective acute inpatient care
						• Offers financial counseling and referral for all care transitions (e.g., residential care)
						• Provides access to geriatric psychiatry, palliative, and neuropalliative specialists across care settings
						• Offers timely referral to home health, LTC, and hospice services when indicated
						• Integrates or coordinates health and community-based services—special emphasis on access and equity
						• Accommodation for language, hearing, vision, mobility, or other difficulties
						• Information, support, and resources for financial, legal, and LTC planning tailored to language, education, and culture as needed

						• Information about modifiable risk factors for poor outcomes (e.g., uncompensated hearing/vision loss, social isolation, physical inactivity, persistent depression, poorly managed comorbid conditions) • Affordable medications, hearing aids, glasses, and durable medical equipment • Affordable home health, respite and other support services
Middle, Moderate Symptoms may include: pronounced memory, mood, behavioral, increasing IADL, and emerging ADL deficits. *Dementia is an organizing principle of care - all care decisions must account for the impact of cognitive impairment.*	• Re-assess and stage cognitive impairment • Revise prognosis as needed • Enroll in regular care management • Update CP/PLWD education and support • Re-assess safety (driving, weapons, home environment) • Consider referral to occupational therapy • Monitor risk/evidence of abuse, neglect, and financial exploitation	• Explain non-volitional nature of many behavior changes ("no-fault" approach) • Watch for and manage emerging behavioral issues • Teach CP how to track symptoms and signs • Coach CP on what and when to report changes to clinical team • Discuss importance of sustained spiritual engagement: e.g. low stimulation spiritual/religious activities, simple meditation, reflection, adapted church services • Establish, simplify, and maintain daily routine reduce over-stimulation, and prioritize pleasant "failure-free" activities • Maintain circadian stimuli (e.g. daytime light exposure)				
Focus: optimizing quality of life while preparing for death						
Late, End-of-life Symptoms and signs include severe decline in function, ADL dependency, predominantly nonverbal communication, and eventual immobility. *Dementia becomes a primary vulnerability factor limiting survival.*	• Assess capacity to communicate feelings/needs • Train CP in understanding nonverbal language • Teach basic nonverbal care skills • Anticipate, compensate for loss of ability to make needs known	• Anticipate terminal delirium, dyspnea, pain, and agitation • Create peaceful environment for comfort • Regulate light, noise, temperature, and visitors based on observed responses • Use multisensory modalities: music, aromatherapy, therapeutic touch, designed environments • Provide comfort medications • Avoid or minimize physical and pharmacological restraints • Offer visiting spiritual or pastoral care	• Be aware of practice guidelines, life expectancy, benefits, and harms of all interventions (including IV hydration, artificial nutrition) • Anticipate and manage pain • Routinely screen for urinary tract infections • Honor patient's expressed wishes for where/how to spend their last days, considering CPs' wishes and readiness • Thoughtfully weigh any changes in care setting	• Educate about dying process and anticipatory grief • Support residential care decisions, transition to hospice • Offer access to 24/7 consultations for questions about symptom management, comfort, and support • Offer bereavement support		

ADL, activities of daily living; EHR, electronic health record; IADL, independent ADL; IV, intravenous; LTC, long-term care; OTC, over the counter; POLST, Physician Orders for Life-Sustaining Treatment.

for future care. This process also includes selecting a surrogate decision maker who can act as a proxy when an individual loses independent decisional capacity. They generally include completing a written document, a national form that has been developed to align nomenclature across states. The "POLST: Portable Medical Orders" is a living document that guides treatment decisions during medical emergencies. This document should be routinely re-evaluated and adjusted as needed. High-quality, regular, flexible, serious illness conversations are associated with improved comfort, satisfaction, and optimal end-of-life dementia care.[20]

The Six Domains of Health

Domain 1. Cognitive Health and Function

Early/Mild-Stage Dementia

Relatively few individuals receive their first dementia diagnosis at early stages when full engagement in care planning is possible. Persons living with dementia at this stage can often process the meaning of their diagnosis, articulate personal goals and preferences, participate in lifestyle changes, and choose to participate in clinical trials.[21] Delayed diagnosis makes people vulnerable to poor financial decisions, family conflict, and, in some cases, abuse and neglect. Primary care settings are ideal for broad, population-based efforts to accelerate the detection and diagnosis of common dementias.[22]

Middle/Moderate-Stage Dementia

Care is principally focused on aligning goals of care with goals of life for both the person and the care partner, accounting for cognitive impairment as a potential limiting factor in all treatment decisions. Adjustment of treatment plans to simplify daily routines, consolidate medication schedules, avoid reliance on memory and planning (which are impaired in dementia), and ensure adequate support at home are vital provisions. At this stage, the presence of dementia is always an influential factor in making healthcare decisions. Other medical or psychiatric comorbidities may temporarily take priority in clinical encounters.

Because of this complexity, a framework for organizing care is so important. In mid-stage dementia, cognitive impairment affects judgment (e.g., forgetting to turn off appliances), sense of time and place (e.g., wandering and getting lost), physical ability (e.g., balance, risk of falls), and senses (e.g., depth perception and temperature sensitivity). Significant behavior problems often emerge at this stage, adding new complexity to everyday care. Risk of abuse, neglect, and financial exploitation tend to increase with patients' increasing dependency on others for care. Nurses can conduct risk appraisals, identify possible harm, and help develop intervention and prevention plans. Because of the escalating complexity of care in mid-stage dementia, the cadence of clinical visits will typically increase, and access to remote communication about emerging symptoms, illness, or injury is essential.

Many care teams prefer to schedule at least quarterly follow-up appointments to assess the well-being of the patient and care partner and identify any needs for additional support; evaluate the safety, risks, and emerging problems; reassess prognosis; and adjust at-home health management. Much of this follow-up can be conducted through telemedicine, including dementia staging. People living with dementia and multiple chronic conditions should be offered regular care management services tightly integrated into team care. Occupational therapy assessment and intervention can enhance function, maintain strengths, optimize home environments, promote relationships and social participation, and provide education and support for care partners.[1]

Late-Stage Dementia and End of Life

The heterogeneity of symptoms, progression, and deficits associated with earlier stages of dementia tend to give way to a more uniform presentation of global deterioration toward the end of life. Impaired thinking is no longer the predominant concern as multiple severe deficits emerge, including progressive frailty, immobility, acute medical complications, and mutism. Small disruptions in health status, such as a minor infection or small stroke, can result in catastrophic, irreversible decline. Care planning must engage care partners as they assume complete responsibility for meeting the needs of their care recipient. At this stage, nonverbal communication predominates as meaningful language deteriorates. Nurses benefit from training to recognize and interpret such communication and can both learn from and support care partners in understanding care recipients' nonverbal communication and behavioral cues. This allows some anticipation of needs that cannot be clearly expressed and can smooth a potentially tumultuous phase.

Hospice Care for People Living with Dementia

Nurses play central roles in end-of-life care because they spend the most time at the bedside of a dying person. Families often lean on nurses for advice, emotional support, reassurance, coaching in optimal symptom management, honoring the dying person's wishes, and providing spiritual and culturally appropriate care. Although hospice is considered the best practice of end-of-life care, general characteristics that qualify an individual with dementia for hospice are those of very advanced decline, such as the inability to ambulate, dress, and maintain hygiene; persistent incontinence; and full or partial mutism. Determining whether death can be expected within 6 months—the general rule for hospice eligibility—is frequently difficult in the context of dementia. Many patients are enrolled in hospice so close to death that the benefits of this care approach for both patients and families cannot be fully realized. In addition, the difficulty of prognosticating helps to explain why rates of hospice disenrollment ("live discharge") are two to four times higher in dementia.[23] Based on a national study, the highest likelihood of disenrollment due to extended prognosis was found among people with dementia who were younger and female, had fewer chronic conditions, and were not nursing home residents. This was attributed to more robust overall health. Another group with high "live discharge" rates included Medicaid recipients, especially those from minoritized racial and ethnic groups, possibly attributable to the use of hospice as the only available means of gaining essential home health services.[23]

Domain 2. Emotional, Behavioral, and Spiritual Health

Early/Mild-Stage Dementia

By the time cognitive impairment is clinically recognized, many persons living with dementia and family members are already aware of changes. Still, they may not have recognized them as part of a pattern that signals the presence of a disorder. As a result, receiving a dementia diagnosis can trigger degrees of shock, sadness, and anticipatory suffering. Persons living with dementia may struggle with worries about diminished personhood as dementia progresses, fears of being a burden to others, and grief over the loss of future possibilities.

In high-income countries and Western cultures, loss of independence and individual abilities loom large.[24] When cognitive impairment is detected during the early stage, persons can usually talk about their reactions and report low mood and feelings of anxiety. They can participate in evaluations of their mental health and benefit from psychotherapy.[25] Some degree of anxiety, sorrow, and anguish on behalf of one's future self may be considered normal and expected by persons living with dementia and care partners, often leading to underreporting and missed opportunities for help. While the essential detection tool is the clinician's awareness, simple screening tools for depression and anxiety (e.g., PhQ-2 and GAD-2)[26] can be used for detection in non-specialist settings. Because most people living with dementia will eventually develop behavioral or neuropsychiatric symptoms that become a focus of caregiver struggle and clinical concern, it helps to prepare persons and care partners to recognize common changes.[25] For example, the care partner can be alerted to apathy and loss of initiative that are features of many dementias; signs and symptoms of anxiety, such as disruptive worry, fear, and agitation; and signs and symptoms of depression, such as sadness, tearfulness, self-deprecation, broken sleep or oversleeping, and expressions of hopelessness or worthlessness. The Cornell Scale for Depression in Dementia is a validated measure incorporating observer- and informant-based information and helps detect clinical depressive syndromes in cognitively impaired persons.[27] Mild depression and anxiety may respond very well to expressive and supportive approaches and behavioral and social activation. Apathy, fears, worry, and existential suffering are best relieved by supporting persons living with dementia to engage in pleasurable cognitive, social, and physical activity and whatever spiritual and religious counseling and practices are meaningful to the individual. Pervasive, lasting mood symptoms may require a combination of medications and psychotherapy.

Middle/Moderate-Stage Dementia: Signs and Symptoms

Neuropsychiatric and behavioral symptoms are ubiquitous but varied during this stage, and not all changes constitute problems. Apathy, amotivation, and loss of initiative are common, underreported, misunderstood symptoms that can be very distressing for care partners, who may interpret them as willful resistance or depression. Apathy can be assessed by asking direct questions. For example, "Does your care recipient seem withdrawn and uninterested in initiating activities?"

A brief informant report, BEHAVE 5+,[28] is a helpful screen for detecting behavioral issues that most often burden care partners and are likely to come to clinical attention. When behavioral problems are identified, the next step is to assess how challenging these symptoms are for care partners to manage. Establishing regular behavioral symptom monitoring at home is essential to mid-stage management; the Neuropsychiatric Inventory–Questionnaire (NPI-Q) is a standardized, valid, and reliable screen for this purpose.[29] New or worsening agitation, aggression, irritability, hallucinations, or delusions in a person living with dementia cause significant suffering for persons and family members and call for urgent evaluation, treatment, and assessment of safety. Most disruptive behaviors in dementia are not subject to volitional control. Causes include the primary effects of neurodegenerative processes on affective and behavioral regulation. Still, they can also reflect the impact of incident medical illness on the brain (e.g., delirium due to incipient pneumonia), medication side effects, unrelieved pain, depression or anxiety, sleep disorder, sensory deficit, and unmet basic needs (e.g., hunger, toileting). Often overlooked are the effects of prior traumatic experiences as behavioral triggers. Dimly recalled or long "forgotten" childhood adverse experiences, intimate partner violence, wartime or political trauma, medical trauma, and bystander (witnessed) trauma can be re-experienced and disrupt behavior even without recollection of the inciting events.

Management of Neuropsychiatric Symptoms

First-line therapies are nonpharmacological in nearly all situations and start with understanding and meeting care recipients' basic needs (e.g., feeding, toileting, pain management, and physical comfort) and working to interpret a person's nonverbal communication and cues accurately. Establishing routines that include pleasurable physical and social activity and finding ways to include the care recipient in household maintenance (e.g., folding laundry, setting the table) are simple stabilizing approaches. Care partners can be coached to describe the behavior, look for triggers, and evaluate their own responses. One example of an integrated assessment/management approach that includes a triad (clinician, care partner, and a person living with dementia) is Describe, Investigate, Create, and Evaluate (DICE).[30] This three-step intervention includes (1) asking the care partner to clearly describe what/where a problem happened and who was involved in the situation when the behavior occurred; (2) requiring the healthcare provider to evaluate all aspects of the person's health, social, and care partner–related factors; (3) collaborating on a careful and regularly evaluated individualized plan. Nonpharmacological interventions include physical activity, music, reminiscence, validation, activity kits, and sensory (e.g., aroma therapy, massage, baking). When nonpharmacological interventions are insufficient, medications can be considered; but they are only sometimes effective in the absence of behavioral management. Long-term use of antipsychotics and sedative-hypnotics is discouraged due to significant side effects that may include cognitive and functional decline and mortality. However, a short trial of antipsychotic medications may be warranted when symptoms are uncomfortable, threaten safety, and do not respond to nonpharmacological interventions. There is no consistent support for the effectiveness of cholinesterase inhibitors, memantine, trazodone, mirtazapine, or selective serotonin reuptake inhibitors in ameliorating neuropsychiatric symptoms in dementia. However, some studies demonstrate moderate efficacy and low side-effect profiles.

Due to the emotionally taxing nature of prolonged caregiving, "emotional contagion" is a risk: care partner and care recipient may both experience difficult-to-control bursts of agitation, anger, or despair. Care partners may want to conceal their own difficulties out of embarrassment or shame, but disclosure with a trusted person who can help is an important step. Nurses can help care partners learn to reflect and self-calm, accept and organize respite care to allow time apart, and foster joint sustained spiritual engagement, all steps that can diminish the likelihood of recurrence. Examples of practical approaches include low-stimulation spiritual/religious activities, simple meditation, reflection, and adapted church services.[31,32]

Late-Stage Dementia/End of Life

During this stage, the focus is on creating a peaceful environment and anticipating and mitigating distressing symptoms such as terminal decline/delirium, dyspnea, and agitation. Persons living with dementia often engage in nonsensical repetitive verbalizations, perseverative behaviors, and reflexive responses (e.g., striking out) and may appear to experience undifferentiated suffering and discomfort. It is essential to avoid or minimize physical and pharmacological restraints. A person can be soothed by comfort medications; regulated light, noise, and temperature; and visitors based on observed responses and tolerance. Multisensory modalities such as music, aromatherapy, therapeutic touch, and calming presence are often helpful. Quality of life and the experience of dying with dementia are greatly benefited by surrounding the dying person with familiar things and people, focusing on the person, avoiding invasive interventions, minimizing care transitions, and providing onsite religious/spiritual services and rituals when meaningful for the dying person and their loved ones.[33]

Domain 3. Physical Health and Function

Early/Mild and Middle/Moderate Stages of Dementia

Care goals during these stages focus on reducing risks and creating strategies for avoiding medical and surgical crises. People living with dementia experience more acute care episodes than other older adults and may have prolonged and complicated stays, poor outcomes, and institutionalization after discharge.[34] Many of these outcomes are multimorbidity effects that are especially common in individuals in their 80s and older. Comprehensive, iterative assessment and proactive, targeted management comprise the cornerstones of best practices in dementia care; but they are even more critical in this group. Integrated care management, regular planned follow-up medical appointments, focused surveillance, medication revision, avoiding over- or undertreatment, crisis prevention, and continuity of care are key to reducing excess disability and maintaining health.[4,5] *Frailty*, a common clinical geriatric syndrome characterized by loss of resilience to physiological and psychological stressors and declining function across multiple systems, is associated with falls, hospitalization, loss of independence, and institutionalization. A recent study summarizes tools that can be used to assess frailty, such as the Frailty Index, which measures the accumulation of age-related deficits, and the Fried Frailty Phenotype, which defines frailty as the presence of weakness, slowness, exhaustion, low physical activity, and unplanned weight loss.[35] *Mobility* assessment and the need for assistive equipment and physical therapy are warranted. Identifying and correcting sensory impairments are particularly important as hearing and vision loss can accelerate interpersonal isolation and functional and cognitive decline.[2] *Pain* is a particularly important cause of behavior change in dementia—it can be difficult to distinguish it from other causes of behavior change when individuals cannot clearly articulate their experience. Interviews with persons living with dementia and care partners, observation, physical exams, and screening tools are used to detect and evaluate pain. Observable signs may include facial expressions, vocalizations of distress, movements/retracting from stimuli, withdrawal, and inconsolable distress. *Sleep disturbances* are common in dementia and detrimental to both dyad members' wellness and quality of life. Common contributors include disruption of sleep-regulating pathways and circadian rhythms, depression, increased sedentary behaviors, inactivity, excessive daytime napping, under- or overstimulation, suboptimal sleep hygiene, nocturia, medication side effects, pain, and symptoms of active medical conditions. Evaluation includes clinical assessment, interview with a person living with dementia and their care partner, evaluation of the environment and sleep hygiene, and diagnostic tests (e.g., sleep apnea).[36]

Late-Stage Dementia/End of Life

As for all terminal conditions during this stage, care for people with dementia focuses on comfort and reducing care transitions and aggressive interventions, whether provided as part of routine care or formal hospice enrollment. Nurses must consider practice guidelines, life expectancy, benefits, and harms of all interventions (including intravenous hydration and artificial nutrition) when creating treatment plans. Maximizing palliative care interventions can reduce suffering and care transitions; improve symptom management, pain, infection, and delirium detection; and increase the likelihood of remaining at home.[37]

Domain 4. Care Partner Capacity and Needs

Early/Mild and Middle/Moderate Dementia Stages

When properly supported, care partners are highly creative, resilient, and expert teachers for healthcare teams, developing insights that can make decisive differences in outcomes. Care partners are always crucial to managing the health and well-being of people living with dementia. Clinical care focuses on establishing and maintaining partnerships and watching for signs that care partners are getting into trouble with fatigue, unmanaged stress, depression, and care demands that exceed their capacities. Despite these well-known risks of caregiving, formal inclusion of care partners in healthcare design has been slow to develop.[4,5,37,38] Failure to engage, coach, and support care partners can contribute to poor outcomes, including potentially preventable hospitalizations, and lead to adverse effects on caregiver health and cognitive function.[39] Ongoing assessment of care partners' needs is integral to high-quality dementia care.[4,5] Care partners have many common concerns, especially finding help with caregiving, navigating day-to-day caregiving tasks, managing medications, monitoring the care recipient's symptoms, and navigating complex and frequently poorly integrated healthcare delivery systems. When these concerns are addressed and care partners are empowered to ask questions, express wishes, and contribute to care planning, they become engaged and activated. *Caregiver activation* is a distinct construct positively related to caregiver mental well-being and preparedness for caregiving and negatively related to stress and anxiety.[40] It starts with acceptance of the caregiving role, recognition of the associated responsibilities as part of the care team, and at least a basic, practical understanding of care recipients' diagnosis, prognosis, and health management needs. Nurses can use simple caregiver needs assessment, for example, Managing Your Loved One's Health (MYLOH), a valid and reliable caregiver-centered tool that measures a core set of healthcare management domains endorsed by clinicians and caregivers as reflecting the broad scope of the caregiving role.[38] Nurses should encourage care partners to engage in regular reflection and self-care activities, seek respite, and maintain connections with friends and spiritual/faith communities. Early preparation of caregivers for a future when the best care for their loved one may be provided in a structured residential setting is an essential component of comprehensive dementia care and relies heavily on sustained, trustworthy partnerships with clinicians.

Late-Stage Dementia/End of Life

During this stage, care partners need support in understanding the dying process, relinquishing unrealistic denial, reconciling conflicting feelings and wishes, and navigating anticipatory grief. Care partners' need for support from the clinical team is crucial during this time as intensive, prolonged caregiving increases the risk of stress-related mental and physical health complications and even premature death.[37] Simple stress monitoring is readily incorporated into routine visits.[28] When higher stress levels are detected, critical sources of stress can be ascertained with detailed interviews, and stress management strategies can be developed. The capacity to provide care at home is often challenged at this stage; conversations that facilitate and support the consideration of residential care options can have dramatic healing effects. When the person is close to death, secure access to 24/7 consultation with the trusted clinical team becomes even more critical in managing the sense of urgency.[37] After death, many care partners benefit from a conversation with members of the care team to help bring closure and from formal bereavement support provided by hospice teams or other skilled professional counselors to work through ways to return to life under radically changed circumstances.

Domain 5. Health-Related Social Needs

All Stages of Dementia

This domain addresses life conditions that affect well-being, health, social connection, and access to supportive care and services. The highest prevalence of dementia is reported among people who live in lower-income areas and have lower levels of education. People from minoritized and marginalized groups report having less frequent access to health services and many missed prevention and care management opportunities.[41,42] Emerging evidence underscores the impact of implicit and explicit bias and stigma against people living with dementia and their family care partners on their well-being and health outcomes.[42] Negative consequences of prejudice and limited access to medical and psychosocial services are especially significant for people living with dementia who do not have family caregivers or are marginalized, including the LGBTQ+, African American, Latinx, and American Indian/Alaska Native communities.[42] It is thereby essential that healthcare teams ask persons living with dementia and care partners about challenges with critical health-related social needs that include housing instability, food insecurity, transportation problems, utility help needs, interpersonal safety, physical safety, financial strain, and family and community support. When needs are identified, timely referrals to community support services can significantly improve persons' and care partners' health and well-being.

Domain 6. Care Delivery Framework

All Stages of Dementia

The care delivery domain encompasses the attributes of dementia-capable healthcare systems. Comprehensive, longitudinal primary care management is accepted as a best practice for people with complex healthcare needs, including dementia, but achieving it continues to pose severe challenges to healthcare systems because many primary care clinicians and the systems and environments they work in are ill-equipped to address chronic disease in the context of cognitive impairment.[43] Dementia-capable healthcare systems incorporate early detection of dementia, identification of care partners in electronic medical records, protocols for individualizing clinical care pathways, organization and function of clinical teams, access to care navigation, linkage to community-based services, and optimal use of available reimbursement and financial resources to persons and families. Existing evidence-based dementia care management models can be grouped into at-home services, primary care consultations and collaborative care, and specialty-based partnerships between health systems and community organizations. Most comprehensive models typically focus on the dyad of the care recipient and care partner. Differences are driven by settings, provider types who serve as care managers, enrollment criteria, and access to outside referrals and resources.[44] Although existing care models demonstrate clinically relevant and statistically significant improvements in selected domains of persons' and care partners' health and well-being, they are not broadly disseminated or integrated into routine care. Making dementia care management models practical, widely available, and sustainable requires new national policies, financial incentives, infrastructure, and healthcare provider training to mitigate the critical shortage of specialists and access to geriatric and palliative care services. Enacting the necessary improvements in health systems depends on preparing a dementia-capable multidisciplinary healthcare workforce.[4] To address this need, in 2020, the US Department of Health and Human Services and the Foundation for the National Institutes of Health commissioned the *Building Evidence for Services and Supports* report, which identified significant gaps in workforce education and training and called for coordinated efforts across academia, professional organizations, and the federal government to specify dementia competencies, develop specialized training programs, and accelerate the development, translation, implementation, evaluation, and scaling-up of evidence-based and evidence-informed services.[45] The 2021 Decadal Survey confirmed and expanded on these priorities and issued a national call for rapid dissemination of best practices in dementia care.[42] To activate dementia capability, adopting the Age-Friendly Health Systems framework[46] can promote basic training in dementia and palliative care principles for all staff. Implementing dementia capability within health systems requires systematic detection and evaluation of all persons living with dementia and their care partners using electronic health record tools, templates, and tracking of simple, relevant measures; flexible scheduling options to accommodate varying degrees of clinical complexity; and integration of care navigation, coordination, transitional care, telemedicine, and specialty and home-based primary care services. Transparency about services covered by a person's insurance plans, incorporating all relevant covered services into routine workflow (e.g., Medicare annual wellness visits, cognitive assessment and care planning, care management, advanced care planning, integrated behavioral health), and providing financial counseling and referral for all care transitions are important elements in assuring equitable access to high-quality, continuous, culturally appropriate, and coordinated health services. These foundational rights guide aspirational goals that can only be realized through integrating accommodations for language, health literacy, hearing, vision, mobility, and other essential access barriers into everyday operations.

Conclusion

The Six Domains of Health framework articulated here can serve as a navigational system to guide nurses toward the most urgent priorities first without losing sight of the overall complexity of care and integrating palliation at every stage. It can also guide health systems toward becoming "dementia-capable."[4] Studies utilizing this framework to drive individualized interventions in advanced illness care[39] have already illustrated its conceptual relevance. Still, its greatest value will be in primary care, where dementia is first detected, care partners can be most readily identified and engaged, and people living with dementia receive most of their healthcare. To succeed, practice improvement efforts must focus on building the human and health information infrastructure that makes comprehensive dementia care feasible and actionable.[5] Nurses, armed with the Six Domains of Health principles, are well positioned to lead the transformation of dementia care.

Acknowledgment

The Six Domains of Health framework was developed by S. Borson, based on an inductive model derived from clinical practice. Although the model has not been independently tested as an integrated whole, each component is supported by empirical studies across a range of clinical and scientific disciplines.

REFERENCES

1. Alzheimer's Disease International. World Alzheimer Report. Life after Diagnosis: Navigating Treatment, Care, and Support. Alzheimer's Disease International; 2022. Accessed February 4, 2023. https://www.alzint.org/resource/world-alzheimer-report-2022/.
2. Livingston G, Huntley J, Sommerlad A, et al. Dementia prevention, intervention, and care: 2020 report of the Lancet Commission. *Lancet*. 2020;396(10248):413–446. https://doi.org/10.1016/S0140-6736(20)30367-6
3. van der Maaden T, van der Steen JT, de Vet HC, et al. Development of a practice guideline for optimal symptom relief for patients with pneumonia and dementia in nursing homes using a Delphi study. *Int J Geriatr Psychiatry*. 2015;30(5):487–496. https://doi.org/10.1002/gps.4167.
4. Borson S, Chodosh J. Developing dementia-capable health care systems: a 12-step program. *Clin Geriatr Med*. 2014;30(3):395–420. https://doi.org/10.1016/j.cger.2014.05.001.
5. Bott NT, Sheckter CC, Yang D, et al. Systems delivery innovation for Alzheimer disease. *Am J Geriatr Psychiatry*. 2019;27(2):149–161. https://doi.org/10.1016/j.jagp.2018.09.015.
6. Schultz SK, Llorente MD, Sanders AE, et al. Quality improvement in dementia care: Dementia Management Quality Measurement Set 2018 implementation update. *Neurology*. 2020;94(5):210–216. https://doi.org/10.1212/WNL.0000000000008678.
7. Yorganci E, Sampson EL, Gillam J, et al. Quality indicators for dementia and older people nearing the end of life: a systematic review. *J Am Geriatr Soc*. 2021;69(12):3650–3660. https://doi.org/10.1111/jgs.17387.
8. Durepos P, Wickson-Griffiths A, Hazzan AA, et al. Assessing palliative care content in dementia care guidelines: a systematic review. *J Pain Symptom Manage*. 2017;53(4):804–813. https://doi.org/10.1016/j.jpainsymman.2016.10.368.
9. Amador S, Sampson EL, Goodman C, Robinson L, Team SR. A systematic review and critical appraisal of quality indicators to assess optimal palliative care for older people with dementia. *Palliat Med*. 2019;33(4):415–429. https://doi.org/10.1177/0269216319834227.
10. Alzheimer's Association. *2019 Alzheimer's Disease Facts and Figures*. Alzheimer's Association; 2019. Accessed February 6, 2023. https://www.alz.org/media/Documents/alzheimers-facts-and-figures-2019-r.pdf.
11. Hagan TL, Xu J, Lopez RP, Bressler T. Nursing's role in leading palliative care: a call to action. *Nurse Educ Today*. 2018;61:216–219. https://doi.org/10.1016/j.nedt.2017.11.037.
12. Hashimie J, Schultz SK, Stewart JT. Palliative care for dementia: 2020 update. *Clin Geriatr Med*. 2020;36(2):329–339. https://doi.org/10.1016/j.cger.2019.11.011.
13. Borson S, Scanlan JM, Chen P, Ganguli M. The Mini-Cog as a screen for dementia: validation in a population-based sample. *J Am Geriatr Soc*. 2003;51(10):1451–1454.
14. Galvin JE, Roe CM, Powlishta KK, et al. The AD8: a brief informant interview to detect dementia. *Neurology*. 2005;65(4):559–564. https://doi.org/10.1212/01.wnl.0000172958.95282.2a.
15. The Gerontological Society of America. *KAER toolkit for brain health*. Retrieved February 4, 2025, from https://gsaenrich.geron.org/kaer-toolkit-for-brain-health
16. Galvin JE. The Quick Dementia Rating System (QDRS): a rapid dementia staging tool. *Alzheimers Dement*. 2015;1(2):249–259. https://doi.org/10.1016/j.dadm.2015.03.003.
17. Sico JJ, Sarwal A, Benish SM, et al. Quality improvement in neurology: Neurology Outcomes Quality Measurement Set. *Neurology*. 2020;94(22):982–990. https://doi.org/10.1212/WNL.0000000000009525.
18. Baile WF, Buckman R, Lenzi R, Glober G, Beale EA, Kudelka AP. SPIKES—a six-step protocol for delivering bad news: application to the patient with cancer. *Oncologist*. 2000;5(4):302–311. https://doi.org/10.1634/theoncologist.5-4-302.
19. Back A, Arnold R, Tulsky J. *Mastering Communication with Seriously Ill Patients: Balancing Honesty with Empathy and Hope*. Cambridge University Press; 2009.
20. Kim H, Cho J, Park WS, Kim SS. Characteristics of advance care planning interventions across dementia stages: a systematic review. *J Nurs Scholarsh*. 2021;53(2):180–188. https://doi.org/10.1111/jnu.12624.
21. Isaacson R, Saif N. A missed opportunity for dementia prevention? Current challenges for early detection and modern-day solutions. *J Prev Alzheimers Dis*. 2020;7(4):291–293. https://doi.org/10.14283/jpad.2020.23.
22. Creavin ST, Noel-Storr AH, Langdon RJ, et al. Clinical judgement by primary care physicians for the diagnosis of all-cause dementia or cognitive impairment in symptomatic people. *Cochrane Database Syst Rev*. 2022;6(6):CD012558. https://doi.org/10.1002/14651858.CD012558.pub2.
23. Hunt LJ, Gan S, Boscardin WJ, et al. A national study of disenrollment from hospice among people with dementia. *J Am Geriatr Soc*. 2022;70(10):2858–2870. https://doi.org/10.1111/jgs.17912.
24. Timmons S, Fox S, Drennan J, Guerin S, Kernohan WG. Palliative care for older people with dementia-we need a paradigm shift in

our approach. *Age Ageing*. 2022;51(3):afac066. https://doi.org/10.1093/ageing/afac066.

25. Mallick A, Biffi A. Diagnostic and management strategies for common neurobehavioral and psychiatric disturbances among patients with cognitive impairment and the dementias. *Clin Geriatr Med*. 2023;39(1):161–175. https://doi.org/10.1016/j.cger.2022.08.004.
26. Staples LG, Dear BF, Gandy M, et al. Psychometric properties and clinical utility of brief measures of depression, anxiety, and general distress: the PHQ-2, GAD-2, and K-6. *Gen Hosp Psychiatry*. 2019;56:13–18. https://doi.org/10.1016/j.genhosppsych.2018.11.003.
27. Park SH. Which of the Cornell Scale for Depression in Dementia or the Geriatric Depression Scale is more useful to screen for depression in older adults? *Asian J Psychiatr*. 2022;72:103147. https://doi.org/10.1016/j.ajp.2022.103147.
28. Borson S, Scanlan JM, Sadak T, Lessig M, Vitaliano P. Dementia Services Mini-Screen: a simple method to identify patients and caregivers in need of enhanced dementia care services. *Am J Geriatr Psychiatry*. 2014;22(8):746–755. https://doi.org/10.1016/j.jagp.2013.11.001.
29. Kaufer DI, Cummings JL, Ketchel P, et al. Validation of the NPI-Q, a brief clinical form of the Neuropsychiatric Inventory. *J Neuropsychiatry Clin Neurosci*. 2000;12(2):233–239. https://doi.org/10.1176/jnp.12.2.233.
30. Kales HC, Gitlin LN, Lyketsos CG, et al. Management of neuropsychiatric symptoms of dementia in clinical settings: recommendations from a multidisciplinary expert panel. *J Am Geriatr Soc*. 2014;62(4):762–769. https://doi.org/10.1111/jgs.12730.
31. Yous ML, Ploeg J, Kaasalainen S, McAiney C, Fisher K. Feasibility, acceptability, and preliminary effectiveness of the adapted Namaste Care program delivered by caregivers of community-dwelling older persons with moderate to advanced dementia: a mixed methods feasibility study. *BMC Geriatr*. 2022;22(1):797. https://doi.org/10.1186/s12877-022-03483-9.
32. Epps F, Moore M, Chester M, et al. The Alter Program: a nurse-led, dementia-friendly program for African American faith communities and families living with dementia. *Nurs Adm Q*. 2022;46(1):72–80. https://doi.org/10.1097/NAQ.0000000000000506.
33. Takahashi Z, Yamakawa M, Nakanishi M, et al. Defining a good death for people with dementia: a scoping review. *Jpn J Nurs Sci*. 2021;18(2):e12402. https://doi.org/10.1111/jjns.12402.
34. Bail K, Goss J, Draper B, Berry H, Karmel R, Gibson D. The cost of hospital-acquired complications for older people with and without dementia; a retrospective cohort study. *BMC Health Serv Res*. 2015;15:91. https://doi.org/10.1186/s12913-015-0743-1.
35. Koria LG, Sawan MJ, Redston MR, Gnjidic D. The prevalence of frailty among older adults living with dementia: a systematic review. *J Am Med Dir Assoc*. 2022;23(11):1807–1814. https://doi.org/10.1016/j.jamda.2022.01.084.
36. Finucane TE. Evidence-based recommendations for the assessment and management of sleep disorders in older persons. *J Am Geriatr Soc*. 2009;57(11):2173–2174. https://doi.org/10.1111/j.1532-5415.2009.02549.x.
37. Hanson E, Hellstrom A, Sandvide A, et al. The extended palliative phase of dementia—an integrative literature review. *Dementia (London)*. 2019;18(1):108–134. https://doi.org/10.1177/1471301216659797.
38. Sadak T, Wright J, Borson S. Managing your loved one's health: development of a new care management measure for dementia family caregivers. *J Appl Gerontol*. 2018;37(5):620–643. https://doi.org/10.1177/0733464816657472.
39. Borson S, Mobley P, Fernstrom K, Bingham P, Sadak T, Britt HR. Measuring caregiver activation to identify coaching and support needs: extending MYLOH to advanced chronic illness. *PLoS One*. 2018;13(10):e0205153. https://doi.org/10.1371/journal.pone.0205153.
40. Sadak T, Korpak A, Borson S. Measuring caregiver activation for health care: validation of PBH-LCI: D. *Geriatr Nurs*. 2015;36(4):284–292.
41. Albaroudi A, Chen J. Consumer assessment of healthcare providers and systems among racial and ethnic minority patients with Alzheimer disease and related dementias. *JAMA Netw Open*. 2022;5(9):e2233436. https://doi.org/10.1001/jamanetworkopen.2022.33436.
42. National Academies of Sciences, Engineering, and Medicine. *Reducing the Impact of Dementia in America: A Decadal Survey of the Behavioral and Social Sciences*. National Academies Press; 2021. https://doi.org/10.17226/26175.
43. Tumlinson A. *A Call For Action: Creating an Optimal System of Brain Health Care in the United States*. Brain Health Partnership; 2019. Accessed November 22, 2020. https://www.usagainstalzheimers.org/sites/default/files/2019-05/BrainHealthOptimalSystemFINAL.pdf.
44. Hovsepian V, Bilazarian A, Schlak AE, Sadak T, Poghosyan L. The impact of ambulatory dementia care models on hospitalization of persons living with dementia: a systematic review. *Res Aging*. 2022;44(7–8):560–572. https://doi.org/10.1177/01640275211053239.
45. U.S. Department of Health and Human Services, Office of the Assistant Secretary for Planning and Evaluation. (n.d.). *National Research Summit on Care, Services, and Supports for Persons with Dementia and Their Caregivers: Final summit report*. Retrieved February 4, 2025, from https://aspe.hhs.gov/reports/national-research-summit-care-services-supports-persons-dementia-their-caregivers-final-summit-0.
46. Institute for Healthcare Improvement. Age-Friendly Health Systems: Guide to Using the 4Ms in the Care of Older Adults. Accessed February 6, 2023. http://www.ihi.org/Engage/Initiatives/Age-Friendly-Health-Systems/Documents/IHIAgeFriendlyHealthSystems_GuidetoUsing4MsCare.pdf.
47. McKhann GM, Knopman DS, Chertkow H, et al. The diagnosis of dementia due to Alzheimer's disease: recommendations from the National Institute on Aging Alzheimer's Association workgroups on diagnostic guideline for Alzheimer's disease. *Alzheimers Dement*. 2011;7:263–269.
48. NINDS–AIREN Criteria for the Diagnosis of Vascular Dementia. The Internet Stroke Center, 2016. http://www.strokecenter.org/professionals/stroke-diagnosis/stroke-assessment-scales/ninds-airen-criteria-for-the-diagnosis-ofvascular-dementia/.
49. McKeith IG, Galasko D, Kosaka K, et al. Consensus guidelines for the clinical and pathologic diagnosis of dementia with Lewy bodies (DLB): report of the consortium on DLB international workshop. *Neurology*. 1996;47:1113–1124.
50. Bang J, Spina S, Miller BL. Frontotemporal dementia. *Lancet*. 2015;386:1672–1682.

49

Palliative Care for Persons with Cirrhosis and Their Family Caregivers

Louise Babikow, Christopher D. Woodrell, and Lissi Hansen

Key Points

- Liver cirrhosis is a severe illness, with difficult symptoms, poor quality of life, fatal complications, and limited treatment options.
- Cirrhosis often coexists with other chronic organ failures and presents numerous difficult-to-manage symptoms.
- Liver disease has a highly unpredictable course, and liver transplants, the only curative treatment, are rarely available.
- In addition to physical symptoms, patients experience significant psychosocial challenges.
- Caregivers of patients with liver cirrhosis experience significant burden that impacts their mental and physical well-being and quality of life.
- Despite the increasing prevalence of liver disease, palliative care for affected individuals is still largely inaccessible.
- Nurses can address the physical, psychosocial, and spiritual needs of patients with cirrhosis, impacting their experience throughout the disease trajectory.
- Early conversations about advance care planning and treatment options can align care with patient wishes and help prepare patients and families for end-of-life and the possibility of death.

Introduction to Palliative Care in Liver Disease

Chronic inflammation of the liver, whether from infectious, toxic, metabolic, or autoimmune causes, can lead to replacement of functional liver by scar tissue, resulting in impaired function and a host of complications.[1] Much like cancer, heart failure, or lung disease, cirrhosis is a serious illness that is characterized by difficult-to-manage symptoms, poor quality of life for those affected and their families, fatal complications, and inadequate treatment options.[2,3] Liver disease can cause other chronic organ-failure illnesses, is associated with numerous difficult-to-manage symptoms, and is highly unpredictable; and few people receive the only curative treatment, a liver transplant.[4] In addition to burdensome physical symptoms, psychosocial issues and caregiver burden and stress are nearly inevitable.[5,6] Patients' everyday lives are significantly impacted. Despite increasing prevalence of liver disease worldwide,[7] palliative care remains largely unavailable to this population.[3]

Liver Disease Can Be Chronic and Invisible

Case Study

A nurse in a gastroenterology practice is seeing a new patient, Ms. M, who was referred from primary care due to a new diagnosis of cirrhosis. Ms. M is a 55-year-old woman with mildly elevated serum transaminases, a Model for End-stage Liver Disease 3.0 (MELD-3.0) score of 6,[8] and a liver elastography reading of F4. Past medical history includes Type 2 diabetes. She has a normal body mass index and no history of alcohol or substance use disorders. The patient lives with her partner, Mr. T, and has minimal family support. Ms. M works as an accountant for a small business and has limited health insurance coverage. She denies having any current symptoms.

Ms. M: I'm not sure why my family doctor sent me to your office.
Nurse: If it's alright, I would like to talk more about that. Could you tell me what you have been told about your liver?

The patient shares that she has a limited understanding of her disease and expresses a wish to learn more, so the nurse provides education on cirrhosis. Educational material (e.g., https://cirrhosiscare.ca/) is also reviewed together.

Nurse: Since this is a new diagnosis for you, I want to make sure you understand it well. Can you tell me in your own words what your take-away points are from our visit?

The patient is able to teach back what she learned about cirrhosis and then states,

Ms. M: The part you mentioned about confusion worries me the most. As long as I don't turn out like my sister. She had no idea what was going on before she died.
Nurse: I'm glad you brought that up. If you feel comfortable sharing, tell me more about what your sister went through (pause). If you ever lose the ability to make your own decisions,

have you considered who you would want making choices about medical treatments for you?

Palliative Care Applications

Any member of a healthcare team can deliver palliative care. Nurses are especially well-equipped to address the physical, psychosocial, and spiritual needs of patients with serious illness. Very few patients and family caregivers will receive specialist palliative care until close to death, if at all.[9] Using a foundational palliative skill set, nurses can positively impact a patient's experience of living with cirrhosis at each stage of the disease trajectory. An important first step in this process is to facilitate illness understanding. The nurse in the case study assessed patient understanding by asking an open-ended question, addressing gaps in knowledge with education materials, and using the teach-back method to probe for understanding.[10] Second, identification of a healthcare agent is key in the early stages of diagnosis. This is ideally completed before additional physical symptoms occur such as hepatic encephalopathy, which is common in decompensated cirrhosis and manifests in neuropsychiatric symptoms ranging from mild confusion to coma.[11] Third, exploration of family caregiver support, beliefs, and values can improve the nurse–patient therapeutic relationship. These communication skills are demonstrated in the care study when the nurse asked a follow-up question regarding the patient's prior experience with illness in her family. The patient's comments are used as a catalyst for discussing appointing a healthcare proxy. Through the use of therapeutic communication techniques and active listening, nurses have the unique opportunity to initiate early palliative care for patients with cirrhosis.

Epidemiology

Approximately 2 million people die worldwide each year from liver disease.[12] In the United States, liver disease is the twelfth most common cause of mortality, with more than 40,000 deaths annually.[13] Cirrhosis is associated with a high mortality rate,[7] significant symptom burden,[6] and resource-intensive care.[14] Cirrhosis-related deaths are predicted to triple by 2030.[15] The main causes of liver damage include viral hepatitis (predominantly hepatitis B and C), and increasingly alcohol use disorder and metabolic dysfunction-associated steatotic liver disease (MASLD), formerly known as nonalcoholic fatty liver disease (NAFLD).[1]

Pathophysiology of Cirrhosis

Fibrosis refers to any degree of replacement of normal liver tissue by collagen, or scar tissue, leading to increased stiffness of the liver, and can result from years of exposure to inflammation or toxic insult. The causes of these insults range from infectious (hepatitis B and C), autoimmune disorders (autoimmune hepatitis, primary sclerosing cholangitis, primary biliary cirrhosis), inherited disorders (hemochromatosis, Wilson's disease, alpha-1 antitrypsin deficiency), chronic alcohol use, and MASLD. As liver disease progresses, fibrosis worsens and causes irregular nodules to replace functional liver tissue. The most severe and advanced pattern of nodular fibrosis is known as cirrhosis.[1] Fibrotic tissue leads to portal hypertension, which is an increase in blood pressure of the portal venous system, or the part of the venous system that carries blood from the gastrointestinal tract to the liver. Depending on the severity, portal hypertension has the potential to cause numerous symptoms including fluid retention, engorged veins or varices, and encephalopathy.

Diagnosis

Diagnosing and predicting the course of cirrhosis remain a challenge for clinicians given the silent and unpredictable nature of the disease.[16] As depicted in the case study, many patients do not have any symptoms early on and can feel well for many years without needing medical interventions. An estimated 630,000 Americans have cirrhosis; however, only one-third are aware of the diagnosis since the liver can continue to function at an adequate level despite severe damage.[13] This is known as "compensated cirrhosis."

Cirrhosis can progress into a "decompensated" state, which occurs when the liver is no longer able to function adequately. Decompensation is characterized by jaundice, ascites, hepatic encephalopathy, hepatorenal syndrome, or variceal hemorrhage. It is not always clear what triggers decompensation; risk factors include ongoing liver injury and the absence of treatment.

Diagnostic tools including blood tests (transaminases, sodium, albumin, bilirubin, international normalized ratio), imaging tests (computerized tomography, magnetic resonance imaging, ultrasound, elastography), or a liver biopsy can be used in the diagnosis of cirrhosis. The stage of fibrosis is important to identify as it will determine prognosis and recommendations for surveillance. Fibrosis exists on a continuum, with the higher stages (F3–F4) indicating a higher chance of clinical complications.[17] In addition to imaging studies, several calculations exist to gauge the degree of severity. The most widely used systems for grading cirrhosis include the Child-Turcotte-Pugh (CTP) and MELD. The CTP score grades cirrhosis from A (mild) to C (severe), while the MELD is a calculation based on blood test results and is particularly helpful for determining when a patient needs a liver transplant.

Assessment

Careful physical assessment is essential, with the most common physical findings listed in Table 49.1. The evaluation of fluid retention and mental functioning is especially important in regard to medication doses and adjustments. In addition to a thorough physical assessment, the clinician should consider psychological symptoms as they can be as impactful as physical symptoms. Further assessment regarding the patient's financial concerns, the challenges of nutritional restrictions, and the ways that cirrhosis impacts lifestyle are valuable to ensure the patient has the support they need. Questions to facilitate these conversations might include:

- What worries you the most about your illness?
- What would be most important to you if your health worsens?
- How has your life changed since you were diagnosed with cirrhosis?
- Who will support you if you need help with medical needs?

In addition to the patient, clinicians should include family caregivers in treatment plans. Support persons of patients with cirrhosis are significantly affected by the disease. They often face psychological and financial challenges. Resources for caregivers could include pastoral care, counseling, support groups, and mental health resources.[5]

Table 49.1 Overview of compensated versus decompensated cirrhosis

	Compensated cirrhosis	Decompensated cirrhosis
Symptoms	Patients may not look or feel sick. Symptoms are mild and include fatigue, weakness, sleep disturbance, decreased appetite, unexplained weight loss, nausea, and mild abdominal discomfort in the right upper quadrant.[6]	Patients can experience debilitating symptoms including abdominal ascites, hepatic encephalopathy, weakness, variceal bleeding, change in mental status, pain, breathlessness, and psychological symptoms.[6]
Physical findings	Little to no physical findings until decompensation occurs.	Jaundice, scleral icterus, asterixis,[a] splenomegaly, abdominal ascites, sarcopenia, esophageal varices, gynecomastia, palmar erythema.[13]
Prognosis	Median survival is 9–12 years. Approximately 5%–7% from this group will develop decompensated cirrhosis each year.[13]	Median survival is 2 years.[13]

[a] Asterixis is involuntary flapping of the hands and can be assessed by asking a patient to extend their arms and dorsiflex their wrists.

Disease Course

The trajectory of cirrhosis is irregular and unique to each patient but in general can be described by a multistate model.[18] This should be clearly communicated with the patient and family caregivers at the time of diagnosis. Median survival for patients with compensated cirrhosis is 12 years, while median survival for patients with decompensated cirrhosis is just 2 years without a liver transplant.[13] Although helpful diagnostic tools exist, a great deal of uncertainty persists regarding the progression and prognosis of cirrhosis. The disease is often silent and asymptomatic until increasing portal hypertension results in overt clinical symptoms. When the disease is advanced, the patient and caregivers frequently struggle to manage the physical and psychosocial challenges. Frequent hospitalizations and healthcare utilization are common among patients with decompensated cirrhosis.[19]

Management: Portal Hypertension and Subsequent Complications

The first step in treatment is to identify the underlying cause and treat it accordingly. This could include treatment for alcohol use disorder, weight loss, or medications for viral hepatitis. As cirrhosis progresses into a decompensated state, additional medications are utilized to manage symptoms.[3] Good physiologic management can translate to palliative management by enhancing the comfort of the patient through minimizing fluid overload and confusion (Table 49.2).

Ascites: A low-sodium diet, 2 g or less per day, is the first treatment recommendation; however, this is rarely sufficient for symptom management. Diuretic medications are frequently used as part of the treatment strategy. Abdominal paracentesis, which involves the insertion of a cannula into the peritoneal cavity to remove fluid, provides quick symptomatic relief in a population for whom diuretic therapy is not sufficient.[20] If repeated paracenteses are required, shunts are another option, which involves inserting a stent to relieve pressure and reduce ascites. Examples include transjugular intrahepatic portosystemic shunts and peritoneovenous shunting. When life expectancy is limited to several months, the use of an indwelling tunneled peritoneal catheter can offer relief from refractory ascites.[21]

Hyponatremia: Defined as serum Na concentration of ≤135 mEq/L, hyponatremia is present in nearly half of patients with ascites from cirrhosis. It is indicative of worsening hemodynamics and advancing disease, and is associated with poor clinical outcomes.[20]

Hepatic hydrothorax: Pleural effusion occurs as a result of portal hypertension. Managemement is similar to ascites, focusing on salt restriction, diuresis, or drainage as needed.

Encephalopathy: Encephalopathy is multifactorial, involving the accumulation of ammonia, which leads to confusion.[22] In addition to confusion, hepatic encephalopathy can manifest as somnolence, agitation, mood symptoms, sleep disturbance, asterixis (muscle twitch created by periodic loss of muscle tone), and, in severe cases, seizures or coma.

Infections: Infections present in approximately one-third of patients with cirrhosis who are hospitalized. A common type is "spontaneous" infections that occur in the absence of any obvious source. A diagnostic paracentesis should be performed as soon as the patient with cirrhosis is hospitalized for any reason, even in the absence of symptoms suggestive of infection or whenever

Table 49.2 Medication management

Symptom	First-line therapy
Ascites	Aldosterone antagonists (e.g., spironolactone) and loop diuretics (e.g., bumetanide, furosemide, torsemide) are used in combination. Doses can be adjusted over time with attempts made to use the lowest dose necessary. Body weight, serum creatinine, and serum sodium should be monitored regularly in patients taking diuretic medications.[20]
Esophageal varices	Nonselective beta-blockers reduce portal pressure and lower the risk of variceal hemorrhage (e.g., carvedilol, nadolol, propranolol, timolol).[23]
Hepatic encephalopathy	Lactulose and rifaximin are used in combination to decrease urease-forming bacteria and ammonia production.
Infection	Common infection is spontaneous bacterial peritonitis (SBP); choice of antibiotic should be based on local rates of bacterial resistance and culture results of ascitic fluid. Patients who have recovered from an episode of SBP are at high risk for recurrence and should be treated prophylactically with long-term daily norfloxacin or ciprofloxacin.[20]

a patient (hospitalized or not) develops signs suggestive of an infection. Long-term prophylaxis is recommended for a subset of patients who are at an increased risk of infection.[20]

Coagulopathy: Decreased synthetic liver function leads to a lack of natural anticoagulants, thus increasing risk of bleeding.

Esophageal varices: Esophageal varices are dilated blood vessels that occur as a result of portal hypertension. Upper endoscopies (esophagogastroduodenoscopy [EGD]) are advised for all cirrhotic patients to screen for varices. Variceal banding can be completed at the time of the EGD. Beta-blocker medications are also recommended to reduce the risk of variceal bleeding.[23]

Hepatorenal syndrome: Hepatorenal syndrome occurs in the setting of decompensated cirrhosis and is related to portal hypertension, reduced blood flow, and intense renal vasoconstriction. Approximately 20% of hospitalized patients with cirrhosis experience hepatorenal syndrome.[1]

Increased risk of liver cancer: Periodic blood tests (serum alpha-fetoprotein) and ultrasound exams every 6 months are recommended for regular cancer screening.[24]

Cirrhosis and Portal Hypertension Can Lead to a Myriad of Symptoms That Affect Appearance and Function and Lead to Family Caregiver Burden

Case Study

Ms. M calls into the clinic to report abdominal and ankle swelling. She also reports "brain fog," several falls, bruising, and fatigue. Mr. T takes the telephone for a minute to state his concerns about several episodes of confusion. An urgent office visit is scheduled for the following day. At the visit, the team orders blood work, lactulose, rifaximin, furosemide, and spironolactone. Additional education is provided to the patient and her partner that these symptoms are signs of progressing disease. A referral is placed to a liver transplant center.

Ms. M: Everything changed so quickly. I didn't think cirrhosis could turn into this.

Nurse: This must be surprising. Tell me more about your concerns.

Palliative Care Applications

As liver disease progresses, symptoms will become more prominent and affect the person's lifestyle to a greater extent. Nurses have the opportunity to continue to offer supportive palliative care interventions at this stage of the disease. First, clear communication regarding disease advancement and prognostic uncertainty is essential. Nurses should use plain language that is easily understood by the patient and family caregivers. In the case study, the patient exhibits signs of decompensation including encephalopathy, weakness, fatigue, and easy bruising.

Advance care planning is the discussion of patient wishes about their healthcare in the event they were to become sicker. While the intersection of advance care planning and serious illness conversation has been debated and serious illness conversations are essential at times of transition and occurrence of complications,[25] early discussions of values and preferences are also important for this population. Specifically, because of the potential for hepatic encephalopathy and/or critical illness that could occur rapidly and unexpectedly, identifying the healthcare agent(s) and encouraging the patient to discuss their wishes with them is important before they lose the ability to do so. In addition, early assessment and documentation of values and preferences, including information preferences (e.g., level of detail and which other parties are to be present) and what activities are valued most by the patient, can help inform information-sharing and medical decision-making in the future. Questions to address patient needs at this stage can include:

- Would it be helpful for you to hear about what to expect in the future?
- What activities are the most difficult for you?
- If you get sicker, what is most important to you?
- Are you experiencing any financial worries?
- How have your family and friends responded to the change in your health?

A multidisciplinary team provides the most effective treatment for patients with cirrhosis. Key members of the healthcare team include chaplains, mental health clinicians, nurses, physical and occupational therapists, physicians, registered dietitians, and social workers. Early referral to a palliative care specialist is correlated with better symptom control and improved mood.[26] Resources and processes may vary by practice setting, so working across specialties to establish case finding procedures for those who need palliative care may be an effective way to connect people with specialist palliative care services.[27]

Common Symptoms in Decompensated Cirrhosis

Symptom management is an essential component of palliative care and often overlooked in patients with decompensated cirrhosis. Several of the most frequently reported symptoms include pain, breathlessness, muscle cramps, pruritus, insomnia, depression and anxiety, and sexual dysfunction due to hypogonadism.

Pain is a particularly difficult symptom to treat for people with cirrhosis given impaired drug metabolism in the liver and risk of sedation and confusion with opioid medications. Analgesic options are limited as major categories of pain medication including acetaminophen, nonsteroidal anti-inflammatory drugs (NSAIDs), cyclooxygenase 2 inhibitors, and opioids are largely metabolized by the liver. NSAIDs are also generally contraindicated because of the risks of kidney injury and bleeding. Furthermore, hepatic encephalopathy poses an additional barrier for the use of opioids given the potential side effects of increased confusion or sedation. Unfortunately, these factors often lead to patients reporting unsatisfactory symptom control. Individualized treatment plans should consider risks and benefits of pain medications as well as the goals of the patient and family.[3]

Pruritus poses another unique challenge in decompensated cirrhosis. It can significantly impact a patient's psychological well-being, and its effects are often underestimated. The exact pathogenesis is unknown; however, the main hypothesis is that increased levels of bile salt accumulate under the skin and cause itching. Bile salt resins, such as cholestyramine, are typically first-line treatment. Severity and responsiveness to medication vary greatly between individuals. Additional symptoms such as muscle cramping and sexual dysfunction can be difficult to treat and at times impossible to completely resolve, but open communication with the patient and their caregivers is essential. Time should be allocated at each visit to address symptoms, functional status, and patient and family concerns and goals. While symptoms can be challenging to manage, numerous beneficial treatment options exist and should be selected based on severity, disease stage, and patient preferences.

Malnutrition in the Cirrhotic Patient

Cirrhosis is a major predisposing condition for the development of malnutrition and occurs in 20% to 60% of patients.[28] Malnutrition occurs as a result of decreased oral intake and impaired nutrient uptake as well as lifestyle and socioeconomic factors. A low serum albumin is common, which further worsens fluid imbalances including abdominal ascites. Poor nutrition leads to sarcopenia and frailty which are both strongly associated with morbidity, mortality, and poor quality of life.[29] All patients with cirrhosis should be screened for malnutrition and referred to a registered dietitian when appropriate. Current guidelines recommend a daily protein intake of 1.0 to 1.5 g/kg of body weight.[28] In addition to nutrition counseling, physical and occupational therapy can be beneficial.

Social Determinants of Health

Social determinants of health are the conditions in which people live, grow, and work. These conditions significantly impact health even before the patient interacts with the healthcare system in their community. Factors such as local laws and politics, community resources, housing stability, food security, financial status, behavioral factors, access to healthcare, and health literacy are considered social determinants of health. Regardless of the etiology, chronic liver disease disproportionately affects racial minorities and low-income communities. Furthermore, inequality extends into the realm of treatment for liver diseases. For example, significant gaps in care exist for incarcerated persons with hepatitis C. Minoritized groups are less likely to receive appropriate variceal screening or be referred for liver transplantation.[30] Low-income patients who rely on public transportation, persons with a history of injecting intravenous drugs, and people with limited support systems are less likely to be referred for liver transplant. The inequalities that exist in hepatology need to be addressed at both the individual and system levels. Nurses have the opportunity to screen patients for systemic barriers, provide education, and connect patients and their caregivers with community resources. On a broader level, healthcare providers can advocate for policy reform that addresses disparities in education, living conditions, and healthcare access.

Decompensating Events Can Occur Unpredictably and Lead to Significant Upheaval of People's Lives

Case Study

Ms. M experiences a minor car accident and cannot afford to repair her car. Due to lack of transportation, she misses follow-up appointments and loses her job. Physical symptoms begin to worsen including ascites, weakness, and encephalopathy. She has a fall at home, and Mr. T takes her to the emergency room. They are overwhelmed with the discharge instructions which include dietary restrictions, medication adjustments, and more appointments. They worry about the growing number of medical bills, and their relationship begins to break down as they navigate these changes. Depression, anxiety, grief, shame, and frustration are felt by both the patient and her partner.

Ms. M: I don't look or feel like myself anymore. I miss how my life used to be. Now I'm just a burden. My partner is struggling to keep up with everything.

Palliative Care Applications

Compensated cirrhosis is often invisible, with minimal symptoms; however, as the disease progresses into a decompensated state, the patient will look and feel different. Symptoms such as jaundice, abdominal ascites, and sarcopenia can significantly affect appearance. Unfortunately, the negative stigma surrounding these symptoms in North American culture can compound psychological impacts for patients and family caregivers. In the case study, the patient communicates dissonance between the present and past versions of herself. These sentiments are common among cirrhotic patients and family members as symptoms become increasingly visible and problematic. At this stage, healthcare providers can offer support to patients and caregivers by continuing to establish a supportive relationship, clarifying the prognosis with simple language, and identifying treatment goals.

A patient with cirrhosis will experience numerous changes and losses as their disease progresses. They will likely grieve the loss of relationships, intimacy, sexual changes, independence, and a sense of self. Exploring the many ways in which the disease is impacting the patient and caregivers will allow the clinician to develop a treatment plan that best meets their needs.

Caregiver Burden

Cirrhosis is a resource-intensive disease, with more than half a million cirrhosis-related hospitalizations each year in the United States. Approximately 70% of the patients who survive their hospitalization will experience a future readmission. This cycle of fluctuating symptoms and frequent hospitalizations can be extremely difficult for caregivers to manage and causes high levels of anxiety, depression, financial stress, and relationship difficulties. A typical patient with cirrhosis requires 9 hours per week of informal caregiving, which is not possible for many families.[31] Feelings of inadequacy or taking responsibility for the patient's decline can further exacerbate depression among family caregivers.[5]

While preventing disease progression is often impossible, there are multiple factors that can help decrease hospitalizations and reduce caregiver burden. The most fundamental element is effective, person-centered communication and education with the patient and family. Including family caregivers during appointments, inquiring about their well-being, and emphasizing the importance of self-care can give them tools to manage the building stress of caring for someone with a progressive disease. While self-care looks different for each individual, encouraging the caregiver to take periods of rest, set boundaries, and continue to engage in meaningful activities will help prevent burnout and promote resilience. Ensuring that patients and caregivers have easy access to a clinic staff member and timely follow-up appointments is also important. Family caregivers should be encouraged to connect with their established support system and have a "back-up caregiver" who could step in if they were to become ill or need a break. New relationships through support groups can also offer support. In addition to benefiting the patient, a multidisciplinary approach will provide more resources for caregivers.

Stigma

Liver disease is often stigmatized because of its association with alcohol and substance use disorders. However, regardless of the etiology, many patients with cirrhosis will experience adverse social judgment due to their medical condition. This stigma can be from friends, family, and medical providers. Studies show that cirrhosis has a low "disease prestige" and that discriminatory feelings among health professionals can cause patients to diminish the severity of their symptoms, delay seeking care, and lead to poor outcomes. Stigmatization frequently leads to isolation, depression, feelings of hopelessness and shame, poor self-image, and reduced quality of life for both the patient and family caregivers.[32]

Recurrent Hospitalizations and Further Functional Decline May Occur as Disease Worsens and Curative Transplant Is Only Available to a Small Fraction of Individuals

Case Study

Ms. M was hospitalized five times in the past 3 months due to generalized weakness, ascites, and encephalopathy. Each time, she seems to quickly improve and returns home, where her only support is her partner. They continue to struggle to organize her medications, coordinate transportation, and afford their bills. Feelings of hopelessness and defeat are present after being told she is not a transplant candidate due to a history of noncompliance and limited social support. Quality of life for both Ms. M and Mr. T has significantly decreased.

Mr. T: I don't understand why this is happening. Isn't there anything else you can do? I'm trying so hard. What am I doing wrong?

Nurse: It was her goal to stay at home with you for as long as possible, and we also want to make sure she has her care needs met. Would it be OK if we talked about services to support both of you in your home?

Palliative Care Application

As the patient nears the end of life, unplanned hospitalizations and healthcare utilization increase. With each admission, the chance of survival decreases. Symptoms typically fluctuate and create an unstable home environment and unpredictable future. Patients and caregivers tend to be more optimistic about the prognosis and chance of survival in comparison to their hepatologists.[33] Lack of communication regarding end-of-life wishes can further prolong a cycle of recurrent hospitalizations that might be misaligned with patient values and inadequate home support. Early elicitation of patient values can help ensure that care setting and intensity are aligned with patient wishes to the extent possible, as they get sicker.[34] Direct conversations about the possibility of death in the near future will help the patient and family prepare. Questions for nurses to ask at this stage could include:

- How do you imagine spending your last months, weeks, and days?
- What does a good day look like?
- What are your fears?

Liver Transplant

Liver transplant is indicated for severe liver disease when medical therapy is no longer sufficient for managing symptoms or complications. The three most common indications for liver transplant in the United States include alcoholic liver disease, MASLD, and hepatitis C (worldwide, hepatitis B is a leading indication).[35] For people with cirrhosis, priority is generally given to those with the most advanced symptoms and highest MELD 3.0 score.[36] Evaluation can be initiated once a patient experiences a sign of decompensation such as ascites, hepatic encephalopathy, or variceal hemorrhage.[37] A MELD 3.0 score of 15 or higher correlates with severe liver dysfunction and would indicate an appropriate time for transplant evaluation.

The transplant evaluation process is extensive, and specific requirements depend on the individual medical center. The patient's medical history, drug and alcohol use, psychological well-being, social support, insurance, and medical compliance are some of the main factors taken into consideration. A multidisciplinary committee reviews each case to determine whether to place a patient on the waiting list. Approximately 14% of patients on a transplant list die annually due to limited organ supply, and another 10% are removed from the list as they become too ill to undergo surgery. Ethical issues continue to be debated including drug and alcohol abstinence requirements before transplant, sex-based disparities, and the transplantation of hepatitis C virus–infected organs.

Palliative Care versus Hospice

Palliative care can be introduced at an early stage and is appropriate for the care of patients with any life-limiting disease. It involves a focus on symptom management in conjunction with ongoing potentially curative therapy, such as patients awaiting a liver transplant. Palliative care is shown to reduce unplanned hospital admissions and improve quality of life for patients with end-stage liver disease and their family caregivers.[26]

Hospice care also focuses on symptom relief but without a curative or life-prolonging intent. Transition to hospice care is appropriate if the medical team believes the patient will die within 6 months, ongoing treatments are no longer beneficial, or the patient and family wish to pursue comfort measures rather than curative treatment. Given the barriers to liver transplantation and limited organ availability, many patients must face the reality that a curative option does not exist. Hospice referrals may occur late and infrequently for people with cirrhosis[38]; intensive disease management related to varices, ascites, and coagulopathy may inform this phenomenon, and more information is needed on alternative strategies like indwelling abdominal catheters.[21]

End of Life Is Fraught with Intense Medical and Social Needs, and Few Individuals Receive Timely Hospice Care

Case Study

After just a couple weeks at home, Ms. M is back in the hospital due to worsening confusion and a fall. She exhibits fluid retention, jaundice, and sarcopenia. Since she has not improved over several days, Mr. T agrees to comfort measures, and she is transferred to an inpatient hospice center.

Mr. T: I wish I could have kept her at home. This doesn't feel anything like our place.

Chaplain: I understand she wanted to die at home and this feels different for you. What are some ways that we could make this space feel more like your home?

Palliative Care Application

Over 70% of patients with end-stage liver disease will die in the hospital.[34] Early palliative care interventions and conversations help patients and family caregivers have the end-of-life experience that they desire. In the case study, the patient was able to die in an inpatient hospice. Inpatient hospice is sometimes used when the patient requires intensive nursing care such as for restlessness, pain, or agitation that would be unmanageable in the home setting. Patients with cirrhosis frequently need this type of intensive care, which can leave caregivers feeling inadequate. Assistance with activities of daily living such as eating and bathing can become exhausting. Encephalopathy, which is common at the end of life, can be particularly difficult to manage. If the patient developed cirrhosis as a result of alcohol or drug use disorder, caregivers may have experienced a traumatic and hurtful relationship previously, which complicates their role. Family caregivers often report pressure to be a "model caregiver" and feel they have failed if the patient does not die at home. Healthcare providers can provide ongoing support to family members through education about what is expected at the end of life. Additionally, taking steps to make the hospital or hospice room feel like a familiar place can be beneficial to both the patient and family caregiver. Questions that a nurse could use at the end of life include:

- How has your family handled death in the past?
- How does the patient want to say goodbye?
- How can we honor spiritual and cultural beliefs and values as death approaches?

Cultural Considerations

The United States continues to become more ethnically diverse, making cultural humility important, given that the background, cultures, and lived experiences of a person have deep implications for the way they receive and experience healthcare. Demonstrating respect for a patient's beliefs and acknowledging the various ways that culture shapes their experience are essential for holistic care. Performing an assessment early in the diagnosis that stems from curiosity, sensitivity, and humility will establish the patient's goals and values at the center of care and inform decision-making. Preferences should not be assumed based on specific attributes since variability exists between individuals.[39] Some patients may want privacy, while others desire many family members to be present at the end of life. Comfort level with discussing death and dying greatly varies between individuals, and healthcare providers should explore how and with whom a person might want these discussions to occur.

Family Caregiver Support

Woven throughout the experience of people confronting cirrhosis is the concept of patient and family caregiver interconnectedness.[40] Liver disease not only significantly impacts the patient; it also places a strain on family members and caregivers. Many hours of unpaid services such as grocery shopping, financial help, and assistance with daily activities are often invisible to healthcare professionals. The stigma associated with cirrhosis makes the journey especially difficult and sets it apart from other chronic diseases, and it may be associated with guilt, fear, frustration, and resentment.[41]

The difficult journey of cirrhosis continues for family caregivers even after their friend, partner, or family member has died. The majority of deaths occur in the hospital setting, which can be traumatic and involve numerous unsuccessful medical interventions.[38] Even if the death occurs in the home or hospice setting, families will still experience a range of emotions. While healthcare workers will not have ongoing contact with caregivers, offering sources of support is appropriate. Chaplains, social workers, and community support groups can provide assistance with processing grief and reflecting on the journey.

Conclusion

Palliative care is a multidisciplinary specialty that focuses on supporting patients facing serious illness and their families. Specialized palliative care teams can offer in-depth services, but all healthcare professionals, including nurses, have the opportunity to utilize palliative care principles when interacting with patients with cirrhosis. The core principals of palliative care include symptom management, discussing information and care preferences that are based on the patient's values, therapeutic communication, and psychosocial, spiritual, and practical support. As depicted in the case study, patients will experience a wide range of physical and psychosocial symptoms as they process the diagnosis and progressive disease. Nurses have the opportunity and skill set to support patients and their caregivers throughout the disease trajectory and make a difficult experience more manageable.

REFERENCES

1. Ginès P, Krag A, Abraldes JG, Solà E, Fabrellas N, Kamath PS. Liver cirrhosis. *Lancet*. 2021;398(10308):1359–1376.
2. Gronkjaer LL, Lauridsen MM. Impact of liver disease on patients' quality of life: a mixed methods systematic review protocol. *JBI Evid Synth*. 2021;19(6):1412–1417.
3. Rogal SS, Hansen L, Patel A, et al. AASLD practice guidance: palliative care and symptom-based management in decompensated cirrhosis. *Hepatology*. 2022;76(3):819–853.
4. Brown CL, Hammill BG, Qualls LG, Curtis LH, Muir AJ. Significant morbidity and mortality among hospitalized end-stage liver disease patients in Medicare. *J Pain Symptom Manage*. 2016;52(3):412–419.e1
5. Woodrell CD, Mitra A, Hamilton A, Hansen L. Burden, quality of life, and palliative care for family caregivers of individuals with advanced liver disease: a systematic literature review. *Curr Hepatol Rep*. 2021;20(3):198–212.
6. Peng JK, Hepgul N, Higginson IJ, Gao W. Symptom prevalence and quality of life of patients with end-stage liver disease: a systematic review and meta-analysis. *Palliat Med*. 2019;33(1):24–36.
7. Ye F, Zhai M, Long J, et al. The burden of liver cirrhosis in mortality: results from the global burden of disease study. *Front Public Health*. 2022;10:909455.
8. Kim WR, Mannalithara A, Heimbach JK, Kamath PS, Asrani SK, Biggins SW, Wood NL, Gentry SE, Kwong AJ. MELD 3.0: The Model for End-Stage Liver Disease Updated for the Modern Era. *Gastroenterology*. 2021 Dec;161(6):1887–1895.e4. doi:10.1053/j.gastro.2021.08.050. Epub 2021 Sep 3. PMID: 34481845; PMCID: PMC8608337.
9. Mazzarelli C, Prentice WM, Heneghan MA, Belli LS, Agarwal K, Cannon MD. Palliative care in end-stage liver disease: time to do better? *Liver Transpl*. 2018;24(7):961–968.
10. Ha Dinh TT, Bonner A, Clark R, Ramsbotham J, Hines S. *The* effectiveness of the teach-back method on adherence and self-management in health education for people with chronic disease: a systematic review. *JBI Database System Rev Implement Rep*. 2016;14(1):210–247.
11. Ferenci P. Hepatic encephalopathy. *Gastroenterol Rep*. 2017;5(2):138–147.
12. Asrani SK, Devarbhavi H, Eaton J, Kamath PS. Burden of liver diseases in the world. *J Hepatol*. 2019;70(1):151–171.
13. Smith A, Baumgartner K, Bositis C. Cirrhosis: diagnosis and management. *Am Fam Physician*. 2019;100(12):759–770.
14. Nguyen MH, Ozbay AB, Liou I, et al. Healthcare resource utilization and costs by disease severity in an insured national sample of US patients with chronic hepatitis B. *J Hepatol*. 2019;70(1):24–32.
15. Tapper EB, Parikh ND. Mortality due to cirrhosis and liver cancer in the United States, 1999-2016: observational study. *BMJ*. 2018;362:k2817.
16. Kimbell B, Boyd K, Kendall M, Iredale J, Murray SA. Managing uncertainty in advanced liver disease: a qualitative, multiperspective, serial interview study. *BMJ Open*. 2015;5(11):e009241.
17. Barr RG, Wilson SR, Rubens D, Garcia-Tsao G, Ferraioli G. Update to the Society of Radiologists in Ultrasound liver elastography consensus statement. *Radiology*. 2020;296(2):263–274.
18. D'Amico G, Morabito A, D'Amico M, et al. Clinical states of cirrhosis and competing risks. *J Hepatol*. 2018;68(3):563–576.
19. Patel AA, Walling AM, Ricks-Oddie J, May FP, Saab S, Wenger N. Palliative care and health care utilization for patients with end-stage liver disease at the end of life. *Clin Gastroenterol Hepatol*. 2017;15(10):1612–1619.e4.
20. Biggins SW, Angeli P, Garcia-Tsao G, et al. Diagnosis, evaluation, and management of ascites, spontaneous bacterial peritonitis and hepatorenal syndrome: 2021 practice guidance by the American Association for the Study of Liver Diseases. *Hepatology*. 2021;74(2):1014–1048.
21. Macken L, Mason L, Evans C, et al. Palliative long-term abdominal drains versus repeated drainage in individuals with untreatable ascites due to advanced cirrhosis: study protocol for a feasibility randomised controlled trial. *Trials*. 2018;19(1):401.
22. Sahney A, Wadhawan M. Encephalopathy in cirrhosis: prevention and management. *J Clin Exp Hepatol*. 2022;12(3):927–936.
23. Turco L, Garcia-Tsao G. Portal hypertension: pathogenesis and diagnosis. *Clin Liver Dis*. 2019;23(4):573–587.
24. Marrero JA, Kulik LM, Sirlin CB, et al. Diagnosis, staging, and management of hepatocellular carcinoma: 2018 practice guidance by the American Association for the Study of Liver Diseases. *Hepatology*. 2018;68(2):723–750.
25. Smith AK. Should we still believe in advance care planning? *J Am Geriatr Soc*. 2022;70(5):1358–1360.
26. Woodland H, Hudson B, Forbes K, McCune A, Wright M; British Association for the Study of the Liver End of Life Special Interest Group. Palliative care in liver disease: what does good look like? *Frontline Gastroenterol*. 2020;11(3):218–227.
27. Courtright KR, Chivers C, Becker M, et al. Electronic health record mortality prediction model for targeted palliative care among hospitalized medical patients: a pilot quasi-experimental study. *J Gen Intern Med*. 2019;34(9):1841–1847.
28. Ge PS, Runyon BA. Treatment of patients with cirrhosis. *N Engl J Med*. 2016;375(21):2104–2105.
29. Tandon P, Montano-Loza AJ, Lai JC, Dasarathy S, Merli M. Sarcopenia and frailty in decompensated cirrhosis. *J Hepatol*. 2021;75(suppl. 1):S147–S162.
30. Kardashian A, Wilder J, Terrault NA, Price JC. Addressing social determinants of liver disease during the COVID-19 pandemic and beyond: a call to action. *Hepatology*. 2021;73(2):811–820.
31. Rakoski MO, McCammon RJ, Piette JD, et al. Burden of cirrhosis on older Americans and their families: analysis of the health and retirement study. *Hepatology*. 2012;55(1):184–191.
32. Carol M, Perez-Guasch M, Sola E, et al. Stigmatization is common in patients with non-alcoholic fatty liver disease and correlates with quality of life. *PLoS One*. 2022;17(4):e0265153.
33. Kaplan A, Comisar L, Ufere NN, et al. Understanding prognosis: discrepancy in prognosis estimates between patients with cirrhosis and their hepatologists. *Clin Gastroenterol Hepatol*. 2023;21(4):1005–1012.e4.
34. Kimbell B, Murray SA, Byrne H, et al. Palliative care for people with advanced liver disease: a feasibility trial of a supportive care liver nurse specialist. *Palliat Med*. 2018;32(5):919–929.
35. Chan WK, Chuah KH, Rajaram RB, Lim LL, Ratnasingam J, Vethakkan SR. Metabolic Dysfunction-Associated Steatotic Liver Disease (MASLD): A State-of-the-Art Review. *J Obes Metab Syndr*. 2023 Sep 30;32(3):197–213. doi:10.7570/jomes23052. Epub 2023 Sep 13. PMID: 37700494; PMCID: PMC10583766.
36. Samuel D, Coilly A. Management of patients with liver diseases on the waiting list for transplantation: a major impact to the success of liver transplantation. *BMC Med*. 2018;16(1):113.

37. Martin P, DiMartini A, Feng S, Brown R Jr, Fallon M. Evaluation for liver transplantation in adults: 2013 practice guideline by the American Association for the Study of Liver Diseases and the American Society of Transplantation. *Hepatology*. 2014;59(3):1144–1165.
38. Jordan RI, ElMokhallalati Y, Corless L, Bennett M. Quality of end-of-life care with non-malignant liver disease: analysis of the VOICES national survey of bereaved people. *Liver Int*. 2023;43(2):308–316.
39. Woodrell CD, Patel AA, Wilder JM, Sundaram V, Chung RT, Ufere NN. Cultural humility and end-of-life communication with people with advanced liver disease. *Clin Liver Dis (Hoboken)*. 2022;20(3):81–85.
40. Hansen L, Chang MF, Lee CS, et al. Physical and mental quality of life in patients with end-stage liver disease and their informal caregivers. *Clin Gastroenterol Hepatol*. 2021;19(1):155–161.e1.
41. Saleh ZM, Salim NE, Nikirk S, Serper M, Tapper EB. The emotional burden of caregiving for patients with cirrhosis. *Hepatol Commun*. 2022;6(10):2827–2835.

50

Palliative Care for Persons Living with Advanced Kidney Disease

Kate Sciacca and Marissa Finger

Key Points

- Persons living with advanced kidney disease have a multitude of symptoms caused by the buildup of toxins, many of which have limited pharmacological treatment options and can be best managed with nonpharmacological treatments.
- While many persons living with chronic kidney disease may elect to initiate dialysis as their kidneys fail, others whose goals do not align with receiving dialysis may choose conservative kidney management, which involves medical and dietary optimization, symptom management, and advance care planning.
- There are specific questions providers can use to attend to a person's discussion of, request for, or communicated decision for withdrawal from dialysis.

Introduction to Kidney Disease

Chronic kidney disease (CKD) and end-stage kidney disease (ESKD) are growing public health concerns in the United States. Approximately 37 million US adults have CKD, and it is the ninth leading cause of death.[1] CKD refers to kidney damage that results in ineffective filtering of blood and removal of fluid. Persons living with CKD have a slow loss of kidney function over time. The two most common causes of kidney disease are diabetes and hypertension.

When the kidneys are no longer able to effectively filter toxins or remove fluid, defined as an estimated glomerular filtration rate (eGFR) of less than 15%, the person has advanced to Stage 5 CKD, or kidney failure.[2] Once a person is on dialysis for at least 3 months or receives a kidney transplant, they are considered to have ESKD.[3] Due to the prevalence of kidney disease, it is important to understand how to care for persons living with this serious illness. In this chapter we will discuss the critical variables to consider when caring for people with kidney disease.

Race Considerations

Blacks, Hispanics, Native Americans, Asian Americans, and Pacific Islanders are at an increased risk to develop kidney disease compared to Caucasian Americans.[4] In addition, Black Americans have an incidence of kidney failure three times that of White Americans. This is largely due to the higher prevalence of diabetes and hypertension caused by social determinants of health and structural racism within our society. Additional contributors to this racial disparity are lack of health insurance, decreased access to healthcare, and delayed treatment.[5] Lack of insurance and access to healthcare lead to limiting of health prevention and promotion measures and delayed referrals and treatment for kidney disease.[6]

Disease Trajectory and Prognosis

The complications of kidney disease affect all organ systems. Many persons who have kidney disease also have other comorbid chronic conditions which impact their quality of life; common comorbid chronic conditions for persons living with kidney disease are diabetes and cardiac disease.[7] The severity of these comorbid chronic conditions has an impact on a person's prognosis.

CKD

Kidney disease progresses at different rates depending on the cause of the kidney disease and treatment. In the United States only 1% of people living with kidney disease end up needing dialysis and/or transplant. CKD is the most expensive of the chronic diseases and reduces a person's life span significantly.[1] The risk for progression to kidney failure can be estimated by looking at a person's GFR and how much albumin is in their urine. In persons aged 85 and older who have CKD Stages 3–5 the risk of death is greater than the risk of progression to kidney failure.[8]

Dialysis

While rates of mortality have decreased for persons receiving renal replacement therapy via dialysis over the years in the United States, being on any form of dialysis indicates a very limited survival: a >25-year loss of life span for men and a >30-year loss of life span for women when compared to the general population. Persons who start dialysis are at high risk of death even within the first year of initiating treatment, with first year mortality at 27% for persons who start hemodialysis (HD) and 35.4% who start peritoneal dialysis (PD). A person on dialysis lives for an average of 48 months for persons on HD and 55 months for persons on PD. In persons on HD the most common cause of death (>50%) is cardiac disease, which closely compares to persons on PD, for whom cardiovascular disease is the cause of death 41.6% of the time.[4]

Calculators have been developed and can be found online (https://qxmd.com/calculate/calculator_135/6-month-mortality-on-hd) to help clinicians to estimate mortality risk for persons on HD. This calculator uses the surprise question ("Would you be surprised if this patient died within the next 6 months?") as well as albumin levels, age, the presence of dementia, and the presence of peripheral vascular disease.[9]

Transplant

Like dialysis rates of mortality, transplant mortality and graft failures have also decreased in the last decade. Kidney transplant is the preferred renal replacement therapy for persons living with ESKD. The risk of death from a kidney transplant is less than that for a person receiving any form of dialysis.[10] There are many different factors that affect how long a transplanted kidney can last. On average, a transplanted kidney lasts approximately 11 years, with living-donor kidney transplants having better outcomes compared to deceased-donor kidney transplants.[11,12]

Medical Management of Kidney Disease

The medical management of kidney disease includes slowing its progression, treating reversible causes of kidney failure, managing complications related to kidney failure, adjusting medication dosages for the patient's eGFR, identifying when renal replacement therapy may soon be needed to prepare the patient, and initiating their preferred treatment option. It is important for the palliative nurse to be able to identify common complications of kidney disease and work with the providers to alleviate these complications in hopes of slowing the progression of kidney disease. Common complications from kidney disease to be aware of include volume overload, hyperkalemia, mineral and bone disorders, metabolic acidosis, hypertension, anemia, dyslipidemia, and sexual dysfunction.[13]

The palliative nurse must be able to identify and educate the person on the common medications associated with kidney disease as well as provide information on diet and other nonpharmacological interventions and preventions of contributing diseases such as hypertension and diabetes. The medications associated with kidney disease include sodium bicarbonate to correct the acid levels in the body, calcium and phosphorus binders to treat hyperphosphatemia and hypocalcemia, potassium binders to treat hyperkalemia, angiotensin-converting enzyme inhibitors and angiotensin receptor blockers to treat hypertension and proteinuria, vitamin D supplements to treat hypovitaminosis D and hyperparathyroidism, and erythropoietin (Epogen) to treat anemia-associated ESKD.[14]

It is recommended that persons living with kidney disease avoid nephrotoxic drugs such as nonsteroidal anti-inflammatory drugs (ibuprofen, naproxen, Aleve), radiographic contrast, and certain antibiotics. Some persons living with kidney disease may require special diets. These diets vary depending upon the eGFR, the type of kidney disease, and the presence of other comorbidities such as diabetes, heart failure, or hypertension.[15]

Symptoms of Advanced Kidney Disease

Persons living with advanced kidney disease suffer from a plethora of symptoms that cause anguish and poor quality of life. These are known as uremic symptoms,' which arise from metabolic disturbances associated with advancing kidney disease.[16] Persons living with advanced kidney disease have as many symptoms as persons living with advanced cancer; however, their symptoms often are unrecognized and undertreated.[17]

Common symptoms and nonpharmacologic treatments are detailed in Table 50.1. Recognizing and understanding these factors that are impacting a person's quality of life are important in the treatment of advanced kidney disease because interventions can be implemented to reduce the person's symptom burden.[18]

Options for Renal Replacement Therapy

There are three main options for renal replacement therapy. These include HD, PD, and renal transplant. It is imperative for the nurse to be familiar with these modalities to provide proper education to the person regarding their options. Each of these modalities needs additional workups. According to current guidelines, persons should receive education regarding their options for renal replacement therapy when their eGFR is 30 mL/min/1.73 m^2. Once informed, the person can receive a referral for kidney transplant evaluation, select their preferred renal replacement therapy, or elect for conservative kidney management (CKM) and have functioning access in place for when the time comes to initiate renal replacement therapy.[19]

Kidney transplant is the preferred renal replacement therapy option when compared with maintenance dialysis. Kidney transplants involve taking a kidney from a deceased or living donor and implanting it in a person whose kidneys are no longer working. It is the preferred modality as it is associated with better quality of life, lower risk of death, fewer dietary restrictions, and lower treatment costs.[20] Although it is the preferred therapy, not everyone is a candidate for a renal transplant, which is why there is such an extensive workup. When educating about transplant the person should be aware that they will need to take several medications to avoid acute rejection for the rest of their life. The person must understand what to report to their transplant provider, such as signs and symptoms of infection, flank pain, sudden weight gain, changes in heart rate or blood pressure, etc.

HD is the process of filtering waste and excess fluid from the body as the kidneys normally would. This can be completed in an outpatient clinic or at the person's home. This type of treatment requires the person to obtain access. There are three types of access, which include central line, graft, and arteriovenous fistula. Each type of access has a different healing time. It is not uncommon for persons to need revisions of their fistula or graft. Standard HD schedules are 4-hour cycles either Monday–Wednesday–Friday or Tuesday–Thursday–Saturday. The scheduling of these sessions is handled by the outpatient HD center.

PD is a treatment that uses the lining of the abdomen to filter the blood in the body. PD requires a day surgery to place a soft tube called a "PD catheter" in the lining of the abdomen. This is usually completed 2 weeks prior to the person initiating dialysis. PD is completed

Table 50.1 Nonpharmacological management of symptoms of end-stage kidney disease

Symptom	Treatment
Nausea/vomiting	• Reduce or eliminate nauseating stimuli • Encourage trial of cold, bland foods • Ginger products (e.g., tea, tablet, ginger ale, candied ginger) • Eat frequent small, high-calorie meals/snacks • Sit upright or recline with head elevated for 30–60 minutes after meals • Apply cool, damp cloth on neck/forehead • Consider relaxation, imagery, acupressure, acupuncture • Wear loose-fitting clothing
Shortness of breath (SOB)	• Pursed-lipped breathing techniques • The use of a fan or position by a window to blow air gently across the face for chronic SOB • Sit in an upright position • Supplemental oxygen, if indicated
Itching	• Low-phosphorus diet, if appropriate • Ultraviolet therapy • Bathe in lukewarm water, do not shower daily • Pat skin dry and moisturize with aqueous emollients within 2 min • Use gentle soap with no fragrances or additives • Keep skin cool • Avoid scratching—maintain short, smooth fingernails
Weakness/lack of energy	• Complete additional assessment (depression, dietary intake, sleep patterns) • Educate on proper sleep hygiene, regular exercise • Educate on energy conservation strategies
Pain	• Exercising, physical therapy • Meditation • Guided imagery • Heat/cold application • Acupuncture • Cognitive behavioral therapy
Constipation	• Encourage fluids, if appropriate • Increase dietary fiber • Encourage physical activity • Recommend probiotics
Dry/sore mouth, taste changes	• Saline spray • Artificial saliva • Ice • Chewing gum, if appropriate • Sugar-free hard candies • Proper dental hygiene • Recommend dental cleaning every 4–6 months
Restless leg syndrome	• Encourage aerobic exercise • Encourage resistant training • Abstinence from stimulants (alcohol, caffeine, nicotine) • Increase mental alertness (puzzles, games) • Optimize sleep hygiene
Poor mobility	• Exercise • SMART goals for exercise • Referral to physical therapy
Poor appetite	• Consume 4–6 small meals/snacks daily • Try cold foods • Eat high-protein foods (eggs, meat, fish, poultry) first • Use calorie/protein supplements if needed, such as Nephro shakes

Source: Reference 33.

in the comfort of the person's home. There are two types of PD, continuous ambulatory PD (CAPD) and automated PD (APD). CAPD is completed manually by the person, and APD is completed by using a mechanical device to assist in the delivery and drainage of the dialysate.[21] APD is typically completed while the person is sleeping. The biggest risk associated with PD is peritonitis, inflammation of the peritoneum. The nurse should educate the person with a PD catheter of signs and symptoms associated with peritonitis.

CKM

CKM is an alternative to dialysis for the treatment of CKD. CKM includes the medical management of CKD, symptom management, and advance care planning. Persons who choose CKM rather than the initiation of dialysis can survive for several years and experience a sustained quality of life up until very close to the end of life.[22] Depending on their age and comorbidities, people may live longer on dialysis; this additional length of life is mostly spent in a medical facility or at a dialysis unit.[23] It is very common for older adults who are on dialysis to have repeat hospital admissions due to complications from the dialysis treatment itself or their dialysis access. In addition, older adults who initiate dialysis experience a functional decline directly after initiation of dialysis and tend to get weaker over time, not stronger, whereas those receiving CKM tend to maintain their physical function level until the very end of life.[24,25] Prognosticating length of life for persons receiving CKM is difficult; however, persons can live for months to years while receiving this type of care.[26]

Despite being endorsed by professional societies and the availability of information on individuals' experiences with CKM, it is not routinely offered or discussed as a treatment option for people living with kidney disease.[27] Nurses, who are often the ones providing education about dialysis modalities and treatments for kidney disease in the outpatient setting, can play a vital role in offering and providing education on CKM. In addition to eliciting a person's goals and values to determine if CKM could be the treatment modality that aligns with their goals, nurses can spearhead initiatives at their institutions to ensure that CKM is discussed on a systematic basis.

Case 1: Person Receiving CKM

Ms. S is a 79-year-old woman with CKD, heart failure, hypertension, and hyperlipidemia. She is Spanish-speaking. She lives at home with her dog and her daughter, who is her healthcare proxy and very involved with her care. She comes into the hospital after falling at home and is found to have worsening of her kidney disease and pneumonia. She is given antibiotics and fluids, and both her pneumonia and kidney function start to improve. She and her daughter meet with the medical team to talk about what to do if her renal function worsens. She states that her sister was on HD, she saw how difficult it was for her, and she has decided that dialysis treatment is not within her preferences if her kidney function gets worse. Her daughter supports her mother in this decision, and they elect for CKM care going forward. Ms. S is discharged home with close follow-up with her nephrologist and palliative care team.

Medical Management

One of the domains of CKM care is medical management of CKD. This care is typically performed by the person's primary nephrologist and can be in collaboration with the palliative care team. In Case 1, the person's primary nephrologist continued to provide nephrology care and order medications to promote kidney health for as long as possible, and the palliative care team focused on symptom management, serious illness communication, and advance care planning.

Symptom Management

Persons receiving CKM may have symptoms of their renal disease or symptoms from another comorbidity or cause. Comprehensive CKM care treats both symptoms of kidney disease as well as other symptoms affecting a person's quality of life. Some of the most common symptoms treated in persons receiving CKM care are fatigue, cold aversion, pruritus, lower torso weakness, and dry skin. Of note, persons who receive CKM care report a comparable symptom burden to those who receive dialysis.[26,27] These symptoms can be treated with both pharmacological and nonpharmacological methods (refer to Table 50.1).

Communication and Advance Care Planning

Understanding a person's goals and values through serious illness conversations and planning for if/when kidney disease progresses, advance care planning, are of the utmost importance for persons receiving CKM care. Ensuring that the person's family is aware of the person's preferences and knowing how to talk about CKM care with other healthcare providers are imperative to ensuring that the person's wishes are upheld and that they receive adequate symptom management. If a person's family is unaware of their preference for CKM care, the person is at risk for being initiated on dialysis in an emergency setting if they are unable to speak for themselves.

CKM care must include discussions with the person and their family about what will happen if the person's kidney function worsens. As described in the example above, a transition to end-of-life care or hospice is most common when the person experiences symptoms that cannot be managed by outpatient providers or their priority is to remain at home.

In addition to family and caregiver awareness about dialysis decision-making, ensuring formal documents such as healthcare proxy forms and resuscitation order forms are filled out and on file is a critical aspect of advance care planning for persons receiving CKM.

Case 1: Person Receiving CKM Continued

Ms. S stays out of the hospital for many months after her discharge. She meets regularly with her nephrologist for medical management of her blood pressure, potassium, and other electrolytes. She develops some pain in her lower back with walking that is treated with lidocaine patches and low-dose gabapentin. She is brought to the hospital one day by her daughter after an episode of fainting and found to be in kidney failure. She had a do-not-resuscitate/intubate form indicating no dialysis, which the hospital staff honored. Home hospice was set up, and she was discharged home. She passed away at home several weeks later.

Important Considerations

There are several important things to consider that determine if a person is appropriate for CKM. Foremost, CKM care is for persons living with progressive CKD, not those with an acute kidney injury whose prognosis will be very limited without the initiation of dialysis; these persons often need rapid initiation of end-of-life/hospice care. Another important consideration is to make sure the person's goals line up with this type of care. For persons who feel that longevity is their primary goal, CKM care may not be the most appropriate pathway. Very few people who elect CKM change their minds and initiate dialysis; however, it is of the utmost importance that persons are given the resources and opportunity to change their preferences. Persons may feel physically or emotionally different over the course of their illness. This leads some persons to alter their care plan from CKM to initiating dialysis. It is important as a clinical provider to act in accordance with their wishes.

CKM is a growing field of practice and research in the United States in both the nephrology and palliative care communities. Palliative care nurses can play a pivotal role in CKM care by encouraging persons to speak with their providers about this type of care if they feel that their goals are in line with CKM, performing symptom management, collaborating with the person's nephrology and other providers, and participating in advance care communication with the person and caregivers.

Withdrawal from HD

Most persons who are on dialysis think about stopping; however, not all persons share these thoughts with a healthcare provider or their families. Of the persons in the United States with known causes of death while on dialysis, withdrawal from dialysis accounts for 19.6% of deaths.[28] It is important to consider that withdrawal may be listed as a cause of death when a non-kidney-related health setback occurs, and the body cannot tolerate further dialysis treatment, meaning that not all the persons made an elective decision to withdraw from dialysis.

Persons may be more open about their thoughts and feelings about stopping dialysis with nursing, and it is important to ensure that these persons feel heard and supported in this conversation and responded to without judgment or panic. If a person vocalizes a desire to stop dialysis, it is important to ask several questions of the person and family to understand the reasons for their request and know what the best course of action is. The set of questions in Table 50.2, used in order, will help to see where the persons is in their decision-making process. The answers to these questions can also serve as a framework to speak with the person's nephrologist and other providers about the person's preferences.

Case 2: Withdrawing from Dialysis

Mr. T is a 63-year-old with ESKD, Type 1 diabetes, hypertension, vascular disease, and coronary artery disease. He has been on dialysis for 8 years. He has been living at home with his wife, who helps to care for him; however, recently he had a long hospital and rehab stay after needing to have a right-sided below-the-knee amputation due to a gangrene infection. His infection comes back, and he makes a comment to you about feeling that he does not want to continue dialysis.

Table 50.2 Questions to ask persons who vocalize consideration of dialysis withdrawal

Question	Rationale
1. What is making the thought of continuing dialysis unbearable?	To understand the root cause of the person's desire
2. Is this the first time you have thought about stopping dialysis?	Gives an idea of how much the person has been contemplating this decision
3. Are you suffering any physical or emotional pain that is causing you to want to stop dialysis?	May reveal a symptom which could be intervened upon
4. Is there anything you can think of to change that would make continuing dialysis acceptable?	Helps determine both how certain the person is and if there is a symptom that could be intervened upon
5. Have you spoken with your nephrologist or other providers about stopping dialysis?	Gives a sense of if the person has taken steps to act on their decision and if the clinician feels this is a reasonable choice
6. Have you spoken with your support system about stopping dialysis? What did they think?	To determine if the person will need assistance navigating family dynamics
7. How sure do you feel about the choice to stop?	Gives an idea of what next steps are in communicating with the rest of the person's clinical team

Many persons talk about or contemplate stopping dialysis over a long period of time rather than decide suddenly. As they experience health setbacks related to complications of the dialysis treatment or other comorbid conditions, their lives may become increasingly physically or cognitively restricted. Some persons will adapt to these changes and reconfigure their lives and views of self to adjust to these changes in their bodies. Others may reach a point in which they feel that dialysis is lowering their quality of life. At this point in their treatment, the person needs to assess their options to decide if dialysis aligns with their current goals. Unfortunately, sometimes a person's body makes this decision for them.

Communication and symptom management are important considerations for the person who decides to withdraw from dialysis. It is imperative that the person has time to consider their decision. This ensures that the person understands their prognosis, symptoms of withdrawal, and support in place to aid them with the withdrawal from dialysis. Having this conversation over time and ensuring the person is not rushed into a decision without the proper information will help to ensure that persons are certain of their decisions, caregivers are prepared, and clinical providers feel included in the decision-making. In persons who have mental health comorbidities, depression, cognitive decline or delay, or confusion, requests to stop dialysis need to be addressed by a multidisciplinary team. This may also include the involvement of social work, psychiatry, and/or ethics.

Prognosis in terms of length of life for persons who choose to stop dialysis (PD or HD) depends on several factors, the most impactful being if the person is anuric (makes no urine) or still produces urine. Persons who make urine, even small amounts, have some residual kidney function, which will help them to regulate the electrolytes in the body; and this prevents them from having a fatal arrythmia. Additional factors that have been shown to indicate shorter life expectancy after stopping dialysis are male sex, referral from a hospital, lower Palliative Performance Scale score, and the presence of peripheral edema.[29] Sometimes it is possible for a nephrologist or other clinician to give a better estimate of time by looking at the person's basic metabolic panel between dialysis sessions; persons whose electrolytes do not fluctuate very much between dialysis and non-dialysis days may live longer off dialysis. The average life expectancy for persons who choose to withdraw from dialysis is around 7 days, with large ranges from person to person.[29]

Case 2: Withdrawal from Dialysis Continued

After going through the questions in Table 50.2 with the person, you learn that it is the thought of being bed-bound in a facility that makes continuing unbearable, he has considered this for 3–4 months since his hospitalization, he is not in any pain or suffering, there is not anything that can be changed to make it acceptable, he has not talked with his nephrologist, he has talked with his wife who was upset but said she will be supportive if that is what he wants, and he feels sure of his choice. You contact the person's primary nephrologist and let them know about your conversation. The person's nephrologist follows up with the person and places a referral for hospice.

Aside from a person making the choice to stop dialysis, there are several criteria the Renal Physicians Association has published to help distinguish in which clinical situations it may be appropriate to withdraw or forgo initiating dialysis.[30] These guidelines can be useful when talking with persons and their loved ones, as well as healthcare providers (Box 50.1).

End of Life in Kidney Disease

End of life due to kidney disease is similar in terms of experienced symptoms for persons who have chosen CKM and those who withdraw from dialysis. When the kidney is no longer functioning, urea builds up in the bloodstream, and the person becomes uremic. The buildup of this toxin as well as the body's inability to rid itself of water are the most common causes of symptoms for persons dying from kidney failure. These symptoms include dyspnea, fatigue, edema, pain, and anorexia and typically require pharmacological management including diuretics, opioids, and other common end-of-life symptom management medications. Dying of kidney disease is not typically associated with significant increases in pain.[31] In persons living with ESKD it is important to dose medications according to guidelines for persons living with impaired renal function.

Box 50.1 Renal Physician Association Shared Decision-Making Guidelines:

If appropriate, forgo (withhold initiating or withdraw ongoing) dialysis for patients with acute kidney injury (AKI), chronic kidney disease (CKD), or end-stage kidney disease (ESKD) in certain, well-defined situations:

- Patients with decision-making capacity who, being fully informed and making voluntary choices, refuse dialysis or request that dialysis be discontinued.
- Patients who no longer possess decision-making capacity who have previously indicated refusal of dialysis in an oral or written advance directive.
- Patients who no longer possess decision-making capacity and whose properly appointed legal agents/surrogates refuse dialysis or request that it be discontinued.
- Patients with irreversible, profound neurological impairment such that they lack signs of thought, sensation, purposeful behavior, and awareness of self and environment.

Consider forgoing dialysis for AKI, CKD, or ESKD patients who have a very poor prognosis or for whom dialysis cannot be provided safely:

- Those whose medical condition precludes the technical process of dialysis because the patient is unable to cooperate (e.g., advanced dementia patient who pulls out dialysis needles) or because the patient's condition is too unstable (e.g., profound hypotension).
- Those who have a terminal illness from non-renal causes (acknowledging that some in this condition may perceive benefit from and choose to undergo dialysis).
- Those with Stage 5 CKD older than 75 years who meet two or more of the following statistically significant very poor prognosis criteria (see Recommendations No. 2 and 3): (1) clinicians' response of "No, I would not be surprised" to the surprise question; (2) high comorbidity score; (3) significantly impaired functional status (e.g., Karnofsky Performance Status score less than 40); and (4) severe chronic malnutrition (i.e., serum albumin less than 2.5 g/dL using the bromocresol green method).

Indications for Hospice

Currently persons living with CKD are only eligible for hospice when they have very advanced kidney disease. For this group of persons, palliative care involvement for many years before hospice transition may be warranted. All persons who withdraw from dialysis should be referred to hospice care as soon as possible after withdrawal or ideally in advance (as they have a prognosis of less than 6 months) to support the person and their family for their end of life as persons who withdraw from dialysis tend to get sick quickly, and families need support to take care of them.

Key Nursing Considerations for Persons Living with Advanced Kidney Disease:

The palliative care nurse should be able to work with the person to prevent or slow the progression of kidney disease by providing education on diet and nephrotoxic medications to avoid and working with the interdisciplinary team to manage risk factors associated with advancing kidney disease. The nurse should have the skills to be able to identify acute changes in kidney function by assessing uremic symptoms, recognizing changes in labs, performing key assessments, and identifying signs and symptoms of adverse events and infection to report to the person's nephrologist. By using therapeutic communication and shared decision-making, the palliative nurse can evaluate the person's understanding of kidney disease, future goals, and treatment options, whether that be transplant, renal replacement therapy, or conservative kidney management. When a person living with CKD progresses to kidney failure, the nurse should focus on promoting the physical and psychosocial well-being of the person.

REFERENCES

1. Centers for Disease Control and Prevention. *Chronic Kidney Disease in the United States, 2021*. US Department of Health and Human Services, Centers for Disease Control and Prevention; 2021.
2. KDIGO 2012 Clinical Practice Guideline for the Evaluation and Management of Chronic Kidney Disease. *Kidney Int Suppl*. 2012;3(1). https://kdigo.org/wp-content/uploads/2017/02/KDIGO_2012_CKD_GL.pdf.
3. Centers for Medicare & Medicaid Services. End-Stage Renal Disease (ESRD). Updated December 1, 2021. Accessed September 30, 2022. https://www.cms.gov/Medicare/Coordination-of-Benefits-and-Recovery/Coordination-of-Benefits-and-Recovery-Overview/End-Stage-Renal-Disease-ESRD/ESRD.
4. *U.S. Renal Data System, USRDS 2016 Annual Data Report: Atlas of Chronic Kidney Disease and End-Stage Renal Disease in the United States*. National Institutes of Health, National Institute of Diabetes and Digestive and Kidney Diseases; 2016.
5. Cerdeña TJ, Grubbs V. *APOL1*, Black race, and kidney disease: turning attention to structural racism. *Am J Kidney Dis*. 2021;77(6):857–860. https://doi.org/10.1053/j.ajkd.2020.11.029.
6. Norton JM, Moxey-Mims MM, Eggers PW, et al. Social determinants of racial disparities in CKD. *J Am Soc Nephrol*. 2016;27(9):2576–2595. https://doi.org/10.1681/ASN.2016010027.
7. Brown E, Murtagh F, Murphy E. *Kidney Disease from Advanced Disease to Bereavement*. Oxford University Press; 2012.
8. O'Hare AM, Choi AI, Bertenthal D, et al. Age Affects Outcomes In Chronic Kidney Disease. *J Am Soc Nephrol*. 2007;18(10):2758–2765. https://doi.org/10.1681/ASN.2007040422.
9. Cohen LM, Ruthazer R, Moss AH, Germain, MJ. Predicting six-month mortality for patients who are on maintenance hemodialysis. *Clin J Am Soc Nephrol*. 2010;5(1):72–79. https://doi.org/10.2215/CJN.03860609
10. Vella J. Kidney Transplantation in Adults: Patient Survival after Kidney Transplantation. UpToDate. June 21, 2021. Accessed September 15, 2022. https://www.uptodate.com/contents/kidney-transplantation-in-adults-patient-survival-after-kidney-transplantation?search=Kidney%20Transplantation%20in%20Adults:%20Patient%20Survival%20After%20Kidney%20Transplantation.%22%20&source=search_result&selectedTitle=1~150&usage_type=default&display_rank=1.
11. Brennan D, DeMarcho MM. Kidney Transplantation in Adults: Kidney Transplantation and the Older Adult Patient. UpToDate. September 29, 2022. https://www.uptodate.com/contents/kidney-transplantation-in-adults-kidney-transplantation-and-the-older-adult-patient?search=transplant%20kidney%20as%20RRT&source=search_result&selectedTitle=7~150&usage_type=default&display_rank=7#H25563782.
12. Pesavento TE. Kidney transplantation in the context of renal replacement therapy. *Clin J Am Soc Nephrol*. 2009;4(12):2035–2039. https://doi.org/10.2215/CJN.05500809.

13. Rosenberg M. Overview of the Management of Chronic Kidney Disease in Adults. UpToDate. April 21, 2022. Accessed September 13, 2022. https://www.uptodate.com/contents/overview-of-the-management-of-chronic-kidney-disease-in-adults?search=medical+management+of+ckd&source=search_result&selectedTitle=1~150&usage_type=default&display_rank=1#H6.
14. KGIGO 2012 Clinical Practice Guideline for the Evaluation and Management of Chronic Kidney Disease. *Nephrol Dial.* 2013:3(1):22–206. https://doi.org/10.28996/1680-4422-2017-1-22-206.
15. Cho M, Srinivasan B. Dietary Recommendations for Patients with Nondialysis Chronic Kidney Disease. UpToDate. Accessed September 13, 2022. https://www.uptodate.com/contents/dietary-recommendations-for-patients-with-nondialysis-chronic-kidney-disease?search=diets%20of%20kidney%20disease&source=search_result&selectedTitle=1~150&usage_type=default&display_rank=1#H1193190951.
16. Zemaitis MR, Foris LA, Katta S, et al. Uremia. In: *StatPearls.* StatPearls Publishing; 2022. https://www.ncbi.nlm.nih.gov/books/NBK441859/.
17. Carswell C, Noble H, Reid J, McKeaveney D. Conservative management of patients with end-stage kidney disease. *Nurs Stand.* 2020;35(6):43–50. https://doi.org/10.7748/ns.2019.e11416.
18. Krishnan A, Teixeira-Pinto A, Lim WH, et al. Health-related quality of life in people across the spectrum of CKD. *Kidney Int Rep.* 2020:5(12):2264–2274.
19. Bleyer A. Indications for Initiation of Dialysis in Chronic Kidney Disease. UpToDate. September 7, 2021. https://www.uptodate.com/contents/indications-for-initiation-of-dialysis-in-chronic-kidney-disease?search=when%20to%20initiate%20dialysis%20education&source=search_result&selectedTitle=2~150&usage_type=default&display_rank=2.
20. Chandraker A, Yeung M. Kidney Transplantation in Adults: Overview of Care of the Adult Kidney Transplant Recipient. UpToDate, November 3, 2021. Accessed September 10, 2022. https://www.uptodate.com/contents/kidney-transplantation-in-adults-overview-of-care-of-the-adult-kidney-transplant-recipient?search=renal+transplant&source=search_result&selectedTitle=1~150&usage_type=default&display_rank=1.
21. National Institute of Diabetes and Digestive and Kidney Diseases. Dialysis. January 2018, https://www.niddk.nih.gov/health-information/kidney-disease/kidney-failure/peritoneal dialysis.
22. Wong SPY, Rubenzik T, Zelnick L, et al. Long-term outcomes among patients with advanced kidney disease who forgo maintenance dialysis: a systematic review. *JAMA Netw Open.* 2022;5(3):e222255. https://doi.org/10.1001/jamanetworkopen.2022.2255.
23. Rachel CC, Juszczak M, Davenport A, et al. Is maximum conservative management an equivalent treatment option to dialysis for elderly patients with significant comorbid disease? *Clin J Am Soc Nephrol.* 2009;4(10):1611–1619.
24. Manjula KT, Covinsky KE, Chertow GM, et al. Functional status of elderly adults before and after initiation of dialysis. *N Engl J Med.* 2009;361(16):1539–1547. https://doi.org/10.1056/NEJMoa0904655.
25. Murtagh FEM, Addington-Hall JM, Higginson IJ. End-stage renal disease: a new trajectory of functional decline in the last year of life. *J Am Geriatr Soc.* 2011;59(2):304–308. https://doi.org/10.1111/j.1532-5415.2010.03248.x.
26. Chou A, Li KC, Brown MA. Survival of Older Patients With Advanced CKD Managed Without Dialysis: A Narrative Review. *Kidney Medicine.* 2022;4(5):100447. doi:10.1016/j.xkme.2022.100447
27. Bursic AE, Schell JO, Ernecoff NC, Bansal AD. Delivery of active medical management without dialysis through an embedded kidney palliative care model. *Kidney360.* 2022;19;3(11):1881–1889. https://doi.org/10.34067/KID.0001352022.
28. Ren SQ, Ma T, Wang, J, et al. Quality of life, symptoms, and sleep quality of elderly with end-stage renal disease receiving conservative management: a systematic review. *Health Qual Life Outcomes.* 2019;17(1):78. https://doi.org/10.1186/s12955-019-1146-5.
29. US Renal Data System. *2021 USRDS Annual Data Report: Epidemiology of kidney disease in the United States.* National Institutes of Health, National Institute of Diabetes and Digestive and Kidney Diseases; 2021.
30. O'Connor NR, Dougherty M, Harris PS, et al. Survival after dialysis discontinuation and hospice enrollment for ESRD. *Clin J Am Soc Nephrol.* 2013;8(12):2117–2122.
31. Renal Physicians Association. *Shared Decision-Making in the Appropriate Initiation of and Withdrawal from Dialysis.* Renal Physicians Association; 2010.
32. Bausewein C, Booth S, Gysels M, Higginson IJ. Non-pharmacological interventions for breathlessness in advanced stages of malignant and non-malignant diseases. *Cochrane Database Syst Rev.* 2013;2013(11):CD005623. https://doi.org/10.1002/14651858.CD005623.pub3.

51

Palliative Care for Persons Living with a Hematologic Malignancy

Ashley Leak Bryant, Lorinda A. Coombs, Samantha Mayo, Argin Malakian, and Tara A. Albrecht

Key Points

- A hematologic malignancy diagnosis can be overwhelming due to the urgent need for treatment.
- Although early integration of palliative care for hematologic malignancies enhances symptoms and quality of life, its incorporation into standard care practices remains minimal.
- From diagnosis onward, oncology nurses should routinely ask patients about their values and preferences and promptly manage disease- and treatment-related side effects and symptoms.
- Nurses can serve as advocates to support the delivery of palliative care to meet the patient's and family's needs while improving their experience across their disease trajectory.

Case Study

This chapter presents a case study of an older adult with a hematologic malignancy and the effect that both treatment and the disease have on their quality of life. "Jake" is a retired 72-year-old who presents to his primary care provider with bruising on his arm and states that he "feels tired." He reports increasing shortness of breath over the past 2 weeks; prior to the bruising and shortness of breath, he was gardening multiple times as week and working part-time. Physical examination identifies tachypnea, tachycardia, and scattered ecchymosis on arms and legs; laboratory results include white blood cell count (WBC) 19.1, hemoglobin 7.4 g/dL, hematocrit 22%, and platelet count 21/μL. WBC differential has 92% blasts, and a peripheral blood smear evaluation reveals large blasts with Auer rods in the cytoplasm. Bone marrow aspirate shows large blasts with irregular nuclear contours. Unfavorable cytogenetics with del(7q), t(3;5), t(6;9) and complex karyotype are present. Jake also has a history of hyperlipidemia and heart disease, including a coronary artery bypass graft 3 years ago and a current left ventricular ejection fraction of 40%.

Hematologic Malignancies

Hematologic malignancies comprise a broad group of cancers originating from the bone marrow and the lymphatic system, heterogenous cells, molecular and morphological characteristics, etiology, clinical presentation, incidence, and prognosis. The three major groups of hematologic malignancies include leukemias, lymphomas, and multiple myeloma. Hematologic malignancies are among the most common cancers globally.[1]

Treatments for hematologic malignancies commonly include chemotherapy, radiation therapy, targeted therapies, immunotherapies, and stem cell transplantation. Newer treatments, such as chimeric antigen receptor T-cell therapy (CART), have shown promise, particularly in the relapsed and refractory settings, with some increasingly integrated as standard of care depending upon subtype.[2,3] For a subset of people undergoing treatment for a hematologic malignancy, their only hope at cure is to undergo either a hematopoietic stem cell transplant (HCT) or CART. Individual treatment regimens are determined based on many considerations, including molecular and morphological features of the underlying disease and patient characteristics (e.g., comorbidities, functional status).[4–7] Patient response to treatment can also vary based on biopsychosocial and contextual factors, including age and available social support. Consequently, people affected by hematologic malignancies may exhibit multisystem symptom profiles and high levels of supportive care needs related to the disease and its management.[8–13] Recent advances have expanded treatment options for hematologic malignancies, especially targeted therapies and low-intensity regimens for acute myeloid leukemia (AML). With the increase in oral chemotherapies to treat hematologic malignancies, barriers to oral adherence have been identified, and interventions have been implemented.[14–17]

There is a clear need for effective palliative care to address symptom management and supportive care needs throughout the disease and treatment trajectory, including at the end of life. Compared to people with solid tumors, those with hematologic malignancies have higher rates of emergency department (ED) utilization,[18,19] hospitalizations,[18] intensive care unit admissions, and ED and hospital deaths[20] and lower rates of referral for palliative and hospice services. Despite clinical recommendations to offer palliative care to manage symptoms from the time of diagnosis,[21–23] only a small number of persons with hematologic malignancies (<5%) receive palliative care from specialty-trained clinicians to manage symptoms and distress and often not until the last 2 weeks of life.[23–25] Persons with hematologic malignancies often experience unplanned hospitalizations as well as an unpredictable and uncertain illness course regardless of treatment regimen.

This chapter aims to provide an overview of common symptoms and supportive care needs experienced by adults affected by hematologic cancers and the assessment and management strategies that nurses can use to address these issues. As hematologic malignancies represent a broad range of diseases and subtypes, the chapter focuses on the most common issues that nurses may encounter. Additionally, the palliative and supportive care of children affected by pediatric hematologic malignancies is outside of the scope of this chapter.

Early Integration of Palliative Care into Hematologic Malignancy Care

Early integration of specialty palliative care has been shown to improve physical and psychosocial outcomes for persons with hematologic malignancies.[26–28] Consequently, in 2017, the American Society of Clinical Oncology (ASCO) published clinical practice guidelines based on strong clinical and research evidence for integrating specialty palliative care into standard oncology care from diagnosis.[25,29] Despite clinical recommendations to offer palliative care to patients and their families early in the disease trajectory,[21–23] very rarely are these recommendations implemented in clinical practice,[23–25] for a variety of reasons including that many hematologic malignancies often have a labile disease trajectory, making it difficult for hematology-oncology teams to initiate a referral to palliative care.[30] Table 51.1 provides examples of common level of symptom burden and optimal timing for integrating specialty palliative care for various common hematologic malignancies.

Case Study

The hematology-oncology provider introduced palliative care to Jake at the time of diagnosis, given the unfavorable stratification of his disease. Per ASCO guidelines, palliative care that is concurrent with treatment should be standard of care for any patient with advanced cancer.[25,29] The clinical team shared with Jake and his family the benefits of palliative care, including improved symptom management, enhanced quality of life, and increased family awareness and attention. Jake also started on a hypomethylating agent plus venetoclax (HMA + VEN), an oral BCL-2 inhibitor for unfit older adults with AML that has demonstrated remarkable effectiveness.[31]

Values Assessment and Values Integration

Many patients diagnosed with a hematologic malignancy want honest, sensitive discussions regarding their prognosis and treatment options; they want to be involved and informed in treatment decision-making.[32,33] Because the patient, their caregiver, and support system will bear the burden of the treatment decision outcomes, it is the ethical responsibility of clinicians to share decision-making.[34] Although hematologic malignancies represent heterogeneous disease processes and outcomes, all individuals with a hematologic malignancy are offered treatment options. Without awareness of patients' values, treatment decisions, and care may not be concordant with their values and goals, resulting in either undesired aggressive treatment or undertreatment.

Clear communication is at the core of patient-centered cancer care and essential to delivering quality palliative care. Patient-centered and interprofessional communication involve providing information that is understandable to the patient, supporting patients' involvement in decision-making, and making decisions consistent with patients' values.[35,36] Breakdowns and barriers in communication

Table 51.1 Trajectories of hematologic malignancies

Disease	Common level of symptom burden	Suggested timing of specialized palliative care	Reference
Aggressive lymphoma	High symptom burden, high mortality	Integration at time of recurrent or refractory disease or when noncurative treatment is initiated	Odejide et al. (2020)
Acute myeloid leukemia	High symptom burden, high mortality	Early integration at time of diagnosis	El-Jawahri et al. (2021)
Chronic graft-versus-host disease	High symptom burden, high mortality	Integration at time of disease	El-Jawahri et al. (2018)
Chronic lymphocytic leukemia	Low symptom burden, long course of the disease, and low mortality	Symptomatic progress	El-Jawahri et al. (2020)
Indolent lymphoma	Low symptom burden, long course of the disease, and low mortality	Symptomatic progress	El-Jawahri et al. (2020)
Multiple myeloma	Intermediation symptom burden, intermediate course of the disease and mortality	Intermediate, per patient-reported outcomes	Ramsenthaler et al. (2019)

Source: Reference 30.

between oncology clinicians and patients are common[37,38]. They can reduce treatment adherence,[39] impact satisfaction with cancer care[40,41] and the patient's trust in their clinician,[41] and widen health disparities in cancer care.[42,43] Values assessment identifies patients' priorities, philosophies, and preferences related to treatment considerations[44] and facilitates treatment decision-making that reflects patients' values, which is helpful for treating hematology–oncology clinicians. Values assessment has also been identified as an essential domain in the National Cancer Institute's patient-centered communication framework and an approach to care that would benefit individuals receiving care for a hematologic malignancy.[45–48]

Cultural, spiritual, and religious beliefs play an important role in guiding medical and end-of-life decisions for some people; for others, it is not as important.[49] Spiritual and religious needs are common in culturally, religious, and linguistically diverse patient populations but may differ by background.[50] Because of the heterogeneity of the palliative care needs of patients with hematologic malignancies, an assessment of values is foundational for goal-concordant care. Decision-making can be influenced by individual values and priorities regarding issues such as living independently at home, receiving aggressive care, being present for significant life events (e.g., a child's birth or wedding), or transitioning to hospice care. Palliative care clinicians are uniquely qualified to participate in these discussions, given their specialized training in communication around goals of care and experience in collaborating with other specialists and the patient's family members.

Case Study

Jake shared with his nurse that he felt shocked and overwhelmed by his new diagnosis. Prompted by his nurse's inquiry into his values and preferences, Jake shared how important his family, especially his, grandchildren, and pets were to him. It was difficult for Jake to make a treatment decision, but his goals of care were shared along with his concerns regarding his prognosis. His nurse ensured Jake knew the importance of sharing his code status and preferences surrounding his care. Jake was aware that treatment needed to be initiated and relied on his family to contribute to the treatment decision.

Unique Challenges Experienced by Individuals Who Receive Hematopoietic Stem Cell Transplant or CART

For a subset of people undergoing treatment for a hematologic malignancy, their only hope at cure is to undergo either a HCT or CART, a newer form of treatment. HCT and CART are intensive treatments that are associated with significant toxicities and risk of death. Early integration of palliative care is critical to support patients and their families in this context.[51,52] In a pilot randomized trial of adults in an inpatient bone marrow transplant unit, daily use of electronic symptom reporting reduced peak symptom burden and improved individual symptoms 2 weeks post-transplant.[53]

HCT offers a potentially curative treatment for hematologic malignancies, in which hematopoietic progenitor (stem) cells are infused to re-establish the recipient's hematopoietic function. HCT can either be autologous (where the patient receives their stem cells) or allogeneic (where the patient receives matched donor cells from another person). Autologous HCT is often used for lymphomas and multiple myeloma, while allogeneic HCT is usually reserved for patients with acute leukemias. HCT first requires an intensive conditioning regimen with high-dose chemotherapy and sometimes total-body irradiation and other immunomodulatory treatments. People treated with HCT, especially allogeneic HCT, experience high levels of symptom burden and functional deficits throughout recovery, resulting from treatment toxicities and HCT complications, such as acute and chronic graft-versus-host disease (GVHD), graft failure, disease relapse, and other late effects. In the United States, an estimated 12,000 autologous and 8,300 allogeneic transplants were administered in 2020.[1] Survival rates vary widely, with 3-year survival probabilities ranging from 30% to 80%, depending on transplant type, primary disease characteristics, and patient-related factors, such as age at time of HCT and comorbidities.[1] In the context of HCT, palliative care plays a role in reducing suffering at the end of life and in managing symptom burden and functional deficits across the treatment trajectory and into long-term survivorship.

Given that the clinical course experienced by people after HCT is often unpredictable and can change rapidly, an integrated approach to palliative care has the potential to relieve symptom burden and bolster physical and psychosocial functioning throughout the clinical trajectory.[2,3] In a recent randomized controlled trial, an inpatient palliative care intervention focusing on physical and psychological symptoms during hospitalization for allogeneic or autologous HCT was associated with benefits to quality of life, mood, and symptom burden as compared to standard care, which lasted up to 6 months after transplant.[4,5] In the extended post-treatment phase, routine follow-up and effective survivorship care that attended to the late and long-term effects persisting in the months to years after HCT was recommended[6]; however, research is needed to support the development and implementation of effective interventions.[7]

Case Study

After 3 months of treatment, the oncologist shared with Jake that he was not eligible for HCT or CART due to his comorbidities and concerns for worsening physical function because of treatment. Jake's family wanted to know more about HCT and CART, and a family meeting was planned to discuss the benefits and barriers to these treatments. After the family meeting, Jake and his family better understood why he was not a candidate for either treatment and that these treatments did not align with his values and preferences.

Symptom Experiences of Those with Hematologic Malignancies

Research has indicated that individuals diagnosed with hematologic malignancies endure a similar or higher level of symptom burden as those with metastatic solid tumors.[54–56] Many patients with hematologic malignancies receive intensive treatments that require prolonged hospitalization soon after their diagnosis.[57–61] In a cross-sectional study of 180 patients with hematologic malignancies at a tertiary care hospital, the average number of symptoms reported was 8.8[62]; the most prevalent symptoms, affecting 40% to 70% of participants, were lack of energy, difficulty with sleep, pain, and dry mouth.[62] Another study, which included 249 patients newly diagnosed or recently relapsed with acute leukemia, reported a median of nine physical symptoms in its sample.[63] The most prevalent physical symptoms were lack of energy, drowsiness, dry mouth, weight loss, and pain.[63]

A recent population-level analysis indicated that individuals diagnosed with leukemia appear to experience higher levels of distress compared to other cancer patients.[64] Others have found that patients with hematologic malignancies commonly experience psychological distress, including depression and anxiety, with rates ranging from 30% to 60% during treatment.[57,62,65–67] Individuals with acute leukemia and those undergoing HCT face acute stress reactions and posttraumatic stress symptoms as they cope with the overwhelming shock of a life-threatening diagnosis and endure prolonged hospitalizations that can be socially isolating.[57,60,68,69]

Case Study

The patient completed several cycles of HMA + VEN in the outpatient clinic. He had three unplanned ED visits and two unplanned hospitalizations due to prolonged myelosuppression, fevers, and gastrointestinal conditions, which were exacerbated by his several chronic conditions. His family accompanied him to the ED and hospital and was able to advocate for his needs and provide a history of his AML journey.

During Survivorship

Individuals who have overcome hematologic malignancies frequently experience quality-of-life issues and persistent effects stemming from both their illness and its treatments.[11,70–74] Several issues can lead to this decreased quality of life, including, but not limited to, fatigue, pain, neuropathy, infertility, cardiomyopathy, cognitive difficulties, psychological distress, fear of cancer returning, and symptoms akin to posttraumatic stress disorder.[11,75–80] GVHD is a significant contributor to morbidity, physical and functional disabilities, symptomatic burden, and reduced quality of life among recipients of allogeneic HCT.[81–85]

Furthermore, it has been observed that even when hematologic malignancies, such as Hodgkin's lymphoma, are highly curable, around 30% of patients face considerable distress long after their treatment has been completed.[86] In a similar vein, patients diagnosed with chronic lymphocytic leukemia, a disease often slow to progress, which patients can live with for over 10 years, have been found to experience poorer emotional well-being when compared to patients diagnosed with more aggressive solid tumors.[87]

Case Study

The patient reported fatigue leading to functional impairment and decline from two cycles of HMA + VEN treatment. The patient has not completed treatment and will have additional cycles of HMA + VEN. The oncology team referred the patient to outpatient occupational and physical therapy to regain skills and function.

At the End of Life

Research underscores that adults with hematologic malignancies at the end of life bear significant physical and psychosocial burdens that can affect their quality of life and care experience.[88,89] One study noted a high prevalence of physical symptoms and psychosocial distress among patients in noncurative settings, including deterioration of general health, pain, and psychological problems.[90] This is comparable to the symptom burden in patients with solid tumor cancers.[65] Another study found that AML patients' symptom burden, quality of life, and psychological distress intensify as death approaches, with the majority of patients requiring hospitalization and blood transfusions.[89]

Patients with hematologic malignancies are a unique population with differing trajectories at the end of life. Symptoms experienced by patients with hematologic malignancies have similarities to those of patients with solid tumors at the end of life.[65,90] Fatigue and loss of appetite were found to be the most troublesome symptoms in these patients, worsening significantly as death approached.[90]

Assessment of Symptoms among Patients with Hematologic Malignancies during Active Treatment

Nurses play a critical role in assessing and monitoring common physical and psychological symptoms as well as intervening to manage distressing symptoms promptly. Routine, systematic assessment of common symptoms using standardized instruments should be used to capture physical, psychological, functional, and subjective changes. Tools such as the Edmonton Symptom Assessment System (ESAS) can rapidly assess the presence and severity of multiple symptoms, making it easily useful in the clinical setting.[91] Modified versions of the ESAS have been tailored for use in the acute leukemia population in a preliminary validation study.[92] Symptoms with high ESAS scores can be further evaluated, communicated to the broader care team, prioritized for management, or even as a way to trigger a palliative care referral.[93] Emotion- and symptom-focused engagement is an integrated psychosocial and palliative care intervention for patients with acute leukemia which incorporates the ESAS and shows promise for effectiveness.[94]

In conjunction with multisymptom tools like the ESAS, symptom-specific assessment tools can be used for in-depth evaluation of distressing symptoms. For example, the Brief Fatigue Inventory is a nine-item tool that evaluates the severity of fatigue and the impact of fatigue on daily functioning.[95] The World Health Organization mucositis grading system is used to assess and grade the severity of mucositis based on observed clinical signs and symptoms.[96] These and other similar instruments can be integrated into routine interactions between patients and nurses to enhance the systematic monitoring of symptoms.

Management of Common Symptoms among Patients with Hematologic Malignancies

Fatigue

Fatigue is a common and challenging symptoms to manage. This is especially true for patients with hematologic malignancy who are commonly experiencing chronic anemia and receiving some intensive chemotherapy treatment. However, some interventions have shown to improve fatigue in these patients. Nurses should encourage their patients to engage in mild aerobic physical activities like walking and strength training, which help reduce fatigue and improve quality of life.[97] Nurses should also be aware that some patients may benefit from working with physical and/or occupational therapy to help support safe engagement in physical activity to manage fatigue and support physical function. Nurses can also teach strategies such as ways to conserve energy by pacing, planning, and prioritizing tasks to manage fatigue.[98] In addition, ensuring adequate nutritional intake and appropriate nutritional counseling are important since they dampen the impact of distressing physical symptoms.[99] Finally, ensuring that other severe and/or distressing symptoms are managed can improve fatigue levels over time. For more detailed information on fatigue management, please see Chapter 25, "Fatigue," of this textbook.

Insomnia

Nurses can help their patients manage insomnia by teaching and reinforcing good sleep hygiene practices. This includes maintaining a regular sleep schedule, limiting daytime naps, and creating a restful sleep environment.[100–103] If sleep disturbances persist, cognitive behavioral therapy for insomnia can be considered an effective intervention delivered by trained nursing staff.[104] Nonpharmacological interventions such as relaxation techniques can also be taught to promote better sleep.[105] Some pharmacological interventions may be needed with prescribed sleep aids. Please see Chapter 26, "Insomnia," for more detailed information regarding the diagnosis and management of this symptom.

Pain

Effective pain management requires a thorough assessment, intervention(s), communication, and education between the clinician, the patient, and often the family. Nonpharmacological pain relief methods, such as heat or cold application, positioning for comfort, massage, and distraction techniques, can be employed by nurses caring for patients with hematologic malignancies.[106–109] Education about how and when to use these techniques can also be provided to informal caregivers who may be able to utilize these skills at later times. Education on pain medication usage, potential side effects, and the importance of regular pain assessment is crucial for patients and their informal caregivers.[110] Persistent or escalating pain may warrant the inclusion of specialty palliative care in the patient's care. Please see Chapter 11, "Pain Management," for more detailed information regarding the diagnosis and management of this symptom.

Xerostomia and Mucositis

Mucositis and xerostomia, common complications in hematologic malignancy treatment, require a multifaceted approach for effective management.[96] Nurses should teach their patients that hydration and meticulous oral hygiene practices are vital preventive strategies, and saliva substitutes, oral lubricants, and medications like pilocarpine can provide symptomatic relief for dry mouth.[96,111] Dietary modifications can further alleviate symptoms, such as avoiding spicy foods and choosing saliva-stimulating options like sugar-free gum or citrus fruits. Per clinical guidelines, regular standardized instrument assessments should monitor these conditions, capturing physical, functional, and subjective changes.[96] Please see Chapter 15, "Dysphagia, Hiccups, and Other Oral Symptoms," for more detailed information regarding the diagnosis and management of these symptoms.

Graft-versus-Host Disease

Managing GVHD in blood and marrow transplantation patients is a complex process requiring comprehensive skills, knowledge, and constant coordination.[112] It is crucial for nurses to possess knowledge of both acute and chronic GVHD symptoms and treatments, understanding expected and less common side effects of treatment.[113] For skin GVHD, nursing care includes hygiene practices, topical and systemic therapies, infection prevention, and steps to alleviate discomfort.[112] Patient education about sun protection, skin assessment, and recognition of risk for skin and oral cancer are essential preventative measures.

In cases of gastrointestinal GVHD, meticulous attention to intake and output, culture procurement, managing fluid and electrolyte imbalances, nutrition, and skin care are required.[112,114] The side effects of GVHD treatment, such as infectious complications, microvascular damage, renal dysfunction, and steroid myopathy resulting from steroid use, also need to be monitored closely. Incorporating physical and occupational therapy consultations, as well as endocrine consultations for diabetes education, are significant considerations.

It is important to prepare patients for all outcomes, including potential end-of-life situations in refractory cases of GVHD. Education and certification of bone marrow transplant nurses play a crucial role in ensuring a knowledgeable workforce is available to care for patients with GVHD and other reported symptoms.[112] Nurses must maintain current knowledge and seek special training to effectively assist patients and caregivers in coping with the intricacies of GVHD management.

Psychosocial Support

Psychosocial support and professional counseling are often beneficial in helping patients cope with the various challenges they face while living with a hematologic malignancy. These challenges may include body image changes, fatigue, cognitive alterations, sleep disorders, anxiety, depression, acute stress disorder, and posttraumatic stress, among others. Nurses can use brief psychotherapeutic techniques to help manage these challenges.[115] These interventions can be integrated within interdisciplinary palliative care teams and implemented as early as the time of diagnosis to provide psychosocial support to patients and their families.[94]

Case Study: Continued

At Jake's clinic visit for cycle 3, he reports to his nurse that he feels tired most of the day, but he is having difficulty falling asleep at night. The nurse asks Jake what he is doing during the day and about his bedtime routine. Jake tells her that he is not doing much at all. He sits and does some crossword puzzles, sometimes plays a video game with his grandchildren, and then likes to watch TV in bed until he can fall asleep. He does not have a schedule. The nurse encourages Jake and his wife to plan a short walk in their neighborhood daily, slowly building up the time they walk. She also discusses sleep hygiene with Jake, which includes avoiding late afternoon and evening naps, no TV in the bedroom, dimming lights 30 minutes to 1 hour prior to desired bedtime, trying to have a consistent bedtime, and avoiding caffeine and chocolate late in the afternoon and evening. Jake and his wife agree to begin walking and trying to apply some of the sleep hygiene tips.

Role of Palliative Care for Individuals with Hematologic Malignancy and Their Families

Hematologic malignancies impact not only the individual but also family and friends. Due to the complicated disease trajectory, frequent hospitalizations, and often burdensome, if not debilitating, symptoms, those diagnosed with a hematologic malignancy usually must rely on family and friends to provide care, transportation, and emotional support.[116] Unfortunately, this level of support and care is often very demanding (physically, emotionally, and/or financially) and can be overwhelming to family and friends, especially when they have had little time to prepare for the role of caregiver.[117] The demands of caregiving negatively affect the physical and emotional health of the individual who fills the caregiving role.[118,119] Not only are patients with hematologic malignancies at risk for adverse effects, but those caring for patients are also at risk for adverse health outcomes, including depression, anxiety, physical health complications, caregiver burden, and a decreased quality of life.[120] Thus, including palliative care for the patient and family is invaluable as the palliative care team is best equipped to provide team-based, family-centered support across a labile disease trajectory. Ultimately, palliative care should not be an afterthought for patients with a hematologic malignancy and their families but an available specialized resource prepared to fill common unmet needs, including symptom management, psychosocial and/or spiritual support, as well as goals-of-care discussions.

The nurse has a critical role in the education of palliative care for individuals with hematologic malignancies and their families. Nurses can encourage and support adults with hematologic malignancies to be more physically active during treatment and beyond. Families spend significant time and energy caring for their loved one[25,117] and frequently lack knowledge and skills[121] to assume a primary care role to respond to the patient's rapid symptom changes, such as fatigue and functional decline.[118,119,122] In an Oncology Care Partner Program for adults with hematologic malignancies, care partners reported positive caregiving outcomes (e.g., physical health, energy levels). Still, they had difficulty providing the patient with symptom, functional, and emotional support.[123] These physical function activities can increase mobility and enhance overall quality of life. In a qualitative inquiry of the Palliative and Collaborative Intervention in a National Institutes of Health–funded pilot study, 14 AML care partners described the following about HMA + VEN cycle 1: (1) AML diagnosis was unexpected and shocking, (2) care provided to the patient included protecting the care partner from illness, and (3) care for an older adult with AML came with complex challenges (e.g., caring for another older adult parent, being an older adult themselves).[122] Thus, AML care partners experience high levels of distress,[118,122] burdens,[118,122,124,] and associated psychological,[118,125,126] physical,[118,125,] and functional harms.[118,125] HMA + VEN treatment is given indefinitely over time, with uncertainty about the "end" of treatment and the potential demands of care partnering activities.[31,127,128] Nurses can facilitate and support adults with hematologic malignancies and their families to maintain their function in their home setting, supporting the need for registered nurse-led and team-based intervention.

Case Study: Continued

Unfortunately, Jake's health continues to worsen after six cycles of HMA + VEN. He has increased healthcare utilization, including both ED visits and hospitalizations. The clinical team and the palliative care team met with Jake and his family to review his care goals. Jake and his family ultimately decided to stop HMA + VEN treatment and focus on his comfort and quality time with his family. The patient's preferences were valued at the time of diagnosis, during treatment, and at the end of life.

Conclusion

Patients with hematologic malignancy often experience multiple severe and distressing co-occurring symptoms that negatively affect their quality of life. In addition, they commonly receive complex intensive treatments that result in a labile disease trajectory. The disease, treatment, and subsequent sequelae are burdensome for the patient and their family. Historically, palliative care has been underutilized in this patient population despite evidence supporting the early integration of palliative care for the patient's and family's benefit. Understanding the unique patient experiences during treatment and beyond provides clear opportunities for delivering palliative care to enhance patients' quality of life. The nurse's critical role is supporting patients with a hematologic malignancy and their families through the complicated treatment journey and the healthcare system. Nurses can serve as advocates to support the delivery of palliative care to meet the patient's and family's dynamic needs while improving their experience across the disease trajectory.

REFERENCES

1. Zhang N, Wu J, Wang Q, et al. Global burden of hematologic malignancies and evolution patterns over the past 30 years. *Blood Cancer J*. 2023;13(1):82. https://doi.org/10.1038/s41408-023-00853-3.
2. Zhang X, Zhu L, Zhang H, Chen S, Xiao Y. CAR-T cell therapy in hematological malignancies: current opportunities and challenges. *Front Immunol*. 2022;13:927153. https://doi.org/10.3389/fimmu.2022.927153.
3. Merino A, Maakaron J, Bachanova V. Advances in NK cell therapy for hematologic malignancies: NK source, persistence and tumor targeting. *Blood Rev*. 2023;60:101073. https://doi.org/10.1016/j.blre.2023.101073.
4. Monteith BE, Sandhu I, Lee AS. Management of multiple myeloma: a review for general practitioners in oncology. *Curr Oncol*. 2023;30(5):4382–4401. https://doi.org/10.3390/curroncol30050334.
5. Poletto S, Novo M, Paruzzo L, Frascione PMM, Vitolo U. Treatment strategies for patients with diffuse large B-cell lymphoma. *Cancer Treat Rev*. 2022;110:102443. https://doi.org/10.1016/j.ctrv.2022.102443.
6. Smyth E, Cheah CY, Seymour JF. Management of indolent B-cell lymphomas: a review of approved and emerging targeted therapies. *Cancer Treat Rev*. 2023;113:102510. https://doi.org/10.1016/j.ctrv.2023.102510.

7. Stubbins RJ, Francis A, Kuchenbauer F, Sanford D. Management of acute myeloid leukemia: a review for general practitioners in oncology. *Curr Oncol.* 2022;29(9):6245–6259. https://doi.org/10.3390/curroncol29090491.
8. Hochman MJ, Yu Y, Wolf SP, Samsa GP, Kamal AH, LeBlanc TW. Comparing the palliative care needs of patients with hematologic and solid malignancies. *J Pain Symptom Manage.* 2018;55(1):82–88.e1. https://doi.org/10.1016/j.jpainsymman.2017.08.030.
9. Hall A, Lynagh M, Bryant J, Sanson-Fisher R. Supportive care needs of hematological cancer survivors: a critical review of the literature. *Crit Rev Oncol Hematol.* 2013;88(1):102–116. https://doi.org/10.1016/j.critrevonc.2013.03.008.
10. Tsatsou I, Konstantinidis T, Kalemikerakis I, Adamakidou T, Vlachou E, Govina O. Unmet supportive care needs of patients with hematological malignancies: a systematic review. *Asia Pac J Oncol Nurs.* 2021;8(1):5–17. https://doi.org/10.4103/apjon.apjon_41_20.
11. Mayo SJ, Brennenstuhl S, Panesar P, Bryant AL. Patterns of concerns among hematological cancer survivors. *Cancer Nurs.* 2022;45(6):447–456.
12. Hall AE, Sanson-Fisher RW, Lynagh MC, Tzelepis F, D'Este C. What do haematological cancer survivors want help with? A cross-sectional investigation of unmet supportive care needs. *BMC Res Notes.* 2015;8:221. https://doi.org/10.1186/s13104-015-1188-7.
13. Leak Bryant A, Lee Walton A, Shaw-Kokot J, Mayer DK, Reeve BB. Patient-reported symptoms and quality of life in adults with acute leukemia: a systematic review. *Oncol Nurs Forum.* 2015;42(2):E91–E101. https://doi.org/10.1188/15.Onf.E91-e101.
14. Bryant AL, Buhlinger K. Role of the advanced practitioner in the management of oral chemotherapy for adults with AML. *J Adv Pract Oncol.* 2022;13(3):333–336. https://doi.org/10.6004/jadpro.2022.13.3.31.
15. Bryant AL, Chan YN, Richardson J, Foster M, Owenby S, Wujcik D. Understanding barriers to oral therapy adherence in adults with acute myeloid leukemia. *J Adv Pract Oncol.* 2020;11(4):342–349. https://doi.org/10.6004/jadpro.2020.11.4.2.
16. Muluneh B. Enhancing the design and evaluation of care delivery for patients on oral anticancer agents. *J Natl Compr Canc Netw.* 2022;20(10):1185–1187. https://doi.org/10.6004/jnccn.2022.7076.
17. Muluneh B, Muir MA, Collins JB, et al. Barriers and facilitators associated with implementing interventions to support oral anticancer agent adherence in academic and community cancer center settings. *PLoS One.* 2023;18(7):e0286630. https://doi.org/10.1371/journal.pone.0286630.
18. Bryant AL, Deal AM, Walton A, Wood WA, Muss H, Mayer DK. Use of ED and hospital services for patients with acute leukemia after induction therapy: one year follow-up. *Leuk Res.* 2015;39(4):406–410. https://doi.org/10.1016/j.leukres.2015.01.006.
19. Mayer DK, Travers D, Wyss A, Leak A, Waller A. Why do patients with cancer visit emergency departments? Results of a 2008 population study in North Carolina. *J Clin Oncol.* 2011;29(19):2683–2688. https://doi.org/10.1200/jco.2010.34.2816.
20. Leak A, Mayer DK, Wyss A, Travers D, Waller A. Why do cancer patients die in the emergency department? An analysis of 283 deaths in NC EDs. *Am J Hosp Palliat Care.* 2013;30(2):178–182. https://doi.org/10.1177/1049909112445306.
21. Kamal AH, LeBlanc TW, Meier DE. Better palliative care for all: improving the lived experience with cancer. *JAMA.* 2016;316(1):29–30. https://doi.org/10.1001/jama.2016.6491.
22. LeBlanc TW, O'Donnell JD, Crowley-Matoka M, et al. Perceptions of palliative care among hematologic malignancy specialists: a mixed-methods study. *J Oncol Pract.* 2015;11(2):e230–e238. https://doi.org/10.1200/jop.2014.001859.
23. LeBlanc TW. Addressing end-of-life quality gaps in hematologic cancers: the importance of early concurrent palliative care. *JAMA Intern Med.* 2016;176(2):265–266. https://doi.org/10.1001/jamainternmed.2015.6994.
24. LeBlanc TW, Ritchie CS, Friedman F, et al. Adherence to measuring what matters items when caring for patients with hematologic malignancies versus solid tumors. *J Pain Symptom Manage.* 2016;52(6):775–782. https://doi.org/10.1016/j.jpainsymman.2016.09.004.
25. Ferrell BR, Temel JS, Temin S, et al. Integration of palliative care into standard oncology care: American Society of Clinical Oncology clinical practice guideline update. *J Clin Oncol.* 2017;35(1):96–112. https://doi.org/10.1200/jco.2016.70.1474.
26. El-Jawahri A, LeBlanc T, VanDusen H, et al. Effect of inpatient palliative care on quality of life 2 weeks after hematopoietic stem cell transplantation: a randomized clinical trial. *JAMA.* 2016;316(20):2094–2103. https://doi.org/10.1001/jama.2016.16786.
27. El-Jawahri A, LeBlanc TW, Kavanaugh A, et al. Effectiveness of integrated palliative and oncology care for patients with acute myeloid leukemia: a randomized clinical trial. *JAMA Oncol.* 2021;7(2):238–245. https://doi.org/10.1001/jamaoncol.2020.6343.
28. El-Jawahri A, Nelson AM, Gray TF, Lee SJ, LeBlanc TW. Palliative and end-of-life care for patients with hematologic malignancies. *J Clin Oncol.* 2020;38(9):944–953. https://doi.org/10.1200/jco.18.02386.
29. Smith TJ, Temin S, Alesi ER, et al. American Society of Clinical Oncology provisional clinical opinion: the integration of palliative care into standard oncology care. *J Clin Oncol.* 2012;30(8):880–887. https://doi.org/10.1200/jco.2011.38.5161.
30. Wedding U. Palliative care of patients with haematological malignancies: strategies to overcome difficulties via integrated care. *Lancet Healthy Longev.* 2021;2(11):e746–e753. https://doi.org/10.1016/s2666-7568(21)00213-0.
31. DiNardo CD, Pratz K, Pullarkat V, et al. Venetoclax combined with decitabine or azacitidine in treatment-naive, elderly patients with acute myeloid leukemia. *Blood.* 2019;133(1):7–17. https://doi.org/10.1182/blood-2018-08-868752.
32. Loh KP, Tsang M, LeBlanc TW, et al. Decisional involvement and information preferences of patients with hematologic malignancies. *Blood Adv.* 2020;4(21):5492–5500. https://doi.org/10.1182/bloodadvances.2020003044.
33. Geerts PAF, van der Weijden T, Moser A, Bos GMJ. The perception of shared decision-making in hematology by patients and physicians seems satisfactory, but important steps are still ahead of us. *Hemasphere.* 2020;4(4):e417. https://doi.org/10.1097/hs9.0000000000000417.
34. Katz SJ, Belkora J, Elwyn G. Shared decision making for treatment of cancer: challenges and opportunities. *J Oncol Pract.* 2014;10(3):206–208. https://doi.org/10.1200/jop.2014.001434.
35. Street RL Jr, Mazor KM, Arora NK. Assessing patient-centered communication in cancer care: measures for surveillance of communication outcomes. *J Oncol Pract.* 2016;12(12):1198–1202. https://doi.org/10.1200/jop.2016.013334.
36. Bryant AL, Van Den Eynde M, Grewe ME, Alderman JT, Zomorodi M, Durham CF. Interprofessional communication in the care of adults with cancer: exploring clinicians' perceptions of team rounding. *J Interprof Care.* 2022;36(6):951–954. https://doi.org/10.1080/13561820.2021.2000374.

37. Parker SM, Clayton JM, Hancock K, et al. A systematic review of prognostic/end-of-life communication with adults in the advanced stages of a life-limiting illness: patient/caregiver preferences for the content, style, and timing of information. *J Pain Symptom Manage.* 2007;34(1):81–93. https://doi.org/10.1016/j.jpainsymman.2006.09.035.
38. Weeks JC, Catalano PJ, Cronin A, et al. Patients' expectations about effects of chemotherapy for advanced cancer. *N Engl J Med.* 2012;367(17):1616–1625. https://doi.org/10.1056/NEJMoa1204410.
39. Jacobs JM, Pensak NA, Sporn NJ, et al. Treatment satisfaction and adherence to oral chemotherapy in patients with cancer. *J Oncol Pract.* 2017;13(5):e474–e485. https://doi.org/10.1200/jop.2016.019729.
40. Thind A, Liu Y, Maly RC. Patient satisfaction with breast cancer follow-up care provided by family physicians. *J Am Board Fam Med.* 2011;24(6):710–716. https://doi.org/10.3122/jabfm.2011.06.100288.
41. Venetis MK, Robinson JD, Turkiewicz KL, Allen M. An evidence base for patient-centered cancer care: a meta-analysis of studies of observed communication between cancer specialists and their patients. *Patient Educ Couns.* 2009;77(3):379–383. https://doi.org/10.1016/j.pec.2009.09.015.
42. Karliner LS, Hwang ES, Nickleach D, Kaplan CP. Language barriers and patient-centered breast cancer care. *Patient Educ Couns.* 2011;84(2):223–228. https://doi.org/10.1016/j.pec.2010.07.009.
43. Fiscella K, Humiston S, Hendren S, et al. Eliminating disparities in cancer screening and follow-up of abnormal results: what will it take? *J Health Care Poor Underserved.* 2011;22(1):83–100. https://doi.org/10.1353/hpu.2011.0023.
44. Lee YK, Low WY, Ng CJ. Exploring patient values in medical decision making: a qualitative study. *PLoS One.* 2013;8(11):e80051. https://doi.org/10.1371/journal.pone.0080051.
45. Eide H, Graugaard P, Holgersen K, Finset A. Physician communication in different phases of a consultation at an oncology outpatient clinic related to patient satisfaction. *Patient Educ Counsel.* 2003;51(3):259–266. https://doi.org/10.1016/s0738-3991(02)00225 2.
46. Eide H, Quera V, Graugaard P, Finset A. Physician–patient dialogue surrounding patients' expression of concern: applying sequence analysis to RIAS. *Soc Sci Med.* 2004;59(1):145–155. https://doi.org/10.1016/j.socscimed.2003.10.011.
47. Beach WA, Easter DW, Good JS, Pigeron E. Disclosing and responding to cancer "fears" during oncology interviews. *Soc Sci Med.* 2005;60(4):893–910. https://doi.org/10.1016/j.socscimed.2004.06.031.
48. Epstein RM, Street RL Jr. *Patient-Centered Communication in Cancer Care: Promoting Healing and Reducing Suffering.* Publication No. 07-6225. National Institutes of Health; 2007.
49. Rego F, Gonçalves F, Moutinho S, Castro L, Nunes R. The influence of spirituality on decision-making in palliative care outpatients: a cross-sectional study. *BMC Palliat Care.* 2020;19(1):22. https://doi.org/10.1186/s12904-020-0525-3.
50. Astrow AB, Kwok G, Sharma RK, Fromer N, Sulmasy DP. Spiritual needs and perception of quality of care and satisfaction with care in hematology/medical oncology patients: a multicultural assessment. *J Pain Symptom Manage.* 2018;55(1):56–64.e1. https://doi.org/10.1016/j.jpainsymman.2017.08.009.
51. Nelson AM, Johnson PC, Kavanaugh AR, et al. Palliative care for patients undergoing stem cell transplant: intervention components and supportive care measures. *Bone Marrow Transplant.* 2021;56(8):1971–1977. https://doi.org/10.1038/s41409-021-01281-2.
52. Mitchell SA. Palliative care during and following allogeneic hematopoietic stem cell transplantation. *Curr Opin Support Palliat Care.* 2018;12(1):58–64. https://doi.org/10.1097/spc.0000000000000327.
53. Bryant AL, Coffman E, Phillips B, et al. Pilot randomized trial of an electronic symptom monitoring and reporting intervention for hospitalized adults undergoing hematopoietic stem cell transplantation. *Support Care Cancer.* 2020;28(3):1223-1231. https://doi.org/10.1007/s00520-019-04932-9.
54. LeBlanc TW, Roeland EJ, El-Jawahri A. Early palliative care for patients with hematologic malignancies: is it really so difficult to achieve? *Curr Hematol Malig Rep.* 2017;12(4):300–308. https://doi.org/10.1007/s11899-017-0392-z.
55. LeBlanc TW, El-Jawahri A. When and why should patients with hematologic malignancies see a palliative care specialist? *Hematology Am Soc Hematol Educ Program.* 2015;2015(1):471–478.
56. El-Jawahri A, Nelson AM, Gray TF, Lee SJ, LeBlanc TW. Palliative and end-of-life care for patients with hematologic malignancies. *J Clin Oncol.* 2020;38(9):944.
57. El-Jawahri AR, Traeger LN, Kuzmuk K, et al. Quality of life and mood of patients and family caregivers during hospitalization for hematopoietic stem cell transplantation. *Cancer.* 2015;121(6):951–959.
58. Gratwohl A, Baldomero H, Frauendorfer K, Urbano-Ispizua A. EBMT activity survey 2004 and changes in disease indication over the past 15 years. *Bone Marrow Transplant.* 2006;37(12):1069–1085.
59. Majhail NS, Mau L-W, Chitphakdithai P, et al. National survey of hematopoietic cell transplantation center personnel, infrastructure, and models of care delivery. *Biol Blood Marrow Transplant.* 2015;21(7):1308–1314.
60. LeBlanc TW, Fish LJ, Bloom CT, et al. Patient experiences of acute myeloid leukemia: a qualitative study about diagnosis, illness understanding, and treatment decision-making. *Psychooncology.* 2017;26(12):2063–2068.
61. Alibhai SM, Leach M, Kermalli H, et al. The impact of acute myeloid leukemia and its treatment on quality of life and functional status in older adults. *Crit Rev Oncol Hematol.* 2007;64(1):19–30.
62. Manitta V, Zordan R, Cole-Sinclair M, Nandurkar H, Philip J. The symptom burden of patients with hematological malignancy: a cross-sectional observational study. *J Pain Symptom Manage.* 2011;42(3):432–442.
63. Zimmermann C, Yuen D, Mischitelle A, et al. Symptom burden and supportive care in patients with acute leukemia. *Leuk Res.* 2013;37(7):731–736.
64. Batty GD, Russ TC, Stamatakis E, Kivimäki M. Psychological distress in relation to site specific cancer mortality: pooling of unpublished data from 16 prospective cohort studies. *BMJ.* 2017;356:j108.
65. Fadul NA, El Osta B, Dalal S, Poulter VA, Bruera E. Comparison of symptom burden among patients referred to palliative care with hematologic malignancies versus those with solid tumors. *J Palliat Med.* 2008;11(3):422–427. https://doi.org/10.1089/jpm.2007.0184.
66. Albrecht TA, Keim-Malpass J, Boyiadzis M, Rosenzweig M. Psychosocial experiences of young adults diagnosed with acute leukemia during hospitalization for induction chemotherapy treatment. *J Hosp Palliat Nurs.* 2019;21(2):167–173. https://doi.org/10.1097/njh.0000000000000545.
67. Albrecht TA, Boyiadzis M, Elswick RK Jr, Starkweather A, Rosenzweig M. Symptom management and psychosocial needs

of adults with acute myeloid leukemia during induction treatment: a pilot study. *Cancer Nurs*. 2017;40(6):E31–E38. https://doi.org/10.1097/ncc.0000000000000428.
68. Rodin G, Yuen D, Mischitelle A, et al. Traumatic stress in acute leukemia. *Psychooncology*. 2013;22(2):299–307.
69. Nissim R, Zimmermann C, Minden M, et al. Abducted by the illness: a qualitative study of traumatic stress in individuals with acute leukemia. *Leuk Res*. 2013;37(5):496–502.
70. Duell T, Van Lint MT, Ljungman P, et al. Health and functional status of long-term survivors of bone marrow transplantation. *Ann Intern Med*. 1997;126(3):184–192.
71. Pidala J, Anasetti C, Jim H. Health-related quality of life following haematopoietic cell transplantation: patient education, evaluation and intervention. *Br J Haematol*. 2010;148(3):373–385.
72. Pidala J, Anasetti C, Jim H. Quality of life after allogeneic hematopoietic cell transplantation. *Blood*. 2009;114(1):7–19.
73. Syrjala KL, Langer SL, Abrams JR, et al. Recovery and long-term function after hematopoietic cell transplantation for leukemia or lymphoma. *JAMA*. 2004;291(19):2335–2343.
74. Altmaier EM, Ewell M, McQuellon R, et al. The effect of unrelated donor marrow transplantation on health-related quality of life: a report of the unrelated donor marrow transplantation trial (T-cell depletion trial). *Biol Blood Marrow Transplant*. 2006;12(6):648–655.
75. Damlaj M, El Fakih R, Hashmi SK. Evolution of survivorship in lymphoma, myeloma and leukemia: metamorphosis of the field into long term follow-up care. *Blood Rev*. 2019;33:63–73.
76. Lee S, Loberiza F, Antin J, et al. Routine screening for psychosocial distress following hematopoietic stem cell transplantation. *Bone Marrow Transplant*. 2005;35(1):77–83.
77. Lee SJ, Fairclough D, Parsons SK, et al. Recovery after stem-cell transplantation for hematologic diseases. *J Clin Oncol*. 2001;19(1):242–252.
78. Chan YN, Betancur S, Conklin JL, et al. Cognitive function in adults with acute myeloid leukemia treated with chemotherapy: a systematic review. *Cancer Nurs*. 2024;47(2):121–131. https://doi.org/10.1097/ncc.0000000000001164.
79. LeBlanc MR, Bryant AL, LeBlanc TW, et al. A cross-sectional observational study of health-related quality of life in adults with multiple myeloma. *Support Care Cancer*. 2022;30(6):5239–5248. https://doi.org/10.1007/s00520-022-06943-5.
80. LeBlanc MR, Zimmerman S, LeBlanc TW, Bryant AL, Hudson KE, Smith SK. Persistent fatigue among long-term non-Hodgkin lymphoma survivors. *Leuk Lymphoma*. 2022;63(2):344–352. https://doi.org/10.1080/10428194.2021.1984450.
81. Mayo SJ, Wozniczka I, Edwards B, et al. A qualitative study of the everyday impacts of cognitive difficulties after stem cell transplantation. *Oncol Nurs Forum*. 2022;49(4):315–325.
82. Socié G, Stone JV, Wingard JR, et al. Long-term survival and late deaths after allogeneic bone marrow transplantation. *N Engl J Med*. 1999;341(1):14–21.
83. Lee SJ, Flowers ME. Recognizing and managing chronic graft-versus-host disease. *Hematology Am Soc Hematol Educ Program*. 2008;2008(1):134–141.
84. Sutherland H, Fyles G, Adams G, et al. Quality of life following bone marrow transplantation: a comparison of patient reports with population norms. *Bone Marrow Transplant*. 1997;19(11):1129–1136.
85. Pidala J, Kurland B, Chai X, et al. Patient-reported quality of life is associated with severity of chronic graft-versus-host disease as measured by NIH criteria: report on baseline data from the Chronic GVHD Consortium. *Blood*. 2011;117(17):4651–4657.
86. Troy JD, Locke SC, Samsa GP, Feliciano J, Richhariya A, LeBlanc TW. Patient-reported distress in Hodgkin lymphoma across the survivorship continuum. *Support Care Cancer*. 2019;27:2453–2462.
87. Shanafelt TD, Bowen D, Venkat C, et al. Quality of life in chronic lymphocytic leukemia: an international survey of 1482 patients. *Br J Haematol*. 2007;139(2):255–264.
88. Malakian A, Rodin G, Widger K, Ali R, Mahendiran AE, Mayo SJ. Patient experience of care near the end of life among adults with acute leukemia: a scoping review. *J Palliat Medi*. 2024;27(2):255–264.
89. Lowe JR, Yu Y, Wolf S, Samsa G, LeBlanc TW. A cohort study of patient-reported outcomes and healthcare utilization in acute myeloid leukemia patients receiving active cancer therapy in the last six months of life. *J Palliat Med*. 2018;21(5):592–597.
90. LeBlanc TW, Smith JM, Currow DC. Symptom burden of haematological malignancies as death approaches in a community palliative care service: a retrospective cohort study of a consecutive case series. *Lancet Haematol*. 2015;2(8):e334–e338.
91. Nekolaichuk C, Watanabe S, Beaumont C. The Edmonton Symptom Assessment System: a 15-year retrospective review of validation studies (1991–2006). *Palliat Med*. 2008;22(2):111–122.
92. Tricou C, Mah K, Malfitano C, et al. *Preliminary Validation of the Edmonton Symptom Assessment Scale–Acute Leukemia (ESAS-AL) in Patients with Acute Leukemia (AL)*. American Society of Clinical Oncology; 2018.
93. Hui D, Bruera E. The Edmonton Symptom Assessment System 25 years later: past, present, and future developments. *J Pain Symptom Manage*. 2017;53(3):630–643. https://doi.org/10.1016/j.jpainsymman.2016.10.370.
94. Rodin G, Malfitano C, Rydall A, et al. Emotion and Symptom-Focused Engagement (EASE): a randomized phase II trial of an integrated psychological and palliative care intervention for patients with acute leukemia. *Support Care Cancer*. 2020;28(1):163–176.
95. Mendoza TR, Wang XS, Cleeland CS, et al. The rapid assessment of fatigue severity in cancer patients: use of the Brief Fatigue Inventory. *Cancer*. 1999;85(5):1186–1196.
96. Quinn B, Potting CM, Stone R, et al. Guidelines for the assessment of oral mucositis in adult chemotherapy, radiotherapy and haematopoietic stem cell transplant patients. *Eur J Cancer*. 2008;44(1):61–72.
97. Bergenthal N, Will A, Streckmann F, et al. Aerobic physical exercise for adult patients with haematological malignancies. *Cochrane Database Syst Rev*. 2014;11:CD009075.
98. Barsevick AM, Dudley W, Beck S, Sweeney C, Whitmer K, Nail L. A randomized clinical trial of energy conservation for patients with cancer-related fatigue. *Cancer*. 2004;100(6):1302–1310.
99. Ravasco P. Nutrition in cancer patients. *J Clin Med*. 2019;8(8):1211.
100. Irish LA, Kline CE, Gunn HE, Buysse DJ, Hall MH. The role of sleep hygiene in promoting public health: a review of empirical evidence. *Sleep Med Rev*. 2015;22:23–36.
101. Galvin KT, Garland SN, Wibowo E. The relationship between sleep hygiene, mood, and insomnia symptoms in men with prostate cancer. *Support Care Cancer*. 2022;30(5):4055–4064.
102. Papadopoulos D, Kiagia M, Charpidou A, Gkiozos I, Syrigos K. Psychological correlates of sleep quality in lung cancer patients under chemotherapy: a single-center cross-sectional study. *Psychooncology*. 2019;28(9):1879–1886.
103. Zupanec S, Jones H, McRae L, Papaconstantinou E, Weston J, Stremler R. A sleep hygiene and relaxation intervention for children with acute lymphoblastic leukemia: a pilot randomized controlled trial. *Cancer Nurs*. 2017;40(6):488.

104. Savard M-H, Savard J. Cognitive-behavioral therapy for insomnia in cancer patients: an update of efficacy evidence and areas for future research. *Curr Sleep Med Rep*. 2017;3:66–75.
105. Demiralp M, Oflaz F, Komurcu S. Effects of relaxation training on sleep quality and fatigue in patients with breast cancer undergoing adjuvant chemotherapy. *J Clin Nurs*. 2010;19(7-8):1073–1083.
106. Ruano A, Garcia-Torres F, Galvez-Lara M, Moriana JA. Psychological and non-pharmacologic treatments for pain in cancer patients: a systematic review and meta-analysis. *J Pain Symptom Manage*. 2022;63(5):e505–e520.
107. Weinrich SP, Weinrich MC. The effect of massage on pain in cancer patients. *Appl Nurs Res*. 1990;3(4):140–145.
108. Kuon C, Wannier R, Harrison J, Tague C. Massage for symptom management in adult inpatients with hematologic malignancies. *Glob Adv Health Med*. 2019;8:2164956119849390.
109. McCaffery M, Wolff M. Pain relief using cutaneous modalities, positioning, and movement. *Hospice J*. 1992;8(1–2):121–153.
110. Vallerand AH, Musto S, Polomano RC. Nursing's role in cancer pain management. *Curr Pain Headache Rep*. 2011;15:250–262.
111. Wiseman LR, Faulds D. Oral pilocarpine: a review of its pharmacological properties and clinical potential in xerostomia. *Drugs*. 1995;49:143–155.
112. Neumann J. Nursing challenges caring for bone marrow transplantation patients with graft versus host disease. *Hematol Oncol Stem Cell Ther*. 2017;10(4):192–194.
113. Dignan FL, Amrolia P, Clark A, et al. Diagnosis and management of chronic graft-versus-host disease. *Br J Haematol*. 2012;158(1):46–61.
114. Woodward S. Management of faecal incontinence in graft-versus-host disease. *Br J Nurs*. 2012;21(2):84–88.
115. Malakian A, Mohammed S, Fazelzad R, Ajaj R, Artemenko A, Mayo SJ. Nursing, psychotherapy and advanced cancer: a scoping review. *Eur J Oncol Nurs*. 2022;56:102090.
116. Gemmill R, Cooke L, Williams AC, Grant M. Informal caregivers of hematopoietic cell transplant patients: a review and recommendations for interventions and research. *Cancer Nurs*. 2011;34(6):E13–E21. https://doi.org/10.1097/NCC.0b013e31820a592d.
117. Kent EE, Rowland JH, Northouse L, et al. Caring for caregivers and patients: research and clinical priorities for informal cancer caregiving. *Cancer*. 2016;122(13):1987–1995. https://doi.org/10.1002/cncr.29939.
118. Albrecht TA, Hoppe R, Winter MA. How caregivers cope and adapt when a family member is diagnosed with a hematologic malignancy: informing supportive care needs. *Cancer Nurs*. 2022;45(6):E849–E855. https://doi.org/10.1097/ncc.0000000000001063.
119. Hoppe R, Winter MA, Graap K, Albrecht TA. Impact of a hematologic malignancy diagnosis and treatment on patients and their family caregivers. *Oncol Nurs Forum*. 2022;49(5):445–453. https://doi.org/10.1188/22.Onf.445-453.
120. Alam S, Hannon B, Zimmermann C. Palliative care for family caregivers. *J Clin Oncol*. 2020;38(9):926–936. https://doi.org/10.1200/jco.19.00018.
121. McCusker J, Yaffe M, Lambert SD, et al. Unmet needs of family caregivers of hospitalized older adults preparing for discharge home. *Chronic Illn*. 2020;16(2):131–145. https://doi.org/10.1177/1742395318789467.
122. Tan KR, Chan YN, Iadonisi K, et al. Perspectives of caregivers of older adults with acute myeloid leukemia during initial hypomethylating agents and venetoclax chemotherapy. *Support Care Cancer*. 2023;31(1):95. https://doi.org/10.1007/s00520-022-07565-7.
123. Creedle C, Leak A, Deal AM, et al. The impact of education on caregiver burden on two inpatient oncology units. *J Cancer Educ*. 2012;27(2):250–256. https://doi.org/10.1007/s13187-011-0302-3.
124. Bellg AJ, Borrelli B, Resnick B, et al. Enhancing treatment fidelity in health behavior change studies: best practices and recommendations from the NIH Behavior Change Consortium. *Health Psychol*. 2004;23(5):443–451. https://doi.org/10.1037/0278-6133.23.5.443.
125. Dionne-Odom JN, Currie ER, Johnston EE, Rosenberg AR. Supporting family caregivers of adult and pediatric persons with leukemia. *Semin Oncol Nurs*. 2019;35(6):150954. https://doi.org/10.1016/j.soncn.2019.150954.
126. Posluszny DM, Bovbjerg DH, Syrjala KL, Agha M, Dew MA. Correlates of anxiety and depression symptoms among patients and their family caregivers prior to allogeneic hematopoietic cell transplant for hematological malignancies. *Support Care Cancer*. 2019;27(2):591–600. https://doi.org/10.1007/s00520-018-4346-3.
127. Mukherjee S, Sekeres, M. Novel therapies in acute myeloid leukemia. *Semin Oncol Nurs*. 2019;35(6):150955.
128. Lachowiez CA, Loghavi S, Kadia TM, et al. Outcomes of older patients with NPM1-mutated AML: current treatments and the promise of venetoclax-based regimens. *Blood Adv*. 2020;4(7):1311–1320. https://doi.org/10.1182/bloodadvances.2019001267.
129. Odejide OO. Strategies for introducing palliative care in the management of relapsed or refractory aggressive lymphomas. *Hematology Am Soc Hematol Educ Program*. 2020;(1):148–153. https://doi.org/10.1182/hematology.2020000100.
130. El-Jawahri A, LeBlanc TW, Kavanaugh A, et al. Effectiveness of integrated palliative and oncology care for patients with acute myeloid leukemia: a randomized clinical trial. *JAMA Oncol*. 2021;7(2):238–245. https://doi.org/10.1001/jamaoncol.2020.6343.
131. El-Jawahri A, Pidala J, Khera N, et al. Impact of psychological distress on quality of life, functional status, and survival in patients with chronic graft-versus-host disease. *Biol Blood Marrow Transplant*. 2018;24(11):2285–2292. https://doi.org/10.1016/j.bbmt.2018.07.020.
132. El-Jawahri A, Nelson AM, Gray TF, Lee SJ, LeBlanc TW. Palliative and end-of-life care for patients with hematologic malignancies. *J Clin Oncol*. 2020;38(9):944–953. https://doi.org/10.1200/JCO.18.02386.
133. Ramsenthaler C, Gao W, Siegert RJ, Edmonds PM, Schey SA, Higginson IJ. Symptoms and anxiety predict declining health-related quality of life in multiple myeloma: a prospective, multicentre longitudinal study. *Palliat Med*. 2019;33(5):541–551. https://doi.org/10.1177/0269216319833588.

52

Palliative Care for Persons Living with Cancer

Denice R. Economou, Alissa A. Ulanday, and Eden R. Brauer

Key Points

- According to the National Cancer Institute and others, a person is considered to be a cancer survivor from the time of diagnosis through the balance of life.
- The palliative care approach to persons living with and beyond cancer includes assessment of physical, psychological, social, and spiritual concerns as well as caregiver needs and concerns across the cancer continuum.
- Palliative care can be delivered concurrently with curative-intent treatment.
- Early integration of palliative care improves quality of life and symptoms, may reduce caregiver burden, and supports patients and families as they make decisions regarding the benefits and burdens of treatments.
- Rehabilitation services can be incorporated into a palliative approach to focus on function and manage common symptoms.
- A comprehensive geriatric assessment can inform the plan of care and help to identify supportive care needs of older adults.
- Nurses can help alleviate suffering by supporting patients and families using a palliative care approach to address multidimensional concerns.

Introduction

With the availability of new therapies and improvements in early detection strategies, the number of cancer survivors is rising rapidly, and people with cancer are living longer. "Cancer survivorship" is a term that includes many different stages along the cancer continuum, and it is difficult to identify the specific needs of cancer survivors based on that singular title. Although the term "cancer survivorship" was historically used to describe the period after completion of curative-intent treatments, it is increasingly recognized that this understanding is too narrow and outdated.[1] To better reflect advancements in treatments and the realities of patients living for long periods after initial diagnosis, a broader, more inclusive definition was needed. According to the National Cancer Institute, American Society Clinical Oncology (ASCO), and others, an individual is considered a cancer survivor from the time of diagnosis through the remainder of life.[2] Therefore, cancer survivorship encompasses the diverse experiences of all persons living with cancer. This chapter describes the role of palliative care in patients living with cancer, the overlapping principles between palliative care and survivorship care, and the use of palliative treatments for patients with advanced cancer. We use the terms "palliative" and "supportive" care interchangeably in this chapter.

The Intersection between Palliative Care and Survivorship Care

Palliative care and survivorship care overlap in their holistic approach and focus on aligning care with patients' values. Both disciplines aim to improve quality of life (QOL) and quality of care for cancer patients and their families by addressing the physical, psychological, social, and spiritual domains of care (Table 52.1).[3,4] Both teams can provide care to a diverse group of individuals living with cancer across the continuum. This includes those who have completed active treatment for curative intent and are surviving with minimal symptoms related to cancer or its treatment as well as those who are dealing with difficult symptoms and require a multidisciplinary approach to relieve their symptoms. Additionally, recent advances in cancer treatment often include long-term oral therapies that lack a clear treatment endpoint.[4] Therefore, palliative management may involve primary and specialty care to address the needs of patients and their families. Specialty care provides management of chronic side effects and of comorbidities associated with chronic disease or aging and is focused on palliation, symptom management, and QOL. For cancer survivorship care, the approach is similar to chronic disease management, where symptoms may improve or become well-controlled but may never be cured.[1]

The multiple models used to provide survivorship care as well as palliative/supportive care vary widely depending on the available resources in individual settings and communities. This is the challenge that organizations face as they attempt to incorporate palliative care into survivorship care.[4] Risk stratification of people who are living

Table 52.1 Comprehensive palliative care assessment and associated palliative care domains

Assessment category	Assessment subcategory examples	Domains of palliative care
Symptoms	Pain Anxiety Demoralization Depression Fatigue Sleep disturbance Sexual function/limitations Nausea Dyspnea Constipation Nutritional status	2: Physical Aspects of Care 3: Psychological and Psychiatric Aspects 7: Care of the Patient Nearing the End of Life
Support	Sources of strength of patient, family, and/or caregiver(s) Physical support from family and/or caregiver(s) Work-related issues Financial constraints Roles and relationships Spiritual and religious preferences Existential distress Guilt Grief and bereavement	3: Psychological and Psychiatric Aspects 4: Social Aspects of Care 5: Spiritual, Religious, and Existential Aspects of Care 6: Cultural Aspects of Care 7: Care of the Patient Nearing the End of Life
Goals of care	Advance care planning and documentation Designation of surrogate decision maker Communication and decision-making preferences What brings the patient joy, gives their life meaning What constitutes an acceptable quality of life Health literacy Prognostic awareness Treatment preferences	5: Spiritual, Religious, and Existential Aspects of Care 6: Cultural Aspects of Care 7: Care of the Patient Nearing the End of Life 8: Ethical and Legal Aspects of Care
Disposition	Referrals may include to services such as outpatient palliative care clinic, hospice, other specialists, rehabilitation services, integrative providers, behavioral health/social workers, chaplains, child life specialists, and nurse navigators	Includes components of all eight domains

Source: Reference 10.

with cancer can provide a guide for deciding how to refer patients to the appropriate healthcare team.[5,6] In this approach, patients are categorized into those with a low risk of developing long-term or late effects of treatment; those who have a moderate risk of developing long-term and late effects of treatment; and those at high risk of developing long term and late effects of treatment or also have complicated chronic illnesses. Triaging care based on treatment-related effects as well as potential for cancer recurrence has been recommended to improve survivorship care access by researchers in the United Kingdom and Australia.[7]

There are unique issues and challenges for cancer patients beginning with early survivorship and continuing through end-of-life (EOL) care. Discussions about palliative care and survivorship support should be included early, at the time of diagnosis, and continue throughout the disease trajectory, with focus on patients at highest risk for long-term side effects and cancer recurrence.[4] There is strong evidence that earlier integration of palliative care improves QOL, depression, and satisfaction with care.[4] The challenge most often is in identifying who is at greatest risk for long-term side effects and at the highest risk for recurrence.[5,7] In order to meet the combined survivorship and palliative care needs, the focus should be on providing the most appropriate services based on the individual needs of the patient and family.[8] Applying this information to a case study will help illustrate these principles for integrating palliative care in the disease trajectory for people living with cancer.

Case Study: A Patient Navigating Cancer Survivorship with Ovarian Cancer

Haley is a 32-year-old female who was initially diagnosed with low-grade serous carcinoma of the ovary and shortly thereafter underwent fertility-sparing surgery with right salpingo-oophorectomy, left ovarian cystectomy, infra-colic omentectomy, and appendectomy. Later that year, she developed a recurrent left adnexal mass and underwent a laparoscopic hysterectomy. She was then lost to follow-up with her oncologist for 2 years due to insurance-related barriers. Eventually, she returned with worsening ascites and carcinomatosis on imaging and underwent further surgical interventions including tumor debulking and lysis of adhesions. It was at this time that the patient was seen by the palliative care service (PCS) in the hospital and then closely followed in the outpatient clinic for symptoms of abdominal pain, nausea, chronic fatigue, and anxiety. Opioids were started via a patient-controlled analgesia pump to control Haley's pain, which was later transitioned to methadone tablets. Multimodal medications were started to manage severe nausea, and Haley was started on escitalopram to address her anxiety. Haley's disease eventually stabilized with chemotherapy, and she was able to resume her educational studies and spend more time with her family and partner. The PCS outpatient clinic continued to follow Haley to manage ongoing chronic pain and symptom issues, as did the oncology social worker to help her process her fear of eventual progression of disease and grief related to the lost ability to bear children.

Outpatient survivorship programs should have dedicated embedded resources to deliver supportive services to complement usual oncology care and can also utilize nurse navigators, geriatric oncology, pain management services, and social workers to provide additional support to meet the patient's needs.[4] Primary palliative care provided by the oncology team is appropriate for patients who have early-stage disease, have a low symptom burden, and/or are receiving minimally complex surveillance care.[6] Specialty palliative care should be reserved for people living with a high risk of recurrence, multiple comorbid diseases, significant symptom burden, treatment-related complications, or unmet needs and/or are in the advanced stages of their disease. The use of specialty palliative care for cancer survivors who have minimal disease and/or low symptom needs adds burden to both the patient as well as the specialty PCS.[5,9] Furthermore, there is an ongoing deficit in the number of specialty trained palliative care clinicians, and this underscores the need to be judicious when referring patients.[10] Increased training opportunities for oncology clinicians to develop palliative care skills will help address some of the barriers to providing primary palliative care or accessing early palliative care in the outpatient setting.[4] Oncology nurses play an important role in identifying patients who are most appropriate for specialized palliative care across the cancer care trajectory.[5,8]

Compared to childhood cancer survivors, less is known about the incidence of symptoms and late and long-term effects in adults living with cancer.[11] People living with cancer experience both physical and psychosocial late or long-term effects that are related to their cancer treatment, age, comorbidities, and genetics and can benefit from engaging in health promotion behaviors such as diet and exercise.[2] As such, nearly all people living with cancer can benefit from the principles of palliative care, through either primary or specialty palliative care.

A communication tool that nurses may find useful to help describe a care pathway where disease management and palliative care are integrated from the time of diagnosis was developed in 2014 (Figure 52.1). It is referred to as "The Bow Tie Model of 21st Century Palliative Care: Palliative care-enhanced model." The model was developed for clinicians to provide a clear conceptual model of disease management that includes the integration of pain and symptom management, palliative care, potential survivorship care, rehabilitation, hospice, and EOL care through bereavement.[12] It provides a clear illustration of how palliative care can be integrated from diagnosis across the disease trajectory.

More evidence is needed to determine optimal care models for this diverse population of individuals living with cancer, but it is clear that one size will not fit all. Discussions related to prognosis, cure, and living well despite a chronic illness can guide much needed conversations for people living with cancer. By focusing on QOL, goals of care, and the management of long-term symptoms and psychosocial issues, these discussions can help clinical teams tailor care to the needs, values and preferences of patients and their families.[1] Clinical models of care include inpatient consultation for management of high pain and symptom burden and complex goals-of-care discussions, outpatient clinics that can provide low to moderate symptom management, and community-based models and hospice care.[9] Studies have shown that palliative care improves QOL, survival, and healthcare costs; but it is not currently feasible for all patients living with cancer to be referred to palliative care services.[7,9,13,14] Further research related to models of care and appropriate referral processes is needed.

Common Concerns, Symptoms, and Assessment Strategies of Persons Living with Cancer across the Cancer Care Trajectory

People living with cancer express multidimensional concerns, and incorporation of the holistic approach of palliative care can improve overall QOL. Although many of the same principles apply, the approach to palliative care for cancer survivors likely to be cured of their cancer differs somewhat from those with advanced or metastatic disease.[3] For example, many individuals will be cured or in remission for extended periods, but they may need support to manage long-term side effects and fears of recurrence.[15] Individuals living with advanced metastatic disease may also need multidisciplinary palliative support in collaboration with other specialized referrals such as a psychologist, chaplain, social worker, or occupational therapist.[16]

The palliative care approach to care for people living with cancer begins with a global assessment of physical, psychological, social, and spiritual concerns. Table 52.1 presents a comprehensive palliative care assessment that focuses on four main categories and their subcategories that align with the domains of palliative care as stated in the National Consensus Project for Quality Palliative Care guidelines.[10] Psychosocial stressors may contribute to or exacerbate physical symptoms,[3] so it is important that a comprehensive assessment includes an evaluation of emotional issues, strain on social and family relationships, and caregiver needs. In Haley's case, she was experiencing multiple symptoms necessitating a comprehensive assessment

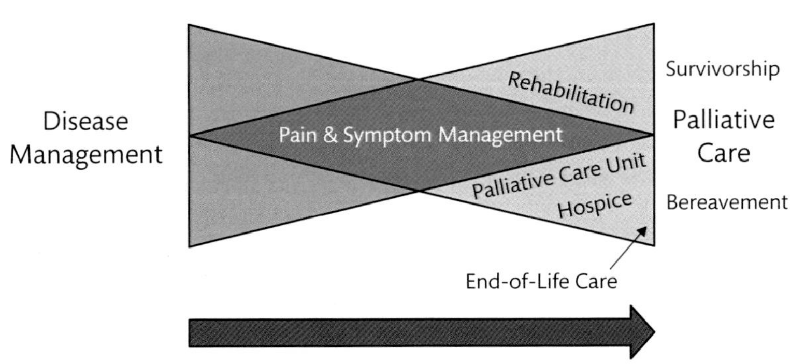

Figure 52.1 Palliative care-enhanced model. *Source*: Reference 12.

that led to multidisciplinary management. A palliative care team can provide symptom management and initiate psychological support through referrals to psychological services and/or initiation of pharmacological management as needed. Nonpharmacologic approaches should be prioritized when possible as the side-effect profiles of some medications may exacerbate other symptoms. In cases where medications are needed, short-term use is preferable to long-term use, and medications should be adjusted and titrated as indicated to provide improved symptomatic relief.[3] The benefits of early palliative care may extend to caregivers by providing techniques to reduce anxiety and improve communication.[17] Supportive interventions for caregivers may include telephone coaching by nurses; education in symptom management, problem-solving, communication skills, and self-care strategies; and referral to behavioral health or support groups.[4]

People living with cancer should receive counseling about nutrition, lifestyle factors, or integrative approaches to support their overall health and manage their long-term symptoms. Despite the known benefits of these healthy lifestyle behaviors, research shows that most people living with cancer do not meet the recommendations of the guidelines. The National Comprehensive Cancer Network (NCCN) survivorship guidelines and the American Cancer Society guidelines provide suggestions for physical activity, nutrition, and weight management.[18,19] In addition, Kleckner and Magnuson provide specific recommendations for screening and managing nutritional needs in older cancer survivors.[20] Additional management resources will be discussed in Chapter 27, "Complementary and Integrative Therapies in Palliative Care."

Rehabilitation is another important aspect of care for patients living with cancer across their disease trajectory. Tailored rehabilitation interventions can be effective in improving function and managing symptoms such as pain, fatigue, disturbed sleep, as well as neuromuscular and cognitive deficits. Rehabilitative interventions can also prevent or reduce chronic issues in individuals with cancer, such as lymphedema. Yet, rehabilitation for people living with cancer is often overlooked, and rehabilitation services are underutilized.[16] Depending on the patient's needs and availability of rehabilitation services in each unique setting, referrals to a physiatrist, physical therapists, and/or occupational therapist may be important to better support physical and cognitive deficits experienced by patients living with cancer.[16,21]

People living with cancer are often concerned about recurrence and managing uncertainty, including understanding the meaning of symptoms and whether they may represent disease recurrence.[3,22] These emotional concerns should be addressed routinely as the circumstances of a patient's disease change over time. In the case study continuation, Haley experiences recurrence and subsequently requires more extensive palliative care intervention and emotional support.

Case Study: A Patient Navigating Cancer Survivorship with Ovarian Cancer (Continued)

After 6 months of stable disease, Haley was hospitalized again and found to have metastatic disease to the lungs. She underwent talc pleurodesis and PleurX catheter placement and was started on targeted drug therapy and hormone-based chemotherapy. She soon again achieved stable disease on imaging but would occasionally be admitted to the hospital with flares in pain or nausea. The PCS was able to remain a source of consistency regarding her pain and symptom management and would recommend to continue pain and nausea medications that have historically been most effective for the patient during each hospitalization. Haley continued to struggle emotionally with her uncertain illness trajectory, as well as relying on her mother and partner as caregivers. Haley was eventually receptive to discuss advance care planning, and the PCS would frequently reassess what constitutes the patient's acceptable QOL. Eventually, Haley married her partner 1 year later and tries to travel and remain active when her pain and symptoms are relatively controlled. Through the integrated approach of the multidisciplinary team of both the inpatient and outpatient PCS and oncology social worker, Haley has continued to remain well-supported on her 5-year journey thus far with cancer.

People living with cancer frequently experience troubling side effects, which may persist during the early survivorship period, or the side effects may eventually become chronic. Common symptoms may include fatigue, sleep disturbance, neuropathy, pain, depression, and anxiety.[19]

Neuropathy

Individuals with cancer who are treated with taxanes, platinum drugs, thalidomide, and bortezomib are at risk of developing chemotherapy-induced peripheral neuropathy (CIPN).[23] CIPN typically manifests as numbness, tingling, or a burning pain in the hands and/or feet and can persist for months to years after treatment. CIPN can negatively affect an individual's balance, gait, and coordination, resulting in limitations in daily activities and increased risk for falls.[24] Ultimately, CIPN can contribute to poorer QOL, functional impairments, and disability.[25,26] CIPN is a difficult symptom to treat, and oncology nurses should not only assess for the presence of CIPN but educate patients on the importance of sharing with their care team if/when these symptoms begin.

The NCCN and ASCO have published guidelines on the management of CIPN in adults with cancer and cancer survivors.[18,27] Currently, the only evidence-based treatment recommended to manage CIPN is duloxetine.[27] However, several small studies have shown modest yet encouraging results using nonpharmacologic approaches such as exercise and acupuncture to manage persistent CIPN.[28–31] In a recent meta-analysis, exercise was found to significantly improve QOL and reduce symptoms of CIPN in patients living with cancer.[32] Multimodal exercise approaches that combine both balance training and muscle strengthening may be most effective, but research is ongoing to explore the effect of tailored exercise prescriptions on CIPN symptoms.[30] Referrals to rehabilitation services may also be considered in the management of CIPN to incorporate individualized exercise plans and strategies to reduce the risk of falls and disability.[32]

Cognitive Impairment

Changes in cognition for people living with cancer are frequently referred to in the literature as "cancer-related cognitive impairment" (CRCI), "cancer-induced cognitive impairment," or "chemo-brain" when related directly to chemotherapy.[33,34] CRCI can be subtle or severe, with the most common complaints related to short-term and working memory, attention, concentration, executive function, and processing speed, which can negatively impact QOL for those affected.[35–38] Recent reviews have found that a history of cancer is associated with a 40% increase in self-reported memory problems. Among individuals with non–central nervous system (CNS) cancers, CRCI is reported in 13% to 75% of people during and after treatment but reaches 90% in those with CNS cancers. For individuals with confirmed CRCI it has been found to persist for up to 20 years post-chemotherapy.[33,35–37] Risk factors for CRCI include age, genetic factors, cognitive reserve, ethnicity, and treatment.[34] Furthermore, newer therapies such as hormone therapy, immunotherapy, and targeted therapy have also been found to affect cognitive functions.

While there are no universally accepted cognitive assessments for the evaluation of CRCI, it is recommended that the comprehensive oncological treatment plan includes an ongoing assessment of cognitive function.[37] Interestingly, people living with cancer often self-report impaired cognition, but results from neuropsychological testing appear within normal limits. This phenomenon is a consequence of both the limitations of available testing methods, which have been largely developed for patients with dementia, as well as important confounding factors in cognitive impairment, such as depression, fatigue, insomnia, medications, and/or anxiety.[36] The International Cancer and Cognition Task Force (2011) recommends utilizing the following neuropsychological measures: the Hopkins Verbal Learning Test—Revised to assess learning and memory, the Controlled Oral Word Association Test to assess executive function, and the Trail Making Test to assess processing speed and executive function.[38] Since these tests can be quite costly and time-consuming, cognitive screening tools are more feasible in the clinical setting. The Montreal Cognitive Assessment (MoCA), the Mini-Mental State Exam, the Clock Draw Test (CDT), and the Functional Assessment of Cancer Therapy—Cognition (FACT-Cog) are frequently utilized.[39–41] The MoCA and CDT appear to be the most objective screening tools.[39,40] While there is limited high-level evidence for interventions to treat CRCI, recommended behavioral interventions include CRCI education, cognitive training, cognitive rehabilitation, exercise, and mindfulness practices to manage insomnia, fatigue, and pain.[35–37,39,42] Referral to a neuropsychologist, speech and language pathologist, physical therapist, or occupational therapist may be useful in some cases to better assess risk factors and the nature of cognitive symptoms.[34] Occupational therapists can provide tools to help patients address memory or attention deficits and improve their ability to perform activities of daily living. Physical therapists can provide training on the role of exercise and physical activity to minimize cognitive challenges. Speech and language pathologists can provide strategies related to word identification and verbal recall.[42] Pharmacologic interventions, including methylphenidate, modafinil, donepezil, and memantine, currently lack widely generalizable indications outside of clinical trials.[35,39,42] Nurses have a significant role in identifying and validating cognitive concerns, monitoring cognitive function over time, and initiating interventions for people with CRCI.

Fatigue, Depression, and Anxiety

Fatigue, depression, and anxiety are all common symptoms experienced by people living with cancer at some point in their disease trajectory and are often underdiagnosed and undertreated.[43,44] Cancer-related fatigue may occur as an isolated symptom or as part of a symptom cluster including depression, pain, menopausal symptoms, and sleep disturbance.[43] Patients should be routinely assessed for fatigue using brief self-report screening measures such as the Brief Fatigue Inventory,[45] the Patient-Reported Outcomes Measurement Information System (PROMIS) Fatigue scale, or other measures that include a fatigue subscale or single item. The NCCN and ASCO provide guidelines on cancer-related fatigue posttreatment.[46,47] Emotional distress can range from normal feelings of vulnerability and fear of cancer recurrence to significant depression, anxiety, and trauma symptoms.[48] Symptoms of anxiety and depression often overlap with other concerns such as cognitive difficulties and fatigue.[49] Factors associated with fear of recurrence included being female, being of a younger age, being from deprived areas, having received chemotherapy, and more recent completion of therapy. Survivors with lower levels of physical activity and current smokers were more likely to experience fear of recurrence.[50] The identification of depression and distress may be improved with the routine incorporation of patient-reported outcome assessments using brief tools. According to the NCCN guidelines for distress management,[48] appropriate instruments may include the NCCN Distress Thermometer, the Hospital Anxiety and Depression Scale, the PROMIS instruments, and the Patient Health Questionnaire (PHQ-2 or 4).[51,52] Furthermore, the incorporation of a comprehensive geriatric assessment (CGA) in follow-up visits may help to identify older patients with depression and other unmet needs.[53] Refer to Chapter 24, "Anxiety and Depression," and Chapter 25, "Fatigue," for more detailed discussion regarding these three symptoms in a broader scope.

In summary, persons living with cancer have a wide variety of supportive care concerns, needs, and ongoing symptoms that are influenced by their unique disease, treatment course, and goals of care. In order to deliver holistic person-centered care, it is imperative that each patient's needs are understood and that appropriate resources and specialists are identified. Additionally, given that over half of people living with cancer are 65 years or older, the unique considerations for older patients are necessary,[11] as indicated in Case Study 2 regarding Max's cancer journey.

Case Study 2: Colorectal Cancer

Max is a 74-year-old male with Stage IIIC colorectal cancer (T4aN2aM0). He was diagnosed and treated 2 years ago with subtotal colectomy and FOLFOX. His chief complaint is increasing diarrhea especially after eating or drinking. He struggles to maintain his weight and is concerned about being too far away from a bathroom due to the diarrhea. This has also limited his activity and socialization, which has in turn negatively impacted his QOL. His spouse of 44 years passed away last year, and he now lives alone in a single-family home. He has two adult sons who live in the area and provide support.

His follow-up plan includes specific surveillance per NCCN guidelines: carcinoembryonic antigen test every 6 months for 5 years, chest/abdominal computed tomography will extend from every 6 months to yearly now at the 2-year mark, colonoscopy yearly.

In addition, a geriatric assessment (G-8) is performed regularly and compared to the patient's established baseline of >14 two-years ago. G-8 screening now is 7.5, and Max is describing a loss of weight, decline in food intake due to concern about diarrhea, reduced mobility for fear of loss of bowel control, and depressive symptoms.

Comprehensive Geriatric Assessment in Older Individuals with Cancer

Individualizing the plan of care for older adults living with cancer is essential to optimize clinical outcomes. In particular, it is important to reduce the risk of polypharmacy and ensure that physical, functional, nutritional, and social support needs are being met.[54] Older adults with cancer often have different reasons for why they would benefit from palliative care. For example, some older adults with cancer may require a referral to specialty palliative care because of their frailty, functional dependence, cognitive impairment, distress, and/or caregiver challenges.[55] A CGA provides an evidence-based approach to determine health concerns and guide treatment decisions and supportive care interventions for older adults with cancer.[55] The CGA typically evaluates functional status, comorbidities, cognition, social and psychological issues, depression, nutrition status, and polypharmacy.[53] Unfortunately, CGA is not routinely implemented in oncology settings.[56] One approach to identifying older adults who might benefit from a more comprehensive assessment is using the shorter G-8 screening tool.[57] When a G-8 is completed, nurses can facilitate referrals to specialty services, communicate with primary care providers, and follow up with patients to assess adherence to recommendations.[56] Ongoing assessments of older adults offer a proactive way that nurses can mitigate risks for complications such as high symptom burden, distress, and polypharmacy and/or identify those who require a referral to specialty palliative care.[58] Case Study 2 provides an illustration of Max, a patient who identified multiple concerns in the CGA over time. This regular assessment provided a mechanism to evaluate changes in Max's functioning and add new support services as needed throughout the trajectory of his cancer experience. Additional strategies for palliative management of the older adult will be discussed in detail in Chapter 71, "Palliative Care for Older Adults."

Social Well-being, Assessment Strategies, and Interventions in Patients Living with Cancer

The intrinsic social needs of people living with cancer can change over the course of their disease along with their life circumstances.[59] An individual's social well-being directly influences their perceived QOL.[59] For people living with cancer, their roles at work and with their family, their relationships, and their finances all influence their social well-being.[4]

Social determinants of health are complex and greatly influence social well-being and thus should be evaluated as part of an overall plan of care.[60] For individuals receiving cancer care, challenges in social well-being may become more problematic as they move beyond acute phases of treatment. Work- and insurance-related issues may arise as treatment plans are developed and modified. For example, a needs assessment conducted in a cross-sectional convenience sample of more than 1,000 cancer survivors found significantly moderate to high concern responses related to finances and medical costs.[59] These changes may require referrals to appropriate social services where assistance with financial, housing, and food insecurities may be provided. For these reasons, it is important for clinical teams and institutions to have well-established community partnerships with such services and be equipped to help patients and families navigate these resources. As treatment ends, the needs of families can also change, and the tasks of informal caregiving can shift once treatments are completed. Patients may be trying to gain back their independence and resume work while still processing the diagnosis and treatment events as well as trying to manage residual symptoms. It is also important to consider that patients may have moderate to high fears of recurrence or developing a second cancer, especially in the first 5 years post-treatment.[59] In the midst of these changes, caregivers may be uncertain of their roles and how to best help their loved one.[61] Case Study 2 identifies Max's concerns about his inability to socialize and his feelings of depression. Here, a referral to psychosocial support is warranted. Ultimately, nurses should include routine assessments of social well-being in the care of their patients.

Spiritual and Existential Concerns, Assessment Strategies, and Interventions in Patients Living with Cancer

Spirituality is an important aspect of QOL for many patients living with cancer.[62] Spirituality is described as how people find meaning and purpose in their lives and the degree of connectedness to themselves, others, the transcendent, or the sacred.[62] Spirituality is accepted to include three components: meaning, peace, and faith.[62,63] Examples of spiritual or existential concerns that arise for survivors include questioning the meaning of their illness or life purpose and dealing with grief, loss, anger, and survivor's guilt, as well as positive outcomes such as forgiveness and gratitude. People living with cancer have described the importance of spirituality in their ability to cope with their illness and strengthen their feelings of hope, meaning, and the purpose of their life.[67] People living with cancer describe treatment completion as a spiritual time, a time when they can reflect on what they have been through and the awareness of what it means for their future.[64] Research exploring spiritual well-being in women with ovarian cancer found that spirituality had a significant impact on positive well-being 1-year post-diagnosis, specifically related to lower rates of depression, anxiety, and total distress as well as greater feelings of peace.[65] In another study, the experience of peace as a part of spiritual growth in people living with cancer positively impacted well-being scores and highlights the importance of supporting spirituality in survivorship follow-up.[64] Nurses can help facilitate improved spiritual well-being, help patients with cancer find meaning in their experience, and promote inner peace by conducting a spiritual assessment and normalizing the importance of spiritual support.[62,66]

Identifying and managing spiritual well-being in people living with cancer can have positive effects on their QOL.[67] Current evidence suggests that patients would like providers to talk to them about their spiritual concerns.[68] It is important to recognize that even patients without a strong history of spiritual or religious affiliation may find spiritual support important or their interest renewed as they face cancer. Cultural identity influences individuals' behaviors and preferences and thus should be considered as nurses tailor approaches of spiritual support for their patients.[69] There are currently several tools available to help nurses initiate discussions about spirituality and assess spiritual well-being in individuals living with cancer. The FICA Spiritual History Tool (*Faith*, belief or meaning; *Importance* of spirituality; individual's spiritual *Community*; and interventions to *Address* spiritual needs) provides a clinically efficient method to screen for spiritual preferences and well-being of patients with cancer while also facilitating opportunities to provide patient-centered care.[68] The Functional Assessment of Chronic Illness Therapy-Spiritual Well-being (FACIT-SP) provides a 12-item tool to measure spirituality with three subscales: meaning, peace, and faith.[63] The NCCN Distress Thermometer is a single-item tool that asks patients to rate their general level of distress from 0 (no distress) to 10 (extreme distress) over the past week.[25] The accompanying Problem List has a section specific to Spiritual or Religious Concerns where patients can indicate concerns with their sense of meaning or purpose; changes in faith or beliefs; death, dying, or afterlife; conflict between beliefs and cancer treatments; relationship with the sacred; and ritual or dietary needs.[48] If spiritual well-being is a concern, referral to a chaplain or other spiritual counselor is needed for a comprehensive assessment of spiritual concerns to strengthen resources for coping. People living with cancer for whom spiritual practices are important can be encouraged to reconnect with religious leaders and community support to build positive coping strategies (mindfulness practices, meditation, meaning-oriented therapy).[68]

Palliative Care in Persons Living with Advanced Cancer

Individuals living with advanced cancer may be receiving continuous treatment to maintain stable disease or palliative chemotherapy for symptom control while also processing their own mortality.[70] Many challenges remain in how and when patients are referred to either palliative or survivorship care teams. Given the ongoing advances in cancer care, even patients with advanced cancer may live for years with their disease. Thus, palliative care teams are often managing a chronic disease while also supporting the complex psychosocial needs of patients living with a terminal diagnosis. In this setting, palliative care teams can focus on symptom management and advance care planning for people experiencing significant needs and an uncertain illness trajectory. With the introduction of new ongoing treatment options for advanced disease, understanding the needs of this population is essential and requires that palliative and survivorship teams work together to identify the unmet needs of these individuals and their families.[70] Nurses are instrumental in supporting this relationship between the teams.

Palliative Care Modalities for Individuals Living with Cancer

Palliative care modalities for people living with cancer are focused on the relief of distressing symptoms while attempting to anticipate, prevent, and/or reduce suffering for patients and their families.[21] Advanced symptom management requires specialty palliative care and an interdisciplinary team approach. Choosing necessary interventions is dependent on the person and patient- and family-specific goals of care.[21] Advanced palliative oncology often includes palliative surgery and palliative chemotherapy, which will be reviewed below.

Palliative Surgery

"Palliative surgery" is defined as any surgical interventions in patients with incurable malignancy; the treatment intent is focused on symptom management and QOL, rather than cure.[71] The field of palliative surgery is rapidly increasing and becoming recognized as a key component of comprehensive cancer care.[72] Current literature suggests that surgery with palliative intent significantly improves physical and functional well-being despite a complication rate of 35%.[72] Shared decision-making is an essential component of advanced palliative modalities.[73]

The decision-making process in palliative surgery should involve perspectives from the patient, family, and healthcare team while considering all dimensions of QOL. Potential benefits and harms, the complexity of the procedure, duration of hospitalization, recovery time, and anticipated disease progression should be discussed.[72] Other factors in decision-making include the social impact of symptoms, preservation of normal bodily functions (i.e., the desire to eat and drink), prolonged life expectancy, and maintenance of hope.[72] Nurses can help patients clarify their questions and concerns in these discussions. Ultimately, palliative surgery has an important role in the symptomatic support of many patients with advanced cancer but requires good communication so that patients and families can make truly informed decisions.

Palliative Chemotherapy

"Palliative chemotherapy," in its broadest sense, is the use of systemic antineoplastic agents in noncurative settings to optimize symptom control and maintain QOL.[74–76] Current literature strongly supports the role of palliative chemotherapy in managing troublesome symptoms and maintaining QOL in advanced pancreatic cancer, non-small-cell lung cancer, and breast cancer.[74] The decision to treat or not to treat is based on patient preferences and important prognostic indicators. Chemotherapy, even when palliative in intent, involves a commitment on the part of the patient and family to travel to the treating institution on a scheduled basis.[77] In addition to chemotherapy administration, repeated hospitalizations, venipunctures, cannulations, and assessments are inevitable consequences of palliative chemotherapy treatment that should be considered. Therefore, discussions with patients and their families regarding values, goals, and treatment preferences should be held when palliative chemotherapy is being considered and especially when considered closer to the end of life. Studies have shown that palliative chemotherapy initiated within 30 days of a patient's death is associated with poorer outcomes, such as reduced QOL, given increased need for hospital admissions, cardiopulmonary resuscitation, death in intensive care, and low rates of hospice use leading to high cost of care at the end of life.[78–80] In terms of key prognostic factors, performance status is key when making decisions regarding palliative chemotherapy.[78] A severely debilitated patient with a restricted performance status is more likely to sustain excessive chemotherapy toxicity. These factors need to be addressed with people living with cancer and their families in an effort to facilitate a collaborative decision-making process.

Nurses are often the first to recognize the need for dialogue between the healthcare team and the patient and family regarding treatment intent and prognosis.[79] Nurses can collaborate with palliative care and oncology services to ensure patients and their families remain well-informed and active participants in their plan of care.

Clinical Trial Participation and Advanced Cancer

Patients with advanced cancer are frequently offered the opportunity to enroll in a phase I clinical trial. It is important to note that phase I studies are designed to determine the toxicity and maximum tolerated dose of potential treatments, mostly for currently incurable cancers. These studies are not designed to have, and do not typically have, a therapeutic effect for participants. In fact, studies have shown that therapeutic effects from cancer investigational therapeutic agents occur in only 2%–4% of subjects enrolled in a phase I clinical trial.[78] The impact of clinical trial participation on physical symptoms related to advanced cancer is complex, and there is a paucity of data regarding the extent of these symptoms. Although the structure and requirement of a clinical trial protocol mandates the inclusion of a plan of action for unexpected physical symptoms, these plans often are focused on pharmacological interventions only. For example, if nausea and/or vomiting is an anticipated or expected side effect, a protocol of which antiemetic agents to use is written into the clinical trial protocol itself. However, the psychological and social distress that participants may experience is not included in the plan. Unfortunately, patients often have expectations for participation in clinical trials including a response to therapy, a reduction in symptoms, and improved and increased communication with their physicians.[13] The current evidence suggests that there is controversy about whether patients with advanced incurable cancers, when faced with decision-making regarding their plan of care, fully understand the choices that are available to them. Many patients report an overwhelming desire to fight their cancer at any cost and do not consider alternative approaches.[80,81] For example, patients who would qualify for hospice services as regulated by Medicare often have very little understanding of admission criteria and services rendered.[82,83] Ferrell et al.[84] completed a randomized controlled trial of patients with solid tumors beginning a phase I clinical trial. They tested a palliative care intervention versus usual care with the hypothesis that a palliative care intervention would improve psychological distress, QOL, symptom management, patient satisfaction, and resource utilization. This study was conducted in two cancer care settings and compared psychological distress, QOL, oncology care satisfaction, and communication between the intervention and control groups at baseline, 6 weeks, and 12 weeks after starting on the clinical trial. The palliative care intervention included an interdisciplinary team–created care plan and two teaching sessions by a nurse following a standardized workbook to improve referrals and communication and completion of evaluation tools FACT-G, Psychological Distress, and FAMCARE communications. Results of the study demonstrated a significant improvement in psychological distress but no significant difference in symptom burden in the palliative care intervention group versus the control group. This could be due to the increase of symptom burden experienced by participants in phase I trials with advancing disease and maximum tolerated doses. Findings from this innovative study indicate that phase I trial participants may benefit from palliative care interventions provided in a consistent manner. A clinical trial protocol generally does not include plans that specifically state the need for referrals to specialty services such as palliative care, and this is important to discuss with patients with incurable disease as they consider clinical trial participation. Offering palliative care referrals and interventions in the context of phase I clinical trials is an emerging and important area where nurses can advocate for patients and families.

The Role of Nurses in Palliative Care of People Living with Cancer

Nursing care is essential in the delivery of primary and specialty palliative care to patients living with cancer. For example, given that patients living with cancer often experience transitions in care, nurses play a vital role in ensuring continuity of care across settings such as the operating room, intensive care units, postoperative surgical units, outpatient clinics, infusions centers, and home care. Nurses also play a crucial role in assessing symptoms, side effects, and complications related to a patient's disease and treatment trajectory. Nurses should monitor and support patients' needs as treatment plans change while collaborating with the multidisciplinary teams. Finally, it is imperative that nurses maintain expert knowledge in pain and symptom management and clinical problem-solving to support the patients and families they care for. These competencies enhance quality of patient care, adherence to treatments, and patient and family satisfaction.

Conclusion

It is imperative to provide patient-centered care to people living with cancer; however, identifying patients who will benefit the most from palliative and supportive care interventions can be challenging. Referral criteria based on symptom burden, patient and caregiver needs, treatment type and intensity, and risk for recurrence are essential. Recognizing that the highest unmet need of many people living with cancer is related to psychosocial concerns can be a starting point for assessment and referrals that can improve care and support.[21] Recent studies of concurrent palliative care with standard oncologic care have demonstrated improved health-related QOL, reduction in symptom burden, and the potential to reduce aggressive treatment at the end of life while still showing improvement in survival.[14] Therefore, patients should have access to palliative care early in the decision-making process and throughout their treatment course.[4]

Ongoing assessment of symptoms and unmet needs is necessary to identify individuals living with cancer who are appropriate candidates for interdisciplinary and specialized palliative/supportive care services. A comprehensive assessment using validated tools should include physical, psychological, social, and spiritual domains and will provide a roadmap to guide supportive care interventions and referrals to appropriate services. Recognizing that people living with cancer and their families have different needs along the trajectory of survivorship from diagnosis to death supports the need for ongoing assessment. Importantly, people living with cancer who are in transition from active treatment or in remission may benefit from early referrals to rehabilitation services to manage symptoms and prevent long-term physical debilitation. Individuals living with metastatic or advanced disease recurrence with high symptom burden may benefit from focused assessment and interdisciplinary planning provided by specialty palliative care teams. Hospitals and community practices should assess their current resources and identify ways to improve or supplement the supportive care services available to their patients and families through strong community partnerships. Oncology nurses can help deliver primary palliative care and facilitate identifying when a referral to specialty palliative care is indicated.[85] Furthermore, additional training in palliative care for oncology nurses and clinicians will help to ensure that people living with cancer receive supportive care services especially in areas where palliative care teams are not readily available or are overburdened.

R

REFERENCES

1. MacDonald C, Theurer J, Doyle P. "Cured" but not "healed": the application of principles of palliative care to cancer survivorship. *Soc Sci Med.* 2021;(275):113802. https://doi.org/10.1016/j.socscimed.2021.113802.
2. Denlinger CS, Sanft T, Baker KS, et al. Survivorship, version 2.2018, NCCN clinical practice guidelines in oncology. *J Natl Compr Canc Netw.* 2018;16(10):1216–1247. https://doi.org/10.6004/jnccn.2018.0078.
3. Dy SM, Isenberg SR, Al Hamayel NA. Palliative care for cancer survivors. *Med Clin North Am.* 2017;101(6):1181–1196. https://doi.org/10.1016/j.mcna.2017.06.009.
4. Ferrell BR, Temel JS, Temin S, et al. Integration of palliative care into standard oncology care: American Society of Clinical Oncology clinical practice guideline update. *J Clin Oncol.* 2017;35(1):96–112. https://doi.org/10.1200/JCO.2016.70.1474.
5. Jacobs LA, Shulman LN. Follow-up care of cancer survivors: challenges and solutions. *Lancet Oncol.* 2017;18(1):e19–e29. https://doi.org/10.1016/S1470-2045(16)30386-2.
6. Mayer DK, Alfano CM. Personalized risk-stratified cancer follow-up care: its potential for healthier survivors, happier clinicians, and lower costs. *J Natl Cancer Inst.* 2019;111(5):442–448. https://doi.org/10.1093/jnci/djy232.
7. Jefford M, Howell D, Li Q, et al. Improved models of care for cancer survivors. *Lancet.* 2022;399(10334):1551–1560. https://doi.org/10.1016/S0140-6736(22)00306-3.
8. Tralongo P, McCabe MS, Surbone A. Challenge for cancer survivorship: improving care through categorization by risk. *J Clin Oncol.* 2017;35(30):3516–3517. https://doi.org/10.1200/JCO.2017.74.3450.
9. Hui D, Bruera E. Models of palliative care delivery for patients with cancer. *J Clin Oncol.* 2020;38(9):852–865. https://doi.org/10.1200/JCO.18.02123.
10. National Consensus Project for Quality Palliative Care. *Clinical practice guidelines for quality palliative care.* 4th ed. National Coalition for Hospice and Palliative Care; 2018.
11. Denlinger CS, Sanft T, Moslehi JJ, et al. NCCN guidelines insights: survivorship, version 2.2020. *J Natl Compr Canc Netw.* 2020;18(8):1016–1023. https://doi.org/10.6004/jnccn.2020.0037.
12. Hawley PH. The bow tie model of 21st century palliative care. *J Pain Symptom Manage.* 2014;47(1):e2–e5. https://doi.org/10.1016/j.jpainsymman.2013.10.009.
13. Ferrell BR, Paterson CL, Hughes MT, Chung V, Koczywas M, Smith TJ. Characteristics of participants enrolled onto a randomized controlled trial of palliative care for patients on phase I studies. *J Palliat Med.* 2017;20(12):1338–1344. https://doi.org/10.1089/jpm.2017.0158.
14. Temel JS, Greer JA, Muzikansky A, et al. Early palliative care for patients with metastatic non-small-cell lung cancer. *N Engl J Med.* 2010;363(8):733–742. https://doi.org/10.1056/NEJMoa1000678.
15. Osman H, Shrestha S, Temin S, et al. Palliative care in the global setting: ASCO resource-stratified practice guideline. *J Glob Oncol.* 2018;4:1–24. https://doi.org/10.1200/JGO.18.00026.
16. Smith SR, Zheng JY. The intersection of oncology prognosis and cancer rehabilitation. *Curr Phys Med Rehabil Rep.* 2017;5(1):46–54. https://doi.org/10.1007/s40141-017-0150-0.
17. Pop RS, Puia A, Mosoiu D. Factors influencing the quality of life of the primary caregiver of a palliative patient: narrative review. *J Palliat Med.* 2022;25(5):813–829. https://doi.org/10.1089/jpm.2021.0322.
18. Cowens-Alvarado R, Sharpe K, Pratt-Chapman M, et al. Advancing survivorship care through the National Cancer Survivorship Resource Center: developing American Cancer Society guidelines for primary care providers. *CA Cancer J Clin.* 2013;63(3):147–150.
19. Tevaarwerk A, Denlinger CS, Sanft T, et al. Survivorship, Version 1.2021. *J Natl Compr Canc Netw.* 2021;19(6):676–685. Published 2021 Jun 30. doi:10.6004/jnccn.2021.0028.
20. Kleckner AS, Magnuson A. The nutritional needs of older cancer survivors. *J Geriatr Oncol.* 2022;13(5):738–741. https://doi.org/10.1016/j.jgo.2021.12.007.
21. National Comprehensive Cancer Network. NCCN Clinical Practice Guidelines in Oncology—Palliative Care. Version 1.2022. Updated March 8, 2022. Accessed October 2, 2022, ///C:/Users/deconomou/Downloads/palliative.pdf.
22. Hall DL, Park ER, Cheung T, Davis RB, Yeh GY. A pilot mind-body resiliency intervention targeting fear of recurrence among cancer survivors. *J Psychosom Res.* 2020;137:110215.
23. Staff NP, Grisold A, Grisold W, Windebank AJ. Chemotherapy-induced peripheral neuropathy: a current review. *Ann Neurol.* 2017;81(6):772–781. https://doi.org/10.1002/ana.24951.
24. Tanay MA, Armes J. Lived experiences and support needs of women who developed chemotherapy-induced peripheral neuropathy following treatment for breast and ovarian cancer. *Eur J Cancer Care (Engl).* 2019;28(3):e13011. https://doi.org/10.1111/ecc.13011.
25. Miaskowski C, Mastick J, Paul SM, et al. Chemotherapy-induced neuropathy in cancer survivors. *J Pain Symptom Manage.* 2017;54(2):204–218.e2. https://doi.org/10.1016/j.jpainsymman.2016.12.342.
26. Winters-Stone KM, Horak F, Jacobs PG, et al. Falls, functioning, and disability among women with persistent symptoms of chemotherapy-induced peripheral neuropathy. *J Clin Oncol.* 2017;35(23):2604–2612. https://doi.org/10.1200/JCO.2016.71.3552.
27. Loprinzi CL, Lacchetti C, Bleeker J, et al. Prevention and management of chemotherapy-induced peripheral neuropathy in survivors of adult cancers: ASCO guideline update. *J Clin Oncol.* 2020;38(28):3325–3348.
28. Kleckner IR, Kamen C, Gewandter JS, et al. Effects of exercise during chemotherapy on chemotherapy-induced peripheral neuropathy: a multicenter, randomized controlled trial. *Support Care Cancer.* 2018;26(4):1019–1028.
29. Zimmer P, Trebing S, Timmers-Trebing U, et al. Eight-week, multimodal exercise counteracts a progress of chemotherapy-induced peripheral neuropathy and improves balance and strength in

metastasized colorectal cancer patients: a randomized controlled trial. *Support Care Cancer*. 2018;26(2):615–624.

30. Kneis S, Wehrle A, Müller J, et al. It's never too late—balance and endurance training improves functional performance, quality of life, and alleviates neuropathic symptoms in cancer survivors suffering from chemotherapy-induced peripheral neuropathy: results of a randomized controlled trial. *BMC Cancer*. 2019;19(1):414.
31. Chien T-J, Liu C-Y, Fang C-J, Kuo C-Y. The efficacy of acupuncture in chemotherapy-induced peripheral neuropathy: systematic review and meta-analysis. *Integr Cancer Ther*. 2019;18:1534735419886662.
32. Guo S, Han W, Wang P, Wang X, Fang X. Effects of exercise on chemotherapy-induced peripheral neuropathy in cancer patients: a systematic review and meta-analysis. *J Cancer Surviv*. 2023;17(2):318–331.
33. Ren X, Boriero D, Chaiswing L, Bondada S, St Clair DK, Butterfield DA. Plausible biochemical mechanisms of chemotherapy-induced cognitive impairment ("chemobrain"), a condition that significantly impairs the quality of life of many cancer survivors. *Biochim Biophys Acta Mol Basis Dis*2019;1865(6):1088–1097. https://doi.org/10.1016/j.bbadis.2019.02.007.
34. Padgett LS, Van Dyk K, Kelly NC, Newman R, Hite S, Asher A. Addressing cancer-related cognitive impairment in cancer survivorship. *Oncol Issues*. 2020;35(1):52–57. https://doi.org/10.1080/10463356.2020.1692601.
35. Allen DH, Myers JS, Jansen CE, Merriman JD, Von Ah D. Assessment and management of cancer- and cancer treatment-related cognitive impairment. *J Nurse Pract*. 2018;14(4):217–224.e5. https://doi.org/10.1016/j.nurpra.2017.11.026.
36. Lange M, Joly F, Vardy J, et al. Cancer-related cognitive impairment: an update on state of the art, detection, and management strategies in cancer survivors. *Ann Oncol*. 2019;30(12):1925–1940. https://doi.org/10.1093/annonc/mdz410.
37. Pendergrass JC, Targum SD, Harrison JE. Cognitive impairment associated with cancer: a brief review. *Innov Clin Neurosci*. 2018;15(1–2):36–44.
38. Wefel JS, Vardy J, Ahles T, Schagen SB. International Cognition and Cancer Task Force recommendations to harmonise studies of cognitive function in patients with cancer. *Lancet Oncol*. 2011;12(7):703–708. https://doi.org/10.1016/S1470-2045(10)70294-1.
39. Hardy SJ, Krull KR, Wefel JS, Janelsins M. Cognitive changes in cancer survivors. *Am Soc Clin Oncol Educ Book*. 2018;38:795–806. https://doi.org/10.1200/EDBK_201179.
40. Rambeau A, Beauplet B, Laviec H, et al. Prospective comparison of the Montreal Cognitive Assessment (MoCA) and the Mini Mental State Examination (MMSE) in geriatric oncology. *J Geriatr Oncol*. 2019;10(2):235–240.
41. Van Dyk K, Crespi CM, Petersen L, Ganz PA. Identifying cancer-related cognitive impairment using the FACT-Cog perceived cognitive impairment. *JNCI Cancer Spectr*. 2020;4(1):pkz099. https://doi.org/10.1093/jncics/pkz099
42. Vardy JL, Bray VJ, Dhillon HM. Cancer-induced cognitive impairment: practical solutions to reduce and manage the challenge. *Future Oncol*. 2017;13(9):767–771. https://doi.org/10.2217/fon-2017-0027.
43. Thong MSY, van Noorden CJF, Steindorf K, Arndt V. Cancer-related fatigue: causes and current treatment options. *Curr Treat Options Oncol*. 2020;21(2):17. https://doi.org/10.1007/s11864-020-0707-5.
44. Bevilacqua LA, Dulak D, Schofield E, et al. Prevalence and predictors of depression, pain, and fatigue in older- versus younger-adult cancer survivors. *Psychooncology*. 2018;27(3):900–907.
45. Mendoza TR, Wang XS, Cleeland CS, et al. The rapid assessment of fatigue severity in cancer patients: use of the Brief Fatigue Inventory. *Cancer*. 1999;85(5):1186–1196.
46. Bower JE, Bak K, Berger A, et al. Screening, assessment, and management of fatigue in adult survivors of cancer: an American Society of Clinical Oncology clinical practice guideline adaptation. *J Clin Oncol*. 2014;32(17):1840–1850. https://doi.org/10.1200/jco.2013.53.4495.
47. Mock V, Atkinson A, Barsevick A, et al. NCCN practice guidelines for cancer-related fatigue. *Oncology (Williston Park)*. 2000;14(11A):151–161.
48. Riba MB, Donovan KA, Ahmed K, et al. NCCN Guidelines® insights: distress management, version 2.2023: featured updates to the NCCN Guidelines. *Journal of the National Comprehensive Cancer Network*. 2023;21(5):450–457.
49. Yi JC, Syrjala KL. Anxiety and depression in cancer survivors. *Med Clin North Am*. 2017;101(6):1099–1113. https://doi.org/10.1016/j.mcna.2017.06.005.
50. Thewes B, Husson O, Poort H, et al. Fear of cancer recurrence in an era of personalized medicine. *J Clin Oncol*. 2017;35(29):3275–3278.
51. Snaith RP, Zigmond AS. The Hospital Anxiety and Depression Scale. *Br Med J (Clin Res Ed)*. 1986;292(6516):344. https://doi.org/10.1136/bmj.292.6516.344.
52. Kroenke K, Spitzer RL, Williams JB, Lowe B. An ultra-brief screening scale for anxiety and depression: the PHQ-4. *Psychosomatics*. 2009;50(6):613–621. https://doi.org/10.1176/appi.psy.50.6.613.
53. Soto-Perez-de-Celis E, Li D, Yuan Y, Lau YM, Hurria A. Functional versus chronological age: geriatric assessments to guide decision making in older patients with cancer. *Lancet Oncol*. 2018;19(6):e305–e316.
54. Cancer and Aging Research Group. Accessed October 2, 2022. http://www.mycarg.org/.
55. Shapiro CL. Cancer survivorship. *N Engl J Med*. 2018;379(25):2438–2450. https://doi.org/10.1056/NEJMra1712502.
56. Overcash J, Momeyer MA. Comprehensive geriatric assessment and caring for the older person with cancer. *Semin Oncol Nurs*. 2017;33(4):440–448. https://doi.org/10.1016/j.soncn.2017.08.006.
57. Bellera CA, Rainfray M, Mathoulin-Pelissier S, et al. Screening older cancer patients: first evaluation of the G-8 geriatric screening tool. *Ann Oncol*. 2012;23(8):2166–2172. https://doi.org/10.1093/annonc/mdr587.
58. Association of Community Cancer Centers. *Practical Application of Geriatric Assessment: A How-to Guide for the Multidisciplinary Care Team*. 2021. https://www.accc-cancer.org/docs/projects/geriatric-patients-with-cancer/practical-application-of-geriatric assessment_a-how-to-guide.pdf?
59. Mazanec S, Gallagher P, Rowehl Miano W, Sattar A, Daly B. Comprehensive assessment of cancer survivors' concerns to inform program development. *J Community Support Oncol*. 2017;15(3):155–162.
60. Alcaraz KI, Wiedt TL, Daniels EC, Yabroff KR, Guerra CE, Wender RC. Understanding and addressing social determinants to advance cancer health equity in the United States: a blueprint for practice, research, and policy. *CA Cancer J Clin*. 2020;70(1):31–46.
61. Kim Y, Carver CS, Ting A. Family Caregivers' Unmet Needs in Long-Term Cancer Survivorship. Elsevier; 2019.
62. Puchalski CM, King SD, Ferrell BR. Spiritual considerations. *Hematol Oncol Clin*. 2018;32(3):505–517.
63. Schultz M, Meged-Book T, Mashiach T, Bar-Sela G. Distinguishing between spiritual distress, general distress, spiritual well-being,

and spiritual pain among cancer patients during oncology treatment. *J Pain Symptom Manage*. 2017;54(1):66–73.

64. Burney S. Psychological issues in cancer survivorship. *Climacteric*. 2019;22(6):584–588.
65. Davis LZ, Cuneo M, Thaker PH, Goodheart MJ, Bender D, Lutgendorf SK. Changes in spiritual well-being and psychological outcomes in ovarian cancer survivors. *Psychooncology*. 2018;27(2):477–483. https://doi.org/10.1002/pon.4485.
66. Minton ME, Isaacson MJ, Varilek BM, Stadick JL, O'Connell-Persaud S. A willingness to go there: nurses and spiritual care. *J Clin Nurs*. 2018;27(1–2):173–181. https://doi.org/10.1111/jocn.13867.
67. Nolan TS, Browning K, Vo JB, Meadows RJ, Paxton RJ. CE: Assessing and managing spiritual distress in cancer survivorship. *Am J Nurs*. 2020;120(1):40–47.
68. Puchalski C. Spiritual care in health care: guideline, models, spiritual assessment and the use of the ©FICA Spiritual History Tool. In: Bussing A, ed. *Spiritual Needs in Research and Practice*. Springer; 2021:27–45.
69. Gudenkauf LM, Clark MM, Novotny PJ, et al. Spirituality and emotional distress among lung cancer survivors. *Clin Lung Cancer*. 2019;20(6):e661–e666.
70. Cottingham AH, Cripe LD, Rand KL, Frankel RM. "My future is now": a qualitative study of persons living with advanced cancer. *Am J Hosp Palliat Med*. 2018;35(4):640–646.
71. Lilley EJ, Cooper Z, Schwarze ML, Mosenthal AC. Palliative care in surgery: defining the research priorities. *Ann Surg*. 2018;267(1):66–72. https://doi.org/10.1097/SLA.0000000000002253.
72. Cohen JT, Miner TJ. Patient selection in palliative surgery: defining value. *J Surg Oncol*. 2019;120(1):35–44.
73. Roodbeen R, Vreke A, Boland G, et al. Communication and shared decision-making with patients with limited health literacy; helpful strategies, barriers and suggestions for improvement reported by hospital-based palliative care providers. *PLoS One*. 2020;15(6):e0234926.
74. Wulff-Burchfield E, Spoozak L, Finlay E. Palliative chemotherapy and the surgical oncologist. *Surg Oncol Clin*. 2021;30(3):545–561.
75. Zhang Z, Chen M-L, Gu X-L, Liu M-H, Zhao W-W, Cheng W-W. Palliative chemotherapy near the end of life in oncology patients. *Am J Hosp Palliat Med*. 2018;35(9):1215–1220.
76. Akhlaghi E, Lehto RH, Torabikhah M, et al. Chemotherapy use and quality of life in cancer patients at the end of life: an integrative review. *Health Qual Life Outcomes*. 2020;18(1):332. https://doi.org/10.1186/s12955-020-01580-0.
77. Wright AA, Keating NL, Ayanian JZ, et al. Family perspectives on aggressive cancer care near the end of life. *JAMA*. 2016;315(3):284–292. https://doi.org/10.1001/jama.2015.18604.
78. Markman M. Why should phase 1 cancer trial participation and optimal end-of-life care be incompatible? *Oncology*. 2017;92(1):1–2. https://doi.org/10.1159/000452161.
79. Ferrell B, Buller H, Paice J, Anderson W, Donesky D. End-of-Life Nursing and Education Consortium communication curriculum for interdisciplinary palliative care teams. *J Palliat Med*. 2019;22(9):1082–1091.
80. Economou D, Walshe C, Brearley SG. Exploring the experience of recurrence with advanced cancer for people who perceived themselves to be cancer free: a grounded theory study. *Support Care Cancer*. 2021;29(7):3885–3894.
81. Hurd TC, Kaplan CD, Cook ED, et al. Building trust and diversity in patient-centered oncology clinical trials: an integrated model. *Clin Trials*. 2017;14(2):170–179. https://doi.org/10.1177/1740774516688860.
82. Mols F, Tomalin B, Pearce A, Kaambwa B, Koczwara B. Financial toxicity and employment status in cancer survivors. A systematic literature review. *Support Care Cancer*. 2020;28(12):5693–5708.
83. Pearce A, Tomalin B, Kaambwa B, et al. Financial toxicity is more than costs of care: the relationship between employment and financial toxicity in long-term cancer survivors. *J Cancer Surviv*. 2019;13(1):10–20.
84. Ferrell B, Chung V, Hughes MT, et al. A palliative care intervention for patients on phase 1 studies. *J Palliat Med*. 2021;24(6):846–856. https://doi.org/10.1089/jpm.2020.0597.
85. Ferrell BR, Paice JA, Coyne PJ, et al. Outcomes of a national training curriculum to advance generalist level palliative care. *J Palliat Med*. 2023;26(2):228–234.

PART VI
Care Near the End of Life

53

Urgent Syndromes at the End of Life*

Christina Feindt and Kelli Gershon

Key Points

- Numerous urgent syndromes can occur in the course of advanced disease, seriously affecting quality of life.
- Urgent syndromes include superior vena cava obstruction, pleural effusion, hemoptysis, spinal cord compression, hypercalcemia, pathological fractures, and bowel obstructions.
- Astute assessment and management skills are crucial to diminish distress and suffering for patients and their loved ones.

Introduction

The end of life is a fragile and significant time; palliative care can diminish distress and suffering for both the patient and the family. This chapter will discuss the following syndromes that may occur urgently at the end of life: superior vena cava obstruction (SVCO), pleural effusion (PE), hemoptysis, spinal cord compression (SCC), hypercalcemia, pathological fractures, and bowel obstructions.

Superior Vena Cava Obstruction

Case Study: A Patient with SVCO

Mr. J, a 57-year-old man, went to the emergency department 1 week ago with shortness of breath and was subsequently diagnosed with non-small-cell lung cancer. Before his first oncologist appointment, his wife noticed that his shortness of breath was increasing and his face was swelling. She called the new oncologist, who advised that Mr. J report to the nearest hospital.

Questions to Consider:

1. Is diagnostic imaging warranted?
2. What is the best treatment option for Mr. J?

Description

SVCO is defined as obstructed blood flow through the superior vena cava (SVC; mechanical), which is part of the venous system responsible for draining the upper extremities and head into the right atrium (see Box 53.1). The severity depends on the cause of the obstruction, which generally develops gradually but can be emergent when SVCO occurs.[1]

Approximately 70% of cases are related to malignancy, while 30% are benign and include device-related causes.[2] Eighty percent of all tumors and infections that induce SVCO occur in the right thoracic region, and SVCO occurs in 5%–10% of patients with infectious damage to a tissue or organ in this region. The most harmful form of SVCO occurs in people aged 40–60 years, with greater risk among males because of their higher rates of smoking-related lung cancer. Benign cases occur in individuals aged 30–40 years, but there are no gender-based differences in frequency. Because incidence rates of lung cancer and lymphoma differ according to race, the distribution of SVCO within the population depends on the prevalence of SVCO-inducing cancers in these communities.[3]

Pathophysiology

Tumor infiltration and thrombosis formation are the primary causes of SVCO. Compression of the SVC can result from intrinsic or extrinsic causes.[4] As a growing tumor occupies thoracic space, pressure inside the SVC increases from 2–8 mm Hg to 20–30 mm Hg. This leads to facial swelling, and the enlargement of the neck and

Box 53.1 Symptoms of Superior Vena Cava Obstruction

- The primary causes of superior vena cava obstruction (SVCO) are lung cancer, lymphomas, thrombus, and stenosis secondary to venous lines.
- Facial and neck swelling commonly present with episodes of shortness of breath.
- Chest X-ray and computed tomography (CT) are used to identify the extent of obstruction, damage, and assist in the development of a treatment plan for SVCO.
- The SVCS grading system and management algorithm are available to guide clinical decisions.

* Acknowledgement to prior authors and content creator, Quinten Robertson.

chest wall become visible. In response to SVC malfunction, the body uses collateral veins located in the thoracic, esophageal, and paraspinal regions—such as the inferior vena cava and the azygos vein—and the patient may experience difficulty breathing or eating. When the collateral veins cannot accommodate the excess pressure, the frequency of the symptoms increases, and the patient may die.[5]

Signs and Symptoms

Signs and symptoms of SVCO depend on the acuity and degree of obstruction. The most notable symptoms are swelling of the nose, face, neck, and chest wall, especially in the morning hours after the patient has been recumbent. The swelling gradually subsides but may remain visible in prolonged cases. Dyspnea—especially when sleeping—hoarseness, constant coughing, lethargy, and head fullness are symptoms of SVCO that may lead to exhaustion. Other clinical signs include facial swelling and abnormally rapid breathing when lying down or bending forward.[6]

Diagnostic Procedures

History and physical examination are adequate to diagnose SVCO. However, diagnostic imaging may be warranted to provide a more subtle assessment of the patient's condition. Initially, chest radiography is performed to reveal any inflammation or added mass in the right thoracic region, which could be the first sign of SVCO.[3] Computed tomography (CT) scan can reveal the exact location of the blockage, whether it is the result of a thrombosis or tumor, and the extent of cavity damage to determine whether thoracic surgery is necessary.[7]

Magnetic resonance imaging (MRI) is often preferred for cancer patients with contrast allergies or renal failure. This approach can show damaged tissue in greater detail and offer different views of the infected area while allowing direct visualization of blood flow to assess pressure inside the SVC. Venography, the most conclusive SVCO diagnostic tool, reveals the full extent of vena cava occlusion and is necessary during preparation for corrective surgery.[8] Contrast venography is the most reliable technique for diagnosis of malignant SVCO; however, if the primary collateral vein—the inferior vena cava—malfunctions due to pressure or tumor necrosis and progresses to venous compression, a radionuclide technetium-99m venography is the preferred alternative.[9]

Treatment

The treatment approach to SVCO is multidisciplinary and may include chemotherapy with or without radiation therapy, surgical bypass, angioplasty, stenting, and catheter-based thrombus removal.

SVC Stenting

Stenting has become the standard of care for SVCO for both benign and malignant origins.[10] Venography is essential during stent placement to determine the necessary length and number of stents to open the obstruction.[11] Stent placement has reportedly produced acceptable outcomes in the management of SVCO.[12] A minor complication associated with endovascular intervention is hematoma at the entry site; major complications may include stent migration, bleeding, and pericardial tamponade.[11]

Thrombolytic Therapies

When a thrombus is identified as the cause of mechanical SVCO, thrombolytic therapies are preferred for medical management to limit thrombus extension. The patient may present with acute symptoms of SVCO, warranting delivery of thrombolytic agents via catheter to remove the thrombus.[11] Thrombolytic therapy should be initiated within 2–5 days of the initial symptoms for optimal outcomes and may not be effective if initiated after the 10th day.[11] Tissue plasminogen activator is the most commonly used thrombolytic medication.

Box 53.2 Superior Vena Cava Obstruction Grading System

- Grade: 0–5
- Category: Asymptomatic to life-threatening
- Definition: Absence of symptoms to death

Source: Reference 2.

Drug Therapy

Though lacking evidence-based research to support their effectiveness, short-term administration of anti-inflammatory steroids such as dexamethasone has been used to treat SVCO.[13] Diuretics may also be used despite lack of evidence supporting their effectiveness.[13]

Medical Management

Clinicians first work to identify the cause of SVCO, which is most often related to cancer or chronic illness. The care team then works to reduce the symptoms[14]; for example, elevating the patient's head may diminish facial swelling. In SVCO resulting from cancers such as non-small-cell lung cancer, the histology of the primary malignant condition is then determined. Radiation therapy may be used when a tumor is the cause of the obstruction. According to Nickloes, chemotherapy is an alternative to radiation therapy for patients with chemotherapy-sensitive tumors.[3]

The increased predominance of SVCO caused by chronic diseases has prompted development of new treatment methods. Endovascular treatment that is effective but less invasive has since become the preferred method for managing SVCO patients in palliative care.[15] The severity of SVC syndrome based on clinical presentation, developed by Yu et al., is a useful tool to guide clinical decision-making in the medical management of SVCO patients.[16]

Nursing Management

Nurses should employ palliative techniques to relieve pain and offer comfort to SVCO patients in tandem with medical management. Nursing assessment using the SVCO grading system is essential to identify clinical manifestations of SVCO (see Box 53.2).

It is vital for nurses to build relationships with the patient and their family to reduce stress and improve the patient's functional status. Nurses should also clarify the goals of treatment to ensure they are consistent with the patient's wishes. In addition, nurses should assess the patient's unique coping needs and provide necessary support, ensuring regular therapy tailored for each patient.[17]

Pleural Effusion

Case Study: A Patient with PE

Mr. S, a 39-year-old geologist who worked as an executive with a large oil and gas company, was diagnosed with Stage III Hodgkin's lymphoma approximately 4 months ago. He started chemotherapy treatment and completed a positron emission tomography (PET) scan 2 weeks later. While at work last week, he noticed that he was having trouble breathing. The shortness of breath was mild at first but gradually intensified until he began to sleep in a recliner because he was unable to lay flat at night. Eventually, the shortness of breath became so severe that Mr. S went to the emergency room, where clinicians detected decreased breath sounds and a chest X-ray confirmed a large PE on the left side.

Questions to Consider:

1. Is PE common with Hodgkin's lymphoma? What other diagnoses frequently develop PEs?
2. Does the PE change Mr. S's prognosis?
3. What is the best treatment option given Mr. S's diagnosis?

Description

PE occurs when too much fluid collects in the pleural space. It is commonly known as "water on the lungs" and is characterized by shortness of breath, chest pain, gastric discomfort, and cough. There are two types of PE: transudative and exudative. A *transudate* is a clear fluid similar to blood serum that forms when the forces that normally produce and remove pleural fluid at the same rate are out of balance, primarily in patients with heart failure, liver disease, or nephrotic syndrome. An *exudate* is cloudy fluid containing cells and large amounts of protein that results from disease in the pleura itself. For example, cancer, infection, and pulmonary embolism would cause exudate pleural effusions.[18]

Epidemiology

Congestive heart failure, cancer, pneumonia, and pulmonary embolism cause the most PEs.[18] More than 175,000 individuals in the United States are affected by malignant PE,[19] most commonly secondary to lung cancer. Approximately 15% of lung cancer patients have malignant PE at diagnosis, but 50% of patients with disseminated lung cancer ultimately develop the condition. Breast cancer is the second most frequent cause of malignant PE; however, it is rare among presenting patients but generally occurs with progressive disease. Hematological malignances (lymphomas and leukemia) are the third most frequent cause of malignant PE.[20] The condition, which is generally associated with widespread disease, has a poor clinical prognosis—particularly in patients with malignancy.[21] Most patients with malignant PE are appropriate candidates for hospice care.

Pathophysiology

Each lung is covered with a serous membrane called the *pleura*, forming a closed cavity between the pleura and the lung surface. The normal pleural space contains approximately 10 mL of fluid, representing a balance between (1) hydrostatic and oncotic forces in the visceral and parietal pleural capillaries and (2) persistent sulcal lymphatic drainage. Osmotic and hydrostatic pressures act to maintain equilibrium between absorption and production of fluid in the pleural space. When this equilibrium is disturbed, fluid can accumulate in the pleural cavity.[22]

Pulmonary effusion is attributed to altered permeability of the pleural membranes caused by multiple conditions including inflammation, malignancy, and pulmonary embolism. In patients with malignancies, it is not uncommon to have multiple simultaneous causes of PE. Hypoalbuminemia can reduce intravascular oncotic pressure and increased capillary permeability, or vascular disruption can result from trauma, malignancy, inflammation, infection, or pulmonary infarction.[22]

Signs and Symptoms

Dyspnea, which may develop suddenly or gradually depending upon how rapidly the fluid accumulates, is the most common symptom of PE and often results in increased anxiety. If the effusion is free-flowing, dyspnea will become more severe while the patient is fully prone; however, shortness of breath will remain constant regardless of the patient's position if the effusion is loculated. A large effusion will cause sudden and severe shortness of breath, whereas onset is more gradual with a small and slowly developing effusion. Patients may experience pleural pain, an intense pain in the chest area that is sometimes confused with cardiac pain.

The patient's inability to expand the lung leads initially to reports of exertional dyspnea. As the effusion volume increases, resting dyspnea, orthopnea, and tachypnea develop. The patient may describe a dry, nonproductive cough and a heaviness or aching pain—often described as dull or pleuritic—in the chest. Physical examination commonly reveals increased respiratory rate and use of accessory muscles for breathing. Auscultation indicates decreased breath sounds on the affected side, and percussion shows dullness in the affected lung field. A large effusion may cause tracheal deviation and mediastinal shift to the affected side.

Diagnostic Procedures

When PE is expected a standard anteroposterior and lateral chest radiography should be performed. A fluid volume of 200 mL will be evident on an anteroposterior film, and costophrenic angle blunting can be seen on a lateral film at an accumulation of only 50 mL.[23] A chest X-ray will reveal whether the fluid is free-flowing versus loculated, which will determine the preferred treatment plan. Ultrasonography is more accurate than auscultation or chest radiography in detecting PE and is more sensitive than CT at detecting pleural fluid separations.[23] CT scanning produces cross-sectional images that are useful for evaluation of complex cases where routine radiography or ultrasonography cannot provide a conclusive assessment. CT scanning can show pleural or lung masses, adenopathy, pulmonary abnormalities such as infiltrates or atelectasis, or distant disease.

Treatment

Medical management of malignant PE depends on multiple factors, including the history of the primary tumor, prior patient history and response to therapy, extent of disease and overall medical condition, goals of care, and severity of symptom distress. It is important to evaluate the underlying cause of the PE and determine whether it can be treated to prevent further accumulation of fluid. This treatment might include systemic therapy (e.g., chemotherapy, antibiotics), hormonal therapy, or radiation therapy. Symptomatic management includes the use of opioids to manage pain and dyspnea, as well as anxiolytics to control concomitant anxiety. The most common treatments for PE include (1) observation to see how it responds to treatment of the underlying disease, (2) thoracentesis,

(3) pleurodesis, (4) indwelling pleural catheter placement, and (5) palliation of symptoms.[24]

Thoracentesis

Thoracentesis is indicated for all patients with more than a minimal PE (i.e., >1 cm in height on lateral decubitus radiography, ultrasonography, or CT scanning) of unknown origin. Larger effusions (>5 cm) on lateral radiography in patients with pneumonia warrant diagnostic aspiration because parapneumonic effusions and empyema can cause nonresponse to treatment. Guidelines recommend that, when possible, thoracentesis is be performed with ultrasound guidance; this increases the likelihood of successful aspiration and decreases the risk of organ puncture.[23]

Thoracentesis has been shown to relieve dyspnea associated with large PEs. Although thoracentesis may produce rapid relief of symptoms, fluid reaccumulates quickly—usually within 3–4 days—and within 30 days in 97% of patients.[25] When fluid reaccumulates, it must be decided whether the risks of repeated thoracentesis outweigh the benefit. Risks include empyema, pneumothorax, unexpandable lung from inadequate drainage and/or loculated fluid, and possible increasing tissue malnutrition from the removal of the protein-rich effusion fluid. If the risks outweigh the benefit, alternative treatments including pleurodesis, pleurectomy, or indwelling catheter must be considered.

Pleurodesis

Pleurodesis is not recommended in patients who have a life expectancy of less than 3 months.[26] Palliative treatment, especially for those with a life expectancy of months rather than weeks, is best accomplished by thoracentesis or pleural catheter placement. The goal of pleurodesis is to drain the pleural cavity completely, expand the lung fully, and instill a chemical agent into the pleural cavity. With a large effusion, only 1,000–1,500 mL should be drained initially to avoid re-expansion pulmonary edema from rapid draining of large volumes as in some cases large hydropneumothorax has resulted from rapid evacuation of large PE fluid volumes.[21]

After placement, the chest tube is connected to a closed-drainage device. To prevent re-expansion pulmonary edema, water-seal drainage and intermittent tube clamping should be used to allow fluid to drain slowly. Complications of chest tube placement include bleeding and development of pneumothorax, which results from rapid fluid removal in patients with an underlying noncompliant lung. The procedure causes pain and requires aggressive pain management with opioids and possible sedation.

The purpose of pleurodesis is to administer agents that cause inflammation and subsequent fibrosis into the pleural cavity to produce long-term adhesion of the visceral and parietal pleural surfaces to prevent reaccumulation of pleural fluid. Sclerosing agents or chemical irritants used to treat malignant PE include talc, tetracycline, minocycline, doxycycline, silver nitrate, bleomycin, cisplatin, recombinant adenoviral human p53, and human tumor necrosis factor (see Table 53.1).[2,28]

For patients experiencing symptomatic malignant pleural effusions PEs, with a confirmed or likely expandable lung, and who have not previously received definitive therapy, chemical pleurodesis can be employed as a primary pleural intervention. Patients may undergo talc pleurodesis, using either talc poudrage or talc slurry, as a definitive approach for managing the condition. [27]

Patients with symptomatic malignant PEs and expandable lung may undergo talc pleurodesis with talc poudrage or talc slurry.[27]

Pleurectomy

Pleurectomy, a surgical stripping of the parietal pleura, is a possible treatment for malignant PE, but this surgery lacks evidence as treatment in comparison to pluerodesis.[21] Video-assisted thoracoscopy and pleurectomy have been performed successfully, but this intervention is generally inappropriate for the palliative care patient at the end of life.

Indwelling Pleural Catheters

Patients with symptomatic, unilateral effusions who have a reasonable performance status may benefit from indwelling pleural catheters, which can be placed under local anesthesia. It has been suggested that tunneled pleural catheters may provide better long-term drainage and symptom control of malignant PE.[21] The tunneled catheter is a small-bore tube attached to a gravity drainage bag or vacuum drainage. Most patients and families can be taught to drain the effusion effectively with few side effects. Rare complications include tumor seeding, obstruction, infection, cellulitis of the tract site, and pain during drainage. This treatment offers the potential for better quality of life (QOL) and reduction of overall healthcare costs.[30]

Nursing Management

Nursing management includes symptom control, education, and communication regarding goals of care. Symptoms most commonly associated with PE are dyspnea, pain, and anxiety, which are treated aggressively with medications, education, and nonpharmacological techniques. Nurses should educate patients and their families about each

Table 53.1 Agents used to treat malignant plural effusion

Agent	Characteristics
Talc	Trilayered, magnesium sheet silicate Most effective and most commonly used
Minocycline and doxycycline	Tetracycline derivatives Less effective than talc
Silver nitrate	Tetracycline derivatives Equal effectiveness to talc
Bleomycin	Less commonly used because of systemic toxicity and cost
Cisplatin	Widely used in patients with lung cancer
Recombinant adenoviral human p53	Higher short-term response rate and fewer side effects than cisplatin Less effective but fewer side effects than talc

procedure, including its purpose, how it is carried out, how pain will be addressed, home care techniques, and possible side effects or complications. A variety of nonpharmacological techniques can be used to relieve dyspnea and pain, including comfortably positioning the patient, using relaxation techniques, and providing oxygenation as appropriate.

Education is a large component of the nursing role in managing patients with PE, including instruction on treatment options and on self-management of interventions. For example, if the patient has a tunneled catheter, the family must recognize the importance of monitoring drainage volume to detect possible spontaneous pleurodesis, which can be identified through increased drainage output over time. Because PE and its associated symptoms are distressing to patients and family members, nurses should encourage open communication about their distress, concerns about advancing disease, and goals of care.

Hemoptysis

Case Study: A Patient with Hemoptysis

Ms. C, a 60-year-old retired waitress, was diagnosed with small-cell lung cancer 3 months ago. Initially hesitant to pursue treatment, she consulted with her family and decided to seek chemotherapy and radiation therapy. While at the clinic for treatment, Ms. C told the oncology nurse that she was concerned because she had been coughing up blood 3–4 days per week for about 2 weeks.

Questions to Consider:

1. What assessment criteria are critical to obtain in Ms. C's case?
2. What are three differential diagnoses to consider?
3. What diagnostic imaging should be ordered for Ms. C?

Hemoptysis, or expectoration of blood, can present in a broad range of conditions and manifestations. The blood can range from small streaks in the sputum from the lungs to a larger volume of blood without any sputum. Hemoptysis can also result from bleeding outside the lungs and the airways.[31] Blood-tinged sputum mixed with blood suggests lung disease; *pseudohemoptysis* is coughing up blood that does not originate from the lungs.[32]

Epidemiology

The cause of hemoptysis varies, with half of cases having unknown etiology. The most common etiologies stem from infectious and inflammatory airway diseases (25.8%) and cancer (17.4%).[33] Blood volume loss from hemoptysis can be minimal to massive or even life-threatening. While the literature is inconsistent regarding volumes of massive hemoptysis, studies identify different volume thresholds ranging from 100 to 1,000 mL over a 24-hour period. Because of this inconsistency, it is recommended to measure blood loss on admission.[34] Mortality risk among patients with massive hemoptysis is greater than 80% without a timely intervention.[34]

Pathophysiology

The pulmonary and bronchial arteries are the two systems of blood supply in the lungs. The pulmonary artery facilitates gas exchange at low pressure, while the bronchial arteries are part of the systemic blood circulation at much higher pressure. The high pressure is partly responsible for the bronchial arteries being the primary source of hemoptysis, although non-bronchial arteries also contribute to the condition. When an infection such as bronchitis increases pulmonary circulation, the increased pressure results in bursting of the thin walls, causing overflow of blood into the alveoli and bronchi, leading to hemoptysis. Similarly, chronic illnesses such as lung cancer can cause blood overflow when a growing tumor or the spread of malignant cells promotes the growth of fragile collateral vessels or the remodeling of other arteries. Lung cancer patients account for 7%–10% of hemoptysis cases.[35] The blood vessels are thin-walled and prone to bursting from the slightest provocation, such as an acute case of vomiting. The bronchial arteries account for 90% of bleeding instances, while the pulmonary artery causes only 5% of cases.[36] The remaining episodes result from the non-bronchial systemic arteries. When blood overflows, it searches for an opening, which accounts for blood in the sputum when coughing or when vomiting.

Signs and Symptoms

The signs and symptoms of hemoptysis are specific to the area of possible involvement. It is difficult to predict the severity and course of hemoptysis[32]; therefore, careful assessment is key. Cardiac signs and symptoms include tachycardia, heart murmur, chest pains, and fixed split S2. Respiratory signs and symptoms include tachypnea, voice hoarseness, wheezing, pursed lip breathing, decreased lung sounds, and shortness of breath.[37] The patient may also present with fever, cachexia, or nausea.

Differential diagnoses are formulated based on assessment findings. For example, findings for bronchogenic tumors may include night sweats, weight loss, and history of heavy smoking. Findings significant to pneumonia are fever, productive cough, decreased breath sounds, and pleuritic chest pain.[37] Because the causes for hemoptysis can be unclear, a thorough and accurate assessment is essential to identify the cause and location of the bleeding.

Diagnostic Procedure

The source of the bleeding causing the hemoptysis must be quickly identified. A medical history and physical examination are completed to collect subjective and objective information that will assist in differentiating whether the patient has hemoptysis, hematemesis, or pseudohemoptysis. Diagnostic testing begins with a lateral chest X-ray; however, X-rays can offer insufficient information, and a chest multiple detector CT (MDCT) may be ordered for patients with blood-streaked sputum and chronic illness such as lung cancer.[37] The MDCT locates the source of the bleeding and indicates the exact presence, number, origin, and trajectory of the bronchial and pulmonary arteries that may be the source of bleeding. The MDCT can detect 70%–88% of cases resulting from bronchial artery overflow and 62%–97% of the non-bronchial arteries that cause bleeding.[35] The MDCT may be followed by a diagnostic bronchoscopy, which is carried out during active hemoptysis or within 24–48 hours after cessation and can detect the source of bleeding in 73%–93% of cases.[35]

Treatment

There are two types of hemoptysis: non-massive and massive. Common goals for the management of either type are to

(1) identify the origin of bleeding, (2) stop the bleeding, (3) treat the underlying cause, and (4) prevent aspiration in patients with massive hemoptysis.[38]

Non-massive Hemoptysis

The treatment plan for patients with non-massive hemoptysis is focused on the cause of the bleeding and the blood volume loss over 24 hours. The blood volume should be scant or minimal as this suggests a self-limiting cause such as pneumonia. This patient will require a standard chest X-ray for diagnosis confirmation and is considered low risk. Treatment is managed in the outpatient setting and involves a normal follow-up appointment. Some patients' hemoptysis may be high risk and require an outpatient CT. Nursing management of non-massive hemoptysis includes establishing patient trust, education, and emotional support.

Massive Hemoptysis

Medical management for the patient with massive hemoptysis begins with airway protection and establishment of hemodynamic stability. Any acquired coagulopathies such as thrombocytopenia, disseminated intravascular coagulation, or drug-induced platelet dysfunctions are then identified and treated.[34]

Hemoptysis has proven to be a difficult and uncertain symptom to manage, but technological advances and newer and better techniques have been evolving. Common treatments for hemoptysis include endoscopic treatment, which is used to locate and identify the cause of bleeding. The goal of this therapy is to ensure adequate gas exchange by clearing the airways of blood. Additionally, use of a cryoprobe to extract large clots in the airway may be considered. Bronchial artery embolization is preferred due to its minimally invasive nature. This treatment stabilizes pressures and reduces the risk of bleeding.[33]

Nursing Management

The patient with massive hemoptysis, which can result in death if not resolved immediately, requires emergent management.[33] Respiratory assessment and vital signs are monitored for significant hemodynamic changes because massive blood loss can lead to sudden cardiovascular instability. This situation can be frightening for the patient as well as the family; therefore, the nurse should provide emotional support if needed. When hemoptysis occurs at the end of life in people with cancer, aggressive therapies such as endoscopy, embolization, or surgery are used depending on the patient's condition, the likelihood of success based on the diagnosis, and the patient's goals of care.[35]

Spinal Cord Compression

Case Study: A Patient with SCC

Ms. S is a 54-year-old woman who was diagnosed with breast cancer 3 years ago and was treated with a resection followed by radiation therapy. On a recent visit with her oncologist, she complained of significant back pain and said that she cannot enjoy her grandkids anymore. Ms. S thought her back was giving out but was informed 2 months ago that cancer was found in her spine.

Questions to Consider:

1. What factors put Ms. S at risk for SCC?
2. What are the four stages of SCC?
3. What is the best treatment option given Ms. S's diagnosis?

Description

SCC is a medical emergency in which the spinal cord is compressed as a result of pressure, for example, from a bone fragment or tumor. SCC can occur anywhere between the cervical and the lumbar regions as a result of wear and tear on the vertebrae, spinal tumor, injury to the spine, bone disease, or infection.[38,39] The condition occurs in 5%–10% of patients with advanced cancer. Rates of occurrence for different cancers are breast malignancies (5.5%), prostate cancer (7.2%), myeloma (7.9%) and nasopharynx (6.5%).[40] This condition qualifies as an end-of-life (EOL) manifestation because of its incidence in patients with terminal illness.

Pathophysiology

The pathophysiology of SCC includes injury as a result of trauma, infection, or inflammatory disease; however, tumors are the primary cause. At the point of epidural intrusion, venous flow in the spine is affected, and the patient may experience sharp irregular pains during activities like walking. As the spread of malignant cells infiltrates the white and gray matter, depending on the level of the terminal illness, the patient experiences tissue death.[40] When the malignancy enters the bony structures of the vertebrae, the cells spread to the bones that support the arms, and patients often experience difficulties walking and maintaining a straight posture. The pelvis, femur, ribs, humerus, and skull are systematically destroyed, significantly impacting motor abilities and causing loss of bowel, bladder, and sexual function, followed by paralysis.[41]

Signs and Symptoms

Symptoms of SCC depend on the affected region of the spinal cord; however, back pain is the first sign of the condition in most cases.[42,43] The pain worsens with specific activities such as coughing, sneezing, or straining while toileting and can lead to difficulties during walking. Other non-pain-related symptoms include loss of bladder control, weak limbs, erection problems, and changes to body sensations.

Signs of SCC occur in four stages starting with pain and weakness and ending with ataxia and sensory loss. Back and neck pain, the earliest and lowest-level symptoms, are the most common signs of SCC. Ataxia and loss of sensation are the highest-level symptoms and are a critical EOL manifestation. Patients with ataxia have abnormal gait and nervous system dysfunction such that they cannot coordinate body movements.[44] During ataxia, the patient cannot receive any treatment, and nurses manage the condition by providing hospice care. In the final stage of the illness before death, symptoms worsen, and compression blocks nerve impulses, leading to paralysis and complete loss of sensation.[44] Hospice management of SCC symptoms at the end of life depends on the patient's pain level and the stage of the condition.[45]

Metastatic SCC (MSCC) warrants intervention as early as possible. These signs and symptoms of MSCC would trigger a referral within

24 hours: (1) pain in the thoracic area, (2) spinal pain aggravated by straining, (3) localized spinal tenderness, and (4) nocturnal pain preventing sleep.[46] Emergent signs and symptoms that warrant an immediate referral in oncology patients are (1) loss of coordination, (2) bladder or bowel dysfunction, and (3) limb weakness and inability to walk.[46]

Diagnostic Procedures

Diagnostic imaging used to identify spinal cord injuries includes spinal X-ray (usually insufficiently sensitive), CT scan, and gadolinium-enhanced MRI, which is the gold standard for its specificity and sensitivity.[41] MRI of the complete spine is useful because tumors are found at multiple sites along the spine in one-third of patients.[42]

Treatments

Important aspects of medical management for the SCC patient are analgesia, corticosteroids, radiation therapy, and decompression surgery.

Analgesia

The SCC patient will at some point experience discomfort and back pain as the spinal cord becomes more compressed.[42] Consequently, continuous pain assessment and management are essential. Several modalities can be used to effectively manage pain, including opioid and non-opioid analgesics and nonpharmacologic techniques. For cases of severe pain in patients with spinal tumors, opioids are the first-line medications to effectively manage pain.[47] When opioids are prescribed, the patient should be placed on a bowel regimen to prevent constipation and prevent any additional triggers of pain by straining. If pain is decreased and managed, opioids should be titrated accordingly.

Corticosteroids

Corticosteroids are essential to reducing edema at the compressed site in patients with SCC, particularly in patients with MSCC, so that optimal radiation therapy can be applied at the tumor site.[42] As the edema around the spinal cord is reduced, compression pain may decrease, and neurological function may improve.[47] Corticosteroids have adverse effects that must be monitored during steroid therapy, including weight gain, fluid retention, increased appetite, and facial puffiness.

Radiation Therapy

Radiation therapy is used to decrease the size of a tumor that is compressing the spinal cord, especially in cases of radiosensitive tumors.[42] Radiation treatment is guided by tumor size, spine stability, and the degree of symptoms related to the spinal cord compression.[41] Radiation therapy may be for palliative reasons if the patient has 6 months or less to live, but the National Institute for Health and Care Excellence recommends single fraction radiation therapy.[48] Patients receiving radiation therapy may encounter side effects specific to the site of therapy, but general symptoms include fatigue, alopecia, nausea, and pain.

Decompression Surgery

Spinal surgery is required to remove a tumor compressing the spinal cord. Spinal surgery for patients with SCC would be the optimal choice if there is spinal instability, but spinal tumor patients with a prognosis of 2–3 months will receive palliative radiation therapy in lieu of surgery.[41]

In the management of SCC, regular exercise strengthens body muscles and keeps the spine flexible. Furthermore, maintaining proper body posture when standing, sitting, and sleeping maintains the natural body and spinal curve to avoid strain. In addition, a reasonable body mass index reduces extra pressure on the spine and minimizes the risk of spinal damage. The administration of body mechanics such as exercise routines, massages, and hot showers can be used to reduce back pains.

Nursing Management

Patients with SCC require consistent pain and neurological assessments to manage pain effectively and prevent additional neurological deficits that could diminish QOL.

Hypercalcemia

Case Study: A Patient with Hypercalcemia

Mr. C is a 54-year-old tree cutter recently diagnosed with metastatic lung cancer. He was in good health until approximately 6 weeks ago when he noticed shortness of breath and fatigue. His primary care doctor treated him for bronchitis, but his doctor ordered a chest X-ray when he did not respond to treatment. The chest X-ray showed a lung mass with enlarged mediastinal lymph nodes. Diagnosis was confirmed by outpatient biopsy, and an oncology appointment was scheduled. Unfortunately, he was admitted to a local emergency room with altered mental status and lethargy before his appointment and was found to have hypercalcemia with ionized calcium.

Questions to Consider:

1. What causes of delirium need to be ruled out other than hypercalcemia?
2. What factors put Mr. C at high risk for hypercalcemia?
3. What is the best treatment option given Mr. C's diagnosis and symptoms?

Description

Hypercalcemia is an excessive amount of ionized calcium in the blood. Patients with a corrected serum calcium level less than 12 mg/dL are considered to have mild hypercalcemia, those with serum calcium levels of 12–14 mg/dL are classified as having moderate hypercalcemia, and those with a calcium level greater than 14 mg/dL are classified as severe.

It is most frequently associated with multiple myelomas and breast cancers but is also observed in patients with squamous cell carcinomas of the head and neck, lung, kidney, and cervix. It is much less common in patients with prostate cancer, small-cell lung cancer, and gastric/large bowel tumors.[49] Incidence ranges from 30% to 40% in breast cancer patients with bone metastases, from 20% to 40% in patients with multiple myeloma, from 12.5% to 35% in those with squamous cell lung carcinomas, and from 2.9% to 25% in patients with head and neck malignancies.[49]

Primary hyperparathyroidism and cancer account for around 90% of hypercalcemia cases. Primary hyperparathyroidism occurs in around 25 people per 100,000 in the general population. Most episodes of malignancy-associated hypercalcemia occur in patients with advanced disease and typically result in a poor prognosis, with 30-day mortality in up to 50% of patients.[50]

Pathophysiology

Hypercalcemia in malignant disease is primarily due to increased mobilization of calcium from bone, although increased renal tubular calcium resorption is also a factor. The most common cause (80%) is humoral hypercalcemia of malignancy (HHM). Parathyroid hormone-related protein (PTHrp) released into systemic circulation by cancer cells is the primary mediator. PTHrP shares significant N-terminal homology with parathyroid hormone (PTH) and stimulates osteoclastic bone resorption and renal tubal calcium reabsorption. In addition to hypercalcemia, PTHrP is important in other aspects of cancer biology including susceptibility and tumor behavior.[51] Twenty percent of cases are due to local osteolytic hypercalcemia (LOH) associated with multiple myeloma and metastatic cancers with large bone burden (e.g., breast, lung). Calcium is mobilized by osteoclasts activated by paracrine products.[52] Both HHM and LOH involve proliferation and activation of osteoclasts that resorb bone and generate hypercalcemia. Activation of vitamin D (seen with lymphomas) and secretion of native PTH are less common causes of hypercalcemia.

The kidneys normally adapt to disturbances in calcium homeostasis. However, in the presence of malignancy, patients may experience treatment- or disease-related side effects including vomiting, mucositis, anorexia, dysphagia, and fever—all of which can lead to volume depletion. This imbalance signals the kidneys to resorb sodium to correct extracellular volume depletion. Calcium and sodium resorption are closely linked in the body; when sodium is resorbed, calcium follows. As calcium ions are resorbed in the kidney, the tubules lose their ability to concentrate urine, leading to high-output polyuria and further dehydration. Poor renal perfusion reduces glomerular filtration and compromises excretion of calcium, leading to a further increase of calcium in the blood and eventual renal failure.

A high calcium level can significantly alter a patient's mental status, which in turn can greatly affect the patient's ability to drink fluids. Cellular dehydration and resulting hypotension are exacerbated by decreased proximal renal tubule reabsorption of sodium, magnesium, and potassium. Bone loss due to immobilization, lack of physical exercise, inappropriate use of thiazide diuretics, poor diet, and general physiological wasting will also increase the amount of free calcium ions in the circulation, further increasing calcium levels.

Signs and Symptoms

Symptoms of hypercalcemia are easily overlooked as they are insidious and nonspecific. Symptoms, their severity, and how quickly they appear vary from patient to patient. Mild symptoms of hypercalcemia include fatigue/lethargy, mental dullness, weakness, anorexia, increased thirst, polyuria, and constipation. Severe symptoms include drowsiness, delirium, nausea, vomiting, confusion, dehydration, and coma.[49] The most common symptoms are gastrointestinal, including nausea, vomiting, anorexia, constipation, and, in extreme cases, ileus. Polyuria and polydipsia are associated with hypercalcemia due to impaired renal tubular concentration.[52] Bone pain can be caused by cancer but may also be a symptom of hypercalcemia. Rare symptoms include bradycardia and shortening of the QTc interval, wide T waves, cardiac arrhythmias, and prolonged PR interval.[49]

Because the symptoms of hypercalcemia can mimic both side effects of cancer treatment and progression of the disease, a thorough assessment is essential to the diagnosis and treatment of hypercalcemia. Many symptoms of hypercalcemia cause the patient to become increasingly dehydrated, which increases the hypercalcemia and creates a spiraling effect.

Ionized calcium concentration is the most important laboratory test in the diagnosis of hypercalcemia and the most accurate indicator of the blood calcium level, although the correlation between total serum calcium level and ionized calcium is fair at best. When ionized calcium cannot be used as a diagnostic tool, the total serum calcium value may be used but must be corrected for serum albumin.[53] The formula is: Corrected Calcium mg /dL = (0.8 * (NormalAlbumin – Pt's)) + Sserum Ca

Treatments

Regardless of the overall goals of care, the active treatment goal for hypercalcemia is to alleviate distressing symptoms. Trial of therapy is warranted in all patients with symptomatic hypercalcemia, if the treatment will not exacerbate their existing symptoms. Hypercalcemia is reversed by replenishing depleted intravascular volume, promoting diuresis of calcium, shutting down osteoclast activity in the bone, inhibiting renal tubular reabsorption of calcium, and promoting patient mobilization to the greatest extent possible.[54] Table 53.2 lists commonly used treatments for hypercalcemia.

Hydration is the first step in effective treatment. Although restoration of fluid volume will aid in diluting the serum calcium concentration, its primary purpose is to increase calcium excretion. Electrolytes and other laboratory values are closely monitored including serum calcium (ionized or corrected), potassium, magnesium, other electrolytes, albumin, and bicarbonate levels. Renal function tests, including blood urea nitrogen and creatinine, are also monitored; and dialysis may be considered in rare cases. In most patients, cardiac effects of hypercalcemia are minimal, and outcomes are not usually affected, so cardiac monitoring is unnecessary.

Bisphosphonate Therapy

After fluid administration, the first-line treatment option for malignant hypercalcemia is intravenous bisphosphonate therapy, an effective therapy for a number of cancers.[55] Bisphosphonates have a high affinity for the mineral component of bone, which allows them to reach very high skeletal concentrations.[53] Three bisphosphonates are currently available in intravenous form (bioavailability 1%–2%), but only pamidronate and zoledronate are approved by the US Food and Drug Administration (FDA) for the treatment of malignancy-associated hypercalcemia.

Both pamidronate and zoledronate are approved by the FDA for the treatment of malignant hypercalcemia; however, zoledronate remains the preferred therapy because of the ease of its use, as a 15-minute infusion, as opposed to 2 hours with pamidronate.[51] Pamidronate is usually given as 90 mg intravenously over 2 hours and has a response rate of 33.3% within 4 days, 63.6% within 7 days,

Table 53.2 Common treatments for hypercalcemia in palliative care

Treatment	Mechanism of action
Hydration with intravenous fluids	Increase urinary calcium excretion and improve kidney function
Bisphosphonates (pamidronate and zoledronate most frequently)	Inhibit osteoclast activity
Denosumab	Monoclonal antibody leading to inhibition of osteoclast differentiation and bone resorption
Calcitonin	Inhibits calcium resorption
Dialysis	Dialyze excess calcium out

and complete response within 18 days. Zoledronate is usually administered as 4 mg intravenously over 15 minutes and has a 45.3% response rate by day 4, an 82.6% response rate by day 7, and a complete response within 32 days.[54] Pamidronate and zoledronate can cause renal toxicity, making evaluation and continued monitoring of kidney function essential before and during administration. Some clinicians may opt to use pamidronate in lower doses over longer durations for renal patients. Bisphosphonates can cause osteonecrosis of the jaw, especially in patients with myeloma who have been treated with pamidronate and zoledronate over a long period of time and those with dental problems.[56] Since hypercalcemia tends to recur, pamidronate or zoledronate must be administered approximately every 4 weeks.

Immediate side effects of pamidronate therapy include low-grade fever appearing within 48 hours of treatment and redness, induration, and swelling at the catheter site. Hypomagnesemia and hypocalcemia may also occur. Rapid administration of intravenous bisphosphonates can cause significant pain and should be avoided. Subcutaneous administration of clodronate has been found to be an efficient treatment for malignant hypercalcemia[56] and may be particularly useful in hospital, home, and hospice settings. This approach reduces patient discomfort and decreases costs associated with transportation and intravenous administration in the hospital environment.

It is important to evaluate the entire clinical picture when choosing a bisphosphonate. Hydration is crucial before using this medication. Careful assessment of the severity of hypercalcemia, fluid volume status, renal function, and disease status should guide which type of bisphosphonate is used.

Calcitonin

Calcitonin inhibits calcium resorption and can rapidly restore normal calcium, often within 2–4 hours of administration; however, it is much less effective than pamidronate. Its role in managing hypercalcemia is limited to short term use of 2–3 days. Side effects are usually mild and may include nausea and vomiting, skin rashes, and flushing. Calcitonin can be an alternative treatment in patients with kidney failure, for whom pamidronate and zoledronate are contraindicated.[56]

Denosumab

Denosumab is a monoclonal antibody that may also be a treatment option for patients with hypercalcemia of malignancy. Limited research suggests that this medication could benefit patients who cannot receive bisphosphates because of renal failure.[57] Denosumab was approved by the FDA in late 2014 for treatment of malignancy-associated hypercalcemia refractory to bisphosphonates based on an open-label, single-arm study of patients diagnosed with malignancy-associated hypercalcemia who were unresponsive to bisphosphonate therapy.[58] However, monoclonal antibodies are extremely costly, and logistics often make them a less than ideal treatment option for emergency management of malignant hypercalcemia.

Dialysis

Removal of calcium by hemodialysis against a low-calcium dialysate bath and continuous renal replacement therapy using citrate as an anticoagulant and a calcium chelator has been reported.[52]

Nursing Management

Hypercalcemia can cause distressing symptoms including bone pain, agitation and confusion, severe constipation, and delirium. Treatment can reduce pain and other symptoms, improve QOL, and reduce hospitalizations. At the end of life, promotion of comfort and symptom management are the primary goals of palliative nursing care. If hypercalcemia cannot be reversed or if the patient decides that the burden of interventions is greater than the benefit, the patient should be offered the option to discontinue treatment.

Hypercalcemia is a life-threatening condition that frequently occurs in end-stage cancer patients. Nurses must be well-versed in the treatment options for hypercalcemia and be able to clearly explain the advantages and disadvantages of each treatment to assist patients and their families in making educated choices. Because hypercalcemia is very symptomatic, it is also important for the nurse to review the symptom management plan with the patient and family. If the patient and/or family decide to withdraw or withhold treatment for hypercalcemia, it is the nurse's responsibility to support them in their decision. Ongoing education is essential to support the patient and family as the patient will eventually die from untreated hypercalcemia.

Bone Metastasis and Pathological Fractures

Case Study: A Patient with Pathological Fracture

Ms. W is a 61-year-old woman who had been receiving treatment for multiple myeloma; however, her treatment was put on hold when her insurance was terminated. Although she was working with the palliative care social worker to re-establish her insurance, she was temporarily without systemic treatment. While sweeping her patio, Ms. W had a sudden onset of severe pain in her upper left arm. After talking with the palliative care team by phone, she was instructed to report to the outpatient clinic. On arrival, she described severe pain in her upper arm with swelling, bruising, and loss of function.

Questions to Consider:

1. What makes Ms. W at high risk for a pathologic fracture?
2. What are the treatment options for Ms. W?
3. Is systemic treatment important to decrease the chances of pathological fractures?

Description

A pathologic fracture is a bone fracture resulting from weakness of the bone structure caused by disease. This process is most commonly due to osteoporosis but may also be caused by other pathologies such as cancer, infection (such as osteomyelitis), inherited bone disorders, or a bone cyst.

Epidemiology

Metastatic disease is the most common bone malignancy, with prostate, breast, lung, kidney, and thyroid cancer accounting for 80% of skeletal metastases.[59] The most common sites of bone metastases are the spine, pelvis, ribs, skull, and proximal femur.[59] It has been reported that 9%–29% of patients who suffer from bone metastases develop pathological fractures,[60] most commonly in the long bones, although the spine is the most common site of skeletal metastases.

There is a 3-year survival rate of patients with bone metastases and pathological fractures as compared to those without pathological fractures (19% vs. 35%).[60] The most commonly reported survival rates across all patients are in the range of only 30%–40% at 1 year. Median time from fracture to death across all patients was only 3.3 months, although the actual times were affected by the type of cancer and Eastern Cooperative Oncology Group score. Breast cancers had the best outcomes, with a median survival time of 6.3 months; prostate cancer had a median survival time of 4.5 months; and lung cancer fared the worst, with a median time of only 2.4 months from fracture to death.[60]

Pathophysiology

Once in the marrow, metastatic cancer cells take advantage of normal marrow physiology to survive away from the primary tumor.[61] Bone marrow is a unique environment that houses both cells of hematopoietic lineage and cells responsible for bone remodeling (osteoblasts and osteoclasts). These disseminated tumor cells (DTCs) also actively influence bone remodeling to create a favorable environment for further recruitment and better survival of DTCs within the marrow.[62] Subsequently, DTCs become dormant and eventually regrow.

Signs and Symptoms

Pain is usually the first sign of bone metastasis and is usually worse at night and may improve with movement. As the bone metastasis progresses, the pain becomes more severe and worsens with activity. Continued weakening of the bone because of the metastasis could eventually lead to a pathological fracture. Signs of pathological fracture are sudden onset of pain in the affected area, in addition to possible swelling, bruising, and loss of function.

Pathological spinal fractures usually cause severe pain or progressive neurological deficits; hence, prevention of pathological fractures is a primary goal in the management of spinal metastasis. However, diagnosis of spinal metastasis is frequently delayed because the onset of symptoms often results from neural tumor invasion or development of pathological fracture, which is the initial manifestation of spinal metastasis in many cases.[63] Hypercalcemia may also result from bone metastasis, causing symptoms that include constipation, nausea, loss of appetite, extreme thirst, fatigue, weakness, sleepiness, and confusion. The high calcium also causes more urine output, leading to dehydration.

Diagnostic Procedures

Bone metastases are sometimes diagnosed when the patient seeks care because of pain or other symptoms. They are also sometimes found during the initial cancer workup or during follow-up imaging to determine response to treatment. In either case, bone metastases are usually found on an X-ray, a bone scan, a CT scan, an MRI, or a PET scan.

In osteolytic or lytic metastases, the cancer cells dissolve the bone, making part of it less dense. If the cancer has destroyed enough of the bone, these changes look like a darker hole in the gray–white bone seen on an X-ray. Osteoblastic or blastic metastases cause an area of the bone to look denser or sclerotic, which appears on X-rays as spots that are whiter than the bone around them. Bone metastases often have both lytic and blastic features.

Occasionally, a blood and/or urine test will be ordered to evaluate for the presence of substances that indicate bone metastasis. A blood test, for example, may reveal high calcium and/or elevated alkaline phosphate. Several substances can be released into the urine when bone is damaged, such as N-telopeptide. Bone metastasis is confirmed through biopsy, frequently guided by CT scan.

Treatments

The goals of treatment for bone metastasis and pathological fractures are to relieve pain and restore function without causing further decline in QOL. Management options for skeletal metastases vary with bone type, anatomical location, and loading condition.[59] Treatments include radiation therapy, systemic treatment, embolization, electrochemotherapy, radiofrequency ablation (RFA), and high-intensity focused ultrasound (HIFU).[59] Treatment of pathological fractures involves surgery and splinting or immobilization.

Bone Metastasis Treatment

Palliative Radiation

Palliative radiation therapy can reduce pain in 60% of patients, with about 25% of patients achieving complete response.[63] Palliative radiation therapy can be administered as conventional external-beam radiation or intravenous bone-seeking radiopharmaceuticals. The goals of palliative radiation therapy are to use a short treatment schedule to minimize the commitment of time for therapy and to achieve rapid symptomatic relief.[59] No significant difference in pain relief has been reported between single and multiple fractions of radiation therapy.[62] Palliative radiation is associated with few side effects, but an increase in bone pain called a "pain flare" occurs immediately after radiation therapy in 2%–44% of cases.[63] Bone-seeking radiopharmaceuticals, such as radium-223 (^{223}Ra), selectively deliver ionized radiation to target areas of amplified osteoblastic activity.[64]

Systemic Treatment

Palliative chemotherapy that is targeted to the treatment of a specific cancer can be used to treat bone metastasis; however, cancer metastasis remains poorly understood in terms of clinical outcome, pathology, and tissue specificity of different tumor types. The predilection of some cancers to target and proliferate in the bone is also unclear.

Palliative Embolization

Embolization is useful for the treatment of metastatic bone disease as an adjunctive procedure to devascularize the tumor, reduce the size of the metastases, cause calcification of the margins of the tumor, and relieve pain. It is typically performed at 4- to 6-week intervals until symptoms improve or until the tumor's vascularity disappears, as indicated by angiography, MRI, or CT scan.[59] Embolization therapy does not appear to improve survival, but it may provide palliation and improve QOL. Previous studies have associated embolization with reduced pain and tumor volume lasting from 1 to 9 months.[59]

Radiofrequency Ablation

RFA is a form of electrosurgery in which an alternating current of high-frequency radio waves passes from an electrode tip into human tissues and dissipates its energy as heat.[65] RFA has emerged as a safe, easy, and predictable technique for thermal ablation in the liver, kidney, heart, prostate, breast, brain, lung, lymph nodes, thyroid and parathyroid glands, nerve ganglia, and bone.[65] In the past two decades, use of RFA for the treatment of primary or metastatic bone disease has increased.

High-Intensity Focused Ultrasound

HIFU has been described as a safe, completely noninvasive, and extracorporeal method to treat primary solid tumors and metastatic bone disease.[66] The treatment rapidly delivers the energy required to raise tissue temperature to a cytotoxic level so that the tissue vasculature does not significantly affect the extent of cell lysis.[59] Although in its infancy, HIFU appears to be a safe, noninvasive, promising treatment approach for cancer patients with bone metastases.

Pathological Fracture Treatments

Because of the high mortality related to pathological fractures, the risk factors associated with metastatic bone disease remain poorly understood. This knowledge is necessary for the prevention, detection, and treatment of pathological fractures. Risk factors for pathological fractures in patients with bone metastasis include increasing pain, radiographic osteolytic appearance, lesion size (>25 cm), axial cortical involvement (>30 mm), and circumferential cortical involvement (>50%).[67]

Surgical treatment is a good option for patients with metastatic or impending pathological fractures and solitary metastatic lesions. Treatment must be tailored individually, considering the estimated life expectancy and general condition of each patient. The treatment goals are to reduce pain and restore function for the duration of the expected life span. A population-based study of patients with femoral metastasis showed that patients who received prophylactic stabilization of metastatic bone disease had better survival outcomes than those who received surgical interventions post-fracture.[68]

Bowel Obstruction

Case Study: A Patient with a Bowel Obstruction

Ms. C is a 52-year-old female who was diagnosed with metastatic ovarian cancer approximately 5 years ago. She is currently on her third chemotherapy regime but has had little response to treatment. She has a 1-day history of abdominal pain, vomiting, and increasing constipation. Due to her inability to keep any fluids down and increased pain, she calls her palliative care providers' 24/7 line. She is instructed to be evaluated in the emergency center.

Questions to Consider:

1. What clinical findings suggest bowel obstruction versus increased constipation?
2. What are the treatment options for bowel obstruction and metastatic ovarian cancer?
3. Does Ms. C's prognosis change with the new bowel obstruction?

Description

Small bowel obstruction (SBO) is a frequent cause of hospital admissions and patient morbidity and mortality. It comprises about 15% of all acute surgical gastrointestinal admissions and about 15% of all emergency admissions for abdominal pain. SBO causes about 30,000 deaths per annum and commonly results in decreased QOL, mostly from chronic postoperative pain or obstructive symptoms.[69]

Epidemiology

Abdominal adhesions remain the most common etiology of SBO (60%–70%). Complications usually result within 1 year of the original operative procedure. Abdominal hernias account for about 10%–15% of SBOs. Crohn's disease accounts for approximately 5%–7% of SBOs, and neoplasms account for 5%–10%.[70] Malignant bowel obstruction (MBO) is a complex issue affecting numerous cancer patients, most notably those with abdominopelvic malignancies. Between 10% and 28% of patients with colorectal cancer and up to 50% of those with ovarian cancer will develop an MBO at some point in the course of their disease.[71,72]

Pathophysiology

Normal small intestine functions include absorption of nutrients, electrolytes, and water from ingested food. Due to an obstruction, the proximal bowel dilates due to accumulation of water and swallowed air. SBOs can be mechanical or functional. Mechanical SBOs can be caused by intraluminal or extraluminal mechanical compression. Most common causes are hernias, malignancy, and/or infectious/inflammatory disorders. Functional obstruction is due to dysfunctional peristalsis or ileus.

Diagnostic Procedures

History and physical examination can provide insights into diagnosis; however, they are not sufficiently sensitive or specific. Imagining is essential for adequate diagnosis and can include plain radiograph, CT, MRI, and ultrasound. CT is the standard of care for imaging; however, plain radiographs are often used in initial stages of diagnosis given their low cost and availability.[73]

Treatments

For the purpose of this palliative care textbook we will focus on MBOs.

Initial treatment should focus on resuscitation and medical stabilization, including attention to major comorbidities. Patients should be made nil per os (NPO) status because food in the gut places greater metabolic stress on the potentially already ischemic gut mucosa. Hydration should occur via intravenous route with either normal saline or lactated Ringer's solution. Antiemetics should be administered intravenously to reduce nausea and vomiting that may lead to aspiration pneumonia.

Little prognostic evidence exists to predict which MBOs will spontaneously resolve and which will require surgical management.[73] Evidence suggests that aggressive medical management alone will facilitate resolution of up to 40% of MBOs.[74]

Prior to surgical intervention, medical management should be attempted. In 2021 the Multinational Association for Supportive Care in Cancer (MASCC) published new guidelines for the medical management of MBO in patients with advanced cancer.[74]

MASCC Recommendations[74]:

1. Octreotide is effective at reducing gastrointestinal secretions and colic, thereby reducing nausea and vomiting.
2. Scopolamine is not as effective as octreotide for treatment of symptoms related to MBO; however, it may be used as a breakthrough medication.
3. Ranitidine plus dexamethasone may be effective at reducing nausea and vomiting from MBO, but evidence is too low to recommend routine use.
4. Olanzapine and metoclopramide are effective at reducing nausea and vomiting secondary to partial bowel obstruction
5. Haloperidol has traditionally been used to treat breakthrough nausea and vomiting for MBO; however, it has not been compared to other antiemetics in randomized control studies.

Surgical intervention is typically left to the surgeon's discretion and rates of resection, bypass, and stoma differ widely across studies. Overall, 18%–48% of patients with MBO of gastrointestinal origin treated with surgery undergo resection, 37%–42% undergo bypass, 19.6%–23% undergo stoma creation, 10% undergo gastrostomy, and 10% undergo exploration with no definitive intervention.[75] If a patient is determined to not be a surgical candidate due to type of obstruction (peritoneal implants) or poor general condition due to metastatic disease, a decompression or venting gastric tube might be an option. Survival estimates after decompression gastric tube should be interpreted with caution as some studies include patients receiving total parenteral nutrition (TPN), while others do not report TPN use.

Nursing Management

MBO is a palliative care emergency and requires quick intervention to prevent symptoms and hopefully resolve the obstruction. The life expectancy of an advanced oncological patient from the diagnosis of inoperable MBO is short, with an estimated mean survival rate no longer than 4 weeks. Even if an MBO is resolved, the patient is at high risk for recurrence of this condition.

Nurses are going to be integral in helping patients and families understand the diagnosis of MBO and possible treatment options that are available to them. These treatment options will vary based on the cause of the obstruction and the prognosis of the patient.[76] Symptom management is crucial, and these patients will require intravenous medications for absorption and to increase small bowel rest. Due to the patient being NPO and frequently having a nasogastric tube, oral care is of utmost importance.

If the patient is not a surgical candidate and the obstruction is not resolved with medication, a venting gastric tube might be beneficial for symptom relief. Education must be provided to the patient and family that the tube is not for hydration or feeding but just to decompress the bowel and relieve pressure/pain. The patient can drink fluids for comfort, but these fluids will be drained via the venting gastric tube, therefore not providing true hydration. Artificial hydration and nutrition will have to be discussed with the patient and family. A patient with unresolved MBO is an ideal hospice candidate, and transition to that level of care should be discussed with the patient and family.

Conclusion

The urgent syndromes presented in this chapter are discussed to educate, empower, and equip current and future palliative care nurses. Because many of these topics are emergent in nature, the palliative care nurse must be prepared to provide optimal patient care specific to the disease and to educate patients and family members. EOL care is all about maintaining hope and dignity even when urgent syndromes affect the patient.

REFERENCES

1. Fisher R, Fay J. Primary care management of palliative care emergencies. *InnovAiT*. 2014;7(10):581–586.
2. Azizi AH, Shafi I, Shah N, et al. Superior vena cava syndrome. *JACC Cardiovasc Interv*. 2020;13(24):2896–2910. https://doi.org/10.1016/j.jcin.2020.08.038.
3. Nickloes TA. Superior Vena Cava Syndrome. Medscape. Updated May 15, 2017. Accessed February 11, 2018. https://emedicine.medscape.com/article/460865-overview#a6.
4. O'Dea J, Schainfeld R. Venous interventions. *Circ Cardiovasc Interv*. 2014;7(2):256–265.
5. Siegel Y, Schallert E, Kuker R. Downhill esophageal varices: a prevalent complication of superior vena cava obstruction from benign and malignant causes. *J Comput Assist Tomogr*. 2015;39(2):149–152.
6. Shah, R. P., Bolaji, O., Duhan, S., Ariaga, A. C., Keisham, B., Paul, T., Aljaroudi, W., & Alraies, M. C.(2023). Superior Vena Cava Syndrome: An Umbrella Review. *Cureus, 15* (7), e42227. https://doi.org/10.7759/cureus.42227.
7. Acton AQ. *Advances in Venae Cavae Research and Application*. Scholarly Editions; 2013.
8. Sonavane SK, Milner DM, Singh SP, Abdel Aal AK, Shahir KS, Chaturvedi A. Comprehensive imaging review of the superior vena cava. *Radiographics*. 2015;35(7):1873–1892.
9. Liu CT, Chu HL, Tsai IH, Chang YL, Lin CY. Clinical application of technetium-99m-labeled red blood cells subcutaneous

radionuclide venography and abdominal/pelvic hybrid SPECT/CT imaging in patients with suspicion of proximal deep vein thrombosis. *J Nucl Med Radiat Ther*. 2016;7:295.

10. Azizi AH, Shafi I, Shah N, et al. (2020). Superior vena cava syndrome. *JACC Cardiovasc Intervent*. 2020;13(24):2896–2910.
11. Rachapalli V, Boucher L. Superior vena cava syndrome: role of the interventionalist. *Can Assoc Radiol J*. 2014;65(2):168–176.
12. Gwon DI, Ko GY, Kim JH, Shin JH, Yoon HK, Sung KB. Malignant superior vena cava syndrome: a comparative cohort study of treatment with covered stents versus uncovered stents. *Radiology*. 2013;266(3):979–987.
13. Danjoux C, Tsao M, Barnes E, Chow E. Superior vena cava syndrome. *J Pain Symptom Manage*. 2015;8(4):283.
14. Kokotsakis J, Chaudhry UA, Tassopoulos D, et al. Surgical management of superior vena cava syndrome following pacemaker lead infection: a case report and review of the literature. *J Cardiothorac Surg*. 2014;9(1):107.
15. del Río Solá ML, Garrido RF, Alonso VG, Puerta CV. Endovascular treatment of superior vena cava syndrome caused by malignant disease. *J Vasc Surg*. 2014;59(6):1705–1706.
16. Yu JB, Wilson LD, Detterbeck FC. Superior vena cava syndrome--a proposed classification system and algorithm for management. J Thorac Oncol. 2008 Aug;3(8):811-4. doi: 10.1097/JTO.0b013e3181804791. PMID: 18670297.
17. Tan WW, McMillan JM. Palliative Cancer Care Guidelines. Medscape. Updated February 2, 2017. Accessed February 18, 2018. https://emedicine.medscape.com/article/2500043-overview.
18. Jany B, Welte T. Pleural effusion in adults—etiology, diagnosis, and treatment. *Dtsch Arztebl Int*. 2019;116:377–386. https://doi.org/10.3238/arztebl.2019.0377.
19. Kastelik JA. Management of malignant pleural effusions. *Lung*. 2013;191(2):165–175.
20. Gomathi RG, Rajagopalan B, Dhanasekar T. Role of bronchoscopy in malignant pleural effusions. *IJMRHS*. 2016;5(4):78–81.
21. Egan AM, McPhillips D, Sarkar S, Breen DP. Malignant pleural effusion. *QJM Int J Med*. 2014;107(3):179–184.
22. Boka K. Pleural Effusion. Medscape. Updated July 21, 2017. Accessed February 11, 2018. https://emedicine.medscape.com/article/299959-overview#a6.
23. Aguilera A, Wyrick K, Hallgren J. Diagnostic approach to pleural effusion. *Am Fam Physician*. 2014;90(2):99–104.
24. Davies HE, Lee YOC. Management of malignant pleural effusions: questions that need answers. *Curr Opin Pulm Med*. 2013;19(4):374–379.
25. Fortin M, Tremblay A. Pleural controversies: indwelling pleural catheter vs pleurodesis for malignant pleural effusions. *J Thorac Dis*. 2015;7(6):1052–1057.
26. Yoon DW, Cho JH, Choi YS, et al. Predictors of survival in patients who underwent video-assisted thoracic surgery talc pleurodesis for malignant pleural effusion. *Thorac Cancer*. 2016;7(4):393–398.
27. Li Q, Sun W, Yuan D, et al. Efficacy and safety of recombinant human tumor necrosis factor application for the treatment of malignant pleural effusion caused by lung cancer. *Thorac Cancer*. 2016;7(1):136–139.
28. Feller-Kopman D, Reddy C, DeCamp M, et al. Management of malignant pleural effusions: an official ATS/STS/STR clinical practice guideline. *Am J Respir Crit Care Med*. 2018;198(7):839–849.
29. McPhillips D, Breen D. Indwelling pleural catheters for malignant pleural effusion. *Int J Palliat Nurs*. 2015;21(6):266–270.
30. Lee MK, Kim SH, Yong SJ, et al. Moderate hemoptysis: recurrent hemoptysis and mortality according to bronchial artery embolization. *Clin Respir J*. 2015;9(1):53–64.
31. Feller_Kopman DJ. Etiology of hemoptysis in adults. In: UpToDate, Post TW (Ed). UpToDate; last updated approximately April 2024. Accessed June 9, 2025.
32. Ittrich H, Bockhorn M, Klose H, Simon M. The diagnosis and treatment of hemoptysis. *Dtsch Arztebl Int*. 2017;114(21):371–381.
33. Gagnon S, Quigley N, Dutau H, Delage A, Fortin M. Approach to hemoptysis in the modern era. *Can Respir J*. 2017;2017:1565030. https://doi.org/10.1155/2017/1565030.
34. Cordovilla R, de Miguel EB, Ares AN, Povedano FJ, Ortega IH, Merchán RJ. Diagnosis and treatment of hemoptysis. *Arch Bronconeumol*. 2016;52(7):368–377.
35. Larici AR, Franchi P, Occhipinti M, et al. Diagnosis and management of hemoptysis. *Diagn Interv Radiol*. 2014;20(4):299.
36. American College of Radiology. ACR appropriateness criteria: hemoptysis. Updated 2019. Accessed June 4, 2025. https://acsearch.acr.org/docs/69449/Narrative.
37. Lechtzin N. Hemoptysis. Merck Manual Professional Version. Updated July 2016. Accessed February 11, 2018. www.merckmanuals.com/professional/pulmonary-disorders/symptoms-of-pulmonary-disorders/hemoptysis.
38. Johns Hopkins Medicine. Overview of Nervous System Disorders. Accessed February 11, 2018. www.hopkinsmedicine.org/healthlibrary/conditions/nervous_system_disorders/overview_of_nervous_system_disorders_85,P00799.
39. Ingledew PA, Tseng J. Spinal Cord Compression: Epidemiology. Learn Oncology. August 15, 2014. Accessed June 4, 2025. https://www.learnoncology.ca/modules/spinal-cord-compression.
40. Ropper AE, Ropper AH. Acute spinal cord compression. *N Engl J Med*. 2017;376(14):1358–1369.
41. Khan UA, Shanholtz CB, McCurdy MT. Oncologic mechanical emergencies. *Hematol Oncol Clin North Am*. 2017;31(6):927–940.
42. White N. Metastatic spinal cord compression: presentation, diagnosis, and management. *Hosp Med Clin*. 2016;5(3):452–465.
43. Rubin M. Compression of the Spinal Cord. MSD Manual: ConsumerVersion. Accessed June 4, 2025. https://www.merckmanuals.com/home/brain-spinal-cord-and-nerve-disorders/spinal-cord-disorders/compression-of-the-spinal-cord.
44. Foran B. Recognition and Treatment of Malignant Spinal Cord Compression. Sheffield Teaching Hospital. May 11, 2017. Accessed February 11, 2018. http://www.sth.nhs.uk/clientfiles/File/Spinal%20cord%20compression%20BHF-%20MSCC%20study%20day%20May%202017%20%20final.pdf.
45. Warnock C, Hodson S, Tod A, et al. Improving care of patients with metastatic spinal cord compression. *Br J Nurs*. 2014;23(suppl 2):S14–S18.
46. Kaplow R, Iyere K. Understanding spinal cord compression. *Nursing*. 2016;46(9):44–51.
47. Nair C, Panikkar S, Ray A. How not to miss metastatic spinal cord compression. *Br J Gen Pract*. 2014;64(626):e596–e598.
48. Pettifer A, Grant S. The management of hypercalcemia in advanced cancer. *Int J Palliat Nurs*. 2013;19(7):327–331.
49. Green T. Hypercalcemia in Emergency Medicine. Medscape. Updated December Apr 26, 2023, 2017. Accessed June 4, 2025. https://emedicine.medscape.com/article/240681-overview emedicine. medscape.com/.
50. Chakhtoura M, Fuleihan G. Treatment of hypercalcemia of malignancy. *Endocrinol Metab Clin North Am*. 2021;50(4):781–792.
51. Fallah-Rad N, Morton R. Managing hypercalcemia and hypocalcemia in cancer patients. *BMJ Support Palliat Care*. 2013;7(3):265–271.
52. Dellay B, Groth, M. Emergency management of malignancy-associated hypercalcemia. *Adv Emerg Nurs J*. 2016;38(1):15–25.

53. Dalkin AC, Rosner MH. Denosumab in the treatment of hypercalcemia secondary to malignancy. *Orphan Drugs Res Rev.* 2015;2015(1):113–121.
54. O'Carrigan, B., Wong, M. H., Willson, M. L., Stockler, M. R., Pavlakis, N., & Goodwin, A. (2017). Bisphosphonates and other bone agents for breast cancer. *The Cochrane database of systematic reviews*, 10 (10), CD003474. https://doi.org/10.1002/14651858.CD003474.pub4.
55. Sternlicht H, Glezerman IG. Hypercalcemia of malignancy and new treatment options. *Ther Clin Risk Manage.* 2015;11:1779.
56. Beach A, de Ber H. Denosumab for tumor induced hypercalcemia complicated by renal failure. *Ann Intern Med.* 2012;156(12):906–907.
57. Hu MI, Glezerman IG, Leboulleux S, et al. Denosumab for treatment of hypercalcemia of malignancy. *J Clin Endocrinol Metab.* 2014;99(9):3144–3152.
58. Mavrogenis AF, Angelini A, Vottis C, et al. Modern palliative treatments for metastatic bone disease: awareness of advantages, disadvantages, and guidance. *Clin J Pain.* 2016;32(4):337–350.
59. Hill T, D'alessandro P, Murray K, Yates P. Prognostic factors following pathological fractures. *ANZ J Surg.* 2015;85(3):159–163.
60. Olechnowicz SW, Edwards CM. Contributions of the host microenvironment to cancer-induced bone disease. *Cancer Res.* 2014;74(6):1625–1631.
61. Tsuzuki S, Park SH, Eber MR, Peters CM, Shiozawa Y. Skeletal complications in cancer patients with bone metastases. *Int J Urol.* 2016;23(10):825–832.
62. Cho JH, Ha JK, Hwang CJ, Lee DH, Lee CS. Patterns of treatment for metastatic pathological fractures of the spine: the efficacy of each treatment modality. *Clin Orthop Surg.* 2015;7(4):476–482.
63. De Felice F, Piccioli A, Musio D, Tombolini V. The role of radiation therapy in bone metastases management. *Oncotarget.* 2017;8(15):25691.
64. Lee FY, Latich I, Toombs C, et al. Minimal invasive image-guided ablation, osteoplasty, reinforcement, and internal fixation (AORIF) for osteolytic lesions in the pelvis and periarticular regions of weight-bearing bones. *J Vasc Interv Radiol.* 2020;23(4):649–658.e1.
65. Huisman M, Lam MK, Bartels LW, et al. Feasibility of volumetric MRI-guided high intensity focused ultrasound (MR-HIFU) for painful bone metastases. *J Ther Ultrasound.* 2014;2(1):16.
66. Choy WS, Kim KJ, Lee SK, et al. Surgical treatment of pathological fractures occurring at the proximal femur. *Yonsei Med J.* 2015;56(2):460–465.
67. Singh G, Lim CT, Jonathan TJ, Nathan SS. Evaluation of the role and cost-effectiveness of end-of-life orthopaedic interventions in cancer patients with skeletal metastases to the hip. *J Palliat Care.* 2013;29(2):83–90.
68. Azagury D, Liu RC, Morgan A, Spain DA. Small bowel obstruction. *J Trauma Acute Care Surg.* 2015;79(4):661–668.
69. Rami-Reddy S, Cappell M. A systemic review of clinical presentation, diagnosis and treatment of small bowel obstructions. *Curr Gastroenterol Rep.* 2017;19:28.
70. Furnes B, Svensen R, Helland H, Ovrebo K. Challenges and outcome of surgery for bowel obstruction in women with gynaecologic cancer. *Int J Surg.* 2016;27:158–164.
71. Chouhan J, Gupta R, Ensor J, et al. Retrospective analysis of systemic chemotherapy and total parenteral nutrition for the treatment of malignant small bowel obstruction. *Cancer Med.* 2016;5(2):239–247.
72. Syrmis W, Richard R, Jenkins-Marsh S, Chia SC, Good P. Oral water soluble contrast for malignant bowel obstruction. *Cochrane Database Syst Rev.* 2018;3:CD012014.
73. Romeo M, de Los LGM, Cuadra Urteaga JL, et al. Outcome prognostic factors in inoperable malignant bowel obstruction. *Support Care Cancer.* 2016;24(11):4577–4586.
74. Mellar D, Hui D, Davis A, et al. Medical management of malignant bowel obstructions in patients with advance cancer: 2021 MASCC guidelines update. *Support Care Cancer.* 2021;(29):8089–8096.
75. Shariff F, Bogach J, Guidolin K, Nadler A. Malignant bowel obstruction management over time: are we doing anything new? A current narrative review. *Ann Surg Oncol.* 2022;29:1995–2005.
76. Long B, Robertson J, Koyfman A. Emergency medicine evaluation and management of small bowel obstruction: evidence-based recommendations. *J Emerg Med.* 2019;56(2):166–176.

54

Sedation for Refractory Symptoms

Sandra Perrotta

Key Points

- Palliative sedation or continuous deep sedation is used during the final days to hours of life to control symptoms such as pain and restlessness, refractory to aggressive palliative treatment.
- Palliative sedation differs from euthanasia in that the medical provider's goal is to relieve refractory symptoms, not to end the patient's life.
- Palliative sedation requires expertise, collaborative decision-making and support, knowledge of ethical and legal issues, ability to understand the dynamics of suffering, informed consent, and a compassionate and therapeutic presence.
- Palliative sedation varies by provider and is an individualized end-of-life care option that focuses on the relief of a patient's unique refractory symptoms by dosing to effect. There is no maximum dose, and there is no one universal treatment plan.
- Palliative sedation effectively addresses the basic ethical principles of dignity, autonomy, fidelity, beneficence, and nonmaleficence.

Introduction

To fully understand the important role palliative sedation can play in the control of intractable pain or refractory symptoms and suffering for a dying patient, one must understand how the body shuts down during the dying process, the legal precedence for the use of palliative sedation, the specific goals of palliative sedation, and the patient's right to define what they perceive as suffering. It is also important for the healthcare professional to examine their own cultural, religious, and personal beliefs and how they may affect the ability to care for a patient undergoing palliative sedation.[1–9]

The Dying Process

During the dying process the body struggles to make the most effective use of available oxygen.[10] Its main focus becomes the preservation of cardiac, pulmonary, and cerebral function. All other systems experience a marked reduction in perfusion and function.[10,11]

- *The gastrointestinal system* undergoes a severe reduction in peristalsis, progressing to the loss of the ability to swallow. This contributes to a normal loss of appetite. Any food or fluid provided can result in vomiting, aspiration, abdominal distension, and pain. The loss of appetite and ability to eat may not be well accepted by a society that embraces food as a form of love and comfort. The fear of starving a loved one to death can result in the use of continuous tube feedings and forced feedings that can hasten death. The feedings may cause the patient to expend precious energy and create the likelihood of aspiration.[10,11]
- *The nervous system* is deeply affected by circulating toxins and waste products from progressively failing organs such as the kidney and liver. These toxins are particularly irritating to the cells of the brain and can result in confusion, agitation, and delirium. This is also heightened by the natural dehydration and hypoperfusion that occur as part of the dying process. The dying will sleep more in an effort to conserve energy and will be less responsive as a result of reduced cerebral perfusion and cellular death. They will not be interactive with family and friends, and cognitive function will become progressively more impaired. Involuntary body functions, such as breathing, will become more dependent upon the involuntary stimulus of the brainstem.[10,11]
- *The respiratory system* undergoes a dramatic change as the brainstem takes over involuntary function. Respirations become agonal and irregular, as the lungs continue to struggle to pull in oxygen. Blood pressure is insufficient to effectively maintain the required pressure gradient for oxygen transport, and fluid begins to accumulate in the lungs, causing the congestive "death rattle" also known as "upper airway secretions." Suctioning does not reduce these secretions; it only deprives the dying patient of more oxygen. High-dose supplemental oxygen will only prolong the dying process.[10,11]
- *The circulatory system* attempts to adjust to a continued drop in blood pressure, resultant loss of oxygen, and the loss of circulating protein. Colloidal osmotic pressure cannot be maintained, so fluids introduced into the circulation have only a short time to influence blood pressure and cellular perfusion before they seep into surrounding tissues and ultimately accumulate in the lungs. Increasing intravenous fluids can result in massive pulmonary edema and cause a patient to die more quickly. The heart begins to fail as its energy needs cannot be met to continue to beat effectively. As cells die, there is an increased release of potassium, and irregular heart rhythms worsen until finally the heart can only

quiver, no blood can circulate, respirations cease, and brain cells continue to die.[10,11]

Legal Precedence for the Use of Palliative Sedation

The concept and use of palliative sedation or continuous deep sedation have evolved over the past 25 years and are no longer called "terminal sedation," a term first coined by Enck in 1991. By 2010, the term "palliative sedation" was used consistently when describing the monitored administration of medications to induce sedation in an effort to control refractory and unendurable symptoms near the end of life.[2] "Palliative sedation is not only a legal act; it is grounded in basic ethical precepts including dignity, autonomy, fidelity, beneficence, nonmaleficence, and the principal of double effect."[2 (p. 397)]

- *Dignity* involves an individual's right to be perceived as worthy of honor and respect. This personal desire involves the ethical concept of autonomy; individuals fear the loss of control over their bodies in the dying process, and this loss of control equates to the loss of dignity.
- *Autonomy*, also referred to as "self-determination," is a core belief in the United States and is based on the principle of respect. It addresses the right of an individual to decide a course of action based on their personal goals and values.
- *Fidelity* is the commitment of healthcare professionals to keep their promises to patients and family members and not to abandon them and their needs, especially during the dying process.
- *Beneficence* involves doing good and caring for patients in a way that they would want. This typically is reflected in the management of their refractory symptoms.
- *Nonmaleficence* is the standard of not causing harm through omission of care or not following a patient's request that could result in a loss of their dignity, diminish their autonomy, result in abandonment, or ignore their care wishes.
- *Principle of double effect* acknowledges that there can be both good and bad consequences to an action, but the action is undertaken with the hope (ethical/moral) or intent that the good consequence will occur.[2] "Potentially causing complication or hastening death is not the means or the intent of the action so the use of palliative sedation is morally permissible."[2 (p. 397)]

The intent of palliative sedation is to control symptoms, not hasten death.[2,3] "Intent," was identified by the US Supreme Court as one of the dominant factors required to be proved when trying to establish a standard for euthanasia.[12,13]

In 1997, the US Supreme Court ruled unanimously that there is no constitutional right to physician-assisted suicide, but palliative sedation is intended for symptom relief and not assisted suicide, and is appropriate in the aggressive practice of palliative care.[12,14,15] The American Nurses Association and the Oncology Nursing Society have position papers opposed to physician-assisted suicide.[16,17] Although neither of the position papers addresses the exact issue of palliative sedation, both support the risk of hastening death through treatments aimed at alleviating suffering or controlling symptoms as ethically and legally acceptable. The Hospice and Palliative Nurses Association has also issued a position paper in support of palliative sedation.[18] The use of palliative sedation to address existential suffering remains controversial.[19]

The use of palliative sedation requires three basic elements: (1) a need for relief of intractable symptoms, (2) death is estimated within days to hours, and (3) there is a need to involve medications to reduce awareness.[4] The concept of *proportionality* is another legal precedent used to justify the amount of medication required to reduce awareness. The patient's consciousness is lowered just enough to relieve refractory suffering.[9,20] Proportionality is also a factor referenced when attempting to clearly separate palliative sedation from euthanasia. The intent of palliative sedation is to allow the patient to die comfortably and peacefully at a pace set by their body,[8] whereas euthanasia involves administering a lethal medication in order to promote death.[21]

The benefits of palliative sedation should be stressed over the concerns of accelerating the dying process. The benefits should be discussed with the terminally ill patient or the durable power of attorney/next of kin, if the patient does not have capacity to make their own needs known.[9,22] Refractory symptoms such as pain, delirium, and existential suffering can be controlled; and concerns over the loss of communication, starvation, dehydration, and fears of euthanasia must be weighed against the comfort benefits obtained from deep sedation and the fact that many of the disadvantages identified with the use of palliative sedation occur naturally during the dying process.[8,9]

An informed consent should be obtained prior to the use of palliative sedation. Ideally, informed consent should be obtained from the terminally ill patient.[2,3,8,9] Often, informed consent is obtained from the family, next of kin, or someone with a durable power of attorney who is designated as able to make decisions for the patient. Advance directives, extensive education, and planning are essential strategies to prepare patients and their families for the end of life; and these can greatly assist with the promotion of a peaceful death.[9]

The Goal of Palliative Sedation

The goal of palliative sedation is to provide a medically induced level of unresponsiveness for relief of refractory suffering during the active dying process.[23,24] Palliative sedation is not intended to accelerate the dying process. Patients and their families should discuss its use as refractory symptoms are identified.[25,26] A plan to use palliative sedation should be an interdisciplinary approach including the patient and family and should be instituted as part of a natural dying process to assist in the promotion of a comfortable, compassionate, and peaceful death.[2,22]

Impact of a Care Provider's Personal, Cultural, and Religious Beliefs

It is essential that the healthcare provider is aware of their personal views and biases regarding palliative sedation.[23,27] If the provider has a spiritual or personal objection, removal from direct patient care should be accommodated. Often the healthcare provider can become more comfortable if the purpose and implementation of palliative sedation are explained. There will continue to be objections for its use, but the requests of the dying patient and their family must take precedence. A semistructured interview–based qualitative research study conducted by De Vries and Plaskota[9] exploring the ethical dilemmas faced by seven hospice nurses when administering palliative sedation to patients with terminal cancer concluded: "Hospice nurses need to be confident, competent, and well supported within the expert palliative care team when faced with making decisions about the use of palliative sedation."[(p. 155)]

The Patient's Right to Define Suffering

Suffering at the end of life may involve physical, psychological, social, or spiritual distress. In most situations, multidisciplinary palliative interventions can effectively comfort, but in some instances, suffering becomes refractory and intolerable.[2,3] Existential suffering (sometimes referred to as "terminal anguish") is a more ethically challenging reason for the use of palliative sedation, but it has an important impact on quality end-of-life care.[19] The ability to empathize, to understand the need for hope and optimism and the desire of an individual to have meaning for their suffering, is often poorly understood by the healthcare professional and can cloud the importance of relieving personal and spiritual suffering.

Case Study: Existential Suffering

Edward was an example of a patient experiencing existential suffering. He was a 38-year-old man who had been fiercely independent all his life. He developed metastatic rectal cancer and now required help with all of his activities of daily living. This was intolerable to him, especially when he required help after his frequent episodes of incontinence. His pain was controlled with opioids, but he began to have terror attacks when he required any assistance. He begged his primary team to sedate him as his strength further declined, and he was finally placed on a continuous midazolam infusion. He died peacefully 3 days later. Was palliative sedation necessary for this man? By his standards, and the emotional suffering he was enduring, it was. The healthcare staff had difficulty sedating him even though his condition met the three basic elements for palliative sedation: (1) a need for relief of intractable symptoms, (2) death was estimated within days to hours, and (3) there was a need to involve medications to reduce awareness.[4] Several nurses declined to care for him after palliative sedation was initiated.

The use of palliative sedation for existential suffering remains challenging from ethical, personal, and professional standpoints. There should always be the option for healthcare staff to request that they not be involved if they hold strong beliefs against the provision of palliative sedation. An important concept to consider is that the goal should always be to provide quality end-of-life care as the patient defines it. For Edward, palliative sedation was the right choice.[12,19,20]

Questions to Consider:

1. In your opinion was it necessary to palliatively sedate this patient? Why or why not?
2. If this patient were on your unit, would you consider caring for him? Why or why not?
3. What information can you, as the nurse, provide to this patient's family and friends as means of education and support?

Medications Routinely Used for Palliative Sedation

Bodnar[7] surveyed 381 physicians regularly caring for hospice/palliative care patients and noted that 84% had moderate to no experience with palliative sedation and that only 88% had participated in palliative sedation in the past 5 years. The option to provide palliative sedation does not occur often, and its implementation can vary greatly by provider. There are varying definitions of the process, and no one standardized procedure exists.[7] Drugs most commonly used for palliative sedation include benzodiazepines, barbiturates, and propofol.[7] Additional agents such as opioids and psychotropic drugs like haloperidol and opioids are incorrectly given for their secondary sedating effects. "In end-of-life-care, medications indicated and used to address specific symptoms with a subsequent reduction in the level of consciousness to a varying degree as a side effect should not be used for sedation."[7 (p. 17)] The most commonly used drug used in palliative sedation is continuously administered midazolam.[22] Haloperidol is the gold standard for delirium therapy and agitation. Opioids are designed to address pain and respiratory distress. Haloperidol is unreliable for complete sedation, and it is possible for some patients to have no response or a paradoxical effect.

In addition to the use of medications not specific to providing sedation, actual levels of sedation can vary. Proportional sedation is recommended as a guideline. It requires that sedation be provided only to the point of symptom relief. In most areas of the United States, palliative sedation is considered deep continuous sedation as the patient is rendered unresponsive.[7,27,28] In other areas of the world, palliative sedation can take two distinct forms: one where the goal is to preserve alertness as much as possible and the other is to sedate to unconsciousness because the patient's intractable symptoms are so profound.[7] In-depth discussions should be held with the patient and family to confirm their wishes for the level of sedation. In most instances, palliative sedation is not discussed until symptoms are too severe and intractable, so deep sedation is typically the standard of practice.

Bodnar noted that the most recommended agents used for palliative sedation are midazolam, lorazepam, diazepam, phenobarbital, and propofol (see Table 54.1).[7]

Midazolam is the most commonly used of the recommended palliative sedation–producing drugs.[7,29] It has a rapid onset of 60 seconds, a peak effect in 2–5 minutes, a half-life of 1–3 hours, and a duration of action of slightly less than 2 hours. There is a ceiling effect for central nervous depression found with all benzodiazepines. This can result in midazolam being ineffective over time. In cases where rapid sedation is required, midazolam can be given in 5–10-mg intravenous doses every 5 minutes to a maximum of 20 mg. Dosing beyond 20 mg has little to no efficacy, and another agent will be needed.

Since duration of effect is an important consideration for effective midazolam use, continuous infusions should always start with a bolus, and rates can be adjusted every 1–2 hours with additional boluses.[7]

Table 54.1 Medications used for palliative/continuous deep sedation

Medication	Effect	Peak effect	Bolus	Infusion	Considerations
Midazolam	1 min	2–5-min bolus 50–60-min infusion	2–5 mg q 5 min, max of 20 mg	1–20 mg/h titrate q 1 h + bolus dose 0.7–10 mg/h	Short half-life, give IV or SQ, central nervous system ceiling, variable effect
Lorazepam	5 min	30 min	4 mg q 4 h repeat q 30 min if no other agents available	20–40 mg in 250 mL 1 mg/h after 4-mg bolus, max 7–10 mg/h	Prolonged time to peak effect, best for prolonged sedation; peak effect lasts 4 h
Diazepam	1 min	2–5 min	5–10 mg q 5 min, max of 30 mg	5 mg in 100 mL will be stable for 24 h	Very rapid onset to peak effect, best for deep sedation; need large dilution for IV precipitates
Phenobarbital	5 min	30 min	200 mg q 30 min, minimum effective dose ~100 mg	None Give 10% of loading dose q 12 h	Often effective with midazolam failure; long half-life, accumulation; difficult to titrate
Propofol	30 s	90 s	0.5–1 mg/kg, may repeat half of loading dose	1 mg/kg/h or 15 mcg/kg/min, titrate 5–10 mcg/kg/min q 20 min	High risk of side effect with large loading dose given rapidly CNS depression ceiling Always effective in sufficient doses

IV, intravenous; SQ, subcutaneous.
Source: Reference 7.

Lorazepam is a favored benzodiazepine for prolonged palliative sedation cases anticipated to extend for greater than 24–48 hours because it begins to retain more than half of its effect after 4 hours of sustained sedation. It is a commonly administered drug, so nurses are more comfortable with its use. Lorazepam requires 20–30 minutes to reach full effect, and initially, all effects will wear off in 1–2 hours unless prolonged sedation is delivered.[7,21,23,30]

Diazepam, is a much older and fast-acting benzodiazepine. Its rapid peak onset of 2–5 minutes makes it a valuable resource when rapid sedation is required. Its duration of effect is half that of midazolam, but the need for large volumes of fluid to dilute, its tendency to precipitate out of solution, and its cumulative effect resulting in a long half-life have caused diazepam to become unsuitable for long-term and continuous sedation. Its use in palliative sedation is primarily as a supplemental agent.[7]

Phenobarbital can be given subcutaneously, like midazolam, although this is not an approved route by the manufacturer. The ability to give this drug subcutaneously makes it a valuable resource for sedation in both the hospital and hospice settings. Phenobarbital is stronger than midazolam and is often used when midazolam has proved ineffective, yet it is not a first-line agent used for palliative sedation because it was originally designed to treat intracranial hypertension and status epilepticus. It has a more extensive accumulation effect with repeated administration and with the use of a continuous infusion that can result in a half-life of 53–120 hours. Dosing in a hospice setting is 200 mg every 30 minutes, followed by intravenous boluses of 260–1250 mg every 8 hours or a continuous infusion of 30–160 mg/hour.[7]

Propofol is slowly gaining popularity as an option for use in palliative sedation. It was specifically designed for sedation and anesthesia. It has no central nervous system depression ceiling effect, a rapid onset and peak effect, a short half-life, and a duration of effectiveness of 2–6 minutes. There are only a few published studies on its use for an estimated 4% of all palliative sedations provided in the United States. Dosages of propofol are significantly smaller for palliative sedation than those required for anesthesia. Yet propofol is not a first choice for many healthcare providers due to policies that prevent its administration in unmonitored areas, requirement for its use only with the failure of other sedating agents, no antidote, and the lack of experience with the drug.

Palliative Sedation Nursing Care

The bedside nurse is an essential part of the palliative sedation team. Each physician will differ with their titrating criteria, but the goal for the provider is to keep the dying patient as comfortable as possible and allow the patient's body to shut down naturally without suffering. Sedation usually includes a continuous opioid infusion and the use of a benzodiazepine. Sedation is proportional in that the amount of sedation is in proportion to the patient's body requirements to be kept deeply and continuously sedated. The bedside nurse may need to stay in close communication with the prescribing physician, nurse practitioner, or physician's assistant for more specific directions or concerns.[31]

Family members become distressed if they feel their loved one is suffering, so the nurse should have orders available to address these concerns. Education and a continued presence are often required. Grieving friends and families of loved ones may not absorb information provided only once, so the bedside nurse should be prepared to re-explain all teaching as necessary. There will be a need to reinforce to friends and family members that palliative sedation is not intended to speed up the dying process, nor is it causing additional suffering because their loved one can no longer eat or drink. The normal course the body takes in shutting down during the dying process should be emphasized, as discussed in an earlier section of this chapter. The dying have a natural loss of appetite, thirst, and desire to communicate. Often the loss of these associated interactions is difficult for grieving families, and they will require frequent reassurance.[32,33]

General care for a patient undergoing palliative sedation becomes much like any other dying patient's care. The sedation has simply allowed them to be less restless and have their intractable symptoms controlled.[31]

> One family member stated that once he was sedated, they were actually able to spend a lot of quality time together. They played music that they played at their wedding, and he was so much more peaceful. She laid on the bed with him, and she slept in the room. And because he was in this state rather than the aggressive one, they were able to spend a few days of some quality time together without his last day of his life being agitated and aggressive.... He was settled and peaceful.[9 (p. 153)]

Nurses have an important role in supporting patients and families in effective end-of-life care. Nurse practices in their role in end-of-life care are essential to ensuring that the patient experiences a dignified death.[34,35]

Conclusion

Many nurses and healthcare professionals remain uncomfortable with palliative sedation. Often, this discomfort can be attributed to a lack of understanding of the ethics that guide the providing of palliative sedation and what transpires in the normal dying process. Patients with intractable symptoms that cause them to suffer on any level as they die need their symptoms to be addressed. Palliative sedation does not speed up the dying process, and it is not a form of slow euthanasia. Healthcare providers may not all agree about how to define a "good death," but there is a general understanding about what constitutes a "bad death." Palliative sedation is a reasonable and ethical option for patients with refractory and intolerable symptoms and suffering at the end of life, and for many it is essential for a compassionate, dignified, and peaceful death.

Acknowledgment

I would like to acknowledge Chandana Banerjee and Bonnie Freeman for their efforts and significant contributions in the previous edition of this chapter that laid the foundation for this version.

REFERENCES

1. Byock I. *Best Care Possible: A Physician's Quest to Transform Care through End-of-Life*. Avery; 2012.
2. Bander, PN. Palliative sedation: when suffering is intractable at end of life. *J Hosp Palliat Nurs*. 2017;19(5):394–401.
3. Sulmasy D, Coyle N. Palliative sedation. In: Doka KJ, Tucci AS, Corr CA, Jennings B, eds. *End-of-Life Ethics: A Case Study Approach*. Hospice Foundation of America; 2012:109–125.
4. Maiser S, Estrada-Stephen K, Sahr N, Gully J, Marks S. A survey of hospice and palliative care clinicians' experiences and attitudes regarding the use of palliative sedation. *J Palliat Med*. 2017;20(9):915–921.
5. Lynch M. Care of the actively dying patient. In: Dahlin CM, Lynch MT, eds. *Core Curriculum for the Advanced Practice Nurse*. 2nd ed. Hospice and Palliative Nurses Association; 2013:573–574.
6. Benitez-Rosario M, Castillo-Padros M, Garrido-Bernet B, Ascanio-Leon B. Quality of care in palliative sedation: audit and compliance monitoring of a clinical protocol. *J Pain Symptom Manage*. 2012;44:532–541.
7. Bodnar J. A review of agents for palliative sedation/continuous deep sedation: pharmacology and applications. *J Pain Palliat Care Pharmacother*. 2017;31(1):16–37.
8. Rich BA. Terminal suffering and the ethics of palliative sedation. *Camb Q Healthc Ethics*. 2012;21:30–39.
9. De Vries K, Plaskota M. Ethical dilemmas faced by hospice nurses when administering sedation to patients with terminal cancer. *Palliat Support Care*. 2017;15:148–157.
10. Edmonds M. What happens during the dying process? HowStuffWorks. March 31, 2010. Accessed October 1, 2018. https://health.howstuffworks.com/diseases-conditions/death-dying/dying-process.htm.
11. King P. When the Human Body Dies of Natural Causes. Quora. Accessed May 27, 2025. https://www.quora.com/When-the-human-body-dies-of-natural-causes-what-is-the-shutdown-sequence-Does-the-brain-tell-different-organs-or-cells-to-stop-working-including-itself.
12. Burt RA. The Supreme Court speaks: not assisted suicide but a constitutional right to palliative care. *N Engl J Med*. 1997;337:1234–1236.
13. Lobato Prado B, Bugano Diniz Gomes D, Luiz Serrano Usón Júnior P, et al. Continuous palliative sedation for patients with advanced cancer at a tertiary care cancer center. *BMC Palliat Care*. 2018;17:13. https://doi.org/10.1186/s12904-017-0264-2.
14. Orentlicher D. The Supreme Court and physician-assisted suicide: rejecting assisted suicide but embracing euthanasia. *N Engl J Med*. 1997;337:1236–1239.
15. Vacco v Quill, 521 U.S. 793 (United States Govt 1997).
16. American Nurses Association. *Code of Ethics for Nurses with Interpretive Statements*. American Nurses Association; 2015.
17. Oncology Nursing Society. Position Statement on the Nurse's Responsibility to the Patient Requesting Assisted Suicide. Accessed October 1, 2018. https://www.ons.org/advocacy-policy/positions.
18. Hospice and Palliative Nurses Association. Position Statement: Palliative Sedation. Accessed October 1, 2018. https://advancingexpertcare.org/position-statements.
19. Cripe LD, Perkins SM, Cottingham A, Tong Y, Kozak MA, Mehta R. Physicians in postgraduate training characteristics and support of palliative sedation for existential distress. *Am J Hospice Palliat Med*. 2017;34(8):697–703.
20. Wiegand DL, Russo MM. Ethical considerations. In: Dahlin CM, Lynch MT, eds. *Core Curriculum for the Advanced Practice Hospice and Palliative Registered Nurse*. 2nd ed. Hospice and Palliative Nurses Association; 2013:52–53.
21. Claessens P, Menten J, Schotsmans P, Broeckaert B. Level of consciousness in dying patients: the role of palliative sedation: a longitudinal prospective study. *Am J Hosp Palliat Care*. 2012;29:195–200.
22. Peereboom K, Coyle N. Facilitating goals of care discussions for patients with life limiting disease: communication strategies for nurses. *J Hosp Palliat Nurs*. 2012;14(4):251–258.
23. Bruinsma S, Rietjens J, van der Heide A. Palliative sedation: a focus group study on the experience of relatives. *J Palliat Med*. 2012;16(4):349–355.
24. Bruinsma SM, Rietjens JAC, Seymour JE, Rotterdam EMC, van der Heide A. The experience of relatives with the practice of palliative sedation: a systematic review. *J Pain Symptom Manage*. 2012;44(3):431–445.

25. Koike K, Terui T, Takajashi Y, et al. Effectiveness of multidisciplinary team conference in decision-making surrounding the application of continuous deep sedation for terminally ill cancer patients. *Palliat Support Care*. 2013;4:1–8.
26. Bobb B. A review of palliative sedation. *Nurs Clin North Am*. 2016;51: 449–457.
27. Morita T, Imai K, Yokomichi N, Mori M, Kizawa Y, Tsuneto S. Continuous deep sedation: a proposal for performing more rigorous empirical research. *J Pain Symptom Manage*. 2017;53(1):146–152.
28. Breura E. Palliative sedation: when and how? *J Clin Oncol*. 2012;31(12):1258–1259.
29. Robijn L, Chambaere K, Kraus K, Rietjens J, Deliens L. Reasons for continuous sedation until death in cancer patients: a qualitative interview study. *Eur J Cancer Care (Engl)*. 2017;26(1):12405. https://doi.org/10.1111/ecc.12405.
30. Eun Y, Hong IW, Bruera E, Kang JH. Qualitative study on the perceptions of terminally ill cancer patients and their family members regarding end-of-life experiences focusing on palliative sedation. *J Pain Symptom Manage*. 2017;53(6):1010–1016.
31. Vayne-Bossert P, Zulian G. Palliative sedation: from the family perspective. *Am J Hosp Palliat Care*. 2013;30(8):786–790.
32. Camartin C, Bjökem-Bergman L. Palliative sedation. The last resort in case of difficult symptom control: a narrative review and experiences from palliative care in Switzerland. *Life (Basel)*. 2022;12(2):298. https://doi.org/10.3390/life12020298.
33. Hwang IC. Current status and future directions of research on palliative sedation. *J Hosp Palliat Care*. 2022;25(4):193–197. https://doi.org/10.14475/jhpc.2022.25.4.193.
34. Nacak UA, Erden Y. End-of-life care and nurse's roles. *Eurasian J Med*. 2002;54:S141–S144. https://doi.org/10.5152/eurasianjmed.2022.22324.
35. American Nurses Association. *Nurses' Roles and Responsibilities in Providing Care and Support at the End of Life*. American Nurses Association; 2016.

55

Withdrawal or Cessation of Life-Sustaining Therapies: Mechanical Ventilation, Hemodialysis, Cardiac Devices

Margaret L. Campbell, Alvin H. Moss, and Sarah E. Schroeder

Key Points

- Patients undergoing ventilator withdrawal are at high risk for developing dyspnea.
- Patients are vulnerable for undetected distress as they may be unable to give a report secondary to altered consciousness.
- The Respiratory Distress Observation Scale is a valid and reliable means for assessment when the patient cannot give a dyspnea self-report.
- Patients undergoing withdrawal of a left ventricular assist device are at risk for dyspnea due to flash pulmonary edema.
- Deactivation of cardiac devices is not well understood by patients and their loved ones, and can cause increased stress and anxiety, in an already stressful situation. Healthcare team members need to be mindful of this with clear understanding of deactivation of the device.
- Dialysis withdrawal is the third most common reason for dialysis patient death after cardiovascular disease and infections.
- Factors associated with dialysis withdrawal include older age, number and severity of comorbidities, longer duration on dialysis, frailty, and cognitive impairment.
- Because multiple complications occur when dialysis is stopped, a comfortable death for a patient with kidney failure requires careful medical management.

Some patients with serious illness who are approaching the end of life are dependent on one or more life-sustaining therapies that may include mechanical ventilation, hemodialysis, pacemaker, cardioverter-defibrillator, left ventricular assist device, and extracorporeal membrane oxygenation. The withdrawal or cessation of these supports is within the patient's right to forgo treatment that is either no longer wanted or no longer beneficial. This chapter will provide evidence-based guidance on care of patients undergoing withdrawal of life-sustaining treatments.

Case Study 1: A Patient on Mechanical Ventilation

Mr. G., a 43-year-old man, presented to the emergency department with difficulty breathing secondary to streptococcal pneumonia. He required intubation, invasive mechanical ventilation, and admission to the medical intensive care unit (MICU). His long MICU course with refractory pneumonia was complicated by deep venous thrombosis, pulmonary embolus, and witnessed cardiac arrest. He sustained anoxic encephalopathy and remained ventilator-dependent with a tracheostomy. After discussion of his poor prognosis, his family decided with the MICU team to forgo further aggressive life-sustaining measures and to withdraw mechanical ventilation. The family was given the opportunity to remain at the bedside or wait in a private area during the withdrawal process.

Questions to Consider:

1. How can we ascertain the patient's risk for developing respiratory distress?
2. Which method (weaning vs. immediate cessation) is most suitable for the patient at risk for developing respiratory distress?
3. Which opioid has the strongest evidence to support its use for reducing dyspnea/respiratory distress?

Ventilator Withdrawal

Ventilator withdrawal is considered as a treatment option when the treatment is more burdensome than beneficial, such as when the patient has a terminal illness or is unconscious or when the patient makes an informed, capable decision to cease treatment because their quality of life is poor. Ventilator withdrawal is conducted to allow a natural death free of tubes and machines. Clinical standards, policies, and procedures about forgoing life-sustaining therapy, including mechanical ventilation, are in wide use and reflect broad agreement about the underlying principles regarding these decisions.

Although withdrawal of ventilation occurs on a frequent basis across settings of care, there is little empiric evidence to guide the process. Review of the evidence to guide ventilator withdrawal found small samples and largely retrospective chart reviews.[1] Only one intervention clinical trial has been conducted, and the effectiveness of an algorithmic approach was supported.[2] This approach will be presented here.

Timing to conduct the withdrawal process is generally negotiated with the patient's family and the healthcare team. This timing will depend on which team members will be present, including support personnel such as a chaplain. The time needs to be communicated to all clinical team members, and, ideally, the assigned nurse should have a reduced assignment to be able to spend one-on-one time with the patient and family.

Neuromuscular blocking agents (NMBAs), such as pancuronium or vecuronium, are being used with less frequency in the intensive care unit (ICU); when in use it is impossible to assess the patient's comfort. Thus, the NMBA should be discontinued with evidence of patient neuromuscular recovery before ventilator withdrawal is undertaken. In some cases, the duration of action of these agents is prolonged, such as when the patient has liver or renal failure and impaired clearance. Therefore, although controversial, withdrawal can proceed with careful attention to ensuring patient comfort if an unacceptable delay in withdrawing mechanical ventilation occurs because of protracted effects of the NMBA.

Measuring Distress

Dyspnea, also known as breathlessness, is a nociceptive phenomenon defined as "a subjective experience of breathing discomfort that consists of qualitatively distinct sensations that vary in intensity."[3(p435)] Dyspnea can be perceived and verified only by the person experiencing it. Many patients who are undergoing ventilator withdrawal are cognitively impaired or unconscious because of underlying neurological lesions or hemodynamic, metabolic, or respiratory dysfunction that produce cognitive impairment or unconsciousness. Respiratory distress is an observable (behavioral) corollary to dyspnea; the physical and emotional suffering that results from the experience of asphyxiation is characterized by behaviors that can be observed and measured.

Most patients undergoing ventilator withdrawal will be unable to provide a self-report about any dyspnea experienced, particularly patients who are unconscious or severely cognitively impaired, as well as infants and neonates. Attempts to elicit a self-report should be made if the patient is conscious. Initiation and escalation of sedatives and opioids should be guided by patient behaviors.

The Respiratory Distress Observation Scale (RDOS) is suitable for assessing the adult patient during the withdrawal of mechanical ventilation; reliability, validity, and intensity cut-points have been established.[4–6] This eight-variable categorical scale is the only known tool for assessing respiratory distress when the patient cannot self-report dyspnea, as typifies most patients undergoing ventilator withdrawal. Each variable is scored from 0 to 2 points, and the points are summed. Scores range from 0 to 16: 0–2 = no distress, 3 signifies mild distress, 4–6 represents moderate distress, and scores of 7 or higher signify severe distress. The goal during withdrawal is to maintain RDOS ≤3.

Premedication for Anticipated Distress

Anticipatory premedication is a sound practice if distress is already evident and if distress can be anticipated. Using the Richmond Agitation and Sedation Scale (RASS), patients with scores of +3 to −3 are likely to experience distress, and patients with RASS scores of −4 or −5 are unlikely. Pre-medication with morphine 4 mg and lorazepam 1 mg is given if RASS is +3 to −3; fentanyl 40 mcg can be substituted. Pre-medication is not needed for RASS −4 or −5 and when the patient is brain-dead. Doses may be adjusted to reflect patient tolerance. After pre-medication, if indicated, the withdrawal method can proceed.

Withdrawal Methods

Terminal extubation is characterized by ceasing ventilatory support and removing the endotracheal tube in one step. *Terminal weaning* is a process of stepwise, gradual reductions in oxygen and ventilation, terminating with placement of a t-piece or with extubation. In a clinical effectiveness trial, patients undergoing terminal extubation experienced more distress than patients with the algorithmic, RDOS-guided approach.[2] Likewise, patients in the terminal extubation arm of a multisite comparison of extubation versus weaning were in more distress than those in the weaning arm.[7] Terminal extubation poses an abrupt change from supported ventilation to spontaneous ventilation in a fragile patient, likely contributing to the distress noted in these studies.

Rapid terminal weaning may afford the clinician the most control because it allows for careful, sequential adjustments to the ventilator with precise titration of medications to ensure patient comfort and is the approach for the patient who can experience distress (Table 55.1). Weaning is paused whenever RDOS is >3, and the patient receives a morphine bolus. Documentation of the RDOS and rationale for dose escalation when RDOS is >3 are important to ensure continuity across professional caregivers and to prevent overmedication and the appearance of hastening death.

Terminal extubation can be used when the patient is unlikely to experience distress or is brain-dead. Assessment with RDOS should be done when the ventilator is turned off and subsequently in case the patient develops unexpected distress.

A continuous opioid infusion may be needed after withdrawal if the patient needed medication during the process and if expected to live longer than minutes. A recommended infusion dose is 50% of the sum of the bolus doses given for pre-medication and during withdrawal.

Extubation Considerations

Patients who are ventilator-dependent for 14 days or more are generally ventilated through a tracheostomy tube. After ventilator withdrawal, a tracheostomy collar with humidified room air or low-flow oxygen can be placed. Patients experiencing acute respiratory failure are ventilated through a nasal or oral endotracheal tube. Adult tubes have a cuff to maintain tube placement and occlude the trachea to prevent air leaking and loss of tidal volume.

Removal of the endotracheal tube should be performed whenever possible because of patient comfort and the aesthetic appearance of the patient. However, in some cases airway compromise

Table 55.1 Sample rapid wean

Process	Steps	Rationale
Pre-medication: Patients able to experience distress (e.g., RASS +3 to −3)	Morphine 4 mg IV bolus	Morphine is effective for treating dyspnea. Comatose patients may not need pre-medication but should be monitored for distress development.
Weaning	1. Turn off PEEP 2. Wean FiO_2 by 0.2 every 1–2 minutes if no distress until FiO_2 = 0.21 (room air) 3. Change ventilator mode to SIMV at a rate of 10 with PSV at 5 cm. 4. Reduce SIMV rate by two breaths every 1–2 minutes if no distress until SIMV rate = 4. 5. Change ventilator mode to CPAP 0 PSV 5 cm 6. Turn off ventilator and remove from patient. 7. Extubate.	Step-wise weaning affords an opportunity to pause the process when distress develops. Patients are given the opportunity to "adjust" to each change rather than rapidly being changed from full ventilation to complete spontaneous breathing.
Assess distress	Measure RDOS at baseline and after every ventilator change.	Patients may develop respiratory distress anywhere along the trajectory from fully supported ventilation to spontaneous breathing.
Treat distress	Morphine 4 mg IV bolus whenever RDOS is ≥4.	RDOS 0–2 = no distress; 3 = mild distress.
Maintain comfort	Morphine infusion if patient needed medication during withdrawal and if predicted survival is more than minutes. Calculate the total morphine given during withdrawal as bolus doses. Begin infusion at a rate = 50% of total bolus doses. Titrate to maintain RDOS ≤3.	Patients may survive longer than minutes and can be triaged to a non-ICU bed. Nurse–patient ratios on non-ICU units do not afford frequent IV bolus dosing.
Treat stridor	Racemic epinephrine in 3cc normal saline as an aerosol treatment. May need to be repeated ×1.	Opioids and benzodiazepines will not treat airway obstruction.

CPAP, continuous positive airway pressure; FiO_2, fraction of inspired oxygen; ICU, intensive care unit; IV, intravenous; PEEP, positive end-expiratory pressure; PSV, pressure support ventilation; RASS, Richmond Agitation Severity Scale; RDOS, Respiratory Distress Observation Scale; SIMV, synchronized intermittent mandatory ventilation.

can be anticipated, such as when the patient has a swollen, protuberant tongue or intrapulmonary hemorrhage. Stridor may develop after extubation, and aerosolized racemic epinephrine is a useful intervention.[8]

Oxygen

When patients are near death and in no distress, oxygen is not necessary.[9] Thus, the patient can be cared for without oxygen following ventilator withdrawal unless there are signs of respiratory distress and hypoxemia. Nasal cannula is better tolerated than a face mask if oxygen is initiated.

Duration of Survival

Triage considerations after ventilator withdrawal may be guided by estimations of duration of survival. As expected, patients with the highest illness severity will die more quickly, particularly if they are also dependent on vasopressors or high levels of oxygen.[2,10,11]

Case Study 2: A Patient Undergoing Hemodialysis

Ms. S is a 74-year-old woman with diabetes, hypertension, heart failure, and kidney failure who has been on dialysis for 7 years. Nine months ago, she had a massive myocardial infarction, had a cardioverter-defibrillator placed for an ejection fraction of 15%, and is a candidate only for medical management without further cardiac interventions. Her dialysis is problematic due to intradialytic hypotension and incomplete volume removal. Intermittently she is hospitalized for fluid overload. The nurses and techs have noted that she says she is "tired" of the "dialysis life." She denies depression. She has shortness of breath from walking across her living room, and she does not have the energy to do things she used to enjoy. Her husband has confided to the dialysis nurses that he is worried about her. Several times recently she has asked not to go to dialysis because she does not feel up to it and even hinted that she might want to stop.

Questions to Consider:

1. If she decides to stop dialysis, based on which of the common reasons for dialysis withdrawal is Ms. S likely to stop?
2. If the patient chooses to continue dialysis, could she be referred to hospice and receive concurrent dialysis and hospice under Medicare?
3. Which symptoms are most common after dialysis withdrawal, and what medications are recommended to manage them?

Dialysis Withdrawal

By most accounts, dialysis has been a dramatically successful life-sustaining therapy. Patients who otherwise would have died from kidney failure if they were not able to receive a preemptive kidney transplant (only 3% do) are able to live for years with either hemodialysis or peritoneal dialysis provided at home or in a dialysis center. For some patients, dialysis serves as a bridge to kidney transplantation. For them, once the patient has successfully completed a transplant workup and is listed, the patient can receive a transplant through a deceased donor from a transplant waiting list or through a living donor. According to the 2021 *Annual Data Report* of the US Renal Data System, which provides data for 2019, there were 134,608 individuals who were newly diagnosed with end-stage renal disease that year; 85% started in-center hemodialysis at one of the over 7,500 dialysis centers in the United States, and 11% started peritoneal dialysis at home. At the end of 2019, 492,096 individuals were receiving in-center hemodialysis, 12,243 were performing home hemodialysis, and 62,275 were performing home peritoneal dialysis.[12]

Although patients may benefit from dialysis for a number of years and be satisfied with their quality of life, dialysis withdrawal (also called "dialysis discontinuation" or "stopping dialysis") is the third most common reason for dialysis patient death after cardiovascular disease and infections, occurs in approximately 10% to 20% of dialysis patients, and appears to be increasing.[12,13] Nephrology professional societies recommend shared decision-making prior to the initiation of dialysis and before dialysis withdrawal to be sure that patient values and preferences play a prominent role in decision-making.[14] Factors associated with dialysis withdrawal include older age, number and severity of comorbidities, longer duration on dialysis, frailty, and cognitive impairment.[15]

In the hospital, especially in the ICU, dialysis withdrawal for acute kidney injury may occur because the patient is dying, usually from multiple organ system failure or from an inability to tolerate the dialysis process. Standard dialysis (also called "intermittent hemodialysis") is a cardiovascular stress because it requires sufficient increased cardiac output to compensate for blood flowing at ~400 mL/minute outside the body through the dialysis circuit. For ICU patients with compromised blood pressure because of cardiogenic or septic shock who cannot tolerate dialysis without going into worsened shock, continuous renal replacement therapy (CRRT) is used preferentially to standard hemodialysis. CRRT is gentler and uses lower blood flow rates (~250 mL/min) and less rapid fluid and solute removal, resulting in less hemodynamic instability. CRRT is only provided in closely monitored healthcare settings with high nurse to patient ratios such as ICUs.

Because dialysis in the ICU for a patient with acute kidney injury may be associated with a mortality exceeding 50%, nephrology professional societies have recommended shared decision-making before dialysis initiation.[14] Studies suggest that such discussions should include the issues of potential high mortality; permanent dialysis dependence, especially in older patients with impaired baseline kidney function; impaired quality of life; and low likelihood of returning home.[16]

Critically ill patients in the ICU who require vasopressors to maintain a sufficient blood pressure to undergo dialysis are appropriate candidates for a time-limited trial of dialysis.[17] If at the end of the time-limited trial, the patient continues to require vasopressors for dialysis, then the patient has failed to improve during the agreed-upon time frame. In such cases, nephrologists in conjunction with intensivists inform the patient if they have decision-making capacity or more often their surrogate decision maker that because dialysis is not feasible outside the ICU, it will be stopped.

Duration of Survival

When dialysis is stopped in a patient with no remaining kidney function, death usually occurs within 7–10 days.[12] It typically is preceded by a buildup of uremic toxins (kidney poisons), and death may occur from hyperkalemia or an infection. Because multiple complications occur when dialysis is stopped, a comfortable death for a patient with kidney failure requires careful medical management (Table 55.2). Since death is anticipated with cardiac arrest prior to death, the patient, if the patient still has decision-making capacity, or the patient's surrogate is asked for consent to a do-not-resuscitate order and other treatment limitations which are appropriate at the end of life such as do not intubate, no bilevel positive airway pressure, do not transfer to the ICU, no tube feedings, and no vasopressors. Once dialysis is stopped, patients are transitioned to comfort-focused care and, if possible, discharged home with hospice or to an inpatient hospice unit.

Case Study 3: A Patient Undergoing Cardiac Device Cessation

Ms. M is a 63-year-old woman, with a prior health history of non-ischemic cardiomyopathy, diabetes, smoking, and end-stage heart failure. She underwent a left ventricular assist device (LVAD) implantation 2.5 years ago. She had an uneventful recovery period but continued to smoke and take her medications infrequently. She presented with an acute stroke with left-sided hemiplegia and aphasia; she was placed in intensive care. There were daily discussions of suspected prognosis, which was felt to be poor from all providers on her case. A family conference was conducted with cardiology, cardiothoracic surgery, the intensivist, and the palliative care teams. The main concern was that she would not recover from the stroke, leading to her husband's request to proceed with end-of-life care.

Table 55.2 Symptoms and treatment after dialysis withdrawal for comfort-focused care

Symptom/sign	Reason	Treatment
Shortness of breath, swelling, and excessive secretions	Fluid overload from intravenous (IV) or oral fluid and medications with no/minimal urine output	Stop IV and enteral fluids; give opioids, preferentially IV fentanyl in kidney failure, for labored breathing with accessory muscle use; limit oral intake if alert to sips and ice chips; ultrafiltration without dialysis for severe symptoms; glycopyrrolate for excessive secretions
Deep, labored, gasping breathing (Kussmaul)	Respiratory compensation for metabolic acidosis	Manage distressing breathing with small doses of IV fentanyl
Confusion, somnolence, and hallucinations	Buildup of uremic toxins	Reassurance; haloperidol for agitated behavior
Myoclonic jerking; rarely seizures	Uremic encephalopathy	IV benzodiazepines to stop jerking
Pain	Typically, musculoskeletal pain, pain from endotracheal tube, chest tube, or intercurrent process	Opioids without renally excreted metabolites, usually fentanyl

Questions to Consider:

1. What should nursing staff expect with care at the end of life in a patient with a durable LVAD?
2. If she would continue support per her husband's request, what type of care would she require?
3. In what scenarios should one consider deactivating the durable LVAD?

Cardiac Device Cessation

Heart disease remains the leading cause of death in the United States, accounting for one in every five deaths.[18] More than 20 million Americans suffer from coronary artery disease, and out-of-hospital cardiac arrests occur in more than 356,000 people annually and are unfortunately 90% fatal.[19] A multitude of devices are utilized in cardiac conditions related to coronary artery disease. Permanent pacemakers (PPMs) are placed in individuals who suffer from symptomatic bradyarrhythmias or other dysfunctions of the electrical conduction system. An implantable cardiac defibrillator (ICD) is used in primary prevention of potentially fatal ventricular arrhythmias when the left ventricular ejection fraction is ≤35% or secondary prevention in those who have previously suffered a prior sudden cardiac arrest, documented ventricular arrhythmias, or unexplained syncope with an ejection fraction ≤35%.[20] An LVAD is used as an option for end-stage heart failure, defined as New York Heart Association Class IV symptoms (at rest or minimal exertive shortness of breath, fatigue, or decreased energy), an ejection fraction ≤25%, life expectancy less than a year, and advanced structural heart changes, despite heart failure guideline–driven medical therapy.[21] One last medical device option for the most critically ill is veno-arterial or veno-venous extracorporeal membranous oxygenation (ECMO). This temporary therapy uses a heart–lung bypass machine as life support in some of the most critical situations, including lung damage from infection, a significant myocardial infarction, or systemic cardiogenic shock. Each one of these types of devices serves a purpose, and careful consideration should be exercised when an individual using one of these devices reaches the end of life. The purpose of this section is to discuss the steps for withdrawal of each of the four devices mentioned, with examples of case studies for PPM, ICD, LVAD, and ECMO.

PPM and ICD

Evidence suggests that there is no indication to deactivate pacemakers during the dying process as the pacemakers are not felt to prolong life through the final stages. However, in rare instances and upon the family member's request, pacemakers may be deactivated through device reprogramming from a cardiologist or pacemaker technician.[22] On the other hand, there is a significant amount of evidence to support the deactivation of the ICD during the end-of-life care of an individual proceeding through the dying process. The purpose of deactivation of the ICD prior to the dying process is to allow for natural processes to occur should the individual go into a fatal ventricular arrhythmia. Cardiac arrhythmias may occur if an individual is transitioning toward death, and the individual may have distress and anxiety should they inadvertently get shocked by the ICD. In an urgent situation, a magnet may be placed in the location of the ICD to deactivate the functionality of the ICD itself. There should be a direct order in the individual's chart to deactivate the ICD therapies. Key instructions to discuss with family members and the patients if they are still aware of the situation include that death is not caused from turning off the ICD and that turning the ICD off does not induce arrhythmias and is not painful.[23] When death is not expected in the next 24 hours, oftentimes device representatives will deactivate the ICD therapies directly themselves to avoid the use of magnets.

LVAD

Oftentimes LVAD patients will die in the hospital setting, therefore stressing the importance of steps to deactivate the device when the situation warrants. Much of the current literature focuses on pre-LVAD advanced care planning, including multiple discussions surrounding the patient's wishes regarding certain scenarios that may occur post-LVAD. During these discussions, there is extreme importance in asking the patient "What makes life worth living" and "If you become sicker, what are your wishes"? Many hospitals and LVAD programs have developed protocols and policies for end-of-life care. Providers need to be clear with patients on what to expect during the dying process.[24] If the patient wishes, family members may be present during the final withdrawal of any support devices. Clinicians should consult with the LVAD coordinator for instructions prior to any deactivation of an LVAD. Deactivation entails disconnecting power sources, silencing alarms, disconnecting the primary percutaneous lead from the controller, and finally deactivating the controller directly to stop alarms.[25]

ECMO

There is increased incidence of withdrawal of short-term ECMO following such things as an anoxic brain injury. When there is quicker than expected decline, healthcare teams need to prepare for potential end-of-life care when using life-sustaining devices in critically ill patients. Following discussions with available family members, if futility has been reached and there is no "bridge to" option, the ECMO circuit should be withdrawn. Generally, the ICU nurse remains at the bedside, along with the respiratory therapist, the cardiothoracic surgeon, and/or the perfusion team to assist in the discontinuation of the ECMO circuits. Death is immediate in nearly all cases following the withdrawal of ECMO due to circulatory arrest and organ failure.[26]

Summary

Withdrawal of life support is done to allow a natural, unencumbered, not prolonged death. Monitoring and treating any distress that may develop are essential. Patients having mechanical ventilation withdrawn are at high risk for developing respiratory distress, and an evidence-based approach is offered. When hemodialysis is stopped, patients may develop a constellation of symptoms from uremia, which can be anticipated and treated. Turning off cardiac devices may not generally lead to patient distress, although the patient should be monitored for the most likely symptoms such as pain or dyspnea.

REFERENCES

1. Efstathiou N, Vanderspank-Wright B, Vandyk A, et al. Terminal withdrawal of mechanical ventilation in adult intensive care units: a systematic review and narrative synthesis of perceptions, experiences and practices. *Palliat Med.* 2020;34(9):1140–1164.
2. Campbell ML, Yarandi HN. Effectiveness of an algorithmic approach to ventilator withdrawal at the end of life: a stepped wedge cluster randomized trial. *J Palliat Med.* 2024;27(2):185–191.
3. Parshall MB, Schwartzstein RM, Adams L, et al. An official American Thoracic Society statement: update on the mechanisms, assessment, and management of dyspnea. *Am J Respir Crit Care Med.* 2012;185(4):435–452.
4. Campbell ML. Psychometric testing of a respiratory distress observation scale. *J Palliat Med.* 2008;11(1):44–50.
5. Campbell ML, Kero KK, Templin TN. Mild, moderate, and severe intensity cut-points for the Respiratory Distress Observation Scale. *Heart Lung.* 2017;46(1):14–17.
6. Campbell ML, Templin T, Walch J. A Respiratory Distress Observation Scale for patients unable to self-report dyspnea. *J Palliat Med.* 2010;13(3):285–290.
7. Robert R, Le Gouge A, Kentish-Barnes N, et al. Terminal weaning or immediate extubation for withdrawing mechanical ventilation in critically ill patients (the ARREVE observational study). *Intensive Care Med.* 2017;43(12):1793–1807.
8. Pluijms WA, van Mook WN, Wittekamp BH, Bergmans DC. Postextubation laryngeal edema and stridor resulting in respiratory failure in critically ill adult patients: updated review. *Critical Care.* 2015;19:295.
9. Campbell ML, Yarandi H, Dove-Medows E. Oxygen is nonbeneficial for most patients who are near death. *J Pain Symptom Manage.* 2013;45(3):517–523.
10. Huynh TN, Walling AM, Le TX, Kleerup EC, Liu H, Wenger NS. Factors associated with palliative withdrawal of mechanical ventilation and time to death after withdrawal. *J Palliat Med.* 2013;16(11):1368–1374.
11. Long AC, Muni S, Treece PD, et al. Time to death after terminal withdrawal of mechanical ventilation: specific respiratory and physiologic parameters may inform physician predictions. *J Palliat Med.* 2015;18(12):1040–1047.
12. US Renal Data System. *USRDS Annual Data Report: Epidemiology of Kidney Disease in the United States.* US Renal Data System; 2021.
13. Schmidt RJ, Moss AH. Dying on dialysis: the case for a dignified withdrawal. *Clin J Am Soc Nephrol.* 2014;9(1):174–180.
14. Renal Physicians Association. *Shared Decision-Making in the Appropriate Initiation of and Withdrawal from Dialysis: Clinical Practice Guidelines.* 2nd ed. Renal Physicians Association; 2010.
15. Wetmore JB, Yan H, Hu Y, Gilbertson DT, Liu J. Factors associated with withdrawal from maintenance dialysis: a case–control analysis. *Am J Kidney Dis.* 2018;71(6):831–841.
16. Moss AH. Integrating supportive care principles into dialysis decision making: a primer for palliative medicine providers. *J Pain Symptom Manage.* 2017;53(3):656–662.e1.
17. Scherer JS, Holley JL. The role of time-limited trials in dialysis decision making in critically ill patients. *Clin J Am Soc Nephrol.* 2016;11(2):344–353.
18. Centers for Disease Control and Prevention. *About Multiple Causes of Death, 1999–2020.* Centers for Disease Control and Prevention; 2022.
19. Tsao CW, Aday AW, Almarzooq ZI, et al. Heart disease and stroke statistics—2022 update: a report from the American Heart Association. *Circulation.* 2022;145(8):e153–e639.
20. Al-Khatib SM, Stevenson WG, Ackerman MJ, et al. 2017 AHA/ACC/HRS guideline for management of patients with ventricular arrhythmias and the prevention of sudden cardiac death: executive summary: a report of the American College of Cardiology/American Heart Association Task Force on Clinical Practice Guidelines and the Heart Rhythm Society. *Heart Rhythm.* 2018;15(10):e190–e252.
21. Writing Committee, Maddox TM, Januzzi JL Jr, et al. 2021 Update to the 2017 ACC expert consensus decision pathway for optimization of heart failure treatment: answers to 10 pivotal issues about heart failure with reduced ejection fraction: a report of the American College of Cardiology Solution Set Oversight Committee. *J Am Coll Cardiol.* 2021;77(6):772–810.
22. Benjamin MM, Sorkness CA. Practical and ethical considerations in the management of pacemaker and implantable cardiac defibrillator devices in terminally ill patients. *Proc (Bayl Univ Med Cent).* 2017;30(2):157–160.
23. Harrington MD, Luebke DL, Lewis WR, Aullisio MP, Johnson MJ. *Implantable Cardioverter-Defibrillators at End of Life.* Palliative Care Network of Wisconsin; 2022.
24. McIlvennen CK, Grady KL, Matlock DD, Helmkamp LJ, Abshire M, Allen LA. End of life care for patients with left ventricular assist devices: insights from INTERMACS. *J Heart Lung Transplant.* 2018;38(4):374–381.
25. Johnson MH, Bass C, Schroeder SE. The fountain of youth will not last forever: End of life in patients receiving mechanical circulatory support. AACN Adv Crit Care. 2021;32(4):452–460.
26. Mulaikal TA, Nakagawa S, Prager KM. Extracorporeal membrane oxygenation bridge to no recovery. *Circulation.* 2019;139(4):428–430.

56

Palliative Care and Requests for Assistance in Dying

Kaveri Roy and Sarah Rossmassler

Key Points

- Medical aid in dying (MAiD) is now available in 10 states and the District of Columbia and has been considered in six more states. Outside the United States, MAiD has been legalized in 12 countries, with euthanasia legalized in nine countries, making it increasingly likely that palliative care clinicians will encounter a request.
- Increasing requests for assistance in dying brings the ethical, legal, and clinical issues to the forefront, requiring more nursing education around this topic. Both the Hospice & Palliative Nurses Association and the American Nurses Association support providing care, education, and advocacy for patients and families who request MAiD.
- There must be a process for conscientious objection. If the clinician is not comfortable discussing MAiD, care should be handed off to another willing clinician who, ideally, is knowledgeable about the MAiD process.
- Although assistance in dying is not a palliative intervention, palliative care clinicians are uniquely prepared to field requests without judgment, assess the concerns underlying the request, and provide much needed guidance.

Introduction

Requests for assistance in dying are becoming increasingly common in the United States due to the successful passing of legislation in New Mexico (2021), Hawaii (2019), Maine (2019), New Jersey (2019), Colorado (2016), California (2015), and the District of Columbia (2016) permitting people with serious illness to request medical aid in dying (MAiD).[1–3] These states joined Oregon (1997) and Washington (2009), which enacted death with dignity acts by referendum, followed by Vermont (2013).[4–7] In a landmark 2009 ruling, the Montana Supreme Court became the first and only judiciary to authorize MAiD by reversing an earlier district court judgment, thus protecting a right to pursue MAiD and effectively shielding from prosecution those physicians who choose to honor a person's request.[8] These states along with the District of Columbia make up 22% of the US population.[9] Outside the United States, assistance in dying is legal in Canada, the Netherlands, Austria, Belgium, Luxembourg, New Zealand, some territories in Australia, Switzerland, Portugal, Spain, Colombia, Germany, Italy, and Ecuador. Germany, Italy, and Ecuador do not yet have legislation or regulations for the implementation of MAiD.

For many nurses, it is only a matter of time before they are confronted with this highly sensitive and personal topic. To address this, the American Nurses Association (ANA) issued a position statement in 2019, stating that nurses could not "abandon or refuse to provide comfort and safety measures" to a patient who has requested MAiD.[10] The ANA made nine recommendations to guide and educate nurses whose patients request MAiD in providing consistent, compassionate, nonjudgmental care. The Hospice and Palliative Nurses Association (HPNA) also made key changes to its position statement in 2024, to better reflect changing attitudes and laws. This position statement outlines five areas of MAiD in which hospice and palliative care nurses must obtain competencies: education, clinical practice, research, policy/advocacy, and leadership. The HPNA, like the ANA, states that patients should receive compassionate and nonjudgmental care and that a nurse must take care of patients who request MAiD or practice conscientious objection. The HPNA position statement goes on to state that if a nurse cannot provide MAiD education to the patient and family, the nurse must connect them to the resources or clinicians who can.[11]

While nurses do not have to agree with the patient's choice to seek MAiD and can follow a process to conscientiously object, they do have to make sure that the patient's and family's goals of care are supported and that they are able to make informed decisions.[12]

Assistance in dying is not considered a palliative intervention. However, Radbruch et al. (2016) point out the complexities behind patient requests for MAiD and many different factors, such as psychosocial, cultural, economic, medical and personal issues may play a role in MAiD requests.[13] Palliative nurses are uniquely trained to assess the hopes, fears, and concerns underlying patient requests for MAiD without agenda or judgment. Patients will have individual goals and values deserving of respect, even when they differ from the values of those providing their care. As a result, some may request assistance in dying despite receiving expert palliative care. To ensure palliative nurses are prepared to handle requests for assistance in dying, this chapter will explore the issues and concepts surrounding such requests.

Definitions

The nomenclature for medical assistance in dying has often been value-laden and intended to sway the reader for or against it, depending on the perspective with which the author writes. The literature elucidates evolution not only of nomenclature but also the underlying philosophy of this topic. Medical assistance in dying is inextricably linked to historical connections to assisted suicide and euthanasia. Definitions are far from standardized and differ based on intent (legal, academic, clinical, societal, and cultural). Therefore, it is necessary to cite important definitions as a foundation for this chapter.

1. *Euthanasia*: A physician (or another person) intentionally ending the life of a person by the administration of drugs, at that person's voluntary and competent request.[13] (Note: In some countries, both euthanasia and MAiD fall under the umbrella of "medical aid in dying.")
2. *Physician-assisted suicide*: A physician intentionally helps a person to terminate their life by providing drugs for self-administration at that person's voluntary and competent request.[13]
3. *MAiD (medical aid in dying, physician aid in dying, physician-assisted dying)*: A physician (or nurse practitioner in Canada) provides, at the patient's request, a prescription for a lethal dose of medication that the patient can self-administer by ingestion with the explicit intention of ending life.[14]
4. *Assistance in dying*: A spectrum of practices including withholding or withdrawing potentially life-sustaining treatment, assisted voluntary stoppage of eating and drinking, and palliative sedation.[15]
5. *Non-treatment decisions*: Withholding or withdrawing treatment from a person either because of medical futility or at that person's voluntary and competent request.[13,16]

History

Better understanding of requests for aid in dying in the present time requires an examination of its history, including the origins of suicide, assisted suicide, and euthanasia in past eras. Probing history brings to light the close entanglement of religious, cultural, social, philosophical, political, legal, and moral codes with sentiments, pragmatics, and legalities of assisted dying. Furthermore, the presence or absence of nurses or other clinicians, status of human rights, and the changing concept of suffering in different eras are all closely linked to stances on requests for assistance in dying. Acceptance, rejection, or indifference to the prospect of voluntary death varies from aboriginal eras through the Middle Ages, classical era to the Enlightenment, and, most recently, the modern to postmodern eras.[17]

The present-day permutations surrounding legal, moral, ethical, and clinical standards occur within dramatic technologic and clinical advances in illness and disease. Religious beliefs often intersect at the bedside with scientific and evidentiary foundations of healthcare.

Noteworthy Historical Events in the Evolution of MAiD

- Aboriginal societies, with principal motivations centering on survival of the clan or tribe, may have invited or allowed practices such as infanticide, abortion, or suicide in efforts to prioritize the well-being of the tribe over an infirm or weakened individual.
- Emerging civilizations that included abstract moral codes, religious tenets, and consideration of life and death began questioning these practices.
- Philosophical and religious thought developed throughout the ancient Greek and Roman civilizations including Judeo–Christian influences throughout the Middle Ages and the Renaissance, broadening from a narrower focus of physical survival to include consideration of sanctity of life, free will, human suffering, and the deliberation of the human condition.
- Influential and timeless arguments and viewpoints of scholars like Socrates, Plato, and Aristotle on the topics of suicide and assistance in suicide intersected with developing legal, political, and social and cultural mores of past eras; many remain central to current philosophical and ethical debates.
- The professionalization of healthcare brought mandates of ethical behavior to the forefront, including the Hippocratic Oath and its provision to "first, do no harm," which was, and continues to be, used by proponents and opponents of MAiD.
- Notable events and people in the twentieth century include Samuel Williams, who first proposed the use of medication to intentionally end life, and Dr. Harry Haiselden, who recommended against surgery for a baby with severe deformities, thus fueling a global ethics debate and inviting formal position statements from interested parties.
- In the second half of the twentieth century, political positioning gave rise to pro-euthanasia advocacy groups, including the Euthanasia Society of America and the Hemlock Society.
- Recent decades have seen the passage of death with dignity acts that have withstood challenges and, with public sentiment and support, have grown over the decades as more US states, several European countries, and Canada have legalized MAiD.
- Canada is the first and only place worldwide where nurse practitioners have been granted rights as providers of MAiD.

United States

The movement toward assisted dying has gained momentum in the United States following the inception of Oregon's Death with Dignity Act (1994), with 51% of voters in favor of the law. Implementation was delayed by legal injunction until 1997, when voters again retained the act, with 60% voting for it.[18] Passage of the law demonstrated a landmark change in attitude and legislation regarding the "right to die" debate in the United States. At that time, the US Supreme Court ruled that MAiD should be determined at the state level.[19]

Prescriptions are permitted based on safeguard criteria allowing adults with mental capacity, who have a prognosis of 6 months or less, to provide informed and voluntary consent. Moreover, consultation with a second clinician is required, and follow-up with mental health professionals is recommended if there are concerns of psychological or psychiatric disorders.[1]

Brittany Maynard, a 29-year-old volunteer in a national right-to-choose advocacy organization who suffered from cancer, brought end-of-life (EOL) discussions into the national spotlight in 2014, when she moved from California to Oregon for access to assisted dying. Her movement sparked controversy and brought a new perspective to a contentious issue that had been primarily associated with the elderly.[20] Hospice is commonly provided concurrently to patients who utilize assisted dying. Reports from 2021 demonstrated that in Oregon 98% and in Washington 90% of MAiD patients received hospice. As of 2021, 3,280 prescriptions were written, and 2,159 people died from ingestion since initiation of the law. The state of Washington (2020) reported 2,277 prescriptions and 2,173 deaths since from 2009 to 2020.[7] However, the relationship between hospice and assisted dying is complex and not entirely sanctioned. Policy does not always reflect clinical practice as some hospice/healthcare agencies prohibit their staff from talking about MAiD.[21] Clinicians have stated that the lack of policies and education about assisted dying has presented challenges. Euthanasia continues to be illegal in the United States; but numerous states have drafted assisted dying legislation bills, and public debate on the implications of MAiD continues.

World View

Assisted dying and euthanasia are often defined differently outside of the United States. Some countries consider euthanasia and MAiD to be equivalent or to have subtle nuances so that incident rates for both are combined. For the purposes of this section, the umbrella term "MAiD" will be used for both assistance in dying and euthanasia.

As of 2024, assisted dying is legal in 15 countries, and euthanasia is legal in nine countries (World Federation of Right to Die Societies [WFRDS], 2024).[2,3,38a] As MAiD legislation is increasingly common worldwide, more research related to practice, geographic attitudes, and the role of palliative care needs to occur. Many countries require voluntary consent, mandatory reporting, physician involvement, and a second opinion. These requirements aim to protect against improprieties in euthanasia and assisted death practices. Though there continues to be fear about misuse of and rising numbers of MAiD, this has not been borne out by the data.[5] However, utilization of aid in dying has increased across Europe and Canada, where MAiD is legal. This may be due to greater access, less stringent policies, and greater education and acceptance of MAiD.[22]

Europe is in the vanguard of policy development regarding assisted dying and euthanasia. The laws of Switzerland, which date to the first Swiss federal penal code of 1918, hold that suicide is not considered a crime if motivated by altruistic reasons.[23] In 1942, assisted suicide was decriminalized, although the law does not recognize euthanasia as legal.[24] The law uniquely permits assisted suicide by nonphysicians. Article 115 of the Swiss penal code stipulates that persons assisting suicide are only committing a crime if the motive is selfish and otherwise condones the act for altruistic considerations.[23]

Patients requesting MAiD have consistently accounted for 1.5% of all deaths in Switzerland.[25] Prior to May 2022, Swiss citizens and foreigners did not have to have a life-limiting condition to request assistance.[4] However, due to the more lenient policies, Switzerland has seen an influx in "suicide tourism," with increasing requests from visitors with life-threatening diagnoses.[26] As a result, the Swiss Medical Association tightened its guidelines to bring them into accord with the guidelines instituted by the Swiss Academy of Medical Sciences in 2018.[27] Now patients seeking MAiD must prove that their suffering is "unbearable" and that all other options are either "unsuccessful" or "unreasonable."[27]

Elsewhere in Europe, assisted dying was legalized in the Netherlands (2001), Belgium (2002), and Luxembourg (2009).[13] Legalization of euthanasia and assisted suicide was sanctioned in the Netherlands through the Termination of Life on Request and Assisted Suicide Act. Minors aged 12–16 can also access the law if the requirement for obtaining parental consent is met.[13] There is also consideration for people with dementia.[28] Data from 2018 showed that patients in the Netherlands requesting MAiD accounted for 4% of total deaths and for around 2.1% in Belgium.[1] The percentage of deaths from MAiD in Belgium increased in 2019, accounting for 2.4% of all deaths. Increased percentages of euthanasia over assisted suicide in countries where both are legal are thought to show a preference for patients to have providers perform the procedure when given a choice. However, research in Belgium and the Netherlands shows that euthanasia and MAiD are not reported consistently. Providers may not view their actions as euthanasia or MAiD, or they may not follow prescribed protocol.[24] A recent study showed that only 60% of MAiD cases were reported, signifying a significant level of underreporting.[29,30]

Belgium legalized MAiD in 2002 as a voluntary act with similar qualifications as the Netherlands. The condition need not be "terminal," but additional process and time requirements are imposed if the person is not terminally ill. The law was extended in 2014 to include minors with parental consent and in certain cases when criteria are met for patients with mental suffering.[28] The extension accounts for a small percentage of total reported cases.[31] Case totality increased significantly between 2003 (0.2% of all deaths) and 2019 (2.4% of all deaths). Notably, Flanders, the Dutch-speaking region of Belgium, had an even higher rate of MAiD utilization (4.6%) than Wallonia, the French-speaking region of Belgium. The rate in Flanders was comparable to MAiD rates in the Netherlands.

Palliative services were provided concurrently in 74% of Belgian cases in 2013.[5,32] A comparison of palliative development between 2005 and 2012 in the Benelux countries, where assisted dying is legal, compared to countries where it is not permitted showed that, despite theories that palliative development would be stunted, services and spending expanded.[33] In fact, Switzerland, the Netherlands, and Belgium are within the top five European countries when it comes to the integration of palliative care into the health system.[18] Furthermore, a recent systematic review suggests that palliative care is offered to 74%–88% of patients who opt for MAiD in these countries.[21] In 2015, the European Association for Palliative Care published a follow-up white paper on assisted dying/euthanasia to provide an ethical framework for the palliative care field.[13] The paper supported palliative care involvement for people considering assisted dying/euthanasia yet stipulated that the practice should not be a part of palliative care. The paper refocused core palliative care tenets as a benefit to comprehensively assess and understand the rationale behind an individual requesting assisted dying.[13]

Canada legalized MAiD in 2015, via a unanimous decision by the Supreme Court of Canada (*Carter v. Canada*), which followed years of consideration by Parliament (aside from Quebec, which passed MAiD legislation in 2014). The court ruled that prohibition of assisted dying was in violation of the Canadian Charter of Rights and Freedoms and spurred legislative development to support assisted dying.[32] The Parliament of Canada passed legislation in 2016 that allowed eligible adults to seek MAiD. Eligibility criteria include mental capacity, voluntary request, and a "grievous and irremediable condition" that causes intolerable suffering. Canadians overwhelmingly supported the ruling, with 78% of those polled in agreement.[18] Canadian law also broadens the role of clinicians who can provide care to include both physicians and nurse practitioners in certain provinces.[34] In 2021, the Canadian government passed revised legislation for MAiD.[35] The changes include:

- Removal of the eligibility requirement that death be "reasonably foreseeable."
- Temporary restriction of eligibility for individuals with only a mental illness diagnosis until an expert review taskforce establishes safe protocols.
- Permission for individuals who are at risk of losing mental capacity (e.g., dementia) the right to waive final consent.
- Permission for federal data collection and monitoring for quality improvement purposes.

Utilization of MAiD in Canada has increased dramatically from its inception in 2016 to 2022. MAiD accounted for 4.1% of all deaths in Canada in 2022, which has led to a debate about how MAiD is being used and whether the criteria need to be tightened.[35a]

The Colombian Constitutional Court initially permitted mercy homicide in 1997 but took almost two decades to develop specific protocols to guide the process.[28] In 2015, the Colombian Ministry of Health formalized the process for MAiD. In 2022, Colombia's Constitutional Court ruled that individuals did not have to have serious illness to access MAiD. The court stated that MAiD was permissible if individuals had a serious illness causing intense physical and/or mental pain and loss of dignity. Patients must express their wish for MAiD, and it must be done under the guidance of an authorized provider of MAiD.[36]

Australia passed legislation in 1996 legalizing both assisted dying and euthanasia in the Northern Territory. It was overturned the following year by Parliament as assisted dying and euthanasia legislation was determined to be a matter for the state parliaments.[10] In late 2017, the Australian state of Victoria passed legislation legalizing assisted dying.[37] The law came into effect in 2019. Western Australia passed a law in 2019 allowing MAiD that took effect in 2021. Tasmania passed a law allowing MAiD in 2021, which took effect in 2022. Queensland, South Australia, and New South Wales have all passed MAiD legislation, which took effect in 2023.[38]

More recently, Spain (in 2021) and Portugal (in 2023) passed assisted dying legislation.[38a] Ecuador, Germany and Italy have legalized MAiD, but their governments have not passed legislation or established protocols for it.[38a–c] Italy's Constitutional Court has ruled that MAiD can only be carried out in exceptional circumstances under strict guidelines.[39]

Case Study 1: A Patient Requesting MAiD

Carla, a 68-year-old Black, married, cis-female (she/her/hers) was diagnosed with metastatic ovarian cancer 3 years ago. She has a master's degree in biochemistry and works for a pharmaceutical company. Carla has completed the standard treatment protocol for her cancer followed by a clinical trial, but her cancer progressed, leading to partial bowel obstructions and generalized edema, rendering her bed-bound. She has been readmitted to the hospital with a recurrent bowel obstruction.

Carla and her wife met with the palliative care team 3 years ago after receiving the cancer diagnosis. At that time, Carla inquired about the MAiD process, but it was not legal in her state of residence. More recently, the state passed death with dignity laws allowing for MAiD. During this recent admission, with her wife at her side, Carla revisited this option with the team, explaining why MAiD appealed to her. She shared that she had lost control and noted the lack of further disease-modifying treatment options, making further decline, suffering, and death inevitable. Carla worried that she was only prolonging the burden of care for her wife and did not see a purpose in continuing to live with the progressive decline. She reminded the team that MAiD had been on her mind for the past few years, and now that this choice was legal in her state of residence, she wanted to proceed with this option.

Questions to Consider:

1. What other information would you, the clinician, want to elicit from Carla and her wife?
2. Does Carla meet the general criteria for MAiD? Why or why not?
3. How would you guide Carla and her wife through the MAiD process? What should you make them aware of?

Ethics of Requests for Assistance in Dying

The ethical deliberations encompassing MAiD are based predominantly on the four pillars of bioethics: autonomy, beneficence, nonmaleficence, and justice.[40] *Autonomy* in decision-making can be defined as a patient's ability to make independent decisions related to their well-being.[41–43] Often, this is further defined as a patient's ability to make a decision without coercion or untreated mental illness and with the ability to rationalize a decision.[44] Autonomy is the foremost ethical concept supporting MAiD requests. It is essential to ensure the patient's autonomy in relation to their decision to request aid in dying.[16,45] There are several threats to autonomy, including, but not limited to, metabolic disturbances, brain metastasis, unmanaged symptom burden, and poorly understood complex care plans. In addition, religious influence and family perception of the situation affect decisions around MAiD.[46] Family beliefs can guide patients to make a decision contradicting their personal choices. If care decisions are made based on family preference, autonomy may be sacrificed.[47] Family preferences warrant consideration at the end of life; however, they currently have little impact on MAiD because of the competency requirements and the inability of surrogate decision makers to select MAiD on behalf of their loved one in most locales.[48]

The autonomy of the care team is also valued. The nurse may object to participation in what they view as the termination of a patient's life and should have the right to do so.[32] Conscientious objection can also be found among other care team members and, if encountered, should be respected.[49,50] Transfer of care to other willing staff should be encouraged.

Beneficence is benefit to the patient, and here MAiD is a major point of contention.[40] Proponents argue that MAiD is beneficial to the individual in the advanced phase of illness by allowing the patient control of their dying process, hence preventing decreased of quality of life (QOL). Opponents argue that improved technologies such as palliative surgery, radiation, or medication management can provide improved QOL. Furthermore, they posit that the availability and engagement of palliative and hospice care invalidate the benefit and need for MAiD. The palliative care and hospice healthcare team provide the standard of care during the advanced phase of a person's illness and are recognized as experts in symptom management, with the primary focus on improving QOL. It is important to recognize that where MAiD has been legalized, the prevailing views of the legal system and public opinion are that MAiD provides benefit to the patient and that choosing MAiD does not preclude receiving palliative or hospice services.[32,42,51]

Nonmaleficence means "first do no harm," another source of debate regarding MAiD.[40] Supporters indicate that, by respecting autonomy, the patient dictates their own course and decline, choosing the time of death in relation to the disease process. MAiD prevents the patient from being harmed by uncontrolled or underaddressed symptoms while avoiding prolonged suffering and loss of dignity or respect. Opponents argue that MAiD brings harm by ending life, potentially depriving people of valuable experiences, both personally and with loved ones.

Justice is viewed as providing what is fair and equitable to a patient.[40] This can be viewed on an individual level as related to patient choice or on a systems level based on resources available. The issue of justice is partially addressed in states and countries where MAiD is legal by making it available to all residents. Unfortunately, socioeconomic status may preclude some from accessing MAiD due to the high cost of filling certain prescriptions. In addition, MAiD is not available in every state, and residency requirements restrict those from requesting it who do not live within the jurisdiction in which it is legal.

Another concern about justice is that providers of MAiD are providing EOL care and, at times, hastening the end of life of patients who, in their view, are suffering.[46] Timothy Quill, in his writing on "The Graying of America," argues this point; whether through withdrawal of treatments, failure to offer treatments, or adjustment of medications with the understanding of the dual effect of these medications with palliative intent, he believes that hastening of death is occurring, although it appears to be "unevenly and unpredictably available."[52] Quill supports legalization of MAiD and making it available to all only after expert palliative care has been obtained and patients have failed to respond adequately with treatment.[52] A study completed in European intensive care units indicated that physicians caring for patients who had treatments withdrawn would intentionally accelerate the dying process in up to 18% of cases. While this supports Quill's concern regarding the justice of MAiD, it also demonstrates the concept of double effect. While these clinicians were attempting to alleviate symptoms, they may have accelerated the patient's death.[46]

Throughout healthcare and legal literature related to MAiD, the terms "suffering" and "dignity" are often referenced.[45,53,54] Each individual is responsible for defining what suffering and dignity mean, and these definitions underlie an individual's narrative and therefore cannot be interpreted by another without exploring the individual's definitions.[43,54,55] For the sake of this discussion, we will discuss and define these terms based on current literature.

There are several types of suffering—physical, psychiatric, emotional, and spiritual, with the latter two characterized as existential.[53,56,57] Physical suffering is addressed with direct management of the identified source of suffering. For example, mixed pain with bone and nerve components secondary to compression fracture may be treated with analgesics and/or kyphoplasty. Existential suffering, on the other hand, can lead to significant treatment challenges due, in part, to a lack of training for clinicians.[56] Existential suffering may include, but is not limited to, loss of dignity, purpose, or meaning. There are validated screening tools available to assist the palliative care team in this area. Unfortunately, the resources allocated to the treatment of existential suffering are often overtasked and understaffed, thus highlighting the importance of a team approach versus an individual one. The interdisciplinary palliative care team focuses on emotional, social, physical, and spiritual aspects of suffering, otherwise known as "total pain," and treats them accordingly.

Palliative clinicians must strive to understand the individual's narrative and how it can modify how they relate to or define suffering.[43] The narrative is not only generated individually but is shaped by surrounding influences. In the past, the question was asked whether those who pursue MAiD are doing so secondary to depression.[57] Today, it is fair to also consider whether it represents an autonomous choice to forego living with a disease and its burden. If an individual demonstrates the ability to understand a disease and its outcome and can rationalize the result of their actions independently and without coercion, it may be considered a valid decision.[44,58,59]

Like suffering, dignity is inherent to the topic of MAiD. Soren Holm, in "Undignified Arguments," notes the frequent use of the term in healthcare, ethical, and legal literature, as well as in rulings associated with malpractice cases.[32,43,45,60] Dignity often relates to the ethical principle of autonomy, which is a direct reflection of an individual's choices. This may be subdivided to include inherited dignity (being a human being) and personal dignity, as well as identifying key areas of focus for dignity, including respect, spiritual peace, and hope.[43,61] The patient is not the only one experiencing the dying process. Family, friends, and the healthcare team of the patient will also perceive the event through the lens of their own individual values and beliefs, each determining whether it was a dignified death. Whether MAiD is applied or not, it is vital to understand the individual's values and beliefs that inform treatment. Consideration should be given to involving palliative care or hospice, usually well-equipped in both training and skills, to meet the needs and goals of the patient and family.

Informed consent in MAiD is also an area of concern. Informed consent must exist if the patient is to exercise autonomous decision-making in treatment choices.[48,52] As the complexity of treatment plans increases, how much the patient and family understand about treatment is often less clear.[55] Within each locality where MAiD is legal, there are various criteria in place, including second opinions, psychiatric evaluations, and documentation of the ability to rationalize the choice, to ensure that the patient is fully capable of consent and fully understands what is being requested.[32]

The World Health Organization (WHO) has not to date issued a formal statement either for, against, or with studied neutrality for MAiD. The WHO does, however, have a strong position about access to palliative care for patients with advanced or serious illness, estimating that worldwide 56 million people are in need of palliative care[35] and that only 12% of those currently have access to it or receive it.[35,62,63] The disparity between the need for and access to high-quality palliative care is linked to concerns that unaddressed suffering may be the reason that some patients explore MAiD, when they may otherwise allow natural death to unfold. Position statements from healthcare organizations often reinforce the importance of access to high-quality palliative care as an alternative to the legal means of hastening death.[11,14,64]

Finally, morality is often brought up in the context of MAiD. Unlike other ethical tenets, which are widely agreed upon within healthcare institutions, moral arguments can be open to interpretation, polarizing, and potentially divisive. In other words, doing what is "right" is a worthy moral imperative but does not, in the domain of the MAiD landscape, clarify what "right" actually encompasses.[65] Traditionally, the domain of philosophy or religion prescribes what is "moral" and what is "immoral," but this risks potential overreach into personal values and cultural beliefs and is best left for people to come to terms with individually and with family.[66]

Legal Issues

One of the first legal cases bringing attention to QOL issues and prolonged dying was the Karen Ann Quinlan case in the 1970s, which became an impetus for discussion around MAiD and withdrawal of life-prolonging interventions. From there, several subsequent treatments that prolonged life began to be addressed.[42] Several cases have been heard by the US Supreme Court, with favorable rulings for patients' or surrogates' right to refuse life-sustaining therapies as well as the states' rights to individually address issues of MAiD.[42,67] Today, these questions continue to be encountered, particularly in the presence of advancing technologies. Although less litigious, these questions can become the charge of local palliative care or ethics teams to address within healthcare systems.

Legalization for MAiD has been accompanied by safeguards to prevent potential misuse of the laws and to protect not only patients but also providers of MAiD. There are concerns that some of the safeguards are not being monitored or enforced with regularity and that MAiD is being carried out in violation of acceptable standards of care. There are also concerns that with increasing legalization, people who are mentally ill and people with disabilities will be coerced into MAiD. This has created some apprehension about a "slippery slope." However, the evidence does not support this concern. Less than 1% of all deaths are due to MAiD, and globally, there has been no disproportionate impact or increase of deaths due to MAiD and no increased risk to vulnerable individuals.[68] Furthermore, strict eligibility criteria have served to limit the number of deaths from MAiD. The most recent revision of criteria was completed by the Physician Aid in Dying Clinical Criteria Committee, convened by the organization Compassion & Choices.[48] By ensuring that safeguards and defined clinical criteria are followed, it has been proven possible to protect both the patient and providers of MAiD.

Of the individuals requesting MAiD, a systematic review found that the majority were nearing the end of life and over 70% had a cancer diagnosis. However, uncontrolled pain and physical symptoms were not the reasons cited for the requests. Rather, it was the loss of autonomy, diminished ability to participate in activities that bring joy, and loss of dignity that led to the requests for MAiD.[24] The review found that patients making MAiD requests were primarily aged 65 years or older, White, assigned male at birth, and college-educated and had a cancer diagnosis.[24] A retrospective study of the experiences of families of patients dying from MAiD in Switzerland, who were cared for by a palliative team, found that existential distress and fear of loss of control were predominant reasons for requests.[69] There continues to be debate over the use of MAiD in cases of pediatric/infant serious illness, psychiatric illness, and cognitive deficits. There are valid concerns about these individuals as they are considered vulnerable populations. The indications, motivations, and competencies of the individuals in making the decision to choose assisted dying must be considered.[29,70] Those with cognitive decline (e.g., dementia) will eventually lose the ability to give consent and need to designate a health proxy to give the final consent, which may lead to future conflicts and issues. There are also varying opinions as to what conditions constitute intractable disease in the context of psychiatric disease.[1] As the number of patients with psychiatric illnesses and cognitive decline utilizing MAiD has gone up, the concern around voluntary consent and MAiD provider psychological stress has grown.[1,29]

Continued high visibility around the issue of MAiD has resulted in a rapid acceleration of attempts and successes in introducing legislation at the state level.[67] These efforts are being driven by public opinion and awareness, as well as by legal action.

Responding to Assisted Dying Requests

Most who request MAiD are individuals who are facing a life-limiting situation. A conversation may be initiated by a patient shortly after hearing the news of having a life-limiting prognosis, sometimes as short as weeks or days. Requests for information about MAiD may occur for several reasons including, but not limited to, curiosity, contingency planning, and fear of lingering or suffering. Requests may also be made as a planning measure to ensure control and provide options for individuals with serious illness who are fearful of potential physical or emotional suffering. Supplementary requests are made with the intent to move forward with MAiD.[55]

Regardless of the clinician's personal position or whether it is legal within the area in which the interaction occurs, it is vital for the clinician to listen to the patient without judgment while offering support.[71] Exploration of the hopes, worries, and concerns of the patient will assist in clarifying the intent of the request while identifying opportunities for palliative intervention with the goal of relieving distress. Clinicians who are willing to listen to patients and openly discuss the option of MAiD foster respect, thus building a therapeutic relationship between the clinician and patient at a critical juncture.[71]

Conversations about MAiD should offer insight into whether the patient possesses decision-making capacity, is adversely affected by psychiatric illness, or is suffering emotional distress, thus allowing for screening and appropriate referral to a mental health professional.[72,73] The clinician should attempt to ascertain how the request correlates with the patient's goals and values.[71] Consistency over time may lend credence to a request, whereas inconsistency may alert the clinician to the need to further explore the request. If feasible, the clinician should also ask for a second opinion from another clinician experienced in EOL care.

The conversation about goals of care should include all EOL options: MAiD, hospice care, palliative sedation, and withdrawal of treatment. Family meetings are highly encouraged, and if the patient is hesitant to include family members, the reason should be explored.[74] Finally, the clinician should document a patient's request for MAiD and ensure patient understanding of the process, the medications used, and the fact that the patient has the right to stop the MAiD process at any time. Patients and families often fear they will be abandoned by their care team; therefore, reassurance that the clinician and the healthcare team will continue to care for them, regardless of whether they choose MAiD or not, is important.[48]

Though the process of obtaining MAiD may differ from region to region, the basic requirements are similar.[1]

- Most jurisdictions have minimum age restrictions and eligibility requirements.
- The request for MAiD must be voluntary, sustained over a period of time, and considered seriously by the care team.
- Most jurisdictions require that the patient has a serious, incurable, and/or life-threatening condition.
- The patient must have intractable physical or psychological symptoms.
- Clinicians must have an open discussion about prognosis and options for treatment with the patient and family. Agreement must be reached that there is no chance of improvement.
- A second opinion by a clinician knowledgeable about EOL care should be obtained.
- There is often a mandatory waiting period between the request for MAiD and it being carried out.
- Euthanasia must be reported for review.

The cost of assisted dying may be a barrier for many. Insurance does not typically cover visits, referrals, and medications associated with MAiD.[22,75] Medications used for MAiD typically include an antiemetic (to decrease nausea), a benzodiazepine (to relax the patient), and then a high dose barbiturate (to cause death). Different combinations of medications are utilized. Medications are often in a powdered form, dissolved in liquid or a slurry. The barbiturate solution must be taken quickly so that the patient does not fall asleep during administration of the medication.[1,48] However, recent shortages of barbiturates have made utilizing them cost-prohibitive for some. To address this, prescribing MAiD providers have come up with combinations of drugs, such as benzodiazepines, cardiac medications (propranolol, digoxin), and opioids, with varying results.[75,76]

Withdrawing Treatment Is Not Equivalent to Assisted Dying

Patients who request MAiD may find barriers blocking access. Some barriers include, but are not limited to, locating a prescriber, waiting the 2- to 3-week period required by law, insufficient finances to purchase the medications, and lack of family support. As a result, patients may consider alternative options to allow for a faster or more natural dying process. It is often possible to meet most patients' needs, resulting in a natural death rather than utilization of MAiD.[52]

Healthcare professionals, including nurses in all roles, may consider the ethical and clinical implications of non-treatment decisions, which may include not initiating potentially beneficial interventions at the request of a patient or discontinuing treatments or interventions that are either non-beneficial (sometimes referred to as "futile") or undesired by the patient. Non-treatment decisions, while legally, ethically, and clinically sound, can be mistaken for actively hastening a patient's death by the clinical team or a patient's family.[77] Discomfort and moral distress on the part of the clinical team during non-treatment decisions should be explored and supported to allow for exploration of complex feelings on the part of the team providing care.

Alternatives to MAiD include the right to refuse or withdraw treatments. For example, a patient with myelodysplastic syndrome converting to acute myeloid leukemia, who is transfusion-dependent, may opt to forego further transfusions. In cases where the patient demonstrates refractory symptoms creating uncontrolled suffering, palliative sedation may be employed. The procedure titrates sedation until symptom relief.[78] Some view palliative sedation as the most intense method of symptom management, carrying with it the recognition that it truly represents the end of the patient's life, unless it is utilized for respite.[79] Finally, voluntary stoppage of eating or drinking is an alternative that is gaining more attention in the literature. This method allows the patient to stop consuming any food or fluids to hasten death.

In all situations, patients with a prognosis of 6 months or less may benefit from hospice care. Hospice benefits offer support and assistance and should be encouraged for every person facing the end of life, whether the patient chooses MAiD or not. The hospice team provides a high quality of pain and symptom management with a focus on the social, emotional, spiritual, and physical aspects that may improve the patient's QOL, while allowing the natural failure of the body from disease.[64] The benefit also offers 13 months of bereavement care to the family, thus allowing for grief support.

Case Study 2: A Clinician Conscientiously Objecting

Mark (he/him) is a registered nurse working in a home-based hospice in Vermont. He has worked in home care for the past 6 years, and prior to this position he worked in various roles in an academic healthcare center for two decades. He values his strong skills in symptom assessment, communication, and med-surg nursing, which has brought him close to many patients over the years. Mark's professional identity is closely intertwined with being an advocate for his patients and helping to relieve suffering in the setting of advanced illness. His work in hospice has been particularly meaningful for him as it has allowed him to practice more independently and to develop relationships with his patients and their families in the home setting.

One of his patients, David (he/him), a 56-year-old man with advanced-stage amyotrophic lateral sclerosis (using bilevel positive airway pressure intermittently and a percutaneous endoscopic gastrostomy tube for nutrition), is interested in MAiD and lives in Vermont, where it is legal. David and his wife let Mark know that he is in the final stages of planning and wish Mark to be present and available at the designated day and time of his death to continue his nursing and personal support. Mark listens to the request and asks for time to consider his response. He loses sleep thinking about being part of assisting with a voluntary death but does not want to abandon his patient. Mark seeks out guidance from the hospice chaplain, the interdisciplinary team, nursing organization position statements, Vermont law, and his own family. Ultimately, he decides he will not be present in a nursing role on David's day of death. Mark carefully explains to his patient that a nurse with expertise in medically assisted dying will be supporting him. A willing nurse colleague steps in to care for the patient, and the interdisciplinary team supports both nurses as the process unfolds.

Questions to Consider:

1. What would be some potential ramifications to Mark if he did not acknowledge his feelings and seek out counsel about David's request?
2. If Mark came to you with his concerns, what are some resources you could offer him, and what guidelines would you use to inform your counsel?
3. Have you ever been involved in a clinical situation where you felt the impulse to conscientiously object? If you had a chance to relive that situation, would you do it differently?

Nursing Role and Implications

Nurses commit to caring for patients throughout the life cycle, including death and dying. Both the ANA and HPNA have made clear that nurses are responsible for providing the support, education, and advocacy needed for patients to access MAiD.[10,11,22] Nurses must support the patient and family in informed decision-making and goals-of-care discussions. However, this does not mean that nurses are compelled to participate. Nurses can conscientiously object, but they must transfer care of the patient to another clinician without displaying disapproval or moral judgment.[50,80] Nurses also have a duty as advocates for healthcare policy to help clarify access and protocols for assisted dying. As the largest segment of healthcare, nurses can make a significant impact.

Now that MAiD has been legalized in an increasing number of jurisdictions, issues around the nursing role in MAiD are cropping up. Many of the patients who access MAiD are on hospice services. Hospices have differing policies around the nursing role in MAiD. However, some hospices do not allow nurses to be present before, during, or after medication ingestion.[21,81–83] This can present a problem as occasionally medication ingestion is unsuccessful, leaving the patient and family in distress. In this case, they will need nursing assistance and support. With a greater nursing voice in healthcare and MAiD polices, such issues can be anticipated and hopefully avoided.

Nurses and advanced practice registered nurses may be called upon to take an active role in prescribing for or participating in MAiD cases.[65] Changes to Canadian law in 2016[34] broadened the types of healthcare clinicians able to participate in MAiD to include the "nurse practitioner" as prescribers in MAiD; additionally, under Canadian law C-14 nurse practitioners may provide an independent second opinion about a patient's eligibility to receive MAiD.[84] It remains to be seen if this expansion of legislative authority will be afforded to advanced practice nurses in other countries or jurisdictions where MAiD is currently legal. Nurse practitioners often take on leadership roles and may also take on responsibility for helping to process the professional feelings, emotions, and well-being of nursing and interdisciplinary colleagues when MAiD intersects with a particular setting or workplace. Finally, nurse practitioners may play a role in policy-level advocacy either for or against further expansion of MAiD.[85]

Conclusion

MAiD is a subject encompassing historical, clinical, legal, and ethical issues. Though not a palliative intervention, palliative clinicians are uniquely prepared to assess the multiple sources of physical, psychological, and existential suffering that led to its consideration, thus leading to appropriate treatment resulting in improved QOL. Some, however, may not be palliated despite expert intervention or may consider MAiD for personal reasons. They may also benefit from palliative consultation as a means of exploring their options without judgment or agenda and with empathy and kindness. Clinicians should access available supports when hastened death requests are sought or considered.

Acknowledgments

Many thanks to our reference librarians, Lindsey Nichols and Jessica Bell, for helping us find the most up to date resources. Also, thanks to Carey T. Ramirez, Kathleen Fundalinski, Judy Knudson, and John Himberger, who wrote the original chapter on MAiD and provided us a wonderful framework to follow.

REFERENCES

1. Mroz S, Dierickx S, Deliens L, Cohen J, Chambaere K. Assisted dying around the world: a status quaestionis. *Ann Palliat Med.* 2021;10(3):3540–3553. https://doi.org/10.21037/apm-20-637.
2. Battin M, Pope T, Shavelson, L. Medical aid in dying: Ethical and legal issues. 2024. Accessed January 11, 2024. https://www.uptodate.com/contents/medical-aid-in-dying-ethical-and-legal-issues
3. Pope TM. Medical aid in dying: key variations among U.S. state laws. *J Health Life Sci Law.* 2020;14(1):25–59. https://doi.org/10.2139/ssrn.3743855.
4. Colorado Department of Public Health & Environment. Medical Aid in Dying. 2022. Accessed September 5, 2022. https://www.colorado.gov/pacific/cdphe/medical-aid-dying.
5. Emanuel EJ, Onwuteaka-Philipsen BD, Urwin JW, Cohen J. Attitudes and practices of euthanasia and physician-assisted suicide in the United States, Canada, and Europe. *JAMA.* 2016;316(1):79–90. https://doi.org/10.1001/jama.2016.8499.
6. Public Health Division, Center for Health Statistics. *Oregon Death with Dignity Act.* Oregon Health Authority; 2021. Accessed September 5, 2022. https://www.oregon.gov/oha/PH/PROVI

DERPARTNERRESOURCES/EVALUATIONRESEARCH/DEATHWITHDIGNITYACT/Documents/year24.pdf.
7. Washington State Department of Health. Death with Dignity Act. 2021. Accessed September 5, 2022. https://doh.wa.gov/sites/default/files/2022-02/422-109DeathWithDignityAct2020.pdf?uid=63151d6584ae2.
8. Compassion & Choices. Montana. Accessed October 4, 2022. https://www.compassionandchoices.org/in-your-state/montana.
9. US Census Bureau. Population by State. 2022. Accessed September 5, 2022. https://www.census.gov/search-results.html?q=state+population&page=1&stateGeo=none&searchtype=web.
10. ANA Center for Ethics and Human Rights. The Nurse's Role When a Patient Requests Medical Aid in Dying. 2019. https://www.nursingworld.org/~49e869/globalassets/practiceandpolicy/nursing-excellence/ana-position-statements/social-causes-and-health-care/the-nurses-role-when-a-patient-requests-medical-aid-in-dying-web-format.pdf.
11. Hospice & Palliative Nurses Association. HPNA Position Statement: Medical Aid in Dying (MAID). August 2024. file:///Users/kaveriroy/Downloads/HPNA_Position_MAiD-Statement-FINAL%20(4).pdf
12. Death with Dignity. Take Action: Death with Dignity around the US. Accessed September 26, 2022. https://www.deathwithdignity.org/take-action/.
13. Radbruch L, Leget C, Bahr P, et al. Euthanasia and physician-assisted suicide: a white paper from the European Association for Palliative Care. *Palliat Med.* 2016;30(2):104–116. https://doi.org/10.1177/0269216315616524.
14. American Academy of Hospice and Palliative Medicine. Statement on Physician-Assisted Dying. 2016. Accessed September 2, 2022. http://aahpm.org/positions/pad.
15. Downie J, Gupta M, Cavalli S, Blouin S. Assistance in dying: a comparative look at legal definitions. *Death Stud.* 2022;46(7):1547–1556. https://doi.org/10.1080/07481187.2021.1926631.
16. Gibson JA, Boerstler JJ, Chase J, Smith C. Withdrawing life-sustaining treatments v euthanasia: the ethical difference. *Nursing (Lond).* 2022;52(7):59–61. https://doi.org/10.1097/01.NURSE.0000832380.26717.3d.
17. Dowbiggin IR. *A Concise History of Euthanasia: Life, Death, God, and Medicine.* Rowman & Littlefield; 2005.
18. Chin AE, Hedberg K, Higginson GK, Fleming DW. *Oregon's Death with Dignity Act: The First Year's Experience.* Department of Human Resources, Oregon Health Division, Center for Disease Prevention and Epidemiology; 1999. Accessed September 30, 2022. https://www.oregon.gov/oha/PH/PROVIDERPARTNERRESOURCES/EVALUATIONRESEARCH/DEATHWITHDIGNITYACT/Documents/year1.pdf.
19. Legal Information Institute. Washington, et al., Petitioners, v. Harold Glucksberg et al. 1997. https://www.law.cornell.edu/supremecourt/text/521/702#writing-USSC_CR_0521_0702_ZS.
20. Maynard B. My Right to Death with Dignity at 29. CNN. November 2, 2014. Accessed September 28, 2022. http://www.cnn.com/2014/10/07/opinion/maynard-assisted-suicide-cancer-dignity/index.html.
21. Gerson SM, Koksvik GH, Richards N, Materstvedt LJ, Clark D. The relationship of palliative care with assisted dying where assisted dying is lawful: a systematic scoping review of the literature. *J Pain Symptom Manage.* 2020;59(6):1287–1303.e1. https://doi.org/10.1016/j.jpainsymman.2019.12.361.
22. Roy K. Medical aid in dying: what every nurse needs to know. *Am J Nurs.* 2022;122(3):30–37. https://doi.org/10.1097/01.NAJ.0000822660.87763.45.
23. Hurst SA. Assisted suicide and euthanasia in Switzerland: allowing a role for non-physicians. *BMJ.* 2003;326(7383):271–273. https://doi.org/10.1136/bmj.326.7383.271.
24. Emanuel E. Euthanasia and physician-assisted suicide: focus on the data. *Med J Aust.* 2017;206(8):339–340. https://doi.org/10.5694/mja16.00132.
25. Bartsch C, Landolt K, Ristic A, Reisch T, Ajdacic-Gross V. Assisted suicide in Switzerland: an analysis of death records from Swiss institutes of forensic medicine. *Dtsch Arztebl Int.* 2019;116(33–34):545–552. https://doi.org/10.3238/arztebl.2019.0545.
26. Gauthier S, Mausbach J, Reisch T, Bartsch C. Suicide tourism: a pilot study on the Swiss phenomenon. *J Med Ethics.* 2015;41(8):611–617. https://doi.org/10.1136/medethics-2014-102091.
27. Swiss Academies of Medical Sciences. Dying and Death. 2022. https://www.samw.ch/en/Ethics/Topics-A-to-Z/Dying-and-death.html.
28. Dyer O, White C, García Rada A. Assisted dying: law and practice around the world. *BMJ.* 2015;2015:351. https://doi.org/10.1136/bmj.h4481.
29. Dierickx S, Deliens L, Cohen J, Chambaere K. Euthanasia for people with psychiatric disorders or dementia in Belgium: analysis of officially reported cases. *BMC Psychiatry.* 2017;17(1):203. https://doi.org/10.1186/s12888-017-1369-0.
30. Raus K, Vanderhaegen B, Sterckx S. Euthanasia in Belgium: shortcomings of the law and its application and of the monitoring of practice. *J Med Philos Forum Bioeth Philos Med.* 2021;46(1):80–107. https://doi.org/10.1093/jmp/jhaa031.
31. Mehlum L, Schmahl C, Berens A, et al. Euthanasia and assisted suicide in patients with personality disorders: a review of current practice and challenges. *Borderline Personal Disord Emot Dysregul.* 2020;7(1):15. https://doi.org/10.1186/s40479-020-00131-9.
32. Landry JT, Foreman T, Kekewich M. Ethical considerations in the regulation of euthanasia and physician-assisted death in Canada. *Health Policy.* 2015;119(11):1490–1498. https://doi.org/10.1016/j.healthpol.2015.10.002.
33. Radbruch L, de Lima L, Lohmann D, Gwyther E, Payne S. The Prague Charter: urging governments to relieve suffering and ensure the right to palliative care. *Palliat Med.* 2013;27(2):101–102. https://doi.org/10.1177/0269216312473058.
34. Government of Canada. Medical Assistance in Dying. Accessed September 30, 2022. https://www.canada.ca/en/health-canada/services/medical-assistance-dying.html.
35. Connor S. *Global Atlas of Palliative Care.* Worldwide Hospice Palliative Care Alliance; 2020.
35a. Health Canada. Fourth Annual Report on Medical Assistance in Dying in Canada 2022. *Canada.ca*, Government of Canada, October 2023. https://www.canada.ca/en/health-canada/services/publications/health-system-services/annual-report-medical-assistance-dying-2022.html.
36. Taylor L. Colombia becomes first Latin American country to decriminalise assisted suicide. *BMJ.* 2022;377:o1219. https://doi.org/10.1136/bmj.o1219.
37. Baidawi A. Euthanasia law passes in Australia for first time. *The New York Times.* November 29, 2017. https://www.nytimes.com/2017/11/29/world/australia/australia-euthanasia-victoria-assisted-dying.html.
38. Queensland University of Technology. End of Life Law for Clinicians. https://end-of-life.qut.edu.au/.

38a. World Federation of Right to Die Societies. World Map. *World Federation of Right to Die Societies*. wfrtds.org/worldmap/. Accessed 11 January 2025.
38b. Delogu G, Morena D, Tortorella V, Perna F, Arcangeli M, Rinaldi R. First Case of Medically Assisted Suicide in Italy Set New Legal Perspectives. *Clin Ter*. 2024 Jan-Feb;175(1):7–10. doi:10.7417/CT.2024.5026. PMID: 38358470.
38c. Taylor L. Ecuador Becomes Second Latin American Country to Decriminalise Euthanasia. *BMJ*. 2024;384:q357. https://doi.org/10.1136/bmj.q357.
39. Povoledo E. Man paralyzed 12 years ago becomes Italy's first assisted suicide. *The New York Times*. June 16, 2022. https://www.nytimes.com/2022/06/16/world/europe/italy-assisted-suicide.html.
40. Farris G. Approach to the medical ethics consultation. *Hosp Med Clin*. 2015;4(1):98–105.
41. Varelius J. On the moral acceptability of physician-assisted dying for non-autonomous psychiatric patients: physician-assisted dying for psychiatric patients. *Bioethics*. 2016;30(4):227–233. https://doi.org/10.1111/bioe.12182.
42. Jackson J. In the matter of Karen Ann Quinlan after 40 years: some personal remembrances from the sidelines of history. *MD Advis*. 2016;9(3):15–20.
43. Holm S. Undignified arguments: a critique. *Camb Q Healthc Ethics*. 2016;25(2):228–238. https://doi.org/10.1017/S0963180115000535.
44. Varelius J. The value of autonomy in medical ethics. *Med Health Care Philos*. 2006;9(3):377–388. https://doi.org/10.1007/s11019-006-9000-z.
45. Malpas PJ, Owens RG. Given that physician-assisted dying is ethical, should it be part of a doctor's role? *Mortality*. 2016;21(4):295–304. https://doi.org/10.1080/13576275.2015.1137279.
46. Lewis D. Assisted dying: a global overview. In: *Palliative Care Nursing: Principles and Evidence for Practice*. 3rd ed. McGraw Hill Education; 2018:391–411.
47. Black BS, Fogarty LA, Phillips H, et al. Surrogate decision makers' understanding of dementia patients' prior wishes for end-of-life care. *J Aging Health*. 2009;21(4):627–650. https://doi.org/10.1177/0898264309333316.
48. Orentlicher D, Pope TM, Rich BA; Physician Aid-in-Dying Clinical Criteria Committee. Clinical criteria for physician aid in dying. *J Palliat Med*. 2016;19(3):259–262. https://doi.org/10.1089/jpm.2015.0092.
49. Goligher EC, Ely EW, Sulmasy DP, et al. Physician-assisted suicide and euthanasia in the ICU: a dialogue on core ethical issues. *Crit Care Med*. 2017;45(2):149–155. https://doi.org/10.1097/CCM.0000000000001818.
50. Lamb C, Pesut B. Conscience and conscientious objection in nursing: a personalist bioethics approach. *Nurs Ethics*. 2021;28(7–8):1319–1328. https://doi.org/10.1177/0969733021996037.
51. Chan B, Somerville M. Converting the "right to life" to the "right to physician-assisted suicide and euthanasia:: an analysis of *Carter v Canada (attorney general)*, Supreme Court of Canada. *Med Law Rev*. 2016;24(2):143–175. https://doi.org/10.1093/medlaw/fww005.
52. Quill TE. Physicians should "assist in suicide" when it is appropriate. *J Law Med Ethics*. 2012;40(1):57–65. https://doi.org/10.1111/j.1748-720X.2012.00646.x.
53. Karsoho H, Fishman JR, Wright DK, Macdonald ME. Suffering and medicalization at the end of life: the case of physician-assisted dying. *Soc Sci Med*. 2016;170:188–196. https://doi.org/10.1016/j.socscimed.2016.10.010.
54. Dees M, Vernooij-Dassen M, Dekkers W, van Weel C. Unbearable suffering of patients with a request for euthanasia or physician-assisted suicide: an integrative review. *Psychooncology*. 2010;19(4):339–352. https://doi.org/10.1002/pon.1612.
55. Lehto RH, Olsen DP, Chan RR. When a patient discusses assisted dying: nursing practice implications. *J Hosp Palliat Nurs*. 2016;18(3):184–191. https://doi.org/10.1097/NJH.0000000000000246.
56. Bates A. Addressing existential suffering. *BC Med J*. 2016;58(5):268–273.
57. van Veen S, Widdershoven G, Beekman A, Evans N. Physician assisted death for psychiatric suffering: experiences in the Netherlands. *Front Psychiatry*. 2022;13:895387. https://doi.org/10.3389/fpsyt.2022.895387.
58. Furfari K, Zehnder N, Abbott J. A case of attempted suicide in Huntington's disease: ethical and moral considerations. *J Clin Ethics*. 2016;27(1):39–42.
59. Campo-Engelstein L, Jankowski J, Mullen M. Should health care providers uphold the DNR of a terminally ill patient who attempts suicide? *HEC Forum*. 2016;28(2):169–174. https://doi.org/10.1007/s10730-015-9289-1.
60. Meisel A. Ethics and law: physician-assisted dying. *J Palliat Med*. 2005;8(3):609–623. https://doi.org/10.1089/jpm.2005.8.609.
61. Hemati Z, Ashouri E, AllahBakhshian M, et al. Dying with dignity: a concept analysis. *J Clin Nurs*. 2016;25(9–10):1218–1228. https://doi.org/10.1111/jocn.13143.
62. World Health Organization. Palliative Care Fact Sheet. August 5, 2020. Accessed August 20, 2022. https://www.who.int/newsroom/fact-sheets/detail/palliative-care.
63. Knaul FM, Farmer PE, Krakauer EL, et al. Alleviating the access abyss in palliative care and pain relief—an imperative of universal health coverage: the Lancet Commission report. *Lancet*. 2018;391(10128):1391–1454. https://doi.org/10.1016/S0140-6736(17)32513-8.
64. De Lima L, Woodruff R, Pettus K, et al. International Association for Hospice and Palliative Care position statement: euthanasia and physician-assisted suicide. *J Palliat Med*. 2017;20(1):8–14. https://doi.org/10.1089/jpm.2016.0290.
65. Schiller CJ, Pesut B, Roussel J, Greig M. But it's legal, isn't it? Law and ethics in nursing practice related to medical assistance in dying. *Nurs Philos Int J Healthc Prof*. 2019;20(4):e12277. https://doi.org/10.1111/nup.12277.
66. Berwick DM. The moral determinants of health. *JAMA*. 2020;324(3):225. https://doi.org/10.1001/jama.2020.11129.
67. Fontalis A, Prousali E, Kulkarni K. Euthanasia and assisted dying: what is the current position and what are the key arguments informing the debate? *J R Soc Med*. 2018;111(11):407–413. https://doi.org/10.1177/0141076818803452.
68. Downie J, Schuklenk U. Social determinants of health and slippery slopes in assisted dying debates: lessons from Canada. *J Med Ethics*. 2021;47(10):662–669. https://doi.org/10.1136/medethics-2021-107493.
69. Gamondi C, Pott M, Payne S. Families' experiences with patients who died after assisted suicide: a retrospective interview study in southern Switzerland. *Ann Oncol*. 2013;24(6):1639–1644. https://doi.org/10.1093/annonc/mdt033.
70. Sheehan K, Gaind KS, Downar J. Medical assistance in dying: special issues for patients with mental illness. *Curr Opin Psychiatry*. 2017;30(1):26–30. https://doi.org/10.1097/YCO.0000000000000298.
71. Quill TE, Back AL, Block SD. Responding to patients requesting physician-assisted death: physician involvement at the very end

of life. *JAMA*. 2016;315(3):245–246. https://doi.org/10.1001/jama.2015.16210.
72. Bryden J. Senate passes bill giving Canadians expanded access to medically assisted dying. *Canadian Press*. March 17, 2021. https://toronto.citynews.ca/2021/03/17/canadians-notnear-death-gain-access-to-assisted-dying-as-senate-passesbill-c-7-2.
73. Hendin H, Foley K. Physician-assisted suicide in Oregon: a medical perspective. *Mich Law Rev*. 2008;106(8):1613–1640.
74. Borasio GD, Jox RJ, Gamondi C. Regulation of assisted suicide limits the number of assisted deaths. *The Lancet*. 2019;393(10175):982–983. https://doi.org/10.1016/S0140-6736(18)32554-6.
75. Riley S. Navigating the new era of assisted suicide and execution drugs. *J Law Biosci*. 2017;4(2):424–434.
76. Dear J. The doctors who invented a new way to help people die. *The Atlantic*. January 22, 2019. Accessed October 4, 2022. https://www.theatlantic.com/health/archive/2019/01/medical-aid-in-dying-medications/580591/.
77. Magelssen M, Kaushal S, Nyembwe KA. Intending, hastening and causing death in non-treatment decisions: a physician interview study. *J Med Ethics*. 2016;42(9):592–596. https://doi.org/10.1136/medethics-2015-103022.
78. ten Have H, Welie JVM. Palliative sedation versus euthanasia: an ethical assessment. *J Pain Symptom Manage*. 2014;47(1):123–136. https://doi.org/10.1016/j.jpainsymman.2013.03.008.
79. Quill TE, Lo B, Brock DW, Meisel A. Last-resort options for palliative sedation. *Ann Intern Med*. 2009;151(6):421–424. https://doi.org/10.7326/0003-4819-151-6-200909150-00007.
80. College of Nurses of Ontario. *Guidance on Nurses' Roles in Medical Assistance in Dying*. College of Nurses of Ontario; 2021. Accessed September 19, 2022. https://www.cno.org/globalassets/docs/prac/41056-guidance-on-nurses-roles-in-maid.pdf.
81. Tahoe Forest Health System. Tahoe Forest Hospice Statement Regarding Medical Aid in Dying Act. 2022. https://www.tfhd.com/medical-aid-dying-act.
82. End of Life Washington. End of Life Attending Physicians Packet. 2022. https://endoflifewa.org/wp-content/uploads/2022/04/EOLWA-AP-Packet_4.11.22.pdf.
83. Campbell CS, Black MA. Dignity, Death, and dilemmas: a study of Washington hospices and physician-assisted death. *J Pain Symptom Manage*. 2014;47(1):137–153. https://doi.org/10.1016/j.jpainsymman.2013.02.024.
84. Canadian Nurses Association. Medical Assistance in Dying. Accessed October 4, 2022. https://www.cna-aiic.ca/en/policy-advocacy/advocacy-priorities/medical-assistance-in-dying#:~:text=Medical%20assistance%20in%20dying%20(MAID,who%20have%20explicitly%20requested%20MAID.
85. Beuthin R, Bruce A. Medical assistance in dying (MAiD): ten things leaders need to know. *Can J Nurs Leadersh*. 2018;31(4):74–81. https://doi.org/10.12927/cjnl.2019.25753.

57 Planning for Death

Reiko Asano

Key Points

- Nurses play a critical role in caring for and meeting the individual needs of patients during their dying process and death—the most vulnerable state for both patients and their families.
- Focus on patient-centered holistic care as the goal of care shifts from curative/aggressive treatment to symptom management, prioritizing comfort, and alleviating pain.
- Offer support to the patient achieving a good death at the end of life by listening to their wishes, honoring their dignity, and respecting their cultural and spiritual beliefs.
- Stay attuned to the unique individual needs of patients and their families by continuing to be their advocate and provide compassionate care, as many terminally ill patients and their families will have a hard time facing and accepting death.

Introduction

Dying and death are inevitable and unavoidable events for all of us. Despite death being part of life, the topic around dying and death often goes unspoken as discussion around death makes most people uncomfortable.[1] The diagnoses that account for approximately 90% of all deaths are considered serious illnesses, such as metastatic or hematologic cancer, interstitial lung disease, chronic obstructive pulmonary disease, end-stage renal failure, heart failure, cirrhosis, diabetes with complications (heart disease, renal disease, peripheral vascular disease), advanced liver disease, amyotrophic lateral sclerosis, multimorbidity, and dementia.[2] The serious illness can be defined as "a health condition that carries a high risk of mortality and either negatively impacts a person's daily function or quality of life, or excessively strains their caregivers."[2(p8)] All humans have to face and go through the process of dying and death at one point in their lives. Dying and death can have so many meanings to each individual and may bring up some strong and complex emotions of fear, uncertainty, the unknown, anxiety, withdrawal, depression, calmness, relief, or acceptance. Oftentimes, the conversation around prognosis and goals of care is not had with patients, family members, and caregivers.[3]

Nurses are privileged to be able to offer support in one of the most significant events, dying and death, which can never be undone. It is important to recognize that there is no second chance to make this process right. A critical role nurses play in this process is providing holistic care to patients and their families. In order to accomplish this role, a nurse "must use her brain, heart, and hands to create healing environments to care for the patient's body, mind and spirit."[4(p1)] However, the discussion of dying and death is considered taboo in many cultures and societies. In these cultures, it can be difficult to talk about death openly for everyone. These discussions of death make people feel unease, uncomfortable, or vulnerable in some situations.[5]

Differences between Hospice and Palliative Care Near the End of Life

Hospice and palliative care have been recognized as healthcare specialties in the United States, United Kingdom, Ireland, Canada, Australia, and New Zealand.[6] While hospice is limited to seriously ill patients with a life expectancy of less than 6 months, palliative care may be initiated at any time of a person's illness while they continue to receive active medical treatments for their illness. Hospice care costs may be covered by Medicare Part A (Hospital Insurance) if the hospice doctor certifies with a life expectancy of fewer than 6 months and the patient opts for comfort care over curative treatment.[7] Additionally, Medicare Part B (Medical Insurance) may cover palliative care costs. The majority of private insurance plans cover the care provided in the hospital, skilled nursing, rehabilitation, hospice/palliative care facilities, or home.[8]

Hospice care is provided to relieve symptoms and pain; support the patient and their family with their emotional, psychological, and spiritual needs; assist in the coordination of care; and improve quality of life. Receiving hospice care means stopping curative active medical treatments for one's physical illness, and the person is expected to die within six months or less. Therefore, the decision to receive hospice care is a hard one for patients and their families. They need guidance and assistance from healthcare professionals in making decisions that best fit their needs. Hospice care is usually provided by an interdisciplinary team consisting of hospice physicians, nurses, social workers, and spiritual care clinicians.

Alternatively, palliative care is "an approach that improves the quality of life of patients and their families facing the problem associated with life-threatening illness, through the prevention and relief of

Table 57.1 Barriers and facilitators of a good death organized by key themes

Barriers	Facilitators
Health care system/delivery models	
Patient preferences not aligned with healthcare delivery models Financial and administrative models of healthcare Healthcare professionals focused on cure	Use of specialized advanced heart failure care program Advance medical planning Educate healthcare professionals about palliative care
Palliative care	
Late referral Healthcare professionals fail to adopt palliative care	Palliative care consultations Initiation of referral to palliative care services Involvement of palliative care teams Effective use of pain medications
Prediction of mortality	
Difficulty predicting mortality Lack of awareness of the proximity of death Lack of awareness of high mortality	Use of more comprehensive predictors of mortality
Health status/disease progression	
Impaired decision-making Severity of illness Change in preferences as the disease progresses toward end of life Very poor functional status of patient	Knowledge and education about the disease process Frequent and close communication with multidisciplinary team Frequent and close communication with family members who make decisions for an impaired patient
Communicating about death	
Lack of communication Lack of advanced care planning Difficulty in approaching the topic (death and dying) for patient, professional, and family member Avoidance of acknowledgment of the potential imminence of dying Avoidance of open awareness of death	Initiation of a conversation about death and dying by healthcare professionals Open discussion about death and dying

Source: Reference 12.

suffering by means of early identification and impeccable assessment and treatment of pain and other problems, physical, psychosocial and spiritual."[9(p17)] The goal of palliative care is to prioritize and enhance the quality of life for patients with a life-limiting illness by identifying and relieving symptom burdens through addressing an individual's physical, psychological, emotional, or spiritual needs. Palliative care is generally provided by an interdisciplinary team consisting of primary physicians, specialists, nurses, social workers, and spiritual care clinicians. In contrast to hospice, persons living with a serious illness can receive palliative care services without forgoing active medical treatments for their illness, and this has some coverage by Medicare.[10]

Yet, according to the World Health Organization, less than 15% of patients worldwide who require palliative care receive it.[9] Palliative care may be provided in a hospital (inpatient or outpatient), assisted living facility, nursing home, or home.

Planning for Death

The meaning and perception of death may vary by culture, belief, religion, and ethnicity. Therefore, it is important to provide culturally appropriate care and be culturally sensitive, especially when patients are at the most vulnerable state both physiologically and psychologically. Similarly, understanding and achieving a good death are important topics. According to the National Academy of Medicine, a good death can be defined as "free from avoidable distress and suffering for patient, family and caregivers, in general accord with the patient's and family's wishes, and reasonably consistent with clinical, cultural and ethical standards."[11(p1)] The perception of a good death may change over time based on the progression of the disease and toward the end of life.[12] In order to achieve a good death, the following factors need to be taken into consideration: minimizing symptom burden, making relational reconciliation, spiritual peacemaking, and decreasing the burden on loved ones by making financial and funeral plans in advance.[12] The research highlights that a good death may be receiving comfort care and dying at home rather than dying in the intensive care unit or in the hospital while receiving invasive life-prolonging procedures.[12] Table 57.1 summarizes the barriers and facilitators of a good death.

Regardless of cultural beliefs about death, it is unknown to all of us and brings uncertainty for the dying person and the family. The planning for death may bring up intense emotions as the dying person and their family face the possibility of dying. Preparing for actual death is one of the hardest times for all involved. It is vital to remember that some patients and family members are more prepared than others.

Nurses are uniquely positioned to provide symptom management and prepare the patient and their family for what to expect as death is nearing. Nurses caring near death must be prepared to offer support throughout the dying process, have difficult conversations, and help patients and families cope with realistic expectations of the dying and death.

Near the End of Life

"End of life" refers to the period of time around death, which varies from hours, days, weeks, to months. Palliative and hospice care may be offered to better support seriously ill patients and their families near the end of life regardless of the settings. Experiences near the end of life differ for each individual. For some patients and their caretakers, death may come suddenly; and for others, it may happen over some period of time. Patients' physical and cognitive functions also vary, where some stay conscious with a clear state of mind through the end of life while others may be less conscious or have an altered state of mind.

Despite the concept of palliative care having been around since the early 1960s, inequity still exists in access and utilization of palliative care depending on diseases and illnesses. Moreover, misunderstanding of palliative care may lead to some healthcare professionals being more reluctant to make referrals to palliative care due to difficult conversations with patients and their families, a sense of failure due to transitioning into comfort care over invasive procedures, or feelings of abandonment.[13]

Research shows that many healthcare professionals feel unprepared to care for patients at the end of life and to have conversations around difficult and complex topics, death and dying, with patients and their families. One of the reasons that healthcare professionals are not equipped to discuss this topic with patients and families is that they received inadequate education and training on topics around death and dying and the purpose of palliative and hospice care. Furthermore, the important emphasis on the integration of palliative care for persons and their families living with serious illnesses is lacking in nursing education.

Culturally Sensitive Care Near the End of Life

When providing near-end-of-life care, it is of utmost importance to consider cultural differences, in order to be able to provide culturally sensitive care across diverse populations.[14] The care of persons and their families as they near the end of life must be provided in a culturally sensitive manner that aligns with their beliefs, values, and preferences for end-of-life care.

In order to provide culturally sensitive palliative care to meet the unique individual needs of patients and families, nurses need to be educated and trained to provide holistic person-centered palliative care.

Support for Family Members and Caregivers Near the End of Life

Family members and caregivers are a crucial part of care as death nears. They may include families, as well as friends, neighbors, church members, or healthcare facility staff. Persons with serious illnesses may be cared for at inpatient hospitals, intensive care units, home settings, nursing homes, residential facilities, assisted living facilities, group homes, or prisons. This poses challenges to some families due to limited space, visiting hours, and privacy. Anticipation of common symptoms and extensive planning may mitigate unexpected challenges for all involved.[15] Many of the family members may hold full-time jobs outside of caring for their loved ones. They may only be able to visit the patients after work or school, which could be outside visiting hours. Some families may be juggling raising young children or caring for other sick family members at home while working full-time or commuting long hours. In these cases, their ability to be involved or present at the bedside may be very limited despite their wishes. In essence, the healthcare team may be the ones spending most of the time at the bedside caring for dying individuals.

Meeting Individual Needs at the End of Life: The Nurses' Role

The following characteristics and traits are important for nurses to consider when providing support and care to persons and their families near the end of life:

- Empathy: The ability to understand the patient's personal experience from their view free from bias or prejudice.[15]
- Authenticity: The ability to carry openness and trustworthiness in a genuine manner rather than a professional facade.[15]
- Person-centered care: The ability to provide care that ensures the patient's wishes are honored. Treat patients with respect, compassion, and dignity. Actively advocate for their wishes[16,17]
- Compassion: The ability to be aware of others' suffering and pain and take nonverbal and verbal cues.[18]
- Comfort: The ability to provide care focused on pain relief, symptom control, and quality of life.[18]
- Dignity: The ability to honor others' sense of self, desire for control, privacy, and autonomy.[19]
- Unconditional positive regard: The ability to accept others without passing judgment, communicate with all respect, and honor the patient's values and needs.[15]
- Attention to detail: The ability to think and assess the situation critically without assumptions. Consider every scenario before making any premature decisions or judgments.[15]

Physical Needs

The majority of patients experience distressing symptoms such as pain, fatigue, and dyspnea that may require extra care, attention, and medications to alleviate as much as possible. The focus of care shifts from fixing problems to monitoring and controlling vital signs closely and tightly; the healthcare team may be more focused on providing comfort care by minimizing discomfort near the end of life.[15] Plans of care at the end of life include weighing between the benefits and burdens of treatment.

At this stage, the interventions are decided based on the patient's distress and discomfort by following their wishes and goals of care. It is important to have plans for the deactivation of implantable cardioverter defibrillators or resuscitation by following their advance directives. In case the patient may not be capable of making decisions, it is important to have them identify a decision maker or healthcare power of attorney in advance to prevent any miscommunication or misunderstanding in making decisions.

A decrease in fluid intake or dry mouth may be observed in patients at the end of life. In order to minimize distressing symptoms caused by dehydration, ice chips or sips of water may be offered as appropriate. In some cases, providing mouth care or spraying normal saline into the mouth may help relieve some discomfort related to dehydration.[15] As the body is slowly shutting down, it may cause patients difficulties in swallowing medications in the form of capsules and tablets. Nurses may need to advocate for the patient's needs by following the principles of providing comfort care to reduce as much discomfort and distress as possible.

Psychological, Emotional, and Spiritual Needs

Patients near the end of life experience complex symptoms with many emotions.[20] The pain they experience may not be related to physiological pains. Some patients experience psychological pain, which is associated with fear of abandonment, pain, or personal value.[20] Some may experience spiritual pain, which can be defined as a "pain deep in one's soul or being that is not physical," in which more than half of patients experience spiritual struggles including conflicts, tensions, and negative emotions while receiving palliative care.[20(p1215)] Spirituality is "a dynamic and intrinsic aspect of humanity through which persons seek ultimate meaning, purpose, and transcendence, and experience relationship to self, family, others, community, society, nature, and the significant or sacred."[20(p1216)] Providing psychosocial, emotional, and spiritual care is an essential component of near-end-of-life care. A lack of spiritual care support by the healthcare professional may lead to patients receiving more aggressive care and experiencing poor quality of life. Consequently, it may lead to the underutilization of hospice in some cases.[20] In order for patients to receive patient-centered end-of-life care, a comprehensive assessment of their psychosocial, emotional, and spiritual needs should be performed by an interdisciplinary team. In addition, complementary alternative therapy such as mindfulness, guided imagery, and cognitive behavioral therapy may be used to facilitate relaxation.[21] These noninvasive therapies can be beneficial to help reduce depression and anxiety.[21] Lastly, it is important to keep in mind that the patient's psychological and spiritual needs may change over time toward the end of dying and death.

Imminent Death

Case Study: Person Nearing Imminent Death

James, 68 years old, was diagnosed with bladder cancer at the age of 64. He had a surgical procedure for a urostomy. He was in remission for 2 years. Then cancer came back. James was raised in the rural south during the pre-Depression and served in World War II in the Pacific theater in the Army. After the war, he returned to his home state of Louisiana and started a career in home improvement and carpentry. He lived with his 64-year-old wife. His older son was living out of state, and his younger son was living near his home. James and his wife had 11 grandchildren who were not living close by.

One day, James' older son received a call from James' attending physician saying his dad was gravely ill and probably will pass within 2 weeks. James' son recalls, "Something told me that I needed to go see him now and not to wait." James' son immediately booked a flight with his daughter and was at James' bedside the very night he received the call.

James was heavily sedated with morphine for his pain. He had periods when he could respond and talk and other periods when he could not stay alert. His son thanked James and told him what a great father he was. He also thanked his father for all the things that he had done for him and told him what a great role model he was.

At one point, his son asked James, "Why didn't you leave mom? She did not treat you right." James and his wife had a troubled marriage, and she treated him very badly. James responded to his son, "I did not want to lose you and your brother."

James had a couple of friends who came to see him in the hospital that evening and left. His son spent all night with James at the bedside and did not leave the hospital. Around midnight, James' son stepped out of the room for no more than 10 minutes to make some phone calls. When his son came back to the room, James had died.

James' son recalls about the night of James' passing, "I was just hollow, I just felt I kind of knew it was coming but you were never prepared until it comes. When I went back to the room, my dad's eyes were open, and he was not breathing. I immediately got on the phone, and I called the doctor. He came to the room and said my dad was gone. So, I called my mom and my brother, and they were at my dad's bedside by 1 a.m., but he had already passed."

He also recalls about the night of passing that "The nurse came in the room, and she gave my dad morphine. Within half an hour he was gone. He was suffering, and he was in a lot of pain."

> I was there with my dad. If I had waited even for a day, that would have been too late. Something said you need to go there immediately. It is a very personal thing when somebody is passing. I did not want my daughter to see my dad dying, so I left her with her grandmother. I didn't know if I wanted to see him dying because it was a personal thing for him. I just wanted to show him how much I appreciated him and thank him for being a great father. I just wanted to thank him for the opportunity to be with him.

Questions to Consider:

1. A patient requests morphine for the intolerable pain; however, his family asks that it not be given to him as they are afraid of losing him. How would you handle this situation?
2. James' son regrets leaving the room and that his dad was alone when he took his last breath. He feels it was his fault. How would you respond to him?
3. James' son feels that the last dose of morphine hastened his dad's death. How would you respond to him?

Imminent death may be predicted by the body's systems slowly shutting down.[15] This means patients may present with gradual hypoxia, metabolic or respiratory acidosis from renal failure, and brain dysfunction related to a hypoxic state. The signs and symptoms of imminent death include a drop in oxygen saturation, weakness, drowsiness, confusion, pale skin, decreased food or fluid intake, difficulty swallowing, and difficulty taking oral medications.[15] Table 57.2 highlights the physiological changes of dying and interventions for patients and caregivers.

Family and Caregiver Needs

Family members and caregivers often experience heightened duties and burdens during end-of-life care.[1] Caring for patients with serious illnesses is burdensome and causes emotional difficulties for family members and caregivers.[22] Moreover, they are at higher risk of developing anxiety, stress, and depression regardless of age, sex, or ethnicity as they care for their loved ones.[22] In reality, the majority of family members and caregivers are responsible for performing tasks such as communicating with healthcare professionals, making decisions, and anticipating loss and grief.[22] As imminent

Table 57.2 Symptoms in the normal progression of dying and suggested interventions

Symptoms	Suggested interventions
Early-stage sensation	
Perception.	Interpret the signs and symptoms to the patient (when appropriate) and family as part of the normal dying process; for example, assure them the patient's "seeing" and even talking to persons who have died is normal and often expected.
Impairment in the ability to grasp ideas and reason; periods of alertness along with periods of disorientation and restlessness are also noted.	Urge family members to look for metaphors for death in speech and conversation (e.g., talk of a long journey, needing maps or tickets, or preparing for a trip in other ways) and use these metaphors as a departure point for conversation with the patient.
	Urge family to take advantage of the patient's periods of lucidity to talk with patient and ensure nothing is left unsaid.
	Encourage family members to touch and speak slowly and gently to the patient without being patronizing.
	Maximize safety; for example, use bedrails and schedule people to sit with the patient.
Some loss of visual acuity.	Keep sensory stimulation to a minimum, including light, sounds, and visual stimulation; reading to a patient who has enjoyed reading in the past may provide comfort.
Increased sensitivity to bright lights while other senses, except hearing, are dulled.	Urge the family to be mindful of what they say "over" the patient because hearing remains present; also continue to urge family to say what they wish not to be left unsaid.
Cardiorespiratory	
Increased pulse and respiratory rate.	Normalize the observed changes by interpreting the signs and symptoms as part of the normal dying process and ensuring the patient's comfort.
Agonal respirations or sounds of gasping for air without apparent discomfort.	Again, normalize the observed changes by interpreting the signs and symptoms as part of the normal dying process and ensuring the patient's comfort; assess and treat respiratory distress as appropriate.
Apnea, periodic, or Cheyne-Stokes respirations.	Assess and treat respiratory distress as appropriate.
Inability to cough or clear secretions efficiently, resulting in gurgling or congested breathing (sometimes referred to as the "death rattle").	Assess use and need for parenteral fluids, tube feedings, or hydration. (It is generally appropriate to either discontinue or greatly decrease these at this point in time.)
	Reposition the patient in a side-lying position with the head of the bed elevated.
	Suctioning is rarely needed, but when appropriate, suction should be gentle and only at the level of the mouth, throat, and nasal pharynx.
	Administer anticholinergic drugs (transdermal scopolamine, hyoscyamine) as appropriate, recognizing and discussing with the family that they will not decrease already existing secretions.
Renal/urinary	
Decreasing urinary output, sometimes urinary incontinence or retention.	Insert catheter and/or use absorbent padding.
	Carefully assess for urinary retention because restlessness can be a related symptom.
Musculoskeletal	
Gradual loss of the ability to move, beginning with the legs, then progressing.	Reposition every few hours as appropriate.
	Anticipate needs such as sips of fluids, oral care, changing of bed pads and linens, and so on.
Late-stage sensation	
Perception	
Unconsciousness.	Interpret the patient's unconsciousness to the family as part of the normal dying process.
Eyes remain half-open, blink reflex is absent; sense of hearing remains intact and may slowly decrease.	
	Provide for total care, including incontinence of urine and stool.
	Encourage family members to speak slowly and gently to the patient, with the assurance that hearing remains intact.
Cardiorespiratory	
Heart rate may double, strength of contractions decrease; rhythm becomes irregular.	Interpret these changes to family members as part of the normal dying process.
Patient feels cool to the touch and becomes diaphoretic.	Frequent linen changes and sponge baths may enhance comfort.
Cyanosis is noted in the tip of the nose, nail beds, and knees; extremities may become mottled (progressive mottling indicates death within a few days); absence of a palpable radial pulse may indicate death within hours.	
Renal/urinary	
A precipitous drop in urinary output.	Interpret to the family the drop in urinary output as a normal sign that death is near, usually 24–72 hours away.
Carefully assess for urinary retention; restlessness can be a related symptom.	

Source: Reference 15.

death approaches, patients are more likely to lose physical function and independence. A recent study highlights the association between the functional independence of the patient and the emotional burden of the caregiver.[23] Therefore, family-centered interventions are crucial to patients achieving a good death. As family members and caregivers are critical components for patients achieving a good death and optimal end-of-life care, the healthcare team needs to be mindful of their coping skills and religious beliefs and provide resources such as referral to pastoral care consult and social work to best support them while they go through one of the most vulnerable and difficult times of their lives in caring for dying patients.[22]

Nursing Caring at the End of Life

Providing care at the end of life can be emotionally demanding and ethically challenging to nurses.[24] In order to best support patients in achieving a good death, nurses themselves need to be prepared mentally, psychologically, and emotionally to best guide and support end-of-life care to patients and their families. It is a privilege and honor for nurses to assist and be part of dying patients' and their families' journeys. To be able to provide compassionate care, it is important to understand the unique needs of our patients and their families at these most difficult and stressful times of their lives. The end-of-life experiences of patients and families can be affected by the words, actions, and care we provide to our patients.[20] Witnessing patients suffer may cause emotional distress to nurses, ultimately leading to compassion fatigue.[25] Up to 30% of palliative care nurses face burnout.[26] The factors associated with burnout include emotional exhaustion, conciliation, workload, and work environment.[26] For more on self-care for palliative and hospice nurses, please see Chapter 73, "Occupation Stress, Burnout, and Self-care in Palliative Nursing."

Conclusion

To be included in this most vulnerable and personal life event is a true privilege. Many terminally ill patients and their families will have a hard time facing and accepting death. While most individuals are not afraid of death, the process of dying is what most affects them. What we can offer as nurses when accompanying dying patients is to honor their wishes. This is also the time for nurses to go back to the most basic nursing principles—be a patient's advocate and provide compassionate care—the core of what nurses are called to do as the most trusted profession.

REFERENCES

1. Oates JR, Maani C v. Death and Dying. 2022. Retrieved February 2, 2025, from https://www.ncbi.nlm.nih.gov/books/NBK536978/
2. Kelley AS, Bollens-Lund E. Identifying the population with serious illness: the "denominator" challenge. *Journal of Palliative Medicine*. 2018;21(S2):S-7.
3. Curtis JR, Downey L, Back AL, et al. Effect of a patient and clinician communication-priming intervention on patient-reported goals-of-care discussions between patients with serious illness and clinicians: a randomized clinical trial. *JAMA Intern Med*. 2018;178(7):930–940.
4. Riegel F, Crossetti MGO, Martini JG, Nes AAG. Florence Nightingale's theory and her contributions to holistic critical thinking in nursing. *Rev Bras Enferm*. 2021;74(2):e20200139.
5. Bergenholtz H, Missel M, Timm H. Talking about death and dying in a hospital setting—a qualitative study of the wishes for end-of-life conversations from the perspective of patients and spouses. *BMC Palliat Care*. 2020;19(1):1–9.
6. Kumar S, Palmed D. Palliative Care and Hospice Outside of the United States. 2023. Retrieved February 2, 2025, from https://www.uptodate.com/contents/palliative-care-and-hospice-outside-of-the-united-states
7. Medicare.gov. Hospice Care. 2023. Accessed June 1, 2023. https://www.medicare.gov/coverage/hospice-care.
8. Centers for Medicare & Medicaid Services. Medicare Hospice Benefits. Retrieved February 2, 2025, from https://www.medicare.gov/publications/02154-medicare-hospice-benefits.pdf
9. Radbruch L, de Lima L, Knaul F, et al. Redefining palliative care—a new consensus-based definition. *J Pain Symptom Manage*. 2020;60(4):754–764.
10. Medicare.org. Does Medicare Cover Palliative Care? 2023. Accessed June 1, 2023. https://www.medicare.org/articles/does-medicare-cover-palliative-care/.
11. Newman T. What Does a "Good Death" Really Mean? 2016. Retrieved June 1, 2023, from https://www.medicalnewstoday.com/articles/308447
12. Asano R, Abshire M, Dennison-Himmelfarb C, Davidson PM. Barriers and facilitators to a "good death" in heart failure: an integrative review. *Collegian*. 2019;26(6):651–665.
13. Hawley P. Barriers to access to palliative care. *Palliat Care*. 2017;10:1178224216688887.
14. Coats H, Downey L, Sharma RK, Curtis JR, Engelberg RA. Quality of communication and trust in patients with serious illness: an exploratory study of the relationships of race/ethnicity, socioeconomic status, and religiosity. *J Pain Symptom Manage*. 2018;56(4):530–540.
15. Berry P, Griffie J. Planning for the actual death. *Social Aspects of Care*. 2019;5:420–431.
16. American Association of Colleges of Nursing. Person-Centered Care. 2023. Accessed February 12, 2023. https://www.aacnnursing.org/5B-Tool-Kit/Themes/Person-Centered-Care.
17. Rodríguez-Prat A, Monforte-Royo C, Porta-Sales J, Escribano X, Balaguer A. Patient perspectives of dignity, autonomy and control at the end of life: systematic review and meta-ethnography. *PLoS One*. 2016;11(3):e0151435.
18. Skorpen Tarberg A, Landstad BJ, Hole T, Thronæs M, Kvangarsnes M. Nurses' experiences of compassionate care in the palliative pathway. *J Clin Nurs*. 2020;29(23–24):4818–4826.
19. Martí-García C, Fernández-Férez A, Fernández-Sola C, et al. Patients' experiences and perceptions of dignity in end-of-life care in emergency departments: a qualitative study. *J Adv Nurs*. 2023;79(1):269–280.
20. Antunes ML, Reis-Pina P. The physician and end-of-life spiritual care: the PALliatiVE approach. *Am J Hosp Palliat Med*. 2022;39(10):1215–1226.
21. Farabelli JP, Kimberly SM, Altilio T, et al. Top ten tips palliative care clinicians should know about psychosocial and family support. *J Palliat Med*. 2020;23(2):280–286.
22. Asano R, Kellogg A, Sulmasy D, Anderson KM, Nolan MT. Religious involvement, depressive symptoms, and burden in caregivers of terminally ill patients. *J Hosp Palliat Nurs*. 2021;23(3):271–276.
23. Soto-Rubio A, Perez-Marin M, Tomas Miguel J, Barreto Martin P. Emotional distress of patients at end-of-life and their caregivers: interrelation and predictors. *Front Psychol*. 2018;9:2199.

24. White D, Meeker MA. Guiding the process of dying: the personal impact on nurses. *J Hosp Palliat Nurs*. 2019;21(5):390–396.
25. Portoghese I, Galletta M, Larkin P, et al. Compassion fatigue, watching patients suffering and emotional display rules among hospice professionals: a daily diary study. *BMC Palliat Care*. 2020;19(1):1–7.
26. Gómez-Urquiza JL, Albendín-García L, Velando-Soriano A, et al. Burnout in palliative care nurses, prevalence and risk factors: a systematic review with meta-analysis. *Int J Environ Res Public Health*. 2020;17(20):7672.

58

Grief and Bereavement

Inge B. Corless and Danai Papadatou

Key Points

- People with a life-threatening condition and their family members experience a wide range of losses, which trigger a grieving process that helps them to reconstruct their life story that has been affected by the illness experience.
- "Anticipatory grief" is common when death is impending or certain. Although painful, it provides patients and families the opportunity to participate in advance care planning that ensures a dignified death in accord with their preferences and values.
- Bereavement is the state of having experienced the death of a significant other.
- The grief process of bereaved families is affected by how people die and how children and adults were informed and supported through the exchange of farewells with the dying. Such factors shape contribute to their subsequent adjustment to loss.
- Grief manifestations which are misperceived and treated as depression may forestall or complicate a person's bereavement
- Most people are supported by their family network and community; some may need grief counseling, and only few require grief therapy. Nurses are in a key position to assess their needs.

We contend that *grieving* through the illness or accident and subsequent death of a person is not merely an intrapsychic process but rather an *intersubjective process* that evolves among the ill/injured person, the family, and their social network, as well as the cultural and religious community. Following the death of the individual, this intersubjective process also includes memories of the deceased who is, in varying degrees, present or absent from the inner world of bereaved individuals and families. To examine these issues, this chapter is divided into two sections: anticipation of the loss and the dying in the first section and post-death bereavement considerations in the second section. Our focus is primarily on adults afflicted with a life-threatening illness, or accident, and the effects on and implications for members of their family and significant others.

Grieving Associated with Impending Death

Toward the end of life, the seriously ill/injured person and family members are confronted with *multiple losses*. These losses involve: the potential loss of wholeness and bodily integrity; the certainty caused by the realization (if the person retains that capacity) that life is coming to an end; the loss of control and freedom to act in familiar ways; losses related to changes in family dynamics; and losses in roles, responsibilities, and relationships at work and in social/family life. These losses trigger a *grieving process* that helps patients and families to adjust to the reality that is imposed by the impending death. Grieving is not a passive but rather a healthy active process which involves the reconstruction of a world of meanings that have been challenged by the diagnosis of a life-threatening illness or accident and the possibility and subsequent certainty of a loved one's mortality.

Meaning-making varies according to the person's family, social and cultural background. The question for healthcare professionals is how to best support the family through their grief and the adjustment to the realities imposed by the death due to the accident or illness.

Sharing "Bad" News

The establishment of a trusted relationship among the dying person, the family, and the healthcare team is affected by how information about the accident's occurrence/illness progression and prognosis is imparted, as well as how through this process patients and families feel understood and supported. To begin with, sharing what most would consider to be bad news is never easy to do. The patient (if conscious) is in a liminal state; that is, they consider alternative outcomes about what the provider will say.

In palliative care, it has been argued that opportunities for discussions about end-of-life (EOL) preferences should occur earlier in the illness trajectory. Knutzen and colleagues note that "most EOL discussions occur approximately 1 month before death."[1(p1)] They attribute this to the treatment style of oncologists who battle on to defeat their foe, the neoplasm. The oncologists in the Knutzen study responded to patient concerns about disease progression or dying with "optimistic future talk . . . or expressed concern over treatment discontinuation."[1(p1)]

The SPIKES and PEWTER frameworks[2] provide pneumonics for nurses and other professionals to use in preparation for the delivery of difficult-to-convey information that is even more difficult to hear

Box 58.1 The SPIKES Framework

The SPIKES framework helps the professional to remember the importance of:

- the *Setting*
- the patient's *Perceptions* of the situation
- the *Invitation/information* the patient and family would like to have
- the *Knowledge* about and when the bad news is to be presented
- the *Empathy* needed when hearing and discussing "bad" news
- the *Summary* and explanation of what has been said

These activities serve as the prelude to discussing the plan of care.[2]

(Box 58.1). This information, often referred to as "bad news," is defined by Buckman as "any information, which adversely and seriously affects an individual's view of his or her future."[3(p15)]

The concepts in the PEWTER model are similar to the SPIKES framework. In a demonstration of the use of the SPIKES and PEWTER models of delivering "bad news," Bumb and colleagues[2] give an example of a physician and nurse entering the room in which the patient begins to cry. Neglecting the patient's tears, they immediately delve into their agenda for the visit. And while the focus of the meeting from the perspective of the providers is breaking bad news to the patient in a humane way following the indicated steps, attention to the tears and the unease of the patient would appear to be of the utmost concern to and for the patient and is part of the initial steps of the model. Inquiring of the patient about the tears is essential if the focus is the person and not the delivery of any news and, especially, what will be perceived by the patient and family as "bad news." And while it is likely the tears are about what the patient fears they will be hearing from the providers, it might be a concern about another family member or some other matter. Unless one inquires to discover what is uppermost on the person's mind at that moment, the opportunity is lost. Listening may reveal important information that will have implications for the ability to engage in shared decision-making regarding one's palliative care and is a part of the steps of the SPIKES model. The example given in the Bumb et al.[2] paper, unfortunately, is what commonly occurs in many practices.

In the event, the tears are about what the patient will hear from the providers; the opportunity is present to learn more about the patient's concerns. This is a golden opportunity in that the presentation of the proposed plan of care can be framed, as much as possible, to meet those concerns. This example highlights the importance of making the priorities of the patient the priorities of the healthcare team to the degree possible. Once the information is shared and the patient's and family's questions are addressed, professionals need to be able to co-create with the patient and family a plan that addresses their concerns, ways of meeting their needs, and the decisions with regard to palliative care, including the amelioration of discomfort. Providing time for the patient and family to ask questions, express hesitations, request a second opinion, and receive counseling with regard to specific concerns is as essential as the information that is presented by the care providers, including how to contact them with questions, concerns, and/or healthcare issues.

1. Absorbing bad news may take more than a few minutes and often involves a psychosocial process extended over several days or longer depending on personal, family, and interpersonal factors. Whatever the case, the role of professionals is to support the patient and family and to help them address the situation in a manner over which they have some control.

Acknowledging Losses and Providing Grief Support

Imparting information about a life-threatening condition is never enough in and of itself. The sensitivity, skills, and compassion with which information is shared affect people's trust in professionals and willingness to share deeper suffering that is triggered by the multiple actual or potential losses experienced throughout the illness trajectory and at the end of a person's life, as illustrated in Table 58.1.

It is worth underscoring that the "loss of the self" is not evoked solely by physical discomfort or malfunction but involves a profound alienation from oneself. "Alienation" refers to being a stranger to oneself, to others, or to one's familiar world. Clinicians and researchers who have studied the suffering of patients[4–8] highlighted the significance of helping the person to voice the suffering evoked by the grieving process over multiple losses and to create narratives about their experiences.

Arthur Frank discusses three narratives that encompass how people may make sense of their illness and related suffering.[9] These narratives have implications for EOL care.

The "restitution" narrative involves accounts about how life was interrupted by the disease and getting back to the way things were prior to the diagnosis of illness. The illness is perceived as an "unlucky breakdown to be fixed" or "a bump in the road to be overcome"; the confrontation with one's mortality is not considered. Restitution narratives are often maintained and reinforced by healthcare professionals because their exclusive focus is on hope for a cure; they never include the consideration "what if things do not go as expected" and one's life-threatening condition deteriorates or leads to death. The tragedy when this happens is that people are left with no story because it has been limited to a "survival" narrative, which was often reinforced by people in their environment.

The "chaos" narrative has no plot, no coherent sequence of events, no structure of a story. For the person, the illness is perceived as a long battle with no perceived end in sight. They are submerged in anxiety over the multiple losses, experience intolerable uncertainty, are unable to reflect upon or put into words their experiences.

Table 58.1 Potential losses

• Loss of one's sense of wholeness and sense of indestructibility
• Loss of bodily integrity
• Loss of familiar self-image
• Loss of familiar world and way of living
• Loss of familiar ways of relating to others
• Loss of certainty and control over one's life
• Loss of family, professional, and social roles and responsibilities
• Loss of goals and life plans as to who one might become
• Loss of freedom to act in ways that give meaning to one's life
• Loss of one's assumptive world
• Loss of one's life story

According to Frank, chaos narratives are "anti-narratives" and, as such, represent a "non-self" story.[9] For this reason, it is important to honor them and acknowledge the person's suffering of a life that is perceived as horrific and meaningless.

In the "quest" narrative, the illness becomes the opportunity to "gain" something that transforms one's view of self and life. In this narrative, meaning is attributed to one's experience. These stories involve accounts of a trajectory through the illness with alternative pathways, including one's mortality; the person acknowledges and grieves over multiple losses and concurrently attributes meaning to hardships in such ways that are indicative of personal growth.

Most healthcare providers reinforce restitution narratives such as "keep thinking that you will get well" and avoid patients offering chaos narratives that evoke increased anxiety and are inspired by people who share quest narratives. When accompanying the dying person and family, it is therefore important to listen and honor their stories and provide a safe space where they can share their suffering, grieve their losses, and attribute a meaning that helps them cope effectively with EOL challenges. It is also essential to avoid correcting, shaping, or idealizing their narratives.

During the pandemic, some attention has been given to the illness narratives of patients with COVID-19 or long COVID. According to Rushforth et al., a unique feature of long COVID narratives was the absence of a professional witness to them.[10] People struggled with a fragmented inner monologue before finding an empathetic audience and other resonant narratives in an online community. Participants provided a rich description of the diverse manifestations of a grave, unknown, and life-threatening illness; a shared account of rejection by the healthcare system; and a powerful call for action to fix the broken story.

Anticipatory Grief and Support at the End of Life

When the person's condition deteriorates, they experience life-in-limbo, given that they are not actively dying but are not able to function with their prior competence. The term "liminality" reflects a condition of being in limbo—neither "here" nor "there"—and not being the accomplished individual the person perceived themself as previously being.

Death is not probable but certain. Grieving in anticipation involves a process of adaptation to the reality of impending death manifested through worries about deterioration and the prospect of death, separation anxiety, emotional withdrawal, concerns about location of care and death, and direct or indirect communication of farewells.[11]

Family members often experience "ambiguous loss" when the individual *is physically present but psychologically absent* due to major changes in physical condition, psychosocial well-being, and ways of relating to others.[12] The nurse's listening ear can help the family express their concerns and their pain when death ceases to be "possible" and becomes "certain" or "impending." Family members do not necessarily lose hope, but the nature of their hope changes when death becomes inevitable. From hoping for a cure or the stabilization of a deteriorating condition, they may now hope for the relief of the dying person's suffering or for conditions that will ensure a good death or for being present at the bedside of their loved one when death occurs.

The realization of one's impending death evokes in both the patient and family members "anticipatory grief," described as a form of grief work that occurs in anticipation of a loved one's death. Coehlo and Barbosa identified two aspects of the anticipatory grief experience, namely *traumatic distress*, related to exposure to life-threatening conditions, and *separation distress*, concerned with losses in the current relationship as well as anticipation of future loss and the adjustment to loss of the relationship.[11]

Anticipatory grief is often disregarded or disenfranchised by healthcare professionals who feel nonplussed as to how to support the grieving family members. However, anticipatory grief actively engages the person and family in defining and ensuring conditions for a "good death" which affects their experience of EOL care and death.[13] Not all people (those dying and/or their loved ones) express anticipatory grief. This is for a variety of reasons. The individual may not understand, be ready, or want to understand the "reality" of the situation as perceived by the healthcare professionals. For healthcare providers, this creates the challenge of assessing whether the patient's or family's lack of professed recognition will preclude engaging in activities and decisions (e.g., care at home vs. hospital vs. hospice) that might otherwise be performed. Consultation with a professional expert in this field will provide the assistance that the staff need to support the patient and family.

The question of whether experiencing anticipatory grief is related to improved bereavement outcomes is disputed, with some researchers such as Nielsen et al.[14] indicating that it may be related to problems in subsequent bereavement, while others such as Rogalla[15] highlight the positive impact of anticipatory grief both in preparation for and at the time of death, as well as throughout bereavement.

An intervention that has been found to positively affect both the dying person and family who are aware of it is advance care planning (ACP). In a qualitative analysis of the literature on the goals of ACP, Fleuren and colleagues identified five components of ACP: "respecting individual patient autonomy, improving quality of care, strengthening relationships, preparing for end-of-life, and reducing overtreatment."[16(p13)] It is clear from these goals that some, if not all, of these objectives apply to the professional caregiving team and their interactions with the patient. Strengthening and maintaining relationships as well as preparation for the end of life have application to the patient and family as well. The researchers underscore the importance of the ACP for the patient, the family, and the healthcare team. Through a shared decision-making process, the best possible care at the end of life is ensured in accord with the patient's and family's values and priorities. Although the ACP may have been discussed and developed long before the current phase of the illness, at the end of life, it may be revised and adapted to the person's condition and current preferences. The development or revision of an ACP brings death to the forefront of the discussion and may evoke grief responses. Therefore, in addition to deciding upon a plan, it is equally important to provide a safe space for the ongoing support of all family members, including the patient, who may be grieving in anticipation of death.

Support at the end of life is most helpful when patients and families are encouraged to engage in a life review and have opportunities for meaningful exchanges and farewells, which entails the sharing of anticipatory grief. Chochinov et al.[17] proposed "dignity therapy" (DT) to facilitate a life review and meaningful exchanges with significant others and as an approach to preserving meaning and hope.

Fitchett and colleagues[18] illustrate some of the core questions for an interview suggested by Chochinov and Cann,[19] including queries such as "What are your most important accomplishments, and what are you most proud of? What are your hopes and dreams for your loved ones? What have you learned about life that you would want to pass along to others?" It is readily apparent why such thought-provoking questions would be helpful for the dying person and the family and a gift each can give the other of memorable and loving responses.

Although the term "dignity therapy" is a misnomer in that there is no "therapy" or "psychotherapy," it was found to be useful for patients in high distress.[20] An earlier review of the literature by Fitchett and colleagues[18] found benefits and high satisfaction by patients receiving DT and their families. In a more recent study, the Patient Dignity Inventory and the Dignity Therapy Patient Feedback questionnaires were used to assess dignity-related distress and feedback from the study participants.[21] Twenty-eight of the 37 patients enrolled completed the study. Although most participants found the intervention to be helpful, no statistically significant reduction in inventory scores occurred. The authors concluded that the participants found a "sense of purpose, continuity of self, and connection with their family."[21(p11)] However, the nurses involved in the study noted that too much time was involved in the process. These professionals had time constraints, making it difficult for them to devote the time required for DT. To implement DT requires specialized training. However, some of the questions involved in a life review may be of value to nurses and other clinicians who support dying people and may facilitate meaningful exchanges with family members. Nurses play a significant role in helping families to develop new and enhance existing resources (Box 58.2).

Box 58.2 Something with a Little Something in It!

One of the co-authors of this chapter (I. C.) was following a patient at the request of the Medical Oncology Service. When visiting her at 7:00 a.m. one Thursday, the patient asked her, "Where's my drink?" The nurse responded, "Where's your drink?" after which the patient replied "Yes, something with a little something in it." The nurse, wanting to be sure she did not jump to the wrong conclusions, asked, "What are your favorite somethings with a little something in it?" After the patient mentioned some of her favorite drinks, the nurse responded, "It sounds like you would like to have a party," to which the patient replied in the affirmative: "What about tomorrow evening?"

Her sister was at the bedside and said she would make the arrangements for a party on Friday evening. On the day of the party, the nurse remained at work until the evening, when she brought some cookies to the patient who wore makeup and was attired in a new bed-jacket. Close family members were there including a young man with a guitar so that there could be music and song. (The patient had performed in professional musical comedy when she was younger.) After greeting everyone, the nurse left so that the family could enjoy this special time together. It was Friday; the patient died the following Tuesday.

Several months later the nurse encountered family members at a local shopping center. After hugs, the family members spoke enthusiastically about the party and said that when they remembered the hospital, they thought of the party. They remembered their loved one at a happy time, even though she was in the hospital.

The something with a little something in it was the music and the family gathering. And the nurse recognized that, in effect, it was the patient's going-away party.

The Challenge of Ensuring a "Good Death"

Ensuring a "good death" according to the priorities, values, and preferences of the dying person and of family members is of critical importance. How people die affects the grieving process of significant others and their subsequent adjustment to loss. A recent study highlights the lack of palliative care in different segments of the world. Connor and colleagues[22] conducted a study estimating the number of people who received palliative care in 2017. Data was obtained by sampling countries as listed in World Bank Income groups. This resulted in respondents from the following: 9 high-income countries (17%); 13 middle-income countries (32%); 10 lower- to middle-income countries (31%); and 7 lower-income countries (33%). Not only the existence of palliative care services in each country but the availability and variability in data collection approaches influenced the number of countries sampled in each region. Thus, in regions with both palliative care services and data collection methodologies, fewer countries were sampled as data was readily available. That was not the case in other parts of the world where the authors found a paucity of both formal palliative care amenities and data collection services. The researchers stressed the challenge of defining what constitutes palliative care in each country and whether generalized or specialized palliative care services were offered. They highlighted the significance of further investigation.

In another cross-country comparison by 181 country experts on the level of quality EOL care in 81 countries, Finkelstein and colleagues focused on five categories of indicators: "Palliative and health care environment, Human resources, Affordability of care, Quality of care," and "Community engagement."[23(pe420)] Managing pain and discomfort was considered of greatest importance with non-medical concerns of least importance. It should also be noted that "clean and safe space" was the second most highly rated indicator and "spiritual needs" the second lowest rated indicator. Clearly, there is room for debate, and the professions of the country experts may have had an influence on the rankings.

There are also distinctions by countries as to how a "good death" is defined. In a study by Sepulveda et al.,[24] of the relative importance of different indicators in India, Kenya, Singapore, the United Kingdom, and the United States, the researchers found that management of pain and discomfort and costs were not a barrier and were more significant for India than the other four countries. Being treated kindly and coping emotionally were more important for the United Kingdom than the comparison countries. A clean and safe space, clear and timely information, and contact with family were more important for Singapore than the United Kingdom, Kenya, India, or the United States. For Kenya, asking enough questions, having coordinated care, and non-medical concerns were more important than these concerns were for comparison countries. Lastly for the United States, preferred place of death and spiritual needs were more significant than for the four comparisons countries. It must be asserted that all of the concerns were important to all of the countries. (The comparison just noted was developed by examining the data provided in the paper.)

The countries ranked most highly for the quality of palliative care in the Finkelstein et al. study[23] were all high-income countries, with the exception of Costa Rica, a middle-income country. Most of the countries that received failing grades were low-income countries, except for two high-income countries that also were considered by their country experts to provide less than adequate care.

Factors that contributed to a low ranking included: EOL care was not recognized as a human right, the lack of an approach making palliative care a national strategy, the high cost of palliative care, and the lack of palliative care training. The authors note that their "effort is intended to provide grounding evidence and build awareness—social, political, and financial of EOL care as an important public health and societal issue."[23(p.e428)]

The data by Finkelstein et al.[23] may be a stimulus to making palliative and EOL care and hospice a policy priority for all countries. That it is not, even for those nations that have been deemed as having high-quality care such as the United Kingdom, gives one pause.[25] The United Kingdom is the home country of Dame Cicely Saunders, the founder of hospice and palliative care services. That Sleeman and her colleagues found that "palliative and end of life care are rarely explicit policy priorities in U.K. health and social care policy"[25(p8)] gives one pause and indicates how much more attention needs to be given to this area of health and illness care.

Studies that have been conducted to identify EOL quality measures have been found not to be applicable for patients in all settings.[26] Holm and colleagues[27] attempted to develop an anticipatory grief scale and found that the subscales Behavioral Reactions and Emotional Reactions emphasized a loss-oriented form of grief with an emphasis on separation from a key figure.[(p16)]

"Questions relating to pain, symptoms, emotional needs, and family concerns" have been found to be the issues of greatest importance for outcome measurement.[28(p451)] European researchers have identified "last days of life, quality of death, pain, fatigue and cachexia" as significant areas of inquiry.[29(p39)] These outcome measures will vary not only by the disease, injury, and pathology of the dying person but by the resources at hand to provide palliation of symptoms and psychosocial support for the patient and family.

Another important issue for the dying and their families is place of death and the congruence between their preference and the actual occurrence.[30] The patient's functional status, treatment-related aspects, marital status, a non-working relative, decision-making capacity, having spoken to a professional about preferred place of death, and caregiver's preference are some of the illness-related, individual, and environmental factors that are related to enhancing congruence between a patient's preference for place of death and the actual place of death. What is interesting is that having spoken with a family member about preferred place of death is not included in this listing, although, clearly, some of the factors listed are key to the opportunity to achieve congruence between one's wishes and the ultimate place of death.

In a paper in which the focus was on studies conducted in the United Kingdom, Canada, Australia, and New Zealand, access to hospice care was investigated.[31] As in other studies, the predominance of patients receiving hospice care were those with a cancer diagnosis. This may be a result of reimbursement methods such as those in Canada, where payment for residential hospice care is prescribed as available for 3 months or less.[32] Given that the progression from advanced illness to death is easier to predict for individuals diagnosed with cancer than for some other diseases, there may be a preference for individuals with this diagnosis by both the patient/family and the providers.

The Grieving Process of the Bereaved Individual

With the death of an individual, those who have the closest blood or legal connections to the deceased are considered bereaved.

> Bereavement confers a special status on the individual, entailing both obligations and special rights. The obligations concern disposition of the body and any attendant ceremonies, as well as disposal of the worldly goods of the deceased unless indicated otherwise in a legal document such as a last will and testament. The rights include dispensation from worldly activities such as work and, to a lesser degree, family roles for variable periods of time. Bereavement entails loss, grief, and recovery, and associated processes.[13(p390)]

Whereas "bereavement" infers the individual has experienced the death of a family member or close friend, "grieving" is the process by which a person adapts to the loss. Meaning attribution is an aspect of grieving whereby the bereaved integrates the loss into their life without the bereaved. Although family members may have been experiencing anticipatory grief at the end of a loved one's life, this does not imply that they will not engage in an active grieving process after the person's death. Some of the most common grief responses as described by Worden[33] are included in Table 58.2.

It should be stressed that the acceptable manifestations of grief vary by the cultural expectations for such expressions. When behaviors occur which are not congruent with these expectations, the person exhibiting them and their responses tend to be pathologized. Problems occur when grief manifestations are misperceived, for example, as depression; and culturally indicated "therapy" may forestall or complicate the person's grieving process.

As noted by Corless et al.,[34] who cite Stroebe et al.,[35] "given the increased risk of mortality associated with bereavement, there is all the more reason for healthcare providers to investigate the occurrence of grief and bereavement in the lives of their patients"[(p135)] and to differentiate it from depression given that different interventions are required. While both grief and depression involve intense sadness and sleep and eating disturbances, the bereaved experiences "waves" of grief manifestations, perceives the external world as cold and empty without the loved one around, manages to cope more or less effectively with daily challenges, and benefits from support when it is perceived as helpful. In contrast, the person who is clinically depressed experiences a pervasive sense of sadness, which is associated with low self-esteem and sense of worthlessness. They perceive their internal world as totally empty and remain unable to seek out or benefit from support. In addition, the person loses interest in all activities and relationships that may have once been enjoyed and experiences pervasive guilt. The guilt that bereaved people may sometimes experience is usually associated with a specific aspect of the loss (e.g., "I could not be present at his bedside" or "I didn't tell her how much I loved her before her death"), rather than experiencing an overall sense of culpability, which is a common symptom in clinical depression.

Clinicians and researchers have proposed various grief models to depict the process that people engage in as they strive to come to terms with the loss of their loved one and adjust to a new reality without them. Sigmund Freud[36,37] was the first to describe the grieving process in terms of an intrapsychic process, which he named the "work of mourning" or "grief work," through which the bereaved "let[s] go" and gradually "withdraws his or her emotional investment in

Table 58.2 Common grief responses

Feelings	Physical sensations	Cognitions
Sadness	Hollowness in the stomach	Disbelief
Anger	Tightness in the chest	Confusion
Anxiety	Tightness in the throat	Preoccupation
Guilt and self-reproach	Oversensitivity to noise	Sense of presence
Loneliness	Sense of depersonalization	Visual or auditory hallucinations
Sense of helplessness	Breathlessness (short of breath)	
Fatigue	Weakness in muscles	
Shock	Lack of energy	
Yearning	Dry mouth	
Emancipation		
Numbness		
Relief		
Behaviors		
Sleep disturbances		
Appetite disturbances		
Absent-minded behavior		
Social withdrawal		
Dreams of the deceased		
Avoiding reminders of the deceased		
Searching and calling out		
Sighing		
Restless hyperactivity		
Crying		
Visiting places reminding of the deceased		
Treasuring objects belonging to the deceased		

the deceased" by transferring it into new relationships. Bowlby,[38,39] who is widely known for his attachment theory and his studies on loss, excluded from the resolution of grief any concept associated with bonds. Maintaining an ongoing bond with the deceased was perceived to be pathological. Klass et al.[40] challenged this assumption and proposed a paradigm shift that affected our knowledge and practices in the field of bereavement. In fact, they supported the idea that investments are not "withdrawn" from the deceased but rather that the bereaved seeks to maintain a "continuing bond" with the deceased person who had a special place in the life of the survivor. In other words, bonds are not severed, but the person maintains an attachment within new life conditions and circumstances.

Grief models which have been supported by research evidence adopt the concept of continuing bonds as a key aspect of the grieving process. Some of the most popular models which have been supported over the past decades by research evidence and have implications in clinical practice with the bereaved are the following.

The Task Model

William Worden[33] describes the grieving process in terms of tasks that bereaved people have to actively undertake in the process of adjusting to loss. These tasks involve (a) accepting the reality of the loss, (b) processing the pain of grief, (c) adjusting to a new reality without the deceased while acknowledging the multiple roles that the person had in one's life, and (d) finding an enduring connection with the deceased in the midst of embarking on a new life. These tasks facilitate both adaptation and integration of loss into the person's life story which is reconstructed. According to Worden, tasks are not linear, with the person going back and forward, addressing them as needed.

The Dual Process of Coping with Loss

Margaret Stroebe and Hunk Schut[41] proposed a dual process model of coping with bereavement. They referred to two types of stressors associated with bereavement: "loss-oriented stressors" (e.g., going through the belongings of the deceased, visiting the grave, looking at photos) and "restoration-oriented stressors" (e.g., learning new skills to adopt the roles previously assumed by the deceased, moving to a smaller apartment, or taking up a job to compensate for reduced income). Coping involves a dynamic process of oscillation between dealing with the one or the other type of stressors, reflecting the effort required to adjust to a new reality. "Bereavement overload" is another aspect of the model, which explains variation in the oscillation process when people feel overburdened, having more than they perceive themselves able to deal with, commonly experienced during the pandemic era.[42]

The Meaning Reconstruction of Loss

Neimeyer et al.[43] adopted a constructivist perspective, which views grieving as a process of reconstructing a world of meaning that has been challenged by loss. They argue that coping effectively with grief involves the rebuilding of previously held assumptions about one's relationship to the deceased, which are renegotiated over time, as well as assumptions about self and one's worldview. Meaning-making, therefore, entails an ability to assimilate or accommodate to the loss, by creating a meaningful self-narrative. When a death is violent, sudden, and unexpected, meaning-making is more challenging given that the bereaved tends to perceive the world to be dangerous, unpredictable, or unjust. Inability to make sense of the death enhances the possibility of manifesting grief complications and the fragmentation of a self-narrative.[43]

The Model of Grief Trajectories through Loss

Bonnano[44] described resilient bereaved individuals who adapt well to the loss and argued that their resilient trajectory through grief is more common than most people believed. Through extensive research, he illuminated some unique trajectories of responses to loss, with some individuals displaying quite resilient responses, others showing improvement in functioning over time, still others experiencing relief following a period of considerable distress due to the burden of caregiving or an oppressive relationship, and still others displaying grief complications, requiring professional help. He challenged the belief that people go through stages and provided evidence about four discrete grief trajectories: (a) the resilience trajectory, (b) the chronic grief trajectory (an onset of depression following loss), (c) the depressed-improved trajectory (high pre-loss depression that decreased following loss), and the (d) preexisting chronic depression trajectory (high depression at all assessments).[45]

In reality, none of the above models support evidence about stages that are relevant to the grieving process. Studies on family grief, although limited, illuminate the social dynamics involved in bereavement and describe the impact that significant others have upon the bereaved.[46] Grieving is negotiated among bereaved family members who engage in an ongoing process of developing narratives about the life and death of the deceased, which affect in positive or negative ways their adjustment to loss. Walter[47] supports the idea that the construction of a durable biography enables the living to integrate the memory of the dead into their ongoing lives through discussions with others who knew the deceased. In other words, grief becomes a social rather than a private experience and a process through which the biography of the bereaved and of the deceased are continually re-created through the eyes and accounts of others. It can be a very enriching process for all concerned.

Factors Affecting the Grieving Process

Grief responses and trajectories vary. Assessment should always take into account a multitude of factors that may facilitate or hinder the person's grieving process. However, to fully understand grief complications or the occurrence of manifestations of psychopathology, healthcare professionals involved in the care of the bereaved must first understand the normal grieving process and the factors that affect it. Some of these factors are depicted in Figure 58.1.

1. *Relationship to the person who died*: (e.g., the loss of a highly dependent attachment bond with the person who died may create more adjustment challenges to the bereaved; or a highly conflictual relationship may evoke guilt and despair over unattended matters)
2. *Meaning attribution to the death*: (e.g., pervasive guilt feelings for having caused or not prevented the death may complicate grief)
3. *Conditions of dying and death*: (e.g., having contributed to a "good death" of one's loved one and having shared farewells throughout the dying process may facilitate grieving by comparison to one's exposure to a sudden death or uncaring/traumatic dying conditions)

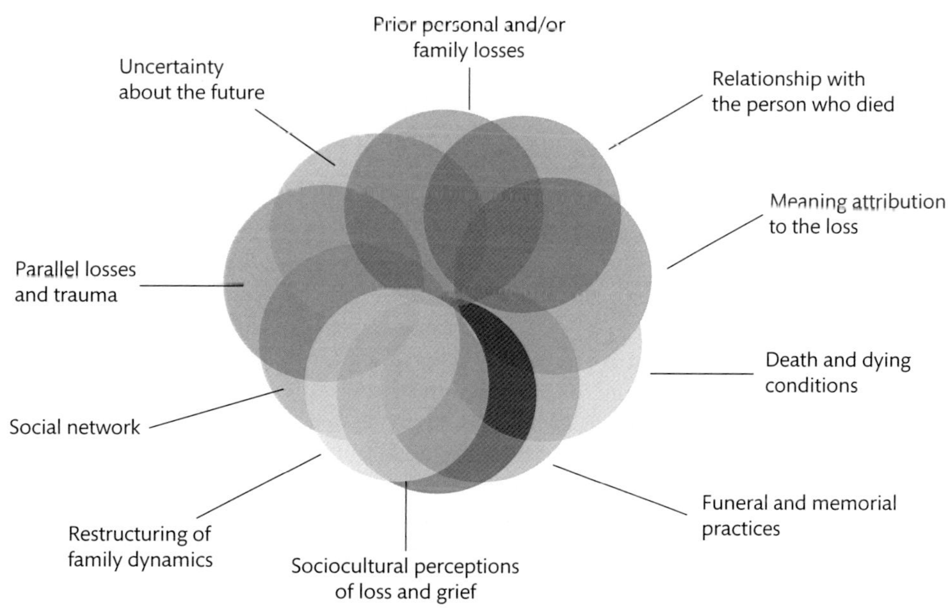

Figure 58.1 Key factors affecting the grieving process

4. *Funeral and memorial practices*: (e.g., attendance to funeral and memorial practices may render the loss real vs. the absence of rituals and the deprivation of honoring the deceased)
5. *Sociocultural and religious perceptions of loss and grief*: (e.g., the stigmatization or marginalization of the bereaved or the disenfranchisement of their grief may affect grieving and deprive the bereaved of support)
6. *Family dynamics*: (e.g., the restructured dynamics may solidify constructive or destructive patterns of communication and interaction throughout the grieving process)
7. *Supportive network*: (e.g., not only the number is important but also the quality and availability of support by family members, friends, co-workers, community members, and mental health professionals)
8. *Parallel losses and/or trauma*: (e.g., additional losses after and because of the loss that involve radical changes in a person's life may complicate the grieving process or cause bereavement overload—change of housing, school, work)
9. *Prior personal and/or family losses*: (e.g., growth and resilience through prior losses or unexplored traumatic losses that have never been addressed)

Case Study

Mr. Fleming, whose 40-year-old wife is dying of cancer, is spending all day at her bedside, after she decided to reject another cycle of chemotherapy and opt for palliative care. He supported her in her decision, in spite of her family's objections. When she is asleep, he has a hard time holding back his tears, thinking of how empty life will be without her. Being aware that her life is coming to an end, Ms. Fleming asked him today to bring their children to the hospice, for one last visit. He confides to you that he does not know how to inform his 7-year-old son and 9-year-old daughter that their mother is dying and has doubts as to whether to encourage them to visit her and include them in their mother's funeral ceremony. He is very concerned whether he will manage to be a "good father" by conveying to his children a model of "strength" in the face of adversity and by helping them to "overcome" such a loss, given his overwhelming sense of devastation. He considers a move to a new apartment so as to avoid all reminders and open up a new chapter in his and the children's lives.

Suggested Approach

Normalize Mr. Fleming's Anticipatory Grief and Highlight His Support to His Wife

Acknowledge the grief that Mr. Fleming is experiencing as a result of his wife's impending death and normalize his thoughts and concerns about her dying as well as about the future of his family. Provide him with positive feedback as to his supportive role at the bedside of his wife, and respect of her choice for palliative care.

Discuss How to Inform Children and Handle Possible Responses

Prepare with Mr. Fleming a plan for the discussion with his children by determining (a) *when* to have a discussion (i.e., avoid evening hours and times he will not be available afterward), (b) *how* to address the topic of the mother's dying, and (c) *how* to invite children to visit their mother at the palliative care setting. Any discussion must begin by exploring what the children understand or suspect about their mother's health condition. It is important to invite them first to raise questions and concerns. Information about her condition and the role of palliative care should be clear and address any misconceptions. Moreover, it should be adjusted to the children's needs and questions. Words such as "dying" and "death" should be used, and euphemisms such as "she is leaving us," "sleeping," or "going to heaven" should be avoided. The visit to their dying mother should be discussed and prepared for so that they will know what to expect.

Mr. Fleming should be encouraged to leave time and space for the expression of concerns and the sharing of feelings and accept, without criticizing, any response (e.g., turning attention to other matters, crying, leaving the room, etc.). It may be helpful to share with him our knowledge from clinical experience and research evidence that children sense when something "wrong" is happening to their family and that when they remain uninformed, they experience increased anxiety, are constantly in a state of alert, and are left alone to cope with an intolerable uncertainty.

Attending the funeral after their mother's death is an issue to be discussed after the death. Children should be informed about *what* to expect during the burial or cremation ceremony, *who* will be at their side should they decide to retreat from the ceremony, and the option of attending or not attending the ceremony should always be available to them. Children who decide not to be present should always be offered the option of sending a symbolic object, letter, or drawing to accompany their mother in the afterlife.

Educate Mr. Fleming about the Grieving Process over the Loss of a Loved Person

Convey some clear message about grieving. For example, that it involves a *natural, healthy*, and *long-lasting process* over a loss which turns a family's world upside down, affecting their daily life. Through this process, he and his children will progressively adapt to the new reality from which his wife is missing and attribute meaning to their loss. Convey to him the message that despite the intensity of suffering, most people successfully cope with their loss and engage in healthy levels of functioning, whereas some may even display personal growth.

Help him to understand that children have different ways of expressing their grief, which is often communicated indirectly or symbolically (e.g., through drawings, choice of play) and through behavioral changes (e.g., sleep difficulties, irritability, withdrawal, separation anxiety). Convery the message that there is no right or wrong way to grieve and that grieving may have peaks and valleys, which are often unpredictable; families need to embrace the differences and leave space for alternative ways of experiencing and expressing sadness, anger, guilt, longing, or remaining silent, without isolating or criticizing a child who may or may not be doing so.

Explore Issues Related to His and the Family's Support System

It is important to encourage Mr. Fleming to explore the nature and quality of the supportive relationships he has in his life. These may include family members, work colleagues, members of his social or community network, etc. Some people will be valued for "being present" to listen and share his grief, whereas others will be valued for helping him to "move away from grief" and enjoy the pleasures of life. Encourage Mr. Fleming to embrace and treasure both types of support. Also, highlight the importance of letting members of his support network know what is helpful and what is unhelpful to him and his children throughout their grieving. Teachers must be informed that the children's mother has died, and an open communication between Mr. Fleming and the school must be established.

Address His Concern of Being a "Good" Parent throughout Bereavement

Explore what "good" parenting means to him. Correct misconceptions about being "strong" for the sake of his children. Suggest that grieving does not imply "being strong," "overcoming" loss, or "forgetting." His spouse and mother of his children will always hold a special place in their hearts, and they will choose their own ways of commemorating and celebrating her existence. It is over time that they will eventually develop a new and comforting bond with her that will help them integrate her loss into their life story. Help him understand that parents who are supportive to their children are able to listen to them, recognize and accept their unique ways of grieving, and do not hide nor impose their grief upon them. Involving them in family decisions regarding the deceased (e.g., what to do with her belongings, how to celebrate the memorial) will enhance their sense of belonging to their family. Such parents are well supported and do not hesitate to seek guidance or grief counseling when in need.

Discuss His Consideration to Move to a New Apartment

Moving to a new apartment immediately after Mrs. Fleming's death will create more problems than it may solve. It will evoke additional losses and grieving in Mr. Fleming and his children, who in addition to the death of their mother, will lose neighborhood friends and classmates in case they change schools and be deprived of an established life that was familiar to them. It is important for Mr. Fleming to understand that reminders of his wife will always exist, and the challenge for him, his children, and significant others is to find ways to integrate the reminders into a shared family story, rather than condemn each member to grieving in isolation.

Support for the Bereaved

Most bereaved people do not need professional help. But some may benefit when they feel stuck and overwhelmed by their loss, unable to function in any aspect of their life; and others may realize that they have rushed too quickly to close the door on their loss and move on with life. In addition, families who have been exposed to a sudden death, which was lived traumatically, may benefit from professional support when they experience serious difficulties adjusting to daily life and reconstructing their world of assumptions which has been shattered by their loss.

The question of who needs bereavement support led to a study in a community sample in Australia.[48] Family members bereaved 6–24 months were asked to complete a questionnaire containing a screening measure for prolonged grief disorder. A public health approach to bereavement support formed the background to this study.[49,50] The model predicted that 60% of the bereaved would be low risk, 30% moderate risk, and 10% high risk for grief complications. Findings were close to the model predictions in that 58.4% of the bereaved were considered low risk, 35.2% were moderate risk, and 6.4% were high risk. The authors advocate the use of the public health model for the allocation of support services.

Penny and Relf[51] also propose three levels of support for the bereaved. Component 1 is comprised of the *support by family and friends* in their existing network. Health professionals currently providing care to the family are also among those offering this basic level of support. Component 2 is composed of selective services which are targeted to the needs of the bereaved and provided by trained volunteers or professionals. Component 3 is operationalized when complex needs are addressed by specialized bereavement practitioners and mental health professionals. Killikelly and colleagues[52] propose the use of specialized services for individuals diagnosed with prolonged grief disorder and underscore the significance of developing consensus protocols for the introduction of prolonged grief disorder to various stakeholders.

Compassionate Communities Supporting the Bereaved

It takes a community for an individual to thrive.[53(p49)] Formal care should be complemented by "community care," not the other way around.[48,54] In the context of a public health approach, palliative and bereavement service providers develop partnerships and collaborations with communities who have in place or develop social initiatives for the support of the person and family before and after the individual's death.

In an investigation of the support strategies found to be most helpful by the bereaved, Aoun and colleagues[55] found that the most frequently mentioned resources were family, friends, funeral provider, general practitioner (physician), and financial or legal services, followed closely by religious or spiritual advisor (in that order). Least frequently mentioned started with psychiatrist, followed by case coordinator, bereavement support group, and psychological and social work support. There may be several reasons for these findings including the most obvious to the authors of this chapter being that most of the people in the study were likely to be in the low-or moderate-risk group where family and friends would be the most salient source of help. Thus, the rankings for bereavement support might vary if there were a cross-tabulation by level of risk.

Aoun and colleagues[55] examined the sources of support by degree of helpfulness. Although all sources of help were considered "very or quite helpful," with percentages ranging from 53.8% to 92%, sources perceived as "little or not helpful" ranged from 8% to 46.2%.[(p1382)] The researchers noted that the lowest proportion of "unhelpfulness" was that which was provided by informal support such as family. However, all levels of support were characterized to some degree by absence, insensitivity, poor advice, lack of empathy, and systemic hindrance.[(p7)] Kellehear and colleagues[56] addressed the importance of compassionate communities in supporting the bereaved. They suggest:

> Unlike most professional systems, including the use of volunteers from within health service, compassionate communities employ the practices of participatory civic action. This means teams of leaders (compassionate cities) or ordinary members of neighborhoods (compassionate communities) come together to identify common problems and solutions for promoting health and wellbeing, as well as tackling the co-morbidities of dying, caregiving and bereavement.[(p.818)]

In a blog, Abel[57] suggested that those providing professional services should participate in inspiring community sources of support "without guiding, without interference, and without taking control."[(p4)]

With an emphasis on the community of those affected by death, namely the bereaved, Phyllis Silverman in her Widow-to-Widow project[58,59] described the development and benefits of a mutual-help and community support program, among bereaved widows. She revealed how intimate sharing of loss experiences, wisdom, tears, and laughter among widows can empower the bereaved to move through the grieving process with the support of their peers. What Silverman described was a project that fit within a public health approach rather than relying solely on professional care. This approach supports the premise that bereavement is not "a problem to be solved" with the help of professional expertise but rather an experience to be engaged in.[48] Indeed, one might consider bereavement a developmental phase that occurs in different phases of one's lives that may result in personal growth. That growth may occur as a consequence of an introspective process involving the redefinition of oneself, worldview, and relation to the deceased but also as a consequence of family, community, and/or professional support or formal care.

Nurses and Clinicians Grieve Too

Caring for seriously ill and dying people and coming to terms with their deaths unavoidably affects all healthcare professionals involved in the person's care and family's support. The stress that is experienced has been the focus of several studies which have described various aspects of the suffering. Burnout, compassion fatigue, secondary posttraumatic stress, and moral distress are some of the conditions that nurses and other healthcare professionals experience under acute or prolonged distress. However, little formal attention has been given to the grief experienced by healthcare providers. Jeanne Quint Benoliel[60] was the first to observe that physicians and nurses who are caring for seriously and terminally ill patients are grieving. Papadatou and colleagues proposed a model about the grieving process of healthcare professionals derived from trans-cultural research evidence involving samples of nurses and physicians who provide services to children in acute care and oncology clinics in Greece and Hong Kong.[61–63] The researchers challenged the preconceived assumption that healthcare professionals do not experience suffering and described the nature of losses that trigger a grieving process: (1) the loss of a personal bond with a patient with whom one held a close relationship; (2) identification with a bereaved relative's suffering over the loss of a valued relationship; (3) the lack of completion of one's professional goals (e.g., to cure or to ensure a dignified death); (4) the loss of long-held assumptions about self and others (e.g., "I should always succeed," "be in control," "save others," "people should always recognize my contributions") and invalidation of the belief that life should be fair; (5) the resurfacing of past, unaddressed personal losses; and (6) awareness of one's mortality and grief over one's future death.

Characteristic of the professionals' grieving process is *a fluctuation* between the *experience of grief responses* over perceived loss(es) and the selective *avoidance or repression of grief responses* so as to address the required tasks and duties without being overwhelmed by loss. This fluctuation is adaptive and healthy and enables healthcare professionals, first, to meet job demands; second, to attribute meaning to the death of each patient; and third, to come to terms with their losses. Meaning attributions to a patient's death are ascribed by individual care providers as well as by teams depending on how they perceive death and what goals they set for the patient's care. Individual and collective meanings are attributed to death, dying, and caregiving, which facilitate, hinder, or prolong grieving in the face of death. However, grieving is also affected by the team's often unspoken rules which determine a set of acceptable and expected behaviors in the face of death (e.g. "Health professionals must not be affected by death"). In this model, grieving is not a private affair but a social process that occurs within teams which use functional or dysfunctional approaches to cope with the suffering that the death evokes in staff members. The organizational culture of the work setting affects whether the professionals' distress is acknowledged and addressed through supportive measures.[61]

Nurses' Grief through the Pandemic

More recently, attention has expanded beyond the various manifestations of nurses' distress (e.g., burnout, moral distress, compassion fatigue) and illuminated their grief over multiple deaths of patients, colleagues, and/or loved ones, under the unprecedented conditions of the COVID pandemic. The number of dying or critically ill patients requiring care at the same time overwhelmed the resources of most institutions. Further, the vulnerability of the front-line providers to infection while caring for their patients increased the distress experienced by these providers, some of whom became infected and died.

McCallum and colleagues[64] suggested that "It is also a form of grief to have anxiety for oneself—nurses have seen COVID-19 take the fit, the healthy, the young."[(p2116)] The combination of feeling helpless as they care for those who are dying and particularly those "dying before their time" and the recognition that they too could be in that situation make the current COVID situation an anomaly for many healthcare providers who acknowledge their grief.

Das and colleagues[65] offer some recommendations for helping the families of front-line workers and note the challenges faced by these workers including the fear of spreading disease to their families and to other healthcare workers and the absence of adequate training for confronting the challenges they faced. All of this could have been expected had the approach to epidemics in other countries been preparation for the possible influx of infected persons to uninfected countries. The dissemination of microbes may be a matter of days, weeks, months or years. A public health approach combined with education, research, and systems preparation applies to governments and healthcare systems including the professions. Data, however, is the foundation for planning given that it provides a basis for responding to unanticipated findings.

Bhatia,[66] cited by McCallum and colleagues,[64] noted that non-white persons are two to three times more likely to die from COVID-19. Furthermore, a higher proportion of deaths among nurses has been reported among Black, Asian, and minority ethnic nurses according to Braithwaite.[67] Whether this is from lack of or the non-use of personal protective equipment or failure to receive vaccinations and boosters rather than some physiological distinction is not examined further by McCallum and colleagues.[64]

Whereas physicians, prior to the COVID pandemic, would hide, deny, or minimize their grief at the death of a patient, although they may have felt guilty or a sense of failure, Rabow and colleagues[68] suggest this may lead to burnout due to the compounding and lack of processing of the grief. The clinical environment is not one where the display of emotions, other than joy at some accomplishment, is the norm. Indeed, as Lathrop observes, "grief in the workplace is unsanctioned."[69(p375)] And one might add that the majority of physicians are still male (although this is changing) and the majority of nurses are female (although the number of male nurses is increasing), which may help account for the stiff upper lip mentality in clinical settings. This is also aggravated by the lack of compassionate role models in educational healthcare institutions.

There is also the sense that tears are the province of the person's family and close friends and that clinicians are there to support the patient. Remarkably, family members are often touched when they see evidence that the clinician, too, is pained at the death of a patient. Indeed, it becomes part of the family folklore and a source of pride that nurse X or doctor Y had tears in their eyes when they spoke of the patient's demise. Rabow et al.[68] not only recognize the grief that healthcare workers confront in their patients and families, their colleagues, and themselves; they normalize it, considering healthcare workers both witnesses and victims. Confronting grief during the COVID pandemic exposed healthcare workers not only to a virus but to the deaths of many people of various ages. Rabow and colleagues provide a road map for changes in the healthcare system, particularly in hospitals and other facilities, and convey the following message to all healthcare providers:

> Through recognition of the risks for complicated or prolonged grief, we have an opportunity to promote both individual and systemic resiliency and resources to address HCW [health care worker] personal and professional grief in the time of COVID-19. Ultimately, competent clinical care requires not just our expertise but our humanity and vulnerability as well. HCWs owe such a comprehensive commitment to our patients, their loved ones, our own loved ones, and to ourselves.[(p654)]

Conclusions

Supporting the dying person, the bereaved family, and the grieving colleague offers healthcare providers the potential of experiencing multiple personal and professional rewards.[70] Growth is reflected in how they perceive themselves, in how they connect with others and become enriched by compassionate relationships, and in how they strive to live in a way that is meaningful and enriching for self and others.

REFERENCES

1. Knutzen KE, Sacks OA, Brody-Bizar OC, et al. Actual and missed opportunities for end-of-life care discussions with oncology patients: a qualitative study. *JAMA Netw Open*. 2021;4(6):e2113193. https://doi.org/10.1001/jamanetworkopen.2021.13193.
2. Bumb M, Keefe J, Miller L, Overcash J. Breaking bad news: an evidence-based review of communication models for oncology nurses. *Clin J Oncol Nurs*. 2017;21(5):573–580. https://doi.org/10.1188/17.CJON.573-580.
3. Buckman R. *How to Break Bad News: A Guide for Health Care Professionals*. Johns Hopkins University Press; 1992.
4. Cassell EJ. Recognizing suffering. *Hastings Rep*. 1991;1(3):24–31.
5. Younger JB. The alienation of the sufferer. *ANS Adv Nurs Sci*. 1995;17(4):53–72. https://doi.org/10.1097/00012272-199506000-00006.
6. Fredrickson L, Eriksson K. The patient's narrative of suffering: a path to health? An interpretive research synthesis on narrative understanding. *Scand J Caring Sci*. 2001;15(1):3–11. https://doi.org/10.1046/j.1471-6712.2001.1510003.x.
7. Morse JM. Toward a praxis theory of suffering. *ANS Adv Nurs Sci*. 2001;24(1):47–59. https://doi.org/10.1097/00012272-200109000-00007.
8. Toombs SK. *The Meaning of Illness: A Phenomenological Account of the Different Perspectives of Physician and Patient*. Kluwer Academic Publishers; 1992.
9. Frank AW. *The Wounded Storyteller: Body, Illness, and Ethics*. University of Chicago Press; 1995.
10. Rushforth A, Ladds E, Wieringa S, Taylor S, Husain L, Greenhalgh T. Long Covid—the illness narratives. *Soc Sci Med*. 2021;286:114326. https://doi.org/10.1016/j.socscimed.2021.114326.
11. Coelho A, Barbosa A. Family anticipatory grief: an integrative literature review. *Am J Hosp Palliat Care*. 2017;34(8):774–785. https://doi.org/10.1177/1049909116647960.
12. Boss, P. *Loss, Trauma and Resilience: Therapeutic Work with Ambiguous Loss*. Norton Professional Books; 2006.
13. Corless IB, Meisenhelder JB. Bereavement. In: Ferrell BR, Paice JA, eds. *Oxford Textbook of Palliative Nursing*. 5th ed. Oxford University Press; 2019:390–404.
14. Nielsen MK, Neergaard MA, Jensen AB, Vedsted P, Bro F, Guldin MB. Preloss grief in family caregivers during end-of-life cancer care: a nationwide population-based cohort study. *Psychooncology*. 2017;26(12):2048–2056. https://doi.org/10.1002/pon.4416.
15. Rogalla KB. Anticipatory grief, proactive coping, social support, and growth: exploring positive experiences of preparing for loss. *Omega (Westport)*. 2020;81(1):107–129. https://doi.org/10.1177/0030222818761461.
16. Fleuren N, Depla MFIA, Janssen DJA, Huisman M, Hertogh CMPM. Underlying goals of advance care planning (ACP): a qualitative analysis of the literature. *BMC Palliat Care*. 2020;19(1).27. https://doi.org/10.1186/s12904-020-0535-1.
17. Cochinov HM, Cann B, Cullihall K, et al. Dignity therapy: a feasibility study of elders in long-term care. *Palliat Support Care*. 2012;10(1):3–15. https://doi.org/10.1017/S1478951511000538.
18. Fitchett G, Emanuel L, Handzo G, Boykin L, Wilkie DJ. Care of the human spirit and the role of dignity therapy: a systematic review of dignity therapy research. *BMC Palliat Care*. 2015;14:8. https://doi.org/10.1186/s12904-015-0007-1.
19. Cochinov HM, Cann BJ. Intervention to enhance the spiritual aspects of dying. *J Palliat Med*. 2005;8(suppl 1):S103–S115. https://doi.org/10.1089/jpm.2005.8.s-103.

20. Martinez M, Arantzamendi M, Belar A. "Dignity therapy", a promising intervention in palliative care: a comprehensive literature review. *Palliat Med*. 2017;31(6):492–509. https://doi.org/10.1177/0269216316665562.
21. Nuziante F, Tanzi S, Alquati S, et al. Providing dignity therapy to patients with advanced cancer: a feasibility study within the setting of a hospital palliative care unit. *BMC Palliat Care*. 2021;20:129. https://doi.org/10.1186/s12904-021-00821-3.
22. Connor SR, Centeno C, Garralda E, Clelland D, Clark D. Estimating the number of patients receiving specialized palliative care globally in 2017. *J Pain Symptom Manage*. 2021;61(4):812–816.
23. Finkelstein EA, Bhadlia A, Goh C, et al. Cross country comparison of expert assessments of the quality of death and dying. *J Pain Symptom Manage*. 2022;63(4):e419–e429. https://doi.org/10.1016/j.jpainsymman.2021.12.015.
24. Sepulveda JMG, Baid D, Johnson FR, Finkelstein EA. What is a good death? A choice experiment on care indicators for patients at end of life. *J Pain Symptom Manage*. 2022;63(4):457–467. https://doi.org/10.1016/j.jpainsymman.2021.11.005.
25. Sleeman KE, Timms A, Gillam J, et al. Priorities and opportunities for palliative and end of life care in United Kingdom health policies: a national documentary analysis. *BMC Palliat Care*. 2021;20:108. https://doi.org/10.1186/s12904-021-00802-6.
26. Hoare S, Antunes B, Kelly MP, Barclay S. End-of-life care quality measures: beyond place of death. *BMJ Support Palliat Care*. 2022;14(e1):e613–e621. https://doi.org/10.1136/spcare-2022-003841.
27. Holm M, Alvariza A, Furst CJ, Ohlen J, Arestedt K. Psychometric evaluation of the anticipatory grief scale in a sample of family caregivers in the context of palliative care. *Health Qual Life Outcomes*. 2019;17:42. https://doi.org/10.1186/s12955-019-1110-4.
28. Higginson IJ, Simon ST, Benali H, et al. Republished: which questions of two commonly used multidimensional palliative care patient reported outcome measures are most useful? Results from the European and African PRISMA survey. *BMJ Support Palliat Care*. 2012;2(1):451–457.
29. Sigurdarfottir KR, Haugen DF, Bausewein CH, et al. A pan-European survey of research in end-of-life cancer care. *Support Cancer Care*. 2012;20:39–48. https://doi.org/10.1007/s00520-010-1048-x.
30. Garcia-Sanjuan S, Fernandez-Alcantara M, Clement-Carbonell V, Campos-Calderon CP, Orts-Beneito N, Cabanero-Martinez MJ. Levels and determinants of place of death congruence in palliative patients: a systematic review. *Front Psychol*. 2022;12:807869. https://doi.org/10.3389/fpsyg.2021.807869.
31. Tobin J, Rogers A, Winterburn I, et al. Hospice care access inequalities: a systematic review and narrative synthesis. *BMJ Support Palliat Care*. 2022;12:142–151. https://doi.org/10.1136/bmjspcare-2020-002719.
32. Canadian Palliative Care Association. Hospice Palliative Care in Canada. 2022 Fact Sheet: Hospice settings of Care. Residential Hospice; 2022:6. https://www.chpca.ca/wp-content/uploads/2022/04/2022-Fact-Sheet-CHPCA-EN.pdf.
33. Worden JW. *Grief Counseling and Grief Therapy: A Handbook for the Mental Health Professional*. 4th ed. Springer Publishing; 2009.
34. Corless IB, Cartier JM, Guarino AJ. Depression and grief: overlapping phenomena or lack of individuation? *Crisis Illness Loss*. 2011;19(2):125–141. https://doi.org/10.2190/IL.19.2.c.
35. Stroebe M, Schut H, Stroebe W. Health outcomes of bereavement. *Lancet*. 2007;370(9603):1960–1973. https://doi.org/10.1016/S0140-6736(07)61816-9.
36. Freud S. *Mourning and Melancholia*. Standard ed. Vol. 14. Hogarth; 1917.
37. Freud S. Mourning and melancholia. In Strache J, ed. *The Standard Edition of the Complete Psychological Works of Sigmund Freud*. Vol. 14. Hogarth Press; 1957.
38. Bowlby J. *Attachment and Loss*. Vol. 111, *Loss, Sadness and Depression*. Basic Books; 1980.
39. Bowlby J. (G)Rief and mourning in infancy and early childhood. *Psychoanalyt Study Child*. 1960;15:9–52. https://doi.org/10.1080/00797308.1960.11822566.
40. Klass D, Silverman PR, Nickman SL, eds. *Continuing Bonds: New Understandings of Grief*. Taylor and Francis; 1996.
41. Stroebe M, Schut H. The dual process model of coping with bereavement: rationale and description. *Death Stud*. 1999;23(3):197–224. https://doi.org/10.1080/074811899201046.
42. Stroebe M, Schut H. Bereavement in times of COVID-19: a review and theoretical framework. *Death Stud*. 2021;82(3):500–522.
43. Neimeyer RA, Prigerson H, Davies B. Mourning and meaning. *Am Behav Sci*. 2002;46:235–251.
44. Bonnano GA. *The Other Side of Sadness: What the New Science of Bereavement Tells Us about Life after Loss*. Basic Books; 2019.
45. Bonanno GA, Wortman CB, Nesse, RM. Prospective patterns of resilience and maladjustment during widowhood. *Psychol Aging*. 2004;19:260–271.
46. Nadeau J. *Families Making Sense of Death*. Sage; 1998.
47. Walter T. A new model on bereavement: bereavement and biography. *Mortality*. 1999;1(1):7–25. https://doi.org/10.1080/713685822.
48. Aoun SM, Breen LJ, Howting DA, Rumbold B, McNamara B, Hegney D. Who needs bereavement support? A population based survey of bereavement risk and support need. *PLoS One*. 2015;10(3):e0121101. https://doi.org/10.1371/journal.pone.0121101.
49. Aoun S, Breen LJ, O'Connor M, Rumbold B, Nordstrom C. A public health approach to bereavement support services in palliative care. *Aust NZJ Public Health*. 2012;36(1):14–16. https://doi.org/10.1111/j.1753-6405.2012.00825.x.
50. Rumbold B, Aoun S. Bereavement and palliative care: a public health perspective: progress in palliative care. *Sci Art Caring*. 2014;22(3):131–135.
51. Penny A, Relf M. *A Guide to Commissioning Bereavement Services in England*. National Bereavement Alliance; 2017.
52. Killikelly C, Smid GE, Wagner B, Boelen PA. Responding to the new International Classification of Diseases-11 prolonged grief disorder during the COVID-19 pandemic: a new bereavement network and three tiered model of care. *Public Health*. 2021;191:85–90. https://doi.org/10.1016/j.puhe.2020.10.034.
53. Abel J, Clarke L. *The Compassion Project: A Case for Hope & Human Kindness from the Town That Beat Loneliness*. Octopus Publishing Group; 2020.
54. Abel J, Walter T, Carey LB, Rosenberg J. Circles of care: should community development redefine the practice of palliative care? *BMJ Support Palliat Care*. 2013;3(4):385–388. https://doi.org/10.1136/bmjspcare-2012-000359.
55. Aoun SM, Breen LJ, White I, Rumbold B, Kellehear A. What sources of bereavement support are perceived helpful by bereaved people and why? Empirical evidence for the compassionate communities approach. *Palliat Med*. 2018;32(8):1378–1388. https://doi.org/10.1177/0269216318774995.
56. Kellehear A, Abel J, Selman L, Aoun S. Bereavement care reimagined. *Annals of Palliative Medicine*. 2023;12(4):816–825.

57. Abel J. Community Sources of Bereavement Support. BMJ Supportive & Palliative Care (blog). October 1, 2021. https://blogs.bmj.com/spcare/2021/10/01/community-sources-of-bereavement-support/.
58. Silverman PR. Widow-to-widow: a mutual help program for the widowed. In: Price RH, Cowen EL, Lorion RP, Ramos-McKay J, eds. *Fourteen Ounces of Prevention: A Casebook for Practitioners*. American Psychological Association; 1998:175–186. https://doi.org/10.1037/10064-014.
59. Silverman P. *Widow to Widow: How the Bereaved Help One Another*. 2nd ed. Routledge; 2004.
60. Benoliel JQ. Anticipatory grief in physicians and nurses. In: Schoenberg B, ed. *Anticipatory Grief*. Columbia University Press; 1974:218–228.
61. Papadatou D. *In the Face of Death: Professionals who Care for the Dying and the Bereaved*. Springer Publishing; 2009.
62. Papadatou D, Martinson I, Chung PM. Caring for dying children: a comparative study of nurses' experiences in Greece and Hong Kong. *Cancer Nurs*. 2001;24(5):402–412.
63. Papadatou D, Bellali T, Papazoglou D, Petraki D. Greek nurse and physicians' grief as a result of caring for children dying of cancer. *Pediatr Nurs*. 2002;28(4):345–353.
64. McCallum KJ, Walthall H, Aveyard H, Jackson D. Grief and nursing: life and death in the pandemic. *J Adv Nurs*. 2021;77(5):2115–2116. https://doi.org/10.1111/Jan.14815.
65. Das S, Singh T, Varma R, Arya YK. Death and mourning process in frontline health care professionals and their families during COVID-19. *Front Psychiatry*. 2021;12:624428. https://doi.org/10.3389/fpsyt.2021.624428.
66. Bhatia M. COVID-19 and BAME group in the United Kingdom. *Int J Community Soc Dev*. 2020;2(2):269–272. https://doi.org/10.1177/2516602620937878.
67. Braithwaite B. Black Lives Matter and the disparities and risk of COVID-19 in BAME nurses. *Health Care Assist*. 2020;14(7):318–320. https://doi.org/10.12968/bjha.2020.14.7.318.
68. Rabow MW, Huang C-HS, White-Hammond GE, Tucker RO. Witnesses and victims both: healthcare workers and grief in the time of COVID-19. *J Pain Symptom Manage*. 2021;62(3):647–656. https://doi.org/10.1016/j.jpainsymman.2021.01.139.
69. Lathrop D. Disenfranchised grief and physician burnout. *Ann Fam Med*. 2017;15(4):375–378. https://doi.org/10.1370/afm.2074.
70. Sourkes B, Liben S, Papadatou D. Witness to suffering: the clinician experience. In: Wolfe J, Hinds P, Sourkes B, eds. *Interdisciplinary Pediatric Palliative Care*. 2nd ed. Oxford University Press; 2022:150–164.

PART VII
Mode of Palliative Care Delivery

59

Hospice and Community-Based Palliative Care

Karen F. Hyden, Maura Lipp, and Tammy Stokes

Key Points

- The number of seriously ill homebound patients is increasing. The goals of care of this population reflect a desire for the quality of days to take precedence over the extension of life. Yet many end up cycling in and out of healthcare facilities and even dying in the hospital when their preference for death is to be at home.
- The number of unpaid caregivers is increasing at a staggering rate. These caregivers are called upon to act as navigators and coordinators of an increasingly siloed and confusing healthcare system. There is an increasing understanding of the gap in care for this hidden, suffering population.
- Palliative care in the community is effective, it decreases hospitalizations, and impacts positively upon symptom burden and caregiver distress. Individuals receiving community-based palliative care are more likely to complete advance care planning documents, to transition to hospice when it is appropriate, and to die at home.
- There is an urgent need for nursing education to prepare a qualified workforce to serve this population. Palliative care nurses at all levels must be trained, qualified, and competent to deliver high-quality palliative care to each suffering patient and family they touch.

Introduction

For centuries, the informal work of palliative care has impacted countless lives in the pursuit of comfort and supportive care. Managing symptoms, advocating for patient goals, and supporting caregivers are within the nurses' scope of practice as well as in their hearts. As the US healthcare system grew and became increasingly industrialized and siloed, these very important aspects of care have often been overlooked. Thankfully, palliative care emerged as its own specialty more than three decades ago offering a more formalized approach. Since that time, palliative care services have evolved, positioning nurses and other members of the interdisciplinary team to positively impact the trajectory of patients and families as they face serious illness. This is particularly critical as the number of unpaid caregivers has grown to approximately 53 million-an increase of nearly 10 million since 2015-hilighting the escalating need for robust support systems for those navigating serious illness.[1]

Additionally, palliative care services within the hospital setting continue to rise, with 94% of hospitals with over 300 beds now reporting having a palliative care team.[2] Despite this growth, the National Academy for State Health Policy reports less than 5% of patients living with serious illness receive palliative care services.[3] At this point, community-based palliative care (CBPC) services vary greatly in availability and standardization. To positively improve patient outcomes, leaders in palliative care must seek to advance CBPC services to promote patient access to high-quality palliative care. This will allow seriously ill patients and their caregivers the chance for better quality of life and care focused on meeting the goals and needs of the patient.

Caregiver Strain

Family caregivers have historically been the mainstay of care in the home for ill members of the family. Today, this care has morphed into a highly complex, stressful, and costly burden. Caregivers often assume responsibility for such things as the administration of medications, wound care, symptom management, decisions regarding patient care, and managing care with various healthcare professionals.

Palliative care in the community has the capability to answer many of the challenges currently being faced by patients with serious illness and the families and caregivers who are struggling to care for them. The demonstrated impact of CBPC programs has improved caregiver burden, maintenance of caregiver quality of life, and family satisfaction.[14,17–19] Palliative care services, utilizing the interdisciplinary team (IDT) model, can assess and intervene with symptom burden, identify and work to decrease caregiver burden, coordinate appropriate community resources, establish goals of care and treatment preferences, coordinate care, and assist in providing a badly needed and critical layer of support.[15,16]

Effectiveness of Palliative Care in the Home

Though more research is needed to validate the effectiveness of CBPC programs, the evidence to date is highly encouraging. CBPC has been shown to enhance symptom management, improve patient quality of life, reduce aggressive care at the end of life, increase advance directive completion, reduce hospitalization rates and emergency room visits, decrease intensive care unit (ICU) length of stay, lower overall healthcare cost, as well as improve patient and family satisfaction scores. However, there is still a high degree of variability among CBPC programs; and, as such, not all are able to demonstrate these outcomes to the same degree.[3,20–23]

A 2016 Cochrane review revealed strong evidence that home palliative care increases the chances of one dying at home if that is the desire. Home palliative care was also found to reduce symptom burden, in particular for patients with cancer, without impacting the grief experienced by the caregiver.[23] What is even more intriguing are the results found by Higginson and colleagues in a small, randomized trial conducted in 2013.[24] These researchers questioned the effectiveness of integrating palliative care early in the disease trajectory of persons with advanced disease and refractory breathlessness. Their results strongly support the early integration of palliative care for persons with serious illness other than cancer and breathlessness, as well as for those with cancer.

Delivery Models of CBPC

Great strides are being made to develop a standardized approach to delivering CBPC services. The Centers for Medicare & Medicaid Innovation's fast-track development of a CBPC demonstration model is one example of the effort to improve outcomes while decreasing unwanted and unnecessary care during the COVID-19 pandemic. The goals of CBPC models are to identity persons with serious illness who are considered high risk earlier in the diagnosis in order to decrease symptom burden and provide education and support while ensuring the needs and goals of those being cared for are being met.

Given the restrictions that often result from a fee-for-service care model, CBPC practices must be smart and creative in order to improve provider productivity, while maintaining valuable care and not creating provider burnout. Some may, for example, decide to focus their geographical catchment in order to minimize expensive drive time for their staff. Practices may see patients in certain zip codes limit their services to specific facilities such as independent living facilities, assisted living facilities, skilled nursing facilities, or senior communities. A short description of various models follows.

Consultative Programs

CBPC programs continue to evolve to better serve a growing number of patients living with serious chronic illness throughout the disease continuum. Consultative models in the inpatient setting have a great responsibility to ensure continuity of care continues after discharge. It is essential for inpatient and community-based models to work together to meet the needs of the patient and their caregivers. In the community setting, often palliative care specialists work closely with the primary care provider (PCP) or referring physician/specialist. The palliative care specialist, a physician or advanced practice registered nurse (APRN), will receive a referral to assess a seriously ill patient and their family, then make recommendations to the primary care team to meet the identified palliative care needs. The CBPC staff functions as a consultant service and does not provide primary care.

Home healthcare agencies may provide primary palliative care to meet the needs of their medically complex patients who may not yet be eligible for hospice or whose goals of care do not reflect the hospice philosophy. Home healthcare agencies are primarily reimbursed through Medicare A, Medicaid, and commercial insurances for episodic care for nursing or therapy needs. Patients must meet criteria for home healthcare and must demonstrate progression toward improvement. Registered nurses (RNs) are reimbursed within the per diem rate, whereas APRNs may bill for their palliative care services under Medicare B, Medicaid, or commercial insurance per visit. Patient and referral source satisfaction lead to increased referrals for the home healthcare agency, increasing revenue and support of the CBPC practice.

Hospice

CBPC may be provided by hospice agencies as a separate service line. For patients who are not currently eligible for the hospice benefit or who are continuing to seek curative or life-prolonging treatment, the hospice agency's palliative care service will deploy APRNs, RNs, and occasionally social workers and chaplains to render these services. APRNs and licensed clinical social workers bill under Medicare B, Medicaid, or commercial insurance, although fee-for-service billing is rarely adequate for a sustainable practice. The hospice agency justifies this service arm by metrics such as earlier referrals to hospice, improvement in quality care, and increased length of hospice stays. CBPC providers are skilled in having goals-of-care discussions with those with serious illness and their families, which often results in a transition to hospice at the appropriate time, allowing for the reception of more hospice benefits over time. Palliative care providers are skilled in identifying hospice appropriateness in their patients. There are key indicators of decline, such as frequent hospitalizations, decreased functionality, and increased dependence in activities of daily living.

Hospice is different from palliative care in that it is for those with a prognosis of 6 months or less. The hospice philosophy is to focus on comfort, and thus any potentially life-prolonging treatments are discontinued, such as chemotherapy, radiation, and dialysis. Infection is considered uncomfortable, so in most cases, infection is still treated. There is further emphasis on de-prescribing in hospice care, but if families have concerns about certain medications or treatments being discontinued, that should be discussed with the hospice director as different programs have different parameters around what they will allow as an expense under the hospice benefit. There are many misconceptions around hospice, which create fear and barriers to transitioning to this appropriate level of care for many with a terminal diagnosis. Nurses are invaluable in their ability to educate and discuss this service in a way that concerns are addressed and the benefits of this care model are understood. Hospice offers 24/7 access to providers, takes over all care so that there is no longer a need for appointments with multiple providers, and has nurses who will come to the home in order to prevent the use of emergency health services.

Private Duty Nursing Agencies

Private duty nursing agencies may offer palliative care provided by certified nursing assistants and RNs, primarily in support of the plan of care developed by palliative care specialists. Payment is through long-term care insurance or as an out-of-pocket expense.

Primary Care Practices

Primary care practice in the home is a growing field that is providing care to people with multiple medical morbidities and complex illness right where they live. There is no medical specialty more appropriately positioned to deliver palliative care than those practicing in the general practice setting. They know the medical, psychosocial, and environmental challenges faced by their patients better than any other provider. As such, general practice APRNs are seeing the demand for addressing palliative care during their home-based primary care visits. Most CBPC programs are reimbursed by Medicare B, Medicaid, and commercial insurance. They are often available 24/7. Home-based primary care programs vary widely from the multistate Veterans Affairs system, which utilizes the physician/APRN model, to solo APRNs making house calls.

Within this construct, those PCPs who are palliative care–trained make a valuable impact on meeting the palliative care needs of their seriously ill patients. However, their approach is somewhat "grass roots" at this moment. PCPs who have advanced their palliative care skills and knowledge are able to identify and address palliative care needs, but the approach is reactive in nature. As this area matures, ways to incorporate the identification and treatment of palliative care needs from a systematic viewpoint will emerge.

Free-Standing Palliative Care

There are palliative care programs that exist without attachment to other service lines. These exist in those hospital systems that often wish to impact negative metrics such as the 30-day rehospitalization metric. Various forms of teams consisting of nurses, social workers, and administration staff work to provide palliative care to their patients after discharge from their hospital setting. Their reimbursement is in the form of fee-for-service billing (if they have clinicians with licensure to bill) or by avoiding the penalties associated with frequent readmission rates.

Another version of the free-standing palliative care model is for-profit, multistate organizations. These companies are reimbursed by insurances on a per-patient per-month basis. The goal is to reduce the hospitalizations and increase hospice referrals for enrollees with high utilization rates. These patients are often defined through an algorithm using data held by the insurance company. APRNs and RNs work in tandem with a physician to manage symptoms, provide education and support, and discuss goals of care and advance care planning.

Pediatric Palliative Care

Pediatric palliative care in the community is complex. Children covered by state Medicaid or the Children's Health Insurance Program and who have a terminal illness are able to receive hospice care and curative therapies simultaneously. A child may be eligible to receive skilled intermittent and 24-hour nursing along with respite care and other therapies. There are few pediatric community care programs in the United States due to cost and payment limits.

Payment for Palliative Care Services in the Community

Reimbursement for palliative care in the community is ever evolving to meet the demand for effective care of the seriously ill, while making palliative services feasible for the organizations offering the care. As the traditional fee-for-service model of paying for services rendered is moved to newer, alternative payment models, such as value-based payment structures and direct contracting agreements with payors, there is increased opportunity for CBPC. Moving to value-based and risk-sharing partnerships may allow for the hiring of a full complement of IDT members, allowing a more comprehensive model of care and supportive services to be delivered to persons with serious illness and their caregivers. In 2020, the administration announced a commitment to three goals for value-based payment: advancing health equity, improving quality of care, and lowering costs.[25] Research suggests that only the defined-scope-of-practice or condition-specific payment models of care are designed to involve low to medium risk across all risk categories for organizations, while providing strong flexibility and revenue stability. Examples of these models are bundled or per-member per-month payment arrangements.[26–31]

Value-based billing made up 38% of all US healthcare payments at the end of 2015.[28–30] Tightly woven into the value-based payment structure is the need to identify, collect, analyze, and report on measurements and metrics of the palliative care programs. Measuring the quality of care delivery is integral to hospice and palliative care programs, as specified by the National Consensus Project's *Clinical Practice Guidelines* and the Joint Commission Advanced Certification Program for Palliative Care, as well as by stakeholders and payers.[27–32] Currently, no national standards for measurement or databases that would support benchmarking exist in palliative care.

The Quality and Practice Standards Committee of the American Academy of Hospice and Palliative Medicine along with the Hospice and Palliative Nurses Association (HPNA) initiated the Measuring What Matters consensus project.[33–35] The overall goal of the project was to recommend a concise portfolio of valid, clinically relevant, cross-cutting performance indicators for internal measurement for hospice and palliative care programs.[34,35] The Measuring What Matters project is now in phase two and will take on more complex tasks, such as creating e-specifications and patient-reported outcome measures; field-testing altered, expanded, or untested measures; and developing a common palliative care denominator. Additionally, they are investigating collaborations, strategic alliances and funding, and developing a companion paper to Measuring What Matters on quality research priorities. The Measuring What Matters development participants also identified six areas of creative tension in developing a quality strategy for the palliative care field: process or outcome measures, specialty focus or primary care focus, perfection or pragmatism, quality improvement or accountability, hospice or palliative care, and medical model or multidisciplinary?[34,35] They recommend that existing palliative organizations take steps to align

Table 59.1 Roles of palliative care interdisciplinary team (IDT) members

Caregivers	Provide daily or around-the-clock custodial care. Often family members or may be paid professionals.
Registered nurses/licensed practical nurses[2]	Deliver skilled care as directed by care plan. Often nurses lead goals-of-care discussions, provide education and support around the diagnosis and prognosis, do medication reconciliation and education regarding medication administration, and provide wound care as needed. Coordination of care is often provided by nurses with other providers or such as home health for skilled services and advanced practice nurses for symptom management.
Advanced practice registered nurses/physician assistants	Coordinate total patient care to complex patients; supervise/delegate to other nurses; assess and diagnose; prescribe medications.
Physical therapists	Deliver skilled care to increase strength and function, assess for assistive devices.
Psychologists	Address stress, body image, depression.
Occupational therapists	Address patients' abilities to perform their everyday tasks with greater independence and efficiency.
Speech therapists	Improve speech and swallowing problems, address hearing loss and language problems.
Chaplains	Address spiritual issues, adjustment to "new normal."
Physicians	Coordinate/oversee nursing and therapist staff, certify care plan.
Nutritionists	Provide diet counseling for special nutritional needs.
Pharmacists	Review medications, make recommendations for adjustments, cost, contraindications.
Volunteers	Assist patients and families in meeting goals, legacy work, socialization.
Home health aides	Perform personal care and basic nursing tasks.
Homemakers	Provide cleaning, tidying, shopping, pet care.
Social workers (MSW/LCSW)	Identify needs of family and patient, refer to community resources, counseling.

with existing quality measurement requirements, identify priorities, and improve.[34,35]

Roles and Responsibilities of the Specialized Palliative Care Team in the Community

There is much discussion in the healthcare literature about how healthcare disciplines, operating in numerous silos, interact to care for patients. However, given the increasing complexity of medical care as well as heightened limitations on a provider's time, care that operates under the traditional model can become disjointed. For those living with a serious illness, which carries a heavy treatment burden, this effect is often amplified. Having to navigate such a landscape can have deleterious effects on the illness experience. It can also create an environment in which ultimately the medical care delivered will be less than ideal.

In palliative care, this issue is recognized; and thus, care coordination is one of the key pillars of the discipline. CBPC is uniquely positioned to fully evaluate one's circumstance and in turn communicate with all members of the healthcare team. Using a consultative model, it seeks to work with, not replace, other disciplines in order to enhance overall care. This model incorporates the multidisciplinary approach, operating through the IDT. This ensures that all aspects of the illness experience (medical, spiritual, psychosocial) are addressed in a way that complements the chosen treatment plan. In this respect, the IDT can fill in the "gaps" in care in ways the traditional model cannot.

IDTs base their function as a team on interdependent interaction, which results in a synergistic effect that happens when the members possessing specific expertise work closely together.[38] Palliative care teams in the community are generally comprised of caregivers, care coordinators, physician medical directors, nurse practitioners, nurses, and social workers, though for completeness, other disciplines do participate in CBPC IDTs. Please refer to Table 59.1 for the roles and responsibilities of the disciplines typically found on a palliative care team.

Professional Issues for Nurses Providing Palliative Care in the Community

State regulations, Medicare, and commercial insurance companies each impact the practice of CBPC nursing. Nurses working in palliative care should work with state legislatures to effect positive change related to palliative care practice within their states. It is important to note that state nurse practice acts vary widely in the scope of practice for RNs and APRNs. It is recommended that nurses familiarize themselves with the state regulations guiding their practice. The National Council of State Boards of Nursing provides resources and can be found at https://www.ncsbn.org/.

Key Takeaways for Nurses Providing Palliative Care in the Community

Palliative care, as its own area of expertise, has grown significantly since the American Board of Medical Specialties approved the creation of hospice and palliative medicine as a subspecialty in 2006. This approach to care is so new that generations of healthcare professionals have had no exposure to it. This presents a significant challenge to palliative care academia to keep up with the demand for quality curriculum and programs to educate its clinicians. In 2000, the End-of-Life Nursing Education Consortium (ELNEC) project was funded by The Robert Wood Johnson Foundation. This national education initiative to improve palliative care developed and delivers nursing curriculum in end-of-life care. This project has been extremely successful in impacting the knowledge curve for all nurses caring for patients living with serious illness. In 2013, ELNEC debuted its curriculum for the APRN community. The ELNEC website states that it has trained "over 21,400 nurses and other healthcare professionals, representing all 50 US states, plus 90 countries."[36]

Outside of this highly contributive body of work, the availability of accredited programs remains small. In 2017, the HPNA's website listed 15 master's and doctoral palliative care graduate programs available and another three with electives in palliative care.[37] Two newly created, innovative programs, one launched at the University of Colorado and another at the University of Maryland, offer interprofessional master's degrees and certifications in palliative care. These programs incorporate students and faculty from all palliative care disciplines.

Although these novel programs and others segregated by discipline are currently developing, schools will require years to graduate the estimated 10,000 educated clinicians this field requires.

While the opening of CBPC programs is hailed as filling a rapidly growing need, there is currently a dearth of trained, qualified palliative care professionals. As the understanding and acceptance of specialty palliative care are increasingly embraced, the appreciation for integrating palliative care earlier in the disease trajectory creates an exploding demand for these nurses and other healthcare professionals.

Community-based agencies struggling to meet the demands of increased referrals have no other choice but to recruit and hire untrained, unqualified clinicians.

Fortunately, leading national palliative care organizations anticipated this need years ago and have published guiding principles for the education of future practitioners. The National Consensus Project for Quality Palliative Care, a subcommittee of the Hospice and Palliative Care Coalition, is one such organization. This project drew upon five major US palliative care organizations to develop clinical guidelines for quality palliative care services. The guidelines, originally released in 2004, have undergone two revisions and are now in their fourth edition, released in 2018.

Specifically for the nursing discipline, the HPNA established standards of care in their important document *HPNA Standards for Clinical Education of Hospice and Palliative Nurses*, originally created in 2005, with the second edition released in 2015.[38]

The Joint Commission, a national accrediting body, launched its certification program for hospital-based palliative care in 2011, closely followed by its certification for CBPC programs in 2016. The Joint Commission requires that clinicians are trained in palliative care.

The Center to Advance Palliative Care is a national organization that has created an in-depth platform of education, mentoring, tools, training, and measurements. These can be found at the Center to Advance Palliative Care website: www.capc.org.

Since 1965, Community Health Accreditation Partners (CHAP) has been working to elevate and standardize care delivered in the community. In 1992, CHAP began a relationship with the Centers for Medicare & Medicaid Services; compliance with CHAP standards can be used by organizations to demonstrate that they meet the conditions of participation for home health, hospice, and home medical equipment Medicare/Medicaid programs.

The establishment of these curricula and position statements is a critical step. Moving to an accepted standard for entry-level palliative care clinicians is the next. It is imperative that agencies ensure that their palliative care clinicians are adequately educated, trained, and supported, as well as having appropriate certification.

CBPC Summary

In the past, when medical care was much simpler, patients were cared for by local family physicians who made house calls. The "house call" itself was deemed imperative as this was the means by which physicians grew to understand all aspects of the illness, most notably the psychosocial aspects. They were granted greater insight into the patient's life and subsequently were the first to provide truly holistic care. With modernization of healthcare, the "house call" was phased out, and part of the art was lost.

The modernization of medical care has led to a great number of scientific advances, and people are living longer than ever as a result. Groundbreaking advances are made every day. The trade-off, however, is increasingly more complex medical care, often difficult for patients to navigate. Persons with serious illness, as a result of living longer, can amass a long list of chronic conditions and an even longer list of specialist physicians. They are often confronted with a plethora of information as well as seemingly endless choices. While that is a positive aspect of modern medical care, it can be overwhelming, particularly for those with a serious, life-limiting illness. Moreover, healthcare decisions are not made in a vacuum. Cultural, spiritual, and psychosocial factors will affect choices as much as, if not more than, the medical facts alone. Yet, in the setting of an office visit, the provider may be limited in how much focus they can place on this important aspect.

CBPC can serve to replace what house calls once provided. IDTs can gain valuable insight into a patient's life by being present in the home. Through effective communication, strong relationships are built. Careful care coordination and collaboration among providers involved in the care result in improved quality of care and health-related quality of life. Introducing palliative care early in the disease trajectory allows time for these processes to occur when appropriate. The palliative care team can, through a holistic view and with a strong relationship, help guide persons with serious illness and their families through the illness journey, attending to any physical and existential distress. When the time is right, if the goal is hospice care, the palliative care team can also assist with a seamless transition to hospice services.

CBPC is not yet universally available; however, it has grown considerably in recent years. With further education of healthcare providers and increased demand it is likely that access to CBPC will continue to evolve and will result in better-quality outcomes.

The Future for Nurses in Palliative Care in the Community

Nurses have been bringing care, including unnamed palliative care, into people's homes since the 1800s. The current move of healthcare back into the community brings with it the opportunity for nursing to continue to positively impact the trajectory of the experience of serious illness. Through exemplary communication skills and a wide-ranging knowledge base, the nursing force is set to deliver multifaceted care while acting as liaisons and guides for those who are seriously ill, attempting to navigate the increasingly complex healthcare system. Nurses, with their ability to respond quickly to changing needs, fill the large unaddressed gap in care. By effectively orchestrating much needed difficult conversations around advance care planning, managing immense symptom burden, intervening with caregiver strain, and coordinating care, nurses impact the very heart of suffering.

Now, more than ever, the need is great for nurses from all backgrounds of healthcare to seek out and obtain advanced education in palliative care. Identifying wishes and goals of care along with treatment preferences, then advocating for these desires, is one of the true callings of the nursing discipline. Ideally, all nurses would be trained, qualified, and competent to deliver high-quality palliative care to each suffering patient and family they touch.

Case Study: A Patient in Palliative Care

Arthur is a 79-year-old man with a history of hypertension, obesity, and severe chronic obstructive pulmonary disease with chronic respiratory failure. He has a history of frequent exacerbations despite having quit smoking several years ago. He has frequently required admission for these exacerbations and over the last few years has only been able to remain out of the hospital for 1 to 2 months at a time. Additionally, Arthur had neither a PCP nor a regular pulmonologist.

He then experienced a prolonged hospital stay, including an ICU stay after contracting COVID-19, which caused pneumonia as well as acute on chronic respiratory failure. He was seen initially by the inpatient palliative care team who, in addition to discussing goals of care, helped to facilitate communication between Arthur, his healthcare team, and his family. This required additional effort given the visitation restrictions enacted during the COVID-19 pandemic.

Fortunately, he did survive his illness but developed significant weakness, found himself debilitated, and experienced ongoing shortness of breath above his usual baseline. He was initially discharged to a short-term care facility for rehabilitation, to be followed by continued rehabilitation at home. At the time of hospital discharge, he was referred to CBPC services. The inpatient palliative care team communicated with the community-based team, ensuring continuity.

The CBPC nurse first met Arthur while he was still residing at the short-term care facility. Further discussions regarding goals of care were undertaken as well as relationship-building. The nurse was also able to help coordinate care between the facility and the receiving home health services and was able to help the patient establish care with a primary care physician as well as pulmonologist. At the time of discharge home, the patient had all the necessary care services in place.

When the patient was discharged, now already being familiar with Arthur, the nurse was able to visit him in his home. She was able to review his medications and provide additional education to both Arthur and his family, who was now able to see Arthur in person for the first time since becoming ill. Goals of care were reviewed again with them all present together, during which time she helped to answer questions, address concerns, and facilitate the family meeting.

Two months had passed, and despite being able to avoid readmission to the hospital, Arthur continued to complain of significant shortness of breath, which markedly affected his quality of life. During a particular follow-up visit, the nurse noted he had developed lower extremity edema. The physical exam also revealed new crackles in the lung bases. Arthur did not previously have a history of congestive heart failure. His goals of care indicated that he was do not resuscitate/intubate and wanted to avoid further hospital admissions.

Working along with his new PCP, diuretics and medications to help with management of refractory dyspnea were initiated. Education was provided. Home health was able to draw lab work at home while diuretics were being titrated. The palliative care nurse visited Arthur frequently, which enabled her to closely monitor his congestive heart failure symptoms and proactively work with his PCP to manage his medication regimen accordingly. His symptoms improved, and Arthur was able to avoid any visits to the hospital, in keeping with his stated wishes.

Arthur was able to enjoy 14 months at home without a single hospital visit. His symptoms remained controlled, and he was even able to engage in some of his favorite hobbies. After 14 months, however, despite maximum medical management, his condition did deteriorate. By this point, the palliative care nurse had a strong relationship with both Arthur and his family. Knowing his wishes well, a plan had been made in advance for how he would like to be cared for when this day came. He wanted to remain at home, with family at his side. Given his condition, however, despite having a large family, they needed additional assistance in caring for Arthur. Hospice services were called. The nurse was able to communicate clearly with the hospice team, and he had a smooth transition without interruption to his current care plan.

The hospice team was able to continue adjusting the medical regimen to meet Arthur's needs. Additionally, they were able to arrange for a hospital bed as well as other necessary medical equipment. They kept his symptoms under control while providing support to his family for the next 3 months until he passed peacefully at home, as he had wished. After his passing, the hospice team was able to provide grief support to his family, helping them through the difficult time.

Case Study Summation

This case study illustrates the multiple ways in which CBPC can improve patient outcomes. Palliative care was initiated during the hospital stay and then continued into the home after hospital discharge, which would otherwise not have been possible. Given the ability of a single provider to see the patient in both the care facility and his home, continuity was maintained. Using the "house call" model, the nurse was able to develop a strong relationship with the patient and his family as well as gain insight into his personal goals and values. The nurse was able to help coordinate care with all other members of Arthur's medical team, including the home health agency. The nurse was instrumental in detecting the change in Arthur's condition, identifying congestive heart failure in a timely manner. Had this not been the case, it is likely that Arthur would have decompensated prior to the next office visit with his PCP, leading to the need for aggressive care. Through collaboration with Arthur's PCP, the condition was managed proactively, avoiding the need for hospital admission. This ensured Arthur's goals were met. Because clear prognostication as well as goals-of-care conversations had continued through every change in his condition, Arthur and his family were prepared for the decline he would eventually face. The nurse had normalized the process for them, which reduced anxiety, helping with the grieving process. He was able to transition seamlessly to hospice services who continued to care for his every need until his peaceful passing. Arthur's family was also cared for during his death as well as after with grief support provided by the hospice team.

Without CBPC, Arthur's disease trajectory might have looked quite different. Given his severe conditions and lack of providers, it is likely he would have frequented the emergency room and required continued hospital admissions. Additionally, his symptoms would not be as well controlled, and his quality of life would suffer as a result. If careful and ongoing goals of care conversations had not taken place, his family could have been blindsided by the severity of Arthur's condition; and decisions would have been made hastily, leading to aggressive interventions including ICU level of care or cardiopulmonary resuscitation, which was something Arthur did not want. Without forethought, hospice services are often introduced very late (if at all) in the disease process, depriving patients and their families of the full benefits hospice can provide. Through education, the disease process was normalized for the patient's family; without this, they would be subject to increased anxiety and a negative grief response.

REFERENCES

1. National Alliance for Caregiving, AARP Public Policy Institute. *Caregiving in the United States 2020 Report*. Published May 14, 2020. Accessed January 22, 2025. https://press.aarp.org/2020-5-14-Caregiving-in-the-US-Report
2. Morrison RS, Augustin R, Souvanna P, Meier DE. America's care of serious illness: a state-by-state report card on access to palliative care in our nation's hospitals. *J Palliat Med*. 2011 Oct;14(10).1094–1096. doi:10.1089/jpm.2011.9634. Epub 2011 Sep 16. PMID: 21923412; PMCID: PMC3391707.
3. National Academy for State Health Policy. *Palliative care checklist: A guide for policymakers to support access and quality*. Published March 2022. Accessed January 22, 2025. https://www.nashp.org/wp-content/uploads/2022/03/NASHP-Palliative-Care-Checklist_March2022.pdf
4. Arias E, Tejada-Vera B, Ahmad F. *Provisional Life Expectancy Estimates for January through June, 2020*. National Center for Health Statistics; 2021. Accessed August 8, 2022.
5. Boersma P, Black LI, Ward BW. Prevalence of multiple chronic conditions among US adults, 2018. *Prev Chronic Dis*. 2020;17:200130. http://dx.doi.org/10.5888/pcd17.200130.
6. American Action Forum. *Chronic disease in the United States: A worsening health and economic crisis*. Published September 15, 2022. Accessed January 22, 2025. https://www.americanactionforum.org/research/chronic-disease-in-the-united-states-a-worsening-health-and-economic-crisis/
7. Association of American Medical Colleges. *Homebound, not hopeless*. Published January 26, 2023. Accessed January 22, 2025. https://www.aamc.org/news/homebound-not-hopeless
8. Centers for Disease Control and Prevention. *Chronic disease: Facts and statistics*. Published n.d. Accessed January 22, 2025. https://www.cdc.gov/chronic-disease/data-research/facts-stats/index.html
9. Cancer Health. *Cancer and quality of life: The importance of patient-centered research*. Published n.d. Accessed January 22, 2025. https://www.cancerhealth.com/article/cancer-quality-life-patientcentered-research
10. AARP. *More Americans are dying at home than in hospitals*. Published December 11, 2019. Accessed January 22, 2025. Available from: https://www.aarp.org/health/conditions-treatments/info-2019/more-dying-at-home-than-hospital.html
11. Colby S, Ortman JM. The Baby Boom Cohort in the United States: 2012 to 2060. Population Estimates and Projections. US Census Bureau. May, 2014. Accessed July 22, 2017. https://www.census.gov/prod/2014pubs/p25-1141.pdf.
12. Lund D, Utz R, Caserta M, et al. Time for living and caring: an intervention to make respite more effective for caregivers. *Int J Aging Hum Dev*. 2014;79(2):157–178.
13. Thomas Hebdon MC, Phan CT, Phillips C, et al. Ethical and policy implications of financial burden in family caregivers. *J Hosp Palliat Nurs*. 2022;24(5):E226–E232. https://doi.org/10.1097/NJH.0000000000000887.
14. Ortega-Galán ÁM, Ruiz-Fernández MD, Carmona-Rega MI, Cabrera-Troya J, Ortíz-Amo R, Ibáñez-Masero O. The experiences of family caregivers at the end of life: suffering, compassion satisfaction and support of health care professionals: experiences of caregivers at the end of life. *J Hosp Palliat Nurs*. 2019;21(5):438–444. https://doi.org/10.1097/NJH.0000000000000586.
15. Arias-Rojas M, Carreño-Moreno S, Arias-Quiroz N. The "PalliActive Caregivers" intervention for caregivers of patients with cancer in palliative care: a feasibility pilot study. *J Hosp Palliat Nurs*. 2020;22(6):495–503. https://doi.org/10.1097/NJH.0000000000000696.
16. Williams N, Jamal S, Guthrie D. The relationship between caregiver burden and depressive symptoms in Ontario home care clients. *Home Health Care Serv Q*. 2018;37(1):60–76.
17. Wu KK, Bos T, Mausbach B, et al. Long-term caregiving is associated with impaired cardiovagal baroreflex. *J Psychosom Res*. 2017;103:29–33.
18. Akyar I, Dionne-Odom JN, Bakitas MA. Supporting Family Caregivers of Turkish Elders: A Systematic Review. *J Hosp Palliat Nurs*. 2016;18(3):256–267. https://doi.org/10.1097/NJH.0000000000000244.
19. Reina-Gamba NC, Medellin-Olaya J, Burbano-Rivera DV, Miranda-Rojas HM, Vargas-Escobar LM, Colmenares-Tovar C. Health-related quality of life in primary caregivers of people receiving palliative home care. *J Hosp Palliat Nurs*. 2022;24(2):E41–E47. https://doi.org/10.1097/NJH.0000000000000832.
20. Davis M, Temel J, Balboni T, Glare P. A review of the trials which examine early integration of outpatient and home palliative care for patients with serious illnesses. *Ann Palliat Med*. 2015;4(3):99–121.
21. Gomes B, Calanzani N, Higginson I. Benefits and costs of home palliative care compared with usual care for patients with advanced illness and their family caregivers. *JAMA*. 2014;311(10):1060–1061.
22. Ventura A, Burney S, Brooker J, Fletcher J, Ricciardelli L. Home-based palliative care: a systematic literature review of the self-reported unmet needs of patients and carers. *Palliat Med*. 2014;28(5):391–402.
23. Gomes B, Calanzani N, Curiale V, et al. Effectiveness and cost-effectiveness of home palliative care services for adults with advanced illness and their caregivers. *Sao Paulo Med J*. 2016;134(1):93–94.

24. Higginson IJ, Bausewein C, Reilly C, et al. An integrated palliative and respiratory care service for patients with advanced disease and refractory breathlessness: a randomised controlled trial. *Lancet Respir Med.* 2014;2(12):979–987.
25. Center to Advance Palliative Care. *CMMI releases more details on direct contracting model opportunities.* Published December 10, 2020. Accessed January 22, 2025. Available from: https://www.capc.org/blog/cmmi-releases-more-details-on-direct-contracting-model-opportunities/
26. Hospice News. *New research proposes sustainable palliative care payment model.* Published June 24, 2022. Accessed January 22, 2025. Available from: https://hospicenews.com/2022/06/24/new-research-proposes-sustainable-palliative-care-payment-model/
27. McKnight's Senior Living. *Palliative care payment model is on the not-so-distant horizon, advocates believe.* Published October 13, 2022. Accessed January 22, 2025. Available from: https://www.mcknightsseniorliving.com/news/palliative-care-payment-model-is-on-the-not-so-distant-horizon-advocates-believe/
28. American Academy of Hospice and Palliative Medicine. *Advocacy and regulatory payment issues.* Published n.d. Accessed January 22, 2025. Available from: https://aahpm.org/advocacy/regulatory-payment/
29. American Journal of Managed Care. *The role of palliative care in accountable care organizations.* Published November 29, 2022. Accessed January 22, 2025. Available from: https://www.ajmc.com/view/the-role-of-palliative-care-in-accountable-care-organizations-
30. American Journal of Managed Care. *Value-based payment, the safety net, and rethinking risk.* Published October 26, 2022. Accessed January 22, 2025. Available from: https://www.ajmc.com/view/value-based-payment-the-safety-net-and-rethinking-risk
31. Meier DE, Silvers A. Payment for palliative care. Center to Advance Palliative Care. 2017. Accessed August 30, 2017. https://www.capc.org/topics/payment/.
32. National Consensus Project for Quality Palliative Care. *Clinical Practice Guidelines for Quality Palliative Care.* 4th ed. National Coalition for Hospice and Palliative Care; 2018.
33. Joint Commission. Certification for Palliative Care Programs. Accessed August 7, 2017. http://www.jointcommission.org/certification/palliative_care.aspx.
34. Dy SM, Kiley KB, Ast K, et al. Measuring what matters: top-ranked quality indicators for hospice and palliative care from the American Academy of Hospice and Palliative Medicine and Hospice and Palliative Nurses Association. *J Pain Symptom Manage.* 2015;49(4):773–781.
35. Advancing Expert Care. *Performance measures.* Published n.d. Accessed January 22, 2025. Available from: https://www.advancingexpertcare.org/practice-research/research/performance-measures/
36. Dahlin CM, Coyne PJ, Paice J, Malloy P, Thaxton CA, Haskamp A. ELNEC-APRN: meeting the needs of advanced practice nurses through education. *J Hosp Palliat Nurs.* 2017;19(3):261–265.
37. Dahlin C. HPNA Graduate Program Listing. Hospice and Palliative Nurses Association. Accessed July 17, 2017. http://hpna.advancingexpertcare.org.

60

Telehealth, Telephonic Care, and Remote Patient Monitoring

Laraine Ann Chiu, Jennifer Curtis, and Inez Brandon

Key Points

- Explore novel approaches to palliative care through the use of telehealth and remote patient monitoring in evidence-based nurse-led telephonic programs.
- Key techniques and skills for practicing palliative telehealth nursing, including the implementation of roles in clinical care coordination, symptom management, and advance care planning.
- Core telehealth nursing principles, challenges, barriers, and legal considerations with implications for nursing practice, education, research, legislation, and policy.

Introduction

A popular anecdote in the literature on the origin story of telehealth relates that the first telehealth encounter occurred on March 10, 1876, when Alexander Graham Bell used his newly patented device, the telephone, to call out to Thomas Watson for medical assistance after spilling sulfuric acid on his clothing in his laboratory. "Mr. Watson, come here! I want to see you."[1,2] Whether legend or fact, the implication is clear: the development of technologies to bridge the distances between us in real time has enabled the deployment of necessary medical services during emergencies and in the delivery of routine care. Over the last 150 years, increasingly more sophisticated telehealth technology has played a major role in enhancing healthcare access in rural, urban, and suburban areas and expanding the delivery of specialty services, including palliative care. This chapter aims to explore the history and practice of telehealth nursing including the use of remote monitoring technologies in palliative care.

The Health Resources and Services Administration (HRSA) defines telehealth as "the use of electronic information and telecommunication technologies to support and promote long-distance clinical healthcare, patient and professional health-related education and public health and health administration."[2] In 1996 the Institute of Medicine (IOM) released its report *Telemedicine: A Guide to Assessing Telecommunications for Health Care*.[3] The IOM noted that telehealth is not a single technology but a collection of clinical practices, technological applications, and organizational arrangements that changes rapidly with the demand for healthcare access and the growth of communication systems for information exchange.[3] The 2011 IOM report *The Future of Nursing: Leading Change, Advancing Health* noted that there is no greater opportunity to transform practice than through technology.[4] The HRSA sponsored the IOM in 2012 to again examine the use of telehealth technology in the US healthcare system. The focus was on extending resources to serve geographically isolated individuals while maintaining the quality and value of healthcare delivery.

The COVID-19 pandemic fueled the need for rapid expansion of telehealth resources including remote patient monitoring (RPM).[2] Prior to the declaration of the public health emergency in March of 2020, Medicare provided reimbursement for telehealth services only to people living in underserved, rural areas and from specific physicians.[5,6] The Centers for Medicare & Medicaid Services' rapid expansion of payment authorization for telehealth in an amount equivalent to an in-person consult in a formal healthcare setting, with private insurers quickly following suit, meant that nearly every individual with the technology to connect to services could access care, from virtual urgent care visits with nurse practitioners and physician assistants to specialty consults from a physician with whom they had no prior relationship.[5,6] The US Congress extended reimbursement for telehealth services regardless of whether the public health emergency ended given the impact on equitable healthcare.[6]

Telehealth Nursing

Nurses are at the forefront of delivering efficient, patient-centered healthcare services through telehealth technology. The expansion of the role of telehealth nursing addresses the growing demand for innovative approaches to equitable healthcare. According to the American Telehealth Association (ATA), telehealth nursing is a tool for delivering nursing care remotely to improve efficiency and patient access to healthcare.[7] Telehealth nurses use telecommunication technology to provide high-quality care for people who need highly specialized services including palliative care. ATA noted that nurses

Table 60.1 American Nurses Association's Core Principles on Connected Health

Principle 1	The use of connected health technologies does not alter the standards of professional practice when delivering healthcare, conducting research, or providing education.
Principle 2	As connected health is a method of healthcare delivery, the healthcare provided is subject to the same healthcare laws and board oversight as the healthcare provided in person.
Principle 3	Healthcare services delivered via connected health technologies should prioritize improving access to quality healthcare that is guided by best available evidence, accepted clinical standards, and best practices.
Principle 4	Professional practice and healthcare delivery, regardless of venue and channel of delivery, mandates that healthcare professionals meet state-specific regulatory and institutional requirements in accordance with scope of practice.
Principle 5	Nursing and other healthcare professions are responsible for developing their own competencies to ensure the safe, effective, and competent delivery of healthcare via connected health technologies using a patient- and family-centered, team-based approach.
Principle 6	Healthcare services delivered via connected health technologies should be congruent with in-person care and must adhere to the best available evidence that represents current and emerging interdisciplinary standards of care, while recognizing the limitations inherent in technology to ensure optimal patient-centered outcomes.
Principle 7	When using connected health technologies, the integrity and therapeutic value of the patient–healthcare professional relationship should be established, maintained, and promoted via connected health.
Principle 8	Safeguards must be taken with the transmission of electronic information and communication conducted using connected health technologies in all practice settings.
Principle 9	Documentation requirements for healthcare services delivered via the utilization of connected health technologies should be consistent with requirements applicable to all other patient encounters.
Principle 10	Patients involved in a connected health encounter should be informed about the process, the inherent risks and benefits, and their rights and responsibilities, in compliance with applicable federal and state laws.
Principle 11	The safety of patients and healthcare professionals must be ensured.
Principle 12	In order to inform connected health and ensure the best outcomes, it is essential that the assessment, evaluation, and study of all aspects of connected health are ongoing and systematic.
Principle 13	Policies governing the practices and reimbursement of healthcare should be continuously updated and modernized to allow for the integration, national adoption, and sustainability of connected health.

Source: Reference 10.

are designers, developers, implementers, administrators, educators, and researchers of telehealth services.[2,7,8] Nurses are positioned to support all aspects of the telehealth continuum in order to have the greatest impact on high-quality patient care.[8]

The National Council of State Boards of Nursing indicated that the practice of nursing delivered through telehealth technology begins with engaging and interacting with a person at a remote location, electronically receiving health status updates for initiating and transmitting therapeutic interventions or regimens, then monitoring and documenting individual responses with nursing care outcomes.[9] The value of telehealth nursing is bringing high-quality, skilled, empathetic, and effective nursing care to persons living with serious illness across distances with limited resources through telecommunication technology. The American Nurses Association (ANA) updated the 1998 ANA Core Principles on Telehealth in 2019 to the ANA Core Principles on Connected Health to help guide practice (see Table 60.1).[10]

Evidence-Based Nurse-Led Telephonic Palliative Care Programs

Nurse-led telephonic palliative care programs have demonstrated positive encounters and outcomes for both seriously ill persons and their caregivers. ENABLE (Educate, Nurture, Advise, Before Life Ends) was an early telephonic palliative care intervention that was adopted at various care settings since 1998.[11] The goal of ENABLE was to alleviate symptoms of disease and treatment, enhance patient–clinician communication, support family caregivers, and address their emotional or spiritual needs including family bereavement. Telephonic palliative care nurse coordinators conducted assessments for symptom management and quality of life across the illness trajectory. The nurse also provided advance care planning to discuss end-of-life care for individualized goals, values, and preferences. ENABLE-CANCER served adults with solid tumors or hematologic malignancies within 60 days of advanced cancer diagnosis as well as their family caregivers.[11]

Most recently, ENABLE-CHF PC (Comprehensive Heartcare for Patients and Caregivers) served persons 50 years or older with New York Heart Association Class III or IV heart failure or American College of Cardiology Stage C or D heart failure.[12] This program was conducted from October 1, 2015, to May 31, 2019, at a large southeastern US academic tertiary medical center and a Veterans Affairs medical center. Nurses led a series of six weekly coaching sessions. Among the 415 individuals, a high proportion were African American with good baseline quality of life who had clinically improved pain intensity and pain interference postintervention.[12] This clinical trial also evaluated 158 family caregivers on quality of life, mood, and burden as primary outcomes, as well as global health and positive aspects of caregiving as secondary outcomes.[13]

The EMPallA (Emergency Medicine Palliative Care Access) trial funded by the Patient-Centered Outcomes Research Institute (PCORI) is a large, multicenter, parallel, two-arm randomized controlled trial comparing two models of palliative care: nurse-led telephonic case management and specialty, outpatient palliative care.[14,15] Nurses provided telehealth services to older adults with serious illness including persons living with advanced cancer, end-stage heart failure with New York Heart Association Class III or IV, end-stage renal disease with glomerular filtration rate <15 mL/min/m^2, and global initiative for chronic obstructive lung disease Stage III, IV, or oxygen-dependent chronic obstructive pulmonary disease.[14,15] Study outcomes included advance care planning, quality of life, healthcare utilization, loneliness, and symptom burden among seriously ill persons, as well as caregiver strain, caregiver quality of life, and bereavement among family caregivers.

Another pilot factorial trial from October 2019 to October 2020 for family caregivers of persons with newly diagnosed advanced cancer is CASCADE (CAre Supporters Coached to be Adept DEcision Partners).[16] CASCADE determined the feasibility, acceptability, and efficacy of an early nurse-led telephonic palliative care decision support training intervention. Caregiver decision support provided by the telephonic nurse included discussions around treatment, surgery, devices, care transitions, care setting, self-care, accessing palliative and hospice care, and life-sustaining treatments. All of these focus on the goals, values, and treatment preferences of persons living with advanced cancer to decrease caregiver distress, burden, or receipt of treatment inconsistent with their wishes. In each of these studies, nurses deliver care coordination, symptom management, advance care planning, and psychoeducational intervention through telephonic care. Furthermore, the implementation of nurse-led telephonic palliative care programs provides accessibility to consultations, education, and collaboration among providers, clinicians, people living with serious illness, and their families and caregivers.

Modalities of Telehealth Technology

Telehealth services are implemented in various ways and determined by intended delivery of services or means for interaction. The most common telehealth application domains are asynchronous, synchronous, mobile health, and RPM.[17] Asynchronous telehealth communication is a real-time encounter through email, text messaging, or online applications as a form of store-and-forward where data is sent and received with a waiting response time period. This modality has commonly been used nationwide in most hospitals and outpatient clinics with the implementation of the electronic medical record and the capability for in and out of network communication between healthcare institutions or agencies. Synchronous telehealth communication is a live, face-to-face encounter through audio–video conferencing which has been shown to improve convenience, accessibility, and efficiency of healthcare delivery.[17]

Studies show that live video visits offer additional benefits compared with telephone visits given the visual contact and the ability to see individuals in their home environment through virtual means.[17] However, it may require more complex training, setup, equipment, video-enabled devices, and broadband internet access. Nevertheless, research studies aim to identify best practices for such innovative programs. Mobile Health or mHealth is the use of mobile technologies including cellular devices, applications, personal digital assistants, and other wireless devices as tools and platforms for health research and healthcare delivery according to the National Institutes of Health's Fogarty International Center.[18]

REACH-PC is a multicenter comparative effectiveness trial also funded by PCORI that uses audio–video conferencing at 20 cancer centers nationwide to provide integrated telehealth palliative care visits for adults with non-small-cell lung cancer.[19] This audio–video service is encrypted and creates a safe virtual clinic for people living with serious illnesses and their family caregivers. Given this new platform, healthcare professional users receive specialized training and address individual learning needs with connectivity during the initial consult visit. Individuals were provided with a tablet computer and cellular service plan for study visits in order to ease participation burden.[19]

Remote Patient Monitoring

RPM is the use of digital health devices to capture and serially monitor vital signs and biometrics. The data captured is uploaded to a digital platform for review by both the individual and the clinical team.[20,21] RPM may include US Food and Drug Administration–approved medical-grade devices that may be implanted, stationary or wearable, such as blood glucose monitors or Holter monitors.[22] Consumer-grade devices include wearable devices such as smartwatches or fitness trackers and home monitoring devices such as blood pressure monitors or pulse oximetry.[21,23] In addition to data that is captured by a device, RPM can include data inputted to a secure platform by an individual or caregiver for viewing by the clinical team.[20] The data gathered may be vital signs taken or questionnaire responses.[23] Smartphone or tablet cameras enable persons or caregivers to upload photographs to secure electronic medical record portals to provide caregivers with important visual information.[24]

Wearable smart devices that collect and transmit data through a wired or wireless network are part of the internet of things (IoT). The IoT is a system of wireless, interrelated, and connected digital devices that collect, send, and store data over a network without human-to-human or human-to-computer interaction.[25] "Health IoT" (HIoT) refers to devices that collect health-related data from an individual.[26] Wearable devices, smartphones, mHealth, semantic devices, and Ambient Assisted Living (AAL) are examples of HIoT.[26] Semantic devices are capable of navigating the environment for visually impaired persons. There are also community-based healthcare platforms that provide the technology to allow nurses to monitor and interact with homebound people in synchronous and asynchronous care coordination.[25] The rapid growth of HIoT to augment the delivery of healthcare is changing clinical practices and provision of care.[26] AAL refers to devices that can be purchased to enable individuals to live in their home independently through the use of cameras, social assistive robots, pill dispensers, and monitors that send emergency alerts in the case of a fall or if a person with memory impairment wanders.[27] AAL has the potential to reduce costs by keeping older adults safely in their homes and well supported.

RPM has been used with a variety of people living with chronic illnesses such as chronic obstructive pulmonary disease, congestive heart failure, peritoneal dialysis, diabetes mellitus, and COVID-19 who are not sick enough to require hospitalization but who have comorbidities that put them at high risk for severe illness or complications.[24] Table 60.2 shows the components of a successful RPM program.[28] One of the first studies that examined

Table 60.2 Components of successful remote patient monitoring programs

Components	Elements
Assess for appropriate population	High risk for readmission Cognitive limitations Lack of interest in their healthcare Technology challenged Physical limitations: hand/eye coordination, visual and auditory acuity
Digital electronic platform	Must be HIPAA-compliant Ensure data is protected from cyber attack Need reliable internet service and mobile device
HIoT monitoring device (blood glucose monitor, pulse oximeter, blood pressure monitor)	Digital literacy Person and caregiver training on device
Clinical alert parameters (severe or worsening symptoms or out-of-range data)	Collaboration with provider to ensure alerts are patient-specific to avoid false alarms
Clinical workforce (monitor and respond to alerts)	Adequate staff Sufficient training on equipment Staff able to act in timely and effective manner
Standardized response (symptom management and out of range data)	Algorithm to guide clinician Measures in place to reach out when patient/caregiver fail to input data or equipment fails

Source: Reference 28.

RPM in palliative care demonstrated the use of a communication and monitoring application in rural North Carolina among people with one or more life-threatening illness.[29] The application was a secure, encrypted, and Health Insurance Portability and Accountability Act (HIPAA)–compliant RPM platform using a smartphone or tablet. The application was tailored to meet individual needs for care plan reminders, symptom review, follow-up, and medication management. The inputted data was transmitted to clinicians through a secure dashboard or team smartphone. The evidence indicates the acceptability, feasibility, and usability of RPM among persons living with serious illness, with improvement in symptom burden, advanced directives, and hospice transitions.[29,30]

Advantages, Disadvantages, and Future Role of RPM

The advantages of RPM are early and real-time detection of illnesses or decline in status and reduction of hospital utilization, as discussed in several studies.[20,24,28,29] RPM also enables persons living with serious illness to remain and be monitored in their own home.[20,23,27,29] In one study, individuals reported a sense of security with someone monitoring them, a sense of connection with the clinical team during the pandemic, and a sense of empowerment through the education they received on their condition.[20]

The disadvantages of RPM are individual and caregiver concerns about the burden of additional time and cost.[31,32] A study on individual expectations and experiences of RPM for chronic diseases revealed that some individuals are reluctant to learn new systems or processes and do not trust new technology.[32] Other individuals reported a fear of losing interpersonal connection and felt that the clinicians paid more attention to the data than to their symptoms or concerns.[32] In the case of patients with serious illness transitioning to hospice, there was a concern that primary caregivers and family would focus on the numbers and have difficulty letting go of the task of monitoring. It is important to have an ongoing conversation to manage caregiver and family expectations as the person with serious illness declines.

RPM technology is improving at a rapid pace. In 2018, the World Health Organization noted that digital health and mHealth have the potential to improve the quality of and access to health information as well as coverage of care.[33] According to the International Telecommunication Union, there are over 7 billion mobile telephone subscriptions in the world, with the majority in low- to middle-income countries.[33] The increase in mobile and digital technology has the potential to improve access to healthcare services through telehealth.

The Practice of Palliative Telehealth Nursing

The foundation of practicing palliative telehealth nursing is interpersonal communication which includes oral, verbal, nonverbal, and listening techniques. The ability of the palliative telehealth nurse to engage in open and effective communication is key to caring for people with serious illnesses and supporting their family caregivers.[34] Palliative telehealth nursing ideally is used to build connections by gathering and sharing information with other clinicians to enhance their ability to have strengthened relationships with the seriously ill person. In an increasingly complex technological environment, conversation remains the backbone of telephonic nursing care. The definition of conversation is the exchange of observations and ideas.[35] A good conversationalist displays empathy with the ability to put one's self in the other person's shoes. In a clinical setting, conversation may be limited and occurring simultaneously during the time needed for a nurse to complete a task such as performing a physical assessment, documenting, or administering medications, whereas in palliative telehealth nursing, conversation is the task in relationship-based care.[36,37]

In the absence of face-to-face interaction or video conferencing, the ability to communicate effectively in order to increase trust, clarity, and rapport is impacted by the nurse's voice, tonation, speech, pauses, and silence. It is also helpful to mirror the individual's tone, pace, and word choice during conversations.

Table 60.3 Comparison of factors affecting nursing communication in different settings

	In-person clinic nurse	Palliative telehealth nurse
Environmental factors	Controlled environment in the presence of healthcare providers Private outpatient clinic rooms and limited companions or presence of family members Opportunity for physical and visual assessment	Engaging with individuals in their own personal safe space Exposure to family dynamics, living situations, and possible stressors (background noise: family, children, pets, construction, verbal conflict) Modified verbal and descriptive assessment based on individual or caregiver reports
Communication	Face-to-face Visual, verbal, and nonverbal cues: body language, facial expressions and gestures	Telephone or virtual platform Verbal, nonverbal and auditory cues: spoken words, voice, tone, pace, pauses, silence, audible signs of illness (cough, breathing, hoarse or weak voice)
Interaction time	Limited conversation with a set amount of time Task-oriented, leading or facilitated questions Appointment time slot per clinic schedules	Flexible time for conversation More time for open-ended questions Meets individuals' schedules

Utilizing communication skills and techniques including return-feedback, clarification, reflection, and summarization at the correct time without interrupting the individual fosters empathetic and therapeutic communication.[38–40] It is important to ask open-ended questions that allow people with serious illness the time to express emotions and feelings. An experienced palliative telehealth nurse can help normalize these feelings and expressions among seriously ill people through conversation. Skillful listening to verbal, nonverbal, and auditory cues is critical in palliative telehealth nursing with the inability to visualize the individual.[41] Through comprehensive active and reflective listening, the palliative telehealth nurse can in turn demonstrate complex reflective responses that elicit deeper conversations. The palliative telehealth nurse must also actively listen for environmental cues that provide further information regarding the individual's home, family dynamics, living situation, and possible stressors (see Table 60.3).[42]

Roles in the Delivery of Palliative Telehealth Nursing

The palliative telehealth nurse performs beyond telephone triage, follow-up, clinical care coordination, or case management (see Figure 60.1).[43,44] Palliative telehealth nursing requires culturally competent, compassionate care and extensive clinical knowledge to accurately identify and meet the needs of those who are seriously ill. The goal is to reduce suffering, provide relief, and improve the quality of life. Due to the possible lack of visual cues such as body language, facial expressions, and gestures on the telephone, a skilled palliative telehealth nurse uses both oral and descriptive assessments.[45] Accurate palliative assessments, decision-making,

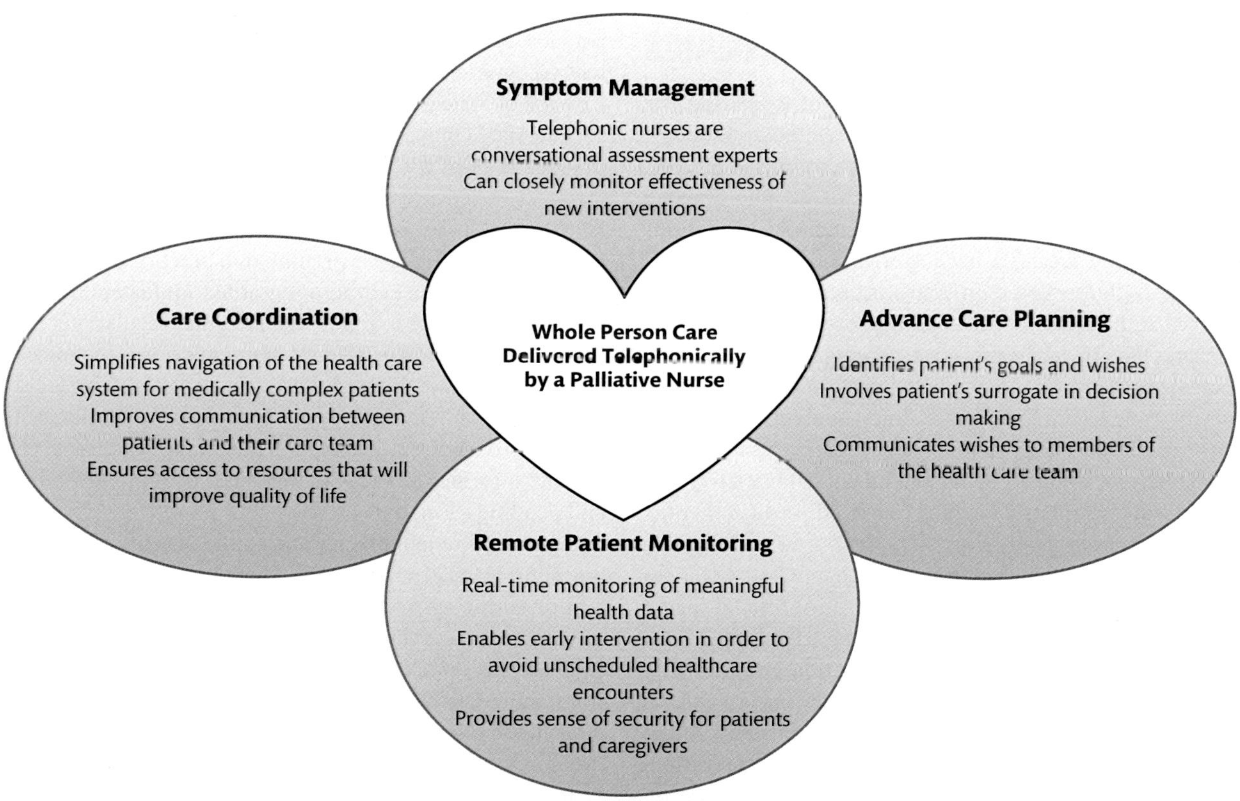

Figure 60.1 The dynamic role of the Registered Nurse in the delivery of palliative telehealth nursing.

and advice on supported self-management, referrals to specialists, or emergency care for distressing symptom issues involve critical thinking.[46] Supported self-management is the process of integrating strategies catered to each individual to cope with their disease or treatment-related symptoms which can reduce physical, psychological, and existential distress during end-of-life care.[47] The capacity to make decisions based on clinical experience, nursing knowledge, and ethical codes allows for the ability to act. Timely action while anticipating barriers to seeking or accessing immediate care for high-risk individuals is critical for palliative telehealth nurses to address urgent issues, problems, or concerns related to symptom management.

Palliative telehealth nurses facilitate meaningful conversations and move advance care planning forward with seriously ill persons and their family caregivers as they navigate through life-threatening illnesses and the end of life. Palliative telehealth nurses engage seriously ill persons outside of the clinical setting and in their homes where they are safe and comfortable to have open discussions of existential experiences.[48,49] This allows for sharing their reflection on the most challenging and emotional experiences of their lives, which may lead to a clearer understanding of their personal goals, values, and preferences for life-sustaining treatment. Persons living with life-threatening illnesses may also have multiple competing needs and less time or energy for conversations on the phone; therefore, involving family or surrogate decision makers is crucial during this time period as primary caregivers and support persons. Last but not least, palliative telehealth nurses share important information from high-quality conversations with the individual's healthcare team so that the team may develop better understanding and stronger connections in person-centered care.

Challenges and Barriers to Delivery

Telehealth nurses are faced with the challenge of delivering the same degree of human compassion through remote technology. Concerns around technology depersonalizing encounters and conflicting with core principles of palliative care or nursing practice have been reported given the value of a nurturing, caring relationship that supports and creates a healing environment for persons living with serious illness. Based on Watson's human caring theory, caring is placed at the center of the nursing process, and reports on therapeutic presence in telehealth are emerging.[50] The ATA position statement on telehealth nursing noted that nurses who achieve competency in using technology demonstrate the ability to perform assessments remotely through audio–video communication, implement care plans for evaluation, and document data in electronic health records while seamlessly meeting care needs in an authentic, respectful, and caring way.[51]

Standardization of guidelines for telehealth nursing practices and training across state lines is a challenge; therefore, ensuring high-quality care through constant monitoring, developing, and improving delivery is central to the safety, satisfaction, and reliability of the services provided. Factors that ensure high-quality care in telehealth nursing include the accessibility and sustainability of the program, the availability of healthcare resources and organization, specialist education and nursing experience, skilled communication and person-centered care, as well as safe, efficient, and competent care.[52] These factors for high-quality care can overcome the barriers to equitable distribution of telehealth services.

Variable technological equipment, device ownership, lack of broadband internet access, and network infrastructure can also cause disparities in the delivery of telehealth services. Network infrastructure includes hardware devices for video visits, software applications for monitoring or management, and network services for connectivity. These barriers are most prominent among individuals with limited English proficiency or digital literacy. National survey data from the Census Bureau revealed disparities in utilization of telehealth modalities by race, ethnicity, age, education, income, and health insurance coverage which disproportionately impact healthcare delivery and access across the United States.[53] Data showed lower rates of telehealth use among historically underserved populations including people with lower household income; adults without a high school degree; older adults; respondents who self-identified as Black, Latino, or Asian; and people without health insurance.[53] To ensure equitable use of telehealth services, considerations for focused education, training, and technical support, as well as adequate mechanisms for obtaining funding, reimbursement, or insurance coverage, are needed to deliver culturally competent care.

Legal Considerations for Nurses

It is essential for nurses to be aware of the legal and regulatory implications of telehealth with evolving changes in nursing practice and the rise of telecommunication services. Licensing, credentialing, and interstate compact agreement statutes are particularly important. Certification in specialty areas may also be recommended or required by employers.

Telehealth nurses work across state lines to virtually meet where persons seeking care and their providers are located. The mutual recognition model of licensure was proposed by the National Council of State Boards of Nursing in 1998 for each state to adopt an interstate compact that establishes legal authority for nurses to practice at both the person's and provider's locations.[54] Therefore, the Nurse Licensure Compact (NLC) was enacted into legislation to allow nurses a multistate license to practice. A nurse licensed in one compact-member state is permitted to practice in another compact-member state. Nurses who are granted multistate licensure privileges must continue to follow the laws and regulations of each state in which they practice. In 2021, 39 jurisdictions recognize multistate licensing and have enacted the NLC legislation. This legislation has made telehealth nursing more feasible. The National Telehealth Policy Resource Center as well as the Nurse Practice Act hold state-specific information on laws, regulations, reimbursement policies, and pending legislation.[55]

In terms of patient privacy and confidentiality, nurses have an important role in keeping protected health information safe and secure by preventing unauthorized access to medical records. Telehealth nurses must meet the requirements of HIPAA as well as individual state privacy laws, organizational or institutional policies, and ethical standards. The use of telecommunication technology, including mHealth applications and RPM devices, will also need to consider cybersecurity protection from data breaches or data theft. Electronic systems that transmit or store patient information electronically, such as audio–video recordings, files, or images, must be monitored by expert technicians in security measures. It is important to collaborate with developers of information technology systems that ensure privacy and security of health information, while also ensuring ease of use and proper information-sharing capabilities.

Case Study: Advance Care Planning, Symptom Management, and Care Coordination in a Telephonic Palliative Care Program

Selma Norwood is a 68-year-old woman who was enrolled in a nurse-led telephonic palliative care program affiliated with a local hospice agency after a brief hospitalization. She did not meet criteria for home health services from a certified home health aide but was identified as a candidate for the palliative care program by a clinical hospital discharge coordinator with a comprehensive knowledge of regional palliative care resources who believed this individual would benefit from an extra layer of support. She met program criteria for enrollment with a qualifying diagnosis of pulmonary arterial hypertension (PAH). She was oxygen-dependent and had been optimized on medical therapy, with a continuous subcutaneous home infusion of treprostinil for the last 9 months.

During the first scheduled call with her certified hospice and palliative care nurse, a complete telephonic assessment was performed across all eight of the palliative care domains. Despite having a New York Heart Association Class III functional level (no dyspnea at rest but severe dyspnea and fatigue with minimal activity), Selma reported that her most troubling symptom was undertreated chronic back pain related to a history of spinal surgery after a car accident in her mid-40s. She told the story of being treated to her satisfaction at a local private pain clinic until they considered her "too medically complex" due to her PAH. The pain clinic continued to prescribe a low dose of a short-acting opioid and had no suggestions for the patient about where to go to receive adequate treatment for her back pain. Selma spoke of growing feelings of hopelessness and despair because "I can't do what I want to do when I want to do it. I sit here all day and try not to move so I don't have back pain!" Further conversation revealed that while she felt loved and supported by her husband and children, she desperately missed attending Sunday services, prayer meetings, and Bible study groups at her local church, all of which had recently resumed in-person services after a year of meetings over Zoom during the pandemic shutdown.

During the first call, the registered nurse (RN) did a review of Selma's medications, comparing it to the After Visit Summary faxed to the agency with the referral. Selma demonstrated a good understanding of her medication regimen, and as she was focused on pain relief, the RN reviewed nonpharmacological pain relief strategies and let Selma know she would work with her medical team to achieve a level of pain relief which would allow her to improve the current quality of her life. During discussion of advance directives, Selma disclosed that she fully understood the seriousness of her illness and knew that "things will only get worse with my breathing, and there aren't any more treatments that will make a difference." She expressed a fear of dying in the intensive care unit, where she had to stay each time she went to the hospital due to her continuous infusion of vasoactive medication. She spoke at length of sleepless nights alone watching staff run from room to room responding to code alarms during the critical period of the COVID pandemic and knowing by the mood on the unit that many of the patients were never going home. Her husband was her designated surrogate; and she knew he would not "keep me going on machines," but she did not know how she might achieve her goal of dying in the "peace and quiet of my own home." The RN provided education on the Medical Orders for Life-Sustaining Treatment (MOLST) form, and Selma expressed surprise that she could make decisions about the end of her life that would be honored whether she was at home or in the hospital. At the conclusion of the call, both parties agreed to weekly calls to prioritize pain relief and the completion of advance directives.

Following the call, the RN completed a personalized care plan for Selma and placed calls to both her primary care provider (PCP) and the pain clinic. A detailed message with a request for a call back was left for the PCP, but the pain clinic staff said they could not disclose any information or engage in any conversation about the person without a physical consent for release of information signed by the individual. At the end of her shift, the RN received a call back from the PCP. He expressed reluctance to take over management of chronic pain, suggesting that the person's PAH team reach out to pain management to discuss her treatment. He was also unaware that Selma had strong feelings about avoiding life-sustaining treatments and medicalized death, suggesting "We aren't anywhere near that point. Why does she need a MOLST?" The following morning the RN placed a call to the PAH team and left a detailed message requesting a call back. After 24 hours without a response, the RN followed agency protocol and sent a HIPAA-compliant encrypted email to the members of that team detailing the nature of her role, her recent conversations with Selma and her PCP, and the inability to get background from the pain clinic in the absence of a physical consent form that would be burdensome to obtain and would delay care.

Unable to make meaningful progress with Selma's providers, the RN scheduled a meeting with the telephonic program's interdisciplinary team to discuss Selma's case and explore Selma's disease process, prognosis, goals, and wishes. It was agreed that if there was no action from her PCP or specialists, then the telephonic team would initiate referral to her health system's outpatient palliative care clinic for symptom management and completion of the MOLST form.

Outcome: Selma was referred to an outpatient palliative care clinic due to her complex needs. Her visits were conducted via video to reduce the burden of travel. A comprehensive pain management plan was implemented, and the telehealth RN continued with frequent calls to Selma for pain assessment and education. With her pain under control, Selma found that she was able to ambulate further distances without experiencing disabling dyspnea. She was monitored closely by staff at the palliative care clinic via RPM installed in her home, which transmitted a set of vitals and answers to a symptom questionnaire to them daily. Her availability for calls with the palliative telehealth RN was reduced as she achieved her goal of a more active engagement in her community. A mutual agreement was reached to conclude the episode of telephonic support during a call when Selma announced she felt well enough to participate in an upcoming multi-day women's conference at a nearby spiritual retreat center. She remained connected to her health system's palliative care team, and a little over a year later they helped her to achieve her end-of-life goal of dying at home.

Conclusion

The widespread adoption of telehealth technologies to deliver nonemergent healthcare during the COVID-19 pandemic placed a spotlight on the ability of nurses to operate at the top of their license as an essential member of the public health effort to decompress acute care settings and support people living with serious illness across the continuum of care. It continues to be demonstrated that nurses have the ability to deliver safe, effective, and affordable patient-centered care through telehealth services. Universal acceptance of telehealth nursing as a valid and cost-effective mode of healthcare delivery guarantees that nurses will continue to develop and facilitate the delivery of equitable healthcare. Competent palliative telehealth nurses are self-directed and proactive with strong assessment and communication skills to care for persons with life-threatening illness. It is essential that we educate all existing and future members of the nursing profession to deliver culturally competent, patient-centered care through existing and emerging palliative telehealth modalities.

REFERENCES

1. Genes N. Alexander Graham Bell and the Birth of Telemedicine. Telemedicine. 2017. Accessed October 1, 2022. http://www.telemedmag.com/article/alexander-graham-bell-and-the-birth-of-telemedicine.
2. Rutledge CM, Gustin T. Preparing nurses for roles in telehealth: now is the time! *Online J Issues Nurs*. 2021;26(1):3. https://doi.org/10.3912/OJIN.Vol26No01Man03.
3. Institute of Medicine. Telemedicine: A Guide to Assessing Telecommunications for Health Care. Washington, DC: National Academy Press; 1996. Accessed August 2, 2022. https://nap.nationalacademies.org/catalog/5296/telemedicine-a-guide-to-assessing-telecommunications-for-health-care
4. National Academy of Sciences, Institute of Medicine. *The Future of Nursing: Leading Change, Advancing Health*. National Academies Press; 2011. Accessed August 2, 2022. https://nap.nationalacademies.org/catalog/12956/the-future-of-nursing-leading-change-advancing-health
5. Centers for Medicare & Medicaid Services. President Trump Expands Telehealth Benefits for Medicare Beneficiaries during Covid-19 Outbreak. 2020. Accessed October 1, 2022. https://www.cms.gov/newsroom/press-releases/president-trump-expands-telehealth-benefits-medicare-beneficiaries-during-covid-19-outbreak
6. Koma W, Cubanski J, Neuman T. Medicare and Telehealth: Coverage and Use during the COVID-19 Pandemic and Options for the Future. Kaiser Family Foundation. May 19, 2021. Accessed October 1, 2022. https://www.kff.org/medicare/issue-brief/medicare-and-telehealth-coverage-and-use-during-the-covid-19-pandemic-and-options-for-the-future/.
7. American Telehealth Association. Telehealth Nursing Fact Sheet: ATA Telehealth Nursing Special Interest Group. 2018. Accessed August 2, 2022. https://www.americantelemed.org/resources/telehealth-nursing-fact-sheet/.
8. Anglea T, Murray C, Cox DL, Mastal MF, Clelland S. *Scope and Standards of Practice for Professional Telehealth Nursing*. 6th ed. American Academy of Ambulatory Care Nursing; 2018.
9. National Council of State Boards of Nursing. NCSBN Position Paper on Telehealth Nursing Practice. 2014. Accessed August 2, 2022. https://www.ncsbn.org/papers/the-ncsbn-position-paper-on-telehealth-nursing-practice
10. American Nurses Association. Core Principles on Connected Health. 2019. Accessed October 1, 2022. https://www.nursingworld.org/globalassets/docs/ana/practice/ana-core-principles-on-connected-health.pdf
11. Bakitas M, Stevens M, Ahles T, et al. Project ENABLE: a palliative care demonstration project for advanced cancer patients in three settings. *J Palliat Med*. 2004;7(2):363–372. Accessed September 30, 2022. https://doi.org/10.1089/109662104773709530
12. Bakitas MA, Dionne-Odom JN, Ejem DB, et al. Effect of an early palliative care telehealth intervention vs usual care on patients with heart failure: the ENABLE CHF-PC randomized clinical trial. *JAMA Intern Med*. 2020;180(9):1203–1213. https://doi.org/10.1001/jamainternmed.2020.2861.
13. Dionne-Odom JN, Ejem DB, Wells R, et al. Effects of a telehealth early palliative care intervention for family caregivers of persons with advanced heart failure: the ENABLE CHF-PC randomized clinical trial. *JAMA Netw Open*. 2020;3(4):e202583. https://doi.org/10.1001/jamanetworkopen.2020.2583.
14. Schmucker AM, Flannery M, Cho J, Goldfeld KS, Grudzen C; EMPallA Investigators. Data from emergency medicine palliative care access (EMPallA): a randomized controlled trial comparing the effectiveness of specialty outpatient versus telephonic palliative care of older adults with advanced illness presenting to the emergency department. *BMC Emerg Med*. 2021;21(1):83. https://doi.org/10.1186/s12873-021-00478-4.
15. Tan AJ, Yamarik R, Brody AA, Chung FR, Grudzen C; EMPallA Telephonic Working Group. Development and protocol for a nurse-led telephonic palliative care program. *Nurs Outlook*. 2021;69(4):626–631. https://doi.org/10.1016/j.outlook.2020.12.011.
16. Dionne-Odom JN, Wells RD, Guastaferro K, et al. An early palliative care telehealth coaching intervention to enhance advanced cancer family caregivers' decision support skills: the CASCADE pilot factorial trial. *J Pain Symptom Manage*. 2022;63(1):11–22. https://doi.org/10.1016/j.jpainsymman.2021.07.023.
17. Fathi JT, Modin HE, Scott JD. Nurses advancing telehealth services in the era of healthcare reform. *Online J Issues Nurs*. 2017;22(2):2. https://doi.org/10.3912/OJIN.Vol22No02Man02.
18. Laranjeira C, Dixe MA, Martinho R, Rijo R, Querido A. Building bridges for "palliative care-in-place": development of a mHealth intervention for informal home care. *Front Psychol*. 2022;13:1–8. https://doi.org/10.3389/fpsyg.2022.862347.
19. Allen Watts K, Malone E, Dionne OJN, et al. Can you hear me now? Improving palliative care access through telehealth. *Res Nurs Health*. 2021;44(1):226–237. https://doi.org/10.1002/nur.22105
20. Daly B, Lauria TS, Holland JC. et al. Oncology patients' perspectives on RPM for COVID-19. *J Clin Oncol*. 2021;17(9):e1278–e1285. https://doi.org/10.1200/JCO.2021.39.15_suppl.1504.
21. Krishnaswami A, Beavers C, Dorsch MP, et al. Gerotechnology for older adults with cardiovascular disease. *J Am Coll Cardiol*. 2020;76(22):2650–2670. https://doi.org/10.1016/jacc.2020.09.606.
22. Lynch KA, Ganz DA, Saliba D, Chang DS, de Peralta SS. Improving HF care and guideline-directed medical therapy through proactive RPM-Home telehealth and pharmacy integration. *BMJ Open Qual*. 2022;11:e001901. https://doi.org/10.1136/bmjoq-2022-001901.
23. Malansinghe LP, Ramzan N, Dahal K. RPM: a comprehensive study. *J Ambient Intell Hum Comput*. 2019;10:57–76. https://doi.org/10.1007/s12652-017-0598-x.
24. Kelly JT, Campbell KL, Gong E, Scuffham P. The internet of things: impact and implications for health care delivery. *J Med Internet Res*. 2020;22(11):e20135. https://doi.org/10.2196/20135.

25. Robert NJ. The promise and perils of health internet of things (HIoT). *Online J Issues Nurs*. 2021;26(3). https://doi.org/10.3912/OJIN.Vol26No03Man01.
26. Cicirelli G, Marani R, Petitti A, Milella A, D'Orazio T. Ambient assisted living: a review of technologies, methodologies and future perspectives for healthy aging of population. *Sensors*. 2021;21(10):3549. https://doi.org/10.3390/s21103549.
27. Thomas EE, Taylor ML, Banbury A, et al. Factors influencing the effectiveness of RPM interventions: a realist review. *BMJ Open*. 2021;11:e051844. https://doi.org/10.1136/bmjopen-2021-051844.
28. Bonsignore L, Bloom N, Steinhauser K, et al. Evaluating the feasibility and acceptability of a telehealth program in a rural PC population: TapCloud for PC. *J Pain Symptom Manage*. 2018;56(1):7–14. https://doi.org/10.1016/j.painsymman.2018.03.013.
29. Sensmeier J. Managing health with remote patient monitoring. *Nurs Manage*. 2021;52(11):13–17. doi:10.1097/01.NUMA.0000795604.69169.51
30. US Food & Drug Administration. Home Health and Consumer Devices. August 25, 2021. Accessed October 1, 2022. https://www.fda.gov/medical-devices/products-and-medical-procedures/home-health-and-consumer-devices.
31. Center for Medicare & Medicaid Services. Final Policy, Payment, and Quality Provisions: Changes to the Physician Fee Schedule for Calendar Year 2021. Accessed October 1, 2022. https://www.cms.gov/newsroom/fact-sheets/final-policy-payment-and-quality-provisions-changes-medicare-physician-fee-schedule-calendar-year-1.
32. Walker RC, Tong A, Howard K, Palmer SC. Patient expectations and experiences of RPM for chronic diseases: systematic review and thematic synthesis of qualitative studies. *Int J Med Inform*. 2019;124:78–85. https://doi.org/10.1016/j.ijmedinf.2019.01.013.
33. World Health Organization. Seventy-first World Health Assembly. mHealth: Use of Appropriate Digital Technologies for Public Health. March 26, 2018. https://apps.who.int/gb/ebwha/pdf_files/WHA71/A71_20-en.pdf.
34. Stockdill ML. Telehealth in palliative care: communication strategies from the COVID-19 pandemic. *Clin J Oncol Nurs*. 2021;25(1):17–22.
35. Merriam-Webster Online Dictionary. Conversation. 2023. https://www.merriam-webster.com/dictionary/conversation.
36. Reilly J, Krause K, Zande CV, Knutzen B. Implementing relationship-based care as a professional practice model: promoting nurses' understanding and confidence to apply in practice. *Creat Nurs*. 2019;25(4):e36–e43.
37. Baines D, Dulhunty A, Charlesworth S. Relationship-based care work, austerity and aged care. *Work Employ Soc*. 2022;36(1):139–155.
38. Lee HJ, Park BM, Shin MJ, Kim DY. Therapeutic communication experiences of nurses caring for patients with hematology. *Healthcare (Basel)*. 2022;10(12):2403. https://doi.org/10.3390/healthcare10122403.
39. Khoir M. Therapeutic communication skills of nurses in hospital. *Int J Nurs Health Serv*. 2020;3(2):275–283.
40. Moore PM, Rivera S, Bravo-Soto GA, Olivares C, Lawrie TA. Communication skills training for healthcare professionals working with people who have cancer. *Cochrane Database Syst Rev*. 2018;7(7):CD003751. https://doi.org/10.1002/14651858.CD003751.pub4.
41. Wanko Keutchafo EL, Kerr J, Jarvis MA. Evidence of nonverbal communication between nurses and older adults: a scoping review. *BMC Nurs*. 2020;19(1):1–3.
42. Duane JN, Blanch-Hartigan D, Sanders JJ, et al. Environmental considerations for effective telehealth encounters: a narrative review and implications for best practice. *Telemed e-Health*. 2022;28(3):309–316.
43. Briggs JK. *Telephone Triage Protocols for Nurses*. 6th ed. Wolters Kluwer; 2021.
44. Martich D. *Telehealth Nursing: Tools and Strategies for Optimal Patient Care*. Springer Publishing; 2017.
45. B.C. Centre for Palliative Care. Inter-professional Palliative Symptom Management Guidelines. 2019. Accessed January 20, 2023. https://bc-cpc.ca/wp-content/uploads/2019/03/BCPCClinicalBestPracticesInteractiveMarch2019.pdf.
46. B.C. Emergency Health Services. Virtual Palliative Assessment CPG. 2020. Accessed January 20, 2023. https://handbook.bcehs.ca/clinical-practice-guidelines/virtual-health-assessments/virtual-palliative-assessments/.
47. Cusimano MC, Sajewycz K, Nelson M, et al. Supported self-management as a model for end-of-life care in the setting of malignant bowel obstruction: a qualitative study. *Gynecol Oncol*. 2020;157(3):745–753.
48. Drillaud F, Saussac C, Keusch F, et al. The existential dimension of palliative care: the mirror effect of death on life. *Omega (Westport)*. 2022;85(4):915–935.
49. Bolton LE, Seymour J, Gardiner C. Existential suffering in the day to day lives of those living with palliative care needs arising from chronic obstructive pulmonary disease (COPD): a systematic integrative literature review. *Palliat Med*. 2022;36(4):567–580.
50. Chammas D. Seeing with my ears. *J Pain Symptom Manage*. 2022;63(5):e563–e564. https://doi.org/10.1016/j.jpainsymman.2020.09.027.
51. Adzhigirey L, Berg J, Bickford C, et al. Telehealth Nursing, Foundations for Governance: A Position Statement. American Telemedicine Association. 2019. Accessed August 1, 2022. https://www.americantelemed.org/resources/telehealth-nursing-foundations-for-governance 2019/.
52. Gustafsson SR, Eriksson I. Quality indicators in telephone nursing—an integrative review. *Nurs Open*. 2021;8(3):1301–1313. https://doi.org/10.1002/nop2.747.
53. Karimi M, Lee EC, Couture SJ, et al. *National Trends in Telehealth Use in 2021: Disparities in Utilization and Audio vs. Video Services*. Research Report No. HP-2022-04. Office of the Assistant Secretary for Planning and Evaluation, US Department of Health and Human Services; 2022. https://aspe.hhs.gov/sites/default/files/documents/4e1853c0b4885112b2994680a58af9ed/telehealth-hps-ib.pdf.
54. Brous E. Legal clinic: legal considerations in telehealth and telemedicine. *Am J Nurs*. 2016;116(9):64–67. https://doi.org/10.1097/01.NAJ.0000494700.78616.d3.
55. Center for Connected Health Policy, National Telehealth Policy Resource Center. State Laws and Reimbursement Policies. 2016. http://cchpca.org/state-laws-and-reimbursement-policies.

61

Palliative Care Nursing in the Outpatient Setting

Nancy A. Robertson and Ami K. Goodnough

Key Points

- The ambulatory setting is an important site for the provision of palliative care as the majority of care for chronic life-limiting illnesses is provided in outpatient clinics.
- Nurses and advanced practice registered nurses play a key role in the provision of palliative care in the outpatient setting.
- A building body of evidence solidly recommends the early involvement of outpatient palliative care in the setting of serious illness to promote quality of life, reduce emergency department visits and hospitalizations, promote earlier hospice enrollment, and possibly prolong life.
- Palliative care in the ambulatory setting is expanding from its initial focus on oncology to other disease settings such as cardiology, pulmonology, nephrology, neuromuscular diseases, and gerontology.
- Primary palliative care is first-line care that should be a part of the management of any serious illness. Nurses in the outpatient setting should be able to provide fundamental symptom management and coaching in basic advance care planning.
- Specialty palliative care should be available for patients with complex pain and symptom problems, high levels of psychosocial distress, or unusual disease characteristics.

Case Study

Ava is a 74-year-old woman who was diagnosed with Parkinson's disease (PD) 3 years ago after experiencing profound fatigue, weakness, and tremors. Since her diagnosis, she has been seen by a PD specialist who titrated her medication regime to include carbidopa/levodopa, rasagiline, and a rotigotine patch. Although her tremors are now less noticeable, Ava has experienced several progressive losses over time, including a weakening of her voice that prevents her from singing, chronic constipation, and a loss of the ability to engage in complex decisions. This resulted in mismanagement of her complicated medication schedule and moments of confusion while driving. Her family recently took over her medication management and convinced her to give up her driving rights. She has had many fainting and falling episodes from hypotensive episodes managed for now by intermittent doses of midodrine throughout the day. She remains independent in her activities of daily living. Ava has been distressed by her many losses of independence and is grappling with the knowledge that she will continue to lose function and ability as her PD progresses. She is easily tearful and is eager to do all she can to preserve as much quality of life (QOL) as possible.

Introduction

Most healthcare in the United States is provided in outpatient ambulatory care clinics. Patients are living longer and with greater disabilities than ever before.[1] In addition to advanced cancer, other serious illnesses that are managed in ambulatory care include end-stage heart failure, chronic lung diseases, advanced cirrhosis, kidney failure, and progressive neurological disorders such as advanced dementia and amyotrophic lateral sclerosis.

Experts agree that the well-defined benefits of inpatient palliative care improve clinical care, QOL, and healthcare utilization. However, it has only been in more recent years that evidence has shown that outpatient palliative care also provides benefits to patients and their families.[2–5] Specifically, the findings of seminal studies have shown that outpatient palliative care improves symptoms, QOL, patient and family satisfaction, and survival and decreases healthcare utilization.[3,6–9] This chapter addresses the provision of palliative care in the adult outpatient setting, with a focus on the role of nurses and advanced practice registered nurses.

Case Study

Ava's neurologist recently referred her to the outpatient palliative care clinic. The clinic is in the same building as her other healthcare providers, so she can see the palliative team on the same day she comes in for a neuro follow-up visit. In her first team visit to the clinic, the team shares that they will work with Ava to manage the many symptoms that accompany her progressive illness.

Models of Care

Outpatient palliative care clinics offer a unique and important entry for access to timely palliative care for individuals living with serious life-limiting illnesses. Variations in outpatient clinics include embedded clinics, stand-alone clinics incorporating nurse-led and telehealth care, and enhanced primary palliative care.[10] The embedded clinic (also known as "integrated" or "concurrent model") is the most prevalent style found in the outpatient setting and has been utilized extensively in the oncology setting.[10] Each outpatient model of care delivery is discussed further below.

In embedded palliative care clinics, the palliative care team takes the lead in managing certain aspects of care, such as tending to distressing symptoms, counseling for existential distress, and facilitating goals-of-care discussions, thus allowing the primary clinician to focus on the overall management of the patient's disease condition. The strength of this model lies in its advantage of specialists from both fields contributing to personalized care and working together to improve QOL in distinct yet complementary roles. The benefits of an embedded clinic are that it creates immediate access to palliative care, minimizes healthcare utilization, facilitates collaboration, and is cost-effective. However, this type of delivery creates difficulties in predicting staffing needs, and follow-ups are challenging to schedule and can cause patient/family fatigue due to additional appointments all in one day.[11] The palliative care team must foster a good relationship with the referring clinician and be flexible and willing to work within the framework of the individual clinician's style of practice.

Stand-alone palliative care clinics vary in who is overseeing the care and the availability of interdisciplinary team (IDT) members. Some clinics are staffed by physicians only or are nurse-led, while other clinics offer a full IDT including nurses, physicians, social workers, chaplains, psychologists, and physical therapists. The use of a specialist palliative care IDT in the clinic setting remains the gold standard, yet challenges to funding limit the widespread use of this model.[12] It is important to note that physician only palliative care clinics have not shown the same benefits for patients as palliative clinics where there is access to an IDT including a nurse.[13]

Nurse-led delivery of palliative care is relatively new and thus is still evolving. In this model of care, it is within the nurse's scope of practice to provide education regarding disease and treatment options, assess symptom burden and other patient-identified needs, provide self-management strategies for common bothersome and distressing symptoms, provide support for family caregivers, and discuss goals of care and advance care planning (ACP). If a full panel of IDT members exists, it may be beneficial to assign specific roles for each member to avoid confusion about responsibilities. The nurse may take lead on elements of care such as assisting the patient in identifying a surrogate decision maker, initiating and documenting ACP conversations, and assessing caregiver burden. This approach streamlines the team and meets patient needs more efficiently. This nurse-focused intervention can occur in person but has been found to be effective via telephonic interaction.[14,15] Nurses then collaborate and share their findings with the members of the IDT.

Enhanced primary palliative care includes the management of basic palliative care needs in addition to management of life-limiting and chronic illnesses, such as dementia, hypertension, and osteoarthritis. An advanced practice provider with additional training in palliative care can assess and manage the distressing symptoms that accompany serious illnesses such as pain, shortness of breath, and fatigue as well as facilitate conversations about goals of care and ACP. If symptoms become advanced or refractory, a referral can be made to a palliative care specialist. The clinician serving in an enhanced primary palliative care role must have a broad knowledge base and access to specialists for formal or informal consultation. This approach offers a great opportunity for all populations, especially those high users of healthcare resources and those medically underserved and vulnerable.[16]

Case Study

Ava is introduced to the social worker and chaplain along with the palliative nurse and physician, who help think through the coming challenges that will likely arise as the PD progresses. Energy conservation is a big concern, so the team works to cluster appointments when Ava has the most energy. The neurologist continues to direct Ava's care but welcomes consultation of the palliative team.

Benefits and Challenges Faced in the Outpatient Setting

The ambulatory setting is ideal for providing palliative care as the pace is less crisis-driven than inpatient care, and patients can benefit from long-term trusting relationships that form with the healthcare team over months and even years. These factors permit dialogues regarding ACP and the patient's goals of care to be held over a series of visits. Ultimately, the ambulatory setting provides opportunities for patients and families to work with the palliative care team to develop plans to enhance their QOL and future care.

Another benefit of the outpatient palliative care team is that they can assist with seamless transitions between inpatient and outpatient care as needed. The palliative care service is available to address ongoing supportive care needs across settings.[10,17] Early involvement of palliative care in the outpatient setting can positively support patients and their families as they navigate a serious life-limiting illness.

Many challenges faced in the outpatient setting are common to palliative care teams in any setting, such as receiving late referrals (when a patient is actively dying) and funding issues. Clinicians caring for individuals with a life-limiting illness either do not understand palliative care or are challenged to identify which of their patients are appropriate for palliative care services. Additionally, the determination of prognosis is difficult with any life-limiting illness but is particularly nuanced for those with heart failure, chronic obstructive pulmonary disease, renal failure, and dementia, making the judgment of when to refer for hospice services uncertain.[3,18] Other challenges specific to the outpatient setting include the need to coordinate outpatient palliative care visits around other provider visits to decrease appointment burden, provide seamless coordination of care, and supply 24-hour on-call services. Limited financial and workforce presence makes meeting these challenges at times insurmountable.

A unique issue faced by some outpatient palliative care programs is referrals for the management of chronic pain not related to the primary diagnosis (e.g., chronic low back pain requiring opioid therapy in a patient with a non-life-limiting illness) or ongoing management of chronic pain in a cancer survivor years after completion of therapy.[19] Most outpatient palliative care programs focus on patients with life-limiting illnesses, thus the long-term management of complex chronic pain syndromes may be beyond the parameters of what a palliative care team can offer and may decrease the availability of the palliative care team to care for patients with serious life-limiting illnesses.

Practical Details in Providing Palliative Care in the Outpatient Setting

Many questions arise when developing or expanding an outpatient palliative care program. This section will address common issues in the implementation of palliative care that includes a compilation of palliative care team members and key aspects of referrals to the palliative care outpatient clinic.

Team Members

The outpatient palliative care team may range from a single part-time nurse to a fully staffed IDT working in a wide range of outpatient settings and with clinic appointments available daily. The most common disciplines comprising the outpatient palliative care team include physicians, nurse practitioners, nurses, social workers, and chaplains.[20] In some instances, there may also be administrative support as well as access to consulting specialists such as pain management providers. Access to pain management specialists is an example of a creative way to support patients with complex chronic pain syndromes that are unrelated to their life-limiting illness.[21]

Palliative Care Referrals

Referrals to outpatient palliative care depend on multiple factors unique to the individual provider, clinic milieu, and organizational setting. Palliative care referral patterns may be influenced by many factors, and there is a continuing need for education and work to improve collaboration and appropriate referrals. Close physical proximity to the referring clinician appears to play a major role in generating consults.[10] However, each referring clinician has different evaluation criteria for who would benefit most from employing the palliative care team.[10] Triggers for referral may be based on diagnosis, symptoms, advancing age, high-risk patients, or psychosocial factors.[22,23] Palliative care nurses can play a key role in the clinic setting by building relationships to foster improvements in patient referrals. Establishing an ongoing referral base is important when building and maintaining a palliative care outpatient clinic. The embedded palliative care practice model creates the most referrals, especially if the team can see a new consult soon after, or even concurrently with, the referring clinician to assist with "bad news" discussions, complex treatment decisions, or complicated symptom management.[24] Palliative care rounds, such as the Schwartz Rounds, in which complex patient cases are discussed, are other sources to generate referrals.[25]

New Patient Referrals

When receiving a palliative care referral in the outpatient setting, it is important to ascertain several key points. Palliative care nurses often assist with coordinating new referrals to the palliative care clinic. Below are several questions that palliative care nurses can ask to better support the patient and the team.

First, *what is the purpose of the consult?* If the referral simply indicates "palliative care, evaluate and treat," it is helpful to speak with the referring team to ask what specifically triggered the request for this patient. Are there signs of psychosocial distress? Are the goals of the patient and caregiver not aligned? Is the patient experiencing ongoing severe symptoms that are negatively affecting their QOL? A few minutes spent clarifying the consult can help the palliative care team determine the appropriateness of the consult and better understand the situation.

Second, *what is the urgency of the consult?* Should the consult be scheduled immediately, or can the initial palliative care visit be held until the next outpatient clinic visit in a few weeks? An important observation is that what is deemed urgent by the referring source may not appear urgent to the palliative care team or the patient.[10] For example, the patient may exhibit high levels of distress to the team, agreeing to receive help as soon as possible, but then decline to schedule a next-day appointment with the outpatient palliative care team.

Third, *are the patient and caregiver aware of the consult?* Even if they are aware, it is surprising how many perceive the palliative care referral as abandonment and ask the scheduler "Is this how Dr. Jones is telling me he's given up on me?" Therefore, when setting up the initial visit, it is important to explain the purpose of the palliative care visit. If there appears to be any confusion or hesitation, the referring team should be notified and asked to assist with communication regarding the referral.

The wait time from referral to the first outpatient palliative care appointment is ideally less than 2 weeks, with urgent consults seen earlier if possible.[11] This may be a challenge for many programs due to provider staffing limitations. If an urgent consult cannot be accommodated as a clinic appointment, a palliative care nurse, if available, can assess the patient's needs in person or by phone and make recommendations to the primary provider until the patient can be scheduled with the outpatient palliative care provider.

Maintaining a Good Relationship with the Referring Provider

Success in providing outpatient palliative care in the collaborative model requires the maintenance of positive relationships with the referring team members. It may be helpful to think of the referring provider as the "customer" and palliative care as the service they are "buying." Close communication and a respectful approach are key, along with negotiation of "who does what" in the care of the patient.[26] It is important for the palliative care team to respect the provider's specialized skills, acknowledging that they have known the particular patient for years, even decades. In addition, it is helpful to recognize that the referring clinician, as the "captain of the ship," may feel a bit threatened when referrals to palliative care are generated by another source, especially if they perceive that symptoms and distress are well managed. Direct voice-to-voice communication with the primary team should be a priority if issues or potential issues arise, such as when the patient voices changes in goals of care. Although this coordination of care can take a significant amount of time, such coordination can help maintain positive relationships, avoid misunderstandings, assure future referrals, and optimize patient-centered care.

Case Study

The palliative care registered nurse (PCRN) is establishing rapport with Ava and learns that Ava is eager to do all she can to increase energy and maintain independence. After consulting with the team, she facilitates a referral to the nutritionist to discuss protein consumption, massage therapy to help with spasticity, and physical therapy to enhance strength and conditioning. Representatives of a few of these disciplines are members of the palliative team and discuss Ava's case during team meetings.

Components of the Palliative Care Visit

Patients living with serious illnesses have many needs impacting their QOL. Determining which issues to address at each outpatient palliative care visit depends on the needs identified by the patient and the stated purpose of the consult. Three key domains are the focus of most outpatient palliative care visits: (1) symptom management, (2) addressing psychosocial and spiritual needs, and (3) discussing future care decisions.[20] At the initial visit, the palliative care provider comes to know the patient outside the illness and builds rapport. The provider introduces the palliative care team's role, shares the referring provider's consult request, and asks the patient about the most important issues they would like addressed during the visit. Thus, the palliative care provider addresses the patient's priorities, with additional issues deferred to follow-up visits.

Length of Palliative Care Visits

The literature indicates a variety of visit lengths for outpatient palliative care, but a key consensus is that providing palliative care takes time; quality care cannot be rushed.[27] Initial visits generally range from 60 to 120 minutes and follow-up visits from 30 to 60 minutes. Disease progression can lead to an increase in the number and intensity of symptoms, news of progressive illness creates worsening distress, and goals of care, ACP, and end-of-life decision-making often are time-intensive. To reduce gaps in care, reduce redundancy, and justify productivity, it is valuable to clarify the goals of the visits and the roles of each member of the team. This is especially important since nurses are not able to bill for their time but add significant support to the entire IDT.

Case Study

In addition to Ava's quarterly appointment with the palliative clinician, the PCRN touches base with Ava every month by phone to follow up with symptoms. During these calls, the PCRN focuses on education on the timing of her complicated PD medication regimen, assesses mood, and continues to coordinate with the IDT. It is during these conversations that the PCRN also helps Ava think through possible surrogate decision makers and goals of care, which enhances the conversations held during the quarterly visits.

Clinical Measures Utilized in Outpatient Palliative Care Visits

The National Consensus Project's *Clinical Practice Guidelines for Quality Palliative Care* recommends routine screening and assessments for all domains of care.[4] A variety of instruments exist for incorporation into palliative care clinic visits. These fall into the major categories of functional scales, global symptom scales, pain scales, psychological and social measures, spiritual assessment, and QOL scales. The Edmonton Symptom Assessment System (ESAS), for example, is a global scale that assesses the severity of common symptoms experienced by patients receiving palliative care. Each symptom is rated on a 0–10 numeric rating scale. This validated instrument is commonly used in palliative care practice as it can be completed relatively quickly by patients and assessed rapidly by clinicians. Routine use of the ESAS in clinical practice has been found to aid in understanding the patient's subjective experience of symptoms as well as facilitating conversations and building rapport.[28] Many clinical practices use a standardized template for palliative care consultation and follow-up visits. It is important to be consistent while using the tools of choice so that symptoms and the impact of interventions can be measured over time. Pediatric tools are not included in this discussion, but it is important to choose tools that meet the cognitive state of the patient population.

Telephone Support and Patient Education

Providing patient support via the telephone is a key function for the palliative care nurse.[29] Telephone visits are a source of patient education, encourage adherence to the plan of care, and provide emotional support. Phone support by palliative care nurses is most often spent intervening with symptom management, assessing medication understanding, assessing clinical updates, and assuring scheduling needs.[29]

Offering patient education is an essential nursing domain and is a significant focus for palliative care services. Topics of education may include strategies to address worsening pain and distressing symptoms, tips to improve sleep, steps to reduce anxiety, or methods to prevent and manage constipation. Preparing written materials on these topics will streamline the educational process and provide a useful resource for patients and caregivers at home. Telephonic interventions can also focus on designating a surrogate decision maker, facilitating ACP conversations, and assessing caregiver burden.[14]

Case Study

At her last palliative appointment, Ava was started on a low-dose benzodiazepine to treat sleep and anxiety. Today when Ava arrived at the clinic, the PCRN performed a routine urine drug screen and discussed the controlled substances contract completed on the initiation of treatment. Ava has a complicated medication regimen with very specific times for each of her therapies. The PCRN used these tools to help educate Ava about the medications, especially timing of dosing and filling the medications on time. Ava notes that she feels supported by the team's attention and concern.

Managing Opioid Analgesics, Benzodiazepines, and Other Controlled Substances in the Outpatient Palliative Care Setting

Opioid analgesics, benzodiazepines, and stimulants are essential for pain and symptom management in palliative care. Approximately 43% of palliative care patients screened are at high risk for opioid misuse.[30] To ensure ongoing and appropriate access to these essential medications, clinicians are obligated to institute strategies to maintain patient safety and prevent misuse and diversion.

In 2020, 59 million Americans aged 12 or older used an illicit drug within the previous year, and 16 million people in the United States misused prescription psychotherapeutic drugs.[31] Patients living with serious illness are a part of this American demographic, with estimates that 1 in 5 cancer patients are at risk of substance use disorder (SUD).[32] Additionally, more than 65% of persons who abuse opioids bought, took, or were given them from family members or friends with a legitimate prescription.[31] Concerns for and actual diversion of prescribed medications have the potential to put palliative care patients at risk of experiencing uncontrolled symptoms.

When a person with a current or history of SUD develops a life-limiting illness, it is not uncommon for maladaptive coping strategies to emerge. "Chemical coping" is a term used to describe the use of opioids or other substances as a method to manage the high level of stress experienced as a result of the associated diagnosis or progression of disease.[33] Current evidence suggests that nearly 1 in 5 individuals with cancer may be classified as chemical copers.[32] These concerns further highlight the essential role the palliative care team has in conducting thorough assessments and providing essential support across the illness trajectory.

The use of universal precautions is a strategy that is highly recommended when opioids and/or other controlled substances are being prescribed.[34] Universal precautions have been found to support opioid medication adherence.[35,36] Universal precautions consider that all patients receiving an opioid or other controlled substance should be screened for risk of drug misuse, provided education on safe use, and regularly monitored. Such screening does not imply that a person with a history of SUD cannot receive opioid therapy. Rather, this is a tool to support the safe prescribing and monitoring of controlled substances and is essential to providing quality care.[34] Common components of universal precautions include assessment of risk for substance misuse, informed consent, patient–provider treatment agreements, urine drug screenings, and review of the state prescription drug monitoring program. All clinic patients should be informed of the screening and monitoring policies, to prevent patients and families from feeling threatened or profiled when universal precautions are used. While successful implementation of universal precautions in the outpatient palliative care clinic is documented,[34] further research is necessary to identify universal precaution components that are most effective.[35]

Nurses play a key role in assisting with patient screening, reviewing prescription monitoring programs, tracking analgesic use, and educating patients on the safe use, storage, and disposal of opioid analgesics. Nurses in the outpatient palliative setting are in a critical position to educate patients on the appropriateness of using opioids. This is important not only for patients who may be at risk for chemical comping and SUD but also to support the many patients and families who may be fearful of taking prescribed opioids.

Conclusion

This is an exciting time of growth in the field of outpatient palliative care. As the discipline continues to grow and mature, attention is turning toward improving the reach of clinics to increase access to patients living with serious illnesses. The imperative of reducing healthcare costs caused by frequent emergency department visits, hospital admissions, and readmissions while improving the QOL for individuals living with life-limiting illnesses can be positively impacted by outpatient palliative care.

Unfortunately, the number of trained specialist palliative care providers, including nurses, is limited. Thus, screening methods should be used to identify those individuals who are in the greatest need of receiving care from a specialized palliative care team. For patients who have a lower symptom burden, healthcare professionals are called upon to learn skills essential to provide primary palliative care in the outpatient setting.

Palliative care nurses play an essential role in the outpatient palliative care clinic. They can facilitate referrals to the clinic, between specialties, and between inpatient and outpatient palliative care services, as well as support and educate patients and their families before, during, and after clinic visits. As the outpatient palliative care clinic need grows, so will the need for well-trained palliative care nurses.

Case Study

Ava continues to follow up with the palliative team for several years. During times of slow progression, she may only come to the clinic every 6 months, with increasing frequency and telephonic interactions during the time of progression and decline. By adding the support of the team earlier in her disease course, Ava made choices to forgo life-sustaining measures near the end of life, leaning on her husband and adult daughter as decision makers.

The palliative team continued to collaborate with her neurologist and worked together to recommend home hospice when the time was appropriate. Her family noted that the palliative team helped her feel heard and respected throughout the journey, but most importantly she felt a sense of companionship as she navigated the effects of the illness.

REFERENCES

1. Grantmakers in Aging. Fast Facts: Aging in America. GIA's Comprehensive Guide to Funding in Aging. Accessed August 17, 2022. https://www.giaging.org/better-with-age
2. Ferrell BR, Paice JA, Coyne PJ, et al. Outcomes of a national training curriculum to advance generalist level palliative care. *J Palliat Med.* 2023;26(2):228–234. https://doi.org/10.1089/jpm.2022.0262.
3. Enguidanos S, Cardenas V, Wenceslao M. Health care provider barriers to patient referral to palliative care. *Am J Hosp Palliat Med.* 2021;38(9):1112–1119.
4. Ferrell BR, Twaddle ML, Melnick A, Meier DE. National Consensus Project Clinical Practice Guidelines for Quality Palliative Care guidelines, 4th edition. *J Palliat Med.* 2018;21(2):1684–1689.
5. Temel J, Greer J, El-Jawahri A, et al. Effects of early integrated palliative care in patients with lung and GI cancer: a randomized clinical trial. *J Clin Oncol.* 2017;35(8):834–841.

6. Temel JS, Greer JA, Muzikansky A, et al. Early palliative care for patients with metastatic non–small-cell lung cancer. *N Engl J Med.* 2010;363(8):733–742. https://doi.org/10.1056/NEJMoa1000678.
7. Hoerger M, Wayser GR, Schwing G, Suzuki A, Perry LM. Impact of interdisciplinary outpatient specialty palliative care on survival and quality of life in adults with advanced cancer: a meta-analysis of randomized controlled trials. *Ann Behav Med.* 2019;53(7):674–685. https://doi.org/10.1093/abm/kay077.
8. Bakitas M, Dionne-Odom JN, Pamboukian SV, et al. Engaging patients and families to create a feasible clinical trial integrating palliative and heart failure care: results of the ENABLE CHF-PC pilot clinical trial. *BMC Palliat Care.* 2017;16(1):45. https://doi.org/10.1186/s12904-017-0226-8.
9. Ora L, Mannix J, Morgan L, Wilkes L. Nurse-led integration of palliative care for chronic obstructive pulmonary disease: an integrative literature review. *J Clin Nurs.* 2019;28(21–22):3725–3733. https://doi.org/10.1111/jocn.15001.
10. Hui D, Bruera E. Models of palliative care delivery for patients with cancer. *J Clin Oncol.* 2020;38(9):852–865. https://doi.org/10.1200/JCO.18.02123.
11. Hui D, Hannon B, Zimmermann C, Bruera E. Improving patient and caregiver outcomes in oncology: team-based, timely, and targeted palliative care. *CA Cancer J Clin.* 2018;68(5):356–376. https://doi.org/10.3322/caac.21490.
12. Hui D. Palliative cancer care in the outpatient setting: which model works best? *Curr Treat Options Oncol.* 2019;20(2):1–13.
13. Scarpi E, Dall Agata M, Zagonel V, et al. Systematic vs. on-demand early palliative care in gastric cancer patients: a randomized clinical trial assessing patient and healthcare service outcomes. *Support Care Cancer.* 2019;27(7):2425–2434.
14. Tan AJ, Yamarik R, Brody AA, Chung FR, Grudzen C. Development and protocol for a nurse-led telephonic palliative care program. *Nurs Outlook.* 2021;69(4):626–631. https://doi.org/10.1016/j.outlook.2020.12.011.
15. Lindell KO, Klein SJ, Veatch MS, et al. Nurse-led palliative care clinical trial improves knowledge and preparedness in caregivers of patients with idiopathic pulmonary fibrosis. *Ann Am Thorac Soc.* 2021;18(11):1811–1821. https://doi.org/10.1513/AnnalsATS.202012-1494OC.
16. Knox Rice T, Xuan L, Wadsworth H, Halm E, Rhodes R. Examining the association between healthcare utilization and clinical characteristics among cancer patients in a safety net health system. *J Palliat Med.* 2019;22(1):80–83. https://doi.org/10.1089/jpm.2018.0202.
17. Rabow MW, Dahlin C, Calton B, Bischoff K, Ritchie C. New frontiers in outpatient palliative care for patients with cancer. *Cancer Control.* 2015;22(4):465–474. https://doi.org/10.1177/107327481502200412.
18. Hui D. Prognostication of survival in patients with advanced cancer: predicting the unpredictable? *Cancer Control.* 2015;22(4):489–497. https://doi.org/10.1177/107327481502200415.
19. Merlin JS, Young SR, Arnold R, et al. Managing opioids, including misuse and addiction, in patients with serious illness in ambulatory palliative care: a qualitative study. *Am J Hosp Palliat Med.* 2020;37(7):507–513. https://doi.org/10.1177/1049909119890556.
20. Rabow M, Parrish M, Kinderman A. Staffing in California public hospital palliative care clinics: a report from the California Health Care Foundation palliative care in public hospitals learning community. *J Palliat Med.* 2021;24(7):1045–1050. https://doi.org/10.1089/jpm.2020.0562.
21. Finlay E, Newport K, Sivendran S, Kilpatrick L, Owens M, Buss M. Models of outpatient palliative care clinics for patients with cancer. *J Oncol Pract.* 2019;15(4):187–193. https://doi.org/10.1200/JOP.18.00634.
22. Hui D, Anderson L, Tang M, Park M, Liu D, Bruera E. Examination of referral criteria for outpatient palliative care among patients with advanced cancer. *Support Care Cancer.* 2020;28(1):295–301. https://doi.org/10.1007/s00520-019-04811-3.
23. Patel B, Secheresiu P, Shah M, et al. Trends and predictors of palliative care referrals in patients with acute heart failure. *Am J Hosp Palliat Med.* 2019;36(2):147–153. https://doi.org/10.1177/1049909118796195.
24. Hui D, Heung Y, Bruera E. Timely palliative care: personalizing the process of referral. *Cancers.* 2022;14(4):1047. https://doi.org/10.3390/cancers14041047.
25. The Schwartz Center for Compassionate Healthcare. Schwartz Rounds. Accessed September 13, 2022. https://www.theschwartzcenter.org/programs/schwartz-rounds/
26. Salins N, Ghoshal A, Hughes S, Preston N. How views of oncologists and haematologists impacts palliative care referral: a systematic review. *BMC Palliat Care.* 2020;19(1):175.
27. Zimmermann C, Ryan S, Hannon B, et al. Team-based outpatient early palliative care: a complex cancer intervention. *BMJ Support Palliat Care.* 2024;14:e700–e709. https://doi.org/10.1136/bmjspcare-2019-001903.
28. Barbera L, Sutradhar R, Seow H, et al. The impact of routine Edmonton Symptom Assessment System (ESAS) use on overall survival in cancer patients: results of a population-based retrospective matched cohort analysis. *Cancer Med.* 2020;9(19):7107–7115. https://doi.org/10.1002/cam4.3374.
29. Valenti V, Rossi R, Scarpi E, et al. Nurse-led telephone follow-up for early palliative care patients with advanced cancer. *J Clin Nurs.* 2023;32(11–12):2846–2853. https://doi.org/10.1111/jocn.16403.
30. Barclay JS, Owens JE, Blackhall LJ. Screening for substance abuse risk in cancer patients using the Opioid Risk Tool and urine drug screen. *Support Care Cancer.* 2014;22(7):1883–1888. https://doi.org/10.1007/s00520-014-2167-6.
31. Richesson D, Hoenig J. *Key Substance Use and Mental Health Indicators in the United States: Results from the 2020 National Survey on Drug Use and Health.* Substance Abuse and Mental Health Services Administration; 2021. Accessed September 14, 2022. https://www.samhsa.gov/data/sites/default/files/reports/rpt35319/2020NSDUHFFR1PDFW102121.pdf.
32. Carmichael AN, Morgan L, Del Fabbro E. Identifying and assessing the risk of opioid abuse in patients with cancer: an integrative review. *Subst Abuse Rehabil.* 2016;2016:71–79. https://doi.org/10.2147/SAR.S85409.
33. Del Fabbro E. Assessment and management of chemical coping in patients with cancer. *J Clin Oncol.* 2014;32(16):1734–1738. https://doi.org/10.1200/JCO.2013.52.5170.
34. Broglio K, Doering A, Bassett E, et al. Universal precautions for opioid prescribing in ambulatory palliative care (FR441D). *J Pain Symptom Manage.* 2018;55(2):617–618. https://doi.org/10.1016/j.jpainsymman.2017.12.125.
35. Paice JA. Cancer pain management and the opioid crisis in America: how to preserve hard-earned gains in improving the quality of cancer pain management. *Cancer.* 2018;124(12):2491–2497. https://doi.org/10.1002/cncr.31303.
36. Bruera E, Paice JA. Cancer pain management: safe and effective use of opioids. *Am Soc Clin Oncol Educ Book.* 2015;35(1):e593–e599. https://doi.org/10.14694/EdBook_AM.2015.35.e593.

62

Long-Term Care

Melissa McClean and Joan G. Carpenter

Key Points

- Many older adults residing in nursing homes will live their final days in this setting.
- While the number of hospice patients living in nursing homes has increased dramatically over the past decade, comprehensive palliative care models have not been widely adopted or tested in nursing homes.
- Hospice and palliative care nurses play critical roles in collaborating with nursing home staff to enhance end-of-life care and outcomes for older adults.

Introduction

The US population is aging at an alarming rate.[1] Adults aged 65 years and older experience a myriad of health changes including an increased incidence of disease and chronic illness, alterations in functional mobility, and dependence on other individuals for care. For much of the last century, receiving care in a nursing home (NH) was standard for older adults and others without family and community support. However, care quality provided in NHs has often been questioned due to safety concerns and inadequate staffing. One suggestion to improve the care provided in these settings, endorsed by both policymakers and healthcare advocates, is incorporating the provision of palliative care.[2] The National Consensus Project for Quality Palliative Care defines palliative care as "... an interdisciplinary care delivery system designed to anticipate, prevent, and manage physical, psychological, social, and spiritual suffering to optimize quality of life (QOL) for patients, their families and caregivers."[3(pii)] As many as 1.3 million older Americans are living and dying in NHs and other long-term care (LTC) settings, and a solution for improving care at the end of life (EOL) is a high priority.[4–6]

LTC Delivery Settings

According to a 2022 analysis conducted by the Kaiser Family Foundation, there are approximately 15,000 certified nursing facilities.[7] These healthcare settings operate as nonprofit, for-profit, or government facilities; and sources of payment include private pay, Medicare (traditional and Advantage plans), and Medicaid. Medicare pays for most short-term skilled nursing care, while private pay and Medicaid covers most long-term NH care. Government facilities such as Federal Veterans Affairs Community Living Centers and State Veterans Homes are owned, operated, and managed by federal and state governments.[8]

LTC

"LTC" refers to a continuum of services and supports the health, personal care, and social service needs for residents experiencing cognitive, physical, or functional impairment. LTC settings can include NHs, assisted living facilities (ALFs), residential care communities, group homes, private homes, and adult day service centers. About two-thirds of people receive LTC services in NHs, though occupancy rates are decreasing.[4,9]

Non-NH Residential LTC Settings

ALFs are residential settings that house individuals who need help coordinating day-to-day healthcare activities and supportive services but do not need 24-hour skilled nursing care. Services include meal planning and preparation, assistance with activities of daily living (ADLs), medication administration and monitoring, and recreational activities.[9,10] State governments certify and regulate ALFs, and there is much variation among states regarding regulations, definitions, and Medicaid support. Residents and/or their families pay most expenses as there is relatively little state or federal government support for ALFs.[11] After residing in assisted living for about 2 years, 60% of residents will move to a nursing facility for a higher level of care.[9] Increasingly, ALFs are becoming a setting of EOL care, and residents in ALF settings often report that they expect to die in this setting. Additionally, some staff in ALF settings report they are unprepared to initiate EOL discussions.[12]

Continuing care retirement communities (CCRCs) are for-profit or not-for-profit organizations that offer a full range of services including independent living, assisted living, and NH care. CCRCs provide different levels of service in one location with a stepwise approach. For example, residents who experience physical or cognitive decline can receive additional services such as assistance with medications and personal care. For short-term skilled care or longer-term nursing care, a resident can move to the CCRC's NH. Most costs are paid out of pocket, and many facilities require that residents have Medicare coverage for skilled nursing care when needed.

Group homes, also called "adult family homes," "boarding homes," "personal care homes," and other names, are small dwellings where residents with similar needs live and receive help with daily care. A notable difference is that residents in group homes do not require 24-hour skilled nursing care. One model of smaller-scale group homes gaining more recent attention is the Green House model. There are currently 300 Green House NHs operating in 32 states across the country.[13] Group homes typically house 8–12 residents in private rooms and therefore care can be individualized with a focus on increasing the quality of care and the residents' QOL. A study conducted by Zimmerman et al. identified that the benefits of these small NHs include lower infection rates and infection-related mortality than traditional NHs with >50 beds.[13]

Skilled Nursing Care

NHs that provide skilled care 24 hours/day are often referred to as "skilled nursing facilities" (SNFs). SNFs can be stand-alone facilities, part of an acute care hospital, or facilities within a larger campus. The purpose of an SNF is to provide a place for residents to receive intensive medical and nursing care such as intravenous fluids, dressing changes, enteral feeding, and/or rehabilitation for a period of days to several weeks with a goal of returning to a more independent level of activity. Following rehabilitation, residents are discharged home or admitted to another care setting for LTC if they are unable to return home. A 2019 report from the US Department of Health and Human Services found that the average length of stay for LTC residents was 485 days, while the average length of stay for residents in an SNF was 28 days. Between 2019 and 2020, total Medicare spending on facility-based skilled nursing care increased 4.4%, and the average length of stay for residents in an SNF increased by 1.6 days.[9]

The LTC Environment

Resident Characteristics

According to the most recent data collected from 2014 to 2016, more than 85% of NH residents are aged 65 years or older, and more than 40% are 85 years or older. The age of residents has remained relatively consistent over the last 30 years; however, recent data suggests that demographics such as gender and race have shifted.[9] Female residents comprise close to 70% of the total NH population, down from 72% in 1985. Additionally, 21% of total NH residents are Black or Hispanic, up from 7.8% in 1985, indicating an increase in residents with racial and ethnic diversity.[9]

Beyond age, gender, and race, residents in NHs are differentiated by physical and cognitive function. Functional decline, exhibited when residents require assistance with ADLs, impacts more NH residents now than compared to 1985.[14] A resident's cognitive function often correlates with physical decline and can range from a mild to severe impairment.[4] Diagnoses such as Alzheimer's disease and related dementias represent the most prevalent chronic conditions in NHs and impact close to half of residents in the LTC setting.[9]

Lastly, residents diagnosed with psychiatric illnesses have increased over the last 30 years, with depression occurring in over 40% of facility-dwelling individuals.[9,14] The prevalence of schizophrenia has increased in the NH population, as has the use of medications to manage psychiatric illnesses including antipsychotics, antidepressants, and anxiolytics.[14] The use of these medications can be associated with adverse events such as falls, which occur in nearly 20% of long-stay residents.[9] Taken collectively, NH residents represent a vulnerable population in which individualized, patient-centered care can benefit.

Interdisciplinary Care Team

Many NH communities employ an interdisciplinary approach for the care of their residents to enhance the likelihood residents receive high-quality resident- and family-centered care. While the interdisciplinary team (IDT) often varies according to setting and the care delivery model, it generally consists of staff in medical, nursing, and ancillary support including physical, occupational, and recreational therapy, and administrative roles. Dietary workers, environmental services personnel, and beauty shop employees also play important roles because they are part of the residents' home.

Medical and nursing staff provide most of the direct care to residents. Medical staff include physicians, nurse practitioners (NPs), and physician assistants (PAs). Though a shortage of primary care physicians exists, research demonstrates that greater NP/PA presence in NHs is associated with better NH care quality.[15,16] Licensed nursing staff, including registered nurses and licensed practical/vocational nurses, are responsible for administering medications, delivering treatments, assessing and managing physical and psychosocial problems, and communicating with primary care providers. Nursing assistants, or direct care workers, represent more than one-third of the staff in NHs and aid with activities such as bathing, dressing, grooming, transferring, and toileting.

Care Considerations

NH routines, regulations, and restrictions result in an environment that is structured according to staff schedules and can impact a resident's autonomous decision-making. Allowing residents choices, especially in directing their own care, is important. Nurses need to advocate for residents' autonomy.

One common and sometimes difficult ethical issue facing residents, families, and IDTs is the decision to provide medically administered nutrition or tube feeding. Not surprisingly, societal and cultural practices may influence a family care partner's decision to continue to feed residents when they are no longer able to safely receive oral nutrition. However, the use of feeding tubes to provide medically administered nutrition has shown no difference in survival and does not improve QOL, prevent aspiration, or promote the healing of pressure ulcers in individuals with end-stage dementia.[17,18]

NH staff can assist families by explaining that it is normal to lose appetite or develop feeding difficulties at the end of life. Encouraging a resident to eat against their will may create more burden than benefit and potentially cause the resident undue distress and discomfort. Nursing staff and family care partners may offer "comfort feeding" with small amounts of favorite foods and drinks. The goal of comfort feeding is to provide the most satisfying type of food during careful handfeeding. Handfeeding offers human interaction and therapeutic touch. Resources on the Choosing Wisely website (http://www.choosingwisely.org/patient-resources/feeding-tubes-for-people-with-alzheimers/) can help guide discussions with family members about feeding tubes and other treatments when dysphagia occurs.[19]

Palliative Care Delivery in NHs

NH residents with access to palliative care demonstrate improved health outcomes including lower rates of hospitalization, reduced burdensome treatments at EOL including intravenous fluids and tube feedings, and more adequate pain management for symptoms of serious illness.[2,6,20] Despite the benefits, creating a culture with a palliative care philosophy and approach in NHs is often difficult. These difficulties include a lack of general understanding of palliative care, unclear consensus on EOL quality measures applicable to the NH setting, and inadequately developed models to guide care providers.[2] Given the challenges, the delivery of high-quality, person-centered palliative care in NHs is possible and reasonable. The following sections will discuss the various models of palliative care delivery, challenges for incorporating palliative care philosophy, and facilitators for improving care for NH residents at EOL.

Models to Deliver Palliative Care in NHs

There are several approaches to delivering palliative care in NHs: hospice–NH partnerships, external palliative care consultation teams, and in-house teams and specialized palliative care units.[6] While hospice care has been associated with better EOL outcomes for NH residents who receive services compared to those who do not,[21,22] there is limited evidence regarding specialized palliative care interventions in enhancing resident and family outcomes.[23]

Hospice Care in NHs

Hospice care is the most common and well-established program for delivering palliative care in US NHs.[2,5] The Medicare Hospice Benefit (MHB) was extended to NHs in 1989, and by 2004, 78% of NHs reported having at least one contract with a hospice agency.[4] In 2013, the Centers for Medicare & Medicaid published requirements for NHs when providing hospice services to residents through a contracted entity. One important regulation requires NHs that do not have a contract with a hospice agency to either (1) arrange for hospice services when appropriate or (2) assist with the resident's transfer to a facility that offers hospice if a resident chooses to use the MHB.[24]

The MHB pays for the hospice agency to oversee the plan of care and provide all medical supplies, IDT visits, and medications related to the terminal condition. The facility continues to deliver 24-hour nursing care for the resident. The MHB does not pay for room and board or for care focused on rehabilitation; as a result, hospice generally serves only LTC residents and not those receiving care under the Medicare SNF benefit unless the hospice terminal condition and SNF diagnosis are unrelated.[4,21,22]

The use of hospice in NHs is associated with improved pain management, fewer hospitalizations, better psychosocial support, and lower healthcare costs for NH residents at EOL.[4] The challenge for hospice agencies, facilities, and providers is that many NH residents have a life-limiting illness with an uncertain trajectory, making it difficult to decide when the illness is "terminal" according to existing guidelines.[25,26] Hospices are required to discharge patients who no longer meet the MHB enrollment guidelines because either they have outlived their 6-month life expectancy or their health unexpectedly improves. This raises serious concerns about the mismatch between the MHB guidelines and the illness trajectories of NH residents. Another challenge with hospice care occurs if there is poor communication or inadequate care coordination between NH and hospice staff.[4] Each must share a resident's plan of care; this can create confusion or misunderstandings over who manages what parts of the resident's care. The result is a potential for gaps or overlaps in care delivery. Bereaved family members report concerns about NH and hospice staff collaboration and communication, including delegation of patients' care tasks (e.g., who is responsible for what care) and information coordination (e.g., timely updates and sharing information).[27]

External Consultation Teams

An increasingly common and practical option for NH palliative care is external palliative care consultation teams, who provide specialized services in NHs and make recommendations for the residents' care. A resident who receives an NH palliative care consultation is more likely to experience a significant reduction in emergency room visits and hospitalizations, as well as fewer depressive symptoms.[28] Consultation teams often are an extension of a hospice agency's services, an existing hospital-based palliative care team, or independent practitioners. Depending on the team and resources, consultations focus on symptom management, advance care planning, or assisting with prognostication and/or hospice entry. Need for a consult is typically identified by clinical staff and/or leadership, then formally requested by the primary care provider. The consultant bills for services under Medicare Part B, and thus the costs for these services are not incurred by the NH. One critical barrier is the lack of specialty palliative care consultants in NHs. In recent years, and specifically during the COVID-19 pandemic, telehealth has grown as a care delivery modality that increases access to specialty care in NHs—including palliative care.[29]

The outcomes of external palliative care consultation depend on several factors. First, the consulting clinician needs to understand the NH environment and have knowledge of interventions that can and cannot be carried out. For example, the ability to administer and titrate intravenous opioids may be limited. Second, implementing recommendations depends on the NH primary care provider being made aware of the consultant's clinical impression and their willingness to accept recommendations. Research has shown that miscommunication between hospital-based palliative care teams and NH providers and staff often results in a failure to implement recommendations.[30] Third, each NH has its unique culture and characteristics, and facility staff may feel EOL care is at odds with the philosophy of a restorative and rehabilitative model of care.[31]

Integrated Palliative Care

Some facilities report that they provide internal palliative care services and train their staff in palliative care knowledge, practice, and skills. In 2016, one-third of NHs reported palliative care interdisciplinary rounds, 50% had instituted comfort-care policies, and 60% had instituted policies for palliative care. Incorporating palliative care into daily routines requires a commitment to person-centered care and improving EOL care. NHs that report higher palliative care knowledge are associated with a lower likelihood of residents being exposed to burdensome treatments and transitions such as artificial feeding tubes and emergency department visits.[32]

A major hindrance to developing internal NH palliative care services is the lack of funding and competing priorities. Baseline findings from a study published in 2017 entitled *Improving Palliative Care through Teamwork* (IMPACTT) suggests that the focus on SNF reimbursement and skilled care inhibits allocation of resources to facility-based palliative care.[33] Another challenge to integrated palliative care is deciphering the palliative care practices that are practical and reasonable for NHs. In a recent Delphi study, researchers used national guidelines to identify preferred practices that were both important and potentially feasible to implement in NHs, but implementation of preferred practices would require ongoing staff education and support.[34] Additional research is needed to verify the usefulness of the findings because guidelines and recommendations, in and of themselves, are unlikely to change practice.

Enhancing Palliative Care in NHs

In addition to, or instead of, comprehensive models, some NHs incorporate specific palliative care approaches. These targeted areas often include the assessment and management of physical and psychosocial aspects of care, incorporating advance care planning, and utilizing interventions to decrease hospitalizations.

Physical and Psychosocial Aspects of Care

The assessment of NH residents, namely those experiencing symptoms of advanced dementia, is difficult when residents cannot clearly communicate their needs. Given the challenges in assessment, pain and other symptoms of physical, psychosocial, and emotional distress are common in NH residents. More than one-third of NH residents have intermittent or persistent pain that often goes inadequately treated.[35,36] Additionally, research suggests that symptoms inherently present in EOL, such as psychosocial and emotional distress, are not widely documented, likely due to an inability to detect.[37] Yet due to the nature of their role, direct care staffs' assessments are integral to a resident's physical, psychosocial, and emotional care.[38] Many excellent resources are available to promote quality palliative care symptom assessment and management in NHs (Table 62.1).

Advance Care Planning

The number of NH residents with advance directives (ADs) increased dramatically since the Patient Self-Determination Act was enacted.[39] When a resident lacks medical decision-making capacity, a resident's family member (acting as an appointed healthcare agent or surrogate decision maker) will ideally use the AD as guidance when making decisions regarding medical treatments and EOL care. Most ADs for older NH residents reflect preferences for less aggressive EOL care. As a result, advance care planning and ADs are associated with decreased hospitalization rates, reduced antibiotic use, and increased likelihood of residents dying in the NH rather than the hospital.[39,40]

Although documented preferences about resuscitation are common, documented preferences about other interventions

Table 62.1 Palliative care resources for nursing home staff and other providers

Resource	Description
End-of-Life Nursing Education Consortium (ELNEC) Geriatric curriculum	Comprehensive training for nurses and nursing assistants, as well as social workers, chaplains, and others working in nursing homes. Also useful for hospice staff who serve nursing homes ELNEC website: http://www.aacnnursing.org/ELNEC; online training website: https://www.relias.com/elnec
Advancing Excellence in America's Nursing Homes	Initiative of the Advancing Excellence in Long-Term Care Collaborative; goal of the campaign is to ensure quality of care and quality of life for nursing home residents. Website contains resources on palliative care topics such as advance care planning and pain assessment and management organized within a quality improvement framework: https://www.nhqualitycampaign.org/default.aspx
Core Curriculum for the Long-Term Care Nurse	Comprehensive curriculum in detailed outline, book format organized by the National Consensus Project domains.[77] Available from the Hospice and Palliative Nurses Association: https://www.hpna.org/HPNA_Item_Details.aspx?ItemNo=978-1-934654-30-9
Palliative Care in the Long-Term Care Setting	Developed for medical directors and primary care providers in nursing homes. Contains a variety of resources to improve palliative and end-of-life care through leadership, education, best-practice guidelines, and quality assurance. Available from the American Medical Directors Association: https://paltc.org/product-store/palliative-care-long-term-care-setting
Geriatric Pain website	Website containing evidence-based materials to guide nurses and other nursing home staff in assessing and managing residents' pain, including those with dementia: https://geriatricpain.org/
Palliative Care for Advanced Dementia	Developed by the Beatitudes Campus Dementia and Aging Research Department and Hospice of the Valley in Phoenix, Arizona, this interdisciplinary program specifically targets the knowledge and skills needed to provide person-centered comfort care to persons with dementia and their families: http://www.comfortmatters.org/
Choosing Wisely website	Website includes clinician and patient/family resources to guide decision-making around several end-of-life issues for nursing home residents including: Feeding tubes: http://www.choosingwisely.org/patient-resources/feeding-tubes-for-people-with-alzheimers/ Hospitalizations: http://www.choosingwisely.org/clinician-lists/amda-aggressive-or-hospital-level-care-for-frail-elder/ Use of lipid-lowering medications: http://www.choosingwisely.org/clinician-lists/amda-lipid-lowering-medications/
Consult Geri_RN	Website with articles and videos relevant to the care of older adults, including pain assessment in nonverbal persons and avoiding restraint use: https://consultgeri.org/

such as medically administered nutrition and hydration, hospitalization, antibiotics, and comfort measures are not.[41] The use of structured advance care planning interventions that result in portable life-sustaining treatment orders (i.e., "POLST") is one way of encouraging discussion about, and documentation of, residents' and families' decisions about specific therapeutic approaches. POLST programs increase concordance between residents'/families' preferences and care received.[42]

Decision aids can increase effective communication about values and goals at the EOL. Hickman et al. demonstrated that a structured approach to discussions about care preferences that includes staff support and resource allocation increased advance care planning conversations and POLST form completion with a focus on preferences for less aggressive treatment.[43] Hanson and colleagues trained staff to use a goals-of-care intervention consisting of a video decision aid, along with a structured discussion guide for family decision makers of NH residents with dementia.[44] Decision makers reported better overall EOL communication, and residents experienced less potentially burdensome transitions.

EOL Transitions

Many NH residents are hospitalized in the final weeks of life to receive rehabilitation-focused care and potentially burdensome treatments with little benefit.[30] EOL hospitalizations are costly and often avoidable.[45] In coordination with the Centers for Medicare & Medicaid Innovations, researchers have implemented quality improvement programs designed to reduce potentially avoidable hospitalizations, decrease healthcare costs, improve medical care, and manage care transitions.[46–49]

Recent evidence highlights the impact of racial disparities in NHs. For example, Black residents diagnosed with Alzheimer's disease and related neurological conditions experience higher rates of hospitalization and potentially burdensome treatments at EOL compared to White residents.[50] Additionally, Hispanic individuals previously residing in NHs are more likely to receive mechanical ventilation in intensive care units compared to White individuals.[51] Understanding hospice utilization and the use of other palliative care interventions is one of the highest research priorities of the National Academies of Sciences, Engineering, and Medicine.[4,52] Therefore, many opportunities exist for NHs to engage more minority populations in advance care planning to limit care not concordant with expressed goals of care.

Challenges and Facilitators to Palliative Care Delivery

Challenges to Palliative Care Delivery

Regulatory structures, reimbursement policies, workforce issues, and resident characteristics hamper the delivery of palliative care services in NHs. For example, regulations tend to favor restorative rather than palliative care.[5] In addition, efforts to administer palliative care are sometimes misinterpreted by facilities and regulators, leading to citations for poor care. For example, NH surveyors often cite facilities for residents' weight loss, which could reflect inattention to nutritional needs in some residents. In many instances, however, weight loss is an inevitable result of the dying process, and aggressive interventions such as tube feeding are ineffective and inappropriate. Therefore, it is essential for IDTs to document residents' progressive conditions, discuss care goals and preferences for life-sustaining treatments, and review and update the care plan accordingly.

Reimbursement also promotes more aggressive therapy. Generally, Medicare and Medicaid pay NHs a per diem for the care they provide. Specifics of care are accounted for in the facility's case mix index, a composite score reflecting the complexity of care delivered to residents. In facilities providing more medical interventions, therapy services, and assistance with ADLs, the case mix index is higher, thereby increasing reimbursement rates to the NH. Therefore, facilities are financially incentivized to accept residents requiring "skilled" treatments. In addition, payment for a resident's room and board at the facility is generally covered under the Medicare SNF benefit for the first 20 days of care, following a qualifying hospitalization.[4] Many seriously ill residents and their family caregivers find this financial assistance advantageous because out-of-pocket spending is reduced. These policies act as incentives to NHs to provide skilled nursing services to residents, and their family caregivers to accept them even though these services may not match the residents' and families' goals of care or improve residents' QOL.[31]

In addition to regulatory and financial pressures, workforce issues are challenging. NH staff tend to lack training in palliative and EOL care and therefore have difficulty recognizing and implementing palliative treatments when needed.[22] With lack of knowledge in EOL care, staff also feel unequipped to manage multiple experiences of grief when residents die, therefore adding emotional burden to staff and increasing risk of burnout and other negative psychological impacts. As a result, staff turnover is staggeringly high. The annual turnover among nursing assistants is 78% and that of licensed practical nurses (LPNs) and registered nurses (RNs) is 53% and 56%, respectively.[14] High turnover is associated with lack of care continuity and poorer care, resulting in a workforce that is constantly changing, overwhelmed, and dissatisfied. Improving the capacity and adaptability of the NH workforce requires offering educational programs on a continual basis to keep knowledge and skills current.[22]

Finally, many residents have complex physical, psychosocial, and spiritual needs that are difficult to assess and manage because of cognitive impairment.[35,38] Severe impairment interferes with residents' ability to provide reliable self-report, thereby hindering pain and symptom assessment and management. When pain and other symptoms are identified, multiple comorbidities and polypharmacy further complicate effective treatment.[35]

Facilitators to Providing Palliative Care

Although there are hindrances, some aspects of the care provided in NHs are consistent with characteristics of palliative care. These factors include the use of federally mandated assessment tools to provide a comprehensive view of the residents' clinical and functional status, the existing team approach to care, and the partnership between care staff and residents' families. Taken together, NHs have a rich infrastructure to support the philosophy of palliative care.

The Minimum Data Set version 3.0 (MDS 3.0) is a mandated assessment tool for Medicare and Medicaid beneficiaries in NHs. Its goal is to create a comprehensive evaluation and to identify opportunities to improve clinical and functional status. The tool is completed by an RN at specified intervals using medical records, staff input, and observation in combination with a resident interview. The resident interview consists of discussions of preferences for routines and activities—including goals of care—and questions about pain, mood, and cognition.[53,54] The MDS 3.0 can be used to identify residents with serious illness who have unmet symptom management and psychosocial and spiritual support needs. Further, several researchers have used elements from the MDS 3.0 to inform a risk index for mortality or adverse outcomes (e.g., rehospitalization) that can prompt a referral for advanced care planning or hospice services.[55,56]

The existing IDT—RNs, LPNs, nursing assistants, social work, rehabilitation specialists, dietitians, and wound care specialists—support the standard interdisciplinary approach to palliative care. NHs are required to schedule quarterly IDT care planning meetings with residents, their family members and/or surrogate decision makers to discuss the comprehensive physical, emotional, mental, and social care plan for each resident. Care plan meetings provide a designated time that the IDT, resident, and/or family can review and share information; discuss values, goals, and treatment preferences; ask and answer questions; and revise the care plan to match the resident's needs.

Partnerships between care staff and a resident's family becomes increasingly important as staff gain insight into the resident's life, habits, preferences, and care needs.[57] This holistic approach is foundational to the palliative care philosophy of patient- and family-centered care. Partnership, as a concept, is viewed as a catalyst for increased staff, resident, and family satisfaction and ultimately leads to more consistency between the resident's goals and the care staff's plan of care.[57,58]

Resources for Palliative Care in NHs

Over the past several years, many professional and industry groups have developed curricula, websites, and other palliative care resources for NHs (Table 62.1). However, a recent systematic review revealed that education alone does not improve staff clinical practice and resident EOL outcomes.[59] Multifaceted programs that include education in addition to leadership support for EOL care processes and capacity-building for comprehensive palliative care delivery are more likely to be effective.

Conclusion

While NHs represent a unique short- and long-term care environment, modifications can help facilities in delivering high-quality EOL care. The NH staff should address the physical, psychological, social, and spiritual needs of all residents. Primary care clinicians need to recognize the regulations and guidelines under which facilities operate. Palliative care delivery models and targeted strategies can be integrated into NHs. The principles of palliative care should be an integral part of NH care.

Case Study

Mr. X is an 87-year-old man with congestive heart failure, a pacemaker for sick sinus syndrome, and mild dementia. He was recently hospitalized with syncope related to anemia and diagnosed with myelodysplastic syndrome. Prior to the hospitalization, he lived in an ALF and was able to care for himself. However, during the hospitalization he experienced confusion, hallucinations, and significant functional decline. Mr. X is now receiving post-acute skilled nursing care and rehabilitation in a local NH. He is not making significant progress in physical therapy, sleeps most of the day, and has a poor appetite. On multiple occasions, he has told the nursing staff he is tired and wants to be left alone. During the most recent MDS assessment, the staff noted his overall decline and worsening cognitive function and contacted the family to discuss his care. Mr. X's children are concerned that the new myelodysplastic syndrome diagnosis is causing his symptoms, and they want to him to pursue "a little bit" of chemotherapy treatment "to see if it will help."

Mr. X has many unmet needs. In this case, the nurse caring for Mr. X in the NH assessed his understanding of his illness and willingness to discuss his diagnosis and its associated symptoms. The nurse discovered that Mr. X did not seem to understand his illness and failed to recall his clinic appointments with the hematology specialist. The primary care provider was consulted to evaluate Mr. X's decision-making status and determined that Mr. X was not able to make his own medical decisions. The family was notified and asked to attend a family meeting with the nurse, primary care provider, and Mr. X. Together they discussed Mr. X's diagnosis, treatment options, current functional status and symptoms, and concurrent medical conditions. Based on Mr. X's previously expressed preferences to not pursue life-sustaining treatments, current decline in status, and fatigue, his family opted to meet with hospice and learn about services. Though the team felt Mr. X met eligibility criteria for hospice admission, Mr. X's family was not ready to initiate services and decided to continue physical and occupational therapy in the hope that his physical condition improved. After several weeks, Mr. X demonstrated little progress in rehabilitation. Mr. X's family met with the care team again and decided to pursue care goals focused on comfort. He was discharged from post-acute care and admitted to hospice care at the NH as an LTC resident. The hospice agency and NH staff worked together to develop a plan of care that focused on supporting Mr. X and his family. The NH staff clarified with the hospice agency what aspects of care each was responsible for and communicated updates weekly and more often as needed.

REFERENCES

1. US Census Bureau. 65 and Older Population Grows Rapidly as Baby Boomers Age. Accessed September 24, 2022. https://www.census.gov/newsroom/press-releases/2020/65-older population-grows.html.
2. Ersek M, Unroe KT, Carpenter JG, Cagle JG, Stephens CE, Stevenson DG. High-quality nursing home and palliative care—one and the same. *J Am Med Dir Assoc.* 2022;23(2):247–252. https://doi.org/10.1016/j.jamda.2021.11.027.
3. National Consensus Project for Quality Palliative Care. *Clinical Practice Guidelines for Quality Palliative Care.* 4th ed. Accessed October 14, 2022. https://nchpc.conferencespot.org/67968-nchpc-1.4266595/t001-1.4266873/f001-1.4266874/a001-1.4266878.
4. National Academies of Sciences, Engineering, and Medicine. *The National Imperative to Improve Nursing Home Quality: Honoring*

Our Commitment to Residents, Families, and Staff. National Academies Press; 2022.

5. Hunt LJ, Stephens CE, Smith AK. Palliative care in the nursing home—shifting paradigms. *JAMA Intern Med*. 2020;180(2):243–244. https://doi.org/10.1001/jamainternmed.2019.5359.
6. Kaasalainen S, Sussman T, McCleary L, et al. Palliative care models in long-term care: a scoping review. *Nurs Leadersh (Tor Ont)*. 2019;32(3):8–26. https://doi.org/10.12927/cjnl.2019.25975.
7. Kaiser Family Foundation. Total Number of Certified Nursing Facilities. Accessed October 16, 2022. https://www.kff.org/other/state-indicator/number-of-nursing-facilities/?currentTimeframe=0&sortModel=%7B%22colId%22:%22Location%22,%22sort%22:%22asc%22%7D.
8. US Department of Veteran Affairs. What Is a State Veterans Home? Accessed October 14, 2022. https://www.va.gov/GERIATRICS/pages/State_Veterans_Homes.asp.
9. Harris-Kojetin L, Sengupta M, Lendon J, Rome V, Valverde R, Caffrey C. *Long-Term Care Providers and Services Users in the United States, 2015–2016*. Vital and Health Statistics. Series 3(43). National Center for Health Statistics; 2019.
10. American Health Care Association. Facts & Figures. Accessed October 14, 2022. https://www.ahcancal.org/Assisted-Living/Facts-and-Figures/Pages/default.aspx.
11. Frey R, Balmer D, Boyd M, Robinson J, Gott M. Palliative care nurse specialists' reflections on a palliative care educational intervention in long-term care: an inductive content analysis. *BMC Palliat Care*. 2019;18(1):103. https://doi.org/10.1186/s12904-019-0488-4.
12. Temkin-Greener H, Mukamel DB, Ladd H, et al. Impact of nursing home palliative care teams on end-of-life outcomes: a randomized controlled trial. *Med Care*. 2018;56(1):11–18. https://doi.org/10.1097/mlr.0000000000000835.
13. Zimmerman S, Dumond-Stryker C, Tandan M, et al. Nontraditional small house nursing homes have fewer COVID-19 cases and deaths. *J Am Med Dir Assoc*. 2021;22(3):489–493. https://doi.org/10.1016/j.jamda.2021.01.069.
14. Fashaw S, Thomas K, McCreedy E, Mor V. Thirty-year trends in nursing home composition and quality since the passage of the omnibus reconciliation act. *J Am Med Dir Assoc*. 2020;21(2):233–239. https://doi.org/10.1016/j.jamda.2019.07.004.
15. Barker RO, Craig D, Spiers G, Kunonga P, Hanratty B. Who should deliver primary care in long-term care facilities to optimize resident outcomes? A systematic review. *J Am Med Dir Assoc*. 2018;19(12):1069–1079. https://doi.org/10.1016/j.jamda.2018.07.006.
16. Mileski M, Pannu U, Payne B, Sterling E, McClay R. The impact of nurse practitioners on hospitalizations and discharges from long-term nursing facilities: a systematic review. *Healthcare (Basel)*. 2020;8(2):114. https://doi.org/10.3390/healthcare8020114
17. Ijaopo EO, Ijaopo RO. Tube feeding in individuals with advanced dementia: a review of its burdens and perceived benefits. *J Aging Res*. 2019;2019:7272067. https://doi.org/10.1155/2019/7272067.
18. Schneider P, Fruchtman C, Indenbaum J, Neuman E, Wilson C, Keville T. Ethical considerations concerning use of percutaneous endoscopic gastrostomy feeding tubes in patients with advanced dementia. *Perm J*. 2021;25(3):20.302. https://doi.org/10.7812/TPP/20.302.
19. Choosing Wisely. Feeding Tubes for People with Alzheimer's. Accessed October 14, 2022. https://www.choosingwisely.org/patient-resources/feeding-tubes-for-people-with-alzheimers/.
20. Lima JC, Miller SC. Palliative care consults in U.S. nursing homes: not just for the dying. *J Palliat Med*. 2018;21(2):188–193. https://doi.org/10.1089/jpm.2017.0099.
21. Miller SC, Lima JC, Mitchell SL. Influence of hospice on nursing home residents with advanced dementia who received Medicare-skilled nursing facility care near the end of life. *J Am Geriatr Soc*. 2012;60(11):2035–2041. https://doi.org/10.1111/j.1532-5415.2012.04204.x.
22. Unroe KT, Cagle JG, Dennis ME, Lane KA, Callahan CM, Miller SC. Hospice in the nursing home: perspectives of front line nursing home staff. *J Am Med Dir Assoc*. 2014;15(12):881–884. https://doi.org/10.1016/j.jamda.2014.07.009.
23. Carpenter JG, Lam K, Ritter AZ, Ersek M. A systematic review of nursing home palliative care interventions: characteristics and outcomes. *J Am Med Dir Assoc*. 2020;21(5):583–596.e2. https://doi.org/10.1016/j.jamda.2019.11.015.
24. Centers for Medicare & Medicaid Services. Medicare and Medicaid Programs; Requirements for Long Term Care Facilities; Hospice Services. Accessed October 14, 2022. https://www.federalregister.gov/documents/2010/10/22/2010-26395/medicare-and-medicaid-programs-requirements-for-long-term-care-facilities-hospice-services.
25. Finucane AM, Stevenson B, Murray SA. Gradual physical decline characterises the illness trajectories of care home residents. *Int J Palliat Nurs*. 2017;23(9):457–461. https://doi.org/10.12968/ijpn.2017.23.9.457.
26. Tatum PE, Mills SS. Hospice and palliative care: an overview. *Med Clin North Am*. 2020;104(3):359–373. https://doi.org/10.1016/j.mcna.2020.01.001.
27. Hwang D, Teno JM, Clark M, et al. Family perceptions of quality of hospice care in the nursing home. *J Pain Symptom Manage*. 2014;48(6):1100–1107. https://doi.org/10.1016/j.jpainsymman.2014.04.003.
28. Miller SC, Lima JC, Intrator O, Martin E, Bull J, Hanson LC. Palliative care consultations in nursing homes and reductions in acute care use and potentially burdensome end-of-life transitions. *J Am Geriatr Soc*. 2016;64(11):2280–2287. https://doi.org/10.1111/jgs.14469.
29. Baxter KE, Kochar S, Williams C, Blackman C, Himmelvo J. Development of a palliative telehealth pilot to meet the needs of the nursing home population. *J Hosp Palliat Nurs*. 2021;23(5):478–483. https://doi.org/10.1097/njh.0000000000000784.
30. Carpenter JG, Berry PH, Ersek M. Nursing home care trajectories for older adults following in-hospital palliative care consultation. *Geriatr Nurs*. 2017;38(6):531–536. https://doi.org/10.1016/j.gerinurse.2017.03.016.
31. Temkin-Greener H, Lee T, Caprio T, Cai S. Rehabilitation therapy for nursing home residents at the end-of-life. *J Am Med Dir Assoc*. 2019;20(4):476–480.e1. https://doi.org/10.1016/j.jamda.2018.07.024.
32. Miller SC, Lima JC, Thompson SA. End-of-life care in nursing homes with greater versus less palliative care knowledge and practice. *J Palliat Med*. 2015;18(6):527–534. https://doi.org/10.1089/jpm.2014.0393.
33. Temkin-Greener H, Ladwig S, Ye Z, Norton SA, Mukamel DB. Improving palliative care through teamwork (IMPACTT) in nursing homes: study design and baseline findings. *Contemp Clin Trials*. 2017;56:1–8. https://doi.org/10.1016/j.cct.2017.01.011.
34. Temkin-Greener H, Ladwig S, Caprio T, et al. Developing palliative care practice guidelines and standards for nursing home-based palliative care teams: a Delphi study. *J Am Med*

Dir Assoc. 2015;16(1):86.e1–e7. https://doi.org/10.1016/j.jamda.2014.10.013.
35. Weisbrod N. Primary palliative care in dementia. *Neurotherapeutics*. 2022;19(1):143–151. https://doi.org/10.1007/s13311-021-01171-x.
36. Hunnicutt JN, Ulbricht CM, Tjia J, Lapane KL. Pain and pharmacologic pain management in long-stay nursing home residents. *Pain*. 2017;158(6):1091–1099. https://doi.org/10.1097/j.pain.0000000000000887.
37. Hermans K, Cohen J, Spruytte N, Van Audenhove C, Declercq A. Palliative care needs and symptoms of nursing home residents with and without dementia: a cross-sectional study. *Geriatr Gerontol Int*. 2017;17(10):1501–1507. https://doi.org/10.1111/ggi.12903.
38. Bolt SR, van der Steen JT, Mujezinović I, et al. Practical nursing recommendations for palliative care for people with dementia living in long-term care facilities during the COVID-19 pandemic: a rapid scoping review. *Int J Nurs Stud*. 2021;113:103781. https://doi.org/10.1016/j.ijnurstu.2020.103781.
39. Manu ER, Mody L, McNamara SE, Vitale CA. Advance directives and care received by older nursing home residents. *Am J Hosp Palliat Care*. 2017;34(2):105–110. https://doi.org/10.1177/1049909115611875
40. Martin RS, Hayes B, Gregorevic K, Lim WK. The effects of advance care planning interventions on nursing home residents: a systematic review. *J Am Med Dir Assoc*. 2016;17(4):284–293. https://doi.org/10.1016/j.jamda.2015.12.017.
41. Hickman SE, Nelson CA, Smith-Howell E, Hammes BJ. Use of the physician orders for life-sustaining treatment program for patients being discharged from the hospital to the nursing facility. *J Palliat Med*. 2014;17(1):43–49. https://doi.org/10.1089/jpm.2013.0097.
42. National POLST. Honoring the Wishes of Those with Serious Illness and Frailty. Accessed October 14, 2022. https://polst.org/.
43. Hickman SE, Unroe KT, Ersek MT, Buente B, Nazir A, Sachs GA. An interim analysis of an advance care planning intervention in the nursing home setting. *J Am Geriatr Soc*. 2016;64(11):2385–2392. https://doi.org/10.1111/jgs.14463.
44. Hanson LC, Zimmerman S, Song MK, et al. Effect of the goals of care intervention for advanced dementia: a randomized clinical trial. *JAMA Intern Med*. 2017;177(1):24–31. https://doi.org/10.1001/jamainternmed.2016.7031.
45. Xing J, Mukamel DB, Temkin-Greener H. Hospitalizations of nursing home residents in the last year of life: nursing home characteristics and variation in potentially avoidable hospitalizations. *J Am Geriatr Soc*. 2013;61(11):1900–1908. https://doi.org/10.1111/jgs.12517.
46. Ingber MJ, Feng Z, Khatutsky G, et al. Initiative to reduce avoidable hospitalizations among nursing facility residents shows promising results. *Health Aff (Millwood)*. 2017;36(3):441–450. https://doi.org/10.1377/hlthaff.2016.1310.
47. Bonner A, Tappen R, Herndon L, Ouslander J. The INTERACT institute: observations on dissemination of the INTERACT quality improvement program using certified interact trainers. *Gerontologist*. 2015;55(6):1050–1057. https://doi.org/10.1093/geront/gnu103.
48. Pathway H. Interventions to Reduce Acute Care Transfers: INTERACT 2017. Accessed October 14, 2022. http://www.pathway-interact.com/.
49. Center for Medicare & Medicaid Services. Initiative to Reduce Avoidable Hospitalizations among Nursing Facility Residents: Phase Two. Accessed October 14, 2022. https://www.cms.gov/priorities/innovation/innovation-models/rahnfr-phase-two
50. Temkin-Greener H, Yan D, Wang S, Cai S. Racial disparity in end-of-life hospitalizations among nursing home residents with dementia. *J Am Geriatr Soc*. 2021;69(7):1877–1886. https://doi.org/10.1111/jgs.17117.
51. Estrada LV, Agarwal M, Stone PW. Racial/ethnic disparities in nursing home end-of-life care: a systematic review. *J Am Med Dir Assoc*. 2021;22(2):279–290.e1. https://doi.org/10.1016/j.jamda.2020.12.005.
52. Lin P-J, Zhu Y, Olchanski N, et al. Racial and ethnic differences in hospice use and hospitalizations at end-of-life among Medicare beneficiaries with dementia. *JAMA Netw Open*. 2022;5(6):e2216260. https://doi.org/10.1001/jamanetworkopen.2022.16260.
53. Saliba D. Making the investment count: revision of the minimum data set for nursing homes, mds 3.0. *J Am Med Dir Assoc*. 2012;13(7):602.
54. Saliba D, Jones M, Streim J, Ouslander J, Berlowitz D, Buchanan J. Overview of significant changes in the minimum data set for nursing homes version 3.0. *J Am Med Dir Assoc*. 2012;13(7):595–601. https://doi.org/10.1016/j.jamda.2012.06.001.
55. Thomas KS, Ogarek JA, Teno JM, Gozalo PL, Mor V. Development and validation of the Nursing Home Minimum Data Set 3.0 Mortality Risk Score (MRS3). *J Gerontol A Biol Sci Med Sci*. 2019;74(2):219–225. https://doi.org/10.1093/gerona/gly044.
56. Burke RE, Hess E, Barón AE, Levy C, Donzé JD. Predicting potential adverse events during a skilled nursing facility stay: a skilled nursing facility prognosis score. *J Am Geriatr Soc*. 2018;66(5):930–936. https://doi.org/10.1111/jgs.15324.
57. Jang HY, Song EO, Ahn JW. Development and validation of the Scale for Staff–Family Partnership in Long-Term Care (SSFPLC). *Int J Older People Nurs*. 2021;17(2):e12426. https://doi.org/10.1111/opn.12426.
58. Carpenter J, Miller SC, Kolanowski AM, et al. Partnership to enhance resident outcomes for community living center residents with dementia: description of the protocol and preliminary findings. *J Gerontol Nurs*. 2019;45(3):21–30. https://doi.org/10.3928/00989134-20190211-03.
59. Anstey S, Powell T, Coles B, Hale R, Gould D. Education and training to enhance end-of-life care for nursing home staff: a systematic literature review. *BMJ Support Palliat Care*. 2016;6(3):353–361. https://doi.org/10.1136/bmjspcare-2015-000956.

63

Palliative Care in the Emergency Department

Rebecca Wright and Benjamin Roberts

Key Points

- Palliative care is still an evolving specialty in the emergency department (ED), requiring further research and development of tailored, interdisciplinary training and education programs and care processes.
- Research has demonstrated that safe and effective delivery of ED-based palliative care is possible, with growing numbers of tools and models to support care delivery and goals-of-care conversations.
- Community-based nurses and other healthcare professionals involved in referring patients with palliative care needs to the ED should encourage ongoing discussions and documentation of preferences and goals of care to support shared decision-making and treatment congruent with patient wishes. Once in the ED, assessments for patients with long-term, incurable conditions should also address palliative care needs, including cultural, social, spiritual, and family needs
- An ED visit can provide an opportunity to identify unmet or exacerbated palliative care needs for patients and families.

Introduction

The emergency department (ED) has not historically been associated with palliative care. The traditional model of "resuscitate, stabilize, transfer" was seemingly at odds with the holistic, in-depth approach of palliative care. This is emphasized by the use of ED visits and acute care utilization as an indicator for poor outcomes and failures in coordinated, community-based care.[1] However, despite efforts to reduce ED visits and return visits by improving provision of palliative care in community settings, a significant number of people with palliative care needs continue to visit the ED in times of crisis, viewing it as a "safety net."[2] Further complicating matters are the growing complexities of caring for an aging population with comorbidities, meaning that some ED visits may be due to underlying, complicated palliative care needs.[3]

The ED serves as the gateway for access to healthcare for many people, and there is a growing consensus that it can and should play a vital role in the provision of palliative care.[4] Despite many challenges, the ED represents a place of safety and refuge in times of crisis. People with complex and unpredictable conditions, along with those who may struggle to access healthcare due to financial challenges and inequalities in healthcare access, particularly benefit. Many nursing roles intersect with the ED and have the potential to support transitions of palliative care across settings at what often represents the most distressing times of illnesses.

This chapter presents the epidemiology of patients who use the ED with or for palliative care needs and reviews the main barriers to provision of ED-based palliative care, drawing on published examples of patient and clinician experiences. These barriers are addressed by outlining facilitators to ED-based palliative care including new models, approaches, and tools. The role of the ED within the wider healthcare context of palliative care is emphasized. To illustrate the challenges for clinicians caring for palliative care patients in the ED and how to address them, a three-part case study will be presented with practice-based discussion points.

Epidemiology: Incidence, Prevalence, Causes

Despite exploration of the incidence and nature of ED patients with palliative care needs, there remains a lack of a uniform definition of palliative care in the ED setting. This presents a challenge in tailoring and delivering care for the ED patient with palliative care needs.[5] Further exacerbating this challenge is the wide range of information generated by numerous site-specific studies regarding the demographics and characteristics of ED patients with palliative care needs, including gender, race, and disease.[6] A small body of qualitative research exploring the experiences of palliative care patients seen in the ED identified common themes triggering visits (see the section "Needs and Experiences of the Palliative Care Patient"). These included uncontrollable symptom burden and inability to cope at home[7] and inability to access or lack of access to community-based care services.[2] Lack of access to care and financial reasons were noted particularly for minority populations in the United States.[8] In some cases, patients were directed to the ED by their community providers, for example, cancer patients receiving chemotherapy in response to a spiking temperature.[2] The notion of the ED as a safety net in times of crisis was raised by patients with some relief but with the caveat that there was also no alternative.[2]

Patients admitted to the ED who then receive palliative care consultation present with a wide variety of traits and conditions. It is critical to reach consensus about these traits in order to identify palliative care needs and provide timely care.[5] This is particularly important given the increasing usage of the ED by patients with palliative care needs.[7] Complicated factors must be addressed; for example, data suggesting different conditions, such as cancer and chronic obstructive pulmonary disease (COPD), have different drivers for ED visits, different palliative care needs, and report different experiences.[2,9]

Still, studies suggest certain trends, such as a common need for symptom management and life-prolonging interventions.[7] Green et al. (2016) found that, within a large urban hospital, the leading causes of ED visits by people with palliative care needs were shortness of breath and pain. Other common complaints included falls, neurological symptoms, nausea and vomiting, fever, dehydration, diarrhea, and fatigue.[10] However, a clear distinction was made to differentiate between these presenting symptoms and the "underlying palliative conditions," such as cancer, COPD, and dementia.[10] Not all palliative care admissions are from complicated causes; in some cases, the reason for the visit is classified as a "palliative emergency"; these are instances occurring in patients with an incurable condition that will lead to death or decreased quality of life (QOL). Common palliative emergencies include uncontrolled pain, acute dyspnea, hemorrhage, hypercalcemia, acute anxiety, and acute loss of function.[11] Many of these trends are found globally, which can enable cross-cultural learning and highlights international gaps in care delivery meeting patient needs.

Drawing this information into the first of a three-part case study, Part 1 highlights the issues outlined in a common ED visit from a patient with underlying palliative care needs. The barriers and facilitators to integration of palliative care in the ED are introduced.

Case Study Part 1: A Patient in the ED

Mary is a 72-year-old Spanish-speaking wife and grandmother with a past medical history of end-stage COPD (GOLD Stage IV) complicated by several ED visits in the past year, left-sided heart failure (ejection fraction 10%–15%), Type 2 diabetes mellitus, depression, and osteoarthritis causing chronic pain to wrists, fingers, and knees, who presents to the ED from home due to 2–3 days of progressively worsening shortness of breath and lower extremity swelling. Mary lives with her husband of the same age, who helps her with basic activities of daily living but is often unable to engage in his own health maintenance due to fatigue. For several months, Mary had neither the energy nor the motivation to pursue her lifelong passion of gardening. Since her recent hospitalization, Mary receives weekly visits from a home health nurse, who assists with medical management and daily care and provides emotional support to both Mary and her husband. On days without her nurse, Mary and her husband made medication errors and did not bathe. Most days, Mary did not go outside. She has presented five times to the ED over the past year, which was an increase from three times the previous year and once the year prior.

In the ED, Mary's SpO_2 rapidly declined as she became dyspneic, tachycardic, and hypotensive. The ED providers ordered multiple large-bore intravenous placements, fluid boluses, stat arterial blood gasses, and 100% nonrebreather facemask. Mary was afraid, in tremendous pain, and confused and felt unable to speak or be spoken for: her husband had not yet arrived, and she had no advance directives (ADs) in place due to her religious belief that illness and death can be planned only by God and not by herself nor her doctors.

A chest X-ray revealed diffuse bilateral congestion and left lower lobe pleural effusion. A chest tube was inserted emergently at bedside, draining purulent fluid. Only 5 cc of local analgesia was administered subcutaneously—no systemic pain control was considered. As the team discussed bilevel positive airway pressure versus emergent intubation, her SaO_2 began to stabilize in the high 80s, her breathing became less labored, and she became calmer and more alert.

Discussion Points

Barriers to palliative care:

- Adequate care at home for frail individuals is expensive and often unavailable, leading to loss of ability to accomplish daily tasks and participate in activities of passion and enjoyment and increased depression.
- The standard ED model focuses on life-saving care, paying less attention to alleviating suffering and increasing QOL.
- Communication of medical preferences is challenging in the ED due in part to rapid stabilization efforts without clear explanation of likely sequelae, language barriers, physical and psychological symptoms, and limited use of ADs.

Ways to integrate palliative care:

- In the case study, notice the recent increase in visits to the ED in the past year. Each ED can pay careful attention to frequent visits, particularly for patients suffering from life-limiting illness, and create automatic triggers for palliative care referral and delivery for these patients.
- Every visit to the ED is an opportunity for education about ADs and advance care planning. No one near the end of life (EOL) need leave the ED for the fifth time in 1 year without a documented patient-centered care plan.

If emergency procedures such as chest tube insertion are to be carried out, the administration of sufficient systemic and local analgesia can be prioritized for the patient with palliative care needs.

Barriers and Challenges to ED Palliative Care

Having outlined the triggers for an ED visit and demonstrated the need for a palliative care–prepared ED, the following is a discussion of the issues that prevent high-quality palliative care delivery. It is important to understand these barriers for effective integration of palliative care into the ED. Current barriers include, but are not limited to, the traditional ED model of care delivery and care processes, the physical environment, changes in the clinical presentations of the population served by the ED, and a lack of evidence supporting best practice. Patient, family caregiver, and clinician experiences are also reviewed because an understanding of their perceptions enables better understanding of how to tailor strategies and implement new models of care to address issues specific to palliative care populations.

The Current ED Model

The ED is a time-sensitive environment, influencing hospital admission and discharge rates and serving as the gateway to healthcare for many people in times of crisis.[12] The current ED emerged from the "casualty" model employed on battlefields, where saving lives was the focus.[13] While there are many successful stories of ED-based palliative care,[14,15] the ED model of care still largely retains the "triage, resuscitate, stabilize, transfer" approach. The "resuscitate, stabilize" focus poses a challenge to ED clinicians when caring for patients with complex needs who require a more holistic and broader assessment.[5] Even when faced with palliative emergencies, ED clinicians require an understanding of the underlying trajectory and plan of care to conduct necessary conversations with patients and families and rapidly focus or refocus treatments.[11] Clinicians require training and education to refocus on symptom control and QOL over life-sustaining measures. As discussed later, this can be acutely distressing for ED clinicians.[16]

The ED model extends to the physical environment, and here, too, there are challenges for delivery of palliative care. In line with the need for practical and immediate, unplanned emergent care, the majority of EDs are brightly lit and contain different treatment areas according to severity of patient need (e.g., minor and major injuries and resuscitation). Even in modern EDs, space is often limited and lacking in privacy.[17] High patient numbers, distressing conditions and sounds, and a constant flow of patients and staff result in a noisy environment. The ED functions as a streamlined department in which its clinicians are highly trained and operating within routines and standardized procedures. However, to many patients, particularly those who are more vulnerable, the constant movement and sound can make it appear chaotic and unorganized.[17] This can exacerbate tensions and concerns for palliative care patients and families whose needs may be prioritized below other more obviously acutely ill patients.[16,18] Indeed, some palliative patients report feeling that they are competing for attention against other patients (see the section "Needs and Experiences of the Palliative Care Patient").

Palliative Care–Specific Patient Complexities

"Traditional" ED patients can be classified as those experiencing "spectacular" medical or surgical crises (e.g., myocardial infarction, shortness of breath, road traffic accidents, falls, and other injuries).[18] However, advances in healthcare delivery, treatments, and improved QOL have seen people living longer with multiple conditions.[19] Some community programs and resources are available, but, as highlighted, people may not be connected to them or are unable to access them.[10] As a result, ED clinicians increasingly care for patients with "subtacular" needs.[18] Coined by Bailey, subtacular patients in the ED include those with EOL or hospice care needs, nontraditional palliative emergencies, and complex psychosocial needs as people approach the EOL.

Clinicians also need to be careful to retain an individual, holistic approach, recognizing different patterns across conditions. Patients with cancer may be more likely to attend the ED having tried alternative routes first, whereas people with COPD may be more likely to bypass other services and seek out emergency care, ensuring that they carry pertinent information with them.[9] Additional complications for ED clinicians trying to identify palliative care needs include multiple conditions, different condition trajectories, and underlying palliative needs not immediately identified in the presenting complaint.[20] In many of these cases, a major barrier is the lack of preexisting clinician–patient relationships.[18] When faced with complicated family relationships and patients with varying degrees of cognition, clinicians may struggle to identify patient goals and preferred care. Many clinicians avoid these complex discussions with patients.[18] Furthermore, use of ADs is not systematically employed, meaning that patients may not have participated in advance care planning or may not know to alert ED clinicians to the existence of this information. This and other gaps in communication between patient, family, and provider could lead to worsened outcomes and conflict surrounding life-sustaining interventions (see the section "Clinician Training and Perceptions").[16]

Needs and Experiences of the Palliative Care Patient

Palliative care research and services aim to support patients and families by identifying and working to meet their goals and preferences. However, there are limited data exploring ED-specific preferences and experiences. This is likely due to the inherent ethical and practical challenges of conducting palliative care research with a vulnerable population in a challenging environment.[21,22] To date, a small number of qualitative studies have sought to explore patient and family caregiver perspectives. There is an increasing global interest in the patient experience, and interestingly the ED structure is consistent across numerous countries and healthcare systems, with similar patient–family experiences reflected throughout. However, the evidence base presently lacks exploration of patient experiences in regard to equity in access to and delivery of palliative care in the ED.

Patient and family experiences in the ED and their reactions to palliative care measures fall broadly into "positive" and "negative" categories, with patients expressing a mixture of "anxiety, uncertainty and relief."[2] Clinicians sending patients to the ED or admitting and caring for them should be aware that the ED can be seen as either a place of reassuring assistance or a regretfully unavoidable outcome.[23] The ED environment, in addition to being challenging for delivery of palliative care, has been cited as hectic and overwhelming.[2] Factors increasing uncertainty are particularly distressing, such as long wait times and a lack of clarity regarding referral processes and navigation between settings.[9,16] Some patients and family caregivers noted that ED care focused more on diagnostics than on symptom management.[2] Patients who recount positive experiences of using the ED when experiencing palliative care needs highlight "soft skill measures," such as communication about wait times and ED processes that were impactful in reducing anxiety.[9,22] Given that symptom control is a major reason for use of the ED, this is a key area for staff training and education in palliative care assessment. Indeed, it may be beneficial to introduce palliative care measures, such as consults or other supportive measures, during long wait times to alleviate distress and promote progress with care planning.[9]

When palliative care was provided, the integration of care sometimes caused concerns when ED staff lacked the training to implement specific measures.[16] When reflecting on ED-initiated referrals to palliative care services or seeing palliative care clinicians in the ED, patients and families had varying responses depending on their familiarity with and understanding of palliative care.[24] Prior knowledge of palliative care meant less concern. General misunderstandings of palliative care can lead some patients to relate it directly to EOL care and a sense of "giving up."[24]

Notably, patients with palliative care needs or certain conditions (such as cancer) may see themselves as being different from other patients due to the severity of their conditions.[24] Coming to the ED meant they needed help but did not mean they wanted all possible treatments.[9] Clinicians should note that this emphasizes the need and opportunity for shared decision-making.[25] Often patients were dealing with their reactions to the intense environment of the ED in conjunction with the changes in their physical condition and personal lives.[22] When considering goals of care, ED clinicians can be mindful that palliative care patients and family caregivers are grappling with multiple changes. The ED visit may often represent unplanned or unmanageable changes in condition, capacity, or disease trajectory, thus triggering further anxiety.[22] Patients with cancer or older patients were most concerned about the potential implications of the ED visit (death, irreversible decline),[9,22] whereas patients with COPD were more likely to find the environment reassuring and be more familiar with the documentation needed to ensure appropriate care.[9]

The implications affect both the patient and the informal caregiver. Clinicians should include caregiver needs as part of their assessment, not least because of their pivotal role as a major source of support and reassurance.[2,22] This role is emphasized in the ED, where caregivers often help maintain a sense of normalcy for the patient.[9] Thus, while the ED may represent a decline in condition or caregiver capacity to cope at home, the visit provides an opportunity for assessment of caregiver burden and referral to support or palliative care services while acknowledging and validating their role.

Clinician Training and Perceptions

Clinician buy-in is essential if palliative care is to be routinely offered in the ED. Palliative care ED training and education for physicians has been developing since the implementation of co-certification in palliative and emergency medicine in the United States in 2006. Importantly for nurses, there is still no standardized certification in ED-based palliative care, although the End-of-Life Nursing Education Consortium (ELNEC) training program does include the ED.[26] While there are a small number of palliative care ED training modules available,[27] most focus on doctors.[28] While these are important programs, the lack of inclusion of an interdisciplinary team (IDT) jeopardizes the opportunity for the collaborative work required for both palliative and ED care. Often, nurses and physicians will seek out palliative care training[29] because standardized palliative care education and training is not routinely provided in most EDs. Generic palliative care training may address emergencies but does not routinely equip clinicians to engage in smooth transfer and care delivery processes. Few programs address some of the more unique challenges of the ED whose solutions will not be possible to implement, despite inventive adaptation. There remains a need for standardized, tailored, IDT, ED-based palliative care training.[30]

In response to the increased presence of palliative patients in the ED and the initiation of palliative care as a subspecialty of emergency medicine, several small-scale qualitative studies have explored ED clinician experiences, perceptions, and beliefs about the provision of ED-based palliative care.[29,31] Again, the focus is predominantly doctors and/or nurses, with very limited inclusion of other members of the IDT (e.g., social workers[32] and administrators[33]). Rarely do studies examine multiple members of the IDT together.[22,31]

Studies have found a mixed response from ED staff considering palliative care. Resistance to palliative care often stems from the desire to provide the best care for patients and concerns that the ED should not encourage palliative care patient visits because it may not be the best location in which to treat such patients.[31] Limited time and space and sound were often cited as barriers to delivery of palliative care by ED clinicians.[29] Some stated that, even if it were appropriate, integration of palliative care into the existing model would be too costly and challenging.[31] Those in favor of integrating palliative care state that it is a core part of the role of the ED and that the ED at its core must respond to the needs of the patients who are seeking care.[30] These clinicians are often highly skilled in palliative care delivery or have a particular interest in the topic. However, even among those in favor of integration of palliative care into the ED, there were concerns about the ability of providers to offer the type of care required under current conditions. Given the algorithmic approach to patient care that supports the ED model, a lack of clarity in such a vital aspect of healthcare delivery must be addressed to support the practice of ED clinicians.

As with patient and family experiences, ED clinicians have witnessed a variety of positive and negative experiences. Beyond these personal experiences, additional challenges include difficulty accessing key information when patients are admitted from the community (e.g., ADs and goals of care).[29,34] ED clinicians expressed concern that care is impeded by limited access to palliative care teams, particularly outside of normal working hours.[34,35] These reflections were tied to a common theme of role confusion over palliative care delivery and questions about who should implement palliative care and if it is part of the role of the ED clinician at all.[29] The frequency of role confusion in several studies suggests this is an area for focus in ED-based palliative care training and education, where clarifications and agreed processes can support practice. Embedded in this role confusion is an issue of significant concern: that there continues to be a lack of agreement and understanding of *what* palliative care actually is.[29,31]

Considering their clinical practice and values, the life-saving focus of the ED means that some ED clinicians struggle with the underlying concepts of palliative care. For some, palliative care means giving up or betraying their patients by taking alternative courses of action that focus on QOL and symptom management as opposed to full resuscitation measures.[16] This sentiment is exacerbated in instances where patients are unknown to ED staff.[16] Inpatient and community nurses can play an important role in supporting ED clinicians, for example, by educating patients and families about what information is required if an emergency visit occurs. This can include completing ADs and care plans with contact details for core care providers that patients can carry with them should they require ED services. A more integrated community ED could also support those ED clinicians who may be reluctant to look beyond the immediate presenting cause. Such actions can be particularly useful in instances when ED clinicians may be reluctant to question current treatment regimens even when verbally requested by patients and families.[16] Standardized or easily accessible documentation could also improve the quality of difficult conversations between ED staff and medical teams overseeing some patients and between ED staff and patients/families.

Limited Knowledge and Research

Increased recognition of patients with palliative and EOL needs in the ED has encouraged a growing field of research and study. Much of this work is still in exploratory stages.[25,29,36] As outlined earlier, a handful of small-scale qualitative studies have provided valuable insight into clinician perceptions and experiences, but these tend not to have an IDT focus. Patient- and family caregiver–centered research is gradually increasing but tends to focus on patients with cancer.[2,37,38] Numerous ethical and feasibility challenges can deter researchers and impact the validity of quantitative research, while some may deem qualitative research overly draining or inappropriate for patients at the EOL.[39] Ultimately, in both clinician and patient–family populations, a limited body of research has moved beyond exploration of perceptions and experiences, although this rich source of data can provide a foundation on which to build. A small number of more rigorous studies have studied the impact of palliative care measures implemented into the ED which demonstrate feasibility and impact (see the section "Facilitators to ED Palliative Care").[14,40] Sadly, patient and family caregiver involvement remains limited, thus decreasing the ability of nurses and other care providers to tailor care or implement new models. Certainly, the current body of knowledge is not yet broad or rigorous enough to conduct comparative effectiveness trials to inform evidence-based best practice guidelines. However, the development of consensus statements and research agendas is beginning to address different aspects of ED-based palliative care, for example, shared decision-making.[25]

To demonstrate the practical implications of these barriers, Part 2 of the case study demonstrates how different approaches to and understandings of palliative care among ED clinicians can confuse and affect the trajectory of a patient's condition. The value in written documentation to support shared decision-making processes is highlighted.

Case Study Part 2: A Patient in the ED

The resident leading the response to Mary's respiratory distress, Dr. Watkins, told her she would need mechanical ventilation if her oxygen saturation began to decline again. Due to stress and systematic barriers such as lack of interpretation services and supportive decision aids, in conjunction with Dr. Watkins' jargon-filled explanation, Mary could not understand what it meant to be "on mechanical ventilation." Feeling she had no other choice, she assented. Mary's husband, Anthony, arrived. Upon hearing she may need to be intubated, Anthony implored the primary registered nurse (RN), Julia, to "slow everything down" as Mary had previously expressed fear around being "on machines." Julia told the husband, "Mary almost needed a breathing machine moments ago, and at any point could become critical again; we have to do everything we can to save your wife." The husband sat with Mary and held her hand. "How are you my love?" he asked. She replied, "More than anything I'm scared. I don't want to die, but I know what happened to my mom—she was never herself again after the breathing machine." Sensing conflict around Mary's goals of care and potential wish to avoid intubation, Julia paged Dr. Watkins to the bedside. When he arrived, he stated, "We are doing everything we can for your wife—she is in very good hands. As you can see, she is already in better condition than she arrived in." Having received an in-service from the inpatient palliative care team last month, Julia asked Mary and Anthony if they had ever heard of palliative care. Anthony asked, "Is that hospice?" Julia was not confident about how to respond but explained that the palliative specialists could discuss Mary's wishes, if a consult were placed. Dr. Watkins rapidly assessed Mary's clinical status, saw her settling respiratory rate and stable SpO_2, and said, "We don't need them! We've got her stabilized, we can send her to the floor in no time. You're not going to die Mary."

Discussion Points

Barriers to palliative care:

- The lack of patient-centered communication and shared decision-making led Mary to agree to a procedure she had previously questioned. Language barriers and health literacy issues may be present in addition to difficulty understanding medical jargon.
- Because of the standard ED model's focus on life-saving and the myth of palliative care as being only useful for actively dying patients, the resident does not see the utility of a palliative care consult for a patient whose emergency is improving.

Facilitators to palliative care:

- The RN is able to begin talking with the family and patient about their treatment goals and introduces the possibility of palliative care.
- This RN is willing to ask the doctor to order a palliative care consult, even though he shows resistance.

Ways to integrate palliative care:

- ED providers can communicate with their patients in clear, nonmedical terms and ask for teach-back to ensure the patient understands. Furthermore, patients with limited English proficiency must be offered formal interpreter services, especially during consenting procedures.
- ED providers can clearly document any preferences and concerns raised by patients to support their transfer and future care.

The ED can incorporate primary palliative care training for all disciplines to both address primary palliative needs and assess the need for specialty palliative consults. With standardized training, all practitioners will have a better sense of when palliative care is appropriate. Nurses are on the front line of patient advocacy and are in a prime position to ensure that both primary and specialty palliative care delivery can occur in a timely and effective manner.

Facilitators to ED Palliative Care

Despite the barriers to ED palliative care, a number of commonalities between the two specialties demonstrate the capacity and potential for integration. Both deal with highly emotive interactions and provide for care of patients of all ages, many with a variety of chronic or life-threatening diseases, often focusing on controlling the presenting and distressing symptoms or cause.[15] Over the past decade, researchers, policymakers, and palliative care and ED clinicians have sought to develop and test different models, approaches, and tools to provide for patients with palliative care needs in the ED. This process is still in its infancy, and currently there is no consensus on the most effective mechanisms for integration.[14] This marks a key challenge for nurses working in and outside of the ED to know how best to support patients and facilitate smooth and appropriate transfers and referrals. Small review studies have now begun to collate the research literature in order to analyze the effects of different models. Thus, while there are no standard or internationally agreed-upon guidelines, some key findings and features that demonstrate innovative ways that nurses can recommend and support patients with palliative care needs in the ED are known.

Models and Approaches

A seminal report published in 2013 by the Improving Palliative Care—Emergency Medicine (IPAL-EM) initiative described 11 clinical demonstrations of ED palliative care integration, focusing on ED-initiated palliative care consultations.[15] The report identified that palliative care integration is on a spectrum ranging from traditional consultation to basic integration, advanced integration, and ED-focused advanced care. The practical delivery within this spectrum ranges from contacting the palliative care team in specific, individual situations to fully integrated care with ED-owned responsibility for palliative care delivery. In the latter case, there may still be a relationship with the palliative care team, but features can include dual-certified ED practitioners, provision of individual case management for high-risk palliative care patients, palliative care training and education from the palliative care team, specific palliative care processes and procedures integrated into routine care, and an IDT approach.[15] Drawing from this report, ED nurses can review their own ED and hospital setting to identify local resources to improve quality of care. Examples of practice that can be adapted include working with in-hospital palliative care and specialty medical teams, developing or improving access to palliative care training programs, and collaboration with ED and community-based members of the IDT to create tailored processes for high-need patients.[15]

Encouraging emerging research is beginning to evaluate the impact of these different mechanisms. On the lower end of the spectrum (traditional consultation), there was one randomized clinical trial that compared QOL, depression, healthcare utilization, and survival in ED patients with advanced cancer between those randomized to ED-initiated palliative care consultation and those to care as usual.[40] Results were statistically significant for QOL, with longer survival rates for those seen by the palliative care team.[40] An example of ED-focused care was conducted in Taiwan.[14] Led by a hospice and palliative medicine specialist, ED nurses and doctors received palliative care training, and residents rotated on hospice wards. Their program included education programs, monthly interdisciplinary meetings with the palliative care team, use of an app to communicate information and experiences, and identifying a specific emergency hospice room for dying patients. The study reports that initiation of do-not-resuscitate orders increased, as did palliative care consultation and ED nurse knowledge, timing, and method of consultation with the palliative care team.[14]

Where ED-focused advanced mechanisms are not possible, ED nurses can make use of different palliative care needs assessment tools to support their practice and improve quality of care. A systematic review of currently available tools, triggers, and criteria for palliative care ED patient assessment found a range of approaches. Nurses can find assessment tools for different patient populations, such as cancer, dementia, and older people.[5] Some draw on the expertise of different members of the IDT, such as social workers, nurses, and physicians.[5] Others can be applied at different points in the process of ED care, for example, at triage, for palliative care consultation while in the ED, to trigger a palliative care evaluation while in the hospital, or to assess for the need for community or hospice services.[5] EDs should identify which tools most suit their patient populations and care processes and draw on the different members of the IDT, including social workers and case managers, to help implement high-quality care. The third and final part of the case study demonstrates in practical terms how such integration can take place.

Case Study Part 3: A Patient in the ED

Julia, the RN, had extra time for Mary, having just admitted a different patient to the hospital. She returned to Mary and her husband, Anthony, who were sitting holding hands. Mary had weaned to 4 L O_2 via nasal cannula, on which her SpO_2 was stable at 87%, nearly her baseline given her COPD. Subjectively, she had improved but continued to report mild dyspnea "like I climbed a few stairs" and moderate anxiety associated with dry mouth and dizziness. She had a sharp pain in her right side from the chest tube, and her lower back was in spasm. Julia knew that, despite the pushback regarding the palliative care consult, she could still provide palliative care directly in the ED. She asked Mary, "Can you tell me a bit about what matters most to you right now?" Mary replied, "Right now, I just want to have less pain, to stay calm, and to have my husband by my side." Julia asked, "What should I know about what specifically helps you be more comfortable?" "I don't take drugs," replied Mary, "but I think I might need some this time." Julia spoke with Dr. Watkins, who ordered PRN analgesia and anxiolytics. She brought these to Mary and offered hot packs, a cool beverage, and a light massage, all of which Mary accepted. Julia asked, "Can you tell me what else you want me to know about you?" Anthony encouraged Mary to ask for an exception to the visitor policy, allowing Mary's children, siblings, and cousins to spend time with her. Mary added, "One more thing—I don't want any more tubes in me. I don't want to go through what my mom went through. I don't want to go like that." Julia noted this in the patient's chart and sent a message to Dr. Watkins. Julia asked Mary about her passion for gardening and what she was currently growing. Mary said, "Oh nothing, just some roses. With my arthritis, I can't grow much else." "They are beautiful roses," said Anthony. Their conversation ended when the transport team arrived to take Mary to the medical inpatient unit. Julia was able to work with the admitting team to order a palliative care consult on admission, paged the palliative care team to ask if they could see her on the unit, and ensured that the primary team knew of Mary's request for no intubation; and a do-not-intubate order was written.

Discussion Points

Facilitators to palliative care:

- This RN has shown determination, enacting fundamental principles of palliative care in her care of Mary despite resistance from her team. She discussed with the patient what interventions she does *not* want during this hospital stay, an important step toward creating her AD and code status.
- The RN engages the patient on a personal level, offering complementary methods of symptom management and investigating what is important to the patient in her life. Education is provided where necessary.
- The RN identifies a provider who is "palliative-friendly" and successfully ensures that Mary will receive a palliative care consult during her inpatient admission.

Ways to integrate palliative care:

- ED practitioners do not need to be palliative care specialists to offer palliative care. Finding out what matters to the patient, taking seriously those priorities even when they conflict with those of the ED, and offering creative solutions to address those needs can be done in any encounter with a patient. Standardized education for all ED practitioners can encourage these smaller-scale incorporations of palliative care.
- Identifying allies, and therefore building support from within the ED team, will be crucial to creating lasting change within the ED setting.

Current Gaps and Next Steps

Despite increasing attention on the role of palliative care in the ED, further steps will be critical to meeting the demands of an aging population with extensive palliative care needs. High-quality research into the costs and comparative effectiveness of implementing palliative care in the ED setting may influence stakeholders to ensure that adequate palliative care consultation services exist. Moreover, while education is lacking for RNs, advanced practice RNs, physician assistants, and physicians alike,[41] there is minimal evidence of multidisciplinary approaches with tailored ED palliative care training, education, and certification.[14] It is recommended that EDs implement a systematized training on the basics of palliative care, as well as a standardized protocol for involving palliative care specialists in patient care. Education will reduce confusion over definitions and roles in palliative care, while increased access to palliative care professionals, including bereavement support services, social work, and homecare services, could eliminate much of the gap between the patients' and the providers' goals.[16] Finally, no palliative care program in an ED will be entirely successful unless the total hospital system also values palliative care. Of particular importance is the negative impact of delaying or avoiding advance care planning on the quality of a person's final months of life.[42] A greater ubiquity of documentation containing information on patient preferences, wishes, or goals-of-care conversations may increase the presence of patient-centered and palliative care delivery in the ED. Being at the front line of direct patient care, nurses are optimal resources for education and advance care planning discussions.

Conclusion

Palliative care in the ED has traditionally been highly challenging for multiple reasons, including the environment and "identity" of the ED and its staff, as well as misunderstandings of what palliative care delivery may entail among clinicians and patients. Despite this, growing numbers of people with palliative care needs are seen in the ED, reflecting a shift in the aging population, as well as people living longer with chronic, life-limiting conditions. While there are numerous challenges, new models of care are emerging and showing good outcomes. ED palliative care will need to continue to evolve as the patient population changes. The nurse needs to be at the forefront of and adaptable to such changes in order to best support patients and their families.

REFERENCES

1. Seow H, Brazil K, Sussman J, et al. Impact of community based, specialist palliative care teams on hospitalisations and emergency department visits late in life and hospital deaths: a pooled analysis. *BMJ*. 2014;348:g3496. https://doi.org/10.1136/bmj.g3496.
2. Philip J, Remedios C, Breen S, et al. The experiences of patients with advanced cancer and caregivers presenting to emergency departments: a qualitative study. *Palliat Med*. 2018;32(2):439–446. https://doi.org/10.1177/0269216317735724.
3. Kirkland SW, Garrido Clua M, Kruhlak M, et al. Comparison of characteristics and management of emergency department presentations between patients with met and unmet palliative care needs. *PLoS One*. 2021;16(9):e0257501. https://doi.org/10.1371/journal.pone.0257501.
4. George N, Bowman J, Aaronson E, Ouchi K. Past, present, and future of palliative care in emergency medicine in the USA. *Acute Med Surg*. 2020;7(1):e497. https://doi.org/10.1002/ams2.497.
5. George N, Phillips E, Zaurova M, Song C, Lamba S, Grudzen C. Palliative care screening and assessment in the emergency department: a systematic review. *J Pain Symptom Manage*. 2016;51(1):108–119.e2. https://doi.org/10.1016/j.jpainsymman.2015.07.017.
6. Amado-Tineo JP, Oscanoa-Espinoza T, Vásquez-Alva R, Huari-Pastrana R, Delgado-Guay MO. Emergency department use by terminally ill patients: a systematic review. *J Pain Symptom Manage*. 2021;61(3):531–543. https://doi.org/10.1016/j.jpainsymman.2020.08.009.
7. Wong J, Gott M, Frey R, Jull A. What is the incidence of patients with palliative care needs presenting to the emergency department? A critical review. *Palliat Med*. 2014;28(10):1197–1205. https://doi.org/10.1177/0269216314543318.
8. Grudzen CR, Stone SC, Mohanty SA, et al. "I want to be taking my own last breath": patients' reflections on illness when presenting to the emergency department at the end of life. J *Palliat Med*. 2011;14(3):293–296. http://dx.doi.org/10.1089/jpm.2010.0306.
9. Green E, Shaw SE, Harris T. "They shouldn't be coming to the ED, should they?" A qualitative study of why patients with palliative care needs present to the emergency department. *BMJ Support Palliat Care*. 2016;9:e29. https://doi.org/10.1136/bmjspcare-2015-000999.
10. Green E, Gott M, Wong J. Why do adults with palliative care needs present to the emergency department? A narrative review of the literature. *Prog Palliat Care*. 2016;24(4):195–203. https://doi.org/10.1080/09699260.2015.1115805.

11. Fisher R, Fay J. Primary care management of palliative care emergencies. *InnovAiT*. 2014;7(10):581–586. https://doi.org/10.1177/1755738014545898.
12. Siegel M, Bigelow S. Palliative care symptom management in the emergency department: the ABC's of symptom management for the emergency physician. *J Emerg Med*. 2018;54(1):25–32. https://doi.org/10.1016/j.jemermed.2017.08.004.
13. Anshuni MK. The history and development of trauma and emergency care in England. *Trauma*. 2014;17(1):52–57. https://doi.org/10.1177/1460408614552514.
14. Weng TC, Yang YC, Chen PJ, et al. Implementing a novel model for hospice and palliative care in the emergency department: an experience from a tertiary medical center in Taiwan. *Medicine*. 2017;96(19):e6943. https://doi.org/10.1097/md.0000000000006943.
15. Quest T, Herr S, Lamba S, Weissman D; IPAL-EM Advisory Board. Demonstrations of clinical initiatives to improve palliative care in the emergency department: a report from the IPAL-EM Initiative. *Ann Emerg Med*. 2013;61:661–667.
16. Di Leo S, Alquati S, Autelitano C, et al. Palliative care in the emergency department as seen by providers and users: a qualitative study. *Scand J Trauma, Resusc Emerg Med*. 2019;27(1):88. https://doi.org/10.1186/s13049-019-0662-y.
17. Liu B, McD Taylor D, L-Y Ling S, MacGibbon P. Non-medical needs of older patients in the emergency department. *Australas J Ageing*. 2016;35(3):174–179. https://doi.org/10.1111/ajag.12265.
18. Bailey C, Murphy R, Porock D. Trajectories of end-of-life care in the emergency department. *Ann Emerg Med*. 2011;57(4):362–369. https://doi.org/10.1016/j.annemergmed.2010.10.010.
19. Heeren P, Hendrikx A, Ceyssens J, et al. Structure and processes of emergency observation units with a geriatric focus: a scoping review. *BMC Geriatr*. 2021;21(1):95. https://doi.org/10.1186/s12877-021-02029-9.
20. Wilson JG, English DP, Owyang CG, et al. End-of-life care, palliative care consultation, and palliative care referral in the emergency department: a systematic review. *J Pain Symptom Manage*. 2020;59(2):372–383.e1. https://doi.org/10.1016/j.jpainsymman.2019.09.020.
21. Higginson IJ. Research challenges in palliative and end of life care. *BMJ Support Palliat Care*. 2016;6(1):2–4. https://doi.org/10.1136/bmjspcare-2015-001091.
22. Wright R, Lowton K, Hansen BR, Grocott P. Older adult and family caregiver preferences for emergency department based-palliative care: an experience-based co-design study. *Int J Nurs Stud Adv*. 2021;3:100016. https://doi.org/10.1016/j.ijnsa.2020.100016.
23. Wright née Blackwell R, Lowton K, Robert G, Grudzen C, Grocott P. Using experience-based co-design with older patients, their families and staff to improve palliative care experiences in the emergency department: a reflective critique on the process and outcomes. *Int J Nurs Stud*. 2017;68:83–94. http://dx.doi.org/10.1016/j.ijnurstu.2017.01.002.
24. Smith AK, Schonberg MA, Fisher J, et al. Emergency department experiences of acutely symptomatic patients with terminal illness and their family caregivers. J *Pain Symptom Manage*. 2010;39(6):972–981. http://dx.doi.org/10.1016/j.jpainsymman.2009.10.004.
25. George NR, Kryworuchko J, Hunold KM, et al. Shared decision making to support the provision of palliative and end-of-life care in the emergency department: a consensus statement and research agenda. *Acad Emerg Med*. 2016;23(12):1394–1402. https://doi.org/10.1111/acem.13083.
26. Duarte CA. End-of-Life Nursing Education Consortium (ELNEC)—Critical Care Curriculum. http://www.aacnnursing.org/ELNEC/About.
27. Wang DH. Beyond code status: palliative care begins in the emergency department. *Ann Emerg Med*. 2017;69(4):437–443. https://doi.org/10.1016/j.annemergmed.2016.10.027.
28. Wright R, Hayward B, Kistler E, Vaughan Dickson V, Grudzen C. That was a game changer: clinical impact of an emergency department-based palliative care communication skills training workshop. *Emerg Med J*. 2020;37(5):262–264. https://doi.org/10.1136/emermed-2019-208567.
29. Wright R, Lowton K, Robert G, Grudzen C, Grocott P. Emergency department staff priorities for improving palliative care provision for older people: a qualitative study. *Palliat Med*. 2017;32(2):417–425. https://doi.org/10.1177/0269216317705789.
30. Aaronson EL, Wright RJ, Ritchie CS, et al. Mapping the future for research in emergency medicine palliative care: a research roadmap. *Acad Emerg Med*. 2022;29(8):963–973. https://doi.org/10.1111/acem.14496.
31. Shearer FM, Rogers IR, Monterosso L, Ross-Adjie G, Rogers JR. Understanding emergency department staff needs and perceptions in the provision of palliative care. *Emerg Med Australas*. 2014;26(3):249–255. https://doi.org/10.1111/1742-6723.12215.
32. Aaronson EL, Greenwald JL, Krenzel LR, Rogers AM, LaPointe L, Jacobsen JC. Adapting the serious illness conversation guide for use in the emergency department by social workers. *Palliat Support Care*. 2021;19(6):681–685. https://doi.org/10.1017/s1478951521000821.
33. Grudzen CR, Richardson LD, Major-Monfried H, Kandarian B, Ortiz JM, Morrison RS. Hospital administrators' views on barriers and opportunities to delivering palliative care in the emergency department. *Ann Emerg Med*. 2013;61(6):654–660. http://dx.doi.org/10.1016/j.annemergmed.2012.06.008.
34. Lamba S, Nagurka R, Zielinski A, Scott S. Palliative care provision in the emergency department: barriers reported by emergency physicians. *J Palliat Med*. 2013;16(2):143–147. https://doi.org/10.1089/jpm.2012.0402.
35. Gips A, Daubman B-R, Petrillo LA, et al. Palliative care in the emergency department: a qualitative study exploring barriers, facilitators, desired clinician qualities, and future directions. *Palliat Support Care*. 2022;20(3):363–368. https://doi.org/10.1017/S1478951521001012.
36. Lamba S, DeSandre PL, Todd KH, et al. Integration of palliative care into emergency medicine: the Improving Palliative Care in Emergency Medicine (IPAL-EM) collaboration. *J Emerg Med*. 2014;46(2):264–270. https://doi.org/10.1016/j.jemermed.2013.08.087.
37. Caswell G, Seymour J, Crosby V, et al. Lung cancer diagnosed following an emergency admission: exploring patient and carer perspectives on delay in seeking help. *Support Care Cancer*. 2017;25(7):2259–2266. https://doi.org/10.1007/s00520-017-3633-8.
38. Wilcock A, Crosby V, Hussain A, et al. Lung cancer diagnosed following an emergency admission: mixed methods study of the management, outcomes and needs and experiences of patients and carers. *Respir Med*. 2016;114:38–45. https://doi.org/10.1016/j.rmed.2016.03.006.
39. Blum D, Inauen R, Binswanger J, Strasser F. Barriers to research in palliative care: a systematic literature review. *Prog Palliat Care*. 2015;23(2):75–84. https://doi.org/10.1179/1743291X14Y.0000000100.

40. Grudzen CR, Richardson LD, Johnson PN, et al. Emergency department–initiated palliative care in advanced cancer: a randomized clinical trial. *JAMA Oncol.* 2016;2(5):591–598. https://doi.org/10.1001/jamaoncol.2015.5252.
41. Siegel M. Palliative care as life support for my career. *J Emerg Med.* 2017;52(1):121–122. https://doi.org/10.1016/j.jemermed.2016.09.019.
42. Brinkman-Stoppelenburg A, Rietjens JA, van der Heide A. The effects of advance care planning on end-of-life care: a systematic review. *Palliat Med.* 2014;28(8):1000–25. https://doi.org/10.1177/0269216314526272.

64

Hospital-Based Palliative Care

Barbara Reville and Anessa M. Foxwell

Key Points

- Hospital-based palliative care (HBPC) teams provide interdisciplinary, specialized palliative care to patients and families affected by serious illness in a variety of delivery models and settings.
- HBPC provides person-centered support to patients and families during hospitalizations, improving the quality of care, decreasing unnecessary intensive care stays, and providing care matched to patient preferences.
- There are myriad roles for nurses—across practice levels—to deliver palliative care to hospitalized patients and their families.
- Nurses can impact access to HBPC for hospitalized patients and their families by assessing needs, advocating for specialty HBPC involvement, and committing to quality improvement and to culturally sensitive, equitable care.

Case: Introducing Rita

Rita is a 62-year-old woman with recently diagnosed acute myeloid leukemia (AML) that was discovered through routine blood work a few weeks ago. Rita is now hospitalized for induction chemotherapy. Prior to this diagnosis, Rita was a relatively healthy woman. She works in school administration and is married to her wife Janet. They do not have children but are close with extended family. This is Rita's first time being in a hospital since her mother's death 8 years ago. She confides in her bedside nurse that she hates hospitals and that she is anxious about whether the chemo will work. On day +4 of induction, Rita's symptoms worsen; she is nauseous all the time despite around-the-clock antiemetics, and her anxiety and insomnia worsen. On rounds, the bedside nurse advocates for a palliative care consult for symptom management and psychosocial support.

Evolution of Hospital-Based Palliative Care

Hospital-based palliative care (HBPC) originated in the 1990s.[1,2] Research that confirmed substantial shortcomings in care for hospitalized seriously ill adults galvanized change.[3] Multiple pioneering institutions including The Cleveland Clinic (Ohio), Memorial Sloan-Kettering Cancer Center (New York), Mount Sinai (New York), Massachusetts General Hospital and Beth Israel Deaconess Medical Center (Massachusetts), Virginia Commonwealth University, Cooper Green Hospital (Alabama), Northwestern Memorial Hospital (Illinois), and the University of Pittsburgh (Pennsylvania) issued a palliative care system case series to describe their programs.[1] Each of these pioneering institutions created an HBPC program based on identified gaps in hospital palliative and end-of-life care delivery. While HBPC remains diverse in origins, makeup, and models, the goal of improving patient-centered palliative care remains at its heart. As the early palliative nursing leader Nessa Coyle opined in 1997, collaborative and comprehensive HBPC "anticipates problems and has a preemptive approach" and "needs an interprofessional team, and that in this way values are realized and suffering minimized."[4(p266)]

Today, HBPC does not have a one-size-fits-all formula but rather, by a myriad of configurations of interdisciplinary team members who provide primary or specialty HBPC as consultative services and/or dedicated units. This chapter will aim to define these types and models of HBPC, the scope of HBPC, and the roles of nurses.

Defining HBPC

The Center to Advance Palliative Care (CAPC) defines HBPC as an interdisciplinary specialized medical team focused on symptom management and intensive person-centered communication that aims to clarify goals of treatment and coordination of care across healthcare settings. HBPC can further be categorized as primary or specialty palliative care. Primary palliative care can be delivered by any healthcare provider prepared in basic palliative care skills, while specialty palliative care is delivered by expert, often specially certified, palliative care clinicians equipped to support complex, chronically ill patients and families (see Table 64.1 for more details).

Scope of HBPC in the United States

CAPC manages the National Palliative Care Registry, which aims to trend palliative care practices and reach nationally. Nearly 90% of hospitals with 300 beds or more have an HBPC team, and 72% of hospitals with a census of 50 or more have an HBPC team.[5,6] Between 2009 and 2015, HBPC service penetration increased by almost 80%.[6] Much of this growth has been associated with the increased presence

Table 64.1 Skill sets of primary and specialty palliative care clinicians

Primary palliative care skill set	Specialty palliative care skill set
Manage pain and symptoms of serious illness.	Manage complex or refractory pain and symptoms during serious illness and at end of life.
Manage anxiety, depression, emotional and spiritual distress associated with serious illness.	Manage complex psychological conditions, anxiety, depression, and grief reactions.
Initiate conversations about advance care planning, elicit illness understanding and preferences about limits of treatment and goals of care.	Assist medical teams during conflict about medical decision-making.
Explain palliative care and hospice care options.	Facilitate complicated care transitions for end-of-life care and provide end-of-life care.

Source: Reference 15.

of advanced practice registered nurses (APRNs) on HBPC teams.[6] In 2015, the mean percentage of patients who received a palliative care consult for all hospital admissions was 4.8%.[6] Forty-four percent of programs have a core interdisciplinary team that includes at least one physician, one nurse (either registered nurse or APRN), a social worker, and a chaplain.[6] The availability of HBPC varies by region, with more accessibility in the regional northeast and west coast. Patients who received HBPC are primarily discharged to home (43.5%), with only a third of those patients discharged home with hospice services.[6]

In terms of patient population served, the most common primary serious illness diagnosis seen in HBPC is cancer (26%), followed by cardiac (13%), then pulmonary (12%), and neurologic diagnoses (8%).[6] This is not surprising given that HBPC consult teams are highly prevalent (90%) in National Cancer Institute–designated cancer centers.[7] More than one-third of Medicare beneficiaries with serious illness—such as cancer, heart failure, chronic lung disease, coronary artery disease, renal failure, peripheral vascular disease, advanced diabetes, chronic liver disease and dementia—experience an average of four transitions in care during the last year of life.[5,8,9] These transitions between home and healthcare settings (i.e., hospitals, rehabilitation, etc.) generally occur with a progression of illness. As serious illnesses worsen, so too do the burden of symptoms and complexity of decision-making. In fact, 29% of Medicare beneficiaries have an intensive care admission within the last 30 days of life.[10] While the proportion of those who die in the hospital has decreased, 1 in 5 Medicare patients died during a hospital admission.[10] HBPC consultation teams support patients during these admissions by providing pain/symptom management and clarifying goals of care. Research has shown that seriously ill hospitalized patients who have an HBPC consult for goals of care have lower future healthcare utilization (i.e., hospital admissions) and overall cost.[11,12] Furthermore, given the wide variation in the characteristics and adoption of HBPC teams at a given hospital, there is potential to influence treatment intensity at the end of life and access to palliative care or hospice services.[13]

Standards for HBPC

The National Consensus Project (NCP) and the National Quality Forum spearheaded the development of quality standards for the palliative care field, while the Joint Commission (TJC) codified the standards for hospital-based palliative care programs.[14] In 2011, TJC launched the Advanced Certification Program for Palliative Care to identify high-quality programs. To attain certification, programs must demonstrate palliative care expertise among the leadership and the interdisciplinary team, adherence to evidence-based practice standards, and processes for routine performance measurement.

Types of HBPC

Primary Palliative Care

Primary palliative care is defined as the basic skills and competencies required of all physicians, nurses, and other healthcare practitioners who encounter persons with serious, life-limiting illness. All clinicians should be competent in basic pain and symptom management, straightforward goals-of-care discussion, assisting with advanced care planning, and providing initial emotional support to patients and families experiencing serious illness (see Table 64.1). There is a growing availability of continuing education, including established academic programs for all disciplines to improve their knowledge of basic palliative care principles. The End-of-Life Nursing Education Consortium (ELNEC) and CAPC online modules offer two comprehensive educational programs on primary palliative care skills. For more details of education programs, refer to Chapter 76, "Nursing Education."

Specialty Palliative Care

Specialty palliative care refers to palliative care delivered by expert palliative care clinicians. These clinicians may provide care through an interdisciplinary team, a specialized palliative care unit, or both. Specialty palliative care clinicians are unable to evaluate and treat every patient with serious illness, and therefore are expertly trained as a resource and guide for their primary palliative care colleagues. Specialists may act as a clinical, educational, and/or research expert in hospitals and health systems to promote, deliver, and develop palliative care. Organizations at different levels may choose among different components of care to incorporate into their model. This may include (1) a clinical component (i.e., an interdisciplinary inpatient consult service, a specialized acute palliative care unit, an outpatient palliative care clinic, or outreach to skilled nursing facilities); (2) an education component (i.e., promote primary palliative care skills through staff education, develop care pathways, or direct an interdisciplinary fellowship training program); (3) a research mission (i.e., tracking patient demographics and needs to advocate for more staffing, developing a quality improvement project, or partnering with palliative care researchers to study patient-specific outcomes).

Models of HBPC

The Inpatient Interdisciplinary Consult Team

A growing literature summarizes the development of palliative care consultation teams within hospitals to offer specialized consultation and expertise to patients, families, and other healthcare providers.[13] American and European HBPC teams have shared the elements of a successful, well-functioning team as an interdisciplinary, responsive consultation model, available during off hours, and able to provide continuity of palliative care.[16–18] The interdisciplinary consultation team generally consists of one or more of the following disciplines: physician, advanced practice nurse, registered nurse, social worker, chaplain, pharmacist, psychologist, child life specialist, and/or art therapist.[19] While this is the gold standard, only 25% of HBPC programs are able to staff a "full" team.[18] Psychosocial, spiritual, or pharmacy providers may be employed by other hospital departments. Alternatively, some HBPC may consist of only a single specialist nurse or APRN. Factors that influence the makeup of the palliative care service (PCS) team include administrative and financial support of the program, availability of professionals, and hospital case mix.

Inpatient interdisciplinary teams are consulted by hospital providers in need of specialty palliative care, whether pain/symptom management, complex goals of care discussions, skilled end-of-life care, or treatment of psychosocial or existential distress for their patients. HBPC teams typically provide recommendations hospital and work with those teams to improve the patient's comfort.

The Acute Palliative Care Unit

When available, a dedicated acute palliative care unit (APCU) admits seriously ill patients with severe symptom distress who need a higher level of care that is directed by palliative care specialists. Resources to support an APCU include an interdisciplinary team and palliative care–trained nursing staff. These resources are more often found in larger hospitals that already support a consultation service.[7] When patients are admitted to the APCU or transferred there during an admission, a change of usual care team can be distressing to the patient and family. Nursing can assist by explaining the rationale for the shift and adjusting expectations.

According to Hui and Bruera[7] 20%–30% of US cancer centers have APCUs. Given the severity of the APCU patient's condition, mortality is 30%–50%.[7] Fewer APCU patients are stable enough to discharge home compared to other units; that is, 40% are discharged to home hospice.[7] Some favorable palliative care outcomes from an APCU stay include an increased rate of advance care planning, goals-of-care discussions, and clarification of code status—most often to avoid resuscitation.[20] Early reports from referring clinicians indicate that they favored the quality of care on an APCU compared to usual end-of-life care; however, there is a lack of randomized controlled trials of patient outcomes.[7]

Case Revisited: Consulting Palliative Care

During Rita's initial hospital stay, the bedside oncology nurse recognized a need for additional support to help with Rita's refractory symptoms, namely nausea, anxiety, and insomnia. The oncology team and bedside nurses had managed Rita's nausea and anxiety with firstline antiemetics and emotional support. This could be categorized as primary palliative care skills. Then, recognizing that Rita's symptoms were refractory, the nurse advocated for further expertise from the palliative care team.

Nursing Is Primary in Care of the Seriously Ill

Nursing care is the primary service provided to individuals during hospital admission. By virtue of their close proximity to patients and families, nurses hear the lived experience of illness and hopes for improved health or a peaceful death.[21] As advocates and leaders, nurses are positioned to influence patient care at the organizational level and in collaboration with specialty palliative care teams.[21–24] For further reading on the role of the nurse in palliative care, see Chapter 2, "Role of Nursing in Palliative Care."

Leveraging Relationships to Support Patient and Family Needs

In the model of relational nursing care, the bedside nurse builds a therapeutic relationship that supports the patient and family during the vulnerability of serious illness; creates a safe atmosphere for expression of concerns or fears, goals, and illness understanding; and closely observes effects of the illness and treatment. Clinical competence, attentive listening, and communication skills are primary palliative care skills the nurse applies to intercede on the patient's and family's behalf with the hospital care team.[25] The nurse integrates information from these ways of knowing and communicates palliative care needs to the hospital team. In collaboration with the nurse, the interdisciplinary team can formulate a patient-centered care plan to optimize symptom control, garner psychosocial or spiritual supports, or clarify patient preferences and values.[23,24,26]

Nurses Influencing Access to Palliative Care

Leading improvements in patient care is a nursing responsibility.[27] Nurses may observe concerning patterns of unmet needs or underutilization of palliative care at the unit level, not just in their individual patients. For example, nurses on an oncology unit caring for patients with advanced cancer notice that palliative care consults are called at a late stage when patients are near the end of life or that staff lack confidence to manage symptoms. Solutions might include developing unit-wide triggers for palliative care consults or an evidence-based order set for common symptoms.[25]

Nurse practice councils or designated palliative care champions aligned with unit nursing leadership can gather data using quality improvement tools to understand the scope of the problem and determine how to intervene for better patient care outcomes and optimal use of resources[28,29] (see Chapter 78, "Developing and Implementing Quality Improvement Programs across Settings"). Palliative care teams and specialty nurses are resources for education efforts, advocacy for institutional change, or mentoring in primary palliative care skills. By working together, nurses can catalyze change and embody palliative nursing leadership.[27]

Palliative Care Nurse Champions

A successful nursing model, the palliative nurse champion, builds unit-based palliative care expertise for select nurses, who then influence improvements in palliative care nursing practice and staff skill set.[28,29] Champions commit to additional palliative care education and join a network of peers from other units in the hospital. Drach et al.[28] describe a pediatric unit's palliative care champion program designed to train bedside experts so that they can support patients and families with palliative care needs, mentor other nurses, and extend the reach of the HBPC specialty team. Their program increased staff's comfort and confidence in providing end-of-life care and helped garner funding for more HBPC staffing.[28]

Nursing Roles in HBPC

The roles that nurses play in care of the seriously ill are as varied as the settings and models of care delivery where they work (see Table 64.2 for examples of nursing roles compiled from NCP guidelines and clinical practice). In the acute care setting, primary palliative nursing involves helping patients and families navigate serious illness and empowering them by offering options and by advocacy.[26,30] The nurse anticipates needs and connects patients between settings or intensity levels of care, between hospital teams, and sometimes even within the family system.[23] The nurse leader responds to the changing needs of the community or institution by shaping policy and practice to achieve best patient outcomes.[27]

Consulting Specialty Palliative Care

Traditionally, HBPC consults are requested by a physician or ordering provider based on their understanding of the patient's prognosis, palliative care needs, and familiarity with specialty palliative care.[32] However, by relying on clinicians alone to identify palliative care needs and refer in a timely fashion, other seriously ill patients are missed, while less appropriate consults add to HBPC staff workload.[33–35] There is evidence of disparities in referral patterns based on disease, admitting service, race, or ethnicity.[35,36] Hospitalized patients deserve access to both skilled primary palliative care clinicians and specialists when needed. There is vigorous debate about which patients need specialty HBPC and which patients are well served by the primary palliative care skills of nurses and hospital teams.[15,32,36] Table 64.3 offers an example of the evolution of primary and specialty palliative care needs.

The need for solutions is growing more urgent given the anticipated shortage of specialty palliative care physicians by 2030 amidst an uptrend in Americans with serious illness.[36,37] Determining when and where specialty palliative care delivers value toward patient outcomes is crucial to understand staffing and training needs. Ongoing efforts to train nurses and other providers in primary palliative care skills are laudable; however, uniform palliative care competency among primary providers cannot be assumed.[28,32,38] Hospitals need evidence-based and scalable models to determine which patients, whether due to prognosis, illness severity, or distress, warrant the resources of specialty palliative care expertise[32,34,36]

Table 64.2 Palliative and hospice nursing roles in hospitals

Nursing role	Role description
Triage nurse	As a member of the palliative care consultation team, the triage nurse is the first contact for incoming palliative care consult requests. Determines urgency of request and assigns to appropriate team member(s), educates hospital staff on consult request process.
Nurse navigator	Provides proactive outreach to patients with chronic illness for the duration of their chronic care condition. Some functions overlap with triage nurses. Liaises between inpatient and outpatient palliative care teams to ensure continuity of care between episodes of hospital care.
Acute palliative care unit (APCU) nurse	Provides bedside care for patients admitted to APCU, including complex symptom management and/or skilled end-of-life care. Unit-based training in palliative care and hospice is required for nurses on this unit.
Palliative care nurse champion	Seeks additional training in primary palliative care as a means to create more nursing experts at the bedside and to extend the reach of the HBPC specialty team. Advocates for specialty referrals, mentors nursing staff, and provides interventions to offload the specialty team.
Hospice liaison nurse	Provides in-hospital informational visits to patients and families by referral; coordinates hospice transitions from hospital to other settings (e.g., home, hospice facility) in collaboration with the hospital team. May be employed by a hospice agency and work by contract with client hospitals.
Hospice nurse	Advises bedside nurses and the hospital team caring for hospitalized hospice patients in the transition to end-of-life care, consults on symptom management, and models effective patient and family communication. The hospice nurse can be employed by either the hospital or the hospice agency.
Nurse manager	Supervises nursing staff of an inpatient unit that admits seriously ill and dying patients and maintains collaborative relationships with disciplines that support patient care. Supports staff development in primary palliative care skills from onboarding to professional advancement. Intervenes when necessary for safety of patients, families, and staff on the unit and oversees quality improvement efforts to improve care.
Clinical educator/clinical nurse specialist	Supports nursing practice at unit level by role-modeling palliative nursing excellence, conducts educational needs assessment, and coordinates in-service education that promulgates evidence-based practice standards. Participates in quality improvement screening and process improvements.
Nurse case manager	Provides initial and ongoing nursing assessments of patient and family needs during the hospital stay and coordinates post-hospital plan of care with hospital team members.
Nurse scientist	Acts as a resource to nursing staff who develop evidence-based practice projects, encourages nursing scholarship, conducts own research, and disseminates relevant findings to nursing staff.

Source: Reference 31.

Table 64.3 Evolution of primary and specialty palliative care needs over successive hospital stays

Patient case: Rita		Primary palliative care needs	Specialty palliative care needs
Hospital Stay 1	Induction chemo	• Nausea regimen	• No specialty needs
	Day 4	• Emotional support • Nausea assessment and medication management	• Symptom management for refractory symptoms: nausea anxiety, insomnia • Psychosocial distress • Engagement of HBPC social worker
Hospital Stay 2	Disease recurrence	• Loss of occupation • Debility • Financial resources with loss of income	• Existential distress • Advance care planning • Psychosocial support and resource access • Family support
Hospital Stay 3	Refractory disease with fungal pneumonia	• Dyspnea • Fatigue • Fever • Severe debility	• Symptom management • Re-engagement of social worker and chaplain • Caregiver burden/distress
	Transfer to ICU	• Worsening dyspnea requiring intubation • Anxiety	• Family meeting to discuss illness understanding, prognosis, values, preferences • Surrogate decision-making support • Time-limited trial of life support

HBPC, hospital-based palliative care; ICU, intensive care unit.

Triggers for Palliative Care Involvement

Palliative care can help during all phases of a serious illness; however, not all patients with a serious illness need a specialist, just as not every patient with hypertension needs a cardiologist unless their condition is refractory to control.[32] Hospital clinicians in collaboration with population health researchers have developed systematic strategies that identify patients at time of admission who, based on a variety of prognostic factors, are likely to benefit from timely intervention by HBPC.[34,36,39]

In one national survey of HBPC teams that routinely use palliative care referral triggers, a large percentage of respondents agreed that triggers promoted earlier referrals, overcame resistance to palliative care among some referring providers, and increased consult volume.[33] However, some of the increased consults were not appropriate. Moreover, PCS clinicians expressed mixed feelings that referral triggers generated more work and hampered team capacity to effectively complete all consults.[33]

Referral triggers tailored to specific patient populations can improve access and serve to educate those subspecialty providers on reasons to consult. For example, cardiologists convened to generate consensus on palliative care referral criteria for patients with serious heart disease.[40] While common prognostic criteria applied to this population (e.g., prognosis of 6 months or less, frequent hospital stays, and severe symptoms), there are other markers specific to serious heart diseases, such as use of advanced heart therapies, cardiac cachexia, cardiorenal syndrome, and consideration of heart transplant.

Computer modeling that automates prognostic prediction may be superior to clinician judgment and would overcome referral bias when integrated into routine care and the electronic medical record.[41] These models have been shown to increase earlier palliative care consults, promote advance care planning documentation, and referral to home-based palliative care.[34] However, they may not fully capture subjective factors or clinician judgment in the referral decision. Therefore, ideal referral criteria models should be developed with interdisciplinary partner input and be designed to allow providers to opt out of the consult if not appropriate.[33,34,41]

Assessing Palliative Care Needs

Nurses at the bedside are the gatekeepers to palliative care access by identifying patients with serious illness who need intervention for pain, symptoms, emotional and spiritual distress, family distress or conflict, and help with medical decision-making.[25,26] Many of these concerns can be addressed by nursing and hospital team intervention or referral to ancillary hospital services such as social work or spiritual care—this is primary palliative care. When those needs are complicated or when initial interventions fall short, consultation by specialty HBPC should be considered.

Making the Case for Palliative Care Intervention

Nurses are usually not authorized to order PCS consults directly; however, they can advocate for involvement of palliative care expertise with the hospital team.[25] Unfortunately, nurses encounter barriers to referrals which may be due to misconceptions about the role of HBPC among patients and families, clinician bias, or missed messaging between the nurse and ordering providers about the potential value of referral.

Lack of knowledge and misconceptions about palliative care are known to be common among some patient populations. In a public opinion survey by CAPC, adults were asked about their overall impression of palliative care. Forty-two percent of respondents were not familiar enough to share an opinion.[42] Once a definition of palliative care was provided, 60% of respondents endorsed wanting palliative care if they or a family member became seriously ill.[42] Enguidanos et al.[43] reported that among hospitalized Hispanics, misunderstandings about hospice are common, which can explain underutilization of these services. Similar misunderstandings, lack of cultural alignment, and mistrust in the medical system due to a history of racism and unauthorized experimentation lead to lower acceptance of hospice and palliative care among other racial and ethnic minoritized groups including African Americans, Indigenous populations, and Asian Americans. When role models who represent diverse patient groups communicate in their language about palliative care, knowledge scores can be boosted.[43]

Broaching the idea of a palliative care consultation to a patient and family is the responsibility of the hospital interdisciplinary team, including nursing. Hospital clinicians may be uncertain how to message this recommendation without eliciting an emotional reaction. Patients are generally unfamiliar with the term "palliative care" or may associate it with end-of-life care. For example, patients who are early in their disease process may wonder why they need a consult.

The nurse can be instrumental in clarifying patient and family expectations in advance of a PCS consultation. Establishing the patient's level of understanding and explaining the role and focus of the palliative care team are important steps prior to the consultation. Adjusting expectations and eliciting concerns can engender trust and allay fears that the primary team is abandoning the patient. While the PCS consults and provides expert guidance to the hospital team their involvement does not supersede the role of the provider team. A neutral description suggested for clinicians to use is: "Palliative care clinicians can help you and your family deal with the changes brought on by your illness." Alternatively, the nurse can explain the specific reason for the consult, for instance, to consult experts on managing pain.[44] Hints on ways to broach a palliative care consult are provided on the Palliative Care Fast Facts website (https://www.mypcnow.org/fast-facts/) and smartphone app Broaching the Topic of a Palliative Care Consultation with Patients and Families.

Case Revisited: Nurse's Role in Helping Rita Understand HBPC

Upon hearing that palliative care is consulted, Rita expresses worry to her nurse that the doctors have given up and that induction chemotherapy is not working. Rita becomes emotional recalling her mother's care by a hospice team in her final days. The nurse reassures her of the team's non-abandonment and explains that the palliative care's involvement does not indicate that Rita's therapy is failing; rather, they will help her hospital team better treat her symptoms and support her. The nurse provides written resources about palliative care to Rita and Janet.

The Initial Palliative Care Consultation

The team concept is integral to PC practice; however, an HBPC team's workflow will differ based on setting, staffing, workload, or reason for the consultation. One clinician may be designated to receive initial consults and organize distribution of work for the day. Another model may require that all new consults are seen first by a medical provider—a physician or advanced practice provider (APRN or physician assistant). The physician serves as the medical resource for the other team members and supervises physician learners, including palliative medicine fellows, as well as trainees from other health professions.

During the initial consultation the clinician(s) will assess needs both within and outside the parameters of the reason for referral (e.g., psychosocial-spiritual distress). These needs may warrant inclusion of other team members who are integrated into the plan of care. For example, a social worker may join the initial consultation if the reason for referral involves emotional distress or assess the patient separately after the initial consult visit (see Table 64.4). HBPC teams have a structure for interdisciplinary review of active consults that inform the plan of care.[31]

The nurse should debrief with the HBPC providers after the initial consultation to learn their perspective, clarify assessments, and discuss the plan of care. The action plan may include medication changes for symptom management, involvement of psychosocial or spiritual providers to address distress, and/or a plan to explore goals of care in a team–family meeting. Ultimately, the HBPC team's client is the hospital team,[32] and any plan of care must be approved by the primary hospital team.

Case Revisited: Initial HBPC Consult and Plan for Follow-up

The palliative care team was helpful in designing an antiemetic regimen during the worst phase of Rita's chemotherapy-induced nausea and vomiting. Since starting a low-dose anti-anxiety medication at bedtime, Rita sleeps better and feels more in control of her emotions. Although the HBPC sees her weekly, Rita continues to meet frequently with the palliative care social worker to talk about her worries about the future of her illness.

Table 64.4 Integration of team members based on reason for palliative care specialty referral

Consult reason	Nurse	APRN/PA	MD	PharmD	SW	Chaplain
Pain management	X	X	X	X		
Physical symptoms	X	X	X	X		
Goals of care and medical decision-making	X	X	X		X	X
Psychosocial distress	X	X	X		X	X
Spiritual/existential distress	X	X	X		X	X
End-of-life issues	X	X	X		X	X
Advance care planning	X	X	X	X	X	X
Access to community resources				X	X	

MD, physician; APRN/PA, advanced practice registered nurse or physician assistant; PharmD, doctor of pharmacy; SW, social worker.

Ongoing Palliative Care Involvement during the Hospital Stay

After an initial consultation, depending on the patient's needs, one or more HBPC team members will make follow-up visits throughout the hospital stay. Some patients may have acute needs, such as uncontrolled pain, that may require daily follow-up visits, while other patients can be seen intermittently until the goal of the initial consultation is achieved. Occasionally, the hospital team may reconsult the HBPC team after completion of a consult for further engagement or to approach a new problem.

Case Revisited: Hospitalization 2

Rita completed her induction chemotherapy, went home, and enjoyed a disease remission lasting 6 months. When she develops new fatigue, bony pain, and abnormal blood work, tests show that the AML has recurred. Due to the new chemotherapy treatment schedule and side effects, Rita took a leave from her job as a school administrator. She worries that her immunocompromised state will preclude her work in a school for the foreseeable future. Rita is admitted to the hospital for the second time with fever and neutropenia since the AML recurrence. Her symptoms of fatigue and bony pain are well managed; however, the nurse advocates to the hospital team to re-engage the palliative care social worker to assist Rita in applying for the school system's long-term disability.

During visits with the palliative care social worker, Rita expresses pessimism about her chances of survival and laments time away from her family during the hospital stays. Whenever Rita broaches the possibility of a bad outcome with her wife, Janet gets tearful and upset, which leaves Rita feeling isolated in her worries. With Rita's permission, the nurse and social worker invite Janet for a conversation about what is important to Rita now and if she becomes sicker. Janet agrees to meet separately with the palliative care social worker for support. The social worker and nurse help Rita complete an advance directive naming Janet as healthcare proxy.

Transitions of Care and Continuity

Continuity is improved dramatically when there is an outpatient follow-up after inpatient HBPC, for example, in a palliative care clinic. In a Canadian study, Webber et al.[45] found that patients seen by specialty HBPC or in an APCU were more apt to be connected to outpatient palliative care after discharge from hospital. This trend was more common for patients with cancer compared to other chronic illnesses (i.e., congestive heart failure, chronic pulmonary or renal conditions, and dementia). Chapters 59, "Hospice and Community-Based Palliative Care," and 61, "Palliative Care Nursing in the Outpatient Setting," discuss community-based and outpatient palliative care delivery models, respectively, in further depth.

Nurses in roles of navigator and care coordinators are key players in offering options to patients and families for post-acute care tailored to their needs. There is a need for better guidance on when to refer to outpatient resources, such as a palliative care clinic. Similar to referral patterns to inpatient HBPC, there is a lack of consensus about which patients benefit most from post-discharge palliative care follow-up.

Oncology guidelines advocate involvement of palliative care for patients who present with advanced illness at time of diagnosis.[7,46,47] Referral criteria developed by a consensus panel of oncology experts were compared to reasons for referral to a palliative oncology clinic.[48] Authors found that 85% of patients met one or more of these referral criteria and were most commonly seen for severe physical distress (pain, fatigue, or insomnia) and less commonly for emotional symptoms, help with decision-making, or neurological deficits.[48] Patients seen had a median survival of 14 months after the first clinic visit, suggesting that broader adoption of uniform outpatient referral criteria would promote earlier involvement of outpatient palliative care.[48]

Case Revisited: Hospitalization 3

Some months have passed since Rita's AML recurrence. The chemotherapy regimens have yielded only short-term remissions. Rita has not returned to work, and Janet is now her full-time caregiver. Then, Rita is readmitted with shortness of breath, fever, neutropenia, and a serious, fungal pneumonia due to her persistent immunocompromised state. She is too debilitated for more chemotherapy, and her impending respiratory failure will necessitate intensive care and intubation on a ventilator. She is unable to participate in medical decision-making. Janet is uncertain about how to proceed without knowing about Rita's chances of getting better.

The nurse suggests that the palliative care team be consulted to assist with decision-making and support of Rita's healthcare proxy. Subsequently, the palliative care social worker coordinates a meeting with Janet, Rita's oncologist, the hospital team, nurse, the intensive care physician, and the palliative care team. The oncologist speaks about limited options for a prolonged remission from the AML even with enrollment in a clinical trial. The intensivist explains that the prognosis from fungal pneumonia is poor and that even with a good outcome, Rita would need to remain on a ventilator for some weeks, followed by transfer to a rehabilitation center.

Janet, supported by the palliative care social worker and nurse, relates Rita's wish to avoid advanced medical technologies if there is no guarantee of getting back to her prior level of function and home. The palliative care team elicits further questions from Janet and any further options from the hospital team and intensivist. Given the uncertain trajectory of Rita's acute illness, the intensivist suggests a time-limited trial of intubation to see if Rita can progress in the next 72 hours. If Rita improves, life support will continue; if her respiratory status does not improve, there will be a second meeting to revisit changing her code status and withdrawing life support. The palliative care team and nurse remain after the meeting to review Janet's understanding of the discussion and to offer further emotional support.

Future Directions for HBPC

Ensuring Culturally Sensitive and Equitable Care

Nurses must collectively reflect on the roots of inequality in the hospital environment, routinely assess the social determinants of health, and expand their connections with community resources for the benefit of patients from underrepresented minorities.[49] The case of Rita threaded through this chapter highlights "seamless" care of a queer adult. Rita's sexual identity and partnership are normalized and accepted as an exemplar of palliative care for LGBTQIA+ individuals. However, many patients have unique care needs to consider based on cultural issues, gender identity, and sexual preferences; for more details, please see Chapter 28, "Cultural Considerations in Palliative Care," and Chapter 67, "Affirmative Palliative Care for LGBTQIA+ Patients and Their Families."

Conclusion

The expansion and evolution of HBPC across US hospitals are mirrored by growing opportunities for nurses at all practice levels to provide palliative nursing. Given the surging numbers of Americans with life-limiting illness amidst an anticipated shortage of palliative care providers, nurses must equip themselves to participate in access, diversity, and resource challenges. Professional associations and national guidelines define state-of-the-art HBPC and offer nurses many paths to expertise in primary or specialty practice. Collaboration, mentoring, and advocacy by nurses aligned with HBPC teams will influence palliative care's reach from the bedside to the health system.

Acknowledgments

Dr. Reville and Dr. Foxwell acknowledge Dr. Patricia Maani-Fogelman and Dr. Maria Bakitas for their contributions to the previous editions of this chapter.

REFERENCES

1. Arnold R, Bailey FA, Billings JA, et al. *Pioneer Programs in Palliative Care: Nine Case Studies*. Milbank Memorial Fund; 2000.
2. Morrison RS. Models of palliative care delivery in the United States. *Curr Opin Support Palliat Care*. 2013;7(2):201–206. https://doi.org/10.1097/spc.0b013e32836103e5.
3. Connors AF, Dawson NV, Desbiens NA, et al. A controlled trial to improve care for seriously ill hospitalized patients. *JAMA*. 1995;274(20):1591–1598. https://doi.org/10.1001/jama.1995.03530200027032.
4. Coyle N. Interdisciplinary collaboration in hospital palliative care: chimera or goal? *Palliat Med*. 1997;11(4):265–266. https://doi.org/10.1177/026921639701100401.
5. Dumanovsky T, Augustin R, Rogers M, Lettang K, Meier DE, Morrison RS. The growth of palliative care in U.S. hospitals: a status report. *J Palliat Med*. 2016;19(1):8–15. https://doi.org/10.1089/jpm.2015.0351.
6. Rogers M, Dumanovsky T. *How We Work: Trends and Insights in Hospital Palliative Care*. Center to Advance Palliative Care; 2017.
7. Hui D, Bruera E. Models of palliative care delivery for patients with cancer. *J Clin Oncol*. 2020;38(9):852–865. https://doi.org/10.1200/JCO.18.02123.
8. Wang SY, Aldridge MD, Gross CP, Canavan M, Cherlin E, Bradley E. End-of-life care transition patterns of Medicare beneficiaries. *J Am Geriatr Soc*. 2017;65(7):1406–1413. https://doi.org/10.1111/jgs.14891.
9. Sullivan DR, Ganzini L, Lapidus JA, et al. Improvements in hospice utilization among patients with advanced-stage lung cancer in an integrated health care system. *Cancer*. 2018;124(2):426–433. https://doi.org/10.1002/cncr.31047.
10. Teno JM, Gozalo P, Trivedi AN, et al. Site of death, place of care, and health care transitions among US Medicare beneficiaries, 2000–2015. *JAMA*. 2018;320(3):264–271. https://doi.org/10.1001/jama.2018.8981.
11. Morrison RS, Dietrich J, Ladwig S, et al. Palliative care consultation teams cut hospital costs for Medicaid beneficiaries. *Health Aff (Millwood)*. 2011;30(3):454–463. https://doi.org/10.1377/hlthaff.2010.0929.
12. O'Connor NR, Junker P, Appel SM, Stetson RL, Rohrbach J, Meghani SH. Palliative care consultation for goals of care and future acute care costs: a propensity-matched study. *Am J Hosp Palliat Med*. 2018;35(7):966–971. https://doi.org/10.1177/1049909117743475.
13. Horton JR, Morrison RS, Capezuti E, Hill J, Lee EJ, Kelley AS. Impact of inpatient palliative care on treatment intensity for patients with serious illness. *J Palliat Med*. 2016;19(9):936–942. https://doi.org/10.1089/jpm.2015.0240.
14. Joint Commission. Palliative Care Certification. Accessed July 24, 2023, https://www.jointcommission.org/what-we-offer/certification/certifications-by-setting/hospital-certifications/palliative-care-certification/.
15. Quill TE, Abernethy AP. Generalist plus specialist palliative care—creating a more sustainable model. *N Engl J Med*. 2013;368(13):1173–1175. https://doi.org/10.1056/nejmp1215620.
16. Dalal S, Bruera E. End-of-life care matters: palliative cancer care results in better care and lower costs. *Oncologist*. 2017;22(4):361–368. https://doi.org/10.1634/theoncologist.2016-0277.
17. Berendt J, Stiel S, Simon ST, et al. Integrating palliative care into comprehensive cancer centers: consensus-based development of best practice recommendations. *Oncologist*. 2016;21(10):1241–1249. https://doi.org/10.1634/theoncologist.2016-0063.
18. Kamal AH, Bowman B, Ritchie CS. Identifying palliative care champions to promote high-quality care to those with serious illness. *J Am Geriatr Soc*. 2019;67(suppl 2):S461–S467. https://doi.org/10.1111/jgs.15799.
19. Center to Advance Palliative Care. *Policies and Tools for Hospital Palliative Care Programs: A Crosswalk of National Quality Forum Preferred Practices*. Center to Advance Palliative Care; 2017. https://media.capc.org/filer_public/88/06/8806cedd-f78a-4d14-a90e-aca688147a18/nqfcrosswalk.pdf.
20. Zhang H, Barysauskas C, Rickerson E, et al. The intensive palliative care unit: changing outcomes for hospitalized cancer patients in an academic medical center. *J Palliat Med*. 2017;20(3):285–289. https://doi.org/10.1089/jpm.2016.0225.
21. Lazenby M. *Caring Matters Most*. Oxford University Press; 2017.
22. Lynch M, Dahlin C, Hultman T, Coakley EE. Palliative care nursing: defining the discipline? *J Hosp Palliat Nurs*. 2011;13(2):106–111. https://doi.org/10.1097/NJH.0b013e3182075b6e.

23. Sekse RJT, Hunskår I, Ellingsen S. The nurse's role in palliative care: a qualitative meta-synthesis. *J Clin Nurs*. 2018;27(1–2):e21–e38. https://doi.org/10.1111/jocn.13912
24. Hospice & Palliative Nurses Association. *Value Statement: Value of Professional Nurse in Palliative Care*. HPNA, 2023. https://www.advancingexpertcare.org/sdc_download/7487/?key=nfd7zgp2owvtl6myaez6hkczm1w94u
25. Coyle N, Kirk TW. Advocacy in palliative nursing. In: Ferrell BR, Paice JA, eds. *Oxford Textbook of Palliative Nursing*. 5th ed. Oxford University Press; 2019:861–876.
26. Fliedner M, Halfens RJG, King CR, Eychmueller S, Lohrmann C, Schols J. Roles and responsibilities of nurses in advance care planning in palliative care in the acute care setting: a scoping review. *J Hosp Palliat Nurs*. 2021;23(1):59–68. https://doi.org/10.1097/NJH.0000000000000715.
27. Hospice & Palliative Nurses Association. Position Statement: Palliative Nursing Leadership. HPNA, 2015. www.advancingexpertcare.org
28. Drach LL, Cook M, Shields S, Burger KJ. Changing the culture of pediatric palliative care at the bedside. *J Hosp Palliat Nurs*. 2021;23(1):20–27. https://doi.org/10.1097/njh.0000000000000707.
29. Witkamp FE, van Zuylen L, van der Rijt CC, van der Heide A. Effect of palliative care nurse champions on the quality of dying in the hospital according to bereaved relatives: a controlled before-and-after study. *Palliat Med*. 2016;30(2):180–188. https://doi.org/10.1177/0269216315588008.
30. Neiman T. Acute care nurses' experiences of basic palliative care. *J Hosp Palliat Nurs*. 2020;22(2):101–107. https://doi.org/10.1097/njh.0000000000000622.
31. National Consensus Project for Quality Palliative Care. *Clinical Practice Guidelines for Quality Palliative Care*. National Coalition for Hospice and Palliative Care; 2018. https://www.nationalcoalitionhpc.org/ncp.
32. Periyakoil VS, von Gunten CF, Bowman B, Emanuel E, Smith TJ. Incentives for palliative care. *J Palliat Med*. 2022;25(7):1024–1030. https://doi.org/10.1089/jpm.2022.0280.
33. Heitner R, Rogers M, Silvers A, Courtright KR, Meier DE. Palliative care team perceptions of standardized palliative care referral criteria implementation in hospital settings. *J Palliat Med*. 2021;24(5):747–750. https://doi.org/10.1089/jpm.2020.0296.
34. Courtright KR, Chivers C, Becker M, et al. Electronic health record mortality prediction model for targeted palliative care among hospitalized medical patients: a pilot quasi-experimental study. *J Gen Intern Med*. 2019;34(9):1841–1847. https://doi.org/10.1007/s11606-019-05169-2.
35. Ehrman S, Lockwood B, Russell D, Bickley M, Myers S, Radwany S. Impact of referring team characteristics on inpatient palliative care consultation rate at a comprehensive cancer center. *J Palliat Med*. 2022;25(9):1413–1417. https://doi.org/10.1089/jpm.2022.0088.
36. Palmer JA, Sullivan JL, Wachterman MW, Sager ZS, Wiener RS. "If you built it, they could come": opportunities to expand access to palliative care. *J Palliat Med*. 2022;25(2):200–204. https://doi.org/10.1089/jpm.2021.0109.
37. Kamal AH, Wolf SP, Troy J, et al. Policy changes key to promoting sustainability and growth of the specialty palliative care workforce. *Health Aff (Millwood)*. 2019;38(6):910–918. https://doi.org/10.1377/hlthaff.2019.00018.
38. Back AL, Fromme EK, Meier DE. Training clinicians with communication skills needed to match medical treatments to patient values. *J Am Geriatr Soc*. 2019;67(suppl 2):S435–S441. https://doi.org/10.1111/jgs.15709.
39. Weissman DE, Meier DE. Identifying patients in need of a palliative care assessment in the hospital setting: a consensus report from the Center to Advance Palliative Care. *J Palliat Med*. 2011;14(1):17–23. https://doi.org/10.1089/jpm.2010.0347.
40. Chang YK, Allen LA, McClung JA, et al. Criteria for referral of patients with advanced heart failure for specialized palliative care. *J Am Coll Cardiol*. 2022;80(4):332–344. https://doi.org/10.1016/j.jacc.2022.04.057.
41. Bange EM, Courtright KR, Parikh RB. Implementing automated prognostic models to inform palliative care: more than just the algorithm. *BMJ Qual Saf*. 2021;30(10):775–778. https://doi.org/10.1136/bmjqs-2021-013510.
42. CAPC. BRIEFING: Key Findings on the Perceptions of Palliative Care. Webinar. August 8, 2019. https://www.capc.org/events/recorded-webinars/briefing-key-findings-perceptions-palliative-care/.
43. Enguidanos S, Storms AD, Lomeli S, van Zyl C. Improving palliative care knowledge among hospitalized Hispanic patients: a pilot study. *J Palliat Med*. 2022;25(8):1179–1185. https://doi.org/10.1089/jpm.2021.0559.
44. Arnold RM, Weissman DE. Broaching the topic of a palliative care consultation with patients and families #42. *J Palliat Med*. 2004;7(3):472–3. https://doi.org/10.1089/1096621041349365.
45. Webber C, Isenberg SR, Scott M, et al. Inpatient palliative care is associated with the receipt of palliative care in the community after hospital discharge: a retrospective cohort study. *J Palliat Med*. 2022;25(6):897–906. https://doi.org/10.1089/jpm.2021.0496.
46. Ferrell BR, Temel JS, Temin S, et al. Integration of palliative care into standard oncology care: American Society of Clinical Oncology clinical practice guideline update. *J Clin Oncol*. 2017;35(1):96–112. https://doi.org/10.1200/JCO.2016.70.1474.
47. Temel JS, Greer JA, Muzikansky A, et al. Early palliative care for patients with metastatic non-small-cell lung cancer. *N Engl J Med*. 2010;363(8):733–742. https://doi.org/10.1056/nejmoa1000678.
48. Hui D, Anderson L, Tang M, Park M, Liu D, Bruera E. Examination of referral criteria for outpatient palliative care among patients with advanced cancer. *Support Care Cancer*. 2020;28(1):295–301. https://doi.org/10.1007/s00520-019-04811-3.
49. Dahlin C, DePace N, Ford J, Maani-Fogelman P, Chow K. Promoting health equity: palliative nurses on the frontlines. *J Hosp Palliat Nurs*. 2022;24(4):218–224. https://doi.org/10.1097/NJH.0000000000000864.

65

The Intensive Care Unit

Jennifer McAdam, Céline Gélinas, and Kathleen Turner

Key Points

- All intensive care unit (ICU) patients deserve palliative care, whether the goal is cure or a peaceful end of life.
- Symptom assessment and management, although challenging in an ICU setting, are primary roles and contributions of the ICU nurse.
- Conducting family meetings early in the ICU stay, establishing goals of care, and helping patients and families with decision-making are important aspects of quality palliative and end-of-life care.
- Optimal family care occurs at any point along the patient's illness trajectory by providing access, information, support, and involvement in caregiving activities.
- Caring for the ICU healthcare professional is essential to prevent moral distress and burnout.

Introduction

An intensive care unit (ICU) is the setting in which the most aggressive care is rendered to hospitalized patients. However, many patients die in ICUs. It is estimated that greater than 500,000 people die after admission to ICUs in the United States each year.[1] In a recent study, researchers reported that one-third of ICU deaths occurred within the first 24 hours of admission.[2] Investigators comparing Medicare beneficiaries' places of care and sites of death reported that 29% of older adults were admitted to the ICU in the last 30 days of their life.[3] In addition, more than 60% of critically ill advanced cancer patients do not survive their ICU stay.[4] Therefore, it is clear that management of the process of dying is common in ICUs.

In the high-technology environment of an ICU, it may be difficult for healthcare professionals and families of dying patients to acknowledge that there are limits to the effectiveness of medical care. However, it is important to focus on providing the type of care that is appropriate for the individual patient and the patient's family. This chapter discusses the provision of palliative care in ICUs, with an emphasis on end-of-life care. Specifically, challenges and barriers to providing such care in ICUs are described, and recommendations are offered for the provision of symptom assessment and management. Current issues related to holding family meetings, establishing patient goals of care, surrogate decision-making, and withholding and withdrawing life-sustaining therapies (LSTs) are covered. Recommendations are offered for attending to the needs of families as well as healthcare providers who care for ICU patients at the end of life. Finally, an unfolding case scenario is utilized to highlight key points (see Case Study Parts 1–5).

Case Study Part 1

Ms. S had spent many years as a nurse providing primary care to underserved communities. When she retired, she and her husband moved near the ocean, where they spent their time swimming, hiking, and walking their dog. Then one day, Ms. S was diagnosed with multiple myeloma, and everything changed. Her days were now spent going from appointment to appointment. During her treatment, she received several courses of chemotherapy. Unfortunately, this resulted in cardiomyopathy and renal failure. As her disease progressed, she continued to pursue aggressive treatment where she received plasmapheresis and hemodialysis in hopes of the possibility of a stem cell transplant. However, her treatment plan was not working, and she was admitted to the ICU with hypotension, fatigue, dyspnea, worsening nausea, edema, and decreased urine output.

The Limitations of End-of-Life Care in ICUs

The ICU is rarely a place that one would choose to die.[5] Healthcare professionals in ICUs, frequently uncertain about whether a patient will live or die, are caught between the opposing goals of preserving life and preparing the patient and family for death. It is important for professionals to realize that a patient's death is not necessarily an indication of ineffective care. Yet, there remain serious limitations to the care provided to seriously ill and dying patients and their families. Communication between physicians, patients, and families may be poor[6]; patients and families may be overly optimistic about the outcomes of cardiopulmonary resuscitation (CPR)[7] and have unrealistic expectations of ICU technological treatments[8]; end-of-life decision-making can be challenging and present conflicts[6,9]; and many hospitalized patients die in moderate to severe pain and with other troubling symptoms.[10,11]

Planning Palliative Care for ICU Patients

Providing comfort to patients should accompany all ICU care, even during aggressive attempts to prolong life. However, if a patient is not expected to survive, the focus shifts to an emphasis on palliative care. A transition period occurs during which healthcare professionals, the patient's family, and sometimes the patient recognize the appropriateness of withdrawing and/or withholding LSTs and begin to make preparations for death. The transition period may be a matter of minutes or hours, or it may be a matter of weeks. Clearly, this time difference must be recognized as a factor that can influence the experience of a patient's family. When patients rapidly approach death, their families may not have time to adjust to the possibility of death. On the other hand, when death is prolonged, family frustration and fatigue may be part of their experience. Healthcare professionals who are sensitive to these different experiences can individualize their approaches and interventions for families.

The transition from aggressive care to death preparation has not been well operationalized. The transition period may be uncomfortable for many healthcare professionals because clinically useful prediction models recognizing which patients have the highest risk of death in the ICU remain elusive.[12] Therefore, it is important for healthcare professionals to integrate palliative care principles early in the patient's ICU stay. The use of palliative care triggers and protocols is associated with higher transitions to do-not-resuscitate orders, an increase in referrals to hospice care, and decreased ICU resource utilization.[13] In addition, palliative care consultations reduced ICU length of stay and costs without impacting mortality.[14] Of equal importance is holding regular patient and family meetings for the purposes of orientating and informing the family to establish trust, establishing goals of care for the patient, and for closure and transition from the ICU.[15]

Case Study Part 2

During her ICU stay, Ms. S had difficulty moving her legs, was unable to eat, and reported significant dyspnea. During hemodialysis, she became acutely hypotensive. The dialysis was stopped, and she was started on continuous renal replacement therapy (CRRT) to correct her electrolyte imbalances while preventing further fluid buildup. She also reported severe pain in her back and legs, uncontrolled nausea and vomiting, and dyspnea. She was miserable but wanted to keep going for her family. The ICU nurse knew it was time to engage the specialized palliative care team.

Symptom Assessment and Management: Essential Components of Palliative Care

Pain Assessment

In spite of advances in pain assessment and management techniques, hospitalized patients continue to receive inadequate pain management.[11] Pain research focusing specifically on dying ICU patients remains scarce, but advances that have been made in the assessment of pain in critically ill patients can be applied to dying patients.[16,17] The patient's report of pain is still considered to be the most valid source. ICU patients, even if they are being mechanically ventilated, may be able to use simple numeric or word rating scales, word quality scales, and body outline diagrams. A 0–10 visually enlarged, numeric rating scale was found to be the most valid and feasible of five pain intensity rating scales.[16]

Many critically ill patients are unable to self-report because of their disease process, technological treatment interventions, or the effects of medications. For example, the use of high doses of benzodiazepine (BZD) or anesthetic (propofol) infusions may make patients too sedated to respond to pain, although pain may still be present. On the other hand, the use of neuromuscular blocking agents such as vecuronium may limit or entirely mask the patient's ability to express or show any behavioral signs of pain. It is essential that clinicians understand that these medications have no analgesic properties, although visible signs of pain disappear during their use. If these agents are used, they must be accompanied by infusions of analgesics, sedatives, or both.[18] In addition, nurses can elicit the assistance of the patient's family to help assess the patient's pain if they feel comfortable doing so.[19]

When patients are too ill to communicate their pain through self-report, behavioral scales are recommended as alternative measures of pain.[10,20] According to a systematic review, the Critical-Care Pain Observation Tool (CPOT) and the Behavioral Pain Scale (BPS), available in 15 to 20 languages, have sound psychometrics[21] and are recommended for pain assessment of critically ill adults unable to self-report by the Society of Critical Care Medicine.[10] A BPS version is also available for non-intubated patients (BPS-NI) in which a vocalization item can be used instead of compliance with mechanical ventilation.[22] Another tool, the Behavior Pain Assessment Tool (BPAT), underwent validation at the international level with translation in 12 languages and testing in 3,851 ICU patients from 28 countries. Its feasibility for use in daily practice continues to be investigated.[23]

Behavioral scales are not applicable in unresponsive patients. In such a situation, no other alternative measures of pain are available. Vital signs are not valid indicators of pain[10,20]; however, recent evidence has shown that they could be considered as adverse events of severe pain.[24] Exploration of other physiologic measures (e.g., pupil dilation reflex) and novel technologies is needed to provide nurses with alternative tools to use in the pain assessment process of this vulnerable population.[25] Another strategy nurses can use is to identify possible sources of pain by asking the question, "Does this patient present a condition that is associated with pain or require care procedures that are known to be painful?" Even if patients are not exhibiting behavioral or physiological signs of pain, it does not mean that they are pain-free.[20]

Procedural Pain

Critically ill patients undergo many diagnostic, treatment, and care procedures. Many of these may be unnecessary, and some procedures, such as central line placements, chest tube removal, and endotracheal suctioning, are quite painful and may be the primary cause of suffering at the end of life.[26] Nurses can act as "gatekeepers" by evaluating the appropriateness of procedures being planned for patients, especially after a decision has been made to withdraw LST; and they can advocate for their omission. Practice guidelines recommend that anticipating and treating pain be part of procedural instructions.[27]

Pharmacological Management of Pain

Numerous categories of analgesics and types of modalities exist for administration to critically ill patients.[28] As in all situations, the selection of analgesics should depend on the specific pain mechanism, and the route and modality should be matched to their predictability of effectiveness. Although no comprehensive survey of pain management techniques used for dying ICU patients has been reported, the most common analgesic intervention is use of intravenous (IV) opioids.[28] Choosing the best opioid and method of delivery will depend on factors such as the patient's body composition (e.g., amount of adipose tissue), development of tolerance, and the adverse effect profiles of the various opioids (see Chapter 11, "Pain Management").[28] Use of a continuous infusion of an opioid allows for titration of the drug to a level of analgesic effectiveness and for maintenance of steady plasma levels within a therapeutic range. Additionally, healthcare professionals may consider the administration of intermittent opioid boluses for breakthrough pain. Table 65.1 provides information on opioids commonly used in the ICU setting.[28]

Concerns about patients becoming tolerant of or dependent on opioids are misplaced during terminal care. What is important is that professionals recognize the development of tolerance, which is the need for larger doses of opioid analgesics to achieve the original effect,[29] and increase the dosage as necessary. There is no ceiling effect from opioids; the dose can be increased until the desired effect is reached or intolerable side effects develop. Opioid-dependent patients are at high risk of developing withdrawal symptoms,[29,30] which would seriously increase their discomfort. In this situation, physical dependence can be addressed by gradually lowering the opioid dose while carefully assessing for signs of pain or withdrawal.[30]

Titration of analgesics to achieve the desired effect is one of the most challenging and important contributions that ICU nurses can make to the comfort care of dying patients. The desired effect can often be described as use of the least amount of medication necessary to achieve the greatest comfort along with the optimum level of tranquil awareness. In ICU settings, there may be concerns that administration of analgesics in the amounts necessary to provide comfort could "cause" death. It is essential that ICU health professionals understand the "double-effect" principle. In brief, the double-effect principle states that administration of analgesics to dying patients in the amounts necessary to decrease pain and suffering—although possibly causing unintentional hastening of death—is an ethically sound way to treat a dying patient.[31] When the ICU patient is approaching death, the most important aim of care should be to make the patient as comfortable as possible.

Nonpharmacological Management of Pain

Nonpharmacological interventions for pain management complement, but do not substitute for, the use of pharmacological interventions. Numerous therapies are available to promote patient comfort, and many of these therapies are low-cost, safe, and easy to implement. Among these, ice therapy, music, massage, and relaxation techniques (e.g., deep breathing) have been suggested for ICU pain management.[10] In addition, if they feel comfortable doing so, family members should be encouraged to participate in pain management and in the delivery of nonpharmacological interventions.[19]

Anxiety, Agitation, and Sedation

An important part of palliative care in the ICU is assessment and treatment of anxiety and agitation (see Chapter 24, "Anxiety and Depression"). Simple numeric rating scales for anxiety can be used if the patient can self-report.[11] Healthcare professionals and patients are familiar with the use of the 0 to 10 numeric rating scales

Table 65.1 Pharmacology of commonly used opioids in the intensive care unit

Agent	Equianalgesic dose (mg)		Onset	Half-life	Intermittent dose	Infusion dose range	Active metabolites	Unique concerns[a]
	IV	oral						
Fentanyl	0.1	N/A	1–2 min	2–4 h	0.35–0.5 µg/kg IV every 0.5–1 h	0.7–10 µg/kg/h	No metabolite, parent accumulates in fatty tissues	Less hypotension than morphine Accumulation in hepatic impairment Muscle rigidity
Hydromorphone	1.5	7.5	5–10 min	2–3 h	0.2–0.6 mg IV every 1–2 h	0.5–3 mg/h	None	May work in patients tolerant to morphine or fentanyl Accumulation in hepatic/renal impairment
Morphine	10	30	5–10 min	3–4 h	2–4 mg IV every 1–2 h	2–30 mg/h	6- and 3-glucuronide metabolite	Bradycardia/hypotension Bronchospasm Accumulation in hepatic/renal impairment
Remifentanil	N/A	N/A	1–3 min	3–10 min	N/A	1.5 µg/kg loading dose, then 0.5–15 µg/kg/h	None	Bradycardia/hypotension No accumulation in hepatic/renal failure Use IBW if >30% IBW

IBW, ideal body weight; IV, intravenous; N/A, not applicable.

[a] Common adverse effects associated with all opioids, such as respiratory and central nervous system depression, are not listed.

Source: Reference 28.

for pain. "Anxiety" word anchors can be substituted for "pain" word anchors so that the numeric rating scales also can be used to quantify the degree of anxiety. Unfortunately, no tool is available to assess anxiety in patients unable to self-report. However, common behavioral or physiological signs of anxiety include trembling, restlessness, sweating, tachycardia, tachypnea, difficulty sleeping, and irritability.[32]

Several agitation/sedation assessment scales are available. It is recommended to use validated scales (e.g., the Richmond Agitation Sedation Scale (RASS) and Sedation Agitation Scale (SAS).[10,32,33] These scales can be printed on the patient flowsheet, on a separate form, or in the electronic medical record and used as a bedside assessment tool. The frequency with which the scales are used depends on the patient's condition and the schedule for evaluating treatment interventions.

Pharmacological Management to Promote Sedation in Anxious or Agitated Patients

Along with opioids, other categories of sedating drugs are frequently used in the ICU, especially for patients who are mechanically ventilated. Guidelines[10] exist regarding the use of analgesics and sedatives. Often, the goal of combined analgesic–sedative therapy is to promote physical and psychological comfort. Practice decisions include choosing the right type and combination of medications, determining whether to use interrupted sedative infusions or continuous infusions, determining appropriate clinical endpoints for pharmacological interventions,[10,34] and evaluating the effectiveness of sedation protocols on practices and outcomes.[35]

The appropriate pharmacological agent to control agitation and anxiety is selected according to the desired effect.[34] BZDs (e.g., midazolam, lorazepam) and non-BZDs (e.g., propofol, dexmedetomidine) are common agents for anxiolysis, but they possess no analgesic or psychological properties. Their concomitant use with opioids may relieve anxiety-provoking symptoms through a synergistic action. When used together, these drugs can be administered in lower doses less frequently, have fewer side effects, and can decrease or delay development of tolerance or dependence. At lower doses, BZDs reduce anxiety without causing central nervous system sedation or a decrease in cognitive or motor function. With increasing dosages, inhibition of motor and cognitive functions as well as central nervous system depression does occur. Sufficiently high doses can induce hypnosis and coma.[34] However, BZDs should be used cautiously in older adults as they can cause acute delirium and other serious side effects (see Chapter 71, "Palliative Care for Older Adults").

The most frequently used BZDs in critical care are midazolam and lorazepam (see Table 65.2).[16,32] Lorazepam gives effective sedation and anxiety relief over a longer period than midazolam. Cardiovascular and respiratory effects occur less frequently with this drug than with other BZDs. It may also act synergistically with haloperidol, a neuroleptic agent. As with opioids, tolerance to BZD effects can develop in critically ill patients. BZD dependence is evidenced by symptoms such as dysphoria, tremor, sweating, anxiety, agitation, muscle cramps, myoclonus, and seizures on abrupt

Table 65.2 Pharmacological symptom management

Symptom	Drug type most frequently used	Method of administration	Usual dose[a]
Pain	Opioids (e.g., morphine, fentanyl, hydrocodone, methadone)	Continuous IV infusions with use of intermittent boluses for procedure-related pain or during treatment withdrawal	Continuous infusion: 1–10 mg/h morphine equivalents
			Bolus: 2–5 mg IV morphine equivalent slow push; titrate to effect
Anxiety/ agitation	Benzodiazepines (e.g., lorazepam, midazolam)	Same as for opioids	Continuous midazolam infusion: 1–20 mg/h
			Bolus midazolam: 2–5 mg IV
			Continuous lorazepam infusion: 1–10 mg/h
			Bolus lorazepam: 2–6 mg IV every 4–6 h
	Propofol	Continuous IV infusion	Continuous: 50–150 μg/kg/min
Dyspnea	Oxygen	Multiple methods (e.g., nasal cannula, mask, ventilator)	Concentration as needed
	Opioids (e.g., morphine)	Continuous IV infusion and/or IV bolus; or per nebulizer	See above for IV doses
			Per nebulizer: 2.5 mg in 3 mL saline (preservative-free) or sterile water every 4 h
	Benzodiazepines	See above	See above
	Bronchodilators (e.g., Alupent)	Per nebulizer	Alupent: 2.5 mL 0.4%–0.6% solution
	Diuretics (e.g., Lasix)	IV bolus, slow push	Bolus Lasix: 20–40 mg IV
	Anticholinergics (e.g., atropine)	Per nebulizer	Atropine: 0.025 mg/kg diluted with 3–5 mL saline three or four times daily; doses not to exceed 2.5 mg

IV, intravenous.

[a] Drug doses are general recommendations. Dosing should be individualized to a particular patient. Under usual circumstances, start with low doses, wait for effect, and titrate to desired effect.

Sources: References 16 and 32.

medication withdrawal.[30] The use of non-BZDs is suggested over BZDs considering that they may be a risk factor in the development of ICU delirium.[34]

Propofol is a highly lipophilic IV sedative/hypnotic agent that has a very rapid onset of action and short duration (see Table 65.2). It is indicated for use in the ICU to control agitation and the stress response in patients who are mechanically ventilated and those who require deep sedation for procedures.[10,34] During initial use of propofol, a drop in systolic blood pressure, mean arterial blood pressure, and heart rate may occur in patients with fluid deficits and in those receiving opioids.[34] The short effective half-life of propofol allows rapid clinical evaluation of the patient's level of consciousness and determination of the minimum dose required for effective sedation. This may make it a useful drug during situations in which intermittent interaction with professionals and families is desired.

Dexmedetomidine is a potent, centrally acting alpha 2-adrenergic agonist that can be used for ICU patients requiring light sedation.[36] Even though this medication does have analgesic properties, most patients will require additional opioids for pain management.[36] Continuous infusions of dexmedetomidine have been associated with bradycardia and hypotension, whereas frequent bolus doses have been associated with hypertension. Due to side effects occurring from rapid bolus dosing, it may not be the preferred choice for patients with acute agitation.[36] In addition, because this medication is metabolized by the liver, it should be used with caution in those with liver disease.[36] Current pain, agitation, and delirium guidelines suggest the use of non-BZD sedatives, such as propofol and dexmedetomidine, as the preferred choice for sedation medications.[10]

It is important that patients in ICUs be routinely assessed for the presence of delirium using validated tools such as the Intensive Care Delirium Screening Checklist (ICDSC) or the Confusion Assessment Method for ICU (CAM-ICU).[11,32,33,37] Haloperidol and other antipsychotic medications are no longer recommended to treat delirium as the risks related to their use outweigh their potential benefits. A multicomponent, nonpharmacological approach is suggested (see Chapter 23, "Acute Delirium"). This approach may include several interventions aimed at reducing modifiable risk factors for delirium such as reorientating the patient and optimizing sleep, mobility, hearing, and vision.[32]

Nonpharmacological Interventions for Anxiety and Agitation

Numerous interventions exist that may promote tranquillity and comfort in a critical care environment. In a recent systematic review, listening to music was associated with reduced anxiety and stress as well as improved sleep quality.[38] The act of physically caring for a patient and providing gentle touch is a major source of comfort for patients in critical care. Taking the time to provide simple measures such as back rubs and massages, repositioning the patient, and providing mouth and eye care promotes comfort and decreases anxiety. For alert patients, increasing opportunities for control is a strategy that can reduce the sense of helplessness that often accompanies patients who are critically ill. Finally, facilitating communication with clergy, psychologists, or psychiatrists, if appropriate, can help to alleviate the distress experienced by both patients and families.

Dyspnea Assessment and Management

Dyspnea is a subjective experience of feeling short of breath and is one of the most distressing symptoms that can be experienced by critically ill patients at high risk for dying.[32] The gold standard for assessing dyspnea is patient self-report. A 0–10 numeric rating scale can also be used to establish the intensity of dyspnea.[39] However, most critical care patients at high risk of dying cannot self-report and give a yes or no answer.[39] In this case, the Respiratory Distress Observation Scale (RDOS) is the only known tool to assess dyspnea in these patients.[16,32,39] Management of dyspnea in patients at high risk of dying includes oxygen therapy, opioids, BZDs, bronchodilators, diuretics, and anticholinergics (see Table 65.2 and Chapter 12, "Dyspnea and Cough").[16,32]

Other Distressing Symptoms

Puntillo and colleagues[11] are among the few investigators studying the self-reported symptom experiences of ICU patients at high risk of dying. These investigators used a 10-item symptom checklist measuring both the intensity and distress of symptoms such as pain, fatigue, shortness of breath, restlessness, anxiety, sadness, hunger, fear, thirst, and confusion. The most prevalent symptoms included fatigue (75%), thirst (71%), and anxiety (56%). Symptoms lower in prevalence but reported to be moderately distressful by patients included shortness of breath, pain, confusion, fear, and sadness. This study demonstrated that a significant proportion of patients at high risk of dying in ICUs experience substantial emotional and physical symptoms. Because nurses are constantly at the bedside, they can assess the presence of the multitude of symptoms patients experience, advocate for effective pharmacological therapy, use additional nursing comfort measures, and provide for continuity of therapy. Symptom management is a special contribution that ICU nurses can make to their patients at the end of life.

Case Study Part 3

The palliative care team worked with Ms. S and determined that her pain appeared to have three main components: bone pain from a lesion in her spine, neuropathic pain emanating from her low back into all extremities, and discomfort due to edema now extending to her pelvis. Ms S. discussed with the palliative care team that she did not want IV medications. Using this information, their recommendation was to start daily methadone, with oxycodone for breakthrough pain. Dexamethasone was also added as adjunctive therapy. For her uncontrolled nausea, the team started around-the-clock haloperidol, with sublingual lorazepam available for breakthrough nausea and vomiting. The dexamethasone was expected to help with her nausea as well. For her dyspnea, oxygen via nasal cannula was continued. Ms. S finally started to feel in control of her care and was relieved to have a plan that may help ameliorate her symptoms.

End-of-Life Practice Issues: Withholding and Withdrawing LSTs

Withholding or withdrawing LSTs in the ICU is common and generally occurs when death is believed to be inevitable despite aggressive interventions. The American College of Physicians[40] supports the right of a competent patient to refuse LSTs. It also notes that there is no moral difference between withholding and withdrawing therapy. In addition, critical care–related professional organizations support patient autonomy regarding withholding and withdrawal decisions.[41,42]

If patients are unable to make treatment decisions, then these decisions must be made on the patient's behalf by surrogates or by the healthcare team.[43] When surrogates are asked to participate in decision-making, the recommendation is that the meeting is interdisciplinary[9] and family-centered[44] and that a shared decision-making approach is used.[43] This approach allows families to arrive at decisions about the patient's goals of care and may help reduce the burden and distress they experience during this time.[6] Because problems with decision-making and communication around end-of-life care are still frequent sources of conflict in the ICU,[6,9] having a guideline to follow for conducting family meetings may be helpful (see Box 65.1 and Chapter 5, "Palliative Nursing Communication").[6,9,15,45]

Box 65.1 Useful Guidelines in Conducting Intensive Care Unit Family Meetings

Plan and Prepare

- Review the patient history, medical problems, and treatment plan to date.
- Coordinate who on the healthcare team will attend the meeting (should be interdisciplinary and include the attending physician, bedside registered nurse, social worker, palliative care clinician[s], and other relevant healthcare team members).
- Discuss goals of the meeting with the healthcare team, confirm understanding of the plan of care, anticipate conflicts and challenges beforehand.
- Identify one team member as meeting leader.
- Discuss which families will be present.
- Arrange a private, quiet location with seating for all.

Open the Meeting

- Introduce all in attendance.
- Provide a succinct summary in easy-to-understand language and allow families the opportunity to correct or provide missing information.
- Establish the overall goal of the meeting and elicit family goals.
- Acknowledge that this is a difficult time and situation.
- Set rules for the discussion (e.g., time frame for the meeting).

Elicit Family Understanding

- Ask questions of families and listen.
- As they respond, think about questions, such as What do they understand? What do they believe will happen? What are their emotions?

Identify Preferences for Decision-Making and Information-Sharing

- Identify how families prefer to receive information and the level of detail they would like to receive.
- Assess the family's preference for their role in decision-making (this can range from letting the physician decide to the family member assuming all responsibility for the decision).

Give Information

- Give brief information (e.g., two points you really want them to understand) and allow time for family to ask questions.
- Avoid medical jargon and try not to talk too much or focus on technical matters.
- Be transparent about uncertainty.
- If the patient is dying, be sure to use the word "death" or "dying."

Respond with Explicit Empathy to Family Emotions

- Don't fight but rather join family statements of hopefulness, using wish statements (e.g., "I wish I could promise that things would get better. I hope he gets better soon too.").
- See if the family can hope for the best but prepare for the worst.
- Use helpful mnemonics:
  - VALUE
    - Value and appreciate what the family has said.
    - Acknowledge family emotions.
    - Listen to the family.
    - Understand the patient as a person through the family.
    - Elicit family's concerns and questions.
  - NURSE
    - Name: "You seem distressed (or angry or worried, etc.)."
    - Understand: "This must be very difficult for you."
    - Respect: "I can see how much you are trying to honor your dad's wishes."
    - Support: "We will be there to help advise you."
    - Explore: "Tell me more about what you are thinking/feeling."
  - Ask-Tell-Ask
    - Ask—the family to explain the situation in their own language
    - Tell—the family the information the team needs to communicate (focus on one or two key points)
    - Ask—check for understanding, "What questions do you have?"

After Giving Information, Ask about Concerns and Questions

- "You just got a lot of information. What questions do you have?"

Elicit Patient and Family Values and Goals

- Ask about the patient's goals, values, and previous discussion about end-of-life care.
- Frame those wishes within the context of the current medical situation.
- Avoid asking family, "What do you think we should do?" Instead, ask what they know about their loved one's preferences and maintain focus on the patient's perspective.
- Identify pertinent cultural, ethnic, or religious beliefs that may influence communication, decision-making, family relationships, and concepts of death and dying.

Deal with Decisions That Need to Be Made

- Make a recommendation based on patient and family goals.
- Time-limited trials with clear endpoints may make sense in certain clinical situations.
- Do not offer treatments that are inappropriate, as when the burdens outweigh the benefits.
- Do not speak of "withdrawing care" or "treatment." Affirm ongoing quality of care and reassure the family that care will never be withdrawn but that the focus of care may change.

Close the Meeting

- Offer a brief summary of what was discussed.
- Offer to answer questions and assure the family that the team is accessible.
- Check in to make sure the family heard what you wanted them to hear.
- Express appreciation and respect for the family.
- Facilitate referrals to support services.

Sources: References 6, 9, 15, and 45.

When a decision to forgo LST is made in the ICU, there should be a concerted effort to evaluate all therapies to assess whether these treatments could make a positive contribution to the patient's comfort. Withdrawal of therapies should be preceded by chart notations of do-not-resuscitate orders and a note documenting the rationale for comfort care and removal of life support.[42] There should be a clear plan of action and provision of information and support to the family.[46] Adequate documentation of patient assessments, withdrawal decisions and plans, therapy withdrawal orders, and patient and family responses during and after withdrawal is essential.[46]

Withdrawal of Ventilator Therapy with Consideration of Analgesic and Sedative Needs

Withdrawal of mechanical ventilation deserves the same clinical preparation as any other ICU procedure.[47] The primary goal during this process should be to ensure that patients and families are as comfortable as possible, both psychologically and physically.[47] Although there is considerable variability regarding the preferred approach to withdrawal, recommendations regarding specific procedures are available.[33] Box 65.2 presents a protocol for withdrawal of mechanical ventilation for the clinician's consideration that includes specific recommendations regarding use of analgesics and sedatives.[32,33,48]

Regardless of the processes used to withdraw LSTs, the critical care nurse plays a major role during the decision and implementation of withdrawal of patients from mechanical ventilation. Specifically, the nurse can be an active member at family meetings where patient prognosis and goals of care are discussed.[9] In addition, the nurse can ensure that a rationale for, and all elements of, the plan have been adequately discussed among the team, patient, and family.[46] The nurse can ensure that adequate time is given to families and their support persons, such as clergy, to reach as good a resolution as possible.[6,9] The family needs reassurance that they and the patient will not be abandoned and that the patient will be kept comfortable with the use of medications and other measures.[46]

Case Study Part 4

One evening, Ms. S revealed to her nurse that she had made all the treatment decisions more for her loved ones than for herself. The nurse sat with Ms. S and listened to her as she talked about her dreams where she could walk in the hills near her home, shop at her local farmer's market, and have boisterous family dinners. She told the nurse she wanted to return home for her last days. Her nurse discussed this with the ICU resident, and a family meeting was initiated for the next day. The nurse prepared Ms. S for the interdisciplinary family meeting and helped her think about the goals she wanted for her remaining time.

Box 65.2 A Protocol for the Withdrawal of Mechanical Ventilation

I. Plan, anticipate, and prevent
   A. Decide on either immediate extubation (i.e., abrupt removal of the patient from ventilator assistance) or terminal weaning (i.e., gradual withdrawal of ventilator assistance). Both have positives and negatives, but immediate extubation is preferable.
   B. Inform and review process in advance with patient (if awake), family, and the healthcare team. Identify goals during withdrawal (e.g., ability to communicate vs. sedation). Arrange a time that allows the family to be present, if they wish, along with a private room if possible. Provide for any special needs (e.g., clergy, bereavement counselor).
   C. Assess and manage distress (e.g., respiratory, pain, agitation, and delirium). Use opioids and/or benzodiazepines[a] to control respiratory distress (i.e., increased respiratory rate, use of accessory muscles, nasal flaring, increase in heart rate or blood pressure, grimacing, clutching). In patients already receiving these agents, dosing should be guided by the current dose.
   D. Discontinue therapies not directed toward patient comfort:
      1. Stop neuromuscular blockade agents (NMBAs) after opioids and/or benzodiazepines have been started or increased.[b] The use of NMBAs makes it almost impossible to assess patient comfort; although the patient appears comfortable, they may be experiencing pain, respiratory distress, or severe anxiety.
      2. Discontinue laboratory tests, radiographs, vital signs. Remove any unnecessary tubes and restraints, silence alarms, and disconnect monitors.

II. Optimize existing function
   A. Administer breathing treatment, if indicated.
   B. Suction out the mouth and hypopharynx. Endotracheal suctioning before withdrawal may or may not be advisable depending on patient distress and family perception. There are no standard recommendations on the routine use of anticholinergic medications (e.g., atropine, scopolamine) for excessive secretions. The use of these medications is individualized for each patient.
   C. Place the patient at least 30 degrees upright, if possible.

III. Discontinuation of ventilation[c]
   A. In general, the sequence and process should be individualized for each patient with comfort as the main goal.
   B. Mechanical ventilation should be withdrawn quickly with the goal to extubate to room air.
   C. Constant re-evaluation for distress is mandatory. A physician and nurse should be present during and immediately after extubation to assess the patient and to titrate medications. Treat distress with additional bolus doses of opioids and/or benzodiazepines as appropriate.
   D. Consider inhaled epinephrine for post-extubation stridor in conscious patients.

[a] Drug doses are difficult to specify because of the enormous variability in body weight and composition, previous exposure, and tolerance. Opioid-naive patients can be started on a bolus of 2 mg intravenous morphine titrated to effect. Patients receiving a continuous infusion of morphine can receive a bolus dose of 2 times the hourly infusion rate every 15 minutes. Patients receiving a continuous infusion of fentanyl can receive a bolus dose equal to the hourly infusion rate every 5 minutes as needed. If a patient receives two bolus doses in an hour of either morphine or fentanyl, it is reasonable to double the infusion rate. Sedatives should be used only after pain and dyspnea are treated. Benzodiazepine-naive patients can receive 2 mg intravenous midazolam, followed by a 1-mg/hour infusion. Patients receiving a continuous infusion of midazolam can receive a bolus dose of 1–2 times the hourly infusion rate and every 5 minutes as needed. If a patient receives two bolus doses in an hour, it is reasonable to double the infusion rate. Propofol can be used as an alternative to benzodiazepines.

[b] Usually the effects of NMBAs can be reversed within a short period, but it may take days to weeks if patients have been receiving NMBAs chronically for management of ventilatory failure. Neuromuscular blockade masks signs of discomfort. Therefore, clinicians should feel that the patient has regained sufficient motor activity to demonstrate discomfort.

[c] There is no one sequence applicable to all patients because their clinical situations are so variable. The pace of changes depends on patient comfort and may proceed as quickly as 5–15 minutes or, in an awake patient to be extubated, over several hours.

Sources: References 32, 33, and 48.

At the family meeting, the team explained that there were no further curative therapies available for Ms. S. They offered that the care should be refocused on maximizing comfort and quality of life. Ms. S shared her wish to not pursue any further aggressive treatment. At her instruction, a "do-not-resuscitate-or-intubate" order was placed in her chart. When asked about her goals, Ms. S discussed the following:

- Remove enough edema to allow her to walk
- Keep her pain and nausea under control
- Be able to swim near her home
- Be able to spend time with her husband and her dog
- Be able to see her second grandchild, due to be born soon

To help accomplish her goals, nephrology increased the CRRT fluid removal rate and discontinued all nonessential lab work. Her one-on-one nursing care continued—fine-tuning doses and frequencies of her pain and nausea medications so that Ms. S would have the best possible regimen on which to discharge home. She received the sacrament of healing from the visiting priest. She and the chaplain took advantage of some down time to reflect and work together on letters to her grandchildren. Ms. S shared with the team that, for the first time, she believed she would make it home.

Care for the Family of the Dying ICU Patient

Although the focus of care in the ICU is on the critically ill patient, comprehensive patient care includes care of the patient's family. A family-centered approach to care is strongly supported by evidence-based guidelines.[44] An ICU experience for families can be stressful (especially when their loved one dies in the ICU) and has been associated with symptoms of posttraumatic stress disorder, anxiety, depression, and complicated grief.[6] Caring for ICU families encompasses major aspects of access, information and support, and involvement in caregiving activities.

Access

A crucial aspect of family care is ensuring that the family can be with their critically ill loved one, especially if their loved one is dying. Historically, critical care settings have restricted family access and discouraged lengthy family visitation. However, providing open visitation is associated with improved patient outcomes (e.g., reduced frequency of delirium) and greater family satisfaction.[49] In addition, visitation of children should be considered when a loved one is dying. Visitation has the potential to help the child cope and gives the child a chance to say goodbye. If ICU clinicians account for the child's developmental status and properly prepare the child, then children can visit a critically ill family member in the ICU without ill effects.[44]

Information and Support

Information has been identified as a crucial component in family coping and satisfaction in critical care settings.[6] Support, in the form of clinicians' caring behaviors and interactions, is enormously influential in shaping the critical care experience for both patients and their families.[6] In the context of caring for a critically ill, dying patient, however, nurses and physicians alike have reported high stress related to notifying families of the patient's death or terminal prognosis.[50] In general, very few healthcare providers feel they have the skills and knowledge necessary to counsel families effectively during this emotionally charged time. However, providing education that includes didactic, practice, and affective elements can be successful in improving clinicians' skills in this area.[50]

Overall satisfaction with end-of-life care has been associated with completeness of information received by families, support and care shown to the patient and family, consistency in staff, and satisfaction with the amount or level of healthcare received.[51] Interdisciplinary family conferences have been used extensively as a means to improve communication between healthcare providers and families. Using best practices in relation to the timing, content, and participants necessary for optimal communication during a family conference has been shown to lower emotional distress for families, maintain consistency with the patient's goals and values, and achieve consistent communication throughout the ICU stay.[6] Other supportive interventions include supporting families to attend rounds and to complete ICU diaries. Both have been shown to improve family satisfaction with communication and may help lower their distress.[44]

Finally, because feelings of grief in surviving families are still commonly unresolved 6 months to 1 year after a loved one's death, many critical care units have organized bereavement programs.[52] These programs may involve providing a bereavement brochure, contacting the surviving family by telephone or mail, sending a condolence card, and holding a memorial service.[52] In addition to remembering and supporting the family, these programs have been shown to help healthcare providers cope with the loss.[52]

Involvement in Caregiving Activities

Research is limited on the effect of family caregiving on critically ill patients, yet families should have the opportunity to be helpful. Allowing family members to provide direct physical care, especially at the end of life, may help bring them peace of mind after the death and help them feel needed and useful. Family caregiving can range from minor activities (such as assisting with oral care or massaging the dying patient's feet) to major activities (assisting with postmortem care). Nurses' facilitation of family involvement in their dying loved one's care is a practical family intervention that should be more widely employed if humane and comprehensive palliative care is desired.[53]

Care for the Caregiver of the Dying ICU Patient

Numerous studies have described the tension and moral distress between the cure-oriented critical care setting and palliative care.[54] The nurse often feels caught between differing perceptions held by physicians and families concerning patient progress and treatment goals.[54] Facilitating and coordinating dialogue and consensus between these groups as well as caring for the dying patient and family can cause conflicts and can be physically and emotionally exhausting.[54] If the dying process is prolonged, the nurse can become frustrated and fatigued. Although healthcare providers often cope with this stress by emotionally disengaging themselves from the charged atmosphere, emotional distancing has been shown to hamper skill acquisition and the development of involvement skills and lead to burnout.[54] This section discusses two strategies to help healthcare providers sustain their caring practices and extend their involvement skills—sharing narratives and end-of-life education.

Sharing Narratives

Debriefing has been used effectively in many settings to discuss and process critical incidents; analyze healthcare providers' performance in terms of skill, knowledge, and efficiency; and learn, both personally and institutionally, from mistakes and system breakdown.[55] Sharing stories or narratives of practice can be used to achieve the same goals, but telling stories from practice also enables clinicians to (1) increase their skill in recognizing patient and family concerns; (2) learn to communicate more effectively with patients, families, and other healthcare providers; (3) reflect on ethical comportment and engaged clinical reasoning; and (4) articulate clinical knowledge development.[56]

End-of-Life Education

Closely coupled with sharing clinical narratives is the use of seminars and other reflective exercises aimed at preparing nurses and other healthcare providers for the care of dying patients and their families. End-of-life education often consists of didactic and experiential classes. Participants in these classes are encouraged to reflect on and share their own perceptions and anxieties about death, as well as their attitudes toward care of the dying patient and their family. This approach has been used with varying degrees of success with nurses and physicians.[57,58] Because many healthcare providers feel ill-prepared to effectively care for terminally ill patients and have also identified barriers to delivering quality end-of-life care, this strategy deserves more implementation and research[50]—mainly, educating critical care staff about palliative care (e.g., principles of shared decision-making, communication techniques, symptom management, and practices of withdrawal of life support) through lectures, workshops, pamphlets, teaching videos, simulation, and role play.[57,58]

Case Study Part 5

Later that day, the ICU teams met with Ms. S and her family. "We're ready to get her home—this is our window of opportunity," noted her family. The oncology and palliative care social workers set up home hospice referral, had durable medical equipment delivered, and located a pharmacy near the small town where the family lived. To each team member, Ms. S and her family expressed their thanks and gratitude for supporting them and helping them through this difficult journey. A little while later, Ms. S went home—to walk, swim, and relax with her dog. She died a week later, in her own bed, on her own terms.

Summary

Striving to relieve suffering from pain and other distressing symptoms and providing a dignified death is the right of all ICU patients. Research has offered some guidance for managing the issues that surround ICU patient deaths. However, Stokes and colleagues[59] present important goals to consider during an ICU patient's dying process: (1) creating a good death by facilitating comfort and being there for the patient and the family; (2) navigating the challenges that arise; and (3) making it work by building relationships, taking care of oneself, and recognizing that this type of care is both rewarding and a privilege.

REFERENCES

1. Angus DC, Barnato AE, Linde-Zwirble WT, et al. Use of intensive care at the end of life in the United States: an epidemiologic study. *Crit Care Med.* 2004;32(3):638–643.
2. Andersen SK, Montgomery CL, Bagshaw SM. Early mortality in critical illness - A descriptive analysis of patients who died within 24 hours of ICU admission. *J Crit Care.* 2020;60:279–284.
3. Teno JM, Gozalo P, Trivedi AN, et al. Site of Death, Place of Care, and Health Care Transitions Among US Medicare Beneficiaries, 2000-2015. *JAMA.* 2018;320(3):264–271.
4. Patel VN, Stone SD. Patients With Advanced Cancer Requiring Intensive Care: Reasons for ICU Admission, Mortality Outcomes, and the Role of Palliative Care. *AACN Adv Crit Care.* 2021;32(3):324–331.
5. Ali M, Capel M, Jones G, Gazi T. The importance of identifying preferred place of death. *BMJ Support Palliat Care.* 2019;9(1):84–91.
6. Rhoads S, Amass T. Communication at the End-of-Life in the Intensive Care Unit: A Review of Evidence-Based Best Practices. *R I Med J (2013).* 2019;102(10):30–33.
7. Ouellette L, Puro A, Weatherhead J, et al. Public knowledge and perceptions about cardiopulmonary resuscitation (CPR): Results of a multicenter survey. *Am J Emerg Med.* 2018;36(10):1900–1901.
8. White DB, Carson S, Anderson W, et al. A Multicenter Study of the Causes and Consequences of Optimistic Expectations About Prognosis by Surrogate Decision-Makers in ICUs. *Crit Care Med.* 2019;47(9):1184–1193.
9. Kentish-Barnes N, Jensen HI, Curtis JR. The legacy of the interprofessional family meeting. *Intensive Care Med.* 2022.
10. Devlin JW, Skrobik Y, Gélinas C, et al. Clinical Practice Guidelines for the Prevention and Management of Pain, Agitation/Sedation, Delirium, Immobility, and Sleep Disruption in Adult Patients in the ICU. *Crit Care Med.* 2018;46(9):e825–e873.
11. Puntillo KA, Arai S, Cohen NH, et al. Symptoms experienced by intensive care unit patients at high risk of dying. *Crit Care Med.* 2010;38(11):2155–2160.
12. Keuning BE, Kaufmann T, Wiersema R, et al. Mortality prediction models in the adult critically ill: A scoping review. *Acta Anaesthesiol Scand.* 2020;64(4):424–442.
13. Ma J, Chi S, Buettner B, et al. Early Palliative Care Consultation in the Medical ICU: A Cluster Randomized Crossover Trial. *Crit Care Med.* 2019;47(12):1707–1715.
14. Kyeremanteng K, Gagnon LP, Thavorn K, Heyland D, D'Egidio G. The Impact of Palliative Care Consultation in the ICU on Length of Stay: A Systematic Review and Cost Evaluation. *J Intensive Care Med.* 2018;33(6):346–353.

15. Kerckhoffs MC, Senekal J, van Dijk D, et al. Framework to Support the Process of Decision-Making on Life-Sustaining Treatments in the ICU: Results of a Delphi Study. *Crit Care Med.* 2020;48(5):645–653.
16. Puntillo K, Nelson JE, Weissman D, et al. Palliative care in the ICU: relief of pain, dyspnea, and thirst--a report from the IPAL-ICU Advisory Board. *Intensive Care Med.* 2014;40(2):235–248.
17. Gélinas C. Pain assessment in the critically ill adult: Recent evidence and new trends. *Intensive Crit Care Nurs.* 2016;34:1–11.
18. Chanques G, Constantin JM, Devlin JW, et al. Analgesia and sedation in patients with ARDS. *Intensive Care Med.* 2020;46(12):2342–2356.
19. Gosselin E, Richard-Lalonde M. Role of Family Members in Pain Management in Adult Critical Care. *AACN Adv Crit Care.* 2019;30(4):398–410.
20. Herr K, Anderson, AR, Arbour C, Ely E, Gélinas C, Manworren RCB. Pain Assessment in the Patient Unable to Self- Report: Clinical Practice Recommendations in Support of the ASPMN 2024 Position Statement. *Pain Manag Nurs.* 2024;25(6):551–568.
21. Gélinas C, Joffe AM, Szumita PM, et al. A Psychometric Analysis Update of Behavioral Pain Assessment Tools for Noncommunicative, Critically Ill Adults. *AACN Adv Crit Care.* 2019;30(4):365–387.
22. Chanques G, Payen JF, Mercier G, et al. Assessing pain in non-intubated critically ill patients unable to self report: an adaptation of the Behavioral Pain Scale. *Intensive Care Med.* 2009;35(12):2060–2067.
23. Gélinas C, Puntillo KA, Levin P, Azoulay E. The Behavior Pain Assessment Tool for critically ill adults: a validation study in 28 countries. *Pain.* 2017;158(5):811–821.
24. de Jong A, Molinari N, de Lattre S, et al. Decreasing severe pain and serious adverse events while moving intensive care unit patients: a prospective interventional study (the NURSE-DO project). *Crit Care.* 2013;17(2):R74.
25. Chanques G, Gélinas C. Monitoring pain in the intensive care unit (ICU). *Intensive Care Med.* 2022;48(10):1508–1511.
26. Puntillo KA, Max A, Timsit JF, et al. Determinants of procedural pain intensity in the intensive care unit. The Europain® study. *Am J Respir Crit Care Med.* 2014;189(1):39–47.
27. Czarnecki ML, Turner HN, Collins PM, Doellman D, Wrona S, Reynolds J. Procedural pain management: a position statement with clinical practice recommendations. *Pain Manag Nurs.* 2011;12(2):95–111.
28. Joffe AM, Hallman M, Gélinas C, Herr DL, Puntillo K. Evaluation and treatment of pain in critically ill adults. *Semin Respir Crit Care Med.* 2013;34(2):189–200.
29. Puntillo KA, Naidu R. Chronic pain disorders after critical illness and ICU-acquired opioid dependence: two clinical conundra. *Curr Opin Crit Care.* 2016;22(5):506–512.
30. Arroyo-Novoa CM, Figueroa Ramos MI, Puntillo KA. Opioid and Benzodiazepine Iatrogenic Withdrawal Syndrome in Patients in the Intensive Care Unit. *AACN Adv Crit Care.* 2019;30(4):353–364.
31. White DB. Withholding and withdrawing ventilatory support in adults in the intensive care unit In: UpToDate, Arnold R, Parsons P, eds. *UpToDate.* Waltham, MA: UpToDate January 25, 2022.
32. Campbell ML. Caring for dying patients in the intensive care unit: managing pain, dyspnea, anxiety, delirium, and death rattle. *AACN Adv Crit Care.* 2015;26(2):110–120; quiz 121–2.
33. Downar J, Delaney JW, Hawryluck L, Kenny L. Guidelines for the withdrawal of life-sustaining measures. *Intensive Care Med.* 2016;42(6):1003–1017.
34. Hughes CG, McGrane S, Pandharipande PP. Sedation in the intensive care setting. *Clin Pharmacol.* 2012;4:53–63.
35. Marra A, Ely EW, Pandharipande PP, Patel MB. The ABCDEF Bundle in Critical Care. *Crit Care Clin.* 2017;33(2):225–243.
36. Reardon DP, Anger KE, Adams CD, Szumita PM. Role of dexmedetomidine in adults in the intensive care unit: an update. *Am J Health Syst Pharm.* 2013;70(9):767–777.
37. Gélinas C, Berube M, Chevrier A, et al. Delirium Assessment Tools for Use in Critically Ill Adults: A Psychometric Analysis and Systematic Review. *Crit Care Nurse.* 2018;38(1):38–49.
38. Chen L, Yin J, Zheng Y, et al. The effectiveness of music listening for critically ill patients: A systematic review. *Nursing in Critical Care.* 2022.
39. Choi J, Campbell ML, Gélinas C, Happ MB, Tate J, Chlan L. Symptom assessment in non-vocal or cognitively impaired ICU patients: Implications for practice and future research. *Heart Lung.* 2017;46(4):239–245.
40. Sulmasy LS, Bledsoe TA; ACP Ethics, Professionalism and Human Rights Committee. American College of Physicians Ethics Manual: seventh edition. *Ann Intern Med.* 2019;170(2_suppl):S1–S32.
41. Kon AA, Shepard EK, Sederstrom NO, et al. Defining futile and potentially inappropriate interventions: a policy statement from the Society of Critical Care Medicine Ethics Committee. *Crit Care Med.* 2016;44(9):1769–1774.
42. Canadian Critical Care Society Ethics Committee; Bandrauk N, Downar J, Paunovic B. Withholding and withdrawing life-sustaining treatment: the Canadian Critical Care Society position paper. *Can J Anaesth.* 2018;65(1):105–122.
43. Michalsen A, Long AC, DeKeyser Ganz F, et al. Interprofessional shared decision-making in the ICU: a systematic review and recommendations from an expert panel. *Crit Care Med.* 2019;47(9):1258–1266.
44. Davidson JE, Aslakson RA, Long AC, et al. Guidelines for family-centered care in the neonatal, pediatric, and adult ICU. *Crit Care Med.* 2017;45(1):103–128.
45. McFarlin J, Tulsky JA, Back AL, Arnold RM. A talking map for family meetings in the intensive care unit. *JCOM.* 2017,24(1):15–22.
46. Wiegand DL, Cheon J, Netzer G. Seeing the patient and family through: nurses and physicians experiences with withdrawal of life-sustaining therapy in the ICU. *Am J Hosp Palliat Care.* 2019;36(1):13–23.
47. Braganza MA, Glossop AJ, Vora AV. Treatment withdrawal and end-of-life care in the intensive care unit. *BJA Educ.* 2017;17(12):396–400.
48. Efstathiou N, Vanderspank-Wright B, Vandyk A, et al. Terminal withdrawal of mechanical ventilation in adult intensive care units: a systematic review and narrative synthesis of perceptions, experiences and practices. *Palliat Med.* 2020;34(9):1140–1164.
49. Nassar Junior AP, Besen B, Robinson CC, Falavigna M, Teixeira C, Rosa RG. Flexible versus restrictive visiting policies in ICUs: a systematic review and meta-analysis. *Crit Care Med.* 2018;46(7):1175–1180.
50. Ganz FD. Improving family intensive care unit experiences at the end of life: barriers and facilitators. *Crit Care Nurse.* 2019;39(3):52–58.
51. Seaman JB, Arnold RM, Scheunemann LP, White DB. An integrated framework for effective and efficient communication with families in the adult intensive care unit. *Ann Am Thorac Soc.* 2017;14(6):1015–1020.
52. Erikson A, McAdam J. Bereavement care in the adult intensive care unit: directions for practice. *Crit Care Nurs Clin North Am.* 2020;32(2):281–294.

53. Hetland B, McAndrew N, Perazzo J, Hickman R. A qualitative study of factors that influence active family involvement with patient care in the ICU: survey of critical care nurses. *Intensive Crit Care Nurs*. 2018;44:67–75.
54. McAndrew NS, Leske J, Schroeter K. Moral distress in critical care nursing: the state of the science. *Nurs Ethics*. 2018;25(5):552–570.
55. Browning ED, Cruz JS. Reflective debriefing: a social work intervention addressing moral distress among ICU nurses. *J Soc Work End Life Palliat Care*. 2018;14(1):44–72.
56. Jun J, Costa DK. Is it me or you? A team approach to mitigate burnout in critical care. *Crit Care Nurs Clin North Am*. 2020;32(3):395–406.
57. Arora S, Shaikh S, Karachi T, et al. End-of-life skills and professionalism for critical care residents in training: the ESPRIT survey. *J Intensive Care Med*. 2021;36(11):1272–1280.
58. Ferrell B, Buller H, Paice J, Anderson W, Donesky D. End-of-Life Nursing and Education Consortium communication curriculum for interdisciplinary palliative care teams. *J Palliat Med*. 2019;22(9):1082–1091.
59. Stokes H, Vanderspank-Wright B, Fothergill Bourbonnais F, Wright DK. Meaningful experiences and end-of-life care in the intensive care unit: a qualitative study. *Intensive Crit Care Nurs*. 2019;53:1–7.

PART VIII

Considerations for Person and Family-Centered Palliative Care

66

Addressing Health Inequalities, Social Determinants of Health, and Underrepresented Individuals in Palliative Care

Binu Koirala, Rebecca Wright, Patricia M. Davidson, Marlena C. Fisher, Katie E. Nelson, Benjamin Roberts, Danetta H. Sloan, and David S. Wu

Key Points

- Although the effect of social determinants of health (SDOH) and those with inequitable distribution of healthcare has been recognized, personal, social, political, economic, and environmental forces that determine health and outcomes are generally not the focus of daily clinical practice, including in palliative care.
- Regardless of age, color, ethnicity, socioeconomic status, or other disparities, all people, families, and communities have the right to access high-quality palliative nursing care.
- Palliative care nurses may use their position, wherever they are, to inspire and equip others to identify and address medical and social healthcare needs, act on health inequality, and develop and tailor the tools and resources needed to promote health equity, address SDOH and improve health outcomes of underrepresented individuals in palliative care.

Introduction

Social determinants of health (SDOH) are the conditions in the environments where people are born, live, learn, work, play, worship, and age that affect a wide range of health, functioning, quality-of-life, health outcomes, and risks.[1] Factors such as access to housing, education, food, transportation, finances, community, and employment impact not just how a person lives but also how they approach and experience the end of their life. Nurses are in a unique position of relationship and trust that can be leveraged when working as part of interdisciplinary teams to provide palliative care. The whole-person and collaborative nature of palliative care means that nurses are remarkably positioned to initiate, undertake, and support assessments; access resources; and advocate across a wide range of challenges and barriers that can result in poor and potentially avoidable experiences for people with palliative care needs.

SDOH can have both positive and negative outcomes on the health and well-being of individuals and communities.[2] Negative outcomes have been specifically seen among individuals identified as "underrepresented," "minority," "historically excluded," "at-risk," "vulnerable," or "marginalized." This chapter will use these terms interchangeably to describe individuals, groups, or communities that have not received equitable access to healthcare, quality of care, and health outcomes. Examples of underrepresented groups include, but are not limited to, Black, Latino, Hispanic, Asian, and Indigenous populations; disabled people; those living in rural communities; LGBTQ+ individuals (see Chapter 67, "Affirmative Palliative Care for LGBTQIA+ Patients and Their Families"); unhoused individuals; individuals who are incarcerated; and persons with complex healthcare needs including those with comorbid substance use disorder (see Chapter 68, "Palliative Care in the Setting of Substance Use Disorder") or serious psychiatric illnesses (see Chapter 69, "Palliative Care in the Setting of Serious Mental Illness").[2] The disparities in healthcare among the underrepresented population have been extending to healthcare for people living with serious illnesses and at the end of life.

It is imperative to look beyond the individual level and to acknowledge the interpersonal, organizational, community/societal, and political factors that may have an impact on the differences in perception and preferences of palliative and end-of-life care. An example of this is the historical context of slavery and racism that has had a justifiable impact on many Black people in the United States and their mistrust of the healthcare system.[3] Additionally, racial and ethnic disparities exist in health and access to palliative care services internationally.[3] High-income countries have increased access to palliative care services.[4] Furthermore, research illustrated that providers are apprehensive about engaging underserved populations in advance care planning conversations and often avoid these conversations.[5] This unfortunate truth perpetuates existing provider bias and potentially inequities in care by placing the responsibility on patients to engage providers in advance care planning conversations. Nurses can be advocates in this area, initiating conversations about implicit bias and the impact it can have on care delivery, in order to promote therapeutic engagement of patients in advance care planning conversations. Ultimately, the patient is the expert themselves and the best person to share their person, social, and cultural preferences for care.

The groups mentioned above are reported to underutilize palliative and end-of-life care.[6] Despite advances in palliative care and acknowledgment of health disparities in palliative care access, quality, and outcomes, there is limited knowledge and there are few evidence-based strategies specifically addressing SDOH and the needs of underserved populations in practice. The chapter highlights the current evidence and tools in addressing health inequalities among underrepresented groups receiving palliative care and warrants change in the healthcare system to meet the needs of the increasingly diverse, and historically underserved, patient population and their family. Further, the chapter emphasizes the role of nurses and their leadership in interdisciplinary palliative care in examining the determinants of health, the quality of palliative care services, and the complex need and preferences of patients living with serious illnesses and their family members addressing health inequalities.

Case Study Part 1: Transition from Emergency Department to Intensive Care

Sheila has experienced a complex cycle of care involving multiple visits to the emergency department (ED) and inpatient hospitalizations in the last 6 months. She is a 60-year-old, African American female with insecure housing. Sheila has a history of chronic obstructive pulmonary disease (COPD) and cigarette use and was recently diagnosed with metastatic lung cancer.

The ED nurse found a documented goals-of-care discussion in Sheila's medical record from a previous visit, where she stated, "I would only want cancer treatment if it cured me. I don't want to stay alive for longer and be in even more pain." She was discharged to a shelter with follow-up appointments scheduled for Outpatient Oncology and Palliative Care; but she did not make them, and the team was not able to reach her.

Presently, Sheila is experiencing shortness of breath, anxiety, and respiratory failure likely due to COPD exacerbation. Her computed tomography (CT) scan shows rapid lung cancer progression with possible brain metastases. She was placed on bilevel positive airway pressure (BiPAP) and posted for a bed in the intensive care unit (ICU). Sheila is lethargic due to her respiratory failure; therefore, the provider is unable to have a thorough discussion with her regarding her code status. As such, she is entered into the system as Full Code.

The ED nurse pauses and says to her colleague: "Sheila said during her last admission that she would only want treatment if it cured her. I don't think there's any cure for this, especially now with potential brain metastases. . . . Are we sure that she would want to be a Full Code and moved to the ICU?"

Background

SDOH: Implications, and Challenges for Palliative Care Nursing

Health and illness are often associated with personal, social, economic, environmental, cultural, and interpersonal factors identified as SDOH. Inequalities in daily living standards and inequitable distribution of resources, money, and power create socially disadvantaged groups who have adverse experiences with illness and worse health outcomes.[7] The opportunity to attain optimal health and well-being is not equitable for all people; no matter where one lives in the world, the risk and outcomes of disease are far more for those with a lower socioeconomic spectrum.[8] Lack of resources such as safe affordable housing, food insecurity, issues with transportation, and less access and utilization of healthcare systems and medicines are related to poorer health outcomes.[9,10] SDOH associated with negative health outcomes may also include personal and social factors such as disability status, race and ethnicity, insurance, income inequality, and many more. SDOH can affect an individual's health and well-being and influence how they perceive and experience care in the healthcare system, community, and home. Although the effect of SDOH and those with inequitable distribution of healthcare has been recognized, personal, social, political, cultural, economic, and environmental forces that determine health and outcomes are generally not the focus of daily clinical practice, including in palliative care.

The National Consensus Project's (NCP's) *Clinical Practice Guidelines for Quality Palliative Care* indicate that best practices in palliative care include all individuals living with serious illness in all settings, across all diagnoses, prognoses, and ages for the attainment of comprehensive care needs of the patients and their family and caregivers.[11] This guideline has been seen as useful in identifying disparities and targeting improvement priorities that can address issues of quality and equity among underrepresented groups with serious illnesses. However, inequalities in palliative care access and outcomes exist among those living with serious illnesses specifically in care system structures (affordability, organizational structure/setting, payment system), processes (communication and trust, acceptability of care, care delivery, and cultural humility and responsiveness), and outcomes (care satisfaction, pain and symptom management and quality of life).[8] Contributing factors to such inequalities in palliative care can also include SDOH, structural racism, economic insecurities, lack of education and employment, nutrition, housing, and social support.[12] Further, communication and language barriers, lack of culturally sensitive care and training, and the resulting mistrust in healthcare systems and care teams can also increase disparities.[12] The persistent lack of knowledge and awareness of the scope of health inequalities in the care for people with serious illnesses generates, upholds, and perpetuates barriers to effective action toward more equitable care across underrepresented, vulnerable groups.[8]

Nurses focus on whole-person care, which means education and practice must go beyond medical needs and should address the behavioral, socioeconomic, cultural, and spiritual issues of the individual including the systemic issues that influence SDOH.[2] It is important in addressing health inequality that nurses and the care team demonstrate the necessary skills and knowledge to be effective partners in the care of those living with serious illnesses, who can advocate for patient needs, provide care that is consistent with the patient's values, and respect wishes and inherent dignity. In palliative nursing, understanding disparities are crucial as they can affect the care an individual received at the time of diagnosis of a serious illness, as their condition progresses, and in their palliative and end-of-life care.[2] Achieving equity in nursing care begins with an understanding of the root causes of inequalities. There are no defined healthcare and/or nursing competencies or frameworks that fully address the promotion of health equity in palliative care.[13,14] Existing tools and evidence can be used as a starting point, yet nurses need to think from a perspective of cultural humility[15] and be open to understanding the context and taking feedback from the people they aim to serve. The lived experiences and individual contexts can not only provide nuanced insights but also help identify the action plans that can impact care and decrease disparities. Regardless of socioeconomic status or outward appearance, maintaining curiosity, graciousness, and cultural humility; respecting commitments; and honoring patients' experiences must remain at the forefront of interactions to enable those who have been underrepresented to develop trust with healthcare professionals and provide quality palliative care.

Context Matters

Knowledge of the history and spread of modern palliative and hospice practices is an important factor for nurses when addressing needs and inequities, particularly recognizing why some groups have been historically underrepresented or why prevailing medical recommendations may be at odds with personal preferences in different populations. The modern hospice movement evolved from work led by Dame Cicely Saunders in the 1960s in the United Kingdom, and the ethos was, and remains, holistic in nature. However, "holism" in this context is still framed from a Western perspective. Therefore, the uptake of palliative care practices and accompanying guidance on standards, best practices, and evaluation of quality of palliative care reflect this cultural understanding and may not always account for different interpretations of holism, or what matters most to one community compared to another.[16] For example, recent discussions about palliative care in Africa have observed a colonizing effect wherein "international standards" and "best practice" can fail to capture, or push against, core end-of-life care practices that have been around for generations within a given community.[16] Another example is the *Quality of Death Index*,[17] a report ranking global palliative care which included 80 countries based on their ability to be measured against five criteria: the palliative and healthcare environment, human resources, the affordability of care, the quality of care, and the level of community engagement. Key recommendations were clear national policies and partnerships between government, academia, and nonprofit groups.[17] A palliative care equity consideration for nurses when interpreting reports such as this is that, though it provides insights into some global practices and highlights barriers that some countries have in accessing and providing resources such as analgesia, the criteria are from a European perspective specifically and may not be sensitive enough to capture historical practices and preferences in caring for those approaching the end of life. Essentially, countries "missing" from reports like this may not have a formal palliative care structure, but there will still be long-held and practiced beliefs, preferences, and wishes about palliative and end-of-life care.

At a local level when considering equity and access to palliative care, nurses need to consider the barriers and inequities that exist within their own context. For example, in the United Kingdom, while there is limited but growing evidence about inequities for Black, Asian, and ethnic minority populations, populations with the least evidence for care preferences or knowledge of equitable access to care include people with disabilities, people from traveler communities, and people in institutions such as long-term hospitals and prisons.[18] Comparatively, in the United States, while there is similar documentation about inequities experienced by Black/African Americans, others, such as those from Asian, Hispanic, or Native American populations, are often far less likely to be included in the evidence base or in work seeking to understand and address inequities in palliative care.[19] Knowledge of why this is, what is the truth behind it, and how systems and structures aid or harm can help provide a pathway for nurses to address different barriers.

Context must also be considered on a personal level as differences in preferences or interpretation of social norms can also vary within a single community. Successful tailoring of palliative care to individual needs is rooted in culturally humble consideration of global, local, and communal contexts and interpretations. The original and driving context of palliative care must be taken into consideration so that the preferences of the patient and family can be fully understood and honored, which may help to negate barriers and challenges in communication and goal-setting. Another area where inequities can occur is in the nondominant culture. Palliative care clinicians should address cultural needs to address inequities and improve access to high-quality care (see Chapter 28, "Cultural Considerations in Palliative Care").

The Evidence Base and Challenges for Palliative Care

While the ethos of the field of palliative care is holistic, there are many areas of care delivery lacking in supporting evidence or guidance that compound or are a direct result of inequities in systems of care. These gaps exist within our understanding of how to tailor palliative care across conditions, populations, settings, and cultures. To ensure safe and transparent care, it is imperative for nurses to be aware of the level and quality of evidence underpinning their practice, particularly as some protocols may have had to depend on expert opinion or anecdotal reports. The following serves as examples of where we have stronger or weaker evidence supporting care but is not an exhaustive list.

Most of the evidence for palliative care stems from research with people with cancers, heart failure, or COPD.[20–23] There is a growing though limited body of palliative care evidence for neuromuscular disorders and end-stage renal failure,[24,25] but many conditions, such as sickle cell disease, and for those living with the competing priorities and demands of multiple chronic conditions are lacking in evidence for the provision of palliative care. In these instances, nurses must often draw from the closest related evidence or expert opinion to determine how to proceed with their care.

Patient and family preferences for care, including perceptions of quality and satisfaction, have been explored to some degree but often from the perspective of standardized metrics and clinician-focused outcomes. This aspect of care is particularly lacking in evidence for how to tailor care from culturally humble and sensitive perspectives, where "culture" is understood as a driving force for communication, rather than a stand-alone or "check-box" factor. Caution must be taken as patient preference work often focuses on a single angle of a person's identity or demographic status, which may not consider the nuances and complexities of a person's intersectionality; for example, people living without fixed homes are rarely included in research that explores their experiences of care beyond being "being homeless." Other challenges for nurses seeking evidence to support their practice are barriers connected to recruitment and retention of palliative care populations in the research itself, for a range of reasons including fluctuating and unpredictable conditions, demands of study participation, cultural beliefs around discussing death and dying, mistrust or concerns about taking part in research, misunderstandings about palliative care, and gatekeeping preventing access.[26] Other factors exist, but nurses should pay close attention to *who* is actually in the evidence base they are drawing from and what factors have been considered in a study's analysis as there may not be consideration of cultural, social, or financial factors.

The evidence for specific palliative care interventions also has strengths and weaknesses, with certain aspects receiving greater or lesser attention, often based on feasibility issues previously mentioned. As certain interventions have received greater or lesser attention, for example, interprofessional palliative care teams and palliative care telehealth,[27] guidance therefore varies for how confident nurses can be in their application.[21] Examples for why this is the case include the challenges in carrying out palliative care–focused research, such as ethical or feasibility factors.[28,29] Obtaining funding, support, and ongoing retention of participants in studies can weaken the ability to determine effectiveness of interventions.[26,28,29] These factors, in combination with high variability in study designs, populations, and specific details of interventions, mean that the prevailing evidence base for many approaches to care delivery and the anticipated outcomes often have mixed or unclear outcomes. [26,28,29]

All of the elements discussed feed into the very crux of how SDOH can be compounded and exacerbated, why there are health inequalities in palliative care, and who some of the underrepresented groups are. As such, we cannot stress enough the importance of the role of the nurse in addressing and working to close some of these gaps through assessment and action considering the needs of underrepresented groups. The section "Role of Nursing in Promoting Health Equity among Underserved Populations" goes into greater detail about the role of the nurse in this area, but we conclude this section by highlighting the power of nursing advocacy through influencing policy and collaboration with, as well as personal development of, academic and research platforms that respond to the gaps directly. This can include reporting gaps in evidence that leave practice decision-making under supported, developing and leading research to generate new evidence, application of local quality improvement and service improvement work, and partnering with local communities across all of these areas.

Assessing and Measuring Patient and Family Needs in Palliative Care for Underrepresented Groups

As the conceptualization of palliative care has evolved, so too have the tools and assessments nurses can use to gauge and support the needs of patients with serious illnesses. The NCP *Clinical Practice Guidelines* provide a blueprint for assessing and intervening on eight broad domains for quality palliative care: (1) Structure and Processes of Care; (2) Physical Aspects of Care; (3) Psychological and Psychiatric Aspects of Care; (4) Social Aspects of Care; (5) Spiritual, Religious, and Existential Aspects of Care; (6) Cultural Aspects of Care; (7) Care of the Patient Nearing the End of Life; and (8) Ethical and Legal Aspects of Care.[11] Many existing tools and assessments have broadly been developed using this framework. Table 66.1 highlights a select few underrepresented groups, as highlighted by the End-of-Life Nursing Education Consortium (ELNEC), and specific tools or strategies that nurses may utilize for assessing patients' and families' needs by palliative care domain.

It is important to evaluate these assessment tools and strategies within the context of their limitations. ElMokhallalati and colleagues (2020) conducted a systematic review to evaluate the accuracy of existing screening tools for identification of patients with advanced progressive diseases who are likely to have palliative care needs in primary healthcare.[35] They commented on the

Table 66.1 Palliative care–focused assessment tools and strategies for nurses

Marginalized/ underserved population	Assessment tool/strategy	Domain/focus	Explicit incorporation/partnership with marginalized/ underserved population
Veteran	Veterans RAND 12-Item Health Survey (VR-12)[30]	Quality of life	Validated in veteran population; not mentioned whether included in development of tool
African American	Making Your Wishes Known: Planning Your Medical Future (MYWK)[31]	Advance care planning	Recruitment led by pastors from predominantly African American churches and MYWK validated among African American participants; not mentioned whether included in development of survey
LGBTQIA+	Nurses' Health Education about LGBTQ Elders (HEALE)[32]	Improving nurse insight	Curriculum designed for nurses by those identifying as LGBTQ+
Unhoused	Thematic analysis to improve access[32]	Improving clinician insight	Qualitative interviews with 19 unhoused individuals with palliative needs
Severe persistent mental illness (SPMI)	Do It Your Way[34]	Advance care planning	Validated in SPMI population; those with SPMI not included in development

performance matrices of most of the existing tools as being poor because they mostly used prognosis or prediction of death or deterioration as a proxy for identifying people with unmet palliative care needs. The only tool identified that explicitly addresses equity was the SPICT—Spanish Language, which was a cross-cultural adaptation of the Supportive & Palliative Care Indicators Tool (SPICT).[36,37] However, there is currently no evidence to support outcomes of the SPICT—Spanish Language tool from a patient perspective.

As stated throughout this chapter, equity considerations for palliative care vary internationally. For example, the seminal consensus statement from the US-based Center to Advance Palliative Care (CAPC) has no mention of diversity, inequity, inequality, SDOH, marginalized, underserved, or underrepresented populations.[38] There is one reference to "culture," but it pertains to "hospital culture" only. Published in 2011, the consensus statement stands in sharp contrast to those institutions focusing on palliative needs among marginalized groups.[38] Meanwhile, in Australia, incremental progress in addressing equity in palliative care is underway, though much of the work is still in review and recognition stages.[39] However, recognition at the systems level is imperative as it can then have a trickle-down effect to organizations, hospitals, units, and individual healthcare staff, for example, identifying gaps in availability and use of assessment tools for underrepresented populations.

Case Study Part 2: Transition from Intensive to Intermediate Care

Sheila's condition stabilized in the ICU without the need for mechanical ventilation. After 24 hours of monitoring, she was transferred to the intermediate care unit (IMC) to receive treatment for COPD exacerbation as well as intravenous antibiotics. Presently, she is still on BiPAP but alert and oriented. She remains short of breath and feels extremely anxious. Sheila has no family or friends listed as emergency contacts. The IMC nurse notices that Sheila is clutching a holy rosary between her swollen hands.

Given Sheila's complicated medical course, the IMC nurse takes the opportunity to go through the Making Your Wishes Known: Planning Your Medical Future (MYWK) tool, a computer-based program that presents clinical scenarios to help the user determine their preferences and articulate desired goals and values. The nurse says, "Ms. Sheila, I notice the beautiful rosary you have in your hands. Is your religion or spirituality important to you?" Sheila shares that she has been distressed about not being able to attend mass each week since she is living on the streets and does not have reliable transportation to church. She lost her husband 4 years ago, at which point her anxiety worsened, and she turned to alcohol to cope with her grief. Sheila then tearfully reiterates, "I don't want to live like this anymore. I am just ready to see my husband again." The nurse sits with Sheila and asks her if there is anyone else in her life other than her late husband. Sheila states, "I have a daughter, but we haven't spoken in years."

The nurse contacts the unit social worker to inform her of Sheila's case and to see about finding her daughter's contact information. The nurse also contacts the covering provider to inform them of Sheila's goals for her care and advocate that they are not currently being met because her symptoms are unmanaged, and she remains a Full Code. Sheila, although improved, is still anxious and dyspneic on exertion. Palliative care could greatly help with management of her symptoms. The provider stated, "I will review her chart, assess the patient, and then address these concerns in interdisciplinary rounds later this afternoon."

The nurse attends interdisciplinary care team rounds later in the shift, where she informs the team that Sheila's main goal is comfort. She advocates for consultations with social work, case management, and palliative care for further support. She also places a request for a chaplain to come pray with Sheila. The provider agrees that even though she is young, the requested consultations are appropriate and realistic for an individual with metastatic disease; he states, "I plan to talk with Sheila after rounds to ensure she understands the ramifications of these decisions."

Example Framework for Tailoring Palliative Care

Conceptual frameworks serve a type of systematic ecosystem in research and practice to help understand a phenomenon, bridging all influences, contexts, theory, and study design together in a meaningful way.[40] To promote health equity, the existing frameworks and/or tools may need tailoring with the evolving evidence and specific need and background of individuals, family, or communities. The authors' team collectively developed a conceptual framework for addressing disparities in access to palliative care using the socio-ecological model as the basis (Figure 66.1).[41]

Our hope was that this framework may be useful for palliative care clinicians and researchers in being able to consider the holistic needs and preferences of patients, while concurrently considering and acknowledging the sociohistorical contexts which may inhibit them from being able to equitably access care. However, when used as a "crutch," conceptual frameworks can limit the extent of questions asked, biases questioned, protocols carried out, etc. Therefore, it is important that they not be generically applied to *all* populations and/or clung to too tightly in cases where they are not applicable. Table 66.2 offers a broad example of how this type of framework may help draw comparisons between groups of people and outlines areas where this specific framework may need to be tailored for specific groups.

Role of Nursing in Promoting Health Equity among Underserved Populations

Unique Role of Nursing

The philosophical premises of palliative care and nursing are closely intertwined, both prioritizing holistic, compassionate, and person-centered care.[7] Nurses are well positioned and should be educated to practice primary or generalist palliative care for all individuals they care for to help improve health outcomes. Primary palliative care focuses on understanding illness trajectories, pain and symptom management, advanced care planning, working with individuals to help identify community resources, and initiating specialist palliative care when necessary.[11] Specialist palliative care focuses on the knowledge of serious illnesses and their trajectories, the management of complex pain and symptoms, difficult conversations, and

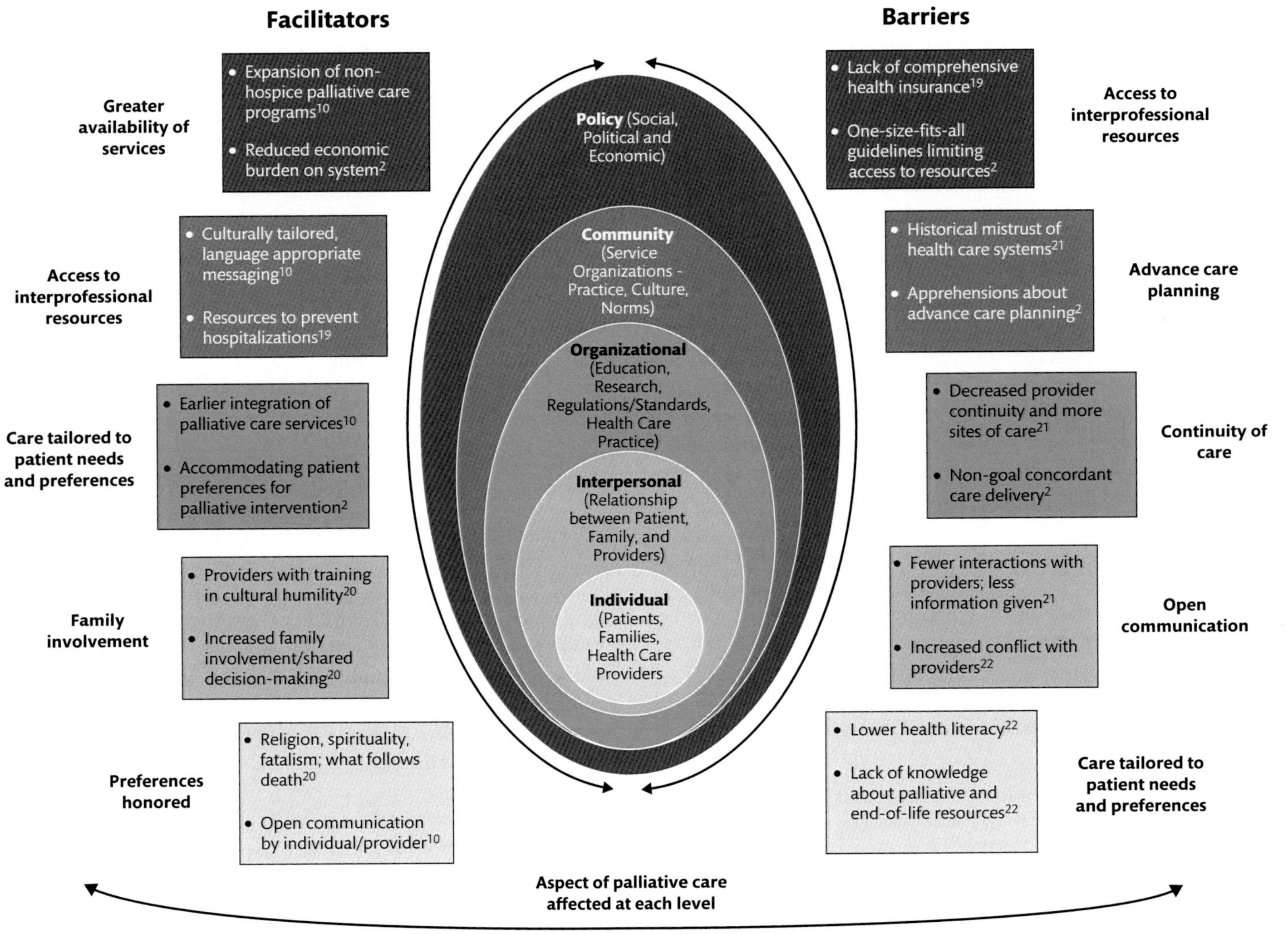

Figure 66.1 Addressing palliative care access disparities framework.
Source: Reference 45.

end-of-life care.[11] Both primary and specialty palliative care nurses can greatly help narrow disparities and promote equitable health services using person-centered, family-centered, and community-centered approaches.[2] Nurses are key stakeholders to ensure the availability, accessibility, and adaptability of palliative care to promote health equity.[8]

Although there is no exact guide on nurses' role in promoting health equity, the palliative care tools/frameworks identified in the previous section and current palliative care nursing competencies that speak to health equity concepts offer a starting point. The above section of this chapter, "Example Framework for Tailoring Palliative Care," warrants the need of tailoring palliative care for underrepresented patients, family, and community considering their need and wishes and existing evidence to address health inequality, limit negative effects of SDOH, and promote health equity in palliative care. Nurses can play a critical role in this by using existing nursing, palliative care, and health equity standards and developing and tailoring innovative approaches to better serve underrepresented population.

The NCP *Clinical Practice Guidelines* identified the demand to assess social and cultural aspects of care to ensure quality palliative care.[11] The American Nurses Association's scope and standard of nursing practice highlights that nurses need to respect all patients, families, and professionals and demonstrate equitable care for all patients in need.[42] Palliative nursing specific competencies identified by the American Association of Colleges of Nursing, in collaboration with the ELNEC project for both undergraduate nursing students (CARES)[43] and graduate nursing students in master's and doctor of nursing practice programs (G-CARES[44]), clearly emphasize the need to (1) respect cultural, spiritual, and other forms of diversity and (2) promote social justice, equity, and equality for patients with serious illness. The Hospice and Palliative Nurses Association also stressed the need for culturally congruent care and nurses' response to diversity through their scope and standard of practice as well as palliative care competencies.[45] These existing resources are valuable for the nursing profession and offer a launchpad for promoting health equity in the context of palliative care—until more specific directives are made publicly available. Enhancing advocacy beyond the bedside is also critical for moving the needle forward. Increased nurse leadership in intersectoral advocacy and interdisciplinary collaborations at local, national, and international

Table 66.2 Tailoring the "palliative care access disparities framework" to underrepresented populations

Goal: advance care planning	Black individuals living with kidney failure		Indigenous, reservation-based individuals	
	Facilitators	**Barriers**	**Facilitators**	**Barriers**
Individual	Having a master's or doctoral degree and accepting the illness of kidney disease increased the likelihood of engaging in informal advance care planning with family.	Those who qualitatively described a discomfort in discussing death often did not engage in any form of advance care planning.	Strong cultural bonds to Creator give many Indigenous peoples peace in the setting of serious illness.	Depending on which tribe or community an individual is from, some are not able to use specific language to discuss death according to traditional Indigenous protocols.
Interpersonal/family	Having a trusted family member who will follow their wishes as outlined, wanting to avoid being a burden on one's family, and having experience as a decision maker for someone who died increased the likelihood of engaging in informal advance care planning with family.	Distrust that their family would follow their wishes at the end of life decreased the likelihood of engaging in informal advance care planning with family.	Many are inclined to partake in advance care planning to avoid burdening their relatives. Helps caregivers proactively plan for the type(s) of funeral a person may want, which is an intense family and community effort in many Indigenous communities.	Many live in multigenerational households, which can make choosing a decision maker difficult.
Organizational	Having a recent hospitalization within the past 6 months increased the likelihood of engaging in informal advance care planning with family.	Reliance on advance directives. *This form of advance care planning does not accommodate all cultures.*	*Per one author's (K. E. N.) community-based participatory research experience working with an Indigenous community, feedback highlighted that this level of the framework felt irrelevant given the absence of organizations in reservation-based communities supporting care during serious illness.*	
Community	The in-center hemodialysis community is a major support. Many who receive hemodialysis in centers witness other people having cardiac events. In many cases this drove them to engage in some form of advance care planning.	The only method of advance care planning in dialysis clinics is an advance directive provided at admission. There is rarely follow-up on someone's psychosocial status or advance care planning needs post-admission.	Collectivistic culture; Indigenous peoples will always be inclined to do something (despite any level of discomfort) if it will benefit their collective peoples.	Indigenous peoples' way of life emphasizes oral storytelling as means of sharing information; therefore, signing formal documentation that outlines their stories/wishes goes against this tradition.
Political	The Patient Self-Determination Act requires hospitals to provide information and ask if a patient has completed an advance directive on admission. The simple act of asking combined with what the person experiences during that hospitalization may increase the likelihood of engaging in some form of advance care planning.	Many rely on Social Security Disability while on dialysis, and it does not provide a living wage (considerable financial strain). *The Patient Self-Determination Act relies on advance directives, which are not the preferable form of advance care planning for many cultures. This is an example where the same concept spans multiple socioecological levels.*	*Per one author's (K. E. N.) community-based participatory research experience working with an Indigenous community, feedback highlighted that this level of the framework may be offensive to some individuals—as if the researcher is making an assumption that the US government has supported their people (when they overwhelmingly have been socially excluded and ignored).*	The US government has broken numerous treaties negotiated between 1778 and 1868, some of which granted them access to healthcare services.

levels may strategically lead to universal access and utilization of palliative care.[11]

Regardless of age, color, ethnicity, socioeconomic status, or other disparities, all people, families, and communities have the right to access high-quality palliative nursing care. Palliative care nurses may use their position to inspire and equip others to identify and address medical and social healthcare needs, act on health equity, and provide the tools and resources needed. Nurses can promote health equity by providing patient-centered care through the SDOH lens. There are a variety of interventions nurses can take specifically to help limit the negative impact of SDOH on palliative care and promote health equity. Nurses can have a unique role in addressing inequality including how to:

- Work to increase awareness of SDOH and the benefits of palliative care among the patients, families, and communities they serve
- Work to increase awareness of SDOH and the benefits of palliative care among nurses, interdisciplinary care team members, community workers, volunteers, and community members
- Assess SDOH and cultural background that can shape individuals' perception of illness, care access, and care utilization
- Develop and practice culturally sensitive care and language
- Be aware of diversity and create and maintain a culture of inclusivity
- Build strong and long-term relationships within underserved communities
- Identify and direct patients with nonmedical needs to local community resources
- Collaborate with interdisciplinary teams to help promote need-based care
- Be prepared to question and alter established practices to address disparities in palliative care access and patient/family experiences to improve health outcomes

Be present, listen, ask, understand, and be flexible with the need and preferences of the patient and their family rather than make assumptions and follow rules.

Interdisciplinary Collaboration in Promoting Health Equity

The interdisciplinary team, using multiple specialized disciplines to support the diversity of patients,[11] is the core of palliative care delivery. The interdisciplinary team, generally consisting of nurses, physicians, nurse practitioners, social workers, pharmacists, spiritual workers (chaplain), allied therapists, hospice aids, and other care team members, can help identify and support the unique needs of patients and their family members' physical, psychological, social, emotional, spiritual, cultural, and practical aspects as well as goals of care. As identified in the above section, "The Evidence Base and Challenges for Palliative Care," current evidence related to interdisciplinary collaboration has proven helpful in improving health outcomes among patients and families receiving palliative and end-of-life care.[27] Interdisciplinary collaboration in palliative care can also help address health inequalities by ensuring that patients receive care congruent with their individual values, principles, and needs. Identifying the intersection of health and social care is critical and can be achieved through interdisciplinary collaboration, which can affect acceptance of palliative care, identify priorities in social needs and treatment goals, and increase access and quality of palliative care among the underrepresented population. To effectively serve underrepresented groups with serious illnesses and their families, healthcare professionals, clerics, and social workers must lead and create multidisciplinary learning opportunities. It is also crucial to provide long-term, community-based palliative care through interdisciplinary teamwork to patients with serious illnesses who can live in their community but deal with the challenges of advanced and progressive illnesses. Nurses can take a leadership role in identifying and connecting patients and their families with interdisciplinary teams and resources.

Case Study Part 3: Transition from Hospital to Hospice

The day after interdisciplinary rounds social work, palliative care and pastoral care come to see Sheila. Social work asks her about her daughter and if she would like to complete a Five Wishes document to express her wishes for the end of her life, specifically regarding her comfort and how she wants to be treated in her final days. A palliative care provider assesses Sheila and writes orders for medications to help with her symptoms of anxiety and shortness of breath. They also engage her in a goals-of-care discussion to assess what care Sheila wants. Sheila mentions that she completed the MYWK tool with her nurse that helped her formulate her goals. Pastoral care came and prayed with her. They also informed her that she can watch mass on the hospital televisions and showed her what channel it is on. Finally, the provider came in to talk with Sheila about her goals and confirmed that she understands that she will die without cancer treatment.

Sheila spent another week in IMC, and she became more and more lethargic. Palliative care continued to manage her symptoms and adjust her medications to ensure she was comfortable. Pastoral care continued to visit her daily and gave her last rights during a period of alertness, because that was important to Sheila. The social worker found contact information for her daughter and called her to see if she would be willing to speak with her mother. Unfortunately, she wasn't willing to speak to her; she was not over what her mother had done. Case management worked on placement for Sheila in an inpatient hospice facility, which proved to be difficult due to Sheila being too young to apply for Medicare hospice benefits. Due to this, Sheila was transferred to the inpatient hospital hospice unit, where her stay was covered by the "charity care" fund at the hospital.

Presently, Sheila is on the hospice unit receiving care and medications to manage her dyspnea and anxiety. Pastoral care continues to visit her daily and prays with and for her even if she is lethargic and unable to participate. She appears comfortable and at peace. The provider called Sheila's daughter to let her know that her mother is dying and is in her final days. The daughter asked if they could put the phone to Sheila's ear so that she could say goodbye.

Summary and Conclusion

There are countless personal, social, political, and economic drivers of vulnerability affecting health around the world. The inequalities in these forces lead to unfair and avoidable health disparities in people's perception of serious illness, chronic diseases, end-of-life care, and how they access and utilize palliative care and services. Health equity aims to minimize and eliminate health disparities that can be avoided. A commitment to health equity in palliative care includes nurses' leadership in examining the determinants of health, access to palliative care among underrepresented groups, and the quality of palliative care services, as well as understanding the complex relationship between patients living with serious illness, their family members, and the community they live in. Nurses can lead multidisciplinary collaboration and use this understanding to develop and practice evidence-based strategies to promote equity in palliative care access and quality and health outcomes.

Authors' Note

Our authorship team wrote this chapter with great care, respect, and humility. This work is written from a culturally humble ethos.[15]We acknowledge and include the work of those who have led work in healthcare inequities—and charted a course for up-and-coming clinicians and researchers—while also acknowledging the limited application and exploration of equity in palliative care to date.[46] The theory of cultural humility acknowledges the differences between us, emphasizes the need for lifelong learning, and recognizes that cultural conflict is normal and to be expected.[15] The authors note that we come from diverse backgrounds including race, ethnicity, nationality, gender, disability, culture, profession, and lived experience. We write this piece from a space of shared learning, and we humbly acknowledge that this work is ultimately incomplete. We offer examples to emphasize our points; however, these lists are not exhaustive—nor do we wish to make any assumptions—as many vulnerable and/or underrepresented groups of people may not even be known or expected due to their unique and nuanced circumstances.

There is no definitive course for moving this evolving work forward, but regardless of the approach, it must involve humility. This was the lens through which the case study woven throughout the chapter was created. Drawn from clinical and research evidence, its purpose is to provide context to the lived experiences of the issues discussed. Though the case centers around a single, fictional patient, the case aims to highlight the myriad of issues any person experiencing challenges in representation and equitable access to care may encounter.

REFERENCES

1. US Department of Health and Human Services, Office of Disease Prevention and Health Promotion. Healthy People 2030: Social Determinants of Health. Accessed October 26, 2022. https://health.gov/healthypeople/objectives-and-data/social-determinants-health.
2. Rivera-Burciaga AR, Palacios M, Kemery SA. Educating for equity in palliative care: implications of the future of nursing 2030 report. *J Prof Nurs.* 2022;42:134–139. https://doi.org/10.1016/j.profnurs.2022.06.012.
3. Cain CL, Surbone A, Elk R, Kagawa-Singer M. Culture and palliative care: preferences, communication, meaning, and mutual decision making. *J Pain Symptom Manage.* 2018;55(5):1408–1419. https://doi.org/10.1016/j.jpainsymman.2018.01.007.
4. Poudel A, Bhuvan KC, Shrestha S, Nissen L. Access to palliative care: discrepancy among low-income and high-income countries. *J Glob Health.* 2019;9(2):020309. https://doi.org/10.7189/jogh.09.020309.
5. Ashana DC, D'Arcangelo N, Gazarian PK, et al. "Don't talk to them about goals of care": understanding disparities in advance care planning. *J Gerontol A Biol Sci Med Sci.* 2022;77(2):339–346. https://doi.org/10.1093/gerona/glab091.
6. Jones T, Luth EA, Lin S-Y, Brody AA. Advance care planning, palliative care, and end-of-life care interventions for racial and ethnic underrepresented groups: a systematic review. *J Pain Symptom Manage.* 2021;62(3):e248–e260. https://doi.org/10.1016/j.jpainsymman.2021.04.025
7. Bharmal N, Derose K, Felician M, Weden M. *Understanding the Upstream Social Determinants of Health.* RAND Corporation; 2015. https://www.resourcebasket.org/wp-content/uploads/2019/01/upstream.pdf.
8. Jones T, Nedjat-Haiem F, Bullock K. Health equity in palliative care. In: Altilio T, Otis-Green S, Cagle JG, eds. *The Oxford Textbook of Palliative Social Work.* 2nd ed. Oxford University Press; 2022.
9. Eckersley R. Beyond inequality: acknowledging the complexity of social determinants of health. *Soc Sci Med.* 2015;147:121–125. https://doi.org/10.1016/j.socscimed.2015.10.052.
10. Havranek EP, Mujahid MS, Barr DA, et al. Social determinants of risk and outcomes for cardiovascular disease: a scientific statement from the American Heart Association. *Circulation.* 2015;132(9):873–898. https://doi.org/10.1161/cir.0000000000000228.
11. National Coalition for Hospice and Palliative Care. *Clinical Practice Guidelines for Quality Palliative Care.* 4th ed. National Coalition for Hospice and Palliative Care; 2018. Accessed October 26, 2022. https://www.nationalcoalitionhpc.org/wp-content/uploads/2020/07/NCHPC-NCPGuidelines_4thED_web_FINAL.pdf.
12. Gardner DS, Doherty M, Bates G, Koplow A, Johnson S. Racial and ethnic disparities in palliative care: a systematic scoping review. *Fam Soc.* 2018;99(4):301–316. https://doi.org/10.1177/1044389418809083.
13. Phan Q, Johnson N, Hillman J, Geller D, Kimble LP, Swan BA. Assessing baccalaureate nursing students' knowledge and attitudes of social determinants of health after a health equity simulation. *Int J Nurs Educ Scholarsh.* 2020;17(1):20200024. https://doi.org/10.1515/ijnes-2020-0024.
14. Ravenna PA, Bream KD, Fancher T, et al. Who, what, and where: transforming primary care education to advance health equity. *J Health Care Poor Underserved.* 2020;31(4 suppl):128–138. https://doi.org/10.1353/hpu.2020.0144.
15. Foronda C. A theory of cultural humility. *J Transcult Nurs.* Jan 2020;31(1):7–12. https://doi.org/10.1177/1043659619875184.
16. Ntizimira C, Deo MS, Dunne M, Krakauer E. Decolonizing end-of-life care: lessons and opportunities. *Ecancermedicalscience.* 2022;16:ed121.
17. Economist Intelligence Unit. *The 2015 Quality of Death Index Ranking Palliative Care across the World.* Economist Intelligence Unit; 2015. https://impact.economist.com/perspectives/sites/default/files/2015%20EIU%20Quality%20of%20Death%20Index%20Oct%2029%20FINAL.pdf.
18. Dixon J, King D, Matosevic T, Clark M, Knapp M. *Equity in the Provision of Palliative Care in the UK: Review of Evidence.* Personal Social Services Research Unit, London School of Economics and Political Science; 2015. https://www.mariecurie.org.uk/globalassets/media/documents/policy/campaigns/equity-palliative-care-uk-report-full-lse.pdf.
19. Nelson KE, Wright R, Peeler A, Brockie T, Davidson PM. Sociodemographic disparities in access to hospice and palliative care: an integrative review. *Am J Hosp Palliat Med.* 2021;38(11):1378–1390. https://doi.org/10.1177/1049909120985419.
20. Frasca M, Galvin A, Raherison C, et al. Palliative versus hospice care in patients with cancer: a systematic review. *BMJ Support Palliat Care.* 2021;11(2):188–199. https://doi.org/10.1136/bmjspcare-2020-002195.
21. Quinn KL, Shurrab M, Gitau K, et al. Association of receipt of palliative care interventions with health care use, quality of life, and symptom burden among adults with chronic noncancer illness: a systematic review and meta-analysis. *JAMA.* 2020;324(14):1439–1450. https://doi.org/10.1001/jama.2020.14205.
22. Fernandes Pedro J, Reis-Pina P. Palliative care in patients with advanced heart failure: a systematic review. *Acta Med Port.* 2022;35(2):111–118. https://doi.org/10.20344/amp.15963.
23. Broese JM, de Heij AH, Janssen DJ, et al. Effectiveness and implementation of palliative care interventions for patients with chronic obstructive pulmonary disease: a systematic review. *Palliat Med.* 2021;35(3):486–502. https://doi.org/10.1177/0269216320981294.
24. de Visser M, Oliver DJ. Palliative care in neuromuscular diseases. *Curr Opin Neurol.* 2017;30(6):686–691. https://doi.org/10.1097/wco.0000000000000493.
25. Imamah NF, Lin HR. Palliative care in patients with end-stage renal disease: a meta synthesis. *Int J Environ Res Public Health.* 2021;18(20):10651. https://doi.org/10.3390/ijerph182010651.
26. Chen EK, Riffin C, Reid MC, et al. Why is high-quality research on palliative care so hard to do? Barriers to improved research from a survey of palliative care researchers. *J Palliat Med.* 2014;17(7):782–787. https://doi.org/10.1089/jpm.2013.0589.
27. Ahluwalia SC, Chen C, Raaen L, et al. A systematic review in support of the National Consensus Project Clinical practice guidelines for quality palliative care, fourth edition. *J Pain Symptom Manage.* 2018;56(6):831–870. https://doi.org/10.1016/j.jpainsymman.2018.09.008.

28. Khalil H, Ristevski E. The challenges of evidence-based palliative care research. *Int J Evid Based Healthc.* 2018;16(3):136–137. https://doi.org/10.1097/xeb.0000000000000153.
29. Higginson IJ. Research challenges in palliative and end of life care. *BM J Support Palliat Care.* 2016;6(1):2–4. https://doi.org/10.1136/bmjspcare-2015-001091.
30. Selim AJ, Rothendler JA, Qian SX, Bailey HM, Kazis LE. The history and applications of the Veterans RAND 12-Item Health Survey (vr-12). *J Ambul Care Manage.* 2022;45(3):161–170. https://doi.org/10.1097/jac.0000000000000420.
31. Markham SA, Levi BH, Green MJ, Schubart JR. Use of a computer program for advance care planning with African American participants. *J Natl Med Assoc.* 2015;107(1):26–32. https://doi.org/10.1016/s0027-9684(15)30006-7.
32. Howard Brown Health. Nurse's Health Education about LGBTQ Elders (HEALE). Accessed October 25, 2022, http://www.nursesheale.org/.
33. De Veer AJE, Stringer B, Van Meijel B, Verkaik R, Francke AL. Access to palliative care for homeless people: complex lives, complex care. *BMC Palliat Care.* 2018;17(1):119. https://doi.org/10.1186/s12904-018-0368-3.
34. Foti ME. "Do It Your Way": a demonstration project on end-of-life care for persons with serious mental illness. *J Palliat Med.* 2004;6(4):661–669. https://doi.org/10.1089/109662103768253830.
35. ElMokhallalati Y, Bradley SH, Chapman E, et al. Identification of patients with potential palliative care needs: a systematic review of screening tools in primary care. *Palliat Med.* 2020;34(8):989–1005. https://doi.org/10.1177/0269216320929552.
36. University of Edinburgh. Supportive & Palliative Care Indicators Tool (SPICT™). Accessed October 23, 2022, https://www.spict.org.uk/.
37. Fachado AA, Martínez NS, Roselló MM, et al. Spanish adaptation and validation of the Supportive & Palliative Care Indicators Tool—SPICT-ES™. *Rev Saude Pública.* 2018;52:3. https://doi.org/10.11606/s1518-8787.2018052000398.
38. Weissman DE, Meier DE. Identifying patients in need of a palliative care assessment in the hospital setting: a consensus report from the Center to Advance Palliative Care. *J Palliat Med.* 2011;14(1):17–23. https://doi.org/10.1089/jpm.2010.0347.
39. Javanparast S, Anaf J, Tieman J. Equity consideration in palliative care policies, programs, and evaluation: an analysis of selected federal and South Australian documents. *BMC Palliat Care.* 2022;21(1):109. https://doi.org/10.1186/s12904-022-00997-2.
40. Ravitch SM, Mittenfelner Carl S. Conceptual frameworks in research. In: Ravitch SM, Mittenfelner CS, eds. *Qualitative Research: Bridging the Conceptual, Theoretical, and Methodological.* 2nd ed. SAGE; 2020.
41. Nelson KE, Wright R, Fisher M, et al. A call to action to address disparities in palliative care access: a conceptual framework for individualizing care needs. *J Palliat Med.* 2021;24(2):177–180. https://doi.org/10.1089/jpm.2020.0435.
42. American Nurses Association. *Nursing: Scope and Standards of Practice. 3rd ed.* American Nurses Association; 2015.
43. Ferrell B, Malloy P, Mazanec P, Virani R. CARES: AACN's new competencies and recommendations for educating undergraduate nursing students to improve palliative care. *J Prof Nurs.* 2016;32(5):327–333. https://doi.org/10.1016/j.profnurs.2016.07.002.
44. Lippe M, Davis A, Stock N, Mazanec P, Ferrell B. Updated palliative care competencies for entry-to-practice and advanced-level nursing students: new resources for nursing faculty. *J Prof Nurs.* 2022;42:250–261. https://doi.org/10.1016/j.profnurs.2022.07.012.
45. American Nurses Association. *Palliative Nursing: Scope and Standards of Practice. 6th ed.* American Nurses Association; 2020.
46. Richards N. The equity turn in palliative and end of life care research: Lessons from the poverty literature. *Sociol Compass.* 2022;16(5):e12969. https://doi.org/10.1111/soc4.12969.

67

Affirmative Palliative Care for LGBTQIA+ Patients and Their Families

Kailey E. Roberts, William E. Rosa, Noelle Marie Javier, Pierce DiMauro, Joshua C. Eyer, and Kristin G. Cloyes

Key Points

- Quality palliative care includes provision of responsive, affirming, and inclusive care to LGBTQIA+ patients and families.
- The LGBTQIA+ community experiences health and healthcare disparities due in large part to discrimination and systemic barriers.
- As frontline clinicians, nurses are well positioned to take steps to addressing these disparities and improving care for LGBTQIA+ patients with serious illness and their families in the ethical/legal, physical, and psychosocial domains of palliative care.

In the United States alone, recent estimates suggest 7.1% of the population identify as lesbian, gay, bisexual, transgender, queer, intersex, or asexual (LGBTQIA+; + represents sexual orientations and gender identities not captured in the listed letters), with the relative proportion increasing notably in younger generations.[1] Yet 50%–70% of LGBTQIA+ individuals have reported receiving poor medical care across a range of clinical settings, including palliative and end-of-life (EOL) care.[2,3] LGBTQIA+ cultural responsiveness is an essential component of nursing practice.[4,5] The ability to provide accessible, inclusive, and affirming care requires being aware of and addressing patients' and families' unique needs, contexts, and experiences, while also working to reduce the pervasive disparities shaped by structural and systemic barriers that limit access to quality healthcare.[2,6] Healthcare education and providers' practices are also shaped by structural barriers and cultural norms, such as cisheteronormativity (see Table 67.1), that can lead to unconscious and conscious biases. Thus, care necessitates not only cultural responsiveness but cultural humility, an important process necessitating nurses to reflect on their own identities and values and how these may impact those receiving care.[7]

This chapter aims to provide nurses with essential information and guidance to empower them to practice LGBTQIA+ responsive and affirming palliative care. We review key concepts and terms, health disparities that impact palliative care needs, ethical considerations, physical care needs, psychosocial and spiritual needs, and the needs of families and caregivers. Throughout the chapter we present a case to illustrate key points nurses need to consider and apply when providing care to LGBTQIA+ patients and families.

Central Concepts and Terms

Responsive, affirming, and inclusive palliative nursing for LGBTQIA+ patients involves recognizing and understanding relevant terms and concepts. This includes assigned sex at birth, gender identity, and sexual orientation (see Table 67.1 for additional terms and concepts). Assigned sex at birth (ASAB) refers to a binary label of male or female typically determined by observing an infant's genitals at birth. Gender is a social construct encompassing both identity and expression; it can be fluid across the life span and influenced by culture and life circumstances.[8] Gender identity is an individual's internal sense of gender, while gender expression refers to one's outward gender presentation, which may or may not match one's gender identity.[5] Gender identity and expression may or may not align with ASAB; however, they can be influenced by and/or conflated with ASAB.

"Transgender" is a term for individuals whose ASAB does not align with their gender identity, whereas "cisgender" refers to individuals whose ASAB aligns with their gender identity. Others may not experience gender according to a masculine/feminine binary and identify as gender-fluid, genderqueer, or nonbinary. Transgender and nonbinary individuals do not always seek gender-affirming surgeries or other forms of body modification and/or may be selective about how they express gender, depending on the setting.[5] It is critical to follow a person's lead on gender identity and not make assumptions about identity or terms based on observed gender expression, body parts, or diagnosis (e.g., cancer location).[5] For example, while a veteran may identify as a trans woman and generally express her gender in a more feminine manner, she may present as masculine when visiting a veteran space because of military cultural expectations and associated safety concerns.

Table 67.1 Key terms and concepts for LGBTQIA+ responsive and affirming care

Term	Definition
Asexuality	A sexual orientation term for someone who does not experience sexual attraction or experiences little sexual attraction. Note asexuality does not necessarily equate to not engaging in sexual behaviors or not having romantic or intimate relationships. Also referred to as "ace."
Assigned sex-at-birth (ASAB)	A binary label of male or female typically determined by observing genitals at birth. ASAB may not align with gender identity
Biological sex	References anatomical, genetic, and physiological characteristics that are used to label individuals as male, female, or intersex. Often conflated with gender.
Bisexual	Refers to individuals who are attracted romantically, sexually, and/or emotionally to more than one gender. The "bi" does not inherently indicate attraction to only cisgender/binary individuals. Some may also or instead refer to themselves as "pansexual."
Chosen family	Kinship formations that do not necessarily correspond to biological or legal familial ties. Can include friends, bio-legal family, neighbors, and other community members. Also referred to as "family of choice" versus "family of origin."
Cisgender	ASAB and gender identity align. Also referred to as "cis."
Cisheteronormativity	Implicit assumptions that being cisgender and heterosexual or straight is the norm and superior. Can manifest as microaggressions toward LGBTQIA+ individuals or explicit discrimination.
Deadname	Name that a transgender or nonbinary person was given at birth but that they no longer use.
Detransition/detransitioning	Process by which a person either by choice or without consent transitions to their ASAB. This can come in the form of stopping treatments such as hormone replacement therapy, changing gender expression, or reversing surgical interventions. Posthumous nonconsensual detransitioning can be a risk if individuals do not document their preferences prior to death.
Disenfranchised grief	Grief that is not acknowledged as "legitimate" by society and that is subsequently ignored or invalidated in some way. Related concepts include stifled or suffocated grief.
Gay	Describes individuals who identify as men who are emotionally, sexually, and/or romantically attracted to other men. Sometimes also used more broadly to capture being part of the LGBTQIA+ community by those in the community.
Gender	A social construct including behaviors, roles, and characteristics on a spectrum of femininity, masculinity, and androgyny. Often conflated with biological sex. Includes gender identity and expression.
Gender-affirming surgery	Surgical interventions that may be performed as part of gender-affirming care. "Bottom surgery" refers to surgery to modify genitals and/or reproductive organs. "Top surgery" refers to surgery performed on the chest area to remove, reduce, or increase tissue.
Gender expression	How an individual expresses or communicates gender through appearance, clothing, and actions. May be on a spectrum of masculinity, femininity, and androgyny. Does not necessarily align with gender identity.
Gender-fluid	A gender identity in which a person's gender may fluctuate day to day. May come across primarily in gender expression.
Gender identity	An individual's internal sense of gender. May or may not align with ASAB.
Gender nonconforming	Used to describe those who identify as genderqueer, nonbinary, gender-fluid, or any identity that does not conform to masculine/feminine binary. Can be considered pathologizing based on its placing of people as "not" falling into a norm.
Heterosexual or straight	Sexual or romantic attraction to those of a different gender or sex.
Homophobia/transphobia	Prejudice and bias toward LGBTQIA+ individuals.
Homosexual	Generally considered outdated, this term was used in the medical and psychological literature to refer to same-gender sexual orientation. Though considered offensive because of its association with pathologizing of LGBTQ+ communities, some individuals, especially older adults, may still use this term to refer to themselves.
Hormone replacement therapy	A gender-affirming treatment involving the taking of either testosterone or estrogen.
Intersex	Some infants are born intersex, which can refer to variations in chromosomes or internal structures or external genitalia. When observable externally, parents typically choose a sex assignment for the child.
Lesbian	Individuals who identify as women who are emotionally, sexually, and/or romantically attracted to other women.
Men who have sex with men	Often used in epidemiological or medical literature to refer to cisgender men who have sex with cisgender men but who do not necessarily identify as gay, bisexual, or queer.
Microaggressions	Microaggressions are defined as verbal or nonverbal messages of discrimination or insult based on a marginalized identity. Typically they are linked to implicit bias, and the person engaging in the microaggression may not be aware they are doing it. Microaggressions toward LGTBQIA+ patients and families in medical settings include cisheteronormative assumptions, blatant misgendering, and misguided assumptions about or lack of recognition of kinships (e.g., not having chosen family recognized).
Minority and minoritized	"Minority" is used to refer to nondominant or marginalized groups. "Minoritized" is increasingly being used to replace the word "minority" to indicate that oppression is not an identity but rather a state imposed on marginalized groups.
Nonbinary/genderqueer	A gender identity in which a person does not identify solely with binary gender (masculine or feminine). "Nonbinary" can overlap with the term "genderqueer," though individuals may have distinctions depending on which term they feel identifies them best. Genderqueer tends to be associated with certain subcultures of LGBTQIA+ communities and/or politized.

Table 67.1 Continued

Term	Definition
Polyamorous	Having multiple, consenting intimate relationships as opposed to monogamy. Typically used to refer to romantic or sexual relationships but not always. Poly partners may maintain separate relationships with their partners, or there may be poly kinships in which multiple partners are in a relationship with each other. Also referred to as "poly," "multi-," and "ethically non-monogamous."
Queer	A reclaimed word historically used in a derogatory manner. Often used as a broad term to capture being part of the LGBTQIA+ community by those in the community. Can also be used to reference a gender identity or sexual orientation that does not align with a binary.
Sexual orientation/identity	An identity connected to whom one is attracted to romantically or sexually, if anyone. Can also be a relational and community orientation more generally. Does not inherently correspond to sexual behavior or expression.
Sexuality	Umbrella term encompassing the intersection of sexual orientation, sexual expression, sexual behaviors, and gender identity.
Transgender	ASAB and gender identity do not align. Also referred to as "trans."
Transgender man	Typically refers to an individual who identifies as a man but whose ASAB was female. Also referred to as "trans man."
Transgender woman	Typically refers to an individual who identifies as a woman but whose ASAB was male. Also referred to as "trans woman."
Transition/transitioning	Process by which individuals affirm their gender identity socially, medically, and/or legally, if it does not align with ASAB. Can involve taking hormones (e.g., testosterone, estrogen), surgeries, as well as name and pronoun changes.
Transexual	Outdated term that formerly referred to individuals whose ASAB does not align with their gender identity. "Transgender" has replaced this term for many; however, particularly older adults may still use this term. It is not appropriate to use this term unless it is what a person wishes to be referred to as because it has been used in a derogatory and/or inaccurate manner.
Two-spirit	Refers to individuals who also identify as Indigenous who experience their gender identity as having both masculine and feminine spirits.

"Sexual orientation" (or "sexual identity") refers to an identity that reflects whom one is attracted to romantically or sexually, yet it also pertains to individuals who identify as asexual and does not inherently correspond to sexual expression or behavior. It is also often experienced more broadly as a relational and/or community orientation and identity.[9] Sexuality, encompassing the intersection of sexual orientation, sexual expression, sexual behaviors, and gender identity, is important to many, though not all, people in circumstances of serious illness.

Sexual orientation and gender identity (SOGI) are not the only factors that may be key to providing responsive, affirming, and inclusive palliative care. The LGBTQIA+ community comprises diverse individuals and groups, with varying experiences based on LGBTQIA+ identity(-ies) as well as race, religion, nationality, age, social networks, health history, life course, and lived experiences. An *intersectionality* framework can guide the understanding of an individual's sociocultural identities and how these impact their experiences of privilege, oppression, and power.[2,10] For example, a 70-year-old socially isolated Black, gay, cisgender man with low income who lived through the HIV/AIDS epidemic brings distinctive histories and experiences that will impact his healthcare needs when facing illness.

Introducing Gerry

Consider the experience of Gerry,* a 65-year-old queer, Black trans man diagnosed with ovarian cancer. At the time of his diagnosis, he had been married to Ana, a 44-year-old bisexual, Latina cis woman, for 16 years. Ana and Gerry have two children, a 15-year-old from Ana's previous marriage and a 10-year-old conceived through in vitro fertilization, both of whom were co-parented with Ana's ex-husband, Victor. Until his cancer diagnosis, Gerry had worked as a high school math teacher, a job he loved, but then went on medical leave. Consequently, they have struggled with finances, relying on Ana's income*.

Gerry had an oophorectomy and hysterectomy after his cancer diagnosis, surgeries that were emotionally charged as he had been considering gender-affirming surgery prior to his diagnosis but had encountered roadblocks to accessing this care. When he began chemotherapy, the oncologist pushed for Gerry to discontinue gender-affirming testosterone hormone therapy. Though this was a devastating decision, Gerry agreed, maintaining hope that it would be temporary and that the chemotherapy would succeed. Gerry was given insufficient information to effectively engage in decision-making around balancing life-extending interventions with quality of life. Together, the cessation of his gender-affirming care, the oncologic surgeries, and chemotherapy heightened his gender dysphoria about his anatomy; paired with his advancing disease, Gerry suffered tremendous emotional and physical pain. Despite his distress, he adaptively coped by drawing on the support of Ana, Victor, their children, his mother, his friend and healthcare proxy Chun, and his faith community.

* Case reflects common experiences among LGBTQIA + patients and families; details do not represent a single individual.

Disparities in Health and Healthcare

LGBTQIA+ individuals are at high risk for developing serious and chronic illnesses that require palliative care,[11,12] such as cardiovascular disease[13] and cancer,[14] although current estimates likely undercount incidence and prevalence because SOGI data is not routinely collected in many medical and research settings.[15,16] Serious and chronic illness prevalence disparities are associated with stigma,[6] discrimination,[17] disparate access to quality healthcare,[18] provider assumptions,[19] and medical mistrust due to personal or collective trauma,[18] all factors that deter LGBTQIA+ individuals from pursuing routine health screening and/or treatment. Within the LGTBQIA+ population, transgender individuals, people of color,[20] older adults,[21] those living with HIV,[22] and those with low income[23] are at significantly higher risk for discrimination and poor care. Gatekeeping access to gender-affirming care[8] also contributes to explicit barriers, as well as potentially perpetuating a lack of agency in those pursuing care.

Barriers to LGTBQIA+ responsive palliative care are numerous and range from basic lack of knowledge or awareness to forms of implicit and explicit bias and discrimination operating at intrapersonal, interpersonal, and institutional levels.[2] Explicit forms of discrimination include physical abuse, neglect, or outright refusal of care; and implicit forms include microaggressions (see Table 67.1), neglect, and unconscious prejudice, such as invoking stereotypes.[2] Institutional factors may also present barriers by setting limitations on visitors, failing to document name changes or preferred pronouns, not collecting SOGI demographic data on all patients, and failing to include patients' chosen care partners in communication and planning.[3,16] Historical and current systemic trauma and discrimination contribute to medical mistrust. Transgender individuals of color, in particular, have expressed fears around being left to die, not receiving equitable or affirming care, concerns about active treatment being taken away because of identity, and fears of being treated violently, often reflecting personal histories of mistreatment and violence.[2,6,24] As a result, they may fail to receive appropriate gender-affirming care and support in the context of serious illness and be forced to detransition.[25] As we saw with Gerry, though he ultimately agreed to discontinue hormone replacement therapy at the recommendation of his provider, he was not given sufficient information about the costs and benefits of doing so.

Despite evidence of barriers to quality care and health disparities in the LGBTQIA+ community, notably, providers may not think that LGBTQIA+ patients or families have unique EOL care needs; they may also believe that they treat all patients and families the same.[26] Palliative and EOL care providers may generalize needs as being universal and lack knowledge of how the history and context of LGBTQIA+ disparities shape individual experiences.[19]

Ethical and Legal Considerations

Foundational to addressing barriers to LGBTQIA+ responsive palliative care is affirming communication and documentation in the context of working with an interdisciplinary team. When engaging in discussions about and documenting advance care planning, healthcare proxy designations, and a living will,[27] nurses and other healthcare professionals should sensitively invite opportunities for disclosure and directly communicate with the patient in a private setting.[2] It is important to be mindful of who should be involved in care discussions with the patient, chosen family, and/or family of origin. There may be complex family dynamics, yet nurses should avoid assuming family discordance just because the patient is LGBTQIA+.

Documentation about communication preferences, including SOGI identifiers and pronouns, should be reflected in the medical records and integrated into all discussions and patient interactions.[2] To ensure consistency of care across patients, nurses who are new to a patient should inquire about how they wish to be referred to by asking their names and gender pronouns. In some cases, a patient may express that they prefer to be referred to in a certain way in clinical spaces while maintaining different identifiers in the medical record because of privacy and safety concerns.[28] For example, a transgender or nonbinary patient may express that they prefer their "deadname" (i.e., name that they were given at birth but no longer use) be used in the medical record but that they would like to be called by their actual name by staff.[28,29] Sensitivity around documentation should also be extended to any in-room charting or posting of the patient's name and/or pronouns. Change-in-shift reports should communicate the patient's preferences and any unique circumstances in which they wish to be referred to differently (e.g., if certain family members are present) including the patient's support system and caregivers.[16,28,29]

Documentation considerations also extend to information about caregivers and family members for both legal purposes (e.g., identifying the patient's healthcare proxy) and the provision of caregiver and bereavement care.[16] Despite legal recognition in some countries of same-sex marriage and associated rights, these laws remain precarious; LGBTQIA+ partners or spouses still face discrimination in healthcare settings.[30] Further, chosen family members who are not legally married or who do not match heteronormative conceptualizations of family (e.g., friends) are often excluded or overlooked despite commonly being in caregiving roles for LGBTQIA+ individuals.[15,31] See Table 67.2 for suggested ways to assess name, pronouns, and family.

Ethical and legal dilemmas may arise around burial and funeral planning when working with LGBTQIA+ patients and families.[32] Transgender or nonbinary individuals who do not legally document their wishes may be at risk for posthumous *detransitioning*,

Table 67.2 Questions to ask to guide an LGBTQIA+ responsive, affirming, and inclusive palliative care assessment

Circumstance/purpose	Question
Inquiry about sex and gender	• What sex were you assigned at birth? • How do you describe your gender?
Establishing name and pronouns	• What name would you like to be called? • What pronouns do you use? • Are there circumstances or settings in which you would like to be referred to by a different name or have other pronouns used?
Determining supports, caregivers, and who should be included in decision-making/care discussions	• Who are the important people in your life? • Who is involved in your care?

which in turn can violate their dignity in death, as well as cause more sorrow for grieving loved ones.[24] While nurses may not be directly involved in bereavement care beyond initial follow-up, they often play an important role in initiating discussions about and documenting the patient's goals of care and EOL wishes. This is an opportunity to inquire about their body disposition and burial preferences, as well as who should be contacted for bereavement follow-up if they die.[32]

In Gerry's case, documentation issues, as well as a lack of understanding about his chosen family contributed to substandard care when he was also grappling with the devastating news that the cancer metastasized. A few weeks after Gerry received the result of metastatic cancer, he and Ana scheduled a consultation with palliative care and had been considering a shift in his goals toward a more comfort-focused approach. However, due to an acute-onset stomach pain, Gerry was admitted, alone, to a local hospital that contained older medical records documenting his deadname and ASAB. Eventually, Ana and Chun arrived at the hospital and advocated for modifications to the record. In the meantime, amidst his excruciating pain, Gerry had become increasingly distressed as he faced correcting each provider who misgendered him and called him by his deadname. Moreover, upon learning that Ana was Gerry's wife, the healthcare team began directing their attention only to Ana, excluding Chun from conversations, despite their role as Gerry's additional caregiver and healthcare proxy. Responsive and affirming care in these circumstances would involve the care team clarifying the documentation issue with each other to remove the burden from Gerry when possible and apologizing for instances of misgendering when corrected. Additionally, in care discussions, the team should respect Gerry's preference that both Ana and Chun be closely involved. Often nurses have close and frequent contact with patients and their families more than other providers and thus can be key conduits for communicating preferences and needs to their interdisciplinary teams.

Physical Care for LGBTQIA+ Patients

While the holistic tradition of palliative nursing may meet some physical needs of LGBTQIA+ patients, nurses may lack formal training on unique physical aspects of care for this population. As with all aspects of palliative nursing, it is important for nurses to work closely with an interdisciplinary team, especially if they lack knowledge about specific LGBTQIA+ needs.[2] For any form of physical care, nurses should be particularly attentive to seeking permission, vocalizing and explaining each step of the care they are providing, and following the lead of the patient as many LGBTQIA+ individuals have had negative experiences in medical settings.[33] In initial encounters it is critical to demonstrate openness and respect in order to cultivate comfort in the encounter and facilitate the physical exam and history-taking.[34]

Though important for all patients, particularly in practice with transgender or nonbinary patients, the nurse should employ cultural humility when addressing patient anatomy and treatment plans to ensure an outcome that considers and validates the patient's identity.[7] A patient's permission should always be obtained when performing physical examinations, allowing patients to lead based on their comfort level. The nurse should allow the patient to provide insight on the naming of their anatomy while avoiding labeling specific body parts using gendered terms.[28,33]

Providing responsive, affirming, and inclusive palliative care for the LGBTQIA+ community also includes acknowledging and supporting the sexual needs and experiences of these patients.[2] Microaggressions are common when discussing sexual health with LGBTQIA+ individuals, such as assuming penetration in sex or assumptions and judgments about having multiple sexual partners. Nurses should not make assumptions about sexual behavior or needs based on sexual orientation or gender identity and should cultivate comfort with addressing sexual health questions for patients. For some LGTBQIA+ patients, physical needs may also include discussions around reproduction and fertility preservation. Nurses should not discount or ignore fertility needs based on gender identity, sexual orientation, or partner status.

Older LGBTQIA+ adults should receive goal-concordant medical care within the appropriate care setting, whether at home or in a facility (see Chapter 71, "Palliative Care for Older Adults"; Chapter 62, "Long-Term Care").[3] While older age can be linked with additional vulnerabilities, palliative nurses can also focus on the strengths and resilience of older LGBTQIA+ adults, many of whom have successfully navigated a lifetime of discrimination impacting health and healthcare. For older LGBTQIA+ adults with an HIV diagnosis, though antiretroviral therapy has dramatically reduced morbidity, palliative nurses should assess symptom burden and collaborate with the patient and interdisciplinary care team to develop care plans addressing pain, symptom distress, and illness trajectory.[2]

Gerry's challenges with ovarian cancer were exacerbated by problematic interactions with providers. Several times providers expressed confusion about his diagnosis of ovarian cancer and his masculine appearance, with several initially treating Ana as if she were the patient with cancer and assuming Gerry was her caregiver. Providers were inconsistently attentive to Gerry's discomfort with medical exams involving gendered body parts. Vaginal ultrasounds were particularly traumatic for him. During one outpatient appointment, Gerry and Ana had hoped to talk to the nurse about genital tissue dryness and recommendations for comfort care as well as sexual health. The nurse appeared uncomfortable, saying "I think we need to prioritize other more important aspects of your care" and quickly suggested that Ana and Gerry "see a specialist to figure that out" but was unable to provide a referral. Given his increasingly poor health, Gerry and Ana did not pursue a referral, leaving Gerry in continued discomfort.

There are several ways Gerry's physical care could have been improved. Providers could have drawn upon trauma-informed approaches to establish a safe encounter by offering choices, collaboration opportunities, validation of his and his families' needs or concerns, and confirmation that their wishes would drive the care planning.[34] Clinicians should use nongendered terms such as "genital opening" rather than "vagina." Gerry's sexual health needs could have been addressed more sensitively by first validating his experiences and then providing a warm handoff to a person more qualified if the nurse was unfamiliar with LGBTQIA+ sexual health.[35]

Psychosocial and Spiritual Needs

The psychosocial needs of LGBTQIA+ palliative care patients are also influenced by their individual life and illness circumstances, as well as by the care given in other domains of palliative care.[6]

LGBTQIA+ individuals may experience stressors that exacerbate and amplify illness-related stressors including discrimination, medical trauma, microaggressions, family conflict, separation from chosen family, and social isolation.[6] Additionally, LGBTQIA+ individuals may have preexisting mental health concerns connected to a lifetime of exposure to stressors and traumas[21] and the resulting lack of social safety.[36] LGBTQIA+ people of color are at particularly high risk for experiencing mental health distress, including suicidal ideation, due to multiple sources of minority stress.[36] Many LGBTQIA+ individuals experience intersectional marginalization from ageism, racism, cis-sexism, financial disenfranchisement, and ableism that can significantly impact their mental health.[6,10,21] Specific psychosocial needs may include coping with risk, stigma, trauma, identity distress, and supporting of resilience.[21]

Psychological Care

Quality psychological palliative care requires careful assessment of the needs and contexts of each patient and addressing patient concerns in a way that is aligned with their cultural and personal preferences.[37] Assessment should be attentive to the possibility of physical causes of psychological distress (e.g., discontinuing gender-affirming hormone therapy). It is also important to avoid assumptions that all of a patient's psychological needs revolve around their sexual orientation or gender identity.[8]

The preservation of a patient's sense of dignity and meaning should guide psychosocial support in palliative care. LGBTQIA+ individuals may have experienced indignities throughout their life, and distress around this can resurge when facing a life-threatening illness.[6] This is particularly the case if healthcare experiences perpetuate or remind them of past medical traumas.[34] For example, we witnessed in Gerry's story that he did not receive sensitive gynecologic or oncologic care, which could be both traumatizing and dehumanizing.[35] Psychological care aimed at maintaining dignity and meaning for the patient can include the delivery of evidence-based interventions such as Meaning-Centered Psychotherapy.[37] A shared element across dignity and meaning-focused interventions is the idea of having one's story witnessed. For LGBTQIA+ individuals, who may have had their stories and sense of worth invalidated repeatedly across their lives, simply pausing to listen to their experiences without judgment and honoring their resilience and personhood can be a powerful intervention.[37]

When delivering psychological interventions that involve the reframing of distressing thoughts or perspective-taking, clinicians should be mindful to avoid invalidating the unique and common stressors and fears LGBTQIA+ individuals experience.[38] These may include fear of bodily violation or disrespect, homophobia, transphobia, discrimination, stereotypes, and stigma. It is equally critical to balance adaptive coping with validation of painful realities.[38] Trauma-informed care should also be drawn upon when working with LGBTQIA+ individuals.[34] Sensitivity to the scope of practice and reasonable limits on what may be addressed in a palliative care context are key (e.g., not pushing patients to disclose trauma and being sensitive to their shifting emotional needs).

While hospitalized, Gerry's condition quickly declined, and he began to be in and out of consciousness. At times he presented as irritable toward staff, at one point shouting when a nurse came to change his catheter at night. The nurse became frustrated and assumed Gerry was "just being difficult." The next day, Ana returned to the hospital and found Gerry highly distressed. He said that he was in pain and that strangers had been touching him in the night. Ana brought this up to the team and was initially met with assertions that Gerry was being "too sensitive." Eventually, it was determined that Gerry was suffering from delirium caused by a urinary tract infection, and it was treated (see Chapter 23, "Acute Delirium"). However, Gerry and Ana were upset at the assumptions that had been made about his psychological presentation. Gerry endured microaggressions as providers invalidated his distress. Black individuals are particularly subject to discrimination when it comes to expressions of pain and mental health distress.[39] In this circumstance, it would be important for the team to be aware of the potential for bias and to draw on a trauma-informed approach to reduce his distress. The nurse could have taken steps to create a safer environment, such as asking permission, explaining the reason for the intervention, and validating his distress. After identifying and treating the delirium, the team could have provided psychoeducation to Gerry and Ana and normalized the distressing nature of the situation.

Spiritual Care

Spiritual care is a critical component of palliative psychosocial support (see Chapter 33, "Addressing Spiritual, Religious, and Existential Needs in Palliative Care"). Though such support should be offered to all patients, nurses working with LGBTQIA+ patients may make assumptions that limit access to spiritual care such as believing that LGBTQIA+ individuals are not religious or have negative views of religion or spirituality.[40,41] Moreover, nurses' own religious views may entail biases that impede them from engaging LGBTQIA+ patients in religious or spiritual assessment.[40,41] Spiritual care should be offered to all patients regardless of identities as part of culturally responsive care. Each person's particular needs should be considered (i.e., their faith, if any, and preferences for chaplains or opportunities to contact other faith leaders outside of the hospital). Considerations should also be made that family and patient spiritual needs may differ.[6]

For example, in Gerry's case, his faith differed from his mother's. In a moment when Gerry was not able to communicate and Ana was taking a needed break at home, his mother and Chun were at his bedside. His mother demanded the nurse bring in a chaplain to provide last rites. Chun expressed that they had already done this with Gerry's queer Unitarian Universalist pastor and that a chaplain was not needed. The nurse, unsure of who to listen to, acquiesced to the mother's request, assuming that Chun was "just" a friend and not realizing that Chun was indeed the healthcare proxy. In this case, it would have been important for the team to assess Gerry's spiritual needs as early in admission as possible and, if he was unable to communicate, to verify the healthcare proxy so as to ensure Gerry's spiritual care wishes were met.

Families and Caregivers

Responsive, affirming, and inclusive palliative care also attends to caregiver and family member needs, both before and after the patient's death.[30] Identifying family in the LGBTQIA+ patient's life involves recognizing that both family of origin and chosen family members may be involved and that their needs and preferences may align or differ.[16] For many LGBTQIA+ people, their primary supports may be friends rather than biological or legal family members. If the patient is able to communicate, it is critical to ask who they consider family and who they want to be involved in their care and medical decision-making.[16]

Some LGTBQIA + individuals, especially those over 80+ years old, may lack supports because of disenfranchisement within the LGBTQIA+ community due to ageism and/or cissexism, generational differences in experiences of intergenerational relationships, and dwindling social support networks.[6] These patients can benefit from assessment of their support system and referral to formal support resources. For patients who do have supports, these individuals may have varying needs and experiences. Family members may identify as LGTBQIA+ and be concerned about or experience stigmatization or discrimination in the context of their loved one's care.[16,42] The experiences of chosen family may also be impacted by their particular relationship with the patient (e.g., partner, friend).[15,31] The ethical and legal ramifications should be considered along with support needs of the individuals involved.

Though Gerry's family generally was united in his care, it was also clear that the identification of each person's role in his care was a challenge that the medical team failed by making assumptions about whose input should be prioritized. During his hospitalization even the most well-meaning of providers engaged in microaggressions, with one nurse expressing to Ana "I'm so sorry about your wife." Another was overheard "joking" about how confusing their family is when Victor was visiting one day with the children and Chun had just been by. Recognizing and addressing biases related to LGBTQIA+ kinship structure is critical to responsive and affirming palliative care.

Bereavement

Bereavement care is an often-overlooked aspect of palliative care, though no less essential.[43] Too often chosen family members do not receive bereavement care, in part due to barriers in being able to know who to contact[16] and due to assumptions that family of origin should be prioritized for bereavement care. LGBTQIA+ bereaved family members may also be at risk for *disenfranchised grief*, or grief that is not acknowledged as "legitimate" by society and that is subsequently ignored or invalidated.[30,32] Bereavement care should begin before the patient's death and particularly when working with LGBTQIA+ patients and families (see Chapter 58, "Grief and Bereavement"). This should include documentation about who the family is and who may need bereavement follow-up should the patient die. This may not be apparent and may necessitate inquiring with the patient prior to their death as part of family-centered care.[16] Further, palliative care nurses are positioned to provide bereavement care both before and immediately after a patient's death including educating and preparing families about EOL processes, conducting bereavement risk screening, and connecting family and supporters to appropriate support services.[43] In the context of caring for LGBTQIA+ patients and their families, factors that can complicate bereavement include family conflict or estrangement, trauma history, and isolation; and these may increase the risk for disenfranchised grief.[32] If conducting condolence calls, nurses should also be mindful of any information documented about the patient's wishes regarding the extent to which they were "out" and to whom. For example, if the patient had requested to be called by their deadname while their family of origin was present, this should be respected in the context of their death even if the care team otherwise referred to them by their actual name.[24]

Though his wish was to die at home with all of his loved ones nearby, Gerry died overnight in the hospital with only Ana by his side. The team offered sympathies to Ana and information about contacting social work for grief support, but Chun and Gerry's mother were not contacted with bereavement follow-up. With his loved ones as fierce advocates, Gerry was fortunate to not face indignities in death such as posthumous misgendering. Further, as his families of choice and of origin generally were on good terms, they united in their grief. However, the EOL experiences of many LGBTQIA+ individuals are fraught. Power dynamics and conflict among the medical team or the patients' family can contribute to potentially traumatic EOL scenarios.[44] Nurses may experience a sense of moral distress amidst structural barriers to providing LGBTQIA+ responsive and affirming care.[44] Thus, institutions must support nurses by offering and incentivizing continuing education for all providers in this area and employing systems-level changes such as consistent documentation of SOGI information.

Conclusion

Throughout this chapter, the unique palliative care needs of LGBTQIA+ patients and families have been highlighted with recommendations for how palliative nurses can practice more responsive, affirming, and inclusive care. While clinical competency guidelines have been developed for LGBTQIA+ responsive care across practice settings,[2,40] gaps remain in the research on clinical care for LGBTQIA+ individuals facing serious illness, as do systemic barriers that produce extensive health and healthcare disparities.[11,12] Nevertheless, individual nurses can be key to improving care for LGBTQIA+ individuals and families by (1) documenting and communicating about care needs, kinship, and SOGI identifiers; (2) engaging in additional training on competencies for LGBTQIA+ care; and (3) continuing to cultivate cultural humility and recognition of biases.[6,40] Responsive and affirming care also involves recognizing the resilience of LGBTQIA+ individuals and how the community has mobilized to care for its members when those in power have failed to do so.[2] Resilience and coping have been exemplified in the community-based caregiving seen during the HIV/AIDS epidemic, in activism for LGBTQIA+ rights, in mutual caregiving among queer people with disabilities,[45] and in the formation of chosen families.[9] Affirming and inclusive palliative care necessitates balancing the recognition and reduction of challenges LGBTQIA+ individuals face in healthcare with honoring the robust interpersonal and intrapersonal resources they may draw upon when facing serious illness.[2]

REFERENCES

1. Jones JM. U.S. LGBT Identification Steady at 7.2%. Gallup. February 22, 2023. Accessed August 1st, 2023. https://news.gallup.com/poll/470708/lgbt-identification-steady.aspx.
2. Javier NM. Palliative care needs, concerns, and affirmative strategies for the LGBTQ population. *Palliat Care Soc Pract.* 2021;15:26323524211039234.

3. Haviland K, Burrows Walters C, Newman S. Barriers to palliative care in sexual and gender minority patients with cancer: a scoping review of the literature. *Health Soc Care Community*. 2021;29(2):305–318.
4. ANA Ethics Advisory Board. ANA position statement: nursing advocacy for LGBTQ+ populations. *Online J Issues Nurs*. 2018;24(1). https://ojin.nursingworld.org/table-of-contents/volume-24-2019/number-1-january-2019/ana-position-statement-advocacy-for-lgbtq/
5. Lippe MP, Eyer JC, Roberts KE, et al. Affirmative palliative care for transgender and gender nonconforming individuals. *Am J Nurs*. 2023;123(4):48–53.
6. Rosa WE, Roberts KE, Baybrook D, et al. Palliative and end-of-life care needs, experiences and preferences of LGBT+ individuals with serious or chronic illness: a systematic review. *Palliat Med*. 2023;37(4):460–474.
7. Sprik P, Gentile D. Cultural humility: a way to reduce LGBTQ health disparities at the end of life. *Am J Hosp Palliat Care*. 2020;37(6):404–408.
8. Chang SC, Singh AA. Affirming psychological practice with transgender and gender nonconforming people of color. *Psychol Sex Orient Gender Divers*. 2016;3(2):140–147.
9. Hammack PL, Frost DM, Hughes SD. Queer intimacies: a new paradigm for the study of relationship diversity. *J Sex Res*. 2019;56(4–5):556–592.
10. Damaskos P, Amaya B, Gordon R, Walters CB. Intersectionality and the LGBT cancer patient. *Semin Oncol Nurs*. 2018;34(1):30–36.
11. Stinchcombe A, Smallbone J, Wilson K, Kortes-Miller K. Healthcare and end-of-life needs of lesbian, gay, bisexual, and transgender (LGBT) older adults: a scoping review. *Geriatrics (Basel)*. 2017;2(1):13.
12. National Academies of Sciences, Engineering, and Medicine. *Understanding the Well-Being of LGBTQI+ Populations*. National Academies Press; 2020.
13. Rosati F, Williams DP, Juster R-P, Thayer JF, Ottaviani C, Baiocco R. The cardiovascular conundrum in ethnic and sexual minorities: a potential biomarker of constant coping with discrimination. *Front Neurosci*. 2021;15:619171.
14. Saunders CL, Meads C, Abel GA, Lyratzopoulos G. Associations between sexual orientation and overall and site-specific diagnosis of cancer: evidence from two national patient surveys in England. *J Clin Oncol*. 2017;35(32):3654–3661.
15. Marsack J, Stephenson R. Barriers to end-of-life care for LGBT persons in the absence of legal marriage or adequate legal documentation. *LGBT Health*. 2018;5(5):273–283.
16. Rosa WE, Banerjee SC, Maingi S. Family caregiver inclusion is not a level playing field: toward equity for the chosen families of sexual and gender minority patients. *Palliat Care Soc Pract*. 2022;16:26323524221092459.
17. Casey LS, Reisner SL, Findling MG, et al. Discrimination in the United States: experiences of lesbian, gay, bisexual, transgender, and queer Americans. *Health Serv Res*. 2019;54 Suppl 2:1454–1466.
18. Martos AJ, Fingerhut A, Wilson PA, Meyer IH. Utilization of LGBT-specific clinics and providers across three cohorts of lesbian, gay, and bisexual people in the United States. *SSM Popul Health*. 2019;9:100505.
19. Reynaga M, Bybee S, Gettens C, et al. "We treat everyone equally": hospice care team members' language use regarding sexual and gender minority patients and caregivers. *Am J Hosp Palliat Care*. 2023;40(6):601–606.
20. Howard SD, Lee KL, Nathan AG, Wenger HC, Chin MH, Cook SC. Healthcare experiences of transgender people of color. *J Gen Intern Med*. 2019;34(10):2068–2074.
21. McCann E, Brown MJ. The mental health needs and concerns of older people who identify as LGBTQ+: a narrative review of the international evidence. *J Adv Nurs*. 2019;75(12):3390–3403.
22. Emlet CA, Fredriksen-Goldsen KI, Kim HJ, Jung H. Accounting for HIV health disparities: risk and protective factors among older gay and bisexual men. *J Aging Health*. 2020;32(7–8):677–687.
23. Gavulic KA, Gonzales G. Health care expenditures and financial burden: a comparison of adults in same-sex couples and different-sex couples. *Med Care Res Rev*. 2022;79(2):281–289.
24. Brooks Whitestone S, Giles H, Linz D. Overcoming ungrievability: transgender expectations for identity after death. *Sociol Inq*. 2020;90(2):316–338.
25. Turban JL, Loo SS, Almazan AN, Keuroghlian AS. Factors leading to "detransition" among transgender and gender diverse people in the United States: a mixed-methods analysis. *LGBT Health*. 2021;8(4):273–280.
26. Cloyes KG, Jones M, Gettens C, et al. Providing home hospice care for LGBTQ+ patients and caregivers: perceptions and opinions of hospice interdisciplinary care team providers. *Palliat Support Care*. 2023;21(1):3–11.
27. Reich AJ, Perez S, Fleming J, et al. Advance care planning experiences among sexual and gender minority people. *JAMA Netw Open*. 2022;5(7):e2222993.
28. Deutsch MB, Feldman JL. Updated recommendations from the world professional association for transgender health standards of care. *Am Fam Physician*. 2013;87(2):89–93.
29. Braybrook D, Bristowe K, Timmins L, et al. Communication about sexual orientation and gender between clinicians, LGBT+ people facing serious illness and their significant others: a qualitative interview study of experiences, preferences and recommendations. *BMJ Qual Saf*. 2023;32(2):109–120.
30. Cloyes KG, Hull W, Davis A. Palliative and end-of-life care for lesbian, gay, bisexual, and transgender (LGBT) cancer patients and their caregivers. *Semin Oncol Nurs*. 2018;34(1):60–71.
31. Anderson JF, Flatt J. Characteristics of LGBT caregivers of older adults: results from the national caregiving in the U.S. 2015 survey. *J Gay Lesbian Soc Serv*. 2018;30(2):103–116.
32. Bristowe K, Marshall S, Harding R. The bereavement experiences of lesbian, gay, bisexual and/or trans* people who have lost a partner: a systematic review, thematic synthesis and modelling of the literature. *Palliat Med*. 2016;30(8):730–744.
33. Chang SC, Singh AA, dickey lm. *A Clinician's Guide to Gender-Affirming Care: Working with Transgender & Gender Nonconforming Clients*. Context Press; 2018.
34. Levenson JS, Craig SL, Austin A. Trauma-informed and affirmative mental health practices with LGBTQ+ clients. *Psychol Serv*. 2023;20(suppl 1):134–144.
35. Stenzel AE, Moysich KB, Ferrando CA, Starbuck KD. Clinical needs for transgender men in the gynecologic oncology setting. *Gynecol Oncol*. 2020;159(3):899–905.
36. Diamond LM, Alley J. Rethinking minority stress: a social safety perspective on the health effects of stigma in sexually-diverse and gender-diverse populations. *Neurosci Biobehav Rev*. 2022;138:104720.
37. Roberts KE, Rogers M, Weinsaft A, Prigerson H. G. Interventions for patients with life-limiting illness and caregivers at the end-of-life. In: Schneiderman N, Antoni M, Pandeo F, Smith T, Anderson N, Revenson T, Abraido-Lanza A, eds. *American Psychological Association Handbook of Health Psychology*. Volume 2. American Psychological Association; 2025:525–542.

38. Austin A, Craig SL, Alessi EJ. Affirmative cognitive behavior therapy with transgender and gender nonconforming adults. *Psychiatr Clin North Am*. 2017;40(1):141–156.
39. Estrada LV, Agarwal M, Stone PW. Racial/ethnic disparities in nursing home end-of-life care: a systematic review. *J Am Med Dir Assoc*. 2021;22(2):279–290.e1.
40. Cloyes KG, Candrian C. Palliative and end-of-life care for sexual and gender minority cancer survivors: a review of current research and recommendations. *Curr Oncol Rep*. 2021;23(4):39.
41. Fair TM. Lessons on older LGBTQ individuals' sexuality and spirituality for hospice and palliative care. *Am J Hosp Palliat Care*. 2021;38(6):590–595.
42. Cloyes KG, Reynaga M, Vega M, et al. The burden of having to wonder: hospice caregiving experiences of LGBTQ+ cancer family caregivers. *Am J Hosp Palliat Care*. 2024;41(1):56–62.
43. Roberts KE, Lichtenthal WG, Ferrell BR. Being a bereavement-conscious hospice and palliative care clinician. *J Hosp Palliat Nurs*. 2021;23(4):293–295.
44. Lippe M, Eyer JC, Rosa WE, et al. Caring for an unconscious transgender patient at the end of life: ethical considerations and implications. *J Hosp Palliat Nurs*. 2021;23(4):300–308.
45. Sharman Z. *The Care We Dream of: Liberatory & Transformative Approaches to LGBTQ+ Health*. Arsenal Pulp Press; 2021.

68

Palliative Care in the Setting of Substance Use Disorder

Peggy Compton, Yu-Ping Chang, and Salimah H. Meghani

Key Points

- With the changing face of cancer and other advanced diseases progressing, patients are living for longer periods of time, which creates new challenges in treating pain and potential substance use disorder issues on an extended basis.
- Identifying substance use disorder in patients with advanced disease can be challenging, and provision of opioid analgesics in the context of the recent opioid crisis requires expansion of the nursing care plan.
- Patients with advanced disease and comorbid substance use disorder can be difficult to manage but can be successfully treated with careful documentation, planning, and a patient-centered approach.
- Remember that the patient with an advanced disease and comorbid substance use disorder may have two conditions in need of concurrent integrated treatment: one of an addiction disorder and one of pain.

Introduction

Substance use disorders (SUDs) are an endemic disease globally, with estimated base rates in the United States of 14.5%.[1] Although higher in certain subgroups, its presence certainly impacts all medically ill patient populations and can negatively affect how pain is treated. Even though national guidelines exist for the treatment of pain disorders such as cancer pain, they continue to be undertreated throughout the palliative care continua; a recent systematic review and meta-analysis found a pooled pain prevalence of 40% among persons undergoing active cancer treatments (95% confidence interval [CI] 0.29–0.51).[2] The prevalence is higher in persons with advanced, metastatic, or terminal cancer, with the prevalence of pain being closer to 66% (95% CI 58%–75%).[3] In some studies, over 90% of patients with advanced cancer or other advanced diseases report unrelieved pain.[4–6] Inadequate treatment of cancer pain is even greater if the patient is a member of a racial or ethnic minority, less educated, or older or has mental health comorbidities.[7] This is particularly likely to be the case in patients with a history of SUD as the primary pharmacologic tool used to treat pain in advanced disease, the opioids, also have a known abuse potential. Stigma and biases associated with SUD (the more correct diagnostic term for addiction or alcoholism) can lead to poor pain management, mutual suspicion and alienation, and unnecessary suffering unless adequately addressed.[8] Although advanced illness does not preclude clinicians from practicing universal precautions related to responsible opioid prescription, such as stratifying risks of opioid misuse and monitoring for aberrant drug-related behaviors,[9–11] clinicians must always remain alert to how conceptions and misconceptions about SUD can ultimately lead to pain undertreatment. Managing pain with opioids in persons with advanced disease when concerns about SUD arise poses a clinical challenge. These concerns have only been amplified in the context of current headlines and public health data demonstrating that opioid use disorder (OUD) and opioid overdose have been significant problems in the United States.[1,12] However, abuse of any substance leading to SUD can complicate the management of pain for patients at the end of life. While specific estimates of the prevalence of addiction in terminally ill patients are limited (see below), evidence supports that SUD is an issue for those with advanced illness, including cancer and hospice patients. Care of terminally ill patients with a history of or an active SUD presents many unique challenges, including poor compliance with therapeutic regimens, reliance on family caregivers to dispense medications, lack of addiction expertise of providers, overarching tendency to rely on controlled substances for symptom management, and the perception that addressing substance misuse or abuse in end-of-life care is unnecessary. Notable is that palliative care populations tend to be excluded from general practice guidelines on the use of opioids to treat acute and ongoing pain,[9,13–17] although there is good evidence that recent guidelines have had a chilling effect on the provision of or access to opioids for patients with cancer.[18–20] This chapter will provide an overview of SUDs, including definitions and terminology, and review what is known about the prevalence of opioid misuse and diversion in palliative care patients. Current clinical evidence surrounding the intersection of SUD and pain management in palliative care patients, including assessment, management, and best practice guidelines, will be presented.

Substance Use, Abuse, and SUD

Drug and alcohol use is a common behavior in the United States, thus is not uncommonly encountered in cancer nursing practice, including among persons receiving hospice and palliative care. The great majority of persons who drink alcohol or use a psychoactive drug do so within a functional or recreational social context and rarely develop problematic use patterns. However, with repeated use, some at-risk persons will develop SUD, a chronic, treatable, neuropsychiatric disease which brings consequences manifest in all life domains (health [physical and psychological], family, employment, financial, spiritual, functional, social). As such, SUD can have a significant impact on patient responses to all aspects of cancer and palliative therapy, most notably in the provision of pain care when medications with an abuse potential (i.e., opioids, benzodiazepines, central nervous system [CNS] stimulants) are used.

In attempting to estimate the prevalence or presence of SUD in patients with advanced diseases, terminology becomes important (see Table 68.1), especially in that lay language describing the disease has historically been notably imprecise. It is increasingly understood that SUD is a behavioral disorder and is not defined by physical dependence and tolerance, which are simply predictable neurophysiologic consequences of repeated use of certain substances. Reflecting this, in the *Diagnostic and Statistical Manual of Mental Disorders*, 5th edition (DSM-5), tolerance and withdrawal are not considered criteria for the SUD diagnosis if a patient is taking an opioid analgesic under medical supervision.[21] Not only does confusing nomenclature complicate the effort to distinguish appropriate from inappropriate drug-taking behaviors in patients with advanced disease; it also impedes the communication that is fundamental for proper pain management and medical care.

Alcohol is the most commonly used and abused drug in the United States. In 2020, 138.5 million Americans aged 12 or older reported current use of alcohol, with nearly half (44.4%) reporting binge alcohol use in the past month and 1 in 8 (12.8%) reporting heavy alcohol use in the past month. Nicotine products (i.e., tobacco products or vaped nicotine) were used by approximately 57.3 million (1 in 5) people aged 12 or older in 2020, indicating that 20.7% of the population are current cigarette smokers, making it the second most commonly used drug in the United States. Among current users of nicotine products, nearly two-thirds of adolescents aged 12 to 17 (63.1%) vaped nicotine but did not use tobacco products, while 88.9% of current nicotine product users aged 26 or older used only tobacco products.[1]

With respect to drug use, an estimated 59.3 million Americans aged 12 or older reported using an abusable drug during the past month. The most commonly used drug was marijuana, which was used by 49.6 million people aged 12 or older. Following in prevalence, approximately 20.6 million people reported misusing prescription medications (pain reliever, tranquilizer or sedative, and stimulant) at least once in the past month, including 9.3 million people (3.3% of the population) who were misusers of prescription pain relievers. Thus, the number of current misusers of pain relievers was second only to marijuana among specific drugs of abuse. Hydrocodone products were the most misused subtype of prescription pain relievers including Vicodin®, Lortab®, Norco®, Zohydro® ER, and generic hydrocodone, followed by oxycodone products including OxyContin®, Percocet®, Percodan®, Roxicodone®, and generic oxycodone.[1]

These figures characterize rates of use and misuse of alcohol and drugs in the United States but do not reflect the numbers of persons suffering from SUD. In 2020, approximately 40.3 million people aged 12 or older met the diagnostic criteria for SUD for alcohol or illicit drugs in the past 12 months as specified in the DSM-5,[21] including 28.3 million people with an alcohol use disorder and

Table 68.1 Terms associated with substance use disorder (SUD)

Term	Definition
SUD	The clinical diagnosis of a problematic pattern of substance use behaviors leading to clinical impairment or distress, including the inability to control use, consequences related to use, and failure to meet major responsibilities at work, school, or home. SUDs are categorized as mild, moderate, or severe to indicate the level of severity and are both preventable and treatable.
Misuse	The intentional or unintentional use of a prescribed medication for nonmedical use or for reasons other than prescribed (i.e., altering dosing, route of administration, or combining substances). Misuse may or may not reflect SUD.
Abuse	A maladaptive pattern of substance use leading to clinically significant impairment or distress (mild to moderate SUD).
Physical dependence	A state of neurophysiological adaptation to substance, evident in a drug class–specific withdrawal syndrome upon abrupt cessation, rapid dose reduction, and/or administration of an antagonist. Physical dependence may or may not reflect SUD.
Tolerance	A state of neurophysiological adaptation in which increased amounts of substance are needed over time to achieve desired effect. Tolerance may or may not reflect SUD.
Addiction	A chronic, relapsing, and progressive disease leading to significant impairment in all life domains (moderate to severe SUD).
Pseudoaddiction	Opioid drug-seeking behaviors secondary to inadequate pain control.
Chemical coping	Misuse of a medication in a nonprescribed way to cope with various stressful events associated with disease or disease management.
Opioid-induced hyperalgesia	A state of nociceptive (pain) sensitization caused by exposure to opioids.
Aberrant drug-use behavior	Taking a medication in a manner that is outside the boundaries of the prescribed treatment plan, such as using multiple pharmacies and prescribers, repeatedly losing medication, or requesting early refills. The presence of these behaviors may or may not reflect SUD.
Diversion	The transfer of a prescribed medication from the person to whom it was prescribed to another person.

Source: Reference 84.

18.4 million people with an illicit drug use disorder. Among those with a drug use disorder, the most common disorder was for marijuana (14.2 million people), followed by an estimated 3 million people with an OUD, which includes 2.3 million people with a prescription pain reliever use disorder and 0.7 million people with a heroin use disorder.[1]

SUDs in Patients with Advanced Disease

Although substance misuse, abuse, and their associated morbidity and mortality are significant problems in the United States, specific estimates of substance abuse in palliative care patients are limited. Whereas concerns about misuse and abuse of prescribed opioids have mainly focused on patients with chronic noncancer pain, similar issues have been described in patients with cancer and other life-limiting illnesses. A systematic review synthesizing 28 articles published between 1995 and 2018 found that the prevalence of SUD among patients with heterogeneous cancer types ranged from 2% to 35%, with a median rate of 25.5% for alcohol misuse and 18% for opioid misuse.[22] Because the metabolites of ethanol are carcinogenic, the prevalence of alcohol misuse in cancer patients may reflect a causal pathway. A recent systematic review of 18 studies conducted in the United States assessing opioid misuse among patients with cancer found that the risk of opioid misuse using self-reported tools was between 6% and 65%, while the actual prevalence of opioid misuse as determined by urine drug test ranged from 6.5% to 24%.[23] Various tools were used in assessing risk for opioid misuse across the studies, which likely explains the rate discrepancy in detecting the risk of opioid misuse.

Today, cancer patients live longer, may have extended exposure to opioids, and exhibit the same risk factors for opioid misuse as patients struggling with chronic but nonmalignant pain. In general, risk factors for inappropriate use of opioids appear to be the same for cancer and noncancer pain patients, with a history of alcohol and illicit drug abuse being the most consistent predictor of current prescription opioid abuse in patients with pain, regardless of age. Other important risk factors for opioid abuse include family history of substance abuse, history of a mood or anxiety disorder (e.g., current depression), pain-related functional limitations, current cigarette smoking, history of child sexual abuse or child neglect, involvement in the legal system, and significant psychosocial stressors.[24,25] The same systematic review found that risk factors of opioid misuse in patients with cancer include younger age, personal or familial mental health history, and history of illicit drug use.[23]

Although few studies have been conducted to evaluate the epidemiology of SUD in patients with advanced illness, reports of opioid misuse among cancer patients have emerged in the literature.[26,27] In an examination of aberrant drug behaviors in cancer patients, Passik and colleagues found in a secondary analysis of a large controlled trial of fentanyl buccal tablet that 17% (n = 1,160) of participants exhibited an aberrant opioid use behavior.[28] A survey of 57 hospice and palliative medicine fellows reported challenging encounters with patients with substance abuse issues, with 77% of fellows having seen at least one such patient and 29% reporting more than two encounters within the past 2 weeks.[29]

Assessment of SUD in Patients with Advanced Disease

The co-occurrence of SUD and advanced disease has a negative impact on therapeutic responses and health outcomes. Illicit drug use, actual or suspected misuse of prescribed medication, or actual SUD creates difficulties in the clinical setting and complicates pain management for patients with advanced disease. Effective management of SUD is fundamental to adherence to medical therapy and safety during treatment, including avoiding risks associated with the toxic effects of drugs and alcohol on body tissues (including overdose)[17] and adverse interactions between illicit drugs, alcohol, and medications prescribed as part of the patient's treatment. Ongoing substance abuse may make it difficult for the patient to adhere to a treatment regimen and alienate or weaken an already tenuous social support network needed to help alleviate the stressors associated with advanced disease and its treatment.

Therefore, it is important to incorporate substance use screening and treatment into palliative care and care coordination for both conditions if needed. The first goal of assessment is to determine whether the patient has a history of substance abuse and then to determine whether the history is active or remote; further, if the history is remote, pain management may differ if the patient is in drug-free recovery or receiving pharmacologic treatment with a medication with opioid activity (e.g., methadone, buprenorphine, or naltrexone) for their SUD.

Multiple standardized screening tools for substance misuse and abuse have been published (see Table 68.2) and are available at the National Institute on Drug Abuse website (https://nida.nih.gov/nidamed-medical-health-professionals/science-to-medicine/screening-substance-use/in-pain-management-setting, https://nida.nih.gov/nidamed-medical-health-professionals/screening-tools-resources/chart-screening-tools); some are generic and used to screen for many types of substance use, while others are used to screen for abuse of a specific substance (e.g., alcohol, tobacco, opioids). Unfortunately, the majority of these tools assess for the presence of so-called aberrant behaviors, which do not necessarily indicate the diagnosis of SUD (see Table 68.1) and may indicate other issues including undertreatment of pain, self-treatment of psychological and spiritual distress, or sleep disturbances.[30–32] Further, a 2021 scoping review of the literature found limited evidence of reliability and validity of these tools in palliative care populations specifically[33]; in fact, a recent expert consensus panel called for evaluation

Table 68.2 Screening tools for opioid misuse in patients with pain

Assessment tool	Length and administration	Reference
Opioid Risk Tool (ORT)	5 items Self-report checklist	94
Screener and Opioid Assessment for Patients with Pain (SOAPP-R®)	24 items Self-report rating scales	95
Opioid Risk Tool of Opioid Use Disorder (ORT-OUD)	9 items Self-report checklist	96
Brief Risk Interview (BRI)	12 items Clinician-administered	97

Box 68.1 Risk Factors in the Development of Substance Use Disorder

Risk Factor
Family history of substance use disorder
Personal history of drug misuse or substance use disorder (including nicotine)
Younger age
Psychiatric illness (depression, anxiety disorder)
Early drug or alcohol misuse (<13 years old)
Childhood physical/sexual/emotional trauma

of the use of screening tools to identify patients with life-limiting illnesses who have OUDs as a "high-priority" research topic.[34] Thus, the findings of these screening tools must be interpreted cautiously in patients receiving palliative care; however, they may be helpful in identifying the known risk factors for SUD in the general population (see Box 68.1).

In an effort to not offend, threaten, or anger patients, clinicians may avoid asking patients about alcohol or drug use. There is often the expectation that patients will not answer truthfully. However, obtaining a detailed history of duration, frequency, and desired effect of drug use is vital. Adopting a nonjudgmental position and communicating in an empathetic and truthful manner is the best strategy when taking patients' substance abuse histories. Patients may misrepresent their drug or alcohol use for logical reasons, such as stigmatization, mistrust of the interviewer, or concerns regarding fears of undertreatment. When taking a patient's substance use history, nurses should use a matter-of-fact approach, acknowledging that alcohol and drug use are common behaviors in society and explaining that drinking alcohol or using certain medications or drugs can influence responses to cancer medications and treatment. It is helpful to explain that in an effort to keep the patient as comfortable as possible, by preventing withdrawal states and prescribing sufficient medication for pain and symptom control, an accurate account of use is necessary.

A careful, graduated-style interview can be beneficial in introducing the assessment of substance abuse. This approach begins with broad and general inquiries regarding the role of legal drugs in the patient's life, such as caffeine, nicotine, alcohol, and, increasingly, cannabis, and gradually proceeds to more specific questions regarding illicit drugs. This interview style can also assist in discerning any coexisting psychiatric disorders, which may result in aberrant drug-taking behaviors. As discussed below, once identified, treatment of comorbid psychiatric disorders can greatly enhance management strategies and decrease the risk of relapse in persons with SUD. Questions regarding substance use patterns (e.g., onset, frequency, types, amounts, circumstances of use), including current use and the last episode of use, should be explored. Family history of addiction, as well as problems indicative of a substance abuse disorder in legal, employment, and social domains, as reflected in the DSM-5 criteria,[21] should be asked. In addition, nurses should take note of obvious signs of intoxication or withdrawal. Other signs of chronic substance use, such as the medical sequelae of abuse (e.g., liver dysfunction, infection), can aid in identification of patients with active SUD.

With patients who are in remission (either in drug-free or on medication-assisted recovery), nurses should ask for how long and under what circumstances they have been in recovery. The primary substance of abuse should be noted, as well as any current relationship with a support/recovery therapy group and/or sponsor. Patients' concerns about exposure to medications with abuse liability (opioids, marijuana, benzodiazepines) over the course of treatment should be explored, with assurance that non-opioid and nonpharmacologic pain management interventions can be offered. For patients on medication for the treatment of OUD (MOUD) who are taking methadone, buprenorphine, or naltrexone, nurses should note the daily dose the patient receives and, with the patient's permission, initiate contact with the clinic or provider to ensure continuity of care. Patients should be assured that pharmacologic therapy for the treatment of SUD will continue throughout palliative care treatment and will not interfere with the provision of adequate analgesia as needed.

Challenges to Assessment

Case Study: A 65-Year-Old Woman with Breast Cancer

Ms. C., a 65-year-old divorced woman with posttraumatic stress disorder related to early life trauma, underwent an uneventful lumpectomy for breast cancer at age 56. Although she responded well to the surgery and chemotherapy, within 3 months of the procedure, she returned to the oncologist's office with significant anxiety related to the recent onset of severe, constant lower back pain. The nurse practitioner on the palliative care team referred her to the pain clinic, and magnetic resonance imaging (MRI) ruled out metastatic disease. The pain was deemed to be of neuropathic origin, exacerbated by a poorly treated anxiety disorder. With significant psychological support, cognitive behavioral therapy, and psychotherapy, her symptoms became well controlled with low doses of oxycodone and clonazepam, and her functionality improved markedly. However, upon her retirement at age 63 and change in insurance plan, her pain care was transferred to a new primary care clinician, who was concerned about her daily opioid use and initiated a slow opioid taper. As the taper progressed, Ms. C.'s pain became increasingly severe and her anxiety worsened, making it difficult to sleep; she began to increase her use of clonazepam to manage these symptoms. A routine visit to her oncologist during this time revealed a recurrence of her breast cancer, necessitating mastectomy. The original palliative care team assumed management of her symptoms at this time, agreed to continue her opioid prescription, but became concerned about the escalation of her clonazepam use, knowing that, combined, the medications put her at high risk for overdose. With several attempts at a clonazepam taper, Ms. C. reported intolerable increases in pain; thus, her opioid dose was increased. A urine toxicology was ordered, and although the benzodiazepine was present, oxycodone was not. When asked, Ms. C. eventually revealed to the palliative care team that she had started skipping oxycodone doses and hoarding them for fear of untreated postoperative pain and that, related to this fear, was considering not undergoing the surgery at all. With reassurances that her postoperative pain would be adequately managed by the palliative care team and the identification of a primary care provider in her insurance network willing to provide ongoing pain medication, Ms. C. was able to return to appropriate and effective patterns of opioid and benzodiazepine use and proceed with the surgery.

Identification of SUD in patients with advanced disease can be challenging related to aspects of the disease process itself, the presence of pain, concurrent psychiatric disorders, sociocultural biases in opioid prescription, and end-of-life psychological responses. Changes induced by advanced disease and disease treatment can result in alterations in physical and behavioral functioning that may be hard to distinguish from the diagnostic indicators of SUD. For example, SUD-related behaviors may be difficult to discern in a patient who develops social withdrawal or cognitive changes after brain irradiation for metastases. Even if diminished cognition is related to pain medication, this effect might simply reflect a narrow therapeutic window rather than aberrant analgesic misuse. Similarly, the presence of mild mental clouding or the amount of time spent in bed may be less indicative of SUD than other behaviors, such as noncompliance with primary therapy or disrupted relationships with physicians, other healthcare professionals, and family members. To accurately assess alcohol or drug-related behaviors in patients with advanced disease, explicit information is required regarding the role of the substance in the patient's life. Varied and repeated observations over time may be necessary to categorize questionable behaviors properly.

Issues other than SUD should also be considered if questionable or aberrant opioid use behaviors arise during pain treatment. As previously reviewed, there is compelling evidence that pain is undertreated in populations with advanced disease,[4–6] and clinical experience indicates that the inadequate management of pain and related symptoms may motivate aberrant drug-taking behaviors, including so-called "drug-seeking". For example, "pseudoaddiction," a term coined by Weissman and Haddox, describes drug-seeking behaviors which occur in the context of unrelieved pain, such as obtaining opioids from multiple sources or hoarding medication.[35,36] A defining characteristic of pseudoaddiction is that the aberrant behaviors cease with sufficient pain relief and control of nociceptive input. A related concept, chemical coping, first described by Passik and colleagues, refers to patients being motivated to seek opioids to self-medicate spiritual and psychosocial distress,[31,32] including symptoms of anxiety, depression, or insomnia or problems of adjustment (including boredom caused by decreased ability to engage in usual activities and hobbies). A Delphi survey of international experts showed high consensus for several warning signs of chemical coping in cancer patients including depression, psychiatric comorbidity, history of substance abuse and alcoholism, and a positive score on the CAGE screening tool for alcoholism.[37] A more recent Delphi study identified the ability to define chemical coping as being one of the most relevant primary addiction medicine skills hospice and palliative medicine physicians should acquire during their training.[38] Unfortunately, pseudoaddiction and chemical coping syndromes pose diagnostic challenges as the boundaries of these two syndromes are not readily discernable; nevertheless, each is unique and requires different approaches for effective treatment.[32,37] Although it may be obvious that drug-related behaviors are aberrant, the meaning of these behaviors may be difficult to discern in the context of unrelieved non-pain symptoms.

There is also strong accumulated evidence that suggests that patients who are members of a racial or ethnic minoritized group are at a greater risk of inadequate treatment of cancer pain due to provider bias, stereotypes, and structural barriers to access to pain care.[39–45] In general, studies have documented that minoritized patients receive insufficient pain treatment compared with patients from majoritized groups for pain caused by a variety of sources and across healthcare settings.[46–48] While being non-White is a risk factor for pain undertreatment, members of certain racialized subgroups, such as Blacks/African Americans, have a disproportionate risks of pain undertreatment in the United States, specially opioid pain management.[48]

An earlier meta-analysis of 20 years of published research found that Blacks were 34% less likely than Whites to be prescribed opioids for pain conditions when a source of pain was not readily identifiable such as backaches or abdominal pain and 14% less likely to receive opioids for pain caused by injuries or surgery.[48] These findings are significant as nonspecific pain is often associated with advanced illness and disease progression. When prescribed opioids, Blacks/African Americans are also less likely to be safely managed with opioids by their clinicians and oncologists. For example, morphine has clinically relevant toxic metabolites that can accumulate in the presence of chronic kidney disease (CKD) and renal insufficiency. In one study, investigators found that patients with CKD who received morphine reported a greater severity of analgesic-related adverse effects than patients who received oxycodone. However, despite controlling for health insurance, African American patients had 71% lower odds of receiving a prescription of oxycodone than White patients. In adjusted analysis, race remained a significant predictor of the prescribed opioid selection despite clinical risks, and type of opioid prescription in turn explained greater burden of opioid-related adverse effects for African Americans with CKD.[43]

Minoritized patients with cancer are also more likely to have negative Pain Management Index scores, indicating inadequacy of cancer pain treatment relative to the level of their reported pain severity.[49] They are also at a greater risk of being mislabeled as drug-seeking or exhibiting aberrant behaviors[50,51] and are more often subject to opioid risk assessment than their White counterparts.[39,50,52] Clinicians should recognize many structural and clinical sources of disparities in serious illness care of persons with actual or assumed SUD and identify relevant drivers to close the gaps in care.

An additional diagnostic challenge is that problematic opioid use may be indicative of an untreated psychiatric symptom or personality disorder, the diagnosis of which has important therapeutic implications. Patients with borderline personality disorders, for example, may impulsively use prescription medications that regulate inner tension or improve boredom and express anger at physicians, friends, or family. Psychiatric assessment is vitally important for both the population without a prior history of substance abuse and the population of known substance abusers who have a high incidence of psychiatric comorbidity.[53] On occasion, aberrant drug-related behaviors appear to be causally remotely related to a mild encephalopathy, reflecting confusion about the appropriate therapeutic regimen. These diagnoses are not mutually exclusive.

Clinical Management of Advanced-Disease in Patients with Substance Use Histories

As patients face end-of-life planning, those with a history of SUD have unique needs. As previously noted, the intrapersonal and interpersonal stressors elicited by physical or emotional states, as well as exposure to medications with an abuse potential (benzodiazepines, opioids, CNS stimulants), may precipitate craving or relapse.

Patients in stable recovery are likely to have good social and family supports in place, but for those with recent or frequent exacerbations of their disease, these may be more tenuous. In addition, all patients with this history are likely to face a certain amount of stigma from healthcare providers and others engaged in their palliative care and may receive suboptimal treatment as a result.[54–56] Although opioid analgesic prescription should always be approached cautiously in patients with an SUD history, it is not uniformly contraindicated. The degree to which the pain interferes with activities of daily living, quality of life, and end-of-life priorities must be balanced with risk for relapse and the effectiveness of non-opioid and multimodal interventions; further, as outlined below, universal precautions to mitigate the risks associated with opioid prescribing for all recipients of palliative care will serve to minimize issues in patients with a history of SUD.

Patients with Untreated SUD: Focus on SUD Treatment

The most challenging issues in caring for patients with advanced disease typically arise from patients who are actively abusing alcohol or other drugs. For these patients, seeking and using drugs are their priority as opposed to adhering to or engaging in the palliative care treatment plan. The sleep disturbances, mood states, and functional losses that accompany SUD, in addition to intermittent withdrawal and craving states, can make symptoms, especially pain, difficult to manage. If pain is undertreated, the risk of bingeing with prescription medications and/or other substances increases for patients with SUD.

Opioids should be used judiciously and under tightly controlled circumstances in patients with pain and active SUD, regardless of type(s) of substance abused. Patients meeting DSM-5 criteria for SUD are, by definition, unable to control their use and achieve the goals of optimal functioning and maximal quality of life. Untreated addiction results in impaired function and diminished engagement in satisfying life activities, thus will necessarily result in poor pain and palliative care outcomes. In many care settings, the ability to provide the comprehensive services necessary to treat patients with both palliative care and SUD are lacking; of 1,144 US cancer centers surveyed in 2021, less than half offered either alcohol or SUD services,[57] and a recent national survey of palliative care providers found that only 27% reported having training or systems in place to address SUD.[58] Thus, these patients must be referred to formal addiction treatment, and it is incumbent upon the palliative care provider to have available a referral network of substance abuse treatment providers willing to collaborate on providing care to patients with advanced illness, pain, and SUD. After referral, the palliative care clinician should continue to work closely with the SUD treatment provider to address pain symptoms and other end-of-life needs.

Patients who are actively abusing prescribed opioids must be seen more frequently (e.g., weekly, if possible) to allow for close monitoring as well as to build therapeutic rapport with staff and afford evaluation of symptom control and SUD-related concerns. Frequent visits allow the opportunity to prescribe small quantities of drugs,[10] which may decrease the temptation to divert as well as provide a motive for attending appointments. Until adequately treated, opioid prescriptions should be limited in length[11] and dispensed by a family member or member of the healthcare team. Abuse-deterrent formulations may be considered, as should shorter-acting agents which contain less opioid than long-acting formulations. Perhaps most importantly, non-opioid (anti-inflammatory, anticonvulsants) and nonpharmacologic pain interventions should be implemented, including acupuncture, massage, mindful meditation, and distraction. These nonpharmacologic approaches will concurrently reinforce SUD treatment interventions as well as be useful for managing pain and other symptoms associated with advanced disease.

Certain palliative care providers (physicians, nurse practitioners, and physician assistants) have the additional ability to independently initiate a highly effective pharmacologic treatment for OUD, buprenorphine.[59–61] This partial opioid agonist produces opioid effects (i.e., euphoria, respiratory depression), however at lower and more limited levels than full opioid agonists such as morphine, methadone, and heroin. When taken as prescribed, buprenorphine has unique pharmacological properties that help to diminish withdrawal symptoms and cravings, while minimizing the risk of misuse and overdose.[61] Although there is no current consensus among palliative care physicians that they should receive training in buprenorphine treatment for patients with OUD,[38] a recent survey found that 13% of palliative care providers currently report having the ability to prescribe buprenorphine.[58] In a 2022 survey of hospice and palliative care providers who expressed interest in prescribing buprenorphine for the treatment of OUD, less than half of those with the ability to prescribe actually did prescribe the medication and cited discomfort managing concurrent pain, buprenorphine, and OUD; concerns about impacts on practice; unsupportive practice culture; insufficient practice support; patient facing challenges; and regulatory policies as barriers to its use in practice.[62] In the midst of the recent opioid overdose crisis, there is an urgent call for opioid prescribers across all specialties, including palliative care, to gain the knowledge and skills necessary to provide this highly effective medication to improve public health.[63,64]

Patients with SUD in Remission: Focus on Relapse Prevention

For individuals with addiction in remission, the goal of treatment is the same as for all palliative care patients: to maximize quality of life, optimize functionality, and manage distressing symptoms, including pain. Indicators of successful pain management include the patient's ability to comply with pain management and palliative care regimens, engage in cognitive behavioral pain management strategies, utilize positive coping skills to manage stress, and establish better social support systems. As noted, management of comorbid psychiatric complications, such as depression or anxiety, is critical to maximize functionality.

The literature provides evidence that patients with successfully treated SUD can be effectively managed with opioids for pain. As noted, for patients with OUD, disease remission may include MOUD, utilizing methadone, buprenorphine, or naltrexone in the context of broader psychosocial treatment. For patients receiving methadone or buprenorphine, it can be erroneously assumed that the treatment opioid will provide pain relief; however, the duration of analgesic action is shorter than effects on withdrawal and craving, so they provide incomplete pain control.[65,66] Further, patients on MOUD typically have developed some degree of opioid analgesic tolerance, thus may require higher opioid doses to appreciate pain relief.[67,68] In addition, studies have provided evidence that methadone and buprenorphine maintenance patients may, in fact, have heightened pain sensitivity (opioid-induced hyperalgesia), and therefore have a higher opioid analgesic requirement than matched controls.[69,70]

Although hospice and palliative care physicians report that the ability to manage patients on buprenorphine or methadone therapy should be a component of their training,[38] and recent data suggests that the majority (74%) of oncology clinicians surveyed express confidence in providing pain management for the patient on MOUD therapy,[15] existing literature does not address how to manage cancer or end-of-life pain in patients on MOUD.[71] Expert consensus in 2021 deemed it appropriate to continue buprenorphine or methadone therapy for OUD, albeit in more frequent divided daily dosing and adding full agonist analgesics titrated for pain control,[71] although the variety of opinion among the experts in palliative care and addiction medicine was notable.[13] Guidance based on empirical evidence is lacking; a recent systematic review of the literature on pain management strategies for patients on methadone maintenance therapy deemed the overall strength of the evidence to be poor,[72] with Bates and colleagues concluding that MOUD has "not been systematically studied for the treatment of opioid use disorder in patients with cancer pain."[73(p349)]

Regardless of the type(s) of substance previously abused, exposure to opioid medications can lead to relapse in patients with a recently or poorly treated SUD. Thus, when providing opioid therapy, the palliative care treatment goals are expanded to include relapse prevention strategies into the plan of care. Relapse is a predictable event in the course of addictive disease and is understood to be a process that does not occur suddenly or spontaneously and is, therefore, preventable.[74] Central to avoiding relapse are learned cognitive and behavioral strategies the patient can employ in the face of high-risk relapse-promoting situations. These include techniques designed to assist the individual in anticipating and effectively coping with these situations and more general self-control approaches designed to reduce relapse risk by promoting positive lifestyle changes. Specific intervention strategies include enhancing self-efficacy by setting achievable behavioral goals and incorporating stress-reduction activities into their daily life, such as exercise or meditation. The overall goal is lifestyle balancing, which increases self-efficacy across life domains and therefore minimizes the risk of relapse.

Provider Challenges to Clinical Management

Challenging the provision of effective palliative care to patients with SUD is a relative lack of training for palliative care providers on the management of SUD and pain in patients with addiction. A 2012 survey of 57 hospice and palliative medicine fellows on their self-perceived competency in caring for patients who misuse opioids found that less than half (47%) reported having a working knowledge of addiction; a minority (37%) believed they knew how to differentiate undertreated pain from addiction, and only 1% agreed that their training prepared them to manage opioid misuse.[29] Furthermore, only 21% were satisfied with how they treat symptoms in this population, and the majority felt uncomfortable dealing with issues such as lost or stolen medications. A decade later these insufficiencies persist, with only 23% to 35% of surveyed cancer care providers reporting adequate knowledge and confidence in managing patients with cancer and OUD;[75] a similar survey of Canadian palliative care providers in 2021 showed that less than half (47%) felt confident in screening for OUD, and only 39% felt confident in recognizing signs of OUD.[15]

Further, palliative care and hospice settings lack policies requiring providers to screen for SUD and diversion in patients and their family members. A national survey regarding the management of substance abuse sent to 94 accredited palliative medicine fellowship program directors found that of the directors who responded (n = 39), less than half (40.5%) had policies for screening patients for SUD, and the use of an opioid risk screening tool was reported infrequently (32.4%). Even fewer reported having policies to deal with opioid diversion (27%) or screened family members for SUD (16.2%).[76] Despite this, more than half of respondents indicated that substance abuse and diversion was an issue for their clinics, with only 25% indicating substance abuse was not an issue. Less than half (47%) of staff received mandatory training for dealing with substance misuse. A similar survey of 23 Virginia hospice agencies found that less than half required mandatory training on substance abuse (43.8%) or had policies on screening for substance abuse in patients (43.5%); fewer reported policies for screening for substance abuse in family members (30.4%). With respect to potential diversion, a minority screened for diversion in patients (21.7%) and families (17.4%). Less than one-third had policies in place to guide the use of opioids in patients with a history of SUD (33.3%) or diversion (30.4%).[77]

This data indicates that current practices for screening for SUD and diversion in palliative care patients and family members is inadequate and that education of hospice workers about SUD is equally insufficient. Despite widespread use of opioids and benzodiazepines as mainstay therapies for pain, dyspnea, anxiety, nausea, and insomnia in terminally ill patients, policies regarding safe use and best practices remain rare. Few guidelines address substance abuse and diversion in oncology, palliative care, or hospice[16,78]; and standard screening tools have not been validated in cancer patients. Consensus guidelines addressing SUD and diversion for palliative patients are needed to address this growing problem.[14,79]

General Guidelines

In 2016, the Centers for Disease Control and Prevention (CDC) released the highly influential guidelines for opioid prescribing in chronic pain.[80] The scope of the guideline included cancer survivors and those beyond active cancer treatment; although patients with terminal disease and those receiving end-of-life care were excluded, there is evidence that the guidelines had a negative effect on opioid provision to recipients of palliative care and caused confusion with existing care guidelines for cancer pain.[81] The revised CDC guideline for opioid prescribing in the United States published in 2022 again excluded persons with cancer from its scope.[82]

The American Cancer Society Cancer Action Network found that cancer patients in 2018 reported more difficulty in accessing opioids than 2016; although the proportion with opioid prescriptions (43%) did not change from 2016 to 2018, there was a substantial increase (from 16% to 41%) in those unable to obtain opioids at the pharmacy.[19] In nearly half, pain treatment options were limited by guidelines, insurance coverage, or laws. When asked how the opioid crisis influenced the treatment of cancer pain, oncologists described three major challenges to safe and effective opioid prescribing: (1)

patients who receive opioids for cancer feel stigmatized by clinicians, pharmacists, and society; (2) patients with cancer-related pain fear becoming addicted, which affects their willingness to accept prescription opioids; and (3) guidelines for safe and effective opioid prescribing are often misinterpreted, leading to access issues.[18] Subsequently, the American Society of Clinical Oncology (ASCO) released its guidelines which address risk stratification and adherence monitoring in cancer patients, including patients with advanced disease.[83] ASCO noted that many current recommendations are based on expert consensus, and research is urgently needed to generate empirical evidence to support long-term opioid prescribing in patients with chronic cancer-related pain, including those with concurrent substance use disorder.

The National Comprehensive Cancer Network (NCCN) annually updates its guidelines for management of cancer pain. These guidelines recommend risk management strategies for all cancer patients receiving opioids including prescribing naloxone for administration by caregivers in case of an emergency, patient and family education on usage of naloxone, calling emergency services (911) if naloxone is administered, instructing patients to maintain pain medication diaries, medication pill counts at outpatient visits or by home health/hospice to assist in correct use of medication, and urine drug testing at baseline and during treatment to detect misuse and diversion.[84]

For high-risk patients, (i.e., patients who exhibit one or more opioid misuse and abuse risk factors) the 2022 NCCN guidelines recommend additional education and support services including cognitive behavioral interventions, an increased frequency of outpatient weekly visits/and or reducing quantity of drug prescribed per prescription, referral to an interventional pain specialist to maximize non-opioid options for pain control and referral to an addiction specialist, and considering utilizing programmable electronic medication dispensers.[84]

The following guidelines broadly reflect the types of interventions that might be considered in this clinical context and can be beneficial whether the patient is actively abusing drugs or is at high risk for SUD.[85] The principles outlined go beyond the general risk mitigation practices now considered standard for all opioid prescribing and assist palliative care clinicians in establishing structure, control, and monitoring of SUD-related behaviors, which may be helpful and necessary at times in all pain treatment.

Multidisciplinary Approach

Pain and symptom management is often complicated by various medical, psychosocial, and administrative issues in the population of advanced patients with SUD. The most effective team may include a physician with expertise in pain/palliative care, nurses, social workers, and a mental healthcare provider, addiction medicine specialist, or health behaviorist with expertise in the area of addiction medicine.

Monitoring for Risk

Patients with a more recent history of SUD, a strong family history of drug or alcohol abuse, or a history of major psychiatric disorders are at the highest risk of opioid misuse.[83] These risks should be monitored monthly, including detailed interview about drug and alcohol use behaviors, checking a prescription drug monitoring program database for evidence of doctor shopping, and urine drug testing (UDT).[10,11] Several tools are available to clinicians to monitor risk, including the COMM™ (Current Opioid Misuse Measure),[86] PDUQ (Prescription Drug Use Questionnaire), and self-report version PDUQ-p,[87,88] and the ABC (Addiction Behaviors Checklist).[89] Note that all of these tools measure aberrant behaviors and behaviors in violation of the written treatment agreement (see below), such as obtaining opioids from multiple providers, using other illicit drugs, or increasing dose or frequency, and are not diagnostic of SUD.

Use of Written Agreements

Written treatment agreements that clearly state the roles of the team members and expectations for the patient with respect to medication use are helpful for patient education and for identifying signs of relapse. These agreements typically stipulate that opioids are obtained from a single provider, that they are taken only as prescribed, procedures for refills and replacement of lost prescriptions, the expectation that patients are engaged in SUD and palliative care treatment, use of regular and random UDT, and the importance of safe storage of medications. Basing the level of restrictions on the patient's behaviors, graded agreements should be enforced that clearly state the consequences of aberrant drug use.[90] Clinicians who are covering for the palliative care provider must be advised of the guidelines that have been established for each patient with a substance abuse history to avoid conflict and disruption of the treatment plan.

Setting Realistic Goals for Therapy

Rates of relapse with SUD are high. The stress associated with advanced illness and the availability of drugs with an abuse liability increase this risk. Therefore, total prevention of relapse may be impossible in this type of setting. Gaining an understanding that complete compliance and abstinence are not realistic goals may decrease conflicts with staff members in terms of management goals. Instead, the goals might be perceived as the creation of a structure for therapy that includes ample social/emotional support and limit-setting to control the harm done by relapse.

Evaluation and Treatment of Comorbid Psychiatric Disorders

As previously noted, high comorbidity of personality disorders, depression, and anxiety disorders exists in alcoholics and other patients with SUD histories.[53] The treatment of depression and anxiety can increase patient comfort and decrease the risk of relapse or aberrant drug-taking behaviors.

Preventing or Minimizing Withdrawal Symptoms

Because patients with SUD histories often use multiple drugs, it is necessary to conduct a complete drug-use history to prepare for the possibility of withdrawal, not only from opioids but also from alcohol and benzodiazepines. Delayed abstinence syndromes, such as those that may occur after use of some long-acting opioids or benzodiazepines, may be particularly diagnostically challenging because they emerge slowly and can last for extended periods of time. It is important to anticipate and prevent these as much as possible because the emergence of withdrawal symptoms can worsen pain, motivate drug or alcohol use, and precipitate relapse.

Applying Pharmacological Principles to Treating Pain

Self-report remains the gold standard upon which to prescribe opioids for pain, with exact dose being individualized to identify a favorable equilibrium between efficacy and side effects. Individualization of the dose without regard to the absolute amount prescribed can be difficult in populations with a history of SUD; however, foregoing the principle of dose individualization may increase the risk of undertreatment in this population. The ASCO guidelines recommend using no more than one opioid (e.g., no prescription of a second short-acting opioid) in patients at high risk of opioid misuse.[83] As noted above, clinicians should likewise consider the possibility if pain can be adequately managed with adjunctive non-opioid therapies.

Use of 12-Step Programs

Depending on the patient's stage of advanced illness and functional capabilities, the clinician may want to consider referring the patient to a 12-step program, or otherwise engage in active recovery treatment, with the stipulation that attendance be documented for ongoing opioid prescription purposes. If the patient has a sponsor, and the patient is agreeable, the clinician may wish to contact the patient's sponsor, depending on the stage of illness and individual capabilities, in an effort to disclose the patient's illness and that medication is required in the treatment of the illness. This contact will also help to decrease the risk of stigmatizing the patient as being noncompliant with the principles of the 12-step program. If the patient is unable to participate in a 12-step program, other psychosocial and/or spiritual team members can provide care that supports sobriety.

Family Sessions and Meetings

As with all palliative care, in an effort to increase support and function, meetings with family members and significant others should be included in the treatment plan. Qualitative study has shown that family caregivers' concerns about perceived "behavioral and physical symptoms of drug addiction" related to pain management at home resulted in disruption in the patient–caregiver relationship, caregiver fatigue, and disruption in pain alleviation; thus, engaging them in these conversations around pain and SUD can be valuable.[91] These meetings will allow the clinician and other team members to become familiar with the family and identify family members who are using substances (see below). These meetings will also assist the team in identifying dependable individuals who can serve as a source of strength and support for the patient during treatment.

Safe Storage and Proper Disposal of Opioid Medication

In the context of the recent opioid crisis in the United States, the importance of safe storage of these prescribed medications deserves special mention. Improper storage and disposal of opioids increase the availability of these medications for abuse, diversion, and accidental poisoning. Among people aged 12 or older who misused pain relievers in the past year, about half (47.2%) indicated that they obtained them from a friend or relative (i.e., given, buying or taking them without asking).[1] Up to 90% of patients with advanced cancer require treatment with opioids,[90] and those with advanced disease are most commonly treated with high-dose opioids, and therefore are a likely source of diversion of these medications into the community. Because cancer patients can experience acute, chronic, and/or breakthrough pain and frequently undergo opioid titrations and rotations to help manage pain and opioid-induced neurotoxicity,[92] they not uncommonly possess multiple unused or expired opioids, which can be diverted.

Limited information is available about the storage, use, and disposal practices of cancer patients receiving opioids. A survey study of 300 cancer patients found that 19% reported unsafe storage, defined as storing opioids in plain sight; 69% kept opioids hidden but unlocked; and only 9% locked their opioids. Seventy-eight patients (26%) reported unsafe use by sharing (9%) or losing (17%) their opioids. Overall, 74% of patients surveyed were unaware of proper opioid disposal methods, and 46% had unused opioids at home.[93] These findings suggest that many cancer patients improperly and unsafely use, store, and dispose of opioids, highlighting the need for patient education and drug take-back programs. In fact, explaining best practices to dispose of unused opioids was identified as an addiction medicine skill palliative medicine physicians should receive during their training,[38] whereas in 2021, 60% of Canadian palliative care providers reported never or rarely providing education on the safe storage or disposal of opioids.[15]

These findings also raise concern regarding family drug diversion; being a familial disease, it is not uncommon to find that relatives of the patient also have a history of or active SUD. Given significant debility in terminal illness, family members are often administering opioid medications. Patient education regarding safe use of opioids should include teaching them to avoid exposing family members with SUD to these medications. However, fewer than 20% of healthcare providers address caregiver history of addiction,[76] which can put the impaired family member, who now has regular access to these drugs, at increased risk. Prescribers who work in palliative care settings have a special responsibility to ensure that these medications are not misused or diverted into the community. Diversion can be difficult to detect, but the UDT can provide evidence that prescribed opioids are not being taken by the patient and perhaps diverted.

Summary

Treating patients with a history of SUD who are experiencing pain from advanced illness is both complicated and challenging because each condition can significantly complicate the other. Patients are living longer with advanced disease and ongoing pain concerns. In the context of the recent opioid crisis, it is no longer acceptable to justify high-dose opioid therapy for pain in a vacuum without actively and knowledgeably assessing and managing the risks of SUD and diversion. The management of pain in a patient who is actively abusing drugs and/or is a member of an ethnic minority is further complicated due to issues of stigma, bias, and cultural differences that may exist. Using a treatment plan that involves a team approach that recognizes and responds to the complex needs of the patient with a history of SUD is the best strategy to facilitate optimal outcomes. Although pain management may continue to be challenging even when all treatment plan procedures are implemented, the healthcare team's goal should be to provide the highest level of pain management for all patients with SUD.

In achievement of pain management goals, patients receiving palliative care are commonly prescribed opioids to treat pain and may have large amounts of controlled substances in their homes. Balancing the mission of pain relief with concerns about SUD and diversion is a difficult issue for palliative care providers. Many providers are not well prepared to screen for these problems in their patients or the family caregivers, and few work in settings with established policies outlining how to care for those with identified problems. Given the enormous public health implications of the high rates of OUD and overdose in the United States, it is imperative that the palliative care community takes an active role in addressing the issue to provide adequate treatment of pain and other symptoms in patients with life-limiting illnesses.

REFERENCES

1. Center for Behavioral Health Statistics and Quality. *2020 National Survey on Drug Use and Health: Detailed Tables*. Substance Abuse and Mental Health Services Administration; 2022. Accessed July 30, 2022. https://www.samhsa.gov/data/release/2020-national-survey-drug-use-and-health-nsduh-releases.
2. Evenepoel M, Haenen V, De Baerdemaecker T, et al. Pain prevalence during cancer treatment: a systematic review and meta-analysis. *J Pain Symptom Manage*. 2022;63:e317–e335.
3. van den Beuken-van Everdingen MH, Hochstenbach LM, Joosten EA, Tjan-Heijnen VC, Janssen DJ. Update on prevalence of pain in patients with cancer: systematic review and meta-analysis. *J Pain Symptom Manage*. 2016;51(6):1070–1090.e9.
4. Mori M, Elsayem A, Reddy SK, Bruera E, Fadul NA. Unrelieved pain and suffering in patients with advanced cancer. *Am J Hosp Palliat Care*. 2012;29(3):236–240.
5. O'Connor M, Weir J, Butcher I, et al. Pain in patients attending a specialist cancer service: prevalence and association with emotional distress. *J Pain Symptom Manage*. 2012;43(1):29–38.
6. Swarm RA, Abernethy AP, Anghelescu DL, et al. Adult cancer pain. *J Natl Compr Canc Netw*. 2013;11(8):992–1022.
7. Stein KD, Alcaraz KI, Kamson C, Fallon EA, Smith TG. Sociodemographic inequalities in barriers to cancer pain management: a report from the American Cancer Society's Study of Cancer Survivors-II (SCS-II). *Psychooncology*. 2016;25(10):1212–1221.
8. Caruso R, Nanni MG, Riba MB, Sabato S, Grassi L. The burden of psychosocial morbidity related to cancer: patient and family issues. *Int Rev Psychiatry*. 2017;29(5):389–402. https://doi.org/10.1080/09540261.2017.1288090.
9. Scarborough BM, Smith CB. Optimal pain management for patients with cancer in the modern era. *CA Cancer J Clin*. 2018;68(3):182–196. https://doi.org/10.3322/caac.21453.
10. Arthur J, Reddy A. Opioid prescribing in an opioid crisis: what basic skills should an oncologist have regarding opioid therapy? *Curr Treat Options Oncol*. 2019;20(5):39. https://doi.org/10.1007/s11864-019-0636-3.
11. Arthur J, Hui D. Safe opioid use: management of opioid-related adverse effects and aberrant behaviors. *Hematol Oncol Clin North Am*. 2018;32(3):387–403. https://doi.org/10.1016/j.hoc.2018.01.003
12. Hedegaard H, Miniño AM, Warner M. Drug overdose deaths in the United States, 1999–2019. NCHS Data Brief, no 394. Centers for Disease Control and Prevention. Last updated December 22, 2020. Accessed June 13, 2022. https://www.cdc.gov/nchs/products/databriefs/db394.htm.
13. Moryl N, Malhotra VT. A case for palliative care and addiction specialists collaboration and joint research. *JAMA Netw Open*. 2021;4(12):e2143436. https://doi.org/10.1001/jamanetworkopen.2021.43436.
14. Jones CA, Kamal AH. From alleviating suffering to avoiding addiction: a call to action to evaluate and mitigate risk in outpatient specialty palliative care. *J Palliat Med*. 2021;24(3):316–317. https://doi.org/10.1089/jpm.2021.0008.
15. Tedesco A, Brown J, Hannon B, Hutton L, Lau J. Managing opioids and mitigating risk: a survey of attitudes, confidence and practices of oncology health care professionals. *Curr Oncol*. 2021;28(1):873–878. https://doi.org/10.3390/curroncol28010086.
16. Copenhaver DJ, Karvelas NB, Fishman SM. Risk management for opioid prescribing in the treatment of patients with pain from cancer or terminal illness: inadvertent oversight or taboo? *Anesth Analg*. 2017;125(5):1610–1615. https://doi.org/10.1213/ANE.0000000000002463.
17. Lowry S. When management of cancer-related pain is complicated by coexisting opioid use disorder: a case review. *J Hosp Palliat Nurs*. 2022;24(2):112–118. https://doi.org/10.1097/NJH.0000000000000828.
18. Schenker Y, Hamm M, Bulls HW, et al. This is a different patient population: opioid prescribing challenges for patients with cancer-related pain. *JCO Oncol Pract*. 2021;17(7):e1030–e1037. https://doi.org/10.1200/OP.20.01041
19. Patel JN, Salib M, Parala-Metz A. Best practices for opioid abuse screening in cancer patients. *BMJ Support Palliat Care*. 2020;10(3):306–309. https://doi.org/10.1136/bmjspcare-2019-001950.
20. Merlin JS, Young SR, Arnold R, et al. Managing opioids, including misuse and addiction, in patients with serious illness in ambulatory palliative care: a qualitative study. *Am J Hosp Palliat Care*. 2020;37(7):507–513. https://doi.org/10.1177/1049909119890556.
21. American Psychiatric Association. *Diagnostic and Statistical Manual of Mental Disorders*. 5th ed. American Psychiatric Association; 2013.
22. Yusufov M, Braun IM, Pirl WF. A systematic review of substance use and substance use disorders in patients with cancer. *Gen Hosp Psychiatry*. 2019;60:128–136. https://doi.org/10.1016/j.genhosppsych.2019.04.016.
23. Keall R, Keall P, Kiani C, Luckett T, McNeill R, Lovell M. A systematic review of assessment approaches to predict opioid misuse in people with cancer. *Support Care Cancer*. 2022;30:5645–5658 https://doi.org/10.1007/s00520-022-06895-w.
24. Sehgal N, Manchikanti L, Smith HS. Prescription opioid abuse in chronic pain: a review of opioid abuse predictors and strategies to curb opioid abuse. *Pain Physician*. 2012;15(3 suppl):ES67–ES92.
25. Jamison RN, Edwards RR. Risk factor assessment for problematic use of opioids for chronic pain. *Clin Neuropsychol*. 2013;27(1):60–80.
26. Barclay JS, Owens JE, Blackhall LJ. Screening for substance abuse risk in cancer patients using the Opioid Risk Tool and urine drug screen. *Supp Care Cancer*. 2014;22(7):1883–1888.
27. Granata R, Bossi P, Bertulli R, Saita L. Rapid-onset opioids for the treatment of breakthrough cancer pain: two cases of drug abuse. *Pain Med*. 2014;15(5):758–761.
28. Passik SD, Messina J, Golsorkhi A, Xie F. Aberrant drug-related behavior observed during clinical studies involving patients taking chronic opioid therapy for persistent pain and fentanyl

buccal tablet for breakthrough pain. *J Pain Symptom Manage.* 2011;41(1):116–125.
29. Childers JW, Arnold RM. "I feel uncomfortable 'calling a patient out'": educational needs of palliative medicine fellows in managing opioid misuse. *J Pain Symptom Manage.* 2012;43:253–260.
30. Kwon JH, Tanco K, Park JC, et al. Frequency, predictors, and medical record documentation of chemical coping among advanced cancer patients. *Oncologist.* 2015;20(6):692–697.
31. Del Fabbro E. Assessment and management of chemical coping in patients with cancer. *J Clin Oncol.* 2014;32(16):1734–1738.
32. Kwon JH, Tanco K, Hui D, Reddy A, Bruera E. Chemical coping versus pseudoaddiction in patients with cancer pain. *Palliat Support Care.* 2014;12(5):413–417.
33. Lau J, Mazzotta P, Fazelzad R, et al. Assessment tools for problematic opioid use in palliative care: a scoping review. *Palliat Med.* 2021;35(7):1295–1322. https://doi.org/10.1177/02692163211015567.
34. Lau J, Mazzotta P, Whelan C, et al. Opioid safety recommendations in adult palliative medicine: a North American Delphi expert consensus. *BMJ Support Palliat Care.* 2022;12(1):81–90. https://doi.org/10.1136/bmjspcare-2021-003178.
35. Weissman DE, Haddox JD. Opioid pseudoaddiction: an iatrogenic syndrome. *Pain.* 1989;36:363–366.
36. Passik SD, Webster L, Kirsh KL. Pseudoaddiction revisited: a commentary on clinical and historical considerations. *Pain Manag.* 2011;1(3):239–248.
37. Kwon JH, Hui D, Bruera E. A pilot study to define chemical coping in cancer patients using the Delphi method. *J Palliat Med.* 2015;18(8):703–706.
38. Chua IS, Fratt E, Ho JJ, Roldan CS, Gundersen DA, Childers J. Primary addiction medicine skills for hospice and palliative medicine physicians: a modified Delphi study. *J Pain Symptom Manage.* 2021;62(4):720–729. https://doi.org/10.1016/j.jpainsymman.2021.02.035.
39. Jones KF, Laury E, Sanders JJ, et al. Top ten tips palliative care clinicians should know about delivering antiracist care to Black Americans. *J Palliat Med.* 2022;25:479–487.
40. Meghani SH, Rosa WE, Chittams J, Vallerand AH, Bao T, Mao JJ. Both race and insurance type independently predict the selection of oral opioids prescribed to cancer outpatients. *Pain Manag Nurs.* 2020;21:65–71.
41. Jefferson K, Quest T, Yeager KA. Factors associated with Black cancer patients' ability to obtain their opioid prescriptions at the pharmacy. *J Palliat Med.* 2019;22(9):1143–1148. https://doi.org/10.1089/jpm.2018.0536.
42. Mack DS, Hunnicutt JN, Jesdale BM, Lapane KL. Non-Hispanic Black–White disparities in pain and pain management among newly admitted nursing home residents with cancer. *J Pain Res.* 2018;11:753–761.
43. Meghani SH, Kang Y, Chittams J, McMenamin E, Mao JJ, Fudin J. African Americans with cancer pain are more likely to receive an analgesic with toxic metabolite despite clinical risks: a mediation analysis study. *J Clin Oncol.* 2014;32:2773–2779.
44. Stephenson N, Dalton JA, Carlson J, Youngblood R, Bailey D. Racial and ethnic disparities in cancer pain management. *J Natl Black Nurses Assoc.* 2009;20:11–18.
45. Anderson KO, Mendoza TR, Valero V, Richman SP, Russell C, Hurley J, et al. Minority cancer patients and their providers. *Cancer.* 2000;88:1929–1938.
46. Burgess DJ, Crowley-Matoka M, Phelan S, Dovidio JF, Kerns R, Roth C, et al. Patient race and physicians' decisions to prescribe opioids for chronic low back pain. *Soc Sci Med.* 2008;67(11):1852–1860.
47. Cintron A, Morrison RS. Pain and ethnicity in the United States: a systematic review. *J Palliat Med.* 2006;9(6):1454–1473.
48. Meghani SH, Byun E, Gallagher RM. Time to take stock: a meta-analysis and systematic review of analgesic treatment disparities for pain in the United States. *Pain Med.* 2012;13(2):150–174.
49. Meghani SH, Thompson AM, Chittams J, Bruner DW, Riegel B. Adherence to analgesics for cancer pain: a comparative study of African Americans and Whites using an electronic monitoring device. *J Pain.* 2015;16(9):825–835.
50. Jones KF, Sager Z, Leiter RE, Sanders JJ. When treatment algorithms fail: a response to the development of a nomogram to determine the frequency of elevated risk for non-medical opioid use in cancer patients. *Palliat Support Care.* 2021;19(5):636–637. https://doi.org/10.1017/S1478951521001255.
51. Becker WC, Starrels JL, Heo M, Li X, Weiner MG, Turner BJ. Racial differences in primary care opioid risk reduction strategies. *Ann Fam Med.* 2011;9:219–225.
52. Hirsh AT, Anastas TM, Miller MM, Quinn PD, Kroenke K. Patient race and opioid misuse history influence provider risk perceptions for future opioid-related problems. *Am Psychol.* 2020;75:784–795.
53. Gros DF, Milanak ME, Brady KT, Back SE. Frequency and severity of comorbid mood and anxiety disorders in prescription opioid dependence. *Am J Addict.* 2013;22(3):261–265.
54. Goodyear K, Haass-Koffler CL, Chavanne D. Opioid use and stigma: the role of gender, language and precipitating events. *Drug Alcohol Depend.* 2018;185:339–346. https://doi.org/10.1016/j.drugalcdep.2017.12.037.
55. Simon R, Snow R, Wakeman S. Understanding why patients with substance use disorders leave the hospital against medical advice: a qualitative study. *Subst Abus.* 2020;41(4):519–525. https://doi.org/10.1080/08897077.2019.1671942.
56. Hoover K, Lockhart S, Callister C, Holtrop JS, Calcaterra SL. Experiences of stigma in hospitals with addiction consultation services: a qualitative analysis of patients' and hospital-based providers' perspectives. *J Subst Abuse Treat.* 2022;138:108708. https://doi.org/10.1016/j.jsat.2021.108708.
57. Niazi SK, Spaulding A, Brennan E, et al. Mental health and chemical dependency services at US cancer centers. *J Natl Compr Canc Netw.* 2021;19(7):829–838. https://doi.org/10.6004/jnccn.2020.7657.
58. Merlin JS, Patel K, Thompson N, et al. Managing chronic pain in cancer survivors prescribed long-term opioid therapy: a national survey of ambulatory palliative care providers. *J Pain Symptom Manage.* 2019;57(1):20–27. https://doi.org/10.1016/j.jpainsymman.2018.10.493.
59. National Institute on Drug Abuse. How Effective Are Medications to Treat Opioid Use Disorder? Last updated December 3, 2021. Accessed June 13, 2022. https://nida.nih.gov/publications/research-reports/medications-to-treat-opioid-addiction/efficacy-medications-opioid-use-disorder.
60. Mattick RP, Breen C, Kimber J, Davoli M. Buprenorphine maintenance versus placebo or methadone maintenance for opioid dependence. *Cochrane Database Syst Rev.* 2014;2:CD002207. https://doi.org/10.1002/14651858.CD002207.pub4.
61. Substance Abuse and Mental Health Services Administration. Buprenorphine. Last updated July 14, 2022. Accessed July 30, 2022. https://www.samhsa.gov/medication-assisted-treatment/medications-counseling-related-conditions/buprenorphine.

62. Janet Ho J, Jones KF, Sager Z, et al. Barriers to buprenorphine prescribing for opioid use disorder in hospice and palliative care. *J Pain Symptom Manage.* 2022;64(2):119–127. https://doi.org/10.1016/j.jpainsymman.2022.05.004.
63. Pergolizzi J, LeQuang J, Breve F. The end of the x-waiver: not a moment too soon! *Cureus.* 2021;13(5):e15123. https://doi.org/10.7759/cureus.15123.
64. Woodruff AE, Tomanovich M, Beletsky L, Salisbury-Afshar E, Wakeman S, Ostrovsky A. Dismantling buprenorphine policy can provide more comprehensive addiction treatment. *NAM Perspect.* 2019;2019:10.31478/201909a.
65. Athanasos P, Smith CS, White JM, Somogyi AA, Bochner F, Ling W. Methadone maintenance patients are cross-tolerant to the antinociceptive effects of very high plasma morphine concentrations. *Pain.* 2006;120(3):267–275.
66. Hay JL, White JM, Bochner F, Somogyi AA. Antinociceptive effects of high-dose remifentanil in male methadone-maintained patients. *Eur J Pain.* 2008;12(7):926–933.
67. Blinderman C, Sekine R, Zhang B, Nillson M, Shaiova L. Methadone as an analgesic for patients with chronic pain in methadone maintenance treatment programs (MMTPs). *J Opioid Manage.* 2009;5(2):107–114.
68. Peles E, Schreiber S, Gordon J, Adelson M. Significantly higher methadone dose for methadone maintenance treatment (MMT) patients with chronic pain. *Pain.* 2005;113(3):340–346.
69. Carullo V, Fitz-James I, Delphin E. Opioid-induced hyperalgesia: a diagnostic dilemma. *J Pain Palliat Care Pharmacother.* 2015;29:378–384.
70. Compton P, Charuvastra VC, Kintaudi K, Ling W. Pain responses in methadone-maintained opioid abusers. *J Pain Symptom Manage.* 2000;20(4):237–245.
71. Merlin JS, Khodyakov D, Arnold R, et al. Expert panel consensus on management of advanced cancer-related pain in individuals with opioid use disorder. *JAMA Netw Open.* 2021;4(12):e2139968. https://doi.org/10.1001/jamanetworkopen.2021.39968.
72. Taveros MC, Chuang EJ. Pain management strategies for patients on methadone maintenance therapy: a systematic review of the literature. *BMJ Support Palliat Care.* 2017;7(4):383–389. https://doi.org/10.1136/bmjspcare-2016-001126.
73. Bates N, Bello JK, Osazuwa-Peters N, Sullivan MD, Scherrer JF. Depression and long-term prescription opioid use and opioid use disorder: implications for pain management in cancer. *Curr Treat Options Oncol.* 2022;23(3):348–358. https://doi.org/10.1007/s11864-022-00954-4.
74. Marlatt GA, Gordon JR. *Relapse Prevention: Maintenance Strategies in the Treatment of Addictive Behaviors.* Guilford Press; 1985.
75. Arthur J, Edwards T, Lu Z, Hui D, Fellman B, Bruera E. Health care provider attitudes, beliefs, and perceived confidence in managing patients with cancer pain and nonmedical opioid use. *J Pain Symptom Manage.* 2021;61(1):128–135.e6. https://doi.org/10.1016/j.jpainsymman.2020.06.040.
76. Tan PD, Barclay JS, Blackhall LJ. Do palliative care clinics screen for substance abuse and diversion? Results of a national survey. *J Palliat Med.* 2015;18(9):752–757.
77. Blackhall LJ, Alfson ED, Barclay JS. Screening for substance abuse and diversion in Virginia hospices. *J Palliat Med.* 2013;16(3):237–242.
78. Anghelescu DL, Ehrentraut JH, Faughnan LG. Opioid misuse and abuse: risk assessment and management in patients with cancer pain. *J Natl Compr Canc Netw.* 2013;11(8):1023–1031.
79. Pergolizzi JV, Zampogna G, Taylor R, Gonima E, Posada J, Raffa RB. A guide for pain management in low and middle income communities. Managing the risk of opioid abuse in patients with cancer pain. *Front Pharmacol.* 2016;7:42. https://doi.org/10.3389/fphar.2016.00042.
80. Dowell D, Haegerich TM, Chou R. CDC guideline for prescribing opioids for chronic pain—United States, 2016. *MMWR Recomm Rep.* 2016;65(1):1–49. http://dx.doi.org/10.15585/mmwr.rr6501e1.
81. Meghani SH, Vapiwala N. Bridging the critical divide in pain management guidelines from the CDC, NCCN, and ASCO for cancer survivors. *JAMA Oncol.* 2018;4:1323–1324.
82. Dowell D, Ragan KR, Jones CM, Baldwin GT, Chou R. CDC Clinical Practice Guideline for Prescribing Opioids for Pain—United States, 2022. *MMWR Recomm Rep.* 2022;71(No. RR-3):1–95. doi:http://dx.doi.org/10.15585/mmwr.rr7103a1
83. Paice JA, Portenoy R, Lacchetti C, et al. Management of chronic pain in survivors of adult cancers: American Society of Clinical Oncology clinical practice guideline. *J Clin Oncol.* 2016;34(27):3325–3345.
84. National Comprehensive Cancer Network. NCCN Guidelines: Adult Cancer Pain. Version 2.2022. Last updated February, 2022. Accessed July 17, 2022. https://www.nccn.org/guidelines/guidelines-detail?category=3&id=1413.
85. Fitzgerald Jones K, Khodyakov D, Arnold R, et al. Consensus-based guidance on opioid management in individuals with advanced cancer-related pain and opioid misuse or use disorder. *JAMA Oncol.* 2022;8(8):1107–1114. https://doi.org/10.1001/jamaoncol.2022.2191.
86. Butler S, Budman S, Fernandez K, et al. Development and validation of the current opioid misuse measure. *Pain.* 2007;130:144–156. https://doi.org/10.1016/j.pain.2007.01.014.
87. Compton P, Darakjian J, Miotto K. Screening for addiction in patients with chronic pain with "problematic" substance use: evaluation of a pilot assessment tool. *J Pain Symptom Manage.* 1988;16:355–363.
88. Compton P, Wu SM, Schieffer B, Pham Q, Naliboff BD. Introduction of self-report version of the Prescription Drug Use Questionnaire and relationship to medication agreement noncompliance. *J Pain Symptom Manage.* 2008;36(4):383–395.
89. Wu S, Compton P, Bolus R, et al. The Addiction Behaviors Checklist: validation of a new clinician-based measure of inappropriate opioid use in chronic pain. *J Pain Symptom Manage.* 2006;32(4):342–351.
90. Caraceni A, Hanks G, Kaasa S, et al. Use of opioid analgesics in the treatment of cancer pain: evidence-based recommendations from the EAPC. *Lancet Oncol.* 2012;13(2):e58–e68. https://doi.org/10.1016/S1470-2045(12)70040-2.
91. Rafii F, Taleghani F, Khatooni M. Barriers to effective cancer pain management in home setting: a qualitative study. *Pain Manag Nurs.* 2021;22(4):531–538. https://doi.org/10.1016/j.pmn.2020.11.003.
92. Reddy A, Yennurajalingam S, Pulivarthi K, et al. Frequency, outcome, and predictors of success within 6 weeks of an opioid rotation among outpatients with cancer receiving strong opioids. *Oncologist.* 2013;18:212–220. https://doi.org/10.1634/theoncologist.2012-0269.
93. Reddy A, de la Cruz M, Rodriguez EM, et al. Patterns of storage, use, and disposal of opioids among cancer outpatients. *Oncologist.* 2014;19(7):780–785.

94. Webster LR, Webster R. Predicting aberrant behaviors in opioid-treated patients: preliminary validation of the Opioid Risk Tool. *Pain Med.* 2005;6(6):432
95. Butler S, Fernandez K, Benoit C, Budman S, Jamison R. Validation of the Revised Screener and Opioid Assessment for Patients with Pain (SOAPP-R). *J Pain.* 2008;9:360–372. https://doi.org/10.1016/j.jpain.2007.11.014.
96. Cheatle MD, Compton P, Dhingra L, Wasser T, O'Brien C. Development of the Revised Opioid Risk Tool to predict opioid use disorder in patients with chronic non-malignant pain. *J Pain.* 2019;20(7):842–851. https://doi.org/10.1016/j.jpain.2019.01.011.
97. Jones T, Moore T. Preliminary data on a new opioid risk assessment measure: the Brief Risk Interview. *J Opioid Manag.* 2013;9(1):19–27. https://doi.org/10.5055/jom.2013.0143.

69

Palliative Care in the Setting of Serious Mental Illness

Lindsey C. Wright

Key Points

- In 2020, of the approximately 52.9 million individuals diagnosed with any mental illness there were an estimated 14.2 million adults with serious mental illness (SMI), or approximately 5.6% of US adults.
- Patients with SMI die approximately 15 to 25 years earlier than those without mental illness and have an all-cause mortality rate 3.7 times higher than that of the general population, highlighting a profound health disparity for this population.
- Nurses are well positioned to bridge gaps between mental healthcare and palliative care for patients with SMI and have a responsibility to do so.

Introduction

In 2020, of the approximately 52.9 million individuals diagnosed with any mental illness (AMI) there were an estimated 14.2 million adults with serious mental illness (SMI), or approximately 5.6% of US adults.[1] Almost half of adults who meet criteria for one mental illness meet criteria for a second, with mood, anxiety, and substance use disorders being the most common comorbid mental illnesses.[1] Those who have SMI are historically underserved in healthcare, including in palliative care.[1–9] In a well-regarded study comparing end-of-life care among individuals with schizophrenia versus matched controls, individuals with schizophrenia were less than half as likely to receive specialty palliative care services, 30% less likely to be prescribed analgesia, and more likely to spend their end of life in nursing homes.[5] Population data from other global health systems supports the finding that individuals with SMI are 2 to 4 times less likely to access palliative care services in the last months of life as compared to those without SMI.[4–6,8] Other studies show that palliative care utilization data in mentally ill patients varies widely, making the understanding of how palliative care is adapted (or not) to meet the needs of patients with SMI difficult to qualify.[1,5–7] Compounding this, there is almost no existing data on the clinical practice of palliative or end-of-life care for these individuals and their families. The current data in this population focuses on questions regarding systems-level access to palliative care and the utilization of services such as hospice. Little focuses on the practice-level standards on how pain and symptom management, including psychiatric symptom management, may differ in patients with SMI and life-threatening illness or best practices on the communication skills necessary to facilitate serious illness conversations with patients and families who live with SMI.[2] It is therefore reasonable to suspect there are care discrepancies in the provision of palliative care nursing for patients with SMI. Nurses are well positioned for bridging palliative care and psychiatric mental healthcare gaps for their patients with SMI and can provide in-scope basic mental healthcare to their patients receiving palliative care.[10] This chapter aims to address these practice disparities through discussion of the clinical manifestations of SMI in palliative care. Future directions for the intersection of palliative care, psychiatry, and nursing are presented at the conclusion of the chapter.

Defining SMI

There are nearly 300 mental health diagnoses classified in the *Diagnostic and Statistical Manual of Mental Health Disorders*, fifth edition, text-revised (DSM5-TR), the clinical manifestations of which lie on spectrums of symptom severity, duration, functional impairment, and clinical distress.[11] SMI, however, is not defined based on a particular diagnostic category or cluster of symptoms or typified by any one disorder but is based on a patient's functioning and quality of life.[1,12] Therefore, SMI is an inherently palliative descriptor for mental health disorders. The definition of SMI is often nebulous and may vary based on context or clinical setting.[2] Often in academic research, mental health disorders are divided in two broad categories: AMI and SMI.[1] The disease burden of AMI is concentrated in patients who experience disability due to SMI.[1] For the purposes of this chapter, we will functionally understand SMI (see Box 69.1) as psychiatric disorders that are chronic, require ongoing treatment, have a significant impact on functioning, and negatively affect quality of life.[2]

Box 69.1 Key Serious Mental Illness Diagnoses

Major depressive disorders
Schizophrenia
Schizoaffective disorder
Bipolar disorder
Obsessive-compulsive disorder
Panic disorder
Posttraumatic stress disorder
Borderline personality disorder
Anorexia nervosa
Bulimia nervosa

Clinical Manifestations of SMI

> It is far more important to know what person the disease has than what disease the person has.
>
> —Hippocrates

Since all mental health disorders have the potential to become SMI, an overview of each clinical presentation of the many disorders or even the most common ones would not do justice to the full understanding of those disorders (for that there is the DSM5-TR and *Kaplan & Sadock's Synopsis of Psychiatry*[13]). However, this section lists and describes the categories of related psychiatric conditions, reviews their common presentations, explains how specific clusters of symptoms impact access to and delivery of palliative care, and provides practical suggestions on how to adapt palliative care interventions to meet the needs of patients with SMI.

Persons with Psychotic Disorders

The psychotic disorders include delusional disorder, brief psychotic disorder, schizophreniform disorder, schizophrenia, schizoaffective disorder bipolar and depressive types, substance- or medication-induced psychotic disorders, and psychotic disorders due to another medical condition.[11] Treatment approaches in SMI due to psychotic disorders are recovery-oriented, rehabilitative, and palliative; and there is no curative treatment for psychotic disorders.[13] Increasingly, studies have found that a palliative approach to treating symptoms of schizophrenia may improve symptom response and decrease the risk of over- or undertreatment, thus improving outcomes for persons living with schizophrenia.[14,15] Thus, standard of care for the provision of palliative care for patients with SMI should include aggressive treatment and symptom management of the SMI itself, unless that treatment becomes too burdensome and is no longer goal-concordant (as can occur in advanced age or at the end of life).[16]

Psychotic disorders are characterized by delusions, hallucinations, disorganized speech and behavior, abnormal motor behavior, and profound changes in motivation and affect known as "negative symptoms."[11] Often patients are repeatedly psychiatrically hospitalized, and nonadherence to medications is frequently problematic.[13] Treatment is multimodal and intensive and generally includes long-term psychiatric management with often high-dose and multiple psychotropic medications, including antipsychotics, mood stabilizers, and antidepressants.[13] A review of psychopharmacological treatment of psychotic disorders is beyond the scope of this chapter (but readers will find *Stahl's Essential Psychopharmacology*[17] to be particularly helpful).

Perceptual disturbances that affect sensory integration, attention and concentration deficits that affect executive functioning, and thought-disordered reasoning are of concern when providing palliative care for patients with SMI due to psychosis. As an example, patients with schizophrenia may have delays in pain management due to reduced sensitivity to pain, which is then complicated by reduced or altered expression of and relation to pain.[18,19] A recent review study demonstrated that this association is only when subjective pain assessment is applied and that the physiological mechanisms associated with pain remain intact.[19] It becomes important for nurses to use additional screening tools for pain (such as the Pain Assessment in Advanced Dementia) and other distressing symptoms such as untreated constipation (which can arise from the anticholinergic burden of many antipsychotics).

Nurses can provide compassionate supportive mental healthcare to patients with psychosis in palliative care through careful assessment of their physical and mental health symptoms using both verbal and behavioral cues, closely monitoring mental status to identify early any fluctuations that may be due to worsening of psychosis, and becoming familiar with the challenges and complications that patients with psychosis may experience. Questions regarding decisional capacity become more complicated in patients with SMI due to psychosis, and the implications of this are high stakes in palliative care.[20] The nurse is positioned to develop a therapeutic relationship with patients and can help advocate for their patient's rights to self-determination and autonomy while also keeping patients with psychosis safe by recognizing that, in some cases, patients are unwell and unable to make decisions for themselves.[20] For readers looking for a comprehensive discussion of the ethical and legal considerations at the intersection of palliative care and psychiatry, please consult the *Oxford Handbook of Psychiatry in Palliative Medicine*.[21]

Persons with Mood Disorders

Mood disorders include the bipolar and related disorders and the depressive disorders: bipolar I disorder, bipolar II disorder, cyclothymic disorder, and bipolar disorder due to another medical condition or substance/medication.[11] The depressive disorders in adults include major depressive disorder, persistent depressive disorder, premenstrual dysphoric disorder, substance- and medication-induced depressive disorder, and depressive disorders due to another medical condition or substance.[11] Major depressive disorder remains the leading cause of disability worldwide.[22]

SMIs due to mood disorders may have a fluctuating course of symptom severity, disease burden, and disability; but some have the potential to resolve, as in the case of a single episode of major depressive disorder.[13] More frequently people with SMIs due to mood disorders experience recurrent mood episodes, rendering the illness chronic and debilitating.[13] Mood disorders arise when normal controls of mood states become dysregulated and manifest clinically as a significant change in the underlying mood state from baseline.[13] Mania is the hallmark example of this, in which patients present with a rapid onset of inflated self-esteem, grandiosity, euphoric or elated mood, giddiness, distractibility, disinhibition, decreased need for sleep, pressured speech, flight of ideas, increase in goal-directed activities, and excessive involvement in pleasurable activities that have high risk for negative consequences (e.g., excessive shopping or sex, uncharacteristic substance use) that lasts 4 or more days and represents a clear change in baseline mood.[11,13] Severe mania can manifest as agitation, severe irritability, restlessness, pacing, hand wringing, mood lability, affect instability, and fulminant psychosis.[13]

Moods that become persistently low are emblematic of a major depressive episode with symptoms of anhedonia, loss of interest in pleasurable activities, hopelessness, helplessness, excessive guilt and shame, lack of energy, difficulty concentrating, hypersomnia or insomnia, loss of appetite or hyperphagia, and, when severe, suicidal ideation, irritability, psychotic features and catatonia.[11,13] Symptom assessment and severity of depression may become more difficult in the setting of life-threatening medical illnesses.[21] As an example, many of the neurovegetative symptoms of depression, such as poor concentration, lack of energy, fatigue, sleep, and appetite disturbances can all be present due to the underlying medical illness (such as cancer).[21] This has led to the diagnosis of major depressive disorder in patients with serious medical illness to become both underdiagnosed (when clinicians dismiss symptoms of depression for those of being normative in the serious illness, as in cancer) and overdiagnosed (when clinicians assume that depression is causing the symptoms where really it is related to the underlying disease state, as can happen in renal failure, chronic obstructive pulmonary disease, or end-stage cardiovascular illness).[22] This led to the proposal of using the Endicott substitution criteria for depression, which replaces change in appetite and weight, sleep disturbance, fatigue and loss of energy, and diminished ability to think or concentrate with tearfulness and depressed appearance, social withdrawal and decreased talkativeness, brooding self-pity and pessimism, and lack of reactivity.[23,24] Additionally, the presence of excessive or inappropriate guilt, shame, hopelessness, helplessness, suicidality, or anhedonia is more sensitive to diagnosing depression in SMI patients and should be weighted more than changes in weight and appetite, for example.[23] However, for all patients one of the most sensitive and specific interview questions to uncover a mood disorder is to simply ask "Are you depressed?"[25] The palliative care nurse can ask this question in a nonjudgmental and curious manner, and if the patient agrees that they have been feeling this way, the nurse can use the Patient Health Questionnaire (PHQ-9) screening tool to further specify the degree of depressive symptoms.

Mood disorders are treated with a combination of psychotropic medication and psychotherapy. Bipolar and related disorders are treated with mood stabilizers, antipsychotics, and lithium, while depressive disorders are treated with antidepressants, augmenting agents (which can include lithium and antipsychotics), and recently esketamine.[17] Mood disorders are also treated symptomatically with medications for sleep or comorbid anxiety, particularly when first initiating maintenance treatment for the underlying disorder as most psychotropic medications for depression require at least 6 weeks of daily dosing before seeing treatment effect.[17] This time course to onset of effect is important to recognize as a consideration in palliative care settings if prognosis is on the order of days to weeks or even weeks to months if the anticipated therapeutic effect may not happen in the patient's life expectancy. In such cases it is appropriate for psychiatric collaborative management, particularly for patients with SMI. Sometimes medications like esketamine and psychostimulants such as methylphenidate may be used for more immediate effect.[26,27] The nurse should recognize when prognosis could impact choice of therapeutic agent and advocate for their patients.

While psychotherapy is a key treatment modality for mood disorders, in palliative care settings it can become challenging, due to the burdens of treatment and illness, as well as the financial burdens. With the emergence of telehealth, some of these barriers to access have been curtailed, though equity and access issues remain. If possible, maintaining connection to a long-standing therapist or clinic can be a major source of support and respite from the burdens of medical care and offer patients opportunities to process their feelings and experiences related to the underlying illness.[25] There are also specific psychotherapies used in palliative care settings including meaning centered psychotherapy (MCP) and dignity therapy (DT); while MCP may be more difficult for patients with SMI, DT was shown to be a valuable intervention for people with SMI.[28]

The palliative care nurse can ask the patient if they have a therapist and, if not, if they ever had been in therapy before. Be curious about what that experience was like for them and engage in motivational interviewing with the patient about whether they might want to return to therapy if there is a treatment lapse. It is helpful to refer to social work to help with bridging gaps in therapy and for linking to appropriate psychotherapy and counseling services. While the psychotherapeutic modalities above are more specific to the mood disorders, the process of therapy described and the considerations for therapy in the context of serious illness can be applied broadly to all patients with SMI.

Persons with Anxiety Disorders and Somatic Symptom and Related Disorders

The anxiety disorders include separation anxiety disorder, selective mutism, specific phobia, agoraphobia, social anxiety disorder, panic disorder, and generalized anxiety disorder, along with unspecified and other specified anxiety disorders and anxiety disorders due to another medical condition or induced by substances or medications.[11] The somatic symptom and related disorders include somatic symptom disorder, illness anxiety disorder, functional neurological symptom disorder, factitious disorder, psychological factors affecting other medical conditions, as well as other specified and unspecified somatic symptom and related disorders.[11] While a separate DSM5 category, somatic symptom and related disorders are included here, given the correlation between anxiety, somatic preoccupation, and the physical symptoms experienced in life-threatening illness.

Anxiety and somatic symptom disorders share clinical features of excessive fear (emotional response to threat), anxiety (anticipation of future threat), or worry and their related behavioral disturbances.[11,13] Fear is associated with autonomic hyperarousal necessary for fight or flight, belief in immediate danger, and escape behaviors (such as eloping or voicing wish for hastened death).[11,13] Anxiety is associated with muscle tension, irritability, vigilance in preparation for future danger, and cautious or avoidant behaviors (such as canceling a surgery or test at the last minute).[11,13] Both fear and anxiety are normative and important responses to danger and are crucial for survival.[13] However, SMI due to anxiety or somatic symptom disorders differs from normative fear and anxiety. As an example, patients with SMI may refuse treatment, including refusing to leave their home due to agoraphobia or severe and recurrent panic attacks, that can be worsened during life-threatening illness. Patients with SMI due to illness anxiety disorder may excessively seek out reassurance and treatment from medical professionals due to fear that they have acquired a serious-life threatening illness.[13] Patients with this underlying disorder who acquire a life-threatening illness may be at higher risk for psychiatric decompensation and debility because the very situation they most fear has now come to fruition. These patients will likely need an extra layer of support from palliative care and psychiatry. Perhaps most disruptive to healthcare providers are those patients who have factitious disorder, where patients fabricate and exaggerate physical and psychiatric symptoms to gain sympathy, attention, and care from medical providers. These patients can present as highly dysregulated and anxious and difficult to console. It is important to realize that factitious disorder is often comorbid with personality disorders, particularly borderline personality disorder.[13] Patients require a team-based approach and collaborative expert psychiatric management.[2,13]

Anxiety and somatic preoccupation can be difficult to assess and treat in palliative care settings due to the complexity of the underlying life-threatening illness; it is normative for people who are diagnosed with life-threatening illness to feel anxious and afraid and become more aware and hypervigilant about their bodies; however, in patients with SMI the degree of anxiety and somatic preoccupation is often persistent, severe, and very distressing to the patient and family and can interfere with the provision of medical and nursing care.[29] It is therefore important to understand how anxiety and somatic preoccupation can be palliated.

Anxiety disorders and somatic symptom disorders are treated with psychotropic medication, often the selective serotonin reuptake inhibitors (SSRIs) and benzodiazepines, and are addressed psychotherapeutically, often through cognitive behavioral therapy (CBT) and other strategies such as exposure and response prevention.[13,17] However, anxiety itself may preclude patients from starting medications in general and psychotropics and palliating medications specifically out of fear that the medications may have adverse outcomes. Reality testing and other CBT strategies are vital to address these concerns, and motivational interviewing can be particularly effective for harnessing the patient's inner strengths to empower change.[30]

As the life-threatening illness progresses and the threat of death and dying looms, patients with SMI due to anxiety and somatic preoccupation may experience panic attacks, which manifest as acute severe feelings of dread and of dying with somatic symptoms such as heart palpitations, diaphoresis, tremors, tunnel vision, tinnitus, flushing or feeling cold, and even nausea and vomiting.[13] Panic attacks can be particularly distressing to the nurse as many serious medical conditions present this way as well (acute coronary syndrome, for example). Panic attacks can occur spontaneously or in response to a known trigger, and in patients with dyspnea from their underlying illness, panic attacks may arise with air hunger.[31] As previously discussed, patients with SMI often have their physical symptoms undertreated.[7] Therefore, patient reports of dyspnea and panic should be taken seriously and addressed. Refractory dyspnea is treated with low-dose opioids, while panic attacks are treated with benzodiazepines (acutely) and SSRIs.[31] Choice of agent must be considered by the palliative care clinician based on the underlying etiology and the indication for the medication. When multiple PRN orders for anxiety pain or dyspnea medications are available to the patient, it becomes important for the nurse to work with the patient to discern if the onset of the panic seems to be temporally related to the exacerbation of dyspnea. If so, it is reasonable to provide the opioid over the benzodiazepine as treatment of reversible causes of psychiatric symptom exacerbation is preferable. However, if panic attacks are contributing to the exacerbation of dyspnea, it may be reasonable to provide benzodiazepines more frequently for patients with recurrent severe panic, particularly near the end of life. In some (rare) cases, patients with refractory panic, anxiety, and existential distress may require palliative sedation at the end of life.[32]

It is important for nurses to understand how to therapeutically respond to patients with SMI who are anxious. Generally, a therapeutic presence, validation of the patient's feelings and experience, reassuring the patient that they are safe, reorienting the patient to the here and now, deploying therapeutic distraction techniques, and reviewing and reinforcing adaptive coping strategies can be particularly helpful to respond to patients who are experiencing anxiety or panic.[13] Fear of death is a complex topic and is frequently manifested by patients with SMI with these disorders. It is important to meet the patient where they are and not to overly challenge patients to understand their prognosis or medical circumstances if their preferred coping strategy is avoidance to maintain emotional well-being. Avoidance does not always equate to denial, and patients may avoid treatment and retain decision capacity. In such cases, it can be helpful to provide psychoeducation about a patient's right not to know specific details related to their serious illness (such as prognosis), to have them assign a healthcare agent as a surrogate decision maker, and to voice their preferences for information-sharing and medical decision-making.[33]

Persons with Obsessive–Compulsive and Related Disorders

The obsessive–compulsive and related disorders include obsessive–compulsive disorder (OCD), body dysmorphic disorder, hoarding disorder, trichotillomania, excoriation disorder, other specified and unspecified obsessive–compulsive and related disorders, and disorders due to another medical condition or substance/medication.[11] People with SMI due to OCD and related disorders struggle with obsessions (intrusive, unwanted, recurrent, persistent thoughts, urges, or images) and compulsions (repetitive behaviors or mental acts a person feels driven to perform in response to an obsession)—the classic example of this is fear of contamination and repeated handwashing.[13] Patients may also have preoccupations and repetitive body behaviors or mental acts in response to preoccupations (as in body dysmorphia or excoriation disorder).[11,13] Patients with OCD are generally treated with high and often heroic dosing of SSRIs and require specific types of psychotherapy for appropriate treatment.[17]

Hoarding

While much of this chapter has focused on the provision of palliative care in acute care settings, patients with SMI due to hoarding disorder are of particular concern for community-based and home-based palliative care nurses and nurses working home hospice who are more likely to encounter hoarding disorder and its challenges in delivering palliative care.[13]

Hoarding disorder is not rare and affects about 2.6% of the US population.[34] Individuals with hoarding disorder feel a need to save or collect objects and experience persistent difficulties discarding possession regardless of their value.[11] Possessions congest and clutter living areas, compromising the use and function of these spaces, which interferes with a patient's functioning and quality of life.[11,13] It can also impact the safety and structural integrity of the home.[13] In extreme hoarding, pests, animals, and biohazardous material may be present. Working appliances, heat, air conditioning, and running water may not be available to patients with SMI in severe cases, making it unfit for them to reside in their homes.[13] Generally, patients with hoarding disorder require substantial support to live and age safely at home. Hoarding, although contributing significantly to disability, is often not of clinical distress to the patient, particularly in SMI.[13] This is often due to individuals having poor or absent insight or delusional thinking about the condition of their home; they may not seek help and are resistant to accepting treatment.

Hospice and home-based palliative care programs may have significant barriers to accessing the home, which often results in patients being moved into skilled nursing facilities, long-term care settings, or residential hospices for the provision of their end-of-life care.[35] Sometimes adult protective services must be called, particularly when there are questions of a patient's safety and decisional capacity. In a subset of cases, patients may need to have a court-appointed guardian to keep them safe and cared for. This is common for patients with SMI and should be a question the nurse asks in the course of a social history.[35] Hoarding behaviors can also manifest in hospital rooms and nursing homes (such as hoarding food) and in such cases the nurse should consult with their psychiatric colleagues for assistance with therapeutic management. Nurse care managers and discharge planners should also have heightened awareness of the impacts of hoarding disorder and consult with community agencies and services and adult protective services.[35]

Treatment for hoarding disorder requires early identification and intervention to mitigate risk and the establishment of expectations and goals with patient and family.[13] Psychoeducation regarding the potential dangers associated with hoarding should be gently and therapeutically provided.[13] Hazards such as fire, falls, unsanitary conditions, and pest infestations are of particular concern for older patients with limited mobility or sensory impairments and become more acutely concerning when being treated for a life-threatening illness that includes immunocompromised states (such as cancer).[13] Often patients are unaware of these potential dangers and may be willing to make changes once the seriousness of risk is explained and the patient's insight is augmented.[13] Identification and involvement of supportive others, when possible, is important as patients with hoarding disorder may be ashamed, isolated, suspicious of the intentions of other (such that they may steal or discard their possessions), or overtly paranoid and unwilling to allow others into their home whatsoever.[13] Trusted support persons can enhance patient engagement with outside agencies, lessen barriers to treatment, and improve access to resources. Treatment also relies on psychiatric evaluation for potential comorbid disorders, such as a major neurocognitive disorder, which may negatively affect response to treatment, or an underlying mood disorder that may respond well to medications and therapy, which can indirectly improve receptivity to treatment for hoarding disorder.[13,34] While there are no medications that are indicated specifically to treat hoarding disorder, antidepressants like venlafaxine and others such as atomoxetine and methylphenidate have some data to support their use.[35–37] Referral to a hoarding disorder specialist for CBT specific for hoarding is ideal; however, patients who are too ill to participate in this level of service could benefit from mutual help or support groups, such as the Buried In Treasure groups and workshops, which may be of particular help for patients and families and contribute to harm reduction and improved quality of life over time.[38–40]

Persons with Trauma and Stressor-Related Disorders

The trauma and stressor-related disorders in adults include, posttraumatic stress disorder (PTSD), complex PTSD, acute stress disorder, adjustment disorder, prolonged grief disorder, and other specified and unspecified trauma and stressor-related disorders. The clinical manifestations for these disorders are similar, although their severity, time course, precipitating factors, and prognosis all vary, making them clinically distinct syndromes. Trauma and stressor-related disorders include disorders where exposure to a trauma is part of the diagnostic criterion.[11] In patients with SMI due to these disorders, instead of responding to trauma or stress with anxiety or fear-based symptoms, the most prominent clinical manifestations are anhedonia; dysphoria; high negative affectivity; externalizing, angry, and aggressive behavior; and dissociative symptoms.[13] Trauma and stressor disorders have a high incidence of medical and psychiatric comorbidity, including substance use disorders, making this cluster of disorders often difficult to treat.[13] These disorders are generally treated with medications (such as the SSRIs) and trauma-informed psychotherapies, peer support groups, and mindfulness-based stress reduction techniques.[13,17]

Trauma informed care is critical when providing palliative care to patients in general and in patients living with SMI, but more sensitivity must be paid to patients who have previously diagnosed trauma and stressor-related disorders as they are at high risk for reactivation of symptoms of stress and trauma while seriously medically ill and under threat of death.[41] A review of trauma informed care is outside the scope of this chapter; however, readers may find tools and resources offered by the National Hospice and Palliative Care Organization and the Center to Advance Palliative Care to be particularly helpful. Of most importance to the palliative care nurse is to understand and respect that patients may not want to be touched, hugged, or engaged with in certain circumstances and may refuse physical exams, lab draws, and other medical interventions out of fear of experiencing trauma-related symptoms, such as flashbacks, nightmares, panic attacks, hyperstartle responses, irritability, persistently negative views about themselves, and in some cases transient paranoid ideation and misperceptions.[13] It is also important to note that patients with SMI due to other disorders may develop PTSD during the course of a life-threatening medical illness, particularly if they had experienced delirium or required life support for critical illness. The nurse should communicate clearly what assessments or interventions they are performing and why, ask for permission to examine or touch a patient, and recognize that information processing and retention is more difficult in patients experiencing active hyperarousal responses or panic when triggered and that repeating information and plans of care may be required.[41] Careful attention should be given to patients who have diagnosed trauma and stressor-related disorders when planning family meetings in palliative care, and psychiatric providers can offer additional assistance with this.[41]

Persons with Personality Disorders

Personality traits are enduring patterns of perceiving, relating to, and thinking about the world and how one relates to it and lie on a continuum of different domains (such as negative affectivity vs. emotional stability or antagonism vs. agreeableness).[11,13] Approaching personality traits as vulnerabilities that are accentuated by stress and that therefore result in the use of predictable coping mechanisms (e.g., Facets) can be a useful way to change stigmatized attitudes toward people with personality disorders (PDs).[13] Please refer to Table 69.1 for review of the classic PD cluster types and hallmark characteristics. PDs develop when enduring maladaptive patterns of behavior, cognition, self-identity and perception, affective orientation, interpersonal functioning, impulsivity, and lack of flexibility in interfacing with themselves, others, and systems.[11] Very often patients who meet criteria for one PD meet criteria for multiple PDs.[11]

People with PDs can present major challenges for medical staff in part because of the maladaptive coping strategies used considering the associated personality traits and in part because of the stigma associated with PDs.[13,42] PDs are enduring patterns of relating, and therefore have latent response to psychiatric treatment (if at all); and while current evidence demonstrates that people with PD can be treated (usually through intensive outpatient programs that utilize specific, evidence-based approaches such as dialectical behavioral therapy) nurses must have realistic expectations for patients with PD as well as their treatment goals and outcomes.[13,42] Currently, there is no medication with a US Food and Drug Administration indication for the treatment of PDs (although there are a few that are in consideration).[13,17] Pharmacotherapy in patients with PD is used either to treat comorbid psychiatric diagnoses that may respond to medication (such as depression) or to palliate severe symptoms, such as the use of lithium for chronic and serious suicidality.[13,42] The primary tool in treating patients living with PDs is the relationship with the psychiatric provider or therapist.[13,42] However, the nurse should anticipate that interpersonal issues with people diagnosed with PDs will arise and are often the most problematic for healthcare providers.[42] People living with these disorders tend to have an increased risk of splitting behaviors, particularly patients with a high degree of borderlinity.[13] Splitting attempts to cause a rift between others so that the patient becomes the focus of the attention of those they have broken apart.[42] Development of a consistent approach will minimize the patient's ability to split staff and minimize the heightened feelings that can arise in caring for this population. It remains important for nurses to be aware of the feelings that the person living with PD brings up for them, which are psychodynamically understood as a countertransference reaction.[13] Patients with PD can evoke strong reactions from staff that may interfere with the delivery of quality care that may require support from and consultation with psychiatric providers.[42]

Psychiatric Emergencies

Psychiatric emergencies are important to recognize, and activation of emergency behavioral response teams (such as behavioral rapid response teams in acute care settings[43]), mobile crisis units, and emergency medical services is crucial whenever a patient becomes a danger to themselves or others; and prompt intervention is lifesaving.[13] Psychiatrists and other psychiatric providers should be immediately consulted when there is concern for a psychiatric

Table 69.1 Overview of specified personality disorders

Cluster and description	DSM5 specified disorder	Hallmark characteristics/traits
Cluster A		
Individuals appear and relate as odd and eccentric	Paranoid	Distrust and suspiciousness of others, motives of others are interpreted as malevolent or persecutory.
	Schizoid	Detachment from social relationships and a restricted range of expression of emotions in interpersonal settings.
	Schizotypal	Social and interpersonal deficits marked by acute discomfort with and reduced capacity for close relationships as well as by cognitive or perceptual distortions and eccentric behavior.
Cluster B		
Individuals appear and relate as dramatic, emotional, and erratic	Antisocial	Disregard for and violating the rights of others, lying, stealing, defaulting on debts, neglect of children or other dependents.
	Borderline	Instability of interpersonal relationships, self-concept, affects and control over impulses, with marked fear of abandonment and extreme efforts to avoid perceived abandonment.
	Histrionic	Excessive emotionality and attention-seeking behavior.
	Narcissistic	Grandiosity, need for admiration, need to be surrounded by success, lack of empathy in interpersonal relationships.
Cluster C		
Individuals appear and relate as fearful, anxious, and rigid	Avoidant	Social inhibition, feelings of inadequacy and hypersensitivity to negative evaluation, rejection sensitivity dysphoria.
	Dependent	Feelings of inadequacy, inability to make own decisions, submissiveness, avoidance of confrontation for fear of losing source of support from others or systems.
	Obsessive–compulsive	Preoccupation with perfectionism, mental and interpersonal control and orderliness at the expense of flexibility, openness, and efficiency.

emergency such as violence, homicidal ideation, and suicidal ideation. Psychiatric providers will work to ensure patients and others are safe, de-escalate the situation, and determine if patients have decisional capacity; they may recommend hospitalization (both voluntary and involuntary) and other interventions such as use of restraints and emergency administration of psychotropic medications (sometimes given over objection when patients are posing acute danger to themselves or others).[13] The least restrictive setting is always the goal. However, in palliative care settings, the nurse may find that there is added complexity in determining what is a psychiatric emergency, particularly related to suicidality as patients consider their life expectancy and adjust to the reality of end of life, with patients voicing wished for hastened death and aid in dying.

Suicidality and Wish for Hastened Death

All patients with SMI are at higher risk for suicidal ideation and attempt as compared to the general population.[1,44] All discussion of suicidal ideation, or a patient's thoughts of taking steps to end their life, should be taken seriously; and a thorough psychiatric assessment should be performed, even when repeated threats of suicide occur. Expression of active suicidal ideation with means (access to lethality), intent (desire to end one's life), and plan (actionable timeline for when suicide will be attempted) requires immediate psychiatric evaluation and intervention. Patients with SMI may have chronic, recurrent suicidality. Nurses should engage in screening of suicidality through the Columbia-Suicide Severity Rating Scale (C-SSRS) when a patient opens up about thoughts of wanting to end their life (see The Lighthouse Project https://cssrs.columbia.edu/). Contracting for safety has fallen out of favor in routine psychiatric practice; however, safety planning and self-management plans are important to help patients cope ahead and anticipate how they might respond to worsening suicidality or triggers for suicidal behavior.[13] Risk for suicide fluctuates over time, with acute suicide risk increasing then decreasing over a short period of time. One particularly helpful tool is the Stanley Brown Safety Plan, which asks patients to create a personalized resource when becoming more suicidal. The goal of safety planning is for patients to augment their self-awareness of their personal warning signs that a suicidal crisis is beginning or escalating so that they or their caregivers can respond before making an attempt or gesture. The nurse should consider these interventions for patients with SMI who are voicing suicidal thoughts.

However, increased preoccupation with death and dying, thoughts of accepting death, and expression of thoughts of dying are common in palliative care patients who are diagnosed with life-threatening illness with and without SMI. Such views should be listened to, validated, reflected on, and responded to in an open, nonjudgmental, and curious manner that fosters further exploration and discussion. It is important to consider the underlying reasons for wish for hastened death, with factors including pain, depression, hopelessness, the feeling of being a burden, loss of autonomy, and loss of dignity.[45] Nurses should not assume that because a patient has a diagnosis consistent with SMI any expression for wish to die in a palliative care setting is equivalent to active suicidality but instead seek to understand why a person might be expressing this thought or feeling at that time in this context.

Conclusion

> [There is] an interpersonal process of therapeutic interactions between an individual who is sick, and a nurse educated to recognize and respond to the need for help.
>
> —Hildegard Peplau

Seriously ill individuals with SMI require special consideration and additional support from healthcare professionals and systems given the disparities in their access to and receiving of palliative care and the limited understanding of when and how to adapt or augment the palliative care intervention to best meet the patient's and family's needs with the goal of alleviation of suffering. To do this, it is incumbent upon nurses to understand how patients with SMI suffer and to advocate for the patient, including ongoing and close collaboration between psychiatry, palliative care, community-based supports, and medicine. Nurses should feel empowered to call these disciplines together in service of their patients with SMI who have life-threatening illness so that care is consistent, cohesive, goal-concordant, compassionate, and in service of the patient.

REFERENCES

1. National Institute of Mental Health. Mental Illness. 2022. https://www.nimh.nih.gov/health/statistics/mental-illness.
2. Shalev D, Fields L, Shapiro PA. End-of-life care in individuals with serious mental illness. *Psychosomatics*. 2020;61(5):428–435. https://doi.org/10.1016/j.psym.2020.06.003.
3. Olfson M, Gerhard T, Huang C, Crystal S, Stroup TS. Premature mortality among adults with schizophrenia in the United States. *JAMA Psychiatry*. 2015;72(12):1172–1181. https://doi.org/10.1001/jamapsychiatry.2015.1737.
4. Kredentser MS, Martens PJ, Chochinov HM, Prior HJ. Cause and rate of death in people with schizophrenia across the lifespan. *J Clin Psychiatry*. 2014;75(02):154–161. https://doi.org/10.4088/jcp.13m08711.
5. Chochinov HM, Martens PJ, Prior HJ, Kredentser MS. Comparative health care use patterns of people with schizophrenia near the end of life: a population-based study in Manitoba, Canada. *Schizophr Res*. 2012;141(2–3):241–246. https://doi.org/10.1016/j.schres.2012.07.028.
6. Spilsbury K, Rosenwax L, Brameld K, Kelly B, Arendts G. Morbidity burden and community-based palliative care are associated with rates of hospital use by people with schizophrenia in the last year of life: a population-based matched cohort study. *PLoS One*. 2018;13(11):e0208220. https://doi.org/10.1371/journal.pone.0208220.
7. Butler H, O'Brien AJ. Access to specialist palliative care services by people with severe and persistent mental illness: a retrospective cohort study. *Int J Ment Health Nurs*. 2017;27(2):737–746. https://doi.org/10.1111/inm.12360.
8. Huang HK, Wang YW, Hsieh JG, Hsieh CJ. Disparity of end-of-life care in cancer patients with and without schizophrenia: a nationwide population-based cohort study. *Schizophr Res*. 2018;195:434–440. https://doi.org/10.1016/j.schres.2017.10.029.
9. Fond G, Salas S, Pauly V, et al. End-of-life care among patients with schizophrenia and cancer: a population-based cohort study from the French national hospital database. *Lancet Public Health*. 2019;4(11):e583–e591. https://doi.org/10.1016/s2468-2667(19)30187-2.

10. Blythe J, White J. Role of the mental health nurse towards physical health care in serious mental illness: an integrative review of 10 years of UK literature. *Int J Ment Health Nurs.* 2012;21(3):193–201. https://doi.org/10.1111/j.1447-0349.2011.00792.x.
11. American Psychiatric Association. *Diagnostic and Statistical Manual of Mental Disorders, Text Revision.* 5th ed. American Psychiatric Association; 2022.
12. Hancq ES. Serious mental illness deserves policy priority. *Health Aff (Millwood).* 2022;41(5):773. https://doi.org/10.1377/hlthaff.2021.02016.
13. Boland RJ, Verduin ML, Ruiz P. *Kaplan & Sadock's Synopsis of Psychiatry*. Wolters Kluwer; 2022.
14. Trachsel M, Irwin SA, Biller-Andorno N, Hoff P, Riese F. Palliative psychiatry for severe persistent mental illness as a new approach to psychiatry? Definition, scope, benefits, and risks. *BMC Psychiatry.* 2016;16(1):260. https://doi.org/10.1186/s12888-016-0970-y.
15. Trachsel M, Irwin SA, Biller-Andorno N, Hoff P, Riese F. Palliative psychiatry for severe and persistent mental illness. *Lancet Psychiatry.* 2016;3(3):200. https://doi.org/10.1016/s2215-0366(16)00005-5.
16. Rosenbaum DMS, Robertson D, Law S. Psychiatric futility and palliative care for a patient with clozapine-resistant schizophrenia. *J Psychiatr Pract.* 2022;28(4):344–348. https://doi.org/10.1097/pra.0000000000000645.
17. Stahl SM, Grady MM, Muntner N. *Stahl's Essential Psychopharmacology: Prescriber's Guide Antidepressants.* Cambridge University Press; 2017.
18. Kudoh A, Ishihara H, Matsuki A. Current perception thresholds and postoperative pain in schizophrenic patients. *Reg Anesth Pain Med.* 2000;25(5):475–479. https://doi.org/10.1097/00115550-200009000-00007.
19. Sakson-Obada O. Pain perception in people diagnosed with schizophrenia: where we are and where we are going. *Psychosis.* 2017;9(4):358–366. https://doi.org/10.1080/17522439.2017.1344294.
20. McGrath PD, Forrester K. Ethico-legal issues in relation to end-of-life care and institutional mental health. *Aust Health Rev.* 2006;30(3):286. https://doi.org/10.1071/ah060286.
21. Chochinov, H. M., & Breitbart, W. (2023). Handbook of psychiatry in palliative medicine: psychosocial care of the terminally ill (Third edition. ed.). Oxford University Press.
22. World Health Organization. Depression. September 13, 2021. https://www.who.int/news-room/fact-sheets/detail/depression.
23. Guan NC, Sulaiman AH, Zainal NZ, Boks MPM, de Wit NJ. Diagnostic criteria for major depressive disorder in cancer patients: a review. *Int J Psychiatry Med.* 2013;45(1):73–82. https://doi.org/10.2190/pm.45.1.f.
24. Kathol RG, Noyes R, Williams J, Mutgi A, Carroll B, Perry P. Diagnosing depression in patients with medical illness. *Psychosomatics.* 1990;31(4):434–440. https://doi.org/10.1016/s0033-3182(90)72140-8.
25. Carlat, D. J. (2024). *The psychiatric interview, 5e.* Lippincott Williams & Wilkins, a Wolters Kluwer business. https://psychiatry.lwwhealthlibrary.com/book.aspx?bookid=3268&sectionid=0
26. Sullivan DR, Mongoue-Tchokote S, Mori M, Goy E, Ganzini L. Randomized, double-blind, placebo-controlled study of methylphenidate for the treatment of depression in SSRI-treated cancer patients receiving palliative care. *Psychooncology.* 2016;26(11):1763–1769. https://doi.org/10.1002/pon.4220.
27. Falk E, Schlieper D, van Caster P, et al. A rapid positive influence of S-ketamine on the anxiety of patients in palliative care: a retrospective pilot study. *BMC Palliat Care.* 2020;19(1):1. https://doi.org/10.1186/s12904-019-0499-1.
28. Grassi L, Nanni MG, Caruso R, et al. A comparison of dignity therapy narratives among people with severe mental illness and people with cancer. *Psychooncology.* 2022;31(4):676–679. https://doi.org/10.1002/pon.5913.
29. Brown R, Chambers S, Rosenberg J. Exploring palliative care nursing of patients with pre-existing serious persistent mental illness. *Prog Palliat Care.* 2019;27(3):117–121. https://doi.org/10.1080/09699260.2019.1619964.
30. Landa A, Makous M, Fallon BA. Treating somatic symptom disorder and illness anxiety in integrated care settings. In: Feinstein RE, Connelly JV, Feinstein MS, eds. *Integrating Behavioral Health and Primary Care.* Oxford University Press; 2017:276–302. https://doi.org/10.1093/med/9780190276201.003.0016.
31. Periyakoil VS, Skultety K, Sheikh J. Panic, anxiety, and chronic dyspnea. *J Palliat Med.* 2005;8(2):453–459. https://doi.org/10.1089/jpm.2005.8.453.
32. Cotogni P, Brazzi L. Palliative sedation: a feasible option to improve end-of-life care in seriously ill dying patients. *Minerva Anestesiol.* 2017;83(5):446–448. https://doi.org/10.23736/s0375-9393.17.11906-1.
33. Davies B. The right not to know and the obligation to know. *J Med Ethics.* 2020;46(5):300–303. https://doi.org/10.1136/medethics-2019-106009.
34. Postlethwaite A, Kellett S, Mataix-Cols D. Prevalence of hoarding disorder: a systematic review and meta-analysis. *J Affect Disord.* 2019;256:309–316. https://doi.org/10.1016/j.jad.2019.06.004.
35. Davies S. How can community and primary care nurses support and treat people with hoarding disorder? February 14, 2020. Accessed February 9, 2021. https://rcni.com/primary-health-care/evidence-and-practice/research-focus/how-can-community-and-primary-care-nurses-support-and-treat-people-hoarding-disorder-157696.
36. Landau D, Iervolino AC, Pertusa A, Santo S, Singh S, Mataix-Cols D. Stressful life events and material deprivation in hoarding disorder. *J Anxiety Disord.* 2011;25(2):192–202. https://doi.org/10.1016/j.janxdis.2010.09.002.
37. Saxena S, Sumner J. Venlafaxine extended-release treatment of hoarding disorder. *Int Clin Psychopharmacol.* 2014;29(5):266–273. https://doi.org/10.1097/yic.0000000000000036.
38. Mathews CA, Mackin RS, Chou CY, et al. Randomised clinical trial of community-based peer-led and psychologist-led group treatment for hoarding disorder. *BJPsych Open.* 2018;4(4):285–293. https://doi.org/10.1192/bjo.2018.30.
39. Frost RO, Ruby D, Shuer LJ. The Buried in Treasures Workshop: waitlist control trial of facilitated support groups for hoarding. *Behav Res Ther.* 2012;50(11):661–667. https://doi.org/10.1016/j.brat.2012.08.004.
40. Rodgers N, McDonald S, Wootton BM. Cognitive behavioral therapy for hoarding disorder: an updated meta-analysis. *J Affect Disord.* 2021;290:128–135. https://doi.org/10.1016/j.jad.2021.04.067.
41. Volpin M. Posttraumatic stress disorder in hospice and palliative care: current knowledge, current practice (S709). *J Pain Symptom Manage.* 2018;55(2):660–661. https://doi.org/10.1016/j.jpainsymman.2017.12.363.
42. Terpstra TL, Williamson S. Palliative care for terminally ill individuals with borderline personality disorder. *J Psychosoc Nurs*

Ment Health Serv. 2019;57(9):24–31. https://doi.org/10.3928/02793695-20190531-01.

43. Smallcomb L, Mack E. Reducing workplace harm through a behavioral rapid response team. *Crit Care Med.* 2021;50(1):654. https://doi.org/10.1097/01.ccm.0000811552.72541.7a.
44. Fu XL, Qian Y, Jin XH, et al. Suicide rates among people with serious mental illness: a systematic review and meta-analysis. *Psychol Med.* 2023;53(2):351–361. https://doi.org/10.1017/s0033291721001549.
45. Monforte-Royo C, Villavicencio-Chávez C, Tomás-Sábado J, Mahtani-Chugani V, Balaguer A. What lies behind the wish to hasten death? A systematic review and meta-ethnography from the perspective of patients. *PLoS One.* 2012;7(5):e37117. https://doi.org/10.1371/journal.pone.0037117.

70

Rural Palliative Care

Richard A. Taylor, J. Nicholas Odom, Erin R. Currie, Chunhong Xiao, and Marie A. Bakitas

Key Points

- Providing palliative care to persons living in rural areas across the globe presents significant barriers including transportation, geographical and economic challenges, and the absence of local palliative care experts and resources to meet the needs of patients with complex, serious illness.
- Telehealth, phone-based care, and specially trained lay community workers are some strategies being applied to increase access to palliative care in rural settings.
- Palliative care research, especially focused on the issues pertinent to rural culture and socioeconomic factors, is needed to address the specific evidence gaps for this unique environment.

Case Study 1: Lack of Access to Advanced Heart Failure Therapies

Denise is a widowed 62-year-old middle school teacher with a history of myocardial infarction, hypertension, and diabetes who was recently diagnosed with Stage D heart failure after an emergent admission for respiratory distress. Denise was flown by helicopter from her rural town's (pop. 5,000) Critical Access Hospital to the tertiary care academic center as there were no cardiac specialists within 3 hours of her town. Denise was in the intensive care unit (ICU) receiving continuous intravenous inotropic support to keep her ejection fraction high enough to maintain her blood pressure and high-dose diuretic therapy. Denise's kidneys were still not perfusing well enough to maintain adequate urine output. The cardiologist believed that the best option to optimize her cardiac output and overcome her prerenal failure was a left ventricular assist device (LVAD). The home health agency serving her rural town was contacted, but they reported that none of their staff was trained in LVAD care. Palliative care had been consulted to discuss goals of care with Denise and her two adult daughters, who lived in a different state. Denise was faced with weighing an LVAD treatment option, including the challenge of navigating the logistical circumstances of living in a rural area and being limited in the available social support needed to manage an LVAD, as well as her other health conditions.

Case Study 2: Lack of Access to Pediatric Specialists in Rural Communities

Jayden is a 2-month-old twin who was born at 37 weeks' gestation. He was hospitalized immediately after birth in his local neonatal ICU; however, Jayden was diagnosed with a critical heart condition requiring a series of complicated surgeries. He was transferred to the only free-standing children's hospital in the state, 2 hours from his home in rural Alabama, and received his first open heart procedure at 3 days old. Jayden suffers from complications such as poor feeding and recurrent infections and has remained hospitalized since birth. He is not a candidate for his next surgery until he is 18 months old, and his medical team does not think he will survive. Jayden's mother, a full-time dental hygienist, and his father, a privately employed mechanic, struggle with visiting Jayden more than 2 hours away from their home while also caring for his twin sister and an older sibling. Because of Jayden's serious illness, he and his family are receiving palliative care and are offered support with difficult decisions. His family would prefer home hospice because his siblings and other family have yet to meet him; however, home hospice is unavailable because there is a lack of specialty-trained pediatric hospice providers in his community. Jayden's family must decide whether to remain at the children's hospital and receive specialized care or transition to a community-based hospital without their trusted cardiology and palliative care teams. This transition would involve establishing trust and rapport at a challenging time when facing end-of-life care planning.

Rural Palliative Care: What Is Different?

Globally, almost half of the population must overcome multiple factors, such as poverty, educational, and employment challenges that

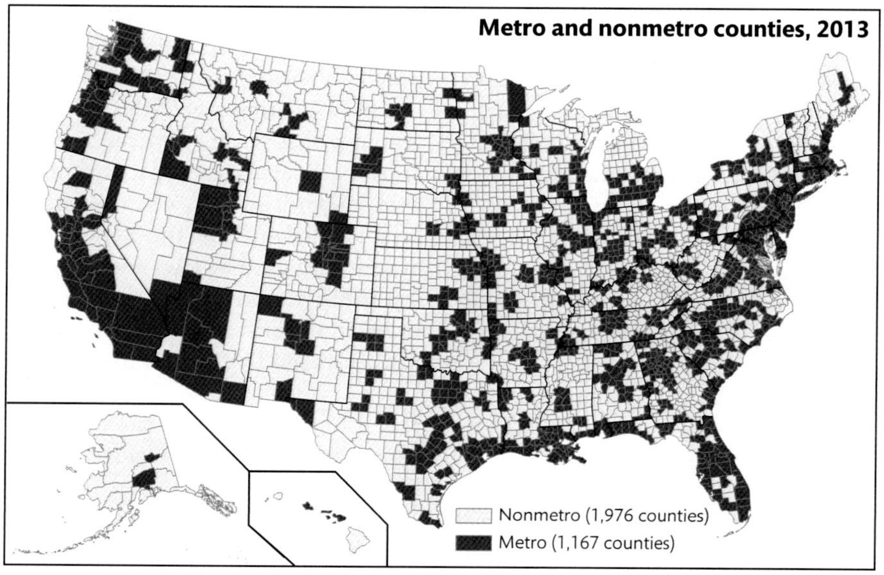

Figure 70.1 Nonmetropolitan counties include some combination of (1) open countryside, (2) rural towns (places with fewer than 2,500 people), and (3) urban areas with populations ranging from 2,500 to 49,999 that are not part of larger labor market areas (metropolitan areas). The US Census Bureau uses much smaller geographic building blocks to define rural areas as open country and settlements with fewer than 2,500 residents. Most counties, whether metro or nonmetro, contain a combination of urban and rural populations.

Source: US Department of Agriculture (2021; map last updated June 17, 2021).

accompany rural living. In 2020, approximately 46 million US residents lived in rural areas, comprising about 14% of the US population.[1] Nearly half (46.7%) of all people living in US rural areas (28 million people) are in the South.[2] The world's rural population has grown since 1950 to 3.4 billion. Africa and Asia remain the most rural continents, accounting for close to 90% of the world's rural population, with India having the largest population, followed by China.[3] Figure 70.1 shows a map of metro and nonmetro counties in the United States.[4]

Sometimes population density is the defining concern; population thresholds used to differentiate rural and urban communities range from 2,500 up to 50,000, depending on the definition. For the 2020 US Census, an "urban" area comprises a densely settled core of census tracts and/or census blocks that meet minimum population density requirements, along with adjacent territory containing nonresidential urban land uses as well as territory with low population density included to link outlying densely settled territory with the densely settled core. The Census Bureau identifies urban areas as 5,000–50,000 or more people[5]; and "rural" encompasses all population, housing, and territory not included within an urban area.[6]

Two main challenges that persons with serious illness residing in a rural locale face are access to and acceptability of palliative care resources.[7–9] A number of reports found that living in US regions served by small rural hospitals puts patients at high risk for limited or no access to hospice and palliative care services.[8,10,11] Approximately 17% of US hospices are located in rural areas, and while hospice programs are increasing in general, hospice programs in rural areas are declining.[12] Even when palliative and hospice services are available, persons in rural and minority groups are less likely to use them, in part due to culturally insensitive healthcare systems, mistrust of healthcare providers, and structural racism.[13–15] Cultural mores about illness and death in Indigenous and Native populations differ significantly from the predominant Caucasian, Western traditions that are at the foundation of many palliative and hospice programs. Caxaj and colleagues'[16] literature review identified priorities and challenges to providing palliative care to rural Indigenous populations such as (1) environmental and contextual issues, (2) institutional barriers, and (3) interpersonal dynamics challenging client–clinician interactions. They recommended recognizing the essential role of family connections in building culturally based community partnerships to increase palliative care capacity. Hence, limited access and lack of culturally acceptable palliative and hospice resources are major challenges to providing equitable care to persons who are seriously ill and dying in rural areas worldwide.

Seriously ill rural patients are particularly vulnerable, may be socially isolated, and are at high risk of experiencing care disparities.[14,17,18] Long distances and low population density impose logistical and financial barriers that can impede specialty care access and diffusion of innovations such as comprehensive hospice and palliative care.[14] Local primary care clinicians are most often multiskilled generalists who may see few seriously ill or dying patients, thus limiting their ability to develop needed palliative care expertise.[14] In small rural communities with scarce palliative care resources, clinicians may face ethical concerns about dual relationships and the challenge of being called on to care for their own family, lifelong friends, and neighbors at their end of life.[14,19]

Rural location has often been related to less and later hospice use and higher rates of hospitalization at the end of life, particularly in rural nursing home residents.[20,21] Most rural patients are unlikely to have access to the "gold standard" interdisciplinary team (IDT) provided by palliative and hospice services.[22,23] Hence, these patients may have to choose between "going without" or being transferred to a distant site for care.[14] Patients transferred to distant tertiary care settings are at high risk of spending their last days or weeks of life far from home and loved ones and without adequate support for themselves and their caregivers. Rural patients with advanced disease, severe pain, or related symptoms who remain in a local facility may suffer during their last weeks of life because state-of-the-art techniques for treating pain or other causes of distress are scarce. The opening cases of this chapter provide vivid examples of the suffering that can occur when local specialty resources are unavailable at the end of life.

Challenges to Providing Palliative Care in Rural Settings

There are numerous challenges and barriers to accessing and providing rural palliative care.[7,14,16,17,24–27] These barriers can include patient, provider, and health system factors (see Box 70.1).

Rural clinicians often receive inadequate training and may not be prepared to provide palliative care.[7,28–30] Therefore, access to distance education, online resources, specialty journals, and textbooks is essential. However, learning complex palliative care communication techniques may be best acquired through in-person and role-play strategies, which may not be readily available.[31] Palliative care education of community-based nurses and lay health workers may close a gap in palliative care of patients in rural areas.

Delivering Rural Palliative Care beyond the United States

Numerous international organizations and bodies have officially recognized and called for providing palliative care as an essential right and component of healthcare.[32] However, according to the World Health Organization, there are an estimated 56.8 million people in need of palliative care globally, and only about 12% of this need is being met.[33] This discrepancy between need and access to palliative care services is even more pronounced in rural areas, particularly rural parts of middle- and low-income countries.[34] Approximately 76% of adults in need of palliative care are from low-income countries.[32] A review by Aregay and colleagues[34] of strategies used by low- and middle-income countries to establish palliative care in rural areas found that significant challenges included national policies not being linked to funding (most palliative care funding coming from nongovernmental organizations), lack of accredited staff that could prescribe and make available medications, lack of staff training and community awareness of palliative care, and lack of palliative care service access and implementation in remote communities. The reader is referred to Chapter 72, "Global Palliative Care in Low- and Middle-Income Countries," for further information.

Box 70.1 Barriers/Challenges to Rural Palliative Care

Patient/Family

- Lack of patient/family knowledge and acceptance of palliative care
- Lack of transportation and long travel distances to palliative care centers (for patients and family/friend visitors)
- Lack of reliable broadband internet coverage to access palliative providers through telehealth
- Patient/family preference to stay in home community for care
- Patient/clinician concerns that they will lose touch with community providers if they seek care at centers far from home
- Mistrust of unfamiliar providers

Provider

- Limited community clinician access to palliative care experts
- Limited community clinician exposure to palliative care patients in their practice (e.g., inadequate primary palliative care skills)
- Limited availability of palliative care education in the community
- Limited scope of practice (e.g., inability of advanced practice practitioners to admit patients to hospice, prescribe opioids)

Health System/Policy/Regulatory

- Poor communication/coordination of care between academic and rural community settings
- Limited evidence of palliative care benefits in rural palliative care
- Lack of availability of technology/techniques used for complex patients (e.g., pain pumps, left ventricular assist devices)
- Scope of practice and regulatory disincentives

Sources: References 4 and 14.

Creative Strategies to Meet the Palliative Care Needs of Rural Patients

Technology-Enabled Healthcare

A major challenge to palliative care delivery in rural areas is the need to provide high-quality care with limited resources. New strategies of technology-enabled approaches have great potential in improving palliative care for rural environments. Technology-enabled health is a synergy between the fields of telehealth, mobile health, electronic health informatics, informatics, and health information exchange. The overall goal is to improve access to and the cost-effectiveness of quality care.[35]

Telehealth is a heterogeneous collection of clinical practices, technologies, and organizational arrangements that can be grouped into three categories: remote patient monitoring, store-and-forward, and real-time audio/video encounters.

Remote monitoring uses devices that transmit data in real time or that can be downloaded to a provider's office or computer. A trial of remote symptom monitoring overseen by a nurse in which cancer patients used a web-based method to report on 12 symptoms was found to improve quality of life (QOL) and 1-year survival in patients with metastatic solid tumors receiving chemotherapy treatments compared with usual cancer care.[36] Community-based models in which providers go to patients' homes to provide palliative care have been developed to address the needs of patients in rural and remote areas.[37] VyncaCare (formerly Resolution Care), a corporation in northern California, provides home-based palliative care via home visits and videoconferencing. It uses an IDT to see patients within a 150-mile radius of a physical office (patients are not seen in the office).[38] It also provides palliative care "telementoring" in partnership with Project ECHO (Extension for Community Healthcare Outcomes) to train healthcare practitioners to provide primary palliative care.[39] Project ECHO is a telehealth model that links rural primary care clinicians with specialists to perform real-time learning using inexpensive videoconferencing technology. The program's novel approach allows physicians, nurse practitioners (NPs), and other clinicians to jointly manage complex illness and promotes the use of best practices while enabling patients to receive treatment in their home communities.

Store-and-forward is the oldest form of telehealth technology. It refers to transmitting images or information from one provider to another. An example of store-and-forward telehealth technology is when a clinician sends a digital image of an X-ray to a radiologist for analysis. State telemedicine reimbursement laws, even in states that require parity for real-time communication, do not always cover store-and-forward telehealth.

Real-time communication is what many consider the most common use of telehealth technology. An example is when a patient is at one location and the provider is at another, and they connect using a video-enabled device and a telephone or computer audio. Detailed information on this topic is provided in Chapter 60, "Telehealth, Telephonic Care and Remote Patient Monitoring."

Monitoring and measuring health data over geographical, social, and cultural distances is being facilitated by smartphones and an explosion of wearable technology, monitoring devices, and mobile applications available for almost any health and illness condition.[40]

Engagement of tele-palliative care for advanced cancer patients increases when a tablet, computer, or smartphone app is the mode of delivery.[41] The COVID-19 pandemic ushered in remote palliative care delivery changes and facilitated a technology-based continuum care plan for cancer patients.[42]

Telehealth strategies are cost-effective and have been associated with high-quality clinical outcomes and patient satisfaction in various pediatric and adult palliative care settings.[43–46] Barriers to telehealth, such as start-up and maintenance costs and concerns over equipment costs, privacy, and security, have begun to decrease. Furthermore, adopting electronic medical records has contributed to staff training and comfort levels with telehealth. Palliative care telehealth approaches being implemented in rural areas around the world can provide access to consultations, education, and collaboration for providers, patients, families, and caregivers.[47,48]

Numerous organizations provide internet-based educational programs and links for patients and caregivers. These include The American Academy of Hospice and Palliative Medicine (AAHPM.org), the Hospice and Palliative Nursing Association (HPNA.org), the National Hospice and Palliative Care Organization, and the Center for the Advancement of Palliative Care (CAPC.org).

Professional Telehealth Programs for Rural Palliative Care

A collaborative model using internet conferencing between a rural palliative care NP and an urban palliative care physician improved symptom management and access for underserved patients and families.[49] A Canadian province developed a 24-hour telephone hotline to provide expert palliative care consultation, which was most frequently accessed by rural communities. This Rural Palliative Telehealth Project received provincial and national funding and examined telehealth to conduct direct palliative care consultations and care conferences with distant primary care teams, deliver staff education, and link rural patients with their urban specialists for palliative care case conferences.[50] Telehealth was beneficial for discharge planning between the urban tertiary palliative care unit and the rural care team when patients with complex issues were being transitioned back to their home communities.[50]

Project ENABLE (Educate, Nurture, Advise, Before Life Ends) was an early use of telehealth to provide oncology palliative care.[51,52] ENABLE, based on the World Health Organization continuum of care and Wagner and McCorkle's chronic illness model of care,[53] which includes face-to-face standardized palliative care consultation and a nurse-coach delivering the standardized "Charting Your Course" curriculum to patients and care partners (see Table 70.1). Approximately 1,000 patients with cancer (and their family caregivers) have participated in ENABLE clinical trials. Published trial results have demonstrated gains in QOL, improvement in symptoms, less depression, and improved survival.[51,54,55] The primary focus of ENABLE is coaching patients to learn new skills of problem-solving, patient empowerment and activation, proactive symptom management, healthcare decision-making, advance care planning, communication, and legacy/life review. Another feature is assisting the patient and family to identify local, community primary care and palliative/hospice resources to reduce dependence on distant care providers and allow them to stay in their home communities. Family caregivers participating in the program report lower depression scores and lower burden.[55] Others have also found telehealth to be an important resource for family caregivers, who have generally expressed satisfaction with this approach.[56]

Telehealth may provide an opportunity for pediatric palliative care providers to educate, consult, and manage seriously ill children in rural areas. For example, a case report of rural pediatric palliative care patients followed by a hospital-based pediatric palliative care team found that patients and families found it helpful to receive counseling that would typically not have been available.[45] Although broadband may not be universally available, many rural communities can obtain internet access in community clinics to access telehealth services.

Strategies to address the palliative care needs of persons in rural areas, especially older adults, must include innovative health

Table 70.1 ENABLE Charting Your Course curriculum

Patient curriculum	Caregiver curriculum
Module 1 (week 1) Behavioral activation/ problem-solving	**Module 1 (week 1)** Caregiver role Creativity, Optimism, Planning, and Expert Advise attitude and problem-solving
Module 2 (week 2) Symptom management	**Module 2 (week 2)** Self-care
Module 3 (week 3) Decision-making, communication, and support	**Module 3 (week 3)** Being a partner in symptom management
Module 4 (week 4) Life accomplishments and goals and life review	**Module (week 4)** Focus on decision-making
Module 5 (week 5) Accomplishments and future goals/forgiveness	Planning for follow-up **Monthly and bereavement follow-up**
Module 6 (week 6) Unfinished business/leaving a legacy	
Monthly follow-up	

services.[29] Lay health workers (community health advisors or community health workers) trained in palliative care have effectively served as a bridge between healthcare institutions and the community by providing psychosocial support, advance care planning, symptom screening, and referral to palliative care.[57] In some areas, community health workers include lay "navigators" to help reduce cancer disparities by encouraging early screening and prevention in high-risk groups.[58,59]

The effectiveness of this approach has been demonstrated in cancer navigation programs. The University of Alabama at Birmingham Health System Cancer Community Network trained nurses and lay navigators (community health advisors) in palliative care principles, including communication skills, decision-making about advanced disease, symptom recognition, and advocacy to reduce barriers to cancer care.[60,61] The program demonstrated improved self-efficacy in the lay navigators, an increase in advance care planning discussions in the African American population, identification and resolution of psychosocial distress, and a statistically significant decline in Medicare spending, emergency room visits, and hospitalization over time.[62,63] In rural regions with high levels of hospice penetration, lay health workers may be engaged as "sitters" who provide individuals with companionship and assistance with activities of daily living. Additionally, hospice and palliative care volunteers in rural regions provide valuable social, emotional, and practical assistance. While evidence supporting lay health workers in palliative care and hospice is sparse, it is expanding in rural regions.[64,65] Important areas for research include defining the role that community health workers or advisors may play in enhancing access to palliative care in rural regions. Defining the role and impact of lay personnel in palliative care and defining the best way to integrate training for this workforce in rural palliative care should be active areas of investigation.

The Role of Critical Access Hospitals

Rural hospitals provide essential healthcare services to nearly 54 million people, including 9 million Medicare beneficiaries, low-income individuals, and Medicaid populations who often need palliative care services. With the closure of 136 rural hospitals between 2010 and 2021 (59% decline between 2015 and 2019),[66] the number of physicians decreased, travel distance to care increased by 24 miles,[67] and 1.7 million people are at higher risk for poor health outcomes due to lack of local access to acute care.[68] Medicare reimbursement issues, workforce shortages, rising healthcare insurance costs, aging rural hospital facilities, and the demand for expensive new information systems all contribute to the daily challenges of providing adequate care in rural settings.[66] To deal with some of these issues, in 1997, through the Balanced Budget Act of 1997, a designation of Critical Access Hospitals (CAHs) was developed to receive cost-based reimbursement. To be designated a CAH, a rural hospital must meet defined criteria, as shown in Box 70.2.[69]

The goal of CAHs can, at times, be at cross-purposes with the goals of palliative care. For example, brief stays have a financial incentive to stabilize and transfer the patient to a larger hospital or academic center.[70] In many cases, for these chronically ill older adults, the more appropriate approach is for these rural hospitals to keep patients for end-of-life care or to stabilize the patient and, if possible, arrange for a return home with hospice care. The nursing and medical staff at the CAH are expert generalists. The nurse may be the first point of contact for the patient and family in the CAH, being responsible for assessing and stabilizing the patient before transfer to the urban hospital. The traditional multidisciplinary specialty palliative care team is rarely available at a CAH, but it is generally available at the urban hospital to guide and coach the rural staff throughout the process. This collaboration is an opportunity to extend palliative care through the local rural providers to the patients they serve.

Box 70.2 Critical Access Hospital Criteria

- Must be rural, located within a state participating in the Medicare Rural Hospital Flexibility program
- Must be more than a 35-mile drive from any other hospital or Critical Access Hospital (CAH; or, in the case of mountainous terrains or in areas where only secondary roads are available, more than 15 miles from any other hospital or CAH)
- Must have 15 or fewer acute inpatient care beds (or, in the case of swing bed facilities, up to 25 inpatient beds that can be used interchangeably for acute or skilled nursing facility-level care, provided no more than 15 beds are used at any one time for acute care) as reported on the cost report
- Must restrict the patient length of stay to no more than 96 hours unless a more extended period is required because of inclement weather or other emergency conditions or a physician review organization or other equivalent entity, on request, waives the 96-hour restriction (the 96-hour length-of-stay limitation was modified in 1999 to a per-patient annual average)
- Must offer 24/7 emergency services
- Must be owned by a public or nonprofit entity (modified in 1999 to extend eligibility to for-profit hospitals)
- Must have and maintain required quality assurance arrangements

Source: Reference 69.

Conclusion

Outstanding efforts have been made in the past two decades to improve standards for the emerging specialty of palliative care.[71] The fourth edition of the National Consensus Project for Quality Palliative Care's *Clinical Practice Guidelines for Quality Palliative Care* has incorporated content and model examples that recognize the unique role of culture and geography that can influence palliative care access. As illustrated in this chapter and described in numerous reviews,[34,72,73] rural populations, in comparison with urban populations, have proportionally more older adults over 65, higher unemployment rates, higher numbers of uninsured, higher numbers of individuals below the poverty line, greater sensitivity to an economic downturn, lower population densities, longer travel distances to healthcare facilities, fewer numbers of healthcare specialists and generalist providers, a narrower scope of available healthcare services, higher rates of chronic disease, and, in the United States, greater dependence on Medicare and Medicaid.

Accounting for these and other unique characteristics of rurality, the question is how palliative care clinicians and researchers should respond. In the case study with Denise, she had limited options as her daughters lived far away, and no one locally was trained to assist her with an LVAD. If there had been a palliative care team at the CAH or in the community where she lived, her options may have been different. The rural perspective of Jayden's case provides another unique challenge. The palliative care team is providing psychosocial support and end-of-life care to the family, but they have the difficult decision to leave him at the hospital for his care or take him home with no hospice services or palliative care available in their community. For palliative care clinicians, any new interaction or consultation with patients, families, and providers should ask about and address any misperceptions about palliative care. Clinicians can initiate regular check-ins with generalist providers in outlying areas to offer expertise and consultation on challenging cases. CAPC now has national Palliative Care Leadership Centers focused on developing community-based palliative care programs beyond the hospital setting. This program provides an online curriculum, webinars, virtual office hours with palliative care experts, on-site training, and more—all focused on incorporating palliative care into the local practice patterns of the community providers.[74]

Palliative care researchers need to address the uncharted terrain of palliative care at the level of living conditions, communities, geography, and social and economic policies and climates.[75,76] Given the growing use, prevalence, and capabilities of communications and other technologies, researchers can test innovative solutions that incorporate such technologies to overcome the geographical obstacles of rural healthcare delivery.[77] Where one lives makes a huge difference in whether a patient and family receive adequate palliative care.

REFERENCES

1. Dobis EA, Krumel TP Jr, Cromartie J, Conley KL, Sander A, Ortiz R. *Rural America at a Glance*. US Department of Agriculture; 2021. Accessed August 11, 2023. https://www.ers.usda.gov/webdocs/publications/102576/eib-230.pdf?v=3149.3.
2. Ratcliffe M, Burd C, Holder K, Field A. *Defining Rural at the U.S. Census Bureau: American Community Survey and Geography Brief* (ACSGEO-1). US Census Bureau; 2016. Accessed August 11, 2023. https://www2.census.gov/geo/pdfs/reference/ua/Defining_Rural.pdf.
3. United Nations, Population Division. *World Urbanization Prospects 2018: Highlights*. United Nations; 2019. Accessed August 11, 2023. https://population.un.org/wup/Publications/Files/WUP2018-Highlights.pdf.
4. US Department of Agriculture. *Broadband*. US Department of Agriculture; 2022. Accessed August 11, 2023. https://www.usda.gov/broadband.
5. Federal Register. Urban Areas for the 2020 Census—Proposed Criteria. Accessed August 9, 2020. https://www.federalregister.gov/documents/2021/02/19/2021-03412/urban-areas-for-the-2020ra-census-proposed-criteria.
6. US Census Bureau. Rural and Urban. Accessed August 9, 2023. https://www.census.gov/programs-surveys/geography/guidance/geo-areas/urban-rural.html.
7. Bakitas M, Allen Watts K, Malone E, et al. Forging a new frontier: providing palliative care to people with cancer in rural and remote areas. *J Clin Oncol*. 2020;38(9):963–973. https://doi.org/10.1200/JCO.18.02432.
8. Center to Advance Palliative Care, National Palliative Care Research Center. America's Care of Serious Illness: A State-by-State Report Card on Access to Palliative Care in Our Nation's Hospitals. 2020. Accessed August 11, 2023. https://www.capc.org/search/?q=America%27s+care+of+serious+illness%3A+A+state-by-state+report+cared+on+access+to+palliative+care+in+our+nation%27s+hospitals.
9. Morin L, Aubry R, Frova L, et al. Estimating the need for palliative care at the population level: a cross-national study in 12 countries. *Palliat Med*. 2017;31(6):526–536. https://doi.org/10.1177/0269216316671280.
10. Center to Advance Palliative Care. Growth of Palliative Care in U.S. Hospitals 2022 Snapshot. Accessed August 11, 2023. https://www.capc.org/documents/1031/?clickthrough_doc_id=core.cmsdocument.1031&clickthrough_req_id=i2nWJClaSf-moGOrAOIopQ&clickthrough.
11. Parajuli J, Tark A, Jao YL, Hupcey J. Barriers to palliative and hospice care utilization in older adults with cancer: a systematic review. *J Geriatric Oncol*. 2020;11(1):8–16. https://doi.org/10.1016/j.jgo.2019.09.017.
12. Medicare Payment Advisory Commission. *Report to the Congress: Medicare Payment Policy*. MedPAC; 2022. Accessed August 11, 2023. https://www.medpac.gov/wp-content/uploads/2022/03/Mar22_MedPAC_ReportToCongress_v2_SEC.pdf.
13. Marcewicz L, Kunihiro SK, Cursee KA, Johnson K, Kavalieratos D. Application of critical race theory in palliative care research: a scoping review. *J Pain Symptom Manage*. 2022;63(6):e667–e684. https://doi.org/10.1016/j.jpainsymman.2022.02.018.
14. Tedder T, Elliott L, Lewis K. Analysis of common barriers to rural patients utilizing hospice and palliative care services: an integrated literature review. *J Am Assoc Nurse Pract*. 2017;29(6):356–362. https://doi.org/10.1002/2327-6924.12475.
15. Umaretiya PJ, Wolfe J, Bona K. Naming the problem: a structural racism framework to examine disparities in palliative care. *J Pain Symptom Manage*. 2022;63(5):e461–e463. https://doi.org/10.1016/j.jpainsymman.2021.07.035.
16. Caxaj CS, Schill K, Janke R. Priorities and challenges for a palliative approach to care for rural Indigenous populations: a scoping review. *Health Soc Care Community*, 2018;26(3):e329–e336. https://doi.org/10.1111/hsc.12469.
17. Rainsford S, MacLeod RD, Glasgow NJ, Phillips CB, Wiles RB, Wilson DM. Rural end-of-life care from the experiences and perspectives of patients and family caregivers: a systematic literature review. *Palliat Med*. 2017;31(10): 895–912. https://doi.org/10.1177/0269216316685234.
18. Wark S, Hussain R, Müller A, Ryan P, Parmenter T. Challenges in providing end-of-life care for people with intellectual disability: health services access. *J Appl Res Intellect Disabil*. 2017;30(6):1151–1159. https://doi.org/10.1111/jar.12408.
19. Wickersham MEE, Sumner JR. The ethics of place: differences in ethical perspectives among urban, suburban, and rural physicians in Georgia. *Online J Health Ethics*. 2015;11(2). https://doi.org/10.18785/ojhe.1102.05
20. Ankuda CK, Mitchell SL, Gozalo P, Mor V, Meltzer D, Teno JM. Association of physician specialty with hospice referral for hospitalized nursing home patients with advanced dementia. *J Am Geriatr Soc*. 2017;65(8):1784–1788. https://doi.org/10.1111/jgs.14888.
21. Quigley DD, Estrada LV, Alexander G, Dick A, Stone PW. Differences in care provided in urban and rural nursing homes in the United States: literature review. *J Gerontol Nurs*. 2021;47(12):48–56. https://doi.org/10.3928/00989134-20211109-09.
22. Bull J, Kamal AH, Harker M, et al. Standardization and scaling of a community-based palliative care model. *J Palliat Med*. 2017;20(11):1237–1243. https://doi.org/10.1089/jpm.2017.0027.
23. Burmeister B, Durão SA, Teves CM, et al. The importance of the interdisciplinary team in running palliative care services in the community. In Silbermann M, ed. *Palliative Care for Chronic*

Cancer Patients in the Community: Global Approaches and Future Applications. Springer International Publishing; 2021:121–130.
24. Bakitas MA, Elk R, Astin M, et al. Systematic review of palliative care in the rural setting. *Cancer Control*. 2015;22(4):450–464. https://doi.org/10.1177/107327481502200411.
25. Jansson M, Dixon K, Hatcher D. The palliative care experiences of adults living in regional and remote areas of Australia: a literature review. *Contemp Nurse*. 2017;53(1):94–104. https://doi.org/10.1080/10376178.2016.1268063.
26. Kirby S, Barlow V, Saurman E, Lyle D, Passey M, Currow D. Are rural and remote patients, families and caregivers needs in life-limiting illness different from those of urban dwellers? A narrative synthesis of the evidence. *Austral J Rural Health*. 2016;24(5):289–299. https://doi.org/10.1111/ajr.12312.
27. Whittall D, Lee S, O'Connor M. Factors affecting rural volunteering in palliative care—an integrated review. *Austral J Rural Health*. 2016;24(6):350–356. https://doi.org/10.1111/ajr.12313.
28. Eriksson G, Bergstedt TW, Melin-Johansson C. The need for palliative care education, support, and reflection among rural nurses and other staff: a quantitative study. *Palliat Support Care*. 2015;13(2):265–274. https://doi.org/10.1017/S1478951513001272.
29. Pesut B, Hooper B, Jacobsen M, Nielsen B, Falk M, O'Connor BP. Nurse-led navigation to provide early palliative care in rural areas: a pilot study. *BMC Palliat Care*. 2017;16(1):37. https://doi.org/10.1186/s12904-017-0211-2.
30. Weng K, Shearer J, Grangaard Johnson L. Developing successful palliative care teams in rural communities: a facilitated process. *J Palliat Med*. 2022;25(5):734–741. https://doi.org/10.1089/jpm.2021.0287.
31. Forbat L, Robinson R, Bilton-Simek R, Francois K, Lewis M, Haraldsdottir E. Distance education methods are useful for delivering education to palliative caregivers: a single-arm trial of an education package (PalliativE Caregivers Education Package). *Palliat Med*. 2018;32(2):581–588. https://doi.org/10.1177/0269216317712849.
32. Worldwide Hospice Palliative Care Alliance. *Global Atlas of Palliative Care*. Worldwide Hospice Palliative Care Alliance; 2020. Accessed August 11, 2023. https://cdn.who.int/media/docs/default-source/integrated-health-services-(ihs)/csy/palliative-care/whpca_global_atlas_p5_digital_final.pdf?sfvrsn=1b54423a_3.
33. World Health Organization. Palliative Care: Key Facts. 2020. Accessed August 11, 2023. https://www.who.int/news-room/fact-sheets/detail/palliative-care.
34. Aregay A, O'Connor M, Stow J, Ayers N, Lee S. Strategies used to establish palliative care in rural low- and middle-income countries: an integrative review. *Health Policy Plan*. 2020;35(8):1110–1129. https://doi.org/10.1093/heapol/czaa051.
35. Barbosa W, Zhou K, Waddell E, Myers T, Dorsey ER. Improving access to care: telemedicine across medical domains. *Annu Rev Pub Health*. 2021;42:463–481. https://doi.org/10.1146/annurev-publhealth-090519-093711.
36. Basch E, Deal AM, Dueck AC, et al. Overall survival results of a trial assessing patient-reported outcomes for symptom monitoring during routine cancer treatment. *JAMA*. 2017;318(2):197–198. https://doi.org/10.1001/jama.2017.7156.
37. Cohn J, Corrigan J, Lynn J, et al. Community-based models of care delivery for people with serious illness. NAM Perspectives. Discussion paper. National Academy of Medicine; 2017. https://doi.org/10.31478/201704b.
38. VyncaCARE. Supportive Care Services. Accessed August 11, 2023. https://www.vyncacare.com/.
39. Arora S, Smith T, Snead J et al. Project ECHO: an effective means of increasing palliative care capacity. *Am J Managed Care*. 2017;23(7 spec no.) Sp267–Sp271.
40. Dimitrov DV. Medical internet of things and big data in healthcare. *Healthc Informat Res*. 2016;22(3):156–163.
41. Goodman W, Bagnall AM, Ashley L, et al. The extent of engagement with telehealth approaches by patients with advanced cancer: systematic review. *JMIR Cancer*. 2022;8(1):e33355. https://doi.org/10.2196/33355.
42. Levoy K, Foxwell A, Rosa WE. Palliative care delivery changes during COVID-19 and enduring implications in oncology nursing: a rapid review. *Curr Opin Support Palliat Care*. 2022;16(3):94–101. https://doi.org/10.1097/spc.0000000000000603.
43. Bradford N, Armfield NR, Young J, Smith AC. The case for home based telehealth in pediatric palliative care: a systematic review. *BMC Palliat Care*.2013;12(1):4. https://doi.org/10.1186/1472-684X-12-4.
44. Bradford NK, Armfield NR, Young J, Smith AC. Paediatric palliative care by video consultation at home: a cost minimisation analysis. *BMC Health Serv Res*. 2014;14(1):328. https://doi.org/10.1186/1472-6963-14-328.
45. Winegard B, Miller EG, Slamon NB. Use of telehealth in pediatric palliative care. *Telemed e-Health*. 2017;23(11):938–940. https://doi.org/10.1089/tmj.2016.0251.
46. Jess M, Timm H, Dieperink KB. Video consultations in palliative care: a systematic integrative review. *Palliat Med*. 2019;33(8):942–958. https://doi.org/10.1177/0269216319854938.
47. Brecher DB. The use of skype in a community hospital inpatient palliative medicine consultation service. *J Palliat Med*. 2013;16(1):110–112. https://doi.org/10.1089/jpm.2012.0022.
48. Namasivayam P, Bui DT, Low C, et al. The use of telehealth in the provision of after-hours palliative care services in rural and remote Australia: a scoping review. *PLoS One*. 2022;17(9):e0274861. https://doi.org/10.1371/journal.pone.0274861.
49. Watanabe SM, Fairchild A, Pituskin E, Borgersen P, Hanson J, Fassbender K. Improving access to specialist multidisciplinary palliative care consultation for rural cancer patients by videoconferencing: report of a pilot project. *Support Care Cancer*. 2013;21(4):1201–1207. https://doi.org/10.1007/s00520-012-1649-7.
50. Spice R, Read Paul L, Biondo PD. Development of a rural palliative care program in the Calgary zone of Alberta Health Services. *J Pain Symptom Manage*. 2012;43(5):911–924. https://doi.org/10.1016/j.jpainsymman.2011.05.019.
51. Bakitas M, Lyons KD, Hegel MT, et al. Effects of a palliative care intervention on clinical outcomes in patients with advanced cancer: the Project ENABLE II randomized controlled trial. *JAMA*. 2009;302(7):741–749. https://doi.org/10.1001/jama.2009.1198.
52. Bakitas MA. On the road less traveled: journey of an oncology palliative care researcher. *Oncol Nurs Forum*. 2017;44(1):87–95. https://doi.org/10.1188/17.ONF.87-95.
53. Wagner E, McCorkle R. Self-management. In: Holland J, Breitbart W, Jacobsen P, Lederberg M, Loscalzo M, McCorkle R, eds. *Psycho-Oncology*. Oxford University Press; 2010:464–468.
54. Bakitas MA, Tosteson TD, Li Z, et al. Early versus delayed initiation of concurrent palliative oncology care: patient outcomes in the ENABLE III randomized controlled trial. *J Clin Oncol*. 2015;33(13):1438–1445. https://doi.org/10.1200/JCO.2014.58.6362.
55. Dionne-Odom JN, Azuero A, Lyons KD, et al. Benefits of early versus delayed palliative care to informal family caregivers of patients with advanced cancer: outcomes from the ENABLE III

randomized controlled trial. *J Clin Oncol*. 2015;33(13):1446–1452. https://doi.org/10.1200/JCO.2014.58.7824
56. Zeng Y, Head BA, Schapmire TJ. A systematic review of telehealth in palliative care: caregiver outcomes. *Telemed e-Health*. 2016;22(4):288–294.
57. Patel MI, Ramirez D, Agajanian R, Agajanian H, Coker T. Association of a lay health worker intervention with symptom burden, survival, health care use, and total costs among Medicare enrollees with cancer. *JAMA Netw Open*. 2020;3(3):e201023. https://doi.org/10.1001/jamanetworkopen.2020.1023.
58. Dickerson JC, Ragavan MV, Parikh DA, Patel MI. Healthcare delivery interventions to reduce cancer disparities worldwide. *World J Clin Oncol*. 2020;11(9):705–722. https://doi.org/10.5306/wjco.v11.i9.705.
59. Campbell C, Baernholdt M. Community health workers' palliative care learning needs and training: Results from a partnership between a US university and a rural community organization in Mpumalanga province, South Africa. *J Health Care Poor Underserved*. 2016;27(2):440–449. https://doi.org/10.1353/hpu.2016.0078.
60. Rocque GB, Dionne-Odom JN, Huang CHS, et al. Implementation and impact of patient lay navigator-led advance care planning conversations. *J Pain Symptom Manage*. 2017;53(4):682–692. https://doi.org/10.1016/j.jpainsymman.2016.11.012.
61. Rocque GB, Partridge EE, Pisu M, et al. The Patient Care Connect Program: transforming health care through lay navigation. *J Oncol Pract*. 2016;12(6):e633–e642. https://doi.org/10.1200/JOP.2015.008896.
62. Rocque GB, Williams CP, Jones MI, et al. Healthcare utilization, Medicare spending, and sources of patient distress identified during implementation of a lay navigation program for older patients with breast cancer. *Breast Cancer Res Treat*. 2017;167:215–223. https://doi.org/10.1007/s10549-017-4498-8.
63. Rocque GB, Taylor RA, Acemgil A, et al. Guiding lay navigation in geriatric patients with cancer using a distress assessment tool. *J Natl Comp Cancer Netw*. 2016;14(4):407–414. https://www.scopus.com/inward/record.uri?eid=2-s2.0-84964344817&partnerID=40&md5=b64110c7f98986dd33a97943ab8601bb.
64. Connell B, Warner G, Weeks LE. The feasibility of creating partnerships between palliative care volunteers and healthcare providers to support rural frail older adults and their families: an integrative review. *Am J Hospice Palliat Med*. 2017;34(8):786–794. https://doi.org/10.1177/1049909116660517.
65. Morris SM, Payne S, Ockenden N, Hill M. Hospice volunteers: bridging the gap to the community? *Health Soc Care Community*. 2017;25(6):1704–1713. https://doi.org/10.1111/hsc.12232.
66. American Hospital Association. *Rural Hospital Closures Threaten Access*. American Hospital Association; 2022. Accessed August 11, 2023. https://www.aha.org/system/files/media/file/2022/09/rural-hospital-closures-threaten-access-report.pdf.
67. US Government Accountability Office. *Rural hospital Closures: Affected Residents Had Reduced Access to Health Care Services*. US Government Accountability Office; 2020. Accessed August 11, 2023. https://www.gao.gov/assets/gao-21-93.pdf.
68. Holmes GM, Kaufman BG, Pink GH. Predicting financial distress and closure in rural hospitals. *J Rural Health*. 2017;33(3):239–249. https://doi.org/10.1111/jrh.12187.
69. Rural Health Information Hub. Critical Access Hospitals (CAHs). 2021. Accessed August 11, 2023. https://www.ruralhealthinfo.org/topics/critical-access-hospitals#:~:text=Congress%20created%20the%20Critical%20Access,the%201980s%20and%20early%201990s.
70. Mayer D, Winters CA. Palliative care in critical access hospitals. *Crit Care Nurse*. 2016;36(1):72–78. https://doi.org/10.4037/ccn2016732.
71. National Consensus Project for Quality Palliative Care. *Clinical Practice Guidelines for Quality Palliative Care*. 4th ed. National Coalition for Hospice and Palliative Care; 2018. Accessed August 11, 2023. https://www.nationalcoalitionhpc.org/ncp.
72. Cai Y, Lalani N. Examining barriers and facilitators to palliative care access in rural areas: a scoping review. *Am J Hosp Palliat Care*. 2022;39(1):123–130. https://doi.org/10.1177/10499091211011145.
73. Suntai Z, Won CR, Noh H. Access barrier in rural older adults' use of pain management and palliative care services: a systematic review. *Am J Hosp Palliat Care*. 2021;38(5):494–502. https://doi.org/10.1177/1049909120959634.
74. Center to Advance Palliative Care. How PCLC Works. 2022. Accessed August 11, 2023. https://www.capc.org/palliative-care-leadership-centers/how-pclc-works/.
75. Grindrod A. Choice depends on options: a public health framework incorporating the social determinants of dying to create options at end of life. *Prog Palliat Care*. 2020;28(2):94–100. https://doi.org/10.1080/09699260.2019.1705539.
76. Quintiens B, D'Eer L, Deliens L, et al. Area-based compassionate communities: a systematic integrative review of existing initiatives worldwide. *Palliat Med*. 2022;36(3):422–442. https://doi.org/10.1177/02692163211067363.
77. Ohta R, Ryu Y. Improvement in palliative care quality in rural nursing homes through information and communication technology-driven interprofessional collaboration. *Rural Remote Health*. 2021;21(2):6450. https://doi.org/10.22605/rrh6450.

71

Palliative Care for Older Adults

Laura Tycon Moreines and Lauren Hunt

Key Points

- Palliative care for the older adult should be patient-centered and carefully weigh risks and benefits.
- Goals of care should be frequently assessed early on while the patient has capacity and should be reassessed as their condition changes.
- A comprehensive geriatric assessment is essential in ensuring a holistic approach to care.
- Informal care partners and other social supports are key partners in the care of the older adult with serious illness.

Introduction

An Aging Population

Around the globe, the population is aging. Due to demographic drivers, the 65 and older population is growing faster than all other age groups. By 2050, one in six people worldwide will be over 65. The population of adults aged 80 and older is growing even more rapidly and is projected to triple from 143 million in 2019 to 426 million in 2050.[1] In the United States, almost 1 in 4 people will be 65 and older and 1 in 20 will be 85 and older by 2060.[2] At the same time, older Americans are becoming more sociodemographically diverse. By 2060, almost 1 in 2 older adults will identify as Black, Hispanic, Asian, or other non-White race.[2] Many older adults face economic challenges, with 15% of adults 65 and older and 20% of adults 80 and older living in poverty.[3]

The Importance of Palliative Care Nursing for Older Adults

As people age, they are more likely to experience chronic and serious illnesses that require palliative care interventions. Aging is the biggest risk factor for most serious illnesses and is a factor in many of the leading causes of death such as cancer, heart failure, and dementia.[4] In addition, many older adults experience significant physical, cognitive, and functional disability in the years leading up to death.[5] Pain and other symptoms are highly prevalent among older adults with serious illness approaching the end of life.[6] Not only does palliative care create value through addressing symptoms to improve quality of life, but research also shows that palliative care intervention may increase the life span at a lower cost than disease-directed interventions.[7]

Trajectories of Serious Illness in Older Adults

Depending on the serious illness(es) they face, older adults may have different functional and healthcare use trajectories at the end of life. These trajectories have been classified into four distinct groups: (1) sudden death, (2) terminal illness, (3) organ failure, and (4) frailty (Figure 71.1).[8]

In the sudden death group, health and function are generally maintained until death, which may be caused by an accident or major health event such as a massive heart attack. The terminal illness trajectory is most typical of cancer patients. These individuals will maintain health and function for a long period of time and then experience a rapid decline in the weeks and months before death. The organ failure trajectory is typical of people with renal or heart failure. For this group, function declines slowly over time, punctuated by periods of exacerbation, followed by partial recovery. The frailty trajectory, which is common among people with advanced dementia, involves a very slow and progressive decline. People with frailty often require long periods of support from others, family caregivers and/or long-term care services; and prognostication in this group is uncertain.

Older adults rarely have just one condition, and evidence indicates substantial variation in end-of-life trajectories among individuals whose cause of death is cancer, organ failure, frailty, and even sudden death.[9] However, this categorization serves as a useful "rule of thumb" for thinking about palliative care needs for older adults with serious illness.

Care Settings and Palliative Care Models

Many older adults state that they prefer to age in place and die in home and community-based settings as opposed to institutional settings like hospitals and nursing homes.[10] Although the number of older adults dying at home has increased in recent years, the majority still die in hospitals and nursing facilities, especially among racial and ethnic minoritized populations. This may be due in part to lack of resources and support for the increasing number of people dying in community-based settings. For those who do die at home, care partners and families often bear the burden of caring for these individuals under challenging circumstances.[11,12]

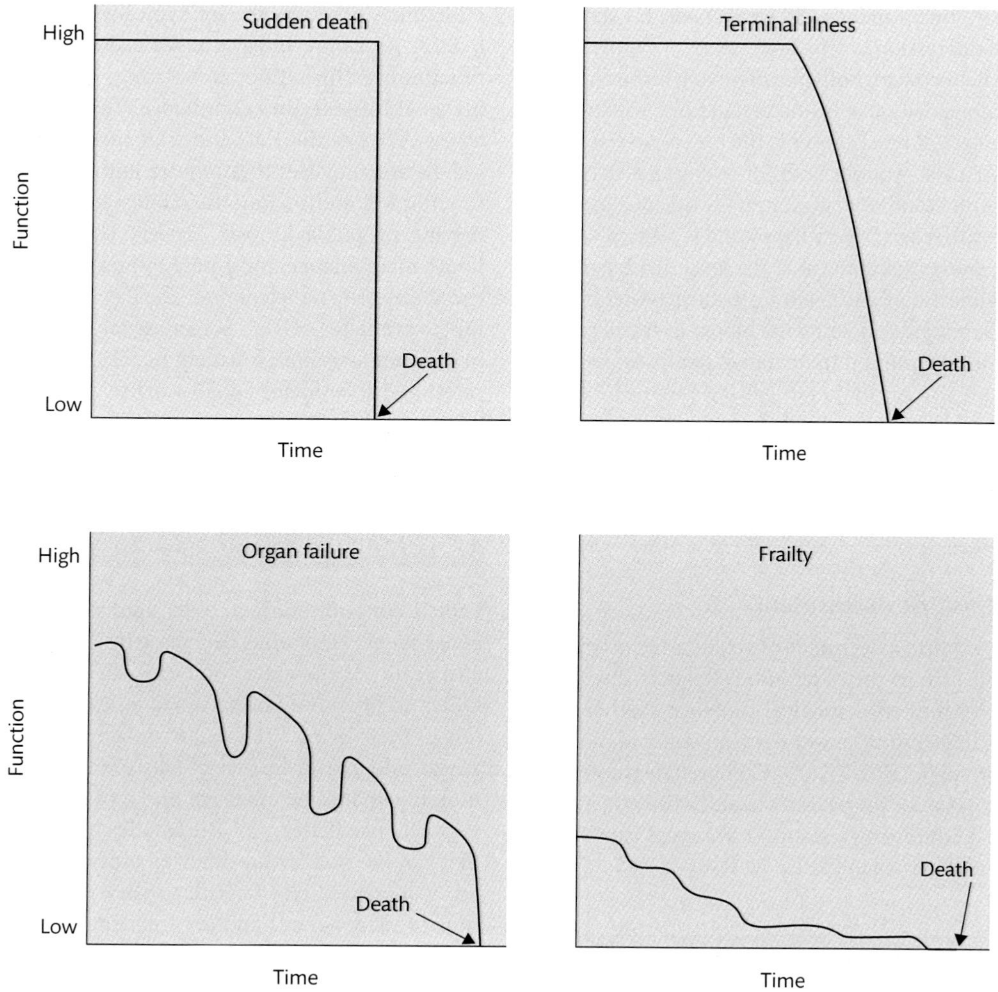

Figure 71.1 Proposed trajectories of dying in older adults.
Source: Reference 8.

The primary model for palliative care delivery for older adults in the United States is the Medicare Hospice Benefit. Hospice eligibility requirements can restrict access to hospice for those with uncertain prognoses, such as people with dementia and people who are reluctant to forgo curative treatments. As a result, there has been growing interest in developing other palliative care models for older adults with serious illness. For older adults, Medicare covers inpatient palliative care, which is now widely available throughout the country.[13] Community-based palliative care in office-based, home, and long-term care settings is growing rapidly; however, Medicare funding for these programs remains limited. Changes in the healthcare payment environment and a shift to value-based care (i.e., managed care and accountable care organizations) may help bolster community-based palliative care programs for older adults.[14]

Case Study

Mr. Wong is an 80-year-old veteran who presents to the geriatric outpatient clinic. He immigrated to the United States from Vietnam and has limited English proficiency. He was diagnosed with moderate dementia about a year ago. He comes to clinic with his brother Ian, who serves as his surrogate decision maker. Mr. Wong has been having fatigue, weight loss, and hematuria for several months. His primary care provider ordered a computed tomographic (CT) scan that revealed a lesion on his right kidney. He was then referred to an oncologist who is now recommending a biopsy. His brother is uncertain whether to proceed with further workup. He is referred to the outpatient geriatric clinic to elicit goals of care and to determine whether proceeding with a medical workup aligns with the patient's goals.

Mr. Wong is ambulatory with a cane. He lives at home alone in affordable housing. He has no children, and his only family is his brother. Ian struggles with decision-making for his brother. On the one hand, Mr. Wong is cheerful and upbeat and seems happy with his quality of life. On the other hand, Ian is unsure whether Mr. Wong fully understands the severity of his illness or the consequences of the treatment options being offered. His wishes had not been discussed prior to his diagnosis with dementia.

The geriatric palliative care nurse conducts a comprehensive geriatric assessment and finds that Mr. Wong is dependent with instrumental activities of daily living (IADLs) and relies solely on his brother for assistance with these activities. He requires assistance with bathing but otherwise is independent with activities of daily living (ADLs). He had two falls in the past year that resulted in mild injuries. He has urinary incontinence and wears pads. He shows no signs or symptoms of depression.

Ian is clearly overwhelmed with both his caregiving responsibilities and the medical decisions that must be made regarding whether further workup of this potential renal cancer is the best course of action for Mr. Wong. In the first visit, you ask both Mr. Wong and his brother what Mr. Wong values most and what gives him the best quality of life. Ian tells you that his brother seems very happy and is pleased with his current life. He most enjoys going to eat at the local diner, going for walks around the neighborhood, and listening to music. After this discussion, the team recommends pursuing the biopsy as it will provide more information about staging and the extent of treatment required.

To help Ian, the team also recommends getting a home health aid to assist Mr. Wong with his ADLs and help Ian with some of his informal caregiving responsibilities. The team involves the social worker to help with service allocation. The geriatric team also refers Ian to the Alzheimer's Association caregiver support group.

Comprehensive Geriatric Assessment

The comprehensive geriatric assessment provides a framework for approaching palliative care in the older adult. It spans several domains including, but not limited to, medical, mobility, psychological, functional, social, and nutritional assessments in concordance with a complementary care plan (Box 71.1).[19] Comprehensive geriatric assessment's aim is to optimize the patient's health while considering their goals of care and addressing current or potential gaps in care with a thorough and inclusive plan (Table 71.1).

Functional Capacity

Functional assessments are ways to assess how patients carry out tasks of daily living and maintain independent functioning.

Box 71.1 Geriatric Syndromes

"Geriatric syndromes" refers to health conditions that result from the accumulated effects of multiple underlying causes which manifest in a single set of observable characteristics, signs, and/or symptoms, or a "phenotype."[15] In contrast to a single disease, geriatric syndromes have many etiologies, often with multiple risk factors and organ systems involved.[16] Geriatric syndromes are very common among older adults and can greatly reduce quality of life and increase risk for poor outcomes, such as nursing home placement and death. Common geriatric syndromes include:

- falls
- incontinence
- pressure ulcers
- dementia
- delirium
- polypharmacy
- frailty

Frailty, for example, affects more than a quarter of adults 85 and older and is characterized by fatigue, weight loss, frequent infections, and general vulnerability to stress.[17] Assessing for the presence of geriatric syndromes should be part of the palliative nurse's approach to care of the older adult.[18] If geriatric syndromes are present, the palliative nurse should modify the care plan accordingly. Depending on the patient's goals of care, this may include taking measures to reverse any treatable causes, addressing any associated symptoms, and providing anticipatory guidance.

Functional assessments are typically subdivided into ADLs and IADLs. ADLs are integral tasks needed to maintain independent functioning, including ambulating, feeding, toileting, dressing, personal hygiene, and continence. The most common tool used to assess ADLs is the Katz Index of Independence of Daily Living.[20] IADLs are activities that require both thinking skills and physical functioning and include the ability to transport oneself either by driving or public transit, grocery shopping, managing finances, home maintenance, meal preparation, managing medications, and the ability to use a telephone. The Lawton Scale is a commonly used tool to evaluate IADLs.[21] Screening for ADLs and IADLs helps determine what assistance a patient needs (if any) in the home to ensure safety and an enhanced quality of life. Anticipatory guidance should be given regularly to the patient and family unit as it is expected that ADL independence will decline as the end of life nears.

Falls/Fall Risk

Falls occur commonly in older adults and can have many negative consequences including decreased functionality, post-fall syndrome, and death. As the older adult ages, the incidence of falls increases.[22] Older adults should be screened annually for their fall risk regardless of their living situation. Risk factors include medications, dizziness, and a prior history of falls, among others. Gait, balance, and mobility should be assessed; one tool for this is the Short Physical Performance Battery.[22,23] The Hendrich Fall Risk model II is one tool that can be used for hospitalized older adults.[24] Patients on hospice are at increased risk for falls as they progressively lose their functional independence and are frequently prescribed medications to alleviate symptoms, such as opiates, which may increase fall risk. Interventions for this population consist of education of patient/caregiver unit on fall prevention, including use of an assistive device if needed, promoting a safe environment, education on proper transfers, and ensuring adequate supervision.[22]

Mood

Major depression is commonly seen in older adults.[25] It is a myth that depression is a normal part of aging. Correctly identifying depression is critical as it can lead to decreased cognitive, physical, and social functioning and impaired quality of life. The Geriatric Depression Screen (GDS) is a validated tool for older adults.[26] Prompt treatment of depression in the older adult is important to ensure optimized quality of life. A multifactorial treatment regimen of both nonpharmacological (e.g., therapy, exercise, mindfulness) and pharmacological treatment is most effective.[27]

Cognition

Up to a third of community-dwelling older adults have mild cognitive impairment, and one-third of all decedents in the United States have dementia at the time of death.[28] Screening for cognitive impairment is important for the older adult receiving palliative care and/or hospice as it can impact many aspects of care including caregiver/patient relationships and affect decision-making about treatment

Table 71.1 Comprehensive geriatric assessment and key nursing interventions

Domain	Assessment	Nursing intervention/key points
Functional capacity	• Activity of daily living: Katz Index of Independence of Daily Living: • Instrumental activity of daily living: Lawton Scale	• Assess a patient's ability to complete tasks necessary to live independently • Help determine what resources/help a patient needs to enhance independence • As disease processes progress, activity of daily living dependence often increases. Anticipatory guidance around expected functional decline to keep patients as independent as possible for as long as possible
Falls	• Community-dwelling adults, the Short Physical Performance Battery • Inpatient setting: Hendrich Fall • Assess for risk factors such as dizziness, medications, and prior falls • Assess gait, balance, and mobility (e.g., Short Physical Performance Battery)	• Falls are common and can have many detrimental ramifications • Prevention is key • Patients on hospice have an increased occurrence of falls • Often polypharmacy and exercise interventions are not possible in this population • Discussions early on with how the patient/family unit would like to handle a fall are important • Environment modification, patient/caregiver education, and proper supervision are important • Gait assessment and consultation for potential assistant device should be performed
Mood	• Geriatric Depression Screen (GDS)	• Multifactorial treatment regimen of both nonpharmacological and pharmacological treatment is most effective
Cognition dementia/delirium	• Montreal Cognitive Assessment (MoCA) • Mini-Mental State Examination (MMSE) • Confusion Assessment Method • Dementia Rating System	• Anticipatory guidance • Caregiver support • Healthcare decisions (artificial nutrition, antibiotics) • Sensory support (e.g., hearing and vision aids)
Incontinence	• Thorough medical evaluation should be completed • Ask patient/proxy about involuntary loss of urine/bowels • Assess for odor and stains • Post-void bladder scan	• Depending on patient's goals and prognosis, aggressive measures such as medication and physical therapy may be appropriate • Use of a bedside commode or urinal • Toilet rounds every 2 hours • For actively dying patients, use of bed pads, undergarments, or Foley catheter if moving patient is painful
Skin	• Braden scale	• Inspection of the skin over the entire body • Assess pressure areas such as the sacrum and heels • Use finger palpation to determine if erythema or discoloration is blanchable
Medication/polypharmacy	• Screening Tool for Older Person's Prescriptions (STOPP)/Screening Tool to Alert to Right Treatment (START) • American Geriatrics Society Beers Criteria	• Medication reconciliations are to be performed with each care transition and at least biannually • Due to physiologic changes in the older adult, there are changes in pharmacokinetics and pharmacodynamics • Certain geriatric syndromes affect the way medications are absorbed, metabolized, and excreted • Polypharmacy ≥5 medications can cause poor outcomes • Due to changes in pharmacodynamics, many medications need to be dose reduced for older adults • Polypharmacy in the older adult receiving hospice and palliative care is often unavoidable • Unnecessary medications need to be stopped
Nutrition and weight	• Mini-Nutritional Assessment (MNA) • Thorough medical workup to be done • Assessment of difficulty chewing, difficulty swallowing, medication-induced nausea, and/or taste	• Eliminating any medications that may be causing symptoms • Providing feeding assistance • Offering appealing foods • Ensuring adequate food availability • Appetite stimulants and supplemental drinks have not been found to be effective • Patient and family education regarding anorexia when patient is at end of life
Hearing	• Hearing screens should be performed	• Use of personal amplifiers if needed • Face-to-face communication • Adequate lighting so patients can see lip movements • Decreasing background noise
Dentition	• If possible, continue dental visits	• When disease has progressed beyond dental visits being feasible, continue bedside oral care
Advanced care planning	• Physician Orders for Life-Sustaining Treatment (POLST)/Medical Orders for Life-Sustaining Treatment (MOLST)	• This process needs to be performed with changes in condition • Important to first establish what the patient/caregiver's perceptions of illness and illness trajectory are • Creating measurable and obtainable goals is important (i.e., "have the energy to have my granddaughter visit weekly") • Treatments are framed within the context of harms, burdens, benefits, and prognosis for each treatment

(*continued*)

Table 71.1 Continued

Domain	Assessment	Nursing intervention/key points
Social support	• Social assessment consisting of who would care for the patient if/when they are unable to care for themselves • Lubben Social Network Scale	• Discussions should be early in the disease course to help with resource allocation • Interventions for loneliness: • Video conferencing • Humor therapy • Mindfulness • Pet therapy • Stress reduction
Informal caregivers	• Caregiver Self-Assessment Questionnaire • Look for signs of caregiver burnout	• Use of interdisciplinary team for services and respite care
Financial concerns	• Asking patients about food and medication availability • Ensuring safe and accessible place to live	• Use of the interdisciplinary team is important for resource allocation
Sexuality	• Permission, Limited Information, Specific Suggestions, and Intensive Therapy (PLISSIT) framework	• Encourage physical touch if desired
Spirituality	• Assessment tools	• Maintaining spirituality is associated with positive outcomes
Elder abuse and mistreatment	• Elder Abuse Suspicion Index (EASI) • Poor hygiene • Bruises in varying stages of healing • Dehydration • Large sums of money missing • Withdrawal from family/friends	• Any suspected abuse to be reported • Older adults with cognitive impairment or functional impairment due to dependency are at high risk

Sources: References 19–26, 28–31, 33–36, 38–53.

plans.[28] There are a number of brief cognitive screening tools, such as the Montreal Cognitive Assessment (MoCA) and the Mini-Mental State Exam (MMSE).[29,30] Staging for dementia can be accomplished with tools such as the Dementia Rating System.[31] It is important to distinguish between cognitive impairment/dementia and delirium since these are often conflated. While dementia is characterized as a chronic and progressive condition, delirium is characterized by acute onset and fluctuating cognition. Tools such as the Confusion Assessment Method can be used to assess for delirium.[32] The palliative nurse's approach to the older adult with cognitive impairment should be focused on addressing functional care needs and providing anticipatory guidance and support to caregivers.[33]

Urinary/Fecal Incontinence

Urinary and/or fecal incontinence, which is defined as the involuntary loss of urine or stool, affects up to a quarter to a half of older adults and is especially common among those with serious illness.[34] Urinary and fecal incontinence can be assessed by asking the patient or caregiver if the older adult has had urinary or fecal incontinence that is bothersome enough that they would like to know how it could be treated. Since some patients may be either reluctant to disclose or may lack the ability to communicate (due to cognitive impairment), the nurse should also observe for odor and stains and demonstrate gentle concern if there are signs of incontinence that the older adult does not disclose. If incontinence is endorsed, a targeted history should assess for onset, duration, characteristics, and triggers. Interventions will vary depending on the type and severity of the incontinence, as well the patient's health status and goals of care. For example, a 65-year-old diagnosed with metastatic breast cancer with urinary stress incontinence during exercise may be a candidate for pelvic floor muscle exercises, while incontinence products and chux may be the most appropriate option for a 95-year-old male with advanced dementia who has urinary and fecal incontinence. Interventions such as a bedside commode and scheduled bathroom times can be helpful with functional incontinence and are often preferred to diapers and indwelling catheters by both patients and caregivers.[35] Overactive bladder, also seen in the medical literature as "OAB," is a condition in which the bladder muscle contracts suddenly, referred to as "detrusor overactivity," causing the bladder to release urine without warning.[36] Consequences of OAB include frequent daytime urination, nocturia, and incontinence; and it must be diagnosed in the absence of a urinary tract infection and other metabolic disorders.[36] Pharmacological management strategies include anticholinergic medications such as oxybutynin. Due to the deleterious side effects in older adults, it is likely best if these medications are avoided. Instead, interventions focusing on nonpharmacological management such as smoking cessation, bowel regulation, avoiding aggravating factors such as caffeine, and bladder retraining are recommended.[36]

Skin

Skin changes as people age: the epidermis thins, skin becomes dryer, sensory perception decreases, and subdermal fat is reduced. These changes can lead to increased vulnerability to skin tears, bruising, and pressure ulcers, particularly in patients who have severe mobility challenges and spend the majority of their day in a chair or bed.[37] Older adults should be assessed for risk factors for skin breakdown and infections, such as poor nutrition, immobility, incontinence, and diabetes. Validated tools such as the Braden Scale should be used to assess for pressure ulcer risk.[38] Comprehensive skin assessments should be conducted regularly. These assessments should include inspection of the skin over the entire body, paying special attention to pressure areas such as the sacrum and heels. Finger palpation can be used to determine if erythema or discoloration is blanchable.

Medications and Polypharmacy

Physiologic changes occur in the older adult that alter pharmacokinetics (how the body absorbs, metabolizes, and excretes medication). These changes include decreased water and lean body mass, increased body fat, decreased hepatic blood flow], decreased first pass metabolism, and decreased renal function. Pharmacodynamics (how the drug interacts with the body) also changes due to many factors causing increased or decreased receptor activity. "Polypharmacy" is the term used when a patient is prescribed more medications than medically necessary or five or more medications.[39] Polypharmacy can be tied to poor outcomes, including falls, hospitalizations, medication errors, adverse drug effects, and drug–drug interactions.[39] Routine and thorough medication reconciliation should be done with every care transition and each biannual appointment, paying special attention to polypharmacy and potentially inappropriate medications. The American Geriatrics Society Beers Criteria is an extensive list of medications that are often poorly tolerated in older adults.[40] The Screening Tool for Older Person's Prescriptions (STOPP)/Screening Tool to Alert to Right Treatment (START) tool can be used to help guide deprescribing in older adults.[41] Deprescribing in collaboration with a physician, nurse practitioner, or physician's associate is a key component of palliative care that nurses can use to improve quality of life for older adults with serious illness while simultaneously simplifying care regimens for caregivers. It is important to note, however, that some of the medications on the Beers Criteria or STOPP and START lists have appropriate uses for the older adult receiving palliative care and hospice.

Nutrition and Weight

Unintentional weight loss in older adults can be due to several causes and warrants a thorough history and medical workup. Issues contributing to weight loss include difficulty chewing and/or swallowing, medication-induced nausea and/or taste changes, financial constraints, and social isolation. The Mini-Nutritional Assessment (MNA) is a tool used to assess nutritional status.[42] Interventions include eliminating medications that may be causing symptoms, providing feeding assistance, offering appealing foods, and help with appropriate resources for food allocation. Appetite stimulants and supplemental drinks have not been found to be effective.[43] As the patient nears the end of life anorexia is expected; therefore, anticipatory guidance to family and the patient is necessary.

Hearing

Hearing loss is common among older adults and can impact the ability to have important discussions at the end of life, such as assessing goals of care and symptom needs. Hearing screens should be performed at regular intervals and interventions to address the issue implemented. Due to the expense of hearing aids, first steps may include personal amplifiers, face-to-face communication, adequate lighting to enable patients to see lip movements, and decreased background noise.[44]

Dentition

Dry mouth and dental carries are problematic for older adults with serious illness. These problems can impact quality of life by limiting certain food choices and hindering nutritional intake. Maintaining hydration and using a humidifier at night can help with dry mouth.[45] Pharmacological interventions include sialagogues. Nonpharmacological measures include mouth moisteners and salivary substitutes that can provide symptomatic relief and are available in mouth rinse/washes, gel, and spray.[46] Depending on the stage of the disease trajectory, dental visits may continue; and as the disease progresses, bedside oral health should be maintained.[47]

Advanced Care Planning

Advanced care planning (ACP) is an important and iterative process that should be frequently revisited at regular intervals and with changes in condition. Patients living with dementia should be encouraged to participate in this process early in their disease course as they may lose decisional capacity once the disease progresses. ACP discussions with the patient caregiver unit treatments can be framed around weighing the harms, burdens, benefits, and prognosis for each treatment. Gaining an understanding of the patient caregiver unit's perceptions of the illness trajectory and disease prognosis is vital.[48] Creating specific goals with the patient family unit that that are both important to the individual and measurable can be helpful. If the patient and caregiver unit are amenable, clear discussion of the expected decline and associated patterns are helpful for anticipatory guidance as the end of life nears. The Physician Orders for Life-Sustaining Treatment (POLST) or Medical Orders for Life-Sustaining Treatment (MOLST) are documents used to record the patient caregiver unit's treatment choices.

Social Support

Social assessments should cover who would care for the patient if/when the patient is unable to care for themselves. These discussions should occur early in the disease course as they can help the healthcare team to understand the patient's needs and be proactive with resources as their illness progresses. Both social isolation and loneliness are detrimental to the health of older adults. A commonly used tool to assess social isolation is the Lubben Social Network Scale (LSNS).[49] Interventions found to be effective to combat loneliness are videoconferencing interventions, humor therapy, mindfulness, pet therapy, and stress reduction.[50]

Informal Caregiving

Informal caregivers are individuals who provide unpaid assistance with ADLs and IADLs for a person with a chronic illness or disability. Informal caregivers, who are usually family members, can have higher levels of emotional, physical, and often financial stress.[51] Due to these negative effects, it is prudent for the medical team to screen informal caregivers for their mental health and help with resource allocation. The American Medical Association has developed a tool called the Caregiver Self-Assessment Questionnaire to assess for caregiver burnout and depression.[52] Several initiatives have been created, including The National Family Caregiver Support Program, to help informal caregivers with financial incentives and provide psychological services such as support groups. In addition, the Lifespan Respite Care Program was passed in 2006 to help with respite care services.

Sexuality

Sexuality remains an important but often overlooked part of life for older adults. Assessment can be performed using the Permission, Limited Information, Specific Suggestions, and Intensive Therapy (PLISSIT) framework.[53] There may be both physiologic and environmental constraints for older adults, making it harder for them to engage in desired sexual activity. Consent is of the utmost importance, particularly in older adults with cognitive impairment. While older adults with severe dementia cannot consent to sexual activity, consent may still be possible in people with mild cognitive dementia or early dementia. The ability to consent to sexual behaviors in individuals and couples should be assessed and discussed openly on an individual basis.[54] Clinicians should monitor for signs of sexual abuse and coercion in individuals without capacity to consent. Physical touch, such as holding hands, hugging, dancing, and caressing, should be encouraged, if desired.[55]

Spirituality

Spirituality in older adults is linked to positive outcomes including improved cognitive function for patients with dementia, improved psychological health, and a decrease in morbidity and mortality.[56] For more information about available tools, see Chapter 33.

Elder Abuse and Mistreatment

Elder abuse is a prevalent and underreported problem. There are six types of abuse: physical abuse, emotional abuse, neglect, abandonment, sexual abuse, and financial abuse. The Elder Abuse Suspicion Index (EASI) can be used to screen for abuse.[57] Signs of abuse include dehydration, poor hygiene, unexplained bruises or bruises in varying stages of healing, withdrawal from family members, and financial mismanagement. If abuse is suspected, this needs to be reported using the approved procedures of the nurses' healthcare organization or state.[58]

Financial Concerns

Asking older adults about their housing situation, food, and medication availability is important to maintain both quality of life and independence. Early recognition of a problem helps the healthcare team with resource allocation such as state or local benefits.

Geriatric Resources

Several geriatric resources exist to help the nurse specializing in geriatric palliative care. The End-of-life Nursing Education Consortium (ELNEC) created a curriculum tailored to the needs of the geriatric patient (https://www.aacnnursing.org/ELNEC/About/ELNEC-Curricula).[59] The Hartford Institute for Geriatric Nursing has online webinars and tutorials (https://hign.org/).

Case Study: Conclusion

It is 6 months later, and Mr. Wong underwent a renal biopsy, which showed widely metastatic disease in both kidneys. Ian and Mr. Wong decided to pursue aggressive treatment, given that he was happy with his current quality of life. He returns to clinic following a prolonged hospital admission for failure to thrive. He has lost 30 pounds, has poor appetite, and is in severe pain. Ian is with the patient and tells you he feels guilty as he does not feel his brother is enjoying his life. Mr. Wong has not been able to go to the local diner, and ambulation has become very difficult (he is now an assist ×2 with a walker). After his most recent hospitalization, many new medications were added to his current regimen. Ian states it is too much of a pill burden and that Mr. Wong seems sleepy most of the time. A medication reconciliation is performed, and Mr. Wong is found to be on 18 medications.

After a lengthy discussion with Ian, the team recommends stopping aggressive treatment given the rapid decline and lack of alignment with patient and family goals. The team places a referral to hospice. A POLST is completed to avoid further aggressive medical care and readmission to the hospital. All duplicative and nonessential medications are discontinued, and his total medication count is reduced to three.

This case illustrates the importance of patient-centered care, frequent assessments of the patient's goals of care, and evaluating the caregiving needs of the patient and burden and stress among caregivers.

REFERENCES

1. United Nations. *World Population Prospects 2019: Highlights.* United Nations; 2019.
2. US Census Bureau Population Division. Projected 5-Year Age Groups and Sex Composition: Main Projection Series for the United States, 2017–2060. Accessed August 31, 2022. https://www.census.gov/data/tables/2017/demo/popproj/2017-summary-tables.html.
3. Cubanski J, Koma W, Damico A, Neuman T. How Many Seniors Live in Poverty? Accessed August 31, 2022. https://www.kff.org/medicare/issue-brief/how-many-seniors-live-in-poverty/.
4. Heron M. Deaths: leading causes for 2017. *Natl Vital Stat Rep.* 2019;68(6):1–77.
5. Smith AK, Walter LC, Miao Y, Boscardin WJ, Covinsky KE. Disability during the last two years of life. *JAMA Intern Med.* 2013;173(16):1506–1513. https://doi.org/10.1001/jamainternmed.2013.8738.
6. Smith AK, Cenzer IS, Knight SJ, et al. The epidemiology of pain during the last 2 years of life. *Ann Intern Med.* 2010;153(9):563–569. https://doi.org/10.7326/0003-4819-153-9-201011020-00005.

7. Temel JS, Greer JA, Muzikansky A, et al. Early palliative care for patients with metastatic non-small-cell lung cancer. *N Engl J Med.* 2010;363(8):733–742. https://doi.org/10.1056/NEJMoa1000678.
8. Lunney JR, Lynn J, Hogan C. Profiles of older Medicare decedents. *J Am Geriatr Soc.* 2002;50(6):1108–1112.
9. Gill TM, Gahbauer EA, Han L, Allore HG. Trajectories of disability in the last year of life. *N Engl J Med.* 2010;362(13):1173–1180. https://doi.org/10.1056/NEJMoa0909087.
10. Barnato AE, Anthony DL, Skinner J, Gallagher PM, Fisher ES. Racial and ethnic differences in preferences for end-of-life treatment. *J Gen Intern Med.* 2009;24(6):695–701. https://doi.org/10.1007/s11606-009-0952-6.
11. Ornstein KA, Wolff JL, Bollens-Lund E, Rahman OK, Kelley AS. Spousal caregivers are caregiving alone in the last years of life. *Health Aff (Millwood).* 2019;38(6):964–972. https://doi.org/10.1377/hlthaff.2019.00087.
12. Mayan I, Yaffe K, James J, Hunt LJ. The association between race and place of death among persons with dementia. *J Pain Symptom Manage.* 2022;64(3):E109–E114. https://doi.org/10.1016/j.jpainsymman.2022.05.010.
13. Rogers M, Meier DE, Heitner R, et al. The National Palliative Care Registry: a decade of supporting growth and sustainability of palliative care programs. *J Palliat Med.* 2019;22(9):1026–1031. https://doi.org/10.1089/jpm.2019.0262.
14. Ankuda CK, Morrison RS, Aldridge MD. The 2021 Medicare Advantage hospice carve-in. *JAMA.* 2021;326(23):2367–2368. https://doi.org/10.1001/jama.2021.21161.
15. Inouye SK, Studenski S, Tinetti ME, Kuchel GA. Geriatric syndromes: clinical, research, and policy implications of a core geriatric concept. *J Am Geriatr Soc.* 2007;55(5):780–791. https://doi.org/10.1111/j.1532-5415.2007.01156.x.
16. Flacker JM. What is a geriatric syndrome anyway? *J Am Geriatr Soc.* 2003;51(4):574–576. https://doi.org/10.1046/j.1532-5415.2003.51174.x.
17. Fried LP, Tangen CM, Walston J, et al. Frailty in older adults: evidence for a phenotype. *J Gerontol A Biol Sci Med Sci.* 2001;56(3):M146–M157. https://doi.org/10.1093/gerona/56.3.m146.
18. Kapo J, Morrison LJ, Liao S. Palliative care for the older adult. *J Palliat Med.* 2007;10(1):185–209. https://doi.org/10.1089/jpm.2006.9989.
19. Parker SG, McCue P, Phelps K, et al. What is comprehensive geriatric assessment (CGA)? An umbrella review. *Age Ageing.* 2018;47(1):149–155. https://doi.org/10.1093/ageing/afx166.
20. Katz S. Assessing self-maintenance: activities of daily living, mobility, and instrumental activities of daily living. *J Am Geriatr Soc* 1983;31(12):721–727. https://doi.org/10.1111/j.1532-5415.1983.tb03391.x.
21. Graf C. The Lawton Instrumental Activities of Daily Living Scale. *Am J Nurs.* 2008;108(4):52–62; quiz 62–63. https://doi.org/10.1097/01.Naj.0000314810.46029.74.
22. Dautzenberg L, Beglinger S, Tsokani S, et al. Interventions for preventing falls and fall-related fractures in community-dwelling older adults: a systematic review and network meta-analysis. *J Am Geriatr Soc.* 2021;69(10):2973–2984. https://doi.org/10.1111/jgs.17375.
23. Welch SA, Ward RE, Beauchamp MK, Leveille SG, Travison T, Bean JF. The Short Physical Performance Battery (SPPB): a quick and useful tool for fall risk stratification among older primary care patients. *J Am Med Dir Assoc.* 2021;22(8):1646–1651. https://doi.org/10.1016/j.jamda.2020.09.038.
24. Ivziku D, Matarese M, Pedone C. Predictive validity of the Hendrich fall risk model II in an acute geriatric unit. *Int J Nurs Stud.* 2011;48(4):468–474. https://doi.org/10.1016/j.ijnurstu.2010.09.002.
25. Blazer DG. Depression in late life: review and commentary. *J Gerontol A Biol Sci Med Sci.* 2003;58(3):M249–M265. https://doi.org/10.1093/gerona/58.3.M249.
26. Yesavage JA, Brink TL, Rose TL, et al. Development and validation of a geriatric depression screening scale: a preliminary report. *J Psychiatr Res.* 1982;17(1):37–49. https://doi.org/10.1016/0022-3956(82)90033-4.
27. Cuijpers P, Reynolds CF III, Donker T, Li J, Andersson G, Beekman A. Personalized treatment of adult depression: medication, psychotherapy, or both? A systematic review. *Depress Anxiety.* 2012;29(10):855–864.
28. Irwin SA, Zurhellen CH, Diamond LC, et al. Unrecognised cognitive impairment in hospice patients: a pilot study. *Palliat Med.* 2008;22(7):842–847. https://doi.org/10.1177/0269216308096907.
29. Nasreddine ZS, Phillips NA, Bédirian V, et al. The Montreal Cognitive Assessment, MoCA: a brief screening tool for mild cognitive impairment. *J Am Geriatr Soc.* 2005;53(4):695–699.
30. Folstein MF, Folstein SE, McHugh PR. "Mini-mental state": a practical method for grading the cognitive state of patients for the clinician. *J Psychiatr Res.* 1975;12(3):189–198. https://doi.org/10.1016/0022-3956(75)90026-6.
31. Galvin JE. The Quick Dementia Rating System (QDRS): a rapid dementia staging tool. *Alzheimers Dement (Amst).* 2015;1(2):249–259. https://doi.org/10.1016/j.dadm.2015.03.003.
32. De J, Wand AP. Delirium screening: a systematic review of delirium screening tools in hospitalized patients. *Gerontologist.* 2015;55(6):1079–1099. https://doi.org/10.1093/geront/gnv100.
33. Harrison KL, Hunt LJ, Ritchie CS, Yaffe K. Dying with dementia: underrecognized and stigmatized. *J Am Geriatr Soc.* 2019;67(8):1548–1551. https://doi.org/10.1111/jgs.15895.
34. Campbell AJ, Reinken J, McCosh L. Incontinence in the elderly: prevalence and prognosis. *Age Ageing.* 1985;14(2):65–70. https://doi.org/10.1093/ageing/14.2.65.
35. Pfisterer MH, Johnson TM 2nd, Jenetzky E, Hauer K, Oster P. Geriatric patients' preferences for treatment of urinary incontinence: a study of hospitalized, cognitively competent adults aged 80 and older. *J Am Geriatr Soc.* 2007;55(12):2016–2022. https://doi.org/10.1111/j.1532-5415.2007.01457.x.
36. Leron E, Weintraub AY, Mastrolia SA, Schwarzman P. Overactive bladder syndrome: evaluation and management. *Curr Urol.* 2018;11(3):117–125. https://doi.org/10.1159/000447205.
37. Holloway S, Jones V. The importance of skin care and assessment. *Br J Nurs.* 2005;14(22):1172 1176. https://doi.org/10.12968/bjon.2005.14.22.20167.
38. Bergstrom N, Braden BJ, Laguzza A, Holman V. The Braden Scale for predicting pressure sore risk. *Nurs Res.* 1987;36(4):205–210.
39. Masnoon N, Shakib S, Kalisch-Ellett L, Caughey GE. What is polypharmacy? A systematic review of definitions. *BMC Geriatr.* 2017;17(1):230. https://doi.org/10.1186/s12877-017-0621-2.
40. 2023 American Geriatrics Society Beers Criteria® Update Expert Panel. American Geriatrics Society 2023 updated AGS Beers Criteria® for potentially inappropriate medication use in older adults. *J Am Geriatr Soc.* 2023;71(7):2052–2081. https://doi.org/10.1111/jgs.18372.
41. O'Mahony D, O'Sullivan D, Byrne S, O'Connor MN, Ryan C, Gallagher P. STOPP/START criteria for potentially inappropriate prescribing in older people: version 2. *Age Ageing.* 2014;44(2):213–218. https://doi.org/10.1093/ageing/afu145.

42. Guigoz Y, Vellas B, Garry PJ. Assessing the nutritional status of the elderly: the Mini Nutritional Assessment as part of the geriatric evaluation. *Nutr Rev*. 1996;54(1):S59.
43. Gaddey HL, Holder K. Unintentional weight loss in older adults. *Am Fam Physician*. 2014;89(9):718–722.
44. Wallhagen MI, Ritchie CS, Smith AK. Hearing loss: effect on hospice and palliative care through the eyes of practitioners. *J Pain Symptom Manage*. 2019;57(4):724–730. https://doi.org/10.1016/j.jpainsymman.2018.12.340.
45. Turner MD, Ship JA. Dry mouth and its effects on the oral health of elderly people. *J Am Dent Assoc*. 2007;138(suppl):15s–20s. https://doi.org/10.14219/jada.archive.2007.0358.
46. Anil S, Vellappally S, Hashem M, Preethanath RS, Patil S, Samaranayake LP. Xerostomia in geriatric patients: a burgeoning global concern. *J Investig Clin Dent*. 2016;7(1):5–12. https://doi.org/10.1111/jicd.12120.
47. Chen X, Kistler CE. Oral health care for older adults with serious illness: when and how? *J Am Geriatr Soc*. 2015;63(2):375–378. https://doi.org/10.1111/jgs.13240.
48. Boyd C, Smith CD, Masoudi FA, et al. Decision making for older adults with multiple chronic conditions: executive summary for the American Geriatrics Society guiding principles on the care of older adults with multimorbidity. *J Am Geriatr Soc*. 2019;67(4):665–673. https://doi.org/10.1111/jgs.15809.
49. Nicholson NR. A review of social isolation: an important but underassessed condition in older adults. *J Prim Prev*. 2012;33(2–3):137–52. https://doi.org/10.1007/s10935-012-0271-2.
50. Gardiner C, Geldenhuys G, Gott M. Interventions to reduce social isolation and loneliness among older people: an integrative review. *Health Soc Care Community*. 2018;26(2):147–157. https://doi.org/10.1111/hsc.12367.
51. Holt Clemmensen T, Hein Lauridsen H, Andersen-Ranberg K, Kaae Kristensen H. Informal carers' support needs when caring for a person with dementia—a scoping literature review. *Scand J Caring Sci*. 2021;35(3):685–700. https://doi.org/10.1111/scs.12898.
52. Epstein-Lubow G, Gaudiano BA, Hinckley M, Salloway S, Miller IW. Evidence for the validity of the American Medical Association's caregiver self-assessment questionnaire as a screening measure for depression. *J Am Geriatr Soc*. 2010;58(2):387–388.
53. Annon JS. The PLISSIT model: a proposed conceptual scheme for the behavioral treatment of sexual problems. *J Sex Educ Ther*. 1976;2(1):1–15. https://doi.org/10.1080/01614576.1976.11074483.
54. Director S. Dementia and concurrent consent to sexual relations. *Hastings Cent Rep*. 2023;53(3):37–45. https://doi.org/10.1002/hast.1489.
55. Morrissey Stahl K, Bower K, Seponski D, Lewis D, Farnham A, Cava Tadik Y. A practitioner's guide to end-of-life intimacy: suggestions for conceptualization and intervention in palliative care. *Omega (Westport)*. 2017;77:003022281769654. https://doi.org/10.1177/0030222817696540.
56. Agli O, Bailly N, Ferrand C. Spirituality and religion in older adults with dementia: a systematic review. *Int Psychogeriatr*. 2015;27(5):715–25. https://doi.org/10.1017/s1041610214001665.
57. Yaffe MJ, Wolfson C, Lithwick M, Weiss D. Development and validation of a tool to improve physician identification of elder abuse: the Elder Abuse Suspicion Index (EASI). *J Elder Abuse Negl*. 2008;20(3):276–300. https://doi.org/10.1080/08946560801973168.
58. van Houten ME, Vloet LCM, Pelgrim T, Reijnders UJL, Berben SAA. Types, characteristics and anatomic location of physical signs in elder abuse: a systematic review: awareness and recognition of injury patterns. *Eur Geriatr Med*. 2022;13(1):53–85. https://doi.org/10.1007/s41999-021-00550-z.
59. Kelly K, Thrane S, Virani R, Malloy P, Ferrell B. Expanding palliative care nursing education in California: the ELNEC Geriatric project. *Int J Palliat Nurs*. 2011;17(4):188–194. https://doi.org/10.12968/ijpn.2011.17.4.188.

72

Global Palliative Care in Low- and Middle-Income Countries

Virginia LeBaron, Thuý Ly Nguyễn, and Usha Thapa

Key Points

- The global landscape of palliative care is evolving rapidly as the world's population ages, more people are diagnosed with noncommunicable diseases, the world is confronted with new, emerging infections, and technology transforms communication and how information is disseminated.
- Quality palliative care is an urgent global need, particularly in low- and middle-income countries where the burden of disease is significant, but resources are often limited.
- Key factors that affect the development and delivery of palliative care in all countries include: (1) shifting demographic and epidemiologic trends; (2) cultural barriers; (3) disparities in access; (4) healthcare policy and payment models; (5) technological advances; and (6) workforce shortages.
- All nurses have a role to play in global palliative care, whether they live and practice in a resource-constrained setting, travel internationally to train and support colleagues, conduct research with global implications, or advocate to reduce disparities within their local community.

Global Palliative Care: An Urgent, Unmet Need

Changing demographics, epidemiological trends, technological advances, economic realities, and evolving cultural and societal norms all intersect to influence palliative care on a global scale. Worldwide, palliative care is growing, but too many countries still lack access even though palliative care and access to pain relief has been recognized as a fundamental human right.[1] In 2014, The World Health Assembly (WHA; the decision-making body of the World Health Organization [WHO], the health-focused branch of the United Nations) passed the landmark Palliative Care Resolution, which officially urged member states to integrate palliative care into their national healthcare systems.[2] Despite this, millions of people experience serious health-related suffering each year (approximately 60 million annually), but most never receive palliative care, especially if they live in a low- or middle-income country (LMIC).[3] The updated *Global Atlas of Palliative Care*[4] reveals that palliative care at the highest level of development is available for only 14% of the global population, the majority in high-resourced European countries (Figure 72.1).[5] Global health emergencies, such as the COVID-19 pandemic, have highlighted the urgent need for palliative care to be integrated within community partnerships in order to reach populations most in need.[6] As the largest frontline workforce, nurses are in a key, and often untapped, strategic position to lead and influence the quality of global palliative care delivery.[7,8]

This chapter recognizes that palliative care is a critical issue for all countries but takes a particular look at palliative care in LMICs—where the greatest burden of disease often coexists with severely constrained health resources and where the need for quality palliative care is arguably the most urgent. An important note regarding terminology: depending on the country, palliative care and hospice can have variable meanings and be operationalized differently. For example, in the United States, the word "hospice" typically refers to a very specific package of healthcare services for patients with a life expectancy of 6 months or less. In other countries, the terms "hospice" and "palliative care" may be used synonymously, or "hospice" may refer to a specific building or location where dying patients receive care. When engaging in global palliative care efforts, it is important to clearly understand how palliative care and hospice are conceptualized and operationalized in a specific practice setting or country. For simplicity, in this chapter, we use the term "palliative care" in its broadest sense to encompass holistic care provided to patients (and their caregivers) with serious illness that has comfort and symptom control as the primary goal.

Key Factors That Influence the Global Delivery of Palliative Care

We propose six key factors that affect the development and delivery of palliative care programs and services in every country, regardless of resources or income: (1) shifting demographic and epidemiologic trends; (2) cultural barriers; (3) disparities in access; (4) healthcare policy and payment models; (5) technological advances; and (6) workforce shortages.

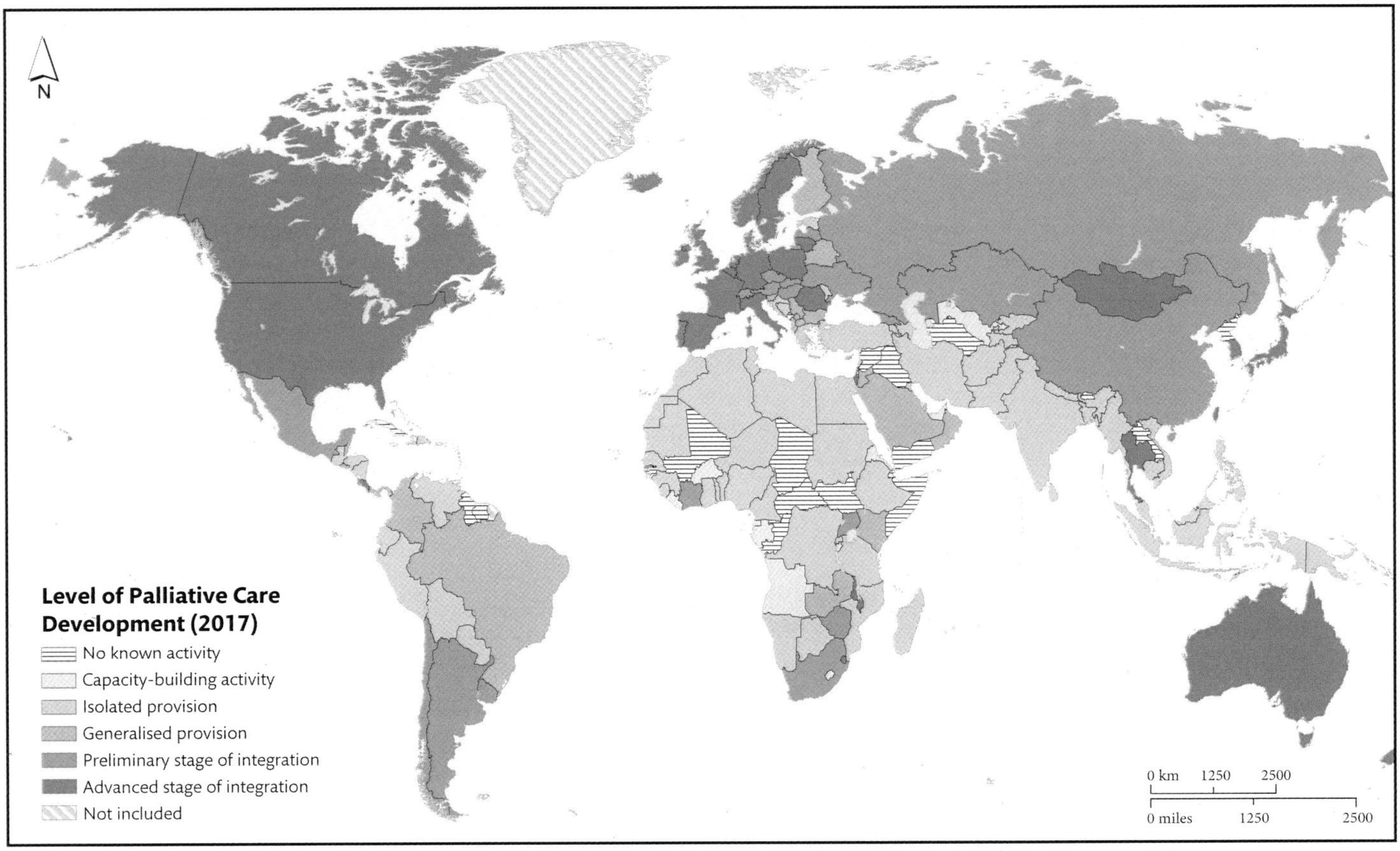

Figure 72.1 Levels of global palliative care development, 2017.
Source: Reference 5.

The first key theme is *shifting demographic and epidemiologic trends* leading to an increased need for palliative care globally. The proportion of older people is growing rapidly. By 2050, the world's population aged 60 years and older is expected to reach 2.1 billion, with two-thirds in LMICs.[9] Additionally, by 2060, an estimated 48 million people will die every year, with 83% of these deaths occurring in LMICs.[10] Relatedly, the number of people diagnosed with noncommunicable diseases (NCDs), such as cardiovascular disease and cancer, is also exploding.[11,12] In fact, prior to the coronavirus disease (COVID-19) pandemic, 68.9% (36.5 million people) of those with palliative care needs among adults were diagnosed with NCDs, such as cardiovascular diseases, cancer, and respiratory diseases.[13] These demographic and epidemiologic realities have serious implications for global health and palliative care as more people around the world live longer with chronic illness and reach the end of their lives in the coming decades.

Second, there are *cultural barriers* that hinder the development or acceptance of palliative care (see Chapter 28, "Cultural Considerations in Palliative Care"). In many countries and cultures, patients are not told their diagnosis or prognosis for fear it will cause despair and hasten death.[14] Additionally, healthcare systems and providers often emphasize "cure" without meaningful discussions regarding goals of care or quality of life. Consequently, even if palliative care services are available, they may not be initiated until the patient's last few weeks of life, if at all. For this to change, there must be a cultural shift from advocating 'cure-at-all-costs' over comfort, greater emphasis on managing chronic illness, effective conversations about the realistic benefits and burdens of treatment, honest dialogue about prognosis, and recognition that death is an inevitable part of life.

Third, there are significant and disturbing *inequities and disparities in access to palliative care*. The vast majority of adults (approximately 80%) in need of palliative care live in LMICs; however, palliative care continues to be underdeveloped in most of the world outside North America, Western Europe, and Australia[4]; and this persistent inequity is projected to worsen.[10] If palliative care services do exist in LMICs, they often focus on the needs of cancer patients and may exclude patients with other chronic diseases or conditions such as congestive heart failure, chronic obstructive pulmonary disease, HIV/AIDS, dementia, or neurodegenerative diseases. Even in countries where palliative care is more established, patients from minoritized racial and ethnic groups and lower socioeconomic status still struggle to obtain care, and palliative care services may be especially difficult to obtain for rural populations, neonatal or pediatric patients, individuals with mental health or substance use disorders, or incarcerated, homeless, LGBTQ+, and Indigenous peoples.[10,15]

A fourth theme affecting global palliative care development and delivery is *a country's healthcare policy and payment models*. According to the WHA, palliative care must be an essential service in a health system and part of universal health coverage of member states. A 2018 Lancet Commission report describes specific components and funding strategies for an "Essential Package" of palliative care services and urges all countries to ensure universal access by

2030.[3] In reality, only a small fraction of the world's population has advanced levels of palliative care integration into health services; almost all are in high-income countries (HIC). When the government does not provide palliative care services, nongovernmental organizations such as religious institutions and philanthropic organizations often fill the void. While these groups provide momentum for the development of palliative care programs, national health systems must include palliative care as an essential service for patients with serious or life-threatening conditions in order to ensure sustainability.[16]

Fifth, *technological advances, such as digital health* (broadly interpreted to mean health-related communications and interventions delivered via mobile technology), continue to transform the delivery of palliative care. With the necessity of physical distancing and increased end-of-life care needs highlighted by the COVID-19 pandemic, the relevance and utility of digital health in palliative care has become even more evident. Digital health technology can be used in palliative care for education, symptom management, information-sharing, point-of-care clinical decision-making, and to support virtual interactions with healthcare practitioners.[17] However, digital health equity is a significant challenge in the context of social and structural disadvantages such as lack of internet/broadband access, limited health and technology literacy, and inefficient infrastructure and must be addressed if the full benefits of digital health technologies are to be achieved.[18]

Finally, perhaps the greatest obstacle to widespread implementation of palliative care services is the *shortage of staff trained to provide this care*. A basic working knowledge of palliative care that includes exposure to clinical research and evidence-based practice is needed by all generalist healthcare providers (HCPs) and should be integrated within baccalaureate curricula for all nurses. Advanced (or specialized) palliative care skills are needed for HCPs who see a large number of patients with palliative care needs or who work in specialized palliative care settings and who train others. The attainment of basic/primary palliative care knowledge and skills can be accomplished through mandatory inclusion of palliative care in medical and nursing curricula and through continuing education programs for practicing HCPs. Programs to provide HCPs with advanced/specialist palliative care skills can be developed once basic palliative care training is established and as country or program demand requires; in many LMICs nurses are the only frontline HCPs available to deliver palliative care[19] (see Case Studies 1 and 2 for examples).

Palliative care training must be adapted to the specific care context and consider available personnel and resources. HCPs in LMICs may include traditional healers, community volunteers, or community health workers. It is vital that palliative care educational initiatives include these individuals as they may be the first, or only, HCP with whom a patient interacts. For example, CHWs in rural areas can be trained in basic palliative care skills to help identify patients in need of specialist palliative care services and then facilitate subsequent referrals. It is critical to remember that in many settings, including most LMICs, the vast majority of patients requiring palliative care are supported by family and friends who usually have not been adequately prepared for such roles. This makes palliative care training to enhance basic capacities for essential symptom management among informal caregivers and the community an urgent and ongoing priority.

Many small countries and LMICs cannot afford a specialized palliative care workforce, and specialty training for nurses may not exist. Barriers to training for nurses can include a lack of qualified trainers, limited recognition or incentive in terms of salary or status for nurses who obtain specialization, a shortage of current and relevant print resources on palliative care, erratic or absent internet access which limits the utility of web-based palliative care training resources, and training that is offered to government/public sector nurses without equal attention to the majority of LMIC nurses who work in private hospitals/institutions. Another key reality is the challenge of palliative care workforce burnout, compassion fatigue, and/or moral distress, all of which can result in compromised patient care and staff attrition.[20,21] Palliative care training programs and institutions should have systems in place to provide emotional support to nurses and other palliative care providers, especially in highly resource-constrained practice settings.

Palliative care workforce training barriers are being addressed, in part, by global initiatives such as the End-of-Life Nursing Education Consortium Training Program (ELNEC-International) and the WHO Collaborating Centers for Palliative Care. ELNEC-International is a structured palliative care curriculum that includes content related to nursing care at the end of life; pain and symptom management; ethical and legal issues; cultural and spiritual considerations; communication; loss, grief, and bereavement; and the final hour/days of life. To date, over 48,000 nurses and other healthcare professionals, representing all 50 United States, plus 115 countries, have completed an ELNEC train-the trainer course.[22] WHO Collaborating Centers are designated by the WHO Director-General to carry out activities in support of WHO programs. There are currently five WHO Collaborating Centers for Palliative Care[23], including one nursing program, the Catholic University of Korea, College of Nursing. These programs are critical to ensure palliative care training for the global heath workforce, especially in LMICs, that can effectively address future palliative care challenges such as greater utilization of digital healthcare, promoting shared decision making between patients and clinicians, and responding to policy and legislative changes.[24]

Case Study 1: Prognosis Disclosure and Honoring End-of-Life Wishes in Vietnam

Lan is a 70-year-old woman in Vietnam with cardiovascular disease and lung cancer, which is no longer responding to curative treatment. When she was in a better state of health, Lan joined the senior club where she could interact with her peers and engage in social activities. She was living with her first son (including his wife and children). Her son decided not to tell his mother about her diagnosis and insisted she continue with aggressive treatment, even though Lan continued to ask her nurse questions about her condition and voiced her concern that she may be dying. The nurse communicated with the primary physician about Lan's wish to be aware of her diagnosis and resume some activities with her family and her friends from the senior club. The care team discussed this with Lan's son, who ultimately agreed Lan should understand her prognosis. Lan's family and primary physician discussed goals of care, clarified Lan's wishes, and reset the goals of care as her needs changed. During the discharge, nurses gave instructions to Lan's family on basic skills to take care of her including mobilizing and engaging in physical therapy to improve strength and reduce infection risk, and educating on pain management including opioid use and nonpharmacological approaches, breathing techniques, and using a portable oxygen concentrator. A palliative care booklet of caring for a person at home was also given to the family members with the physician's and nurse's phone numbers for direct contact if needed. After discharge, a home care nurse from a palliative care program run by a local hospital visited her regularly to check Lan's vital signs and symptoms and routinely facilitate the telehealth consultations with Lan's primary physician to revise essential medications. During the home visits, the nurse identified Lan's evolving needs, provided counseling, and trained family members for adjustment to her illness. With ongoing involvement of the palliative care team and the family's care, Lan's pain, dyspnea, and anxiety improved; and she could receive her peers from the senior club when they visited her at home. The palliative care education for her family helped her control symptoms at home and spend quality time with her family and friends thus, meeting the needs that she voiced and honoring her wishes.

Case Study 2: An Example of a Nurse-Led Outpatient Palliative Care Clinic in Nepal

The nurses' roles in palliative care is expanding from direct, inpatient care to running outpatient palliative care clinics. In Nepal, nurses play a critical role in leading palliative care clinics, especially in central and referral cancer hospitals. The palliative care clinics operate all working days as other outpatient departments of the hospital, and patients are referred from other outpatient departments and inpatient units for pain and symptom management. Sometimes patients are directly referred from other nearby hospitals. The clinic is jointly run by palliative physicians and nurses, and specially trained palliative care nurses are assigned to run the clinic. Duties and responsibilities of nurses include: (1) assessment of pain and discussion with the physician about medicine including opioids (after getting morphine from the hospital pharmacy, the nurse will teach the patient and family how to take morphine at home regarding doses and time of taking the regular and breakthrough dose, side effects, and the need for laxatives); (2) provide support and counseling to the patient as well as to the family to cope with the illness; (3) counseling to patient and family regarding the need for admission in hospice for end-of-life care and symptom management, especially for pain, breathlessness, wound care, and nutritional management (nurses also need to explain about services available in the palliative care unit because in Nepal people believe that palliative care is provided only for dying patients, so the family are often reluctant to admit their loved ones to the hospice and palliative care unit); (4) plan and make appointments for home visits/ bereavement care for those patients who are discharged from the hospice/ palliative unit or pass away; and (5) involvement in consultation services in other inpatient departments of the hospital as members of the interdisciplinary team.

Key Factors That Influence Palliative Care Implementation: Specific Challenges in LMICs

Despite the need, palliative care has only recently been recognized as a public health priority in many countries. Palliative care development using a public health framework includes key elements, such as: (1) appropriate government policies and plans; (2) availability of essential medicines; (3) education of HCPs, policymakers, and civil society; and (4) implementation of palliative care at all levels of healthcare provision. Many LMICs face challenges in each of these areas.

Appropriate government policies and plans. The provision of quality palliative care is facilitated by healthcare policies and guidelines that provide a roadmap for the development and implementation of services.[16] Few LMICs have integrated palliative care into public healthcare policy, strategic health plans, NCD plans, and/or cancer control plans. Government progress in addressing the palliative care needs of its citizens is often hampered by leadership changes within the ministries of health and a lack of champions able to advocate for palliative care as a healthcare priority. Another challenge is the lack of national health insurance plans in many LMICs (and in some HICs, such as the United States). If a plan exists, it rarely includes coverage for palliative care services.

Availability of essential medicines. National policy also affects the availability of essential medicines that are critical for palliative care. Essential medicines are defined by the WHO as medications that every country should have in adequate supply at all times, at a reasonable cost, to meet the needs of the population.[25] In 2007, the International Association for Hospice and Palliative Care, working in collaboration with other international stakeholder organizations, developed a list of essential medicines for palliative care.[26–28] Opioids are classified as essential medicines, but worldwide, 83% of countries have low or nonexistent access to opioids for pain relief.[29] In fact, more than 90% of the world's medicinal morphine supply is used by approximately 1% of the world's wealthiest countries.[3,30,31] As a result, millions suffer and die in agony without access to basic pain relief (Figure 72.2). The reasons for this are complicated but involve a combination of restrictive regulations and bureaucracy, lack of supply (further exacerbated by serious supply-chain issues during emergencies, such as the COVID-19 pandemic[32]), inefficient or erratic distribution and dispensing systems, limitations on prescribers, inflated medication costs, unavailability of oral opioid formulations, and general opioid fears among HCPs and the lay public, fueled in part by the 'opioid epidemic' in the United States which has had a disproportionate impact on international opioid policy.[29] A balanced approach to opioids is recommended to ensure that risks are mitigated while also ensuring access for those with legitimate medical need.[33] Palliative care associations must advocate with their respective ministries of health and national authorities to ensure they are aware of the recommended essential medicines and maintain sufficient buffer stocks using simplified control procedures.

Education of civil society. Countries need HCPs knowledgeable in palliative care to deliver services to citizens and to educate policymakers about the benefits of palliative care and advocate for inclusion of palliative care into health policies. Raising awareness among the lay public is also necessary to overcome stigma and misconceptions about palliative care and to create a demand for services that, in turn, will drive development of palliative care programs and favorable healthcare policies.

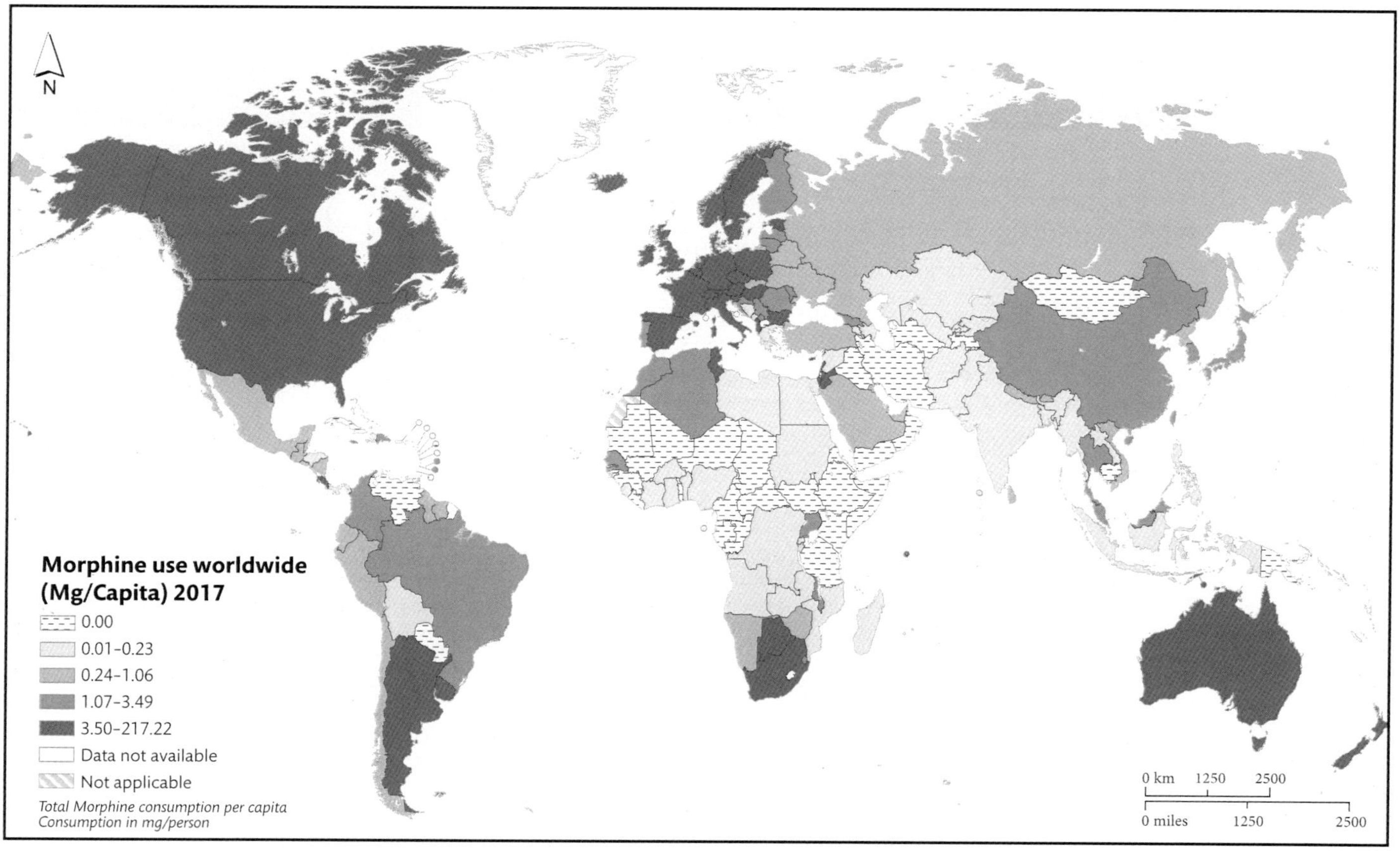

Figure 72.2 Morphine use worldwide.
Source: Reference 4.

Delivery of palliative care at all levels of healthcare provision. Countries organize health services, including palliative care, at the national, provincial/state, or district level; however, there can be wide variability in what is provided, especially at the provincial or district level. In an effort to help standardize service delivery, recommended basic packages of palliative care services have been proposed, offering cost-effective solutions to reduce patient and family suffering.[3] It is critical that palliative care services, regardless of service delivery level, are culturally and contextually congruent. In other words, effective palliative care services must be sensitive to a country's or region's societal and cultural norms; religious and spiritual practices; beliefs regarding illness, disease, and death; and expectations related to patient–family and patient–HCP communication, especially regarding disclosure of diagnosis, discussion of prognosis, and delivering difficult news. Local resources, such as the availability of essential medicines, must also be taken into account. In rural areas or in countries beginning to develop palliative care services, community-based delivery models may be more suitable and easier to implement than hospital-based models.

Implementing Evidence-Based Palliative Care Practices

The highest-quality palliative care is informed by evidence and regularly evaluated. This requires palliative care nurses to take an active role in establishing evidence-based standards and competencies to support their practice and document the impact of their work.[34] However, generating evidence and evaluating outcomes, especially in resource-constrained settings, can be hindered by a lack of trained researchers and mentors, scarce funding and resources, the inherent difficulties of conducting research with acutely ill and dying patients, lack of consensus regarding what "counts" as evidence, unpredictable infrastructure, and inadequate documentation. It is crucial that evidence used to guide palliative care practice is contextual and resource-relevant, such as when including traditional or complementary approaches to palliative care that are utilized in many LMICs. In essence, what works or is needed in an HIC, such as detailed protocols for opioid rotations or withdrawal from ventilator support, may not be feasible or helpful in an LMIC. One example of an organization actively working to develop palliative care evidence specific to its region and context is the African Palliative Care Research Network (Table 72.1).

Specific Challenges Faced by Palliative Care Nurses in LMICs

Role expectations and the status of nurses vary tremendously worldwide. In some countries, palliative care nurses independently care for patients, prescribe opioids, and are viewed as critical members of a collaborative, interdisciplinary team. In other countries, nursing is a low-status position, and nurses are expected to take a passive role in patient management and are criticized or disciplined for questioning physician orders. This can be especially problematic in palliative care as care delivery is seriously compromised if nurses

Table 72.1 Examples of international and regional palliative care organizations and key activities

World Health Organization region/country	Organization	Description*	Activity Highlights
International	International Association for Hospice and Palliative Care (IAHPC)	IAHPC serves as a global platform to inspire, inform, and empower individuals, governments, and organizations to increase access and optimize the practice of palliative care. IAHPC works with United Nations agencies, governments, associations, and individuals to increase access to essential medicines for palliative care; foster opportunities in palliative care education, research, and training; and increase service provision around the globe. https://hospicecare.com/home/	Maintains a global directory of palliative care services, hospices, and organizations as well as a global directory of educational programs in palliative care. Offers financial assistance to palliative care professionals to attend events that will enable them to improve palliative care in their settings; preference given to applicants living in low- or middle-income countries.
International	International Children's Palliative Care Association (ICPCA)	ICPCA seeks to achieve the best quality of life and care for children and young people with life-limiting conditions, their families, and caregivers worldwide by raising awareness of children's palliative care, lobbying for the global development of children's palliative care services, and sharing expertise, skills, and knowledge. http://www.icpcn.org/	Offers multiple resources related to pediatric palliative care services and organizations, as well as resources and information for clinicians.
International	Worldwide Hospice Palliative Care Association (WHPCA)	WHPCA is a network of national and regional hospice and palliative care organizations and affiliate organizations that focuses on hospice and palliative care development worldwide. http://www.thewhpca.org/	Offers a palliative care toolkit for implementation in low-resource settings. Publishes the *Global Atlas of Palliative Care*, which provides a comprehensive summary of palliative care development and progress globally.
African region	African Palliative Care Association (APCA)	A pan-African organization ensuring that palliative care is widely understood, integrated into health systems at all levels, and underpinned by evidence in order to reduce pain and suffering across Africa. https://www.africanpalliativecare.org/	Developed the *APCA Atlas of Palliative Care in Africa*, quality standards, a core curriculum, a framework of core competencies, and an advocacy toolkit for palliative care in Africa.
Region of the Americas: Latin America and the Caribbean	Caribbean Palliative Care Association (CARIPALCA)	This organization with both health professional and civil society membership advocates on behalf of the region and individual countries in terms of education, capacity building, research, access to medicines, linkages to other regional and international bodies, and sharing of policy initiatives. https://www.caripalca.org/	Offers a variety of palliative care educational resources, including a tele-mentoring platform (ECHO) that connects interdisciplinary providers in the Caribbean with palliative care specialists.
Region of the Americas: Latin America and the Caribbean	Asociacion Latinoamericana de Cuidados Paliativos (ALCP) (Latin American Association for Palliative Care)	A nongovernmental organization for the development and advancement of palliative care in Latin America that unites people who work in palliative care or are interested in palliative care. http://cuidadospaliativos.org/	Provides palliative care information and resources in Spanish. This organization headed the development of *The Atlas of Palliative Care in Latin America* in cooperation with IAHPC.
Region of the Americas: Northern America, Canada	Canadian Hospice Palliative Care Association (CHPCA) (Association Canadienne do Soins Palliatifs)	CHPCA is the national leader in the pursuit of quality hospice palliative care in Canada through public policy, education, knowledge translation, awareness, and collaboration. http://www.chpca.net/	Provides a national directory of palliative care programs and services across Canada, as well as a repository of useful palliative care resources for healthcare providers, caregivers, volunteers, patients, researchers, and policymakers.
Region of the Americas: Northern America, United States	American Academy of Hospice and Palliative Medicine (AAHPM) Hospice and Palliative Care Nurses Association (HPNA) National Hospice and Palliative Care Organization (NHPCO)	Professional organization for physicians and other healthcare providers specializing in hospice and palliative care dedicated to advancing hospice and palliative medicine and improving the care of patients with serious illness. www.aahpm.org Professional palliative care organization with a focus on supporting hospice and palliative care nurses. https://advancingexpertcare.org/ NHPCO is a membership organization for providers and professionals who care for people affected by serious and life-limiting illness. NHPCO represents the interests of its members and the general public with legislative advocacy that helps to enhance and expand access to care that addresses holistic health and the well-being of communities. https://www.nhpco.org/	AAHPM activities focus on education and training, resources, networking, and advocacy. AAHPM and HPNA jointly hold an annual, interdisciplinary meeting. HPNA offers a large number of educational, leadership, and research resources, including opportunities for specialty nursing certification in palliative care. NHPCO offers a large number of educational and regulatory resources, some of which are for members only.
Southeast Asia Region: India	Indian Association of Palliative Care (IAPC)	Established in consultation with the World Health Organization and the government of India as a national forum to connect, support, and motivate individuals and institutions involved in palliative care. http://palliativecare.in/	Offers many certificate training programs, including one for nurses in essentials of palliative care. IAPC has been involved in many advocacy projects, including those to improve opioid availability and ensure ethical and legal standards in end-of-life care.

Table 72.1 Continued

World Health Organization region/country	Organization	Description*	Activity Highlights
European region	European Association for Palliative Care (EAPC)	A membership organization dedicated to the promotion and development of palliative care throughout Europe. https://eapcnet.eu/about-us/	Maintains a directory of national palliative care guidelines in Europe by country, as well as a directory of reference group and task force experts for palliative care–related practice and research topics and EU-funded palliative care research projects.
Eastern Mediterranean: Lebanon	Lebanese Centre for Palliative Care—Balsam	Lebanese Centre for Palliative Care—Balsam is a nongovernmental organization working in palliative care development in Lebanon and across the region through patient care, advocacy, training, capacity building, and research. http://www.balsam-lb.org/index.php	Developed the *Atlas of Palliative Care in the Eastern Mediterranean Region* in collaboration with the ATLANTES Research Program.
Western Pacific region	Asia Pacific Hospice Palliative Care Network (APHPCN)	APHPCN is dedicated to promoting hospice and palliative care in Asia and the Pacific. APHPCN promotes education and skills development, enhances awareness and communication, and fosters research and collaboration to encourage established programs to assist less experienced and more isolated colleagues. http://aphn.org/	APHPCN and the Lien Foundation (Singapore) co-developed the *Lien Collaborative for Palliative Care* to enhance palliative care leadership and capacity in developing countries.
Western Pacific region: Australia	Palliative Care Australia	Palliative Care Australia is the national body for palliative care and represents all those who work toward high-quality palliative care for all Australians. Works closely with consumers, member organizations, and the palliative care workforce to improve access to, and promote the need for, palliative care. http://palliativecare.org.au/	Offers a variety of palliative care resources, including those specifically tailored to Indigenous and multicultural communities.
Western Pacific region: China	Committee of Rehabilitation and Palliative Care of China Anti-cancer Association (CRPC)	The CRPC has been the national voice for hospice palliative care in China and works to support research, promote education and training, and improve public awareness. http://www.caca.org.cn/english/	CRPC has helped support a national program to establish pilot units for standard management for cancer patients with pain in general and specialized hospitals. Also, has led advocacy efforts to improve access to essential pain medicines and expand access to community-based hospice care.
Western Pacific region: New Zealand	Hospice New Zealand	Hospice New Zealand exists to lead and support the hospice movement in New Zealand, working to ensure equality of access and consistent delivery of palliative and end-of-life care for New Zealanders. http://www.hospice.org.nz/about-hospice-nz	Offers educational and leadership opportunities and general resources, including the Māori Palliative Care Framework for Hospices.

* *Note*: Descriptions are restatements or brief summaries of mission and/or vision statements from the organization's website.

are not taught, expected, or encouraged to advocate for quality symptom management. Similarly, professional development and advanced practice opportunities for nurses in LMICs may be limited or nonexistent. Another key challenge is that nurses in LMICs are often assigned in a frequent rotating fashion to a variety of units and wards, making it difficult to develop specialization and practice expertise related to palliative care.

Another key challenge faced by nurses who provide palliative care in LMICs involves the reality of *limited material resources and supplies*. Government/public hospitals, where the majority of the LMIC population typically seeks care, are seriously overcrowded and underresourced. Basic supplies, infrastructure (e.g., running water or electricity), essential medicines (such as opioids), and personal protective equipment may be erratically available or completely absent. Patients typically present with late-stage disease and a very high symptom burden. For example, managing large malignant wounds and extensive lymphedema is especially relevant for palliative care nurses in LMICs but often complicated by limited resources and training.[35]

Nurses in LMICs often face the additional challenge of caring for seriously ill patients in unstable situations. For example, nurses in LMICs may find themselves providing palliative care in high-conflict settings/war zones, after devastating natural disasters, with disrupted transportation or communication infrastructure, or in the context of rapidly emerging infectious epidemics and pandemics (e.g., Ebola, COVID-19). Each of these issues presents profound challenges and stressors for the palliative care nurse that must be acknowledged, anticipated, and managed at a systems level to ensure feasible delivery of palliative care services and protection of nurses.

Global and Regional Palliative Care Initiatives

The internet and mobile technology are rapidly changing the way HCPs communicate and collaborate across the globe. Palliative care providers practicing in isolated settings, or novice providers with questions, now have access to a host of resources and support, assuming they have reliable internet service (which, of course, is not always the case). A few examples of excellent, globally focused electronic palliative care resources include E-Hospice, Palliative Care Network, and Palliverse. E-Hospice (https://ehospice.com/) is a global news and information resource for those with a professional or personal interest in palliative care. Palliative Care Network (https://www.palliativecarenetwork.com/) and Palliverse (https://palliverse.com/) are interactive websites that provide opportunities to facilitate the global exchange of knowledge and ideas related to palliative care, promote collaboration among palliative care professionals, and disseminate funding opportunities.

International and regional palliative care organizations also play an important role globally by working to raise the profile of palliative care and ensure palliative care is reflected in international or regional priorities. Most of these organizations do not provide direct patient care services; instead, they focus on advancing palliative care policies, education and training, advocacy, leadership, and research. Excellent initiatives and programs have been undertaken by numerous and varied regional champions, institutions, and organizations to improve the global delivery of palliative care. It is beyond the scope of this chapter to discuss individual programs and initiatives, which are in a constant state of dynamic and rapid evolution. Instead, key international and regional palliative care umbrella organizations, summarized by WHO regions, can be found in Table 72.1; interested readers are encouraged to explore the links for the most up-to-date detailed information and activities.

Nursing's Role in Global Palliative Care

All nurses have a role to play in global palliative care, whether they live and practice in an LMIC, periodically travel internationally to train and support colleagues, conduct research, or advocate to reduce disparities within their local community.[7,36] Now, more than ever, palliative care nursing is truly a "glocal" endeavor, meaning that global issues are also local issues; and universal considerations such as access to pain relief and workforce education are interconnected and can inform each other. For example, learning about strategies to successfully deliver rural palliative care in one country can help inform effective interventions to expand palliative care services in another. This section discusses ways that all palliative care nurses can engage "glocally."

Training and Curriculum Development

The need for a nursing workforce well-versed in palliative care is paramount. At both the basic/primary level and the specialty level, nurses with palliative care and educational experience are often tapped to design and implement training programs. In many countries, palliative care education is heavily physician-/medically oriented; nurses play an essential role by creating or adapting existing curricula to ensure relevance for nursing. The most effective palliative care nursing curricula (1) are attuned to the contextual and cultural realities of practice, (2) take into account available resources and the role expectations of nurses (which can vary widely across the globe), (3) are vetted by on-the-ground clinicians most familiar with the practice environment, and (4) have a plan to evaluate the impact of the training on clinical practice.

Policy and Advocacy

Whether at a family or neighborhood gathering, through membership in a regional organization, or by testifying before a national legislative body, all nurses can advocate for palliative care and its crucial role within healthcare systems and institutions. Nurses contribute significantly to the advancement of palliative care each and every time they take the opportunity to dispel myths and misconceptions, advocate for its importance in policy documents (such as pain management prescribing guidelines), and accept leadership positions where they have a seat at the table to be a strong voice on behalf of palliative care and the role of the nurse.

Cultural Exchange and Mentorship

There are numerous opportunities for nurses to engage with palliative care providers from different countries and cultures. Traditionally, this has most often involved nurses from HICs traveling to LMICs to engage in educational or clinical practice development programs or by partnering or "twinning" an HIC organization with an organization in another (typically LMIC) country. These experiences offer unique and potentially powerful opportunities to learn from each other, share information and strategies, and provide essential role-modeling and nurse mentorship. There is a growing awareness of the importance of the bidirectional aspect of nursing cultural exchange programs and of thoughtful participation to ensure that efforts and initiatives are optimally and mutually beneficial.[37–39]

Advocating for Disproportionately Impacted Populations

All nurses ideally advocate for vulnerable populations and strive to ensure equitable access to quality healthcare for all people. Perhaps nowhere is the nurse's role in advocating for vulnerable populations more vital than with patients who are seriously ill and dying. Regardless of whether nurses practice as clinicians, managers/administrators, educators, or researchers, there are many ways to alleviate suffering experienced by the most vulnerable. For example, nurses can deliver compassionate end-of-life care to populations typically unseen in healthcare systems, such as those coping with housing insecurity; design educational programs that include substantive content about disparities in access to palliative care and pain relief; or conduct research that aims to improve the care of seriously ill patients and their caregivers at a policy and systems level.

Conclusion

The global landscape of palliative care is evolving rapidly as the world's population ages, more people are diagnosed with NCDs, and technology transforms communication and how information is disseminated. The development of palliative care and the role of palliative care nursing, particularly in LMICs, have made significant progress in the past decade; but there is still much to be done. Too many people, especially those who are the most socially, economically, and geographically vulnerable, continue to suffer and die without access to basic palliative care services and pain relief. Continued progress will require demand from the public, advocacy from HCPs, and the political will of national governments and the global health community. Most importantly, all nurses, regardless of role or geographic location, must recognize and leverage the critical role they play in influencing palliative care on a global scale. Health system strengthening *now* is essential to ensure we can meet the rapidly approaching future needs for quality global palliative care.

REFERENCES

1. Human Rights Watch. Global State of Pain Treatment: Access to Palliative Care as a Human Right. 2011. https://www.hrw.org/report/2011/06/02/global-state-pain-treatment/access-medicines-and-palliative-care.
2. World Health Assembly. Palliative Care Resolution. 2014. https://apps.who.int/gb/ebwha/pdf_files/WHA67/A67_R19-en.pdf?ua=1.

3. Knaul FM, Farmer PE, Krakauer EL, et al. Alleviating the access abyss in palliative care and pain relief—an imperative of universal health coverage: the Lancet Commission report. *Lancet*. 2018;391(10128):1391–1454.
4. Connor S. *Global Atlas of Palliative Care*, 2nd ed. Worldwide Hospice Palliative Care Alliance; 2020. Accessed June 27, 2022. http://www.thewhpca.org/resources/global-atlas-on-end-of-life-care.
5. Clark D, Baur N, Clelland D, et al. Mapping levels of palliative care development in 198 countries: the situation in 2017. *J Pain Symptom Manage*. 2020;59(4):794–807.e4. https://doi.org/10.1016/j.jpainsymman.2019.11.009.
6. Mills J, Abel J, Kellehear A, Patel M. Access to palliative care: the primacy of public health partnerships and community participation. *Lancet Public Health*. 2021;6(11):e791–e792. https://doi.org/10.1016/S2468-2667(21)00213-9.
7. Rosa WE, de Campos AP, Abedini NC, et al. Optimizing the global nursing workforce to ensure universal palliative care access and alleviate serious health-related suffering worldwide. *J Pain Symptom Manage*. 2022;63(2):e224–e236. https://doi.org/10.1016/j.jpainsymman.2021.07.014.
8. Hagan TL, Xu J, Lopez RP, Bressler T. Nursing's role in leading palliative care: a call to action. *Nurse Educ Today*. 2018;61:216–219. https://doi.org/10.1016/j.nedt.2017.11.037.
9. World Health Organization. Ageing and Health. Accessed October 30, 2022. https://www.who.int/news-room/fact-sheets/detail/ageing-and-health.
10. Sleeman KE, de Brito M, Etkind S, et al. The escalating global burden of serious health-related suffering: projections to 2060 by world regions, age groups, and health conditions. *Lancet Glob Health*. 2019;7(7):e883–e892. https://doi.org/10.1016/S2214-109X(19)30172-X.
11. Partridge EE, Mayer-Davis EJ, Sacco RL, Balch AJ. Creating a 21st century global health agenda: the General Assembly of the United Nations high level meeting on non-communicable diseases. *CA Cancer J Clin*. 2011;61(4):209–211.
12. World Health Organization. Non-communicable Disease Fact Sheet. 2018. https://www.who.int/news-room/fact-sheets/detail/noncommunicable diseases.
13. Verne J. Demographic and epidemiological challenges. In: Abel J, Kellehear A, Abel J, Kellehear A, eds. *Oxford Textbook of Public Health Palliative Care*. Oxford University Press; 2022:7–13. https://doi.org/10.1093/med/9780198862994.003.0002.
14. Sarafis P, Tsounis A, Malliarou M, Lahana E. Disclosing the truth: a dilemma between instilling hope and respecting patient autonomy in everyday clinical practice. *Glob J Health Sci*. 2013;6(2):128–137. https://doi.org/10.5539/gjhs.v6n2p128.
15. Tobin J, Rogers A, Winterburn I, et al. Hospice care access inequalities: a systematic review and narrative synthesis. *BMJ Support Palliat Care*. 2022;12(2):142–151. https://doi.org/10.1136/bmjspcare-2020-002719.
16. Callaway MV, Connor SR, Foley KM. World Health Organization public health model: a roadmap for palliative care development. *J Pain Symptom Manage*. 2018;55(2):S6–S13. https://doi.org/10.1016/j.jpainsymman.2017.03.030.
17. Finucane AM, O'Donnell H, Lugton J, Gibson-Watt T, Swenson C, Pagliari C. Digital health interventions in palliative care: a systematic meta-review. *NPJ Digit Med*. 2021;4(1):64. https://doi.org/10.1038/s41746-021-00430-7.
18. Crawford A, Serhal E. Digital health equity and COVID-19: the innovation curve cannot reinforce the social gradient of health. *J Med Internet Res*. 2020;22(6):e19361. https://doi.org/10.2196/19361.
19. Brant JM, Al-Zadjali M, Al-Sinawi F, et al. Palliative care nursing development in the Middle East and northeast Africa: lessons from Oman. *J Cancer Educ*. 2021;36(suppl 1):69–77. https://doi.org/10.1007/s13187-021-02044-9.
20. Cross LA. Compassion fatigue in palliative care nursing. *J Hosp Palliat Nurs*. 2019;21(1):21–28. https://doi.org/10.1097/NJH.0000000000000477.
21. Wolf AT, White KR, Epstein EG, Enfield KB. Palliative care and moral distress: an institutional survey of critical care nurses. *Crit Care Nurse*. 2019;39(5):38–49. https://doi.org/10.4037/ccn2019645.
22. AACN. End-of-Life Nursing Education Consortium (ELNEC). 4. https://www.aacnnursing.org/elnec/about
23. World Health Organization. WHO Collaborating Centres. Accessed October 30, 2022. https://apps.who.int/whocc/List.aspx?W70b7VyKAskHZ/zMJcvZLeiT6L7wCBkmjM9bSaaa1TQ=.
24. Phillips JL, Currow D. Challenges and future directions of palliative care. In: MacLeod RD, Van den Block L, eds. *Textbook of Palliative Care*. Springer International Publishing; 2019:111–130. https://doi.org/10.1007/978-3-319-77740-5_5.
25. World Health Organization. WHO model list of essential medicines—22nd list. 2021. Accessed October 30, 2022. https://www.who.int/publications-detail-redirect/WHO-MHP-HPS-EML-2021.02.
26. De Lima L, Krakauer EL, Lorenz K, Praill D, MacDonald N, Doyle D. Ensuring palliative medicine availability: the development of the IAHPC list of essential medicines for palliative care. *J Pain Symptom Manage*. 2007;33(5):521–526.
27. Lima LD. Key concepts in palliative care: the IAHPC list of essential medicines in palliative care. *Eur J Hosp Pharm*. 2012;19(1):34–37. https://doi.org/10.1136/ejhpharm-2011-000044.
28. De Lima L, Radbruch L. The International Association for Hospice and Palliative Care: advancing hospice and palliative care worldwide. *J Pain Symptom Manage*. 2018;55(2 suppl):S96–S103. https://doi.org/10.1016/j.jpainsymman.2017.03.023.
29. Miyachi T, Ozaki A, Saito H, Sawano T, Tanimoto T, Crump A. Opioids: a "crisis" of too much or not enough—or simply how rich you are and where you live? *Eur J Pain*. 2021;25(6):1181–1194. https://doi.org/10.1002/ejp.1767.
30. Cleary JF, Maurer MA. Pain and policy studies group: two decades of working to address regulatory barriers to improve opioid availability and accessibility around the world. *J Pain Symptom Manage*. 2018;55(2 suppl):S121–S134. https://doi.org/10.1016/j.jpainsymman.2017.03.029.
31. Cleary JF, Husain A, Maurer M. Increasing worldwide access to medical opioids. *Lancet*. 2016;387(10028):1597–1599.
32. Pettus K, Cleary JF, de Lima L, Ahmed E, Radbruch L. Availability of internationally controlled essential medicines in the COVID-19 pandemic. *J Pain Symptom Manage*. 2020;60(2):e48–e51. https://doi.org/10.1016/j.jpainsymman.2020.04.153.
33. National Academies of Sciences, Engineering, Medicine. *Pain Management and the Opioid Epidemic: Balancing Societal and Individual Benefits and Risks of Prescription Opioid Use*. National Academies Press; 2017. http://nationalacademies.org/hmd/Reports/2017/pain-management-and-the-opioid-epidemic.aspx.
34. Fitch MI, Fliedner MC, O'Connor M. Nursing perspectives on palliative care 2015. *Ann Palliat Med*. 2015;4(3):150–155. https://doi.org/10.3978/j.issn.2224-5820.2015.07.04
35. LeBaron V. *Caring in Context: An Ethnography of Cancer Nursing in India*. Routledge Press, New York; 2024.

36. Challinor JM, Galassi AL, Al-Ruzzieh MA, et al. Nursing's potential to address the growing cancer burden in low-and middle-income countries. *J Glob Oncol*. 2016;2(3):154–163.
37. LeBaron V, Palat G, Sinha S, et al. Recommendations to support nurses and improve the delivery of oncology and palliative care in India. *Indian J Palliat Care*. 2017;23(2):188–198.
38. LeBaron V, Iribarren S, Perri S, Beck SL. A practical fieldguide to conducting nursing research in low and middle-income countries. *Nurs Outlook*. 2015;63(4):462–473.
39. Galassi A, Pradhan R, Palat G, LeBaron VT. Global oncology volunteering: making an effective contribution. *Oncol Nurs Forum*. 2017;44(5):530–533. https://doi.org/10.1188/17.ONF.530-533

PART IX

Special Considerations for Palliative Care Nurses

73

Occupational Stress, Burnout, and Self-Care in Palliative Nursing

Erica Frechman and Patricia Wright

Personal Reflection

The greatest gift we can give patients and families is NURSE.

N ever
U nderestimate
R eally
S howing up with
E mpathy, compassion, and our whole selves.

Showing up matters. How we show up as nurses caring for patients and families dealing with serious illness is essential in optimizing quality of life while providing people living with serious illness relief of the symptoms and stressors. As a young nurse, I took this concept for granted. I focused on the illness, the task I had to perform, whether administering the blood transfusion or changing the wound dressing, fulfilling the mechanics of my nursing role. Working in oncology, I witnessed the realities of suffering and found myself often taking on secondary traumatic stress, moral injury, and compassion fatigue associated with the patients I cared for so deeply. When I transitioned into palliative care nursing, I felt that I had a firsthand opportunity to be part of the solution, helping with the suffering I witnessed, but also to provide attention to the physical, psychological, social, cultural, and spiritual aspects of care. I started recognizing how showing up mattered, whether that was for the patients who needed pain relief, the families who needed reassurance and support, the referring consultants that needed immediate assistance with a difficult situation, the bedside nurses who needed guidance and a listening ear, or my palliative care teammates who shouldered this work on a daily basis.

Our palliative care program grew with increasing numbers of patients year after year, coupled with administrative demands and pressures, staffing changes and deficits, and leadership challenges. The work was incessant, demanding, and all-encompassing. The overall team morale started to take a hit, our spirits slowly deflated, and showing up became more and more difficult. In order to take back control of our work, we prioritized team health and self-care. We instituted biannual team retreats and monthly wellness activities that focused on connection, purpose, resilience, and optimizing team efficiency. We prioritized ourselves and team wellness, as we recognized that in order to be the best palliative care providers, we had to honor ourselves by taking time to heal, grieve, grow, reflect, and plan.

During the COVID-19 pandemic, the insurmountable levels of deaths, trauma, uncertainties, and emotional heaviness that many palliative care providers and teams witnessed were overwhelming. My memories of that time include our daily interdisciplinary team huddles where we planned care for our patients who were critically ill with COVID-19. I felt helpless listening to my teammates cry out in despair due to the difficulties of the work, the buildup of burnout, and the lack of "feeling heard and understood" by our administration. We stopped, we paused, and we took action. We recognized our ability to show up was limited, we sought help from our Employee Assistance Program, we took time away from the bedside, and we implemented a team wellness activity at the beginning of each morning team huddle to cultivate connection and joy in the workplace.

Throughout my nursing career, I have grown to prioritize my personal dimension of self-care and well-being so that I can be my best authentic self and show up as my whole self in my palliative nursing practice. Giving myself permission to recognize the demands of the work and time to heal my body, mind, and spirit and establishing a self-care practice that is meaningful to me are crucial to my longevity and effectiveness in the specialty. And, most importantly, it allows me to give my very best in showing up for patients living with serious illness and their families as a palliative care NURSE.

—Erica Frechman

Key Points

- Burnout rates across all healthcare settings are steadily rising.
- Occupational stress and burnout in palliative care settings is related to role-specific stressors, short-staffing, and organizational and managerial issues.
- Signs of burnout include: diminished compassion, emotional lability, irritability, sadness, apathy, depression, isolation, overwhelming fatigue, and work dread.
- Strategies to prevent and mitigate burnout should occur on individual (self-care) and organizational levels (workplace strategies that support nurses).

Introduction

High-quality palliative care delivery that is safe, evidence-based, and patient- and family-centered depends on the workforce's well-being, health, and safety.[1,2] Increasing evidence demonstrates the value of palliative care teams in the care of people living with serious illness through improved outcomes for patients, caregivers, and the overall healthcare system.[3] Yet, mounting research and pragmatic realities expose a looming workforce shortage[4] and high levels of burnout.[5–8] Nursing is the nation's largest healthcare profession,[9] and burnout was on the rise even prior to the COVID-19 pandemic, with studies noting burnout rates for palliative care nurses (PCNs) of 24%–73%.[10–12] High burnout rates along with the great resignation drew attention to the pressing need to safeguard nurses in the workforce,[13] to elevate their voices, and to recognize their value in addressing health inequities and improving health and well-being for all.[14] In particular, there is heightened awareness of the stressors involved in the care of those with serious illness, specifically PCNs.[15]

This chapter describes sources of occupational stress in PCNs, signs and symptoms of burnout, and ways that individuals and organizations can promote wellness and self-care. We recognize the great impact that the COVID-19 pandemic has had on nurses and provide recommendations on building and sustaining a healthy palliative care nursing workforce.

Occupational Stress in Palliative Care Nursing

PCNs are generally very proud of the work they do and find great intrinsic rewards in developing relationships with patients and families, alleviating suffering, and honoring patients' wishes.[16] Although PCNs generally report high levels of satisfaction with their work, there are inherent stressors and triggers for burnout related to the care of seriously ill individuals and their families. When job-related stressors are perceived as being greater than an individual's ability to cope, occupational stress occurs, which leads to role dissatisfaction and intent to leave.[17] For PCNs, specifically, role-specific stressors, short-staffing, and organizational and managerial issues are key sources of occupational stress.[17–20] Each of these factors will be discussed in the following sections.

Role-Specific Stressors

Role-specific stressors are related to the essential functions of PCNs. In particular, repeated exposure to suffering and dying is psychologically taxing as it heightens nurses' awareness of their own mortality, their own personal losses, and their own vulnerability.[17,18,20] Nurses may be deeply affected by the deaths of their patients and experience rumination, profound grief, and a sense of injustice, particularly following the death of a younger patient.[20–22] Further, death work prompts examination of the meaning of life, and death and can challenge or strengthen religious and spiritual beliefs.[20,23,24]

Working at the nexus of life and death, PCNs care for patients and families facing life-altering circumstances who may exhibit a variety of uncharacteristic behaviors such as becoming demanding, uncooperative, frustrated, accusatory, and depressed. Facing challenging family dynamics can leave nurses feeling powerless, overwhelmed, frustrated, and exhausted.[25] Additionally, some nurses may self-censor or suppress their emotions, particularly when patients or families have unrealistic beliefs and/or expectations.[20,25,26] Navigating complex situations in palliative care is further complicated by language barriers; religious, spiritual, and cultural norms; and the unpredictable medical needs of patients and families.[20]

Short-Staffing

Palliative care involves a holistic approach to the patient and family focused equally on physical, mental, spiritual, and emotional support. Providing such comprehensive care requires time and focused attention. Yet, many PCNs report that their time with patients is limited due to short-staffing.[17,20] Workforce demands in palliative care have surged over the past 20 years and are expected to further increase as demographic shifts create a greater need for the care of older adults living with serious illness.[4,27,28]

The COVID-19 pandemic worsened staffing shortages in palliative care as morbidity and mortality rates rose exponentially,[18] rapidly and unexpectedly expanding the need for palliative care services. The unprecedented demands for symptom control and patient comfort necessitated overtime and diminished recovery time for professionals.[18,20] Increased patient volume, morbidity, and mortality coupled with resource scarcity and ongoing uncertainty of the pandemic[29] left palliative care staff strained, harrowed, and exhausted.[30,31]

Organizational and Managerial Issues

Within the workplace, primary sources of occupational stress for PCNs include factors that interrupt or impair workflow, such as limited resources, unbalanced work distribution, contradictory messaging regarding work responsibilities, and inadequate or ambiguous communication, which diminish autonomy, impair nurses' ability to provide the type and quality of care they wish to provide, and reduce trust in superiors. Lack of trust in managers and other superiors, specifically, contributes to occupational stress and is part of a host of occupational factors that contribute to job dissatisfaction and intent to leave.[17] Other occupational stressors that are related to the operation of the organization include lack of support from managers, organizational change, office politics, mismatch between organizational goals and individual goals, and lack of organizational support.[17,20] Since occupational stressors are related to individual role stressors, strategies to address occupational stress must be centered not only on the individual but also on how organizations can create a healthy work environment to protect employees from burnout.

Signs of Burnout

Burnout is sometimes associated with other terms that convey a sense of work-related emotional, physical, or mental burden (see Table 73.1). Burnout is defined as a syndrome caused by chronic workplace stress characterized by three domains: emotional exhaustion, increased mental distancing (depersonalization) from one's job, and reduced professional efficacy and accomplishment.[41] Burnout may be episodic and involve emotional lability, irritability, sadness, apathy, depression, isolation, overwhelming fatigue, and work dread. Nurses experiencing burnout may feel like they are failing at their jobs, which is further exacerbated by feelings of disempowerment and a belief that things will not change.[42] Nurses experiencing burnout may exhibit less compassion, make more medication errors, and provide lower-quality patient care.[8,43–46] The serious consequences of burnout affect nurses as individuals, patients and families, and organizations. Proactive burnout prevention strategies are necessary to mitigate burnout and to prevent future episodes of burnout from occurring (see Figure 73.1). Burnout prevention strategies that can be undertaken by individuals and organizations will be discussed in the following sections.

Burnout Prevention

Individual Interventions

PCNs can promote self-care, resilience, and well-being by cultivating an intentional daily practice aimed at fostering connection to one's purpose in nursing. Normalizing the importance of self-care is an important component of one's professionalism that has been codified by the American Nurses Association.[47] In fact, nurses are expected to care for their own well-being with the same significant ethical obligation that they place on caring for others.[48] Self-care must be individualized, however. For example, one nurse may find fulfillment in the practice of self-care through alone time reading a book, while another nurse may enjoy listening to music while on an outdoor walk, and another nurse may delight in the physical demands of rock-climbing. Investing the time and effort to write your own "prescription" for self-care is the first step to adopting a healthy work style, resisting burnout, and building resilience.

Personal care strategies that can be included in a "self-care prescription" include mindfulness, meditation, good sleep hygiene, proper nutrition, avoidance of alcohol and drugs, exercise, development of daily routines, increased self-awareness, maintaining a healthy work/life balance with emotional and physical distancing, reflection, hobbies, leisure time, social support, and participation in religious/spiritual practices.[20,49,50] Some research indicates that personal factors such as emotional intelligence, personal coping skills, and resilience training also buffer the effects of burnout and involve the development of learned skills.[49,50] Individual attention to self-care is important in withstanding the demands of palliative care work. However, recent research also emphasizes the role of organizations in developing and sustaining healthy work environments that promote employee well-being.

Organizational Interventions

Organizational interventions that protect employees' mental health include providing chaplaincy services to hospice staff, developing reflective practices such as Schwartz rounds, and instituting support teams (which can be virtual), to reduce isolation.[20,49,50] Strategies aimed at emotional support, open communication, and reducing isolation are particularly important for team members who work independently completing home visits in the community.[17,19]

Despite the isolating aspects of end-of-life work, team dynamics are preeminently important for reducing employee stress and creating a positive, caring, and supportive workplace. The general climate of an organization, or what is commonly known as "the tone at the top," should ideally value cooperative conflict management styles, which reduce competition and foster trust and commitment

Table 73.1 Terms associated with occupational stressors

Term	Definition
Occupational stress	A harmful physical and emotional response that occurs when work demands and pressures do not match the capabilities, resources, or needs of the worker.[32]
Emotional labor	The act of managing feelings when one's work role indicates particular emotions should be displayed while others should be hidden. For example, nurses who have intensive contact with patients are required to deliver compassionate care often under challenging circumstances.[33]
Compassion fatigue	A state of physical, emotional, and spiritual depletion associated with caring for patients with significant emotional pain and physical distress.[34]
Secondary traumatic stress	The result of stress reactions and symptoms from exposure to another individual's traumatic experience, rather than from exposure directly from a traumatic event. For nurses, this can be considered as a "cost of caring."[35]
Moral injury	A psychological and emotional effect that arises when actions run in opposition to one's personal beliefs and moral values.[36]
Moral distress	An emotional state that occurs when clinicians are unable to prevent medical actions that they deem to be ethically inappropriate.[37]
Self-care	A process of taking steps to engage in activities that promote and maintain health and well-being. This includes activities that foster nurse resilience and reduce emotional labor.[38]
Resilience	The ability to adapt to challenges presented in one's life. Resilience occurs when personal resources can rise above to meet work demands.[39]
Well-being	A state that encompasses physical, mental, and social domains in one's life satisfaction. Clinician well-being is focused on promoting ways to improve patient–clinician relationships, a high-functioning care team, and an engaged workforce that delivers care finding professional fulfillment in work.[40]

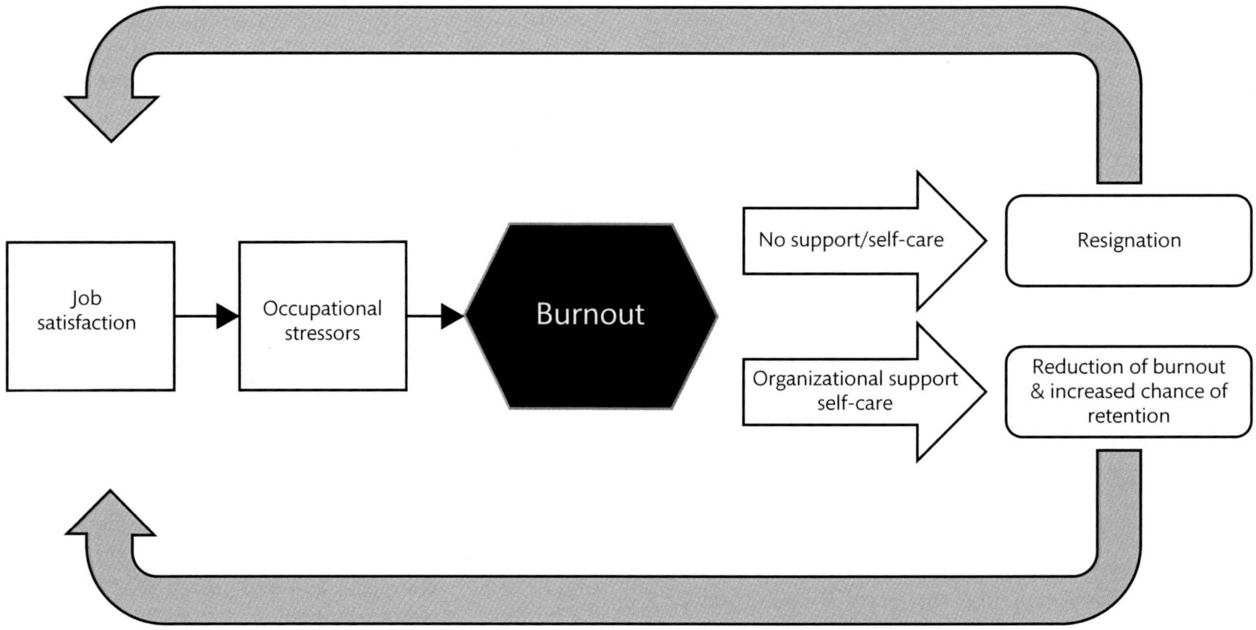

Figure 73.1 Cycles of Burnout

among employees.[51] Further, organization leaders must master, model, and teach conflict resolution skills to provide a positive and safe and comfortable work environment for staff.[17] Taking steps toward improving nurses' work environments and authentically advocating for input, participation, and community-building can help reduce burnout and nurse turnover.[52]

Conclusion

Palliative care work is rewarding, but repeated exposure to suffering and death is demanding and emotionally challenging.[53] Caring for patients and families dealing with serious illness and myriad complex multidimensional needs requires proactive approaches to prioritizing self-care, developing a healthy palliative care workforce, and addressing burnout. Individual nurses must commit to identifying and implementing self-care strategies aimed at building resistance to occupational stressors. At the same time, organizations must take responsibility for developing healthy workplaces where employee well-being is prioritized. PCNs and employers can partner to create compassionate and caring environments for patients as well as clinicians. Although some research has been conducted on the types of interventions that work best for mitigating and preventing burnout, models of care delivery that enhance the well-being of PCNs are desperately needed to build and sustain the palliative care workforce.

REFERENCES

1. National Academies of Sciences, Engineering, and Medicine. *Taking Action against Clinician Burnout: A Systems Approach to Professional Well-Being*. National Academies Press; 2019. https://doi.org/10.17226/25521.
2. Ferrell BR, Twaddle ML, Melnick A, Meier DE. National Consensus Project clinical practice guidelines for quality palliative care guidelines. *J Palliat Med*. 2018;21(12):1684–1689. https://doi.org/10.1089/jpm.2018.0431.
3. Kavalieratos D, Corbelli J, Zhang DI, et al. Association between palliative care and patient and caregiver outcomes: a systematic review and meta-analysis. *JAMA*. 2016;316(20):2104–2114. https://doi.org/10.1001/jama.2016.16840.
4. Kamal AH, Wolf SP, Troy J, et al. Policy changes key to promoting sustainability and growth of the specialty palliative care workforce. *Health Aff (Millwood)*. 2019;38(6):910–918. https://doi.org/10.1377/hlthaff.2019.00018.
5. Kavalieratos D, Siconolfi DE, Steinhauser KE, et al. It is like heart failure. It is chronic … and it will kill you": a qualitative analysis of burnout among hospice and palliative care clinicians. *J Pain Symptom Manage*. 2017;53(5):901–910. https://doi.org/10.1016/j.jpainsymman.2016.12.337.
6. Mills J, Wand T, Fraser JA. Exploring the meaning and practice of self-care among palliative care nurses and doctors: a qualitative study. *BMC Palliat Care*. 2018;17(1):63. https://doi.org/10.1186/s12904-018-0318-0.
7. Orellana-Rios CL, Radbruch L, Kern M, et al. Mindfulness and compassion-oriented practices at work reduce distress and enhance self-care of palliative care teams: a mixed-method evaluation of an "on the job" program. *BMC Palliat Care*. 2018;17(1):3. https://doi.org/10.1186/s12904-017-0219-7.
8. Koh MYH, Khoo HS, Gallardo MD, Hum A. How leaders, teams and organisations can prevent burnout and build resilience: a thematic analysis. *BMJ Support Palliat Care*. 2020;14(e1):e827–e836. https://doi.org/10.1136/bmjspcare-2020-002774.
9. Smiley RA, Ruttinger C, Oliveira CM, et al. The 2020 National Nursing Workforce Survey. *J Nurs Regul*. 2021;12(suppl 1):S1–S48. https://doi.org/10.1016/S2155-8256(21)00027-2.
10. Kamal AH, Bull JH, Wolf SP, et al. Prevalence and predictors of burnout among hospice and palliative care clinicians in the US. *J Pain Symptom Manage*. 2020;59(5):6–13. https://doi.org/10.1016/j.jpainsymman.2019.11.017.
11. Koh MYH, Chong PH, Neo PSH, et al. Burnout, psychological morbidity and use of coping mechanisms among palliative care

practitioners: a multi-centre cross-sectional study. *Palliat Med.* 2015;29(7):633–642. https://doi.org/10.1177/0269216315575850.
12. Lowe MA, Prapanjaroensin A, Bakitas MA, et al. An exploratory study of the influence of perceived organizational support, coworker social support, the nursing practice environment, and nurse demographics on burnout in palliative care nurses. *J Hosp Palliat Nurs.* 2020;22(6):465–472. https://doi.org/10.1097/NJH.0000000000000686.
13. Boston-Fleischhauer C. Reversing the great resignation in nursing: more things to consider. *J Nurs Adm.* 2022;52(6):324–326. https://doi.org/10.1097/NNA.0000000000001155.
14. National Academies of Sciences, Engineering, and Medicine. *The Future of Nursing 2020–2030: Charting a Path to Achieve Health Equity*. National Academies Press; 2021. https://doi.org/10.17226/25982.
15. May S, Gabb F, Ignatyev Y, et al. Mental and physical well-being and burden in palliative care nursing: a cross-setting mixed-methods study. *Int J Environ Res Public Health.* 2022;19(10):6240. https://doi.org/10.3390/ijerph19106240.
16. Head B, Middleton A, Zeigler C. Work satisfaction among hospice and palliative nurses. *J Hosp Palliat Nurs.* 2019;21(5):E1–E11. https://doi.org/10.1097/NJH.0000000000000562.
17. Dos Santos NA, dos Santos J, da Silva VR, Passos JP. Occupational stress in palliative care in oncology. Article in Portuguese. *Cogitare Enferm.* 2017;22(4):e50686. https://doi.org/10.5380/ce.v22i4.50686.
18. Cunha DA, Fuly PD, Siqueira AS, et al. Stress in palliative care nursing staff while coping with COVID-19. *Acta Paul Enferm.* 2021;34:eAPE001915. https://doi.org/10.37689/acta-ape/2021AO001915.
19. Park SA, Park HJ. The relationships between oncology nurses' attitudes toward a dignified death, compassion competence, resilience, and occupational stress in South Korea. *Semin Oncol Nurs.* 2021;37(3):151147. https://doi.org/10.1016/j.soncn.2021.151147.
20. Kagee A, Vasileiou K, Smith P. Experiences of work-related stress and coping among palliative care staff in South Africa: a qualitative study. *S Afr J Psychol.* 2020;50(3):425–437. https://doi.org/10.1177/0081246320902300.
21. Carton ER, Hupcey JE. The forgotten mourners: addressing health care provider grief—a systematic review. *J Hosp Palliat Nurs.* 2014;16(5):291–303. https://doi.org/10.1097/NJH.0000000000000067.
22. Plante J, Cyr C. Health care professionals' grief after the death of a child. *Paediatr Child Health.* 2011;16(4):213–216. https://doi.org/10.1093/pch/16.4.213.
23. Kudubes AA, Akıl ZK, Bektas M, Bektas I. Nurses' attitudes towards death and their effects on spirituality and spiritual care. *J Relig Health.* 2021;60:153–161. https://doi.org/10.1007/s10943-019-00927-2.
24. Stephenson PS, Sheehan D, Hansen D, Mayo MM. Spiritual uncertainty among hospice providers: "there were tensions." *J Hosp Palliat Nurs.* 2019;21(1):90–95. https://doi.org/10.1097/NJH.0000000000000485
25. Dobrina R, Chialchia S, Palese A. "Difficult patients" in the advanced stages of cancer as experienced by nursing staff: a descriptive qualitative study. *Eur J Oncol Nurs.* 2020;46:101766. https://doi.org/10.1016/j.ejon.2020.101766.
26. Pejoski N, Skaczkowski G, Moran J, Hodgson H, Wilson C. Confronting behaviour in palliative care: a qualitative study of the lived experience of nursing staff. *Int J Palliat Nurs.* 2021;27(5):245–253. https://doi.org/10.12968/ijpn.2021.27.5.245.
27. Hughes MT, Smith TJ. The growth of palliative care in the United States. *Annu Rev Public Health.* 2014;35:459–475. https://doi.org/10.1146/annurev-publhealth-032013-182406.
28. Cassel JB, Bowman B, Rogers M, Spragens LH, Meier DE. Palliative care leadership centers are key to the diffusion of palliative care innovation. *Health Aff (Millwood).* 2018;37(2):231–239. https://doi.org/10.1377/hlthaff.2017.1122.
29. Sinclair S. We Are in a War: Mitigating Burnout in COVID-19. Center to Advance Palliative Care. Updated July 13, 2020. Accessed March 7, 2023. https://www.capc.org/blog/we-are-in-a-war-mitigating-burnout-in-covid-19/?clickthrough_doc_id=blog.blogpostpage.1605&clickthrough_req_id=tmqU77CYTuWsTdFzqsGOgw&clickthrough_query=burnout.
30. Davis A, Repar P, Wilson M, De Luca E, Doutrich D, Thanasilp S. Transforming nurse self-care through integration of spirituality: lessons from an international collaboration in palliative care. *J Transcult Nurs.* 2023;34(1):91–99. https://doi.org/10.1177/10436596221134814.
31. Janssen DJ. Palliative care in COVID-19. *Curr Opin Support Palliat Care.* 2021;15(4):199–204. https://doi.org/10.1097/SPC.0000000000000567.
32. World Health Organization. Occupational Health: Stress at the Workplace. Updated October 19, 2020. Accessed March 7, 2023. https://www.who.int/news-room/questions-and-answers/item/ccupational-health-stress-at-the-workplace#:~:text=Work%2Drelated%20stress%20is%20the,challenge%20their%20ability%20to%20cope.
33. Kinman G, Leggetter S. Emotional labour and wellbeing: what protects nurses? *Healthcare.* 2016;4(4):89. https://doi.org/10.3390/healthcare4040089.
34. Figley C. *Compassion Fatigue: Coping with Secondary Traumatic Stress Disorder in Those Who Treat the Traumatized.* Brunner-Routledge; 1995.
35. Gee PM, Weston MJ, Harshman T, Kelly LA. Beyond burnout and resilience: the disillusionment phase of COVID-19. *AACN Adv Crit Care.* 2022;33(2):134–142. https://doi.org/10.4037/aacnacc2022248.
36. Hossain F, Clatty A. Self-care strategies in response to nurses' moral injury during COVID-19 pandemic. *Nurs Ethics.* 2021;1:23–32. https://doi.org/10.1177/0969733020961825.
37. Hamric AB, Borchers CT, Epstein EG. Development and testing of an instrument to measure moral distress in healthcare professionals. *AJOB Prim Res.* 2012;3(2):1–9. https://doi.org/10.1080/21507716.2011.652337.
38. Delgado C, Upton D, Ranse K, Furness T, Foster K. Nurses' resilience and the emotional labour of nursing work: an integrative review of empirical literature. *Int J Nurs Stud.* 2017;70:71–88. https://doi.org/10.1016/j.ijnurstu.2017.02.008.
39. Back AL, Steinhauser KE, Kamal AH, Jackson VA. Building resilience for palliative care clinicians: an approach to burnout prevention based on individual skills and workplace factors. *J Pain Symptom Manage.* 2016;52(2):284–291. https://doi.org/10.1016/j.jpainsymman.2016.02.002.
40. National Academy of Medicine. Action Collaborative on Clinician Well-Being and Resilience. Accessed March 7, 2023. https://nam.edu/initiatives/clinician-resilience-and-well-being/.
41. Maslach C, Schaufeli WB, Leiter MP. Job burnout. *Annu Rev Psychol.* 2001;52(1):397–422. https://doi.org/10.1146/annurev.psych.52.1.397.
42. Centers for Disease Control and Prevention. Emergency responders: Tips for taking care of yourself. Updated March 19,

2018. Accessed March 7, 2023. https://emergency.cdc.gov/coping/responders.asp.
43. Aiken LH, Clarke SP, Sloane SP, Sochalski J, Silber JH. Hospital nurse staffing and patient mortality, nurse burnout, and job dissatisfaction. *JAMA*. 2002;288:1987–1993 https://doi.org/10.1001/jama.288.16.1987.
44. Copeland D. Brief workplace interventions addressing burnout, compassion fatigue, and teamwork: a pilot study. *West J Nurs Res*. 2021;43(2):130–137. https://doi.org/10.1177/0193945920938048.
45. Koh MYH, Hum AYM, Khoo HS, et al. Burnout and resilience after a decade in palliative care: what survivors have to teach us. A qualitative study of palliative care clinicians with more than 10 years of experience. *J Pain Symptom Manage*. 2020;59(1):105–115. https://doi.org/10.1016/j.jpainsymman.2019.08.008.
46. Frechman E, Wright PM. Nurse burnout in hospice and palliative care: a scoping review. *Illn Crisis Loss*. 2023;31(1):137–150. https://doi.org/10.1177/10541373211039825.
47. American Nurses Association. Code of Ethics for Nurses with Interpretive Statements. 2001. https://www.nursingworld.org/practice-policy/nursing-excellence/ethics/code-of-ethics-for-nurses/
48. Fowler M. *Guide to the Code of Ethics for Nurses with Interpretive Statements: Development, Interpretation, and Application*. 2nd ed. American Nurses Association; 2015.
49. Cedar SH, Walker G. Protecting the wellbeing of nurses providing end-of-life care. *Nurs Times*. 2020;116(2):36–40.
50. Horn DJ, Johnston CB. Burnout and self care for palliative care practitioners. *Med Clin North Am*. 2020;104(3):561–572. https://doi.org/10.1016/j.mcna.2019.12.007.
51. Wong A, Wang X, Wang X, Tjosvold D. Ethical leaders manage conflict to develop trust. *Leadersh Organ Dev J*. 2020;41(1):133–146. https://doi.org/10.1108/LODJ-10-2018-0363.
52. Fitzpatrick B, Bloore K, Blake N. Joy in work and reducing nurse burnout: from triple aim to quadruple aim. *AACN Adv Crit Care*. 2019;30(2):185–188. https://doi.org/10.4037/aacnacc2019833.
53. Oldenburger E, De Roo ML. Burnout of healthcare professionals in supportive and palliative care: a summary of recent literature. *Curr Opin Support Palliat Care*. 2023;17(1):77–83. https://doi.org/10.1097/SPC.0000000000000638.

74

Palliative Care and Social Media

Dana Hansen and Amy Petrinec

Key Points

- Social media provides a modern venue for people with serious illness to tell their illness stories and seek online resources and support.
- Social media provides a venue for people with serious illness and their families to receive support from others.
- Social media provides another way for people with serious illness and their families to communicate with others.

Brief History and Impact of Social Media

With Web 2.0 came the creation of user-generated content and web-based interaction, leading to development of a variety of social media platforms.[1] The advent of this technology has influenced human interaction for individuals and communities; individuals now interact in ways not imagined just 15 years ago. As the technology evolved, algorithms were developed which facilitated interconnection of platforms by social networking sites to create a culture of connectivity.[2] Social media frequently provides a venue for hospice and palliative care nurses, families, and patients with serious illness seeking information and support.

Over the past 15 years, internet and social media use has skyrocketed. Today, around 32% of the world's population has internet connection; in 1995, it was less than 1%. The first billion internet users was reached in 2005.[3] At the time of this writing (September 2022), more than 8 million blogs and nearly 1 billion tweets were written or sent, and over 3 trillion people viewed videos on YouTube. Current examples of social media include X, Facebook, YouTube, Instagram, Snapchat, TikTok, and Pinterest. To further define social media, Carrigan[4] and Van Dijck[2] offered the categories listed in Table 74.1. Hootsuite, a social media management platform, offers additional categories to facilitate understanding of these sites and why they are used.[5] It is important for palliative care teams to be aware of various types of social media available to patients and families because of their importance as a method for communication and source of supportive resources during serious illness.

Social media affects multiple aspects of modern life, including words used and their associated meanings. Most people know what is meant by "social media," "Googling," or "tweeting." Words like "friending," "sharing," and "liking" have newly understood meanings.[4] The term "well-connected" used to refer to a person of a certain social status; now, it may refer to how many followers are on one's Facebook page. On social media, these followers indicate "connections" or "friends" and do not discriminate between a close friend and an acquaintance. For example, a Facebook "friend" may be an acquaintance from high school with whom there is very little interaction in real time. In addition, many close friends and family may be denoted as "friends" on a Facebook page. In this way, there is no differentiation between family, close friends, and acquaintances with whom there is no face-to-face interaction.

Social media continues to change and evolve the nature and structure of communication and interpersonal connectivity while serving as a method for obtaining social support, especially during times of crisis or difficulty. The internet allows for interpersonal, participative, and interactive exchanges of information in a variety of ways, including blogs, Facebook, and X. A theoretical view provides more insight into the evolution of social media related to health and healthcare.

Theoretical View

Despite an explosion of research examining digital interaction and networks, this growing body of knowledge has occurred without theoretical structures developed specifically for digital interactions.[6] Much of the theoretical framework used was developed for face-to-face interactions, which may or may not be adequate for examining digital interaction. In an attempt to strengthen the theoretical "scaffolding" used to study digital networks, Lewis identifies five characteristics of digital social networks that differentiate them from face-to-face networks.[6] Digital communication obviates the need for physical presence; loosens the constraints of time, enabling asynchronous interaction; allows for anonymity; can remain invisible to others; and has limited social presence (lacks nonverbal communication cues). Lewis argues that theoretical frameworks derived from face-to-face network interactions may be insufficient for study of digital networks, and further development is needed to achieve solid theoretical underpinnings.[6] Nonetheless, researchers have adopted many different theoretical frameworks to study the impact of social media on everyday life.[7] Frequently cited theories in this category

Table 74.1 Categories of social media

Category	Purpose	Examples (not an exhaustive list)
Social audio platforms	Listening to live conversations on specific topics	Clubhouse, Spotify, X Spaces
Disappearing content formats	Ephemeral messages privately and timely, in-the-moment content	Snapchat, Instagram Stories, Facebook Stories, LinkedIn Stories
Social media live streams	Broadcasting live video	Twitch, YouTube, Instagram Live Rooms, Facebook Live, TikTok
Business social media platforms	Interpersonal, professional connections	LinkedIn, X, Research Gate
Closed/private community social media platforms	Creating communities, some require registration or screening of members	Discourse, Slack, Facebook Groups
Video social media platforms and formats	Support creativity and exchange for driving brand awareness and bringing products to life, capturing attention	YouTube, Instagram Stories and Reels, TikTok, Facebook Watch
Inspirational social media platforms	Searching for information and inspiration, for example, recipes and travel	Pinterest, YouTube, Instagram, blogs
Discussion forums	Older type of social media Used to find, discuss, and share news, information, and opinions	Reddit, Quora, and Digg
Blogging and publishing networks	Regularly updated website or web page Maintained by an individual or small group Can be personal updates and reflections, photos, etc. Often written in a diary style (blogs)	Wordpress, Tumblr, and Medium
Shoppable social media platforms and features	Discover, save, share, and discuss new and trending content, brands, and media	Pinterest Product Pins, Facebook Shops, Instagram Shops, TikTok, Shopify, Douyin, Taobao
Trading and marketing sites or social shopping networks	Exist to exchange products Provide comments and experiences from other shoppers	Amazon, Fancy, and eBay
Interest-based networks	Connect with others around a shared hobby or interest	Goodreads, Houzz, Last.fm
Consumer review networks	Find, review, and share information about brands, products, and services as well as restaurants and travel destinations	TripAdvisor, Yelp
Play and game sites	Host games that are social	Angry Birds, Farm Ville

include social aspects theory, social capital theory, and social power theory. Although an exhaustive review of theoretical considerations for studying digital networks is beyond the scope of the present discussion, social capital theory will be presented to illuminate the role of social media for illness, including research of serious illness such as cancer.

Social Capital Theory

Broadly speaking, social capital is the amount of resources accumulated through relationships among people.[8] Social capital theory describes three types of relationships: bridging, bonding, and linking. "Bonding social capital" represents relationships between and within homogenous groups, while "bridging social capital" refers to relationships between relatively inhomogeneous groups. Finally, "linking relationships" refers to relationships between people who interact across power or authority hierarchies, such as the relationship between teacher and student or physician and patient. Ultimately, the more social capital one has, the more resources and personal relationships one enjoys. The underlying idea of social capital is based on forming social networks characterized by some level of trust. Therefore, people join social networks to form systems such as social support during serious illness which they were unable to attain on their own.

The importance of social capital relies on the ability to access and use resources within a social network. This, in turn, facilitates flow of information, influences decision-making, and provides different forms of support for an individual as a member of a social group sharing similar interests and resources. Therefore, the more people one knows and the more relationships and connections one has within a social network, the more resources one can access through higher levels of social capital. More importantly, quality matters more than the number of relationships and resources available within a social network, consistent with the proverb "It's not what you know but who you know that counts." The dynamic interactions of social capital theory can offer insight into the capabilities of a social structure to influence people's behavior within a social network.

Social Media and Social Capital

Social media usage for enhancing personal relationships is a remarkable revolution of the modern era. Social media provides a rich venue for people to share and exchange their experiences, interests, or views regardless of their racial, sexual, or religious identities. Many internet-based social media applications are available such as Facebook, blogs, X, or Instagram. These applications allow people to share and exchange information using different platforms from texting to photo- or video-sharing. Therefore, social media can be beneficial in building social capital via social networking and has been studied within the social capital framework.[9] Furthermore, social capital has been studied in various health outcomes.[10] Social media has the potential to develop social capital by allowing people with a serious illness to establish and form new social relationships with others or strengthen preexisting relationships within a social network. This may lead to greater levels of social connectedness, social support, self-esteem, experience-sharing, management of burdens, decision-making, and life satisfaction, all of which are important outcomes for both the person with a serious illness and their family. More importantly, social media provides another venue for people with a serious illness and their family to receive support, providing new ways to experience intimacy, friendship, and identity in which people can share their experiences with each other in a public forum. This type of social support network is emerging as a valuable resource for the person with a serious illness and their family.

The Power of Storytelling through Expressive Writing

Human beings are storytellers by nature, and the benefits of storytelling in healthcare are increasingly being recognized.[11,12] Storytelling as a fundamental component of nursing knowledge is a long-standing tradition, and storytelling in social media is a form of expressive writing.[13] Expressive writing assists people with reconceptualizing traumatic experiences such as the serious illness of a loved one. Through the expression of thoughts and feelings, a person creates a story of meaning for the traumatic event.[14] In the case of serious illness, the patient and family receive supportive and often useful comments from their social network in response to the story they are publicly sharing on social media.

As an expressive writing communication strategy, storytelling is useful in understanding experiences and communicating health information in an understandable manner with therapeutic health benefits for the writer and the listener.[15] Therapeutic benefits of storytelling through expressive writing for persons with serious illness include being heard and creating a shared sense of purpose and connection to others. The sense of purpose (or sense-making) comes when the person with a serious illness and their family find a new purpose, sometimes described as "new self," through the sharing of the story.[16] Expressive writing offers initial relief from traumatic experiences; however, a significant cognitive shift may occur at later stages.[17] Within this rationale, writing on social media offers the ability to reflect over time and, therefore, offers opportunities for healing. While sadness is a normal reaction to a loved one's diagnosis of serious illness, it is also a powerful emotion that can lead to a cognitive change when properly guided.[18]

Social Media and Engagement Characteristics

Despite negative aspects and related challenges, social media is an ongoing presence that cannot be ignored. When interacting with patients and their families, it is imperative for nurses to understand typical characteristics of social media that attract users. Researchers have found a direct link between content characteristics (communication processes) and preferences by social media users for a highly engaged site.[19] Sites may invoke both positive and negative emotions, from joy or happiness to envy or even anger.[20]

The influence of social media engagement on users is an important concept for nurses to understand when communicating with patients. Since patient and family engagement with social media can be mediated by their emotional response, clinicians should discuss what the patient and family are finding on social media so that open and transparent communication between the clinician, patient, and family can occur. For example, researchers found that Facebook was the most common platform used by parents to search for a cure for brain tumors.[21] Patients and families are not the only ones who seek knowledge on social media. A recent study found that healthcare researchers and clinicians viewed blogs in their area of interest; the impact of this use is unknown.[22] However, Khan and colleagues found social media use among clinicians at work to be high (91.9%), and a large portion were visiting sites with medical information.[23]

Types of Social Media Used in Illness

Illness Blog

The use of social media in healthcare has also grown rapidly among patients and caregivers. A quick Google search for cancer blogs elicited 172,000,000 results, indicating that even difficult and stressful conversations occur on social media. Blogs initiated by patients or caregivers during treatment of a serious illness have increasingly become a way for individuals to give voice to their unique experiences as well as seek support from others in similar circumstances.[24] An illness blog is the story of one's illness posted on a social media platform which, when read and/or responded to by the family, has the potential to increase the social network and support for both the patient and family by increasing their social capital or resources.[25] Writing about one's illness on a blog has shown positive results for bloggers, including increased connection with others, decreased isolation, and more opportunities to tell their illness stories.[26] In addition, illness blogs have been found to promote accountability (to self and others) and create opportunities for making meaning and gaining insights from the experience of illness, nurturing a sense of purpose, and furthering understanding of their illness.[27]

Facebook

Facebook is a Web 2.0 interface designed as a gathering place for its subscribers, where people who may be no more than acquaintances or even strangers become friends. For example, Gage-Bouchard and colleagues reported that interaction on Facebook provided a venue to express cancer-related stories, promote advocacy, and obtain social support.[28] Interestingly, Facebook social support was significantly related to general social support.[29] Participants valued the support they received from Facebook friends and followers as much as the support received by family and friends in their daily lives. Facebook also offers an opportunity for online support groups, including groups for hospice family caregivers, with positive results such as decreased depression and improved emotional support.[30,31] Online support was found to be useful and as effective as face-to-face support groups, especially when the online support is private.[32] Furthermore, social support in many forms has been found to benefit cancer patients. Valle and colleagues found that Facebook is a beneficial way for young cancer survivors to exchange health information and receive support, especially for promoting physical activity.[33]

X

Seeking health information and online support is commonplace and has been studied from numerous perspectives, including health information–seeking behaviors, predictors of eHealth usage, and the use of X to disseminate health information.[34,35] X is considered "microblogging" because it allows only short messages; therefore, the stated content is often simple. However, a good tweet invokes both emotion and information. X offers a place to garner the views of others, with heightened use during the COVID-19 pandemic in which families were separated from seriously ill loved ones. To understand the role of palliative care during the COVID-19 pandemic, researchers examined X and found there was a recognized value of palliative care during the pandemic. They also found that palliative care was the responsibility of all health professionals, with palliative specialists guiding and supporting all other health professionals.[36] Researchers also analyzed the influence of cancer conversations on X and found they resulted in cancer organizations geared toward patients.[37] Based on current health-related internet research, X is a rich source of health information used by its members to seek health information, change health behaviors, and engage in illness-related discussions.

Social Media and the Family

Social media connects families in many ways. There is some evidence that social media can be a mechanism to enhance certain aspects of family interaction. Discussion about one's serious illness over social media can help open doors for difficult conversations imperative for relationship healing at end of life, which increases opportunities for a peaceful death of the patient and effective grieving for the family.[38,39] The illness blog also provides a charted course of what has happened over the duration of the illness and leads to new avenues of support for and from others, as shown in this example:

> And so it was just like oh, you know, that's my man, you know, and that was one of the most amazing things about it was that in that dark time when he was being stripped of everything, there was this one thing that had grown (his writing); it wasn't going away, it was coming, this new skill had been created or discovered.[26]

Enhancing Family Communication

While healthcare professionals often think of difficult conversations taking place between the healthcare team and the patient and/or the family, difficult conversations also occur between the person living with a serious illness and their family caregivers. When individuals write about their own fears regarding their illness, it can evoke the same emotion in the family caregivers. Examining communication as a factor in the patient–caregiver dyad is crucial to the patient's and caregiver's quality of life.[40,41] However, the illness story also opens doors for further communication, as illustrated by the following participant comments:

> Reading about his fear kind of made that more real for me; there was something about reading when he would write about this thought that makes me really scared and would clue me into what was really bothering him if he hadn't been able to articulate it to me.[26]

Reading a loved one's comments on an illness blog allows the family caregiver to reflect on the message before reacting to the written words, unlike a face-to-face conversation in which an immediate response is usually required. Other interpersonal behaviors, such as involvement of the family caregiver with the person living with a serious illness, may also affect how difficult conversations are initiated and continued throughout the illness trajectory. Some research suggests that when communication and sharing occur among these social networks, there is a sense of relief from emotional turmoil or even the desire to rebuild a crumbled relationship.[42,43] Hansen and colleagues found that patients valued family members who were highly involved with their care during their illness and reported high levels of comfort with a highly involved family caregiver.[42] Furthermore, low-energy activities are better tolerated and appreciated by patients with a serious illness; therefore, interacting through social media may be well accepted as an intervention.

Difficult conversations are filled with a variety of emotions that are challenging, albeit critical, to patient and family caregiver well-being. When a family caregiver has a first glimpse of how their loved one is coping with the illness or approaching decisions that lie ahead, it can open a door for further face-to-face conversations. One participant shared that "sometimes it is easier to write it than to talk about," indicating that the written story makes problems related to the illness easier to talk about later after both the patient and the caregiver have a chance to think about what was written.[26] Another participant remarked how his wife would write about her "feelings, fears, and what was going on," which they would discuss after her posts. This interaction is comforting and presents one way for family caregivers to feel like part of the team.

Facilitating Sense-Making

The written word detailing the illness story on social media becomes a document that tracks events in addition to experiences. These stories offer a method for developing interpretations of events.[44] The development of interpretations facilitates sense-making through a sequential interlacing of past, present, and future events. Stories also facilitate dialogue around the meaning and purpose of the illness.[39] Hansen and colleagues found that participants appreciated the written "track record" as a valuable aspect of the illness blog.[26]

When faced with uncertainty, the ability to create meaning or make sense out of a difficult situation becomes paramount.[45] As patients and family caregivers navigate their way through the disease trajectory, they face uncertainties ranging from initial diagnosis to the prognosis, treatment, and side effects. When patients and family caregivers use their stories to make sense of what is happening, they gain clarity and meaning.

Garnering Social Support

Typically, the end of life is thought to be shadowed by isolation and loneliness; however, caregivers find that through social support, a balance of caregiving and burden is found because the ability to cope is improved.[16,26,40,41] In addition, research on social support demonstrates that close personal relationships assist in improving well-being, even in the absence of stress.[40,41] One method of support is through sharing experiences via social media.

Support can also be derived from others who have shared similar experiences on social media. For example, one family caregiver stated, "the most important thing I think captured on this blog is how it helped other cancer victims and patients."[26] Kim and Gillham reported the experiences of young adult cancer patients as described through online narratives via the website Planet Cancer.[46] Over a 1-month period, they collected and analyzed 168 blog posts written by 12 males and 34 females. Ten main themes were reported from topics ranging from physical and psychological isolation to cancer survivorship. Researchers concluded that online blogs provided a venue for sharing stories with those of similar ages and situations.

Additionally, blogs served as a medium to combat social isolation when faced with physical disfigurement. A study using a sample of young women with cancer examined the use of complementary therapies.[47] Through analysis of illness blog content, the authors reported the emergence of positive themes regarding complementary therapy use for symptom burden. This method of online communication provided an avenue to share information about complementary therapies and glean social support from women of similar ages with a cancer diagnosis.

Another study examined 24 illness blogs from Australia, Canada, the United Kingdom, and the United States written by men and women of different ages and with a range of cancer diagnoses.[48] One of the most distinguishing features of the blogs was the production and management of personal affect through self-expression about the impact of illness on the body and everyday life. The authors also describe the value of the blogs not only as a "communicative labor" but also as a "network-enabling and social" labor. Bloggers generate online spaces where experiences can be shared, which ultimately impacts broader social understanding of their illness.

Leaving a Legacy

As another means for support, social media may serve as a living memorial after a person dies, also known as a "continued bond." Continued bonds assist those mourning the deceased with creating meaning out of their loss and adjusting to life without their beloved family member or friend.[41] Digital legacies are becoming more popular; however, in a survey of 10 hospices, most clinicians are not discussing the creation of digital legacies with patients and families in hospice.[49] Some research has identified the importance of creating a digital legacy with children living with serious illnesses.[50] Keim-Malpass, Adelstein, and Kavalieratos found that posthumous responses on illness blogs serve both legacy-making and grief-processing functions.[47] For example, the posthumous responses included expressions of grief such as videos, obituaries, and communication via X. Other studies support the use of social media in maintaining a continued relationship with the deceased, such as the written communication on deceased individuals' Facebook pages serving the function of sense-making and continued bonding for family members.[51]

Social Media and Healthcare Professionals

Healthcare professionals use social media for both personal and professional objectives, with usage rates approaching 90%.[52] Although there is a great deal of variability in the use of and engagement with social media in the course of their professional duties, a smaller majority of clinicians (67%) use social media in a professional capacity. The driver of professional use has been online professional communities aimed at sharing domain knowledge, keeping up with new developments, communicating with colleagues, or listening to experts.[53] This type of professional interaction and sharing was formerly reserved for regional and national professional meetings that occurred infrequently and required travel. The use of social media for professional education and collaboration has diminished geographic and time restrictions for dissemination of knowledge, collegial discussions, and networking.

Attitudes of healthcare professionals toward the use of social media in communicating with patients and families vary. In general, younger practitioners are more likely than older practitioners to have a favorable view of social media and use it to interact with patients.[54,55] Furthermore, there is some discordance in motives for using social media in healthcare for professionals and patients.[56] Professionals tend to use social media for communicating with colleagues and marketing, whereas patients tend to access social media for healthcare information, advice, and social support. Regardless of usage motives, a majority of healthcare clinicians perceive social media as beneficial to their patients. Some identified benefits of social media use include increased interactions with others, easily accessible and tailored information, social and emotional support, and public health surveillance.[57] The nature of social media involvement by healthcare professionals can vary from direct engagement with patients for the purpose of communication to participation in online health networks dedicated to specific health and wellness issues.[52] Additionally, clinicians can guide patients and families to use social media during the illness trajectory in order to maximize the benefits of their use such as self-management of chronic conditions.[58] A systematic review of the effects of social media on patients and their relationships with healthcare professionals concluded that patient empowerment through the use of social media equalized the power imbalance between patients and healthcare professionals, leading to increased quality of clinical decision-making.[59] Additionally, patients' use of social media positively impacted their perception of their relationship with their healthcare clinician and improved their sense of empowerment.[60] Furthermore, social media interventions have shown some promise for cancer prevention and management by providing combinations of targeted, reliable information and social support.[61] Social media may also be a source of feedback to clinicians. For example, a study conducted in Japan in 2015 concentrated on Japanese men and women with a diagnosis of lung cancer in various stages.[62] Through analysis of 100 blog posts, the authors identified several themes. In general, the content focused on feelings of dissatisfaction and anxiety in patients with cancer and their families and relationships with medical staff, insights not assessed in previous surveys. Most notably, researchers concluded that when comparing illness blog content to voluntary records from previous surveys conducted by the healthcare institution, illness blogs were predicted to be more representative of patients' true thoughts and feelings.

Case Study: Facebook and Useful Resources

A registered nurse (RN) on a pediatric oncology unit was caring for a 10-year-old newly diagnosed with neuroblastoma. The parents of this child were overwhelmed with fear and anxiety and were having a difficult time tracking conversations with the doctors and the nurses caring for their child. They expressed a desire to learn more about this diagnosis and about available resources; however, they did not know where to begin. The RN thought that online resources may be a good place to start because the parents could review the information at their own pace. The RN did some research and even got the hospital librarian involved and found a Facebook support group for parents whose child has been diagnosed with cancer. This site contained all the elements the parents voiced needing. The parents were given this information and voiced appreciation.

The following week the child was admitted to the unit for follow-up with treatment. The same RN was assigned to care for them and entered the room. The parents were notably calmer and came with a list of questions and concerns. They thanked her for the information about the Facebook page and expressed that they have been connected to needed resources.

Questions to Consider:

1. What are some advantages to recommending a social media site to the parents rather than a "medical" website for information?
2. What are some potential drawbacks or concerns in recommending a social media site to the parents?
3. How can the RN work with the unit or manager to ensure that all parents have access to valuable networking sites?

Ethical Considerations

The adoption of social media use among healthcare professionals also carries ethical and professional implications.[63] Concerns have arisen regarding the blurring of professional and personal lines, inadvertent discussion of protected health information, financial conflicts of interest, advertising, and exploitation of patients. Various professional organizations have published recommendations to guide ethical social media use by healthcare practitioners.[64] Additionally, clinicians have a duty to counsel patients and families about potential pitfalls of social media use such as difficulty establishing the reliability of information as well as risks of confidentiality and privacy breach.[57,65] Organizations have an obligation to verify the accuracy of information presented on their sites and disclose conflicts of interest. A conceptual model has been proposed to guide healthcare professionals when identifying and correcting health misinformation on social media.[66] Healthcare professionals have an obligation to maintain appropriate professional boundaries and protect patient privacy. A recent analysis of X data suggests that nearly half of tweet content shared by healthcare professionals about living patients may contain personally identifiable patient information.[67] Chretien and Kind [63] have published guidelines examining the ethical considerations for healthcare clinicians engaging with social media. The authors concluded that clinicians who successfully incorporate the use of social media while maintaining trust and integrity "will be poised to lead this social revolution in healthcare."[63(p1419)]

Conclusion

Social media provides many opportunities for individuals to connect with one another. These connections are important in leveraging social capital, especially during an illness experience. Current research supports the use of social media as a method for public storytelling, with many benefits to the person with serious illness and family members. Benefits for the persons with serious illness include mustering social support, combating isolation, comparing and sharing information with others in similar circumstances, and providing a venue for self-expression. Family members may benefit in terms of facilitating sense-making, garnering social support, enhancing family communication, and, in the event of death, leaving a legacy.

REFERENCES

1. Gavilanes JM, Flatten TC, Brettel M. Content strategies for digital consumer engagement in social networks: why advertising is an antecedent of engagement. *J Advert.* 2018;47(1):4–23. https://doi.org/10.1080/00913367.2017.1405751.
2. Van Dijck J. *The Culture of Connectivity: A Critical History of Social Media.* Oxford University Press; 2013.
3. Internet Live Stats—Internet Usage & Social Media Statistics. Accessed September 21, 2022. https://www.internetlivestats.com/.
4. Carrigan M. *Social Media for Academics.* Sage; 2019.
5. Wong L. 9 Types of Social Media and How Each Can Benefit Your Business. Social Media Marketing & Management Dashboard. September 2, 2021. Accessed October 1, 2022. https://blog.hootsuite.com/types-of-social-media/.
6. Lewis K. Digital networks: elements of a theoretical framework. *Soc Netw.* 2024;77:31–42. https://doi.org/10.1016/j.socnet.2021.12.002.
7. Ngai EW, Tao SS, Moon KK. Social media research: theories, constructs, and conceptual frameworks. *Int J Inf Manag.* 2015;35(1):33–44. https://doi.org/10.1016/j.ijinfomgt.2014.09.004.
8. Dubos R. *Social Capital: Theory and Research.* Routledge; 2017.
9. Poecze F, Strauss C. Social capital on social media—concepts, measurement techniques and trends in operationalization. *Information.* 2020;11(11):515. https://doi.org/10.3390/info11110515.
10. Ehsan A, Klaas HS, Bastianen A, Spini D. Social capital and health: a systematic review of systematic reviews. *SSM Popul Health.* 2019;8:100425. https://doi.org/10.1016/j.ssmph.2019.100425.
11. Rieger KL, West CH, Kenny A, et al. Digital storytelling as a method in health research: a systematic review protocol. *Syst Rev.* 2018;7(1):41. https://doi.org/10.1186/s13643-018-0704-y.
12. Pennebaker JW, Seagal JD. Forming a story: the health benefits of narrative. *J Clin Psychol.* 1999;55(10):1243–1254. https://doi.org/10.1002/(SICI)1097-4679(199910)55:10<1243::AID-JCLP6>3.0.CO;2-N.
13. Valkenburg PM. Understanding self-effects in social media. *Hum Commun Res.* 2017;43(4):477–490. https://doi.org/10.1111/hcre.12113.
14. Gerger H, Werner CP, Gaab J, Cuijpers P. Comparative efficacy and acceptability of expressive writing treatments compared with psychotherapy, other writing treatments, and waiting list control for adult trauma survivors: a systematic review and network meta-analysis. *Psychol Med.* 2022;52(15):3484–3496. https://doi.org/10.1017/S0033291721000143.
15. Zachariae R, O'Toole MS. The effect of expressive writing intervention on psychological and physical health outcomes in cancer patients—a systematic review and meta-analysis. *Psychooncology.* 2015;24(11):1349–1359. https://doi.org/10.1002/pon.3802.
16. Lee H, Fawcett J, DeMarco R. Storytelling/narrative theory to address health communication with minority populations. *Appl Nurs Res.* 2016;30:58–60. https://doi.org/10.1016/j.apnr.2015.09.004.
17. Nicholls S. Beyond expressive writing: evolving models of developmental creative writing. *J Health Psychol.* 2009;14(2):171–180. https://doi.org/10.1177/1359105308100201.

18. Karnaze MM, Levine LJ. Sadness, the architect of cognitive change. In: Lench HC, ed. *The Function of Emotions: When and Why Emotions Help Us*. Springer International Publishing; 2018:45–58. https://doi.org/10.1007/978-3-319-77619-4_4.
19. Schreiner M, Fischer T, Riedl R. Impact of content characteristics and emotion on behavioral engagement in social media: literature review and research agenda. *Electron Commer Res*. 2021;21(2):329–345. https://doi.org/10.1007/s10660-019-09353-8.
20. Syrdal HA, Briggs E. Engagement with social media content: a qualitative exploration. *J Mark Theory Pract*. 2018;26(1–2):4–22. https://doi.org/10.1080/10696679.2017.1389243.
21. Miller TT, Maurer SH, Felker JT. Searching for a cure on Facebook: patterns of social media use amongst caregivers of children with brain tumors. *Cancer Med*. 2022;11(17):3323–3331. https://doi.org/10.1002/cam4.4693.
22. Rukundo A, Fox S, Guerin S, et al. How blogs support the transfer of knowledge into practice in the field of dementia palliative care: a survey of facilitators and barriers. *BMC Palliat Care*. 2022;21(1):117. https://doi.org/10.1186/s12904-022-01001-7.
23. Khan MN, Faraz A, Jamal AB, et al. A study to see the effect of social media usage among healthcare providers. *Cureus*. 2021;13(7):e16350. https://doi.org/10.7759/cureus.16350.
24. Heilferty CM. "Hopefully this will all make sense at some point": meaning and performance in illness blogs. *J Pediatr Oncol Nurs*. 2018;35(4):287–295. https://doi.org/10.1177/104345421 8764880.
25. Heilferty CM. Toward a theory of online communication in illness: concept analysis of illness blogs. *J Adv Nurs*. 2009;65(7):1539–1547. .https://doi.org/10.1111/j.1365-2648.2009.04996.x.
26. Hansen DM, Sheehan D, Stephenson P. The caregiver's experience with an illness blog: a pilot study. *J Hosp Palliat Nurs*. 2016;18(5):464–469. https://doi.org/10.1097/NJH.000000000 0000276.
27. Rains SA, Keating DM. Health blogging: an examination of the outcomes associated with making public, written disclosures about health. *Commun Res*. 2015;42(1):107–133. https://doi.org/ 10.1177/0093650212458952
28. Gage-Bouchard EA, LaValley S, Mollica M, Beaupin LK. Cancer communication on social media: examining how cancer caregivers use Facebook for cancer-related communication. *Cancer Nurs*. 2017;40(4):332–338. https://doi.org/10.1097/NCC.00000 00000000418.
29. Gilmour J, Machin T, Brownlow C, Jeffries C. Facebook-based social support and health: a systematic review. *Psychol Pop Media*. 2020;9:328–346. https://doi.org/10.1037/ppm0000246.
30. Benson JJ, Parker Oliver D, Washington KT, et al. Online social support groups for informal caregivers of hospice patients with cancer. *Eur J Oncol Nurs*. 2020;44:101698. https://doi.org/10.1016/ j.ejon.2019.101698.
31. Parker Oliver D, Washington KT, Benson J, et al. Facebook online support groups for hospice family caregivers of advanced cancer patients: protocol, facilitation skills and promising outcomes. *J Soc Work End Life Palliat Care*. 2022;18(2):146–159. https://doi.org/ 10.1080/15524256.2022.2046236.
32. Buehler EM, Youngvorst LJ. Online support-seeking in the context of grief: how support-seeking message content and communication channels shape support providers' impressions of the bereaved. *Comput Hum Behav*. 2022;137:107428. https://doi.org/ 10.1016/j.chb.2022.107428.
33. Valle CG, Tate DF, Mayer DK, Allicock M, Cai J. A randomized trial of a Facebook-based physical activity intervention for young adult cancer survivors. *J Cancer Surviv*. 2013;7(3):355–368. https://doi.org/10.1007/s11764-013-0279-5.
34. Halwas N, Griebel L, Huebner J. eHealth literacy, internet and eHealth service usage: a survey among cancer patients and their relatives. *J Cancer Res Clin Oncol*. 2017;143(11):2291–2299. https://doi.org/10.1007/s00432-017-2475-6.
35. Tennant B, Stellefson M, Dodd V, et al. eHealth literacy and Web 2.0 health information seeking behaviors among baby boomers and older adults. *J Med Internet Res*. 2015;17(3):e70. https://doi. org/10.2196/jmir.3992.
36. Singh GK, Rego J, Chambers S, Fox J. Health professionals' perspectives of the role of palliative care during COVID-19: content analysis of articles and blogs posted on Twitter. *Am J Hosp Palliat Med*. 2022;39(4):487–493. https://doi.org/10.1177/1049909121 1024202.
37. Jain N, Zachary I, Boren S. Who influences cancer conversations on Twitter?: a comparative surveillance of cancer communications. In: *MEDINFO 2021: One World, One Health—Global Partnership for Digital Innovation*. IOS Press; 2022:719–723. https://doi.org/ 10.3233/SHTI220172.
38. Generous MA, Keeley MP. Exploring the connection between end-of-life relational communication and personal growth after the death of a loved one. *Omega (Westport)*. 2022;84(3):792–810. https://doi.org/10.1177/0030222820915312.
39. Keeley MP, Generous MA. Final conversations: overview and practical implications for patients, families, and healthcare workers. *Behav Sci*. 2017;7(2):17. https://doi.org/10.3390/bs7020017.
40. Sterba KR, Zapka J, Cranos C, Laursen A, Day TA. Quality of life in head and neck cancer patient-caregiver dyads: a systematic review. *Cancer Nurs*. 2016;39(3):238–250. https://doi.org/10.1097/ NCC.0000000000000281.
41. Wittenberg E, Buller H, Ferrell B, Koczywas M, Borneman T. *Understanding Family Caregiver Communication to Provide Family-Centered Cancer Care*. Elsevier; 2017.
42. Hansen DM, Higgins PA, Warner CB, Mayo MM. Exploring family relationships through associations of comfort, relatedness states, and life closure in hospice patients: a pilot study. *Palliat Support Care*. 2015;13(2):305–311. https://doi.org/10.1017/S147895151 4000133.
43. Sheehan DK, Draucker CB. Interaction patterns between parents with advanced cancer and their adolescent children. *Psychooncology*. 2011;20(10):1108–1115. https://doi.org/10.1002/ pon.1831.
44. Cunliffe A, Coupland C. From hero to villain to hero: making experience sensible through embodied narrative sensemaking. *Hum Relat*. 2012;65(1):63–88. https://doi.org/10.1177/001872671 1424321.
45. Stephenson PS, Sheehan D, Hansen D, Mayo MM. Uncertainties experienced by family members when one parent is dying. *Int J Palliat Nurs*. 2015;21(10):488–494. https://doi.org/10.12968/ ijpn.2015.21.10.488.
46. Kim B, Gillham DM. The experience of young adult cancer patients described through online narratives. *Cancer Nurs*. 2013;36(5):377–384. https://doi.org/10.1097/NCC.0b013e318 291b4e9.
47. Keim-Malpass J, Adelstein K, Kavalieratos D. Legacy making through illness blogs: online spaces for young adults approaching the end-of-life. *J Adolesc Young Adult Oncol*. 2015;4(4):209–212. https://doi.org/10.1089/jayao.2015.0003.
48. McCosker A, Darcy R. Living with cancer: affective labour, self-expression and the utility of blogs. *Inf Commun*

Soc. 2013;16(8):1266–1285. https://doi.org/10.1080/1369118X.2012.758303.
49. Coop H, Marlow C. Do we prepare patients for their digital legacy? A survey of palliative care professionals. *Palliat Med.* 2019;33(1):114–115. https://doi.org/10.1177/0269216318802748.
50. Akard TF, Dietrich MS, Friedman DL, et al. Randomized clinical trial of a legacy intervention for quality of life in children with advanced cancer. *J Palliat Med.* 2021;24(5):680–688. https://doi.org/10.1089/jpm.2020.0139.
51. Degroot JM. Maintaining relational continuity with the deceased on Facebook. *Omega (Westport).* 2012;65(3):195–212. https://doi.org/10.2190/OM.65.3.c.
52. Bornkessel A, Furberg R, Lefebvre RC. Social media: opportunities for quality improvement and lessons for providers—a networked model for patient-centered care through digital engagement. *Curr Cardiol Rep.* 2014;16(7):504. https://doi.org/10.1007/s11886-014-0504-5.
53. Guerra F, Linz D, Garcia R, et al. The use of social media for professional purposes by healthcare professionals: the #intEHRAct survey. *Europace.* 2022;24(4):691–696. https://doi.org/10.1093/europace/euab244.
54. Adilman R, Rajmohan Y, Brooks E, et al. ReCAP: social media use among physicians and trainees: results of a national medical oncology physician survey. *J Oncol Pract.* 2015;12(1):79–80. https://doi.org/10.1200/JOP.2015.006429.
55. Antheunis ML, Tates K, Nieboer TE. Patients' and health professionals' use of social media in health care: motives, barriers and expectations. *Patient Educ Couns.* 2013;92(3):426–431. https://doi.org/10.1016/j.pec.2013.06.020.
56. Rolls K, Hansen M, Jackson D, Elliott D. How health care professionals use social media to create virtual communities: an integrative review. *J Med Internet Res.* 2016;18(6):e166. https://doi.org/10.2196/jmir.5312.
57. Moorhead SA, Hazlett DE, Harrison L, Carroll JK, Irwin A, Hoving C. A new dimension of health care: systematic review of the uses, benefits, and limitations of social media for health communication. *J Med Internet Res.* 2013;15(4):e85. https://doi.org/10.2196/jmir.1933.
58. De Angelis G, Wells GA, Davies B, et al. The use of social media among health professionals to facilitate chronic disease self-management with their patients: a systematic review. *Digit Health.* 2018;4:2055207618771416. https://doi.org/10.1177/2055207618771416.
59. Smailhodzic E, Hooijsma W, Boonstra A, Langley DJ. Social media use in healthcare: a systematic review of effects on patients and on their relationship with healthcare professionals. *BMC Health Serv Res.* 2016;16(1):442. https://doi.org/10.1186/s12913-016-1691-0.
60. Benetoli A, Chen TF, Aslani P. How patients' use of social media impacts their interactions with healthcare professionals. *Patient Educ Couns.* 2018;101(3):439–444. https://doi.org/10.1016/j.pec.2017.08.015.
61. Han CJ, Lee YJ, Demiris G. Interventions using social media for cancer prevention and management: a systematic review. *Cancer Nurs.* 2018;41(6):E19–E31. https://doi.org/10.1097/NCC.0000000000000534.
62. Sato A, Aramaki E, Shimamoto Y, Tanaka S, Kawakami K. Blog posting after lung cancer notification: content analysis of blogs written by patients or their families. *JMIR Cancer.* 2015;1(1):e5. https://doi.org/10.2196/cancer.3883.
63. Chretien KC, Kind T. Social media and clinical care: ethical, professional, and social implications. *Circulation.* 2013;127(13):1413–1421. https://doi.org/10.1161/CIRCULATIONAHA.112.128017.
64. Hennessy CM, Smith CF, Greener S, Ferns G. Social media guidelines: a review for health professionals and faculty members. *Clin Teach.* 2019;16(5):442–447. https://doi.org/10.1111/tct.13033.
65. Wang Y, McKee M, Torbica A, Stuckler D. Systematic literature review on the spread of health-related misinformation on social media. *Soc Sci Med.* 2019;240:112552. https://doi.org/10.1016/j.socscimed.2019.112552.
66. Bautista JR, Zhang Y, Gwizdka J. Healthcare professionals' acts of correcting health misinformation on social media. *Int J Med Inf.* 2021;148:104375. https://doi.org/10.1016/j.ijmedinf.2021.104375.
67. Ahmed W, Jagsi R, Gutheil TG, Katz MS. Public disclosure on social media of identifiable patient information by health professionals: content analysis of Twitter data. *J Med Internet Res.* 2020;22(9):e19746. https://doi.org/10.2196/19746.

75

Career Advancement in Palliative Care

Katherine Stackhouse

Key Points

- Career advancement starts with continuing education, knowledge, and sharing experiences, which promote continuous growth and learning.
- Professional development is essential for quality, consistent, evidence-based hospice and palliative care nursing practice.
- Mentorship in hospice and palliative nursing can lead to positive professional growth, improved job performance, increased research productivity, and promotions.
- Maintaining professional boundaries will ensure dignity and equity of care for all members of the patient and team members.

> Let us never consider ourselves finished nurses. We must be learning all of our lives.
>
> —Florence Nightingale

Career advancement in palliative care can be achieved through a combination of education, experience, and professional networking. Palliative care nursing professionals typically have a degree in nursing, social work, or another healthcare-related field. There are also advanced degrees such as a master of science in palliative care, to gain specialized knowledge and skills. Additionally, obtaining certification as a certified hospice and palliative nurse or advanced certified hospice and palliative nurse can demonstrate your expertise and commitment to the field. Palliative care nurses gain experience in a variety of settings which broaden their knowledge and skills and develop a more comprehensive understanding of the needs of patients and families living with serious illness. Building a professional network and participating as a mentee or mentor can help the nurse stay up to date on the latest trends and best practices in palliative care. Attending conferences, workshops, professional organizations, and online forums and discussion groups can build and maintain a network within the hospice and palliative care community. Seeking out leadership opportunities can expand responsibilities, lead to mentoring others, and contribute to the impact of palliative care. Keeping up with the latest research, policies, and trends in palliative care is essential for advancing your career. Subscribing and reading academic journals, attending conferences, and participating in continuing education programs will allow the hospice and palliative nurse to stay informed and engaged. Continual advancement in a career in palliative care can make a positive impact on the lives of patients and families facing serious illness.

Career advancement is a requirement for nurses to continue to flourish and develop in their profession. Education is a primary driver for safe, high-quality patient care. Hospice and palliative nurses need fundamental knowledge and skills in palliative care.[1,2] Ongoing professional development and engaging in lifelong learning are imperative for nurses. Nurses need to reach the level of practice that they are capable of, which depends on their competence and success.[3] One evidence-based process for professional development is performing a needs assessment of your current knowledge and understanding that pulls out what strengths and weaknesses there are to improve on. This will provide a general gauge of current knowledge and skills.[4]

Many national and international resources are available, which include professional organizations, formal structured educational programs, palliative and hospice research journals, and conferences.

Novice and competent learners look to experts for guidance and mentorship. Consider being present at regional, national, or international conferences. Certificate, advanced degree, and fellowship programs can provide a structured approach to professional development.[4] Collaborate with peers and members of the interdisciplinary team by participating in research, community services, and professional organizations that provide opportunities to obtain roles in committee membership and chair and board appointments, which will include networking, developing professional relationships, and collaboration with interdisciplinary members of the team. If you are interested in becoming a voice for change, consider servicing on a policymaking board. Start with a list of what matters most to you and then research agencies that serve that population. Be able to articulate why you want to serve on a board. Network and tell others that you are interested in serving on a board, and ask for their assistance in getting nominated. Consider signing up for board opportunities such as https://www.nursesonboardscoalition.org/[5] as they aim to help the health of communities and the nation through the services of nurses on boards and other bodies. Lastly, consider certificate, advanced degree, and fellowship programs that can provide a structured approach to professional development.[4]

Professional development in hospice and palliative nursing involves five pillars of excellence: advocacy, research and scholarship, education/continuing professional development, continuing competence, and leadership.[6] Professional development is essential for implementation of quality, consistent, evidence-based hospice and palliative nursing practice. Nurses require a complex skill set that ranges from personal to organizational levels to achieve career advancement.[3] Professional development can be compared to Benner's novice to expert continuum. With Benner's seminal work *From Novice to Expert* (1982), a structure for nurses' skill acquisition was created, which is an adaptation of the Dreyfus and Dreyfus (1980) competency model.[4] Benner's novice to expert model is one of the most useful conceptual frameworks that guides the professional development of nurses in individualized care perceptions and practices throughout their clinical experiences.[7] There is a continuum of growth depending on the level of nursing practice that includes novice, advanced beginner, competent, proficient, and expert.[4] Some areas of professional development may include management and leadership training, advancing skills in advanced technology, teamwork and interpersonal skills training, taking a management/leadership position, and obtaining professional certifications or advanced nursing degrees.

There are many benefits, challenges, and processes for engaging in professional development. One of the largest barriers to professional development that can lead to career advancement is lack of time and limited resources. Depending on nursing setting and workload structure, time to develop and refine a skill set that will augment the nurse's practice may be limited. Lack of success and growth limited educators and mentors also contribute to lack of success and growth in an individual's nursing practice.[4] Technical skills gradually shift to interpersonal skill sets that eventually lead to better performance and promotion. Different professional levels of nursing require a variety of organizational expectations and are not always clearly defined. Interpersonal and social interactions influence how and when promotions happen. Identification of the skills required for promotion and career advancement is best done by connecting with a mentor.[3]

Invest in Professional Development

Hospice and palliative care nursing maintains a holistic philosophy of care that focuses on delivering care to individuals with serious illness and their families, individuals within specific disease populations, and those with palliative care needs within the healthcare system and society.[8]

Pursuing professional development and career advancement in hospice and palliative care includes gaining valuable clinical experience, earning continuing nursing education, and pursuing certification in a specialty area. When working on professional development, focus on identifying your passions and interests. Start with a global goal and break it down into smaller stepping stones to arrive at the finish line. Set milestones to keep motivated. Some methods to facilitate professional development include maintaining competency in healthcare technology and software, pursuing a higher degree or certificate, joining a professional organization, attending or leading leadership workshops, and becoming a speaker or presenter at a local, regional, or national conference on a topic that you are passionate about.[9]

Hospice and Palliative Care Specialty Certification

Professional certification is a measure of distinctive nursing practice that validates advanced knowledge in a specialty and implies ongoing high achievement through recertification.[10] Among certified nurses, 95% report a change in their nursing practice after becoming certified, which has a positive effect on the quality of patient care, demonstrates value to healthcare stakeholders, decreases nursing turnover and vacancy rates, and increases patient satisfaction scores.[10]

Specialty certification is a voluntary and self-directed endeavor with intrinsic and extrinsic values. Intrinsic values associated with specialty certification include personal accomplishment, validation of knowledge, personal commitment, satisfaction and growth, professional credibility, and challenge, which enhances confidence and autonomy. Extrinsic values associated with specialty certification include increased marketability, employer recognition, professional and peer recognition, consumer confidence, and salary.[10]

A few identified barriers to specialty certification include eligibility, cost of exams and continuing education to recertify, lack of institutional reward, lace of access to preparation courses or materials, not enough time to prepare for the exam, test-taking anxiety, fear of failure, no desire or interest in certification, and failing the first attempt.[10] To overcome these barriers, nurses can schedule time with study groups or attend review courses provided on behalf of the employer. Look into hospice and palliative nursing education that is on-demand, which is easier to access than a live, synchronous class. Request reimbursement and salary increase from an employer as this may have not been part of the financial budget prior to the request.

Hospice and palliative nurses should maintain competencies to ensure a high standard of care by following clinical practice guidelines for quality palliative care, which promote quality through organized and structured evaluation of care.[1,11] The guidelines include criteria for outcome data and promote the use of sound instruments, serving not only as a resource for all palliative care practitioners but also as a comprehensive blueprint for high-quality palliative care services across healthcare settings and populations. The guidelines emphasize professional competence (achieved by education) and specialty certification (achieved by assessing education and practice) at the program and individual levels.[1,11] Hospice and palliative nurses ensure quality by facilitating its implementation within their work settings. They must champion high-quality care by supporting and driving continuous quality, which will lead to personal accomplishment and satisfaction, validation of specialty nursing knowledge, professional credibility, increased marketability and employer recognition, professional growth, and promotion of hospice and palliative care.

Mentorship has been proven in the literature to support professional development and offer a path to success for both the mentor and mentee. There are many benefits of mentorship, which can include personal or professional rewards. Personal benefits include a chance to share knowledge and experience leading to fulfillment when witnessing the mentee's successes. Professional benefits include professional growth, improved job performance, increased research productivity and promotions, and the opportunity to create new collaboration with others.[12]

Mentorship in hospice and palliative care enhances mentees' clinical skills, instills appropriate attitudes and practices in caring for dying patients, and advances the reputation of the organization.[8] The majority of clinicians in hospice and palliative care spend most of their time in clinical practice and teaching, which lends itself to unique struggles related to academic and career advancement.[13] Building a portfolio of scholarly work is important when seeking advancement or promotion.[13] There are barriers in hospice and palliative care to effective mentoring, which include protected time, availability of mentors, and different expectations of the stakeholders involved.[12] Hospice and palliative clinicians risk burnout from the demands of emotionally intense clinical work and high expectations of scholarly productivity.[14] Pressures are particularly applicable to female clinicians, individuals from underrepresented cultural groups, and those who act as primary caregivers for family members.[14] In order to maintain resiliency, hospice and palliative clinicians require the support of effective mentors. Mentors can include a formal relationship or a less hierarchical relationship called "friendtorship." Friendtors are peers with shared interests who enjoy a personal connection while also intentionally supporting each other's career development.[14] These relationships are found to have more honest and frequent feedback, which leads to a deeper authentic discussion of personal and professional challenges.[14] These relationships may be invaluable to the hospice and palliative clinician as they face shifting personal and professional priorities throughout the career trajectory.[14]

To serve as a mentor and example to others in the hospice and palliative specialty, coach and mentor others through feedback, observation, ongoing education, and support. Contribute to a supportive and healthy work environment by sharing knowledge and skills with colleagues. Provide peers with constructive feedback, and interact with colleagues regarding their performance. Participate in the development and implementation of educational programs for peers, interdisciplinary team members, and the community you serve. Consider participating in hospice and palliative fellowship programs, which often assist in initiating a relationship between the mentor and mentee. Many nurses have been paired with preceptors but not necessarily mentors in their workplace. What makes mentors different is that they most often do not work in the same place as the mentee and do not have direct supervision over their performance. Mentorship is a confidential relationship and can be for a short or long period of time. The mentee and mentor agree upon designation of goals, objectives, a timetable, and outcomes together, which often involves either in-person or virtual face-to-face interactions.[15]

Develop Your Skill Set

Developing new skills can enhance your success and create the opportunity for career advancement. To gain confidence and experience, build upon your clinical skills. According to the American Organization for Nursing Leadership, advancing new skills involves three key domains: "The Science" (Leadership/Business Skills), "The Art" (Leading Your Audience), and "The Leader Within." These domains encompass essential skills ranging from financial management and strategic planning to personal accountability and conflict resolution, all aimed at fostering success and career growth in nursing leadership.[9] Table 75.1 outlines in detail each of these three key domains.

Achieve practice excellence by ensuring the accuracy of the information you practice and mentor others with. Keep clinical reference books published within the last 5 years, and share best practices with others. Research and use electronic resources that provide current and accurate information in your clinical setting. Review Box 75.1 for reputable hospice and palliative care websites.

Know and follow your facility policies, and seek answers to those parts you do not understand to better observe areas of current practice that do not match the facilities policies. In hospice and palliative care, the Centers for Medicare & Medicaid Services provide important regulations that are imperative to follow to ensure compliance. Understanding these regulations and how they impact the care of hospice and palliative patients can clarify how the business must operate and how you can assist in modeling hospice and palliative standards of care to all patients and families.[9]

Many nurses struggle to find a network of experts they can rely on for advice and mentoring. Look to your specialty hospice and palliative nursing organizations to grow your network of those who are willing to support your professional growth. Volunteer for projects particularly with other expert nurses whom you can observe to further develop your skill set throughout the completion of the project. Even finding mentors with different skill sets can be beneficial in that you can use these interactions to broaden your sphere of influence in your practice.

Professional Boundaries

Hospice and palliative care clinicians are commonly faced with high-intensity emotional situations while working in a team-based system which can easily blur boundaries between patient and clinician or the care team and become compromised.[16] According to the *Future of Nursing 2020-2030* report, 2021, attention needs to focus

Table 75.1 Develop your skill set for career advancement

The science—leadership/business skills	Financial management, human resource management, performance improvement, foundational thinking skills, technology, strategic management, and clinical practice knowledge
The art—leading your audience	Staff development skills Relationship management including influencing behaviors, diversity, and shared decision-making
The leader within	Creating the leader within yourself Personal and professional accountability, career planning, personal journey disciplines, optimizing the leader within Conflict resolution

Source: Reference 9.

Box 75.1 National and International Resources

National Hospice and Palliative Care Organization: https://www.nhpco.org/
National Coalition for Hospice and Palliative Care: https://www.nationalcoalitionhpc.org/
Hospice and Palliative Nurses Association: https://www.advancingexpertcare.org/
American Academy of Hospice and Palliative Medicine: https://aahpm.org/
Coalition to Transform Advanced Care: https://thectac.org/
National Association for Home Care & Hospice: https://www.nahc.org/
Oncology Nursing Society: https://www.ons.org/
Center to Advance Palliative Care: https://www.capc.org/
American Nurses Association: https://www.nursingworld.org/
American Association of Nurse Practitioners: https://www.aanp.org/
Centers for Medicare & Medicaid Services: https://www.cms.gov/
National Institutes of Health: https://www.nih.gov/
World Health Organization: https://www.who.int/

on mechanisms for prioritizing and sharing continuing education and skill-training resources focused on nurses' health, well-being, resilience, and self-care to ensure a healthy nursing workforce.[17] Limiting emotional and physical relationships between patients and clinicians can foster healthy boundaries which lead to a trusting patient–clinician relationship. Ensuring that professional boundaries are adhered to will foster maintaining appropriate roles and ensuring dignity and equity of care for all members involved. Boundaries may also become blurred as the clinician strives to protect personal time and relationships in the setting of demanding professional work. Early-career hospice and palliative care clinicians are particularly vulnerable to these challenges, which ultimately lead to burnout.[16]

Some examples to guide the establishment and maintenance of professional boundaries are to consider the cultural aspects of gift giving, taking care to always serve the patient and not the nurse.[6] Maintain social boundaries such as avoiding social media discussions about a patient or patient experience. Avoid having a personal relationship outside of the work setting. Keep your social relationship focused on the patient. Lastly, consider if your actions will be included in the documentation; if not, they may be crossing professional boundaries.[6]

There are six domains of self-care strategies that can assist in the development of resiliency and sustainability in hospice and palliative nursing practice. Those six domains consist of physical, professional, relational, emotional, psychological, and spiritual realms. Practice personal and professional self-care by being wary of providing excessive empathy, which may manifest as exhaustion, insomnia, physical indicators, and decreased endurance. Do not allow the care of patients to invade personal and emotional space with excessive worry.[6] Self-care and stress management include recognizing that self-care is the cornerstone of clinical practice. Compassion fatigue, moral distress, and burnout are some of the most common triggers of poor self-care and stress. Some examples to guide strategies for increasing self-care and decreasing stress are to ensure one's well-being by eating healthy and taking personal leave during periods of illness. Limit excessive work hours due to limited resources and ensure that expectations are clear.[6]

Maintain Continuing Education

After initial nursing training and certified education, continue education opportunities through in-service training as required by federal, state, and agency regulations. Attend specific in-services and competency evaluations related to hospice and palliative care nursing. Immerse yourself in optional opportunities to read professional newsletters and websites, watch educational videos, and attend classes and regional and national Hospice and Palliative Nurses Association conferences.

Networking

Networking is making a professional connection with others from your interdisciplinary team. Networking provides opportunities to discuss similar problems and solutions and decrease feelings of isolation and can occur in many settings.

Advocate for patients, families, and nurses by reminding other team members and the community about the important role of nursing on the hospice and palliative team. Support fellow nurses when improvements are suggested in the care of the seriously ill and dying and their families.

Plan Your Promotion with Professionalism

Personal, interpersonal, and functional skills are required for promotions in nursing, and evidence shows that the more skilled a nurse is in each of these domains, the higher the rate of promotion.[3] Personal skills include attachment to the importance of work and commitment to professional values. Interpersonal capabilities include establishing positive interactions with colleagues and others in your organization, sensitivity to workplace problems, having the desire and ability to guide others as a mentor, and conducting yourself according to professional ethics. Lastly, career competency or functional skills include experience with tirelessness; and practical commitment to professional duties, work discipline, caring about the profession, and patient care follow-up are all indicators of a nurse's work experience.[3]

To plan your promotion with professionalism, there are a few key actions you can take to get started[8,9]:

- Know your role and responsibilities, and prioritize them. Be aware of your own limitations and flexible to learning new things.
- Be professional, respectful, and open to feedback. Work together with patients, families, and members of the interdisciplinary team.
- When a problem is identified, come up with a resolution prior to discussing it with leadership.
- Accept responsibility for your actions. Be transparent when a situation does not go as planned, and come up with a plan to prevent a similar situation from happening in the future. Maintain an environment that is healing and supportive.
- Engage in socialization with coworkers outside of work to strengthen relationships.
- Be available to help others when least expected.

Plan your promotion by developing leadership and identity as a nurse leader. Surround yourself with colleagues who inspire you.

Box 75.2 Career Advancement Strategies

1. Obtain necessary education and certifications
2. Gain experience in different settings of hospice and palliative care to broaden knowledge and skills to develop more comprehensive understanding of the needs of patients and families.
3. Build a professional network
4. Seek out leadership opportunities
5. Stay informed and engaged

Identify with those individuals you strive to be like—role models, in other words. As you find mentors, spend time with them and build strong, lasting relationships. Use social media to build a professional network and a forum to talk to other nurses. Community is the key to career advancement; surround yourself with nurses who want to go where you are going and who have been where you are going (Box 75.2).[18]

Conclusion

Consider career advancement as a conscious and serious process. Like nursing, leadership is a calling and a commitment. Identify what you are passionate about, and align with an organization that will allow you to achieve these goals. Motivation is a key component in career development, and the abilities to think strategically, transform culture, and have organizational impact are major parts of any leadership role.[19] Consider your strengths in addition to areas for growth. This will help align career advancement decisions from an objective perspective and ensure success in a role that is a match for one's passion and experience.[19]

Continue your career advancement by participating in continuous research, leadership, and mentorship. Hospice and palliative nursing leadership is a vital skill demonstrated across all levels and settings of palliative nursing practice. It is demonstrated by actions to promote access, remove disparities, and ensure quality of care, which is advanced by hospice and palliative nurse involvement with national nursing associations; local, regional, and national healthcare initiative; and other healthcare professionals to enhance the quality of care. Hospice and palliative nursing leadership is transformative, leading to improved care of patients with advanced serious illness and influencing the values of care across all healthcare delivery settings.[20–22]

REFERENCES

1. Hospice and Palliative Nurses Association. HPNA Value Statement Assuring High Quality in Hospice and Palliative Care 2021.https://www.advancingexpertcare.org/education-events/publications/. Accessed March 5, 2023
2. American Association of Colleges of Nursing. CARES: Competencies and Recommendations for Educating Undergraduate Nursing Students: Preparing Nurses to Care for the Seriously Ill and Their Families. 2016. Retrieved February 9, 2023. https://www.sciencedirect.com/science/article/abs/pii/S8755722316300850
3. Sheikhi MR, Fallahi-Khoshnab M, Mohammadi F, Oskouie F. Skills required for nursing career advancement: a qualitative study. *Nurs Midwifery Stud*. 2016;5(2):e30777. https://www.ncbi.nlm.nih.gov/pmc/articles/PMC4993070/.
4. Watts PI, Hallmark BF, Beroz S. Professional development for simulation education. *Annu Rev Nurs Res*. 2020;39(1):201–221. https://doi.org/10.1891/0739-6686.39.201.
5. Nurses on Boards Coalition. (n.d.). *Nurses on Boards Coalition: Improving health through the power of nursing leadership*. Retrieved January 29, 2023, from https://www.nursesonboardscoalition.org/
6. Hospice and Palliative Nurses Association (HPNA). (2015). *Core curriculum for the hospice and palliative registered nurse*, 4th ed. Kendall Hunt Publishing.
7. Özdemir NG. The development of nurses' individualized care perceptions and practices: Benner's novice to expert model perspective. *International Journal of Caring Sciences*. 2019;12(2):1239–1245. Retrieved February 4, 2023 from https://internationaljournalofcaringsciences.org/docs/81_ozdemir_special_12_2.pdf.
8. Hospice and Palliative Nurses Association (HPNA). (2024). *Core curriculum for the hospice and palliative nursing assistant and study guide*, 5th ed. HPNA.
9. Dewald G, Reddy N. Becoming a successful nurse manager. *Nephrol Nurs J*. 2020;47(3):259–265. https://pubmed.ncbi.nlm.nih.gov/32639128/.
10. Garrison E, Schulz C, Nelson C, Lindquist C. Specialty certification: nurses perceived value and barriers. *Nurs* Manage. 2018;49(5):42–47. https://www.doi.org/10.1097/01.NUMA.0000532328.69992.fc.
11. National Consensus Project for Quality Palliative Care. *Clinical Practice Guidelines for Quality Palliative Care*. 4th ed. National Hospice and Palliative Care Coalition; 2018. https://www.nationalcoalitionhpc.org/ncp/.
12. Krishna LKR, Tan LHE, Ong YT, Lui GTC, Lim SY, Phua GC, Yee ACN. Enhancing mentoring in palliative care: An evidence-based mentoring framework. *Palliative Medicine Reports*. 2020;1(1):262–273. https://doi.org/10.1177/2382120520957649
13. Lamba S. Standing tall: Advancing your career as an academic clinician and educator in hospice and palliative medicine. *Journal of Pain and Symptom Management*. 2019;57(1):173–177. https://doi.org/10.1016/j.jpainsymman.2018.11.002
14. Lawton AJ, Daubman BR, Rosenberg LB. #Friendtorship: Cultivating peer mentor relationships in hospice and palliative medicine. *Journal of Pain and Symptom Management*. 2023;65(3):273–276. https://doi.org/10.1016/j.jpainsymman.2022.12.001
15. O'Neill Hewlett P, Santolla J, Devi Persaud S. Investing in nursing's future: mentoring across the profession. *Am J Nurs*. 2020;120(8):58–63. https://doi.org/10.1097/01.naj.0000694592.98888.10.
16. Gierisch JL, Gierisch JL. Where do we draw the line? Navigating personal and professional boundaries. *Journal of Pain and Symptom Management*. 2018;56(5):757–758. https://doi.org/10.1016/j.jpainsymman.2018.08.004
17. National Academies of Sciences, Engineering, and Medicine. *The Future of Nursing 2020–2030: Charting a Path to Achieve Health Equity*. National Academies Press; 2021. https://doi.org/10.17226/25982
18. Three Steps for Career Advancement. https://www.yumpu.com/en/document/read/65169229/georgia-nursing-january-2021.
19. Foster R. Tips for coaching career advancement. *Nurs Manage*. 2021;52(1):56. https://doi.org/10.1097/01.NUMA.0000724924.01297.66.
20. Hospice and Palliative Nurses Association. (n.d.). *HPNA value statement: Hospice and palliative nursing*. Hospice and Palliative Nurses Association. Retrieved February 18, 2023, from https://

www.advancingexpertcare.org/practice-research/statements-hpna/

21. American Nurses Association, Hospice and Palliative Nurses Association. Call for Action: Nurses Lead and Transform Palliative Care. Accessed June 9, 2021. https://www.nursingworld.org/~497158/globalassets/practiceandpolicy/healthpolicy/palliativecareprofessionalissuespanelcallforaction.pdf.
22. Dahlin C. Palliative nursing leadership intensive. *J Pain Symptom Manage*. 2018;55(2):548–549. https://doi.org/10.1016/j.jpainsymman.2017.11.063.

76

Nursing Education

Andra Davis and Megan Lippe

Key Points

- There is a need for palliative nursing care education at all levels of preparation.
- Curricular guidelines and competencies for palliative care provide direction for nursing faculty and students.
- Ongoing evolutions in nursing practice and credentialing impact quality palliative care for patients with serious illness and their families across all care settings.

Introduction

More than 56 million people worldwide need palliative care, yet unmet needs persist for individuals with serious, life-threatening illnesses or injuries and their families (of origin or chosen).[1] The needs of a world population living longer with more chronic comorbidities are met with an insufficiently prepared workforce.[1] Palliative care, an inherent human right for persons of all ages,[2] is optimally provided by an interdisciplinary team to promote quality of life throughout the illness trajectory, including physical, psychological, social, and spiritual domains.[3–5] Nurse educators must redesign curricula that use a palliative care lens to prepare prelicensure and graduate nursing students as well as nurses in practice to truly impact and transform nursing practice and quality of life for persons living with serious illness and their families.[6]

Palliative care education can be considered an important public health approach to providing quality and holistic care to persons with serious illness and their families. Studies have demonstrated the relationship between palliative care education and improved knowledge, self-efficacy, attitudes, competence, and comfort in caring for persons with serious illness among nursing students and nurse generalists practicing across settings.[7–16]

Nurses, who spend more time with patients and their families than any other discipline, assess and care for patients with increasingly complex needs. There are over 3 million employed nurses in the United States, representing the largest sector of the healthcare workforce.[17] Nurses need to be prepared to proactively help patients and families navigate the unique needs of living with serious illness and minimize preventable suffering and crisis use of the healthcare system. Reported in 2018, over half of adults in the United States have at least one chronic condition, with over 27% reporting multiple chronic conditions.[18] The number of people in the 65-years-and-older category continues to grow at an extraordinary pace, with people living longer than ever before. By 2050 approximately 83.7 million will be age 65 and older.[19] Children as well live with a current or lifelong health condition chronic illness, with up to 40% living with one or more lifelong health conditions including asthma, blood disorders, heart conditions, and mental health challenges.[20]

This chapter will present a historical review of palliative care nursing education, followed by an exploration of current practices in educating undergraduate and graduate students, registered nurses, advanced practice registered nurses (APRNs), faculty, and interprofessional teams in palliative care. Finally, we discuss certification opportunities that align with effective palliative care educational preparation.

History of Palliative Care Education in Nursing

Nurses have always cared for persons with serious illness and lead efforts to develop policies and guidelines in palliative and end-of-life (EOL) care. This section will present a historical view of the efforts of nurses to advance palliative care education over recent decades.

1998–2010: Recognizing Nurses' Central Role in EOL Care

The landscape of palliative nursing care education has drastically changed since the late 1990s, with a major shift toward greater inclusion of palliative care within nursing education. Findings in those early years substantiate the long-standing belief that gaps existed in palliative and EOL content in nursing education.

Palliative care nurse leaders recognized the critical need for nursing education interventions to prepare students and the workforce to care for patients with serious illness and their families. In 2000, a team of leaders established the End-of-Life Nursing Education Consortium (ELNEC) and developed evidence-based education, initially targeting practicing generalist nurses. This began a long-standing collaboration between City of Hope in Duarte, California, and ELNEC to improve palliative care through education. The first curriculum, ELNEC-Core, was originally funded by the Robert Wood Johnson Foundation (RWJF) and debuted in 2001.

While progress was being made to integrate palliative and EOL education within practice settings, a gap in standardized generalist or primary palliative nursing care (PPNC) education remained in the academic arena. PPNC is defined as care built on foundational nursing education and expected of all nurses regardless of practice setting.[5] PPNC is holistic person- and family-centered care provided by generalist nurses to optimize quality of life by anticipating and intervening in the human response to serious illness.[5] It is distinguished from specialty palliative care in that PPNC contains the core, fundamental skills needed by all clinicians, including basic assessment and management of pain and symptoms and improving communication skills related to advance care planning and setting goals of care.[5] Specialty palliative care refers to providers equipped with advanced education and certification in this care, addressing more complex and refractory symptoms, possessing advanced communication and conflict-resolution skills, and providing care across settings.[21]

A 2006 survey of graduate nursing faculty revealed that, despite the value of palliative care education, they saw their own programs being only moderately effective in promoting and providing the content.[22] Without proper educational preparation, nurses practiced with limited knowledge of how to attend to the suffering of patients living with serious illness and their families or facing EOL considerations.[23]

The recognition of nurses' expertise and central role in caring for persons with serious illness and their families continued with the release of the Institute of Medicine (IOM) report in 2010 *The Future of Nursing: Leading Change, Advancing Health*, which highlighted key areas for nursing transformation in an effort to meet these tremendous needs.[24] The result of a 2-year initiative by the RWJF Campaign for Action outlined four key messages that significantly affect the future of nursing[24]:

1. Nurses should practice to the full extent of their education and training.
2. Nurses should achieve higher levels of education and training through an improved education system that promotes seamless academic progression.
3. Nurses should be full partners with physicians and other healthcare professionals in redesigning healthcare in the United States.
4. Effective workforce planning and policymaking require better data collection and information infrastructure.

2010–2015: Palliative and EOL Education Expands

During ensuing years, ELNEC obtained funding from various federal and foundational organizations to develop courses that addressed the unique needs of caring for persons in various populations. These curricula are delivered through in-person or online platforms, with some offered in both formats (Table 76.1). In-person ELNEC curricula offerings utilize a train-the-trainer format in which attendees learn content and obtain skills and resources to teach the content in their home institutions and communities. The in-person programs deliver content through lectures, case study reviews, role plays, videos, and breakout sessions for interactive application-focused activities. The online curricula content is delivered through digital modules that contain interactive information, case studies, questions to test understanding, and videos. The majority of ELNEC curricula are structured in topical module format based on key concepts of palliative care. A few newer curricula organize content by National Consensus Project of Palliative Care domains of palliative care[5] (Table 76.1). Beginning in 2004, ELNEC has been expanding their curriculum internationally. Leaders across the globe have adapted ELNEC Core content to fit cultural needs of nurses within their countries, with current translation into 12 languages—Albanian, Armenian, Chinese, Czech, German, Hindi, Hungarian, Japanese, Korean, Romanian, Russian, and Spanish.[25] A growing cohort of international nurse leaders continues to advance education in their countries in an effort to address the significant burden of poor access to palliative care throughout the world.[26]

Since 2000, ELNEC has hosted train-the-trainer sessions with nearly 46,000 nurses and other health-related professionals attending from across the United States. These trainers return to their communities to host courses in clinical and educational settings. It is estimated that 1.4 million nurses and other health-related professionals have completed an ELNEC course, highlighting the profound impacts of ELNEC educational initiatives in advancing palliative care across the world.[25]

Nursing faculty, continuing education providers, and staff development educators consider the ELNEC curriculum as the primary evidence-based curriculum used to teach this vital care.[27–32] Each of the ELNEC curricula is updated every 3 years to reflect the most current practice guidelines and evidence.

In 2015, the IOM requested an assessment of progress toward implementing *The Future of Nursing* report recommendations.[33] The 2015 report found that significant strides had been made in educating more nurses at all levels of practice. The report called out the need to develop and evaluate the transition-to-practice programs, especially their effect on patient outcomes.[33] In addition, the report recommended incentives for expansion of programs to prepare nurses with doctorate of nursing practice (DNP) or doctorate of philosophy (PhD) degrees as well as lifelong learning opportunities. Finally, the report emphasized the need for interprofessional education (IPE) and collaboration.

2016–2019: Primary Palliative Care Education Addressed for Schools of Nursing

PPNC education started to move upstream into academia, to support schools of nursing to integrate this material into their curricula. An important document advancing PPNC education was published by the American Nurses Association and Hospice and Palliative Nurses Association (HPNA) in 2017, who jointly issued a call to action recommending that nurses lead and transform palliative care.[3] The directive states that "seriously ill and injured patients, families, and communities should receive quality palliative care in all care settings. This is achieved by the delivery of primary palliative nursing by every nurse, regardless of setting."[3 (p. 3)]

Recognizing that the long-standing scarcity of PPNC education within prelicensure programs persisted, ELNEC designed a curriculum aligned with developmental needs of undergraduate nursing students. In 2015, funded by Cambia Health Foundation, the ELNEC project assessed the current state of palliative care education in undergraduate nursing programs and developed an online prelicensure ELNEC curriculum. Using the original 1998 EOL competencies and Peaceful Death document as a template, the new Competencies And Recommendations for Educating undergraduate

Table 76.1 End-of-Life Nursing Education Consortium (ELNEC) Curricula Content

Module	ELNEC curricula								
	CORE[a]	UG/NEW GRAD[b]	GRAD[b]	APRN[c]	EOA[c,d]	COMM[c,d]	CRIT CARE[a]	PEDS[a]	GERO[a]
Curricula by ELNEC module number									
Palliative Nursing Care	1	1	1	1			1	1	1
Pain Management	2	3	3	2			2	6	2
Symptom Management	3	4	4	3			3	7	3
Ethical/Legal Issues	4	*e*	*e*	*e*			4	4	4
Cultural/Spiritual Considerations	5	*e*	*e*	*e*			5	5	5
Communication	6	2	2	4			6	3	6
Loss/Grief/Bereavement	7	5	*e*	*e*			7	9	7
Final Hours	8	6	5	5			8	8	8
Leadership			6	9					
Finances				6					
Quality				7					
Education				8					
Perinatal and Neonatal PC								2	
Curricula by National Consensus Project (2018) Domain of Palliative Care number									
Structure and Processes					1	1			
Physical Aspects					2	2			
Psychological and Psychiatric Aspects					3	3			
Social Aspects					4	4			
Spiritual, Religious, and Existential Aspects					5	5			
Cultural Aspects					6	6			
Care of the Patient Nearing the End of Life					7	7			
Ethical and Legal Aspects					8	8			
Communication					*f*	*f*			
Responsible Conduct of Research					*f*				

[a] Core; Critical Care; Pediatric; Geriatric (in-person and online offerings).
[b] Undergraduate/New Graduate; Graduate (online offerings only).
[c] Advanced Practice Registered Nurse (in-person offerings only).
[d] Oncology Advanced Practice Registered Nurse; Communication (course implementation based upon grant funding).
[e] Content threaded throughout curriculum.
[f] Module not numbered by National Consensus Project domain.

nursing Students (CARES) was developed and unanimously approved by the American Association of Colleges of Nursing (AACN) in 2016.[34] The CARES document listed 17 competencies for all undergraduate students to achieve by graduation and makes recommendations for how to incorporate them into core nursing courses.[34]

At the urging of nurse faculty, in 2018, ELNEC and AACN convened an expert panel to develop similar competency statements for graduate education known as Graduate Competencies And Recommendations for Educating Nursing Students (G-CARES).[35] These 13 competencies (eight for all graduate students and five for those providing direct patient care) defined the palliative nursing care professional expectations of master's and DNP students.

PPNC education is not reserved for those in undergraduate or graduate programs. Novice and experienced nurses care for a growing population of persons with chronic serious illnesses and their families. Therefore, in 2019, the ELNEC Undergraduate curriculum was updated to support the needs of nurses already caring for patients at the bedside and reflect rapid changes in palliative nursing care, resulting in the ELNEC Undergraduate/New Graduate curriculum.[15,36]

In summary, recent decades have seen a transformation in both the scope and depth of palliative care education for both practicing nurses and nursing students. Future directions for palliative nursing care education hold great promise for even greater achievements.

Current Landscape of Palliative Nursing Education

The past decade has seen a burgeoning of effort and development of PPNC education. Unfortunately, despite great advances, there is still much to be done to support faculty in preparing the workforce to provide PPNC.[37] The message from the IOM in 2010 is still true today. Schools of nursing must develop and promote competencies in "leadership, health policy, system improvement and change, research and evidence-based practice, and teamwork and collaboration" in order to provide quality care beyond acute care settings and inclusive of the community, public health, and long-term care settings.[24 (p. 6)]

This section will summarize contemporary strategies to support advancing PPNC education for students (undergraduate and graduate) and nurses in practice.

Educating Nursing Students

Education-focused recommendations suggest that PPNC education for undergraduate (prelicensure) and graduate degree–seeking students, and continuing education for practicing nurses and APRNs, be based on the ELNEC curricula.[3] The positioning of hospice/palliative/supportive care as one of the four "spheres of care" in the 2021 AACN *Essentials: Core Concepts for Professional Nursing Education* was a pivotal opportunity.[38] Palliative nurse educators, clinicians, and researchers recognized the responsibility to support this landmark moment by sharing "expertise to build on nursing schools' palliative care educational efforts."[39 (p. 1)] These new guidelines call for schools of nursing to include palliative and hospice (including EOL) care in curricula for both undergraduate (Level 1—Entry-Level) and graduate (Level 2—Advanced-Level) nursing students and have established competencies and subcompetencies needed for future practice. Competence is viewed as a construct that develops over time through education, experience, and professional orientation.[38 (p. 15)]

Revised Palliative Care Competencies

As faculty across the country began studying the new AACN Essentials, an ELNEC-appointed team of palliative nursing care experts and faculty in schools of nursing reviewed CARES (2016) and G-CARES (2019) for alignment with the Essentials document.[34,35,40] The team paid careful attention to refining the CARES and G-CARES statements to reflect diversity, equity, and inclusion as well as other intentional language changes that align with the AACN Essentials. The net result was a reduction from 17 original CARES statements to 15 new statements.[40] The new statements are listed in Box 76.1. The G-CARES revision integrated the original set of eight indirect care and five direct care competency statements into a set of 12 global PPNC statements, mirroring the organization of AACN Essential Level 2 competencies and subcompetencies.[40] These new statements are listed in Box 76.2.

The entire process resulted in updated competency statements that were endorsed by ELNEC and the AACN board of directors. The original intention of the CARES and G-CARES statements, which outline the expected competencies of nursing students upon graduation, remains unchanged with the revised statements. Schools of nursing may use these as guides to incorporating PPNC material into didactic courses, simulation, and off-campus practice-focused experiences.[41]

Box 76.1 Competencies And Recommendations for Educating Nursing Students (CARES, 2nd ed.) for Entry-Level Professional Nursing

Entry-level professional nurses should achieve the following by the end of their formal nursing education:

1. Advocate for and promote integration of palliative care for patients with serious illness or injury and their families across the disease trajectory as essential to quality care.
2. Consider the complex and evolving socioeconomic factors that influence equitable palliative care delivery within healthcare systems.
3. Reflect on one's ethical, cultural, and spiritual values and their influence on relationships in palliative care.
4. Demonstrate respect for diversity, equity, and inclusion as essential for the delivery of culturally sensitive, quality palliative care.
5. Communicate effectively, respectfully, and compassionately with patients, families, interprofessional team members, and the public about palliative care.
6. Collaborate effectively within the interprofessional team to coordinate the delivery of high-quality palliative care across healthcare settings.
7. Demonstrate respect for person-centered care by aligning the plan of care with patient and family values, beliefs, preferences, and goals of care.
8. Apply ethical principles, social justice, and moral courage in the care of patients with serious illness, their families, and communities.
9. Comply with state and federal laws and institutional policies relevant to the care of patients with serious illness and their families.
10. Utilize evidence-based tools to perform a holistic health assessment of pain and other symptoms, considering physical, psychological, social, and spiritual needs.
11. Synthesize assessment data to develop and implement plans of care that address physical, psychological, social, and spiritual needs, utilizing holistic, evidence-based approaches.
12. Conduct ongoing reassessment and evaluation of patient outcomes, modifying the plan of care as needed to be consistent with goals of care.
13. Provide culturally sensitive care that is responsive to rapidly changing physical, psychological, social, and spiritual needs during the dying process and after death.
14. Support patients, families, and team members to cope with suffering, grief, loss, and bereavement.
15. Implement self-care behaviors to cope with the experience of caring for seriously ill and dying patients and their families.

Source: Reference 40.

Supporting Innovative Strategies Integrating Palliative Nursing into Curricula

Nursing as a relational and health-based profession is inherently in need of adaptability, and nursing education must be innovative and responsive to multiple forces including changing accreditation guidelines, an evolving healthcare environment, and advances in technologies, all situated within unique communities. For many schools of nursing, curricular guidelines are moving to a competency-based, rather than content-focused, approach with demonstrated efficiencies in streamlining course material and an enhanced interactive, student-centered learning environment.[38,42] AACN defines competency-based education as "a system of instruction, assessment, feedback, self-reflection, and academic reporting that is based on students demonstrating that they have learned the knowledge, attitudes, motivations, self-perceptions,

Box 76.2 Graduate Competencies And Recommendations for Educating Nursing Students (G-CARES, 2nd ed.) for Advanced-Level Nursing

Advanced-level nurses should achieve the following by the end of their formal nursing education:

1. Articulate the value of palliative care to patients, families, interprofessional team members, and the public.
2. Facilitate access to palliative care as standard practice across the disease trajectory and healthcare settings for persons with serious illness and their families.
3. Respond to dynamic changes in population demographics, socioeconomic factors, the healthcare system, and emerging technologies to improve outcomes for persons with serious illness and their families.
4. Demonstrate leadership guided by principles of ethics, social justice, equity, and moral courage in the advancement of quality palliative care.
5. Engage in strategic partnerships with interprofessional colleagues and community stakeholders to influence policies and quality improvement activities related to primary palliative care.
6. Contribute to the development and translation of evidence-based palliative care practice in clinical, administrative, and academic settings.
7. Utilize advanced palliative care communication skills with patients, families, and team members as appropriate to one's functional area of nursing practice and the professional context.
8. Promote delivery of care that supports holistic assessment and management of pain and symptoms common in serious illness at the full scope of practice.
9. Collaborate with healthcare team members to coordinate culturally sensitive, patient-centered, and family-focused palliative care across care settings.
10. Consult with specialty services for complex palliative care issues that exceed one's functional area of practice and educational preparation.
11. Advocate for environments of care that uphold the dignity of the patient and family during the dying process and after death through culturally sensitive and compassionate end-of-life care.
12. Contribute to an environment that fosters well-being for self, patients, families, and team members to cope with suffering, grief, loss, and bereavement.

Source: Reference 40.

and skills expected of them as they progress through their education."[43 (para. 1)] New resources are available to aid faculty in developing skills in competency-based teaching as well as how to address the spheres of care in curriculum development. Here we report on resources related to PPNC education. For more information, visit AACN Essentials at https://www.aacnnursing.org/AACN-Essentials.

There are notable challenges to incorporating even generalist palliative care concepts, which have included perceived lack of faculty expertise, low priority among faculty colleagues, lack of teaching time, curricular saturation, committee barriers, and costs.[29,37] For faculty less versed in PPNC concepts, the ELNEC-Undergraduate/New Graduate curriculum described above is a resource that can be incorporated in existing courses. The curriculum's supplemental faculty content can be used as exemplars of concepts being taught, such as chronic illness, communication, or nursing ethics.

In response to the new AACN Essentials, schools of nursing are examining ways to overcome barriers and strategies to integrate PPNC education. Through a Cambia Health Foundation grant, ELNEC is engaging schools of nursing to advance excellence in palliative care education.[25] Through peer-led leadership and outreach, faculty have access to webinars and teaching resources available through the ELNEC Schools of Nursing Faculty Corner. ELNEC encourages faculty to explore teaching/learning resources, including simulations and evaluation tools to support PPNC education. For more information, go to https://www.aacnnursing.org/elnec/elnec-faculty-corner.

Furthermore, nurses prepared to provide palliative care in advanced practice roles are also needed. Nurses have many options for furthering their education on the graduate level (i.e., master of science in nursing, DNP, PhD, doctor of nursing science, doctor of education). The demand for doctoral nursing education is growing rapidly in the United States. There is evidence of steady increases in DNP programs, nearly fourfold in the last 10 years, and enrolled students are highly satisfied with their education.[44,45]

The AACN Essentials outline the Level 2 subcompetencies, which are written to address nursing education programs that are preparing graduates for practice in advanced positions.[38] Nurse faculty must prepare both master's degree and DNP students in PPNC. APRNs are particularly poised to lead many aspects of PPNC such as addressing policies to support such care, creating effective environments of care, and overseeing clinical care for uncomplicated palliative care needs.[31] ELNEC-Graduate as well as other ELNEC courses such as ELNEC Pediatric, APRN, or Geriatric can provide valuable training to that end in addition to content already included within graduate education.[25] Beyond PPCN, advance practice nurses can specialize in palliative care at the graduate level including master- and doctoral-level education. Such programs prepare nurses to function as experts in palliative care, providing more specialized direct care to persons with complex serious illness and their families.

Nurses are leaders in providing care across the spectrum of health and illness, and they have an impact on quality, access, and delivery of affordable care. As the population ages and care grows in complexity, PPNC continues to gain momentum in the narrative of care. Nurses will need to be well-educated and positioned to participate and lead in these changes and to promote policies that outline excellent palliative care. Educators must be poised to meet these challenges. Schools of nursing are increasingly standardizing and embedding PPNC content into curriculum and program outcomes for both undergraduate and graduate education.

Educating Nurses in Interprofessional Clinical Practice

Nurses across care settings identify palliative and EOL care as integral to their professional nursing practice when caring for patients with serious illness and their families.[46] Yet, upon entering the profession, new nurses have variable prelicensure preparation and competence to implement PPNC within their practice.[47–49] The extant literature highlights specific areas within PPNC that require further educational preparation such as symptom management beyond pain, supporting patients and families with grief and loss, and similarities and differences between palliative care and hospice.[50] Communication is consistently identified as an area of weakness for new graduate nurses, including engaging in difficult conversations, navigating uncertainty, and advocating within interdisciplinary teams.[48,51] Nurses working with neonates also report feeling uncomfortable discussing palliative care with families.[30] It is well established that negative attitudes, such as feeling scared when facing death (fear of death) and death avoidance behaviors, can coexist in reluctant and avoidant behavior in caring for dying patients and their families.[52–56] Nurses and students both report that these perceptions often stem from lack of education.[57–59]

The need for education and its positive impact is supported throughout the literature. Among themes identified by a large cohort of health professionals ($N = 425$), including 52% nurses, 60% listed education as an identified concern—for families and providers.[60] When surveyed, respondents working in different clinical settings indicate the importance of palliative care as a core concept in nursing education to prepare them to care for patients with serious illness and their families across the life span.[61] Education about palliative and EOL care can facilitate reflection on personal beliefs and encourage transformation through knowledge and experience.[62] A recent systematic and meta-analysis found that for EOL care specifically, educational interventions have demonstrated effectiveness in improving attitudes toward death and caring for dying persons.[63] Standardized educational practices in clinical settings continue to be highly varied, although there is evidence of progress. The need remains to educate practicing nurses across care settings in PPNC and EOL care practices and principles to improve knowledge, confidence, attitudes, and behaviors.[13,64]

Palliative care is inherently interdisciplinary and a well-established exemplar of team-based care.[5] Therefore, educational initiatives should prepare students and healthcare professionals to function as effective members of the interdisciplinary team. Opportunities to provide IPE are embraced in both academic and practice settings. The IPE narrative began in the early 1970s by encouraging academic centers to provide team-based experiences. Head and colleagues summarized the discourse and magnitude of the imperative, which gained traction in 2010 with reports from the IOM and the World Health Organization.[65]

IPE in palliative care can be informed by several key resources. The roles and responsibilities of palliative care interprofessional team members are identified within the National Consensus Project document.[5] The CARES and G-CARES (2nd ed.) statements also provide guidance for the expectations of entry- and advanced-level nurses when working within interprofessional teams.[40] The Interprofessional Education Collaborative has established four core competence domains for IPE across all care contexts: values/ethics, roles/responsibilities, interprofessional communication, teams and teamwork.[66] The new AACN Essentials that inform nursing curricula have an entire domain dedicated to interprofessional partnerships, with interprofessional collaboration threaded throughout the domains, competencies, subcompetencies, and concepts.[38] A Delphi study conducted by Donesky et al. established that high-quality postlicensure IPE initiatives should thoughtfully attend to six characteristics: competence, content, educational strategies, interprofessional focus, evaluation, and systems integration.[67] Each characteristic has definitions and subcategories to further guide IPE initiative development. Dyess and colleagues developed an interdisciplinary framework for palliative and hospice education and practice that emphasizes autonomy, self-actualization, dignity, and community as guiding values for collaboration.[68] Development and implementation of IPE activities are not without their challenges, but several scholars have offered pragmatic solutions to overcome these barriers, such as adjusting activities to meet the needs of all participating disciplines and gaining administrative buy-in or support.[69–71]

Recent, promising trends in extant literature suggest that IPE is expanding within palliative care education. Studies reveal that IPE is a useful platform for engaging students and healthcare professionals in collaborative learning experiences to develop their discipline-specific and cross-discipline knowledge, skills, and competencies.[9,65,69,71–84] Learning together fosters appreciation of the unique and synergistic contributions of each profession and presents opportunities to break down barriers. Many IPE activities are particularly useful in developing individuals' confidence and competence in communicating with patients with serious illness and their families as well as with members of the interdisciplinary team. IPE activities include one-time workshops, simulation, clinical care experiences, case studies, formal academic courses (required or elective), threaded content throughout curricula, and online modules and webinars. Successful IPE initiatives have been delivered in person, online, and hybrid.

While many studies report IPE interventions with nursing (students, nurses, and APRNs), medicine (students, fellows, clinicians), social work, and chaplaincy/divinity, there is a growing body of literature that reflects intentional efforts to include diverse members of the palliative care team, including pharmacy, allied health professions, public health, and counseling/psychology.[9,65,69,71–84] Impacts of IPE initiatives vary across disciplines, warranting careful consideration by educators to ensure the objectives and activities meet the needs of all represented professions. All IPE activities should be developed and implemented by educators and faculty representing each included profession with intentional integration of discipline-specific palliative care competencies into the overall program design.

Despite the advances in IPE, most healthcare provider programs and practice settings still lack formal curricular integration of these concepts.[65] It will take normalization of care and communication within the training milieu before the paradigm in practice can shift. As von Gunten and Ferrell remind us, "the greatest mistake in medical and nursing education and training is to view it as a cognitive exercise."[85 (p. 226)] There is an imperative for academia and clinical practice settings to provide evidence-based knowledge and role-model the skills and practices of palliative care for interdisciplinary team members.[40,86,87]

Palliative Care Organizational Membership and Certifications

The 2018 National Consensus Project's *Clinical Practice Guidelines for Quality Palliative Care* is a roadmap used by numerous nursing educators, clinicians, and researchers to develop palliative care programs, curricula, research studies, protocols, and annual competencies. Now in its fourth edition, the guidelines expand ways to "improve access to quality palliative care for all people with serious illness, regardless of setting, diagnosis, prognosis, or age."[5 (p. v)]

Because of these guidelines and their direction in practice, nurses have a clearer understanding of the importance of becoming better educated and even seeking certification in palliative nursing. Belonging to an organization where nurses can meet and learn from each other is critical to professional growth. The HPNA provides position statements, conferences, and support to registered nurses, APRNs, licensed practical/vocational nurses, nursing assistants, and administrators in advancing their palliative care practice.[88] HPNA educational resources and opportunities include continuing education via webinars, ELNEC train-the-trainer courses, special interest groups, online chats, and published resource books. In addition, national hospice and palliative care conferences provide opportunities to network with other nurses and members of the interprofessional team. Nurses can stay updated on the latest evidence-based practice through articles found in the *Journal of Hospice and Palliative Nursing* and an online subscription to the *Journal of Palliative Medicine*. For more information regarding HPNA, go to www.advancingexpertcare.org.

One of two affiliated organizations within HPNA is the Hospice and Palliative Credentialing Center (HPCC; http://hpcc.advancingexpertcare.org/), the only organization that provides specialty certification for all levels of hospice and palliative nursing. There are currently six certification exams offered by HPCC: Advanced Certified Hospice and Palliative Nurse, Certified Hospice and Palliative Nurse, Certified Hospice and Palliative Pediatric Nurse, Certified Hospice and Palliative Licensed Nurse, Certified Hospice and Palliative Nursing Assistant, and Certified in Perinatal Loss Care.[89] The second organization affiliated with HPNA is the Hospice and Palliative Nurses Foundation (HPNF), which is committed to raising awareness and funding ways to support professional development of hospice and palliative nurses. As a 501(c)(3), HPNF provides scholarships for education, research, conferences, and certification.[88] For further information on HPNF, go to http://hpnf.advancingexpertcare.org/.

Conclusion

Education is an essential component of facilitating quality and holistic PPNC for patients living with serious illness and those who are dying. Without such foundational knowledge and skills, nurses are limited in their ability to advocate, develop resources to create environments, provide access, and sustain systems of care conducive to providing palliative care for persons of any age and across settings.

Rosa and colleagues reinforce the critical impact that PPNC education has on shaping the narrative around the world as well as influencing advocacy and policy.[26] It is imperative that palliative care education continue to move upstream, normalizing the role palliative care has in improving the quality of life of millions of people living with serious illness and their families.

REFERENCES

1. World Palliative Care Alliance. *Global Atlas of Palliative Care*. World Palliative Care Alliance; 2020. http://www.thewhpca.org/resources/global-atlas-on-end-of-life-care.
2. Rosa WE, Ferrell BR, Mason DJ. Integration of palliative care into all serious illness care as a human right. *JAMA Health Forum*. 2021;2(4):e211099. https://doi.org/10.1001/jamahealthforum.2021.1099.
3. American Nurses Association, Hospice and Palliative Nurses Association. Call for Action: Nurses Lead and Transform Palliative Care. 2017. Accessed February 5, 2021. https://www.nursingworld.org/globalassets/practiceandpolicy/health-policy/palliativecareprofessionalissuespanelcallforaction.pdf.
4. Hagan TL, Xu J, Lopez RP, Bressler T. Nursing's role in leading palliative care: a call to action. *Nurse Educ Today*. 2018;61:216–219. https://doi.org/10.1016/j.nedt.2017.11.037.
5. National Consensus Project for Quality Palliative Care. *Clinical Practice Guidelines for Quality Palliative Care*. 4th ed. National Coalition for Hospice and Palliative Care; 2018. Accessed October 8, 2020. https://www.nationalcoalitionhpc.org/ncp.
6. Rosa WE, Ferrell BR, Mazanec P. Global integration of palliative nursing education to improve health crisis preparedness. *J Contin Educ Nurs*. 2021;52(3):130–135. https://doi.org/10.3928/00220124-20210216-07.
7. Smith MB, Macieira TGR, Bumbach MD, et al. The use of simulation to teach nursing students and clinicians palliative care and end-of-life communication: a systematic review. *Am J Hosp Palliat Care*. 2018;35(8):1140–1154. https://doi.org/10.1177/1049909118761386.
8. Ratislavová K, Bužgová R, Vejvodová J. Perinatal palliative care education: an integrative review. *Nurse Educ Today*. 2019;82:58–66. https://doi.org/10.1016/j.nedt.2019.08.003.
9. Lippe M, Johnson B, Mohr S, Kraemer K. Palliative care educational interventions for pre-licensure healthcare students: an integrative review. *Am J Hosp Palliat Med*. 2018;35(9):1235–1244. https://doi.org/10.1177/1049909118754494.
10. Lippe MP, Carter P. End-of-life care teaching strategies in prelicensure nursing education: an integrative review. *J Hosp Palliat Nurs*. 2015;17(1):31–39. https://doi.org/10.1097/NJH.0000000000000118.
11. Gillan PC, van der Riet PJ, Jeong S. End of life care education, past and present: a review of the literature. *Nurse Educ Today*. 2014;34(3):331–342. https://doi.org/10.1016/j.nedt.2013.06.009.
12. Condry HM, Kirkpatrick AJ. Simulation in end-of-life nursing education: a literature review. *Clin Simul Nurs*. 2021;59:98–110. https://doi.org/10.1016/j.ecns.2021.06.005.
13. Li WW, Chhabra J, Singh S. Palliative care education and its effectiveness: a systematic review. *Public Health*. 2021;194:96–108. https://doi.org/10.1016/j.puhe.2021.02.033.
14. Clark SB, Lippe MP. Vicarious learning and communication self-efficacy: a pediatric end-of-life simulation for pre-licensure nursing students. *J Prof Nurs*. 2022;43:107–116. https://doi.org/10.1016/j.profnurs.2022.09.008.
15. Mazanec P, Ferrell B, Virani R, Alayu J, Ruel NH. Preparing new graduate RNs to provide primary palliative care. *J Contin Educ Nurs*. 2020;51(6):280–286. https://doi.org/10.3928/00220124-20200514-08.
16. Mason H, Burgermeister D, Harden K, Price D, Roth R. A multimodality approach to learning: educating nursing students in palliative care. *J Hosp Palliat Nurs*. 2020;22(1):82–89. https://doi.org/10.1097/NJH.0000000000000619.
17. US Bureau of Labor Statistics. Registered Nurses. Occupational Employment and Wage Statistics. 2022. Accessed October 17, 2022. https://www.bls.gov/oes/current/oes291141.htm.
18. Boersma P. Prevalence of multiple chronic conditions among US adults, 2018. *Prev Chronic Dis*. 2020;17:200130. https://doi.org/10.5888/pcd17.200130.
19. US Census Bureau. An Aging Nation: The Older Population in the United States. Accessed October 19, 2022. https://www.census.gov/library/publications/2014/demo/p25-1140.html.
20. Child and Adolescent Health Measurement Initiative. 2018 National Survey of Children's Health (NSCH) Data Query. Accessed October 19, 2022. https://www.childhealthdata.org/browse/survey/archive2021/results?q=7344&r=1.

21. Dahlin CM, ed. *Palliative Nursing Scope and Standards of Practice*. 6th ed. Hospice and Palliative Nurses Association; 2021. https://www.hpna.org/HPNA_Item_Details.aspx?ItemNo=9781558105393.
22. Wholihan D, Tilley C. Fundamental skills and education for the palliative advanced practice registered nurse. In: Dahlin C, Coyne P, Ferrell B, eds. *Advanced Practice Palliative Nursing*. Oxford University Press; 2016:13–22.
23. Achora S, Labrague LJ. An integrative review on knowledge and attitudes of nurses toward palliative care: implications for practice. *J Hosp Palliat Nurs*. 2019;21(1):29–37. https://doi.org/10.1097/NJH.0000000000000481.
24. Institute of Medicine. *The Future of Nursing: Leading Change, Advancing Health*. National Academies Press; 2011. https://doi.org/10.17226/12956.
25. End of Life Nursing Education Consortium. About ELNEC. 2022. Accessed September 9, 2022. https://www.aacnnursing.org/ELNEC/About.
26. Rosa WE, Parekh de Campos A, Abedini NC, et al. Optimizing the global nursing workforce to ensure universal palliative care access and alleviate serious health-related suffering worldwide. *J Pain Symptom Manage*. 2022;63(2):e224–e236. https://doi.org/10.1016/j.jpainsymman.2021.07.014.
27. Grant M, Wiencek C, Virani R, et al. End-of-life care education in acute and critical care: the California ELNEC project. *AACN Adv Crit Care*. 2013;24(2):121–129. https://doi.org/10.1097/NCI.0b013e3182832a94.
28. Ferrell BR, Paice JA, Coyne PJ, et al. Outcomes of a national training curriculum to advance generalist level palliative care. *J Palliat Med*. 2023;26(2):228–234. https://doi.org/10.1089/jpm.2022.0262.
29. Davis A, Lippe M, Glover TL, McLeskey N, Shillam C, Mazanec P. Integrating the ELNEC undergraduate curriculum into nursing education: lessons learned. *J Prof Nurs*. 2021;37(2):286–290. https://doi.org/10.1016/j.profnurs.2020.12.003.
30. Ferrell B, Thaxton CA, Murphy H. Preparing nurses for palliative care in the NICU. *Adv Neonatal Care*. 2020;20(2):142–150. https://doi.org/10.1097/anc.0000000000000705.
31. Mazanec P, Ferrell B, Malloy P, Virani R, Cormack C. Preparing advanced practice registered nursing students to provide primary palliative care. *Nurse Educ*. 2021;46(4):221–224. https://doi.org/10.1097/NNE.0000000000000928.
32. Harwell JH, Lippe M. Impact of ELNEC-undergraduate curriculum on associate degree nursing student primary palliative care knowledge. *Teach Learn Nurs*. 2021;16(3):210–214.
33. Altman SH, Butler AS, Shern L, Committee for Assessing Progress on Implementing the Recommendations of the Institute of Medicine report The Future of Nursing: Leading Change. In: *Assessing Progress on the Institute of Medicine Report The Future of Nursing*. National Academies Press; 2016. https://doi.org/10.17226/21838.
34. American Association of Colleges of Nursing. *CARES—Competencies And Recommendations for Educating Undergraduate Nursing Students: Preparing Nurses to Care for the Seriously Ill and Their Families*. American Association of Colleges of Nursing; 2016.
35. American Association of Colleges of Nursing. Preparing Graduate Nursing Students to Ensure Quality Palliative Care for the Seriously Ill & Their Families. 2019. Accessed 10/13/21. https://www.aacnnursing.org/Portals/42/ELNEC/PDF/Graduate-CARES.pdf.
36. American Association of Colleges of Nursing. ELNEC Fact Sheet. 2022. Accessed May 27, 2022. https://www.aacnnursing.org/Portals/42/ELNEC/PDF/ELNEC-Fact-Sheet.pdf.
37. Nilsson S, Gibson J, Paterson C, Crookes P. Evidence informed generalist palliative care content for undergraduate nursing curriculum: an integrative review. *Nurse Educ Pract*. 2022;64:103447. https://doi.org/10.1016/j.nepr.2022.103447.
38. American Association of Colleges of Nursing. *The Essentials: Core Competencies for Professional Nursing Education*. American Association of Colleges of Nursing; 2021. https://www.aacnnursing.org/Portals/42/AcademicNursing/pdf/Essentials-2021.pdf.
39. Ferrell B, Davis A, Lippe M. On becoming "Essential." *J Hosp Palliat Nurs*. 2022;24(1):1. https://doi.org/10.1097/NJH.0000000000000830.
40. American Association of Colleges of Nursing. *Primary Palliative Care Competencies for Undergraduate and Graduate Nursing Students (CARES/G-CARES)*. 2nd ed. American Association of Colleges of Nursing; 2021. Accessed September 21, 2022. https://www.aacnnursing.org/Portals/42/ELNEC/PDF/ELNEC-Cares-and-G-CARES-2nd-Edition.pdf.
41. Lippe M, Davis A, Stock N, Mazanec P, Ferrell B. Updated palliative care competencies for entry-to-practice and advanced-level nursing students: new resources for nursing faculty. *J Prof Nurs*. 2022;42:250–261. https://doi.org/10.1016/j.profnurs.2022.07.012.
42. Repsha CL, Quinn BL, Peters AB. Implementing a concept-based nursing curriculum: a review of the literature. *Teach Learn Nurs*. 2020;15(1):66–71. https://doi.org/10.1016/j.teln.2019.09.006.
43. American Association of Colleges of Nursing. What is competency-based education? American Association of Colleges of Nursing; 2022. Accessed January 8, 2025. https://www.aacnnursing.org/essentials/tool-kit/competency-based-education#:~:text=AACN%20defines%20competency%2Dbased%20education,they%20progress%20through%20their%20education.
44. American Association of Colleges of Nursing. AACN Issues New Report on Doctor of Nursing Practice Education. 2022. Accessed October 17, 2022. https://www.aacnnursing.org/news-data/all-news/article/new-report-on-dnp-education-2022.
45. McCauley LA, Broome ME, Frazier L, et al. Doctor of nursing practice (DNP) degree in the United States: reflecting, readjusting, and getting back on track. *Nurs Outlook*. 2020;68(4):494–503. https://doi.org/10.1016/j.outlook.2020.03.008.
46. Croxon L, Deravin L, Anderson J. Dealing with end of life—new graduated nurse experiences. *J Clin Nurs*. 2018;27(1–2):337–344. https://doi.org/10.1111/jocn.13907.
47. Cleary AS. Graduating nurses' knowledge of palliative and end-of-life care. *Int J Palliat Nurs*. 2020;26(1):5–12. https://doi.org/10.12968/ijpn.2020.26.1.5.
48. Neiman T. Acute care nurses' experiences of basic palliative care. *J Hosp Palliat Nurs*. 2020;22(2):101–107. https://doi.org/10.1097/NJH.0000000000000622.
49. Malone LD, Anderson J, Croxon L. Are newly graduated nurses ready to deal with death and dying? A literature review. *Nurs Palliat Care*. 2016;1(4):89–93.
50. Price DM, Strodtman L, Montagnini M, et al. Palliative and end-of-life care education needs of nurses across inpatient care settings. *J Contin Educ Nurs*. 2017;48(7):329–336. https://doi.org/10.3928/00220124-20170616-10.
51. Hendricks-Ferguson VL, Sawin KJ, Montgomery K, et al. Novice nurses' experiences with palliative and end-of-life communication. *J Pediatr Oncol Nurs*. 2015;32(4):240–252. https://doi.org/10.1177/1043454214555196.
52. Peters L, Cant R, Payne S, et al. How death anxiety impacts nurses' caring for patients at the end of life: a review of literature. *Open*

Nurs J. 2013;7:14–21. https://doi.org/10.2174/1874434601307010014.
53. Cevik B, Kav S. Attitudes and experiences of nurses toward death and caring for dying patients in Turkey. *Cancer Nurs*. 2013;36(6):E58–E65. https://doi.org/10.1097/ncc.0b013e318276924c.
54. Glaser BG, Strauss AL. *Awareness of Dying*. Taylor & Francis; 2017. https://doi.org/10.4324/9781351327923.
55. Cheong CY, Ha NHL, Tan LLC, Low JA. Attitudes towards the dying and death anxiety in acute care nurses—can a workshop make any difference? A mixed-methods evaluation. *Palliat Support Care*. 2020;18(2):164–169. https://doi.org/10.1017/S1478951519000531.
56. Duran S, Polat S. Nurses' attitudes towards death and its relationship with anxiety levels. *Omega (Westport)*. 2024;88(4):1530–1544. https://doi.org/10.1177/00302228211065963.
57. Tüzer H, Kirca K, Özveren H. Investigation of nursing students' attitudes towards death and their perceptions of spirituality and spiritual care. *J Relig Health*. 2020;59(4):2177–2190. https://doi.org/10.1007/s10943-020-01004-9.
58. Xu F, Huang K, Wang Y, Xu Y, Ma L, Cao Y. A questionnaire study on the attitude towards death of the nursing interns in eight teaching hospitals in Jiangsu, China. *BioMed Res Int*. 2019;2019:e3107692. https://doi.org/10.1155/2019/3107692.
59. Giles TM, Hammad K, Breaden K, et al. Nurses' perceptions and experiences of caring for patients who die in the emergency department setting. *Int Emerg Nurs*. 2019;47:100789. https://doi.org/10.1016/j.ienj.2019.100789.
60. Price D, Strodtman L, Montagnini M, Smith H, Ghosh B. Health professionals perceived concerns and challenges in providing palliative and end-of-life care: a qualitative analysis. *Am J Hosp Palliat Care*. 2019;36(4):308–315. https://doi.org/10.1177/1049909118812193.
61. Kyc SJ, Bruno CJ, Shabanova V, Montgomery AM. Perceptions of neonatal palliative care: similarities and differences between medical and nursing staff in a level IV neonatal intensive care unit. *J Palliat Med*. 2020;23(5):662–669. https://doi.org/10.1089/jpm.2019.0523.
62. Barnett MD, Reed CM, Adams CM. Death attitudes, palliative care self-efficacy, and attitudes toward care of the dying among hospice nurses. *J Clin Psychol Med Settings*. 2021;28(2):295–300. https://doi.org/10.1007/s10880-020-09714-8.
63. Chua J, Shorey S. Effectiveness of end-of-life educational interventions at improving nurses and nursing students' attitude toward death and care of dying patients: a systematic review and meta-analysis. *Nurse Educ Today*. 2021;101:104892. https://doi.org/10.1016/j.nedt.2021.104892.
64. Iida K, Ryan A, Hasson F, Payne S, McIlfatrick S. Palliative and end-of-life educational interventions for staff working in long-term care facilities: an integrative review of the literature. *Int J Older People Nurs*. 2021;16(1):e12347. https://doi.org/10.1111/opn.12347.
65. Head BA, Schapmire T, Hermann C, et al. The Interdisciplinary Curriculum for Oncology Palliative Care Education (iCOPE): meeting the challenge of interprofessional education. *J Palliat Med*. 2014;17(10):1107–1114.
66. Interprofessional Education Collaborative. *Core Competencies for Interprofessional Collaborative Practice: 2016 Update*. Interprofessional Education Collaborative; 2016.
67. Donesky D, de Leon K, Bailey A, et al. Excellence in postlicensure interprofessional palliative care education: consensus through a Delphi survey. *J Hosp Palliat Nurs*. 2020;22(1):17–25. https://doi.org/10.1097/NJH.0000000000000602.
68. Dyess SM, Prestia AS, Levene R, Gonzalez F. An interdisciplinary framework for palliative and hospice education and practice. *J Holist Nurs*. 2020;38(3):320–330. https://doi.org/10.1177/0898010119899496.
69. Lippe M, Stanley A, Ricamato A, Halli-Tierney A, McKinney R. Exploring end-of-life care team communication: an interprofessional simulation study. *Am J Hosp Palliat Care*. 2020;37(1):65–71. https://doi.org/10.1177/1049909119865862.
70. Hermann CP, Head BA, Black K, Singleton K. Preparing nursing students for interprofessional practice: the Interdisciplinary Curriculum for Oncology Palliative Care Education. *J Prof Nurs*. 2016;32(1):62–71. https://doi.org/10.1016/j.profnurs.2015.06.001.
71. Kukimoto Y, Maeda K, Yasui N, Nakamura M. Impact of palliative and end of life care interprofessional education for pre-licensure healthcare students: an integrated review. *Am J Hosp Palliat Care*. 2023;40(2):202–215. https://doi.org/10.1177/10499091221108344.
72. Borchers P, Bortz M, Hoffmann H, Seele K, Schübel J. A mixed-methods evaluation of interprofessional education in palliative care: changes in student attitudes towards health professions. *GMS J Med Educ*. 2021;38(6):Doc104. https://doi.org/10.3205/zma001500.
73. Bradway C, Cotter VT, Darrah NJ, et al. An interprofessional education simulation workshop: health professions learning palliative care communication. *J Nurs Educ*. 2018;57(8):493–497. https://doi.org/10.3928/01484834-20180720-08.
74. Balogun SA, Rose K, Thomas S, Owen J, Brashers V. Innovative interprofessional geriatric education for medical and nursing students: focus on transitions in care. *QJM*. 2015;108(6):465–471. https://doi.org/10.1093/qjmed/hcu226.
75. Donesky D, Anderson WG, Joseph RD, Sumser B, Reid TT. TeamTalk: interprofessional team development and communication skills training. *J Palliat Med*. 2020;23(1):40–47. https://doi.org/10.1089/jpm.2019.0046.
76. Ellman MS, Schulman-Green D, Blatt L, et al. Using online learning and interactive simulation to teach spiritual and cultural aspects of palliative care to interprofessional students. *J Palliat Med*. 2012;15(11):1240–1247. https://doi.org/10.1089/jpm.2012.0038.
77. Houle SKD, Lillie E, Richard CL, Slivecka J, Miller A. The design and impact of an interprofessional education event among pharmacy and nursing students in palliative care-RnRx. *J Hosp Palliat Nurs*. 2020;22(4):292–297. https://doi.org/10.1097/NJH.0000000000000657.
78. Pereira J, Meadows L, Kljujic D, et al. Learner experiences matter in interprofessional palliative care education: a mixed methods study. *J Pain Symptom Manage*. 2022;63(5):698–710. https://doi.org/10.1016/j.jpainsymman.2021.12.034.
79. Saylor J, Vernoony S, Selekman J, Cowperthwait A. Interprofessional education using a palliative care simulation. *Nurse Educ*. 2016;41(3):125–129. https://doi.org/10.1097/NNE.0000000000000228.
80. Schapmire TJ, Head BA, Furman CD, et al. The interprofessional education exchange: the impact of a faculty development program in interprofessional palliative oncology education on trainee competencies, skills, and satisfaction. *Palliat Med Rep*. 2021;2(1):296–304. https://doi.org/10.1089/pmr.2021.0045.
81. Starks H, Coats H, Paganelli T, et al. Pilot study of an interprofessional palliative care curriculum: course content and

participant-reported learning gains. *Am J Hosp Palliat Care.* 2018;35(3):390–397. https://doi.org/10.1177/1049909117725042.

82. Thomas S, Calderon B, Ackerman C, Moote R. End of life simulation to improve interprofessional competencies: a mixed methods study. *Curr Pharm Teach Learn.* 2021;13(4):423–428. https://doi.org/10.1016/j.cptl.2020.11.017.
83. Kozhevnikov D, Morrison LJ, Ellman MS. Simulation training in palliative care: state of the art and future directions. *Adv Med Educ Pract.* 2018;9:915–924. https://doi.org/10.2147/AMEP.S153630.
84. Lalloo C, Osei-Twum JA, Rapoport A, et al. Pediatric Project ECHO®: a virtual community of practice to improve palliative care knowledge and self-efficacy among interprofessional health care providers. *J Palliat Med.* 2021;24(7):1036–1044. https://doi.org/10.1089/jpm.2020.0496.
85. von Gunten C, Ferrell B. Medical and nursing education & training. In: Kelley A, Meier D, eds. *Meeting the Needs of Older Adults with Serious Illness: Challenges and Opportunities in the Age of Health Care Reform.* Springer; 2014:225–236.
86. Lappen K. Credentialing, certification, and scope of practice issues for the palliative advanced practice registered nurse. In: Dahlin C, Coyne P, Ferrell B, eds. *The Advanced Practice Palliative Nurse.* Oxford University Press; 2016:23–30.
87. Worldwide Hospice Palliative Care Alliance. About Us. 2015. Accessed October 12, 2022. https://www.thewhpca.org/about-us-3.
88. Hospice and Palliative Nurses Association. About Us. Hospice and Palliative Nurses Association. Accessed October 12, 2022. https://advancingexpertcare.org/HPNA/HPNA/About_Us/About.aspx.
89. Hospice & Palliative Credentialing Center. Certification. Accessed October 12, 2022. https://advancingexpertcare.org/HPNA/HPCC/CertificationWeb/Certification.aspx?hkey=993a4764-2575-4c2e-ac38-203812fc7a0f.

77

Nursing Research

Micah A. Skeens, Amy R. Newman, and Kathleen E. Montgomery

Key Points

- The goal of nursing research is to improve care for patients and their families.
- Nurses have been instrumental in the field of palliative care research and are in ideal roles to be involved in or lead palliative care research.
- Palliative nursing research includes sensitive topics such as suffering, quality of life, communication about death, and life meaning.
- Nurse researchers face many challenges in conducting palliative care research, such as clinician gatekeeping, ethical concerns, financial/time constraints, and openly discussing end-of-life issues with patients and families.

Palliative nursing research should include an international focus to optimize understanding, maximize value and advance the field of palliative care.

Introduction

The ultimate goal of nursing research is to increase the evidence base to support practice and thereby improve quality of care. Palliative care science develops strategies to decrease suffering and enhance quality of life for individuals across the life span living with, suffering from, and dying of serious illness. With their focus on holistic and person-centered care, nurses are poised to not only be a part of palliative care research teams but also to serve as leaders in the field to advance the science of palliative care.

Nurses led some of the earliest palliative care research contributions.[1] Pioneering work by Benoliel and others raised awareness of deficiencies in the care of the dying.[2,3] Early descriptive studies documented the influence of nursing attitudes and beliefs about death on the care provided to patients. Influential studies documented the benefits of different palliative care models and interventions that enhanced patient and family outcomes among vulnerable populations.[4–6] Nurse investigators have addressed aspects of palliative care such as symptom management, bereavement, communication, decision-making, and care of special populations including children and older adults. In addition, considerable work has been done, in an evidence-based manner, to develop robust curricula for training nursing students, nurses including advance practice nurses, and other healthcare professionals in palliative and end-of-life (EOL) care.[7]

In 1997, the National Academy of Science (previously the Institute of Medicine) published a landmark report calling for research to address significant knowledge gaps around care at EOL.[8] In response to this and the growing recognition of the need to further develop palliative care science, several initiatives within the United States were developed to increase palliative and EOL care research. In 1997, the National Institutes of Health (NIH) designated the National Institute of Nursing Research (NINR) as the lead institute of palliative and EOL care research. Table 77.1 highlights organizations supporting palliative and EOL care. In 2006, through philanthropic support, the National Palliative Care Research Center (NPCRC) was developed to provide a foundation on which to develop evidence-based palliative care programs and ensure the provision of high-quality palliative care. Resources within the NPCRC support early career investigators including nurse researchers to obtain the knowledge and skills necessary to build programs of research around palliative care. In addition, pilot grants were made available for researchers to conduct preliminary work, laying the foundation for them to successfully compete for federal research grants including NIH funding.[9] The NPCRC is closely aligned with the Center to Advance Palliative Care, which aims to increase the availability of palliative care to all people with serious illness (www.capc.org). Together they aim to more quickly translate research findings into practice. In 2010, the Palliative Care Research Cooperative (PCRC) Group was established by a group of interdisciplinary palliative care researchers to advance the field of palliative care through collaborative, multi-site research. Similar to the NPCRC, the PCRC provides training and mentorship to early career scientists and funds pilot study work.[10] Through these efforts, palliative and EOL research has increased significantly, as has federal funding.[11,12] Despite these gains, more research needs to be done to continue to advance the science, raise awareness of what palliative care is among the general population, and ensure that more diverse populations of patients living with serious illnesses have access to palliative care.

Goals of Palliative Care Research

Goals of nursing research in palliative care ultimately focus on capturing evidence to improve the outcomes of patients living with

Table 77.1 Organizations supporting palliative and end-of-life care

Organization name/website	
Center to Advance Palliative Care (CAPC) www.capc.org.	A national organization dedicated to increasing the availability of quality, equitable healthcare for people living with serious illness. CAPC provides healthcare professionals and organizations with the training, tools, and technical assistance necessary to effectively meet this need.
Hospice and Palliative Nurses Association (HPNA) www.advancingexpertcare.org	The national professional organization that represents the specialty of palliative nursing, which includes hospice and palliative nurses. HPNA supports the profession through education programs, research initiatives, and advocacy.
National Palliative Care Research Center (NPCRC) www.npcrc.org	The NPCRC aims to strengthen the evidence-based foundation needed for health policy and clinical practice in palliative care medicine by growing and supporting the community of palliative care research scientists and stimulating expanded research and innovation.
Palliative Care Research Cooperative Group (PCRC) www.palliativecareresearch.org	The PCRC aims to develop palliative care research capacity by (1) supporting investigators at all levels of experience in the conduct of clinical studies; (2) conducting nationally representative, multi-institutional studies that include diverse populations; (3) leveraging standardized data elements and a de-identified palliative care study data repository that amplifies the impact of any single study; and (4) providing methodologic resources, participant access/recruitment, and the expertise of PCRC investigators from multiple disciplines.

serious illness. More specifically, research aims to minimize suffering (physical, emotional, and spiritual); enhance care delivery within complex healthcare systems; improve communication among patients, families, and members of the healthcare team; and reduce strain among family caregivers and support systems. A number of national organizations help to establish research goals and priorities for palliative care nursing research. One prominent organization is the Hospice and Palliative Nurses Association (HPNA), a national palliative care organization for nurse clinicians, researchers, and academics. Every 4 years the HPNA Research Committee queries its members and convenes an expert panel to establish research priorities for the future. Once established, these priorities provide focus for nurse researchers, funders, and other palliative care stakeholders.[13]

Priority Research Areas in Palliative Care

Palliative care research priorities were historically established by leading institutes and professional organizations, including the Institute of Medicine, NIH, NINR, NPCRC, and HPNA. Research conducted in response to these priorities led to advancements in symptom management, integration of palliative care in health systems, cultural considerations in palliative care, quality of life of patients and their caregivers, needs of caregivers, and emotional and spiritual aspects of living with a serious illness.[14] With an increasing evidence base and perceived value of palliative care by clinicians, palliative care research priorities have evolved to support a vision of promoting an individual's access to high-quality palliative care.[15] Specifically, there is support for research that (1) optimizes efficiency and scalability of palliative care programming[15]; (2) expands access to palliative care programming across the life span, including pediatrics[13,16,17]; (3) builds the economic evidence base in palliative care and identifies the costs and benefits of palliative care[18]; and (4) addresses racial and ethnic disparities in palliative care.[19] Despite the advancements in palliative care research and early integration of palliative care in clinical care, awareness of palliative care among adults within the United States remains low.[20] Limited awareness of palliative care may threaten future advancements in palliative care research and presents an opportunity for researchers. For example, in a survey of 3,445 adults in the United States, 71% had never heard of palliative care.[20] Adults who knew a little bit about palliative care or could explain palliative care were more likely to be women, to be White, and to have completed at least high school and some college.[20] As palliative care research seeks to increase access to high-quality palliative care, there is an opportunity for researchers to address individual-level factors to increase palliative care awareness and, subsequently, the impact of palliative care research.

The shift in palliative care research priorities is also responsive to changes in the priorities of the NIH and NINR. In 2011, the NINR led The Science of Compassion: Future Directions in End of Life and Palliative Care Research Summit to assess the gaps in knowledge in EOL and palliative care and to further the agenda for future research. Some of the proposed research agenda items at that time were ethical aspects of palliative care, early versus delayed access to care across disease processes, integrated models of palliative care, improved communication, more community involvement, and a need for more longitudinal studies.[21,22] In the most recent NINR strategic plan, palliative care is not explicitly included as a research priority. However, the case for palliative care research remains strong as research that addresses programming, accessibility, scalability, and racial and ethnic disparities may align with one or more of the NINR research lenses. In their 2022–2026 Strategic Plan, the NINR identified five research lenses to promote multilevel approaches, interprofessional collaboration, and community engagement in research.[23] The lenses are (1) health equity, (2) social determinants of health, (3) population and community health, (4) prevention and health promotion, (5) and systems and models of care. Palliative care researchers have potential to apply a single lens or a combination of lenses in their study designs.[23] For example, palliative care research that aims to improve quality of life and decision-making through early palliative care integration for individuals and communities who may be more likely to be diagnosed with illness, have limited access to healthcare, and experience disparate outcomes aligns with the lenses of health equity, social determinants of health, prevention and health promotion, and systems of and models of care.

The HPNA's 2023–2026 Research Agenda[24] identifies several recommendations across five priority areas (Box 77.1). A major priority is supporting research that promotes equitable palliative care. This priority mirrors the NINR's research lens of health equity and

Box 77.1 Hospice and Palliative Nurses Association Research Agenda Priorities

1. Equitable palliative care
2. Local, national, and global disaster/emergency response in palliative and hospice care
3. Well-being of palliative care and hospice clinicians: self-care and workforce development
4. Pediatric palliative and hospice research priorities
5. Transitions in care

incorporates the social determinants of health lens. In addition to equitable access to palliative care, the HPNA set priorities focused on disaster and emergency response in palliative and hospice care in local, national, and global settings; the well-being of palliative care and hospice clinicians; pediatric palliative and hospice; and transitions in care.[24]

As the palliative care evidence base continues to grow, synthesizing literature and assessing readiness for translation of evidence into practice are important research contributions. Literature reviews of all types can be useful in answering research questions important to nurses in palliative care in order to identify gaps in current research and inform future research.[25–28] In one example, researchers conducted an integrative review to examine the evidence regarding patient and care involvement in palliative care research and identify the facilitators, barriers, impacts, and gaps in the evidence base.[29] In another example, researchers conducted a systematic review to report the benefits and burdens of palliative research participation on children, siblings, parents, clinicians, and researchers.[17] Together, the findings of these reviews highlight the need for researchers to engage with patients, family members, and clinicians to illuminate multiple perspectives and strengthen palliative care research.

The continued interest in palliative care research is evidence that there is room for discovery in what nurse scientists know about palliative care and room for improvement in how the information is translated into best practice. The evolving research focus areas reflect significant gaps in the palliative care literature to date and should be used to guide future research directions. Nurse scientists and clinicians must collaborate to identify best strategies to translate findings into practice in a meaningful way if palliative care practice is to evolve and improve based on emerging research.

Benefits and Challenges in Palliative Care Research

Although research agendas exist to strengthen palliative care research and impact, the state of the science has progressed relatively slowly, suggesting the presence of considerable challenges in the field.[30] Research in palliative care includes unique benefits and challenges. Overall benefits of research are ultimately the enhancement of palliative care for those at EOL, yet challenges exist in ensuring they are protected from unnecessary burdens.

While a mention of conducting research with patients who have received a life-threatening diagnosis raises concerns related to their vulnerability, there are also benefits to participants in research during this difficult journey. In fact, studies have shown an underestimation of research benefit and overestimation of research burden at EOL.[17] Specifically in pediatrics, patients, siblings, and parents report more benefit than burden associated with palliative care research. Even when patients feel most vulnerable, having an opportunity to help others through enhancing healthcare providers' awareness and understanding of best practices, symptom management, and access to care is often very rewarding. Participating in research may offer an opportunity to derive some meaning from their experiences and to feel their suffering may even benefit others.[31] Participants may derive therapeutic benefits from telling their stories. In studies involving interviews with bereaved parents and siblings, parents frequently offered positive feedback and thanks to researchers for caring enough to listen to their stories and working toward improving the care of families after the death of a loved one.[32]

Balancing benefit with potential burden of research participation is one challenge. Researchers may encounter this challenge when engaging in the institutional review board (IRB) approval process, with interdisciplinary clinicians, or both. For example, an IRB may have concerns about the impact, including potential for psychosocial distress from talking about sensitive topics, of research participation on vulnerable patients and families.[33] Researchers should be prepared to address potential IRB concerns by describing any previous and future research processes to anticipate and respond to unexpected harm (e.g., psychosocial distress) of participants, use existing literature to support protocol elements, and engage early with the IRB during the regulatory approval process. Researchers may also encounter challenges within their institution, clinical departments, or individual clinicians when recruiting eligible patients. This process, also known as "gatekeeping," is rooted in the assumption of vulnerability of patients,[34] is a prevalent challenge facing palliative care researchers, and has potential to impede scientific advancements.[33] To address this challenge, researchers should engage with clinicians early and throughout the research process to elicit concerns and feedback, while also sharing literature demonstrating the value and benefit of research participation for patients and families.

Staying true to the ethical principles of beneficence and nonmaleficence, as clinicians, nurses strive to enhance a patient's well-being and quality of life while, as researchers, they must be careful not to confound data. Another ethical principle, autonomy, plays into the challenges of gaining informed consent from debilitated and declining patients as nurses strive to protect patient and family independence. Potential research participants may feel obligated to agree to engage in the research, particularly when they are the recipients of high-quality care and feel indebted to providers. While all patients receiving palliative care are vulnerable, some groups, such as children, those with cognitive impairment, the poor, and the elderly, are particularly at risk.[32,35] Funding and time limitations are often barriers to palliative care research. For example, from 2011 to 2015, only 0.2% of all NIH funding supported palliative care research.[12] Telephone interviews with 61 leading researchers in palliative care identified funding and institutional capacity as barriers that limit progress in the field of palliative care.[30] Respondents described a limited number of funding sources and the review process of proposals as blocks to funding. Although community-based palliative care is growing, few outpatient palliative care services exist or have the capacity to conduct research. Palliative care services often are integrated into departments of geriatrics or oncology and may have few dedicated resources for internal research activities. Nurses often serve in roles of recruiters or data collectors for studies. A nurse may have difficulty balancing the role of a researcher with the role of a clinician, wanting to mitigate symptoms rather than assess them.

Design concerns may manifest as challenges to conducting palliative care research. These challenges include, but are not limited to, recruitment and retention of research participants, inconsistent use of terms across studies, access to psychometrically tested measures specific to the context of palliative and hospice care, and challenges associated with longitudinal studies.[36] Potential attrition needs to be considered in determining sample sizes and becomes a real concern when longitudinal studies are proposed, which are definitely needed in palliative care research. Both qualitative[37] and quantitative[38] approaches are useful in the emerging science of palliative care. Definitions of palliative care are disparate and may not be understood by the general population, leading to misunderstandings and potential conflicts. Another challenge is that palliative care is not generally revenue-producing, and its status may not measure up to specialties such as cardiovascular surgery. A research team with members who are passionate about palliative care, knowledgeable, caring, and insightful must be recruited to conduct the research; and burnout remains a constant threat. Interdisciplinary collaboration is a key to success with these complex patients. Finally, serious illnesses are shared experiences, and including families in the research enriches the benefits of palliative care research.[39]

Global Considerations in Palliative Care Research

In the last decade, despite substantial progress in the development of palliative care worldwide, there are still important and significant gaps to be bridged. Specifically, there is increasing evidence and debate on palliative care research priorities and the international research agenda.[40] Priority-setting is recognized as an essential task to help direct finite resources to support research.[41] Priorities are integral to the research process to guide and stimulate funding and to strengthen the role of stakeholders in establishing the research agenda. In palliative care, a range of priority-setting processes have been conducted internationally across different countries, organizations, and networks.[40,42]

Recognizing the need for internationally relevant evidence, initiatives such as the European Palliative Care Research Collaborative have emerged to facilitate the implementation of European evidence-based guidelines in palliative care.[43] Researchers from high-income regions, such as Europe and North America, are undertaking research in low- and middle-income regions of the world, such as Africa. The United States and United Kingdom are the most productive countries in terms of the number of palliative papers published; however, weak collaborations have been observed between low-income or middle-income countries and high-income countries.[44] As research capacity in low- and middle-income countries is low, it is important for researchers in other settings to produce evidence which has international relevance. The extent to which Western researchers in palliative care are supplementing research evidence in other settings is unknown. Thus, there is an urgent need for research collaboration between low- and high-resource countries.[45]

The internationalization of palliative care research raises new issues for researchers, particularly for those from wealthier countries who are conducting studies in poorer regions. Challenges are multifaceted and include a range of ethical issues, such as ensuring the relevance of research to local populations, conducting research to international ethical standards regardless of national regulations, and involving local people and researchers to ensure that research is participatory, with informed consent.[43] Additionally, the lack of palliative care services in some countries offers opportunities to examine human suffering caused by the absence of access to such care. As an example, comparative effectiveness research could be used to examine the differences in patient, family, and system outcomes between regions with and without services.[40]

Palliative care is a field of healthcare with historically a small proportion of research funding[46]; therefore, it is essential to ensure that research value is maximized. International cooperation in health research, specifically palliative care, is a method for promoting knowledge, increasing research capacity, and advancing the field.[44] More international research and cross-institutional cooperation can address more global palliative care issues, potentially leading to higher-quality or more impactful studies. Strengthening the international palliative care evidence base has potential to promote equitable access to high-quality palliative care for all individuals living with serious illness. Thus, there is an urgent need to establish an international network, share ideas, and ensure transparency for increasing partnerships and setting research agendas in palliative care research.[43]

Conclusion

Research is essential to advance the science of palliative care, inform practice, and ensure equitable EOL care across the life span. National organizations establish goals and priorities for palliative care nursing research. Despite continued advancements, awareness, access to care, and research funding for palliative care remain low. Numerous opportunities are available to fund rigorous studies that will significantly impact the field of palliative care and ultimately improve patient care. The palliative care research community is interdisciplinary and collaborative in nature. Nurse scientists should work closely with clinicians to translate evidence into practice and improve palliative care for all. Additionally, a focus on international collaboration and research efforts is necessary. We should continue efforts to support and develop the next generation of nurses to become leading independent palliative care researchers. Nurses are vital to advancing the science of palliative care research and are in ideal roles to not only support but also lead innovative palliative care research that will enhance life and decrease suffering for the patients and families that we serve.

REFERENCES

1. Bailey C, Froggatt K, Field D, Krishnasamy M. The nursing contribution to qualitative research in palliative care 1990–1999: a critical evaluation. *J Adv Nurs*. 2002;40(1):48–60.
2. Benoliel JQ. Death influence in clinical practice: a course for graduate students. *Death Educ*. 1981;5(4):327–346.
3. Benoliel JQ. Health care providers and dying patients: critical issues in terminal care. *Omega (Westport)*. 1988;18(4):341–363.

4. Bakitas MA, Tosteson TD, Li Z, et al. Early versus delayed initiation of concurrent palliative oncology care: patient outcomes in the ENABLE III randomized controlled trial. *J Clin Oncol.* 2015;33(13):1438.
5. Campbell ML, Frank RR. Experience with an end-of-life practice at a university hospital. *Crit Care Med.* 1997;25(1):197–202.
6. Strumpf N, Tuch H, Stillman D, Parrish P, Morrison N. Implementing palliative care in the nursing home. *Ann Long-Term Care.* 2004;12(11):35–41.
7. Ferrell B, Malloy P, Virani R. The end of life nursing education nursing consortium project. *Ann Palliat Med.* 2015;4(2):61–69.
8. Field MJ, Cassel CK. Approaching death: improving care at the end of life. *Palliative Care: Transforming the Care of Serious Illness.* 2010;79.
9. Morrison RS, Meier DE. The National Palliative Care Research Center and the Center to Advance Palliative Care: a partnership to improve care for persons with serious illness and their families. *J Pediatr Hematol Oncol.* 2011;33(suppl 2):S126–S131.
10. Palliative Care Research Cooperative Group. About Us: The PCRC Continues Its Mission and Vision through New Members and Expanding Disciplines. Accessed November 14, 2022. https://palliativecareresearch.org/about-us.
11. National Institute of Nursing Research. Building Momentum: The Science of End-of-Life and Palliative Care. A Review of Research Trends and Funding, 1997–2010. 2013. https://www.ninr.nih.gov/sites/default/files/docs/NINR-Building-Momentum-508.pdf.
12. Brown E, Morrison RS, Gelfman LP. An update: NIH research funding for palliative medicine, 2011–2015. *J Palliat Med.* 2018;21(2):182–187.
13. Romo RD, Carpenter JG, Crescenz CMJ, et al. HPNA 2019–2022 research agenda: development and rationale. *J Hosp Palliat Nurs.* 2019;21(4):E17.
14. Ferrell BR, Coyle N, Paice J. *Oxford Textbook of Palliative Nursing*, 4th ed. Oxford University Press; 2014.
15. Courtright KR, Cassel JB, Halpern SD. A research agenda for high-value palliative care. *Ann Intern Med.* 2018;168(1):71–72.
16. Feudtner C, Rosenberg AR, Boss RD, et al. Challenges and priorities for pediatric palliative care research in the US and similar practice settings: report from a pediatric palliative care research network workshop. *J Pain Symptom Manage.* 2019;58(5):909–917.e3.
17. Weaver MS, Mooney-Doyle K, Kelly KP, et al. The benefits and burdens of pediatric palliative care and end-of-life research: a systematic review. *J Palliat Med.* 2019;22(8):915–926. https://doi.org/10.1089/jpm.2018.0483.
18. Jacobson M, May P, Morrison RS. Improving care of people with serious medical illness—an economic research agenda for palliative care. *JAMA Health Forum.* 2022;3(1):e214464.
19. Gardner DS, Doherty M, Bates G, Koplow A, Johnson S. Racial and ethnic disparities in palliative care: a systematic scoping review. *Fam Soc.* 2018;99(4):301–316.
20. Trivedi N, Peterson EB, Ellis EM, Ferrer RA, Kent EE, Chou W-YS. Awareness of palliative care among a nationally representative sample of US adults. *J Palliat Med.* 2019;22(12):1578–1582.
21. Aziz NM, Miller JL, Curtis JR. Palliative and end-of-life care research: embracing new opportunities. *Nurs Outlook.* 2012;60(6):384–390.
22. Lanctôt A. National Institute of Nursing Research to hold summer conference—The Science of Compassion: Future Directions in End-of-life and Palliative Care. *Altern Ther Health Med.* 2011;17(3):12.
23. National Institute of Nursing Research. The National Institute of Nursing Research 2022–2026 Strategic Plan. Accessed May 9, 2022.
24. Hospice and Palliative Nurses Association. *Hospice and Palliative Nurses Association Research Agenda 2023–2026.* 2022. https://advancingexpertcare.org/research-agenda/.
25. Pollock D, Davies EL, Peters MD, et al. Undertaking a scoping review: a practical guide for nursing and midwifery students, clinicians, researchers, and academics. *J Adv Nurs.* 2021;77(4):2102–2113.
26. Smith J, Noble H. Reviewing the literature. *Evid Based Nurs.* 2016;19(1):2–3.
27. Fink A. *Conducting Research Literature Reviews: From the Internet to Paper*. Sage; 2019.
28. Toronto CE, Remington R. *A Step-by-Step Guide to Conducting an Integrative Review*. Springer; 2020.
29. Chambers E, Gardiner C, Thompson J, Seymour J. Patient and carer involvement in palliative care research: an integrative qualitative evidence synthesis review. *Palliat Med.* 2019;33(8):969–984.
30. Chen EK, Riffin C, Reid MC, et al. Why is high-quality research on palliative care so hard to do? Barriers to improved research from a survey of palliative care researchers. *J Palliat Med.* 2014;17(7):782–787.
31. Alexander S, Pillay R, Smith B. A systematic review of the experiences of vulnerable people participating in research on sensitive topics. *Int J Nurs Stud.* 2018;88:85–96.
32. Akard TF, Skeens MA, Fortney CA, et al. Changes in siblings over time after the death of a brother or sister to cancer. *Cancer Nurs.* 2019;42(1):E20.
33. Mooney-Doyle K, Pyke-Grimm KA, Lanzel AF, et al. Balancing protection and progress in pediatric palliative care research: stakeholder perspectives. *Pediatrics.* 2022;150(4):e2022057502.
34. Kars MC, van Thiel GJ, van der Graaf R, Moors M, de Graeff A, van Delden JJ. A systematic review of reasons for gatekeeping in palliative care research. *Palliat Med.* 2016;30(6):533–548.
35. Blum D, Inauen R, Binswanger J, Strasser F. Barriers to research in palliative care: a systematic literature review. *Prog Palliat Care.* 2015;23(2):75–84.
36. Antonacci R, Barrie C, Baxter S, et al. Gaps in hospice and palliative care research: a scoping review of the North American literature. *J Aging Res.* 2020;2020:3921245.
37. Coats H, Crist JD, Berger A, Sternberg E, Rosenfeld AG. African American elders' serious illness experiences: narratives of "God did," "God will," and "Life is better." *Qual Health Res.* 2017;27(5):634–648.
38. Akard TF, Dietrich MS, Friedman DL, et al. Digital storytelling: an innovative legacy-making intervention for children with cancer. *Pediatr Blood Cancer.* 2015;62(4):658–665.
39. Ciemins EL, Brant J, Kersten D, Mullette E, Dickerson D. A qualitative analysis of patient and family perspectives of palliative care. *J Palliat Med.* 2015;18(3):282–285.
40. Hasson F, Nicholson E, Muldrew D, Bamidele O, Payne S, McIlfatrick S. International palliative care research priorities: a systematic review. *BMC Palliat Care.* 2020;19(1):1–16.
41. Knaul FM, Farmer PE, Krakauer EL, et al. Alleviating the access abyss in palliative care and pain relief-an imperative of universal health coverage: the Lancet Commission report. *Lancet.* 2018;391(10128):1391–1454. https://doi.org/10.1016/s0140-6736(17)32513-8.
42. Spence M, Spencer R, Diffin J, Mellor P, Grande G. Priority setting for end-of-life care. *BMJ Support Palliat Care.* 2016;6(3):399. https://doi.org/10.1136/bmjspcare-2016-001204.39.

43. Clark J, Gardiner C, Barnes A. International palliative care research in the context of global development: a systematic mapping review. *BMJ Support Palliat Care*. 2018;8(1):7–18.
44. Abu-Odah H, Molassiotis A, Liu JYW. Global palliative care research (2002–2020): bibliometric review and mapping analysis. *BMJ Support Palliat Care*. 2021;12(4):376–387.
45. Akinremi TO. Research collaboration with low resource countries: overcoming the challenges. *Infect Agent Cancer*. 2011;6(suppl 2):S3. https://doi.org/10.1186/1750-9378-6-S2-S3.
46. Higginson IJ. Research challenges in palliative and end of life care. *BMJ Support Palliat Care*. 2016;6(1):2–4. https://doi.org/10.1136/bmjspcare-2015-001091.

78

Developing and Implementing Quality Improvement Programs across Settings

Sean M. Reed

Key Points

- Palliative care programs must demonstrate value through a comprehensive equation that balances quality (consistency in care), safety (harm prevention), service (stakeholder engagement), and cost/resource utilization. This framework helps justify and improve palliative care initiatives.
- Programs should develop SMART metrics (Specific, Measurable, Achievable, Realistic, Time-bound) that align with National Consensus Project guidelines. These metrics should be tracked through dashboards that visually display performance data and facilitate programmatic decision-making.
- Quality improvement requires protected time for data collection and analysis, utilizing Plan-Do-Study-Act cycles for systematic program enhancement. Starting with baseline data and realistic metrics helps ensure sustainable improvements.
- Programs must meet regulatory requirements while demonstrating value to stakeholders through consistent data collection, analysis, and reporting. This includes tracking outcomes through electronic health records, satisfaction surveys, and resource utilization measures.

Introduction

An important aspect in articulating the value of palliative care is to develop consistent and reliable processes aimed to measure quality, safety, service, and cost or resources. The National Consensus Project (NCP) published in 2018 is a document outlining clinical practice guidelines for palliative care.[1] These evidence-based guidelines support quality palliative care for all persons coping with a serious illness. The guidelines can also be integrated into a variety of healthcare settings (e.g., acute, post-acute, ambulatory). One of the challenges for palliative care nurses is learning how to translate the NCP guidelines into measurable and practically relevant indicators of good or effective care for their program and setting.[2] Indeed, learning the process of evaluating a palliative care program is essential to starting a new program or expanding a current program, to bend and flex with the changing population and healthcare needs. A key element in developing a QI (quality improvement) program in palliative care is to articulate the value of the program to stakeholders.

Evaluating a Program

The *value equation*[3] is an excellent starting point and framework which guides the palliative care nurse in developing metrics that demonstrate the value of palliative care (Figure 78.1). Essentially, this abstract equation can be stated by saying, the value of palliative care is reflected by the *quality*, *safety*, and *service* provided, for a *specific cost or resource*.

$$\text{Value} = \frac{\text{Quality} + \text{Safety} + \text{Service}}{\text{Cost or Resources}}$$

Figure 78.1 Value Equation

Quality

Quality, in the value equation, represents the reduction in the variation of care delivery and implementation of evidence-based practices.[4] In other words, quality means upholding a high standard of *consistency* when delivering palliative care. For example, when working with all patients, the palliative care nurse implements evidence-based tools or protocols to screen and assess for pain and comfort. The question around quality emerges when we ask a person suffering from pain, how often does the nurse screen and assess for pain? Is it 50% of the time? Perhaps screening and assessing for pain is completed for only 75% of the patients seen. More importantly, perhaps the nurse is screening and assessing but fails to document their findings. The goal for quality in this case is to achieve an acceptable rate of consistency in the provision of screening and assessing for level of comfort with each patient encounter and then documenting in the patient's electronic health record (EHR). While this example describes pain, many other symptoms (e.g., dyspnea, nausea, fatigue, etc.) are equally important and more relevant in some instances. The concept around consistency differs from the concept of outcomes. In the value equation, safety and service are considered outcomes.

Safety

Safety is the prevention of harm and suffering.[5,6] For the ideal palliative care situation, the nurse screens and assesses for pain in each patient encounter, then documents their findings; what happens when an intervention is needed to combat pain? For example, after completing a comprehensive assessment, the palliative care nurse recommends the use of prescribed morphine. Taking into consideration that safety is the prevention of harm and suffering, the palliative care nurse also recommends a bowel regimen to prevent constipation. Here then is the difference between quality (consistency) and safety (an outcome). Consistency in recommending a bowel regimen is a quality indicator; the effectiveness of the bowel regimen becomes the safety outcome. See Table 78.1 for examples of quality and safety concepts. As a safety metric, the palliative care nurse might measure the percentage of patients on opioid treatments who are not constipated.

Service

Service is the active patient, family, and stakeholder partnership and engagement integrated as a human experience.[7] The service element in the value equation is separate and distinct from quality and safety measures. Key to success is understanding how the palliative care nurse impacts patient/family satisfaction and stakeholder partnerships. Most in healthcare today can identify with the importance of patient/family satisfaction surveys (e.g., Consumer Assessment of Healthcare Providers and Systems (CAHPS)[8] or Press Ganey[9]) as a way to measure overall patient/family healthcare experiences. However, less commonly looked at is the importance of collecting data that informs service lines and programs (i.e., palliative care) on the degree to which their stakeholders, such as referral sources (physicians, nurses, case managers) and leadership within an organization (chief executives, directors, managers), are satisfied with their services. This is especially critical if a palliative care program relies on referrals for survival. It goes without saying, if referral sources are dissatisfied with the performance of the palliative care nurse or team, fewer referrals will occur. As a service metric, the palliative care nurse might measure the percentages of "top-box" in patient/family and stakeholder survey scores. "Top-box" refers to the highest (best) possible score given on a survey question.

Table 78.1 Examples of quality and safety concepts

Quality measures	Safety measurement
Screening *(all signs)*	Outcomes
Assessing *(all symptoms)*	Effectiveness
Interventions *(repositioning)*	Appropriateness
Treatments *(prescribing)*	Prevention
Timeliness *(response)*	Reduction
Efficiency *(processes)*	Elimination
Implementation *(evidence-based practices)*	Understanding
Communicating *(care planning)*	
Educating *(treatment options)*	
Cultural sensitivity *(use of translator)*	

Cost or Resources Used

The final element of the value equation is centered on the cost or resources necessary to deliver the quality, safety, and service of the palliative care program. Costs and resources are not to be confused with "cost savings" or "cost avoidance." Instead, for this component of the value equation, compute how much it costs (direct and indirect) to provide palliative care. Direct costs are those that are related to direct patient care (e.g., salaries, wages, benefits, supplies), while indirect costs are those that are necessary but may not be directly patient-related (e.g., administration, human resources, payroll, information technology). The palliative care nurse collaborates with the manager or supervisor to assist in gathering information associated with costs or resources needed to operate the program.

Hospice Quality Reporting

The Hospice Quality Reporting Program (HQRP) was established by the Social Security Act (Section 1814(i)(5)) that requires hospice agencies to report quality measures related to patient care delivery.[10] Hospice nurses are encouraged to regularly visit the website and sign up for listservs related to HQRP by visiting the Provider and Stakeholder Engagement webpage. The HQRP includes data submitted by hospices thorough the Hospice Item Set collection tool, data from Medicare hospice claims, and the experience of care provided through the CAHPS. Noncompliance with the HQRP results in a 4% reduction to the Annual Payment Update for the corresponding fiscal year.

The Joint Commission Advanced Certification Program

The Joint Commission's Advanced Certification Program for Palliative Care acknowledges hospital inpatient programs that deliver superior patient- and family-centered care while improving the quality of life for patients with serious illness.[11] The Joint Commission has selected performance measures deemed vital through the Measuring What Matters initiative of the American Academy of Hospice and Palliative Care and the Hospice and Palliative Nurses Association.[12,13] The current five selected performance measures are: (1) pain screening, (2) pain assessment, (3) dyspnea screening, (4) treatment preferences and goals of care, and (5) treatment preferences for discharge documentation. Palliative care nurses are encouraged to review the Joint Commission's chart abstracted measure for details in documenting quality outcomes in preparation for this voluntary advanced certification.

Developing SMART Metrics

Many palliative care nurses receive annual performance reviews where SMART goals are used to set benchmarks for the following. The SMART model was originally developed as a way to write goals and objectives in a specific, measurable, achievable, realistic, and time-bound way.[3] However, the palliative care nurse can use this model to develop programmatic goals and objectives that demonstrate the value of palliative care while using a dashboard to disseminate the program's outcomes (Table 78.2). In reflecting on the value equation, each element (quality, safety, service, and cost or resources used) should have associated SMART metrics. Each metric should be original and specific to palliative care, not duplicative.

Table 78.2 SMART metric guidelines

S	Specific	Not generalized, abstract or vague; clear
M	Measurable	Quantifiable, computable; concise
A	Achievable	Realistic, reasonable, feasible; obtainable
R	Relevant	Applicable, aligned with organization, important; significant
T	Time-bound	Within a reasonable and appropriate time period; date-driven

"Non-duplicative" in this context refers to palliative care measures not simultaneously measured by another department or entity within the organization.

Data Sources

One of the greatest challenges in developing metrics is obtaining data. The readiness with which data can be collected on a timely and consistent basis is key to any measurement. The palliative care nurse may have the best-constructed measures; however, inconsistent data capturing may impede articulating the value of palliative care. To start, identify the source of the data. Quality and safety measures can usually be obtained through the EHR. Collecting data might be as simple as working with a nurse informaticist to initiate routine reporting (e.g., monthly, quarterly) on specific data points within the EHR. Alternatively, the palliative care nurse can collect data through manual chart review. Manual collection of data through the EHR is a time-consuming process, requiring ample protected time.

Service or satisfaction data can be labor-intensive as well. Outside of developing a homegrown palliative care patient/family satisfaction survey that is mailed out on a timely and routine basis, the palliative care nurse might have alternatives. There are benefits to organically developing such a survey: (1) data is specific to the performance of the palliative care nurse or team; (2) questions are tailored to the human experience of illness, death, and dying; and (3) measures can be constructed in such a way that they are collecting quality data simultaneously. Consider developing a brief survey using a standardized Likert five point scale that aligns with the NCP guidelines (Table 78.3).

Keep surveys simple and easy for the patient/family to respond. If the best method for patient satisfaction is via US mail, then provide a self-addressed stamped envelope in the survey as well.

With regard to collecting data around the satisfaction of referral sources and other stakeholders in the organization, a simple electronic survey through SurveyMonkey (Momentive Inc., San Mateo, CA, USA) can be easily e-mailed to physicians, case managers, and other referral sources. Data collection from web-based questionnaires is quick and easy for analyses. Similar to the patient/family satisfaction survey, a five-point scale Likert can be used to keep the survey simple. Other options for satisfaction surveys include face-to-face or telephone interviews (which are labor- and cost-intensive).

Collecting data for the cost or resources element usually requires assistance from accounting, decision support, and/or direct supervisors. As mentioned earlier, the palliative care nurse will want to identify the cost of human capital—that is, the total salaries, wages, and benefits for the palliative care team. Then a summation of the direct and indirect costs associated with the palliative care program should be computed. For example, what is the allocated cost to have a computer, phone, office space, supplies, malpractice insurance, and other resources needed to have a palliative care program? For those in a home palliative care program, factor in the cost for mileage, cellular phone, laptop computer, etc. Those in an ambulatory setting should consider the cost for having a meeting or exam room, scheduling, and EHR modules. Essentially you will want all data associated with costs or resources needed to provide the palliative care program (as measured by quality, safety, and service). Common metrics around cost or resources reflect the cost per patient and/or cost per patient encounter.

Methodology

Determining the method of data collection and/or computation is key to any measurement. For example, the palliative care nurse may have identified a metric that requires reviewing manually the EHR. For example, assume the palliative care program had 50 consults in a single month. If each consult resulted in an average of 3 visits, that would be 150 records to evaluate. Instead of reviewing every record, the palliative care nurse could randomly select 10%–20% or a reasonable number of patient records. That would require (a) less time to review and (b) fewer records to examine. However, to incorporate best practices for the evaluation of chosen metrics, the SMART metric should be identified a priori and the process of data collection should be kept consistent.

Frequency

When developing SMART metrics around quality, safety, service, and cost or resources, the palliative care nurse must be consistent in collecting data. Determining the frequency of data collection is necessary and usually relates to the consistency in dissemination of findings. Most organizations report metrics on a quarterly basis. However, programs that rely on or require more timely information for decision support may need data collection monthly. Regardless of the frequency, staying consistent in data collection is as important as disseminating findings and outcomes.

Weak Metrics versus SMART Metrics

Developing SMART metrics take time and should not be done hastily. Table 78.4 provides examples of weak metrics contrasted with SMART metrics. Notice the fundamental differences between the two types of metrics. Each metric aligns with the element i.e., quality focuses on consistency, safety and service focus on outcomes, and cost or resources focuses on the actual cost of delivering palliative care. However, the SMART metrics meet the criteria of being specific, measurable, achievable, relevant, and time-bound.

Starting Out

Common questions that emerge for any palliative care nurse are: *Where do I begin*? or *What metrics should I measure? How many metrics should be measured?* These questions are important regardless of whether the palliative care program is well established or just beginning to be settled. First, when possible, always collect data that represents a baseline. This could be simply collecting data needed for the metric from the past 3–6 months. Identifying what the metric will be, collecting the data, and understanding the numerator and denominator is an excellent start. Once a baseline is established, you can alter the metric to a statement of increase or decrease. For example, assume you collected baseline data that

Table 78.3 Example patient/family satisfaction survey

National Consensus Project domain	Satisfaction question	Strongly disagree	Disagree	Neither agree nor disagree	Agree	Strongly agree	Not applicable
		1	2	3	4	5	
Structure and Processes of Care	The palliative care nurse was timely in seeing you.						
Physical Aspects of Care	Goals for pain and other symptoms were achieved after the palliative care nurse began seeing you.						
Psychological and Psychiatric Aspects of Care	Understanding of your illness was improved after the palliative care nurse began seeing you.						
Social Aspects of Care	The palliative care nurse worked with you in developing your care plan.						
Spiritual, Religious, and Existential Aspects of Care	The palliative care nurse assisted you with spiritual concerns.						
Cultural Aspects of Care	The palliative care nurse assisted you with cultural concerns related to your illness.						
Ethical and Legal Aspects of Care	The palliative care nurse respected your wishes regarding choosing or discontinuing treatments.						

Table 78.4 Example weak metrics versus SMART metrics

Element	Weak metric	SMART metric
Quality	Increased documented advance directives	95% of patients will have a documented advance directive within 24 hours of being seen by the palliative care nurse
Safety	Reduction in rehospitalizations	90% of patients seen by the palliative care nurse will not have an unscheduled readmission within 30 days of discharge
Service	Improved patient/family satisfaction	30 days after discharge, 75% of patients/families engaged with the palliative care nurse will rate overall satisfaction in the top-box
Cost or resources	The cost for the palliative care nurse will be 1.0 full-time equivalent	Each month, the average cost per patient visit by the palliative care nurse will be <$109

suggests the current trend of documented advance directives in the intensive care unit is 75%. A SMART metric to address this safety issue might be: *90 days following a competency-based training program, there will be an increase of documented advance directives (from 75% to 90%) in patient's EHR.* In this example the metric meets all the SMART criteria while identifying (a) the baseline (75%) and (b) the goal (90%). When baseline information is not available (e.g., a new palliative care program), develop the SMART metrics and begin collecting data.

In general, it is best to have measures that align with national standards of palliative care. For example, the NCP guidelines can be used to develop measures of clinical practice. This is a good place to start if a current program has not been collecting and analyzing data or a new program is going to launch. Review the NCP guidelines by domain and identify a single metric that corresponds with that domain. For example, Domain 2, guideline 2.2.2 states: "Attention is given to assessing the onset, quality, severity, provoking and relieving factors, response to prior treatment, level of burden, impact on functionality and quality of life, and meaning of distressing symptoms as well as the patient's goals of care."[1 (p. 14)] This guideline describes a comprehensive pain assessment. A quality SMART metric might be: *90% of patients consulted by the palliative care nurse will have a documented comprehensive pain assessment within 24 hours of being seen.*

Developing SMART metrics can be overwhelming. However, consider using the NCP guidelines as a starting point, and develop one metric per domain. Because palliative care is a holistic approach to the human experience by means of physical, psych/social, spiritual/cultural, and legal/ethical aspects of care, the NCP guidelines can be utilized to develop SMART metrics aligned with the value equation. Keep the number of measurements realistic, and ensure adequate protected time is available to collect, measure, and report the findings and outcomes.

Developing the Dashboard

A dashboard is a simple and direct method of organizing metrics into a visual display, summarizing the impact of the palliative care program for the organization. Dashboards may be designed for the benefit of leaders, administrators, or clinicians and are intended to identify patterns, make sense of data, and facilitate decision-making through data visualization.[14] In particular, performance dashboards, which visually display performance metrics against benchmarks or targets, are increasingly common in healthcare.[14] A dashboard specifically derived from the NCP guidelines (Table 78.5) includes the domains SMART metric, method and frequency, and targets.

Targets provide parameters of meeting the SMART metric goal. Akin to performance tiers, the highest level represents meeting the goal (>90%), the middle tier represents almost meeting the goal (89%-80%), and the lowest tier represents being far away from the goal (≤79%). For example, if the goal is 90% and after the palliative care nurse collects and analyzes data and determines the outcome to be 83%, then the smart metric result would fall in the middle tier; similarly, if the outcome is 60%, the result would fall in the lowest tier. Keep in mind when developing any dashboards to use clear visual distinctions beyond just color to ensure accessibility for all users, including those with visual impairments; for instance, it is estimated that 8% of men and 0.5% of women have red-green color blindness.[15] Finally, the SMART metric should be realistic; although all palliative care programs should strive for 100% in their goals, it is not entirely realistic. Keep goals at 90% or above for each metric.

QI Projects

Protected Time

Protected time is necessary to perform data collection, analyses, and dissemination. It is essential the palliative care nurse negotiates with leadership to have "carved" time allocated to perform QI projects.[16] Equally important is the understanding that protected time for QI should not be addressed or identified as "non-productive time." Rather, protected time for QI projects should be deemed as an investment in the provision of palliative care services. In fact, the NCP guidelines clearly outline continuous QI as a standard of Domain 1: Structure and Process of Care.

Plan-Do-Study-Act Rapid Cycle

Developing a dashboard that identifies SMART metrics provides the palliative care nurse with information on what and how to prioritize QI projects. For example, if data supports the need for enhanced spiritual assessments at the initial consult, than developing a QI project is key to reaching the designated goal. One common method for employing QI in healthcare is to initiate a rapid-cycle Plan–Do–Study–Act (PDSA) program.[17] The method allows for small tests of change in a stepwise controlled fashion before permanent changes are made.[18]

This four-step cycle shown in Table 78.6, with a logical sequence of repetitive steps needed to lead to an exponential improvement.

Using the example of enhancing spiritual assessment during the initial palliative care consult, the palliative care nurse starts with the *Plan* phase. In this phase, the ideas for improvement are detailed, tasks are assigned, and measures for improvement are selected. In the *Do* phase, the plan is implemented, and any deviation from the plan is detailed and documented. During the *Study*

Table 78.5 Example palliative care dashboard

National Consensus Project domain	SMART metric	Method and frequency	Target(s)
Structure and Processes of Care	90% of patients seen receive a documented physical examination including identification of current symptoms and functional status within 24 hours of the initial consult	10% of patients are randomly selected for manual chart review each month	≥90% 89%–80% ≤79% Outcome:
Physical Aspects	90% of patients consulted by the palliative care nurse will have a documented comprehensive pain assessment within 24 hours of being seen	10% of patients are randomly selected for manual chart review each month	≥90% 89% 80% ≤79% Outcome:
Psycho/ Psychiatric Aspects	Following the initial consult, 90% of patients have an ongoing and documented plan to monitor and address psychological responses, emotions, and/or changes in cognition as prognosis and goals of care evolve	10% of patients are randomly selected for manual chart review each month	≥90% 89%–80% ≤79% Outcome:
Social Aspects	90% of patients seen by the palliative care nurse have a comprehensive assessment on functional limitations that impact activities of daily living, instrumental activities of daily living, and cognition within 24 hours of the initial consult	10% of patients are randomly selected for manual chart review each month	≥90% 89%–80% <79% Outcome:
Spiritual, Religious, and Existential	90% of patients screened positive for spiritual distress will be seen by a chaplain within 24 hours	10% of patients are randomly selected for manual chart review each month	≥90% 89%–80% ≤79% Outcome:
Cultural Aspects	95% of non-English-speaking patients/families will have a medical interpreter to reduce likelihood of communication issues and misunderstandings prior to meeting with the patient/family	20% of patients are randomly selected for manual chart review each month	≥95% 94%–90% ≤89% Outcome:
Care for the Patient at the End of Life	95% of patients actively dying have the medications, supplies, and equipment needed for a comfortable death	20% of patients are randomly selected for manual chart review each month	≥95% 94%–90% ≤89% Outcome:
Ethical Legal Aspects of Care	90% of patients seen have a documented advance directive in their electronic health record within 24 hours of the initial consult	10% of patients are randomly selected for manual chart review each month	≥90% 89%–80% ≤79% Outcome:

Table 78.6 Plan-do-study-act (PDSA) cycles

I	Plan	• State the objective of the test • Make predictions • Develop plan to carry out the PDSA cycle
II	Do	• Carry out the test • Document problems, expected and unexpected observations • Begin data analyses
III	Study	• Complete the analysis of the collected data • Compare the data to the predictions • Summarize what was learned in this PDSA cycle
IV	Act	• Determine what changes are necessary • Prepare for the next PDSA cycle

Source: Reference 19.

phase, data is collected, analyzed, and interpreted. For example, if the palliative care nurse identified a specific tool to use as part of the spiritual assessment, and it was not utilized consistently, questions around the appropriateness of the tool should be answered (e.g., is the tool challenging to implement, does it take time to complete/is it time-consuming to complete, are patients open to the assessment). In the *Act* phase, decisions are made for changes (e.g., change the spiritual assessment tool), and the PDSA cycle repeats. This process continues until the right solution is found and implemented, monitored, and presented as sustainable. Depending on the project, it could be weeks to months before sustainable palliative care practice is achieved, and a new QI project begins.

Summary

Palliative care programs continue to grow as a specialty within the acute, post-acute, and ambulatory settings. It is essential palliative care nurses ensure high standards of quality, safety, and service are met through QI initiatives. Further, developing SMART (specific, measurable, achievable, and relevant) metrics to measure effectiveness provides evidence of the palliative care program's impact in healthcare settings. Calculating the direct and indirect costs needed for the delivery of palliative care is equally important to understand what resources are necessary to operate the program. Finally, the palliative care nurse should consistently monitor metrics and, where needed, initiate PDSA cycles for continuous QI within the palliative care program.

REFERENCES

1. National Coalition for Hospice and Palliative Care. *Clinical Practice Guidelines for Quality Palliative Care*. 4th ed. National Coalition for Hospice and Palliative Care; 2018. Accessed September 1, 2022. https://www.nationalcoalitionhpc.org/ncp/.
2. Amador S, Sampson EL, Goodman C, Robinson L, SEED Research Team. A systematic review and critical appraisal of quality indicators to assess optimal palliative care for older people with dementia. *Palliat Med*. 2019;33(4):415–429. https://doi.org/10.1177/0269216319834227.
3. Reed SM. President's message: the value proposition of the CNS. *Clin Nurse Spec*. 2020;34(6):239–243. https://doi.org/10.1097/NUR.0000000000000561.
4. Sutherland K, Levesque J. Unwarranted clinical variation in health care: definitions and proposal of an analytic framework. *J Eval Clin Pract*. 2020;26(3):687–696. https://doi.org/10.1111/jep.13181.
5. Crandall WV, Davis JT, McClead R, Brilli RJ. Is preventable harm the right patient safety metric? *Pediatr Clin North Am*. 2012;59(6):1279–1292. https://doi.org/10.1016/j.pcl.2012.09.003.
6. Nabhan M, Elraiyah T, Brown DR, et al. What is preventable harm in healthcare? A systematic review of definitions. *BMC Health Serv Res*. 2012;12:128. https://doi.org/10.1186/1472-6963-12-128.
7. Wolf J, Niederhauser V, Marshburn D, LaVela S. Defining patient experience. *Patient Exp J*. 2014;1(1):7–19.
8. Consumer Assessment of Healthcare Providers and Systems (CAHPS). Accessed October 16, 2022. https://www.ahrq.gov/cahps/index.html.
9. Press Ganey. Healthcare Experience Analytics. Accessed October 16, 2022. https://www.pressganey.com/.
10. Centers for Medicare & Medicaid Services. Hospice Quality Reporting Program. Accessed January 13, 2023. https://www.cms.gov/medicare/quality-initiatives-patient-assessment-instruments/hospice-quality-reporting.
11. Joint Commission. Palliative Care Measures. Accessed January 13, 2023. https://www.jointcommission.org/measurement/measures/palliative-care/.
12. American Academy of Hospice and Palliative Medicine. Measuring What Matters. Accessed January 13, 2023. https://aahpm.org/quality/measuring-what-matters.
13. Hospice and Palliative Nurses Association. Measuring What Matters. Accessed January 13, 2023. https://advancingexpertcare.org/HPNA/HPNAweb/Research/Measuring_What_Matters.aspx.
14. Ruppel H, Oliver A, Chandrasekhar S, et al. Developing a unit profile dashboard to inform nursing care delivery based on unique needs of patients. *J Nurs Adm*. 2022;52(6):332–337. https://doi.org/10.1097/NNA.0000000000001165.
15. Roskoski R. Guidelines for preparing color figures for everyone including the colorblind. *Pharmacol Res*. 2017;119:240–241. https://doi.org/10.1016/j.phrs.2017.02.005.
16. Hunt DF, Dunn M, Harrison G, Bailey J. Ethical considerations in quality improvement: key questions and a practical guide. *BMJ Open Qual*. 2021;10(3):e001497. https://doi.org/10.1136/bmjoq-2021-001497.
17. Agency for Healthcare Research and Quality. Plan–Do–Study–Act (PDSA) Directions and Examples. Updated 2020. Accessed January 16, 2023. https://www.ahrq.gov/health-literacy/improve/precautions/tool2b.html.
18. Adams D. Quality improvement; part 1: introduction and overview. *BJA Educ*. 2018;18(3):89–94. https://doi.org/10.1016/j.bjae.2017.12.002.
19. Institute for Healthcare Improvement. Science of Improvement: Testing Changes. 2023. Accessed January 16, 2023. https://www.ihi.org:443/resources/Pages/HowtoImprove/ScienceofImprovementTestingChanges.aspx.

Index

For the benefit of digital users, indexed terms that span two pages (e.g., 52–53) may, on occasion, appear on only one of those pages.

Tables, figures, and boxes are indicated by an italic *t*, *f*, and *b* following the page number.

5 As, sexual health framework, 345, 346*t*
12-step programs, substance use disorder, 728

Academic Consortium for Integrative Medicine and Health, 280
Academy of Consultation-Liaison Psychiatry, 251
accountable care, 11
accountable care organizations (ACOs), 11
  variation on value-based care (VBC), 59–60
acetaminophen
  pain management, 92, 93*t*
  treatment of mild pain, 381*t*
acquired immune deficiency syndrome (AIDS), 119, 519
  See also people living with HIV (PLWH)
ACS. *See* anorexia/cachexia syndrome (ACS)
acupuncture
  dyspnea, 110
  gastrointestinal symptoms, 285–86
  mind-body approaches for pain, 283
  mood and sleep, 285
  nausea and vomiting, 138*t*
acute confusion, 243
  See also delirium
acute delirium. *See* delirium
acute palliative care unit (APCU), 681
acute symptom management, end-of-life, 472–74
Addison's disease, sexual function, 342
adjuvant analgesics, 97*t*
  antidepressants, 96
  antiepilepsy drugs, 96–97
  cannabinoids, 99
  capsaicin, 98–99
  corticosteroids, 97
  local anesthetics, 97
  NMDA antagonists-ketamine, 97–98
  See also pain management
adolescents
  culture, 298–99
  grief at end of life, 483
  grief support for, 489
  observed pain behaviors, 379*t*
adolescents and young adults (AYA)
  advance care planning (ACP), 450–51
  case study, 447
  coping and well-being, 448–50
  crisis management, 451
  disease implications, 448
  end-of-life care, 452
  fertility, 448
  hospice, 451–52
  implications on family unit, 450
  living with chronic illness and/or long-term treatment, 451
  methods and example phrases for engaging in conversation, 449*t*
  special population considerations, 452
  symptom management, 448
  timing, 447–48
adsorbent agents, diarrhea, 158
adults. *See* adolescents and young adults (AYA); older adults
advance care planning (ACP), 13, 14, 49, 56, 416
  adolescents and young adults, 447, 449*t*, 450–51
  case of conversation at hospital admission, 55
  case of end-of-life decision-making, 55
  communication, 38
  completing advance directives (AD), 52–53
  consensus definition, 50*b*
  conservative kidney management (CKM), 552
  contextual background of, 49–50
  continuum of, 52*f*
  definitions, 50
  documentation of goals of care and, 418
  dying person and family, 625
  ethical dilemma, 352–53
  family caregiver resources, 323
  having goals-of-care conversations, 53
  heart failure, 513
  making upstream and inclusive, 51
  medical orders for life-sustaining treatment, 54
  meetings, 36
  naming surrogate decision maker, 52
  neurological care, 238–39
  nursing homes, 665–66
  older adults, 753*t*, 755
  pediatric serious illness, 416–18, 417*t*, 418*t*
  people living with HIV, 523–25
  Portable Orders for Life-Sustaining Treatment (POLST) and, 54, 54*t*
  process, tools, and strategies facilitating, 51–55
  resources and tools for, 53*t*
  role of caregiver in, 322
  role of nurse in goals of care, 418, 418*t*
  roles and responsibilities of nurses in, 55–56
  shifting focus from legal forms to conversations, 50
  shifting focus from treatment choices to patients' values, 50–51
  tools for pediatric, 417–18, 417*t*
  trending for system and team approach, 51
  use in end-of-life decision-making, 54–55
advance directives (AD), 352, 416
  advance care planning (ACP), 52*f*, 52–53
  pediatric serious illness, 410
  people living with HIV, 523–25
  phrases to avoid and consider, 354*t*
Advanced Certified Hospice and Palliative Care Nurse, 3
advanced disease
  clinical management with substance use histories, 724–26
  natural fluid deficits in, 166
  substance use disorder (SUD) in patients with, 722–24
  See also medically administered nutrition (MAN)
advanced kidney disease (AKD)
  nursing considerations for persons living with, 554
  symptoms, 550
  See also kidney disease
advanced lung disease, managing, 500–1
advanced practice registered nurse (APRN), 7–8
  interdisciplinary palliative care team, 68
  team role, 78*t*
Affordable Care Act (2009), 11, 59
aftercare, pediatric patient at end of life, 475
afterload, 505–6
age
  sexuality and sexual function across life span, 344–45
  spiritual development by, 431, 431*t*
age and developmental stage, culture, 298–99
Age-Friendly Health Systems, 537–38
Aging with Dignity, 462
agitation, hydration, 169
agitation/delirium, end-of-life symptom management, 474*t*
air hunger, 105
airway, clearance techniques, 144
airway obstruction, 106
airway restriction, 106
ALARM, sexual health framework, 345, 346*t*
alcohol use, 721
  See also substance use disorders (SUDs)
alienation, 624
alpha 1 anti trypsin deficiency, 496*b*
alternative medicine, term, 281
Alzheimer's disease, 310–11, 528–29
  case study, 530–31
  diagnostic criteria, 529*t*
  Parkinson's disorder behind, 236
Ambient Assisted Living (AAL), 649
ambiguous loss, 625
ambulatory palliative care model, 66, 67*t*, 72–73
  team roles in model, 80*t*
American Academy of Hospice and Palliative Medicine, 3, 13, 68
American Academy of Pediatrics, 298, 384–85, 440–41, 447
  informed consent, 425
  Policy Statement on Pediatric Palliative and Hospice Care Commitments, Guidelines and Recommendations, 411
American Association of Colleges of Nursing, 706–7
American Board of Medical Specialties, 3

American Cancer Society, cancer-related fatigue, 265
American Cancer Society Cancer Action Network, 726–27
American College of Lifestyle Medicine, 281
American College of Obstetricians and Gynecologists (ACOG), 437
American College of Physicians, 693
American Heart Association, 354
American Holistic Health Association, 281
American Medical Association (AMA), Council on Ethical and Judicial Affairs, 351–52
American Nurses Association (ANA), 6, 55, 130, 356, 594, 605, 648
  Code of Ethics, 27, 419–20, 424
  core principles on connected health, 648*t*
  Nursing Scope and Standards of Practice, 27
American Organization for Nursing Leadership, 787
American Society of Clinical Oncology (ASCO), 130, 252, 495–96, 566, 569, 726–27
American Telehealth Association (ATA), 647–48
American Thoracic Society (ATS), 105, 110–11, 495–96
amyotrophic lateral sclerosis (ALS)
  artificial nutrition, 143–44
  case study, 142, 143–45
  Lou Gehrig's disease, 235
  neurological disorder, 235–36
  new hiccups, 144–45
  oral symptoms, 145
  resources for people living with, 236*t*
analgesics, malignant bowel obstruction, 153
ancillary disciplines/consultants, interdisciplinary palliative care team, 69, 71–72
anorexia, 119, 126
anorexia/cachexia syndrome (ACS)
  assessment, 121–23, 122*b*
  cancer-related (C-ACS), 120, 120*t*
  case study, 119, 122–23, 125
  disease states with, 120*t*
  enteral and parenteral nutrition, 123–25
  exogenous/secondary symptom management, 123
  interventions, 123–25
  management, 119, 120, 126
  mechanisms and effects of, 120*t*
  medications commonly used in, 125*t*
  multimodal approach, 125*b*, 125
  nutritional support, 123
  oral issues, 121
  pathophysiology, 120
  pharmacological interventions, 124–25
  physical symptoms, 121
  primary, 120–21
  psychological and/or spiritual distress, 121
  psychosocial support, 125
  secondary, 121
  term, 120
  treatment side effects, 121
anticholinergics
  diarrhea, 158
  malignant bowel obstruction, 155
anticipatory grief, 623, 625
  end of life, 625–26
anticonvulsants, 96–97, 97*t*
antidepressants, 97*t*
  pain management, 96
antiemetics
  classes of, for nausea and vomiting, 134*b*, 134
  malignant bowel obstruction, 155
antiepilepsy drugs, pain management, 96–97, 97*t*
antihistaminic agents, nausea and vomiting, 135
antiretroviral therapy (ART), 520
antisecretory agents
  diarrhea, 158
  malignant bowel obstruction, 155
anxiety
  commonly prescribed medications, 257*t*
  considerations in children, 256–59
  definition, 251
  diagnosis, 253
  disorders, 255
  factors for consideration in diagnosis, 255
  medication considerations, 256
  patient and family education, 259
  patients living with cancer, 570–71
  pharmacological treatment, 256
  prevalence and scope, 251–52
  psychiatric disorders with, 253*t*
  psychotherapy treatment, 255–56
  screening, 252–53
  treatment considerations, 255
anxiety disorders, persons with, 735–36
appetite issues, pediatric palliative care, 395–96
Arnica gel, pain, 284
aromatherapy
  mind-body approaches for pain, 283
  mood and sleep, 284–85
  nausea and vomiting, 138*t*
artifacts, 28
artificial nutrition, patient with ALS, 143–44
ascites
  assessment, 159
  case of patient with nonalcoholic steatohepatitis cirrhosis, 159, 161
  catheters, 160
  definition, 159
  diagnostic studies, 159–60
  history, 159
  laparoscopy, 159–60
  nursing interventions, 160
  paracentesis, 159–60
  pathophysiology, 159
  pharmacologic management, 160
  physical examination, 159
  prevalence, 159
  procedural and surgical management, 160–61
  shunts, 160
  supportive care, 160
  therapeutic paracentesis, 160
  See also bowel management
asexuality, 712*t*
Ask Suicide Screening Questions, 258
Ask-Tell-Ask, communication strategy, 34*b*, 34
Aspirin, pain management, 92, 93*t*
assigned sex at birth (ASAB), 711, 712*t*
assistance in dying, 606
assisted living facilities (ALFs), 662
atypical antipsychotics, nausea and vomiting, 135
Australia, assisted dying and euthanasia, 608
autoimmune illnesses, physical impact on sexual function, 342
automatic internal cardiac defibrillators (AICD), cardiovascular device, 359
autonomy, 171
  assistance in dying, 608–9
  infringement, 424
  palliative sedation, 594
  pediatric medical decision-making, 424–25
  pediatric palliative care, 424–25
autopsy, end-of-life, 475
AYA. *See* adolescents and young adults (AYA)

Baby Doe, 360
baclofen, 97*t*
beauty, ethos of palliative nursing, 85
Beck Anxiety Inventory (BAI) scale, 284
Beck Hopelessness Scale, 258
Behavioral Pain Scale (BPS), 689
Behavior Pain Assessment Tool (BPAT), 689
Belgium, assisted dying and euthanasia, 607–8
Bell, Alexander Graham, 647
beneficence, 171
  medical aid in dying, 609
  palliative sedation, 594
Benoliel, Jeanne Quint, 632
benzodiazepines, 96
  managing in outpatient setting, 660
  nausea and vomiting, 135
bereavement, 623
  compassionate communities supporting, 631–32
  grief and, 479
  hospital programs, 490
  interventions and support in, 486–90
  keepsake checklist, 442*f*
  LGBTQIA+ patients, 717
  pediatric, 441
  pediatric palliative and hospice care (PPHC), 464
  support for the bereaved, 631
  term, 480, 627
  See also grief
bereavement coordinator, interdisciplinary palliative care team, 69, 72
bereavement course, clinician impact on, 401–2
bereavement overload, 628
Best Interest Standard, definition, 425
BETTER, sexual health framework, 345, 346*t*
Better Breathers Club, 500
Bifidobacterium animalis, 153
biological sex, 712*t*
bisexual, 712*t*
bisphosphonates, pain management, 98
bladder cancer, case study, 178
bladder spasms, 182
bleeding/bleeds
  end-of-life symptom management, 474*t*
  pediatric palliative care, 396–97
body image, impact of serious illness on sexuality, 343
bonding social capital, 778
bone metastasis and pathological fractures
  bone metastasis treatment, 588–89
  case study for pathological fracture, 587–88
  description, 588
  diagnostic procedures, 588
  epidemiology, 588
  high-intensity focused ultrasound, 589
  palliative embolization, 589
  palliative radiation, 588
  pathological fracture treatments, 589
  pathophysiology, 588
  radiofrequency ablation, 589
  signs and symptoms, 588
  systemic treatment, 589
  treatments, 588–89
  See also urgent syndromes at end of life
bowel management
  ascites, 159–61
  constipation, 150–53
  diarrhea, 156–59
  malignant bowel obstruction, 153–56
bowel obstruction
  case study, 589
  description, 589
  diagnostic procedures, 589–90
  epidemiology, 589
  nursing management, 590
  pathophysiology, 589
  treatments, 590
Bow Tie Model, disease management and palliative care, 568*f*, 568
brain tumors, 179–80
breathing, 104
  discomfort, 105
  end-of-life symptom management, 474*t*
breathing, thinking, functioning (BTF) model, dyspnea management, 107–11, 108*f*
breathlessness, 105

schematic of outline of genesis of, 106*f*
support for caregivers, family and patient with chronic, 111–12
bridging social capital, 778
Brophy, Paul, 360
Buffalo Delirium Scale, 245
Building Evidence for Services and Supports, 537–38
bulk laxatives, constipation, 152
buprenorphine, pain management, 95
burial, end-of-life decisions, 433
burnout, 774*f*
individual interventions, 773
organizational interventions, 773–74
prevention, 773–74
signs, 773
butyrophenones, nausea and vomiting, 134

cachexia, 119, 126
definition, 119
stage D heart failure, 513
word, 119
See also anorexia/cachexia syndrome (ACS)
calciphylaxis, 198–99
treatment, 213–14
wound care, 213–14
calendula, gastrointestinal symptoms, 286
California, 12, 465, 605, 607
medical aid in dying (MAID), 357–58
CAM tool, delirium, 245
Canada, 608
cancer
barriers to pain management, 90*b*, 90
diarrhea, 157
fatigue, 265*b*
fatigue related to, 264
physical impact on sexual function, 342
Cancer Dyspnea Scale (CDS), 107
cancer patients
case of patient navigating survivorship with ovarian cancer, 567, 569
case with colorectal cancer, 570–71
clinical trial participation and advanced cancer, 573
cognitive impairment, 569–70
fatigue, depression, and anxiety, 570–71
geriatric assessment in older individuals, 571
nausea and vomiting, 131
neuropathy, 569
palliative care and survivorship care, 568–71
palliative care assessment and domains, 567*t*
palliative care for advanced, 572
palliative care modalities, 572–73
palliative chemotherapy, 572–73
palliative surgery, 572
role of nurses in palliative care, 573
social well-being, assessment and interventions, 571
spiritual and existential concerns, assessment and interventions, 571–72
symptoms and assessment strategies, 568–71
Candida infection, 169
cannabinoids
anorexia/cachexia syndrome (ACS), 124, 125*t*
nausea and vomiting, 136
neuropathic and chronic pain syndromes, 384*t*
pain management, 99
cannabis, pain, 284
capacity, 354–55
capsaicin, 97*t*
pain, 284
pain management, 98–99
cardiac device cessation
case study of patient undergoing, 602–3
extracorporeal membranous oxygenation (ECMO), 603
implantable cardiac defibrillator (ICD), 603
left ventricular assist device (LVAD), 602, 603
permanent pacemakers (PPMs), 603
cardiac output, 505–6
cardiac population, fatigue, 265*b*
cardiopulmonary resuscitation (CPR), 40, 49, 353
cardiorespiratory, symptoms in normal progression in dying, 620*t*
cardiovascular illnesses
implantable electronic devices, 359
physical impact on sexual function, 342
care delivery framework, dementia, 530, 537–38
care partner capacity and needs, dementia, 530, 536–37
care plans, dementia diagnosis and creating, 531
care team
barriers to teamwork, 43
characterizing effective, 42–43
communication and collaboration, 42–45
conflict about members, 43
conflict resolution, 44*b*, 44–45
meetings, 36–37, 37*b*
nurse and physician, 43–44
career advancement, 785–86, 789
continuing education, 788
developing skill set, 787, 787*t*
mentorship, 786–87
national and international resources, 788*b*
networking, 788
professional boundaries, 787–88
professional development, 785–86
promotion with professionalism, 788–89
specialty certification, 786–87
strategies, 789*b*
caregivers
care for, of dying ICU patient, 695–96
communication barriers, 31
LGBTQ, 310
LGBTQIA+ patients, 716–17
needs at imminent death, 619–21
racially diverse, 309–10
strain, 639
strategies to support LGBTQ, 310
strategies to support racially diverse, 310
support for, near end of life, 618
supporting patient with chronic breathlessness, 111–12
Carer Support Needs Assessment Tool (CSNAT), 319
CASCADE (Care Supporters Coached to be Adept Decision Partners), 649
catheters, ascites, 160
Catholic University of Korea, 761
Center for Medicare and Medicaid Innovation (CMMI), 11
Center to Advance Palliative Care (CAPC), 66, 643, 679, 705, 737–38
Centers for Disease Control and Prevention (CDC), 14, 60, 519, 726
Centers for Medicare & Medicaid Innovations, 666
Centers for Medicare & Medicaid Services (CMS), 10, 60, 647
cerebrovascular accident, 179–80
certifications, palliative care, 796–97
Certified Hospice and Palliative Pediatric Nurse, 3
chaos narrative, 624–25
chaplain(s)
interdisciplinary palliative care team, 67–68, 69–70
limited coverage, 433
spiritual support, 433
team role, 78*t*
chemical coping, term, 660
chemotherapy, pain management, 98
chemotherapy-induced peripheral neuropathy (CIPN), 569
CHEST Expert Cough Panel, 112–13
child and grandparents, grief, 482
child and parent, grief, 481–82
child life specialist (CLS), interdisciplinary palliative care team, 71, 72
children
culture and school-aged, 298
depression and anxiety in, 256–59
end-of-life considerations, 258
grief at end of life, 483
grief support for, 489
integrative therapies, 258–59
observational pain scales, 378*t*
observed pain behaviors, 379*t*
spirituality in, 431
suicide, 258
See also pediatric pain
Children's Health Insurance Program, 455, 641
chimeric antigen receptor T-cell therapy (CART), 549, 558
chloride channel activators, constipation, 153
cholestatic pruritus (CP), 228–30
Choosing Wisely, 663–64
chosen family, 712*t*
chronic breathlessness, support for caregivers, family and patient with, 111–12
chronic breathlessness syndrome, 105
chronic dyspnea, 104–5
chronic illness, adolescents and young adults, 451
chronic kidney disease (CKD), 549
case of value-based care (VBC) in action, 62
See also kidney disease
chronic obstructive pulmonary disease (COPD), 104–5, 119, 264, 496*b*
dyspnea and, 105
fatigue, 265*b*
toll of serious illness on persons and family/caregiver, 500
chronic pain, medications for treatment, 384*t*
chronic symptom management, end-of-life, 474
CIM. *See* complementary and integrative medicine (CIM)
circulatory system, dying process, 593–94
cirrhosis
ascites, 542, 542*t*
assessment, 541
caregiver burden, 544–45
coagulopathy, 543
compensated vs decompensated, 542*t*
diagnosis, 541
disease course, 542
encephalopathy, 542
esophageal varices, 542*t*, 543
hepatic hydrothorax, 542
hepatorenal syndrome, 543
hyponatremia, 542
infections, 542–43, 542*t*
malnutrition, 544
pathophysiology, 541
portal hypertension and, 543–44
risk of liver cancer, 543
social determinants of health, 544
stigma, 545
symptoms in decompensated, 543–44
See also liver disease
cisgender, 711, 712*t*
cisheteronormativity, 712*t*
Clinical Practice Guidelines for Quality Palliative Care, 21, 22, 24, 38
clinical trial participation, advanced cancer and, 573
clinicians, grieving process, 632
Clock Draw Test (CDT), 570
clonazepam, 96
Clostridioides difficile, diarrhea, 157, 158–59
Clostridium difficile, diarrhea, 156, 157
Clostridium difficile infection, urinary tract infections (UTIs), 183
code status, 40
codeine, pain management, 95
cognition, older adults, 752–54, 753*t*

cognitive-behavioral therapy for insomnia (CBTi), 276–77
cognitive deficits, palliative patients, 216–17
cognitive distraction, nausea and vomiting, 138*t*
cognitive health and function, dementia, 530, 534
cognitive impairment, patients living with cancer, 569–70
collaboration
  team communication and, 42–45
  value-based care and, across care settings, 61–62
Colorado, 605
  medical aid in dying (MAID), 357–58
colorectal cancer, patients with, 570–71
Columbia, 608
Columbia Suicide Risk Assessment, 258
COMFORT approach, dyspnea, 110–11
comfort feeding only (CFO), 174
communication
  adolescents and young adults, 449*t*
  advance care planning, 38
  care meetings, 36–37, 37*b*
  case study for care at end of life, 41–42
  case study for cultural aspects of care, 34
  case study for imparting information, 32
  case study gathering information, 33
  case study on goals of care, 38
  conflict resolution, 44*b*, 44–45
  core elements of nurse, 32–35
  cultural aspects of care, 34
  cultural assessment questions, 35*b*
  cultural concept in palliative care, 302, 303*b*
  family and caregiver barriers, 31
  family meetings, 36–37, 37*b*
  foundation of palliative nursing, 28
  goals-of-care conversations, 411
  imparting information, 32–33
  information-gathering, 33
  information needs of patients and families, 35–36
  life-sustaining treatment discussions, 40–41
  listening, 34–35
  nurse and physician, 43–44
  nursing, 28–29
  nursing barriers, 31–32
  nursing intervention, 335
  ongoing discussions of goals of care, 38–42, 39*b*
  open-ended questions for initiating discussions, 33*b*
  overview, 28–29
  palliative nursing, 45
  pediatric goals of care, 404, 410–16
  pediatric palliative and hospice care (PPHC), 460
  pediatric palliative care, 392–93
  prognosis, 39–40
  prognosis at end of life, 468
  questions addressing patient and family coping, 38*b*
  questions for changing goals of care, 41*b*
  scheduled meetings and nursing presence, 37–38
  serious news discussions, 39, 40*b*
  social media enhancing family, 780
  stages, 34*b*
  team collaboration and, 42–45
  telehealth, 32
  themes for patients and families, 29*t*
  transition to death, 41–42
  translation of healthcare to lay language, 31*t*
communication frameworks, sexual health, 345, 346*t*
community-based palliative care (CBPC), 639
  case study of patient, 644–45
  consultative programs, 640
  delivery models, 640–41
  free-standing palliative care, 641
  future for nurses, 643–45
  hospice, 640
  key takeaways for nurses in, 642–43
  model, 66, 67*t*, 73
  payment for services, 641–42
  pediatric palliative care, 641
  primary care practices, 641
  private duty nursing agencies, 641
  professional issues for nurses providing care, 642
  roles and responsibilities of specialized care team, 642
  summary, 643
  team roles in model, 80*t*
community care, supporting the bereaved, 631–32
Community Health Accreditation Partners (CHAP), 643
community settings, family caregivers in, 319–20
compassion, 85
compassionate presence, 430
compassion fatigue
  definition, 773*t*
  ethics, 362
  term, 362
compensated cirrhosis, 541
  overview, 542*t*
competence, 354–55
Competencies and Recommendations for Educating Undergraduate Nursing Students (CARES), 792–93, 794, 796
competency, 84
complementary and integrative medicine (CIM), 280
  applications in palliative care, 282
  chronic pain, 282–84
  gastrointestinal symptoms, 285–86
  mood and sleep, 282–85
  prevalence in palliative care, 280–81
  resources, 286–87, 286*t*, 287*t*
  terminology, 281–82
complementary health approaches, term, 281
complete decongestive therapy (CDT), 192
complicated grief, 480
compression bandages, lymphedema, 192–93
compression garments, lymphedema, 193
concentrated ascites reinfusion therapy (CART), 161
concurrent care, 11
Concurrent Care for Children Implementation Toolkit, 455
condolences, staff commemoration at end-of-life, 475–76
conflict resolution, care team, 44*b*, 44–45
confusion, hydration, 169
Confusion Assessment Method for ICU (CAM-ICU), 692
congenital heart defect/ hydrocephalus, case study of patient with, 404
congestive heart failure (CHF), 119
conscious breathing, 104
Consensus Sleep Diary, 275
consequentialist theories, ethics, 349
conservative kidney management (CKM)
  advance care planning, 552
  alternative to dialysis, 551–52
  case of person receiving, 551, 552
  communication, 552
  medical management, 552
  symptom management, 552
constipation
  adverse effect of opioid analgesics, 95
  assessment, 151–52
  assessments, 152*b*
  bulk laxatives, 152
  case study of patient with, 395
  chloride channel activators, 153
  definitions, 150
  diagnostic studies, 152
  guanylate cyclase-C receptor agonists, 153
  history, 151–52
  impact, 150
  nursing interventions, 152
  opioid-induced, 151, 151*t*
  osmotic laxatives, 153
  pathophysiology and risk factors, 150–51
  pediatric palliative care, 395
  peripherally acting mu opioid receptor antagonists, 153
  pharmacological management, 152–53
  physical examination, 152
  prevalence, 150
  probiotics, 153
  Rome IV diagnostic criteria, 150, 151*t*
  secondary causes, 151*t*
  selective serotonin agonists, 153
  stimulant laxatives, 153
  supportive care, 152
  surfactant laxatives, 153
  See also bowel management
consultative programs, community-based palliative care, 640
containment products, incontinence and, 181–82, 181*t*
continence. *See* wound, ostomy, and continence (WOC) care
continent and incontinent fecal and urinary diversions
  assessment, 216
  descriptions, 215, 216*t*
continuing care retirement communities (CCRCs), 662–63
continuous renal replacement therapy (CRRT), 602
contractility, 505–6
Controlled Oral Word Association Test, 570
controlled substances, managing in outpatient setting, 660
coping with loss, dual process of, 628
Coptic Orthodox Church, 432
corticobasal syndrome (CBS)
  neurological disorder, 237
  resources for people living with, 236*t*
corticosteroids, 97*t*
  nausea and vomiting, 135
  pain management, 97
cough, 104, 112–13
  interventions, 112–13
  measurement, 112
  pathophysiology, 112
  pharmacological treatments, 113
  suppressants, 113
  See also dyspnea
cough hypersensitivity syndrome, 112
Cough Severity Diary, 112
Cough Specific Quality of Life Questionnaire, 112
Courageous Parents Network, 417–18, 443*t*
COVID-19 pandemic, 6–7
  advanced lung disease and, 495
  allocating scarce resources, 362–63
  caregiver burnout, 772
  community-based palliative care, 640
  global health emergencies, 19, 759, 761, 762
  global palliative care, 293–94
  healthcare spending after, 59
  illness narrative, 625
  nurses' grief through, 632–33
  respiratory disease, 496*b*
  skin manifestations, 198–99, 214–15
  staffing shortages, 772
  technology-enabled healthcare, 745
  telehealth, 654, 664
  telehealth expansion, 647
Coyle, Nessa, 679
crisis management, adolescents and young adults, 451
Critical-Care Pain Observation Tool (CPOT), 689
Crohn's disease, sexual function, 342
Cruzan, Nancy, 171–72, 360
cultural aspects of care
  assessment questions, 35*b*

case study, 34
communication, 34
cultural assessment, conducting, 297
cultural awareness, 295
cultural competence, 22, 297
cultural desire, 296–97
cultural encounter, 296
cultural humility, 297
cultural knowledge, 295
cultural sensitivity, 296
cultural skill, 295–96
culture
age and developmental stage, 298–99
case study of cultural considerations of family, 295
case study of impact of, on palliative, 302
communication skills and best practices for palliative care, 303*b*
components of, 297–302
definition, 293
disability status, 302
diversity in United States, 294
end-of-life (EOL) rituals, 304
ethnicity, 298
gender, 299–300
as global palliative care issue, 293–94
historically excluded groups with neglected access to palliative care, 294*b*
homeless individuals, 301
impact on health outcomes, 294
key assessment questions, 296*b*
language, 300
neonatal palliative care practices, 440
nutrition, 304
palliative care and, 294–95, 295*b*
place of residence, 301
prisons, 301
race, 297–98
religion and spirituality, 300
social determinants of health (SDOH), 300
socioeconomic status, 300–1
striving to understand, 295–97
US ethnic group consensus estimates (2021), 294*t*
web-based resources, 296*b*
Curcuma longa (turmeric), pain, 284
Cushing's disease, sexual function, 342
cyberknife, 98
cypercoping, 337
cystic fibrosis/bronchiectasis, 496*b*

dashboard, palliative care, 810–11, 811*t*
deadname, 712*t*
death
care at the time of, 463
communication at transition to, 41–42
developmental stages and perceptions, 459*t*
ethics of hastening, 357–58
grieving associated with impending, 623
mental health and wish for hastened, 739
preparing for, 315, 316*t*
religious considerations, 434*t*
sharing "bad" news, 623–24
unanticipated pediatric, 433
See also end of life; good death; planning for death
death rattle, 169
death rituals and practices, cultural assessment questions, 296*b*
Death with Dignity Act (1994), Oregon, 358, 606–7
Decadal Survey, 537–38
decision-making
adolescents and young adults, 448, 449*t*
autonomy in pediatric medical, 424–25
family caregiver resources, 323
guidelines for healthcare team assisting with end-of-life, 419*b*
pediatric serious illness, 409–10
professional organizations' support of nurse's role in, 419–20
quality as metric, 399
role of caregiver in, 322
supporting parental, 425
value-based, for pediatric goal of care, 404–5
decompensated cirrhosis, 541
caregiver burden, 544–45
common symptoms in, 543–44
overview, 542*t*
decongestive lymphatic therapy, 192
dehydration, 168
case study, 174
fluid retention and, 169
Delaware, 500
delirium
acute confusion, 243
assessment, 245–46, 246*t*
case study, 243, 248
challenges in diagnosis and classification, 244
diagnosis criteria, 244
etiology, 245
goal-setting and plan of care, 247–48
hydration, 169
informant-based assessments, 245
laboratory and diagnostic tests, 246*t*
lab results, 246
management, 246–48
mnemonic DELIRIUMS, 245*t*
nursing interventions, 247*t*
pathophysiology, 244
prevalence, 243–44
prognosis, 244
resources for assessment, 246
risk factors, 244–45
screening tools, 246*t*
subtypes, 244
Delirium Observation Screening Scale, 245
dementia, 179–80, 309
care delivery framework, 530, 537–38
care partner capacity and needs, 530, 536–37
case study of Alzheimer's disease, 530–31
cognitive health and function, 530, 534
delirium superimposed on, 245
diagnosis and creating care plans, 531
domains and palliative approaches to supporting people with, 533*t*
emotional, behavioral, and spiritual health, 530, 534–36
health-related social needs, 530, 537
physical health and function, 530, 536
principles of palliative care in, 529*b*
recognizing and staging, 531
serious illness conversations in, 531–34
Six Domains of Health framework, 528, 530*b*, 538
dentition, older adults, 753*t*, 755
deontological theories, ethics, 349
Department of the Army, Pain Management Task Force, 280
depression
commonly prescribed medications, 257*t*
considerations in children, 256–59
definition, 251
diagnosis, 253
disorders, 254
factors for consideration in diagnosis, 254
medication considerations, 256
patient and family education, 259
patients living with cancer, 570–71
pharmacological treatment, 256
prevalence and scope, 251–52
psychiatric disorders with, 253*t*
psychotherapy treatment, 255–56
screening, 252–53
stage D heart failure, 513
treatment considerations, 255
Depression Cancer Consensus Group, 252
detransition/detransitioning, 712*t*, 714–15
dexmedetomidine, sedation in ICU patients, 691*t*, 692
diabetes mellitus, sexual function, 342
Diagnostic and Statistical Manual of Mental Disorders 5th edition (DSM-5), 253, 721
Diagnostic and Statistical Manual of Mental Disorders fifth edition, Text Revision (DSM-5-TR), 244, 733
dialysis, 549–50
discontinuation, 602
See also kidney disease
dialysis withdrawal, 601–3
case study of patient undergoing hemodialysis, 601
duration of survival, 602–3
symptoms and treatment after, for comfort care, 602*t*
diarrhea
adsorbent agents, 158
anticholinergics, 158
antisecretory agents, 158
assessment, 157–58
cancer-associated, 157
case of patient with lung cancer, 156, 158–59
causes, 157
definition, 156
diagnostic studies, 158
history, 157
iatrogenic, 157
infection-related, 156–57
nursing interventions, 158
opioid agonists, 158
pathophysiology and risk factors, 156–57
pharmacological management, 158–59
physical examination, 158
prevalence and impact, 156
prevention, 158
supportive care, 158
See also bowel management
diazepam, palliative sedation, 596, 596*t*
diffusion capacity of the lungs for carbon monoxide (DLCO), 499
dignity therapy, 337, 625–26
palliative sedation, 594
term, 626
disability status, culture, 302
disease coping, people living with HIV, 522
disenfranchised grief, 480, 712*t*
distraction, nursing intervention, 336
distress, 328
definition, 330
existential, 330–31, 330*t*
grief, 331
intensive care unit (ICU), 692
measuring, 600
premedication for anticipated, 600
psychological, 330
serious illness, 331
spiritual, 330
Distress Thermometer, 570, 571–72
District of Columbia, 605
medical aid in dying (MAID), 357–58
medical marijuana, 124
District of Columbia Pediatric Palliative Care Collaborative, 455
diversity, nursing assessment, 334
Dobbs v. Jackson Women's Health Organization, 441
do-not-attempt-resuscitation (DNAR), ethical dilemma, 353–54
dopamine receptor antagonists, nausea and vomiting, 134–35
dry mouth, thirst and, 169
durable power of attorney for healthcare (DPAHC), 352–53
dying patient
care for caregiver of, 695–96
care for family of, 695
dying process, 593–94
dysgeusia
etiology, 147
nursing assessment, 147
nursing interventions, 148
pathophysiology, 147
See also oral symptoms

dysphagia
airway clearance techniques, 144
assessment, 143–42
clinical examination of swallowing, 143
definition, 142
etiology, 143
indications of swallowing disorder, 143*b*
management, 143–44
medically administered nutrition (MAN), 167
neurological disorders, 241
oral feeding suggestions, 144*b*, 144
physiology and pathophysiology of swallowing, 142–43
postural modifications, 144, 144*t*
screening of swallowing function, 143
See also hiccups; oral symptoms
dyspnea, 104, 113
assessment and management, 692
balancing benefit with harm, 110
breathing thinking functioning model, 107–11, 108*f*
case of patient with idiopathic pulmonary fibrosis (IPF), 104, 108, 111–12, 113
case of patient with respiratory distress, 393
empathy exercise, 496*b*
end-of-life symptom management, 474*t*
final common pathway of, 106–7
as "first vital symptom," 104
management, 107–11
management of crisis, 110–11
measurement of, 107
noninvasive ventilation (NIV), 110
online resources for management, 111
outline of genesis of breathlessness, 106*f*
pathophysiology, 105–6
patient experience, 105
pediatric palliative care, 393–94
physiology, 105–7
pulmonary-palliative care, 496
specific interventions, 108–9
stage D heart failure, 512
summary of interventions for management, 109–11, 109*t*
transcutaneous electrical nerve stimulation (TENS), 110
See also cough
Dyspnea-12 (D-12), 107
Dyspnea-ALS Scale, 107

early adulthood, sexuality and sexual function, 344
Eastern Cooperative Oncology Group (ECOG) scale, 21, 22*t*
ECHO (Extension for Community Healthcare Outcomes) project, 744–45
edema, 187, 195
anatomy, physiology, and pathophysiology, 187
comparison of lymphedema and, 186*t*
definition, 186
prevalence and risk factors, 187
stage D heart failure, 512–13
See also lymphedema
Edmonton Symptom Assessment Scale, 25
Edmonton Symptom Assessment Survey (ESAS), 107
Edmonton Symptom Assessment System (ESAS), 659
Edmonton Symptom Assessment System Revised, 133
education
nursing students, 794
pediatric palliative and hospice care (PPHC), 464–65
pediatric palliative care, 393
See also nursing education
E-Hospice, 765–66
ejection fraction, 505–6
heart failure, 506
elder abuse/mistreatment, older adults, 753*t*, 756
electronic health records (EHRs), 18–19, 62
electronic medical records (EMRs), 62
Ellison, Neil, 501
emergency department (ED)
barriers and challenges to palliative care, 671–74
case study of patient in, 671, 674, 675
clinician training and perceptions, 673–74
current ED model, 672
current gaps and next steps, 676
epidemiology of palliative care, 670–71
facilitators to palliative care, 674–75
limited knowledge and research, 674
needs and experiences of palliative care patient, 672–73
palliative care in, 670
palliative care-specific patient complexities, 672
Emergency Medical Treatment and Labor Act, 301–2
Emery-Dreifuss muscular dystrophy, adolescent case study, 447
emotion acknowledgement, nursing intervention, 335
emotional, behavioral, and spiritual health, dementia, 530, 534–36
emotional coping, people living with HIV, 522–23
emotional distress, pediatric palliative care, 397
emotional labor, definition, 773*t*
EMPallA (Emergency Medicine Palliative Care Access), 648–49
empathetic listening, 430
ENABLE (Educate, Nurture, Advise, Before Life Ends)
rural palliative care, 745, 745*t*
telephonic palliative care, 648
end-diastolic volume, 505–6
ending phase, nurse-patient relationship, 30–31, 30*t*
endocrine illnesses, physical impact on sexual function, 342
end of life (EOL)
adolescents and young adults, 452
anticipatory grief and support, 625–26
case of person nearing imminent death, 619
case of wound, ostomy and continence (WOC) care, 199, 215, 221
considerations in children, 258
culturally sensitive care, 618
culture and rituals, 304
differences between hospice and palliative care, 616–17
education, 696
family and caregiver needs, 619–21
hematologic malignancies, 559
imminent death, 619–21
late-stage dementia, 534, 536, 537
liver disease, 546
nurses' role in meeting individual needs at, 618–19
nursing care at, 621
nursing homes, 666
organizations supporting, 802*t*
physical needs, 618
psychological, emotional, and spiritual needs, 619
support for family members and caregivers, 618
symptoms in normal progression in dying, 620*t*
term, 617–18
See also death; intensive care unit (ICU); pediatric patient at end of life; urgent syndromes at end of life
end-of-life decision-making
advance care planning, 52*f*, 54–55
case on facilitating, 55
guidelines for healthcare team assisting, 419*b*
end-of-life decisions
burial, 433
pediatric spiritual assessment, 433
postmortem care, 433
end-of-life huddle, 472, 473*f*
End-of-Life Nursing Education Consortium (ELNEC), 441, 464–65, 501, 642–43, 680, 704, 791, 792
curricula content, 793*t*
End-of-Life Nursing Education Consortium Training Program (ELNEC-International), 761
end-stage kidney disease (ESKD), nonpharmacological management, 551*t*
end-stage renal disease, 119
energy medicine, mood and sleep, 285
enteral nutrition, anorexia/cachexia syndrome (ACS), 123–24
Erikson, Erik, 431
Escherichia coli, diarrhea, 156
esophageal dysfunction, swallowing disorder, 143*b*
ethical climate, 424
ethical dilemmas
advance care planning, 352–53
alternative terminology, 360–61
anticipatory grief and bereavement, 464
cardiovascular implantable electronic devices, 359
care at time of death, 463
case for determining decisional capacity, 350–51
case for withdrawal of life support in ICU, 357
creating a sacred space, 463
declining treatment for children, 426
do-not-attempt-resuscitation (DNAR), 353–54
hastening death, 357–58
medical aid in dying (MAID), 357–58
medically administered nutrition and hydration (MANH), 351, 356–57
medically inappropriate and nonbeneficial treatments, 360–61
palliative sedation, 359–60
pediatric palliative care, 425–26
pediatric serious illness, 410
perinatal palliative care, 462–63
proxy decision-making, 354–55
refusal of pain and symptom management, 355–56
self-care, 463–64
voluntarily stop eating and drinking (VSED), 356, 361–62
ethical reasoning
coping skills and duty to self, 424
cultivating reflective practice, 423–24
fostering a positive ethical climate, 424
pediatric nursing competencies in, 423–24
steps analyzing challenging situations, 423, 423*t*
ethics
allocation of scarce resources, 362–63
compassion fatigue, 362
definition, 349
framework, 350*b*
moral distress, 362
moral reasoning and, 349
nursing issues, 362
social media, 782
steps of ethical problem-solving, 350*b*
term, 424
See also ethical dilemmas
ethics consultation, interdisciplinary palliative care team, 71
ethics of care, 350
ethnicity
cultural assessment questions, 296*b*
culture, 298
See also race; underrepresented groups
ethos of palliative nursing, 83, 703
beauty, 85

case study, 83–84
imagination, 84–85
presence, 85–86
space, 85
trustworthiness, 84
Europe, assisted dying and euthanasia, 607
European Association for Palliative Care, 607–8
euthanasia, 357, 606
excessive secretions
case study of patient with, 394
pediatric palliative care, 394
exemplary practice model
pediatric palliative care, 484–86, 485*f*
reflection and self-awareness for nurses, 486
windmill model, 484–86
existential distress, 330–31, 330*t*, 397
Existential Distress Scale, 371*t*
existential needs. *See* spiritual, religious, and existential (S/R/E) needs
existential pain, assessment findings and therapy, 91*t*
existential suffering, 609
case study, 595
Ex-PLISSIT, sexual health framework, 345, 346*t*
extracorporeal membrane oxygenation (ECMO)
cessation, 603
ethics of initiating, 426
extubation, 600–1
exudate, 106

Facebook, 777, 779
case study, 781–82
faith, Fowler's life-span stages of, 431, 431*t*
faith, import, community, address (FICA), 371*t*
falls and fall risk, older adults, 752, 753*t*
families
adolescents and young adults, 450
being present with bereaved, 488
care for, of dying ICU patient, 695
child and adolescents at the end of life, 483
child and grandparents, 482
child and parent, 481–82
child and siblings, 482–83
communication barriers, 31
communication themes, 29*t*
grief assessment, 484
impact of dynamics on relationship, 482–83
information needs of, 35–36
LGBTQIA+ patients, 716–17
meetings, 36–37, 37*b*
needs at imminent death, 619–21
pain management, 90
palliative care, 309
preparing for uncertainty, 405–6
questions addressing coping, 38*b*
social media and, 780–81
substance use disorder, 728
support for, near end of life, 618
supporting patient with chronic breathlessness, 111–12
value-based care (VBC) and, 63–64
families of choice, 309
families of origin, 309
family caregiver
assessment in palliative care, 317–19
heterogeneous needs and diversity of, 311*f*
in home and community, 319–20
in hospital, 320
in intensive care unit (ICU), 320
in long-term care setting, 321*f*, 321
needs in palliative care, 318*t*
in perioperative setting, 320–21
quality of life, 317
resources, 323
resources for palliative care nurses, 323*t*
role in decision-making and advance care planning, 322
See also family experiences
family-centered care, pediatric palliative and hospice care (PPHC), 458
family-centered palliative care, 309
Family Confusion Assessment Methods (FAM-CAM), delirium, 245
family education, depression and anxiety, 259
family experiences
burdening, 313–14
case study on difficulty of witnessing health changes, 313
contending with change, 314
dimensions of fading away, 316*t*
dimensions of transition of fading away, 311–17
family caregiving in palliative care, 315–17
living day to day, 315
preparing for death, 315
redefining, 311–13
redefining case study, 311–12
resistance to letting go case study, 312
searching for meaning, 314–15
struggling with paradox, 314
transition of fading away, 310–17
See also family caregiver
fatigue, 264, 270–71
assessment, 267–68, 268*b*
cancer-related, 264
case study, 264, 266, 267, 268
definitions, 265
factors influencing, 266–67
hematologic malignancies, 559–60
impact of, 267
management and treatment, 268–69
measurement tools, 268
nonpharmacological interventions, 269–70
nursing interventions, 270*t*
pathophysiology, 266
patients living with cancer, 570–71
pharmacological and herbal interventions, 269
populations at risk, 265*b*
prevalence, 265*b*, 265–66
risk factors associated with, 266*b*
stage D heart failure, 512
Fatigue Observation Checklist, 268
Fatigue Scale, 268
Federal Veterans Affairs Community Living Centers, 662
feeding difficulties, pediatric palliative care, 395–96
fee-for-service (FFS) payment, Medicare, 11
feminist ethics, 350
fentanyl
acute pain treatment, 382*t*
pain management, 93–94
transdermal, pain management, 94
Ferrell, Betty, 496
fertility, adolescents and young adults, 448
fever
diagnostic evaluation, 230–31
nonpharmacologic treatment options, 231
nursing assessment, 230–31
pharmacologic treatment options, 231
underlying mechanism, 230
unknown origin (FUO), 230
See also sweats
FICA model, spiritual history, 430*t*
fidelity, palliative sedation, 594
financial concerns, older adults, 753*t*, 756
financial literacy, 301
fistulas, 219–20
ABCs of persistent, 219*b*
characteristics of effluent, 220*t*
commonly occurring complications, 219*b*
diagnosis and assessment, 220
nutrition management, 221
palliative management, 220–21, 220*t*
pharmacological management, 221
terminology, 219*t*
Five Wishes, 462
fluid buildup, 106
fluid retention, dehydration and, 169
Foldi, Michael, 192
food texture and consistency, swallowing, 144
Four Seasons Consulting, 501
Frank, Arthur, 624
Frankl, Viktor, 329
Frechman, Erica, 771–72
free-standing palliative care, 641
Freud, Sigmund, 627–28
From Novice to Expert (Benner), 785–86
frontotemporal dementia, 528–29, 529*t*
Fry, Sara, 350
Functional Assessment of Anorexia/Cachexia Therapy, 122
Functional Assessment of Cancer Therapy-Cognition (FACT-Cog), 570
functional medicine, term, 281
futility
concept of, 360
medically inappropriate and nonbeneficial treatments, 360–61
term, 360
Future of Nursing, The (IOM), 647, 792
Future of Nursing 2020-2030, The, 300, 787–88

gabapentin, neuropathic and chronic pain syndromes, 384*t*
gait, case study of mobility, 239*b*, 240
gamma knife radiosurgery, 98
gastrointestinal symptoms
mind-body approaches for, 285–86
natural products for, 286
pediatric palliative care, 394–96
gastrointestinal system, dying process, 593
gate keepers, family for adolescents, 448
gay, 712*t*
Geisinger Medical Center, 496–97, 501–2
gender, 712*t*
cultural assessment questions, 296*b*
culture, 299–300
term, 341
gender-affirming surgery, 712*t*
gender expression, 712*t*
gender-fluid, 712*t*
gender identity, 299–300, 712*t*
General Anxiety Disorder scale, 23
Generalized Anxiety Disorder (GAD-7), 252, 253
geriatric assessment, cancer patients, 571
geriatrics. *See* older adults
German Society for Palliative Care, 281
Giardia lamblia, diarrhea, 156
Gilligan, Carol, 85, 350
ginger (*Zingiber officinale*)
gastrointestinal symptoms, 286
nausea, 137
Global Atlas of Palliative Care, 759
global palliative care, 759
case of nurse-led outpatient clinic in Nepal, 762
case of prognosis and end-of-life wishes in Vietnam, 761–62
cultural exchange and mentorship, 766
disproportionately impacted populations, 766
evidence-based practices, 763
factors influencing delivery, 759–62
factors influencing implementation in low- or middle-income countries (LMICs), 762–63
initiatives, 765–66
international and regional organizations, 764*t*
levels of development (2017), 763*f*
morphine use worldwide, 763*f*
nursing role in, 766
policy and advocacy, 766
research considerations, 804

global palliative care (*cont.*)
  specific challenges by nurses in LMICs, 763–65
  training and curriculum development, 766
Global Strategy for the Diagnosis, Management, and Prevention of Chronic Obstructive Pulmonary Disease (GOLD), 495
glucocorticoids, anorexia/cachexia syndrome (ACS), 124, 125*t*
L-glutamine, gastrointestinal symptoms, 286
goals of care
  case study, 38
  case study on care at end of life, 41–42
  life-sustaining treatment discussions, 40–41
  medically administered hydration and nutrition, 41
  ongoing discussions, 38–42
  prognosis, 39–40
  questions for changing, 41*b*
  questions for discussing ongoing care, 39*b*
  serious news discussions, 39, 40*b*
  transition to death, 41–42
  transition to palliative care/hospice, 41
  See also pediatric goals of care; pediatric serious illness
goals-of-care conversations, advance care planning (ACP), 52*f*, 53
good death, 625
  barriers and facilitators of, 617*t*
  challenge of ensuring, 626–27
  definition, 617, 626
Graduate Competencies and Recommendations for Educating Undergraduate Nursing Students (G-CARES), 793, 794, 795*b*, 796
graft-versus-host disease, hematologic malignancies, 560
grandparents
  grief of child and, 482
  supporting bereaved, 489
grief, 23, 331
  assessing throughout the trajectory of care, 483–84
  bereavement and, 479, 480
  case study of adolescent palliative care nurse, 488
  child and grandparents, 482
  child and healthcare team, 483
  child and parent, 481–82
  child and siblings, 482–83
  children and adolescents at end of life, 483
  factors affecting experience, 484
  family assessment, 484
  impact of family dynamics on relationship, 482–83
  interventions and supporting the bereaved, 484–90
  mourning and, 480
  pediatric palliative and hospice care (PPHC), 464
  potential losses, 624*t*
  as process, 479
  relationship context, 481–82
  ritual and meaning-making, 490*b*, 490
  term, 480
  theories and models, 480–81, 481*t*
grief and bereavement support, family caregiver resources, 323
grief distress, death of a child, 483
grief process, 623
grief support, acknowledging losses and providing, 624–25, 624*t*
grief trajectories through loss, model, 629
grieving process, 623, 627
  bereaved individual, 627–29
  case study, 630–31
  common responses, 628*t*
  dual process of coping with loss, 628
  factors affecting, 629*f*, 629–31
  meaning reconstruction of loss, 629
  model of grief trajectories through loss, 629
  nurses and clinicians, 632
  nurses' grief through the pandemic, 632–33
  task model, 628
guanylate cyclase-C receptor agonists, constipation, 153
guardians, pediatric palliative and hospice care (PPHC), 458
guided imagery
  gastrointestinal symptoms, 286
  mind-body approaches for pain, 283
guided participation for clinical practice
  case study of adolescent palliative care nurse, 488
  joining and maintaining attention, 487
  middle-range theory, 486–88, 487*f*
Guidelines for Quality Palliative Care, 67
GUIDE talking map, goals of care, 412, 413*t*
Guillain-Barré syndrome, 179–80

HAND, HIV-associated neurocognitive disorders, 520–21
haptics, 28
Harm Principle, definition, 425
Harvard University, 17
Hawaii, 12, 605
  medical aid in dying (MAID), 357–58
Healing Touch (HT), energy medicine, 285
health, six domains of, 530*b*
health equity
  addressing palliative care access, 706*f*
  interdisciplinary collaboration in promoting, 708
  public policy and, 14
  role of nursing promoting, in underserved populations, 705–8
  See also underrepresented groups
Health Insurance Portability and Accountability Act (HIPAA), 300, 649–50, 652–53
health literacy, 300
health literacy, health numeracy, and financial literacy, culture, 300–1
health numeracy, 300–1
Health Resources and Services Administration (HRSA), 647
healthcare cost, value-based care (VBC) and, 63
healthcare language, translation to lay language, 31, 31*t*
healthcare power of attorney (HCPOA), 18
healthcare professionals
  social media and, 781–82
  supporting grieving of, 489–90
healthcare proxy, 352–53
healthcare settings
  barriers to cancer pain management, 90*b*
  pain management, 90
healthcare team, grief for child and, 483
health-related social needs, dementia, 530, 537
hearing, older adults, 753*t*, 755
heart disease, 309
heart failure, 505
  advance care planning, 513
  assessment and medical management in stage D, 507–12
  case study of patient with, 514–15
  classification systems, 507, 508*t*
  common medications, 510*t*
  comorbidity, 505
  disease trajectory and prognosis, 507
  end-of-life care, 513–15
  left ventricular assist device deactivation, 514*b*
  management of symptoms in stage D, 512–13
  pathogenesis, 505–7
  primary palliative care, 513
  reduced *vs* preserved ejection fraction, 506
  right *vs* left ventricular dysfunction, 506–7
  type, 506*t*
  withdrawal of life-sustaining therapies, 513–15
heart failure, stage D
  health history, 507–8
  heart transplantation, 511–12
  implantable cardioverter-defibrillators (ICDs), 509
  intravenous inotrope therapy, 512
  laboratory data and diagnostic tests, 509
  lifestyle recommendations, 509
  mechanical circulatory support, 509–11
  pharmacologic treatment, 509
  physical exam, 508–9
  renal replacement therapies, 512
  treatment, 509–12
heart rate, 505–6
hematologic malignancies, 556–57
  assessment of symptoms during active treatment, 559
  case study, 556, 557, 558, 559, 560–61
  chimeric antigen receptor T-cell therapy (CART), 549, 558
  during survivorship, 559
  early integration of palliative care into care, 557
  at end of life, 559
  fatigue, 559–60
  graft-versus-host disease, 560
  hematopoietic stem cell transplant (HCT) challenges, 558
  insomnia, 560
  management of common symptoms, 559–61
  mucositis, 560
  pain, 560
  psychosocial support, 560–61
  role of palliative care for individuals with, 561
  symptom experiences, 558–59
  trajectories, 557*t*
  values assessment and integration, 557–58
  xerostomia, 560
hematopoietic stem cell transplant (HCT), 549
  challenges by individuals receiving, 558
hematopoietic stem cell transplantation, case study of patient undergoing, 400–1
hemodialysis (HD)
  case of patient undergoing, 601
  case of withdrawing from, 552, 553
  questions to ask persons considering withdrawal, 553*t*
  withdrawal from, 552–53
  See also kidney disease
hemoptysis
  case study of patient with, 583
  diagnostic procedure, 583
  epidemiology, 583
  massive, 584
  non-massive, 584
  pathophysiology, 583
  signs and symptoms, 583
  treatment, 583–84
  See also urgent syndrome at end of life
hemorrhagic cystitis, 182–83
heterosexual or straight, 712*t*
hiccups
  case study, 144–45
  case study of patient with ALS, 144–45
  etiology, 145
  nursing assessment, 145
  nursing interventions, 145
  pathophysiology, 145
High Needs ACO Realizing Equity, Access, and Community Health program, 60
Hippocrates, 734
HIV/AIDS
  fatigue, 265*b*
  See also people living with HIV
hoarding, 736–38
holistic medicine, 281

Holm, Soren, 609
home setting
  effectiveness of palliative care, 640
  family caregivers in, 319–20
  palliative nursing in, 7
homeless individuals, culture, 301
homeostasis, 166
homophobia/transphobia, 712*t*
homosexual, 712*t*
honesty, 84
hope, 328
  context of serious illness, 331–33
  nursing intervention, 336
  preserving, 432, 462
  reframing, 332–33
  sources of, in seriously ill adults, 332*b*
  See also meaning and purpose
HOPE model, spiritual history, 430*t*
Hopkins Verbal Learning Test-Revised, 570
hormone replacement therapy, 712*t*
hospice
  adolescents and young adults, 451–52
  chronic kidney disease (CKD), 554
  community-based palliative care (CBPC), 640
  conversations about transition to, 41
  term, 759
  See also pediatric hospice
Hospice and Palliative Care Coalition, 643
Hospice and Palliative Credentialing Center, 84, 797
Hospice and Palliative Nurses Association (HPNA), 3, 6, 14–15, 55, 84, 108, 356, 357, 419–20, 605, 641–42, 706–7, 792, 801–3
  research agenda priorities, 803*b*
hospice care
  nursing homes (NHs), 664
  palliative model, 66–67, 67*t*, 73
  people living with dementia, 534
  team roles in model, 80*t*
  term, 454–55
hospice carve-in, 12
Hospice Quality Reporting Program (HQRP), 808
hospital
  critical access, 746*b*, 746
  family caregivers in, 320
hospital admission, case of advance care planning conversation, 55
Hospital Anxiety and Depression Scale, 570
hospital-based palliative care (HBPC)
  acute palliative care unit (APCU), 681
  assessing palliative care needs, 683
  case of Rita, 679, 681, 684, 685
  consulting specialty palliative care, 682–83
  definition, 679
  evolution, 679–81
  evolution of palliative care needs, 683*t*
  future directions for, 686
  initial palliative care (PC) consultation, 684
  inpatient interdisciplinary consult team, 681
  integration for team members, 684*t*
  nursing care of seriously ill, 681–82
  nursing roles in, 682–84
  ongoing PC involvement during stay, 685
  palliative and hospice nursing roles, 682*t*
  palliative care intervention, 683–84
  primary palliative care, 680
  scope of, in United States, 679–80
  specialty palliative care, 680
  standards for, 680
  transitions of care and continuity, 685
  triggers for PC involvement, 683
  types of, 680
hospital bereavement programs, 490
Hospital Elder Life Program (HELP), 248
hospital patient survey, 14
hospital setting, palliative nursing in, 6–7
human immunodeficiency virus (HIV)
  pruritus origin and treatment, 230
  See also people living with HIV (PLWH)
human immunodeficiency virus/acquired immunodeficiency syndrome (HIV/AIDS), 11
hunger, medically administered nutrition (MAN), 167
Huntington's disease (HD)
  neurological disorder, 237–38
  resources for people living with, 236*t*
  symptoms by stage, 237*t*
Huntington's Disease Society of America (HDSA), 237–38
hydration
  benefits and burdens, 168–69
  delirium, confusion, agitation, 169
  literature review, 169–70
  medically administered nutrition (MAN), 167–68
  methods of administration, 168
  myoclonus, 170
  quality of death, 170
  quality of life (QOL), 170
  routes for medically administered, 168*t*
  survival benefit, 170
  thirst and dry mouth, 169
  See also medically administered nutrition (MAN); medically administered nutrition and hydration (MANH)
hydrocodone, pain management, 95
hydromorphone
  acute pain treatment, 382*t*
  pain management, 94
hydroxytryptophan (5HTP), mood and sleep, 285
hypercalcemia, case study, 585
hypercalcemia
  bisphosphonate therapy, 586–87
  calcitonin, 587
  case study, 585
  denosumab, 587
  description, 585–86
  dialysis, 587
  nursing management, 587
  pathophysiology, 586
  signs and symptoms, 586
  treatment, 587*t*
  treatments, 586–87
  See also urgent syndrome at end of life
hyperthermic intraperitoneal chemotherapy (HIPEC), 160–61
hyperthyroidism, sexual function, 342
hypnosis
  gastrointestinal symptoms, 286
  mood and sleep, 285
  nausea and vomiting, 138*t*
hypodermoclysis, 168, 168*t*
hydration, conversations about medically administered, 41

ibuprofen
  pain management, 92, 93*t*
  treatment of mild pain, 381*t*
idiopathic pulmonary fibrosis (IPF), 498, 500
  case of patient with, 104, 108, 111–12, 113
Illinois, 12, 465
illness information, family caregiver resources, 323
imagination, ethos of palliative nursing, 84–85
immigration status, culture, 301–2
immunotherapy, pain management, 98
implantable cardiac defibrillator (ICD), cessation, 603
Implicit Association Test (IAT), 17
Improving Palliative Care through Teamwork (IMPACTT), 665
incompetency, term, 354–55
incontinence, older adults, 753*t*, 754
incontinence-associated dermatitis (IAD), 198–99
  management, 222
  palliative settings, 221–22
  prevention, 222
infants/toddlers
  culture, 298
  observational pain scales, 378*t*
  observed pain behaviors, 379*t*
Infectious Diseases Society of America, 156–57
informal caregiving, older adults, 753*t*, 755–56
Informant Assessment of Geriatric Delirium, 245
information
  communication in gathering, 33
  communication in imparting, 32–33
  needs of patients and families, 35–36
information on specific illnesses, family caregiver resources, 323
information sharing, ethics in pediatric palliative care, 425
informed consent
  American Academy of Pediatrics, 425
  medical aid in dying, 609–10
  palliative sedation, 360
initial phase, nurse-patient relationship, 30, 30*t*
Initiative for Pediatric Palliative Care, 464–65
innovations in patient monitoring, value-based care (VBC) and, 62–63
inotropy, 505–6
inpatient consult service
  palliative care model, 66, 67*t*, 72
  team roles in model, 80*t*
inpatient interdisciplinary consult team, 681
insomnia, 273, 278
  assessment for physical factors, 275*b*, 275
  case study of patient with, 274
  cognitive and emotional factors, 275–76
  cognitive behavioral interventions, 276–77
  cognitive-behavioral therapy for (CBTi), 276–77
  contributing factors, 274–76, 275*b*
  definition, 273
  diagnosis, 273
  environmental factors contributing, 276
  hematologic malignancies, 560
  nonpharmacologic therapies for, 277*t*
  nursing interventions, 275*b*, 275
  over-the-counter preparations, 278
  pathophysiology, 274
  pharmacological interventions, 277–78, 278*t*
  physical factors, 274–75, 275*b*
  prevalence and impact, 273–74
  taking a history about, 275*t*
  treatment, 276–78
inspiratory muscle training (IMT), dyspnea, 109*t*, 110
Institute of Medicine (IoM), 3, 259, 495–96, 647, 792
  When Children Die, 456
Integrated Palliative Care Outcome Scale, 25
integrative health, term, 281
integrative medicine
  case study, 282
  critical role of nurses, 280
  nausea and vomiting, 136–37, 138*t*
  resources, 287, 287*t*
  See also complementary and integrative medicine (CIM)
integrative nursing, resources, 287, 287*t*
integrative therapies, considerations in children, 258–59
Intensive Care Delirium Screening Checklist (ICDSC), 692
intensive care unit (ICU)
  anxiety, agitation, and sedation, 690–91
  care for caregiver of dying patient, 695–96
  care for family of dying patient, 695
  case study, 688, 689, 692, 694, 696

intensive care unit (ICU) (*cont.*)
case study on withdrawal of life support, 357
distressing symptoms, 692
dyspnea assessment and management, 692
end-of-life education, 696
end-of-life practice issues, 693–94
essential components of palliative care, 689–91
family caregivers in, 320
guidelines for family meetings, 693*b*
limitations of end-of-life (EOL) care, 688–89
nonpharmacological interventions for anxiety and agitation, 692
nonpharmacological management of pain, 690
pain assessment, 689
pharmacological management for sedation, 691–92
pharmacological management of pain, 690
pharmacologic of commonly used opioids, 690*t*
planning palliative care for, 689
procedural pain, 689–90
sharing narratives, 696
withdrawal of ventilator therapy, 694–95
withholding and withdrawing life-sustaining treatments (LSTs), 693–94
interdisciplinary legacy work, nursing intervention, 336–37
interdisciplinary palliative care team, 66, 67, 74, 77–78
advanced practice registered nurse (APRN), 68
ancillary disciplines/consultants, 69, 71–72
bereavement coordinator, 69, 72
building, 73–74
care continuum, 79–81
case study demonstrating member contributions, 69
case study with multiple chronic conditions, 79–81
chaplain, 67–68
child life specialist (CLS), 71, 72
ethics consultation, 71
models, 66–67, 67*t*, 72–73
nurses' role in, 78*t*, 79
palliative care chaplain, 69–70
palliative care nurse (PCN), 68, 70
palliative care physician, 70
palliative care social worker, 70–71
physical and occupational therapy, 71
physician, 68
registered dietitian/nutritionist, 72
respiratory therapy, 71
roles of, 78–79, 78*t*
social worker, 68–69
speech-language pathology, 71
sustaining a healthy, functioning, 74
team roles across models, 80*t*
volunteers, 69, 71
interdisciplinary team (IDT), 10, 13, 17
long-term care (LTC), 663
roles of palliative care members, 642*t*
spiritual assessments, 429–30, 433–34
intermittent pneumatic compression devices, lymphedema, 193
International Association for the Study of Pain (IASP), 99
International Cancer and Cognitive Task Force, 570
International Classification of Diseases, 244, 253, 267
International Classification of Sleep Disorders, 273
International Telecommunication Union, 650
internet of things (IoT), health IoT, 649
interpersonal relationships, impact of serious illness on sexual function, 343–44
Interprofessional Spiritual Care Education Curriculum for Pediatrics (ISPEC-Peds), 433
intersectionality, 713
intersex, 712*t*
interstitial lung diseases, 496*b*
intersubjective process, 623
interventional therapies, pain management, 99
intervention strategies, sexual health, 345–46
introductory phase, nurse-patient relationship, 30, 30*t*

Joint Commission Advanced Certification Program, 808
Joint Commission Advanced Certification Program for Palliative Care, 641
Joint Commission on Mental Health of Children, 256–58
Journal of Hospice and Palliative Nursing, 796–97
Journal of Palliative Medicine, 796–97
justice, medical aid in dying, 609

Kaiser Family Foundation, 662
Kant, Immanuel, 84
Kennedy terminal ulcers (KTUs), 198–99
ketamine, 97*t*
neuropathic and chronic pain syndromes, 384*t*
pain management, 97–98
Kickstart, Assess, Evaluate, Refer (KAER model), 531
kidney disease, 309, 549
case of person receiving conservative kidney management, 551
case withdrawing from dialysis, 552, 553
chronic kidney disease (CKD), 549
communication and advance care planning for CKM, 552
conservative kidney management (CKM), 550, 551–52
end of life in, 553
end-stage (ESKD), 549
hemodialysis (HD), 549–50
hospice indications, 554
medical management, 550
medical management of CKM, 552
nonpharmacological management of symptoms of end-stage, 551*t*
nursing considerations for persons living with AKD, 554
race considerations, 549
renal physician association shared decision-making guidelines, 554*b*
renal replacement therapy, 550–51
symptom management of CKM, 552
symptoms of advanced, 550
trajectory and prognosis, 549–50
transplant, 549
withdrawal from HD, 552–53, 553*t*
knowledge management (KM), value-based care (VBC) and, 64
Kohlberg, Lawrence, 431

labored breathing, 105
Lactobacillus acidophilus, 153
Lactobacillus casei, 153
Lancet Commission, 760–61
language
culture, 300
nursing assessment of hope and meaning, 333*t*
laxatives
malignant bowel obstruction, 155
See also constipation
left ventricular assist device (LVAD)
cardiovascular device, 359
cessation, 602, 603
legacy, social media, 781
legacy documents, 337
Leicester Cough Monitor, 112
Leicester Cough Questionnaire, 112
lesbian, 712*t*
leukemia case, pediatric palliative care, 422–23, 426
levorphanol, pain management, 95
Lewy body dementia, 528–29, 529*t*
LGBTQ community/people
advance care planning (ACP), 51
culture, 299–300
LGBTQIA+ individuals, 711
bereavement, 717
case of Gerry, 713
central concepts and terms, 711–13
disparities in health and healthcare, 714
ethical and legal considerations, 714–15
families and caregivers, 716–17
palliative care needs, 711, 717
physical care for, 715
psychosocial and spiritual needs, 715–16
questions for guiding palliative care assessment, 714*t*
sexuality and sexual function of, 344–45
social determinants of health (SDOH), 701
terms and concepts for responsive and affirming care, 712*t*
See also underrepresented groups
Life of Breath project, 104
life review, 337
life span, sexuality and sexual function across, 344–45
life support, case study on withdrawal of, in ICU, 357
life-sustaining therapies withdrawal, heart failure, 513–15
life-sustaining therapy
cardiac device cessation, 602–3
dialysis withdrawal, 601–3
ventilator withdrawal, 599–601
life-sustaining treatments
discussion of, 40–41
medical orders for, 52*f*, 54
lifestyle medicine, term, 281
liminality, term, 625
listening, communication, 34–35
listening for hope, nursing intervention, 336
liver disease
assessment, 541
case study, 540, 543, 544, 545, 546
cirrhosis and portal hypertension, 543–44
course of cirrhosis, 542
cultural considerations, 546
decompensating events and upheaval of lives, 544–45
diagnosis, 541
end-of-life and hospice care, 546
epidemiology, 541
family caregiver support, 546
liver transplant, 545
management, 542–43
medication management, 542*t*
palliative care, 540, 541, 543, 544, 545, 546
palliative care vs hospice, 545–46
pathophysiology of cirrhosis, 541
recurrent hospitalizations, 545–46
See also cirrhosis
living will, 352–53
local anesthetics, 97*t*
pain management, 97
long-acting bronchodilator inhalation therapy, dyspnea, 109, 109*t*
long-term care (LTC)
advance care planning, 665–66
care considerations, 663–64
case study, 667
challenges to palliative care delivery, 666
delivery settings, 662–63
end of life (EOL) transitions, 666
enhancing palliative care in nursing homes (NHs), 665–66
external consultation teams, 664
facilitators to providing palliative care, 666–67
family caregivers in, 321*f*, 321
hospice care in NHs, 664
integrated palliative care, 664–65
interdisciplinary team (IDT), 663
models to delivery palliative care in NHs, 664–65

non-nursing home (NH) residential settings, 662–63
nursing homes (NH) and, 662
palliative care delivery in NHs, 664
palliative care resources for NH staff and providers, 665*t*
palliative nursing in, 7–8
physical and psychosocial aspects of care, 665
resident characteristics, 663
resources for palliative care in NHs, 667
skilled nursing care, 663
lorazepam, 96
palliative sedation, 596, 596*t*
sedation in ICU patients, 691–92, 691*t*
loss of the self, 624
Lou Gehrig's disease, 235
See also amyotrophic lateral sclerosis (ALS)
Loving Kindness Meditation (LKM), 282
lung cancer, case of diarrhea for patient with, 156, 158–59
lung disease, 309
lymphedema, 185, 187–88
anatomy, physiology, and pathophysiology, 187–88
assessment of symptoms, 189
bandages and garments, 192–93
best practice, 188
bioelectrical impedance analysis (BIA), 190*f*, 190
case study, 185–86
comparison of edema and, 186*t*
complete decongestive therapy (CDT), 192
definitions, 186
impact, 187
infection prevention and treatment, 193
infrared perometry, 190*f*, 190
management, 193*b*, 193–94
pneumatic (mechanical) pumps, 193
precision assessment and diagnosis, 188–89
prevalence and risk factors, 187
prevention of infection and skin trauma, 191
quantification, 189–90
risk reduction, 191–92
safe physical exercise, 194
secondary to cancer of head and neck, 195*b*
self-care, 194
sequential circumferential arm measurements, 190
sequential components of assessment, 189*b*
skin care, 194
surgical approach, 192
symptom experience index, 189*t*
symptom management, 194–95
tape measurement, 190*f*
treatment, 192–93
unusual lymphedemas, 194–95
Maani-Fogelman, Patricia, 501
magnesium, gastrointestinal symptoms, 286
MAHN. *See* medically administered hydration and nutrition (MAHN); medically administered nutrition and hydration (MANH)
Maine, 605
medical aid in dying (MAID), 357–58
malignant bowel obstruction
analgesics, 155–56
anticholinergics, 155
antiemetics, 155
antisecretory agents, 155
assessment, 154
case of ovarian cancer patient, 153
definition, 154
diagnostic studies, 154
history, 154
laxatives, 155
nursing interventions, 154
ovarian cancer patient, 153, 156
pathophysiology and risk factors, 154
pharmacologic management, 155–56
physical examination, 154
prevalence, 154
procedural management, 155
supportive care, 154
surgical management, 155
See also bowel management
malignant fungating wounds (MFWs), 198–99, 211*f*, 211–12
assessment, 212
metastatic vulvar cancer, 213*f*
psychosocial and spiritual aspects of care, 212
wound care considerations, 212
MAN. *See* medically administered nutrition (MAN)
MANH. *See* medically administered nutrition and hydration (MANH); medically administered hydration and nutrition (MAHN)
Man's Search for Meaning (Frankl), 329
Marjolin's ulcers, 198–99
skin pathologies giving rise to, 213*b*
treatment, 213
wound care, 212–13
Mary J. Labyak Institute for Innovation, 455
Massachusetts, 465
massage, nausea and vomiting, 138*t*
massage therapy, mind-body approaches for pain, 283
Maynard, Brittany, 607
meaning, 328–30
case study (Mr. M), 329–30, 334–35
case study (Ms. R), 328, 331
case study (Mx. S), 332
loss of, 329–30
nursing intervention, 336
purpose and, 328–30
See also hope; purpose
meaning in illness
assessing diversity, 334
nursing assessment, 333–34, 333*t*
nursing interventions, 335–37
nursing role, 334–37
See also nursing interventions
meaning reconstruction of loss, 629
Measuring What Matters project, 641–42
Medicaid, 12, 60, 66–67, 455, 641
facts, 12*t*
public policy and health equity, 14
medical adhesive-related skin injuries (MARSIs), 198–99
chronic critical limb ischemia with gangrene, 211
risk factors and prevention, 210–11
skin tears and, 209–11, 210*t*
treatment, 211
medical aid in dying (MAID), 605–6
case of clinician conscientiously objecting, 611–12
case of patient requesting, 608
ethics of requests for, 608–10
hastening death, 357–58
historical evolution of, 606
legal issues, 610
medications in, 611
nursing role and implications in, 612
professional position statements, 358
responding to requests, 610–11
United States, 606–7
withdrawing treatment versus, 611–12
world view, 607–8
medical device-related pressure injuries (MDRPIs), 198–99, 206–9
risk factors, risk assessment, and risk reduction, 206
treatment, 206–9
medical emergencies, end-of-life, 474
medical marijuana, pediatrics, 384–85
Medical Oncology Service, 626*b*
Medical Orders for Life-Sustaining Treatment (MOLST/MOST), 54, 353, 418, 653
medical power of attorney (MPOA), 450–51
medically administered hydration and nutrition (MAHN)
conversations, 41
professional position statements, 358
medically administered nutrition (MAN)
benefits and burdens, 166–67
dysphagia, 167
hunger, 167
malnutrition, anorexia, and cachexia, 166–67
medical intervention, 166
potential complications of enteral support, 166*t*
pressure ulcers, 167
quality of life (QOL), 167
survival time, 167
medically administered nutrition and hydration (MANH), 165
advanced illness or end of life in key studies, 171*t*
alternatives, 173–74
case study, 174
comfort feeding only, 174
decision-making and, 170–72
disease-specific guidelines, 170*t*
engaging in conversations and goals of care, 172–73
ethical dilemma, 351, 356–57
ethical issues, 171
initiating and withdrawing/withholding, 174
legal precedent, 171–72
position statements and guidelines, 170
religious and cultural issues, 172
religious beliefs about, 173*t*
voluntary stopping of eating and drinking, 173–74
Medicare, 60, 66–67, 642
basics, 10, 10*t*
MA value-based insurance design, 12
operation of, 10–11
Part A, 10
parts of, 11*t*
payment, 11
public policy and health equity, 14
series illness models, 11–12
Medicare Advantage (MA), 10, 11
Medicare Care Choices Model (MCCM), 11–12
Medicare Hospice Benefit (MHB), 11, 664
Medicare Part A, 616
Medicare Part B, 13, 616
Medicare Part D, opioid overutilization program, 14
Medicare Payment Advisory Commission (MedPAC), 10–11
medications
impact on sexual function, 342*t*
older adults, 753*t*, 755
melatonin, mood and sleep, 285
membrane stabilizers, 96–97
Memorial Delirium Assessment Scale, 245
Memorial Symptom Assessment Scale, 107, 389
mental illness. *See* serious mental illness (SMI)
mentorship, career advancement, 786–87
men who have sex with men, 712*t*
methadone
acute pain treatment, 382*t*
neuropathic and chronic pain syndromes, 384*t*
pain management, 94
methicillin-resistant *Staphylococcus aureus*, urinary tract infections (UTIs), 183
metoclopramide, anorexia/cachexia syndrome (ACS), 125*t*
Michigan, 465
microaggressions, 712*t*

midazolam, 96
palliative sedation, 595, 596*t*
sedation in ICU patients, 691–92, 691*t*
middle adulthood, sexuality and sexual function, 344
middle phase, nurse-patient relationship, 30, 30*t*
mind-body approaches
gastrointestinal symptoms, 285–86
mood and sleep, 284–85
pain, 283
mind-body practices, 282
term, 282
mindfulness, mind-body approaches for pain, 283
Mini-Mental State Exam, 570
minority or minoritized, 712*t*
mobility
case study, 239*b*, 240
gain impairment and falls, 240
myoclonus, 239–40
neurological care, 239–40
spasticity, 239
Montana, medical aid in dying (MAID), 357–58
Montreal Cognitive Assessment (MoCA), 570
mood, older adults, 752, 753*t*
mood and sleep
mind and body approaches, 284–85
natural products, 285
mood disorders, persons with, 734–35
moral character, 83
See also ethos of palliative nursing
moral dilemmas, 349
moral distress, 349
death of a child, 483
definition, 773*t*
ethics, 362
phenomenon, 362
moral injury, definition, 773*t*
moral reasoning, 349–50
ethics and, 349
moral uncertainty, 349
morality, 349
term, 424
morphine
acute pain treatment, 382*t*
pain management, 93
use worldwide, 763*f*
motor and sensory deficits
palliative patients, 217–18
stoma care considerations for patients, 217*t*
motor neuron disease, 309
mourning
grief, bereavement and, 480
term, 480
See also grief
mucositis, hematologic malignancies, 560
Multidimensional Assessment of Fatigue, 268
Multidimensional Dyspnea Profile (MDP), 107
multimorbidity
aging with HIV, 521
case of patient with AIDS and, 524–25
Multinational Association for Supportive Care in Cancer (MASCC), 155, 590
multiple sclerosis (MS), 179–80
fatigue, 265*b*
neurological disorder, 238
resources for people living with, 236*t*
musculoskeletal, symptoms in normal progression in dying, 620*t*
music therapy
mind-body approaches for pain, 283
nausea and vomiting, 138*t*
Mycobacterium avium complex, diarrhea, 156
myoclonus
adverse effect of opioid analgesics, 96
hydration, 170
My Wishes, 462

nalbuphine, limited use in pediatrics, 380–81
naproxen, treatment of mild pain, 381*t*
narrative ethics, 350
National Academies of Sciences, Engineering, and Medicine, 300, 666
National Academy for State Health Policy, 639
National Academy of Medicine, 617
National Academy of Science, 801
National Alliance of Grieving Children, 489
National Association of Neonatal Nurses (NANN), 298, 440–41, 443*t*
National Cancer Institute, 566
toxicity criteria in diarrhea, 156*b*
National Center for Care at the End of Life, 455
National Coalition for Hospice and Palliative Care, 13, 17, 367–68
National Committee for Quality Assurance, 12
National Comprehensive Cancer Network (NCCN), 130, 137, 265, 267, 269, 270, 569, 570, 727
defining distress, 330
Distress Thermometer, 570, 571–72
National Consensus Project (NCP), 38, 67, 78, 294, 429, 495–96, 680
Clinical Practice Guidelines, 641
Clinical Practice Guidelines for Quality Palliative Care, 702
Guidelines for Quality Palliative Care, 456
National Consensus Project for Quality Palliative Care, 345, 662, 746
National Consensus Project for Quality Palliative Care guidelines, 568–69
National Council of State Boards of Nursing, 642, 648, 652
National Healthcare Disparities Report, 298
National Health Expenditures report, 60
National Health Interview Survey (NHIS), 281
National Hospice and Palliative Care Organization (NHPCO), 298, 455, 457, 737–38
National Institute of Nursing Research (NINR), 801
National Institutes of Health (NIH), 281, 801
Building Evidence for Services and Supports, 537–38
Fogarty International Center, 649
National Palliative Care Registry, 679–80
National Palliative Care Research Center (NPCRC), 801
National Pressure Injury Advisory Panel, pressure injury staging system, 207*t*
National Quality Forum (NQF), 12
National Suicide Prevention Lifeline, 258
National Telehealth Policy Resource Center, 652
natural products, 281
gastrointestinal symptoms, 286
mood and sleep, 285
pain, 284
resources, 286–87, 286*t*
nausea
adverse effect of opioid analgesics, 96
antihistaminic agents, 135
assessment, 132–34
benzodiazepines, 135
biological therapies, 137
cancer population, 131
cannabinoids, 136
case study, 130, 136, 137–38
causes, 132
classes of antiemetics, 134*b*
corticosteroids, 135
dopamine receptor antagonists, 134–35
emetic pathways, 132*f*
epidemiology of, in palliative care, 130–31
integrative medicine, 136–37
nonbiological therapies, 137, 138*t*
noncancer population, 131
nonpharmacological approach, 136–37
nursing interventions, 137–38
pediatric palliative care, 394–95
pharmacological management, 134–36
physiological mechanisms, 131–32
prokinetic agents, 134
Rhodes and McDaniel recommended criteria, 133*b*
selective 5HT3 receptor antagonists, 135
self-management, 136, 137*b*
somatostatin analogues, 135–36
substance P antagonists (NK1 receptor antagonists), 136
syndromes involving, in palliative care, 133*b*
term, 131
terminology, 131
tools for measuring, 133*t*
See also vomiting
negotiation, conflict resolution, 44*b*, 44–45
Neonatal Comfort Care Program, 443*t*
neonatal intensive care unit (NICU), 436
bereavement support services, 441
case study of Coco in, 437–38
cultural influences of palliative care practices, 440
palliative care principles in, 438–39
palliative guidelines, 440–41
role of neonatal nurse in palliative care, 439
neonatal palliative care
bereavement keepsake checklist, 442*f*
bereavement support services, 441
nonpharmacologic measures to promote comfort, 444
perinatal resources for education, training, and advocacy, 443*t*
pharmacologic and nonpharmacologic measures, 444*t*
pharmacologic measures for promoting comfort, 441–44
principles of, 438–39
promoting comfort for patients, 441–44
role of labor and delivery nurse, 439–40, 439*t*
nervous system, dying process, 593
networking, career advancement, 788
neurodegenerative diseases, 309
neurological disorders
advance care planning and serious illness communication, 238–39
amyotrophic lateral sclerosis (ALS), 235–36, 236*t*
case study of mobility, 239*b*, 240
case study of speech and swallowing, 240*b*
corticobasal syndrome (CBS), 236*t*, 237
dysphagia, 241
gait impairment and falls, 240
Huntington's disease (HD), 236*t*, 237–38, 237*t*
impaired communication, 240–41
key points for optimizing communication, 236*b*
mobility symptom cluster, 239–40
multiple sclerosis (MS), 236*t*, 238
myoclonus, 239–40
neuropalliative care, 236*t*, 238–41
Parkinson's disease (PD), 236–37, 236*t*
progressive supranuclear palsy (PSP), 236*t*, 237
spasticity, 239
speech and swallowing, 240–41
neurological symptoms, pediatric palliative care, 396*b*, 396

neurologic illnesses, physical impact on sexual function, 342
neuropathic pain
  assessment findings and therapy, 91*t*
  medications for treatment, 384*t*
  pediatric, 383*b*, 383
neuropathy, patients living with cancer, 569
neuropsychiatric symptoms, dementia and management of, 535–36
New Jersey, 500, 605
  medical aid in dying (MAID), 357–58
New Mexico, 605
  medical aid in dying (MAID), 357–58
New York Heart Association, 648–49, 653
Nightingale, Florence, 777
NK1 receptor antagonists, nausea and vomiting, 136
N-methyl-d-aspartate (NMDA) antagonists, 97*t*
  pain management, 97–98
Nodding, Nel, 350
nonalcoholic steatohepatitis cirrhosis, case of patient with, 159, 161
nonbinary/genderqueer, 712*t*
noncancer population, nausea and vomiting, 131
noninvasive ventilation (NIV), 498–99
  dyspnea, 109*t*, 110
nonmaleficence, 171
  medical aid in dying, 609
  palliative sedation, 594
nonpharmacological therapies, pain management, 99
nonsteroidal anti-inflammatory drugs (NSAIDs), 380, 381
  pain management, 92–95, 93*t*
non-treatment decisions, 606
nonverbal communication, 28
nonverbal communication skills, nursing intervention, 335
nurse(s)
  characteristics, 29
  grieving process, 632
  palliative care of people living with cancer, 573
  personal reflection (Frechman), 771–72
  professional issues for providing palliative care in community, 642–43
  roles and responsibilities in advance care planning (ACP), 55–56
  self-appraisal, 337
  self-care for, 337
Nurse Licensure Compact (NLC), 652
NURSE mnemonic, 771
  dementia, 531
NURSE model, communication strategy, 34*b*, 34
nurse-patient-family, fostering therapeutic relationship, 337
Nurse Practice Act, 652
Nurses' Roles and Responsibilities in Providing Care and Support at the End of Life, 40, 419–20
nurse-to-patient communication, 30
  stages of relationship, 30–31, 30*t*
nursing
  communication, 28–29
  communication at end of life, 470
  communication barriers, 31–32
  difficult questions asked of, 471*t*
  prognosis at end of life, 468–70
  role in global palliative care, 766
  scheduled meetings and presence of, 37–38
  telehealth, 647–48
  See also pediatric patient at end of life
nursing care
  end of life, 621
  palliative sedation, 596–97
Nursing Care and Do Not Resuscitate (DNR) Decisions, 40, 419–20
nursing considerations, pediatric palliative care, 457
Nursing Delirium Screening Scale, 245
nursing education
  current landscape, 794–96
  history of, 791–93
  innovative strategies in curricula, 794–95
  interprofessional clinical practice, 795–96
  palliative care organizational membership and certifications, 796–97
  revised palliative care competencies, 794*b*, 794
nursing homes (NHs)
  advance care planning, 665–66
  end-of-life (EOL) transitions, 666
  external consultation teams, 664
  hospice care, 664
  integrated palliative care, 664–65
  palliative care in, 664
  palliative care resources, 665*t*
  physical and psychosocial aspects of care, 665
  skilled nursing care, 663
  See also long-term care (LTC)
nursing interventions
  acknowledging emotions, 335
  distraction, 336
  interdisciplinary legacy work, 336–37
  listening for hope, 336
  nonverbal communication skills, 335
  positive self-talk, 336
  reappraisal of meaning, purpose and hope, 336
  reframing, 335–36
  silence, 335
  supporting spirituality, 336
  symptom management, 336
  therapeutic presence, 335
nursing practice, integrating sexual health into, 345
nursing professionals, team roles, 80*t*
nursing research
  goal, 801
  See also palliative care research
nutrition
  conversations about medically administered, 41
  culture and, 304
  older adults, 753*t*, 755
  See also medically administered hydration and nutrition (MAHN); medically administered nutrition and hydration (MANH)
nutritional support, anorexia/cachexia syndrome (ACS), 123

obsessive-compulsive and related disorders, persons with, 736
occupational stress
  definition, 773*t*
  organizational and managerial issues, 772
  palliative care nursing, 772
  role-specific stressors, 772
  short-staffing, 772
  terms, 773*t*
occupational therapy, interdisciplinary palliative care team, 71
Ohio, 465
older adults
  advanced care planning, 753*t*, 755
  aging population, 750
  care settings and palliative care models, 750–52
  case study, 751–52, 756
  cognition, 752–54, 753*t*
  comprehensive geriatric assessment, 752
  culture, 299
  dentition, 753*t*, 755
  elder abuse and mistreatment, 753*t*, 756
  falls and fall risk, 752, 753*t*
  financial concerns, 753*t*, 756
  functional capacity, 752, 753*t*
  geriatric resources, 756
  geriatric syndromes, 752*b*
  hearing, 753*t*, 755
  importance of palliative care nursing for, 750
  incontinence, 753*t*, 754
  informal caregiving, 753*t*, 755–56
  medications/polypharmacy, 753*t*, 755
  mood, 752, 753*t*
  nutrition and weight, 753*t*, 755
  sexuality, 344, 753*t*, 756
  skin, 753*t*, 754–55
  social support, 753*t*, 755
  spirituality, 753*t*, 756
  trajectories of serious illness, 750, 751*f*
omega-3 fatty acid, pain, 284
Oncology Nursing Society, 108, 594
oncology team, pediatric case study, 422–23, 426
O'Neill, Onora, 84
opioid(s)
  CDC clinical practice guideline for prescribing, 14
  limited or no use in pediatrics, 380–83
  pediatric patient at end of life, 472
  public policies, 13
  safe storage and proper disposal, 728
  See also substance use disorders (SUDs)
opioid agonists, diarrhea, 158
opioid analgesics
  alternative routes of administration, 95
  buprenorphine, 95
  codeine, 95
  constipation, 95–96
  fentanyl, 93–94
  hydrocodone, 95
  hydromorphone, 94
  levorphanol, 95
  managing in outpatient setting, 660
  methadone, 94
  morphine, 93
  myoclonus, 96
  nausea and vomiting, 96
  oxycodone, 94
  oxymorphone, 94
  pain management, 92–94
  preventing and treating adverse effects, 95–96
  pruritus, 96
  respiratory depression, 96
  sedation, 95–96
  tapentadol, 95
  tramadol, 95
  See also pain management
opioid-induced bowel dysfunction (OIBD), 151, 151*t*
opioid-induced pruritus, 230
opioid use disorder (OUD), 720
oral feeding, suggestions, 144*b*, 144
oral-pharyngeal dysfunction, swallowing disorder, 143*b*
oral symptoms
  case study of ALS patient, 145
  dysgeusia, 147–48
  sialorrhea (excess oral secretions), 145–46
  xerostomia (dry mouth), 146–47, 147*t*
  See also dysphagia; hiccups
Oregon, 605, 607
  Death with Dignity Act (DWDA), 358, 606–7
  medical aid in dying (MAID), 357–58
organizational memberships, palliative care, 796–97
organ/tissue donation, end-of-life, 475
Osher Collaborative, 281
osmotic laxatives, constipation, 153
ostomy. *See* wound, ostomy, and continence (WOC) care
outpatient setting, 656
  ambulatory, 656
  benefits and challenges in, 657–58
  case study, 656, 657, 659, 660
  clinical measures in palliative care visits, 659
  components of palliative care visit, 659
  length of palliative care visits, 659
  managing medication in, 660

outpatient setting (*cont.*)
models of care, 657
new patient referrals, 658
palliative care referrals, 658
providing palliative care in, 658–60
relationship with referring provider, 658–59
team members, 658
telephone support and patient education, 659
ovarian cancer
case study patient assessment, 20, 23, 24
patient navigating survivorship, 567, 569
patient with, 153, 156
Oxford Handbook of Psychiatry in Palliative Medicine, 734
oxycodone
acute pain treatment, 382*t*
pain management, 94
oxygen therapy, dyspnea, 109, 109*t*
oxymorphone, pain management, 94

pacemakers, cardiovascular device, 359
pain, 89
assessment and common syndromes, 91–92, 91*t*
assessment and management, 303–4
barriers to cancer pain management, 90*b*
barriers to relief, 90
case study, 89, 98, 99, 100
effects of unrelieved, 91
end-of-life symptom management, 474*t*
healthcare settings, 90
hematologic malignancies, 560
mind-body approaches for, 283
natural products for, 284
prevalence of, 89
stage D heart failure, 512
pain history
OLDCARTS mnemonic for obtaining, 378*b*
self-reporting scales, 377–78
pain management
acetaminophen, 92, 93*t*
adjunct analgesics, 98–99
adjuvant analgesics, 96–98, 97*t*
alternative administration of opioid analgesics, 95
bisphosphonates, 98
buprenorphine, 95
cancer directed therapies, 98
codeine, 95
ethical dilemma of refusal, 355–56
fentanyl, 93–94
fentanyl, transdermal, 94
healthcare settings, 90
hydrocodone, 95
hydromorphone, 94
interventional therapies, 99
levorphanol, 95
methadone, 94
morphine, 93
non-opioid analgesics, 92
nonpharmacological therapies, 99
nonpharmacologic interventions, 380*t*
nonsteroidal anti-inflammatory drugs (NSAIDs), 92–95, 93*t*
opioid analgesics, 92–94
opioids (other), 95
oxycodone, 94
oxymorphone, 94
palliative care setting, 89, 100
patients and families, 90
pediatric palliative and hospice care (PPHC), 460–62, 461*t*
pharmacological, in advanced disease, 92
preventing adverse effects of opioid analgesics, 95–96
principles of, 99–100
radiation therapy and radiopharmaceuticals, 98
tapentadol, 95
tramadol, 95
See also adjunct analgesics; opioid analgesics
Palliative and Hospice Nursing Professional Issues Panel, 6
palliative care
benefits and challenges in research, 803–4
brief history as specialty, 3
building a team, 73–74
case study, 5
conversations about transition to, 41
critical role of nurses, 280
cultural aspects of care, 295*b*
cultural concepts, 302–3
definition, 662
effectiveness in home, 640
evidence base and challenges, 703–4
family caregiver assessment, 317–19
family caregiver resources, 323
family-centered, 309
global research considerations, 804
hematologic malignancies, 561
historically excluded groups with neglected access, 294*b*
interdisciplinary teams (IDTs), 66
LGBTQ caregivers, 310
models of, 66–67, 67*t*, 72–73
organizations supporting, 802*t*
persons living with advanced cancer, 572
priority research areas, 802–3, 803*b*
racially diverse caregivers, 309–10
research goals, 801–2
sedation use in, 359–60
social determinants of health (SDOH), 702–3
sustaining a healthy, functioning team, 74
term, 454–55, 759
See also community-based palliative care (CBPC); rural palliative care; spiritual, religious, and existential (S/R/E) needs
Palliative Care Leadership Centers, 746–47
Palliative Care Network, 765–66
palliative care nurse (PCN)
interdisciplinary palliative care team, 68, 70
team role, 78*t*
palliative care nursing, 3
palliative care programs
cost or resources, 808
dashboard, 810–11, 811*t*
data sources, 809
developing SMART metrics, 808–10, 809*t*
evaluation, 807–8
frequency, 809
hospice quality reporting, 808
Joint Commission Advanced Certification Program, 808
methodology, 809
Plan-Do-Study-Act rapid cycle, 811–12, 812*t*
quality, 807–8, 808*t*
quality improvement projects, 811–12
safety, 808, 808*t*
satisfaction survey, 810*t*
service, 808
weak metrics vs SMART metrics, 809, 810*t*
palliative care referrals, outpatient setting, 658
palliative care registered nurse (PCRN), 659
palliative care research
global considerations, 804
goals, 801–2
Palliative Care Research Cooperative (PCRC) Group, 801
Palliative Care Resolution, 759
palliative care setting, nursing approach to sexual health, 345–46
palliative chemotherapy, patients living with cancer, 572–73
palliative nurse, topics of self-inquiry, 17*b*
palliative nursing
communication as foundation of, 28
communication overview, 28–29
evolving role of, 6
home setting, 7
hospital setting, 6–7
long-term care setting, 7–8
nurse-patient relationship, 30–31, 30*t*
patients and families, 29–31
role of, 5–8
term, 6
Palliative Performance Scale (PPS), 21, 22*t*
palliative sedation, 593
case study of existential suffering, 595
goal, 594–95
impact of care provider's personal, cultural, and religious beliefs, 594–95
legal precedence for use, 594
medications used for, 595–96, 596*t*
nursing care, 596–97
professional position statements, 358
term, 594
palliative sedation to unconscious (PSU), 359–60
palliative surgery, patients living with cancer, 572
palliative telehealth nursing
dynamic role of Registered Nurse in, 651*f*
practice, 650–52
roles in the delivery, 651–52
palliative wound care
calciphylaxis, 213–14
COVID-19 skin manifestations, 214–15
debridement methodologies, 204*t*
etiology of wound pain, 201*b*
factors influencing choice of wound debridement method, 203*b*
interventions for wound-specific bleeding, 205*t*
Kennedy terminal ulcers (KTUs), 198–99, 201
key components to wound bed preparation, 203*b*
malignant fungating wounds (MFWs), 198–99, 211–12
Marjolin's ulcers, 212–13, 213*b*
medical device-related pressure injuries (MDRPI), 206–9
odor- and exudate-absorbent dressings, antimicrobials, and topical antiseptics, 204*t*
periwound moisture-associated skin damage (MASD), 202, 205–6
periwound skin protection, 203*t*
pressure injuries (PIs), 198–99, 201, 206–9
radiation dermatitis, 214
SCALE consensus statements, 200*t*
skin changes at life's end and skin failure, 200–1
skin tears and MARSI, 209–11
systematic approach to, 200*b*
systematic wound assessment, 206*b*
total pain management, 202*b*
Trombley-Brennan terminal tissue injury (TB-TTI), 198–99, 201
wound assessment principles, 206
wound-specific symptoms in complex and nonhealing wounds, 201–5
See also wound, ostomy, and continence (WOC) care
Palliverse, 765–66
paracetamol, pain management, 92
parent(s)
advocates for pediatric palliative care, 457–58
grief of child and, 481–82
pediatric palliative and hospice care (PPHC), 458
preparing bereaved, for grief experience, 488–89
parent outlook and understanding, goal of care, 401
parental influence, spirituality in children, 431

parenteral nutrition, anorexia/cachexia syndrome (ACS), 123–24
Parkinson's disease (PD), 27, 179–80, 309
- case of patient with, 150, 153
- case study, 656, 657, 660
- neurological disorder, 236–37
- resources for people living with, 236*t*
- sexual function, 342

PARTNER trial, meetings, 37
paternalism, 351
patient(s)
- barriers to cancer pain management, 90*b*
- communication themes, 29*t*
- information needs of, 35–36
- pain management, 90
- questions addressing coping, 38*b*
- value-based care (VBC) and, 63–64
- VBC team, 62

patient assessment, 17–18
- best practice tip, 25*b*
- case study (Mary), 18, 20, 23, 24
- electronic health record (EHR), 18–19
- end-of-life, 475
- family and, 17
- initial encounter, 19–20
- physical, 20*b*, 20–21
- psychosocial, 22–23, 23*b*
- review of systems, 21*b*
- spiritual, 23–24, 24*b*

Patient-Centered Outcomes Research Institute (PCORI), 648–49
Patient Dignity Inventory, 626
patient education
- depression and anxiety, 259
- empowerment and self-management, 259
- follow-up on chronic conditions, 259
- outpatient setting, 659

Patient Health Questionnaire (PHQ-2 or 4), 570
Patient Health Questionnaire (PHQ-9), 23, 252, 735
Patient Protection and Affordable Healthcare Act, 455
patient referrals, outpatient setting, 658
Patient-Reported Outcomes Measurement Information System (PROMIS) Fatigue scale, 570
Patient Self-Determination Act (1990), 13, 50, 351
Patient Self-Determination Act (1991), 171–72, 302–3
PAUSE talking map, early goals of care, 412–14, 415*t*
Pediatric Division, 443*t*
pediatric goals of care
- benefit-finding processes during follow-up meetings, 403*t*
- case study for patient's QOL, 399–400
- case study for patient undergoing hematopoietic stem cell transplantation, 400–1
- case study for patient with evolving trajectory of care, 405–6
- case study of patient with congenital heart defect and hydrocephalus, 404
- clinician challenges when leading through uncertainty, 406
- clinician impact on bereavement course, 401–2
- communication and impact on outcomes, 404
- communication throughout the trajectory, 402–4
- continuing bond manifestations during follow-up meetings, 403*t*
- guiding with uncertainty, 400–1
- identifying reconstruction process during follow-up meetings, 403*t*
- outcome considerations, 400
- parent outlook and understanding, 401
- power of social networking, 400
- preparing families for uncertainty, 405–6
- quality, 399
- sense-making processes during follow-up meetings, 402*t*
- value-based decision-making, 404–5

pediatric hospice
- case study, 454, 455, 458, 459–60, 462, 464
- palliative care and, 454–55
- *See also* pediatric palliative and hospice care (PPHC)

pediatric nurses, competencies in ethical reasoning, 423–24
pediatric pain
- acute pain, 380, 381*t*, 382*t*
- assessing neurologic impairment, 379
- case study, 379
- case study of patient in pain crisis, 381
- case study of patient with chronic pain, 384
- case study of patient with peripheral neuropathy, 383
- case study varying route of medication delivery, 381–82
- chronic pain, 383–84, 384*t*
- history and self-reporting pain scales, 377–85
- medical marijuana in pediatrics, 384–85
- medications for neuropathic pain and chronic pain syndromes, 384*t*
- motivations for underreporting and overreporting of pain, 378*t*
- neuropathic pain, 383, 384*t*
- nonpharmacologic interventions, 380*t*
- observational pain scales, 378*t*
- observed pain behaviors, 379*t*
- opioids with limited or no use, 380–83
- physical exam and observational assessment of pain intensity, 377–78
- polypharmacy, 385
- procedural pain management, 379–80
- self-reporting pain scales, 377–78, 378*t*
- sensory abnormalities in neuropathic pain syndromes, 383*b*
- treatment for individual child, 382–83
- treatment of acute pain (mild), 381*t*
- treatment of acute pain (moderate to severe), 382*t*
- using two-step strategy, 380

pediatric palliative and hospice care (PPHC)
- anticipatory grief and bereavement, 464
- barriers to accessing, 457–58
- care at time of death, 463
- communication, 460, 461*t*
- comparing PPC and, 454–55
- components of care, 460–62
- concurrent care, 455
- considerations for, 458–60
- creating a sacred space, 463
- developmental stages and perceptions of death, 459*t*
- education, 464–65
- ethical considerations, 462–64
- family-centered care, 458
- future unfolding for, 465
- interaction with schools, 459–60
- nursing care issues for, 464–65
- nursing considerations, 457
- pain and symptom management, 460–62
- parents as advocates, 457–58
- preserving hope, 462
- progress and challenges, 455–58
- psychological symptoms and suffering, 460–61
- questions for accessing psychosocial factors, 461*t*
- religious/spiritual and cultural considerations, 461, 461*t*
- self care, 463–64
- social aspects, 461, 461*t*
- support for parents/guardians, 458
- support for siblings, 459
- training, 464–65

pediatric palliative care (PPC), 387
- appetite issues, 395–96
- autonomy in, 424–25
- case of leukemia patient, 422–23, 426
- case of patient with constipation, 395
- case of patient with dyspnea and panic, 393
- case of patient with excessive secretions, 394
- case of patient with multiple symptoms, 395–96
- case of patient with nausea, 394
- case of Trevor, 388–89, 390
- communication and care coordination, 392–93
- community-based, 641
- constipation, 395
- creating a treatment/management plan, 389–93
- definition, 454
- description of events surrounding, 456*f*
- documentation and support tools, 392
- dyspnea/respiratory distress, 393–94
- education of child and family, 393
- emotional and existential distress, 397
- essential elements in, 458*f*
- ethical dilemmas encountered in, 425–26
- excessive secretions, 394
- feeding difficulties, 395–96
- gastrointestinal symptoms, 394–96
- hospice service availability and, 457
- nausea/vomiting, 394–95
- neurological symptoms, 396*b*, 396
- OPQRSTUV mnemonic, 389, 389*t*
- overview of symptom assessment and factors, 388–89
- pharmacologic interventions, 390–91, 391*f*
- pharmacological, physical, and psychological (3 P approach) interventions, 387, 391*f*
- physical interventions, 391*f*, 391–92
- psychological interventions, 391*f*, 391
- questions to consider, 390*b*
- reassessment and monitoring, 392
- refractory symptoms, 397
- rollercoaster treatment, 456*f*
- setting for, 456–57
- severe bleeds, 396–97
- shared decision-making in symptom management, 390
- symptom guidelines, 392*f*
- symptom management, 390
- useful websites, 388*b*
- wish, worry, wonder framework, 390*b*
- *See also* adolescents and young adults (AYA)

pediatric patient at end of life
- acute symptom management, 472–74
- aftercare, 475
- autopsy, 475
- care at and after death, 475
- caring for the dying child, 470
- case study, 467, 468, 469, 470, 476
- chronic symptom management, 474
- communicating progress, 468
- difficult questions for nurse, 471*t*
- end-of-life considerations, 475
- end-of-life huddle, 472, 473*f*
- end-of-life period (days to weeks), 469
- end-of-life period (hours to days), 469
- end-of-life period (moments to hours), 469–70
- end-of-life period (weeks to months), 468

pediatric patient at end of life (*cont.*)
  end-of-life symptom management, 472, 474*t*
  interventions, 472
  location of care, 467–68
  medical emergencies, 474
  nursing communication, 470
  opioids and, 472
  organ/tissue donation, 475
  patient assessment, 475
  physiologic changes, 470–72
  prognosis and defining end-of-life period, 468–70
  staff commemoration and condolences, 475–76
pediatric serious illness
  advance care planning, 416–18, 417*t*, 418*t*
  advance directive conversations, 410
  case study of Aniya, 408, 411–12, 413–14, 415–16
  decision-making for, 409–10
  essential core functions of clinician-child/parent communication, 409*t*
  ethical and legal considerations in goals of care, 410
  goals-of-care conversations, 411
  GUIDE talking map, 412, 413*t*
  if family wants to "do everything," 415
  NURSES mnemonic, 411
  parent themes from definition of being a good parent, 410*b*
  PAUSE talking map for early goals of care, 412–14, 414*t*
  regoaling, 415–16
  REMAP talking map for later goals-of-care discussions, 414–15, 415*t*
  responding to emotion, 411–12
  talking maps for goals of care, 412–15
Pennsylvania, 465
people living with HIV (PLWH), 519–20
  advance care planning and advance directives, 523–25
  case of long-term AIDS survivor, 524
  case of patient diagnosed with AIDS, 524
  case of patient with AIDS and multimorbidities, 524–25
  chronic pain management, 521*t*
  coping dimensions by long-term survivors, 521*t*
  disease coping, 522
  emotional coping, 522–23
  living and coping with HIV, 521–25
  multimorbidity and aging, 521
  palliative care in, 520–21
  practical coping, 522
  selected resources, 525*t*
  social support, 523
Peplau, Hildegard, 739
perception, symptoms in normal progression in dying, 620*t*
perinatal death, 439
Perinatal Hospice & Palliative Care, 443*t*
Perinatal Loss and Infant Death Alliance (PLIDA), 443*t*
perinatal palliative care, ethical considerations, 462–63
perioperative setting, family caregivers in, 320–21
peripherally acting mu opioid receptor antagonists (PAMORAs), constipation, 153
peristomal complications
  changes in abdominal planes, 218
  mucocutaneous separation, 218*f*, 218–19
  palliative patients, 218–19
  peristomal MASD, 219
  peristomal varices, 218*f*, 219
permanent pacemakers (PPMs), cessation, 603
personality disorders, persons with, 738–39, 738*t*
PEWTER model, sharing "bad news," 624
pharmacologic interventions, pediatric palliative care, 390–91, 391*f*
phenobarbital, palliative sedation, 596, 596*t*
phenothiazines, nausea and vomiting, 134–35
physical activity
  mind-body approaches for pain, 283
  yoga for mood and sleep, 284
physical assessment
  LGBTQIA+ patients, 715
  patient, 20*b*, 20–21
physical exercise, safe for lymphedema, 194
physical health and function, dementia, 530, 536
physical interventions
  nursing homes, 665
  pediatric palliative care, 391*f*, 391–92
physical therapy, interdisciplinary palliative care team, 71
physician
  interdisciplinary palliative care team, 68, 70
  team role, 78*t*
physician-assisted suicide, 606
Physician Orders for Life-Sustaining Treatment (POLST), 18, 353, 418
Piaget, Jean, 431
Pittsburgh Sleep Quality Index (PSQI), 284
place of residence, culture, 301
Plan-Do-Study-Act rapid cycle, 811–12, 812*t*
planning for death, 617
planning for the future, family caregiver resources, 323
PLEASURE, sexual health framework, 345, 346*t*
pleural effusion
  agents to treat malignant, 582*t*
  case study, 580–81
  description, 581
  diagnostic procedures, 581
  epidemiology, 581
  indwelling pleural catheters, 582
  nursing management, 582–83
  pathophysiology, 581
  pleurectomy, 582
  pleurodesis, 582
  signs and symptoms, 581
  thoracentesis, 582
  treatment, 581–82
  See also urgent syndrome at end of life
PLISSIT, sexual health framework, 345, 346, 346*t*
PLWH. *See* people living with HIV (PLWH)
pneumatic (mechanical) pumps, lymphedema, 193
pneumatic compression devices (PCDs), lymphedema, 193
polyamorous, 712*t*
polypharmacy
  older adults, 753*t*, 755
  pediatrics, 385
population health, 12
Portable Orders for Life-Sustaining Treatment (POLST), advance directives (AD) and, 54, 54*t*
positive self-talk, nursing intervention, 336
postmortem care, end-of-life decisions, 433
posttraumatic stress disorder (PTSD), 737
  grief, 480, 489
postural modifications, swallowing, 144, 144*t*
PPC. *See* pediatric palliative care (PPC)
PPHC. *See* pediatric palliative and hospice care (PPHC)
practical coping, people living with HIV, 522
PRAM model, support for grieving, 489
pregabalin, neuropathic and chronic pain syndromes, 384*t*
preload, 505–6
prematurity complications, pediatric palliative care, 425–26
presence, ethos of palliative nursing, 85–86
pressure injuries (PIs), 198, 206–9
  palliative considerations in treatment, 210*t*
  risk assessment tools, 209*t*
  risk factors, risk assessment, and risk reduction, 206, 209*t*
  risk reduction strategies, 209*t*
  staging system, 207*t*
  treatment, 206–9
pressure ulcers, medically administered nutrition (MAN), 167
primary care practices, 641
primary disease management team, team roles, 78–79, 78*t*, 80*t*
primary palliative care
  definition, 680
  evolution, 683*t*
  integration of team members, 684*t*
principle of double effect, palliative sedation, 360, 594
principlist approach, ethics, 349–50
prisons, culture, 301
private duty nursing agencies, 641
probiotics, constipation, 153
problem-solving, steps of ethical, 350*b*
proctoclysis, 168, 168*t*
professional development, 785–86
progestational agents, anorexia/cachexia syndrome (ACS), 124, 125*t*
prognosis, discussions, 39–40
progressive muscle relaxation (PMR)
  gastrointestinal symptoms, 286
  nausea and vomiting, 138*t*
progressive supranuclear palsy (PSP)
  neurological disorder, 237
  resources for people living with, 236*t*
prokinetic agents, nausea and vomiting, 134
prolonged grief, 480
propofol
  palliative sedation, 596, 596*t*
  sedation in ICU patients, 691*t*, 692
proportionality, concept, 594
proportionate palliative sedation (PPS), 359–60
proxemics, 28
proxy decision-making, ethical dilemma, 354–55
pruritus, 227–30
  adverse effect of opioid analgesics, 96
  case study of hemodialysis patient with, 228
  cholestatic origin, 228–30
  classification, 227
  definition, 227
  HIV origin, 230
  medications in management, 229*t*
  nonpharmacological treatment, 228–30
  nursing assessment, 227–28
  opioid-induced, 230
  pharmacological treatment, 228
  uremic origin, 228
psychiatric emergencies, 738–39
psychological care, LGBTQIA+ patients, 716
psychological distress, 330
psychological intervention, pediatric palliative care, 391*f*, 391
psychosocial assessment
  LGBTQIA+ patients, 715–16
  patient, 22–23, 23*b*
psychosocial impact, serious illness on sexuality, 343–44
psychosocial support
  hematologic malignancies, 560–61
  nursing homes, 665
psychotherapy, 626
psychotic disorders, persons with, 734–36
public policy
  advance care planning, 13
  case study, 10, 14–15
  CDC clinical practice guideline for prescribing opioids, 14

health equity and, 14
hospital patient survey, 14
Medicaid, 12
Medicare, 10–12
Medicare Part D opioid overutilization program, 14
opioid, 13
quality measurement, 13
serious illness population, 12
pulmonary cancers, 496*b*
pulmonary edema, 106
pulmonary hypertension, 496*b*
pulmonary-palliative care, 495–96
advanced lung disease, 497, 497*t*
advanced pulmonary disease, 498
advanced ventilatory technology, 498–99
BODE index (body mass index, airflow obstruction, dyspnea, and exercise), 499
case study of COPD and secondary pulmonary hypertension, 502–3
common lung diseases, 496*b*
dyspnea, 496*b*, 496
End-of-Life Nurse Education Consortium (ELNEC), 501
forecasting, 499
Four Seasons Consulting, 501
GAP index, 499
Geisinger Medical Center, 501–2
medication dilemmas, 498
new construct, 496–97
patient, caregiver and provider advocacy, 500–2
toll of serious illness on persons and family/caregiver, 500
uncertainty in prognosis and disease trajectory, 497–98
We Be-LUNG Together, 501
purpose, 328–30
loss of, 329–30
meaning and, 328–30
See also meaning

quality
concepts, 808*t*
measurement, 13
metric for decision-making, 399
palliative care program, 807*f*, 807–8
See also palliative care programs
quality of death, hydration, 170
Quality of Death Index, 703
quality of life (QOL), 23, 28, 66
anorexia/cachexia syndrome (ACS), 120
case study for patient's, 399–400
ethical analysis, 352
family caregiver, 317
hydration, 170
medically administered nutrition (MAN), 167
pruritus, 227
queer, 712*t*
quest narrative, 625
Quick Dementia Rating System (QDRS), 531
Quill, Timothy, 609
Quinlan, Karen Ann, 171–72, 360, 610

race
cultural assessment questions, 296*b*
culture, 297–98
kidney disease, 549
See also ethnicity, underrepresented groups
racially diverse caregivers, 309–10
strategies to support, 310
radiation dermatitis, 198–99
breast cancer, 214*f*
treatment, 214
wound care, 214
radiation therapy, pain management, 98
radiopharmaceuticals, pain management, 98
RAND Corporation, 13
REACH-PC trial, 649
Reasonable Person Standard, definition, 425
referring providers, outpatient setting, 658–59
refractory breathlessness, 105
reframing, nursing intervention, 335–36
refusal of pain and symptom management, ethical dilemma, 355–56
registered dietitian/nutritionist, interdisciplinary palliative care team, 72
rehabilitation facility, 5
Reiki, energy medicine, 285
relational team communication, 44
relationship, 28
reliability, 84
religion
cultural assessment questions, 296*b*
culture, 300
See also spiritual, religious, and existential (S/R/E) needs; spirituality
REMAP talking map, later goals of care, 414–15, 417*t*
remote patient monitoring (RPM)
advantages, disadvantages, and future role of, 650
components of successful programs, 650*t*
digital health, 649–50
renal, symptoms in normal progression in dying, 620*t*
renal disease, fatigue, 265*b*
resilience, definition, 773*t*
respiratory cluster, 104–5
respiratory depression, adverse effect of opioid analgesics, 96
Respiratory Distress Observation Scale (RDOS), 599, 600, 692
respiratory system, dying process, 593
respiratory therapy, interdisciplinary palliative care team, 71
restitution narrative(s), 624, 625
retching, term, 131
retrovirus, 519
Richmond Agitation and Sedation Scale (RASS), 245
Richmond Agitation and Sedation Scale--Palliative Version (RASS-PAL), 245
rituals, meaning-making and, 490*b*, 490
Robert Wood Johnson Foundation (RWJF), 642–43, 791
rural palliative care, 742–44
barriers and challenges, 744*b*
case of lack of access to advanced heart failure therapies, 742
case of lack of access to pediatric specialists, 742
challenges to providing, 744
creative strategies, 744–45
critical access hospitals, 746*b*, 746
delivering, beyond United States, 744
ENABLE (Educate, Nurture, Advise, Before Life Ends) project, 745, 745*t*
nonmetropolitan counties, 743*f*
technology-enabled healthcare, 744–45
telehealth programs, 745–46

sacred space, creation of, 463
S-adenosyl-L-methionine (SAMe), mood and sleep, 285
safety
concepts, 808*t*
palliative care program, 807*f*, 808
St. John's wort, mood and sleep, 285
Salmonella enterica, diarrhea, 156
Sao Paulo Cancer Institute, 283
Saunders, Cicely, 3, 22, 429, 627, 703
Scarry, Elaine, 85
Schiavo, Terri, 360
school-aged children, culture, 298
schools, pediatric palliative and hospice care (PPHC), 459–60
Schut, Hunk, 628
secondary traumatic stress, definition, 773*t*
secretions, end-of-life symptom management, 474*t*
sedation
adverse effect of opioid analgesics, 95–96
palliative, 593
palliative care, 359–60
pharmacological management promoting, 691–92, 691*t*
See also palliative sedation
seizures, end-of-life symptom management, 474*t*
selective 5HT3 receptor antagonists, nausea and vomiting, 135
selective serotonin agonists, constipation, 153
self-assessment, culture, 297
self-care
definition, 773*t*
lymphedema, 194
nurse, 337
pediatric palliative and hospice care (PPHC), 463–64
self-concept, impact of serious illness on sexuality, 343
self-management
nausea and vomiting, 136, 137*b*
patient empowerment and, 259
self-reporting pain scales, pediatric, 377–78, 378*t*
separation distress, 625
serious illness
case study on impact of, on sexual health, 341–42, 343–44, 346–47
conversations in dementia, 531–34
distress in, 331
hope in context, 331–33, 332*b*
physical impact on sexuality and sexual health, 341–43
serious illness care, fostering therapeutic nurse-patient-family relationship, 337
serious illness communication, neurological care, 238–39
serious illness population, 12
definition, 12*b*
serious mental illness (SMI), 733
clinical manifestations, 734
defining, 733
diagnoses, 734*b*
hoarding, 736–38
overview of specified personality disorders, 738*t*
persons with anxiety disorders and somatic symptom disorders, 735–36
persons with mood disorders, 734–35
persons with obsessive-compulsive and related disorders, 736
persons with personality disorders, 738–39
persons with psychotic disorders, 734–36
persons with trauma and stressor-related disorders, 737–38
psychiatric emergencies, 738–39
suicidality and wish for hastened death, 739
serious news, discussions, 39, 40*b*
serotonin norepinephrine reuptake inhibitors (SRNIs), neuropathic and chronic pain syndromes, 384*t*
service, palliative care program, 807*f*, 808
sex, term, 341
sexual function
common medications and impacts on, 342*t*
physical impact of serious illness on, 341–43
psychosocial impact of serious illness on, 343–44
term, 341
sexual health
case of impact of serious illness on, 341–42, 343–44, 346–47
communication frameworks, 345, 346*t*
concept, 341
nursing approach to, in palliative care setting, 345–46
sexual orientation/identity, 712*t*, 713
sexuality, 341, 712*t*
older adults, 753*t*, 756
physical impact of serious illness on, 341–43
psychosocial impact of serious illness on, 343–44
sexual function and, across the life span, 344–45

shared decision-making, cultural concept in palliative care, 302–3
Short Form 36 Health Survey, 284
shortness of breath, 105
shunts, ascites, 160
sialorrhea
  etiology, 145–46
  excess oral secretions, 145–46
  neurological care, 241
  nursing assessment, 146
  nursing interventions, 146
  pathophysiology, 145–46
  See also oral symptoms
siblings
  bereavement support groups for, 489
  pediatric palliative and hospice care (PPHC), 459
silence, nursing intervention, 335
Silverman, Phyllis, 632
Simonelli, Paul, 501
singultus, 145
  See also hiccups
Sjogren's syndrome, sexual function, 342
Skilled Nursing Facility (SNF), 61
skin, older adults, 753*t*, 754–55
skin care, lymphedema, 194
skin changes at end of life (SCALE), 198–99
SMART metrics (Specific, Measurable, Achievable, Realistic, Time-bound), 807, 808–10, 809*t*
  weak metrics *vs*, 809, 810*t*
social capital theory, 778
social determinants of health (SDOH), 293, 701, 702
  culture, 300
  implications and challenges for palliative care nursing, 702–3
  nursing role in promoting health equity, 706, 707
  See also underrepresented groups
social media, 777
  case study of Facebook and resources, 781–82
  categories, 778*t*
  engagement characteristics and, 779
  ethical considerations, 782
  Facebook, 779
  facilitating sense-making, 780
  family and, 780–81
  healthcare professionals and, 781–82
  history and impact, 777
  illness blog, 779
  leaving a legacy, 781
  power of storytelling through expressive writing, 779–80
  social capital and, 778–79
  social capital theory, 778
  social support and, 780–81
  terms, 777
  theoretical view, 777–79
  Twitter, 779–80
social networking, power of, 400
social support
  older adults, 753*t*, 755
  people living with HIV, 523
  social media garnering, 780–81
social well-being, patients living with cancer, 571
social worker
  interdisciplinary palliative care team, 68–69, 70–71
  team role, 78*t*
Society of Critical Care Medicine, 689
socioeconomic status, culture, 300–1
SOLER model, communication strategy, 34*b*, 34
somatic pain, assessment findings and therapy, 91*t*
somatic symptom and related disorders, persons with, 735–36
somatostatin analogues, nausea and vomiting, 135–36
Sour Seven, 245
space, ethos of palliative nursing, 85
specialist palliative care disciplinary team, team roles, 80*t*
specialty palliative care
  consulting, 682–83
  definition, 680
  evolution, 683*t*
speech and swallowing
  case study, 241
  neurological disorders, 240–41
speech-language pathology, interdisciplinary palliative care team, 71
SPIKES framework, sharing "bad news," 623–24, 624*b*
SPIKES model
  communication strategy, 34*b*, 34
  dementia, 531
spina bifida, 179–80
spinal cord compression (SCC)
  analgesia, 585
  case study, 584
  corticosteroids, 585
  decompression surgery, 585
  description, 584
  diagnostic procedures, 585
  nursing management, 585
  pathophysiology, 584
  radiation therapy, 585
  signs and symptoms, 584–85
  treatments, 585
  See also urgent syndrome at end of life
spiral of disability, 106, 107
SPIRIT model, spiritual history, 430*t*
spiritual, religious, and existential (S/R/E) needs, 367
  assessment, 368–70
  case study navigating disbelief and divine abandonment, 367
  case study on being spiritual while "none and done," 368
  definition, 368
  description, 368
  interventions for attending to, 370–72
  manifestation, 368
  persons receiving palliative care, 369*t*
  prompts/responses indicating need for chaplain referral, 371*t*
  screening and histories, 369–70
  screening questions, 370*t*
  tools and measures for, 371*t*
spiritual and existential concerns, patients living with cancer, 571–72
spiritual assessment, 430
  barriers to obtaining, 433
  history, 430
  LGBTQIA+ patients, 715–16
  patient, 23*b*, 23–24
  screening tools, 430
spiritual care
  compassionate presence, 430
  definition, 430
  education supporting the development of, 434
  empathetic listening, 430
  LGBTQIA+ patients, 716
  providing prayer and support, 430
Spiritual Care Checklist, 371*t*
spiritual distress, 330, 433
spiritual history, 430
  comparing models, 430, 430*t*
Spiritual Injury Scale, 371*t*
Spiritual Needs Questionnaire, 371*t*
Spiritual Pain Assessment Sheet, 371*t*
Spiritual/Religious Struggles Scale-Short Form (RSSS-SF), 371*t*
spiritual support, nursing intervention, 336
spirituality
  case honoring religious beliefs and cultural humility, 432
  chaplains, 433
  in children, 431
  cultural assessment questions, 296*b*
  culture, 300
  definition, 429–30
  older adults, 753*t*, 756
  parental influence, 431
  rituals and cultural traditions, 432
  spiritual development by age, 431, 431*t*
  support for patients and families, 432–33
  See also religion; spiritual, religious, and existential (S/R/E) needs
staff commemoration, end-of-life, 475–76
staging dementia, 531
State Veterans Homes, 662
stereotactic body radiation therapy, 98
stimulant laxatives, constipation, 153
stopping dialysis, 602
storytelling, expressive writing, 779–80
Stroebe, Margaret, 628
stroke volume, 505–6
Subjective Global Assessment for Nutrition (SGA), 122
substance P antagonists, nausea and vomiting, 136
substance use disorders (SUDs), 660, 720
  applying pharmacological principles to treating pain, 728
  assessment in patients with advanced disease, 722–24
  case study of woman with breast cancer, 723
  challenges to assessment, 723–24
  clinical management of advanced-disease patients, 724–26
  drug and alcohol use, 721
  evaluation and treatment of comorbid psychiatric disorders, 727
  family sessions and meetings, 728
  focusing on relapse prevention, 725–26
  focusing on SUD treatment, 725
  general guidelines, 726–27
  monitoring for risk, 727
  multidisciplinary approach, 727
  patients with advanced disease, 722
  preventing/minimizing withdrawal symptoms, 727
  provider challenges to clinical management, 726
  risk factors for development, 723*b*
  safe storage and proper disposal of opioid medication, 728
  screen tools for opioid misuse, 722*t*
  setting realistic goals for therapy, 727
  substance use, abuse and, 721–22
  terms associated with, 721*t*
  treating patients with, 728–29
  use of 12-step programs, 728
  use of written agreements, 727–28
Substituted Judgment standard, 425
sudden breathlessness, COMFORT approach, 110–11, 111*f*
suffering
  case study of existential suffering, 595
  concept, 330
  definition, 609
  medical aid in dying, 609
  patient's right to define, 595
suicide
  considerations in children, 258
  serious mental illness, 739
Suicide Crisis Lifeline, 258
superior vena cava obstruction (SVCO)
  case study, 579
  description, 568–71
  diagnostic procedures, 580
  drug therapy, 580
  grading system, 580*b*
  medical management, 580
  nursing management, 580
  pathophysiology, 569
  SVC stenting, 580
  symptoms, 579*b*, 580
  thrombolytic therapies, 580
  treatment, 580
  See also urgent syndrome at end of life
Supporting & Palliative Care Indicators Tool (SPICT), 704–5
Supreme Court of Canada, 608
surfactant laxatives, constipation, 153
surrogate decision maker
  advance care planning (ACP), 52*f*, 52
  case on not knowing the right, 52
  characteristics for patients choosing, 50*b*

survival benefit, hydration, 170
survival time, medically administered nutrition (MAN), 167
survivorship, case of patient with ovarian cancer, 567
survivorship care, palliative care and, 568–71
swallowing
  clinical examination, 143
  compensatory strategies, 144
  indications of disorder, 143*b*
  physiology and pathophysiology, 142–43
  screening function, 143
  See also dysphagia
sweats, 231
  nonpharmacological treatment options, 231–32
  nursing assessment, 231
  pharmacological treatment options, 232
  See also fever
Swiss Medical Association, 607
symptom cluster(s), 104–5, 106, 130–31
Symptom Distress Scale, 268
symptom management
  ethical dilemma of refusal, 355–56
  nursing intervention, 336
systematic desensitization, nausea and vomiting, 138*t*
systemic sclerosis, sexual function, 342

tapentadol, pain management, 95
task communication, 44
task model, grieving process, 628
technology, value-based care (VBC) and, 62–63
teens, grief support for, 489
telehealth, 647
  case of telephonic palliative care program, 653
  challenges and barriers to delivery, 652
  factors affecting nursing communication, 651*t*
  legal considerations for nurses, 652–53
  modalities of technology, 649
  nursing, 647–48
  practice of palliative nursing, 650–52, 651*f*
  remote patient monitoring (RPM), 649–50, 650*t*
  rural palliative care, 745–46
  technology-enabled healthcare, 744–45
tele-palliative care, model, 66, 73
telephone support, outpatient setting, 659
telephonic palliative care, nurse-led programs, 648–49
terminal extubation, 600
terminal restlessness, 169
terminal weaning, 600
termination, nurse-patient relationship, 30–31, 30*t*
therapeutic presence, nursing intervention, 335
Therapeutic Touch, energy medicine, 285
Thirst, dry mouth and, 169
toddlers
  culture, 298
  observed pain behaviors, 379*t*
toileting aids, incontinence and, 181–82, 181*t*
total dyspnea, concept of, 110
total pain, 609
Traditional Chinese Medicine (TCM), 282
Trail Making Test, 570
training, pediatric palliative and hospice care (PPHC), 464–65
tramadol, pain management, 95
transcutaneous electrical nerve stimulation (TENS), dyspnea, 110
transgender, 712*t*
  term, 711
  See also LGBTQIA+ individuals
transgender man, 712*t*
transgender woman, 712*t*
transition of fading away, 310–11
  burdening, 313–14, 316*t*
  case study of redefining, 319–24
  case study of resistance to letting go, 312
  case study of witnessing health changes, 313
  contending with change, 314, 316*t*
  dimensions of, 316*t*
  family caregiving in palliative care, 315–17
  living day to day, 315, 316*t*
  preparing for death, 315, 316*t*
  redefining, 311–13, 316*t*
  searching for meaning, 314–15, 316*t*
  struggling with paradox, 314, 316*t*
transition/transitioning, 712*t*
transjugular intrahepatic portosystemic shunt (TIPS), 160
trauma, pediatric deaths, 433
trauma and stressor-related disorders, persons with, 737–38
traumatic brain injury, 179–80
traumatic distress, 625
traumatic grief, 480
traumatic spinal cord injury, 179–80
treatment decline, ethics in pediatric palliative care, 426
tricyclic antidepressants, neuropathic and chronic pain syndromes, 384*t*
triple diagnosis, 520
Trombley-Brennan terminal tissue injury (TB-TTI), 198–99
trustworthiness, ethos of palliative nursing, 84
Twitter, 777, 779–80
two-spirit, 712*t*

ulcerative colitis, sexual function, 342
uncertainty
  clinician challenges when leading through, 406
  guiding with, 400–1
underrepresented groups
  addressing palliative care access disparities framework, 706*f*
  assessing and measuring patient and family needs in palliative care, 704–5, 704*t*
  case of transition from emergency to ICU, 702
  case of transition from hospital to hospice, 708
  case of transition from intensive to intermediate care, 705
  framework for tailoring palliative care, 705, 707*t*
  role of nursing in promoting health equity, 705–8
  See also 701
University of Alabama, 746
University of Colorado, 643
University of Maryland, 643
University of North Carolina Palliative Care Program, 357
University of Virginia, 17
University of Washington, 17
uremic pruritus (UP), 228
  pharmacological treatments, 228
  See also pruritus
urgent syndromes at end of life
  bone metastasis and pathological fractures, 587–89
  bowel obstruction, 589–90
  hemoptysis, 583–84
  hypercalcemia, 585–87
  pleural effusion, 580–83
  spinal cord compression, 584–85
  superior vena cava obstruction (SVCO), 579–80
urinary, symptoms in normal progression in dying, 620*t*
urinary dysfunction, 178
  causes, 178
  explanation, 179–80
urinary tract disorders, 178
  assessment, 180
  bladder management, 183
  bladder spasm, 182
  case study, 178
  common bladder disorders and emergencies, 182–83
  containment products, 181*t*
  explanation of dysfunction, 179–80
  hemorrhagic cystitis, 182–83
  incontinence and toileting, 181–82
  pathophysiology and risk factors, 178–79
  psychosocial factors and care environment, 183
  risk factors, 178–79, 179*t*
  toileting aids, 181*t*
  urinary tract infections (UTIs), 183
  voiding dysfunction, 180–81
urinary tract infections (UTIs), 178–79, 183
US Census Bureau, diversity, 294
US Food and Drug Administration (FDA), 134, 158
  bisphosphonate therapy, 586–87
  cannabinoids, 124
  fatigue treatment, 269
  insomnia treatment, 277
  marijuana use, 384–85
  opioids in children, 381
  remote patient monitoring (RPM), 649
US Supreme Court, palliative sedation, 594

Vacco v. Quill, 171–72
valerian root, mood and sleep, 285
value-based care (VBC), 59
  Affordable Care Act, 59
  barriers to implementation, 64
  case study of VBC in action, 62
  collaboration across care settings, 61–62
  documentation and data for, 62–63
  from volume to value, 59–60
  healthcare cost and, 63
  messaging for patients and families, 63–64
  patient-centered outcomes, 63
  patients as part of team, 62
  stakeholders, 60–61
value-based decision-making, pediatric goal of care, 404–5
value equation, 807
vascular dementia, 528–29
  diagnostic criteria, 529*t*
ventilator withdrawal, 599–601
  case of patient on mechanical ventilation, 599
  duration of survival, 601
  extubation considerations, 600–1
  intensive care unit (ICU), 694–95
  measuring distress, 600
  oxygen, 601
  premedication for anticipated distress, 600
  protocol for, 694*b*
  sample rapid wean, 601*t*
  withdrawal methods, 600
Vermont, 605
  medical aid in dying (MAID), 357–58
Veterans Affairs, 66–67
Veteran's Health Administration (VHA), 61
Virginia Health Care Decisions Act, 351–52
visceral pain, assessment findings and therapy, 91*t*
vision deficits, palliative patients, 216
Visual Analog Scale for Fatigue, 268
VitaloJAK, 112
vitamin D, pain, 284
vlogging, 337
vocalics, 28
Voicing My Choices, 450–51, 462
volume depletion, 168
voluntary stopping of eating and drinking (VSED)
  ethical dilemmas, 356, 361–62
  patient with autonomy, 173–74
volunteers, interdisciplinary palliative care team, 69, 71
vomiting
  adverse effect of opioid analgesics, 96
  term, 131
  See also nausea
VyncaCare, 744–45

Washington, 605
  medical aid in dying (MAID), 357–58

We Be-LUNG Together, 501
well-being, definition, 773*t*
Wescoe Foundation for Pulmonary Fibrosis, 500
Wescoe Singley, Jennifer, 500
When Children Die (Institute of Medicine), 456
whole healing traditions, 282
Widow-to-Widow project, 632
windmill model, pediatric palliative care, 484–86, 485*f*
Worden, William, 628
working phase, nurse-patient relationship, 30, 30*t*
World Bank Income groups, 626
World Health Assembly, 759
World Health Organization (WHO), 6, 293–94, 380, 502, 617, 744, 759
  digital health, 650
  medical aid in dying, 610
  pediatric palliative care, 454
  sexual health, 341
  spiritual care, 429
  See also 156
World Hospice and Palliative Care Day, 294
wound, ostomy, and continence (WOC) care, 198–99
  case study at end of life, 199, 215, 221
  specialist-level palliative nurse role, 199*b*, 199

xerostomia
  dry mouth, 146–47
  etiology, 146
  hematologic malignancies, 560
  nursing assessment, 146
  nursing interventions, 146–47, 147*t*
  pathophysiology, 146
  See also oral symptoms

young adulthood. *See* adolescents and young adults (AYA)
young and middle-aged adulthood, culture, 299

Zone of Parental Discretion, 425